# Drug Information *for* Mental Health

**2001**

**Matthew A. Fuller**
**Martha Sajatovic**

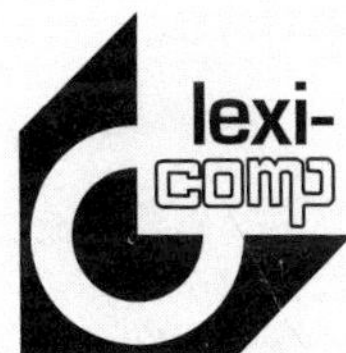


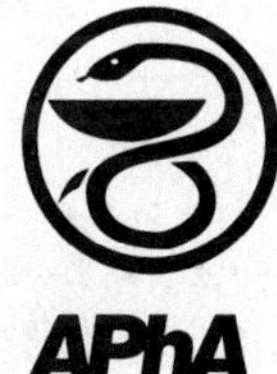

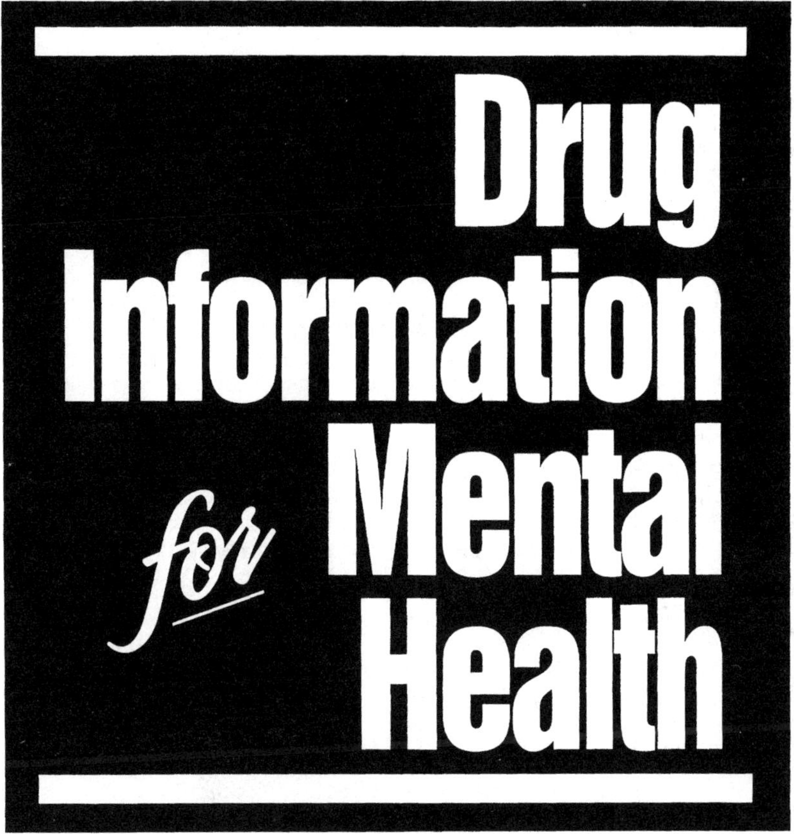


# 2001

**Matthew A. Fuller, PharmD, BCPS, BCPP, FASHP**
*Clinical Pharmacy Specialist, Psychiatry*
Cleveland Department of Veterans Affairs Medical Center
Brecksville, Ohio
*Associate Clinical Professor of Psychiatry*
*Clinical Instructor of Psychology*
Case Western Reserve University
Cleveland, Ohio
*Adjunct Associate Professor of Clinical Pharmacy*
University of Toledo
Toledo, Ohio

**Martha Sajatovic, MD**
*Associate Professor of Psychiatry*
Case Western Reserve University
Cleveland, Ohio

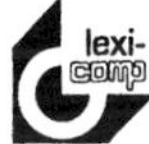


**LEXI-COMP, INC**
**Hudson (Cleveland), OH**

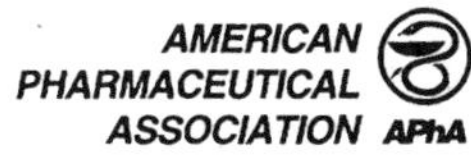

**NOTICE**

This book is intended to serve the user as a handy quick reference and not as a complete drug information resource. It does not include information on every therapeutic agent available. The publication covers commonly used drugs and is specifically designed to present certain important aspects of drug data in a more concise format than is generally found in medical literature or product material supplied by manufacturers.

The nature of drug information is that it is constantly evolving because of ongoing research and clinical experience and is often subject to interpretation. While great care has been taken to ensure the accuracy of the information presented, the reader is advised that the authors, editors, reviewers, contributors, and publishers cannot be responsible for the continued currency of the information or for any errors, omissions, or the application of this information, or for any consequences arising therefrom. Therefore, the author(s) and/or the publisher shall have no liability to any person or entity with regard to claims, loss, or damage caused, or alleged to be caused, directly or indirectly, by the use of information contained herein. Because of the dynamic nature of drug information, readers are advised that decisions regarding drug therapy must be based on the independent judgment of the clinician, changing information about a drug (eg, as reflected in the literature and manufacturer's most current product (information), and changing medical practices. The editors are not responsible for any inaccuracy of quotation or for any false or misleading implication that may arise due to the text or formulas as used or due to the quotation of revisions no longer official.

The editors, authors, and contributors have written this book in their private capacities. No official support or endorsement by any federal agency or pharmaceutical company is intended or inferred.

The publishers have made every effort to trace the copyright holders for borrowed material. If they have inadvertently overlooked any, they will be pleased to make the necessary arrangements at the first opportunity.

If you have any suggestions or questions regarding any information presented in this handbook, please contact our drug information pharmacist at

**1-800-837-LEXI (5394)**



This manual was produced using the FormuLex™ Program — a complete publishing service of Lexi-Comp Inc.

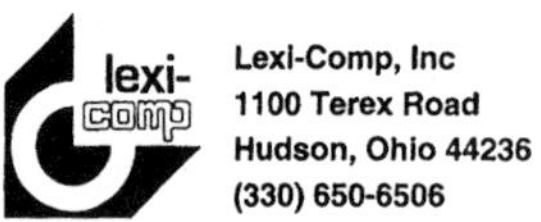


Lexi-Comp, Inc
1100 Terex Road
Hudson, Ohio 44236
(330) 650-6506

ISBN 0-930598-39-4

# TABLE OF CONTENTS

# ABOUT THE AUTHORS

**MATTHEW A. FULLER, PharmD**

Dr Fuller received his Bachelor of Science in Pharmacy from Ohio Northern University and then earned a Doctor of Pharmacy degree from the University of Cincinnati. A residency in hospital pharmacy was completed at Bethesda hospital in Zanesville, Ohio. After completion of his training, Dr Fuller accepted a position at the Veterans Affairs Medical Center in Cleveland, Ohio

Dr Fuller has over 15 years of experience in psychiatric psychopharmacology in a variety of clinical settings including acute care and ambulatory care. Dr Fuller is currently a Clinical Pharmacy Specialist in Psychiatry at the Veterans Affairs Medical Center in Cleveland, Ohio. He is also an Associate Clinical Professor of Psychiatry and Clinical Instructor of Psychology at Case Western Reserve University in Cleveland, Ohio and Adjunct Associate Professor of Clinical Pharmacy at the University of Toledo in Toledo, Ohio. In this position, Dr Fuller is responsible for providing service, education and research. He is also the Director of the ASHP accredited Psychopharmacy Residency Program.

Dr Fuller has received several awards including the Upjohn Excellence in Research Award and the OSHP Hospital Pharmacist of the Year Award in 1994. In 1996 he received the CSHP Evelyn Gray Scott Award (Pharmacist of the Year).

Dr Fuller is Board Certified by the Board of Pharmaceutical Specialties in both Pharmacotherapy and Psychopharmacy. He speaks regularly on the topic of psychotropic use and has published articles and abstracts on various issues in psychiatric psychopharmacology. His research interests include the psychopharmacologic treatment of schizophrenia and bipolar disorder.

Dr Fuller is a member of numerous professional organizations, including the American Society of Health-System Pharmacists (ASHP), where he was recently designated as a fellow. He completed his term as a member of the Commission on Therapeutics and is a member of the Clinical Specialist Section; Ohio Society of Health-System Pharmacists (OSHP) where he has served as an Educational Affairs Division member and a House of Delegates member; American College of Clinical Pharmacy (ACCP), Ohio College of Clinical Pharmacy where he currently serves as secretary/treasurer, Cleveland Society of Health-System Pharmacist (CSHP) where he has served as the education chair and treasurer. He is a member of the National Alliance for the Mentally Ill (NAMI) and also serves as a reviewer for pharmacy and psychiatric journals.

**MARTHA SAJATOVIC, MD**

Dr Sajatovic is Associate Professor of Psychiatry at Case Western Reserve University School of Medicine in Cleveland, Ohio. She is a clinician and researcher with particular interest in health outcome treatment for individuals with serious mental illness. She also has a strong interest in assessment instruments in psychiatry, and frequently serves as a consultant to pharmaceutical companies for rating scales training, as well as publishing in this area.

Dr Sajatovic received her BS in biology at Ohio State University and completed medical school at the Medical College of Ohio at Toledo. She completed her residency training in psychiatry at University Hospitals of Cleveland where she was Chief Resident in Research. Following completion of her residency, Dr Sajatovic was a Clinical Director of Inpatient Schizophrenia Research at University Hospitals of Cleveland, and later, was the Associate Chief of Psychiatry and Chief of the Mood Disorders Program at the Cleveland Veterans Affairs Medical Center in Cleveland, Ohio. Dr Sajatovic has extensive experience with the management of serious mental illness through her work as a state hospital Chief Clinical Officer (Cleveland Campus Northcoast Behavioral Healthcare), in her own private practice, and in consulting with agencies providing community services to the seriously mentally ill.

Dr Sajatovic has published a number of original papers on treatment of serious mental illness and treatment outcomes including work with special populations such as the elderly, women with psychosis, and individuals with developmental disorder. She has been a guest lecturer at numerous academic and community settings including speaking to consumer and family advocacy groups for individuals with psychiatric illness. Dr Sajatovic has a long-standing commitment to education including supervision of medical students and residents in psychiatry, lecturing at Case Western Reserve University School of Medicine, psychiatric resident supervision, and seminar teaching for residents in psychiatry.

# EDITORIAL ADVISORY PANEL

## EDITORIAL ADVISORY PANEL *(Continued)*

# PREFACE

This is the first edition of our new book *Drug Information for Mental Health.* We have taken our second edition of the *Drug Information Handbook for Psychiatry* and have modified it to allow for what we think is a much more user-friendly book. The obvious change is the size. Given the feedback that we have received of the desire for greater ease in finding drug information and the realization that the handbook was most often used as a desk reference, we felt that enlarging the size of the book was justified. Further, we have added dictionary style indexing to allow for more rapid and easier acquisition of drug information.

We continue to strive to make the book a useful, up-to-date tool for the clinician. To this end, we have added several hundred new drugs and much care has been taken to keep this book current with regard to new indications, warnings/precautions, contraindications, adverse reactions, dosing, and dosage forms. In addition, the drug interaction field has been further enhanced to allow for rapid access to detailed drug information.

We have condensed many monographs of infrequently-used compounds or ones not likely to be used by the mental healthcare practitioner. Therefore, all information fields are not included in all drug monographs. The sections of the treatment of medically ill patients and behavioral symptoms and treatment of older adults in particular have been expanded and revised. Herbal monographs have been included as in the past.

This book is not a psychotropic drug handbook, but rather a complete drug information source designed for mental healthcare practitioners. For this purpose, and being aware of the need, we have published the *Psychotropic Drug Information Handbook*, which is currently available in its second edition.

We hope this first edition proves to be a useful tool for the mental healthcare professional when evaluating clients' medication needs. More than ever, your comments are encouraged and appreciated, as we consider these suggestions for future editions, allowing us to better serve your needs.

— Matthew A. Fuller and Martha Sajatovic

# ACKNOWLEDGMENTS

*Drug Information for Mental Health* exists in its present form as the result of the concerted efforts of the following individuals: Robert D. Kerscher, publisher and president of Lexi-Comp Inc; Lynn D. Coppinger, managing editor; Barbara F. Kerscher, production manager; David C. Marcus, director of information systems; and Julian I. Graubart, American Pharmaceutical Association (APhA), Director of Books and Electronic Products.

Special acknowledgment goes to all Lexi-Comp staff for their contributions to this handbook.

Much of the material contained in this book was a result of pharmacy contributors throughout the United States and Canada. Lexi-Comp has assisted many medical institutions to develop hospital-specific formulary manuals that contains clinical drug information as well as dosing. Working with these clinical pharmacists, hospital pharmacy and therapeutics committees, and hospital drug information centers, Lexi-Comp has developed an evolutionary drug database that reflects the practice of pharmacy in these major institutions.

Special thanks from Dr Fuller to his parents, Raymond and Mary Fuller, who afforded him the opportunity to write this book; and to his wife and son, Jeanette and Samuel, who generously gave of their time and support.

A special thanks from Dr Sajatovic goes to her parents, Nick and Martha Sajatovic, to her husband, Douglas N. Flagg, MD, and to her sons, Alexander and Andrew for their continuous patience and support.

# DESCRIPTION OF FIELDS AND SECTIONS

*Drug Information for Mental Health* is divided into five sections.

The first section is a compilation of introductory text pertinent to the use of this book.

The drug information section of the handbook, in which all drugs are listed alphabetically, details information appropriate to each drug. Extensive cross-referencing is provided by brand names and synonyms.

The third section is comprised of several text chapters dealing with various subjects and issues relevant to the management of the psychiatric patient.

The fourth section is an invaluable appendix with charts, tables, nomograms, algorithms, management guidelines, and conversion information which can be helpful for patient care.

The last section of this handbook incorporates three indexes, a pharmacologic category index, an alphabetical index which includes generic names, brand names, synonyms, text chapter headings, and appendix listings; and an international index which lists brand names for 20 different countries.

The **Alphabetical Listing of Drugs** is presented in a consistent format and provides the following fields of information:

| | |
|---|---|
| Generic Name | U.S. adopted name |
| Pronunciation | Phonetic pronunciation guide |
| Related Information | Cross-reference to other pertinent drug information found elsewhere in this handbook |
| U.S. Brand Names | U.S. trade names (manufacturer-specific) |
| Canadian Brand Names | Trade names found in Canada |
| Synonyms | Other names or accepted abbreviations of the generic drug |
| Pharmacologic Category | Unique systematic classification of medications |
| Generic Available | Indicates if a generic form is available for psychotropic medications |
| Use | Information pertaining to appropriate indications of the drug. Includes both FDA approved and non-FDA approved indications. |
| Effect on Mental Status | Pertinent drug effects which may affect or alter a patient's mental status |
| Effect on Psychiatric Treatment | Information relative to the impact on psychiatric treatment |
| Restrictions | The controlled substance classification from the Drug Enforcement Agency (DEA). U.S. schedules are I-V. Schedules vary by country and sometimes state (ie, Massachusetts uses I-VI) |
| Pregnancy Risk Factor | Five categories established by the FDA to indicate the potential of a systemically absorbed drug for causing birth defects |
| Pregnancy/Breast-Feeding Implications | Information pertinent to or associated with the use of the psychotropic drug as it relates to clinical effects on the fetus, breast-feeding/lactation, and clinical effects on the infant |
| Contraindications | Information pertaining to inappropriate use of the drug |
| Warnings/Precautions | Precautionary considerations, hazardous conditions related to use of the drug, and disease states or patient populations in which the drug should be cautiously used |
| Adverse Reactions | Side effects are grouped by percentage of incidence (if known) and/or body system; <1% of incidence are strung and are not listed in most nonpsychotropic drugs |
| Overdosage/Toxicology | Comments and/or considerations are offered when appropriate and include signs/symptoms of excess drug and suggested management of the patient |
| Drug Interactions | Description of the interaction between the drug listed in the monograph and other drugs or drug classes. May include possible mechanisms and effect of combined therapy. May also include a strategy to manage the patient on combined therapy (ie, quinidine). |
| Stability | Information regarding reconstitution, storage, and compatibility is supplied for the psychotropic medications. |
| Mechanism of Action | How the drug works in the body to elicit a response |
| Pharmacodynamics/Kinetics | The magnitude of a drug's effect depends on the drug concentration at the site of action. The pharmacodynamics are expressed in terms of onset of action and duration of action. Pharmacokinetics are expressed in terms of absorption, distribution (including appearance in breast milk and crossing of the placenta), protein binding, metabolism, bioavailability, half-life, time to peak serum concentration, and elimination. |
| Usual Dosage | The amount of the drug to be typically given or taken during therapy for children and adults; also includes any dosing adjustment/comments for renal impairment or hepatic failure |

## DESCRIPTION OF FIELDS AND SECTIONS *(Continued)*

| | |
|---|---|
| Dietary Considerations | Information is offered, when appropriate, regarding food, nutrition, and/or alcohol |
| Administration | Information regarding the recommended final concentrations, rates of administration for parenteral drugs, or other guidelines when giving the psychotropic medications |
| Monitoring Parameters | Laboratory tests and patient physical parameters that should be monitored for safety and efficacy of psychotropic drug therapy |
| Reference Range | Therapeutic and toxic serum concentrations listed for psychotropic agents including peak and trough levels |
| Test Interactions | Listing of assay interferences when relevant;<br>(B) = Blood; (S) = Serum; (U) = Urine |
| Patient Information | Specific information pertinent for the patient |
| Nursing Implications | Includes additional instructions for the administration of the drug and monitoring tips from the nursing perspective |
| Additional Information | Information about sodium content and/or pertinent information about specific brands |
| Dosage Forms | Information with regard to form, strength, and availability of the drug |

# FDA PREGNANCY CATEGORIES

Throughout this book there is a field labeled Pregnancy Risk Factor (PRF) and the letter A, B, C, D, or X immediately following which signifies a category. The FDA has established these five categories to indicate the potential of a systemically absorbed drug for causing birth defects. The key differentiation among the categories rests upon the reliability of documentation and the risk:benefit ratio. Pregnancy Category X is particularly notable in that if any data exists that may implicate a drug as a teratogen and the risk:benefit ratio is clearly negative, the drug is contraindicated during pregnancy.

These categories are summarized as follows:

- A — Controlled studies in pregnant women fail to demonstrate a risk to the fetus in the first trimester with no evidence of risk in later trimesters. The possibility of fetal harm appears remote.
- B — Either animal-reproduction studies have not demonstrated a fetal risk but there are no controlled studies in pregnant women, or animal-reproduction studies have shown an adverse effect (other than a decrease in fertility) that was not confirmed in controlled studies in women in the first trimester and there is no evidence of a risk in later trimesters.
- C — Either studies in animals have revealed adverse effects on the fetus (teratogenic or embryocidal effects or other) and there are no controlled studies in women, or studies in women and animals are not available. Drugs should be given only if the potential benefits justify the potential risk to the fetus.
- D — There is positive evidence of human fetal risk, but the benefits from use in pregnant women may be acceptable despite the risk (eg, if the drug is needed in a life-threatening situation or for a serious disease for which safer drugs cannot be used or are ineffective).
- X — Studies in animals or human beings have demonstrated fetal abnormalities or there is evidence of fetal risk based on human experience, or both, and the risk of the use of the drug in pregnant women clearly outweighs any possible benefit. The drug is contraindicated in women who are or may become pregnant.

## DRUGS IN PREGNANCY

### Analgesics

**Acceptable:** Acetaminophen, meperidine, methadone

**Controversial:** Codeine, propoxyphene

**Unacceptable:** Nonsteroidal anti-inflammatory agents, salicylates, phenazopyridine

### Antimicrobials

**Acceptable:** Penicillins, 1st and 2nd generation cephalosporins, erythromycin (base and EES), clotrimazole, miconazole, nystatin, isoniazid*, lindane, acyclovir, metronidazole

**Controversial:** 3rd generation cephalosporins, aminoglycosides, nitrofurantoin†

**Unacceptable:** Erythromycin estolate, chloramphenicol, sulfa, tetracyclines

### ENT

**Acceptable:** Diphenhydramine*, dextromethorphan

**Controversial:** Pseudoephedrine

**Unacceptable:** Brompheniramine, cyproheptadine, dimenhydrinate

### GI

**Acceptable:** Trimethobenzamide, antacids*, simethicone, other $H_2$-blockers, psyllium, bisacodyl, docusate

**Controversial:** Metoclopramide, prochlorperazine

### Neurologic

**Controversial:** Phenytoin, phenobarbital

**Unacceptable:** Carbamazepine, valproic acid, ergotamine

### Pulmonary

**Acceptable:** Theophylline, metaproterenol, terbutaline, inhaled steroids

**Unacceptable:** Epinephrine, oral steroids

### Psychiatric

**Controversial:** Hydroxyzine*, lithium*, tricyclics, SSRIs, antipsychotics, stimulants

**Unacceptable:** Anticonvulsants

### Other

**Acceptable:** Heparin, insulin

**Unacceptable:** Warfarin, sulfonylureas

*Do not use in first trimester
†Do not use in third trimester

# SAFE WRITING

Health professionals and their support personnel frequently produce handwritten copies of information they see in print; therefore, such information is subjected to even greater possibilities for error or misinterpretation on the part of others. Thus, particular care must be given to how drug names and strengths are expressed when creating written healthcare documents.

The following are a few examples of safe writing rules suggested by the Institute for Safe Medication Practices, Inc.*

1. There should be a space between a number and its units as it is easier to read. There should be no periods after the abbreviations mg or mL.

| Correct | Incorrect |
|---|---|
| 10 mg | 10mg |
| 100 mg | 100mg |

2. Never place a decimal and a zero after a whole number (2 mg is correct and 2.0 mg is **incorrect**). If the decimal point is not seen because it falls on a line or because individuals are working from copies where the decimal point is not seen, this causes a tenfold overdose.
3. Just the opposite is true for numbers less than one. Always place a zero before a naked decimal (0.5 mL is correct, .5 mL is **incorrect**).
4. Never abbreviate the word unit. The handwritten U or u, looks like a 0 (zero), and may cause a tenfold overdose error to be made.
5. IU is not a safe abbreviation for international units. The handwritten IU looks like IV. Write out international units or use int. units.
6. Q.D. is not a safe abbreviation for once daily, as when the Q is followed by a sloppy dot, it looks like QID which means four times daily.
7. O.D. is not a safe abbreviation for once daily, as it is properly interpreted as meaning "right eye" and has caused liquid medications such as saturated solution of potassium iodide and Lugol's solution to be administered incorrectly. There is no safe abbreviation for once daily. It must be written out in full.
8. Do not use chemical names such as 6-mercaptopurine or 6-thioguanine, as sixfold overdoses have been given when these were not recognized as chemical names. The proper names of these drugs are mercaptopurine or thioguanine.
9. Do not abbreviate drug names (5FC, 6MP, 5-ASA, MTX, HCTZ, CPZ, PBZ, etc) as they are misinterpreted and cause error.
10. Do not use the apothecary system or symbols.
11. Do not abbreviate microgram as µg; instead use mcg as there is less likelihood of misinterpretation.
12. When writing an outpatient prescription, write a complete prescription. A complete prescription can prevent the prescriber, the pharmacist, and/or the patient from making a mistake and can eliminate the need for further clarification. The legible prescriptions should contain:

    a. patient's full name

    b. for pediatric or geriatric patients: their age (or weight where applicable)

    c. drug name, dosage form and strength; if a drug is new or rarely prescribed, print this information

    d. number or amount to be dispensed

    e. complete instructions for the patient, including the purpose of the medication

    f. when there are recognized contraindications for a prescribed drug, indicate to the pharmacist that you are aware of this fact (ie, when prescribing a potassium salt for a patient receiving an ACE inhibitor, write "K serum level being monitored")

*From "Safe Writing" by Davis NM, PharmD and Cohen MR, MS, Lecturers and Consultants for Safe Medication Practices, 1143 Wright Drive, Huntington Valley, PA 19006. Phone: (215) 947-7566.

# ALPHABETICAL LISTING OF DRUGS

- **A-200™ Shampoo [OTC]** *see* Pyrethrins *on page 480*
- **A-64077** *see* Zileuton *on page 592*
- **A and D™ Ointment [OTC]** *see* Vitamin A and Vitamin D *on page 586*

## Abacavir (a BAK a veer)

**U.S. Brand Names** Ziagen™

**Pharmacologic Category** Antiretroviral Agent, Reverse Transcriptase Inhibitor (Nucleoside)

**Use** Treatment of HIV infections in combination with other antiretroviral agents

**Effects on Mental Status** May cause fatigue, lethargy, malaise, insomnia, and headache

**Effects on Psychiatric Treatment** Side effects mimic depressive symptoms; caution with benzodiazepines or other CNS depressants and antidepressants

**Pregnancy Risk Factor** C

**Contraindications** Prior hypersensitivity to abacavir (or carbovir) or any component of the formulation; do not rechallenge patients who have experienced hypersensitivity to abacavir

**Warnings/Precautions** Should always be used as a component of a multidrug regimen. Fatal hypersensitivity reactions have occurred. **Patients exhibiting symptoms of fever, skin rash, fatigue, respiratory symptoms (eg, pharyngitis, dyspnea, cough) and GI symptoms (eg, abdominal pain, nausea, vomiting) should discontinue therapy immediately and call for medical attention. Abacavir SHOULD NOT be restarted because more severe symptoms may occur within hours, including LIFE-THREATENING HYPOTENSION AND DEATH. Fatal hypersensitivity reactions have occurred following the reintroduction of abacavir in patients whose therapy was interrupted (interruption in drug supply, temporary discontinuation while treating other conditions). Reactions occurred within hours. In some cases, signs of hypersensitivity may have been previously present, but attributed to other medical conditions (acute onset respiratory diseases, gastroenteritis, reactions to other medications). If abacavir is restarted following an interruption in therapy, evaluate the patient for previously unsuspected symptoms of hypersensitivity. Do not restart if hypersensitivity is suspected. To report these events on abacavir hypersensitivity, a registry has been established (1-800-270-0425).** Use with caution in patients with hepatic dysfunction; prior liver disease, prolonged use, and obesity may be risk factors for development of lactic acidosis and severe hepatomegaly with steatosis.

**Adverse Reactions Note:** Hypersensitivity reactions, which may be fatal, occur in ~5% of patients. Symptoms may include anaphylaxis, fever, rash, fatigue, diarrhea, abdominal pain, nausea and vomiting. Less common symptoms may include edema, lethargy, malaise, myalgia, shortness of breath, mouth ulcerations, conjunctivitis, lymphadenopathy, hepatic failure and renal failure.

Rates of adverse reactions were defined during combination therapy with lamivudine. Adverse reaction rates attributable to abacavir alone are not available.

Adults:
- Central nervous system: Insomnia (7%)
- Gastrointestinal: Anorexia (11%), diarrhea (12%), nausea (47%), pancreatitis, vomiting (16%)
- Neuromuscular & skeletal: Weakness
- Endocrine & metabolic: Hyperglycemia, hypertriglyceridemia (25%)
- Miscellaneous: Elevated transaminases

Children:
- Central nervous system: Fever (19%), headache (16%)
- Dermatologic: Rash (11%)
- Gastrointestinal: Anorexia (9%), diarrhea (16%), nausea (38%), vomiting (38%)

**Drug Interactions**
- Ethanol may increase the risk of toxicity
- Abacavir increases the AUC of amprenavir

**Usual Dosage** Oral:
- Children: 3 months to 16 years: 8 mg/kg body weight twice daily (maximum 300 mg twice daily) in combination with other antiretroviral agents
- Adults: 300 mg twice daily in combination with other antiretroviral agents

**Patient Information** This is not a cure for AIDS or AIDS complex, nor will it reduce the risk of transmission to others. Long-term effects are not known. You will need frequent blood tests to adjust dosage for maximum therapeutic effect. Take as directed, for full course of therapy; do not discontinue (even if feeling better). You may experience headache or muscle pain or weakness. Report skin rash, acute headache, severe nausea or vomiting, or difficulty breathing.

**Dosage Forms**
- Solution, oral (strawberry-banana flavored): 20 mg/mL (240 mL)
- Tablet: 300 mg

- **Abbokinase® Injection** *see* Urokinase *on page 577*
- **Abbreviations and Measurements** *see page 685*
- **ABCD** *see* Amphotericin B Cholesteryl Sulfate Complex *on page 40*

## Abciximab (ab SIK si mab)

**U.S. Brand Names** ReoPro®

**Synonyms** C7E3; 7E3

**Pharmacologic Category** Platelet Aggregation Inhibitor

**Use** Abciximab in for the prevention of acute cardiac ischemic complications in patients at high risk for abrupt closure of the treated coronary vessel; an adjunct with heparin to prevent cardiac ischemic complications in patients with unstable angina not responding to conventional therapy when a percutaneous coronary intervention is scheduled within 24 hours

**Effects on Mental Status** None reported

**Effects on Psychiatric Treatment** None reported

**Pregnancy Risk Factor** C

**Contraindications** Hypersensitivity to abciximab or to murine proteins; active internal hemorrhage or recent (within 6 weeks) clinically significant GI or GU bleeding; history of cerebrovascular accident within 2 years or cerebrovascular accident with significant neurological deficit; clotting abnormalities or administration of oral anticoagulants within 7 days unless prothrombin time (PT) is ≤1.2 times control PT value; thrombocytopenia (<100,000 cells/µL); recent (within 6 weeks) major surgery or trauma; intracranial tumor, arteriovenous malformation, or aneurysm; severe uncontrolled hypertension; history of vasculitis; use of dextran before PTCA or intent to use dextran during PTCA; concomitant use of another parenteral GP IIb/IIIa inhibitor

**Warnings/Precautions** Administration of abciximab is associated with increased frequency of major bleeding complications including retroperitoneal bleeding, spontaneous GI or GU bleeding, and bleeding at the arterial access site and in the following: patients weighing <75 kilograms, elderly patients (>65 years of age), history of previous GI disease, recent thrombolytic therapy.

The risk of major bleeds may increase with concurrent use of thrombolytics. In serious, uncontrolled bleeding, abciximab and heparin should be stopped.

Increased risk of hemorrhage during or following angioplasty is associated with unsuccessful PTCA, PTCA procedure >70 minutes duration, or PTCA performed within 12 hours of symptom onset for acute myocardial infarction.

There is no data concerning the safety or efficacy of readministration of abciximab. Administration of abciximab may result in human antichimeric antibody formation that can cause hypersensitivity reactions (including anaphylaxis), thrombocytopenia, or diminished efficacy. Anticoagulation, such as with heparin, may contribute to the risk of bleeding.

**Adverse Reactions**

>10%:
- Cardiovascular: Hypotension
- Central nervous system: Pain
- Gastrointestinal: Nausea
- Hematologic: Major bleeding episodes

1% to 10%:
- Cardiovascular: Bradycardia, peripheral edema
- Hematologic: Anemia, minor bleeding episodes, thrombocytopenia
- Respiratory: Pleural effusion

**Drug Interactions**
- Heparin and aspirin: Use with aspirin and heparin may increase bleeding over aspirin and heparin alone. However, aspirin and heparin were used concurrently in the majority of patients in the major clinical studies of abciximab
- Monoclonal antibodies: Allergic reactions may be increased in patients who have received diagnostic or therapeutic monoclonal antibodies due to the presence of HACA antibodies
- Thrombolytic agents theoretically may increase the risk of hemorrhage; use with caution
- Warfarin and oral anticoagulants: Risk of bleeding may be increased during concurrent therapy
- Other IIb/IIIa antagonists: Avoid concomitant use of other glycoprotein IIb/IIIa antagonists (see Contraindications)

**Usual Dosage** I.V.: 0.25 mg/kg bolus administered 10-60 minutes before the start of intervention followed by an infusion of 0.125 mcg/kg/minute (to a maximum of 10 mcg/minute) for 12 hours

Patients with unstable angina not responding to conventional medical therapy and who are planning to undergo percutaneous coronary intervention within 24 hours may be treated with abciximab 0.25 mg/kg intravenous bolus followed by an 18- to 24-hour intravenous infusion of 10 mcg/minute, concluding 1 hour after the percutaneous coronary intervention.

**Dosage Forms** Injection: 2 mg/mL (5 mL)

- **Abelcet™ Injection** *see* Amphotericin B, Lipid Complex *on page 42*
- **Absinthe** *see* Wormwood *on page 588*
- **Absorbine® Antifungal [OTC]** *see* Tolnaftate *on page 555*
- **Absorbine® Antifungal Foot Powder [OTC]** *see* Miconazole *on page 364*

♦ **Absorbine® Jock Itch [OTC]** *see* Tolnaftate *on page 555*

♦ **Absorbine Jr.® Antifungal [OTC]** *see* Tolnaftate *on page 555*

♦ **AC-4464** *see* Torsemide *on page 557*

## Acarbose (AY car bose)

**Related Information**
Diabetes Mellitus Treatment *on page 782*
Hypoglycemic Drugs and Thiazolidinedione Information *on page 714*

**U.S. Brand Names** Precose®

**Canadian Brand Names** Pradnase®

**Pharmacologic Category** Antidiabetic Agent (Miscellaneous)

**Use**
Monotherapy, as indicated as an adjunct to diet to lower blood glucose in patients with noninsulin-dependent diabetes mellitus (NIDDM) whose hyperglycemia cannot be managed on diet alone
Combination with a sulfonylurea, metformin, or insulin in patients with NIDDM when diet plus acarbose do not result in adequate glycemic control

**Effects on Mental Status** May cause drowsiness

**Effects on Psychiatric Treatment** Antipsychotics and tricyclic antidepressants may decrease the effects of acarbose. Monoamine oxidase inhibitors, SSRIs, and nefazodone may increase the effects of acarbose.

**Pregnancy Risk Factor** B

**Contraindications** Known hypersensitivity to the drug and in patients with diabetic ketoacidosis or cirrhosis; patients with inflammatory bowel disease, colonic ulceration, partial intestinal obstruction or in patients predisposed to intestinal obstruction; patients who have chronic intestinal diseases associated with marked disorders of digestion or absorption and in patients who have conditions that may deteriorate as a result of increased gas formation in the intestine

**Warnings/Precautions** Hypoglycemia: Acarbose may increase the hypoglycemic potential of sulfonylureas. Oral glucose (dextrose) should be used in the treatment of mild to moderate hypoglycemia. Severe hypoglycemia may require the use of either intravenous glucose infusion or glucagon injection.

Elevated serum transaminase levels: Treatment-emergent elevations of serum transaminases (AST and/or ALT) occurred in 15% of acarbose-treated patients in long-term studies. These serum transaminase elevations appear to be dose related. At doses >100 mg 3 times/day, the incidence of serum transaminase elevations greater than 3 times the upper limit of normal was 2-3 times higher in the acarbose group than in the placebo group. These elevations were asymptomatic, reversible, more common in females, and, in general, were not associated with other evidence of liver dysfunction.

When diabetic patients are exposed to stress such as fever, trauma, infection, or surgery, a temporary loss of control of blood glucose may occur. At such times, temporary insulin therapy may be necessary.

**Adverse Reactions**
>10%:
Gastrointestinal: Abdominal pain (21%) and diarrhea (33%) tend to return to pretreatment levels over time, and the frequency and intensity of flatulence (77%) tend to abate with time
Hepatic: Elevated liver transaminases
<1%: Erythema, headache, severe gastrointestinal distress, sleepiness, urticaria, vertigo, weakness

**Overdosage/Toxicology**
Signs and symptoms: An overdose will not result in hypoglycemia; an overdose may result in transient increases in flatulence, diarrhea, and abdominal discomfort which shortly subside
Treatment: Hypoglycemia must be treated with oral or injectable glucose or injectable glucagon, but not sucrose (cane sugar)

**Drug Interactions** Decreased effect: Thiazides and other diuretics, corticosteroids, phenothiazines, thyroid products, estrogens, oral contraceptives, phenytoin, nicotinic acid, sympathomimetics, calcium channel-blocking drugs, isoniazid, intestinal adsorbents (eg, charcoal), digestive enzyme preparations (eg, amylase, pancreatin)

**Usual Dosage** Oral:
Adults: Dosage must be individualized on the basis of effectiveness and tolerance while not exceeding the maximum recommended dose
**Initial dose:** 25 mg 3 times/day with the first bite of each main meal
**Maintenance dose:** Should be adjusted at 4- to 8-week intervals based on 1-hour postprandial glucose levels and tolerance. Dosage may be increased from 25 mg 3 times/day to 50 mg 3 times/day. Some patients may benefit from increasing the dose to 100 mg 3 times/day.
Maintenance dose ranges: 50-100 mg 3 times/day.
**Maximum dose:**
≤60 kg: 50 mg 3 times/day
>60 kg: 100 mg 3 times/day
**Patients receiving sulfonylureas:** Acarbose given in combination with a sulfonylurea will cause a further lowering of blood glucose and may increase the hypoglycemic potential of the sulfonylurea. If hypoglycemia occurs, appropriate adjustments in the dosage of these agents should be made.
**Dosing adjustment in renal impairment:** $Cl_{cr}$ <25 mL/minute: Peak plasma concentrations were 5 times higher and AUCs were 6 times larger than in volunteers with normal renal function; however, long term clinical trials in diabetic patients with significant renal dysfunction have not been conducted and treatment of these patients with acarbose is not recommended

**Patient Information** Take this medication exactly as directed, with the first bite of each main meal. Do not change dosage or discontinue without first consulting prescriber. Do not take other medications with or within 2 hours of this medication unless so advised by prescriber. It is important to follow dietary and lifestyle recommendations of prescriber. You will be instructed in signs of hypo-/hyperglycemia by prescriber or diabetic educator. If combining acarbose with other diabetic medication (eg, sulfonylureas, insulin), keep source of glucose (sugar) on hand in case hypoglycemia occurs. You may experience mild side effects during first weeks of acarbose therapy (eg, bloating, flatulence, diarrhea, abdominal discomfort); these should diminish over time. Report severe or persistent side effects, fever, extended vomiting or flu, or change in color of urine or stool.

**Dosage Forms** Tablet: 50 mg, 100 mg

♦ **Accolate®** *see* Zafirlukast *on page 589*

♦ **Accupril®** *see* Quinapril *on page 484*

♦ **Accutane®** *see* Isotretinoin *on page 297*

♦ **ACE** *see* Captopril *on page 89*

## Acebutolol (a se BYOO toe lole)

**Related Information**
Beta-Blockers Comparison Chart *on page 709*

**U.S. Brand Names** Sectral®

**Canadian Brand Names** Monitan®; Rhotral

**Pharmacologic Category** Antiarrhythmic Agent, Class II; Beta Blocker (with Intrinsic Sympathomimetic Activity)

**Use** Treatment of hypertension, ventricular arrhythmias, angina

**Effects on Mental Status** Drowsiness/fatigue is common; may cause insomnia, depression, abnormal dreams, and polyuria

**Effects on Psychiatric Treatment** Additive hypotensive and/or sedative effects may be seen with concurrent use of antipsychotics, antidepressants, or benzodiazepines

**Pregnancy Risk Factor** B (per manufacturer); D (in second and third trimester, based on expert analysis)

**Contraindications** Hypersensitivity to beta-blocking agents; uncompensated congestive heart failure; cardiogenic shock; bradycardia or second- and third-degree heart block (except in patients with a functioning artificial pacemaker); sinus node dysfunction; pregnancy (2nd and 3rd trimesters)

**Warnings/Precautions** Abrupt withdrawal of drug **should be avoided.** May result in an exaggerated cardiac responsiveness such as tachycardia, hypertension, ischemia, angina, myocardial infarction, and sudden death. It is recommended that patients be gradually tapered off beta-blockers (over a 2-week period) rather than via abrupt discontinuation. Although acebutolol primarily blocks $beta_1$-receptors, high doses can result in $beta_2$-receptor blockage. Use with caution in diabetic patients. Beta-blockers may impair glucose tolerance, potentiate hypoglycemia, and/or mask symptoms of hypoglycemia in a diabetic patient. Use with caution in bronchospastic lung disease and renal dysfunction (especially the elderly). Beta-blockers with intrinsic sympathomimetic activity do not appear to be of benefit in congestive heart failure and should be avoided. See Usual Dosage - Renal/Hepatic Impairment.

**Adverse Reactions**
>10%: Central nervous system: Fatigue
1% to 10%:
Cardiovascular: Bradycardia, chest pain, edema, hypotension
Central nervous system: Abnormal dreams, depression, dizziness, headache, insomnia
Dermatologic: Rash
Gastrointestinal: Constipation, diarrhea, dyspepsia, flatulence, nausea
Genitourinary: Polyuria
Neuromuscular & skeletal: Arthralgia, myalgia
Ocular: Abnormal vision
Respiratory: Cough, dyspnea, rhinitis
<1%: Anorexia, cold extremities, facial edema, heart block, heart failure, impotence, urinary retention, ventricular arrhythmias, xerostomia

**Overdosage/Toxicology**
Signs and symptoms: Bradycardia, A-V block, hypotension, asystole
Treatment: Initiate support with fluids, epinephrine or dopamine may be useful; glucagon may be particularly effective for reversing cardiac manifestations

**Drug Interactions**
Alpha-blockers (prazosin, terazosin): Concurrent use of beta-blockers may increase risk of orthostasis
Clonidine: Hypertensive crisis after or during withdrawal of either agent
(Continued)

## Acebutolol *(Continued)*

Drugs which slow AV conduction (digoxin): Effects may be additive with beta-blockers

Glucagon: Acebutolol may blunt the hyperglycemic action of glucagon

Insulin and oral hypoglycemics: Acebutolol masks the tachycardia from hypoglycemia

NSAIDs (ibuprofen, indomethacin, naproxen, piroxicam) may reduce the antihypertensive effects of beta-blockers

Salicylates may reduce the antihypertensive effects of beta-blockers

Sulfonylureas: Beta-blockers may alter response to hypoglycemic agents

Verapamil or diltiazem may have synergistic or additive pharmacological effects when taken concurrently with beta-blockers

**Usual Dosage** Oral:

Adults:

Hypertension: 400-800 mg/day (larger doses may be divided); maximum: 1200 mg/day

Ventricular arrhythmias: Initial: 400 mg/day; maintenance: 600-1200 mg/day in divided doses

Elderly: Initial: 200-400 mg/day; dose reduction due to age related decrease in $Cl_{cr}$ will be necessary; do not exceed 800 mg/day

**Dosing adjustment in renal impairment:**

$Cl_{cr}$ 25-49 mL/minute/1.73 $m^2$: Reduce dose by 50%

$Cl_{cr}$ <25 mL/minute/1.73 $m^2$: Reduce dose by 75%

**Dosing adjustment in hepatic impairment:** Use with caution

**Patient Information** Take exactly as directed; do not increase, decrease, or adjust dosage without consulting prescriber. Take pulse daily, prior to medication, and follow prescriber's instruction about holding medication. Do not take with antacids. Do not use alcohol and OTC medications such as cold remedies without consulting prescriber. If diabetic, monitor serum sugars closely (may alter glucose tolerance or mask signs of hypoglycemia). May cause fatigue, dizziness (use caution when driving or engaging in tasks that require alertness until response to drug is known); postural hypotension (use caution when changing position from lying or sitting to standing or when climbing stairs); or alteration in sexual performance (reversible). Report chest pain or palpitations, unresolved swelling of extremities or unusual weight gain, difficulty breathing or new cough, skin rash, unresolved fatigue, unresolved constipation or diarrhea, unusual muscle weakness, or CNS disturbances.

**Dosage Forms** Capsule, as hydrochloride: 200 mg, 400 mg

♦ **Aceon®** *see* Perindopril Erbumine *on page 431*

♦ **Acephen® [OTC]** *see* Acetaminophen *on page 14*

♦ **Aceta® [OTC]** *see* Acetaminophen *on page 14*

## Acetaminophen (a seet a MIN oh fen)

**U.S. Brand Names** Acephen® [OTC]; Aceta® [OTC]; Apacet® [OTC]; Aspirin Free Anacin® Maximum Strength [OTC]; Children's Dynafed® Jr [OTC]; Children's Silapap® [OTC]; Extra Strength Dynafed® E.X. [OTC]; Feverall™ [OTC]; Feverall™ Sprinkle Caps [OTC]; Genapap® [OTC]; Halenol® Children's [OTC]; Infants Feverall™ [OTC]; Infants' Silapap® [OTC]; Junior Strength Panadol® [OTC]; Liquiprin® [OTC]; Mapap® [OTC]; Maranox® [OTC]; Neopap® [OTC]; Panadol® [OTC]; Redutemp® [OTC]; Ridenol® [OTC]; Tempra® [OTC]; Tylenol® [OTC]; Tylenol® Extended Relief [OTC]; Uni-Ace® [OTC]

**Canadian Brand Names** Abenol®; A.F. Anacin®; Atasol®; Pediatrix; Tantaphen®

**Synonyms** APAP; N-Acetyl-P-Aminophenol; Paracetamol

**Pharmacologic Category** Analgesic, Miscellaneous

**Use** Treatment of postoperative and mild to moderate pain and fever; does not have antirheumatic effects (analgesic)

**Effects on Mental Status** None reported

**Effects on Psychiatric Treatment** Barbiturates and carbamazepine may increase the hepatotoxic potential of acetaminophen

**Pregnancy Risk Factor** B

**Contraindications** Patients with known G-6-PD deficiency; hypersensitivity to acetaminophen

**Warnings/Precautions** May cause severe hepatic toxicity on overdose; use with caution in patients with alcoholic liver disease; chronic daily dosing in adults of 5-8 g of acetaminophen over several weeks or 3-4 g/day of acetaminophen for 1 year have resulted in liver damage

**Adverse Reactions** Percentage unknown: May increase chloride, bilirubin, uric acid, glucose, ammonia, alkaline phosphatase; may decrease sodium, bicarbonate, calcium

<1%: Analgesic nephropathy, anemia, blood dyscrasias (neutropenia, pancytopenia, leukopenia), hypersensitivity reactions (rare), nausea, nephrotoxicity with chronic overdose, rash, vomiting

**Overdosage/Toxicology**

Signs and symptoms include hepatic necrosis, transient azotemia, renal tubular necrosis with acute toxicity, anemia, and GI disturbances with chronic toxicity

Treatment: Acetylcysteine 140 mg/kg orally (loading) followed by 70 mg/kg every 4 hours for 17 doses; therapy should be initiated based upon laboratory analysis suggesting high probability of hepatotoxic potential. Activated charcoal is very effective at binding acetaminophen.

**Drug Interactions** CYP1A2 enzyme substrate (minor), CYP2E1 and 3A3/4 enzyme substrate

Decreased effect: Rifampin can interact to reduce the analgesic effectiveness of acetaminophen

Increased toxicity: Barbiturates, carbamazepine, hydantoins, sulfinpyrazone can increase the hepatotoxic potential of acetaminophen; chronic ethanol abuse increases risk for acetaminophen toxicity; effect of warfarin may be enhanced

**Usual Dosage** Oral, rectal (if fever not controlled with acetaminophen alone, administer with full doses of aspirin on an every 4- to 6-hour schedule, if aspirin is not otherwise contraindicated):

Children <12 years: 10-15 mg/kg/dose every 4-6 hours as needed; do **not** exceed 5 doses (2.6 g) in 24 hours; alternatively, the following age-based doses may be used.

0-3 months: 40 mg
4-11 months: 80 mg
1-2 years: 120 mg
2-3 years: 160 mg
4-5 years: 240 mg
6-8 years: 320 mg
9-10 years: 400 mg
11 years: 480 mg

Adults: 325-650 mg every 4-6 hours or 1000 mg 3-4 times/day; do **not** exceed 4 g/day

**Dosing interval in renal impairment:**

$Cl_{cr}$ 10-50 mL/minute: Administer every 6 hours

$Cl_{cr}$ <10 mL/minute: Administer every 8 hours (metabolites accumulate)

Hemodialysis: Moderately dialyzable (20% to 50%)

**Dosing adjustment/comments in hepatic impairment:** Appears to be well tolerated in cirrhosis; serum levels may need monitoring with long-term use

**Dietary Considerations**

Food: May slightly delay absorption of extended-release preparations; rate of absorption may be decreased when given with food high in carbohydrates

Alcohol: Excessive intake of alcohol may increase the risk of acetaminophen-induced hepatotoxicity; avoid or limit alcohol intake

**Patient Information** Take exactly as directed (do not increase dose or frequency); most adverse effects are related to excessive use. Take with food or milk. While using this medication, avoid alcohol and other prescription or OTC medications that contain acetaminophen. Maintain adequate hydration (2-3 L/day of fluids unless instructed to restrict fluid intake). This medication will not reduce inflammation; consult prescriber for anti-inflammatory, if needed. Report unusual bleeding (stool, mouth, urine) or bruising; unusual fatigue and weakness; change in elimination patterns; or change in color of urine or stool.

**Nursing Implications**

Suppositories: Do not freeze

Suspension, oral: Shake well before pouring a dose

**Dosage Forms**

Caplet: 160 mg, 325 mg, 500 mg

Caplet, extended: 650 mg

Capsule: 80 mg

Drops: 48 mg/mL (15 mL); 60 mg/0.6 mL (15 mL); 80 mg/0.8 mL (15 mL); 100 mg/mL (15 mL, 30 mL)

Elixir: 80 mg/5 mL, 120 mg/5 mL, 160 mg/5 mL, 167 mg/5 mL, 325 mg/5 mL

Liquid, oral: 160 mg/5 mL, 500 mg/15 mL

Solution: 100 mg/mL (15 mL); 120 mg/2.5 mL

Suppository, rectal: 80 mg, 120 mg, 125 mg, 300 mg, 325 mg, 650 mg

Suspension, oral: 160 mg/5 mL

Suspension, oral drops: 80 mg/0.8 mL

Tablet: 325 mg, 500 mg, 650 mg

Tablet, chewable: 80 mg, 160 mg

♦ **Acetaminophen and Butalbital Compound** *see* Butalbital Compound and Acetaminophen *on page 80*

## Acetaminophen and Codeine
(a seet a MIN oh fen & KOE deen)

**U.S. Brand Names** Capital® and Codeine; Phenaphen® With Codeine; Tylenol® With Codeine

**Canadian Brand Names** Atasol® 8, 15, 30 With Caffeine; Empracet® 30, 60; Emtec-30®; Lenoltec No 1, 2, 3, 4; Novo-Gesic-C8; Novo-Gesic-C15; Novo-Gesic-C30

**Pharmacologic Category** Analgesic, Narcotic

**Use** Relief of mild to moderate pain

**Effects on Mental Status** Sedation is common; less commonly, codeine may produce euphoria or dysphoria

**Effects on Psychiatric Treatment** Codeine may produce physical and psychological dependence. Antipsychotics, tricyclic antidepressants, monoamine oxidase inhibitors, barbiturates, benzodiazepines, and anticonvulsants may increase the toxicity of codeine. Barbiturates and carbamazepine may increase the hepatotoxic potential of acetaminophen. Diminution of pain relief may occur with the SSRIs.

**Restrictions** C-III; C-V

**Usual Dosage** Doses should be adjusted according to severity of pain and response of the patient. Adult doses ≥60 mg codeine fail to give commensurate relief of pain but merely prolong analgesia and are associated with an appreciably increased incidence of side effects. Oral:

Children: Analgesic:
- Codeine: 0.5-1 mg codeine/kg/dose every 4-6 hours
- Acetaminophen: 10-15 mg/kg/dose every 4 hours up to a maximum of 2.6 g/24 hours for children <12 years
  - 3-6 years: 5 mL 3-4 times/day as needed of elixir
  - 7-12 years: 10 mL 3-4 times/day as needed of elixir
  - >12 years: 15 mL every 4 hours as needed of elixir

Adults:
- Antitussive: Based on codeine (15-30 mg/dose) every 4-6 hours
- Analgesic: Based on codeine (30-60 mg/dose) every 4-6 hours
  - 1-2 tablets every 4 hours to a maximum of 12 tablets/24 hours

**Dosing adjustment in renal impairment:** Refer to individual monographs for Acetaminophen and Codeine

**Dosage Forms**

Capsule:
- #2: Acetaminophen 325 mg and codeine phosphate 15 mg (C-III)
- #3: Acetaminophen 325 mg and codeine phosphate 30 mg (C-III)
- #4: Acetaminophen 325 mg and codeine phosphate 60 mg (C-III)

Elixir: Acetaminophen 120 mg and codeine phosphate 12 mg per 5 mL with alcohol 7% (C-V)

Suspension, oral, alcohol free: Acetaminophen 120 mg and codeine phosphate 12 mg per 5 mL (C-V)

Tablet: Acetaminophen 500 mg and codeine phosphate 30 mg (C-III); acetaminophen 650 mg and codeine phosphate 30 mg (C-III)

Tablet:
- #1: Acetaminophen 300 mg and codeine phosphate 7.5 mg (C-III)
- #2: Acetaminophen 300 mg and codeine phosphate 15 mg (C-III)
- #3: Acetaminophen 300 mg and codeine phosphate 30 mg (C-III)
- #4: Acetaminophen 300 mg and codeine phosphate 60 mg (C-III)

## Acetaminophen and Dextromethorphan

(a seet a MIN oh fen & dex troe meth OR fan)

**U.S. Brand Names** Bayer® Select® Chest Cold Caplets [OTC]; Drixoral® Cough & Sore Throat Liquid Caps [OTC]

**Pharmacologic Category** Cough Preparation

**Use** Treatment of mild to moderate pain and fever; symptomatic relief of coughs caused by minor viral upper respiratory tract infections or inhaled irritants; most effective for a chronic nonproductive cough

**Effects on Mental Status** May cause drowsiness or depression

**Effects on Psychiatric Treatment** Use with MAOIs may cause hypertension crisis; avoid combination

**Usual Dosage** Oral:
- Children: 10-15 mg/kg/dose every 4-6 hours as needed; do **not** exceed 5 doses in 24 hours
- Adults: 325-650 mg every 4-6 hours or 1000 mg 3-4 times/day; do **not** exceed 4 g/day

**Dosage Forms**
- Caplet: Acetaminophen 500 and dextromethorphan hydrobromide 15 mg
- Capsule: Acetaminophen 325 and dextromethorphan hydrobromide 15 mg

## Acetaminophen and Diphenhydramine

(a seet a MIN oh fen & dye fen HYE dra meen)

**U.S. Brand Names** Arthritis Foundation® Nighttime [OTC]; Excedrin® P.M. [OTC]; Midol® PM [OTC]

**Pharmacologic Category** Analgesic, Miscellaneous

**Use** Relief of mild to moderate pain; sinus headache

**Effects on Mental Status** Drowsiness is common

**Effects on Psychiatric Treatment** Concurrent use with CNS depressant may result in additive CNS depression. MAOI may cause additive anticholinergic effects.

**Usual Dosage** Oral: Adults: Take 2 caplets or 5 mL of liquid at bedtime or as directed by physician; do not exceed recommended dosage; not for use in children <12 years of age

**Dosage Forms**

Caplet:
- Excedrin® P.M.: Acetaminophen 500 mg and diphenhydramine citrate 30 mg
- Arthritis Foundation® Nighttime, Midol® PM: Acetaminophen 500 mg and diphenhydramine 25 mg

Liquid (wild berry flavor) (Excedrin® P.M.): Acetaminophen 1000 mg and diphenhydramine hydrochloride 50 mg per 30 mL (180 mL)

♦ **Acetaminophen and Hydrocodone** *see* Hydrocodone and Acetaminophen *on page 272*

♦ **Acetaminophen and Oxycodone** *see* Oxycodone and Acetaminophen *on page 414*

## Acetaminophen and Phenyltoloxamine

(a seet a MIN oh fen & fen il to LOKS a meen)

**U.S. Brand Names** Percogesic® [OTC]

**Pharmacologic Category** Analgesic, Non-narcotic

**Use** Relief of mild to moderate pain

**Effects on Mental Status** None reported

**Effects on Psychiatric Treatment** Barbiturates and carbamazepine may increase the hepatotoxic potential of acetaminophen

**Usual Dosage** Adults: Oral: 1-2 tablets every 4 hours

**Dosage Forms** Tablet: Acetaminophen 325 mg and phenyltoloxamine citrate 30 mg

## Acetaminophen and Pseudoephedrine

(a seet a MIN oh fen & soo doe e FED rin)

**U.S. Brand Names** Allerest® No Drowsiness [OTC]; Bayer® Select Head Cold Caplets [OTC]; Coldrine® [OTC]; Dristan® Cold Caplets [OTC]; Dynafed®, Maximum Strength [OTC]; Ornex® No Drowsiness [OTC]; Sinarest®, No Drowsiness [OTC]; Sine-Aid®, Maximum Strength [OTC]; Sine-Off® Maximum Strength No Drowsiness Formula [OTC]; Sinus Excedrin® Extra Strength [OTC]; Sinus-Relief® [OTC]; Sinutab® Without Drowsiness [OTC]; Tylenol® Sinus, Maximum Strength [OTC]

**Canadian Brand Names** Dristan® ND, Extra Strength

**Pharmacologic Category** Alpha/Beta Agonist; Analgesic, Miscellaneous

**Effects on Mental Status** Anxiety, insomnia, excitability common; hallucination may be seen rarely

**Effects on Psychiatric Treatment** Hypertensive crisis may result with MAOI, effects of CNS depressants may be lessened

**Dosage Forms** Tablet:
- Allerest® No Drowsiness; Coldrine®, Tylenol® Sinus, Maximum Strength; Ornex® No Drowsiness, Sinus-Relief®: Acetaminophen 325 mg and pseudoephedrine hydrochloride 30 mg
- Bayer® Select Head Cold; Dristan® Cold; Dynafed®, Maximum Strength; Sinarest®, No Drowsiness; Sine-Aid®, Maximum Strength; Sine-Off® Maximum Strength No Drowsiness Formula; Sinus Excedrin® Extra Strength; Sinutab® Without Drowsiness; Tylenol® Sinus, Maximum Strength: Acetaminophen 500 mg and pseudoephedrine hydrochloride 30 mg

## Acetaminophen, Aspirin, and Caffeine

(a seet a MIN oh fen, AS pir in, & KAF een)

**U.S. Brand Names** Excedrin®, Extra Strength [OTC]; Gelpirin® [OTC]; Goody's® Headache Powders

**Pharmacologic Category** Analgesic, Miscellaneous

**Use** Relief of mild to moderate pain

**Effects on Mental Status** May cause anxiety, insomnia, and excitability

**Effects on Psychiatric Treatment** Effects of CNS depressants may be lessened by caffeine component

**Usual Dosage** Adults: Oral: 1-2 tablets every 2-6 hours as needed for pain

**Dosage Forms**
- Geltab: Acetaminophen 250 mg, aspirin 250 mg, and caffeine 65 mg
- Powder: Acetaminophen 250 mg, aspirin 520 mg, and caffeine 32.5 mg per dose
- Tablet: Acetaminophen 125 mg, aspirin 240 mg, and caffeine 32 mg; acetaminophen 250 mg, aspirin 250 mg, and caffeine 65 mg

## Acetaminophen, Chlorpheniramine, and Pseudoephedrine

(a seet a MIN oh fen, klor fen IR a meen, & soo doe e FED rin)

**U.S. Brand Names** Alka-Seltzer® Plus Cold Liqui-Gels Capsules [OTC]; Aspirin-Free Bayer® Select® Allergy Sinus Caplets [OTC]; Co-Hist® [OTC]; Sinutab® Tablets [OTC]

**Canadian Brand Names** Tylenol® Allergy & Sinus

**Pharmacologic Category** Analgesic, Miscellaneous; Antihistamine

**Use** Temporary relief of sinus symptoms

**Effects on Mental Status** Sedation with chlorpheniramine is countered by the excitability associated with pseudoephedrine; one effect may predominate in any particular patient

**Effects on Psychiatric Treatment** Usually none; sedative effect of chlorpheniramine may be potentiated by other CNS depressants and MAOIs

**Usual Dosage** Adults: Oral: 2 tablets every 6 hours

**Dosage Forms**
- Caplet: Acetaminophen 500 mg, chlorpheniramine maleate 2 mg, and pseudoephedrine hydrochloride 30 mg
- Capsule: Acetaminophen 250 mg, chlorpheniramine maleate 2 mg, and pseudoephedrine hydrochloride 30 mg

(Continued)

## Acetaminophen, Chlorpheniramine, and Pseudoephedrine *(Continued)*

Tablet: Acetaminophen 325 mg, chlorpheniramine maleate 2 mg, and pseudoephedrine hydrochloride 30 mg

## Acetaminophen, Dextromethorphan, and Pseudoephedrine

(a seet a MIN oh fen, deks troe meth OR fan, & soo doe e FED rin)

**U.S. Brand Names** Alka-Seltzer® Plus Flu & Body Aches Non-Drowsy Liqui-Gels [OTC]; Comtrex® Maximum Strength Non-Drowsy [OTC]; Sudafed® Severe Cold [OTC]; Theraflu® Non-Drowsy Formula Maximum Strength [OTC]; Tylenol® Cold No Drowsiness [OTC]; Tylenol® Flu Maximum Strength [OTC]

**Canadian Brand Names** Contac® Day & Night Cold and Flu System

**Pharmacologic Category** Antihistamine; Antitussive

**Effects on Mental Status** Sedation with dextromethorphan tends to be countered by the excitability associated with pseudoephedrine; one effect may predominate in any particular patient

**Effects on Psychiatric Treatment** Increased toxicity and hypertensive crisis may be seen with concurrent use of MAOIs and CNS depressants, effects of CNS depressants may be lessened

**Dosage Forms** Tablet:

Alka-Seltzer® Plus Flu & Body Aches Non-Drowsy: Acetaminophen 500 mg, dextromethorphan hydrobromide 10 mg, and pseudoephedrine hydrochloride 30 mg

Tylenol® Cold No Drowsiness: Acetaminophen 325 mg, dextromethorphan hydrobromide 15 mg, and pseudoephedrine hydrochloride 30 mg

Comtrex® Maximum Strength Non-Drowsy; Sudafed® Severe Cold; Theraflu® Non-Drowsy Formula Maximum Strength; Tylenol® Flu Maximum Strength: Acetaminophen 500 mg, dextromethorphan hydrobromide 15 mg, and pseudoephedrine hydrochloride 30 mg

## Acetaminophen, Isometheptene, and Dichloralphenazone

(a seet a MIN oh fen, eye soe me THEP teen, & dye KLOR al FEN a zone)

**U.S. Brand Names** Isocom®; Isopap®; Midchlor®; Midrin®; Migratine®

**Pharmacologic Category** Analgesic, Miscellaneous

**Use** Relief of migraine and tension headache

**Effects on Mental Status** May cause drowsiness or dizziness

**Effects on Psychiatric Treatment** Contraindicated with MAOI

**Usual Dosage** Adults: Oral: 2 capsules at first sign of headache, followed by 1 capsule every 60 minutes until relieved, up to 5 capsules in a 12-hour period

**Dosage Forms** Capsule: Acetaminophen 325 mg, isometheptene mucate 65 mg, dichloralphenazone 100 mg

## Acetazolamide (a set a ZOLE a mide)

**Related Information**

Glaucoma Drug Therapy *on page 712*

**U.S. Brand Names** Diamox®; Diamox Sequels®

**Canadian Brand Names** Acetazolam®; Apo®-Acetazolamide; Novo-Zolamide

**Pharmacologic Category** Anticonvulsant, Miscellaneous; Carbonic Anhydrase Inhibitor; Diuretic, Carbonic Anhydrase Inhibitor; Ophthalmic Agent, Antiglaucoma

**Use** Lowers intraocular pressure to treat glaucoma, also as a diuretic, adjunct treatment of refractory seizures and acute altitude sickness; centrencephalic epilepsies (sustained release not recommended for anticonvulsant)

**Effects on Mental Status** Drowsiness is common, may produce depression less commonly

**Effects on Psychiatric Treatment** Can rarely cause bone marrow suppression use cautiously with clozapine and carbamazepine; may increase the excretion of lithium

**Pregnancy Risk Factor** C

**Contraindications** Hypersensitivity to sulfonamides or acetazolamide, patients with hepatic disease or insufficiency; patients with decreased sodium and/or potassium levels; patients with adrenocortical insufficiency, hyperchloremic acidosis, severe renal disease or dysfunction, or severe pulmonary obstruction; long-term use in noncongestive angle-closure glaucoma

**Warnings/Precautions**

Use in impaired hepatic function may result in coma; use with caution in patients with respiratory acidosis and diabetes mellitus; impairment of mental alertness and/or physical coordination may occur

I.M. administration is painful because of the alkaline pH of the drug

Drug may cause substantial increase in blood glucose in some diabetic patients; malaise and complaints of tiredness and myalgia are signs of excessive dosing and acidosis in the elderly

**Adverse Reactions**

>10%:

Central nervous system: Malaise

Gastrointestinal: Anorexia, diarrhea, metallic taste

Genitourinary: Polyuria

Neuromuscular & skeletal: Muscular weakness

1% to 10%: Central nervous system: Mental depression, drowsiness

<1%: Fever, fatigue, rash, hyperchloremic metabolic acidosis, hypokalemia, hyperglycemia, black stools, GI irritation, dryness of the mouth, dysuria, bone marrow suppression, blood dyscrasias, paresthesia, myopia, renal calculi

**Overdosage/Toxicology**

Signs and symptoms include low blood sugar, tingling of lips and tongue, nausea, yawning, confusion, agitation, tachycardia, sweating, convulsions, stupor, and coma

Treatment: Hypoglycemia should be managed with 50 mL I.V. dextrose 50% followed immediately with a continuous infusion of 10% dextrose in water (administer at a rate sufficient enough to approach a serum glucose level of 100 mg/dL). The use of corticosteroids to treat the hypoglycemia is controversial, however, the addition of 100 mg of hydrocortisone to the dextrose infusion may prove helpful.

**Drug Interactions**

Decreased effect: Increased lithium excretion and altered excretion of other drugs by alkalinization of urine (such as amphetamines, quinidine, procainamide, methenamine, phenobarbital, salicylates); primidone serum concentrations may be decreased

Increased toxicity: Cyclosporine trough concentrations may be increased resulting in possible nephrotoxicity and neurotoxicity; salicylate use may result in carbonic anhydrase inhibitor accumulation and toxicity including CNS depression and metabolic acidosis; digitalis toxicity may occur if hypokalemia is untreated

**Usual Dosage Note:** I.M. administration is not recommended because of pain secondary to the alkaline pH

Neonates and Infants: Hydrocephalus: To slow the progression of hydrocephalus in neonates and infants who may not be good candidates for surgery, acetazolamide I.V. or oral doses of 5 mg/kg/dose every 6 hours increased by 25 mg/kg/day to a maximum of 100 mg/kg/day, if tolerated, have been used. Furosemide was used in combination with acetazolamide.

Children:

Glaucoma:

Oral: 8-30 mg/kg/day or 300-900 mg/m$^2$/day divided every 8 hours

I.M., I.V.: 20-40 mg/kg/24 hours divided every 6 hours, not to exceed 1 g/day

Edema: Oral, I.M., I.V.: 5 mg/kg or 150 mg/m$^2$ once every day

Epilepsy: Oral: 8-30 mg/kg/day in 1-4 divided doses, not to exceed 1 g/day; sustained release capsule is not recommended for treatment of epilepsy

Adults:

Glaucoma:

Chronic simple (open-angle): Oral: 250 mg 1-4 times/day or 500 mg sustained release capsule twice daily

Secondary, acute (closed-angle): I.M., I.V.: 250-500 mg, may repeat in 2-4 hours to a maximum of 1 g/day

Edema: Oral, I.M., I.V.: 250-375 mg once daily

Epilepsy: Oral: 8-30 mg/kg/day in 1-4 divided doses; **sustained release capsule is not recommended for treatment of epilepsy**

Altitude sickness: Oral: 250 mg every 8-12 hours (or 500 mg extended release capsules every 12-24 hours)

Therapy should begin 24-48 hours before and continue during ascent and for at least 48 hours after arrival at the high altitude

Urine alkalinization: Oral: 5 mg/kg/dose repeated 2-3 times over 24 hours

Elderly: Oral: Initial: 250 mg twice daily; use lowest effective dose

**Dosing adjustment in renal impairment:**

$Cl_{cr}$ 10-50 mL/minute: Administer every 12 hours

$Cl_{cr}$ <10 mL/minute: Avoid use → ineffective

Hemodialysis: Moderately dialyzable (20% to 50%)

Peritoneal dialysis: Supplemental dose is not necessary

**Patient Information** Take as directed; do not chew or crush long-acting capsule (contents may be sprinkled on soft food). You will need periodic ophthalmic examinations while taking this medication. You may experience drowsiness, dizziness, or weakness (use caution when driving or engaging in tasks that require alertness until response to drug is known); nausea, loss of appetite, or altered taste (small frequent meals, frequent mouth care, sucking lozenges, or chewing gum may help). Monitor serum glucose closely (may cause altered blood glucose in some diabetic patients, or unusual response to some forms of glucose testing); increased sensitivity to sunlight (use sunblock, protective clothing, and avoid exposure to direct sunlight). Report unusual and persistent tiredness; numbness, burning, or tingling of extremities or around mouth, lips, or anus; muscle weakness; black stool; or excessive depression.

**Dosage Forms**
Capsule, sustained release: 500 mg
Injection: 500 mg
Tablet: 125 mg, 250 mg

## Acetohexamide (a set oh HEKS a mide)

**Related Information**
Hypoglycemic Drugs and Thiazolidinedione Information *on page 714*
**U.S. Brand Names** Dymelor®
**Pharmacologic Category** Antidiabetic Agent (Sulfonylurea)
**Use** Adjunct to diet for the management of mild to moderately severe, stable, noninsulin-dependent (type 2) diabetes mellitus
**Effects on Mental Status** Dizziness is common
**Effects on Psychiatric Treatment** Can rarely cause bone marrow suppression use cautiously with clozapine and carbamazepine; MAOIs and TCAs may potentiate hypoglycemic effects
**Pregnancy Risk Factor** D
**Contraindications** Diabetes complicated by ketoacidosis, therapy of type 1 diabetes, hypersensitivity to sulfonylureas
**Warnings/Precautions**
Patients should be properly instructed in the early detection and treatment of hypoglycemia. Use caution in renal impairment.

Product labeling states oral hypoglycemic drugs may be associated with an increased cardiovascular mortality as compared to treatment with diet alone or diet plus insulin. Data to support this association are limited, and several studies, including a large prospective trial (UKPDS) have not supported an association.

**Adverse Reactions**
>10%:
Central nervous system: Dizziness, headache
Gastrointestinal: Anorexia, constipation, diarrhea, epigastric fullness, heartburn
1% to 10%: Dermatologic: Photosensitivity, rash, urticaria

**Overdosage/Toxicology**
Signs and symptoms: Low blood sugar, tingling of lips and tongue, nausea, yawning, confusion, agitation, tachycardia, sweating, convulsions, stupor, and coma
Treatment: Hypoglycemia should be managed with 50 mL I.V. dextrose 50% followed immediately with a continuous infusion of 10% dextrose in water (administer at a rate sufficient enough to approach a serum glucose level of 100 mg/dL)

**Drug Interactions** Monitor patient closely; large number of drugs interact with sulfonylureas
Decreased effect: Decreases hypoglycemic effect when coadministered with cholestyramine, diazoxide, hydantoins, rifampin, thiazides, loop or thiazide diuretics, and phenylbutazone
Increased effect: Increases hypoglycemia when coadministered with salicylates or beta-adrenergic blockers; MAO inhibitors; oral anticoagulants, NSAIDs, sulfonamides, phenylbutazone, insulin, clofibrate, fluconazole, gemfibrozil, $H_2$-antagonists, methyldopa, tricyclic antidepressants

**Usual Dosage** Adults: Oral (elderly patients may be more sensitive and should be started at a lower dosage initially):

Initial: 250 mg/day; increase in increments of 250-500 mg daily at intervals of 5-7 days up to 1.5 g/day. Patients on ≤1 g/day can be controlled with once daily administration. Patients receiving 1.5 g/day usually benefit from twice daily administration before the morning and evening meals. Doses >1.5 g daily are not recommended.

**Dosing adjustment in renal impairment:** $Cl_{cr}$ <50 mL/minute: Acetohexamide is not recommended in patients with renal insufficiency due to the increased potential for developing hypoglycemia

**Dosing adjustment in hepatic impairment:** Initiate therapy at lower than recommended doses; further dosage adjustment may be necessary because acetohexamide is extensively metabolized but no specific guidelines are available

**Patient Information** If nausea or stomach upset occurs, may be taken with food; take at the same time each day; avoid alcohol
**Dosage Forms** Tablet: 250 mg, 500 mg

♦ **Acetomorphine** *see* Heroin *on page 267*

## Acetophenazine (a set oh FEN a zeen)

**Related Information**
Antipsychotic Medication Guidelines *on page 751*
Clinical Issues in the Use of Antipsychotics *on page 630*
Patient Information - Antipsychotics (General) *on page 646*
**Generic Available** No
**Synonyms** Acetophenazine Maleate
**Pharmacologic Category** Antipsychotic Agent, Phenothazine, Piperazine
**Use** Management of manifestations of psychotic disorders
**Pregnancy Risk Factor** C
**Contraindications** Blood dyscrasias and bone marrow suppression, patients in coma or brain damage, known hypersensitivity to acetophenazine
**Adverse Reactions**
>10%:
Cardiovascular: Hypotension, orthostatic hypotension
Central nervous system: Pseudoparkinsonism, akathisia, dystonias, tardive dyskinesia, dizziness
Gastrointestinal: Constipation
Ocular: Pigmentary retinopathy
Respiratory: Nasal congestion
Miscellaneous: Diaphoresis (decreased)
1% to 10%:
Dermatologic: Increased sensitivity to sun, rash
Endocrine & metabolic: Changes in menstrual cycle, breast pain, changes in libido
Gastrointestinal: Weight gain, nausea, vomiting, stomach pain
Genitourinary: Difficulty in urination, ejaculatory disturbances
Neuromuscular & skeletal: Trembling fingers
<1%:
Central nervous system: Neuroleptic malignant syndrome (NMS), impairment of temperature regulation, lowering of seizures threshold
Dermatologic: Discoloration of skin (blue-gray)
Endocrine & metabolic: Galactorrhea
Genitourinary: Priapism
Hematologic: Agranulocytosis, leukopenia
Hepatic: Cholestatic jaundice, hepatotoxicity
Ocular: Cornea and lens changes, pigmentary retinopathy

**Drug Interactions**
Aluminum salts: May decrease the absorption of phenothiazines; monitor
Amphetamines: Efficacy may be diminished by antipsychotics. In addition, amphetamines may increase psychotic symptoms; avoid concurrent use.
Anticholinergics: May inhibit the therapeutic response to phenothiazines and excess anticholinergic effects may occur; includes benztropine, trihexyphenidyl, biperiden, and drugs with significant anticholinergic activity (TCAs, antihistamines, disopyramide)
Antihypertensives: Concurrent use of phenothiazines with an antihypertensive may produce additive hypotensive effects (particularly orthostasis)
Bromocriptine: Phenothiazines inhibit the ability of bromocriptine to lower serum prolactin concentrations
CNS depressants: Sedative effects may be additive with phenothiazines; monitor for increased effect; includes barbiturates, benzodiazepines, narcotic analgesics, ethanol, and other sedative agents
CYP inhibitors: Serum level and/or toxicity of acetophenazine may be increased; profile has not been established; monitor for increased effect
Enzyme inducers: May enhance the hepatic metabolism of phenothiazines; larger doses may be required; includes rifampin, rifabutin, barbiturates, phenytoin, and cigarette smoking
Epinephrine: Chlorpromazine (and possibly other low potency antipsychotics) may diminish the pressor effects of epinephrine
Guanethidine and guanadrel: Antihypertensive effects may be inhibited by chlorpromazine
Levodopa: Chlorpromazine may inhibit the antiparkinsonian effect of levodopa; avoid this combination
Lithium: Chlorpromazine may produce neurotoxicity with lithium; this is a rare effect
Phenytoin: May reduce serum levels of phenothiazines; phenothiazines may increase phenytoin serum levels
Propranolol: Serum concentrations of phenothiazines may be increased; propranolol also increases phenothiazine concentrations
Polypeptide antibiotics: Rare cases of respiratory paralysis have been reported with concurrent use of phenothiazines
QTc prolonging agents: Effects on QTc interval may be additive with phenothiazines, increasing the risk of malignant arrhythmias; includes type Ia antiarrhythmics, TCAs, and some quinolone antibiotics (sparfloxacin, moxifloxacin and gatifloxacin)
Sulfadoxine-pyrimethamine: May increase phenothiazine concentrations
Tricyclic antidepressants: Concurrent use may produce increased toxicity or altered therapeutic response
Trazodone: Phenothiazines and trazodone may produce additive hypotensive effects
Valproic acid: Serum levels may be increased by phenothiazines

**Stability** Protect from light; dispense in amber or opaque vials
**Mechanism of Action** Antagonizes the effects of dopamine in the basal ganglia and limbic areas of the forebrain; this activity appears responsible for the antipsychotic efficacy, as well as the production of extrapyramidal symptoms; increases the secretion of prolactin and has a marked suppressive effect on the chemoreceptor trigger zone; also produces peripheral blockade of cholinergic neurons
**Pharmacodynamics/kinetics**
Onset: 2-4 hours
Duration: ~24 hours, permitting daily dosing
Absorption: Tissue saturation, particularly in high lipid tissues such as the central nervous system
Serum half-life: Range: 20-40 hours
**Usual Dosage** Adults: Oral: 20 mg 3 times/day up to 60-120 mg/day
(Continued)

## Acetophenazine *(Continued)*

Hospitalized schizophrenic patients may require doses as high as 400-600 mg/day

Hemodialysis: Not dialyzable (0% to 5%)

**Patient Information** Do not take antacid within 1 hour of taking drug; may cause drowsiness, avoid alcohol; avoid excess sun exposure (use sun block); rise slowly from recumbent position; use of supportive stockings may help prevent orthostatic hypotension

**Nursing Implications** Observe for tremor and abnormal movement or posturing (extrapyramidal symptoms), increased confusion or psychotic behavior, constipation, urinary retention, abnormal gait

**Dosage Forms** Tablet, as maleate: 20 mg

♦ **Acetophenazine Maleate** *see* Acetophenazine *on page 17*

♦ **Acetoxymethylprogesterone** *see* Medroxyprogesterone *on page 336*

## Acetylcholine (a se teel KOE leen)

**U.S. Brand Names** Miochol-E®

**Pharmacologic Category** Cholinergic Agonist; Ophthalmic Agent, Miotic

**Use** Produces complete miosis in cataract surgery, keratoplasty, iridectomy and other anterior segment surgery where rapid miosis is required

**Effects on Mental Status** None reported

**Effects on Psychiatric Treatment** Intraocular product; should not impact psychiatric drug treatment

**Usual Dosage** Adults: Intraocular: 0.5-2 mL of 1% injection (5-20 mg) instilled into anterior chamber before or after securing one or more sutures

**Dosage Forms** Powder, intraocular, as chloride: 1:100 [10 mg/mL] (2 mL, 15 mL)

## Acetylcysteine (a se teel SIS teen)

**U.S. Brand Names** Mucomyst®; Mucosil™

**Canadian Brand Names** Parvolex®

**Synonyms** Mercapturic Acid; NAC; *N*-Acetylcysteine; *N*-Acetyl-L-cysteine

**Pharmacologic Category** Antidote; Mucolytic Agent

**Use** Adjunctive mucolytic therapy in patients with abnormal or viscid mucous secretions in acute and chronic bronchopulmonary diseases; pulmonary complications of surgery and cystic fibrosis; diagnostic bronchial studies; antidote for acute acetaminophen toxicity

**Effects on Mental Status** May cause drowsiness

**Effects on Psychiatric Treatment** Sedative effects may be potentiated by psychotropic agents

**Pregnancy Risk Factor** B

**Contraindications** Known hypersensitivity to acetylcysteine

**Warnings/Precautions** Since increased bronchial secretions may develop after inhalation, percussion, postural drainage and suctioning should follow; if bronchospasm occurs, administer a bronchodilator; discontinue acetylcysteine if bronchospasm progresses

**Adverse Reactions**

>10%:
- Gastrointestinal: Vomiting
- Miscellaneous: Unpleasant odor during administration

1% to 10%:
- Central nervous system: Chills, drowsiness
- Gastrointestinal: Nausea, stomatitis
- Local: Irritation
- Respiratory: Bronchospasm, hemoptysis, rhinorrhea
- Miscellaneous: Clamminess

<1%: Skin rash

**Overdosage/Toxicology** Treatment of acetylcysteine toxicity is usually aimed at reversing anaphylactoid symptoms or controlling nausea and vomiting. The use of epinephrine, antihistamines, and steroids may be beneficial.

**Drug Interactions** Adsorbed by activated charcoal; clinical significance is minimal, though, once a pure acetaminophen ingestion requiring N-acetylcysteine is established; further charcoal dosing is unnecessary once the appropriate initial charcoal dose is achieved (5-10 g:g acetaminophen)

**Usual Dosage**

Acetaminophen poisoning: Children and Adults: Oral: 140 mg/kg; followed by 17 doses of 70 mg/kg every 4 hours; repeat dose if emesis occurs within 1 hour of administration; therapy should continue until all doses are administered even though the acetaminophen plasma level has dropped below the toxic range

Inhalation: Acetylcysteine 10% and 20% solution (Mucomyst®) (dilute 20% solution with sodium chloride or sterile water for inhalation); 10% solution may be used undiluted

- Infants: 1-2 mL of 20% solution or 2-4 mL 10% solution until nebulized given 3-4 times/day
- Children: 3-5 mL of 20% solution or 6-10 mL of 10% solution until nebulized given 3-4 times/day
- Adolescents: 5-10 mL of 10% to 20% solution until nebulized given 3-4 times/day

**Note:** Patients should receive an aerosolized bronchodilator 10-15 minutes prior to acetylcysteine

Meconium ileus equivalent: Children and Adults: 100-300 mL of 4% to 10% solution by irrigation or orally

**Patient Information** Pulmonary treatment: Prepare solution (may dilute with sterile water to reduce concentrate from impeding nebulizer) and use as directed. Clear airway by coughing deeply before using aerosol. Wash face and face-mask after treatment to remove any residual. You may experience drowsiness (use caution when driving) or nausea or vomiting (small frequent meals may help). Report persistent chills or fever, adverse change in respiratory status, palpitations, or extreme anxiety or nervousness.

**Dosage Forms** Solution, as sodium: 10% [100 mg/mL] (4 mL, 10 mL, 30 mL); 20% [200 mg/mL] (4 mL, 10 mL, 30 mL, 100 mL)

♦ **Acetylsalicylic Acid** *see* Aspirin *on page 49*

♦ **Achromycin® Ophthalmic** *see* Tetracycline *on page 537*

♦ **Achromycin® Topical** *see* Tetracycline *on page 537*

♦ **Aciphex™** *see* Rabeprazole *on page 487*

## Acitretin (a si TRE tin)

**U.S. Brand Names** Soriatane™

**Pharmacologic Category** Retinoid-like Compound

**Use** Treatment of severe psoriasis (includes erythrodermic and pustular types) and other disorders of keratinization

**Effects on Mental Status** None reported

**Effects on Psychiatric Treatment** None reported

**Pregnancy Risk Factor** X

**Contraindications** Pregnancy; retinoids are known to cause severe birth defects in a very high percentage of infants exposed to them in utero

Acitretin is contraindicated in females of childbearing potential unless all of the following conditions apply:

1. The patient has severe psoriasis or other severe disorders of keratinization
2. The patient is reliable in understanding and carrying out instructions
3. The patient is able to comply with mandatory contraceptive measures
4. The patient has received, and acknowledged understanding of, a careful oral and printed explanation of the hazards of fetal exposure to acitretin and the risk of possible contraception failure; this explanation may include showing a line drawing to the patient of an infant with the characteristic external deformities resulting from retinoid exposure during pregnancy

**Warnings/Precautions** See Contraindications; the use of systemic retinoids in humans has been associated with congenital abnormalities. There is an extremely high risk that major human fetal abnormalities will occur if pregnancy occurs during treatment with acitretin. Potentially any exposed fetus can be affected; major fetal abnormalities associated with retinoid administration during pregnancy have been reported including meningomyelocele, meningoencephalocele, multiple synostosis, facial dysmorphia, anophthalmia, syndactyly, absence of terminal phalanges, malformations of hip, ankle and forearm, low set ears, high palate, decreased cranial volume, and alterations of the skull and cervical vertebrae on x-ray.

It is strongly recommended that all female patients of childbearing potential treated with acitretin have monthly pregnancy tests during treatment and at regular intervals for an undetermined period of time of at least 2 years duration after the discontinuation of treatment these pregnancy tests will:

a) Serve primarily to reinforce to the patient the necessity of avoiding pregnancy

b) In the event of accidental pregnancy, provide the physician and patient an immediate opportunity to discuss the serious risk to the fetus from this exposure to acitretin and the desirability of continuing the pregnancy in view of the potential teratogenic effect of acitretin

**Drug Interactions**

Concomitant administration of vitamin A and other systemic retinoids must be avoided due to the risk of possible additive toxic effects

The concomitant administration of methotrexate and etretinate has been associated with hepatitis, a similar increased hepatitis risk may be expected with the combined use of acitretin and methotrexate

Preliminary studies indicated that acitretin does not influence the endogenous progesterone plasma concentrations induced by oral contraceptives

Concomitant administration of phenprocoumon and acitretin does not alter the hypothrombinemic effect of phenprocoumon or the plasma disposition of acitretin

The pharmacokinetics of acitretin and digoxin are not altered by concomitant multiple dose regimens of these two drugs

Concomitant administration of cimetidine did not alter the oral bioavailability of acitretin or the isomerization to its 13-cis form; single oral doses of acitretin did not affect the steady-state plasma concentration or renal clearance of cimetidine

Limited data which could not be duplicated, indicated that acitretin treatment either increased insulin sensitivity directly or interacted with glyburide to do so; careful supervision of diabetic patients under treatment with acitretin is recommended

**Usual Dosage** Adults: Oral: Individualization of dosage is required to achieve maximum therapeutic response while minimizing side effects

Initial therapy: Therapy should be initiated at 25 mg/day, given as a single dose with the main meal; if by 4 weeks the response is unsatisfactory, and in the absence of toxicity, the daily dose may be gradually increased to a maximum of 75 mg/day; the dose may be reduced, if necessary, to minimize side effects

Maintenance doses of 25 to 50 mg/day may be given after initial response to treatment; the maintenance dose should be based on clinical efficacy and tolerability; it may be necessary in some cases to increase the dose to a maximum of 75 mg/day

**Dosage Forms** Capsule: 10 mg, 25 mg

- **Aclovate® Topical** *see* Alclometasone *on page 22*

## Acrivastine and Pseudoephedrine
(AK ri vas teen & soo doe e FED rin)

**U.S. Brand Names** Semprex®-D

**Pharmacologic Category** Antihistamine

**Use** Temporary relief of nasal congestion, decongest sinus openings, running nose, itching of nose or throat, and itchy, watery eyes due to hay fever or other upper respiratory allergies

**Effects on Mental Status** Drowsiness is common; may produce anxiety and insomnia

**Effects on Psychiatric Treatment** Hypertensive crisis may result with MAOI; effects of CNS depressants may be lessened

**Usual Dosage** Adults: 1 capsule 3-4 times/day

**Dosing comments in renal impairment:** Do not use

**Dosage Forms** Capsule: Acrivastine 8 mg and pseudoephedrine hydrochloride 60 mg

- **Actagen-C®** *see* Triprolidine, Pseudoephedrine, and Codeine *on page 572*
- **Actagen® Syrup [OTC]** *see* Triprolidine and Pseudoephedrine *on page 572*
- **Actagen® Tablet [OTC]** *see* Triprolidine and Pseudoephedrine *on page 572*
- **ACTH** *see* Corticotropin *on page 140*
- **Acthar®** *see* Corticotropin *on page 140*
- **Acticin® Cream** *see* Permethrin *on page 432*
- **Actidose-Aqua® [OTC]** *see* Charcoal *on page 106*
- **Actidose® With Sorbitol [OTC]** *see* Charcoal *on page 106*
- **Actifed® Allergy Tablet (Day) [OTC]** *see* Pseudoephedrine *on page 478*
- **Actifed® Allergy Tablet (Night) [OTC]** *see* Diphenhydramine and Pseudoephedrine *on page 175*
- **Actigall™** *see* Ursodiol *on page 577*
- **Actimmune®** *see* Interferon Gamma-1b *on page 290*
- **Actiq® Oral Transmucosal** *see* Fentanyl *on page 221*
- **Activase®** *see* Alteplase *on page 27*
- **Activated Carbon** *see* Charcoal *on page 106*
- **Activated Charcoal** *see* Charcoal *on page 106*
- **Activated Dimethicone** *see* Simethicone *on page 512*
- **Activated Ergosterol** *see* Ergocalciferol *on page 198*
- **Activated Methylpolysiloxane** *see* Simethicone *on page 512*
- **Activella™** *see* Estradiol and Norethindrone *on page 205*
- **Actonel™** *see* Risedronate *on page 495*
- **Actos™** *see* Pioglitazone *on page 447*
- **Actron® [OTC]** *see* Ketoprofen *on page 302*
- **ACU-dyne® [OTC]** *see* Povidone-Iodine *on page 456*
- **Acular® Ophthalmic** *see* Ketorolac Tromethamine *on page 303*
- **Acumen®** *see* Deanol *on page 152*
- **Acutrim® 16 Hours [OTC]** *see* Phenylpropanolamine *on page 440*
- **Acutrim® II, Maximum Strength [OTC]** *see* Phenylpropanolamine *on page 440*
- **Acutrim® Late Day [OTC]** *see* Phenylpropanolamine *on page 440*

## Acyclovir (ay SYE kloe veer)

**U.S. Brand Names** Zovirax®

**Canadian Brand Names** Avirax™

**Pharmacologic Category** Antiviral Agent

**Use** Treatment of initial and prophylaxis of recurrent mucosal and cutaneous herpes simplex (HSV-1 and HSV-2) infections; herpes simplex encephalitis; herpes zoster; genital herpes infection; varicella-zoster infections in healthy, nonpregnant persons >13 years of age, children >12 months of age who have a chronic skin or lung disorder or are receiving long-term aspirin therapy, and immunocompromised patients; for herpes zoster, acyclovir should be started within 72 hours of the appearance of the rash to be effective; acyclovir will not prevent postherpetic neuralgias

**Effects on Mental Status** May see lethargy, confusion, or agitation; rarely may see depression or insomnia

**Effects on Psychiatric Treatment** Usually not a problem, may see additive sedation with sedating psychotropics

**Pregnancy Risk Factor** C

**Contraindications** Hypersensitivity to acyclovir, valacyclovir, or any component

**Warnings/Precautions** Use with caution in patients with pre-existing renal disease or in those receiving other nephrotoxic drugs concurrently; maintain adequate urine output during the first 2 hours after I.V. infusion; use with caution in patients with underlying neurologic abnormalities, serious hepatic or electrolyte abnormalities, or substantial hypoxia. Use with caution in immunocompromised patients; thrombocytopenic purpura/hemolytic uremic syndrome (TTP/HUS) has been reported

**Adverse Reactions**

>10%: Local: Inflammation at injection site

1% to 10%:

- Central nervous system: agitation, coma, confusion, dizziness, headache, lethargy, seizures
- Dermatologic: Rash
- Gastrointestinal: Nausea, vomiting
- Neuromuscular & skeletal: Tremor
- Renal: Impaired renal function

<1%: Anemia, anorexia, hallucinations, insomnia, leukopenia, LFT elevation, mental depression, sore throat, thrombocytopenia

**Drug Interactions** Increased CNS side effects with zidovudine and probenecid

**Usual Dosage**

Dosing weight should be based on the smaller of lean body weight or total body weight

**Treatment of herpes simplex virus infections:** Children >12 years and Adults: I.V.:

- Mucocutaneous HSV or severe initial herpes genitalis infection: 750 mg/m²/day divided every 8 hours or 5 mg/kg/dose every 8 hours for 5-10 days
- HSV encephalitis: 1500 mg/m²/day divided every 8 hours or 10 mg/kg/dose for 10 days

**Treatment of genital herpes simplex virus infections:** Adults:

- Oral: 200 mg every 4 hours while awake (5 times/day) for 10 days if initial episode; for 5 days if recurrence (begin at earliest signs of disease)
- Topical: ½" ribbon of ointment for a 4" square surface area every 3 hours (6 times/day)

**Treatment of varicella-zoster virus (chickenpox) infections:**

- Oral:
  - Children: 10-20 mg/kg/dose (up to 800 mg) 4 times/day for 5 days; begin treatment within the first 24 hours of rash onset
  - Adults: 600-800 mg/dose every 4 hours while awake (5 times/day) for 7-10 days or 1000 mg every 6 hours for 5 days
- I.V.: Children and Adults: 1500 mg/m²/day divided every 8 hours or 10 mg/kg/dose every 8 hours for 7 days

**Treatment of herpes zoster (shingles) infections:**

- Oral:
  - Children (immunocompromised): 250-600 mg/m²/dose 4-5 times/day for 7-10 days
  - Adults (immunocompromised): 800 mg every 4 hours (5 times/day) for 7-10 days
- I.V.:
  - Children and Adults (immunocompromised): 10 mg/kg/dose or 500 mg/m²/dose every 8 hours
  - Older Adults (immunocompromised): 7.5 mg/kg/dose every 8 hours
  - If nephrotoxicity occurs: 5 mg/kg/dose every 8 hours

**Prophylaxis in immunocompromised patients:**

- Varicella zoster or herpes zoster in HIV-positive patients: Adults: Oral: 400 mg every 4 hours (5 times/day) for 7-10 days
- Bone marrow transplant recipients: Children and Adults: I.V.:
  - Allogeneic patients who are HSV seropositive: 150 mg/m²/dose (5 mg/kg) every 12 hours; with clinical symptoms of herpes simplex: 150 mg/m²/dose every 8 hours
  - Allogeneic patients who are CMV seropositive: 500 mg/m²/dose (10 mg/kg) every 8 hours; for clinically symptomatic CMV infection, consider replacing acyclovir with ganciclovir

(Continued)

## Acyclovir *(Continued)*

**Chronic suppressive therapy for recurrent genital herpes simplex virus infections:** Adults: 200 mg 3-4 times/day or 400 mg twice daily for up to 12 months, followed by re-evaluation

**Dosing adjustment in renal impairment:**

Oral: HSV/varicella-zoster:

$Cl_{cr}$ 10-25 mL/minute: Administer dose every 8 hours

$Cl_{cr}$ <10 mL/minute: Administer dose every 12 hours

I.V.:

$Cl_{cr}$ 25-50 mL/minute: 5-10 mg/kg/dose: Administer every 12 hours

$Cl_{cr}$ 10-25 mL/minute: 5-10 mg/kg/dose: Administer every 24 hours

$Cl_{cr}$ <10 mL/minute: 2.5-5 mg/kg/dose: Administer every 24 hours

Hemodialysis: Dialyzable (50% to 100%); administer dose postdialysis

Peritoneal dialysis: Dose as for $Cl_{cr}$ <10 mL/minute

Continuous arteriovenous or venovenous hemofiltration (CAVH/CAVHD) effects: Dose as for $Cl_{cr}$ <10 mL/minute

**Patient Information** This is not a cure for herpes (recurrences tend to appear within 3 months of original infection), nor will this medication reduce the risk of transmission to others when lesions are present. Take as directed for full course of therapy; do not discontinue even if feeling better. Maintain adequate hydration (2-3 L/day of fluids unless instructed to restrict fluid intake) to prevent renal complications. Avoid use of other topical creams, lotions, or ointments unless approved by prescriber. You may experience nausea or vomiting (small frequent meals, frequent mouth care, sucking lozenges, or chewing gum may help); lightheadedness or dizziness (use caution when driving or engaging in tasks that require alertness until response to drug is known); headache, fever, muscle pain (an analgesic may be recommended). Report persistent lethargy, acute headache, severe nausea or vomiting, confusion or hallucinations, rash, or difficulty breathing.

**Nursing Implications** Wear gloves when applying ointment for self-protection

**Dosage Forms**

Capsule: 200 mg

Powder for Injection: 500 mg (10 mL); 1000 mg (20 mL)

Ointment, topical: 5% [50 mg/g] (3 g, 15 g)

Suspension, oral (banana flavor): 200 mg/5 mL

Tablet: 400 mg, 800 mg

- **Adagen™** *see* Pegademase Bovine *on page 422*
- **Adalat®** *see* Nifedipine *on page 393*
- **Adalat® CC** *see* Nifedipine *on page 393*
- **Adamantanamine Hydrochloride** *see* Amantadine *on page 28*

## Adapalene (a DAP a leen)

**U.S. Brand Names** Differin®

**Pharmacologic Category** Acne Products

**Use** Treatment of acne vulgaris

**Effects on Mental Status** None reported

**Effects on Psychiatric Treatment** None reported

**Usual Dosage** Children >12 years and Adults: Topical: Apply once daily at bedtime; therapeutic results should be noticed after 8-12 weeks of treatment

**Dosage Forms**

Cream, topical (Differin®): 0.1%

Gel, topical (alcohol free): 0.1% (15 g, 45 g)

Solution, topical: 0.1% (30 mL)

- **Adapin® Oral** *see* Doxepin *on page 183*
- **Adderall®** *see* Dextroamphetamine and Amphetamine *on page 160*
- **Addiction Treatments** *see page 772*

## Adefovir (a DEF o veer)

**Generic Available** No

**U.S. Brand Names** Preveon™

**Pharmacologic Category** Antiretroviral Agent, Reverse Transcriptase Inhibitor (Nucleoside)

**Use** Investigational (8/1/98); treatment of HIV infections in combination with at least two other antiretroviral agents; also has some activity against hepatitis B virus and herpes viruses

**Pregnancy Risk Factor** Not available

**Adverse Reactions**

Endocrine & metabolic: Elevation of transaminases, hot flashes

Gastrointestinal: GI symptoms

Genitourinary: Urethritis

Hematologic: Elevation of hemoglobin

**Usual Dosage** Oral:

HIV: 125 mg once daily

Hepatitis B: 125 mg once daily

**Patient Information** This is not a cure for AIDS or AIDS complex, nor will it reduce the risk of transmission to others. Long-term effects are not known. You may need frequent blood tests to adjust dosage for maximum therapeutic effect. Take as directed, for full course of therapy; do not discontinue (even if feeling better). You may experience hot flashes (cool environment or cool clothes may help); nausea or vomiting (small, frequent meals, chewing gum, or sucking on lozenges may help); difficulty breathing; or rash. Inform prescriber if you are or intend to be pregnant. Do not breast-feed.

- **Adenocard®** *see* Adenosine *on page 20*

## Adenosine (a DEN oh seen)

**U.S. Brand Names** Adenocard®

**Pharmacologic Category** Antiarrhythmic Agent, Class IV

**Use**

Adenocard®: Treatment of paroxysmal supraventricular tachycardia (PSVT) including that associated with accessory bypass tracts (Wolff-Parkinson-White syndrome); when clinically advisable, appropriate vagal maneuvers should be attempted prior to adenosine administration; **not effective in atrial flutter, atrial fibrillation, or ventricular tachycardia**

Adenoscan®: Pharmacologic stress agent used in myocardial perfusion thallium-201 scintigraphy

**Effects on Mental Status** May rarely see anxiety

**Effects on Psychiatric Treatment** Use caution with carbamazepine and tricyclic antidepressants, may increase heart block

**Usual Dosage**

Adenocard®: **Rapid I.V. push (over 1-2 seconds) via peripheral line:**

Neonates: Initial dose: 0.05 mg/kg; if not effective within 2 minutes, increase dose by 0.05 mg/kg increments every 2 minutes to a maximum dose of 0.25 mg/kg or until termination of PSVT

Maximum single dose: 12 mg

Infants and Children: Pediatric advanced life support (PALS): Treatment of SVT: 0.1 mg/kg; if not effective, administer 0.2 mg/kg

Alternatively: Initial dose: 0.05 mg/kg; if not effective within 2 minutes, increase dose by 0.05 mg/kg increments every 2 minutes to a maximum dose of 0.25 mg/kg or until termination of PSVT; medium dose required: 0.15 mg/kg

Maximum single dose: 12 mg

Adults: 6 mg; if not effective within 1-2 minutes, 12 mg may be given; may repeat 12 mg bolus if needed

Maximum single dose: 12 mg

Follow each I.V. bolus of adenosine with normal saline flush

**Note:** Preliminary results in adults suggest adenosine may be administered via a central line at lower doses (ie, initial adult dose: 3 mg).

Adenoscan®: Continuous I.V. infusion via peripheral line: 140 mcg/kg/minute for 6 minutes using syringe or columetric infusion pump; total dose: 0.84 mg/kg. Thallium-201 is injected at midpoint (3 minutes) of infusion.

Hemodialysis: Significant drug removal is unlikely based on physiochemical characteristics.

Peritoneal dialysis: Significant drug removal is unlikely based on physiochemical characteristics.

**Note:** Patients who are receiving concomitant theophylline therapy may be less likely to respond to adenosine therapy.

**Note:** Higher doses may be needed for administration via peripheral versus central vein.

**Dosage Forms**

Diagnostic use: 60 mg/20 mL and 90 mg/30 mL single-dose vials

Injection, preservative free: 3 mg/mL (2 mL)

- **ADH** *see* Vasopressin *on page 581*
- **Adipex-P®** *see* Phentermine *on page 438*
- **Adlone® Injection** *see* Methylprednisolone *on page 359*
- **Adrenalin®** *see* Epinephrine *on page 195*
- **Adrenaline** *see* Epinephrine *on page 195*
- **Adrenocorticotropic Hormone** *see* Corticotropin *on page 140*
- **Adriamycin PFS™** *see* Doxorubicin *on page 185*
- **Adriamycin RDF®** *see* Doxorubicin *on page 185*
- **Adrucil® Injection** *see* Fluorouracil *on page 231*
- **Adsorbent Charcoal** *see* Charcoal *on page 106*
- **Adsorbocarpine® Ophthalmic** *see* Pilocarpine *on page 445*
- **Adsorbotear® Ophthalmic Solution [OTC]** *see* Artificial Tears *on page 48*
- **Adult ACLS Algorithms** *see page 762*
- **Advanced Formula Oxy® Sensitive Gel [OTC]** *see* Benzoyl Peroxide *on page 62*
- **Advil® [OTC]** *see* Ibuprofen *on page 280*

♦ **Advil® Cold & Sinus Caplets [OTC]** *see* Pseudoephedrine and Ibuprofen *on page 479*

♦ **Advil® Migraine Liqui-Gels [OTC]** *see* Ibuprofen *on page 280*

♦ **AeroBid®-M Oral Aerosol Inhaler** *see* Flunisolide *on page 230*

♦ **AeroBid® Oral Aerosol Inhaler** *see* Flunisolide *on page 230*

♦ **Aerodine® [OTC]** *see* Povidone-Iodine *on page 456*

♦ **Aerolate®** *see* Theophylline Salts *on page 539*

♦ **Aerolate III®** *see* Theophylline Salts *on page 539*

♦ **Aerolate JR®** *see* Theophylline Salts *on page 539*

♦ **Aerolate SR®** *see* Theophylline Salts *on page 539*

♦ **Aeroseb-Dex®** *see* Dexamethasone *on page 157*

♦ **Aeroseb-HC®** *see* Hydrocortisone *on page 273*

♦ **Aerosporin® Injection** *see* Polymyxin B *on page 452*

♦ **Afrin® Children's Nose Drops [OTC]** *see* Oxymetazoline *on page 415*

♦ **Afrin® Sinus [OTC]** *see* Oxymetazoline *on page 415*

♦ **Afrin® Tablet [OTC]** *see* Pseudoephedrine *on page 478*

♦ **Aftate® for Athlete's Foot [OTC]** *see* Tolnaftate *on page 555*

♦ **Aftate® for Jock Itch [OTC]** *see* Tolnaftate *on page 555*

♦ **Agenerase™** *see* Amprenavir *on page 43*

♦ **Agents for Treatment of Extrapyramidal Symptoms** *see page 638*

♦ **Aggrastat®** *see* Tirofiban *on page 550*

♦ **Aggrenox™** *see* Aspirin and Extended-Release Dipyridamole *on page 50*

♦ **Agrylin™** *see* Anagrelide *on page 44*

♦ **A-hydroCort®** *see* Hydrocortisone *on page 273*

♦ **Airet®** *see* Albuterol *on page 22*

♦ **Akarpine® Ophthalmic** *see* Pilocarpine *on page 445*

♦ **AKBeta®** *see* Levobunolol *on page 311*

♦ **AK-Chlor® Ophthalmic** *see* Chloramphenicol *on page 109*

♦ **AK-Cide® Ophthalmic** *see* Sulfacetamide Sodium and Prednisolone *on page 523*

♦ **AK-Con® Ophthalmic** *see* Naphazoline *on page 383*

♦ **AK-Dex® Ophthalmic** *see* Dexamethasone *on page 157*

♦ **AK-Dilate® Ophthalmic Solution** *see* Phenylephrine *on page 439*

♦ **AK-Homatropine® Ophthalmic** *see* Homatropine *on page 268*

♦ **Akineton®** *see* Biperiden *on page 68*

♦ **AK-Nefrin® Ophthalmic Solution** *see* Phenylephrine *on page 439*

♦ **Akne-Mycin® Topical** *see* Erythromycin, Ophthalmic/Topical *on page 202*

♦ **AK-Neo-Dex® Ophthalmic** *see* Neomycin and Dexamethasone *on page 388*

♦ **AK-Pentolate®** *see* Cyclopentolate *on page 145*

♦ **AK-Poly-Bac® Ophthalmic** *see* Bacitracin and Polymyxin B *on page 57*

♦ **AK-Pred® Ophthalmic** *see* Prednisolone *on page 459*

♦ **AKPro® Ophthalmic** *see* Dipivefrin *on page 176*

♦ **AK-Spore® H.C. Ophthalmic Ointment** *see* Bacitracin, Neomycin, Polymyxin B, and Hydrocortisone *on page 57*

♦ **AK-Spore® H.C. Ophthalmic Suspension** *see* Neomycin, Polymyxin B, and Hydrocortisone *on page 389*

♦ **AK-Spore® H.C. Otic** *see* Neomycin, Polymyxin B, and Hydrocortisone *on page 389*

♦ **AK-Spore® Ophthalmic Ointment** *see* Bacitracin, Neomycin, and Polymyxin B *on page 57*

♦ **AK-Spore® Ophthalmic Solution** *see* Neomycin, Polymyxin B, and Gramicidin *on page 389*

♦ **AK-Sulf® Ophthalmic** *see* Sulfacetamide *on page 522*

♦ **AK-Taine®** *see* Proparacaine *on page 473*

♦ **AKTob® Ophthalmic** *see* Tobramycin *on page 551*

♦ **AK-Tracin® Ophthalmic** *see* Bacitracin *on page 56*

♦ **AK-Trol®** *see* Neomycin, Polymyxin B, and Dexamethasone *on page 389*

♦ **Akwa Tears® Solution [OTC]** *see* Artificial Tears *on page 48*

♦ **Ala-Cort®** *see* Hydrocortisone *on page 273*

♦ **Alamast™** *see* Pemirolast *on page 423*

♦ **Ala-Scalp®** *see* Hydrocortisone *on page 273*

♦ **Albalon-A® Ophthalmic** *see* Naphazoline and Antazoline *on page 383*

♦ **Albalon® Liquifilm® Ophthalmic** *see* Naphazoline *on page 383*

## Albendazole (al BEN da zole)

**U.S. Brand Names** Albenza®

**Pharmacologic Category** Anthelmintic

**Use** Treatment of parenchymal neurocysticercosis and cystic hydatid disease of the liver, lung, and peritoneum; albendazole has activity against *Ascaris lumbricoides* (roundworm), *Ancylostoma duodenale* and *Necator americanus* (hookworms), *Enterobius vermicularis* (pinworm), *Hymenolepis nana* and *Taenia* sp (tapeworms), *Opisthorchis sinensis* and *Opisthorchis viverrini* (liver flukes), *Strongyloides stercoralis* and *Trichuris trichiura* (whipworm); activity has also been shown against the liver fluke *Clonorchis sinensis*, *Giardia lamblia*, *Cysticercus cellulosae*, *Echinococcus granulosus*, *Echinococcus multilocularis*, and *Toxocara* sp.

**Effects on Mental Status** None reported

**Effects on Psychiatric Treatment** May rarely cause bone marrow suppression; use caution with clozapine and carbamazepine. Carbamazepine may increase the metabolism of albendazole.

**Usual Dosage** Oral:

Neurocysticercosis:

<60 kg: 15 mg/kg/day in 2 divided doses (maximum: 800 mg/day) with meals for 8-30 days

≥60 kg: 400 mg twice daily for 8-30 days

Note: Give concurrent anticonvulsant and steroid therapy during first week

Hydatid:

<60 kg: 15 mg/kg/day in 2 divided doses with meals (maximum: 800 mg/day) for three 28-day cycles with 14-day drug-free interval in-between

≥60 kg: 400 mg twice daily for 3 cycles as above

Strongyloidiasis/tapeworm:

≤2 years: 200 mg/day for 3 days; may repeat in 3 weeks

>2 years and Adults: 400 mg/day for 3 days; may repeat in 3 weeks

Giardiasis: Adults: 400 mg/day for 3 days

Hookworm, pinworm, roundworm:

≤2 years: 200 mg as a single dose; may repeat in 3 weeks

>2 years and Adults: 400 mg as a single dose; may repeat in 3 weeks

**Dosage Forms** Tablet: 200 mg

♦ **Albenza®** *see* Albendazole *on page 21*

## Albumin (al BYOO min)

**U.S. Brand Names** Albuminar®; Albumisol®; Albunex®; Albutein®; Buminate®; Plasbumin®

**Synonyms** Normal Human Serum Albumin; Normal Serum Albumin (Human); Salt Poor Albumin; SPA

**Pharmacologic Category** Blood Product Derivative; Plasma Volume Expander, Colloid

**Use** Plasma volume expansion and maintenance of cardiac output in the treatment of certain types of shock or impending shock; may be useful for burn patients, ARDS, and cardiopulmonary bypass; other uses considered by some investigators (but not proven) are retroperitoneal surgery, peritonitis, and ascites; unless the condition responsible for hypoproteinemia can be corrected, albumin can provide only symptomatic relief or supportive treatment; nutritional supplementation is not an appropriate indication for albumin

**Effects on Mental Status** None reported

**Effects on Psychiatric Treatment** None reported

**Pregnancy Risk Factor** C

**Contraindications** Patients with severe anemia or cardiac failure, known hypersensitivity to albumin; avoid 25% concentration in preterm infants due to risk of idiopathic ventricular hypertrophy

**Warnings/Precautions** Use with caution in patients with hepatic or renal failure because of added protein load; rapid infusion of albumin solutions may cause vascular overload. All patients should be observed for signs of hypervolemia such as pulmonary edema. Use with caution in those patients for whom sodium restriction is necessary. Rapid infusion may cause hypotension.

**Adverse Reactions** 1% to 10%:

Cardiovascular: Hypervolemia, precipitation of congestive heart failure or hypotension, tachycardia

Central nervous system: Chills, fever

Dermatologic: Rash

Gastrointestinal: Nausea, vomiting

Respiratory: Pulmonary edema

**Overdosage/Toxicology** Signs and symptoms: Hypervolemia, congestive heart failure, pulmonary edema

(Continued)

## Albumin *(Continued)*

**Usual Dosage** I.V.:

**5%** should be used in hypovolemic patients or intravascularly-depleted patients

**25%** should be used in patients in whom fluid and sodium intake must be minimized

**Dose depends on condition of patient:**

Children:

Emergency initial dose: 25 g

Nonemergencies: 25% to 50% of the adult dose

Adults: Usual dose: 25 g; no more than 250 g should be administered within 48 hours

Hypoproteinemia: 0.5-1 g/kg/dose; repeat every 1-2 days as calculated to replace ongoing losses

Hypovolemia: 0.5-1 g/kg/dose; repeat as needed; maximum dose: 6 g/kg/day

**Dosage Forms** Injection, as human: 5% [50 mg/mL] (50 mL, 250 mL, 500 mL, 1000 mL); 25% [250 mg/mL] (10 mL, 20 mL, 50 mL, 100 mL)


- ♦ **Albuminar®** *see* Albumin *on page 21*
- ♦ **Albumisol®** *see* Albumin *on page 21*
- ♦ **Albunex®** *see* Albumin *on page 21*
- ♦ **Albutein®** *see* Albumin *on page 21*


## Albuterol (al BYOO ter ole)

**U.S. Brand Names** Airet®; Proventil®; Proventil® HFA; Ventolin®; Ventolin® Rotocaps®; Volmax®

**Canadian Brand Names** Apo®-Salvent; Novo-Salmol; Sabulin

**Synonyms** Salbutamol

**Pharmacologic Category** $Beta_2$ Agonist

**Use** Bronchodilator in reversible airway obstruction due to asthma or COPD

**Effects on Mental Status** May produce CNS stimulation resulting in anxiety, tremor, and insomnia

**Effects on Psychiatric Treatment** Effect of propranolol may be reduced; cardiovascular effects (tachycardia, palpitations) may be increased with MAOIs, TCAs, and amphetamines

**Pregnancy Risk Factor** C

**Contraindications** Hypersensitivity to albuterol, adrenergic amines or any ingredients

**Warnings/Precautions** Use with caution in patients with hyperthyroidism, diabetes mellitus, or sensitivity to sympathomimetic amines; cardiovascular disorders including coronary insufficiency or hypertension; excessive use may result in tolerance

Some adverse reactions may occur more frequently in children 2-5 years of age than in adults and older children

Because of its minimal effect on $beta_1$-receptors and its relatively long duration of action, albuterol is a rational choice in the elderly when a beta agonist is indicated. All patients should utilize a spacer device when using a metered dose inhaler. Oral use should be avoided in the elderly due to adverse effects.

**Adverse Reactions**

>10%:

Cardiovascular: Palpitations, pounding heartbeat, tachycardia

Gastrointestinal: GI upset, nausea

1% to 10%:

Cardiovascular: Flushing of face, hypertension or hypotension

Central nervous system: CNS stimulation, dizziness, drowsiness, headache, hyperactivity, insomnia, lightheadedness, nervousness

Gastrointestinal: Heartburn, unusual taste, vomiting, xerostomia

Genitourinary: Dysuria

Neuromuscular & skeletal: Muscle cramping, tremor, weakness

Respiratory: Coughing

Miscellaneous: Diaphoresis (increased)

<1%: Chest pain, loss of appetite, paradoxical bronchospasm, unusual pallor

**Overdosage/Toxicology**

Signs and symptoms: Hypertension, tachycardia, angina, hypokalemia

Treatment: Hypokalemia and tachyarrhythmias, prudent use of a cardioselective beta-adrenergic blocker (eg, atenolol or metoprolol); keep in mind the potential for induction of bronchoconstriction in an asthmatic; dialysis has not been shown to be of value in the treatment of an overdose with this agent.

**Drug Interactions**

Decreased effect: Beta-adrenergic blockers (eg, propranolol)

Increased therapeutic effect: Inhaled ipratropium may increase duration of bronchodilation, nifedipine may increase FEV-1

Increased toxicity: Cardiovascular effects are potentiated in patients also receiving MAO inhibitors, tricyclic antidepressants, sympathomimetic agents (eg, amphetamine, dopamine, dobutamine), inhaled anesthetics (eg, enflurane)

**Usual Dosage**

Oral:

Children:

2-6 years: 0.1-0.2 mg/kg/dose 3 times/day; maximum dose not to exceed 12 mg/day (divided doses)

6-12 years: 2 mg/dose 3-4 times/day; maximum dose not to exceed 24 mg/day (divided doses)

Children >12 years and Adults: 2-4 mg/dose 3-4 times/day; maximum dose not to exceed 32 mg/day (divided doses)

Elderly: 2 mg 3-4 times/day; maximum: 8 mg 4 times/day

Inhalation MDI: 90 mcg/spray:

Children <12 years: 1-2 inhalations 4 times/day using a tube spacer

Children ≥12 years and Adults: 1-2 inhalations every 4-6 hours; maximum: 12 inhalations/day

Exercise-induced bronchospasm: 2 inhalations 15 minutes before exercising

Inhalation: Nebulization: 0.01-0.05 mL/kg of 0.5% solution every 4-6 hours; intensive care patients may require more frequent administration; minimum dose: 0.1 mL; maximum dose: 1 mL diluted in 1-2 mL normal saline; continuous nebulized albuterol at 0.3 mg/kg/hour has been used safely in the treatment of severe status asthmaticus in children; continuous nebulized doses of 3 mg/kg/hour ± 2.2 mg/kg/hour in children whose mean age was 20.7 months resulted in no cardiac toxicity; the optimal dosage for continuous nebulization remains to be determined.

Hemodialysis: Not removed

Peritoneal dialysis: Significant drug removal is unlikely based on physiochemical characteristics

**Patient Information** Use exactly as directed. Do not use more often than recommended. Maintain adequate hydration (2-3 L/day of fluids unless instructed to restrict fluid intake). You may experience nervousness, dizziness, or fatigue (use caution when driving or engaging in hazardous activities until response to drug is known); dry mouth, unpleasant taste, stomach upset (frequent small meals, frequent mouth care, chewing gum, or sucking lozenges may help); or difficulty urinating (always void before treatment). Report unresolved GI upset, dizziness or fatigue, vision changes, chest pain or palpitations, persistent inability to void, nervousness or insomnia, muscle cramping or tremor, or unusual cough.

**Administration:** Self-administered inhalation: Store canister upside down; do not freeze. Shake canister before using. Sit when using medication. Close eyes when administering albuterol to avoid spray getting into eyes. Exhale slowly and completely through nose; inhale deeply through mouth while administering aerosol. Hold breath for 1-3 seconds after inhalation. Wait at least 1 full minute between inhalations. Wash mouthpiece between use. If more than one inhalation medication is used, use albuterol first and wait 5 minutes between medications.

Self-administered nebulizer: Wash hands before and after treatment. Wash and dry nebulizer after each treatment. Twist open the top of one unit dose vial and squeeze contents into nebulizer reservoir. Connect nebulizer reservoir to the mouthpiece or face-mask. Connect nebulizer to compressor. Sit in comfortable, upright position. Place mouthpiece in your mouth or put on face mask and turn on compressor. If face-mask is used, avoid leakage around the mask to avoid mist getting into eyes which may cause vision problems. Breath calmly and deeply until no more mist is formed in nebulizer (about 5 minutes). At this point treatment is finished.

**Nursing Implications** Before using, the inhaler must be shaken well; assess lung sounds, pulse, and blood pressure before administration and during peak of medication; observe patient for wheezing after administration, if this occurs, call physician

**Additional Information** ~1% as active as penicillin as an antibiotic; number one over-the-counter drug in Germany; enteric-coated products may demonstrate best results

**Dosage Forms**

Aerosol: 90 mcg/dose (17 g) [200 doses]

Proventil®, Ventolin®: 90 mcg/dose (17 g) [200 doses]

Aerosol, chlorofluorocarbon free (Proventil® HFA): 90 mcg/dose (17 g)

Capsule for oral inhalation (Ventolin® Rotacaps®): 200 mcg [to be used with Rotahaler® inhalation device]

Solution, inhalation: 0.083% (3 mL); 0.5% (20 mL)

Airet®: 0.083%

Proventil®: 0.083% (3 mL); 0.5% (20 mL)

Ventolin®: 0.5% (20 mL)

Syrup, as sulfate: 2 mg/5 mL (480 mL)

Proventil®, Ventolin®: 2 mg/5 mL (480 mL)

Tablet, as sulfate: 2 mg, 4 mg

Proventil®, Ventolin®: 2 mg, 4 mg

Tablet, extended release:

Proventil® Repetabs®: 4 mg

Volmax®: 4 mg, 8 mg


- ♦ **Alcaine®** *see* Proparacaine *on page 473*


## Alclometasone (al kloe MET a sone)

**Related Information**

Corticosteroids Comparison Chart *on page 711*

**U.S. Brand Names** Aclovate® Topical
**Pharmacologic Category** Corticosteroid, Topical
**Use** Treats inflammation of corticosteroid-responsive dermatosis (low potency topical corticosteroid)
**Effects on Mental Status** None reported
**Effects on Psychiatric Treatment** None reported
**Usual Dosage** Topical: Apply a thin film to the affected area 2-3 times/day. Therapy should be discontinued when control is achieved; if no improvement is seen, reassessment of diagnosis may be necessary.
**Dosage Forms**
Cream, as dipropionate: 0.05% (15 g, 45 g, 60 g)
Ointment, topical, as dipropionate: 0.05% (15 g, 45 g, 60 g)

- **Alconefrin® Nasal Solution [OTC]** *see* Phenylephrine *on page 439*
- **Aldactazide®** *see* Hydrochlorothiazide and Spironolactone *on page 271*
- **Aldactone®** *see* Spironolactone *on page 518*
- **Aldara™** *see* Imiquimod *on page 284*

## Aldesleukin (al des LOO kin)

**U.S. Brand Names** Proleukin®
**Pharmacologic Category** Biological Response Modulator
**Use** Treatment of metastatic renal cell carcinoma; also, investigated in tumors known to have a response to immunotherapy, such as melanoma; has been used in conjunction with LAK cells, TIL cells, IL-1, and interferon
**Effects on Mental Status** Sedation, disorientation, delusions, and cognitive changes are common, reversible, and dose related
**Effects on Psychiatric Treatment** Propranolol potentiates hypotensive effects. Interaction may occur with other psychotropic given aldesleukin's effect on mental status.
**Usual Dosage** Refer to individual protocols; all orders must be written in million international units (million IU)

Adults: Metastatic renal cell carcinoma (RCC):
Treatment consists of two 5-day treatment cycles separated by a rest period. 600,000 units/kg (0.037 mg/kg)/dose administered every 8 hours by a 15-minute I.V. infusion for a total of 14 doses; following 9 days of rest, the schedule is repeated for another 14 doses, for a maximum of 28 doses per course
**Dose modification:** In high-dose therapy of RCC, see manufacturer's guidelines for holding and restarting therapy; hold or interrupt a dose - DO NOT DOSE REDUCE; or refer to specific protocol
**Retreatment:** Patients should be evaluated for response approximately 4 weeks after completion of a course of therapy and again immediately prior to the scheduled start of the next treatment course; additional courses of treatment may be given to patients only if there is some tumor shrinkage or stable disease following the last course and retreatment is not contraindicated. Each treatment course should be separated by a rest period of at least 7 weeks from the date of hospital discharge; tumors have continued to regress up to 12 months following the initiation of therapy
**Investigational regimen:** S.C.: 11 million units (flat dose) daily x 4 days per week for 4 consecutive weeks; repeat every 6 weeks
**Dosage Forms** Powder for injection, lyophilized: 22 x $10^6$ international units [18 million international units/mL = 1.1 mg/mL when reconstituted]

- **Aldoclor®** *see* Chlorothiazide and Methyldopa *on page 112*
- **Aldomet®** *see* Methyldopa *on page 356*
- **Aldoril®** *see* Methyldopa and Hydrochlorothiazide *on page 357*

## Alendronate (a LEN droe nate)

**U.S. Brand Names** Fosamax®
**Pharmacologic Category** Bisphosphonate Derivative
**Use** Treatment of osteoporosis in postmenopausal women, Paget's disease of the bone; treatment of glucocorticoid-induced osteoporosis in males and females with low bone mineral density who are receiving a daily dosage ≥7.5 mg of prednisone (or equivalent)
**Effects on Mental Status** None reported
**Effects on Psychiatric Treatment** None reported
**Pregnancy Risk Factor** C
**Contraindications** Hypersensitivity to bisphosphonates or any component of the product; hypocalcemia; abnormalities of the esophagus which delay esophageal emptying such as stricture or achalasia; inability to stand or sit upright for at least 30 minutes
**Warnings/Precautions** Use caution in patients with renal impairment; hypocalcemia must be corrected before therapy initiation with alendronate; ensure adequate calcium and vitamin D intake to provide for enhanced needs in patients with Paget's disease in whom the pretreatment rate of bone turnover may be greatly elevated.
**Adverse Reactions Note:** Incidence of adverse effects increases significantly in patients treated for Paget's disease at 40 mg/day, mostly GI adverse effects
1% to 10%:
Central nervous system: Headache (2.6%); pain (4.1%)
Gastrointestinal: Abdominal distention (1%), acid regurgitation (2%), dysphagia (1%), esophagitis ulcer (1.5%), flatulence (2.6%)
<1%: Erythema (rare), gastritis (0.5%), rash
**Overdosage/Toxicology**
Signs and symptoms: Hypocalcemia, hypophosphatemia; upper GI adverse events (upset stomach, heartburn, esophagitis, gastritis or ulcer)
Treatment: Treat with milk or antacids to bind alendronate; dialysis would not be beneficial
**Drug Interactions** Ranitidine (by increasing gastric pH) can double the bioavailability of alendronate
**Usual Dosage** Oral: Alendronate must be taken with plain water first thing in the morning and ≥30 minutes before the first food, beverage, or other medication of the day. Patients should be instructed to take alendronate with a full glass of water (6-8 oz) and not lie down for at least 30 minutes to improve alendronate absorption.
Adults: Patients with osteoporosis or Paget's disease should receive supplemental calcium and vitamin D if dietary intake is inadequate
**Osteoporosis in postmenopausal women:**
Prophylaxis: 5 mg once daily
Treatment: 10 mg once daily
**Paget's disease of bone:** 40 mg once daily for 6 months
Retreatment: Relapses during the 12 months following therapy occurred in 9% of patients who responded to treatment. Specific retreatment data are not available. Retreatment with alendronate may be considered, following a 6-month post-treatment evaluation period, in patients who have relapsed based on increases in serum alkaline phosphatase, which should be measured periodically. Retreatment may also be considered in those who failed to normalize their serum alkaline phosphatase.
Treatment of glucocorticoid-induced osteoporosis: 5 mg once daily. A dose of 10 mg once daily should be used in postmenopausal women who are not receiving estrogen. Patients treated with glucocorticoids should receive adequate amounts of calcium and vitamin D.
Elderly: No dosage adjustment is necessary
**Dosage adjustment in renal impairment:**
$Cl_{cr}$ 30-60 mL/minute: None necessary
$Cl_{cr}$ <35 mL/minute: Alendronate is not recommended due to lack of experience
**Dosage adjustment in hepatic impairment:** None necessary
**Patient Information** Take as directed, with a full glass of water. Stay in sitting or standing position for 30 minutes following administration to reduce potential for esophageal irritation. Avoid aspirin- or aspirin-containing medications. Consult prescriber to determine necessity of lifestyle changes or dietary supplements of calcium or dietary vitamin D. You may experience GI upset (eg, flatulence, bloating, nausea, acid regurgitation); small frequent meals may help. Report acute headache or gastric pain, unresolved GI upset, or acid stomach.
**Dosage Forms** Tablet, as sodium: 5 mg, 10 mg, 40 mg

- **Alesse™** *see* Ethinyl Estradiol and Levonorgestrel *on page 211*
- **Aleve® [OTC]** *see* Naproxen *on page 384*
- **Alfenta® Injection** *see* Alfentanil *on page 23*

## Alfentanil (al FEN ta nil)

**Related Information**
Narcotic Agonists Comparison Chart *on page 720*
**U.S. Brand Names** Alfenta® Injection
**Pharmacologic Category** Analgesic, Narcotic
**Use** Analgesic adjunct given by continuous infusion or in incremental doses in maintenance of anesthesia with barbiturate or $N_2O$ or a primary anesthetic agent for the induction of anesthesia in patients undergoing general surgery in which endotracheal intubation and mechanical ventilation are required
**Effects on Mental Status** Sedation is common, may see depression or confusion, rarely may cause seizures or delirium
**Effects on Psychiatric Treatment** CNS depressant and beta-blockers may increase toxicity; phenothiazines may antagonize analgesic effect
**Restrictions** C-II
**Usual Dosage** Doses should be titrated to appropriate effects; wide range of doses is dependent upon desired degree of analgesia/anesthesia

Children <12 years: Dose not established
Adults: Dose should be based on ideal body weight
**Dosage Forms** Injection, preservative free, as hydrochloride: 500 mcg/mL (2 mL, 5 mL, 10 mL, 20 mL)

- **Alferon® N** *see* Interferon Alfa-n3 *on page 289*

## Alglucerase (al GLOO ser ase)

**U.S. Brand Names** Ceredase®
(Continued)

## Alglucerase *(Continued)*

**Synonyms** Glucocerebrosidase
**Pharmacologic Category** Enzyme
**Use Orphan drug**: Treatment of Gaucher's disease
**Effects on Mental Status** None reported
**Effects on Psychiatric Treatment** None reported
**Pregnancy Risk Factor** C
**Contraindications** Hypersensitivity to any component
**Warnings/Precautions** Prepared from pooled human placental tissue that may contain the causative agents of some viral diseases
**Adverse Reactions**
>10%: Local: Burning, discomfort, and edema at the site of injection
<1%: Abdominal discomfort, chills, fever, nausea, vomiting
**Overdosage/Toxicology** No obvious toxicity was detected after single doses of up to 234 units/kg
**Usual Dosage** Usually administered as a 20-60 unit/kg I.V. infusion given with a frequency ranging from 3 times/week to once every 2 weeks
**Patient Information** Treatment is required for life
**Dosage Forms** Injection: 10 units/mL (5 mL); 80 units/mL (5 mL)

- **Alinam®** *see* Chlormezanone *on page 111*

## Alitretinoin (a li TRET i noyn)

**U.S. Brand Names** Panretin®
**Pharmacologic Category** Antineoplastic Agent, Miscellaneous
**Use** Topical treatment of cutaneous lesions in AIDS-related Kaposi's sarcoma; not indicated when systemic therapy for Kaposi's sarcoma is indicated
**Effects on Mental Status** Pain is common
**Effects on Psychiatric Treatment** May be photosensitizing; caution with psychotropics
**Usual Dosage** Topical: Apply gel twice daily to cutaneous Kaposi's sarcoma lesions
**Dosage Forms** Gel: 0.1% (60 g)

- **Alkaban-AQ®** *see* Vinblastine *on page 584*
- **Alka-Mints® [OTC]** *see* Calcium Carbonate *on page 84*
- **Alka-Seltzer® Plus Cold Liqui-Gels Capsules [OTC]** *see* Acetaminophen, Chlorpheniramine, and Pseudoephedrine *on page 15*
- **Alka-Seltzer® Plus Flu & Body Aches Non-Drowsy Liqui-Gels [OTC]** *see* Acetaminophen, Dextromethorphan, and Pseudoephedrine *on page 16*
- **Alkeran®** *see* Melphalan *on page 339*
- **Allbee® With C [OTC]** *see* Vitamin B Complex With Vitamin C *on page 586*
- **Allegra®** *see* Fexofenadine *on page 225*
- **Allegra-D™** *see* Fexofenadine and Pseudoephedrine *on page 225*
- **Aller-Chlor® [OTC]** *see* Chlorpheniramine *on page 113*
- **Allercon® Tablet [OTC]** *see* Triprolidine and Pseudoephedrine *on page 572*
- **Allerest® 12 Hour Capsule [OTC]** *see* Chlorpheniramine and Phenylpropanolamine *on page 114*
- **Allerest® 12 Hour Nasal Solution [OTC]** *see* Oxymetazoline *on page 415*
- **Allerest® Eye Drops [OTC]** *see* Naphazoline *on page 383*
- **Allerest® Maximum Strength [OTC]** *see* Chlorpheniramine and Pseudoephedrine *on page 114*
- **Allerest® No Drowsiness [OTC]** *see* Acetaminophen and Pseudoephedrine *on page 15*
- **Allerfrin® Syrup [OTC]** *see* Triprolidine and Pseudoephedrine *on page 572*
- **Allerfrin® Tablet [OTC]** *see* Triprolidine and Pseudoephedrine *on page 572*
- **Allerfrin® w/Codeine** *see* Triprolidine, Pseudoephedrine, and Codeine *on page 572*
- **Allergefon®** *see* Carbinoxamine *on page 92*
- **AllerMax® Oral [OTC]** *see* Diphenhydramine *on page 174*
- **Allerphed Syrup [OTC]** *see* Triprolidine and Pseudoephedrine *on page 572*
- ***Allium savitum*** *see* Garlic *on page 246*

## Allopurinol (al oh PURE i nole)

**U.S. Brand Names** Aloprim™; Zyloprim®
**Canadian Brand Names** Apo®-Allopurinol; Novo-Purol; Purinol®
**Pharmacologic Category** Xanthine Oxidase Inhibitor
**Use**
Oral: Prevention of attack of gouty arthritis and nephropathy; also used to treat secondary hyperuricemia which may occur during treatment of tumors or leukemia, and to prevent recurrent calcium oxalate calculi
Intravenous: Management of patients with leukemia, lymphoma, and solid tumor malignancies who are receiving cancer chemotherapy which causes elevations of serum and urinary uric acid levels and who cannot tolerate oral therapy
**Effects on Mental Status** May cause drowsiness
**Effects on Psychiatric Treatment** Rarely may cause bone marrow suppression; use caution with clozapine and carbamazepine
**Pregnancy Risk Factor** C
**Contraindications** Not to be used in pregnancy or lactation, or in patients with a previous severe allergy reaction to allopurinol or any component
**Warnings/Precautions** Do not use to treat asymptomatic hyperuricemia. Discontinue at first signs of rash; reduce dosage in renal insufficiency, reinstate with caution in patients who have had a previous mild allergic reaction, use with caution in children; monitor liver function and complete blood counts before initiating therapy and periodically during therapy, use with caution in patients taking diuretics concurrently. Risk of skin rash may be increased in patients receiving amoxicillin or ampicillin. The risk of hypersensitivity may be increased in patients receiving thiazides, and possibly ACE inhibitors.
**Adverse Reactions** The most common adverse reaction to allopurinol is a skin rash (usually maculopapular; however, more severe reactions, including Stevens-Johnson syndrome, have also been reported). While some studies cite an incidence of these reactions as high as >10% of cases (often in association with ampicillin or amoxicillin), the product labeling cites a much lower incidence, reflected below. Allopurinol should be discontinued at the first appearance of a rash or other sign of hypersensitivity.
>1%:
Dermatologic: Rash (1.5%)
Gastrointestinal: Nausea (1.3%), vomiting (1.2%)
Renal: Renal failure/impairment (1.2%)
<1%: Acute tubular necrosis, agranulocytosis, angioedema, aplastic anemia, bronchospasm, cataracts, dyspepsia, epistaxis, exfoliative dermatitis, granuloma anulare, granulomatous hepatitis, gynecomastia, hypersensitivity syndrome, increased alkaline phosphatase or hepatic transaminases, interstitial nephritis, macular retinitis, nephrolithiasis, neuritis, pancreatitis, paresthesia, peripheral neuropathy, Steven's Johnson syndrome, TEN, toxic pustuloderma, vasculitis
**Overdosage/Toxicology**
Signs and symptoms: If significant amounts of allopurinol are thought to have been absorbed, it is a theoretical possibility that oxypurinol stones could be formed, but no record of such occurrence in overdose exists
Treatment: Alkalinization of urine and forced diuresis can help prevent potential xanthine stone formation
**Drug Interactions** Hepatic enzyme inhibitor
Decreased effect: Alcohol decreases effectiveness, uricosurics
Increased toxicity:
Allopurinol prolongs half-life of oral anticoagulants; allopurinol increases serum half-life of theophylline; allopurinol may compete for excretion in renal tubule with chlorpropamide and increases chlorpropamide's serum half-life
Cyclosporine levels may be increased
Hepatic iron uptake may be increased with iron supplements
Inhibits metabolism of azathioprine and mercaptopurine (reduce to 1/3 or 1/4 of usual dose)
Thiazide diuretics enhance toxicity, monitor renal function; thiazide diuretics and captopril (possibly other ACE inhibitors) may increase risk of hypersensitivity
Urinary acidification with large amounts of vitamin C may increase kidney stone formation
Use with ampicillin or amoxicillin may increase the incidence of skin rash
Vidarabine neurotoxicity may be enhanced
**Usual Dosage**
Oral:
Children ≤10 years: 10 mg/kg/day in 2-3 divided doses **or** 200-300 mg/m$^2$/day in 2-4 divided doses, maximum: 800 mg/24 hours
Alternative: <6 years: 150 mg/day in 3 divided doses; 6-10 years: 300 mg/day in 2-3 divided doses
Children >10 years and Adults: Daily doses >300 mg should be administered in divided doses
Myeloproliferative neoplastic disorders: 600-800 mg/day in 2-3 divided doses for prevention of acute uric acid nephropathy for 2-3 days starting 1-2 days before chemotherapy
Gout: Mild: 200-300 mg/day; Severe: 400-600 mg/day
Elderly: Initial: 100 mg/day, increase until desired uric acid level is obtained
**Dosing adjustment in renal impairment:** Must be adjusted due to accumulation of allopurinol and metabolites; removed by hemodialysis.

Adult maintenance doses of allopurinol* (mg) based on creatinine clearance (mL/minute):
- $Cl_{cr}$ 140 mL/minute: 400 mg daily
- $Cl_{cr}$ 120 mL/minute: 350 mg daily
- $Cl_{cr}$ 100 mL/minute: 300 mg daily
- $Cl_{cr}$ 80 mL/minute: 250 mg daily
- $Cl_{cr}$ 60 mL/minute: 200 mg daily
- $Cl_{cr}$ 40 mL/minute: 150 mg daily
- $Cl_{cr}$ 20 mL/minute: 100 mg daily
- $Cl_{cr}$ 10 mL/minute: 100 mg every 2 days
- $Cl_{cr}$ 0 mL/minute: 100 mg every 3 days

*Doses based on a standard maintenance dose of 300 mg of allopurinol per day for a patient with a creatinine clearance of 100 mL/minute.

Hemodialysis: Administer dose posthemodialysis or administer 50% supplemental dose

I.V.: Intravenous daily dose can be given as a single infusion or in equally divided doses at 6-, 8-, or 12-hour intervals. A fluid intake sufficient to yield a daily urinary output of at least 2 L in adults and the maintenance of a neutral or, preferably, slightly alkaline urine are desirable.
- Children: Starting dose: 200 mg/m²/day
- Adults: 200-400 mg/m²/day (max: 600 mg/day)

**Dosing adjustment in renal impairment: I.V.:**
- $Cl_{cr}$ 10-20 mL/minute: 200 mg/day
- $Cl_{cr}$ 3-10 mL/minute: 100 mg/day
- $Cl_{cr}$ <3 mL/minute: 100 mg/day at extended intervals

**Patient Information** Take as directed. Maintain adequate hydration (2-3 L/day of fluids unless instructed to restrict fluid intake) to avoid possible adverse renal problems. While using this medication, do not use alcohol, other prescription or OTC medications, or vitamin substances without consulting prescriber. You may experience drowsiness (use caution when driving or engaging in tasks requiring alertness until response to drug is known); nausea, vomiting, or heartburn (small frequent meals, frequent mouth care, chewing gum, or sucking lozenges may help); hair loss (reversible). Report skin rash or lesions; painful urination or blood in urine or stool; unresolved nausea or vomiting; numbness of extremities; pain or irritation of the eyes; swelling of lips, mouth, or tongue; unusual fatigue; easy bruising or bleeding; yellowing of skin or eyes; or any change in color of urine or stool.

**Dosage Forms**
- Injection: 500 mg
- Tablet: 100 mg, 300 mg


- ♦ **All-*trans*-Retinoic Acid** *see* Tretinoin, Oral *on page 561*
- ♦ **Alocril™** *see* Nedocromil *on page 385*
- ♦ **Alomide® Ophthalmic** *see* Lodoxamide Tromethamine *on page 322*
- ♦ **Aloprim™** *see* Allopurinol *on page 24*
- ♦ **Alor® 5/500** *see* Hydrocodone and Aspirin *on page 272*
- ♦ **Alora™ Transdermal** *see* Estradiol *on page 203*


## Alosetron (a LOE se tron)

**U.S. Brand Names** Lotronex®

**Pharmacologic Category** 5-$HT_3$ Receptor Antagonist

**Use** Treatment of irritable bowel syndrome (IBS) in women whose predominant bowel symptom is diarrhea; use in males with IBS has not been substantiated

**Unlabeled use:** Alosetron has demonstrated effectiveness as an antiemetic for a wide variety of causes of emesis

**Effects on Mental Status** May cause depression or sleep abnormalities; may rarely cause anxiety or sedation

**Effects on Psychiatric Treatment** Constipation is common; use caution with TCAs and clozapine

**Pregnancy Risk Factor** B

**Contraindications** Patients who are constipated; history of severe or chronic constipation; history of ischemic colitis, intestinal obstruction, stricture, toxic megacolon, gastrointestinal perforation and/or adhesions; active diverticulitis; Crohn's disease; ulcerative colitis; hypersensitivity to alosetron or any component

**Warnings/Precautions** Constipation is a frequent, dose-related side effect. Serious complications of constipation have been reported infrequently (obstruction, perforation, impaction, toxic megacolon, secondary ischemia). Discontinue immediately if constipation is severe. Non-severe constipation may be managed by temporarily interrupting therapy or treating with a laxative. Carefully monitor the patient and discontinue treatment permanently if constipation does not resolve within 4 days. Acute ischemic colitis has been reported during alosetron treatment. Discontinue immediately in patients who experience rectal bleeding or a sudden worsening of abdominal pain, and do not restart therapy if ischemic colitis is diagnosed. Safety and efficacy have not been established in pediatric or male patients.

**Adverse Reactions**

>10%: Gastrointestinal: Constipation (28%)

1% to 10%:
- Central nervous system: Sleep disorders (3%), depression (2%)
- Cardiovascular: Hypertension (2%)
- Gastrointestinal: Nausea (7%), gastrointestinal discomfort and pain (5%), abdominal discomfort and pain (5%), gastrointestinal gaseous symptoms (3%), viral infections (2%), dyspepsia (3%), abdominal distention (2%), hemorrhoids (2%)
- Otic: Bacterial ear infection (1%)
- Respiratory: Allergic rhinitis (2%); throat and tonsil discomfort and pain (1%); bacterial ear, nose and throat infection (1%)

<1%: Elevated hepatic transaminases (0.5%), acute ischemic colitis, arrhythmias, contusions, hematomas, photophobia, proctitis, abnormal bilirubin levels, breathing disorders, cough, sedation and abnormal dreams, allergies, allergic reactions, unusual odors and taste, anxiety, menstrual disorders, sexual function disorders, acne, folliculitis, urinary infections, polyuria, diuresis

Case report: Hepatitis, ischemic colitis, intestinal perforation, impaction, bowel obstruction, toxic megacolon

**Overdosage/Toxicology** There is not a specific antidote for overdose; manage with appropriate supportive therapy

**Drug Interactions** CYP2C9, CYP3A4, and CYP1A2 enzyme substrate; inhibits CYP1A2, 2E1 only at extremely high concentrations (no clinical significance)

Inducers or inhibitors of these enzymes theoretically may change the clearance of alosetron, but this has not been evaluated. Alosetron inhibits N-acetyltransferase which may influence the metabolism of drugs such as isoniazid, procainamide, and hydralazine but there has not been any investigation of this.

**Usual Dosage**

Adults: Female: Oral: 1 mg twice daily with or without food. Patients who experience constipation may need to interrupt therapy. Discontinue if no improvement is seen after 4 weeks.

**Dosage modification for constipation:**
- Do not start therapy in patients who are constipated (also see contraindications)
- Patients who develop severe constipation: Discontinue immediately and do not resume.
- Patients who develop non-severe constipation: Monitor closely; may interrupt therapy or treat with laxatives. Discontinue and do not resume if constipation does not resolve within 4 days.

**Dosage adjustment in renal impairment:** No dosage adjustment is recommended for patients with $Cl_{cr}$ 4-56 mL/minute; use in $Cl_{cr}$ <4 mL/minute or hemodialysis patients has not been studied

**Dosage adjustment in hepatic impairment:** Specific guidelines are not available

Elderly: Dosage adjustment is not required

**Dietary Considerations** Take with or without food

**Patient Information** Take with or without food. Do not take if you are frequently constipated; constipation is a side effect associated with this medication mad may lead to serious complications. Call your healthcare provider if you become constipated. If you have sudden worsening of abdominal pain, severe constipation, or blood in your stool call your healthcare provider immediately, and stop taking this medication while you are waiting to talk to your health care provider. Notify your healthcare provider if you are pregnant, plan on becoming pregnant, or if you are breast-feeding.

**Nursing Implications** Monitor for improvement in cramping abdominal pain, abdominal discomfort, urgency and diarrhea; notify prescriber if sudden worsening of abdominal pain or blood in stool, or if constipation is noted. Discontinue immediately if severe constipation is noted.

**Dosage Forms** Tablet: 1 mg


- ♦ **Alphagan®** *see* Brimonidine *on page 72*


## Alpha-Lipoic Acid

**Pharmacologic Category** Nutritional Supplement

**Use** Diabetes; diabetic neuropathy; HIV; glaucoma; hypercholesterolemia; other neuropathies

**Warnings/Precautions** Use with caution in individuals who may be predisposed to hypoglycemia (including patients receiving antidiabetic agents). Rare dermatologic reactions (rashes) have been reported with alpha-lipoic acid.

**Usual Dosage** Range: 20-600 mg/day; adult RDA, ODA, and RDI have not been established; most common dosage: 25-50 mg twice daily

**Additional Information** Alpha-lipoic acid is one of the most potent known antioxidants. It is fat-soluble, facilitating transfer to a variety of physiologic environments, prompting some to refer to it as the "universal" antioxidant. Alpha-lipoic acid also functions as a cofactor in key energy-producing metabolic reactions. It has been investigated for its ability to limit oxidative damage resulting in diabetic neuropathy, improve glucose utilization, block viral transcription, and in the treatment of ophthalmologic conditions (cataracts and glaucoma).

(Continued)

## Alpha-Lipoic Acid *(Continued)*

There is no deficiency syndrome associated with alpha-lipoic acid. Since it may be synthesized in the human body, it is not classified as an essential nutrient.

**Dosage Forms** Capsule, tablet

♦ **Alphamin®** *see* Hydroxocobalamin *on page 276*

♦ **AlphaNine® SD** *see* Factor IX Complex (Human) *on page 217*

♦ **Alphatrex®** *see* Betamethasone *on page 65*

## Alprazolam (al PRAY zoe lam)

**Related Information**

Anxiety Disorders *on page 606*
Anxiolytic/Hypnotic Use in Long-Term Care Facilities *on page 754*
Benzodiazepines Comparison Chart *on page 708*
Clinical Issues in the Use of Anxiolytics and Sedative/Hypnotics *on page 634*
Federal OBRA Regulations Recommended Maximum Doses *on page 756*
Patient Information - Anxiolytics & Sedative Hypnotics (Benzodiazepines) *on page 653*

**Generic Available** Yes

**U.S. Brand Names** Xanax®

**Canadian Brand Names** Apo®-Alpraz; Novo-Alprazol; Nu-Alprax

**Pharmacologic Category** Benzodiazepine

**Use** Treatment of anxiety disorder (GAD); panic disorder, with or without agoraphobia; anxiety associated with depression; alcohol withdrawal

**Restrictions** C-IV

**Pregnancy Risk Factor** D

**Pregnancy/Breast-Feeding Implications** Alprazolam is assumed to be capable of causing an increased risk of congenital abnormalities when administered to a pregnant woman during the first trimester; use during this period should be avoided

**Contraindications** Hypersensitivity to this drug or any component of its formulation (cross-sensitivity with other benzodiazepines may exist); narrow angle glaucoma; concurrent use of ketoconazole and itraconazole; pregnancy

**Warnings/Precautions** Rebound or withdrawal symptoms, including seizures may occur 18 hours to 3 days following abrupt discontinuation or large decreases in dose (more common in patients receiving >4 mg/day or prolonged treatment). Dose reductions or tapering must be approached with extreme caution. Between dose, anxiety may also occur. Use with caution in patients receiving concurrent CYP3A4 inhibitors, particularly when these agents are added to therapy. Has weak uricosuric properties, use with caution in renal impairment or predisposition to urate nephropathy. Use with caution in elderly or debilitated patients, patients with hepatic disease (including alcoholics), renal impairment, or obese patients.

Causes CNS depression (dose-related) resulting in sedation, dizziness, confusion, or ataxia which may impair physical and mental capabilities. Patients must be cautioned about performing tasks which require mental alertness (ie, operating machinery or driving). Use with caution in patients receiving other CNS depressants or psychoactive agents. Effects with other sedative drugs or ethanol may be potentiated. Benzodiazepines have been associated with falls and traumatic injury and should be used with extreme caution in patients who are at risk of these events (especially the elderly). Use with caution in patients with respiratory disease or impaired gag reflex.

Use caution in patients with depression, particularly if suicidal risk may be present. Episodes of mania or hypomania have occurred in depressed patients treated with alprazolam. May cause physical or psychological dependence - use with caution in patients with a history of drug dependence. Acute withdrawal, including seizures, may be precipitated in patients after administration of flumazenil to patients receiving long-term benzodiazepine therapy.

Benzodiazepines have been associated with anterograde amnesia. Paradoxical reactions, including hyperactive or aggressive behavior, have been reported with benzodiazepines, particularly in adolescent/pediatric or psychiatric patients. Does not have analgesic, antidepressant, or antipsychotic properties.

**Adverse Reactions**

>10%:
- Central nervous system: Drowsiness, fatigue, ataxia, lightheadedness, memory impairment, dysarthria, irritability
- Endocrine & metabolic: Decreased libido, menstrual disorders
- Gastrointestinal: Xerostomia, decreased salivation, increased or decreased appetite, weight gain or loss
- Genitourinary: Micturition difficulties

1% to 10%:
- Cardiovascular: Hypotension
- Central nervous system: Confusion, dizziness, disinhibition, akathisia, increased libido
- Dermatologic: Dermatitis, rash
- Gastrointestinal: Increased salivation
- Genitourinary: Sexual dysfunction, incontinence
- Neuromuscular & skeletal: Rigidity, tremor, muscle cramps
- Otic: Tinnitus
- Respiratory: Nasal congestion

**Overdosage/Toxicology**

Signs and symptoms: Somnolence, confusion, coma, and diminished reflexes; treatment for benzodiazepine overdose is supportive

Treatment: Rarely is mechanical ventilation required; flumazenil has been shown to selectively block the binding of benzodiazepines to CNS receptors, resulting in a reversal of benzodiazepine-induced sedation; however, its use may not alter the course of overdose

**Drug Interactions** CYP3A3/4 enzyme substrate

CNS depressants: Sedative effects and/or respiratory depression may be additive with CNS depressants. Includes ethanol, barbiturates, narcotic analgesics, and other sedative agents; monitor for increased effect

Enzyme inducers: Metabolism of some benzodiazepines may be increased, decreasing their therapeutic effect; consider using an alternative sedative/hypnotic agent. Potential inducers include phenobarbital, phenytoin, carbamazepine, rifampin, and rifabutin.

CYP3A3/4 inhibitors: Serum level and/or toxicity of some benzodiazepines may be increased. Inhibitors include amiodarone, cimetidine, clarithromycin, erythromycin, delavirdine, diltiazem, dirithromycin, disulfiram, fluoxetine, fluvoxamine, grapefruit juice, indinavir, itraconazole, ketoconazole, nefazodone, nevirapine, propoxyfene, quinupristin-dalfopristin, ritonavir, saquinavir, verapamil, zafirlukast, zileuton; monitor for altered benzodiazepine response

Oral contraceptives: May decrease the clearance of some benzodiazepines (those which undergo oxidative metabolism); monitor for increased benzodiazepine effect

Theophylline: May partially antagonize some of the effects of benzodiazepines; monitor for decreased response; may require higher doses for sedation

**Mechanism of Action** Binds to stereospecific benzodiazepine receptors on the postsynaptic GABA neuron at several sites within the central nervous system, including the limbic system, reticular formation. Enhancement of the inhibitory effect of GABA on neuronal excitability results by increased neuronal membrane permeability to chloride ions. This shift in chloride ions results in hyperpolarization (a less excitable state) and stabilization.

**Pharmacodynamics/kinetics**

Distribution: $V_d$: 0.9-1.2 L/kg; distributes into breast milk
Protein binding: 80%
Metabolism: Extensive in the liver; major metabolite is inactive
Half-life: 12-15 hours
Time to peak serum concentration: Within 1-2 hours
Elimination: Excretion of metabolites and parent compound in urine

**Usual Dosage** Oral:

Children <18 years: Safety and dose have not been established

Adults:
- Anxiety: Effective doses are 0.5-4 mg/day in divided doses; the manufacturer recommends starting at 0.25-0.5 mg 3 times/day; titrate dose upward; maximum: 4 mg/day
- Depression: Average dose required: 2.5-3 mg/day in divided doses
- Alcohol withdrawal: Usual dose: 2-2.5 mg/day in divided doses
- Panic disorder: Many patients obtain relief at 2 mg/day, as much as 10 mg/day may be required

**Dosing adjustment in hepatic impairment:** Reduce dose by 50% to 60% or avoid in cirrhosis

**Note:** Treatment >4 months should be re-evaluated to determine the patient's need for the drug

**Dietary Considerations** Alcohol: May have additive CNS effects, avoid use

**Administration** Can be given sublingually with comparable onset and completeness of absorption

**Monitoring Parameters** Respiratory and cardiovascular status

**Test Interactions** ↑ alkaline phosphatase

**Patient Information** Avoid alcohol and other CNS depressants; avoid activities needing good psychomotor coordination until CNS effects are known; drug may cause physical or psychological dependence; avoid abrupt discontinuation after prolonged use

**Nursing Implications** Assist with ambulation during beginning therapy, raise bed rails and keep room partially illuminated at night; monitor for CNS respiratory depression

**Additional Information** Not intended for management of anxieties and minor distresses associated with everyday life; treatment longer than 4 months should be re-evaluated to determine the patient's need for the drug. Patients who become physically dependent on alprazolam tend to have a difficult time discontinuing it; withdrawal symptoms may be severe. To minimize withdrawal symptoms, taper dosage slowly; do not discontinue abruptly.

**Dosage Forms** Tablet: 0.25 mg, 0.5 mg, 1 mg, 2 mg

## Alprostadil (al PROS ta dill)

**U.S. Brand Names** Caverject® Injection; Edex™; Muse® Pellet

**Pharmacologic Category** Prostaglandin

**Use** Temporary maintenance of patency of ductus arteriosus in neonates with ductal-dependent congenital heart disease until surgery can be performed. These defects include cyanotic (eg, pulmonary atresia, pulmonary stenosis, tricuspid atresia, Fallot's tetralogy, transposition of the great vessels) and acyanotic (eg, interruption of aortic arch, coarctation of aorta, hypoplastic left ventricle) heart disease; diagnosis and treatment of erectile dysfunction of vasculogenic, psychogenic, or neurogenic etiology; adjunct in the diagnosis of erectile dysfunction

**Unlabeled use:** Treatment of pulmonary hypertension in infants and children with congenital heart defects with left-to-right shunts

**Effects on Mental Status** May cause dizziness; rarely may produce irritability

**Effects on Psychiatric Treatment** May cause seizures; use caution with clozapine and bupropion

**Usual Dosage**

**Patent ductus arteriosus** (Prostin VR Pediatric®):

I.V. continuous infusion into a large vein, or alternatively through an umbilical artery catheter placed at the ductal opening: 0.05-0.1 mcg/kg/minute with therapeutic response, rate is reduced to lowest effective dosage; with unsatisfactory response, rate is increased gradually; maintenance: 0.01-0.4 mcg/kg/minute

$PGE_1$ is usually given at an infusion rate of 0.1 mcg/kg/minute, but it is often possible to reduce the dosage to $^1/_2$ or even $^1/_{10}$ without losing the therapeutic effect. The mixing schedule is shown in the table.

**Alprostadil**

| Add 1 Ampul (500 mcg) to: | Concentration (mcg/mL) | Infusion Rate | |
|---|---|---|---|
| | | mL/min/kg Needed to Infuse 0.1 mcg/kg/min | mL/kg/24 h |
| 250 mL | 2 | 0.05 | 72 |
| 100 mL | 5 | 0.02 | 28.8 |
| 50 mL | 10 | 0.01 | 14.4 |
| 25 mL | 20 | 0.005 | 7.2 |

Therapeutic response is indicated by increased pH in those with acidosis or by an increase in oxygenation ($pO_2$) usually evident within 30 minutes

**Erectile dysfunction**

Caverject®, Edex®:

Vasculogenic, psychogenic, or mixed etiology: Individualize dose by careful titration; usual dose: 2.5-60 mcg (doses >60 mcg are not recommended); initiate dosage titration at 2.5 mcg, increasing by 2.5 mcg to a dose of 5 mcg and then in increments of 5-10 mcg depending on the erectile response until the dose produces an erection suitable for intercourse, not lasting >1 hour; if there is absolutely no response to initial 2.5 mcg dose, the second dose may increased to 7.5 mcg, followed by increments of 5-10 mcg

Neurogenic etiology (eg, spinal cord injury): Initiate dosage titration at 1.25 mcg, increasing to a doses of 2.5 mcg and then 5 mcg; increase further in increments 5 mcg until the dose is reached that produces an erection suitable for intercourse, not lasting >1 hour

**Note:** Patient must stay in the physician's office until complete detumescence occurs; if there is no response, then the next higher dose may be given within 1 hour; if there is still no response, a 1-day interval before giving the next dose is recommended; increasing the dose or concentration in the treatment of impotence results in increasing pain and discomfort

Muse® Pellet: Intraurethral: Administer as needed to achieve an erection; duration of action is about 30-60 minutes; use only two systems per 24-hour period

**Dosage Forms**

Injection:

Caverject®: 5 mcg, 10 mcg, 20 mcg

Edex® Injection: 5 mcg, 10 mcg, 20 mcg, 40 mcg

Prostin VR Pediatric®: 500 mcg/mL (1 mL)

Pellet, urethral: 125 mcg, 250 mcg, 500 mcg, 1000 mcg

♦ **AL-R® [OTC]** *see* Chlorpheniramine *on page 113*

♦ **Alrex™** *see* Loteprednol *on page 327*

♦ **Alsadorm®** *see* Doxylamine *on page 186*

♦ **Altace™** *see* Ramipril *on page 487*

♦ **Altamisa** *see* Feverfew *on page 224*

## Alteplase (AL te plase)

**U.S. Brand Names** Activase®

**Canadian Brand Names** Lysatec-rt-PA®

**Pharmacologic Category** Thrombolytic Agent

**Use**

Management of acute myocardial infarction for the lysis of thrombi in coronary arteries; management of acute massive pulmonary embolism (PE) in adults

Acute myocardial infarction (AMI): Chest pain ≥20 minutes, ≤12-24 hours; S-T elevation ≥0.1 mV in at least two EKG leads

Acute pulmonary embolism (APE): Age ≤75 years: As soon as possible within 5 days of thrombotic event. Documented massive pulmonary embolism by pulmonary angiography or echocardiography or high probability lung scan with clinical shock.

Acute ischemic stroke (rule out hemorrhagic courses before administering)

**Effects on Mental Status** None reported

**Effects on Psychiatric Treatment** None reported

**Usual Dosage**

Coronary artery thrombi: I.V.: Front loading dose: Total dose is 100 mg over 1.5 hours (for patients who weigh <65 kg, use 1.25 mg/kg/total dose). Add this dose to a 100 mL bag of 0.9% sodium chloride for a total volume of 200 mL. Infuse 15 mg (30 mL) over 1-2 minutes; infuse 50 mg (100 mL) over 30 minutes. Begin heparin 5000-10,000 unit bolus followed by continuous infusion of 1000 units/hour. Infuse the remaining 35 mg (70 mL) of alteplase over the next hour. For ≤67 kg: 15 mg I.V. bolus over 1-2 minutes. Infuse 0.75 mg/kg (not to exceed 50 mg) over next 30 minutes and then 0.5 mg/kg over next 60 minutes (not to exceed 35 mg).

Acute pulmonary embolism: 100 mg over 2 hours

Acute ischemic stroke: Doses should be given within the first 3 hours of the onset of symptoms. Load with 0.09 mg/kg as a bolus, followed by 0.81 mg/kg as a continuous infusion over 60 minutes; maximum total dose should not exceed 90 mg.

**Dosage Forms** Powder for injection, lyophilized (recombinant): 20 mg [11.6 million units] (20 mL); 50 mg [29 million units] (50 mL); 100 mg [58 million units] (100 mL)

♦ **ALternaGEL® [OTC]** *see* Aluminum Hydroxide *on page 28*

## Altretamine (al TRET a meen)

**U.S. Brand Names** Hexalen®

**Pharmacologic Category** Antineoplastic Agent, Miscellaneous

**Use** Palliative treatment of persistent or recurrent ovarian cancer following first-line therapy with a cisplatin- or alkylating agent-based combination

**Effects on Mental Status** Neurotoxicity is common; rarely may produce depression

**Effects on Psychiatric Treatment** Bone marrow suppression may be seen; use caution with carbamazepine and clozapine; may produce seizures caution with bupropion and clozapine; may cause severe orthostatic hypotension when administered with MAOIs

**Usual Dosage** Adults: Oral (refer to protocol): 4-12 mg/kg/day in 3-4 divided doses for 21-90 days

Alternatively: 240-320 mg/m$^2$/day in 3-4 divided doses for 21 days, repeated every 6 weeks

Alternatively: 260 mg/m$^2$/day for 14-21 days of a 28-day cycle in 4 divided doses

Temporarily discontinue (for ≥14 days) & subsequently restart at 200 mg/m$^2$/day if any of the following occurs:

if GI intolerance unresponsive to symptom measures

WBC <2000/mm$^3$

granulocyte count <1000/mm$^3$

platelet count <75,000/mm$^3$

progressive neurotoxicity

**Dosage Forms** Capsule: 50 mg

♦ **Alu-Cap® [OTC]** *see* Aluminum Hydroxide *on page 28*

## Aluminum Carbonate (a LOO mi num KAR bun ate)

**U.S. Brand Names** Basaljel® [OTC]

**Pharmacologic Category** Antacid

**Use** Hyperacidity; hyperphosphatemia

**Effects on Mental Status** None reported

**Effects on Psychiatric Treatment** Constipation is common; use with low potency antipsychotics and TCAs will likely result in additive effects

**Usual Dosage** Adults: Oral:

Antacid: 2 tablets/capsules or 10 mL of suspension every 2 hours, up to 12 times/day

Hyperphosphatemia: 2 tablets/capsules or 12 mL of suspension with meals

**Dosage Forms**

Capsule: Equivalent to 500 mg aluminum hydroxide

Suspension: Equivalent to 400 mg/5 mL aluminum hydroxide

Tablet: Equivalent to 500 mg aluminum hydroxide

## Aluminum Chloride Hexahydrate

(a LOO mi num KLOR ide heks a HYE drate)

**U.S. Brand Names** Drysol™

**Pharmacologic Category** Topical Skin Product

**Use** Astringent in the management of hyperhidrosis

**Effects on Mental Status** None reported

**Effects on Psychiatric Treatment** None reported

**Usual Dosage** Adults: Topical: Apply at bedtime

**Dosage Forms** Solution, topical: 20% in SD alcohol 40 (35 mL, 37.5 mL)

## Aluminum Hydroxide (a LOO mi num hye DROKS ide)

**U.S. Brand Names** ALternaGEL® [OTC]; Alu-Cap® [OTC]; Alu-Tab® [OTC]; Amphojel® [OTC]; Dialume® [OTC]; Nephrox Suspension [OTC]

**Canadian Brand Names** Basaljel®

**Pharmacologic Category** Antacid; Antidote

**Use** Treatment of hyperacidity; hyperphosphatemia

**Effects on Mental Status** None reported

**Effects on Psychiatric Treatment** Constipation is common and may be additive when used with psychotropics; may decrease the absorption of benzodiazepines and phenothiazines

**Usual Dosage** Oral:

Peptic ulcer disease:

Children: 5-15 mL/dose every 3-6 hours or 1 and 3 hours after meals and at bedtime

Adults: 15-45 mL every 3-6 hours or 1 and 3 hours after meals and at bedtime

Prophylaxis against gastrointestinal bleeding:

Infants: 2-5 mL/dose every 1-2 hours

Children: 5-15 mL/dose every 1-2 hours

Adults: 30-60 mL/dose every hour

Titrate to maintain the gastric pH >5

Hyperphosphatemia:

Children: 50-150 mg/kg/24 hours in divided doses every 4-6 hours, titrate dosage to maintain serum phosphorus within normal range

Adults: 500-1800 mg, 3-6 times/day, between meals and at bedtime; best taken with a meal or within 20 minutes of a meal

Antacid: Adults: 30 mL 1 and 3 hours postprandial and at bedtime

**Dosage Forms**

Capsule:

Alu-Cap®: 400 mg

Dialume®: 500 mg

Liquid: 600 mg/5 mL

ALternaGEL®: 600 mg/5 mL

Suspension, oral: 320 mg/5 mL; 450 mg/5 mL; 675 mg/5 mL

Amphojel®: 320 mg/5 mL

Tablet:

Amphojel®: 300 mg, 600 mg

Alu-Tab®: 500 mg

## Aluminum Hydroxide and Magnesium Carbonate

(a LOO mi num hye DROKS ide & mag NEE zhum KAR bun nate)

**U.S. Brand Names** Gaviscon® Liquid [OTC]

**Pharmacologic Category** Antacid

**Use** Temporary relief of symptoms associated with gastric acidity

**Effects on Mental Status** None reported

**Effects on Psychiatric Treatment** None reported

**Usual Dosage** Adults: Oral: 15-30 mL 4 times/day after meals and at bedtime

**Dosage Forms** Liquid: Aluminum hydroxide 95 mg and magnesium carbonate 358 mg per 15 mL

## Aluminum Hydroxide and Magnesium Hydroxide

(a LOO mi num hye DROKS ide & mag NEE zhum hye DROK side)

**U.S. Brand Names** Maalox® [OTC]; Maalox® Therapeutic Concentrate [OTC]

**Pharmacologic Category** Antacid

**Use** Antacid, hyperphosphatemia in renal failure

**Effects on Mental Status** None reported

**Effects on Psychiatric Treatment** None reported

**Usual Dosage** Oral: 5-10 mL 4-6 times/day, between meals and at bedtime; may be used every hour for severe symptoms

**Dosage Forms**

Suspension:

Maalox®: Aluminum hydroxide 225 mg and magnesium hydroxide 200 mg per 5 mL

High potency (Maalox® TC): Aluminum hydroxide 600 mg and magnesium hydroxide 300 mg per 5 mL

## Aluminum Hydroxide and Magnesium Trisilicate

(a LOO mi num hye DROKS ide & mag NEE zhum trye SIL i kate)

**U.S. Brand Names** Gaviscon®-2 Tablet [OTC]; Gaviscon® Tablet [OTC]

**Pharmacologic Category** Antacid

**Use** Temporary relief of hyperacidity

**Effects on Mental Status** None reported

**Effects on Psychiatric Treatment** None reported

**Usual Dosage** Adults: Oral: Chew 2-4 tablets 4 times/day or as directed by physician

**Dosage Forms** Tablet, chewable:

Gaviscon®: Aluminum hydroxide 80 mg and magnesium trisilicate 20 mg

Gaviscon®-2: Aluminum hydroxide 160 mg and magnesium trisilicate 40 mg

## Aluminum Hydroxide, Magnesium Hydroxide, and Simethicone

(a LOO mi num hye DROKS ide, mag NEE zhum hye DROKS ide, & sye METH i kone)

**U.S. Brand Names** Gas-Ban DS® [OTC]; Magalox Plus® [OTC]; Maximum Strength Maalox® [OTC]; Mylanta® Liquid [OTC]; Mylanta® Maximum Strength Liquid [OTC]

**Pharmacologic Category** Antacid; Antiflatulent

**Use** Temporary relief of hyperacidity associated with gas; may also be used for indications associated with other antacids

**Effects on Mental Status** None reported

**Effects on Psychiatric Treatment** Constipation is common; use with low potency antipsychotics and TCAs will likely result in additive effects

**Usual Dosage** Adults: 10-20 mL or 2-4 tablets 4-6 times/day between meals and at bedtime; may be used every hour for severe symptoms

**Dosage Forms**

Liquid:

Mylanta®: Aluminum hydroxide 200 mg, magnesium hydroxide, 200 mg, and simethicone 20 mg per 5 mL

Maximum Strength Maalox®: Aluminum hydroxide 500 mg, magnesium hydroxide 450 mg, and simethicone 40 mg per 5 mL (30 mL, 180 mL)

Mylanta® Maximum Strength: Aluminum hydroxide 400 mg, magnesium hydroxide 400 mg, and simethicone 40 mg per 5 mL (150 mL, 360 mL)

Tablet, chewable:

Magalox Plus®: Aluminum hydroxide 200 mg, magnesium hydroxide 200 mg, and simethicone 25 mg

♦ **Aluminum Sucrose Sulfate, Basic** *see* Sucralfate *on page 521*

## Aluminum Sulfate and Calcium Acetate

(a LOO mi num SUL fate & KAL see um AS e tate)

**U.S. Brand Names** Bluboro® [OTC]; Boropak® [OTC]; Domeboro® Topical [OTC]; Pedi-Boro® [OTC]

**Pharmacologic Category** Topical Skin Product

**Use** Astringent wet dressing for relief of inflammatory conditions of the skin and to reduce weeping that may occur in dermatitis

**Effects on Mental Status** None reported

**Effects on Psychiatric Treatment** None reported

**Usual Dosage** Topical: Soak affected area in the solution 2-4 times/day for 15-30 minutes or apply wet dressing soaked in the solution 2-4 times/day for 30-minute treatment periods; rewet dressing with solution every few minutes to keep it moist

**Dosage Forms**

Powder, to make topical solution: 1 packet/pint of water [1:40 solution]

Tablet, effervescent: 1 tablet/pint [1:40 dilution]

♦ **Alupent®** *see* Metaproterenol *on page 347*

♦ **Alu-Tab® [OTC]** *see* Aluminum Hydroxide *on page 28*

## Amantadine (a MAN ta deen)

**Related Information**

Agents for Treatment of Extrapyramidal Symptoms *on page 638*

Antiparkinsonian Agents Comparison Chart *on page 705*

Clinical Issues in the Use of Antipsychotics *on page 630*

Discontinuation of Psychotropic Drugs - Withdrawal Symptoms and Recommendations *on page 798*

Patient Information - Agents for Treatment of Extrapyramidal Symptoms *on page 657*

Special Populations - Pregnant and Breast-Feeding Patients *on page 668*

Substance-Related Disorders *on page 609*

**Generic Available** Yes

**U.S. Brand Names** Symadine®; Symmetrel®

**Canadian Brand Names** Endantadine®; PMS-Amantadine

**Synonyms** Adamantanamine Hydrochloride; Amantadine Hydrochloride

**Pharmacologic Category** Anti-Parkinson's Agent (Dopamine Agonist); Antiviral Agent

**Use** Prophylaxis and treatment of influenza A viral infection; treatment of parkinsonism; treatment of drug-induced extrapyramidal reactions

**Pregnancy Risk Factor** C

**Contraindications** Hypersensitivity to amantadine or any component

**Warnings/Precautions** Use with caution in patients with liver disease, history of recurrent and eczematoid dermatitis, uncontrolled psychosis or severe psychoneurosis, seizures, and in those receiving CNS stimulant drugs; reduce dose in renal disease. When treating Parkinson's disease, do not discontinue abruptly. In many patients, the therapeutic benefits of amantadine are limited to a few months. Elderly patients may be more susceptible to CNS effects (using 2 divided daily doses may minimize this effect). Has been associated with neuroleptic malignant syndrome (associated with dose reduction or abrupt discontinuation). Use with caution in patients with CHF, peripheral edema, or orthostatic hypotension. Avoid in angle closure glaucoma.

**Adverse Reactions**

1% to 10%:

Cardiovascular: Orthostatic hypotension, peripheral edema

Central nervous system: Insomnia, depression, anxiety, irritability, dizziness, hallucinations, ataxia, headache, somnolence, nervousness, dream abnormality, agitation, fatigue, confusion

Dermatologic: Livedo reticularis

Gastrointestinal: Nausea, anorexia, constipation, diarrhea, xerostomia

Respiratory: Dry nose

<1%: Amnesia, congestive heart failure, decreased libido, dyspnea, eczematoid dermatitis, euphoria, hyperkinesis, hypertension, instances of convulsions, leukopenia, neutropenia, oculogyric episodes, psychosis, rash, slurred speech, urinary retention, visual disturbances, vomiting, weakness

**Overdosage/Toxicology**

Signs and symptoms: Nausea, vomiting, slurred speech, blurred vision, lethargy, hallucinations, seizures, myoclonic jerking

Treatment: Should be directed at reducing the CNS stimulation and at maintaining cardiovascular function; minimize or discontinue use of other psychotropics that may contribute to adverse effects. Seizures can be treated with diazepam 5-10 mg I.V. every 15 minutes as needed; up to a total of 30 mg in adults (0.25-0.4 mg/kg/dose I.V. every 15 minutes as needed up to a total of 10 mg for children) while a lidocaine infusion may be required for the cardiac dysrhythmias

**Drug Interactions**

Anticholinergics may potentiate CNS side effects of amantadine; monitor for altered response. Includes benztropine and trihexyphenidyl, as well as agents with anticholinergic activity such as quinidine, tricyclics, and antihistamines.

Thiazide diuretics: Hydrochlorothiazide has been reported to increase the potential for toxicity with amantadine (limited documentation); monitor response

Triamterene: Has been reported to increase the potential for toxicity with amantadine (limited documentation); monitor response

Trimethoprim: Has been reported to increase the potential for toxicity with amantadine (limited documentation); monitor for acute confusion

**Stability** Protect from freezing

**Mechanism of Action** As an antiviral, blocks the uncoating of influenza A virus preventing penetration of virus into host; antiparkinsonian activity may be due to its blocking the reuptake of dopamine into presynaptic neurons or by increasing dopamine release from presynaptic fibers

**Pharmacodynamics/kinetics**

Onset of antidyskinetic action: Within 48 hours

Absorption: Well absorbed from GI tract

Distribution: To saliva, tear film, and nasal secretions; in animals, tissue (especially lung) concentrations higher than serum concentrations, crosses blood-brain barrier

$V_d$:

Normal: 4.4±0.2 L/kg

Renal failure: 5.1±0.2 L/kg

Protein binding:

Normal renal function: ~67%

Hemodialysis patients: ~59%

Metabolism: Not appreciable, small amounts of an acetyl metabolite identified

Half-life:

Normal renal function: 2-7 hours

End-stage renal disease: 7-10 days

Time to peak: 1-4 hours

Elimination: 80% to 90% excreted unchanged in urine by glomerular filtration and tubular secretion

**Usual Dosage**

Children: Influenza:

1-9 years: (<45 kg): 5-9 mg/kg/day in 1-2 divided doses to a maximum of 150 mg/day

10-12 years: 100-200 mg/day in 1-2 divided doses

Influenza prophylaxis: Administer for 10-21 days following exposure if the vaccine is concurrently given or for 90 days following exposure if the vaccine is unavailable or contraindicated and re-exposure is possible

Adults:

Drug-induced extrapyramidal reactions: 100 mg twice daily; may increase to 300-400 mg/day, if needed

Parkinson's disease: 100 mg twice daily as sole therapy; may increase to 400 mg/day if needed with close monitoring; initial dose: 100 mg/day if with other serious illness or with high doses of other anti-Parkinson drugs

Influenza A viral infection: 200 mg/day in 1-2 divided doses

Influenza prophylaxis: Minimum 10-day course of therapy following exposure if the vaccine is concurrently given or for 90 days following exposure if the vaccine is unavailable or contraindicated and re-exposure is possible

Elderly patients should take the drug in 2 daily doses rather than a single dose to avoid adverse neurologic reactions

**Dosing interval in renal impairment:**

$Cl_{cr}$ 50-60 mL/minute: Administer 200 mg alternating with 100 mg/day

$Cl_{cr}$ 30-50 mL/minute: Administer 100 mg/day

$Cl_{cr}$ 20-30 mL/minute: Administer 200 mg twice weekly

$Cl_{cr}$ 10-20 mL/minute: Administer 100 mg 3 times/week

$Cl_{cr}$ <10 mL/minute: Administer 200 mg alternating with 100 mg every 7 days

Hemodialysis: Slightly hemodialyzable (5% to 20%); no supplemental dose is needed

Peritoneal dialysis: No supplemental dose is needed

Continuous arterio-venous or venous-venous hemofiltration (CAVH/CAVHD): No supplemental dose is needed

**Monitoring Parameters** Renal function, Parkinson's symptoms, mental status, influenza symptoms, blood pressure

**Reference Range** Toxic and potentially fatal: 4-23 µg/mL

**Patient Information** Do not abruptly discontinue therapy, it may precipitate a parkinsonian crisis; may impair ability to perform activities requiring mental alertness or coordination. Must take throughout flu season or for 2 weeks following vaccination for effective prophylaxis.

**Nursing Implications** If insomnia occurs, the last daily dose should be given several hours before retiring; assess parkinsonian symptoms prior to and throughout course of therapy

**Additional Information** Patients with intolerable CNS side effects often do better with rimantadine

**Dosage Forms**

Syrup, as hydrochloride: 50 mg/5 mL (480 mL)

Tablet, as hydrochloride: 100 mg


- **Amantadine Hydrochloride** *see* Amantadine *on page 28*
- **Amaphen®** *see* Butalbital Compound and Acetaminophen *on page 80*
- **Amaryl®** *see* Glimepiride *on page 250*


## Ambenonium (am be NOE nee um)

**U.S. Brand Names** Mytelase® Caplets®

**Pharmacologic Category** Cholinergic Agonist

**Use** Treatment of myasthenia gravis

**Effects on Mental Status** May produce drowsiness

**Effects on Psychiatric Treatment** None reported; the cholinergic effects may counteract the anticholinergic effects of psychotropics

**Usual Dosage** Adults: Oral: 5-25 mg 3-4 times/day

**Dosage Forms** Tablet, as chloride: 10 mg


- **Amber Touch-and-Feel** *see* St Johns Wort *on page 519*
- **Ambi 10® [OTC]** *see* Benzoyl Peroxide *on page 62*
- **Ambien™** *see* Zolpidem *on page 594*
- **Ambi® Skin Tone [OTC]** *see* Hydroquinone *on page 276*
- **AmBisome®** *see* Amphotericin B, Liposomal *on page 42*


## Amcinonide (am SIN oh nide)

**Related Information**

Corticosteroids Comparison Chart *on page 711*

**U.S. Brand Names** Cyclocort®

**Pharmacologic Category** Corticosteroid, Topical

**Use** Relief of the inflammatory and pruritic manifestations of corticosteroid-responsive dermatoses (high potency corticosteroid)

**Effects on Mental Status** None reported

**Effects on Psychiatric Treatment** None reported

**Usual Dosage** Adults: Topical: Apply in a thin film 2-3 times/day. Therapy should be discontinued when control is achieved; if no improvement is seen, reassessment of diagnosis may be necessary.

**Dosage Forms**

Cream: 0.1% (15 g, 30 g, 60 g)

Lotion: 0.1% (20 mL, 60 mL)

Ointment, topical: 0.1% (15 g, 30 g, 60 g)

- **Amcort®** *see* Triamcinolone *on page 563*
- **Amen® Oral** *see* Medroxyprogesterone *on page 336*
- **Amerge®** *see* Naratriptan *on page 385*
- **Americaine® [OTC]** *see* Benzocaine *on page 61*
- **A-methaPred® Injection** *see* Methylprednisolone *on page 359*
- **Amethopterin** *see* Methotrexate *on page 353*
- **Amfepramone** *see* Diethylpropion *on page 167*
- **Amicar®** *see* Aminocaproic Acid *on page 31*
- **Amidate® Injection** *see* Etomidate *on page 216*

## Amifostine (am i FOS teen)

**U.S. Brand Names** Ethyol®

**Pharmacologic Category** Antidote

**Use** Reduce the incidence of moderate to severe xerostomia in patients undergoing postoperative radiation treatment for head and neck cancer, where the radiation port includes a substantial portion of the parotid glands. Reduce the cumulative renal toxicity associated with repeated administration of cisplatin in patients with advanced ovarian cancer or nonsmall cell lung cancer. In these settings, the clinical data does not suggest that the effectiveness of cisplatin-based chemotherapy regimens is altered by amifostine.

**Effects on Mental Status** Drowsiness is common

**Effects on Psychiatric Treatment** Hypotension is common and may be additive with psychotropics

**Usual Dosage** Adults: I.V. (refer to individual protocols): 910 mg/m$^2$ administered once daily as a 15-minute I.V. infusion, starting 30 minutes prior to chemotherapy

Reduction of xerostomia from head and neck radiation: 200 mg/m$^2$ I.V. (as a 3-minute infusion) once daily, starting 15-30 minutes before standard fraction radiation therapy

**Note:** 15-minute infusion is better tolerated than more extended infusions. Further reductions in infusion times have not been systematically investigated. The infusion of amifostine should be interrupted if the systolic blood pressure decreases significantly from the baseline value. See table.

**Decrease in Systolic Blood Pressure**

| Baseline systolic blood pressure (mm Hg) | <100 | 100–119 | 120–139 | 140–179 | ≥180 |
|---|---|---|---|---|---|
| Decrease in systolic blood pressure during infusion of amifostine (mm Hg) | 20 | 25 | 30 | 40 | 50 |

Mean onset of hypotension is 14 minutes into the 15-minute infusion and the mean duration was 6 minutes. Hypotension should be treated with fluid infusion and postural management of the patient (supine or Trendelenburg position). If the blood pressure returns to normal within 5 minutes and the patient is asymptomatic, the infusion may be restarted so that the full dose of amifostine may be administered. If the full dose of amifostine cannot be administered, the dose of amifostine for subsequent cycles should be 740 mg/m$^2$.

**Dosage Forms** Injection: 500 mg

## Amikacin (am i KAY sin)

**Related Information**

Serum Drug Concentrations Commonly Monitored: Guidelines *on page 759*

**U.S. Brand Names** Amikin® Injection

**Canadian Brand Names** Amikin®

**Pharmacologic Category** Antibiotic, Aminoglycoside

**Use** Treatment of serious infections due to organisms resistant to gentamicin and tobramycin including *Pseudomonas, Proteus, Serratia,* and other gram-positive bacilli (bone infections, respiratory tract infections, endocarditis, and septicemia); documented infection of mycobacterial organisms susceptible to amikacin

**Effects on Mental Status** May cause drowsiness; case reports of delirium and psychosis

**Effects on Psychiatric Treatment** None reported

**Usual Dosage** Individualization is critical because of the low therapeutic index

**Use of ideal body weight (IBW) for determining the mg/kg/dose appears to be more accurate than dosing on the basis of total body weight (TBW)**

In morbid obesity, dosage requirement may best be estimated using a dosing weight of IBW + 0.4 (TBW - IBW)

Initial and periodic peak and trough plasma drug levels should be determined, particularly in critically ill patients with serious infections or in disease states known to significantly alter aminoglycoside pharmacokinetics (eg, cystic fibrosis, burns, or major surgery)

Infants, Children, and Adults: I.M., I.V.: 5-7.5 mg/kg/dose every 8 hours

Some clinicians suggest a daily dose of 15-20 mg/kg for all patients with normal renal function. This dose is at least as efficacious with similar, if not less, toxicity than conventional dosing.

**Dosing interval in renal impairment:** Some patients may require larger or more frequent doses if serum levels document the need (ie, cystic fibrosis or febrile granulocytopenic patients)

$Cl_{cr}$ ≥60 mL/minute: Administer every 8 hours
$Cl_{cr}$ 40-60 mL/minute: Administer every 12 hours
$Cl_{cr}$ 20-40 mL/minute: Administer every 24 hours
$Cl_{cr}$ <20 mL/minute: Loading dose, then monitor levels

Hemodialysis: Dialyzable (50% to 100%); administer dose postdialysis or administer ⅔ normal dose as a supplemental dose postdialysis and follow levels

Peritoneal dialysis: Dose as $Cl_{cr}$ <20 mL/minute: Follow levels

Continuous arteriovenous or venovenous hemodiafiltration (CAVH) effects: Dose as for $Cl_{cr}$ 10-40 mL/minute and follow levels

**Dosage Forms** Injection, as sulfate: 50 mg/mL (2 mL, 4 mL); 250 mg/mL (2 mL, 4 mL)

- **Amikin® Injection** *see* Amikacin *on page 30*

## Amiloride (a MIL oh ride)

**U.S. Brand Names** Midamor®

**Pharmacologic Category** Diuretic, Potassium Sparing

**Use** Counteracts potassium loss induced by other diuretics in the treatment of hypertension or edematous conditions including CHF, hepatic cirrhosis, and hypoaldosteronism; usually used in conjunction with more potent diuretics such as thiazides or loop diuretics

**Unlabeled use:** Cystic fibrosis; reduction of lithium induced polyuria

**Effects on Mental Status** May cause drowsiness; rarely may cause insomnia and depression

**Effects on Psychiatric Treatment** May cause impotence and orthostatic hypotension which may be exacerbated by psychotropics; effective agent for the treatment of lithium induced diabetes insipidus

**Pregnancy Risk Factor** B

**Contraindications** Hypersensitivity to amiloride or any component; presence of elevated serum potassium levels (>5.5 mEq/L); if patient is receiving other potassium-conserving agents (eg, spironolactone, triamterene) or potassium supplementation (medicine, potassium-containing salt substitutes, potassium-rich diet); anuria; acute or chronic renal insufficiency; evidence of diabetic nephropathy. Patients with evidence of renal impairment or diabetes mellitus should not receive this medicine without close, frequent monitoring of serum electrolytes and renal function.

**Warnings/Precautions** May cause hyperkalemia (patients with renal impairment, diabetes and the elderly are at greatest risk). Should be stopped at least 3 days before glucose tolerance testing. Use caution in severely ill patients in whom respiratory or metabolic acidosis may occur.

**Adverse Reactions**

1% to 10%:

Central nervous system: Dizziness, fatigue, headache
Endocrine & metabolic: Dehydration, gynecomastia, hyperchloremic metabolic acidosis, hyperkalemia, hyponatremia
Gastrointestinal: Abdominal pain, appetite changes, constipation, diarrhea, gas pain, nausea, vomiting
Genitourinary: Impotence
Neuromuscular & skeletal: Muscle cramps, weakness
Respiratory: Cough, dyspnea

<1%: Alopecia, angina pectoris, arrhythmias, arthralgia, back pain, bladder spasms, chest pain, decreased libido, depression, dyspepsia, dysuria, flatulence, GI bleeding, heartburn, increased intraocular pressure, insomnia, jaundice, neck/shoulder pain, nervousness, orthostatic hypotension, palpitations, polyuria, pruritus, rash or dryness, shortness of breath, thirst, tremor, vertigo

**Overdosage/Toxicology**

Signs and symptoms: Clinical signs are consistent with dehydration and electrolyte disturbance; severe hyperkalemia (>6.5 mEq/L). Ingestion of large amounts of potassium-sparing diuretics may result in life-threatening hyperkalemia.

Treatment: This can be treated with I.V. insulin and glucose (dextrose 25% in water), with concurrent I.V. sodium bicarbonate (1 mEq/kg up to 44 mEq/dose). If needed, Kayexalate® oral or rectal solutions in sorbitol may also be useful.

**Drug Interactions**

Amoxicillin's absorption may be reduced; avoid concurrent use or observe for clinical response

Angiotensin-converting enzyme inhibitors can cause hyperkalemia, especially in patients with renal impairment, potassium-rich diets, or on other drugs causing hyperkalemia; avoid concurrent use or monitor closely

Potassium supplements may further increase potassium retention and cause hyperkalemia; avoid concurrent use

Quinidine and amiloride together may increase risk of malignant arrhythmias; avoid concurrent use

**Usual Dosage** Oral:
Children: Although safety and efficacy have not been established by the FDA in children, a dosage of 0.625 mg/kg/day has been used in children weighing 6-20 kg.
Adults: 5-10 mg/day (up to 20 mg)
Elderly: Initial: 5 mg once daily or every other day
**Dosing adjustment in renal impairment:**
$Cl_{cr}$ 10-50 mL/minute: Administer at 50% of normal dose.
$Cl_{cr}$ <10 mL/minute: Avoid use.

**Patient Information** Take as directed, preferably early in day. Do not increase dietary intake of potassium unless instructed by prescriber (too much potassium can be as harmful as too little). You may experience dizziness or fatigue; use caution when driving or engaging in tasks that require alertness until response to drug is known. You may experience constipation (increased dietary fluid, fiber, or fruit may help), impotence (reversible), or loss of head hair (rare). Report muscle cramping or weakness, unresolved nausea or vomiting, palpitations, or difficulty breathing.

**Nursing Implications** Assess fluid status via daily weights, I & O ratios, standing and supine blood pressures; observe for hyperkalemia; if ordered once daily, dose should be given in the morning

**Dosage Forms** Tablet, as hydrochloride: 5 mg

## Amiloride and Hydrochlorothiazide
(a MIL oh ride & hye droe klor oh THYE a zide)

**U.S. Brand Names** Moduretic®
**Canadian Brand Names** Apo®-Amilzide; Moduret®; Novamilor; Nu-Amilzide
**Pharmacologic Category** Diuretic, Combination
**Use** Potassium-sparing diuretic; antihypertensive
**Effects on Mental Status** May cause drowsiness; rarely may cause insomnia and depression
**Effects on Psychiatric Treatment** May cause impotence and orthostatic hypotension which may be exacerbated by psychotropics; effective agent for the treatment of lithium induced diabetes insipidus
**Usual Dosage** Adults: Oral: Start with 1 tablet/day, then may be increased to 2 tablets/day if needed; usually given in a single dose
**Dosage Forms** Tablet: Amiloride hydrochloride 5 mg and hydrochlorothiazide 50 mg

♦ **2-Amino-6-Mercaptopurine** *see* Thioguanine *on page 542*

♦ **2-Amino-6-Trifluoromethoxy-benzothiazole** *see* Riluzole *on page 494*

## Aminocaproic Acid (a mee noe ka PROE ik AS id)

**U.S. Brand Names** Amicar®
**Pharmacologic Category** Hemostatic Agent
**Use** Treatment of excessive bleeding from fibrinolysis
**Effects on Mental Status** May cause drowsiness
**Effects on Psychiatric Treatment** May cause hypotension which may be exacerbated by psychotropics; rarely may cause seizures; use caution with clozapine and bupropion
**Usual Dosage** In the management of acute bleeding syndromes, oral dosage regimens are the same as the I.V. dosage regimens in adults and children

Chronic bleeding: Oral, I.V.: 5-30 g/day in divided doses at 3- to 6-hour intervals
Acute bleeding syndrome:
Children: Oral, I.V.: 100 mg/kg or 3 g/m$^2$ during the first hour, followed by continuous infusion at the rate of 33.3 mg/kg/hour or 1 g/m$^2$/hour; total dosage should not exceed 18 g/m$^2$/24 hours
Traumatic hyphema: Oral: 100 mg/kg/dose every 6-8 hours
Adults:
Oral: For elevated fibrinolytic activity, administer 5 g during first hour, followed by 1-1.25 g/hour for approximately 8 hours or until bleeding stops
I.V.: 4-5 g in 250 mL of diluent during first hour followed by continuous infusion at the rate of 1-1.25 g/hour in 50 mL of diluent, continue for 8 hours or until bleeding stops
Maximum daily dose: Oral, I.V.: 30 g
**Dosing adjustment in renal impairment:** Oliguria or ESRD: Reduce to 15% to 25% of usual dose

**Dosage Forms**
Injection: 250 mg/mL (20 mL, 96 mL, 100 mL)
Syrup: 1.25 g/5 mL (480 mL)
Tablet: 500 mg

♦ **Amino-Cerv™ Vaginal Cream** *see* Urea *on page 576*

## Aminoglutethimide (a mee noe gloo TETH i mide)

**U.S. Brand Names** Cytadren®
**Pharmacologic Category** Antineoplastic Agent, Miscellaneous
**Use** Suppression of adrenal function in selected patients with Cushing's syndrome; also used successfully in postmenopausal patients with advanced breast carcinoma and in patients with metastatic prostate carcinoma as salvage (third-line hormonal agent)
**Effects on Mental Status** Drowsiness is common
**Effects on Psychiatric Treatment** May cause hypotension which may be exacerbated by psychotropics; may cause bone marrow suppression; use caution with clozapine and carbamazepine; propranolol may increase the risk of drowsiness
**Usual Dosage** Adults: Oral:
250 mg every 6 hours may be increased at 1- to 2-week intervals to a total of 2 g/day; administer in divided doses, 2-3 times/day to reduce incidence of nausea and vomiting. Follow adrenal cortical response by careful monitoring of plasma cortisol until the desired level of suppression is achieved.
Mineralocorticoid (fludrocortisone) replacement therapy may be necessary in up to 50% of patients. If glucocorticoid replacement therapy is necessary, 20-30 mg hydrocortisone orally in the morning will replace endogenous secretion.
**Dosing adjustment in renal impairment:** Dose reduction may be necessary
**Dosage Forms** Tablet, scored: 250 mg

## Aminolevulinic Acid (a mee noe le vu LIN ik AS id)

**U.S. Brand Names** Levulan® Kerastick™
**Pharmacologic Category** Photosensitizing Agent, Topical; Topical Skin Product
**Use** Treatment of nonhyperkeratotic actinic keratoses of the face or scalp; to be used in conjunction with blue light illumination
**Effects on Mental Status** None reported
**Effects on Psychiatric Treatment** None reported
**Usual Dosage** Adults: Topical: Apply to actinic keratoses (**not** perilesional skin) followed 14-18 hours later by blue light illumination. Application/treatment may be repeated at a treatment site after 8 weeks.
**Dosage Forms** Solution, topical: 20% (with applicator)

♦ **Amino-Opti-E® [OTC]** *see* Vitamin E *on page 586*

♦ **Aminophyllin™** *see* Theophylline Salts *on page 539*

♦ **Aminophylline** *see* Theophylline Salts *on page 539*

## Aminosalicylate Sodium
(a MEE noe sa LIS i late SOW dee um)

**U.S. Brand Names** Sodium P.A.S.
**Canadian Brand Names** Tubasal®
**Pharmacologic Category** Salicylate
**Use** Adjunctive treatment of tuberculosis used in combination with other antitubercular agents; has also been used in Crohn's disease
**Effects on Mental Status** None reported
**Effects on Psychiatric Treatment** May cause bone marrow suppression; use caution with clozapine and carbamazepine
**Pregnancy Risk Factor** C
**Contraindications** Hypersensitivity to aminosalicylate sodium
**Warnings/Precautions** Use with caution in patients with hepatic or renal dysfunction, patients with gastric ulcer, patients with CHF, and patients who are sodium restricted
**Adverse Reactions**
1% to 10%: Gastrointestinal: Abdominal pain, diarrhea, nausea, vomiting
<1%: Agranulocytosis, fever, goiter with or without myxedema, hemolytic anemia, hepatitis, jaundice, leukopenia, skin eruptions, thrombocytopenia, vasculitis
**Overdosage/Toxicology**
Signs and symptoms: Acute overdose results in crystalluria and renal failure, nausea, and vomiting
Treatment: Alkalinization of the urine with sodium bicarbonate and forced diuresis can prevent crystalluria and nephrotoxicity
**Drug Interactions** Decreased levels of digoxin and vitamin $B_{12}$
**Usual Dosage** Oral:
Children: 150 mg/kg/day in 3-4 equally divided doses
Adults: 150 mg/kg/day in 2-3 equally divided doses (usually 12-14 g/day)
**Dosing adjustment in renal impairment:**
$Cl_{cr}$ 10-50 mL/minute: Administer 50% to 75% of dose
$Cl_{cr}$ <10 mL/minute: Administer 50% of dose
Administer after hemodialysis
**Patient Information** May be taken with food. Do not take tablets that are discolored (brown or purple); see pharmacist for new prescription. Do not stop taking without consulting prescriber. Report persistent sore throat, fever, unusual bleeding or bruising, persistent nausea or vomiting, or abdominal pain.
**Nursing Implications** Do not administer if discolored
**Dosage Forms** Tablet: 500 mg

♦ **5-Aminosalicylic Acid** *see* Mesalamine *on page 344*

## Amiodarone (a MEE oh da rone)

**U.S. Brand Names** Cordarone®; Pacerone®

**Pharmacologic Category** Antiarrhythmic Agent, Class III

**Use**

Oral: Management of life-threatening recurrent ventricular fibrillation (VF) or hemodynamically unstable ventricular tachycardia (VT)

I.V.: Initiation of treatment and prophylaxis of frequency recurring VF and unstable VT in patients refractory to other therapy. Also, used for patients for whom oral amiodarone is indicated but who are unable to take oral medication.

**Effects on Mental Status** Insomnia, nightmares, and fatigue are common

**Effects on Psychiatric Treatment** May cause hypotension which may be exacerbated by psychotropics; may cause hypothyroidism; use caution with lithium

**Pregnancy Risk Factor** D

**Contraindications** Hypersensitivity to amiodarone or any component; severe sinus-node dysfunction; second- and third-degree heart block (except in patients with a functioning artificial pacemaker); bradycardia causing syncope (except in patients with a functioning artificial pacemaker);cisapride, ritonavir, sparfloxacin, moxifloxacin, gatifloxacin; pregnancy

**Warnings/Precautions** Not considered first line therapy due to toxicity profile especially with large doses. Reserve for use in arrhythmias refractory to other therapy. Monitor for pulmonary toxicity, liver toxicity, or exacerbation of the arrhythmia. Use very cautiously and with close monitoring in patients with thyroid or liver disease. Significant heart block or sinus bradycardia can occur. Patients should be hospitalized when amiodarone is initiated. Pre-existing pulmonary disease does not increase risk of developing pulmonary toxicity, but if pulmonary toxicity develops then the prognosis is worse. Due to complex pharmacokinetics, it is difficult to predict when an arrhythmia or interaction with a subsequent treatment will occur following discontinuation of amiodarone. May cause optic neuropathy and/or optic neuritis, usually resulting in visual impairment.

**Adverse Reactions** With large dosages (≥400 mg/day), adverse reactions occur in ~75% patients and require discontinuance in 5% to 20%

>10%:

- Cardiovascular: Hypotension (especially with I.V. form)
- Central nervous system: Ataxia, dizziness, fatigue, headache, insomnia, malaise, nightmares
- Dermatologic: Photosensitivity
- Gastrointestinal: Nausea, vomiting
- Neuromuscular & skeletal: Muscle weakness, paresthesias, tremor
- Respiratory: Interstitial pneumonitis, pulmonary fibrosis (cough, fever, dyspnea, malaise),
- Miscellaneous: Alveolitis

1% to 10%:

- Cardiovascular: Cardiac arrhythmias (atropine-resistant bradycardia, heart block, sinus arrest, paroxysmal ventricular tachycardia), congestive heart failure, edema, flushing, myocardial depression
- Central nervous system: Fever, sleep disturbances
- Dermatologic: Solar dermatitis
- Endocrine & metabolic: Decreased libido, hypothyroidism or hyperthyroidism (less common)
- Gastrointestinal: Abdominal pain, abnormal salivation, abnormal taste (oral form), anorexia, constipation,
- Hematologic: Coagulation abnormalities
- Hepatic: Abnormal LFTs
- Local: Phlebitis with concentrations >3 mg/mL
- Neuromuscular & skeletal: Paresthesia
- Ocular: Visual disturbances
- Miscellaneous: Abnormal smell (oral form)

<1%: Alopecia, atrial fibrillation, cardiogenic shock, cirrhosis, corneal microdeposits, discoloration of skin (slate blue), epididymitis, hyperglycemia, hypertriglyceridemia, hypotension (with oral form), increased ALT/AST, increased Q-T interval, optic neuritis, photophobia, pseudotumor cerebri, rash, severe hepatotoxicity (potentially fatal hepatitis), Stevens-Johnson syndrome, thrombocytopenia, vasculitis, ventricular fibrillation

**Overdosage/Toxicology**

Signs and symptoms: Extensions of pharmacologic effect, sinus bradycardia and/or heart block, hypotension and Q-T prolongation; patients should be monitored for several days following ingestion

Treatment: Intoxication with amiodarone necessitates EKG monitoring. When bradycardia occurs atropine may be given, however, atropine-resistant bradycardia has been reported. In cases of difficult to treat amiodarone-induced bradycardia, injectable isoproterenol or a temporary pacemaker may be required.

**Drug Interactions** CYP3A3/4 enzyme substrate; CYP3A3/4, CYP2C9, CYP2D6 enzyme inhibitor

**Note:** Due to the long half-life of amiodarone, drug interactions may take one or more weeks to develop

- Beta-blockers may cause excessive AV block; monitor response
- Cholestyramine may decrease amiodarone blood levels
- Cimetidine may increase amiodarone blood levels
- Cisapride and amiodarone may increase risk of malignant arrhythmias; concurrent use is contraindicated
- Clonazepam effects may be increased by amiodarone
- Codeine: Analgesic efficacy may be reduced
- Cyclosporine blood levels may be increased by amiodarone
- Digoxin levels may be increased by amiodarone; consider reducing digoxin dose by 50% and monitor digoxin blood levels closely
- Diltiazem may cause additive/excessive AV block; monitor response
- Drugs which prolong the Q-T interval include amitriptyline, astemizole, bepridil, disopyramide, erythromycin, haloperidol, imipramine, quinidine, pimozide, procainamide, sotalol, and thioridazine; effect/toxicity increased; use with caution
- Fentanyl: Concurrent use may lead to bradycardia, sinus arrest, and hypotension
- Flecainide blood levels may be increased; consider reducing flecainide dose by 25% to 33% with concurrent use
- Metoprolol blood levels may be increased; monitor response
- Phenytoin blood levels may be increased by amiodarone; amiodarone blood levels may be decreased by phenytoin
- Procainamide and NAPA plasma levels may be increased; consider reducing procainamide dosage by 25% with concurrent use
- Propranolol blood levels may be increased
- Quinidine blood levels may be increased; monitor quinidine trough concentration
- Rifampin may decrease amiodarone blood levels
- Ritonavir and amprenavir may increase amiodarone levels and toxicity; concurrent use is contraindicated
- Sparfloxacin, gatifloxacin, and moxifloxacin may result in additional prolongation of the Q-T interval; concurrent use is contraindicated
- Theophylline blood levels may be increased
- Thyroid supplements: Amiodarone may alter thyroid function; monitor closely
- Verapamil may cause additive/excessive AV block; monitor response
- Warfarin: Hypoprothrombinemic response increased; monitor INR closely when amiodarone is initiated or discontinued; reduce warfarin's dose when amiodarone is started

**Usual Dosage**

Oral:

Children (calculate doses for children <1 year on body surface area): Loading dose: 10-15 mg/kg/day or 600-800 mg/1.73 $m^2$/day for 4-14 days or until adequate control of arrhythmia or prominent adverse effects occur (this loading dose may be given in 1-2 divided doses/day). Dosage should then be reduced to 5 mg/kg/day or 200-400 mg/1.73 $m^2$/day given once daily for several weeks. If arrhythmia does not recur, reduce to lowest effective dosage possible. Usual daily minimal dose: 2.5 mg/kg/day; maintenance doses may be given for 5 of 7 days/week.

Adults: Ventricular arrhythmias: 800-1600 mg/day in 1-2 doses for 1-3 weeks, then when adequate arrhythmia control is achieved, decrease to 600-800 mg/day in 1-2 doses for 1 month; maintenance: 400 mg/day. Lower doses are recommended for supraventricular arrhythmias.

I.V.:

First 24 hours: 1000 mg according to following regimen

- Step 1: 150 mg (100 mL) over first 10 minutes (mix 3 mL in 100 mL $D_5W$)
- Step 2: 360 mg (200 mL) over next 6 hours (mix 18 mL in 500 mL $D_5W$): 1 mg/minute
- Step 3: 540 mg (300 mL) over next 18 hours: 0.5 mg/minute

After the first 24 hours: 0.5 mg/minute utilizing concentration of 1-6 mg/mL

Breakthrough VF or VT: 150 mg supplemental doses in 100 mL $D_5W$ over 10 minutes

**Note:** When switching from I.V. to oral therapy, use the following as a guide:

- <1-week I.V. infusion → 800-1600 mg/day
- 1- to 3-week I.V. infusion → 600-800 mg/day
- >3-week I.V. infusion → 400 mg/day

**Recommendations for conversion to intravenous amiodarone after oral administration:** During long-term amiodarone therapy (ie, ≥4 months), the mean plasma-elimination half-life of the active metabolite of amiodarone is 61 days. Replacement therapy may not be necessary in such patients if oral therapy is discontinued for a period <2 weeks, since any changes in serum amiodarone concentrations during this period may **not** be clinically significant.

**Dosing adjustment in hepatic impairment:** Probably necessary in substantial hepatic impairment.

Hemodialysis: Not dialyzable (0% to 5%); supplemental dose is not necessary.

Peritoneal dialysis effects: Not dialyzable (0% to 5%); supplemental dose is not necessary.

**Patient Information** Emergency use: Patient condition will determine amount of patient education. Oral: May be taken with food to reduce GI disturbance, but be consistent. Always take with food or always take without food. Do not change dosage or discontinue drug without consulting prescriber. Regular blood work, ophthalmic exams, and cardiac assessment will be necessary while taking this medication on a long-term basis. You may experience dizziness, weakness, or insomnia (use caution when driving, climbing stairs, or engaging in tasks requiring alertness until response to drug is known); hypotension (use caution changing position - rising from sitting or lying); nausea, vomiting, loss of appetite, or stomach discomfort, abnormal taste (small frequent meals, frequent mouth care, chewing gum, or sucking lozenges may help); photosensitivity (use sunscreen, wear protective clothing and eyewear, and avoid direct sunlight); or decreased libido (reversible). Report persistent dry cough or shortness of breath; chest pain, palpitations, irregular or slow heartbeat; unusual bruising or bleeding; blood in urine, feces (black stool), vomitus; pain, swelling, or warmth in calves; muscle tremor, weakness, numbness, or changes in gait; skin rash or irritation; or changes in urinary patterns.

**Nursing Implications** Muscle weakness may present a great hazard for ambulation

**Dosage Forms**

Injection, as hydrochloride: 50 mg/mL with benzyl alcohol (3 mL)

Tablet, scored, as hydrochloride: 200 mg

♦ **Ami-Tex LA®** *see* Guaifenesin and Phenylpropanolamine *on page 257*

♦ **Amitone® [OTC]** *see* Calcium Carbonate *on page 84*

## Amitriptyline (a mee TRIP ti leen)

**Related Information**

Antidepressant Agents Comparison Chart *on page 704*

Clinical Issues in the Use of Antidepressants *on page 627*

Discontinuation of Psychotropic Drugs - Withdrawal Symptoms and Recommendations *on page 798*

Federal OBRA Regulations Recommended Maximum Doses *on page 756*

Patient Information - Antidepressants (TCAs) *on page 640*

Serum Drug Concentrations Commonly Monitored: Guidelines *on page 759*

Teratogenic Risks of Psychotropic Medications *on page 812*

**Generic Available** Yes

**U.S. Brand Names** Elavil®; Enovil®

**Canadian Brand Names** Apo®-Amitriptyline; Levate®; Novo-Tryptin

**Synonyms** Amitriptyline Hydrochloride

**Pharmacologic Category** Antidepressant, Tricyclic (Tertiary Amine)

**Use** Relief of symptoms of depression

**Unlabeled uses:** Analgesic for certain chronic and neuropathic pain; prophylaxis against migraine headaches

**Pregnancy Risk Factor** D

**Pregnancy/Breast-Feeding Implications** Although a causal relationship has not been established, there have been a few reports of adverse events, including CNS effects, limb deformities, or developmental delays in infants whose mothers had taken amitriptyline during pregnancy. Use only if the potential benefit to the mother outweighs the risk to the fetus.

**Contraindications** Hypersensitivity to amitriptyline (cross-sensitivity with other tricyclics may occur); use of monoamine oxidase inhibitors within past 14 days; recovery from acute myocardial infarction

**Warnings/Precautions** Often causes drowsiness/sedation, resulting in impaired performance of tasks requiring alertness (ie, operating machinery or driving). Sedative effects may be additive with other CNS depressants and/or ethanol. The degree of sedation is very high relative to other antidepressants. May worsen psychosis in some patients or precipitate a shift to mania or hypomania in patients with bipolar disease. May cause hyponatremia/SIADH. May increase the risks associated with electroconvulsive therapy. This agent should be discontinued, when possible, prior to elective surgery. Therapy should not be abruptly discontinued in patients receiving high doses for prolonged periods.

May cause orthostatic hypotension; the risk of this problem is very high relative to other antidepressants. Use with caution in patients at risk of hypotension or in patients where transient hypotensive episodes would be poorly tolerated (cardiovascular disease or cerebrovascular disease). The degree of anticholinergic blockade produced by this agent is very high relative to other cyclic antidepressants; use with caution in patients with urinary retention, benign prostatic hypertrophy, narrow-angle glaucoma, xerostomia, visual problems, constipation, or a history of bowel obstruction. May alter glucose control - use with caution in patients with diabetes.

Use caution in patients with depression, particularly if suicidal risk may be present. Use with caution in patients with a history of cardiovascular disease (including previous MI, stroke, tachycardia, or conduction abnormalities). The risk of conduction abnormalities with this agent is high relative to other antidepressants. May lower seizure threshold - use caution in patients with a previous seizure disorder or condition predisposing to seizures such as brain damage, alcoholism, or concurrent therapy with other drugs which lower the seizure threshold. Use with caution in hyperthyroid patients or those receiving thyroid supplementation. Use with caution in patients with hepatic or renal dysfunction and in elderly patients. Not recommended for use in patients <12 years of age.

**Adverse Reactions** Anticholinergic effects may be pronounced; moderate to marked sedation can occur (tolerance to these effects usually occurs)

Cardiovascular: Orthostatic hypotension, tachycardia, nonspecific EKG changes, changes in A-V conduction

Central nervous system: Restlessness, dizziness, insomnia, sedation, fatigue, anxiety, impaired cognitive function, seizures, extrapyramidal symptoms

Dermatologic: Allergic rash, urticaria, photosensitivity

Gastrointestinal: Weight gain, xerostomia, constipation

Genitourinary: Urinary retention

Ocular: Blurred vision, mydriasis

Miscellaneous: Diaphoresis

**Overdosage/Toxicology**

Signs and symptoms: Agitation, confusion, hallucinations, urinary retention, hypothermia, hypotension, ventricular tachycardia, seizures

Treatment: Following initiation of essential overdose management, toxic symptoms should be treated. Ventricular arrhythmias often respond to phenytoin 15-20 mg/kg (adults) with concurrent systemic alkalinization (sodium bicarbonate 0.5-2 mEq/kg I.V.). Arrhythmias unresponsive to this therapy may respond to lidocaine 1mg/kg I.V. followed by a titrated infusion. Physostigmine (1-2 mg I.V. slowly for adults or 0.5 mg I.V. slowly for children) may be indicated in reversing cardiac arrhythmias that are due to vagal blockade or for anticholinergic effects, but should only be used as a last measure in life-threatening situations. Seizures usually respond to diazepam I.V. boluses (5-10 mg for adults up to 30 mg or 0.25-0.4 mg/kg/dose for children up to 10 mg/dose). If seizures are unresponsive or recur, phenytoin or phenobarbital may be required.

**Drug Interactions** CYP1A2, 2C9, 2C19, 2D6, and 3A3/4 enzyme substrate

Altretamine: Concurrent use may cause orthostatic hypertension

Amphetamines: TCAs may enhance the effect of amphetamines; monitor for adverse CV effects

Anticholinergics: Combined use with TCAs may produce additive anticholinergic effects

Antihypertensives: Amitriptyline inhibits the antihypertensive response to bethanidine, clonidine, debrisoquin, guanadrel, guanethidine, guanabenz, guanfacine; monitor BP; consider alternate antihypertensive agent

Beta-agonists: When combined with TCAs may predispose patients to cardiac arrhythmias

Bupropion: May increase the levels of tricyclic antidepressants. Based on limited information; monitor response

Carbamazepine: Tricyclic antidepressants may increase carbamazepine levels; monitor

Cholestyramine and colestipol: May bind TCAs and reduce their absorption; monitor for altered response

Clonidine: Abrupt discontinuation of clonidine may cause hypertensive crisis, amitriptyline may enhance the response (also see note on antihypertensives)

CNS depressants: Sedative effects may be additive with TCAs; monitor for increased effect; includes benzodiazepines, barbiturates, antipsychotics, ethanol, and other sedative medications.

CYP1A2 inhibitors: Metabolism of amitriptyline may be decreased; increasing clinical effect or toxicity; inhibitors include cimetidine, ciprofloxacin, fluvoxamine, isoniazid, ritonavir, and zileutin

CYP2C8/9 inhibitors: Serum levels and/or toxicity of some tricyclic antidepressants may be increased; inhibitors include amiodarone, cimetidine, fluvoxamine, some NSAIDs, metronidazole, ritonavir, sulfonamides, troglitazone, valproic acid, and zafirlukast; monitor for increased effect/toxicity

CYP2C19 inhibitors: Serum levels of amitriptyline may be increased; inhibitors include cimetidine, felbamate, fluconazole, fluoxetine, fluvoxamine, omeprazole, teniposide, tolbutamide, and troglitazone

CYP2D6 inhibitors: Serum levels and/or toxicity of some tricyclic antidepressants may be increased; inhibitors include amiodarone, cimetidine, delavirdine, fluoxetine, paroxetine, propafenone, quinidine, and ritonavir; monitor for increased effect/toxicity

CYP3A3/4 inhibitors: Serum level and/or toxicity of some tricyclic antidepressants may be increased. Inhibitors include amiodarone, cimetidine, clarithromycin, erythromycin, delavirdine, diltiazem, dirithromycin, disulfiram, fluoxetine, fluvoxamine, grapefruit juice, indinavir, itraconazole, ketoconazole, nefazodone, nevirapine, propoxyfene, quinupristin-dalfopristin, ritonavir, saquinavir, verapamil, zafirlukast, zileuton. Monitor for altered effects; a decrease in TCA dosage may be required

Enzyme inducers: May increase the metabolism of amitriptyline resulting in decreased effect; includes carbamazepine, phenobarbital, phenytoin, and rifampin; monitor for decreased response

Epinephrine (and other direct alpha-agonists): The pressor response to I.V. epinephrine, norepinephrine, and phenylephrine may be enhanced in patients receiving TCAs; this combination is best avoided

Fenfluramine: May increase tricyclic antidepressant levels/effects

Hypoglycemic agents (including insulin): TCAs may enhance the hypoglycemic effects of tolazamide, chlorpropamide, or insulin; monitor for changes in blood glucose levels; reported with chlorpropamide, tolazamide, and insulin

(Continued)

## Amitriptyline *(Continued)*

Levodopa: Tricyclic antidepressants may decrease the absorption (bioavailability) of levodopa; rare hypertensive episodes have also been attributed to this combination

Linezolid: Hyperpyrexia, hypertension, tachycardia, confusion, seizures, and **deaths have been reported** with agents which inhibit MAO (serotonin syndrome); this combination should be avoided

Lithium: Concurrent use with a TCA may increase the risk for neurotoxicity

MAO inhibitors: Hyperpyrexia, hypertension, tachycardia, confusion, seizures, and **deaths have been reported** (serotonin syndrome); this combination should be avoided

Methylphenidate: Metabolism of amitriptyline may be decreased

Phenothiazines: Serum concentrations of some TCAs may be increased; in addition, TCAs may increase concentration of phenothiazines; monitor for altered clinical response

QTc prolonging agents: Concurrent use of tricyclic agents with other drugs which may prolong QTc interval may increase the risk of potentially fatal arrhythmias; includes type Ia and type III antiarrhythmics agents, selected quinolones (sparfloxacin, gatifloxacin, moxifloxacin, grepafloxacin), cisapride, and other agents

Sucralfate: Absorption of tricyclic antidepressants may be reduced with coadministration

Sympathomimetics, indirect-acting: Tricyclic antidepressants may result in a decreased sensitivity to indirect-acting sympathomimetics; includes dopamine and ephedrine; also see interaction with epinephrine (and direct-acting sympathomimetics)

Valproic acid: May increase serum concentrations/adverse effects of some tricyclic antidepressants

Warfarin (and other oral anticoagulants): Amitriptyline may increase the anticoagulant effect in patients stabilized on warfarin; monitor INR

**Stability** Protect injection and Elavil® 10 mg tablets from light

**Mechanism of Action** Increases the synaptic concentration of serotonin and/or norepinephrine in the central nervous system by inhibition of their reuptake by the presynaptic neuronal membrane

**Pharmacodynamics/kinetics**

Onset of therapeutic effect: 7-21 days

Desired therapeutic effect (for depression) may take as long as 4-6 weeks

When used for migraine headache prophylaxis, therapeutic effect may take as long as 6 weeks; a higher dosage may be required in a heavy smoker because of increased metabolism

Distribution: Crosses placenta; enters breast milk

Metabolism: In the liver to nortriptyline (active), hydroxy derivatives, and conjugated derivatives; metabolism may be impaired in the elderly

Half-life: Adults: 9-25 hours (15-hour average)

Time to peak serum concentration: Within 4 hours

Elimination: Renal excretion of 18% as unchanged drug; small amounts eliminated in feces by bile

**Usual Dosage**

Adolescents: Oral: Initial: 25-50 mg/day; may administer in divided doses; increase gradually to 100 mg/day in divided doses

Adults:

Depression:

Oral: 50-150 mg/day single dose at bedtime or in divided doses; dose may be gradually increased up to 300 mg/day

I.M.: 20-30 mg 4 times/day

Pain management: Oral: Initial: 25 mg at bedtime; may increase as tolerated to 100 mg/day

**Dosing interval in hepatic impairment:** Use with caution and monitor plasma levels and patient response

Hemodialysis: Nondialyzable

**Dietary Considerations** Alcohol: Additive CNS effects, avoid use

**Administration** Not recommended for I.V.

**Monitoring Parameters** Monitor blood pressure and pulse rate prior to and during initial therapy; evaluate mental status; monitor weight; EKG in older adults

**Reference Range** Therapeutic: Amitriptyline and nortriptyline 100-250 ng/mL (SI: 360-900 nmol/L); Toxic: >0.5 µg/mL; plasma levels do not always correlate with clinical effectiveness

**Test Interactions** ↑ glucose

**Patient Information** Avoid alcohol ingestion; do not discontinue medication abruptly; may cause urine to turn blue-green; may cause drowsiness; full effect may not occur for 3-6 weeks; dry mouth may be helped by sips of water, sugarless gum, or hard candy

**Nursing Implications** Evaluate mental status; monitor weight, may increase appetite and possibly induce a craving for sweets; do not administer intravenously; monitor blood pressure and pulse rate prior to and during initial therapy

**Dosage Forms**

Injection, as hydrochloride: 10 mg/mL (10 mL)

Tablet, as hydrochloride: 10 mg, 25 mg, 50 mg, 75 mg, 100 mg, 150 mg

## Amitriptyline and Chlordiazepoxide

(a mee TRIP ti leen & klor dye az e POKS ide)

**Related Information**

Clinical Issues in the Use of Antidepressants *on page 627*

Patient Information - Antidepressants (TCAs) *on page 640*

**Generic Available** Yes

**U.S. Brand Names** Limbitrol®

**Synonyms** Chlordiazepoxide and Amitriptyline

**Pharmacologic Category** Antidepressant, Tricyclic (Tertiary Amine)

**Use** Treatment of moderate to severe anxiety and/or agitation and depression

**Restrictions** C-IV

**Pregnancy Risk Factor** D

**Contraindications** Depression of CNS; MAO inhibitors; acute recovery phase following myocardial infarction; angle-closure glaucoma

**Adverse Reactions** See individual agents

**Drug Interactions** See individual agents

**Usual Dosage** Initial: 3-4 tablets in divided doses; this may be increased to 6 tablets/day as required; some patients respond to smaller doses and can be maintained on 2 tablets

**Dosage Forms** Tablet:

5-12.5: Amitriptyline hydrochloride 12.5 mg and chlordiazepoxide 5 mg

10-25: Amitriptyline hydrochloride 25 mg and chlordiazepoxide 10 mg

## Amitriptyline and Perphenazine

(a mee TRIP ti leen & per FEN a zeen)

**Related Information**

Clinical Issues in the Use of Antidepressants *on page 627*

Patient Information - Antidepressants (TCAs) *on page 640*

**Generic Available** Yes

**U.S. Brand Names** Etrafon®; Triavil®

**Canadian Brand Names** Elavil Plus®; Apo®-Peram; PMS-Levazine; Proavil

**Synonyms** Perphenazine and Amitriptyline

**Pharmacologic Category** Antidepressant, Tricyclic (Tertiary Amine)

**Use** Treatment of patients with moderate to severe anxiety and depression

**Pregnancy Risk Factor** D

**Contraindications** Pregnancy and lactation; hypersensitivity to amitriptyline, perphenazine, or any component, cross-sensitivity with other phenothiazines may exist; angle-closure glaucoma; bone marrow depression; severe liver or cardiac disease

**Warnings/Precautions** Safe use of tricyclic antidepressants in children <12 years of age has not been established; amitriptyline should not be abruptly discontinued in patients receiving high doses for prolonged periods; do not drink alcoholic beverages

**Adverse Reactions**

Cardiovascular: Arrhythmias, hypotension

Central nervous system: Dizziness, drowsiness, headache, confusion, delirium, insomnia, nervousness, restlessness, parkinsonian syndrome, hallucinations, anxiety, seizures

Dermatologic: Alopecia, photosensitivity

Endocrine & metabolic: Sexual dysfunction, breast enlargement, galactorrhea, SIADH

Gastrointestinal: Constipation, xerostomia, increased appetite, nausea, weight gain, unpleasant taste, diarrhea, heartburn, trouble with gums, decreased lower esophageal sphincter tone may cause GE reflux

Genitourinary: Dysuria, testicular edema

Hematologic: Agranulocytosis, leukopenia, eosinophilia

Hepatic: Cholestatic jaundice, increased liver enzymes

Neuromuscular & skeletal: Weakness, fine muscle tremors

Ocular: Blurred vision, eye pain, increased intraocular pressure

Otic: Tinnitus

Miscellaneous: Diaphoresis (excessive), allergic reactions

**Drug Interactions** See individual agents

**Usual Dosage** Oral: 1 tablet 2-4 times/day

**Monitoring Parameters** Blood pressure and pulse rate prior to and during initial therapy; evaluate mental status; monitor weight

**Reference Range** Metabolism may be impaired in the elderly; Toxic: >0.5 µg/mL

**Patient Information** Do not drink alcoholic beverages

**Nursing Implications** May increase appetite and possibly a craving for sweets; offer patient sugarless hard candy for dry mouth

**Dosage Forms** Tablet:

2-10: Amitriptyline hydrochloride 10 mg and perphenazine 2 mg

4-10: Amitriptyline hydrochloride 10 mg and perphenazine 4 mg

2-25: Amitriptyline hydrochloride 25 mg and perphenazine 2 mg

4-25: Amitriptyline hydrochloride 25 mg and perphenazine 4 mg

4-50: Amitriptyline hydrochloride 50 mg and perphenazine 4 mg

♦ **Amitriptyline Hydrochloride** *see* Amitriptyline *on page 33*

## Amlexanox (am LEKS an oks)

**U.S. Brand Names** Aphthasol™
**Pharmacologic Category** Anti-inflammatory, Locally Applied
**Use** Treatment of aphthous ulcers (ie, canker sores); has been investigated in many allergic disorders
**Effects on Mental Status** None reported
**Effects on Psychiatric Treatment** None reported
**Usual Dosage** Administer (0.5 cm - 1/4") directly on ulcers 4 times/day following oral hygiene, after meals, and at bedtime
**Dosage Forms** Paste: 5% (5 g)

## Amlodipine (am LOE di peen)

**Related Information**
Calcium Channel Blocking Agents Comparison Chart *on page 710*
**U.S. Brand Names** Norvasc®
**Pharmacologic Category** Calcium Channel Blocker
**Use** Treatment of hypertension and angina
**Effects on Mental Status** May cause drowsiness; rarely may produce insomnia and nervousness
**Effects on Psychiatric Treatment** None reported
**Pregnancy Risk Factor** C
**Contraindications** Hypersensitivity to amlodipine or any component
**Warnings/Precautions** Increased angina and/or MI has occurred with initiation or dosage titration of calcium channel blockers. Use caution in severe aortic stenosis. Use caution in patients with severe hepatic impairment. Safety and efficacy in children have not been established. Dosage titration should occur after 7-14 days on a given dose.
**Adverse Reactions**
>10%: Cardiovascular: Peripheral edema (1.8%-14.6% dose-related)
1% to 10%:
Cardiovascular: Flushing, palpitations
Central nervous system: Dizziness, fatigue, headache, somnolence (1% to 2%)
Dermatologic: Dermatitis, rash (1% to 2%); pruritus, urticaria (1% to 2%)
Endocrine & metabolic: Sexual dysfunction (1% to 2%)
Gastrointestinal: Abdominal pain (1% to 2%), nausea
Respiratory: Shortness of breath (1% to 2%)
Neuromuscular & skeletal: Muscle cramps (1% to 2%)
<1%: Abnormal EKG, alopecia, anorexia, arrhythmias, bradycardia, constipation, cough, diaphoresis, diarrhea, epistaxis, flatulence, hypotension, insomnia, joint stiffness, malaise, micturition disorder, nasal congestion, nervousness, paresthesia, petechiae, psychiatric disturbances, syncope, tachycardia, tinnitus, tremor, ventricular extrasystoles, vomiting, weakness, weight gain, xerostomia
**Overdosage/Toxicology**
Signs and symptoms: Hypotension, myocardial depression, bradycardia, A-V block
Treatment: Ipecac-induced emesis can hypothetically worsen calcium antagonist toxicity, since it can produce vagal stimulation. Supportive and symptomatic treatment, including I.V. fluids and Trendelenburg positioning, should be initiated as intoxication may cause hypotension. Although calcium (calcium chloride I.V. 1-2 g in adults or 10-30 mg/kg in children over 5-10 minutes with repeats as needed) has been used as an "antidote" for acute intoxications, there is limited experience to support its routine use and should be reserved for those cases where definite signs of myocardial depression are evident. Heart block may respond to isoproterenol, glucagon, atropine and/or calcium, although a temporary pacemaker may be required.
**Drug Interactions** CYP3A3/4 enzyme substrate
Azole antifungals may inhibit calcium channel blocker metabolism; avoid this combination. Try an antifungal like terbinafine (if appropriate) or monitor closely for altered effect of the calcium channel blocker.
Calcium may reduce the calcium channel blocker's effects, particularly hypotension
Rifampin increases the metabolism of calcium channel blockers; adjust the dose of calcium channel blocker to maintain efficacy
**Usual Dosage** Adults: Oral:
Hypertension: Initial dose: 2.5-5 mg once daily; usual dose: 5 mg once daily; maximum dose: 10 mg once daily. In general, titrate in 2.5 mg increments over 7-14 days.
Angina: Usual dose: 5-10 mg; use lower doses for elderly or those with hepatic insufficiency (eg, 2.5-5 mg).
Dialysis: Hemodialysis and peritoneal dialysis does not enhance elimination. Supplemental dose is not necessary.
**Dosage adjustment in hepatic impairment:** Administer 2.5 mg once daily.
**Patient Information** Take as prescribed; do not stop abruptly without consulting prescriber. You may experience headache (if unrelieved, consult prescriber), nausea or vomiting (frequent small meals may help), or constipation (increased dietary bulk and fluids may help). May cause drowsiness; use caution when driving or engaging in tasks that require alertness until response to drug is known. Report unrelieved headache, vomiting, constipation, palpitations, peripheral or facial swelling, weight gain >5 lb/week, or respiratory changes.
**Dosage Forms** Tablet: 2.5 mg, 5 mg, 10 mg

## Amlodipine and Benazepril
(am LOE di peen & ben AY ze pril)

**U.S. Brand Names** Lotrel®
**Pharmacologic Category** Antihypertensive Agent, Combination
**Use** Treatment of hypertension
**Effects on Mental Status** May cause drowsiness; rarely may produce insomnia and nervousness
**Effects on Psychiatric Treatment** May decrease lithium clearance resulting in an increase in serum lithium levels and potential lithium toxicity; monitor serum lithium levels
**Usual Dosage** Adults: Oral: 1 capsule daily
**Dosage Forms** Capsule:
Amlodipine 2.5 mg and benazepril hydrochloride 10 mg
Amlodipine 5 mg and benazepril hydrochloride 10 mg
Amlodipine 5 mg and benazepril hydrochloride 20 mg

## Amobarbital (am oh BAR bi tal)

**Related Information**
Anxiolytic/Hypnotic Use in Long-Term Care Facilities *on page 754*
Clinical Issues in the Use of Anxiolytics and Sedative/Hypnotics *on page 634*
Federal OBRA Regulations Recommended Maximum Doses *on page 756*
Patient Information - Anxiolytics & Sedative Hypnotics (Barbiturates) *on page 654*
Psychiatric Emergencies - Catatonia *on page 660*
**Generic Available** Yes: Capsule
**U.S. Brand Names** Amytal®
**Canadian Brand Names** Amobarbital; Novambarb®
**Synonyms** Amylobarbitone
**Pharmacologic Category** Barbiturate
**Use**
Oral: Hypnotic in short-term treatment of insomnia; to reduce anxiety and provide sedation preoperatively
I.M., I.V.: Control status epilepticus or acute seizure episodes. Also used to control acute episodes of agitated behavior in psychosis and in "Amytal® Interviewing" for narcoanalysis
**Restrictions** C-II
**Pregnancy Risk Factor** D
**Contraindications** Hypersensitivity to barbiturates or any component of the formulation; marked hepatic impairment; dyspnea or airway obstruction; porphyria
**Warnings/Precautions** Safety has not been established in children <6 years of age. Use with caution in patients with CHF, hepatic or renal impairment, hypovolemic shock; when administered I.V., respiratory depression and hypotension are possible, have equipment and personnel available; this I.V. medication should be given only to hospitalized patients. Do not administer to patients in acute pain. Use caution in elderly, debilitated, renally impaired, hepatic impairment, or pediatric patients. May cause paradoxical responses, including agitation and hyperactivity, particularly in acute pain and pediatric patients. Use with caution in patients with depression or suicidal tendencies, or in patients with a history of drug abuse. Tolerance, psychological and physical dependence may occur with prolonged use. May cause CNS depression, which may impair physical or mental abilities. Patients must be cautioned about performing tasks which require mental alertness (ie, operating machinery or driving). Effects with other sedative drugs or ethanol may be potentiated. Use with caution in patients with hypoadrenalism.
**Adverse Reactions**
>10%:
Central nervous system: Dizziness, lightheadedness, "hangover" effect, drowsiness, CNS depression, fever
Local: Pain at injection site
1% to 10%:
Central nervous system: Confusion, mental depression, unusual excitement, nervousness, faint feeling, headache, insomnia, nightmares
Gastrointestinal: Nausea, vomiting, constipation
<1%: Agranulocytosis, apnea, exfoliative dermatitis, hallucinations, hypotension, laryngospasm, megaloblastic anemia, rash, respiratory depression, Stevens-Johnson syndrome, thrombocytopenia, thrombophlebitis, urticaria
**Overdosage/Toxicology**
Signs and symptoms: Unsteady gait, slurred speech, confusion, jaundice, hypothermia, fever, hypotension
Treatment: If hypotension occurs, administer I.V. fluids and place the patient in the Trendelenburg position. If unresponsive, an I.V. vasopressor (eg, dopamine, epinephrine) may be required. Forced alkaline diuresis is of no value in the treatment of intoxications with short-acting barbiturates. Charcoal hemoperfusion or hemodialysis may be useful in

(Continued)

## Amobarbital *(Continued)*

the harder to treat intoxications, especially in the presence of very high serum barbiturate levels.

**Drug Interactions Note:** Barbiturates are cytochrome P-450 enzyme inducers. Patients should be monitored when these drugs are started or stopped for a decreased or increased therapeutic effect respectively.

Acetaminophen: Barbiturates may enhance the hepatotoxic potential of acetaminophen overdoses

Antiarrhythmics: Barbiturates may increase the metabolism of antiarrhythmics, decreasing their clinical effect; includes disopyramide, propafenone, and quinidine

Anticonvulsants: Barbiturates may increase the metabolism of anticonvulsants; includes ethosuximide, felbamate (possibly), lamotrigine, phenytoin, tiagabine, topiramate, and zonisamide; does not appear to affect gabapentin or levetiracetam

Antineoplastics: Limited evidence suggests that enzyme-inducing anticonvulsant therapy may reduce the effectiveness of some chemotherapy regimens (specifically in ALL); teniposide and methotrexate may be cleared more rapidly in these patients

Antipsychotics: Barbiturates may enhance the metabolism (decrease the efficacy) of antipsychotics; monitor for altered response; dose adjustment may be needed

Beta-blockers: Metabolism of beta-blockers may be increased and clinical effect decreased; atenolol and nadolol are unlikely to interact given their renal elimination

Calcium channel blockers: Barbiturates may enhance the metabolism of calcium channel blockers, decreasing their clinical effect

Chloramphenicol: Barbiturates may increase the metabolism of chloramphenicol and chloramphenicol may inhibit barbiturate metabolism; monitor for altered response

Cimetidine: Barbiturates may enhance the metabolism of cimetidine, decreasing its clinical effect

CNS depressants: Sedative effects and/or respiratory depression with barbiturates may be additive with other CNS depressants; monitor for increased effect; includes ethanol, sedatives, antidepressants, narcotic analgesics, and benzodiazepines

Corticosteroids: Barbiturates may enhance the metabolism of corticosteroids, decreasing their clinical effect

Cyclosporine: Levels may be decreased by barbiturates; monitor

Doxycycline: Barbiturates may enhance the metabolism of doxycycline, decreasing its clinical effect; higher dosages may be required

Estrogens: Barbiturates may increase the metabolism of estrogens and reduce their efficacy

Felbamate may inhibit the metabolism of barbiturates and barbiturates may increase the metabolism of felbamate

Griseofulvin: Barbiturates may impair the absorption of griseofulvin, and griseofulvin metabolism may be increased by barbiturates, decreasing clinical effect

Guanfacine: Effect may be decreased by barbiturates

Immunosuppressants: Barbiturates may enhance the metabolism of immunosuppressants, decreasing its clinical effect; includes both cyclosporine and tacrolimus

Loop diuretics: Metabolism may be increased and clinical effects decreased; established for furosemide, effect with other loop diuretics not established

MAOIs: Metabolism of barbiturates may be inhibited, increasing clinical effect or toxicity of the barbiturates

Methadone: Barbiturates may enhance the metabolism of methadone resulting in methadone withdrawal

Methoxyflurane: Barbiturates may enhance the nephrotoxic effects of methoxyflurane

Oral contraceptives: Barbiturates may enhance the metabolism of oral contraceptives, decreasing their clinical effect; an alternative method of contraception should be considered

Theophylline: Barbiturates may increase metabolism of theophylline derivatives and decrease their clinical effect

Tricyclic antidepressants: Barbiturates may increase metabolism of tricyclic antidepressants and decrease their clinical effect; sedative effects may be additive

Valproic acid: Metabolism of barbiturates may be inhibited by valproic acid; monitor for excessive sedation; a dose reduction may be needed

Warfarin: Barbiturates inhibit the hypoprothrombinemic effects of oral anticoagulants via increased metabolism; this combination should generally be avoided

**Stability** Hydrolyzes when exposed to air; use contents of vial within 30 minutes after constitution; use only clear solution

**Mechanism of Action** Interferes with transmission of impulses from the thalamus to the cortex of the brain resulting in an imbalance in central inhibitory and facilitatory mechanisms

**Pharmacodynamics/kinetics**

Onset of action:
- Oral: Within 1 hour
- I.V.: Within 5 minutes

Distribution: Readily crosses the placenta; small amounts appear in breast milk

Metabolism: Chiefly in the liver by microsomal enzymes

Half-life, biphasic:
- Initial: 40 minutes
- Terminal: 20 hours

**Usual Dosage**

Children: Oral:
- Sedation: 6 mg/kg/day divided every 6-8 hours
- Insomnia: 2 mg/kg or 70 mg/m²/day in 4 equally divided doses
- Hypnotic: 2-3 mg/kg

Adults:
- Insomnia: Oral: 65-200 mg at bedtime
- Sedation: Oral: 30-50 mg 2-3 times/day
- Preanesthetic: Oral: 200 mg 1-2 hours before surgery
- Hypnotic:
  - Oral: 65-200 mg at bedtime
  - I.M., I.V.: 65-500 mg, should not exceed 500 mg I.M. or 1000 mg I.V.
- Amobarbital interview: I.V.: 50 mg/minute for total dose up to 300 mg

**Dietary Considerations** Alcohol: Avoid use

**Administration** Drug should be injected within 30 minutes after opening vial because of hydrolysis

I.M. injection: Should be deep to prevent against pain, sterile abscess, and sloughing; vital signs should be monitored during injection and for several hours after administration

When administered I.V.: Respiratory depression and hypotension are possible, have equipment and personnel available; this I.V. medication should be given only to hospitalized patients

**Monitoring Parameters** Vital signs should be monitored during injection and for several hours after administration

**Reference Range** Therapeutic: 1-5 μg/mL (SI: 4-22 μmol/L); Toxic: >10 μg/mL (SI: >44 μmol/L)

**Test Interactions** ↑ ammonia (B); ↓ bilirubin (S)

**Patient Information** Avoid alcohol ingestion; physical dependency may result when used for an extended period of time (1-3 months); do not try to get out of bed without assistance, will cause drowsiness

**Nursing Implications** Raise bed rails at night

**Dosage Forms**
- Capsule, as sodium: 65 mg, 200 mg
- Injection, as sodium: 250 mg, 500 mg
- Tablet: 30 mg, 50 mg, 100 mg

## Amobarbital and Secobarbital

(am oh BAR bi tal & see koe BAR bi tal)

**Related Information**

Clinical Issues in the Use of Anxiolytics and Sedative/Hypnotics *on page 634*

Patient Information - Anxiolytics & Sedative Hypnotics (Barbiturates) *on page 654*

**Generic Available** No

**U.S. Brand Names** Tuinal®

**Synonyms** Secobarbital and Amobarbital

**Pharmacologic Category** Barbiturate

**Use** Short-term treatment of insomnia

**Restrictions** C-II

**Pregnancy Risk Factor** D

**Contraindications** CNS depression; hypersensitivity to secobarbital or amobarbital; marked liver impairment; latent porphyria

**Warnings/Precautions** Safety has not been established in children <6 years of age; potential for drug dependency exists; avoid alcoholic beverages; use with caution in patients with CHF, hepatic or renal impairment, hypovolemic shock

**Adverse Reactions**

>10%:
- Central nervous system: Dizziness, lightheadedness, drowsiness, "hangover" effect
- Local: Pain at injection site

1% to 10%:
- Central nervous system: Confusion, mental depression, unusual excitement, nervousness, faint feeling, headache, insomnia, nightmares
- Gastrointestinal: Constipation, nausea, vomiting

<1%: agranulocytosis, dermatitis, exfoliative, hallucinations, hypotension, megaloblastic anemia, respiratory depression, skin rash, Stevens-Johnson syndrome, thrombocytopenia, thrombophlebitis

**Drug Interactions Note:** Barbiturates are cytochrome P-450 enzyme inducers. Patients should be monitored when these drugs are started or stopped for a decreased or increased therapeutic effect respectively.

Acetaminophen: Barbiturates may enhance the hepatotoxic potential of acetaminophen overdoses

Antiarrhythmics: Barbiturates may increase the metabolism of antiarrhythmics, decreasing their clinical effect; includes disopyramide, propafenone, and quinidine

Anticonvulsants: Barbiturates may increase the metabolism of anticonvulsants; includes ethosuximide, felbamate (possibly), lamotrigine, phenytoin, tiagabine, topiramate, and zonisamide; does not appear to affect gabapentin or levetiracetam

Antineoplastics: Limited evidence suggests that enzyme-inducing anticonvulsant therapy may reduce the effectiveness of some chemotherapy regimens (specifically in ALL); teniposide and methotrexate may be cleared more rapidly in these patients

Antipsychotics: Barbiturates may enhance the metabolism (decrease the efficacy) of antipsychotics; monitor for altered response; dose adjustment may be needed

Beta-blockers: Metabolism of beta-blockers may be increased and clinical effect decreased. Atenolol and nadolol are unlikely to interact given their renal elimination.

Calcium channel blockers: Barbiturates may enhance the metabolism of calcium channel blockers, decreasing their clinical effect

Chloramphenicol: Barbiturates may increase the metabolism of chloramphenicol and chloramphenicol may inhibit barbiturate metabolism; monitor for altered response

Cimetidine: Barbiturates may enhance the metabolism of cimetidine, decreasing its clinical effect

CNS depressants: Sedative effects and/or respiratory depression with barbiturates may be additive with other CNS depressants; monitor for increased effect; includes ethanol, sedatives, antidepressants, narcotic analgesics, and benzodiazepines

Corticosteroids: Barbiturates may enhance the metabolism of corticosteroids, decreasing their clinical effect

Cyclosporine: Levels may be decreased by barbiturates; monitor

Doxycycline: Barbiturates may enhance the metabolism of doxycycline, decreasing its clinical effect; higher dosages may be required

Estrogens: Barbiturates may increase the metabolism of estrogens and reduce their efficacy

Felbamate may inhibit the metabolism of barbiturates and barbiturates may increase the metabolism of felbamate

Griseofulvin: Barbiturates may impair the absorption of griseofulvin, and griseofulvin metabolism may be increased by barbiturates, decreasing clinical effect

Guanfacine: Effect may be decreased by barbiturates

Immunosuppressants: Barbiturates may enhance the metabolism of immunosuppressants, decreasing its clinical effect; includes both cyclosporine and tacrolimus

Loop diuretics: Metabolism may be increased and clinical effects decreased; established for furosemide, effect with other loop diuretics not established

MAOIs: Metabolism of barbiturates may be inhibited, increasing clinical effect or toxicity of the barbiturates

Methadone: Barbiturates may enhance the metabolism of methadone resulting in methadone withdrawal

Methoxyflurane: Barbiturates may enhance the nephrotoxic effects of methoxyflurane

Oral contraceptives: Barbiturates may enhance the metabolism of oral contraceptives, decreasing their clinical effect; an alternative method of contraception should be considered

Theophylline: Barbiturates may increase metabolism of theophylline derivatives and decrease their clinical effect

Tricyclic antidepressants: Barbiturates may increase metabolism of tricyclic antidepressants and decrease their clinical effect; sedative effects may be additive

Valproic acid: Metabolism of barbiturates may be inhibited by valproic acid; monitor for excessive sedation; a dose reduction may be needed

Warfarin: Barbiturates inhibit the hypoprothrombinemic effects of oral anticoagulants via increased metabolism; this combination should generally be avoided

**Usual Dosage** Adults: Oral: 1-2 capsules at bedtime

**Test Interactions** Increases ammonia (B); decreases bilirubin (S)

**Dosage Forms** Capsule:

100: Amobarbital 50 mg and secobarbital 50 mg

200: Amobarbital 100 mg and secobarbital 100 mg

## Amoxapine (a MOKS a peen)

**Related Information**

Antidepressant Agents Comparison Chart *on page 704*

Clinical Issues in the Use of Antidepressants *on page 627*

Discontinuation of Psychotropic Drugs - Withdrawal Symptoms and Recommendations *on page 798*

Federal OBRA Regulations Recommended Maximum Doses *on page 756*

Patient Information - Antidepressants (TCAs) *on page 640*

Teratogenic Risks of Psychotropic Medications *on page 812*

**Generic Available** Yes

**U.S. Brand Names** Asendin®

**Pharmacologic Category** Antidepressant, Tricyclic (Secondary Amine)

**Use** Treatment of depression, psychotic depression, depression accompanied by anxiety or agitation

**Pregnancy Risk Factor** C

**Contraindications** Hypersensitivity to amoxapine; use of monoamine oxidase inhibitors within past 14 days; recovery from acute myocardial infarction

**Warnings/Precautions** May cause sedation, resulting in impaired performance of tasks requiring alertness (ie, operating machinery or driving). Sedative effects may be additive with other CNS depressants and/or ethanol. The degree of sedation is moderate relative to other antidepressants. May worsen psychosis in some patients or precipitate a shift to mania or hypomania in patients with bipolar disease. May increase the risks associated with electroconvulsive therapy. This agent should be discontinued, when possible, prior to elective surgery. Therapy should not be abruptly discontinued in patients receiving high doses for prolonged periods.

May cause extrapyramidal reactions, including pseudoparkinsonism, acute dystonic reactions, akathisia, and tardive dyskinesia (risk of these reactions is low). May be associated with neuroleptic malignant syndrome.

May cause orthostatic hypotension (risk is moderate relative to other antidepressants) - use with caution in patients at risk of hypotension or in patients where transient hypotensive episodes would be poorly tolerated (cardiovascular disease or cerebrovascular disease). The degree of anticholinergic blockade produced by this agent is moderate relative to other cyclic antidepressants - use caution in patients with urinary retention, benign prostatic hypertrophy, narrow-angle glaucoma, xerostomia, visual problems, constipation, or history of bowel obstruction.

Use caution in patients with depression, particularly if suicidal risk may be present. Use with caution in patients with a history of cardiovascular disease (including previous MI, stroke, tachycardia, or conduction abnormalities). The risk conduction abnormalities with this agent is moderate relative to other antidepressants. May lower seizure threshold - use caution in patients with a previous seizure disorder or condition predisposing to seizures such as brain damage, alcoholism, or concurrent therapy with other drugs which lower the seizure threshold. Use with caution in hyperthyroid patients or those receiving thyroid supplementation. Use with caution in patients with hepatic or renal dysfunction and in elderly patients.

**Adverse Reactions**

>10%:

Central nervous system: Drowsiness

Gastrointestinal: Xerostomia, constipation

1% to 10%:

Central nervous system: Dizziness, headache, confusion, nervousness, restlessness, insomnia, ataxia, excitement, anxiety

Dermatologic: Edema, skin rash

Endocrine: Elevated prolactin levels

Gastrointestinal: Nausea

Neuromuscular & skeletal: Tremor, weakness

Ocular: Blurred vision

Miscellaneous: Diaphoresis

<1%: Abdominal pain, abnormal taste, agranulocytosis, allergic reactions, breast enlargement, delayed micturition, diarrhea, elevated liver enzymes, epigastric distress, extrapyramidal symptoms, flatulence, galactorrhea, hypertension, hypotension, impotence, incoordination, increased intraocular pressure, increased or decreased libido, lacrimation, leukopenia, menstrual irregularity, mydriasis, nasal stuffiness, neuroleptic malignant syndrome, numbness, painful ejaculation, paresthesia, photosensitivity, seizures, SIADH, syncope, tachycardia, tardive dyskinesia, testicular edema, tinnitus, urinary retention, vomiting

**Overdosage/Toxicology**

Signs and symptoms: Grand mal convulsions, acidosis, coma, renal failure

Treatment: Following initiation of essential overdose management, toxic symptoms should be treated. Ventricular arrhythmias often respond to phenytoin 15-20 mg/kg (adults) with concurrent systemic alkalinization (sodium bicarbonate 0.5-2 mEq/kg I.V.). Arrhythmias unresponsive to this therapy may respond to lidocaine 1mg/kg I.V. followed by a titrated infusion. Physostigmine (1-2 mg I.V. slowly for adults or 0.5 mg I.V. slowly for children) may be indicated in reversing cardiac arrhythmias that are due to vagal blockade or for anticholinergic effects, but should only be used as a last measure in life-threatening situations. Seizures usually respond to diazepam I.V. boluses (5-10 mg for adults up to 30 mg or 0.25-0.4 mg/kg/dose for children up to 10 mg/dose). If seizures are unresponsive or recur, phenytoin or phenobarbital may be required.

**Drug Interactions** CYP1A2, 2C9, 2C19, 2D6, and 3A3/4 enzyme substrate

Anticholinergics: Combined use with TCAs may produce additive anticholinergic effects

Altretamine: Concurrent use may cause orthostatic hypertension

Amphetamines: TCAs may enhance the effect of amphetamines; monitor for adverse CV effects

Antihypertensives: Amitriptyline inhibits the antihypertensive response to bethanidine, clonidine, debrisoquin, guanadrel, guanethidine, guanabenz, guanfacine; monitor BP; consider alternate antihypertensive agent

Beta-agonists: When combined with TCAs may predispose patients to cardiac arrhythmias

Bupropion: May increase the levels of tricyclic antidepressants; based on limited information; monitor response

Carbamazepine: Tricyclic antidepressants may increase carbamazepine levels; monitor

(Continued)

## Amoxapine *(Continued)*

Cholestyramine and colestipol: May bind TCAs and reduce their absorption; monitor for altered response

Clonidine: Abrupt discontinuation of clonidine may cause hypertensive crisis, amitriptyline may enhance the response

CNS depressants: Sedative effects may be additive with TCAs; monitor for increased effect; includes benzodiazepines, barbiturates, antipsychotics, ethanol and other sedative medications

CYP1A2 inhibitors: Metabolism of amoxapine may be decreased, increasing clinical effect or toxicity; inhibitors include cimetidine, ciprofloxacin, fluvoxamine, isoniazid, ritonavir, and zileutin

CYP2C8/9 inhibitors: Serum levels and/or toxicity of some tricyclic antidepressants may be increased; inhibitors include amiodarone, cimetidine, fluvoxamine, some NSAIDs, metronidazole, ritonavir, sulfonamides, troglitazone, valproic acid, and zafirlukast; monitor for increased effect/toxicity

CYP2C19 inhibitors: Serum levels of some cyclic antidepressants may be increased; inhibitors include cimetidine, felbamate, fluconazole, fluoxetine, fluvoxamine, omeprazole, teniposide, tolbutamide, and troglitazone

CYP2D6 inhibitors: Serum levels and/or toxicity of some tricyclic antidepressants may be increased; inhibitors include amiodarone, cimetidine, delavirdine, fluoxetine, paroxetine, propafenone, quinidine, and ritonavir. Monitor for increased effect/toxicity

CYP3A3/4 inhibitors: Serum level and/or toxicity of some tricyclic antidepressants may be increased; inhibitors include amiodarone, cimetidine, clarithromycin, erythromycin, delavirdine, diltiazem, dirithromycin, disulfiram, fluoxetine, fluvoxamine, grapefruit juice, indinavir, itraconazole, ketoconazole, nevirapine, propoxyfene, quinupristin-dalfopristin, ritonavir, saquinavir, verapamil, zafirlukast, zileuton; monitor for altered effects; a decrease in TCA dosage may be required

Enzyme inducers: May increase the metabolism of amitriptyline resulting in decreased effect; includes carbamazepine, phenobarbital, phenytoin, and rifampin; monitor for decreased response

Epinephrine (and other direct alpha-agonists): The pressor response to I.V. epinephrine, norepinephrine, and phenylephrine may be enhanced in patients receiving TCAs; this combination is best avoided

Fenfluramine: May increase tricyclic antidepressant levels/effects

Hypoglycemic agents (including insulin): TCAs may enhance the hypoglycemic effects of tolazamide, chlorpropamide, or insulin; monitor for changes in blood glucose levels; reported with chlorpropamide, tolazamide, and insulin

Levodopa: Tricyclic antidepressants may decrease the absorption (bioavailability) of levodopa; rare hypertensive episodes have also been attributed to this combination

Linezolid: Hyperpyrexia, hypertension, tachycardia, confusion, seizures, and **deaths have been reported** with agents which inhibit MAO (serotonin syndrome); this combination should be avoided

Lithium: Concurrent use with a TCA may increase the risk for neurotoxicity

MAO inhibitors: Hyperpyrexia, hypertension, tachycardia, confusion, seizures, and **deaths have been reported** (serotonin syndrome); this combination should be avoided

Methylphenidate: Metabolism of amitriptyline may be decreased

Phenothiazines: Serum concentrations of some TCAs may be increased; in addition, TCAs may increase concentration of phenothiazines; monitor for altered clinical response

QTc prolonging agents: Concurrent use of tricyclic agents with other drugs which may prolong QTc interval may increase the risk of potentially fatal arrhythmias; includes type Ia and type III antiarrhythmics agents, selected quinolones (sparfloxacin, gatifloxacin, moxifloxacin, grepafloxacin), cisapride, and other agents

Sucralfate: Absorption of tricyclic antidepressants may be reduced with coadministration.

Sympathomimetics, indirect-acting: Tricyclic antidepressants may result in a decreased sensitivity to indirect-acting sympathomimetics; includes dopamine and ephedrine; also see interaction with epinephrine (and direct-acting sympathomimetics)

Valproic acid: May increase serum concentrations/adverse effects of some tricyclic antidepressants

Warfarin (and other oral anticoagulants): Amitriptyline may increase the anticoagulant effect in patients stabilized on warfarin; monitor INR

**Mechanism of Action** Reduces the reuptake of serotonin and norepinephrine. The metabolite, 7-OH-amoxapine has significant dopamine receptor blocking activity similar to haloperidol.

**Pharmacodynamics/kinetics**

Onset of antidepressant effect: Usually occurs after 1-2 weeks, but may require 4-6 weeks

Absorption: Oral: Rapidly and well absorbed

Distribution: $V_d$: 0.9-1.2 L/kg; distributes into breast milk

Protein binding: 80%

Metabolism: Extensive in the liver

Half-life:

- Parent drug: 11-16 hours
- Active metabolite (8-hydroxy): Adults: 30 hours

Time to peak serum concentration: Within 1-2 hours

Elimination: Excretion of metabolites and parent compound in urine

**Usual Dosage** Oral:

Children: Not established in children <16 years of age

Adolescents: Initial: 25-50 mg/day; increase gradually to 100 mg/day; may administer as divided doses or as a single dose at bedtime

Adults: Initial: 25 mg 2-3 times/day, if tolerated, dosage may be increased to 100 mg 2-3 times/day; may be given in a single bedtime dose when dosage <300 mg/day

Elderly: Initial: 25 mg at bedtime increased by 25 mg weekly for outpatients and every 3 days for inpatients if tolerated; usual dose: 50-150 mg/day, but doses up to 300 mg may be necessary

Maximum daily dose:

- Inpatient: 600 mg
- Outpatient: 400 mg

**Dietary Considerations** Alcohol: Avoid use

**Monitoring Parameters** Monitor blood pressure and pulse rate prior to and during initial therapy evaluate mental status; monitor weight; EKG in older adults

**Reference Range** Therapeutic: Amoxapine: 20-100 ng/mL (SI: 64-319 nmol/L); 8-OH amoxapine: 150-400 ng/mL (SI: 478-1275 nmol/L); both: 200-500 ng/mL (SI: 637-1594 nmol/L)

**Test Interactions** ↑ glucose

**Patient Information** Dry mouth may be helped by sips of water, sugarless gum, or hard candy; avoid alcohol; very important to maintain established dosage regimen; photosensitivity to sunlight can occur, do not discontinue abruptly; full effect may not occur for 4-6 weeks; full dosage may be taken at bedtime to avoid daytime sedation

**Nursing Implications** May increase appetite and possibly a craving for sweets; recognize signs of neuroleptic malignant syndrome and tardive dyskinesia

**Additional Information** Extrapyramidal reactions and tardive dyskinesia may occur

**Dosage Forms** Tablet: 25 mg, 50 mg, 100 mg, 150 mg

## Amoxicillin (a moks i SIL in)

**U.S. Brand Names** Amoxil®; Biomox®; Trimox®; Wymox®

**Canadian Brand Names** Apo®-Amoxi; Novamoxin®; Nu-Amoxi; Pro-Amox®

**Pharmacologic Category** Antibiotic, Penicillin

**Use** Treatment of otitis media, sinusitis, and infections caused by susceptible organisms involving the respiratory tract, skin, and urinary tract; prophylaxis of bacterial endocarditis in patients undergoing surgical or dental procedures; approved in combination with clarithromycin and lansoprazole for eradication of *H. pylori*; in patients with active duodenal ulcer disease or a 1-year history of duodenal ulcer. The combined use of lansoprazole and amoxicillin is approved for patients unable to take clarithromycin.

**Effects on Mental Status** Rarely large doses may produce confusion, hallucinations, and depression; penicillins have been reported to cause apprehension, illusions, agitation, insomnia, depersonalization, and encephalopathy

**Effects on Psychiatric Treatment** Disulfiram may increase amoxicillin levels

**Pregnancy Risk Factor** B

**Contraindications** Hypersensitivity to amoxicillin, penicillin, or any component

**Warnings/Precautions** In patients with renal impairment, doses and/or frequency of administration should be modified in response to the degree of renal impairment; a high percentage of patients with infectious mononucleosis have developed rash during therapy with amoxicillin; a low incidence of cross-allergy with other beta-lactams and cephalosporins exists

**Adverse Reactions**

1% to 10%:

- Central nervous system: Fever
- Dermatologic: Rash, urticaria
- Miscellaneous: Allergic reactions (includes serum sickness, rash, angioedema, bronchospasm, hypotension, etc)

<1%: Anxiety, confusion, depression (with large doses or patients with renal dysfunction), hallucinations, interstitial nephritis, jaundice, leukopenia, nausea, neutropenia, seizures, thrombocytopenia, vomiting

**Overdosage/Toxicology**

Signs and symptoms: Neuromuscular sensitivity, many beta-lactam containing antibiotics have the potential to cause neuromuscular hyperirritability or convulsive seizures

Treatment: Hemodialysis may be helpful to aid in the removal of the drug from the blood, otherwise most treatment is supportive or symptom directed.

**Drug Interactions**

Decreased effect: Efficacy of oral contraceptives may be reduced

Increased effect: Disulfiram, probenecid may increase amoxicillin levels

Increased toxicity: Allopurinol theoretically has an additive potential for amoxicillin rash

**Usual Dosage** Oral:

Children: 20-50 mg/kg/day in divided doses every 8 hours

Subacute bacterial endocarditis prophylaxis: 50 mg/kg 1 hour before procedure

Adults: 250-500 mg every 8 hours or 500-875 mg twice daily; maximum dose: 2-3 g/day

Endocarditis prophylaxis: 2 g 1 hour before procedure

*Helicobacter pylori*: 250-500 mg 3 times/day or 500-875 mg twice daily; clinically effective treatment regimens include triple therapy with amoxicillin or tetracycline, metronidazole, and bismuth subsalicylate; amoxicillin, metronidazole, and an $H_2$-receptor antagonist; amoxicillin, lansoprazole, and clarithromycin.

**Dosing interval in renal impairment:**

$Cl_{cr}$ 10-50 mL/minute: Administer every 12 hours

$Cl_{cr}$ <10 mL/minute: Administer every 24 hours

Dialysis: Moderately dialyzable (20% to 50%) by hemo- or peritoneal dialysis; approximately 50 mg of amoxicillin per liter of filtrate is removed by continuous arteriovenous or venovenous hemofiltration (CAVH); dose as per $Cl_{cr}$ <10 mL/minute guidelines

**Dietary Considerations** Food: May be taken with food

**Patient Information** Take entire prescription, even if you are feeling better. Take at equal intervals around-the-clock; may be taken with milk, juice, or food. You may experience nausea or vomiting (small frequent meals, frequent mouth care, sucking lozenges, or chewing gum may help). If diabetic, drug may cause false tests with Clinitest® urine glucose monitoring; use of glucose oxidase methods (Clinistix®) or serum glucose monitoring is preferable. This drug may interfere with oral contraceptives; an alternate form of birth control should be used. Report rash; unusual diarrhea; vaginal itching, burning, or pain; unresolved vomiting or constipation; fever or chills; unusual bruising or bleeding; or if condition being treated worsens or does not improve by the time prescription is completed.

**Dosage Forms**

Capsule, as trihydrate: 250 mg, 500 mg

Powder for oral suspension, as trihydrate: 125 mg/5 mL (5 mL, 80 mL, 100 mL, 150 mL, 200 mL); 250 mg/5 mL (5 mL, 80 mL, 100 mL, 150 mL, 200 mL)

Powder for oral suspension, drops, as trihydrate: 50 mg/mL (15 mL, 30 mL)

Tablet, chewable, as trihydrate: 125 mg, 250 mg

Tablet, film coated: 500 mg, 875 mg

## Amoxicillin and Clavulanate Potassium

(a moks i SIL in & klav yoo LAN ate poe TASS ee um)

**U.S. Brand Names** Augmentin®

**Canadian Brand Names** Clavulin®

**Synonyms** Amoxicillin and Clavulanic Acid

**Pharmacologic Category** Antibiotic, Penicillin

**Use** Treatment of otitis media, sinusitis, and infections caused by susceptible organisms involving the lower respiratory tract, skin and skin structure, and urinary tract; spectrum same as amoxicillin with additional coverage of beta-lactamase producing *B. catarrhalis*, *H. influenzae*, *N. gonorrhoeae*, and *S. aureus* (not MRSA). The expanded coverage of this combination makes it a useful alternative when amoxicillin resistance is present and patients cannot tolerate alternative treatments.

**Effects on Mental Status** Penicillins have been reported to cause apprehension, illusions, agitation, insomnia, depersonalization, and encephalopathy

**Effects on Psychiatric Treatment** Disulfiram may increase amoxicillin levels

**Pregnancy Risk Factor** B

**Contraindications** Known hypersensitivity to amoxicillin, clavulanic acid, or penicillin; concomitant use of disulfiram

**Warnings/Precautions** In patients with renal impairment, doses and/or frequency of administration should be modified in response to the degree of renal impairment; high percentage of patients with infectious mononucleosis have developed rash during therapy; a low incidence of cross-allergy with cephalosporins exists; incidence of diarrhea is higher than with amoxicillin alone. Hepatic dysfunction, although rare, is more common in elderly and/or males, and occurs more frequently with prolonged treatment.

**Adverse Reactions**

1% to 10%:

Dermatologic: Rash, urticaria

Gastrointestinal: Diarrhea, nausea, vomiting

Genitourinary: Vaginitis

<1%: Abdominal discomfort, flatulence, headache

**Overdosage/Toxicology**

Signs and symptoms: Neuromuscular hypersensitivity (agitation, hallucinations, asterixis, encephalopathy, confusion, and seizures) and electrolyte imbalance with potassium or sodium salts, especially in renal failure

Treatment: Hemodialysis may be helpful to aid in the removal of the drug from the blood, otherwise most treatment is supportive or symptom directed

**Drug Interactions**

Decreased effect: Efficacy of oral contraceptives may be reduced

Increased effect: Disulfiram, probenecid may increase amoxicillin levels, increased effect of anticoagulants

Increased toxicity: Allopurinol theoretically has an additive potential for amoxicillin rash

**Usual Dosage** Oral:

Children ≤40 kg: 20-40 mg (amoxicillin)/kg/day in divided doses every 8 hours or 45 mg/kg in divided doses every 12 hours

Children >40 kg and Adults: 250-500 mg every 8 hours or 875 mg every 12 hours

**Note:** Augmentin® 200 suspension or chewable tablets 200 mg dosed every 12 hours is considered equivalent to Augmentin® "125" dosed every 8 hours; Augmentin® 400 suspension and chewable tablets may be similarly dosed every 12 hours and are equivalent to Augmentin® "250" every 8 hours

**Dosing interval in renal impairment:**

$Cl_{cr}$ 10-30 mL/minute: Administer every 12 hours

$Cl_{cr}$ <10 mL/minute: Administer every 24 hours

Hemodialysis: Moderately dialyzable (20% to 50%)

Amoxicillin/clavulanic acid: Administer dose after dialysis

Peritoneal dialysis: Moderately dialyzable (20% to 50%)

Amoxicillin: Administer 250 mg every 12 hours

Clavulanic acid: Dose for $Cl_{cr}$ <10 mL/minute

Continuous arteriovenous or venovenous hemofiltration (CAVH) effects:

Amoxicillin: ~50 mg of amoxicillin/L of filtrate is removed

Clavulanic acid: Dose for $Cl_{cr}$ <10 mL/minute

**Patient Information** Take entire prescription, even if you are feeling better. Take at equal intervals around-the-clock; may be taken with milk, juice, or food. You may experience nausea or vomiting (small frequent meals, frequent mouth care, sucking lozenges, or chewing gum may help). If using oral contraceptives, use additional contraceptive measures; amoxicillin may reduce effectiveness of your oral contraceptive. Report rash; unusual diarrhea; vaginal itching, burning, or pain; unresolved vomiting or constipation; fever or chills; unusual bruising or bleeding; or if condition being treated worsens or does not improve by the time prescription is completed.

**Nursing Implications** Two 250 mg tablets are not equivalent to a 500 mg tablet (both tablet sizes contain equivalent clavulanate); potassium content: 0.16 mEq of potassium per 31.25 mg of clavulanic acid

**Dosage Forms**

Suspension, oral:

125 (banana flavor): Amoxicillin trihydrate 125 mg and clavulanate potassium 31.25 mg per 5 mL (75 mL, 150 mL)

200: Amoxicillin 200 mg and clavulanate potassium 28.5 mg per 5 mL (50 mL, 75 mL, 100 mL)

250 (orange flavor): Amoxicillin trihydrate 250 mg and clavulanate potassium 62.5 mg per 5 mL (75 mL, 150 mL)

400: Amoxicillin 400 mg and clavulanate potassium 57 mg per 5 mL (50 mL, 75 mL, 100 mL)

Tablet:

250: Amoxicillin trihydrate 250 mg and clavulanate potassium 125 mg

500: Amoxicillin trihydrate 500 mg and clavulanate potassium 125 mg

875: Amoxicillin trihydrate 875 mg and clavulanate potassium 125 mg

Tablet, chewable:

125: Amoxicillin trihydrate 125 mg and clavulanate potassium 31.25 mg

200: Amoxicillin trihydrate 200 mg and clavulanate potassium 28.5 mg

250: Amoxicillin trihydrate 250 mg and clavulanate potassium 62.5 mg

400: Amoxicillin trihydrate 400 mg and clavulanate potassium 57 mg

♦ **Amoxicillin and Clavulanic Acid** *see* Amoxicillin and Clavulanate Potassium *on page 39*

♦ **Amoxil®** *see* Amoxicillin *on page 38*

## Amphetamine (am FET a meen)

**Related Information**

Hallucinogenic Drugs *on page 713*

Patient Information - Stimulants *on page 652*

Sleep Disorders *on page 620*

Special Populations - Children and Adolescents *on page 663*

Stimulant Agents Used for ADHD *on page 728*

Substance-Related Disorders *on page 609*

**Generic Available** Yes

**Synonyms** Amphetamine Sulfate; Racemic Amphetamine Sulfate

**Pharmacologic Category** Stimulant

**Use** Treatment of narcolepsy; attention deficit/hyperactivity disorder (ADHD); exogenous obesity

**Unlabeled uses:** Potential augmenting agent for antidepressants; abnormal behavioral syndrome in children (minimal brain dysfunction)

**Restrictions** C-II

**Pregnancy Risk Factor** C

**Contraindications** Known hypersensitivity or idiosyncrasy to amphetamine or other sympathomimetic amines. Patients with advanced arteriosclerosis, symptomatic cardiovascular disease, moderate to severe hypertension (stage II or III), hyperthyroidism, glaucoma, diabetes mellitus, agitated states, patients with a history of drug abuse, and during or within

(Continued)

## Amphetamine *(Continued)*

14 days following MAO inhibitor therapy. Stimulant medications are contraindicated for use in children with attention deficit/hyperactivity disorders and concomitant Tourette's syndrome or tics.

**Warnings/Precautions** Use with caution in patients with bipolar disorder, cardiovascular disease, seizure disorders, insomnia, porphyria, or mild hypertension (stage I). May exacerbate symptoms of behavior and thought disorder in psychotic patients. Potential for drug dependency exists - avoid abrupt discontinuation in patients who have received for prolonged periods. Stimulant use in children has been associated with growth suppression.

**Adverse Reactions**

Cardiovascular: Arrhythmia (high dose), palpitations, elevation in blood pressure, tachycardia, chest pain

Central nervous system: Overstimulation, restlessness, insomnia, dizziness, euphoria, dyskinesia, dysphoria, headache, exacerbation of motor incoordination, tics, Tourette's syndrome; may rarely see psychosis

Dermatologic: Urticaria

Endocrine & metabolic: Changes in libido

Gastrointestinal: Xerostomia, unpleasant taste, diarrhea, constipation; anorexia and weight loss may occur as undesirable effects when amphetamines aroused for other than anorectic effect

Genitourinary: Impotence

Neuromuscular & skeletal: Tremor

Miscellaneous: Delayed bone growth

**Overdosage/Toxicology** Treatment: There is no specific antidote for amphetamine intoxication and the bulk of the treatment is supportive. Hyperactivity and agitation usually respond to reduced sensory input; however, with extreme agitation, haloperidol (2-5 mg I.M. for adults) may be required. Hyperthermia is best treated with external cooling measures, or when severe or unresponsive, muscle paralysis with pancuronium may be needed. Hypertension is usually transient and generally does not require treatment unless severe. For diastolic blood pressures >110 mm Hg, a nitroprusside infusion should be initiated. Seizures usually respond to diazepam IVP and/or phenytoin maintenance regimens.

**Drug Interactions** CYP2D6 enzyme substrate

Acidifiers: Very large doses of potassium acid phosphate or ammonium chloride may increase the renal elimination of amphetamines due to urinary acidification

Alkalinizers: Large doses of sodium bicarbonate or other alkalinizers may increase renal tubular reabsorption (decreased elimination) and diminish the effect of amphetamine; includes potassium or sodium citrate and acetate

Antipsychotics: Efficacy of amphetamines may be decreased by antipsychotics; in addition, amphetamines may induce an increase in psychotic symptoms in some patients

CYP2D6 inhibitors: Metabolism of amphetamine may be decreased, increasing clinical effect or toxicity; inhibitors include amiodarone, cimetidine, delavirdine, fluoxetine, paroxetine, propafenone, quinidine, and ritonavir; monitor for increased effect/toxicity

Enzyme inducers: Metabolism of amphetamine may be increased, decreasing clinical effect; inducers include barbiturates, carbamazepine, phenytoin, and rifampin

Furazolidine: Amphetamines may induce hypertensive episodes in patients receiving furazolidone

Guanethidine: Amphetamines inhibit the antihypertensive response to guanethidine; probably also may occur with guanadrel

MAOIs: Severe hypertensive episodes have occurred with amphetamine when used in patients receiving MAOIs; concurrent use or use within 14 days is contraindicated

Norepinephrine: Amphetamines may enhance the pressor response to norepinephrine

Sibutramine: Concurrent use of sibutramine and amphetamines may cause severe hypertension and tachycardia; use is contraindicated in product

SSRIs: Amphetamines may increase the potential for serotonin syndrome when used concurrently with selective serotonin reuptake inhibitors (including fluoxetine, fluvoxamine, paroxetine, and sertraline)

Tricyclic antidepressants: Concurrent of amphetamines with TCAs may result in hypertension and CNS stimulation; avoid this combination

**Mechanism of Action** The amphetamines are noncatecholamine sympathomimetic amines with CNS stimulant activity. They require breakdown by monoamine oxidase for inactivation; produce central nervous system and respiratory stimulation, a pressor response, mydriasis, bronchodilation, and contraction of the urinary sphincter; thought to have a direct effect on both alpha- and beta-receptor sites in the peripheral system, as well as release stores of norepinephrine in adrenergic nerve terminals. The central nervous system action is thought to occur in the cerebral cortex and reticular activating system. The anorexigenic effect is probably secondary to the CNS-stimulating effect; the site of action is probably the hypothalamic feeding center.

**Usual Dosage** Oral:

Narcolepsy:

Children:

6-12 years: 5 mg/day, increase by 5 mg at weekly intervals

>12 years: 10 mg/day, increase by 10 mg at weekly intervals

Adults: 5-60 mg/day in 2-3 divided doses

Attention deficit/hyperactivity disorder: Children:

3-5 years: 2.5 mg/day, increase by 2.5 mg at weekly intervals for maximum dose of 40 mg/day

>6 years: 5 mg/day, increase by 5 mg at weekly intervals not to exceed 40 mg/day

Short-term adjunct to exogenous obesity: Children >12 years and Adults: 10 mg or 15 mg long-acting capsule daily, up to 30 mg/day; or 5-30 mg/day in divided doses (immediate release tablets only)

**Monitoring Parameters** CNS

**Reference Range** Therapeutic: 20-30 ng/mL; Toxic: >200 ng/mL

**Patient Information** Take during day to avoid insomnia; do not discontinue abruptly, may cause physical and psychological dependence with prolonged use; sometimes used only during school year to minimize potential long-term effects

**Nursing Implications** Monitor CNS, dose should not be given in evening or at bedtime

**Dosage Forms** Tablet, as sulfate: 5 mg, 10 mg


- **Amphetamine Sulfate** *see* Amphetamine *on page 39*
- **Amphojel® [OTC]** *see* Aluminum Hydroxide *on page 28*
- **Amphotec®** *see* Amphotericin B Cholesteryl Sulfate Complex *on page 40*


## Amphotericin B Cholesteryl Sulfate Complex

(am foe TER i sin bee kole LES te ril SUL fate KOM plecks)

**U.S. Brand Names** Amphotec®

**Synonyms** ABCD; Amphotericin B Colloidal Dispersion

**Pharmacologic Category** Antifungal Agent, Parenteral

**Use** Treatment of invasive aspergillosis in patients who have failed amphotericin B deoxycholate treatment, or who have renal impairment or experience unacceptable toxicity which precludes treatment with amphotericin B deoxycholate in effective doses.

**Effects on Mental Status** None reported

**Effects on Psychiatric Treatment** May cause bone marrow suppression; use caution with clozapine and carbamazepine

**Pregnancy Risk Factor** B

**Contraindications** Hypersensitivity to amphotericin B or its components

**Warnings/Precautions** Anaphylaxis has been reported with other amphotericin B-containing drugs. Facilities for cardiopulmonary resuscitation should be available during administration due to the possibility of anaphylactic reaction. If severe respiratory distress occurs, the infusion should be immediately discontinued. During the initial dosing, the drug should be administered under close clinical observation. Infusion reactions, sometimes, severe, usually subside with continued therapy - manage with decreased rate of infusion and pretreatment with antihistamines/corticosteroids; pulmonary reactions may occur in neutropenic patients receiving leukocyte transfusions; separation of the infusions as much as possible is advised.

**Adverse Reactions**

>10%: Central nervous system: Chills, fever

1% to 10%:

Cardiovascular: Hypotension, tachycardia

Central nervous system: Headache

Dermatologic: Rash

Endocrine & metabolic: Hypokalemia, hypomagnesemia

Gastrointestinal: Nausea, diarrhea, abdominal pain

Hematologic: Thrombocytopenia

Hepatic: LFT change

Neuromuscular & skeletal: Rigors

Renal: Elevated creatinine

Respiratory: Dyspnea

**Overdosage/Toxicology**

Symptoms of overdose include renal dysfunction, anemia, thrombocytopenia, granulocytopenia, fever, nausea, vomiting

Treatment is supportive

**Drug Interactions**

Increased nephrotoxicity: Aminoglycosides, cyclosporine, other nephrotoxic drugs

Potentiation of hypokalemia: Corticosteroids, corticotropin

Increased digitalis and neuromuscular-blocking agent toxicity due to hypokalemia

Decreased effect: Pharmacologic antagonism may occur with azole antifungal agents (eg, miconazole, ketoconazole)

Pulmonary toxicity has occurred with concomitant administration of amphotericin B and leukocyte transfusions

**Usual Dosage** Children and Adults: I.V.:

Premedication: For patients who experience chills, fever, hypotension, nausea, or other nonanaphylactic infusion-related immediate reactions, premedicate with the following drugs, 30-60 minutes prior to drug administration: a nonsteroidal (eg, ibuprofen, choline magnesium trisalicylate, etc) with or without diphenhydramine; or acetaminophen with diphenhydramine; or hydrocortisone 50-100 mg. If the patient experiences rigors during the infusion, meperidine may be administered.

Range: 3-4 mg/kg/day (infusion of 1 mg/kg/hour); maximum: 7.5 mg/kg/day

**Patient Information** This medication can only be administered by infusion and therapy may last several weeks. Maintain good hydration (2-3 L/day of fluids unless instructed to restrict fluid intake). You may experience postural hypotension (use caution when changing from lying or sitting position to standing or when climbing stairs); nausea or vomiting (small frequent meals, frequent mouth care, sucking lozenges, or chewing gum may help). Report chest pain or palpitations; skin rash; chills or fever; persistent nausea, vomiting, or abdominal pain; sore throat; excessive fatigue; swelling of extremities or unusual weight gain; difficulty breathing; pain at infusion site; muscle cramping or weakness; or other adverse reactions.

**Nursing Implications** May premedicate with acetaminophen and diphenhydramine 30 minutes prior to infusion; meperidine may help reduce rigors; avoid injection faster than 1 mg/kg/hour

**Dosage Forms** Suspension for injection: 50 mg (20 mL); 100 mg (50 mL)

♦ **Amphotericin B Colloidal Dispersion** *see* Amphotericin B Cholesteryl Sulfate Complex *on page 40*

## Amphotericin B (Conventional)

(am foe TER i sin bee kon VEN shun al)

**U.S. Brand Names** Fungizone®

**Synonyms** Amphotericin B Desoxycholate

**Pharmacologic Category** Antifungal Agent, Parenteral; Antifungal Agent, Topical

**Use** Treatment of severe systemic and central nervous system infections caused by susceptible fungi such as *Candida* species, *Histoplasma capsulatum, Cryptococcus neoformans, Aspergillus* species, *Blastomyces dermatitidis, Torulopsis glabrata,* and *Coccidioides immitis*; fungal peritonitis; irrigant for bladder fungal infections; and topically for cutaneous and mucocutaneous candidal infections; used in fungal infection in patients with bone marrow transplantation, amebic meningoencephalitis, ocular aspergillosis (intraocular injection), candidal cystitis (bladder irrigation), chemoprophylaxis (low-dose I.V.), immunocompromised patients at risk of aspergillosis (intranasal/nebulized), refractory meningitis (intrathecal), coccidioidal arthritis (intra-articular/I.M.).

Low-dose amphotericin B 0.1-0.25 mg/kg/day has been administered after bone marrow transplantation to reduce the risk of invasive fungal disease. Alternative routes of administration and extemporaneous preparations have been used when standard antifungal therapy is not available (eg, inhalation, intraocular injection, subconjunctival application, intracavitary administration into various joints and the pleural space).

**Effects on Mental Status** Sedation is common; may cause delirium

**Effects on Psychiatric Treatment** May cause bone marrow suppression; use caution with clozapine and carbamazepine

**Pregnancy Risk Factor** B

**Contraindications** Hypersensitivity to amphotericin or any component

**Warnings/Precautions** Anaphylaxis has been reported with other amphotericin B-containing drugs. During the initial dosing, the drug should be administered under close clinical observation. Avoid additive toxicity with other nephrotoxic drugs; drug-induced renal toxicity usually improves with interrupting therapy, decreasing dosage, or increasing dosing interval. I.V. amphotericin is used primarily for the treatment of patients with progressive and potentially fatal fungal infections; topical preparations may stain clothing. Infusion reactions are most common 1-3 hours after starting the infusion and diminish with continued therapy. Use amphotericin B with caution in patients with decreased renal function. Pulmonary reactions may occur in neutropenic patients receiving leukocyte transfusions; separation of the infusions as much as possible is advised.

**Adverse Reactions**

>10%:

- Central nervous system: Chills, fever, generalized pain, headache, malaise
- Endocrine & metabolic: Hypokalemia, hypomagnesemia
- Gastrointestinal: Anorexia
- Hematologic: Anemia
- Renal: Nephrotoxicity

1% to 10%:

- Cardiovascular: Flushing, hypertension, hypotension
- Central nervous system: Arachnoiditis, delirium, pain along lumbar nerves
- Gastrointestinal: Nausea, vomiting
- Genitourinary: Urinary retention
- Hematologic: Leukocytosis
- Local: Thrombophlebitis
- Neuromuscular & skeletal: Paresthesia (especially with I.T. therapy)
- Renal: Renal failure, renal tubular acidosis

<1%: Acute liver failure, agranulocytosis, anuria, bone marrow suppression, cardiac arrest, coagulation defects, convulsions, dyspnea, hearing loss, leukopenia, maculopapular rash, thrombocytopenia, vision changes

**Overdosage/Toxicology**

Signs and symptoms: Renal dysfunction, anemia, thrombocytopenia, granulocytopenia, fever, nausea, and vomiting

Treatment: Supportive

**Drug Interactions**

Increased nephrotoxicity: Aminoglycosides, cyclosporine, other nephrotoxic drugs

Potentiation of hypokalemia: Corticosteroids, corticotropin

Increased digitalis and neuromuscular-blocking agent toxicity due to hypokalemia

Decreased effect: Pharmacologic antagonism may occur with azole antifungal agents (eg, miconazole, ketoconazole)

Pulmonary toxicity has occurred with concomitant administration of amphotericin B and leukocyte transfusions

**Usual Dosage**

I.V.: Premedication: For patients who experience chills, fever, hypotension, nausea, or other nonanaphylactic infusion-related immediate reactions, premedicate with the following drugs, 30-60 minutes prior to drug administration: a nonsteroidal (eg, ibuprofen, choline magnesium trisalicylate, etc) with or without diphenhydramine; or acetaminophen with diphenhydramine; or hydrocortisone 50-100 mg. If the patient experiences rigors during the infusion, meperidine may be administered.

Infants and Children:

Test dose: I.V.: 0.1 mg/kg/dose to a maximum of 1 mg; infuse over 30-60 minutes. Many clinicians believe a test dose is unnecessary.

Maintenance dose: 0.25-1 mg/kg/day given once daily; infuse over 2-6 hours. Once therapy has been established, amphotericin B can be administered on an every-other-day basis at 1-1.5 mg/kg/dose; cumulative dose: 1.5-2 g over 6-10 week

Adults:

Test dose: 1 mg infused over 20-30 minutes. Many clinicians believe a test dose is unnecessary.

Maintenance dose: Usual: 0.25-1.5 mg/kg/day; 1-1.5 mg/kg over 4-6 hours every other day may be given once therapy is established; aspergillosis, mucormycosis, rhinocerebral phycomycosis often require 1-1.5 mg/kg/day; do not exceed 1.5 mg/kg/day

Duration of therapy varies with nature of infection: Usual duration is 4-12 weeks or cumulative dose of 1-4 g

I.T.: Meningitis, coccidioidal or cryptococcal:

Children.: 25-100 mcg every 48-72 hours; increase to 500 mcg as tolerated

Adults: Initial: 25-300 mcg every 48-72 hours; increase to 500 mcg to 1 mg as tolerated; maximum total dose: 15 mg has been suggested

Oral: 1 mL (100 mg) 4 times/day

Topical: Apply to affected areas 2-4 times/day for 1-4 weeks of therapy depending on nature and severity of infection

Bladder irrigation: Candidal cystitis: Irrigate with 50 mcg/mL solution instilled periodically or continuously for 5-10 days or until cultures are clear

**Dosing adjustment in renal impairment:** If renal dysfunction is due to the drug, the daily total can be decreased by 50% or the dose can be given every other day; I.V. therapy may take several months

Dialysis: Poorly dialyzed; no supplemental dosage necessary when using hemo- or peritoneal dialysis or CAVH/CAVHD

Administration in dialysate: Children and Adults: 1-2 mg/L of peritoneal dialysis fluid either with or without low-dose I.V. amphotericin B (a total dose of 2-10 mg/kg given over 7-14 days). Precipitate may form in ionic dialysate solutions.

**Patient Information** Take/use as directed; complete full regimen of treatment (most skin lesions may take 1-3 weeks of therapy). Maintain adequate hydration (2-3 L/day of fluids unless instructed to restrict fluid intake). You may experience nausea, vomiting, or anorexia (small frequent meals, frequent mouth care, sucking lozenges, or chewing gum may help); generalized muscle or joint paint (mild analgesic may help); hypotension (use caution when rising from sitting or lying position or when climbing stairs). Report severe muscle cramping or weakness, chest pain or palpitations, CNS disturbances, skin rash, change in urinary patterns or difficulty voiding, black stool, or unusual bruising or bleeding; (I.V. report pain at infusion site).

Topical: Amphotericin cream may slightly discolor skin and stain clothing; use gloves when applying. Avoid covering topical application with occlusive bandages. Most skin lesions require 1-3 weeks of therapy. Maintain good personal hygiene to reduce the spread and recurrence of lesions.

**Nursing Implications** May be infused over 2-6 hours

**Dosage Forms**

- Cream: 3% (20 g)
- Lotion: 3% (30 mL)
- Ointment, topical: 3% (20 g)
- Powder for injection, lyophilized, as desoxycholate: 50 mg
- Suspension, oral: 100 mg/mL (24 mL with dropper)

♦ **Amphotericin B Desoxycholate** *see* Amphotericin B (Conventional) *on page 41*

## Amphotericin B, Lipid Complex
(am foe TER i sin bee LIP id KOM pleks)

**U.S. Brand Names** Abelcet™ Injection

**Pharmacologic Category** Antifungal Agent, Parenteral

**Use** Treatment of aspergillosis or any type of progressive fungal infection in patients who are refractory to or intolerant of conventional amphotericin B therapy

**Orphan drug**: Cryptococcal meningitis

**Effects on Mental Status** Sedation is common; may cause delirium

**Effects on Psychiatric Treatment** May cause bone marrow suppression; use caution with clozapine and carbamazepine

**Usual Dosage** Children and Adults: I.V.:

Premedication: For patients who experience chills, fever, hypotension, nausea, or other nonanaphylactic infusion-related immediate reactions, premedicate with the following drugs, 30-60 minutes prior to drug administration: a nonsteroidal (eg, ibuprofen, choline magnesium trisalicylate, etc) with or without diphenhydramine; or acetaminophen with diphenhydramine; or hydrocortisone 50-100 mg. If the patient experiences rigors during the infusion, meperidine may be administered.

Range: 2.5-5 mg/kg/day as a single infusion

**Dosing adjustment in renal impairment:** None necessary; effects of renal impairment are not currently known

Hemodialysis: No supplemental dosage necessary

Peritoneal dialysis: No supplemental dosage necessary

Continuous arteriovenous or venovenous hemofiltration (CAVH/CAVHD): No supplemental dosage necessary

**Dosage Forms** Injection: 5 mg/mL (20 mL)

## Amphotericin B, Liposomal
(am foe TER i sin bee lye po SO mal)

**U.S. Brand Names** AmBisome®

**Pharmacologic Category** Antifungal Agent, Parenteral

**Use** Empirical therapy for presumed fungal infection in febrile, neutropenic patients. Treatment of patients with *Aspergillus* species, *Candida* species and/or *Cryptococcus* species infections refractory to amphotericin B desoxycholate, or in patients where renal impairment or unacceptable toxicity precludes the use of amphotericin B desoxycholate. Treatment of visceral leishmaniasis. In immunocompromised patients with visceral leishmaniasis treated with amphotericin B, liposomal, relapse rates were high following initial clearance of parasites.

**Effects on Mental Status** Sedation is common; may cause delirium

**Effects on Psychiatric Treatment** May cause bone marrow suppression; use caution with clozapine and carbamazepine

**Usual Dosage** Children and Adults: I.V.:

Premedication: For patients who experience chills, fever, hypotension, nausea, or other nonanaphylactic infusion-related immediate reactions, premedicate with the following drugs, 30-60 minutes prior to drug administration: a nonsteroidal (eg, ibuprofen, choline magnesium trisalicylate, etc) with or without diphenhydramine; or acetaminophen with diphenhydramine; or hydrocortisone 50-100 mg. If the patient experiences rigors during the infusion, meperidine may be administered.

Empiric therapy: Recommended initial dose: 3 mg/kg/day

Systemic fungal infections (*Aspergillus, Candida, Cryptococcus*): Recommended initial dose of 3-5 mg/kg/day

Treatment of visceral leishmaniasis: Amphotericin B liposomal achieved high rates of acute parasite clearance in immunocompetent patients when total doses of 12-30 mg/kg were administered. Most of these immunocompetent patients remained relapse-free during follow-up periods of 6 months or longer. While acute parasite clearance was achieved in most of the immunocompromised patients who received total doses of 30-40 mg/kg, the majority of these patients were observed to relapse in the 6 months following the completion of therapy.

**Dosing adjustment in renal impairment:** None necessary; effects of renal impairment are not currently known

Hemodialysis: No supplemental dosage necessary

Peritoneal dialysis effects: No supplemental dosage necessary

Continuous arteriovenous or venovenous hemofiltration (CAVH/CAVHD): No supplemental dosage necessary

**Dosage Forms** Injection: 50 mg

## Ampicillin (am pi SIL in)

**U.S. Brand Names** Marcillin®; Omnipen®; Omnipen®-N; Polycillin-N®; Principen®; Totacillin®; Totacillin®-N

**Canadian Brand Names** Ampicin® Sodium; Apo®-Ampi Trihydrate; Jaa Amp® Trihydrate; Nu-Ampi Trihydrate; Pro-Ampi® Trihydrate; Taro-Ampicillin® Trihydrate

**Pharmacologic Category** Antibiotic, Penicillin

**Use** Treatment of susceptible bacterial infections (nonbeta-lactamase-producing organisms); susceptible bacterial infections caused by streptococci, pneumococci, nonpenicillinase-producing staphylococci, *Listeria*, meningococci; some strains of *H. influenzae*, *Salmonella*, *Shigella*, *E. coli*, *Enterobacter*, and *Klebsiella*

**Effects on Mental Status** Large I.V. doses may rarely produce encephalopathy; penicillins have been reported to cause apprehension, illusions, agitation, insomnia, depersonalization, and encephalopathy

**Effects on Psychiatric Treatment** Rarely may cause bone marrow suppression; use caution with clozapine and carbamazepine

**Pregnancy Risk Factor** B

**Contraindications** Known hypersensitivity to ampicillin or other penicillins

**Warnings/Precautions** Dosage adjustment may be necessary in patients with renal impairment; a low incidence of cross-allergy with other beta-lactams exists; high percentage of patients with infectious mononucleosis have developed rash during therapy with ampicillin. Appearance of a rash should be carefully evaluated to differentiate a nonallergic ampicillin rash from a hypersensitivity reaction. Ampicillin rash occurs in 5% to 10% of children receiving ampicillin and is a generalized dull red, maculopapular rash, generally appearing 3-14 days after the start of therapy. It normally begins on the trunk and spreads over most of the body. It may be most intense at pressure areas, elbows, and knees.

**Adverse Reactions**

>10%: Local: Pain at injection site

1% to 10%:

Dermatologic: Rash (appearance of a rash should be carefully evaluated to differentiate, if possible; nonallergic ampicillin rash from hypersensitivity reaction; incidence is higher in patients with viral infections, *Salmonella* infections, lymphocytic leukemia, or patients that have hyperuricemia)

Gastrointestinal: Abdominal cramps, diarrhea, oral candidiasis, vomiting

Miscellaneous: Allergic reaction (includes serum sickness, urticaria, angioedema, bronchospasm, hypotension, etc)

<1%: Anemia, decreased lymphocytes, eosinophilia, granulocytopenia, hemolytic anemia, interstitial nephritis (rare), leukopenia, penicillin encephalopathy, seizures (with large I.V. doses or patients with renal dysfunction), thrombocytopenia, thrombocytopenic purpura

**Overdosage/Toxicology**

Signs and symptoms: Neuromuscular hypersensitivity (agitation, hallucinations, asterixis, encephalopathy, confusion, and seizures) and electrolyte imbalance with potassium or sodium salts, especially in renal failure

Treatment: Hemodialysis may be helpful to aid in the removal of the drug from the blood, otherwise most treatment is supportive or symptom directed

**Drug Interactions**

Decreased effect: Efficacy of oral contraceptives may be reduced

Increased effect: Disulfiram, probenecid may increase penicillin levels, increased effect of anticoagulants

Increased toxicity: Allopurinol theoretically has an additive potential for amoxicillin (ampicillin) rash

**Usual Dosage**

Neonates: I.M., I.V.:

Postnatal age ≤7 days:

≤2000 g: Meningitis: 50 mg/kg/dose every 12 hours; other infections: 25 mg/kg/dose every 12 hours

>2000 g: Meningitis: 50 mg/kg/dose every 8 hours; other infections: 25 mg/kg/dose every 8 hours

Postnatal age >7 days:

<1200 g: Meningitis: 50 mg/kg/dose every 12 hours; other infections: 25 mg/kg/dose every 12 hours

1200-2000 g: Meningitis: 50 mg/kg/dose every 8 hours; other infections: 25 mg/kg/dose every 8 hours

>2000 g: Meningitis: 50 mg/kg/dose every 6 hours; other infections: 25 mg/kg/dose every 6 hours

Infants and Children: I.M., I.V.: 100-400 mg/kg/day in doses divided every 4-6 hours

Meningitis: 200 mg/kg/day in doses divided every 4-6 hours; maximum dose: 12 g/day

Children: Oral: 50-100 mg/kg/day in doses divided every 6 hours; maximum dose: 2-3 g/day

Adults:

Oral: 250-500 mg every 6 hours

I.M.: 500 mg to 1.5 g every 4-6 hours

I.V.: 500 mg to 3 g every 4-6 hours; maximum dose: 12 g/day

Sepsis/meningitis: 150-250 mg/kg/24 hours divided every 3-4 hours

**Dosing interval in renal impairment:**

$Cl_{cr}$ 30-50 mL/minute: Administer every 6-8 hours

$Cl_{cr}$ 10-30 mL/minute: Administer every 8-12 hours

$Cl_{cr}$ <10 mL/minute: Administer every 12 hours

Hemodialysis: Moderately dialyzable (20% to 50%); administer dose after dialysis

Peritoneal dialysis: Moderately dialyzable (20% to 50%)

Administer 250 mg every 12 hours

Continuous arteriovenous or venovenous hemofiltration (CAVH) effects: Dose as for $Cl_{cr}$ 10-50 mL/minute; ~50 mg of ampicillin per liter of filtrate is removed

**Dietary Considerations** Food: Decreases drug absorption rate; decreases drug serum concentration. Take on an empty stomach 1 hour before or 2 hours after meals.

**Patient Information** Take entire prescription, even if you are feeling better. Take at equal intervals around-the-clock; preferably on an empty stomach with a full glass of water (1 hour before or 2 hours after meals). Maintain adequate hydration (2-3 L/day of fluids unless instructed to restrict fluid intake). You may experience nausea or vomiting (small frequent meals, frequent mouth care, sucking lozenges, or chewing gum may help). If diabetic, drug may cause false tests with Clinitest® urine glucose monitoring; use of glucose oxidase methods (Clinistix®) or serum glucose monitoring is preferable. This drug may interfere with oral contraceptives; an alternate form of birth control should be used. Report rash; unusual diarrhea; unusual vaginal discharge, itching, burning, or pain; mouth sores; unresolved vomiting or constipation; fever or chills; unusual bruising or bleeding; or if condition being treated worsens or does not improve by the time prescription is completed.

**Nursing Implications** Ampicillin and gentamicin should not be mixed in the same I.V. tubing or administered concurrently

**Dosage Forms**

Capsule, as anhydrous: 250 mg, 500 mg

Capsule, as trihydrate: 250 mg, 500 mg

Powder for injection, as sodium: 125 mg, 250 mg, 500 mg, 1 g, 2 g, 10 g

Powder for oral suspension, as trihydrate: 125 mg/5 mL (5 mL unit dose, 80 mL, 100 mL, 150 mL, 200 mL); 250 mg/5 mL (5 mL unit dose, 80 mL, 100 mL, 150 mL, 200 mL); 500 mg/5 mL (5 mL unit dose, 100 mL)

Powder for oral suspension, drops, as trihydrate: 100 mg/mL (20 mL)

## Ampicillin and Probenecid (am pi SIL in & proe BEN e sid)

**U.S. Brand Names** Probampacin®

**Pharmacologic Category** Antibiotic, Penicillin

**Use** Uncomplicated infections caused by susceptible strains of *Neisseria gonorrhoeae* in adults

**Effects on Mental Status** Large I.V. doses may rarely produce encephalopathy; penicillins have been reported to cause apprehension, illusions, agitation, insomnia, depersonalization, and encephalopathy

**Effects on Psychiatric Treatment** Rarely may cause bone marrow suppression; may rarely produce seizures; use caution with clozapine, carbamazepine, antidepressants, abruptly discontinued benzodiazepines

**Usual Dosage** Administer entire contents of bottle as a single one time dose

**Dosage Forms** Powder for oral suspension: Ampicillin 3.5 g and probenecid 1 g per bottle

## Ampicillin and Sulbactam (am pi SIL in & SUL bak tam)

**U.S. Brand Names** Unasyn®

**Synonyms** Sulbactam and Ampicillin

**Pharmacologic Category** Antibiotic, Penicillin

**Use** Treatment of susceptible bacterial infections involved with skin and skin structure, intra-abdominal infections, gynecological infections; spectrum is that of ampicillin plus organisms producing beta-lactamases such as *S. aureus*, *H. influenzae*, *E. coli*, *Klebsiella*, *Acinetobacter*, *Enterobacter*, and anaerobes

**Effects on Mental Status** Large I.V. doses may rarely produce encephalopathy; penicillins have been reported to cause apprehension, illusions, agitation, insomnia, depersonalization, and encephalopathy

**Effects on Psychiatric Treatment** Rarely may cause bone marrow suppression; use caution with clozapine and carbamazepine

**Pregnancy Risk Factor** B

**Contraindications** Hypersensitivity to ampicillin, sulbactam or any component, or penicillins

**Warnings/Precautions** Dosage adjustment may be necessary in patients with renal impairment; a low incidence of cross-allergy with other beta-lactams exists; high percentage of patients with infectious mononucleosis have developed rash during therapy with ampicillin. Appearance of a rash should be carefully evaluated to differentiate a nonallergic ampicillin rash from a hypersensitivity reaction. Ampicillin rash occurs in 5% to 10% of children receiving ampicillin and is a generalized dull red, maculopapular rash, generally appearing 3-14 days after the start of therapy. It normally begins on the trunk and spreads over most of the body. It may be most intense at pressure areas, elbows, and knees.

**Adverse Reactions**

>10%: Local: Pain at injection site (I.M.)

1% to 10%:

Dermatologic: Rash

Gastrointestinal: Diarrhea

Local: Pain at injection site (I.V.)

Miscellaneous: Allergic reaction (may include serum sickness, urticaria, bronchospasm, hypotension, etc)

<1%: Chest pain, chills, decreased hemoglobin and hematocrit, dysuria, enterocolitis, fatigue, hairy tongue, headache, increased BUN/creatinine, increased liver enzymes, interstitial nephritis (rare), itching, leukopenia, malaise, nausea, neutropenia, penicillin encephalopathy, pseudomembranous colitis, seizures (with large I.V. doses or patients with renal dysfunction), thrombocytopenia, thrombophlebitis, vaginitis, vomiting

**Overdosage/Toxicology**

Signs and symptoms: Neuromuscular hypersensitivity (agitation, hallucinations, asterixis, encephalopathy, confusion, and seizures) and electrolyte imbalance with potassium or sodium salts, especially in renal failure

Treatment: Hemodialysis may be helpful to aid in the removal of the drug from the blood, otherwise most treatment is supportive or symptom directed

**Drug Interactions**

Decreased effect: Efficacy of oral contraceptives may be reduced

Increased effect: Disulfiram, probenecid results in increased ampicillin levels

Increased toxicity: Allopurinol theoretically has an additive potential for ampicillin rash

**Usual Dosage** Unasyn® (ampicillin/sulbactam) is a combination product. Each 3 g vial contains 2 g of ampicillin and 1 g of sulbactam. Sulbactam has very little antibacterial activity by itself, but effectively extends the spectrum of ampicillin to include beta-lactamase producing strains that are resistant to ampicillin alone. Therefore, dosage recommendations for Unasyn® are based on the ampicillin component.

I.M., I.V.:

Children (3 months to 12 years): 100-200 mg ampicillin/kg/day (150-300 mg Unasyn®) divided every 6 hours; maximum dose: 8 g ampicillin/day (12 g Unasyn®)

Adults: 1-2 g ampicillin (1.5-3 g Unasyn®) every 6-8 hours; maximum dose: 8 g ampicillin/day (12 g Unasyn®)

**Dosing interval in renal impairment:**

$Cl_{cr}$ 15-29 mL/minute: Administer every 12 hours

$Cl_{cr}$ 5-14 mL/minute: Administer every 24 hours

**Patient Information** Take entire prescription, even if you are feeling better. Take at equal intervals around-the-clock; preferably on an empty stomach with a full glass of water (1 hour before or 2 hours after meals). Maintain adequate hydration (2-3 L/day of fluids unless instructed to restrict fluid intake). You may experience nausea or vomiting (small frequent meals, frequent mouth care, sucking lozenges, or chewing gum may help). If diabetic, drug may cause false tests with Clinitest® urine glucose monitoring; use of glucose oxidase methods (Clinistix®) or serum glucose monitoring is preferable. This drug may interfere with oral contraceptives; an alternate form of birth control should be used. Report rash; unusual diarrhea; vaginal discharge, itching, burning, or pain; mouth sores; unresolved vomiting or constipation; fever or chills; unusual bruising or bleeding; or if condition being treated worsens or does not improve by the time prescription is completed.

**Nursing Implications** Ampicillin and gentamicin should not be mixed in the same I.V. tubing or administered concurrently

**Dosage Forms** Powder for injection: 1.5 g [ampicillin sodium 1 g and sulbactam sodium 0.5 g]; 3 g [ampicillin sodium 2 g and sulbactam sodium 1 g]

## Amprenavir (am PRE na veer)

**U.S. Brand Names** Agenerase™

**Pharmacologic Category** Antiretroviral Agent, Protease Inhibitor

**Use** Treatment of HIV infections in combination with at least two other antiretroviral agents; oral solution should only be used when capsules or other protease inhibitors are not therapeutic options

**Effects on Mental Status** Depression is common; may cause headache and fatigue

**Effects on Psychiatric Treatment** Contraindicated with midazolam and triazolam. Concurrent use with vitamin E and sildenafil should be avoided. May increase concentrations of alprazolam, clorazepate, diazepam, flurazepam, sildenafil, carbamazepine, and pimozide. May increase adverse effects of TCAs (monitor serum levels).

**Pregnancy Risk Factor** Unknown

**Contraindications** Hypersensitivity to amprenavir or any component; concurrent therapy with rifampin, astemizole, bepridil, cisapride, dihydroergotamine, ergotamine, midazolam, triazolam, lovastatin, and simvastatin; severe previous allergic reaction to sulfonamides; oral solution is contraindicated in infants or children <4 years of age, pregnant women, patients with renal or hepatic failure, and patients receiving concurrent metronidazole or disulfiram

**Warnings/Precautions** Because of hepatic metabolism and effect on cytochrome P-450 enzymes, amprenavir should be used with caution in combination with other agents metabolized by this system (see Contraindications and Drug Interactions). Use with caution in patients with diabetes mellitus, sulfonamide allergy, hepatic impairment, or hemophilia. Redistribution of fat may occur (eg, buffalo hump, peripheral wasting, cushingoid appearance). Additional vitamin E supplements should be avoided. Concurrent use of sildenafil should be avoided. Certain ethnic populations (Asians, Eskimos, Native Americans) may be at increased risk of propylene glycol-associated adverse effects; use of of the oral solution of amprenavir should be avoided. Use oral solution only when capsules or other protease inhibitors are not options.

**Adverse Reactions** Protease inhibitors cause dyslipidemia which includes elevated cholesterol and triglycerides and a redistribution of body fat

(Continued)

## Amprenavir *(Continued)*

centrally to cause "protease paunch," buffalo hump, facial atrophy, and breast enlargement. These agents also cause hyperglycemia.

>10%:

Dermatologic: Rash (28%)

Endocrine & metabolic: Hyperglycemia (37% to 41%), hypertriglyceridemia (38% to 27%)

Gastrointestinal: Diarrhea (33% to 56%), nausea (38% to 73%), vomiting (20% to 29%)

Miscellaneous: Perioral tingling/numbness

1% to 10%:

Central nervous system: Depression (4% to 15%), fatigue, headache, paresthesia

Dermatologic: Stevens-Johnson syndrome (1% of total, 4% of patients who develop a rash)

Gastrointestinal: Taste disorders (1% to 10%)

**Drug Interactions** CYP3A4 inhibitor and substrate

Increased effect/toxicity: Abacavir, clarithromycin, indinavir, ketoconazole, and zidovudine increase the AUC of amprenavir. Nelfinavir had no effect on AUC, but increased the $C_{min}$ of amprenavir. Amprenavir increased the AUC of ketoconazole, rifabutin, and zidovudine during concurrent therapy. Amprenavir may enhance the toxicity of astemizole, bepridil, cisapride, dihydroergotamine, ergotamine, midazolam, and triazolam - concurrent therapy with these drugs and amprenavir is contraindicated. May increase serum concentration of HMG CoA reductase inhibitors (avoid concurrent use with those metabolized by CYP3A4), diltiazem, nicardipine, nifedipine, nimodipine, alprazolam, clorazepate, diazepam, flurazepam, itraconazole, dapsone, erythromycin, loratadine, sildenafil, carbamazepine, and pimozide. May also increase the toxic effect of amiodarone, lidocaine, quinidine, warfarin, and tricyclic antidepressants. Serum concentration monitoring of these drugs is necessary. Metronidazole and disulfiram may block the metabolism of propylene glycol (present only in the oral solution formulation of amprenavir), leading to potential toxicity. Concurrent use with this formulation is contraindicated.

**Usual Dosage** Oral:

Capsules:

Children 4-12 years and older (<50 kg): 20 mg/kg twice daily or 15 mg/kg 3 times daily; maximum: 2400 mg/day

Children >13 years (>50 kg) and Adults: 1200 mg twice daily

Solution:

Children 4-12 years or older (up to 16 years weighing <50 kg): 22.5 mg/kg twice daily or 17 mg/kg 3 times daily; maximum: 2800/day

Children 13-16 years (weighing at least 50 kg) or >16 years: 1400 mg twice daily

**Dosage adjustment in hepatic impairment:**

Child-Pugh score between 5-8: 450 mg twice daily

Child-Pugh score between 9-12: 300 mg twice daily

**Patient Information** Amprenavir is not a cure for HIV, nor has it been found to reduce transmission of HIV. Take as directed, with or without food. Maintain adequate fluid intake (2-3 L/day of fluids unless instructed to restrict fluid intake) and adequate nutritional intake (small, frequent meals may help). You will be more susceptible to infection (avoid crowds or exposure to contagious diseases or infection). You may experience headache or confusion (use caution when driving or engaging in tasks requiring alertness until response to drug in known); headache (mild analgesic may help); nausea, vomiting, or increase flatulence (small frequent meals, may help); diarrhea (increased dietary fiber, exercise, or boiled milk may help). Inform prescriber if you experience muscle numbness or tingling; unresolved persistent vomiting, diarrhea, or abdominal pain; difficulty breathing or chest pain; unusual skin rash; or change in color of stool or urine. Avoid alcohol if taking oral solution.

**Additional Information** Capsules contain 109 international units of vitamin E per capsule; oral solution contains 46 international units of vitamin E per mL

**Dosage Forms**

Capsule: 50 mg, 150 mg

Solution, oral: 15 mg/mL (240 mL)

- **AMPT** *see* Metyrosine *on page 363*

## Amyl Nitrite (AM il NYE trite)

**Pharmacologic Category** Antidote; Vasodilator

**Use** Coronary vasodilator in angina pectoris; adjunct in treatment of cyanide poisoning; used to produce changes in the intensity of heart murmurs

**Effects on Mental Status** May cause headache

**Effects on Psychiatric Treatment** None reported

**Usual Dosage** Nasal inhalation:

Cyanide poisoning: Children and Adults: Inhale the vapor from a 0.3 mL crushed ampul every minute for 15-30 seconds until I.V. sodium nitrite infusion is available

Angina: Adults: 1-6 inhalations from 1 crushed ampul; may repeat in 3-5 minutes

**Dosage Forms** Inhalant, crushable glass perles: 0.18 mL, 0.3 mL

- **Amylobarbitone** *see* Amobarbital *on page 35*
- **Amytal®** *see* Amobarbital *on page 35*
- **Anabolin® Injection** *see* Nandrolone *on page 383*
- **Anacin® [OTC]** *see* Aspirin *on page 49*
- **Anadrol®** *see* Oxymetholone *on page 415*
- **Anafranil®** *see* Clomipramine *on page 131*

## Anagrelide (an AG gre lide)

**U.S. Brand Names** Agrylin™

**Pharmacologic Category** Platelet Aggregation Inhibitor

**Use** Agent for essential thrombocythemia (ET); treatment of thrombocytopenia secondary to myeloproliferative disorders

**Effects on Mental Status** May impair ability to concentrate and produce bad dreams

**Effects on Psychiatric Treatment** May cause hypotension which may be exacerbated by psychotropics; may cause heart block; use caution with TCAs

**Usual Dosage** Adults: Oral: 0.5 mg 4 times/day or 1 mg twice daily

Maintain for ≥1 week, then adjust to the lowest effective dose to reduce and maintain platelet count <600,000 µL ideally to the normal range; the dose must not be increased by >0.5 mg/day in any 1 week; maximum dose: 10 mg/day or 2.5 mg/dose

**Dosage Forms** Capsule: 0.5 mg, 1 mg

- **Anamine® Syrup [OTC]** *see* Chlorpheniramine and Pseudoephedrine *on page 114*
- **Anaplex® Liquid [OTC]** *see* Chlorpheniramine and Pseudoephedrine *on page 114*
- **Anaprox®** *see* Naproxen *on page 384*
- **Anaspaz®** *see* Hyoscyamine *on page 279*

## Anastrozole (an AS troe zole)

**U.S. Brand Names** Arimidex®

**Pharmacologic Category** Antineoplastic Agent, Miscellaneous

**Use** Treatment of advanced breast cancer in postmenopausal women with disease progression following tamoxifen therapy. Patients with ER-negative disease and patients who did not respond to tamoxifen therapy rarely responded to anastrozole.

**Effects on Mental Status** Drowsiness, confusion, insomnia, and anxiety are common

**Effects on Psychiatric Treatment** None reported

**Usual Dosage** Breast cancer: Adults: Oral (refer to individual protocols): 1 mg once daily

**Dosage adjustment in renal impairment:** Because only about 10% is excreted unchanged in the urine, dosage adjustment in patients with renal insufficiency is not necessary

**Dosage adjustment in hepatic impairment:** Plasma concentrations in subjects with hepatic cirrhosis were within the range concentrations in normal subjects across all clinical trials; therefore, no dosage adjustment is needed

**Dosage Forms** Tablet: 1 mg

- **Anatuss® [OTC]** *see* Guaifenesin, Phenylpropanolamine, and Dextromethorphan *on page 258*
- **Anatuss® DM [OTC]** *see* Guaifenesin, Pseudoephedrine, and Dextromethorphan *on page 259*
- **Anbesol® [OTC]** *see* Benzocaine *on page 61*
- **Anbesol® Maximum Strength [OTC]** *see* Benzocaine *on page 61*
- **Ancef®** *see* Cefazolin *on page 97*
- **Ancobon®** *see* Flucytosine *on page 228*
- **Andec®** *see* Carbinoxamine *on page 92*
- **Androderm® Transdermal System** *see* Testosterone *on page 536*
- **Andro/Fem® Injection** *see* Estradiol and Testosterone *on page 205*
- **AndroGel®** *see* Testosterone *on page 536*
- **Android®** *see* Methyltestosterone *on page 360*
- **Andro-L.A.® Injection** *see* Testosterone *on page 536*
- **Androlone®-D Injection** *see* Nandrolone *on page 383*
- **Androlone® Injection** *see* Nandrolone *on page 383*
- **Andropository® Injection** *see* Testosterone *on page 536*
- **Anectine® Chloride Injection** *see* Succinylcholine *on page 521*
- **Anectine® Flo-Pack®** *see* Succinylcholine *on page 521*
- **Anestacon®** *see* Lidocaine *on page 317*

♦ **Aneurine Hydrochloride** *see* Thiamine *on page 542*

♦ **Anexsia®** *see* Hydrocodone and Acetaminophen *on page 272*

♦ **Angiotensin-Related Agents Comparison Chart** *see page 700*

♦ **Anhydron®** *see* Cyclothiazide *on page 147*

## Anisotropine (an iss oh TROE peen)

**U.S. Brand Names** Valpin® 50
**Canadian Brand Names** Miradon®
**Pharmacologic Category** Anticholinergic Agent
**Use** Adjunctive treatment of peptic ulcer
**Effects on Mental Status** Rarely may produce confusion and memory impairment
**Effects on Psychiatric Treatment** Anticholinergic effects may be exacerbated by psychotropic with anticholinergic activity (benztropine, TCAs)
**Usual Dosage** Adults: Oral: 50 mg 3 times/day
**Dosage Forms** Tablet, as methylbromide: 50 mg

## Anistreplase (a NISS tre plase)

**U.S. Brand Names** Eminase®
**Pharmacologic Category** Thrombolytic Agent
**Use** Management of acute myocardial infarction (AMI) in adults; lysis of thrombi obstructing coronary arteries, reduction of infarct size; and reduction of mortality associated with AMI
**Effects on Mental Status** None reported
**Effects on Psychiatric Treatment** May cause hypotension which may be exacerbated by psychotropics
**Usual Dosage** Adults: I.V.: 30 units injected over 2-5 minutes as soon as possible after onset of symptoms
**Dosage Forms** Powder for injection, lyophilized: 30 units

♦ **Anodynos-DHC®** *see* Hydrocodone and Acetaminophen *on page 272*

♦ **Anoquan®** *see* Butalbital Compound and Acetaminophen *on page 80*

♦ **Ansaid® Oral** *see* Flurbiprofen *on page 236*

♦ **Ansamycin** *see* Rifabutin *on page 492*

♦ **Antabuse®** *see* Disulfiram *on page 178*

♦ **Antagon®** *see* Ganirelix *on page 246*

♦ **Antazoline-V® Ophthalmic** *see* Naphazoline and Antazoline *on page 383*

♦ **Anthra-Derm®** *see* Anthralin *on page 45*

## Anthralin (AN thra lin)

**U.S. Brand Names** Anthra-Derm®; Drithocreme®; Drithocreme® HP 1%; Dritho-Scalp®
**Canadian Brand Names** Anthraforte®; Anthranol®; Anthrascalp®
**Pharmacologic Category** Antipsoriatic Agent; Keratolytic Agent
**Use** Treatment of psoriasis (quiescent or chronic psoriasis)
**Effects on Mental Status** None reported
**Effects on Psychiatric Treatment** None reported
**Usual Dosage Adults: Topical:** Generally, apply once a day or as directed. The irritant potential of anthralin is directly related to the strength being used and each patient's individual tolerance. Always commence treatment for at least one week using the lowest strength possible.

Skin application: Apply sparingly only to psoriatic lesions and rub gently and carefully into the skin until absorbed. Avoid applying an excessive quantity which may cause unnecessary soiling and staining of the clothing or bed linen.
Scalp application: Comb hair to remove scalar debris and, after suitably parting, rub cream well into the lesions, taking care to prevent the cream from spreading onto the forehead
Remove by washing or showering; optimal period of contact will vary according to the strength used and the patient's response to treatment. Continue treatment until the skin is entirely clear (ie, when there is nothing to feel with the fingers and the texture is normal)

**Dosage Forms**
Cream: 0.1% (50 g, 65 g); 0.2% (65 g); 0.25% (50 g); 0.4% (65 g); 0.5% (50 g); 1% (50 g, 65 g)
Ointment, topical: 0.1% (42.5 g); 0.25% (42.5 g); 0.4% (60 g); 0.5% (42.5 g); 1% (42.5 g)

## Anthrax Vaccine Adsorbed
(AN thraks vak SEEN ad SORBED)

**Pharmacologic Category** Vaccine
**Use** Recommended for individuals who may come in contact with animal products which come from anthrax endemic areas and may be contaminated with *Bacillus anthracis* spores; recommended for high-risk persons such as veterinarians and other handling potentially infected animals. Routine immunization for the general population is not recommended.

The Department of Defense is implementing an anthrax vaccination program against the biological warfare agent anthrax, which will be administered to all active duty and reserve personnel.

**Effects on Mental Status** May rarely produce malaise or fatigue
**Effects on Psychiatric Treatment** None reported
**Usual Dosage**
Primary immunization: S.C.: Three injections of 0.5 mL each given 2 weeks apart followed by three additional S.C. injections given at 6, 12, and 18 months
Subsequent booster injections: 0.5 mL at 1-year intervals are recommended for immunity to be maintained
**Dosage Forms** Injection: 5 mL (10 doses each)

♦ **AntibiOtic® Otic** *see* Neomycin, Polymyxin B, and Hydrocortisone *on page 389*

♦ **Anticholinergic Effects of Common Psychotropic Agents** *see page 702*

♦ **Anticonvulsants by Seizures Type** *see page 703*

♦ **Antidepressant Agents Comparison Chart** *see page 704*

♦ **Antidiuretic Hormone** *see* Vasopressin *on page 581*

## Antihemophilic Factor (Human)
(an tee hee moe FIL ik FAK tor HYU man)

**U.S. Brand Names** Hemofil® M; Humate-P®; Koāte®-HP; Koāte®-HS; Monoclate-P®; Profilate® OSD; Profilate® SD
**Pharmacologic Category** Antihemophilic Agent; Blood Product Derivative
**Use** Management of hemophilia A in patients whom a deficiency in factor VIII has been demonstrated. Can be of significant therapeutic value in patients with acquired factor VII inhibitors not exceeding 10 Bethesda units/mL.
**Orphan drug status:** von Willebrand disease and prevention of bleeding from surgery in hemophilia A
**Effects on Mental Status** None reported
**Effects on Psychiatric Treatment** None reported
**Usual Dosage** I.V.: Individualize dosage based on coagulation studies performed prior to and during treatment at regular intervals; 1 AHF unit is the activity present in 1 mL of normal pooled human plasma; dosage should be adjusted to actual vial size currently stocked in the pharmacy.

Hospitalized patients: 20-50 units/kg/dose; may be higher for special circumstances; dose can be given every 12-24 hours and more frequently in special circumstances
Surgery patients: The factor VIII level should be raised to approximately 100% by giving a preoperative dose of 50 international units/kg, to maintain hemostatic levels, repeat infusions may be necessary every 6-12 hours initially and for a total of 10-14 days until healing is complete
**Formula to approximate percentage increase in plasma antihemophilic factor:**
Units required = desired level increase (desired level - actual level) x plasma volume (mL)
Total blood volume (mL blood/kg) = 70 mL/kg (adults); 80 mL/kg (children)
Plasma volume = total blood volume (mL) x [1 - Hct (in decimals)]
Example: For a 70 kg adult with a Hct = 40%: plasma volume = [70 kg x 70 mL/kg] x [1 - 0.4] = 2940 mL
To calculate number of units of factor VIII needed to increase level to desired range (highly individualized and dependent on patient's condition):
Number of units = desired level increase [desired level - actual level] x plasma volume (in mL)
Example: For a 100% level in the above patient who has an actual level of 20% the number of units needed = [1 (for a 100% level) - 0.2] x 2940 mL = 2352 units
**Dosage Forms** Injection: 10 mL, 20 mL, 30 mL

## Antihemophilic Factor (Porcine)
(an tee hee moe FIL ik FAK ter POR seen)

**U.S. Brand Names** Hyate®:C
**Pharmacologic Category** Antihemophilic Agent
**Use** Treatment of congenital hemophiliacs with antibodies to human factor VIII:C and also for previously nonhemophiliac patients with spontaneously acquired inhibitors to human factor VIII:C; patients with inhibitors who are bleeding or who are to undergo surgery
**Effects on Mental Status** None reported
**Effects on Psychiatric Treatment** None reported
**Usual Dosage** Clinical response should be used to assess efficacy rather than relying upon a particular laboratory value for recovery of factor VIII:C.
(Continued)

## Antihemophilic Factor (Porcine) *(Continued)*

Initial dose:

Antibody level to human factor VIII:C <50 Bethesda units/mL: 100-150 porcine units/kg (body weight) is recommended

Antibody level to human factor VIII:C >50 Bethesda units/mL: Activity of the antibody to porcine factor VIII:C should be determined; **an anti-porcine antibody level** >20 Bethesda units/mL indicates that the patient is unlikely to benefit from treatment; for lower titers, a dose of 100-150 porcine units/kg is recommended

If a patient has previously been treated with Hyate:C®, this may provide a guide to his likely response and, therefore, assist in estimation of the preliminary dose

Subsequent doses: Following administration of the initial dose, if the recovery of factor VIII:C in the patient's plasma is not sufficient, a further higher dose should be administered; if recovery after the second dose is still insufficient, a third and higher dose may prove effective

**Dosage Forms** Powder for injection, lyophilized: 400-700 porcine units to be reconstituted with 20 mL sterile water

## Antihemophilic Factor (Recombinant)

(an tee hee moe FIL ik FAK tor ree KOM be nant)

**U.S. Brand Names** Bioclate®; Helixate®; Kogenate®; Recombinate™

**Pharmacologic Category** Antihemophilic Agent

**Use** Management of hemophilia A in patients whom a deficiency in factor VIII has been demonstrated

**Effects on Mental Status** None reported

**Effects on Psychiatric Treatment** None reported

**Usual Dosage** I.V.: Individualize dosage based on coagulation studies performed prior to and during treatment at regular intervals. One AHF unit is the activity present in 1 mL of normal pooled human plasma; dosage should be adjusted to actual vial size currently stocked in the pharmacy.

Hospitalized patients: 20-50 units/kg/dose; may be higher for special circumstances; dose can be given every 12-24 hours and more frequently in special circumstances

**Formula to approximate percentage increase in plasma antihemophilic factor:**

Units required = desired level increase (desired level - actual level) x plasma volume (mL)

Total blood volume (mL blood/kg) = 70 mL/kg (adults); 80 mL/kg (children).

Plasma volume = total blood volume (mL) x [1 - Hct (in decimals)]

ie, for a 70 kg adult with a Hct = 40% : plasma volume = [70 kg x 70 mL/kg] x [1 - 0.4] = 2940 mL

To calculate number of units of factor VIII needed to increase level to desired range (highly individualized and dependent on patient's condition):

Number of units = desired level increase [desired level - actual level] x plasma volume (in mL)

ie, for a 100% level in the above patient who has an actual level of 20% the number of units needed = [1 (for a 100% level) - 0.2] x 2940 mL = 2352 units

**Dosage Forms** Injection: 250 units, 500 units, 1000 units

♦ **Antihist-1® [OTC]** *see* Clemastine *on page 128*

♦ **Antihist-D®** *see* Clemastine and Phenylpropanolamine *on page 128*

## Anti-inhibitor Coagulant Complex

(an tee-in HI bi tor coe AG yoo lant KOM pleks)

**U.S. Brand Names** Autoplex® T; Feiba VH Immuno®

**Pharmacologic Category** Antihemophilic Agent; Blood Product Derivative

**Use** Patients with factor VIII inhibitors who are to undergo surgery or those who are bleeding

**Effects on Mental Status** None reported

**Effects on Psychiatric Treatment** None reported

**Usual Dosage** Dosage range: 25-100 factor VIII correctional units per kg depending on the severity of hemorrhage

**Dosage Forms** Injection:

Autoplex® T, with heparin 2 units: Each bottle is labeled with correctional units of Factor VIII

Feiba VH Immuno®, heparin free: Each bottle is labeled with correctional units of Factor VIII

♦ **Antilirium®** *see* Physostigmine *on page 444*

♦ **Antiminth® [OTC]** *see* Pyrantel Pamoate *on page 480*

♦ **Antiparkinsonian Agents Comparison Chart** *see page 705*

♦ **Antipsychotic Agents Comparison Chart** *see page 706*

♦ **Antipsychotic Medication Guidelines** *see page 751*

## Antirabies Serum (Equine)

(an tee RAY beez SEER um EE kwine)

**Pharmacologic Category** Immune Globulin

**Use** Rabies prophylaxis

**Effects on Mental Status** None reported

**Effects on Psychiatric Treatment** None reported

**Usual Dosage** 1000 units/55 lb in a single dose, infiltrate up to 50% of dose around the wound

**Dosage Forms** Injection: 125 units/mL (8 mL)

♦ **Antispas® Injection** *see* Dicyclomine *on page 165*

## Antithrombin III (an tee THROM bin three)

**U.S. Brand Names** ATnativ®; Thrombate III®

**Pharmacologic Category** Anticoagulant; Blood Product Derivative

**Use** Agent for hereditary antithrombin III deficiency

**Unlabeled use:** Has been used effectively for acquired antithrombin III deficiencies related to DIC, pre-eclampsia, liver disease, shock and surgery complicated by DIC

**Effects on Mental Status** None reported

**Effects on Psychiatric Treatment** None reported

**Usual Dosage** After first dose of antithrombin III, level should increase to 120% of normal; thereafter maintain at levels >80%. Generally, achieved by administration of maintenance doses once every 24 hours; initially and until patient is stabilized, measure antithrombin III level at least twice daily, thereafter once daily and always immediately before next infusion. 1 unit = quantity of antithrombin III in 1 mL of normal pooled human plasma; administration of 1 unit/1 kg raises AT-III level by 1% to 2%; assume plasma volume of 40 mL/kg

Initial dosage (units) = [desired AT-III level % - baseline AT-III level %] x body weight (kg) divided by 1%/units/kg, eg, if a 70 kg adult patient had a baseline AT-III level of 57%, the initial dose would be (120% - 57%) x 70/ 1%/units/kg = 4,410 units

Measure antithrombin III preceding and 30 minutes after dose to calculate *in vivo* recovery rate; maintain level within normal range for 2-8 days depending on type of surgery or procedure

**Dosage Forms** Powder for injection: 500 units (50 mL)

## Antithymocyte Globulin (Rabbit)

(an te THY moe site GLOB yu lin (RAB bit)

**Pharmacologic Category** Immune Globulin

**Use** Treatment of renal transplant acute rejection in conjunction with concomitant immunosuppression

**Effects on Mental Status** None reported

**Effects on Psychiatric Treatment** Leukopenia and thrombocytopenia are common; use caution with clozapine, carbamazepine, and valproic acid

**Usual Dosage** I.V.: 1.5 mg/kg/day for 7-14 days

**Dosage Forms** Injection: 25 mg vials (with diluent)

♦ **Anti-Tuss® Expectorant [OTC]** *see* Guaifenesin *on page 256*

♦ **Antivert®** *see* Meclizine *on page 335*

♦ **Antizol®** *see* Fomepizole *on page 240*

♦ **Antrizine®** *see* Meclizine *on page 335*

♦ **Anturane®** *see* Sulfinpyrazone *on page 525*

♦ **Anucort-HC® Suppository** *see* Hydrocortisone *on page 273*

♦ **Anuprep HC® Suppository** *see* Hydrocortisone *on page 273*

♦ **Anusol® HC 1 [OTC]** *see* Hydrocortisone *on page 273*

♦ **Anusol® HC 2.5% [OTC]** *see* Hydrocortisone *on page 273*

♦ **Anusol-HC® Suppository** *see* Hydrocortisone *on page 273*

♦ **Anusol® Ointment [OTC]** *see* Pramoxine *on page 457*

♦ **Anxanil®** *see* Hydroxyzine *on page 278*

♦ **Anxiety Disorders** *see page 606*

♦ **Anxiolytic/Hypnotic Use in Long-Term Care Facilities** *see page 754*

♦ **Anzemet®** *see* Dolasetron *on page 181*

♦ **Apacet® [OTC]** *see* Acetaminophen *on page 14*

♦ **APAP** *see* Acetaminophen *on page 14*

♦ **Apatate® [OTC]** *see* Vitamin B Complex *on page 586*

♦ **Aphrodyne™** *see* Yohimbine *on page 589*

♦ **Aphthasol™** *see* Amlexanox *on page 35*

♦ **A.P.L.®** *see* Chorionic Gonadotropin *on page 122*

♦ **Aplisol®** *see* Tuberculin Purified Protein Derivative *on page 575*

♦ **Aplitest®** *see* Tuberculin Purified Protein Derivative *on page 575*

## Apomorphine (a poe MOR feen)

**U.S. Brand Names** Uprima™
**Pharmacologic Category** Dopamine Agonist; Impotency Agent
**Use Unlabeled use:** Treatment of erectile dysfunction
**Effects on Mental Status** May cause dizziness or sedation; may rarely cause agitation, confusion, anxiety, insomnia, depression, or euphoria
**Effects on Psychiatric Treatment** Nausea is common, caution with the SSRIs
**Usual Dosage** Adults and Elderly: Sublingual: Initial dose: 2 mg; subsequent doses may be adjusted to a maximum of 4 mg; onset of erection usually occurs within 15-25 minutes; allow at least 8 hours between doses

**Dosage adjustment in renal impairment:** Bioavailability is increased with decreased renal function, however, maximum plasma levels are not significantly changed; begin with 2 mg/dose; any dosage increases should be made with caution

**Dosage adjustment in hepatic impairment:** Half-life and plasma levels are increased with hepatic impairment; use in patients with severe hepatic impairment only if benefits outweigh the risk; begin with 2 mg/dose; any dosage increases should be made with caution

**Additional Information** Apomorphine has little structural similarity to opiates and no narcotic activity.

**Note:** On June 30, 2000, TAP Pharmaceutical Products Inc announced they have voluntarily withdrawn their New Drug Application (NDA) for Uprima® (apomorphine). Uprima® was being studied to treat erectile dysfunction. The company stated that ongoing studies are currently underway to clarify the medications safety and efficacy. According to another news source, one of the side effects reported in the product information, the decrease in blood pressure, was of most concern. TAP is hoping to resubmit the NDA at some point in the future.

**Dosage Forms** Tablet, sublingual: 2 mg, 3 mg, 4 mg

## Apraclonidine (a pra KLOE ni deen)

**U.S. Brand Names** Iopidine®
**Pharmacologic Category** $Alpha_2$ Agonist, Ophthalmic
**Use** Prevention and treatment of postsurgical intraocular pressure elevation
**Effects on Mental Status** May cause drowsiness
**Effects on Psychiatric Treatment** Dry mouth may be exacerbated by concurrent use of psychotropics
**Usual Dosage** Adults: Ophthalmic:

0.5%: Instill 1-2 drops in the affected eye(s) 3 times/day; since apraclonidine 0.5% will be used with other ocular glaucoma therapies, use an approximate 5-minute interval between instillation of each medication to prevent washout of the previous dose

1%: Instill 1 drop in operative eye 1 hour prior to anterior segment laser surgery, second drop in eye immediately upon completion of procedure

**Dosing adjustment in renal impairment:** Although the topical use of apraclonidine has not been studied in renal failure patients, structurally related clonidine undergoes a significant increase in half-life in patients with severe renal impairment; close monitoring of cardiovascular parameters in patients with impaired renal function is advised if they are candidates for topical apraclonidine therapy

**Dosing adjustment in hepatic impairment:** Close monitoring of cardiovascular parameters in patients with impaired liver function is advised because the systemic dosage form of clonidine is partially metabolized in the liver

**Dosage Forms** Solution, ophthalmic, as hydrochloride: 0.5% (5 mL); 1% (0.1 mL, 0.25 mL)

♦ **Apresazide®** *see* Hydralazine and Hydrochlorothiazide *on page 270*

♦ **Apresoline®** *see* Hydralazine *on page 270*

♦ **Apri®** *see* Ethinyl Estradiol and Desogestrel *on page 211*

♦ **Aprodine® Syrup [OTC]** *see* Triprolidine and Pseudoephedrine *on page 572*

♦ **Aprodine® Tablet [OTC]** *see* Triprolidine and Pseudoephedrine *on page 572*

♦ **Aprodine® w/C** *see* Triprolidine, Pseudoephedrine, and Codeine *on page 572*

## Aprotinin (a proe TYE nin)

**U.S. Brand Names** Trasylol®
**Pharmacologic Category** Blood Product Derivative; Hemostatic Agent
**Use** Reduction or prevention of blood loss in patients undergoing coronary artery bypass surgery when a high risk of excessive bleeding exists, including open heart reoperation, pre-existing coagulopathies, operations on the great vessels, and when a patient's beliefs prohibit blood transfusions
**Effects on Mental Status** May cause confusion
**Effects on Psychiatric Treatment** May cause renal dysfunction; use caution with lithium and gabapentin; may rarely cause seizures; use caution with clozapine
**Usual Dosage** least 10 minutes prior to the loading dose to assess the potential for allergic reactions

Regimen A (standard dose):
2 million units (280 mg) loading dose I.V. over 20-30 minutes
2 million units (280 mg) into pump prime volume
500,000 units/hour (70 mg/hour) I.V. during operation

Regimen B (low dose):
1 million units (140 mg) loading dose I.V. over 20-30 minutes
1 million units (140 mg) into pump prime volume
250,000 units/hour (35 mg/hour) I.V. during operation

**Dosage Forms** Injection: 1.4 mg/mL [10,000 units/mL] (100 mL, 200 mL)

♦ **Aquacare® Topical [OTC]** *see* Urea *on page 576*

♦ **Aquachloral® Supprettes®** *see* Chloral Hydrate *on page 107*

♦ **AquaMEPHYTON® Injection** *see* Phytonadione *on page 444*

♦ **Aquaphyllin®** *see* Theophylline Salts *on page 539*

♦ **AquaSite® Ophthalmic Solution [OTC]** *see* Artificial Tears *on page 48*

♦ **Aquasol A®** *see* Vitamin A *on page 585*

♦ **Aquasol E® [OTC]** *see* Vitamin E *on page 586*

♦ **Aquatensen®** *see* Methyclothiazide *on page 356*

♦ **Aqueous Testosterone** *see* Testosterone *on page 536*

♦ **Aquest®** *see* Estrone *on page 208*

♦ **Aralen® Phosphate** *see* Chloroquine Phosphate *on page 111*

♦ **Aralen® Phosphate With Primaquine Phosphate** *see* Chloroquine and Primaquine *on page 111*

♦ **Aramine®** *see* Metaraminol *on page 347*

♦ **Arava™** *see* Leflunomide *on page 308*

## Ardeparin (ar dee PA rin)

**U.S. Brand Names** Normiflo®
**Pharmacologic Category** Low Molecular Weight Heparin
**Use** Prevention of deep vein thrombosis (DVT) which may lead to pulmonary embolism following knee replacement surgery
**Effects on Mental Status** Rare reports of confusion
**Effects on Psychiatric Treatment** None reported
**Usual Dosage** Adults: S.C.: DVT prophylaxis: 50 anti-Xa units/kg every 12 hours

If the ardeparin formulation used contains 5000 anti-Xa units/0.5 mL (recommended for patients up to 100 kg or 220 lb), the volume to be administered is calculated as follows:

Patient's weight (kg) x 0.005 mL/kg = volume (mL)

If the ardeparin formulation used contains 10,000 anti-Xa units/0.5 mL (recommended for patients >100 kg or 220 lb), the volume to be administered is calculated as follows:

Patient's weight (kg) x 0.0025 mL/kg = volume (mL)

**Dosage adjustment in renal impairment:** No adjustment is necessary, although there is limited experience in this population.

Not dialyzable

**Dosage Forms** Injection, as sodium: 5000 anti-Xa units (0.5 mL); 10,000 anti-Xa units (0.5 mL)

♦ **Arduan®** *see* Pipecuronium *on page 447*

♦ **Aredia™** *see* Pamidronate *on page 418*

♦ **Argesic®-SA** *see* Salsalate *on page 503*

## Arginine (AR ji neen)

**U.S. Brand Names** R-Gene®
**Pharmacologic Category** Diagnostic Agent, Pituitary Function
**Use** Pituitary function test (growth hormone); management of severe, uncompensated, metabolic alkalosis (pH ≥7.55) **after** optimizing therapy with sodium and potassium supplements
**Effects on Mental Status** None reported
**Effects on Psychiatric Treatment** None reported
**Usual Dosage** I.V.:

Pituitary function test:
Children: 500 mg kg/dose administered over 30 minutes
Adults: 30 g (300 mL) administered over 30 minutes
(Continued)

## Arginine *(Continued)*

Inborn errors of urea synthesis: Initial: 0.8 g/kg, then 0.2-0.8 g/kg/day as a continuous infusion

Metabolic alkalosis: Children and Adults: ***Arginine hydrochloride is a fourth-line treatment for uncompensated metabolic alkalosis after sodium chloride, potassium chloride, and ammonium chloride supplementation has been optimized.***

Arginine dose (G) = weight (kg) x 0.1 x ($HCO_3^-$ - 24) where $HCO_3^-$ = the patient's serum bicarbonate concentration in mEq/L

Give 1/2 to 1/3 dose calculated then re-evaluate

**Note:** Arginine hydrochloride should never be used as an alternative to chloride supplementation but used in the patient who is unresponsive to sodium chloride or potassium chloride supplementation

Hypochloremia: Children and Adults: Arginine dose (mL) = 0.4 x weight (kg) x (103-$Cl^-$) where $Cl^-$ = the patient's serum chloride concentration in mEq/L

Give 1/2 to 1/3 dose calculated then re-evaluate

**Dosage Forms** Injection, as hydrochloride: 10% [100 mg/mL = 950 mOsm/L] (500 mL)


- **8-Arginine Vasopressin** *see* Vasopressin *on page 581*
- **Aricept®** *see* Donepezil *on page 181*
- **Arimidex®** *see* Anastrozole *on page 44*
- **Aristocort®** *see* Triamcinolone *on page 563*
- **Aristocort® A** *see* Triamcinolone *on page 563*
- **Aristocort® Forte** *see* Triamcinolone *on page 563*
- **Aristocort® Intralesional** *see* Triamcinolone *on page 563*
- **Aristospan® Intra-Articular** *see* Triamcinolone *on page 563*
- **Aristospan® Intralesional** *see* Triamcinolone *on page 563*
- **Arm-a-Med® Isoetharine** *see* Isoetharine *on page 294*
- **Arm-a-Med® Isoproterenol** *see* Isoproterenol *on page 295*
- **Arm-a-Med® Metaproterenol** *see* Metaproterenol *on page 347*
- **A.R.M.® Caplet [OTC]** *see* Chlorpheniramine and Phenylpropanolamine *on page 114*
- **Armour® Thyroid** *see* Thyroid *on page 547*
- **Aromasin®** *see* Exemestane *on page 217*
- **Arrestin®** *see* Trimethobenzamide *on page 569*
- **Artane®** *see* Trihexyphenidyl *on page 568*
- ***Artemisia absinthium*** *see* Wormwood *on page 588*
- **Artha-G®** *see* Salsalate *on page 503*
- **Arthritis Foundation® Nighttime [OTC]** *see* Acetaminophen and Diphenhydramine *on page 15*
- **Arthritis Foundation® Pain Reliever [OTC]** *see* Aspirin *on page 49*
- **Arthrotec®** *see* Diclofenac and Misoprostol *on page 164*
- **Articulose-50® Injection** *see* Prednisolone *on page 459*


## Artificial Tears (ar ti FISH il tears)

**U.S. Brand Names** Adsorbotear® Ophthalmic Solution [OTC]; Akwa Tears® Solution [OTC]; AquaSite® Ophthalmic Solution [OTC]; Bion® Tears Solution [OTC]; Comfort® Tears Solution [OTC]; Dakrina® Ophthalmic Solution [OTC]; Dry Eye® Therapy Solution [OTC]; Dry Eyes® Solution [OTC]; Dwelle® Ophthalmic Solution [OTC]; Eye-Lube-A® Solution [OTC]; HypoTears PF Solution [OTC]; HypoTears Solution [OTC]; Isopto® Plain Solution [OTC]; Isopto® Tears Solution [OTC]; Just Tears® Solution [OTC]; Lacril® Ophthalmic Solution [OTC]; Liquifilm® Tears Solution [OTC]; Liquifilm® Forte Solution [OTC]; LubriTears® Solution [OTC]; Moisture® Ophthalmic Drops [OTC]; Murine® Solution [OTC]; Murocel® Ophthalmic Solution [OTC]; Nature's Tears® Solution [OTC]; Nu-Tears® Solution [OTC]; Nu-Tears® II Solution [OTC]; OcuCoat® Ophthalmic Solution [OTC]; OcuCoat® PF Ophthalmic Solution [OTC]; Puralube® Tears Solution [OTC]; Refresh® Ophthalmic Solution [OTC]; Refresh® Plus Ophthalmic Solution [OTC]; Tear Drop® Solution [OTC]; TearGard® Ophthalmic Solution [OTC]; Teargen® Ophthalmic Solution [OTC]; Tearisol® Solution [OTC]; Tears Naturale® Free Solution [OTC]; Tears Naturale® II Solution [OTC]; Tears Naturale® Solution [OTC]; Tears Plus® Solution [OTC]; Tears Renewed® Solution [OTC]; Ultra Tears® Solution [OTC]; Viva-Drops® Solution [OTC]

**Pharmacologic Category** Ophthalmic Agent, Miscellaneous

**Use** Ophthalmic lubricant; for relief of dry eyes and eye irritation

**Effects on Mental Status** None reported

**Effects on Psychiatric Treatment** None reported

**Usual Dosage** Use as needed to relieve symptoms, 1-2 drops into eye(s) 3-4 times/day

**Dosage Forms** Solution, ophthalmic: 15 mL and 30 mL with dropper


- **A.S.A. [OTC]** *see* Aspirin *on page 49*
- **ASA** *see* Aspirin *on page 49*
- **5-ASA** *see* Mesalamine *on page 344*
- **Asacol® Oral** *see* Mesalamine *on page 344*


## Ascorbic Acid (a SKOR bik AS id)

**U.S. Brand Names** Ascorbicap® [OTC]; C-Crystals® [OTC]; Cebid® Timecelles® [OTC]; Cecon® [OTC]; Cevalin® [OTC]; Cevi-Bid® [OTC]; Ce-Vi-Sol® [OTC]; Dull-C® [OTC]; Flavorcee® [OTC]; N'ice® Vitamin C Drops [OTC]; Vita-C® [OTC]

**Canadian Brand Names** Apo®-C; Ascorbic 500; Redoxon®; Revitalose-C-1000®

**Pharmacologic Category** Vitamin, Water Soluble

**Use** Prevention and treatment of scurvy and to acidify the urine

**Unlabeled use:** In large doses to decrease the severity of "colds"; dietary supplementation; a 20-year study was recently completed involving 730 individuals which indicates a possible decreased risk of death by stroke when ascorbic acid at doses ≥45 mg/day was administered

**Effects on Mental Status** Rare reports of drowsiness; usually well tolerated

**Effects on Psychiatric Treatment** May decrease fluphenazine levels; clinical significance unknown but likely not problematic

**Usual Dosage** Oral, I.M., I.V., S.C.:

Recommended daily allowance (RDA):
- <6 months: 30 mg
- 6 months to 1 year: 35 mg
- 1-3 years: 40 mg
- 4-10 years: 45 mg
- 11-14 years: 50 mg
- >14 years and Adults: 60 mg

Children:
- Scurvy: 100-300 mg/day in divided doses for at least 2 weeks
- Urinary acidification: 500 mg every 6-8 hours
- Dietary supplement: 35-100 mg/day

Adults:
- Scurvy: 100-250 mg 1-2 times/day for at least 2 weeks
- Urinary acidification: 4-12 g/day in 3-4 divided doses
- Prevention and treatment of colds: 1-3 g/day
- Dietary supplement: 50-200 mg/day

**Dosage Forms**

Capsule, timed release: 500 mg
Crystals: 4 g/teaspoonful (100 g, 500 g); 5 g/teaspoonful (180 g)
Injection: 250 mg/mL (2 mL, 30 mL); 500 mg/mL (2 mL, 50 mL)
Liquid, oral: 35 mg/0.6 mL (50 mL)
Lozenges: 60 mg
Powder: 4 g/teaspoonful (100 g, 500 g)
Solution, oral: 100 mg/mL (50 mL)
Syrup: 500 mg/5 mL (5 mL, 10 mL, 120 mL, 480 mL)
Tablet: 25 mg, 50 mg, 100 mg, 250 mg, 500 mg, 1000 mg
Tablet:
- Chewable: 100 mg, 250 mg, 500 mg
- Timed release: 500 mg, 1000 mg, 1500 mg


- **Ascorbicap® [OTC]** *see* Ascorbic Acid *on page 48*
- **Ascriptin® [OTC]** *see* Aspirin *on page 49*
- **ASE-136BS** *see* Dirithromycin *on page 177*
- **Asendin®** *see* Amoxapine *on page 37*
- **Asmalix®** *see* Theophylline Salts *on page 539*


## Asparaginase (a SPIR a ji nase)

**U.S. Brand Names** Elspar®

**Canadian Brand Names** Kidrolase®

**Pharmacologic Category** Antineoplastic Agent, Miscellaneous

**Use** Treatment of acute lymphocytic leukemia, lymphoma; used for induction therapy

**Effects on Mental Status** Rare reports of depression, disorientation, and hallucinations

**Effects on Psychiatric Treatment** May cause myelosuppression; use caution with clozapine and carbamazepine

**Usual Dosage** Refer to individual protocols; dose must be individualized based upon clinical response and tolerance of the patient

I.M. administration is **preferred** over I.V. administration; I.M. administration may decrease the risk of anaphylaxis

Asparaginase is available from two different microbiological sources: One is from *Escherichia coli* and the other is from *Erwinia carotovora*; the *Erwinia* is restricted to patients who have sustained allergic reactions to the *E. coli* preparation

I.M., I.V.: 6000 units/m$^2$ every other day for 3-4 weeks or daily doses of 1000-20,000 units/m$^2$ for 10-20 days; other induction regimens have been utilized

Hemodialysis: Significant drug removal is unlikely based on physiochemical characteristics

Peritoneal dialysis: Significant drug removal is unlikely based on physiochemical characteristics

Desensitization should be performed before administering the first dose of asparaginase to patients who developed a positive reaction to the intradermal skin test or who are being retreated; one schedule begins with a total of 1 unit given I.V. and doubles the dose every 10 minutes until the total amount given in the planned dose for that day

For example, if a patient was to receive a total dose of 4000 units, he/she would receive injections 1 through 12 during the desensitization

**Dosage Forms** Injection:
10,000 units/10 mL
10,000 units/vial (*Erwinia*)

♦ **A-Spas® S/L** *see* Hyoscyamine *on page 279*

♦ **Aspergum® [OTC]** *see* Aspirin *on page 49*

## Aspirin (AS pir in)

**U.S. Brand Names** Anacin® [OTC]; Arthritis Foundation® Pain Reliever [OTC]; A.S.A. [OTC]; Ascriptin® [OTC]; Aspergum® [OTC]; Asprimox® [OTC]; Bayer® Aspirin [OTC]; Bayer® Buffered Aspirin [OTC]; Bayer® Low Adult Strength [OTC]; Bufferin® [OTC]; Buffex® [OTC]; Cama® Arthritis Pain Reliever [OTC]; Easprin®; Ecotrin® [OTC]; Ecotrin® Low Adult Strength [OTC]; Empirin® [OTC]; Extra Strength Adprin-B® [OTC]; Extra Strength Bayer® Enteric 500 Aspirin [OTC]; Extra Strength Bayer® Plus [OTC]; Halfprin® 81® [OTC]; Heartline® [OTC]; Regular Strength Bayer® Enteric 500 Aspirin [OTC]; St Joseph® Adult Chewable Aspirin [OTC]; ZORprin®

**Canadian Brand Names** Apo®-ASA; ASA®; Asaphen; Entrophen®; MSD® Enteric Coated ASA; Novasen

**Synonyms** Acetylsalicylic Acid; ASA

**Pharmacologic Category** Salicylate

**Use** Treatment of mild to moderate pain, inflammation, and fever; prophylaxis for myocardial infarction and transient ischemic episodes; management of rheumatoid arthritis, rheumatic fever, osteoarthritis, and gout (high dose)

**Effects on Mental Status** May cause drowsiness

**Effects on Psychiatric Treatment** May cause leukopenia; use caution with clozapine and carbamazepine; may displace valproic acid from binding sites resulting in an increase of unbound drug; monitor for toxicity

**Pregnancy Risk Factor** C (D if full-dose aspirin in 3rd trimester)

**Contraindications** Hypersensitivity to salicylates or other NSAIDs; asthma; rhinitis; nasal polyps; inherited or acquired bleeding disorders (including factor VII and factor IX deficiency); pregnancy (in 3rd trimester especially); do not use in children (<16 years of age) for viral infections (chickenpox or flu symptoms), with or without fever, due to a potential association with Reye's syndrome

**Warnings/Precautions** Use with caution in patients with platelet and bleeding disorders, renal dysfunction, dehydration, erosive gastritis, or peptic ulcer disease. Heavy alcohol use (>3 drinks/day) can increase bleeding risks. Avoid use in severe renal failure or in severe hepatic failure. Discontinue use if tinnitus or impaired hearing occurs. Caution in mild-moderate renal failure (only at high dosages). Patients with sensitivity to tartrazine dyes, nasal polyps and asthma may have an increased risk of salicylate sensitivity. Surgical patients should avoid ASA if possible, for 1-2 weeks prior to surgery, to reduce the risk of excessive bleeding.

### Salicylates

| Toxic Symptoms | Treatment |
|---|---|
| Overdose | Induce emesis with ipecac, and/or lavage with saline, followed with activated charcoal |
| Dehydration | I.V. fluids with KCl (no $D_5W$ only) |
| Metabolic acidosis (must be treated) | Sodium bicarbonate |
| Hyperthermia | Cooling blankets or sponge baths |
| Coagulopathy/hemorrhage | Vitamin K I.V. |
| Hypoglycemia (with coma, seizures, or change in mental status) | Dextrose 25 g I.V. |
| Seizures | Diazepam 5-10 mg I.V. |

**Adverse Reactions**
>10%: Gastrointestinal: Dyspepsia, epigastric discomfort, heartburn, nausea, stomach pains, vomiting

1% to 10%:
Central nervous system: Fatigue
Dermatologic: Rash, urticaria
Gastrointestinal: Gastrointestinal ulceration
Hematologic: Hemolytic anemia
Neuromuscular & skeletal: Weakness
Respiratory: Dyspnea
Miscellaneous: Anaphylactic shock

<1%: Anemia, bronchospasm, hepatotoxicity, impaired renal function, insomnia, iron deficiency, jitters, leukemia, nervousness, occult bleeding, prolongation of bleeding time, thrombocytopenia

**Overdosage/Toxicology**
Signs and symptoms of overdose include tinnitus, headache, dizziness, confusion, metabolic acidosis, hyperpyrexia, hypoglycemia, coma

Treatment: Based upon symptomatology

**Drug Interactions**
ACE inhibitors: The effects of ACE inhibitors may be blunted by aspirin administration, particularly at higher dosages

Buspirone increases aspirin's free % *in vitro*

Carbonic anhydrase inhibitors and corticosteroids have been associated with alteration in salicylate serum concentrations

Heparin and low molecular weight heparins: Concurrent use may increase the risk of bleeding

Methotrexate serum levels may be increased; consider discontinuing aspirin 2-3 days before high-dose methotrexate treatment or avoid concurrent use

NSAIDs may increase the risk of gastrointestinal adverse effects and bleeding. Serum concentrations of some NSAIDs may be decreased by aspirin

Platelet inhibitors (IIb/IIa antagonists): Risk of bleeding may be increased

Probenecid effects may be antagonized by aspirin

Sulfonylureas: The effects of older sulfonylurea agents (tolazamide, tolbutamide) may be potentiated due to displacement from plasma proteins. This effect does not appear to be clinically significant for newer sulfonylurea agents (glyburide, glipizide, glimepiride).

Valproic acid may be displaced from its binding sites which can result in toxicity

Verapamil may potentiate the prolongation of bleeding time associated with aspirin

Warfarin and oral anticoagulants may increase the risk of bleeding

**Usual Dosage**
Children:
Analgesic and antipyretic: Oral, rectal: 10-15 mg/kg/dose every 4-6 hours, up to a total of 60-80 mg/kg/24 hours

Anti-inflammatory: Oral: Initial: 60-90 mg/kg/day in divided doses; usual maintenance: 80-100 mg/kg/day divided every 6-8 hours, maximum dose: 3.6 g/day; monitor serum concentrations

Kawasaki disease: Oral: 80-100 mg/kg/day divided every 6 hours; after fever resolves: 8-10 mg/kg/day once daily; monitor serum concentrations

Antirheumatic: Oral: 60-100 mg/kg/day in divided doses every 4 hours

Adults:
Analgesic and antipyretic: Oral, rectal: 325-650 mg every 4-6 hours up to 4 g/day

Anti-inflammatory: Oral: Initial: 2.4-3.6 g/day in divided doses; usual maintenance: 3.6-5.4 g/day; monitor serum concentrations

TIA: Oral: 1.3 g/day in 2-4 divided doses

Myocardial infarction prophylaxis: 160-325 mg/day; a lower aspirin dosage has been recommended in patients receiving ACE inhibitors

**Dosing adjustment in renal impairment:** $Cl_{cr}$ <10 mL/minute: Avoid use.

Hemodialysis: Dialyzable (50% to 100%)

**Dosing adjustment in hepatic disease:** Avoid use in severe liver disease.

**Dietary Considerations**
Alcohol: Combination causes GI irritation, possible bleeding; avoid or limit alcohol. Patients at increased risk include those prone to hypoprothrombinemia, vitamin K deficiency, thrombocytopenia, thrombotic thrombocytopenia purpura, severe hepatic impairment, and those receiving anticoagulants.

Food: May decrease the rate but not the extent of oral absorption. Drug may cause GI upset, bleeding, ulceration, perforation. Take with food or large volume of water or milk to minimize GI upset.

Folic acid: Hyperexcretion of folate; folic acid deficiency may result, leading to macrocytic anemia. Supplement with folic acid if necessary.

Iron: With chronic aspirin use and at doses of 3-4 g/day, iron deficiency anemia may result; supplement with iron if necessary

Sodium: Hypernatremia resulting from buffered aspirin solutions or sodium salicylate containing high sodium content. Avoid or use with caution in CHF or any condition where hypernatremia would be detrimental.

Curry powder, paprika, licorice, Benedictine liqueur, prunes, raisins, tea and gherkins: Potential salicylate accumulation. These foods contain 6 mg salicylate/100 g. An ordinarily American diet contains 10-200 mg/day of salicylate. Foods containing salicylates may contribute to aspirin hypersensitivity. Patients at greatest risk for aspirin hypersensitivity include those with asthma, nasal polyposis or chronic urticaria.

Fresh fruits containing vitamin C: Displaces drug from binding sites, resulting in increased urinary excretion of aspirin. Educate patients regarding the potential for a decreased analgesic effect of aspirin with consumption of foods high in vitamin C.

**Patient Information** If self-administered, use exactly as directed (do not increase dose or frequency); adverse reactions can occur with overuse. Take with food or milk. Do not use aspirin with strong vinegar-like odor. Do not crush or chew extended release products. While using this medication,

(Continued)

## Aspirin *(Continued)*

avoid alcohol, excessive amounts of vitamin C, or salicylate-containing foods (curry powder, prunes, raisins, tea, or licorice), other prescription or OTC medications containing aspirin or salicylate, or other NSAIDs without consulting prescriber. Maintain adequate hydration (2-3 L/day of fluids unless instructed to restrict fluid intake). You may experience nausea, vomiting, gastric discomfort (frequent mouth care, small frequent meals, sucking lozenges, or chewing gum may help). GI bleeding, ulceration, or perforation can occur with or without pain. May discolor stool (pink/red). Stop taking aspirin and report ringing in ears; persistent pain in stomach; unresolved nausea or vomiting; difficulty breathing or shortness of breath; unusual bruising or bleeding (mouth, urine, stool); or skin rash.

**Nursing Implications** Do not crush sustained release or enteric coated tablet

**Dosage Forms**

Capsule: 356.4 mg and caffeine 30 mg

Suppository, rectal: 60 mg, 120 mg, 125 mg, 130 mg, 195 mg, 200 mg, 300 mg, 325 mg, 600 mg, 650 mg, 1.2 g

Tablet: 65 mg, 75 mg, 81 mg, 325 mg, 500 mg

Tablet: 400 mg and caffeine 32 mg

Tablet:

- Buffered: 325 mg and magnesium-aluminum hydroxide 150 mg; 325 mg, magnesium hydroxide 75 mg, aluminum hydroxide 75 mg, buffered with calcium carbonate; 325 mg and magnesium-aluminum hydroxide 75 mg
- Chewable: 81 mg
- Controlled release: 800 mg
- Delayed release: 81 mg
- Enteric coated: 81 mg, 325 mg, 500 mg, 650 mg, 975 mg
- Gum: 227.5 mg
- Timed release: 650 mg

♦ **Aspirin and Butalbital Compound** *see* Butalbital Compound and Aspirin *on page 80*

## Aspirin and Codeine (AS pir in & KOE deen)

**U.S. Brand Names** Empirin® With Codeine

**Canadian Brand Names** Coryphen® Codeine; 222® Tablets; 282® Tablets; 292® Tablets

**Pharmacologic Category** Analgesic, Narcotic

**Use** Relief of mild to moderate pain

**Effects on Mental Status** Sedation is common; may produce euphoria or dysphoria

**Effects on Psychiatric Treatment** May cause leukopenia; use caution with clozapine and carbamazepine; may displace valproic acid from binding sites resulting in an increase of unbound drug; monitor for toxicity; codeine is a CNS depressant; monitor for additive effects with concurrent psychotropic use

**Restrictions** C-III

**Usual Dosage** Oral:

Children:

- Aspirin: 10 mg/kg/dose every 4 hours
- Codeine: 0.5-1 mg/kg/dose every 4 hours

Adults: 1-2 tablets every 4-6 hours as needed for pain

**Dosing adjustment in renal impairment:**

- $Cl_{cr}$ 10-50 mL/minute: Administer 75% of dose
- $Cl_{cr}$ <10 mL/minute: Avoid use

**Dosing interval in hepatic disease:** Avoid use in severe liver disease

**Dosage Forms** Tablet:

- #2: Aspirin 325 mg and codeine phosphate 15 mg
- #3: Aspirin 325 mg and codeine phosphate 30 mg
- #4: Aspirin 325 mg and codeine phosphate 60 mg

♦ **Aspirin and Dipyridamole** *see* Aspirin and Extended-Release Dipyridamole *on page 50*

## Aspirin and Extended-Release Dipyridamole

(dye peer ID a mole & AS pir in)

**U.S. Brand Names** Aggrenox™

**Synonyms** Aspirin and Dipyridamole; Dipyridamole and Aspirin

**Pharmacologic Category** Antiplatelet Agent

**Use** Reduction in the risk of stroke in patients who have had transient ischemia of the brain or completed ischemic stroke due to thrombosis

**Effects on Mental Status** May cause amnesia, fatigue, and confusion

**Effects on Psychiatric Treatment** Effect of antidepressants may be blunted due to sedation and fatigue; rare reports of pancytopenia; use caution with clozapine and carbamazepine

**Pregnancy Risk Factor** B (dipyridamole); D (aspirin)

**Contraindications** Hypersensitivity to dipyridamole, aspirin, or any component; allergy to NSAIDs; patients with asthma, rhinitis, and nasal polyps; bleeding disorders (factor VII or IX deficiencies); children <16 years of age with viral infections; pregnancy (especially 3rd trimester)

**Warnings/Precautions** Patients who consume ≥3 alcoholic drinks per day are at risk of bleeding. Cautious use in patients with inherited or acquired bleeding disorders including those of liver disease or vitamin K deficiency. Watch for signs and symptoms of GI ulcers and bleeding. Avoid use in patients with active peptic ulcer disease. Discontinue use if dizziness, tinnitus, or impaired hearing occurs. Stop 1-2 weeks before elective surgical procedures to avoid bleeding. Use caution in the elderly who are at high risk for adverse events. Cautious use in patients with hypotension, patients with unstable angina, recent MI, and hepatic dysfunction. Avoid in patients with severe renal failure. Safety and efficacy in children have not been established.

**Adverse Reactions**

>10%:

- Central nervous system: Headache (38.2%)
- Gastrointestinal: Dyspepsia, abdominal pain (17.5%), nausea (16%), diarrhea (12.7%)

1% to 10%:

- Central nervous system: Pain (6.4%), seizures (1.7%), fatigue (5.8%), malaise (1.6%), syncope (1%), amnesia (2.4%), confusion (1.1%), somnolence (1.2%)
- Cardiovascular: Cardiac failure (1.6%)
- Dermatologic: Purpura (1.4%)
- Gastrointestinal: Vomiting (8.4%), bleeding (4.1%), rectal bleeding 1.6%, hemorrhoids (1%), hemorrhage 1.2%, anorexia (1.2%)
- Hematologic: Anemia (1.6%)
- Neuromuscular & skeletal: Back pain (4.6%), weakness (1.8%), arthralgia (5.5%), arthritis (2.1%), arthrosis (1.1%), myalgia (1.2%)
- Respiratory: Cough (1.5%), upper respiratory tract infections (1%), epistaxis (2.4%)

<1% (limited to life-threatening or important symptoms): Intracranial hemorrhage (0.6%), allergic reaction, fever, hypotension, coma, dizziness, paresthesia, cerebral hemorrhage, subarachnoid hemorrhage, gastritis, ulceration, perforation, tinnitus, deafness, tachycardia, palpitations, arrhythmia, supraventricular tachycardia, cholelithiasis, jaundice, hepatic function abnormality, hyperglycemia, thirst, hematoma, gingival bleeding, agitation, uterine hemorrhage, hyperpnea, asthma, bronchospasm, hemoptysis, pulmonary edema, taste loss, pruritus, urticaria, renal insufficiency and failure, hematuria, flushing, hypothermia, chest pain, angina pectoris, cerebral edema, pancreatitis, Reye's syndrome, hematemesis, hearing impairment, anaphylaxis, laryngeal edema, hepatitis, hepatic failure, rhabdomyolysis, hypoglycemia, dehydration, prolonged PT time, disseminated intravascular coagulation, coagulopathy, thrombocytopenia, prolonged pregnancy and labor, stillbirths, lower weight infants, antepartum and postpartum bleeding, tachypnea, dyspnea, rash, alopecia, angioedema, Stevens-Johnson syndrome, interstitial nephritis, papillary necrosis, proteinuria, allergic vasculitis, anemia (aplastic), pancytopenia, thrombocytosis

**Overdosage/Toxicology** Symptoms of dipyridamole overdose might predominate because of the ratio of dipyridamole to aspirin. Symptoms may include hypotension and peripheral vasodilation. Treatment would include I.V. fluids and possibly vasopressors. Careful medical management is necessary.

**Drug Interactions**

Increased effects: Plasma levels and cardiovascular effects of adenosine are increased; decrease adenosine dose. Use of aspirin-dipyridamole with anticoagulants (heparin, low molecular weight heparins, warfarin) or antiplatelet agents (NSAIDs, IIb/IIIa antagonists) may increase the risk of bleeding. Serum concentrations and and toxicity of methotrexate may be increased when used concurrently with aspirin; avoid concurrent use. Serum concentrations of acetazolamide, phenytoin or valproic acid may be increased with aspirin. Concurrent use of verapamil may prolong bleeding times.

Decreased effect: Angiotensin-converting enzyme inhibitors may have diminished pharmacologic effect with aspirin (at higher dosages). The effect of cholinesterase inhibitors may be reduced with concurrent aspirin-dipyridamole therapy; avoid concurrent use. Aspirin may diminish the effect of diuretics, probenecid, and sulfinpyrazone.

**Usual Dosage** Adults: Oral: 1 capsule (200 mg dipyridamole, 25 mg aspirin) twice daily.

**Dosage adjustment in renal impairment:** Avoid use in patients with severe renal dysfunction ($Cl_{cr}$ <10 mL/minute). Studies have not been done in patients with renal impairment.

**Dosage adjustment in hepatic impairment:** Avoid use in patients with severe hepatic impairment; studies have not been done in patients with varying degrees of hepatic impairment

Elderly: Plasma concentrations were 40% higher, but specific dosage adjustments have not been recommended

**Patient Information** Swallow capsule whole without chewing or crushing; monitor for signs and symptoms of bleeding or another stroke or transient ischemic attack

**Nursing Implications** Monitor for signs and symptoms of bleeding or another stroke or transient ischemic attack

**Dosage Forms** Capsule: 200 mg dipyridamole, 25 mg aspirin

## Aspirin and Meprobamate (AS pir in & me proe BA mate)

**U.S. Brand Names** Equagesic®

**Canadian Brand Names** 292 MEP®

**Pharmacologic Category** Antianxiety Agent, Miscellaneous

**Use** Adjunct to treatment of skeletal muscular disease in patients exhibiting tension and/or anxiety

**Effects on Mental Status** Sedation is common

**Effects on Psychiatric Treatment** May cause leukopenia; use caution with clozapine and carbamazepine; may displace valproic acid from binding sites resulting in an increase of unbound drug; monitor for toxicity; meprobamate is a CNS depressant; monitor for additive effects with concurrent psychotropic use

**Restrictions** C-IV

**Usual Dosage** Oral: 1 tablet 3-4 times/day

**Dosage Forms** Tablet: Aspirin 325 mg and meprobamate 200 mg


- **Aspirin Free Anacin® Maximum Strength [OTC]** *see* Acetaminophen *on page 14*
- **Aspirin-Free Bayer® Select® Allergy Sinus Caplets [OTC]** *see* Acetaminophen, Chlorpheniramine, and Pseudoephedrine *on page 15*
- **Asprimox® [OTC]** *see* Aspirin *on page 49*
- **Assessment of Renal Function** *see page 696*
- **Astelin®** *see* Azelastine *on page 55*
- **Asthma Guidelines** *see page 773*
- **AsthmaHaler®** *see* Epinephrine *on page 195*
- **Astramorph™ PF Injection** *see* Morphine Sulfate *on page 374*
- **Atacand™** *see* Candesartan *on page 87*
- **Atarax®** *see* Hydroxyzine *on page 278*


## Atenolol (a TEN oh lole)

**Related Information**

Beta-Blockers Comparison Chart *on page 709*

Clozapine-Induced Side Effects *on page 780*

Special Populations - Pregnant and Breast-Feeding Patients *on page 668*

**U.S. Brand Names** Tenormin®

**Canadian Brand Names** Apo®-Atenol; Novo-Atenol; Nu-Atenol; Taro-Atenol®

**Pharmacologic Category** Beta Blocker, Beta$_1$ Selective

**Use** Treatment of hypertension, alone or in combination with other agents; management of angina pectoris, postmyocardial infarction patients

**Unlabeled use:** Acute alcohol withdrawal, supraventricular and ventricular arrhythmias, and migraine headache prophylaxis

**Effects on Mental Status** May cause fatigue, insomnia, and confusion which can clinically look like depression

**Effects on Psychiatric Treatment** Concurrent use with other psychotropics may produce an additive hypotensive response (especially low potency antipsychotics and TCAs)

**Pregnancy Risk Factor** D

**Contraindications** Hypersensitivity to atenolol or any component; sinus bradycardia; sinus node dysfunction; heart block greater than first-degree (except in patients with a functioning artificial pacemaker); cardiogenic shock; uncompensated cardiac failure; pulmonary edema; pregnancy

**Warnings/Precautions** Administer cautiously in compensated heart failure and monitor for a worsening of the condition (efficacy of atenolol in heart failure has not been established). Avoid abrupt discontinuation in patients with a history of CAD; slowly wean while monitoring for signs and symptoms of ischemia. Use caution with concurrent use of beta-blockers and either verapamil or diltiazem; bradycardia or heart block can occur. Avoid concurrent I.V. use of both agents. Beta-blockers should be avoided in patients with bronchospastic disease and peripheral vascular disease (may aggravate arterial insufficiency). Atenolol, with B1 selectivity, has been used cautiously in bronchospastic disease with close monitoring. Use cautiously in diabetics - may mask hypoglycemic symptoms. May mask signs of thyrotoxicosis. May cause fetal harm when administered in pregnancy. Use cautiously in the renally impaired (dosage adjustment required). Use care with anesthetic agents which decrease myocardial function. Caution in myasthenia gravis.

**Adverse Reactions**

1% to 10%:

Cardiovascular: Hypotension (4%), persistent bradycardia (3%), Raynaud's phenomenon (rare), second or third degree A-V block (0.7% to 1.7%),

Central nervous system: Confusion (rare), dizziness (4% to 13%), fatigue (3% to 6%), lethargy (1% to 3%), mental impairment (rare)

Gastrointestinal: Diarrhea (2% to 3%), nausea (3% to 4%)

Genitourinary: Impotence (rare)

Respiratory: Dyspnea (especially with large doses), wheezing (0% to 3%)

Miscellaneous: Cold extremities (<10%)

<1%: Depression, headache, nightmares

**Overdosage/Toxicology**

Signs and symptoms of intoxication include cardiac disturbances, CNS toxicity, bronchospasm, hypoglycemia and hyperkalemia. The most common cardiac symptoms include hypotension and bradycardia; atrioventricular block, intraventricular conduction disturbances, cardiogenic shock, and asystole may occur with severe overdose, especially with membrane-depressant drugs (eg, propranolol); CNS effects include convulsions, coma, and respiratory arrest (commonly seen with propranolol and other membrane-depressant and lipid-soluble drugs).

Treatment: Symptomatic treatment of seizures, hypotension, hyperkalemia, and hypoglycemia; bradycardia and hypotension resistant to atropine, isoproterenol, or pacing may respond to glucagon; wide QRS defects caused by the membrane-depressant poisoning may respond to hypertonic sodium bicarbonate; repeat-dose charcoal, hemoperfusion, or hemodialysis may be helpful in removal of only those beta-blockers with a small $V_d$, long half-life, or low intrinsic clearance (acebutolol, atenolol, nadolol, sotalol)

**Drug Interactions**

Alpha-blockers (prazosin, terazosin): Concurrent use of beta-blockers may increase risk of orthostasis

Ampicillin, in single doses of 1 gram, decrease atenolol's pharmacologic actions

Antacids (magnesium-aluminum, calcium antacids or salts) may reduce the bioavailability of atenolol

Clonidine: Hypertensive crisis after or during withdrawal of either agent

Drugs which slow AV conduction (digoxin): Effects may be additive with beta-blockers

Glucagon: Atenolol may blunt the hyperglycemic action of glucagon

Insulin and oral hypoglycemics: Atenolol masks the tachycardia that usually accompanies hypoglycemia

NSAIDs (ibuprofen, indomethacin, naproxen, piroxicam) may reduce the antihypertensive effects of beta-blockers

Salicylates may reduce the antihypertensive effects of beta-blockers

Sulfonylureas: Beta-blockers may alter response to hypoglycemic agents

Verapamil or diltiazem may have synergistic or additive pharmacological effects when taken concurrently with beta-blockers

**Usual Dosage**

Oral:

Children: 0.8-1 mg/kg/dose given daily; range of 0.8-1.5 mg/kg/day; maximum dose: 2 mg/kg/day

Adults:

Hypertension: 50 mg once daily, may increase to 100 mg/day. Doses >100 mg are unlikely to produce any further benefit

Angina pectoris: 50 mg once daily, may increase to 100 mg/day. Some patients may require 200 mg/day

Postmyocardial infarction: Follow I.V. dose with 100 mg/day or 50 mg twice daily for 6-9 days postmyocardial infarction

I.V.: Postmyocardial infarction: Early treatment: 5 mg slow I.V. over 5 minutes; may repeat in 10 minutes. If both doses are tolerated, may start oral atenolol 50 mg every 12 hours or 100 mg/day for 6-9 days postmyocardial infarction.

**Dosing interval for oral atenolol in renal impairment:**

$Cl_{cr}$ 15-35 mL/minute: Administer 50 mg/day maximum

$Cl_{cr}$ <15 mL/minute: Administer 50 mg every other day maximum

Hemodialysis: Moderately dialyzable (20% to 50%) via hemodialysis; administer dose postdialysis or administer 25-50 mg supplemental dose

Peritoneal dialysis: Elimination is not enhanced; supplemental dose is not necessary

**Patient Information** Take exactly as directed. Do not increase, decrease, or adjust dosage without consulting prescriber. Take pulse daily, prior to medication and follow prescriber's instruction about holding medication. Do not take with antacids. Do not use alcohol or OTC medications (eg, cold remedies) without consulting prescriber. If diabetic, monitor serum sugars closely (may alter glucose tolerance or mask signs of hypoglycemia). May cause fatigue, dizziness, or postural hypotension; use caution when changing position from lying or sitting to standing, when driving, or when climbing stairs until response to medication is known. May cause alteration in sexual performance (reversible). Report unresolved swelling of extremities, difficulty breathing or new cough, unresolved fatigue, unusual weight gain, unresolved constipation, or unusual muscle weakness.

**Dosage Forms**

Injection: 0.5 mg/mL (10 mL)

Tablet: 25 mg, 50 mg, 100 mg

## Atenolol and Chlorthalidone

(a TEN oh lole & klor THAL i done)

**U.S. Brand Names** Tenoretic®

**Pharmacologic Category** Antihypertensive Agent, Combination

**Use** Treatment of hypertension with a cardioselective beta-blocker and a diuretic

(Continued)

## Atenolol and Chlorthalidone *(Continued)*

**Effects on Mental Status** May cause fatigue, insomnia, and confusion which can clinically look like depression

**Effects on Psychiatric Treatment** Concurrent use with other psychotropics may produce an additive hypotensive response (especially low potency antipsychotics and TCAs)

**Usual Dosage** Adults: Oral: Initial: One (50) tablet once daily, then individualize dose until optimal dose is achieved

**Dosage Forms** Tablet:
50: Atenolol 50 mg and chlorthalidone 25 mg
100: Atenolol 100 mg and chlorthalidone 25 mg

♦ **Atgam®** *see* Lymphocyte Immune Globulin *on page 329*

♦ **Ativan®** *see* Lorazepam *on page 325*

♦ **ATnativ®** *see* Antithrombin III *on page 46*

♦ **Atolone®** *see* Triamcinolone *on page 563*

## Atorvastatin (a TORE va sta tin)

**Related Information**
Lipid-Lowering Agents Comparison Chart *on page 717*

**U.S. Brand Names** Lipitor®

**Pharmacologic Category** Antilipemic Agent (HMG-CoA Reductase Inhibitor)

**Use** Adjunct to diet for the reduction of elevated total and LDL cholesterol, apolipoprotein B, and triglyceride levels in patients with hypercholesterolemia (Type IIA, IIB, and IIC); adjunctive therapy to diet for treatment of elevated serum triglyceride levels (Type IV); treatment of primary dysbetalipoproteinemia (Type III) in patients who do not respond adequately to diet; to increase HDL cholesterol in patients with primary hypercholesterolemia and mixed dyslipidemia. Also may be used in hypercholesterolemic patients without clinically evident heart disease to reduce the risk of myocardial infarction, to reduce the risk for revascularization, and reduce the risk of death due to cardiovascular causes

**Effects on Mental Status** Rare reports of euphoria

**Effects on Psychiatric Treatment** None reported

**Pregnancy Risk Factor** X

**Contraindications** Hypersensitivity to atorvastatin or any component; active liver disease; unexplained persistent elevations of serum transaminases; pregnancy

**Warnings/Precautions** Liver function must be monitored by periodic laboratory assessment. Rhabdomyolysis with acute renal failure has occurred. Risk is increased with concurrent use of clarithromycin, danazol, diltiazem, fluvoxamine, indinavir, nefazodone, nelfinavir, ritonavir, verapamil, troleandomycin, cyclosporine, fibric acid derivatives, erythromycin, niacin, or azole antifungals. Weigh the risk versus benefit when combining any of these drugs with atorvastatin. Discontinue in any patient experiencing an acute or serious condition predisposing to renal failure secondary to rhabdomyolysis.

**Adverse Reactions**
>1%:
Central nervous system: Headache
Gastrointestinal: Abdominal pain (2% to 3%), diarrhea, flatulence,
Neuromuscular & skeletal: Myalgia (1% to 5%)
<1%: Euphoria, giddiness, impaired short-term memory, mild confusion, mild LFT increases, pharyngitis, rhinitis

**Overdosage/Toxicology**
Signs and symptoms: Few symptoms anticipated
Treatment: Supportive

**Drug Interactions** CYP3A3/4 enzyme substrate
Inhibitors of CYP3A3/4 (clarithromycin, cyclosporine, diltiazem, fluvoxamine, erythromycin, fluconazole, itraconazole, ketoconazole, miconazole, nefazodone,amprenavir, indinavir, nelfinavir, ritonavir, saquinavir, troleandomycin, and verapamil) increase atorvastatin blood levels; may increase the risk of atorvastatin-induced myopathy and rhabdomyolysis. The risk of myopathy and rhabdomyolysis due to concurrent use of a CYP3A3/4 inhibitor with atorvastatin is probably less than lovastatin or simvastatin.
Cholestyramine reduces absorption of several HMG-CoA reductase inhibitors; separate administration times by at least 4 hours
Cholestyramine and colestipol (bile acid sequestrants): Cholesterol-lowering effects are additive
Clofibrate and fenofibrate may increase the risk of myopathy and rhabdomyolysis
Niacin may increase the risk of myopathy and rhabdomyolysis

**Usual Dosage** Adults: Oral: Initial: 10 mg once daily, titrate up to 80 mg/day if needed
**Dosing adjustment in renal impairment:** No dosage adjustment is necessary
**Dosing adjustment in hepatic impairment:** Do not use in active liver disease

**Patient Information** May take with meals at any time of day. Maintain adequate hydration (2-3 L/day of fluids unless instructed to restrict fluid intake). You will need laboratory evaluation during therapy. May cause headache (mild analgesic may help); diarrhea (yogurt or buttermilk may help); euphoria, giddiness, confusion (use caution when driving or engaging in tasks that require alertness until response to medication is known). Report unresolved diarrhea, excessive or acute muscle cramping or weakness, changes in mood or memory, yellowing of skin or eyes, easy bruising or bleeding, and unusual fatigue.

**Dosage Forms** Tablet: 10 mg, 20 mg, 40 mg

## Atovaquone (a TOE va kwone)

**U.S. Brand Names** Mepron™

**Pharmacologic Category** Antiprotozoal

**Use** Acute oral treatment of mild to moderate *Pneumocystis carinii* pneumonia (PCP) in patients who are intolerant to co-trimoxazole; prophylaxis of PCP in patients intolerant to co-trimoxazole; treatment/suppression of *Toxoplasma gondii* encephalitis, primary prophylaxis of HIV-infected persons at high risk for developing *Toxoplasma gondii* encephalitis

**Effects on Mental Status** May cause anxiety

**Effects on Psychiatric Treatment** May cause anemia and neutropenia; use caution with clozapine and carbamazepine

**Pregnancy Risk Factor** C

**Contraindications** Life-threatening allergic reaction to the drug or formulation

**Warnings/Precautions** Has only been indicated in mild to moderate PCP; use with caution in elderly patients due to potentially impaired renal, hepatic, and cardiac function

**Adverse Reactions Note:** Adverse reaction statistics have been compiled from studies including patients with advanced HIV disease; consequently, it is difficult to distinguish reactions attributed to atovaquone from those caused by the underlying disease or a combination, thereof.

>10%:
Central nervous system: Anxiety, fever, headache, insomnia
Dermatologic: Rash
Gastrointestinal: Diarrhea, nausea, vomiting
Respiratory: Cough

1% to 10%:
Central nervous system: Dizziness
Dermatologic: Pruritus
Endocrine & metabolic: Hypoglycemia, hyponatremia
Gastrointestinal: Abdominal pain, anorexia, constipation, dyspepsia, increased amylase
Hematologic: Anemia, leukopenia, neutropenia
Hepatic: Elevated liver enzymes
Neuromuscular & skeletal: Weakness
Renal: Elevated BUN/creatinine
Miscellaneous: Oral moniliasis

**Drug Interactions** Decreased effect: Rifamycins used concurrently decrease the steady-state plasma concentrations of atovaquone
**Note:** Possible increased toxicity with other highly protein bound drugs

**Usual Dosage** Adults: Oral: 750 mg twice daily with food for 21 days

**Patient Information** Take as directed. Take with high-fat meals. You may experience dizziness or lightheadedness; use caution when driving or engaging in tasks that require alertness until response to drug is known. Small meals may help reduce nausea. Report unresolved diarrhea, fever, mouth sores (use good mouth care), unresolved headache or vomiting.

**Dosage Forms** Suspension, oral (citrus flavor): 750 mg/5 mL (210 mL)

## Atovaquone and Proguanil (a TOE va kwone & pro GWA nil)

**U.S. Brand Names** Malarone™

**Pharmacologic Category** Antimalarial Agent

**Use** Prevention or treatment of acute, uncomplicated *P. falciparum* malaria

**Effects on Mental Status** None reported

**Effects on Psychiatric Treatment** Significant adverse GI effects; use caution with SSRIs

**Usual Dosage** Oral (doses given in mg of atovaquone and proguanil):
Children (dosage based on body weight):
Prevention of malaria: Start 1-2 days prior to entering a malaria-endemic area, continue throughout the stay and for 7 days after returning; take as a single dose, once daily
11-20 kg: Atovaquone/proguanil 62.5 mg/25 mg
21-30 kg: Atovaquone/proguanil 125 mg/50 mg
31-40 kg: Atovaquone/proguanil 187.5 mg/75 mg
>40 kg: Atovaquone/proguanil 250 mg/100 mg
Treatment of acute malaria: Take as a single dose, once daily for 3 consecutive days
11-20 kg: Atovaquone/proguanil 250 mg/100 mg
21-30 kg: Atovaquone/proguanil 500 mg/200 mg
31-40 kg: Atovaquone/proguanil 750 mg/300 mg
>40 kg: Atovaquone/proguanil 1 g/400 mg

Adults:

Prevention of malaria: Atovaquone/proguanil 250 mg/100 mg once daily; start 1-2 days prior to entering a malaria-endemic area, continue throughout the stay and for 7 days after returning

Treatment of acute malaria: Atovaquone/proguanil 1 g/400 mg as a single dose, once daily for 3 consecutive days

**Dosage adjustment in renal impairment:** No information available, use with caution

**Dosage adjustment in hepatic impairment:** No information available

Elderly: Use with caution due to possible decrease in renal and hepatic function, as well as possible decreases in cardiac function, concomitant diseases, or other drug therapy

**Dosage Forms**

Tablet: Atovaquone 250 mg and proguanil hydrochloride 100 mg

Tablet, pediatric: Atovaquone 62.5 mg and proguanil hydrochloride 25 mg

♦ **Atozine®** *see* Hydroxyzine *on page 278*

## Atracurium (a tra KYOO ree um)

**U.S. Brand Names** Tracrium®

**Pharmacologic Category** Neuromuscular Blocker Agent, Nondepolarizing

**Use** Drug of choice for neuromuscular blockade in patients with renal and/or hepatic failure; eases endotracheal intubation as an adjunct to general anesthesia and relaxes skeletal muscle during surgery or mechanical ventilation; does not relieve pain

**Effects on Mental Status** None reported

**Effects on Psychiatric Treatment** None reported

**Usual Dosage** I.V. (not to be used I.M.):

Children 1 month to 2 years: 0.3-0.4 mg/kg initially followed by maintenance doses of 0.3-0.4 mg/kg as needed to maintain neuromuscular blockade

Children >2 years to Adults: 0.4-0.5 mg/kg then 0.08-0.1 mg/kg 20-45 minutes after initial dose to maintain neuromuscular block

Infusions (require use of an infusion pump): 0.2 mg/mL or 0.5 mg/mL in $D_5W$ or NS

Continuous infusion: Initial: 9-10 mcg/kg/minute followed by 5-9 mcg/kg/minute maintenance

**Dosing adjustment for hepatic/renal impairment:** Not necessary

**Dosage Forms**

Injection, as besylate: 10 mg/mL (5 mL, 10 mL)

Injection, preservative-free, as besylate: 10 mg/mL (5 mL)

♦ **Atrohist® Plus** *see* Chlorpheniramine, Phenylephrine, Phenylpropanolamine, and Belladonna Alkaloids *on page 115*

♦ **Atrol®** *see* Deanol *on page 152*

♦ **Atromid-S®** *see* Clofibrate *on page 130*

♦ **Atropair® Ophthalmic** *see* Atropine *on page 53*

## Atropine (A troe peen)

**U.S. Brand Names** Atropair® Ophthalmic; Atropine-Care® Ophthalmic; Atropisol® Ophthalmic; Isopto® Atropine Ophthalmic; I-Tropine® Ophthalmic; Ocu-Tropine® Ophthalmic

**Pharmacologic Category** Anticholinergic Agent; Anticholinergic Agent, Ophthalmic; Antidote; Antispasmodic Agent, Gastrointestinal; Ophthalmic Agent, Mydriatic

**Use** Preoperative medication to inhibit salivation and secretions; treatment of sinus bradycardia; management of peptic ulcer; treat exercise-induced bronchospasm; antidote for organophosphate pesticide poisoning; produce mydriasis and cycloplegia for examination of the retina and optic disc and accurate measurement of refractive errors; uveitis

**Effects on Mental Status** May cause drowsiness; rarely may produce anticholinergic toxicity presenting as confusion, delirium, memory loss, restlessness, and hallucinations

**Effects on Psychiatric Treatment** May decrease the effects of phenothiazines. concurrent use with psychotropics may result in additive anticholinergic side effects (dry mouth, blurred vision, constipation)

**Usual Dosage Note**: Doses <0.1 mg have been associated with paradoxical bradycardia

Neonates, Infants, and Children:

Preanesthetic: Oral, I.M., I.V., S.C.:

<5 kg: 0.02 mg/kg/dose 30-60 minutes preop then every 4-6 hours as needed; use of a minimum dosage of 0.1 mg in neonates <5 kg will result in dosages >0.02 mg/kg; there is no documented minimum dosage in this age group

>5 kg: 0.01-0.02 mg/kg/dose to a maximum 0.4 mg/dose 30-60 minutes preop; minimum dose: 0.1 mg

Bradycardia: I.V., intratracheal: 0.02 mg/kg, minimum dose 0.1 mg, maximum single dose: 0.5 mg in children and 1 mg in adolescents; may repeat in 5-minute intervals to a maximum total dose of 1 mg in children or 2 mg in adolescents. (**Note:** For intratracheal administration, the dosage must be diluted with normal saline to a total volume of 1-2 mL); when treating bradycardia in neonates, reserve use for those patients unresponsive to improved oxygenation and epinephrine.

Children:

Bronchospasm: Inhalation: 0.03-0.05 mg/kg/dose 3-4 times/day

Preprocedure: Ophthalmic: 0.5% solution: Instill 1-2 drops twice daily for 1-3 days before the procedure

Uveitis: Ophthalmic: 0.5% solution: Instill 1-2 drops up to 3 times/day

Adults (doses <0.5 mg have been associated with paradoxical bradycardia):

Asystole: I.V.: 1 mg; may repeat every 3-5 minutes as needed

Preanesthetic: I.M., I.V., S.C.: 0.4-0.6 mg 30-60 minutes preop and repeat every 4-6 hours as needed

Bradycardia: I.V.: 0.5-1 mg every 5 minutes, not to exceed a total of 2 mg or 0.04 mg/kg; may give intratracheal in 1 mg/10 mL dilution only, intratracheal dose should be 2-2.5 times the I.V. dose

Neuromuscular blockade reversal: I.V.: 25-30 mcg/kg 30 seconds before neostigmine or 10 mcg/kg 30 seconds before edrophonium

Organophosphate or carbamate poisoning: I.V.: 1-2 mg/dose every 10-20 minutes until atropine effect (dry flushed skin, tachycardia, mydriasis, fever) is observed, then every 1-4 hours for at least 24 hours; up to 50 mg in first 24 hours and 2 g over several days may be given in cases of severe intoxication

Bronchospasm: Inhalation: 0.025-0.05 mg/kg/dose every 4-6 hours as needed (maximum: 5 mg/dose)

Ophthalmic solution: 1%:

Preprocedure: Instill 1-2 drops 1 hour before the procedure

Uveitis: Instill 1-2 drops 4 times/day

Ophthalmic ointment: Apply a small amount in the conjunctival sac up to 3 times/day; compress the lacrimal sac by digital pressure for 1-3 minutes after instillation

**Dosage Forms**

Injection, as sulfate: 0.1 mg/mL (5 mL, 10 mL); 0.3 mg/mL (1 mL, 30 mL); 0.4 mg/mL (1 mL, 20 mL, 30 mL); 0.5 mg/mL (1 mL, 5 mL, 30 mL); 0.8 mg/mL (0.5 mL, 1 mL); 1 mg/mL (1 mL, 10 mL)

Ointment, ophthalmic, as sulfate: 0.5%, 1% (3.5 g)

Solution, ophthalmic, as sulfate: 0.5% (1 mL, 5 mL); 1% (1 mL, 2 mL, 5 mL, 15 mL); 2% (1 mL, 2 mL); 3% (5 mL)

Tablet, as sulfate: 0.4 mg

♦ **Atropine and Diphenoxylate** *see* Diphenoxylate and Atropine *on page 175*

♦ **Atropine-Care® Ophthalmic** *see* Atropine *on page 53*

♦ **Atropisol® Ophthalmic** *see* Atropine *on page 53*

♦ **Atrovent®** *see* Ipratropium *on page 291*

♦ **A/T/S® Topical** *see* Erythromycin, Ophthalmic/Topical *on page 202*

## Attapulgite (at a PULL gite)

**U.S. Brand Names** Children's Kaopectate® [OTC]; Diasorb® [OTC]; Kaopectate® Advanced Formula [OTC]; Kaopectate® Maximum Strength Caplets; Rheaban® [OTC]

**Canadian Brand Names** Kaopectate®

**Pharmacologic Category** Antidiarrheal

**Use** Symptomatic treatment of diarrhea

**Effects on Mental Status** None reported

**Effects on Psychiatric Treatment** Concurrent use with psychotropics may produce additive GI effects (constipation)

**Contraindications** Hypersensitivity to attapulgite or any component

**Warnings/Precautions** Use with caution in patients <3 years or >60 years of age or in presence of high fever

**Adverse Reactions** The powder, if chronically inhaled, can cause pneumoconiosis, since it contains large amounts of silica

1% to 10%: Gastrointestinal: Constipation (dose related)

**Overdosage/Toxicology**

Signs and symptoms: Attapulgite is physiologically inert; upon oral ingestion it swells into a mass that can be up to 12 times the volume of the dry powder, which may cause intestinal obstruction

Treatment: With an oral ingestion of the dry powder, dilution with 4-8 oz of water for adults (no more than 15 mL/kg in children) along with saline catharsis (magnesium citrate 4 mL/kg) usually prevents any powder-induced intestinal obstruction

**Drug Interactions** Decreased GI absorption of orally administered clindamycin, tetracyclines, penicillamine, digoxin

**Usual Dosage** Oral:

Children:

<3 years: Not recommended

3-6 years: 750 mg/dose up to 2250 mg/24 hours

6-12 years: 1200-1500 mg/dose up to 4500 mg/24 hours

Adults: 1200-1500 mg after each loose bowel movement or every 2 hours; 15-30 mL up to 8 times/day, up to 9000 mg/24 hours

**Patient Information** If diarrhea is not controlled in 48 hours, contact a physician

(Continued)

## Attapulgite *(Continued)*

**Dosage Forms**

Liquid, oral concentrate: 600 mg/15 mL (180 mL, 240 mL, 360 mL, 480 mL); 750 mg/15 mL (120 mL)

Tablet: 750 mg

Tablet, chewable: 300 mg, 600 mg

- **Attention-Deficit Hyperactivity Disorder** *see page 624*
- **Atypical Antipsychotics** *see page 707*
- **Augmentin®** *see* Amoxicillin and Clavulanate Potassium *on page 39*

## Auranofin (au RANE oh fin)

**U.S. Brand Names** Ridaura®

**Pharmacologic Category** Gold Compound

**Use** Management of active stage of classic or definite rheumatoid arthritis in patients that do not respond to or tolerate other agents; psoriatic arthritis; adjunctive or alternative therapy for pemphigus

**Effects on Mental Status** None reported

**Effects on Psychiatric Treatment** May rarely produce agranulocytosis; use caution with clozapine and carbamazepine

**Usual Dosage** Oral:

Children: Initial: 0.1 mg/kg/day divided daily; usual maintenance: 0.15 mg/kg/day in 1-2 divided doses; maximum: 0.2 mg/kg/day in 1-2 divided doses

Adults: 6 mg/day in 1-2 divided doses; after 3 months may be increased to 9 mg/day in 3 divided doses; if still no response after 3 months at 9 mg/day, discontinue drug

**Dosing adjustment in renal impairment:**

$Cl_{cr}$ 50-80 mL/minute: Reduce dose to 50%

$Cl_{cr}$ <50 mL/minute: Avoid use

**Dosage Forms** Capsule: 3 mg [29% gold]

- **Aureomycin®** *see* Chlortetracycline *on page 119*
- **Auro® Ear Drops [OTC]** *see* Carbamide Peroxide *on page 92*
- **Aurolate®** *see* Gold Sodium Thiomalate *on page 254*

## Aurothioglucose (aur oh thye oh GLOO kose)

**U.S. Brand Names** Solganal®

**Pharmacologic Category** Gold Compound

**Use** Adjunctive treatment in adult and juvenile active rheumatoid arthritis; alternative or adjunct in treatment of pemphigus; psoriatic patients who do not respond to NSAIDs

**Effects on Mental Status** None reported

**Effects on Psychiatric Treatment** May rarely produce agranulocytosis; use caution with clozapine and carbamazepine

**Usual Dosage** I.M.: Doses should initially be given at weekly intervals

Children 6-12 years: Initial: 0.25 mg/kg/dose first week; increment at 0.25 mg/kg/dose increasing with each weekly dose; maintenance: 0.75-1 mg/kg/dose weekly not to exceed 25 mg/dose to a total of 20 doses, then every 2-4 weeks

Adults: 10 mg first week; 25 mg second and third week; then 50 mg/week until 800 mg to 1 g cumulative dose has been given; if improvement occurs without adverse reactions, administer 25-50 mg every 2-3 weeks, then every 3-4 weeks

**Dosage Forms** Injection, suspension: 50 mg/mL [gold 50%] (10 mL)

- **Autoplex® T** *see* Anti-inhibitor Coagulant Complex *on page 46*
- **Avandia®** *see* Rosiglitazone *on page 501*
- **Avapro®** *see* Irbesartan *on page 292*
- **Avapro® HCT** *see* Irbesartan and Hydrochlorothiazide *on page 292*
- **AVC™ Cream** *see* Sulfanilamide *on page 525*
- **AVC™ Suppository** *see* Sulfanilamide *on page 525*
- **Avelox™** *see* Moxifloxacin *on page 375*
- **Aventyl®** *see* Nortriptyline *on page 400*
- **Avita®** *see* Tretinoin, Topical *on page 563*
- **Avlosulfon®** *see* Dapsone *on page 151*
- **Avonex™** *see* Interferon Beta-1a *on page 289*
- **Awa** *see* Kava *on page 301*
- **Axid®** *see* Nizatidine *on page 398*
- **Axid® AR [OTC]** *see* Nizatidine *on page 398*
- **Axocet®** *see* Butalbital Compound and Acetaminophen *on page 80*

## Ayahuasca

**Pharmacologic Category** Herb

**Use** Religious purposes in South America (as a sacrament)

**Adverse Reactions** Central nervous system: Hallucinations

**Overdosage/Toxicology**

Decontamination: Do **not** induce emesis; lavage within 60 minutes/activated charcoal with cathartic

Treatment: Supportive therapy; benzodiazepines may be useful for sedation

**Drug Interactions** Although this interaction has not been described, use of this tea with specific serotonin reuptake inhibitors may precipitate the serotonin syndrome

**Usual Dosage** 2 mL/kg of the tea

**Additional Information** Average levels of DMT and tetrahydroharmine following a dose of 2 mL/kg: ~15.8 ng/mL and 90.8 ng/mL respectively

- **Aygestin®** *see* Norethindrone *on page 398*

## Azacitidine (ay za SYE ti deen)

**U.S. Brand Names** Mylosar®

**Pharmacologic Category** Antineoplastic Agent, Miscellaneous

**Use** Refractory acute lymphocytic and myelogenous leukemia

**Effects on Mental Status** High doses may produce coma

**Effects on Psychiatric Treatment** Leukopenia is common; use caution with clozapine and carbamazepine

**Usual Dosage** Children and Adults: I.V., S.C.: 50-200 mg/m$^2$/day for 5-10 days, repeated at 2- to 3-week intervals **or** 75 mg/m$^2$/day for 7 days every 4 weeks

**Dosage Forms** Injection: 100 mg

- **Azactam®** *see* Aztreonam *on page 56*

## Azatadine (a ZA ta deen)

**U.S. Brand Names** Optimine®

**Pharmacologic Category** Antihistamine

**Use** Treatment of perennial and seasonal allergic rhinitis and chronic urticaria

**Effects on Mental Status** Drowsiness is common; rare reports of depression

**Effects on Psychiatric Treatment** Contraindicated with MAOIs; may produce additive CNS depressant effect with concurrent psychotropic use

**Pregnancy Risk Factor** B

**Contraindications** Hypersensitivity to azatadine or to other related antihistamines including cyproheptadine; patients taking monoamine oxidase inhibitors should not use azatadine

**Warnings/Precautions** Sedation and somnolence are the most commonly reported adverse effects

**Adverse Reactions**

>10%:

Central nervous system: Slight to moderate drowsiness

Respiratory: Thickening of bronchial secretions

1% to 10%:

Central nervous system: Dizziness, fatigue, headache, nervousness

Gastrointestinal: Abdominal pain, appetite increase, diarrhea, nausea, weight gain, xerostomia

Neuromuscular & skeletal: Arthralgia

Respiratory: Pharyngitis

<1%: Angioedema, bronchospasm, depression, edema, epistaxis, hepatitis, myalgia, palpitations, paresthesia, photosensitivity, rash

**Overdosage/Toxicology**

Signs and symptoms: CNS depression or stimulation, dry mouth, flushed skin, fixed and dilated pupils, apnea

Treatment: No specific treatment for antihistamine overdose, however, most of its clinical toxicity is due to anticholinergic effects. Anticholinesterase inhibitors may be useful by reducing acetylcholinesterase; anticholinesterase inhibitors include physostigmine, neostigmine, pyridostigmine, and edrophonium. For anticholinergic overdose with severe life-threatening symptoms, physostigmine 1-2 mg (0.5 or 0.02 mg/kg for children) I.V., slowly may be given to reverse these effects.

**Drug Interactions** Increased effect/toxicity: Procarbazine, CNS depressants, tricyclic antidepressants, alcohol

**Usual Dosage** Children >12 years and Adults: Oral: 1-2 mg twice daily

**Dietary Considerations** Alcohol: Additive CNS effects, avoid use

**Patient Information** Take as directed; do not exceed recommended dose. Avoid use of other depressants, alcohol, or sleep-inducing medications unless approved by prescriber. You may experience drowsiness or dizziness (use caution when driving or engaging in tasks requiring alertness until response to drug is known); or dry mouth, abdominal pain, or nausea (frequent small meals, frequent mouth care, chewing gum, or sucking hard candy may help). Report persistent sore throat, difficulty breathing, or expectorating (thick secretions); excessive sedation or mental stimulation;

frequent nosebleeds; unusual joint or muscle pain; or lack of improvement or worsening or condition.

**Dosage Forms** Tablet, as maleate: 1 mg

## Azatadine and Pseudoephedrine

(a ZA ta deen & soo doe e FED rin)

**U.S. Brand Names** Rynatan®; Trinalin®

**Pharmacologic Category** Antihistamine/Decongestant Combination

**Use** Perennial and seasonal allergic rhinitis and other allergic symptoms including urticaria

**Effects on Mental Status** Drowsiness is common; rare reports of depression

**Effects on Psychiatric Treatment** Contraindicated with MAOIs; may produce additive CNS depressant effect with concurrent psychotropic use

**Usual Dosage** Adults: 1-2 mg twice daily

**Dosage Forms** Tablet: Azatadine maleate 1 mg and pseudoephedrine sulfate 120 mg

## Azathioprine (ay za THYE oh preen)

**U.S. Brand Names** Imuran®

**Pharmacologic Category** Immunosuppressant Agent

**Use** Adjunct with other agents in prevention of rejection of solid organ transplants; also used in severe active rheumatoid arthritis unresponsive to other agents; other autoimmune diseases (ITP, SLE, MS, Crohn's Disease); **azathioprine is an imidazolyl derivative of 6-mercaptopurine**

**Effects on Mental Status** None reported

**Effects on Psychiatric Treatment** May produce pancytopenia; use caution with clozapine and carbamazepine

**Pregnancy Risk Factor** D

**Contraindications** Hypersensitivity to azathioprine or any component; pregnancy and lactation

**Warnings/Precautions** Chronic immunosuppression increases the risk of neoplasia; has mutagenic potential to both men and women and with possible hematologic toxicities; use with caution in patients with liver disease, renal impairment; monitor hematologic function closely

**Adverse Reactions** Dose reduction or temporary withdrawal allows reversal

>10%:
- Central nervous system: Chills, fever
- Gastrointestinal: Anorexia, diarrhea, nausea, vomiting
- Hematologic: Anemia, leukopenia, thrombocytopenia
- Miscellaneous: Secondary infection

1% to 10%:
- Dermatologic: Rash
- Hematologic: Pancytopenia
- Hepatic: Hepatotoxicity

<1%: Alopecia, aphthous stomatitis, arthralgias (which include myalgias), dyspnea, hypotension, maculopapular rash, rare hypersensitivity reactions, retinopathy, rigors

**Overdosage/Toxicology**

Signs and symptoms of overdose include nausea, vomiting, diarrhea, hematologic toxicity

Treatment: Following initiation of essential overdose management, symptomatic and supportive treatment should be instituted. Dialysis has been reported to remove significant amounts of the drug and its metabolites, and should be considered as a treatment option in those patients who deteriorate despite established forms of therapy.

**Drug Interactions** Increased toxicity: Allopurinol (decreases azathioprine dose to $^1/_3$ to $^1/_4$ of normal dose)

**Usual Dosage I.V. dose is equivalent to oral dose** (dosing should be based on ideal body weight):

Children and Adults: Solid organ transplantation: Oral, I.V.: 2-5 mg/kg/day to start, then 1-2 mg/kg/day maintenance

Adults: Rheumatoid arthritis: Oral: 1 mg/kg/day for 6-8 weeks; increase by 0.5 mg/kg every 4 weeks until response or up to 2.5 mg/kg/day

**Dosing adjustment in renal impairment:**
- $Cl_{cr}$ 10-50 mL/minute: Administer 75% of normal dose daily
- $Cl_{cr}$ <10 mL/minute: Administer 50% of normal dose daily

Hemodialysis: Slightly dialyzable (5% to 20%)
- Administer dose posthemodialysis

CAPD effects: Unknown

CAVH effects: Unknown

**Patient Information** Take as prescribed (may take in divided doses or with food if GI upset occurs).

Rheumatoid arthritis: Response may not occur for up to 3 months; do not discontinue without consulting prescriber.

Organ transplant: Azathioprine will usually be prescribed with other antirejection medications.

You will be susceptible to infection (avoid vaccinations unless approved by prescriber) and avoid crowds or infected persons or persons with contagious diseases. You may experience nausea, vomiting, loss of appetite (small frequent meals, frequent mouth care, chewing gum, or sucking lozenges may help). Report abdominal pain and unresolved gastrointestinal upset (eg, persistent vomiting or diarrhea); unusual fever or chills, bleeding or bruising, sore throat, unhealed sores, or signs of infection; yellowing of skin or eyes; or change in color of urine or stool.

**Dosage Forms**
- Injection, as sodium: 100 mg (20 mL)
- Tablet (scored): 50 mg

♦ **Azdone®** *see* Hydrocodone and Aspirin *on page 272*

## Azelaic Acid (a zeh LAY ik AS id)

**U.S. Brand Names** Azelex®

**Pharmacologic Category** Topical Skin Product, Acne

**Use** *Acne vulgaris*: Topical treatment of mild to moderate inflammatory acne vulgaris

**Effects on Mental Status** None reported

**Effects on Psychiatric Treatment** None reported

**Usual Dosage** Adults: Topical: After skin is thoroughly washed and patted dry, gently but thoroughly massage a thin film of azelaic acid cream into the affected areas twice daily, in the morning and evening. The duration of use can vary and depends on the severity of the acne. In the majority of patients with inflammatory lesions, improvement of the condition occurs within 4 weeks.

**Dosage Forms** Cream: 20% (30 g)

## Azelastine (a ZEL as teen)

**U.S. Brand Names** Astelin®; Optivar™

**Pharmacologic Category** Antihistamine

**Use**

Nasal spray: Treatment of the symptoms of seasonal allergic rhinitis such as rhinorrhea, sneezing, and nasal pruritus in adults and children ≥5 years of age

Ophthalmic: Treatment of itching of the eye associated with seasonal allergic conjunctivitis

**Effects on Mental Status** Drowsiness is common; rare reports of anxiety and nervousness

**Effects on Psychiatric Treatment** Concurrent use with psychotropics may produce additive sedation

**Usual Dosage**

Nasal spray: Children ≥5 years and Adults: 2 sprays (137 mcg/spray) each nostril twice daily. Before initial use, the delivery system should be primed with 4 sprays or until a fine mist appears. If 3 or more days have elapsed since last use, the delivery system should be reprimed.

Ophthalmic: Instill 1 drop into affected eye(s) twice daily

**Dosage Forms** Solution, nasal: 1 mg/mL (137 mcg/spray) (17 mL)

♦ **Azelex®** *see* Azelaic Acid *on page 55*

♦ **Azidothymidine** *see* Zidovudine *on page 592*

## Azithromycin (az ith roe MYE sin)

**U.S. Brand Names** Zithromax™

**Pharmacologic Category** Antibiotic, Macrolide

**Use**

Children: Treatment of acute otitis media due to *H. influenzae, M. catarrhalis*, or *S. pneumoniae*; pharyngitis/tonsillitis due to *S. pyogenes*

Adults:
- Treatment of mild to moderate upper and lower respiratory tract infections, infections of the skin and skin structure, and sexually transmitted diseases due to susceptible strains of *C. trachomatis, M. catarrhalis, H. influenzae, S. aureus, S. pneumoniae, Mycoplasma pneumoniae*, and *C. psittaci*; community-acquired pneumonia, pelvic inflammatory disease (PID)
- For preventing or delaying the onset of infection with *Mycobacterium avium* complex (MAC)
- Prophylaxis of bacterial endocarditis in patients who are allergic to penicillin and undergoing surgical or dental procedures

**Effects on Mental Status** Macrolides have been reported to cause nightmares, confusion, anxiety, and mood lability

**Effects on Psychiatric Treatment** Contraindicated with pimozide; may increase concentration of bromocriptine, carbamazepine and triazolam

**Pregnancy Risk Factor** B

**Contraindications** Hepatic impairment, known hypersensitivity to azithromycin, other macrolide antibiotics, or any azithromycin components; use with pimozide

**Warnings/Precautions** Use with caution in patients with hepatic dysfunction; hepatic impairment with or without jaundice has occurred chiefly in older children and adults; it may be accompanied by malaise, nausea, vomiting, abdominal colic, and fever; discontinue use if these occur; may mask or delay symptoms of incubating gonorrhea or syphilis, so appropriate culture and susceptibility tests should be performed prior to initiating

(Continued)

## Azithromycin *(Continued)*

azithromycin; pseudomembranous colitis has been reported with use of macrolide antibiotics; safety and efficacy have not been established in children <6 months of age with acute otitis media and in children <2 years of age with pharyngitis/tonsillitis

**Adverse Reactions**

1% to 10%: Gastrointestinal: Abdominal pain, cramping, diarrhea, nausea, vomiting (especially with high single-dose regimens)

<1%: Allergic reactions, angioedema, cholestatic jaundice, dizziness, headache, hypertrophic pyloric stenosis, elevated LFTs, eosinophilia, fever, nephritis, ototoxicity, rash, thrombophlebitis, vaginitis, ventricular arrhythmias

**Overdosage/Toxicology**

Signs and symptoms: Nausea, vomiting, diarrhea, prostration

Treatment: Supportive and symptomatic

**Drug Interactions** May inhibit CYP3A3/4 enzyme (mild)

Decreased peak serum levels: Aluminum- and magnesium-containing antacids by 24% but not total absorption

Increased effect/toxicity: Azithromycin may increase levels of tacrolimus, phenytoin, ergot alkaloids, alfentanil, astemizole, terfenadine, bromocriptine, carbamazepine, cyclosporine, digoxin, disopyramide, and triazolam; azithromycin did not affect the response to warfarin or theophylline although caution is advised when administered together

Avoid use with pimozide due to significant risk of cardiotoxicity

**Usual Dosage**

Oral:

Children ≥6 months: Otitis media and community-acquired pneumonia: 10 mg/kg on day 1 (maximum: 500 mg/day) followed by 5 mg/kg/day once daily on days 2-5 (maximum: 250 mg/day)

Children ≥2 years: Pharyngitis, tonsillitis: 12 mg/kg/day once daily for 5 days (maximum: 500 mg/day)

Children: *M. avium*-infected patients with acquired immunodeficiency syndrome: Not currently FDA approved for use; 10-20 mg/kg/day once daily (maximum: 40 mg/kg/day) has been used in clinical trials; prophylaxis for first episode of MAC: 5-12 mg/kg/day once daily (maximum: 500 mg/day)

Adolescents ≥16 years and Adults:

Respiratory tract, skin and soft tissue infections: 500 mg on day 1 followed by 250 mg/day on days 2-5 (maximum: 500 mg/day)

Uncomplicated chlamydial urethritis/cervicitis or chancroid: Single 1 g dose

Gonococcal urethritis/cervicitis: Single 2 g dose

Prophylaxis of disseminated *M. avium* complex disease in patient with advanced HIV infection: 1200 mg once weekly (may be combined with rifabutin)

Prophylaxis for bacterial endocarditis: 500 mg 1 hour prior to the procedure

I.V.: Adults:

Community-acquired pneumonia: 500 mg as a single dose for at least 2 days, follow I.V. therapy by the oral route with a single daily dose of 500 mg to complete a 7-10 day course of therapy

Pelvic inflammatory disease (PID): 500 mg as a single dose for 1-2 days, follow I.V. therapy by the oral route with a single daily dose of 250 mg to complete a 7 day course of therapy

**Dietary Considerations** Food: Rate and extent of GI absorption decreased; take on an empty stomach

Azithromycin suspension, not tablet form, has significantly increased absorption (46%) with food

**Patient Information** Take as directed. Take all of prescribed medication. Do not discontinue until prescription is completed. Take suspension 1 hour before or 2 hours after meals; tablet form may be taken with meals to decrease GI effects. Do not take with aluminum- or magnesium-containing antacids. May cause transient abdominal distress, diarrhea, headache. Report signs of additional infections (eg, sores in mouth or vagina, vaginal discharge, unresolved fever, severe vomiting, or diarrhea).

**Dosage Forms**

Capsule: 250 mg

Capsule (Z-Pak™): 6 caps/pkg

Powder for injection: 500 mg

Powder for oral suspension, as dihydrate: 100 mg/5 mL (15 mL); 200 mg/5 mL (15 mL, 22.5 mL); 1 g (single-dose packet)

Tablet, as dihydrate: 250 mg, 600 mg


- **Azmacort™** *see* Triamcinolone *on page 563*
- **Azolid®** *see* Phenylbutazone *on page 439*
- **Azopt™** *see* Brinzolamide *on page 72*
- **Azo-Standard® [OTC]** *see* Phenazopyridine *on page 433*
- **Azo-Sulfisoxazole** *see* Sulfisoxazole and Phenazopyridine *on page 526*
- **AZT** *see* Zidovudine *on page 592*


## Aztreonam (AZ tree oh nam)

**U.S. Brand Names** Azactam®

**Pharmacologic Category** Antibiotic, Miscellaneous

**Use** Treatment of patients with urinary tract infections, lower respiratory tract infections, septicemia, skin/skin structure infections, intra-abdominal infections, and gynecological infections caused by susceptible gram-negative bacilli; often useful in patients with allergies to penicillins or cephalosporins

**Effects on Mental Status** May rarely produce confusion

**Effects on Psychiatric Treatment** Rarely produces leukopenia and neutropenia; use caution with clozapine and carbamazepine

**Usual Dosage**

Neonates: I.M., I.V.:

Postnatal age ≤7 days:

<2000 g: 30 mg/kg/dose every 12 hours

>2000 g: 30 mg/kg/dose every 8 hours

Postnatal age >7 days:

<1200 g: 30 mg/kg/dose every 12 hours

1200-2000 g: 30 mg/kg/dose every 8 hours

>2000 g: 30 mg/kg/dose every 6 hours

Children >1 month: I.M., I.V.: 90-120 mg/kg/day divided every 6-8 hours

Cystic fibrosis: 50 mg/kg/dose every 6-8 hours (ie, up to 200 mg/kg/day); maximum: 6-8 g/day

Adults:

Urinary tract infection: I.M., I.V.: 500 mg to 1 g every 8-12 hours

Moderately severe systemic infections: 1 g I.V. or I.M. or 2 g I.V. every 8-12 hours

Severe systemic or life-threatening infections (especially caused by *Pseudomonas aeruginosa*): I.V.: 2 g every 6-8 hours; maximum: 8 g/day

**Dosing adjustment in renal impairment:** Adults:

$Cl_{cr}$ >50 mL/minute: 500 mg to 1 g every 6-8 hours

$Cl_{cr}$ 10-50 mL/minute: 50% to 75% of usual dose given at the usual interval

$Cl_{cr}$ <10 mL/minute: 25% of usual dosage given at the usual interval

Hemodialysis: Moderately dialyzable (20% to 50%); administer dose postdialysis or supplemental dose of 500 mg after dialysis

Peritoneal dialysis: Administer as for $Cl_{cr}$ <10 mL/minute

Continuous arteriovenous or venovenous hemofiltration (CAVH/CAVHD): Dose as for $Cl_{cr}$ 10-50 mL/minute

**Dosage Forms** Powder for injection: 500 mg (15 mL, 100 mL); 1 g (15 mL, 100 mL); 2 g (15 mL, 100 mL)


- **Azulfidine® EN-tabs®** *see* Sulfasalazine *on page 525*
- **Azulfidine® Tablets** *see* Sulfasalazine *on page 525*
- **Babee® Teething® [OTC]** *see* Benzocaine *on page 61*


## Bacampicillin (ba kam pi SIL in)

**U.S. Brand Names** Spectrobid®

**Pharmacologic Category** Antibiotic, Penicillin

**Use** Treatment of susceptible bacterial infections involving the urinary tract, skin structure, upper and lower respiratory tract; activity is identical to that of ampicillin

**Effects on Mental Status** Penicillins have been reported to cause apprehension, illusions, agitation, insomnia, depersonalization, and encephalopathy

**Effects on Psychiatric Treatment** May produce agranulocytosis; use caution with clozapine and carbamazepine

**Usual Dosage** Oral:

Children <25 kg: 25-50 mg/kg/day in divided doses every 12 hours

Children >25 kg and Adults: 400-800 mg every 12 hours

**Dosing interval in renal impairment:**

$Cl_{cr}$ 10-30 mL/minute: Administer every 24 hours

$Cl_{cr}$ <10 mL/minute: Administer every 36 hours

**Dosage Forms**

Powder for oral suspension, as hydrochloride: 125 mg/5 mL [chemically equivalent to ampicillin 87.5 mg per 5 mL] (70 mL)

Tablet, as hydrochloride: 400 mg [chemically equivalent to ampicillin 280 mg]


- **Bachelor's Buttons** *see* Feverfew *on page 224*
- **Bacid® [OTC]** *see Lactobacillus acidophilus* and *Lactobacillus bulgaricus on page 305*
- **Baciguent® Topical [OTC]** *see* Bacitracin *on page 56*
- **Baci-IM® Injection** *see* Bacitracin *on page 56*
- **Bacillus Calmette-Guérin (BCG) Live** *see* BCG Vaccine *on page 58*


## Bacitracin (bas i TRAY sin)

**U.S. Brand Names** AK-Tracin® Ophthalmic; Baciguent® Topical [OTC]; Baci-IM® Injection

**Canadian Brand Names** Bacigvent; Bacitin

**Pharmacologic Category** Antibiotic, Ophthalmic; Antibiotic, Topical; Antibiotic, Miscellaneous

**Use** Treatment of susceptible bacterial infections mainly has activity against gram-positive bacilli; due to toxicity risks, systemic and irrigant uses of bacitracin should be limited to situations where less toxic alternatives would not be effective; oral administration has been successful in antibiotic-associated colitis and has been used for enteric eradication of vancomycin-resistant enterococci (VRE)

**Effects on Mental Status** None reported

**Effects on Psychiatric Treatment** None reported

**Usual Dosage** Children and Adults (**do not administer I.V.**):

Infants: I.M.:

≤2.5 kg: 900 units/kg/day in 2-3 divided doses

>2.5 kg: 1000 units/kg/day in 2-3 divided doses

Children: I.M.: 800-1200 units/kg/day divided every 8 hours

Adults: Antibiotic-associated colitis: Oral: 25,000 units 4 times/day for 7-10 days

Topical: Apply 1-5 times/day

Ophthalmic, ointment: Instill 1/4" to 1/2" ribbon every 3-4 hours into conjunctival sac for acute infections, or 2-3 times/day for mild to moderate infections for 7-10 days

Irrigation, solution: 50-100 units/mL in normal saline, lactated Ringer's, or sterile water for irrigation; soak sponges in solution for topical compresses 1-5 times/day or as needed during surgical procedures

**Dosage Forms**

Injection: 50,000 units

Ointment:

Ophthalmic: 500 units/g (1 g, 3.5 g, 3.75 g)

Topical: 500 units/g (1.5 g, 3.75 g, 15 g, 30 g, 120 g, 454 g)

## Bacitracin and Polymyxin B

(bas i TRAY sin & pol i MIKS in bee)

**U.S. Brand Names** AK-Poly-Bac® Ophthalmic; Betadine® First Aid Antibiotics + Moisturizer [OTC]; Polysporin® Ophthalmic; Polysporin® Topical

**Canadian Brand Names** Bioderm®; Polytopic

**Pharmacologic Category** Antibiotic, Ophthalmic; Antibiotic, Topical

**Use** Treatment of superficial infections caused by susceptible organisms

**Effects on Mental Status** None reported

**Effects on Psychiatric Treatment** None reported

**Usual Dosage** Children and Adults:

Ophthalmic ointment: Instill 1/2" ribbon in the affected eye(s) every 3-4 hours for acute infections or 2-3 times/day for mild to moderate infections for 7-10 days

Topical ointment/powder: Apply to affected area 1-4 times/day; may cover with sterile bandage if needed

**Dosage Forms**

Ointment:

Ophthalmic: Bacitracin 500 units and polymyxin B sulfate 10,000 units per g (3.5 g)

Topical: Bacitracin 500 units and polymyxin B sulfate 10,000 units per g in white petrolatum (15 g, 30 g)

Powder: Bacitracin 500 units and polymyxin B sulfate 10,000 units per g (10 g)

## Bacitracin, Neomycin, and Polymyxin B

(bas i TRAY sin, nee oh MYE sin, & pol i MIKS in bee)

**U.S. Brand Names** AK-Spore® Ophthalmic Ointment; Medi-Quick® Topical Ointment [OTC]; Mycitracin® Topical [OTC]; Neomixin® Topical [OTC]; Neosporin® Ophthalmic Ointment; Neosporin® Topical Ointment [OTC]; Ocutricin® Topical Ointment; Septa® Topical Ointment [OTC]; Triple Antibiotic® Topical

**Canadian Brand Names** Neotopic

**Pharmacologic Category** Antibiotic, Ophthalmic; Antibiotic, Topical

**Use** Helps prevent infection in minor cuts, scrapes and burns; short-term treatment of superficial external ocular infections caused by susceptible organisms

**Effects on Mental Status** None reported

**Effects on Psychiatric Treatment** None reported

**Usual Dosage** Children and Adults:

Ophthalmic: Ointment: Apply 1/2" into the conjunctival sac every 3-4 hours for 7-10 days for acute infections; apply 1/2" 2-3 times/day for mild to moderate infections for 7-10 days

Topical: Apply 1-5 times/day to infected area and cover with sterile bandage as needed

**Dosage Forms** Ointment:

Ophthalmic: Bacitracin 400 units, neomycin sulfate 3.5 mg, and polymyxin B sulfate 10,000 units and per g

Topical: Bacitracin 400 units, neomycin sulfate 3.5 mg, and polymyxin B sulfate 5000 units per g

## Bacitracin, Neomycin, Polymyxin B, and Hydrocortisone

(bas i TRAY sin, nee oh MYE sin, pol i MIKS in bee & hye droe KOR ti sone)

**U.S. Brand Names** AK-Spore® H.C. Ophthalmic Ointment; Cortisporin® Ophthalmic Ointment; Cortisporin® Topical Ointment; Neotricin HC® Ophthalmic Ointment

**Pharmacologic Category** Antibiotic, Ophthalmic; Antibiotic, Otic; Antibiotic, Topical; Corticosteroid, Ophthalmic; Corticosteroid, Otic; Corticosteroid, Topical

**Use** Prevention and treatment of susceptible superficial topical infections

**Effects on Mental Status** None reported

**Effects on Psychiatric Treatment** None reported

**Usual Dosage** Children and Adults:

Ophthalmic:

Ointment: Instill 1/2" ribbon to inside of lower lid every 3-4 hours until improvement occurs

Topical: Apply sparingly 2-4 times/day. Therapy should be discontinued when control is achieved; if no improvement is seen, reassessment of diagnosis may be necessary.

**Dosage Forms** Ointment:

Ophthalmic: Bacitracin 400 units, neomycin sulfate 3.5 mg, polymyxin B sulfate 10,000 units, and hydrocortisone 10 mg per g (3.5 g)

Topical: Bacitracin 400 units, neomycin sulfate 3.5 mg, polymyxin B sulfate 10,000 units, and hydrocortisone 10 mg per g (15 g)

## Bacitracin, Neomycin, Polymyxin B, and Lidocaine

(bas i TRAY sin, nee oh MYE sin, pol i MIKS in bee & LYE doe kane)

**U.S. Brand Names** Clomycin® [OTC]

**Pharmacologic Category** Antibiotic, Topical

**Use** Prevention and treatment of susceptible superficial topical infections

**Effects on Mental Status** None reported

**Effects on Psychiatric Treatment** None reported

**Usual Dosage** Adults: Topical: Apply 1-4 times/day to infected areas; cover with sterile bandage if needed

**Dosage Forms** Ointment, topical: Bacitracin 500 units, neomycin base 3.5 g, polymyxin B sulfate 5000 units, and lidocaine 40 mg per g (28.35 g)

## Baclofen (BAK loe fen)

**U.S. Brand Names** Lioresal®

**Canadian Brand Names** Alpha-Baclofen®; PMS-Baclofen

**Pharmacologic Category** Skeletal Muscle Relaxant

**Use** Treatment of reversible spasticity associated with multiple sclerosis or spinal cord lesions

**Unlabeled use:** Intractable hiccups, intractable pain relief, and bladder spasticity

**Effects on Mental Status** Drowsiness and insomnia are common; rare reports of depression, euphoria, and hallucinations

**Effects on Psychiatric Treatment** Concurrent use with psychotropics may produce additive sedation; concurrent use with MAOIs may potentiate their hypotensive effects

**Pregnancy Risk Factor** C

**Contraindications** Hypersensitivity to baclofen or any component

**Warnings/Precautions** Use with caution in patients with seizure disorder, impaired renal function; avoid abrupt withdrawal of the drug; elderly are more sensitive to the effects of baclofen and are more likely to experience adverse CNS effects at higher doses.

**Adverse Reactions**

>10%:

Central nervous system: Ataxia, drowsiness, hypotonia, insomnia, psychiatric disturbances, slurred speech, vertigo

Neuromuscular & skeletal: Weakness

1% to 10%:

Cardiovascular: Hypotension

Central nervous system: Confusion, fatigue, headache

Dermatologic: Rash

Gastrointestinal: Nausea, constipation

Genitourinary: Polyuria

<1%: Abdominal pain, abnormal taste, anorexia, chest pain, depression, diarrhea, dyspnea, dysuria, enuresis, euphoria, excitement, hallucinations, hematuria, impotence, inability to ejaculate, nocturia, palpitations, paresthesia, syncope, urinary retention, vomiting, xerostomia

**Overdosage/Toxicology**

Signs and symptoms: Vomiting, muscle hypotonia, salivation, drowsiness, coma, seizures, respiratory depression

Treatment: Atropine has been used to improve ventilation, heart rate, blood pressure, and core body temperature. Following initiation of essential overdose management, symptomatic and supportive treatment should be instituted.

(Continued)

## Baclofen *(Continued)*

**Drug Interactions**

Increased effect: Opiate analgesics, benzodiazepines, hypertensive agents

Increased toxicity: CNS depressants and alcohol (sedation), tricyclic antidepressants (short-term memory loss), clindamycin (neuromuscular blockade), guanabenz (sedation), MAO inhibitors (decrease blood pressure, CNS, and respiratory effects)

**Usual Dosage**

Oral (avoid abrupt withdrawal of drug):

Children:

2-7 years: Initial: 10-15 mg/24 hours divided every 8 hours; titrate dose every 3 days in increments of 5-15 mg/day to a maximum of 40 mg/day

≥8 years: Maximum: 60 mg/day in 3 divided doses

Adults: 5 mg 3 times/day, may increase 5 mg/dose every 3 days to a maximum of 80 mg/day

Hiccups: Adults: Usual effective dose: 10-20 mg 2-3 times/day

Intrathecal:

Test dose: 50-100 mcg, doses >50 mcg should be given in 25 mcg increments, separated by 24 hours

Maintenance: After positive response to test dose, a maintenance intrathecal infusion can be administered via an implanted intrathecal pump. Initial dose via pump: Infusion at a 24-hour rate dosed at twice the test dose.

**Dosing adjustment in renal impairment:** It is necessary to reduce dosage in renal impairment but there are no specific guidelines available

Hemodialysis: Poor water solubility allows for accumulation during chronic hemodialysis. Low-dose therapy is recommended. There have been several case reports of accumulation of baclofen resulting in toxicity symptoms (organic brain syndrome, myoclonia, deceleration and steep potentials in EEG) in patients with renal failure who have received normal doses of baclofen.

**Patient Information** Take this drug as prescribed. Do not discontinue without consulting prescriber (abrupt discontinuation may cause hallucinations). Do not take any prescription or OTC sleep-inducing drugs, sedatives, antispasmodics without consulting prescriber. Avoid alcohol use. You may experience transient drowsiness, lethargy, or dizziness; use caution when driving or engaging in tasks requiring alertness until response to drug is known. Frequent small meals or lozenges may reduce GI upset. Report unresolved insomnia, painful urination, change in urinary patterns, constipation, or persistent confusion.

**Nursing Implications** Epileptic patients should be closely monitored; supervise ambulation; avoid abrupt withdrawal of the drug

**Dosage Forms**

Injection, intrathecal, preservative free: 500 mcg/mL (20 mL); 2000 mcg/mL (5 mL)

Tablet: 10 mg, 20 mg


- ♦ **Bactocill®** *see* Oxacillin *on page 408*
- ♦ **BactoShield® Topical [OTC]** *see* Chlorhexidine Gluconate *on page 111*
- ♦ **Bactrim™** *see* Co-Trimoxazole *on page 142*
- ♦ **Bactrim™ DS** *see* Co-Trimoxazole *on page 142*
- ♦ **Bactroban®** *see* Mupirocin *on page 376*
- ♦ **Bactroban® Nasal** *see* Mupirocin *on page 376*
- ♦ **Baking Soda** *see* Sodium Bicarbonate *on page 514*
- ♦ **Baldex®** *see* Dexamethasone *on page 157*
- ♦ **BAL in Oil®** *see* Dimercaprol *on page 173*
- ♦ **Bancap HC®** *see* Hydrocodone and Acetaminophen *on page 272*
- ♦ **Banocide®** *see* Diethylcarbamazine *on page 167*
- ♦ **Banophen® Decongestant Capsule [OTC]** *see* Diphenhydramine and Pseudoephedrine *on page 175*
- ♦ **Banophen® Oral [OTC]** *see* Diphenhydramine *on page 174*
- ♦ **Banthine®** *see* Methantheline *on page 350*
- ♦ **Barbidonna®** *see* Hyoscyamine, Atropine, Scopolamine, and Phenobarbital *on page 279*
- ♦ **Barbita®** *see* Phenobarbital *on page 435*
- ♦ **Barc™ Liquid [OTC]** *see* Pyrethrins *on page 480*
- ♦ **Baridium® [OTC]** *see* Phenazopyridine *on page 433*
- ♦ **Basaljel® [OTC]** *see* Aluminum Carbonate *on page 27*
- ♦ **Base Ointment** *see* Zinc Oxide *on page 593*


## Basiliximab (ba si LIKS i mab)

**U.S. Brand Names** Simulect®

**Pharmacologic Category** Monoclonal Antibody

**Use** Prophylaxis of acute organ rejection in renal transplantation

**Effects on Mental Status** Dizziness, headache, and insomnia are common. May cause agitation, anxiety, depression, malaise, or fatigue

**Effects on Psychiatric Treatment** Side effects mimic depressive symptoms; effects of benzodiazepines and antidepressants may be altered

**Usual Dosage** I.V.:

Children 2-15 years of age: 12 mg/m$^2$ (maximum: 20 mg) within 2 hours prior to transplant surgery, followed by a second dose of 12 mg/m$^2$ (maximum: 20 mg/dose) 4 days after transplantation

Adults: 20 mg within 2 hours prior to transplant surgery, followed by a second 20 mg dose 4 days after transplantation

**Dosing adjustment/comments in renal or hepatic impairment:** No specific dosing adjustment recommended

**Dosage Forms** Powder for injection: 20 mg


- ♦ **Baycol™** *see* Cerivastatin *on page 105*
- ♦ **Bayer® Aspirin [OTC]** *see* Aspirin *on page 49*
- ♦ **Bayer® Buffered Aspirin [OTC]** *see* Aspirin *on page 49*
- ♦ **Bayer® Low Adult Strength [OTC]** *see* Aspirin *on page 49*
- ♦ **Bayer® Select® Chest Cold Caplets [OTC]** *see* Acetaminophen and Dextromethorphan *on page 15*
- ♦ **Bayer® Select Head Cold Caplets [OTC]** *see* Acetaminophen and Pseudoephedrine *on page 15*
- ♦ **Bayer® Select® Pain Relief Formula [OTC]** *see* Ibuprofen *on page 280*
- ♦ **Bayotensin®** *see* Nitrendipine *on page 396*
- ♦ **Baypresol®** *see* Nitrendipine *on page 396*
- ♦ **Baypress®** *see* Nitrendipine *on page 396*


## BCG Vaccine (bee see jee vak SEEN)

**U.S. Brand Names** TheraCys®; TICE® BCG

**Canadian Brand Names** ImmuCyst®; Oncotice™; Pacis™

**Synonyms** Bacillus Calmette-Guérin (BCG) Live

**Pharmacologic Category** Biological Response Modulator; Vaccine

**Use** Immunization against tuberculosis and immunotherapy for cancer; treatment of bladder cancer

BCG vaccine is not routinely recommended for use in the U.S. for prevention of tuberculosis

BCG vaccine is strongly recommended for infants and children with negative tuberculin skin tests who:

are at high risk of intimate and prolonged exposure to persistently untreated or ineffectively treated patients with infectious pulmonary tuberculosis, and

cannot be removed from the source of exposure, and

cannot be placed on long-term preventive therapy

are continuously exposed with tuberculosis who have bacilli resistant to isoniazid and rifampin

BCG is also recommended for tuberculin-negative infants and children in groups in which the rate of new infections exceeds 1% per year and for whom the usual surveillance and treatment programs have been attempted but are not operationally feasible

BCG should be administered with caution to persons in groups at high risk for HIV infection or persons known to be severely immunocompromised. Although limited data suggest that the vaccine may be safe for use in asymptomatic children infected with HIV, BCG vaccination is not recommended for HIV infected adults or for persons with symptomatic disease. Until further research can clearly define the risks and benefits of BCG vaccination for this population, vaccination should be restricted to persons at exceptionally high risk for tuberculosis infection. HIV infected persons thought to be infected with *Mycobacterium tuberculosis* should be strongly recommended for tuberculosis preventive therapy.

**Effects on Mental Status** None reported

**Effects on Psychiatric Treatment** None reported

**Pregnancy Risk Factor** C

**Contraindications** Tuberculin-positive individual, hypersensitivity to BCG vaccine or any component, immunocompromized, AIDS and burn patients

**Warnings/Precautions** Protection against tuberculosis is only relative, not permanent, nor entirely predictable; for live bacteria vaccine, proper aseptic technique and disposal of all equipment in contact with BCG vaccine as a biohazardous material is recommended; systemic reactions have been reported in patients treated as immunotherapy for bladder cancer

**Adverse Reactions All serious adverse reactions must be reported to the U.S. Department of Health and Human Services (DHHS) Vaccine Adverse Event Reporting System (VAERS) 1-800-822-7967.**

1% to 10%:

Genitourinary: Bladder infection, dysuria, polyuria, prostatitis

Miscellaneous: Flu-like syndrome

<1%: Abscesses, hematuria, lymphadenitis, rarely anaphylactic shock in infants, skin ulceration, tuberculosis in immunosuppressed patients

**Drug Interactions** Decreased effect: Antimicrobial or immunosuppressive drugs may impair response to BCG or increase risk of infection; antituberculosis drugs

**Usual Dosage** Children >1 month and Adults:

Immunization against tuberculosis (Tice® BCG): 0.2-0.3 mL percutaneous; initial lesion usually appears after 10-14 days consisting of small red papule at injection site and reaches maximum diameter of 3 mm in 4-6 weeks; conduct postvaccinal tuberculin test (ie, 5 TU of PPD) in 2-3 months; if test is negative, repeat vaccination

Immunotherapy for bladder cancer:

Intravesical treatment: Instill into bladder for 2 hours

TheraCys®: One dose diluted in 50 mL NS (preservative free) instilled into bladder once weekly for 6 weeks followed by one treatment at 3, 6, 12, 18, and 24 months after initial treatment

Tice® BCG: One dose diluted in 50 mL NS (preservative free) instilled into the bladder once weekly for 6 weeks followed by once monthly for 6-12 months

**Patient Information** Notify physician of persistent pain on urination or blood in urine

**Dosage Forms** Freeze-dried suspension for reconstitution

Injection: 50 mg (2 mL)

Injection, intravesical: 27 mg (3 vials)

♦ **B-D Glucose® [OTC]** *see* Glucose, Instant *on page 252*

## Becaplermin (be KAP ler min)

**U.S. Brand Names** Regranex®

**Pharmacologic Category** Growth Factor, Platelet-derived; Topical Skin Product

**Use** Debridement adjunct for the treatment of diabetic ulcers that occur on the lower limbs and feet

**Effects on Mental Status** None reported

**Effects on Psychiatric Treatment** None reported

**Usual Dosage** Adults: Topical:

Diabetic ulcers: Apply appropriate amount of gel once daily with a cotton swab or similar tool, as a coating over the ulcer

The amount of becaplermin to be applied will vary depending on the size of the ulcer area. To calculate the length of gel applied to the ulcer, measure the greatest length of the ulcer by the greatest width of the ulcer in inches. Tube size will determine the formula used in the calculation. For a 15 or 7.5 g tube, multiply length x width x 0.6. For a 2 g tube, multiply length x width x 1.3.

**Note:** If the ulcer does not decrease in size by ~30% after 10 weeks of treatment or complete healing has not occurred in 20 weeks, continued treatment with becaplermin gel should be reassessed.

**Dosage Forms** Gel, topical: 0.01% (2 g, 7.5 g, 15 g)

♦ **Because® [OTC]** *see* Nonoxynol 9 *on page 398*

## Beclomethasone (be kloe METH a sone)

**Related Information**

Asthma Guidelines *on page 773*

**U.S. Brand Names** Beclovent® Oral Inhaler; Beconase® AQ Nasal Inhaler; Beconase® Nasal Inhaler; Vancenase® AQ Inhaler; Vancenase® Nasal Inhaler; Vanceril® Oral Inhaler

**Canadian Brand Names** Beclodisk®; Becloforte®; Propaderm®

**Pharmacologic Category** Corticosteroid, Oral Inhaler; Corticosteroid, Nasal

**Use**

Oral inhalation: Treatment of bronchial asthma in patients who require chronic administration of corticosteroids

Nasal aerosol: Symptomatic treatment of seasonal or perennial rhinitis and nasal polyposis

**Effects on Mental Status** None reported

**Effects on Psychiatric Treatment** None reported

**Pregnancy Risk Factor** C

**Contraindications** Status asthmaticus; hypersensitivity to the drug or fluorocarbons, oleic acid in the formulation, systemic fungal infections

**Warnings/Precautions** Not to be used in status asthmaticus; safety and efficacy in children <6 years of age have not been established; avoid using higher than recommended dosages since suppression of hypothalamic, pituitary, or adrenal function may occur

Controlled clinical studies have shown that inhaled and intranasal corticosteroids may cause a reduction in growth velocity in pediatric patients. Growth velocity provides a means of comparing the rate of growth among children of the same age.

In studies involving inhaled corticosteroids, the average reduction in growth velocity was approximately 1 cm (about 1/3 of an inch) per year. It appears that the reduction is related to dose and how long the child takes the drug.

FDA's Pulmonary and Allergy Drugs and Metabolic and Endocrine Drugs advisory committees discussed this issue at a July 1998 meeting. They recommended that the agency develop class-wide labeling to inform healthcare providers so they would understand this potential side effect and monitor growth routinely in pediatric patients who are treated with inhaled corticosteroids, intranasal corticosteroids or both.

Long-term effects of this reduction in growth velocity on final adult height are unknown. Likewise, it also has not yet been determined whether patients' growth will "catch up" if treatment in discontinued. Drug manufacturers will continue to monitor these drugs to learn more about long-term effects. Children are prescribed inhaled corticosteroids to treat asthma. Intranasal corticosteroids are generally used to prevent and treat allergy-related nasal symptoms.

Patients are advised not to stop using their inhaled or intranasal corticosteroids without first speaking to their healthcare providers about the benefits of these drugs compared to their risks.

**Adverse Reactions**

>10%:

Local: Growth of *Candida* in the mouth, irritation and burning of the nasal mucosa

Respiratory: Cough, hoarseness

1% to 10%:

Gastrointestinal: Xerostomia

Local: Nasal ulceration

Respiratory: Epistaxis

<1%: Bronchospasm, dysphagia, headache, nasal congestion, nasal septal perforations, rash, rhinorrhea, sneezing

**Overdosage/Toxicology**

Signs and symptoms: Irritation and burning of the nasal mucosa, sneezing, intranasal and pharyngeal *Candida* infections, nasal ulceration, epistaxis, rhinorrhea, nasal stuffiness, headache. When consumed in excessive quantities, systemic hypercorticism and adrenal suppression may occur

Treatment: In those cases when systemic hypercorticism and adrenal suppression occur, discontinuation and withdrawal of the corticosteroid should be done judiciously

**Drug Interactions** No data reported

**Usual Dosage** Nasal inhalation and oral inhalation dosage forms are not to be used interchangeably

Aqueous inhalation, nasal:

Vancenase® AQ, Beconase® AQ: Children ≥6 years and Adults: 1-2 inhalations each nostril twice daily

Vancenase® AQ 84 mcg: Children ≥6 years and Adults: 1-2 inhalations in each nostril once daily

Intranasal (Vancenase®, Beconase®):

Children 6-12 years: 1 inhalation in each nostril 3 times/day

Children ≥12 years and Adults: 1 inhalation in each nostril 2-4 times/day or 2 inhalations each nostril twice daily; usual maximum maintenance: 1 inhalation in each nostril 3 times/day

Oral inhalation (doses should be titrated to the lowest effective dose once asthma is controlled):

Beclovent®, Vanceril®:

Children 6-12 years: 1-2 inhalations 3-4 times/day (alternatively: 2-4 inhalations twice daily); maximum dose: 10 inhalations/day

Children ≥12 years and Adults: 2 inhalations 3-4 times/day (alternatively: 4 inhalations twice daily); maximum dose: 20 inhalations/day; patients with severe asthma: Initial: 12-16 inhalations/day (divided 3-4 times/day); dose should be adjusted downward according to patient's response

Vanceril® 84 mcg double strength:

Children 6-12 years: 2 inhalations twice daily; maximum dose: 5 inhalations/day

Children ≥12 years and Adults: 2 inhalations twice daily; maximum dose: 10 inhalations/day; patients with severe asthma: Initial: 6-8 inhalations/day (divided twice daily); dose should be adjusted downward according to patient's response

NIH Guidelines (NIH, 1997) (give in divided doses):

Children:

"Low" dose: 84-336 mcg/day (42 mcg/puff: 2-8 puffs/day or 84 mcg/puff: 1-4 puffs/day)

"Medium" dose: 336-672 mcg/day (42 mcg/puff: 8-16 puffs/day or 84 mcg/puff: 4-8 puffs/day)

"High" dose: >672 mcg/day (42 mcg/puff: >16 puffs/day or 84 mcg/puff >8 puffs/day)

Adults:

"Low" dose: 168-504 mcg/day (42 mcg/puff: 4-12 puffs/day or 84 mcg/puff: 2-6 puffs/day)

"Medium" dose: 504-840 mcg/day (42 mcg/puff: 12-20 puffs/day or 84 mcg/puff: 6-10 puffs/day)

"High" dose: >840 mcg/day (42 mcg/puff: >20 puffs/day or 84 mcg/puff: >10 puffs/day)

**Patient Information** Use as directed; do not increase dosage or discontinue abruptly without consulting prescriber. It may take 1-4 weeks for you to realize full effects of treatment. Review use of inhaler or spray with prescriber or follow package insert for directions. Keep oral inhaler clean and unobstructed. Always rinse mouth and throat after use of inhaler to

(Continued)

## Beclomethasone *(Continued)*

prevent opportunistic infection. If you are also using an inhaled bronchodilator, wait 10 minutes before using this steroid aerosol. Report adverse effects such as skin redness, rash, or irritation; pain or burning of nasal mucosa; white plaques in mouth or fuzzy tongue; unresolved headache; or worsening of condition or lack of improvement.

**Nursing Implications** Take drug history of patients with perennial rhinitis, may be drug related; check mucous membranes for signs of fungal infection

**Dosage Forms**

Nasal, as dipropionate:

Inhalation: (Beconase®, Vancenase®): 42 mcg/inhalation [200 metered doses] (16.8 g)

Spray, as dipropionate (Vancenase® AQ Nasal): 0.084% [120 actuations] (19 g)

Spray, aqueous, nasal, as dipropionate (Beconase® AQ, Vancenase® AQ): 42 mcg/inhalation [≥200 metered doses] (25 g); 84 mcg/inhalation [≥200 metered doses] (25 g)

Oral: Inhalation, as dipropionate:

Beclovent®, Vanceril®: 42 mcg/inhalation [200 metered doses] (16.8 g)

Vanceril® Double Strength: 84 mcg/inhalation (5.4 g - 40 metered doses, 12.2 g - 120 metered doses)

- **Beclovent® Oral Inhaler** *see* Beclomethasone *on page 59*
- **Beconase® AQ Nasal Inhaler** *see* Beclomethasone *on page 59*
- **Beconase® Nasal Inhaler** *see* Beclomethasone *on page 59*
- **Becotin® Pulvules®** *see* Vitamins, Multiple *on page 587*
- **Beepen-VK®** *see* Penicillin V Potassium *on page 426*
- **Belix® Oral [OTC]** *see* Diphenhydramine *on page 174*

## Belladonna (bel a DON a)

**Related Information**

Perspectives on the Safety of Herbal Medicines *on page 736*

**Pharmacologic Category** Anticholinergic Agent

**Use** Decrease gastrointestinal activity in functional bowel disorders; delay gastric emptying as well as decrease gastric secretion

**Effects on Mental Status** May cause drowsiness; rare reports of confusion

**Effects on Psychiatric Treatment** Concurrent use with psychotropics may produce additive sedation; may decrease the effects of phenothiazines; concurrent use with psychotropics may result in additive anticholinergic side effects (dry mouth, blurred vision, constipation)

**Usual Dosage** Tincture: Oral:

Children: 0.03 mL/kg 3 times/day

Adults: 0.6-1 mL 3-4 times/day

**Dosage Forms** Tincture: Belladonna alkaloids (principally hyoscyamine and atropine) 0.3 mg/mL with alcohol 65% to 70% (120 mL, 480 mL, 3780 mL)

## Belladonna and Opium (bel a DON a & OH pee um)

**U.S. Brand Names** B&O Supprettes®

**Canadian Brand Names** PMS-Opium & Beladonna

**Pharmacologic Category** Analgesic, Narcotic

**Use** Relief of moderate to severe pain associated with rectal or bladder tenesmus that may occur in postoperative states and neoplastic situations; pain associated with ureteral spasms not responsive to non-narcotic analgesics and to space intervals between injections of opiates

**Effects on Mental Status** None reported

**Effects on Psychiatric Treatment** Constipation and dry mouth are common; use with low potency antipsychotics and TCAs will likely result in additive effects

**Restrictions** C-II

**Usual Dosage** Adults: Rectal: 1 suppository 1-2 times/day, up to 4 doses/day

**Dosage Forms** Suppository:

#15 A: Belladonna extract 15 mg and opium 30 mg

#16 A: Belladonna extract 15 mg and opium 60 mg

- **Bellatal®** *see* Hyoscyamine, Atropine, Scopolamine, and Phenobarbital *on page 279*
- **Benadryl® Decongestant Allergy Tablet [OTC]** *see* Diphenhydramine and Pseudoephedrine *on page 175*
- **Benadryl® Injection** *see* Diphenhydramine *on page 174*
- **Benadryl® Oral [OTC]** *see* Diphenhydramine *on page 174*
- **Benadryl® Topical** *see* Diphenhydramine *on page 174*
- **Ben-Allergin-50® Injection** *see* Diphenhydramine *on page 174*
- **Ben-Aqua® [OTC]** *see* Benzoyl Peroxide *on page 62*

## Benazepril (ben AY ze pril)

**Related Information**

Angiotensin-Related Agents Comparison Chart *on page 700*

**U.S. Brand Names** Lotensin®

**Pharmacologic Category** Angiotensin-Converting Enzyme (ACE) Inhibitors

**Use** Treatment of hypertension, either alone or in combination with other antihypertensive agents; treatment of left ventricular dysfunction after myocardial infarction

**Effects on Mental Status** May cause drowsiness

**Effects on Psychiatric Treatment** May decrease lithium clearance resulting in an increase in serum lithium levels and potential lithium toxicity; monitor serum lithium levels

**Pregnancy Risk Factor** C (1st trimester); D (2nd & 3rd trimester)

**Contraindications** Hypersensitivity to benazepril or any component; angioedema or serious hypersensitivity related to previous treatment with an ACE inhibitor; bilateral renal artery stenosis; primary hyperaldosteronism; patients with idiopathic or hereditary angioedema; pregnancy (2nd and 3rd trimesters)

**Warnings/Precautions** Anaphylactic reactions can occur. Angioedema can occur at any time during treatment (especially following first dose). Careful blood pressure monitoring with first dose (hypotension can occur especially in volume depleted patients). Dosage adjustment needed in renal impairment. Use with caution in hypovolemia; collagen vascular diseases; valvular stenosis (particularly aortic stenosis); hyperkalemia; or before, during, or immediately after anesthesia. Avoid rapid dosage escalation which may lead to renal insufficiency. Hypersensitivity reactions may be seen during hemodialysis with high-flux dialysis membranes (eg, AN69). Deterioration in renal function can occur with initiation. Use with caution in unilateral renal artery stenosis and pre-existing renal insufficiency.

**Adverse Reactions**

1% to 10%:

Central nervous system: Dizziness, fatigue, headache

Gastrointestinal: Nausea (1% to 2%)

Respiratory: Transient cough

<1%: Angioedema, arthralgia, arthritis, asthma, anxiety, bronchitis, constipation, diaphoresis, dyspnea, gastritis, hyperkalemia, hypertonia, hypotension, impotence, insomnia, melena, myalgia, nervousness, paresthesia, photosensitivity, rash, sinusitis, tachycardia, urinary tract infection, vomiting, weakness

**Overdosage/Toxicology**

Signs and symptoms: Mild hypotension has been the only toxic effect seen with acute overdose; bradycardia may also occur. Hyperkalemia occurs even with therapeutic doses, especially in patients with renal insufficiency and those taking NSAIDs.

Treatment: Following initiation of essential overdose management, toxic symptom treatment and supportive treatment should be initiated. Hypotension usually responds to I.V. fluids or Trendelenburg positioning.

**Drug Interactions**

Alpha$_1$ blockers: Hypotensive effect increased

Aspirin: The effects of ACE inhibitors may be blunted by aspirin administration, particularly at higher dosages

Diuretics: Hypovolemia due to diuretics may precipitate acute hypotensive events or acute renal failure

Insulin: Risk of hypoglycemia may be increased

Lithium: Risk of lithium toxicity may be increased; monitor lithium levels

NSAIDs may decrease ACE inhibitor efficacy and/or increase adverse renal effects

Potassium-sparing diuretics or potassium supplements (amiloride, potassium, spironolactone, triamterene): Increased risk of hyperkalemia

Trimethoprim (high dose) may increase the risk of hyperkalemia

**Usual Dosage** Adults: Oral: Initial: 10 mg/day in patients not receiving a diuretic; 20-40 mg/day as a single dose or 2 divided doses; base dosage adjustments on peak (2-6 hours after dosing) and trough responses.

**Dosing interval in renal impairment:** $Cl_{cr}$ <30 mL/minute: Administer 5 mg/day initially; maximum daily dose: 40 mg.

Hemodialysis: Moderately dialyzable (20% to 50%); administer dose postdialysis or administer 25% to 35% supplemental dose.

Peritoneal dialysis: Supplemental dose is not necessary.

**Patient Information** Take exactly as directed; do not discontinue without consulting prescriber. Take first dose at bedtime. Take all doses on an empty stomach (30 minutes before or 2 hours after meals). This drug does not eliminate need for diet or exercise regimen as recommended by prescriber. May cause dizziness, fainting, lightheadedness (use caution when driving or engaging in tasks that require alertness until response to drug is known); postural hypotension (use caution when rising from lying or sitting position or climbing stairs); nausea, vomiting, abdominal pain, dry mouth, or transient loss of appetite (small frequent meals, frequent mouth care, sucking lozenges, or chewing gum may help) - report if these persist. Report mouth sores; fever or chills; swelling of extremities, face, mouth, or tongue; difficulty in breathing or unusual cough; or other persistent adverse reactions.

**Nursing Implications** Watch for hypotensive effect within 1-3 hours of first dose or new higher dose; discontinue therapy immediately if angioedema of the face, extremities, lips, tongue, or glottis occurs

**Dosage Forms** Tablet, as hydrochloride: 5 mg, 10 mg, 20 mg, 40 mg

## Benazepril and Hydrochlorothiazide

(ben AY ze pril & hye droe klor oh THYE a zide)

**U.S. Brand Names** Lotensin® HCT

**Pharmacologic Category** Antihypertensive Agent, Combination

**Use** Treatment of hypertension

**Effects on Mental Status** May cause drowsiness

**Effects on Psychiatric Treatment** May decrease lithium clearance resulting in an increase in serum lithium levels and potential lithium toxicity; monitor serum lithium levels

**Usual Dosage** Dose is individualized

**Dosage Forms** Tablet:

Benazepril 5 mg and hydrochlorothiazide 6.25 mg
Benazepril 10 mg and hydrochlorothiazide 12.5 mg
Benazepril 20 mg and hydrochlorothiazide 12.5 mg
Benazepril 20 mg and hydrochlorothiazide 25 mg

## Bendroflumethiazide (ben droe floo meth EYE a zide)

**U.S. Brand Names** Naturetin®

**Pharmacologic Category** Diuretic, Thiazide

**Use** Management of mild to moderate hypertension, edema associated with congestive heart failure, pregnancy, or nephrotic syndrome; reportedly does not alter serum electrolyte concentrations appreciably at recommended doses

**Effects on Mental Status** May cause drowsiness

**Effects on Psychiatric Treatment** May produce orthostatic hypotension; use caution with concurrent psychotropic use; rare reports of agranulocytosis; caution with clozapine and carbamazepine; may decrease lithium clearance resulting in an increase in serum lithium levels and potential lithium toxicity; monitor serum lithium levels

**Contraindications** Hypersensitivity to thiazides or sulfonamide-derived drugs; anuria; renal decompensation; pregnancy

**Warnings/Precautions** Use with caution in severe renal disease. Electrolyte disturbances (hypokalemia, hypochloremic alkalosis, hyponatremia) can occur. Use with caution in severe hepatic dysfunction; hepatic encephalopathy can be caused by electrolyte disturbances. Gout can be precipitate in certain patients with a history of gout, a familial predisposition to gout, or chronic renal failure. Cautious use in diabetics; may see a change in glucose control. Hypersensitivity reactions can occur. Can cause SLE exacerbation or activation. Use with caution in patients with moderate or high cholesterol concentrations. Photosensitization may occur.

**Adverse Reactions** 1% to 10%:

Cardiovascular: Orthostatic hypotension
Endocrine & metabolic: Hypokalemia, hyponatremia
Gastrointestinal: Anorexia, diarrhea, upset stomach

**Overdosage/Toxicology**

Signs and symptoms: Hypermotility, diuresis, lethargy, confusion, muscle weakness

Treatment: Following GI decontamination, therapy is supportive with I.V. fluids, electrolytes, and I.V. pressors if needed

**Drug Interactions**

Angiotensin-converting enzyme inhibitors: Increased hypotension if aggressively diuresed with a thiazide diuretic

Beta-blockers increase hyperglycemic effects in Type 2 diabetes mellitus

Cyclosporine and thiazides can increase the risk of gout or renal toxicity; avoid concurrent use

Digoxin toxicity can be exacerbated if a thiazide induces hypokalemia or hypomagnesemia

Lithium toxicity can occur by reducing renal excretion of lithium; monitor lithium concentration and adjust as needed

Neuromuscular blocking agents can prolong blockade; monitor serum potassium and neuromuscular status

NSAIDs can decrease the efficacy of thiazides reducing the diuretic and antihypertensive effects

**Usual Dosage** Oral:

Children: Initial: 0.1-0.4 mg/kg/day in 1-2 doses; maintenance dose: 0.05-0.1 mg/kg/day in 1-2 doses; maximum dose: 20 mg/day

Adults: 2.5-20 mg/day or twice daily in divided doses

**Patient Information** May be taken with food or milk; take early in day to avoid nocturia; take the last dose of multiple doses no later than 6 PM unless instructed otherwise. A few people who take this medication become more sensitive to sunlight and may experience skin rash, redness, itching, or severe sunburn, especially if sun block SPF ≥15 is not used on exposed skin areas.

**Dosage Forms** Tablet: 5 mg, 10 mg

- **BeneFix™** *see* Factor IX Complex (Human) *on page 217*
- **Benemid®** *see* Probenecid *on page 463*
- **Benoxyl®** *see* Benzoyl Peroxide *on page 62*
- **Bentyl® Hydrochloride Injection** *see* Dicyclomine *on page 165*
- **Bentyl® Hydrochloride Oral** *see* Dicyclomine *on page 165*
- **Benylin® Cough Syrup [OTC]** *see* Diphenhydramine *on page 174*
- **Benylin DM® [OTC]** *see* Dextromethorphan *on page 160*
- **Benylin® Expectorant [OTC]** *see* Guaifenesin and Dextromethorphan *on page 257*
- **Benylin® Pediatric [OTC]** *see* Dextromethorphan *on page 160*
- **Benzac AC® Gel** *see* Benzoyl Peroxide *on page 62*
- **Benzac AC® Wash** *see* Benzoyl Peroxide *on page 62*
- **Benzac W® Gel** *see* Benzoyl Peroxide *on page 62*
- **Benzac W® Wash** *see* Benzoyl Peroxide *on page 62*
- **5-Benzagel®** *see* Benzoyl Peroxide *on page 62*
- **10-Benzagel®** *see* Benzoyl Peroxide *on page 62*
- **Benzamycin®** *see* Erythromycin and Benzoyl Peroxide *on page 201*
- **Benzashave® Cream** *see* Benzoyl Peroxide *on page 62*
- **Benzathine Benzylpenicillin** *see* Penicillin G Benzathine *on page 425*
- **Benzathine Penicillin G** *see* Penicillin G Benzathine *on page 425*
- **Benzene Hexachloride** *see* Lindane *on page 318*
- **Benzhexol Hydrochloride** *see* Trihexyphenidyl *on page 568*
- **Benzmethyzin** *see* Procarbazine *on page 465*

## Benzocaine (BEN zoe kane)

**U.S. Brand Names** Americaine® [OTC]; Anbesol® [OTC]; Anbesol® Maximum Strength [OTC]; Babee® Teething® [OTC]; Benzocol® [OTC]; Benzodent® [OTC]; Chiggertox® [OTC]; Cylex® [OTC]; Dermoplast® [OTC]; Foille® [OTC]; Foille® Medicated First Aid [OTC]; Hurricaine®; Lanacane® [OTC]; Maximum Strength Anbesol® [OTC]; Maximum Strength Orajel® [OTC]; Mycinettes® [OTC]; Numzitdent® [OTC]; Numzit Teething® [OTC]; Orabase®-B [OTC]; Orabase®-O [OTC]; Orajel® Brace-Aid Oral Anesthetic [OTC]; Orajel® Maximum Strength [OTC]; Orajel® Mouth-Aid [OTC]; Orasept® [OTC]; Orasol® [OTC]; Rhulicaine® [OTC]; Rid-A-Pain® [OTC]; Slim-Mint® [OTC]; Solarcaine® [OTC]; Spec-T® [OTC]; Tanac® [OTC]; Trocaine® [OTC]; Unguentine® [OTC]; Vicks Children's Chloraseptic® [OTC]; Vicks Chloraseptic® Sore Throat [OTC]; Zilactin®-B Medicated [OTC]

**Pharmacologic Category** Local Anesthetic

**Use** Temporary relief of pain associated with local anesthetic for pruritic dermatosis, pruritus, minor burns, acute congestive and serous otitis media, swimmer's ear, otitis externa, toothache, minor sore throat pain, canker sores, hemorrhoids, rectal fissures, anesthetic lubricant for passage of catheters and endoscopic tubes; nonprescription diet aide

**Effects on Mental Status** None reported

**Effects on Psychiatric Treatment** None reported

**Usual Dosage**

Children and Adults:

- Mucous membranes: Dosage varies depending on area to be anesthetized and vascularity of tissues
- Oral mouth/throat preparations: Do not administer for >2 days or in children <2 years of age, unless directed by a physician; refer to specific package labeling
- Topical: Apply to affected area as needed

Adults: Nonprescription diet aid: 6-15 mg just prior to food consumption, not to exceed 45 mg/day

**Dosage Forms**

Mouth/throat preparations:

- Cream: 5% (10 g)
- Gel: 6.3% (7.5 g); 7.5% (7.2 g, 9.45 g, 14.1 g); 10% (6 g, 9.45 g, 10 g, 15 g); 15% (10.5 g); 20% (9.45 g, 14.1 g)
- Liquid: (3.7 mL); 5% (8.8 mL); 6.3% (9 mL, 22 mL, 14.79 mL); 10% (13 mL); 20% (13.3 mL)
- Lotion: 0.2% (15 mL); 2.5% (15 mL)
- Lozenges: 5 mg, 6 mg, 10 mg, 15 mg
- Ointment: 20% (30 g)
- Paste: 20% (5 g, 15 g)

Nonprescription diet aid:

- Candy: 6 mg
- Gum: 6 mg

Topical for mucous membranes:

- Gel: 6% (7.5 g); 20% (2.5 g, 3.75 g, 7.5 g, 30 g)
- Liquid: 20% (3.75 mL, 9 mL, 13.3 mL, 30 mL)

Topical for skin disorders:

- Aerosol, external use: 5% (92 mL, 105 g); 20% (82.5 mL, 90 mL, 92 mL, 150 mL)
- Cream: (30 g, 60 g); 5% (30 g, 1 lb); 6% (28.4 g)
- Lotion: (120 mL); 8% (90 mL)

(Continued)

## Benzocaine *(Continued)*

Ointment: 5% (3.5 g, 28 g)
Spray: 5% (97.5 mL); 20% (20 g, 60 g, 120 g, 13.3 mL, 120 mL)

## Benzocaine, Butyl Aminobenzoate, Tetracaine, and Benzalkonium Chloride

(BEN zoe kane, BYOO til a meen oh BENZ oh ate, TET ra kane, & benz al KOE nee um KLOR ide)

**U.S. Brand Names** Cetacaine®
**Pharmacologic Category** Local Anesthetic
**Use** Topical anesthetic to control pain or gagging
**Effects on Mental Status** None reported
**Effects on Psychiatric Treatment** None reported
**Usual Dosage** Apply to affected area for approximately 1 second or less
**Dosage Forms** Aerosol: Benzocaine 14%, butyl aminobenzoate 2%, tetracaine 2%, and benzalkonium chloride 0.5% (56 g)

## Benzocaine, Gelatin, Pectin, and Sodium Carboxymethylcellulose

(BEN zoe kane, JEL a tin, PEK tin, & SOW dee um kar box ee meth il SEL yoo lose)

**U.S. Brand Names** Orabase® With Benzocaine [OTC]
**Pharmacologic Category** Local Anesthetic
**Use** Topical anesthetic and emollient for oral lesions
**Effects on Mental Status** None reported
**Effects on Psychiatric Treatment** None reported
**Usual Dosage** Apply 2-4 times/day
**Dosage Forms** Paste: Benzocaine 20%, gelatin, pectin, and sodium carboxymethylcellulose (15 g, 5 g)

♦ **Benzocol® [OTC]** *see* Benzocaine *on page 61*
♦ **Benzodent® [OTC]** *see* Benzocaine *on page 61*
♦ **Benzodiazepines Comparison Chart** *see page 708*

## Benzoic Acid and Salicylic Acid

(ben ZOE ik AS id & sal i SIL ik AS id)

**U.S. Brand Names** Whitfield's Ointment [OTC]
**Pharmacologic Category** Antifungal Agent, Topical
**Use** Treatment of athlete's foot and ringworm of the scalp
**Effects on Mental Status** None reported
**Effects on Psychiatric Treatment** None reported
**Usual Dosage** Apply 1-4 times/day
**Dosage Forms**
Lotion, topical:
Full strength: Benzoic acid 12% and salicylic acid 6% with isopropyl alcohol 70% (240 mL)
Half strength: Benzoic acid 6% and salicylic acid 3% with isopropyl alcohol 70% (240 mL)
Ointment, topical: Benzoic acid 12% and salicylic acid 6% in anhydrous lanolin and petrolatum (30 g, 454 g)

## Benzonatate (ben ZOE na tate)

**U.S. Brand Names** Tessalon® Perles
**Pharmacologic Category** Antitussive
**Use** Symptomatic relief of nonproductive cough
**Effects on Mental Status** May cause drowsiness
**Effects on Psychiatric Treatment** May potentiate sedative effects of sedating psychotropics
**Pregnancy Risk Factor** C
**Contraindications** Known hypersensitivity to benzonatate or related compounds (such as tetracaine)
**Adverse Reactions** 1% to 10%:
Central nervous system: Dizziness, headache, sedation
Dermatologic: Rash
Gastrointestinal: GI upset
Neuromuscular & skeletal: Numbness in chest
Ocular: Burning sensation in eyes
Respiratory: Nasal congestion
**Overdosage/Toxicology**
Signs and symptoms: Restlessness, tremor, CNS stimulation. The drug's local anesthetic activity can reduce the patient's gag reflex and, therefore, may contradict the use of ipecac following ingestion, this is especially true when the capsules are chewed.
Treatment: Gastric lavage may be indicated if initiated early on following an acute ingestion or in comatose patients. The remaining treatment is supportive and symptomatic.
**Drug Interactions** No data reported
**Usual Dosage** Children >10 years and Adults: Oral: 100 mg 3 times/day or every 4 hours up to 600 mg/day
**Patient Information** Take only as prescribed; do not exceed prescribed dose or frequency. Do not break or chew capsule. Maintain adequate hydration (2-3 L/day of fluids unless instructed to restrict fluid intake). Avoid use of other depressants, alcohol, or sleep-inducing medications unless approved by prescriber. You may experience drowsiness, impaired coordination, blurred vision, or increased anxiety (use caution when driving or engaging in tasks requiring alertness until response to drug is known); or upset stomach or nausea (frequent small meals, frequent mouth care, chewing gum, or sucking hard candy may help). Report persistent CNS changes (dizziness, sedation, tremor, or agitation), numbness in chest or feeling of chill, visual changes or burning in eyes, numbness of mouth or difficulty swallowing, or lack of improvement or worsening or condition.
**Nursing Implications** Change patient position every 2 hours to prevent pooling of secretions in lung; capsules are not to be crushed
**Dosage Forms** Capsule: 100 mg

## Benzoyl Peroxide (BEN zoe il peer OKS ide)

**U.S. Brand Names** Advanced Formula Oxy® Sensitive Gel [OTC]; Ambi 10® [OTC]; Ben-Aqua® [OTC]; Benoxyl®; Benzac AC® Gel; Benzac AC® Wash; Benzac W® Gel; Benzac W® Wash; 5-Benzagel®; 10-Benzagel®; Benzashave® Cream; BlemErase® Lotion [OTC]; Brevoxyl® Gel; Clear By Design® Gel [OTC]; Clearsil® Maximum Strength [OTC]; Del Aqua-5® Gel; Del Aqua-10® Gel; Desquam-E™ Gel; Desquam-X® Gel; Desquam-X® Wash; Dryox® Gel [OTC]; Dryox® Wash [OTC]; Exact® Cream [OTC]; Fostex® 10% BPO Gel [OTC]; Fostex® 10% Wash [OTC]; Fostex® Bar [OTC]; Loroxide® [OTC]; Neutrogena® Acne Mask [OTC]; Oxy-5® Advanced Formula for Sensitive Skin [OTC]; Oxy-5® Tinted [OTC]; Oxy-10® Advanced Formula for Sensitive Skin [OTC]; Oxy 10® Wash [OTC]; PanOxyl®-AQ; PanOxyl® Bar [OTC]; Perfectoderm® Gel [OTC]; Peroxin A5®; Peroxin A10®; Persa-Gel®; Theroxide® Wash [OTC]; Vanoxide® [OTC]
**Pharmacologic Category** Topical Skin Product; Topical Skin Product, Acne
**Use** Adjunctive treatment of mild to moderate acne vulgaris and acne rosacea
**Effects on Mental Status** None reported
**Effects on Psychiatric Treatment** None reported
**Usual Dosage** Children and Adults:
Cleansers: Wash once or twice daily; control amount of drying or peeling by modifying dose frequency or concentration
Topical: Apply sparingly once daily; gradually increase to 2-3 times/day if needed. If excessive dryness or peeling occurs, reduce dose frequency or concentration; if excessive stinging or burning occurs, remove with mild soap and water; resume use the next day.
**Dosage Forms**
Bar: 5% (113 g); 10% (106 g, 113 g)
Cream: 5% (18 g, 113.4 g); 10% (18 g, 28 g, 113.4 g)
Gel: 2.5% (30 g, 42.5 g, 45 g, 57 g, 60 g, 90 g, 113 g); 5% (42.5 g, 45 g, 60 g, 80 g, 90 g, 113.4 g); 10% (30 g, 42.5 g, 45 g, 56.7 g, 60 g, 90 g, 113.4 g, 120 g); 20% (30 g, 60 g)
Liquid: 5% (120 mL, 150 mL, 240 mL); 10% (120 mL, 150 mL, 240 mL)
Lotion: 5% (25 mL, 30 mL); 5.5% (25 mL); 10% (12 mL, 29 mL, 30 mL, 60 mL)
Mask: 5% (30 mL, 60 mL, 60 g)

## Benzoyl Peroxide and Hydrocortisone

(BEN zoe il peer OKS ide & hye droe KOR ti sone)

**U.S. Brand Names** Vanoxide-HC®
**Pharmacologic Category** Topical Skin Product; Topical Skin Product, Acne
**Use** Treatment of acne vulgaris and oily skin
**Effects on Mental Status** None reported
**Effects on Psychiatric Treatment** None reported
**Usual Dosage** Shake well; apply thin film 1-3 times/day, gently massage into skin
**Dosage Forms** Lotion: Benzoyl peroxide 5% and hydrocortisone alcohol 0.5% (25 mL)

## Benzphetamine (benz FET a meen)

**U.S. Brand Names** Didrex®
**Pharmacologic Category** Anorexiant
**Use** Short-term adjunct in exogenous obesity
**Restrictions** C-III
**Pregnancy Risk Factor** X
**Contraindications** Known hypersensitivity or idiosyncrasy to sympathomimetic amines. Patients with advanced arteriosclerosis, symptomatic cardiovascular disease, moderate to severe hypertension (stage II or III), hyperthyroidism, glaucoma, agitated states, patients with a history of drug abuse, pregnancy, and during or within 14 days following MAO inhibitor

therapy. Concurrent use with other anorectic agents; stimulant medications are contraindicated for use in children with attention deficit/hyperactivity disorders and concomitant Tourette's syndrome or tics.

**Warnings/Precautions** Cardiovascular disease, nephritis, angina pectoris, hypertension, glaucoma, patients with a history of drug abuse

**Adverse Reactions**

Cardiovascular: Hypertension, palpitations, tachycardia, chest pain, T-wave changes, arrhythmias, pulmonary hypertension, valvalopathy

Central nervous system: Euphoria, nervousness, insomnia, restlessness, dizziness, anxiety, headache, agitation, confusion, mental depression, psychosis, CVA, seizure

Dermatologic: Alopecia, urticaria, skin rash, ecchymosis, erythema

Endocrine & metabolic: Changes in libido, gynecomastia, menstrual irregularities, porphyria

Gastrointestinal: Nausea, vomiting, abdominal cramps, constipation, xerostomia, metallic taste

Genitourinary: Impotence

Hematologic: Bone marrow depression, agranulocytosis, leukopenia

Neuromuscular & skeletal: Tremor

Ocular: Blurred vision, mydriasis

**Overdosage/Toxicology** Treatment: There is no specific antidote for amphetamine intoxication and the bulk of the treatment is supportive. Hyperactivity and agitation usually respond to reduced sensory input, however, with extreme agitation haloperidol (2-5 mg I.M. for adults) may be required. Hyperthermia is best treated with external cooling measures, or when severe or unresponsive, muscle paralysis with pancuronium may be needed. Hypertension is usually transient and generally does not require treatment unless severe. For diastolic blood pressures >110 mm Hg, a nitroprusside infusion should be initiated. Seizures usually respond to diazepam IVP and/or phenytoin maintenance regimens.

**Drug Interactions** CYP3A3/4 enzyme substrate

Acidifiers: Very large doses of potassium acid phosphate or ammonium chloride may increase the renal elimination of amphetamines due to urinary acidification

Alkalinizers: Large doses of sodium bicarbonate or other alkalinizers may increase renal tubular reabsorption (decreased elimination) and diminish the effect of amphetamine; includes potassium or sodium citrate and acetate

Antipsychotics: Efficacy of amphetamines may be decreased by antipsychotics; in addition, amphetamines may induce an increase in psychotic symptoms in some patients

CYP3A3/4 inhibitors: Serum level and/or toxicity of some tricyclic antidepressants may be increased. Inhibitors include amiodarone, cimetidine, clarithromycin, erythromycin, delavirdine, diltiazem, dirithromycin, disulfiram, fluoxetine, fluvoxamine, grapefruit juice, indinavir, itraconazole, ketoconazole, nefazodone, nevirapine, propoxyfene, quinupristin-dalfopristin, ritonavir, saquinavir, verapamil, zafirlukast, zileuton. Monitor for altered effects; a decrease in amphetamine dosage may be required.

Enzyme inducers: Metabolism of amphetamine may be increased, decreasing clinical effect; inducers include barbiturates, carbamazepine, phenytoin, and rifampin

Furazolidine: Amphetamines may induce hypertensive episodes in patients receiving furazolidone

Guanethidine: Amphetamines inhibit the antihypertensive response to guanethidine; probably also may occur with guanadrel

MAOIs: Severe hypertensive episodes have occurred with amphetamine when used in patients receiving MAOIs; concurrent use or use within 14 days is contraindicated

Norepinephrine: Amphetamines may enhance the pressor response to norepinephrine

Sibutramine: Concurrent use of sibutramine and amphetamines may cause severe hypertension and tachycardia; use is contraindicated in product

SSRIs: Amphetamines may increase the potential for serotonin syndrome when used concurrently with selective serotonin reuptake inhibitors (including fluoxetine, fluvoxamine, paroxetine, and sertraline)

Tricyclic antidepressants: Concurrent of amphetamines with TCAs may result in hypertension and CNS stimulation; avoid this combination

**Mechanism of Action** Noncatechol sympathomimetic amines with pharmacologic actions similar to ephedrine; require breakdown by monoamine oxidase for inactivation; produce central nervous system and respiratory stimulation, a pressor response, mydriasis, bronchodilation, and contraction of the urinary sphincter; thought to have a direct effect on both alpha- and beta-receptor sites in the peripheral system, as well as release stores of norepinephrine in adrenergic nerve terminals; central nervous system action is thought to occur in the cerebral cortex and reticular activating system; anorexigenic effect is probably secondary to the CNS-stimulating effect; the site of action is probably the hypothalamic feeding center

**Usual Dosage** Adults: Oral: Initial: 25-50 mg once daily; increase according to response; maximum dose: 50 mg 3 times/day

**Patient Information** Take during the day to avoid insomnia; do not discontinue abruptly, may be addicting with prolonged use

**Dosage Forms** Tablet, as hydrochloride: 25 mg, 50 mg

## Benzthiazide (benz THYE a zide)

**U.S. Brand Names** Exna®

**Pharmacologic Category** Diuretic, Thiazide

**Use** Management of mild to moderate hypertension; treatment of edema in congestive heart failure and nephrotic syndrome

**Effects on Mental Status** May cause drowsiness

**Effects on Psychiatric Treatment** May produce orthostatic hypotension; use caution with concurrent psychotropic use; rare reports of agranulocytosis; caution with clozapine and carbamazepine; may decrease lithium clearance resulting in an increase in serum lithium levels and potential lithium toxicity; monitor serum lithium levels

**Pregnancy Risk Factor** C (per manufacturer); D (based on expert analysis)

**Contraindications** Hypersensitivity to benzthiazide or any component, other thiazides, or sulfonamide-derived drugs; anuria; renal decompensation; pregnancy

**Warnings/Precautions** Use with caution in severe renal disease. Electrolyte disturbances (hypokalemia, hypochloremic alkalosis, hyponatremia) can occur. Use with caution in severe hepatic dysfunction; hepatic encephalopathy can be caused by electrolyte disturbances. Gout can be precipitate in certain patients with a history of gout, a familial predisposition to gout, or chronic renal failure. Cautious use in diabetics; may see a change in glucose control. Hypersensitivity reactions can occur. Use with caution in patients with moderate or high cholesterol concentrations. Photosensitization may occur. Correct hypokalemia before initiating therapy.

**Adverse Reactions**

1% to 10%:

Cardiovascular: Orthostatic hypotension

Endocrine & metabolic: Hypokalemia, hyponatremia

Gastrointestinal: Anorexia, diarrhea, upset stomach

<1%: Agranulocytosis, allergic reactions, aplastic anemia, drowsiness, hemolytic anemia, hepatic function impairment, hepatitis, hyperuricemia, leukopenia, nausea, paresthesia, polyuria, thrombocytopenia, uremia, vomiting

**Overdosage/Toxicology**

Signs and symptoms: Hypermotility, diuresis, lethargy, confusion, muscle weakness

Treatment: Following GI decontamination, therapy is supportive with I.V. fluids, electrolytes, and I.V. pressors if needed

**Drug Interactions**

Angiotensin-converting enzyme inhibitors: Increased hypotension if aggressively diuresed with a thiazide diuretic

Beta-blockers increase hyperglycemic effects in Type 2 diabetes mellitus

Cyclosporine and thiazides can increase the risk of gout or renal toxicity; avoid concurrent use

Digoxin toxicity can be exacerbated if a thiazide induces hypokalemia or hypomagnesemia

Lithium toxicity can occur by reducing renal excretion of lithium; monitor lithium concentration and adjust as needed

Neuromuscular blocking agents can prolong blockade; monitor serum potassium and neuromuscular status

NSAIDs can decrease the efficacy of thiazides reducing the diuretic and antihypertensive effects

**Usual Dosage** Adults: Oral:

Edema: 50-200 mg/day; maintenance: 50-150 mg/day; use divided doses after morning and evening meal if total dose exceeds 100 mg

Hypertension: 50-100 mg/day; maintenance: individualize dose (maximum effective dose: 200 mg/day)

**Patient Information** Take early in the day and take last dose in early evening to avoid frequent night urination. Take with food to reduce GI upset. Weigh yourself on a regular basis (same time, same clothes). Report unresolved weight gain (more than 3-5 pounds in 3 days). You may experience dizziness or drowsiness; change positions slowly and use caution when driving or engaging in tasks that require alertness until response to drug is known. May cause photosensitivity; use sunscreen wear protective clothing and eyewear, and avoid direct sunlight. You may experience decreased sexual function; this will resolve when medication is discontinued. Report increased swelling of ankles, fingers, dizziness or trembling, cramps, or muscle pain.

**Nursing Implications** Take blood pressure with patient lying down and standing

**Dosage Forms** Tablet: 50 mg

## Benztropine (BENZ troe peen)

**Related Information**

Agents for Treatment of Extrapyramidal Symptoms *on page 638*
Antiparkinsonian Agents Comparison Chart *on page 705*
Clozapine-Induced Side Effects *on page 780*
Discontinuation of Psychotropic Drugs - Withdrawal Symptoms and Recommendations *on page 798*
Patient Information - Agents for Treatment of Extrapyramidal Symptoms *on page 657*
(Continued)

## Benztropine *(Continued)*

**Generic Available** Yes: Tablet

**U.S. Brand Names** Cogentin®

**Canadian Brand Names** PMS-Benztropine

**Synonyms** Benztropine Mesylate

**Pharmacologic Category** Anticholinergic Agent; Anti-Parkinson's Agent (Anticholinergic)

**Use** Adjunctive treatment of Parkinson's disease; also used in treatment of drug-induced extrapyramidal reactions

**Pregnancy Risk Factor** C

**Contraindications** Children <3 years of age; hypersensitivity to benztropine or any component of the formulation; pyloric or duodenal obstruction, stenosing peptic ulcers; bladder neck obstructions; achalasia; myasthenia gravis

**Warnings/Precautions** Use with caution in older children (dose has not been established). Use with caution in hot weather or during exercise. May cause anhydrosis and hyperthermia, which may be severe. The risk is increased in hot environments, particularly in the elderly, alcoholics, patients with CNS disease, and those with prolonged outdoor exposure.

Elderly patients frequently develop increased sensitivity and require strict dosage regulation - side effects may be more severe in elderly patients with atherosclerotic changes. Use with caution in patients with tachycardia, cardiac arrhythmias, hypertension, hypotension, prostatic hypertrophy (especially in the elderly), any tendency toward urinary retention, liver or kidney disorders, and obstructive disease of the GI or GU tract. When given in large doses or to susceptible patients, may cause weakness and inability to move particular muscle groups.

May be associated with confusion or hallucinations (generally at higher dosages). Intensification of symptoms or toxic psychosis may occur in patients with mental disorders. Benztropine does not relieve symptoms of tardive dyskinesia.

**Adverse Reactions**

Cardiovascular: Tachycardia
Central nervous system: Confusion, disorientation, memory impairment, toxic psychosis, visual hallucinations
Dermatologic: Rash
Endocrine & metabolic: Heat stroke, hyperthermia
Gastrointestinal: Xerostomia, nausea, vomiting, constipation, ileus
Genitourinary: Urinary retention, dysuria
Ocular: Blurred vision, mydriasis
Miscellaneous: Fever

**Overdosage/Toxicology**

Signs and symptoms: CNS depression, confusion, nervousness, hallucinations, dizziness, blurred vision, nausea, vomiting, hyperthermia
Treatment: For anticholinergic overdose with severe life-threatening symptoms, physostigmine 1-2 mg (0.5 or 0.02 mg/kg for children) I.V. or S.C., slowly may be given to reverse these effects. Anticholinergic toxicity is caused by strong binding of the drug to cholinergic receptors. Anticholinesterase inhibitors reduce acetylcholinesterase, the enzyme that breaks down acetylcholine and thereby allows acetylcholine to accumulate and compete for receptor binding with the offending anticholinergic.

**Drug Interactions**

Amantadine, rimantadine: Central and/or peripheral anticholinergic syndrome can occur when administered with amantadine or rimantadine
Anticholinergic agents: Central and/or peripheral anticholinergic syndrome can occur when administered with narcotic analgesics, phenothiazines and other antipsychotics (especially with high anticholinergic activity), tricyclic antidepressants, quinidine and some other antiarrhythmics, and antihistamines
Atenolol: Anticholinergics may increase the bioavailability of atenolol (and possibly other beta-blockers); monitor for increased effect
Cholinergic agents: Anticholinergics may antagonize the therapeutic effect of cholinergic agents; includes tacrine and donepezil
Digoxin: Anticholinergics may decrease gastric degradation and increase the amount of digoxin absorbed by delaying gastric emptying
Levodopa: Anticholinergics may increase gastric degradation and decrease the amount of levodopa absorbed by delaying gastric emptying
Neuroleptics: Anticholinergics may antagonize the therapeutic effects of neuroleptics

**Mechanism of Action** Possesses both anticholinergic and antihistaminic effects. *In vitro* anticholinergic activity approximates that of atropine; *in vivo* it is only about half as active as atropine. Animal data suggest its antihistaminic activity and duration of action approach that of pyrilamine maleate. May also inhibit the reuptake and storage of dopamine and thereby, prolong the action of dopamine.

**Pharmacodynamics/kinetics**

Onset of action:
Oral: Within 1 hour
I.M./I.V.: Within 15 minutes
Duration of action: 6-48 hours (wide range)

**Usual Dosage** Use in children <3 years of age should be reserved for life-threatening emergencies

Drug-induced extrapyramidal reaction: Oral, I.M., I.V.:
Children >3 years: 0.02-0.05 mg/kg/dose 1-2 times/day
Adults: 1-4 mg/dose 1-2 times/day
Acute dystonia: Adults: I.M., I.V.: 1-2 mg
Parkinsonism: Oral:
Adults: 0.5-6 mg/day in 1-2 divided doses; if one dose is greater, administer at bedtime; titrate dose in 0.5 mg increments at 5- to 6-day intervals
Elderly: Initial: 0.5 mg once or twice daily; increase by 0.5 mg as needed at 5-6 days; maximum: 4 mg/day

**Dietary Considerations** Alcohol: Additive CNS effects, avoid use

**Monitoring Parameters** Symptoms of EPS or Parkinson's, pulse, anticholinergic effects

**Patient Information** Take after meals or with food if GI upset occurs; do not discontinue drug abruptly; notify physician if adverse GI effects, rapid or pounding heartbeat, confusion, eye pain, rash, fever, or heat intolerance occurs. Observe caution when performing hazardous tasks or those that require alertness such as driving, as may cause drowsiness. Avoid alcohol and other CNS depressants. May cause dry mouth - adequate fluid intake or hard sugar-free candy may relieve. Difficult urination or constipation may occur - notify physician if effects persist; may increase susceptibility to heat stroke.

**Nursing Implications** No significant difference in onset of I.M. or I.V. injection, therefore, there is usually no need to use the I.V. route except in those individuals who have laryngospasms as a manifestation of a dystonic reaction. Improvement is sometimes noticeable a few minutes after injection.

**Additional Information** I.V. route should be reserved for situations when oral or I.M. are not appropriate

**Dosage Forms**

Injection, as mesylate: 1 mg/mL (2 mL)
Tablet, as mesylate: 0.5 mg, 1 mg, 2 mg

♦ **Benztropine Mesylate** *see* Benztropine *on page 63*

♦ **Benzylpenicillin Benzathine** *see* Penicillin G Benzathine *on page 425*

## Bepridil (BE pri dil)

**Related Information**

Calcium Channel Blocking Agents Comparison Chart *on page 710*

**U.S. Brand Names** Vascor®

**Canadian Brand Names** Bapadin®

**Pharmacologic Category** Calcium Channel Blocker

**Use** Treatment of chronic stable angina; due to side effect profile, reserve for patients who have been intolerant of other antianginal therapy; bepridil may be used alone or in combination with nitrates or beta-blockers

**Effects on Mental Status** May cause nervousness; rare reports of akathisia

**Effects on Psychiatric Treatment** Concurrent use with beta-blockers may decrease AV nodal conduction

**Pregnancy Risk Factor** C

**Contraindications** History of serious ventricular or atrial arrhythmias (especially tachycardia or those associated with accessory conduction pathways), uncompensated cardiac insufficiency, congenital Q-T interval prolongation, patients taking other drugs that prolong the Q-T interval, history of hypersensitivity to bepridil or any component, calcium channel blockers, or adenosine; concurrent administration with ritonavir, amprenavir, or sparfloxacin

**Warnings/Precautions** Use with great caution in patients with history of IHSS, second or third degree A-V block, cardiogenic shock; reserve for patients in whom other antianginals have failed. Carefully titrate dosages for patients with impaired renal or hepatic function; use caution when treating patients with congestive heart failure, significant hypotension, severe left ventricular dysfunction, hypertrophic cardiomyopathy (especially obstructive), concomitant therapy with beta-blockers or digoxin, edema, or increased intracranial pressure with cranial tumors; do not abruptly withdraw (may cause chest pain); elderly may experience hypotension and constipation more readily.

If dosage reduction does not maintain the Q-T within a safe range (not to exceed 0.52 seconds during therapy), discontinue the medication; has class I antiarrhythmic properties and can induce new arrhythmias, including VT/VF; it can also cause torsade de pointes type ventricular tachycardia due to its ability to prolong the Q-T interval; avoid use in patients in the immediate period postinfarction.

**Adverse Reactions**

>10%:
Central nervous system: Dizziness
Gastrointestinal: Dyspepsia, nausea

1% to 10%:
Cardiovascular: Bradycardia, edema, palpitations
Central nervous system: Nervousness, headache (7% to 13%), drowsiness, psychiatric disturbances (<2%), insomnia (2% to 3%)
Dermatologic: Rash (≤2%)
Endocrine & metabolic: Sexual dysfunction
Gastrointestinal: Diarrhea, anorexia, xerostomia, constipation, abdominal pain, dyspepsia, flatulence

Neuromuscular & skeletal: Weakness (6.5% to 14%), tremor (<9%), paresthesia (2.5%)
Ocular: Blurred vision
Otic: Tinnitus
Respiratory: Rhinitis, dyspnea (≤8.7%), cough (≤2%)
Miscellaneous (≤2%): Flu syndrome, diaphoresis

<1%: Abnormal taste, akathisia, altered behavior, arthritis, fever, hypertension, pharyngitis, prolonged Q-T intervals, syncope, ventricular premature contractions

**Overdosage/Toxicology**

Signs and symptoms: The primary cardiac symptoms of calcium blocker overdose includes hypotension and bradycardia. The hypotension is caused by peripheral vasodilation, myocardial depression, and bradycardia. Bradycardia results from sinus bradycardia, second or third degree atrioventricular block, or sinus arrest with junctional rhythm. Intraventricular conduction is usually not affected so QRS duration is normal (verapamil does prolong the P-R interval and bepridil prolongs the Q-T and may cause ventricular arrhythmias, including torsade de pointes).

The noncardiac symptoms include confusion, stupor, nausea, vomiting, metabolic acidosis and hyperglycemia. Following initial gastric decontamination, if possible, repeated calcium administration may promptly reverse the depressed cardiac contractility (but not sinus node depression or peripheral vasodilation); glucagon, epinephrine, and inamrinone may treat refractory hypotension; glucagon and epinephrine also increase the heart rate (outside the U.S., 4-aminopyridine may be available as an antidote); dialysis and hemoperfusion are not effective in enhancing elimination although repeat-dose activated charcoal may serve as an adjunct with sustained-release preparations.

**Drug Interactions** CYP3A3/4 enzyme substrate

Increased toxicity/effect/levels:

Bepridil and cyclosporine may increase cyclosporine levels (other calcium channel blockers have been shown to interact)
Bepridil and digitalis glycoside may increase digitalis glycoside levels
Use with ritonavir, amprenavir and other protease inhibitors may increase risk of bepridil and sparfloxacin toxicity, especially its cardiotoxicity
Coadministration with beta-blocking agents may result in increased depressant effects on myocardial contractility or A-V conduction
Severe hypotension or increased fluid volume requirements may occur with concomitant fentanyl

**Usual Dosage** Adults: Oral: Initial: 200 mg/day, then adjust dose at 10-day intervals until optimal response is achieved; usual dose: 300 mg/day; maximum daily dose: 400 mg

**Patient Information** Take as directed (may be taken with food to reduce gastric side effects). Do not discontinue without consulting prescriber. Regular EKGs and follow-up with prescriber may be required. If taking potassium supplements or potassium-sparing diuretics, serum potassium monitoring will be required. May cause dizziness, shakiness, visual disturbances, or headache; use caution when driving or engaging in tasks that require alertness until response to drug is known. Report irregular or pounding heartbeat, respiratory difficulty, swelling of hands or feet, unresolved headache, dizziness, constipation, or any unusual bleeding or bruising.

**Nursing Implications** EKG required; patient should be hospitalized during initiation or escalation of therapy

**Dosage Forms** Tablet, as hydrochloride: 200 mg, 300 mg, 400 mg

## Beractant (ber AKT ant)

**U.S. Brand Names** Survanta®

**Pharmacologic Category** Lung Surfactant

**Use** Prevention and treatment of respiratory distress syndrome (RDS) in premature infants

Prophylactic therapy: Body weight <1250 g in infants at risk for developing or with evidence of surfactant deficiency
Rescue therapy: Treatment of infants with RDS confirmed by x-ray and requiring mechanical ventilation (administer as soon as possible - within 8 hours of age)

**Effects on Mental Status** None reported

**Effects on Psychiatric Treatment** None reported

**Usual Dosage**

Prophylactic treatment: Administer 100 mg phospholipids (4 mL/kg) intratracheal as soon as possible; as many as 4 doses may be administered during the first 48 hours of life, no more frequently than 6 hours apart. The need for additional doses is determined by evidence of continuing respiratory distress; if the infant is still intubated and requiring at least 30% inspired oxygen to maintain a $PaO_2$ ≤80 torr.
Rescue treatment: Administer 100 mg phospholipids (4 mL/kg) as soon as the diagnosis of RDS is made; may repeat if needed, no more frequently than every 6 hours to a maximum of 4 doses

**Dosage Forms** Suspension: 200 mg (8 mL)

- **Berocca®** *see* Vitamin B Complex With Vitamin C and Folic Acid *on page 586*
- **Beta-2®** *see* Isoetharine *on page 294*
- **Beta-Blockers Comparison Chart** *see page 709*

## Beta-Carotene (BAY tah KARE oh teen)

**Pharmacologic Category** Vitamin, Fat Soluble

**Use** Reduces severity of photosensitivity reactions in patients with erythropoietic protoporphyria (EPP)

**Unlabeled use:** Prophylaxis and treatment of polymorphous light eruption and prophylaxis against photosensitivity reactions in erythropoietic protoporphyria

**Effects on Mental Status** None reported

**Effects on Psychiatric Treatment** None reported

**Usual Dosage** Oral:

Children <14 years: 30-150 mg/day
Adults: 30-300 mg/day

**Dosage Forms** Capsule: 15 mg, 30 mg

- **Betachron E-R®** *see* Propranolol *on page 475*
- **Betadine® [OTC]** *see* Povidone-Iodine *on page 456*
- **Betadine® 5% Sterile Ophthalmic Prep Solution** *see* Povidone-Iodine *on page 456*
- **Betadine® First Aid Antibiotics + Moisturizer [OTC]** *see* Bacitracin and Polymyxin B *on page 57*
- **Betagan® [OTC]** *see* Povidone-Iodine *on page 456*
- **Betagan® Liquifilm®** *see* Levobunolol *on page 311*

## Betaine Anhydrous (BAY tayne an HY drus)

**Related Information**

Natural Products, Herbals, and Dietary Supplements *on page 742*

**U.S. Brand Names** Cystadane®

**Pharmacologic Category** Homocystinuria, Treatment Agent

**Use** Treatment of homocystinuria to decrease elevated homocysteine blood levels; included within the category of homocystinuria are deficiencies or defects in cystathionine beta-synthase (CBS), 5,10-methylenetetrahydrofolate reductase (MTHFR), and cobalamin cofactor metabolism (CBL).

**Effects on Mental Status** None reported

**Effects on Psychiatric Treatment** None reported

**Usual Dosage**

Children <3 years: Dosage may be started at 100 mg/kg/day and then increased weekly by 100 mg/kg increments
Children ≥3 years and Adults: Oral: 6 g/day administered in divided doses of 3 g twice daily. Dosages of up to 20 g/day have been necessary to control homocysteine levels in some patients.
Dosage in all patients can be gradually increased until plasma homocysteine is undetectable or present only in small amounts

**Dosage Forms** Powder: 1 g/1.7 mL (180 g)

## Betamethasone (bay ta METH a sone)

**Related Information**

Corticosteroids Comparison Chart *on page 711*

**U.S. Brand Names** Alphatrex®; Betatrex®; Celestone®; Celestone® Soluspan®; Cel-U-Jec®; Diprolene®; Diprolene® AF; Diprosone®; Maxivate®; Teladar®; Valisone®

**Canadian Brand Names** Betnesol® [Disodium Phosphate]; Diprolene® Glycol [Dipropionate]; Occlucort®; Rhoprolene; Rhoprosone; Taro-Sone; Topilene; Topisone

**Synonyms** Betamethasone Dipropionate; Betamethasone Dipropionate, Augmented; Betamethasone Sodium Phosphate; Betamethasone Valerate; Flubenisolone

**Pharmacologic Category** Corticosteroid, Oral; Corticosteroid, Parenteral; Corticosteroid, Topical

**Use** Inflammatory dermatoses such as seborrheic or atopic dermatitis, neurodermatitis, anogenital pruritus, psoriasis, inflammatory phase of xerosis

**Effects on Mental Status** Insomnia is common

**Effects on Psychiatric Treatment** Enzyme inducers (barbiturates) may decrease the effects of corticosteroids

**Pregnancy Risk Factor** C

**Contraindications** Systemic fungal infections; hypersensitivity to betamethasone or any component

**Warnings/Precautions** Fatalities have occurred due to adrenal insufficiency in asthmatic patients during and after transfer from systemic corticosteroids to aerosol steroids; several months may be required for recovery of this syndrome; during this period, aerosol steroids do **not** provide the systemic steroid needed to treat patients having trauma, surgery, or infections; use with caution in patients with hypothyroidism, cirrhosis, ulcerative colitis; do not use occlusive dressings on weeping or exudative lesions and general caution with occlusive dressings should be observed; discontinue if skin irritation or contact dermatitis should occur; do not use in patients with decreased skin circulation

(Continued)

## Betamethasone *(Continued)*

**Adverse Reactions**

>10%:

Central nervous system: Insomnia

Gastrointestinal: Increased appetite, indigestion

Ocular: Temporary mild blurred vision

1% to 10%:

Dermatologic: Erythema, itching

Endocrine & metabolic: Diabetes mellitus

Local: Dryness, irritation, papular rashes, burning

Ocular: Cataracts

<1%: Acneiform eruptions, confusion, convulsions, cushingoid state, glaucoma, headache, hyperpigmentation or hypertrichosis, hypertension, hypopigmentation, impaired wound healing, maceration of skin, miliaria, myalgia, osteoporosis, peptic ulcer, perioral dermatitis, skin atrophy, sodium retention, sterile abscess, striae, sudden blindness, thin fragile skin, vertigo

**Overdosage/Toxicology**

Signs and symptoms: When consumed in excessive quantities for prolonged periods, systemic hypercorticism and adrenal suppression may occur

Treatment: In those cases, discontinuation and withdrawal of the corticosteroid should be done judiciously

**Drug Interactions** CYP3A enzyme substrate

Decreased effect (corticosteroid) by barbiturates, phenytoin, rifampin

**Usual Dosage** Base dosage on severity of disease and patient response

Children: Use lowest dose listed as initial dose for adrenocortical insufficiency (physiologic replacement)

I.M.: 0.0175-0.125 mg base/kg/day divided every 6-12 hours **or** 0.5-7.5 mg base/m$^2$/day divided every 6-12 hours

Oral: 0.0175-0.25 mg/kg/day divided every 6-8 hours **or** 0.5-7.5 mg/m$^2$/day divided every 6-8 hours

Adolescents and Adults:

Oral: 2.4-4.8 mg/day in 2-4 doses; range: 0.6-7.2 mg/day

I.M.: Betamethasone sodium phosphate and betamethasone acetate: 0.6-9 mg/day (generally, $^1/_3$ to $^1/_2$ of oral dose) divided every 12-24 hours

Foam: Apply twice daily, once in the morning and once at night

**Dosing adjustment in hepatic impairment:** Adjustments may be necessary in patients with liver failure because betamethasone is extensively metabolized in the liver

Intrabursal, intra-articular, intradermal: 0.25-2 mL

Intralesional: Rheumatoid arthritis/osteoarthritis:

Very large joints: 1-2 mL

Large joints: 1 mL

Medium joints: 0.5-1 mL

Small joints: 0.25-0.5 mL

Topical: Apply thin film 2-4 times/day. Therapy should be discontinued when control is achieved; if no improvement is seen, reassessment of diagnosis may be necessary.

**Patient Information** Take exactly as directed; do not increase dose or discontinue abruptly, consult prescriber. Take oral medication with or after meals. Limit intake of caffeine or stimulants. Prescriber may recommend increased dietary vitamins, minerals, or iron. Diabetics should monitor glucose levels closely (antidiabetic medication may need to be adjusted). Inform prescriber if you are experiencing greater than normal levels of stress (medication may need adjustment). Some forms of this medication may cause GI upset (oral medication may be taken with meals to reduce GI upset; small frequent meals and frequent mouth care may reduce GI upset). You may be more susceptible to infection (avoid crowds and persons with contagious or infective conditions). Report promptly excessive nervousness or sleep disturbances; signs of infection (sore throat, unhealed injuries); excessive growth of body hair or loss of skin color; changes in vision; excessive or sudden weight gain (>3 lb/week); swelling of face or extremities; difficulty breathing; muscle weakness; change in color of stools (tarry) or persistent abdominal pain; or worsening of condition or failure to improve.

Topical: For external use only, Not for eyes or mucous membranes or open wounds. Apply in a thin layer (may rub in lightly). Apply light dressing (if necessary) to area being treated. Do not use occlusive dressing unless so advised by prescriber. Avoid prolonged or excessive use around sensitive tissues, genital, or rectal areas. Inform prescriber if condition worsens (redness, swelling, irritation, open sores) or fails to improve.

**Nursing Implications** Apply topical sparingly to areas; not for use on broken skin or in areas of infection; do not apply to wet skin unless directed; do not apply to face or inguinal area. Not for alternate day therapy; once daily doses should be given in the morning; do not administer injectable sodium phosphate/acetate suspension I.V.

**Dosage Forms**

Base (Celestone®), Oral:

Syrup: 0.6 mg/5 mL (118 mL)

Tablet: 0.6 mg

Dipropionate (Diprosone®)

Aerosol: 0.1% (85 g)

Cream: 0.05% (15 g, 45 g)

Lotion: 0.05% (20 mL, 30 mL, 60 mL)

Ointment: 0.05% (15 g, 45 g)

Dipropionate augmented (Diprolene®)

Cream: 0.05% (15 g, 45 g)

Gel: 0.05% (15 g, 45 g)

Lotion: 0.05% (30 mL, 60 mL)

Ointment, topical: 0.05% (15 g, 45 g)

Valerate (Betatrex®, Valisone®)

Cream: 0.01% (15 g, 60 g); 0.1% (15 g, 45 g, 110 g, 430 g)

Lotion: 0.1% (20 mL, 60 mL)

Ointment: 0.1% (15 g, 45 g)

Valerate (Beta-Val®)

Cream: 0.01% (15 g, 60 g); 0.1% (15 g, 45 g, 110 g, 430 g)

Lotion: 0.1% (20 mL, 60 mL)

Valerate (Luxiq™): Foam: 100 g aluminum can (box of 1)

Injection: Sodium phosphate (Celestone® Phosphate, Cel-U-Jec®): 4 mg betamethasone phosphate/mL (equivalent to 3 mg betamethasone/mL) (5 mL)

Injection, suspension: Sodium phosphate and acetate (Celestone® Soluspan®): 6 mg/mL (3 mg of betamethasone sodium phosphate and 3 mg of betamethasone acetate per mL) (5 mL)

## Betamethasone and Clotrimazole

(bay ta METH a sone & kloe TRIM a zole)

**U.S. Brand Names** Lotrisone®

**Canadian Brand Names** Lotriderm®

**Pharmacologic Category** Antifungal Agent, Topical

**Use** Topical treatment of various dermal fungal infections

**Effects on Mental Status** None reported

**Effects on Psychiatric Treatment** None reported

**Usual Dosage** Apply twice daily

**Dosage Forms** Cream: Betamethasone dipropionate 0.05% and clotrimazole 1% (15 g, 45 g)


- **Betamethasone Dipropionate** *see* Betamethasone *on page 65*
- **Betamethasone Dipropionate, Augmented** *see* Betamethasone *on page 65*
- **Betamethasone Sodium Phosphate** *see* Betamethasone *on page 65*
- **Betamethasone Valerate** *see* Betamethasone *on page 65*
- **Betapace®** *see* Sotalol *on page 516*
- **Betapace AF®** *see* Sotalol *on page 516*
- **Betapen®-VK** *see* Penicillin V Potassium *on page 426*
- **Betasept® [OTC]** *see* Chlorhexidine Gluconate *on page 111*
- **Betaseron®** *see* Interferon Beta-1b *on page 290*
- **Betatrex®** *see* Betamethasone *on page 65*


## Betaxolol (be TAKS oh lol)

**Related Information**

Beta-Blockers Comparison Chart *on page 709*

Glaucoma Drug Therapy *on page 712*

**U.S. Brand Names** Betoptic® Ophthalmic; Betoptic® S Ophthalmic; Kerlone® Oral

**Pharmacologic Category** Beta Blocker, Beta$_1$ Selective; Ophthalmic Agent, Antiglaucoma

**Use** Treatment of chronic open-angle glaucoma and ocular hypertension; management of hypertension

**Effects on Mental Status** May cause drowsiness; rare reports of depression and hallucinations

**Effects on Psychiatric Treatment** Has been used to treat akathisia; propranolol preferred

**Pregnancy Risk Factor** C (per manufacturer); D (in second and third trimester, based on expert analysis)

**Contraindications** Hypersensitivity to betaxolol or any component; sinus bradycardia; heart block greater than first-degree (except in patients with a functioning artificial pacemaker); cardiogenic shock; uncompensated cardiac failure; pulmonary edema; pregnancy (2nd and 3rd trimester)

**Warnings/Precautions** Administer cautiously in compensated heart failure and monitor for a worsening of the condition. Avoid abrupt discontinuation in patients with a history of CAD; slowly wean while monitoring for signs and symptoms of ischemia. Use caution with concurrent use of beta-blockers and either verapamil or diltiazem; bradycardia or heart block can occur. Use caution in patients with PVD (can aggravate arterial insufficiency). In general, beta-blockers should be avoided in patients with bronchospastic disease. Betaxolol, with B1 selectivity, should be used cautiously in bronchospastic disease with close monitoring. Use cautiously in diabetics because it can mask prominent hypoglycemic symptoms. Can mask signs of thyrotoxicosis. Can cause fetal harm when administered in pregnancy. Dosage adjustment required in severe renal impairment and those on dialysis. Use care with anesthetic agents which decreases myocardial function.

**Adverse Reactions**

1% to 10%:

Cardiovascular: Bradycardia, palpitations, edema, congestive heart failure

Central nervous system: Dizziness, fatigue, lethargy, headache

Dermatologic: Erythema, itching

Ocular: Mild ocular stinging and discomfort, tearing, photophobia, decreased corneal sensitivity, keratitis

Miscellaneous: Cold extremities

<1%: Chest pain, depression, hallucinations, nervousness, thrombocytopenia

**Overdosage/Toxicology**

Signs and symptoms: Cardiac disturbances, CNS toxicity, bronchospasm, hypoglycemia and hyperkalemia. The most common cardiac symptoms include hypotension and bradycardia; atrioventricular block, intraventricular conduction disturbances, cardiogenic shock, and asystole may occur with severe overdose, especially with membrane-depressant drugs (eg, propranolol); CNS effects include convulsions, coma, and respiratory arrest (commonly seen with propranolol and other membrane-depressant and lipid-soluble drugs).

Treatment: Symptomatic treatment of seizures, hypotension, hyperkalemia, and hypoglycemia; bradycardia and hypotension resistant to atropine, isoproterenol, or pacing may respond to glucagon; wide QRS defects caused by the membrane-depressant poisoning may respond to hypertonic sodium bicarbonate; repeat-dose charcoal, hemoperfusion, or hemodialysis may be helpful in removal of only those beta-blockers with a small $V_d$, long half-life, or low intrinsic clearance (acebutolol, atenolol, nadolol, sotalol)

**Drug Interactions** CYP1A2 and 2D6 enzyme substrate

Alpha-blockers (prazosin, terazosin): Concurrent use of beta-blockers may increase risk of orthostasis

Clonidine; Hypertensive crisis after or during withdrawal of either agent

Drugs which slow AV conduction (digoxin): Effects may be additive with beta-blockers

Glucagon: Betaxolol may blunt the hyperglycemic action of glucagon

Insulin and oral hypoglycemics: May mask tachycardia from hypoglycemia

NSAIDs (ibuprofen, indomethacin, naproxen, piroxicam) may reduce the antihypertensive effects of beta-blockers

Salicylates may reduce the antihypertensive effects of beta-blockers

Sulfonylureas: Beta-blockers may alter response to hypoglycemic agents

Verapamil or diltiazem may have synergistic or additive pharmacological effects when taken concurrently with beta-blockers

**Usual Dosage** Adults:

Ophthalmic: Instill 1 drop twice daily.

Oral: 10 mg/day; may increase dose to 20 mg/day after 7-14 days if desired response is not achieved. Initial dose in elderly: 5 mg/day.

**Dosage adjustment in renal impairment:** Administer 5 mg/day. Can increase every 2 weeks up to a maximum of 20 mg/day.

$Cl_{cr}$ <10 mL/minute: Administer 50% of usual dose.

**Patient Information**

Oral: Use as directed; do not increase dose unless directed by prescriber. You may experience dizziness or blurred vision (use caution when driving engaging in tasks requiring alertness until response to drug is known); nausea or vomiting (small frequent meals, frequent mouth care, sucking lozenges, or chewing gum may help). Report persistent GI response (nausea, vomiting, diarrhea, or constipation); chest pain or palpitations; unusual cough, difficulty breathing, swelling or coolness of extremities; or unusual mental depression.

Ophthalmic: Shake well before using. Tilt head back and instill in eye. Keep eye open; do not blink for 30 seconds. Apply gentle pressure to corner of eye for 1 minute. Wipe away excess from skin. Do not touch applicator to eyes or contaminate tip of applicator. Report if condition does not improve or if you experience eye pain, vision disturbances, or other adverse eye response.

**Nursing Implications** Monitor for systemic effect of beta-blockade

**Dosage Forms**

Solution, ophthalmic, as hydrochloride (Betoptic®): 0.5% (2.5 mL, 5 mL, 10 mL)

Suspension, ophthalmic, as hydrochloride (Betoptic® S): 0.25% (2.5 mL, 10 mL, 15 mL)

Tablet, as hydrochloride (Kerlone®): 10 mg, 20 mg

♦ **Betaxon®** *see* Levobetaxolol *on page 311*

## Bethanechol (be THAN e kole)

**U.S. Brand Names** Duvoid®; Myotonachol™; Urecholine®

**Canadian Brand Names** PMS-Bethanechol Chloride

**Pharmacologic Category** Cholinergic Agonist

**Use** Nonobstructive urinary retention and retention due to neurogenic bladder; treatment and prevention of bladder dysfunction caused by phenothiazines; diagnosis of flaccid or atonic neurogenic bladder; gastroesophageal reflux

**Effects on Mental Status** None reported

**Effects on Psychiatric Treatment** Contraindicated in Parkinson's disease

**Pregnancy Risk Factor** C

**Contraindications** Hypersensitivity to bethanechol; do not use in patients with mechanical obstruction of the GI or GU tract or when the strength or integrity of the GI or bladder wall is in question. It is also contraindicated in patients with hyperthyroidism, peptic ulcer disease, epilepsy, obstructive pulmonary disease, bradycardia, vasomotor instability, atrioventricular conduction defects, hypotension, or parkinsonism; **contraindicated for I.M. or I.V. use due to a likely severe cholinergic reaction**

**Warnings/Precautions** Potential for reflux infection if the sphincter fails to relax as bethanechol contracts the bladder; avoid use in breast-feeding women; safety and efficacy in children <5 years of age have not been established; syringe containing atropine should be readily available for treatment of serious side effects; for S.C. injection only; do not administer I.M. or I.V.

**Adverse Reactions**

Oral: <1%: Hypotension, cardiac arrest, flushed skin, abdominal cramps, diarrhea, nausea, vomiting, salivation, bronchial constriction, diaphoresis, vasomotor response

Subcutaneous: 1% to 10%:

Cardiovascular: Hypotension, cardiac arrest, flushed skin

Gastrointestinal: Abdominal cramps, diarrhea, nausea, vomiting, salivation

Respiratory: Bronchial constriction

Miscellaneous: Diaphoresis, vasomotor response

**Overdosage/Toxicology**

Signs and symptoms: Nausea, vomiting, abdominal cramps, diarrhea, involuntary defecation, flushed skin, hypotension, bronchospasm

Treatment: Atropine is the treatment of choice for intoxications manifesting with significant muscarinic symptoms; atropine I.V. 0.6 mg every 3-60 minutes (or 0.01 mg/kg I.V. every 2 hours if needed for children) should be repeated to control symptoms and then continued as needed for 1-2 days following the acute ingestion. Epinephrine 0.1-1 mg S.C. may be useful in reversing severe cardiovascular or pulmonary sequel.

**Drug Interactions**

Decreased effect: Procainamide, quinidine

Increased toxicity: Bethanechol and ganglionic blockers → critical fall in blood pressure; cholinergic drugs or anticholinesterase agents

**Usual Dosage**

Children:

Oral:

Abdominal distention or urinary retention: 0.6 mg/kg/day divided 3-4 times/day

Gastroesophageal reflux: 0.1-0.2 mg/kg/dose given 30 minutes to 1 hour before each meal to a maximum of 4 times/day

S.C.: 0.15-0.2 mg/kg/day divided 3-4 times/day

Adults:

Oral: 10-50 mg 2-4 times/day

S.C.: 2.5-5 mg 3-4 times/day, up to 7.5-10 mg every 4 hours for neurogenic bladder

**Patient Information** Oral: Take as directed, on an empty stomach to avoid nausea or vomiting. Do not discontinue without consulting prescriber. Maintain adequate hydration (2-3 L/day of fluids unless instructed to restrict fluid intake). May cause dizziness or hypotension (rise slowly from sitting or lying position and use caution when driving or climbing stairs); vomiting or loss of appetite (frequent small meals, frequent mouth care, sucking lozenges, or chewing gum may help). Report persistent abdominal discomfort; significantly increased salivation, sweating, tearing, or urination; flushed skin; chest pain or palpitations; acute headache; unresolved diarrhea; excessive fatigue, insomnia, dizziness, or depression; increased muscle, joint, or body pain; vision changes or blurred vision; or respiratory difficulty or wheezing.

**Nursing Implications** Have bedpan readily available, if administered for urinary retention

**Dosage Forms**

Injection, as chloride: 5 mg/mL (1 mL)

Tablet, as chloride: 5 mg, 10 mg, 25 mg, 50 mg

♦ **Betimol® Ophthalmic** *see* Timolol *on page 549*

♦ **Betoptic® Ophthalmic** *see* Betaxolol *on page 66*

♦ **Betoptic® S Ophthalmic** *see* Betaxolol *on page 66*

## Bexarotene (beks AR oh teen)

**U.S. Brand Names** Targretin®

**Pharmacologic Category** Antineoplastic Agent, Miscellaneous

**Use**

Treatment of cutaneous manifestations of cutaneous T-cell lymphoma in patients who are refractory to at least one prior systemic therapy

Topical: Treatment of cutaneous lesions in patients with cutaneous T-cell lymphoma (stage 1A and 1B) who have refractory or persistent disease after other therapies or who have not tolerated other therapies

(Continued)

## Bexarotene *(Continued)*

**Effects on Mental Status** May cause insomnia, agitation, confusion, and depression

**Effects on Psychiatric Treatment** Leukopenia is common; use caution with clozapine and carbamazepine; effects of psychotropics may be altered secondary to the insomnia, confusion, agitation, and depression seen with bexarotene

**Usual Dosage**

Adults: Oral: 300 mg/m²/day taken as a single daily dose. If there is no tumor response after 8 weeks and the initial dose was well tolerated, then an increase to 400 mg/m²/day can be made with careful monitoring. Maintain as long as the patient is deriving benefit.

If the initial dose is not tolerated, then it may be adjusted to 200 mg/m²/day, then to 100 mg/m²/day or temporarily suspended if necessary to manage toxicity

**Dosing adjustment in renal impairment:** No studies have been conducted; however, renal insufficiency may result in significant protein binding changes and alter pharmacokinetics of bexarotene

**Dosing adjustment in hepatic impairment:** No studies have been conducted; however, hepatic impairment would be expected to result in decreased clearance of bexarotene due to the extensive hepatic contribution to elimination

Gel: Apply once every other day for first week, then increase on a weekly basis to once daily, 2 times/day, 3 times/day, and finally 4 times/day, according to tolerance

**Dosage Forms**

Capsule: 75 mg

Gel, topical: 1% (60 g)



- ♦ **Bexophene®** *see* Propoxyphene and Aspirin *on page 475*
- ♦ **Bextra®** *see* Bucindolol *on page 74*
- ♦ **Biaxin™** *see* Clarithromycin *on page 127*
- ♦ **Biaxin™ XL** *see* Clarithromycin *on page 127*



## Bicalutamide (bye ka LOO ta mide)

**U.S. Brand Names** Casodex®

**Pharmacologic Category** Androgen

**Use** In combination therapy with LHRH agonist analogues in treatment of advanced prostatic carcinoma

**Effects on Mental Status** May produce anxiety, depression, and confusion

**Effects on Psychiatric Treatment** None reported

**Pregnancy Risk Factor** X

**Contraindications** Known hypersensitivity to drug or any components of the product; pregnancy

**Adverse Reactions**

>10%: Endocrine & metabolic: Hot flashes (49%)

≥2% to <5%:

Cardiovascular: Angina pectoris, congestive heart failure, edema

Central nervous system: Anxiety, depression, confusion, somnolence, nervousness, fever, chills

Dermatologic: Dry skin, pruritus, alopecia

Endocrine & metabolic: Breast pain, diabetes mellitus, decreased libido, dehydration, gout

Gastrointestinal: Anorexia, dyspepsia, rectal hemorrhage, xerostomia, melena, weight gain

Genitourinary: Polyuria, urinary impairment, dysuria, urinary retention, urinary urgency

Hepatic: Alkaline phosphatase increased

Neuromuscular & skeletal: Myasthenia, arthritis, myalgia, leg cramps, pathological fracture, neck pain, hypertonia, neuropathy

Renal: Creatinine increased

Respiratory: Cough increased, pharyngitis, bronchitis, pneumonia, rhinitis, lung disorder

Miscellaneous: Sepsis, neoplasma

<1%: Diarrhea (0.5%)

**Overdosage/Toxicology**

Signs and symptoms: Hypoactivity, ataxia, anorexia, vomiting, slow respiration, lacrimation

Treatment: Supportive, dialysis not of benefit; induce vomiting

**Drug Interactions** *In vitro* displacement of warfarin by bicalutamide

**Usual Dosage** Adults: Oral: 1 tablet once daily (morning or evening), with or without food. It is recommended that bicalutamide be taken at the same time each day; start treatment with bicalutamide at the same time as treatment with an LHRH analog.

**Dosage adjustment in renal impairment:** None necessary as renal impairment has no significant effect on elimination

**Dosage adjustment in liver impairment:** Limited data in subjects with severe hepatic impairment suggest that excretion of bicalutamide may be delayed and could lead to further accumulation. Use with caution in patients with moderate to severe hepatic impairment.

**Patient Information** Take as directed and do not alter dose or discontinue without consulting prescriber. Take at the same time each day with or without food. Void before taking medication. Diabetics should monitor serum glucose closely and notify prescriber of changes; this medication can alter hypoglycemic requirements. You may lose your hair and experience impotency. May cause dizziness, confusion, or drowsiness (use caution when driving or engaging in tasks that require alertness until response to drug is known); nausea or vomiting (small frequent meals, frequent mouth care, sucking lozenges, or chewing gum may help); or constipation (increased dietary fiber, fruit, or fluid and increased exercise may help). Report easy bruising or bleeding; yellowing of skin or eyes; change in color of urine or stool; unresolved changes in CNS (nervousness, chills, insomnia, somnolence); skin rash, redness, or irritation; chest pain or palpitations; difficulty breathing; urinary retention or inability to void; muscle weakness, tremors, or pain; persistent nausea, vomiting, diarrhea, or constipation; or other unusual signs or adverse reactions.

**Dosage Forms** Tablet: 50 mg



- ♦ **Bicillin® C-R 900/300 Injection** *see* Penicillin G Benzathine and Procaine Combined *on page 425*
- ♦ **Bicillin® C-R Injection** *see* Penicillin G Benzathine and Procaine Combined *on page 425*
- ♦ **Bicillin® L-A** *see* Penicillin G Benzathine *on page 425*
- ♦ **BiCNU®** *see* Carmustine *on page 94*
- ♦ **Bigumalum** *see* Proguanil *on page 468*
- ♦ **Biltricide®** *see* Praziquantel *on page 458*
- ♦ **Biocef** *see* Cephalexin *on page 103*
- ♦ **Bioclate®** *see* Antihemophilic Factor (Recombinant) *on page 46*
- ♦ **Biodine [OTC]** *see* Povidone-Iodine *on page 456*
- ♦ **Biohist-LA®** *see* Carbinoxamine and Pseudoephedrine *on page 92*
- ♦ **Biomox®** *see* Amoxicillin *on page 38*
- ♦ **Bion® Tears Solution [OTC]** *see* Artificial Tears *on page 48*
- ♦ **Bio-Tab® Oral** *see* Doxycycline *on page 186*



## Biperiden (bye PER i den)

**Related Information**


Antiparkinsonian Agents Comparison Chart *on page 705*

Discontinuation of Psychotropic Drugs - Withdrawal Symptoms and Recommendations *on page 798*

Patient Information - Agents for Treatment of Extrapyramidal Symptoms *on page 657*


**Generic Available** No

**U.S. Brand Names** Akineton®

**Synonyms** Biperiden Hydrochloride; Biperiden Lactate

**Pharmacologic Category** Anticholinergic Agent; Anti-Parkinson's Agent (Anticholinergic)

**Use** Adjunct in the therapy of all forms of Parkinsonism; control of extrapyramidal symptoms secondary to antipsychotics

**Pregnancy Risk Factor** C

**Contraindications** Narrow angle glaucoma; GI or GU obstruction, megacolon; hypersensitivity to biperiden

**Warnings/Precautions** Use with caution in patients with narrow angle glaucoma, peptic ulcer, urinary tract obstruction, hyperthyroidism; some preparations contain sodium bisulfite; syrup contains alcohol

**Adverse Reactions**

Cardiovascular: Orthostatic hypotension, bradycardia (I.V.)

Central nervous system: Drowsiness, euphoria, disorientation, agitation

Gastrointestinal: Constipation, xerostomia

Genitourinary: Urinary retention

Ocular: Blurred vision

**Overdosage/Toxicology**

Signs and symptoms: CNS stimulation or depression; overdose may result in death in infants and children

Treatment: No specific treatment for overdose, however, most of its clinical toxicity is due to anticholinergic effects; anticholinesterase inhibitors may be useful by reducing acetylcholinesterase. Anticholinesterase inhibitors include physostigmine, neostigmine, pyridostigmine and edrophonium; for anticholinergic overdose with severe life-threatening symptoms, physostigmine 1-2 mg (0.5 or 0.02 mg/kg for children) I.V., slowly may be given to reverse these effects.

**Drug Interactions**

Amantadine, rimantadine: Central and/or peripheral anticholinergic syndrome can occur when administered with amantadine or rimantadine

Anticholinergic agents: Central and/or peripheral anticholinergic syndrome can occur when administered with narcotic analgesics, phenothiazines and other antipsychotics (especially with high anticholinergic activity), tricyclic antidepressants, quinidine and some other antiarrhythmics, and antihistamines

Atenolol: Anticholinergics may increase the bioavailability of atenolol (and possibly other beta-blockers); monitor for increased effect

Cholinergic agents: Anticholinergics may antagonize the therapeutic effect of cholinergic agents; includes tacrine and donepezil

Digoxin: Anticholinergics may decrease gastric degradation and increase the amount of digoxin absorbed by delaying gastric emptying

Levodopa: Anticholinergics may increase gastric degradation and decrease the amount of levodopa absorbed by delaying gastric emptying

Neuroleptics: Anticholinergics may antagonize the therapeutic effects of neuroleptics

**Mechanism of Action** Biperiden is a weak peripheral anticholinergic agent with nicotinolytic activity. The beneficial effects in Parkinson's disease and neuroleptic-induced extrapyramidal reactions are believed to be due to the inhibition of striatal cholinergic receptors.

**Pharmacodynamics/kinetics**

Bioavailability: 29%

Half-life: 18.4-24.3 hours

Time to peak serum concentration: 1-1.5 hours

**Usual Dosage** Adults:

Parkinsonism: Oral: 2 mg 3-4 times/day

Extrapyramidal.

Oral: 2 mg 1-3 times/day

I.M., I.V.: 2 mg every 30 minutes up to 4 doses or 8 mg/day

**Administration** I.V. must be given slowly

**Monitoring Parameters** Symptoms of EPS or Parkinson's, pulse, anticholinergic effects (ie, CNS, bowel, and bladder function)

**Reference Range** After a 4 mg oral dose, peak plasma levels range from 3.9-6.3 ng/mL

**Patient Information** May cause drowsiness

**Nursing Implications** No significant difference in onset of I.M. or I.V. injection, therefore, there is usually no need to use the I.V. route. Improvement is sometimes noticeable a few minutes after injection. Do not discontinue drug abruptly.

**Dosage Forms**

Injection, as lactate: 5 mg/mL (1 mL)

Tablet, as hydrochloride: 2 mg

♦ **Biperiden Hydrochloride** *see* Biperiden *on page 68*

♦ **Biperiden Lactate** *see* Biperiden *on page 68*

♦ **Biphenabid** *see* Probucol *on page 463*

♦ **Bisac-Evac® [OTC]** *see* Bisacodyl *on page 69*

## Bisacodyl (bis a KOE dil)

**Related Information**

Laxatives, Classification and Properties *on page 716*

**U.S. Brand Names** Bisac-Evac® [OTC]; Bisacodyl Uniserts®; Bisco-Lax® [OTC]; Carter's Little Pills® [OTC]; Clysodrast®; Dacodyl® [OTC]; Deficol® [OTC]; Dulcolax® [OTC]; Feen-A-Mint® [OTC]; Fleet® Laxative [OTC]

**Canadian Brand Names** Apo®-Bisacodyl; PMS-Bisacodyl

**Pharmacologic Category** Laxative, Stimulant

**Use** Treatment of constipation; colonic evacuation prior to procedures or examination

**Effects on Mental Status** None reported

**Effects on Psychiatric Treatment** None reported

**Pregnancy Risk Factor** C

**Contraindications** Abdominal pain, obstruction, nausea or vomiting; do not administer bisacodyl tannex enema to children <10 years of age

**Warnings/Precautions** Bisacodyl tannex should be used with caution in patients with ulceration of the colon and during pregnancy or lactation; safety of bisacodyl tannex usage in children <10 years of age has not been established

**Adverse Reactions** <1%: Electrolyte and fluid imbalance (metabolic acidosis or alkalosis, hypocalcemia), mild abdominal cramps, nausea, rectal burning, vertigo, vomiting

**Overdosage/Toxicology** Signs and symptoms: Diarrhea, abdominal pain, electrolyte disturbances

**Drug Interactions** Decreased effect: Milk, antacids; decreased effect of warfarin

**Usual Dosage**

Children:

Oral: >6 years: 5-10 mg (0.3 mg/kg) at bedtime or before breakfast

Rectal suppository:

<2 years: 5 mg as a single dose

>2 years: 10 mg

Adults:

Oral: 5-15 mg as single dose (up to 30 mg when complete evacuation of bowel is required)

Rectal suppository: 10 mg as single dose

Tannex:

Enema: 2.5 g in 1000 mL warm water

Barium enema: 2.5-5 g in 1000 mL barium suspension

Do not administer >10 g within 72-hour period

**Patient Information** Onset of action occurs 6-10 hours after oral dose or 15-60 minutes after a rectal dose; swallow tablets whole, do **not** crush or chew; do not take antacid or milk within 1 hour of taking drug

**Dosage Forms**

Powder, as tannex: 2.5 g packets (50 packet/box)

Suppository, rectal: 5 mg, 10 mg

Tablet, enteric coated: 5 mg

♦ **Bisacodyl Uniserts®** *see* Bisacodyl *on page 69*

♦ **Bisco-Lax® [OTC]** *see* Bisacodyl *on page 69*

♦ **Bishydroxycoumarin** *see* Dicumarol *on page 165*

♦ **Bismatrol® [OTC]** *see* Bismuth *on page 69*

## Bismuth (BIZ muth)

**U.S. Brand Names** Bismatrol® [OTC]; Devrom® [OTC]; Pepto-Bismol® [OTC]; Pink Bismuth® [OTC]

**Pharmacologic Category** Antidiarrheal

**Use** Symptomatic treatment of mild, nonspecific diarrhea; indigestion, nausea, control of traveler's diarrhea (enterotoxigenic *Escherichia coli*); an adjunct with other agents such as metronidazole, tetracycline, and an $H_2$-antagonist in the treatment of *Helicobacter pylori*-associated duodenal ulcer disease

**Effects on Mental Status** May rarely cause anxiety, confusion, or depression

**Effects on Psychiatric Treatment** None reported

**Contraindications** Influenza or chickenpox because of risk of Reye's syndrome; hypersensitivity to salicylates; history of severe GI bleeding; history of coagulopathy

**Usual Dosage** Oral:

Nonspecific diarrhea: Subsalicylate:

Children: Up to 8 doses/24 hours:

3-6 years: 1/3 tablet or 5 mL every 30 minutes to 1 hour as needed

6-9 years: 2/3 tablet or 10 mL every 30 minutes to 1 hour as needed

9-12 years: 1 tablet or 15 mL every 30 minutes to 1 hour as needed

Adults: 2 tablets or 30 mL every 30 minutes to 1 hour as needed up to 8 doses/24 hours

Prevention of traveler's diarrhea: 2.1 g/day or 2 tablets 4 times/day before meals and at bedtime

*Helicobacter pylori*: Chew 2 tablets 4 times/day with meals and at bedtime with other agents in selected regiment (eg, an $H_2$-antagonist, tetracycline and metronidazole) for 14 days

Subgallate: 1-2 tablets 3 times/day with meals

**Dosing adjustment in renal impairment:** Should probably be avoided in patients with renal failure

**Dosage Forms**

Liquid, as subsalicylate (Pepto-Bismol®, Bismatrol®): 262 mg/15 mL (120 mL, 240 mL, 360 mL, 480 mL); 524 mg/15 mL (120 mL, 240 mL, 360 mL)

Tablet:

Chewable, as subsalicylate (Pepto-Bismol®, Bismatrol®): 262 mg

Chewable, as subgallate (Devrom®): 200 mg

## Bismuth Subsalicylate, Metronidazole, and Tetracycline

(BIZ muth sub sa LIS i late, me troe NI da zole, & tet ra SYE kleen)

**U.S. Brand Names** Helidac™

**Pharmacologic Category** Antidiarrheal

**Use** In combination with an $H_2$-antagonist, used to treat and decrease rate of recurrence of active duodenal ulcer associated with *H. pylori* infection

**Effects on Mental Status** Dizziness common; metronidazole has been reported to cause depression, insomnia, confusion, panic, delusions, hallucinations, and exacerbation of schizophrenia; tetracycline has been reported to produce memory disturbances as well as mood stabilizing and antidepressant effects

**Effects on Psychiatric Treatment** Metronidazole and tetracycline may increase serum lithium levels and produce lithium toxicity; monitor serum lithium levels

**Contraindications** Pregnancy or lactation; children; significant renal/hepatic impairment; hypersensitivity to salicylates, bismuth, metronidazole, tetracycline, or any component

**Warnings/Precautions** See individual monographs

**Adverse Reactions** See individual monographs

>1%:

Central nervous system: Dizziness

Gastrointestinal: Nausea, diarrhea, abdominal pain, vomiting, anal discomfort, anorexia

Neuromuscular & skeletal: Paresthesia

**Overdosage/Toxicology** The most concerning agent with this combination in overdosage is bismuth subsalicylate due to the salicylate component. **Note:** Each 262.4 mg tablet of bismuth subsalicylate contains an equivalent of 130 mg aspirin (150 mg/kg of aspirin is considered to be toxic; serious life-threatening toxicity occurs with >300 mg/kg).

(Continued)

## Bismuth Subsalicylate, Metronidazole, and Tetracycline *(Continued)*

Signs and symptoms of salicylate intoxication: Hyperpnea, nausea, vomiting, tinnitus, hyperpyrexia, metabolic acidosis/ respiratory alkalosis, tachycardia, and confusion; seizures in severe OD, pulmonary or cerebral edema, respiratory failure, cardiovascular collapse, coma, and death

Treatment: Gastrointestinal decontamination (activated charcoal for immediate release formulations (10 x dose of ASA in g), whole bowel irrigation for enteric coated tablets or when serially increasing ASA plasma levels indicate the presence of an intestinal bezoar), supportive and symptomatic treatment with emphasis on correcting fluid, electrolyte, blood glucose, and acid-base disturbances; elimination is enhanced with urinary alkalization (sodium bicarbonate infusion with potassium), multiple-dose activated charcoal, and hemodialysis.

**Drug Interactions** See individual monographs

Decreased effect: A theoretical reduction in tetracycline systemic absorption due to an interaction with bismuth or calcium carbonate, an excipient of bismuth subsalicylate has, as yet, been unproven to occur or to have any clinical bearing

**Usual Dosage** Adults: Chew 2 bismuth subsalicylate 262.4 mg tablets, swallow 1 metronidazole 250 mg tablet, and swallow 1 tetracycline 500 mg capsule plus an $H_2$-antagonist 4 times/day at meals and bedtime for 14 days; follow with 8 oz of water

**Patient Information** Drink adequate amounts of fluid, particularly with the bedtime tetracycline dose to reduce the risk of esophageal irritation and ulceration; if a dose is missed, continue the normal regimen until the medication is gone; do not take double doses; see your physician if more than 4 doses are missed or if ringing in the ears occur; avoid alcoholic beverages during therapy and for at least 1 day afterward; avoid concurrent use of oral contraceptives (use an alternative method) since tetracyclines may make birth control pills less effective; use protective clothing and avoid prolonged exposure to the sun and ultraviolet light; a temporary and harmless darkening of the tongue and a black stool may occur.

**Dosage Forms**

Tablet:

Bismuth subsalicylate: Chewable: 262.4 mg

Metronidazole: 250 mg

Capsule: Tetracycline: 500 mg

## Bisoprolol (bis OH proe lol)

**Related Information**

Beta-Blockers Comparison Chart *on page 709*

**U.S. Brand Names** Zebeta®

**Pharmacologic Category** Beta Blocker, $Beta_1$ Selective

**Use** Treatment of hypertension, alone or in combination with other agents

**Unlabeled use:** Angina pectoris, supraventricular arrhythmias, PVCs

**Effects on Mental Status** Fatigue is common; may cause insomnia, confusion, and depression

**Effects on Psychiatric Treatment** Barbiturates may decrease the effects of beta-blockers

**Pregnancy Risk Factor** C (per manufacturer); D (in second and third trimester, based on expert analysis)

**Contraindications** Hypersensitivity to bisoprolol or any component; sinus bradycardia; heart block greater than first-degree (except in patients with a functioning artificial pacemaker); cardiogenic shock; uncompensated cardiac failure; pulmonary edema; pregnancy (2nd and 3rd trimesters)

**Warnings/Precautions** Administer cautiously in compensated heart failure and monitor for a worsening of the condition. Avoid abrupt discontinuation in patients with a history of CAD; slowly wean while monitoring for signs and symptoms of ischemia. Use caution in patients with PVD (can aggravate arterial insufficiency). Use caution with concurrent use of beta-blockers and either verapamil or diltiazem; bradycardia or heart block can occur. In general, beta-blockers should be avoided in patients with bronchospastic disease. Bisoprolol, with B1 selectivity, should be used cautiously in bronchospastic disease with close monitoring. Use cautiously in diabetics because it can mask prominent hypoglycemic symptoms. Can mask signs of thyrotoxicosis. Can cause fetal harm when administered in pregnancy. Dosage adjustment is required in patients with significant hepatic or renal dysfunction. Use care with anesthetic agents which decrease myocardial function.

**Adverse Reactions**

>10%: Central nervous system: Fatigue, lethargy

1% to 10%:

Cardiovascular: Hypotension, chest pain, heart failure, Raynaud's phenomenon, heart block, edema, bradycardia

Central nervous system: Headache, dizziness, insomnia, confusion, depression, abnormal dreams

Dermatologic: Rash

Gastrointestinal: Constipation, diarrhea, dyspepsia, nausea, flatulence, anorexia

Genitourinary: Polyuria, impotence, urinary retention

Hepatic: Increased LFTs

Neuromuscular & skeletal: Arthralgia, myalgia

Ocular: Abnormal vision

Respiratory: Dyspnea, rhinitis, cough

**Overdosage/Toxicology**

Signs and symptoms of intoxication: Cardiac disturbances, CNS toxicity, bronchospasm, hypoglycemia, and hyperkalemia. The most common cardiac symptoms include hypotension and bradycardia; atrioventricular block, intraventricular conduction disturbances, cardiogenic shock, and asystole may occur with severe overdose, especially with membrane-depressant drugs (eg, propranolol); CNS effects include convulsions, coma, and respiratory arrest (commonly seen with propranolol and other membrane-depressant and lipid-soluble drugs).

Treatment: Symptomatic treatment of seizures, hypotension, hyperkalemia, and hypoglycemia; bradycardia and hypotension resistant to atropine, isoproterenol, or pacing may respond to glucagon; wide QRS defects caused by the membrane-depressant poisoning may respond to hypertonic sodium bicarbonate; repeat-dose charcoal, hemoperfusion, or hemodialysis may be helpful in removal of only those beta-blockers with a small $V_d$, long half-life, or low intrinsic clearance (acebutolol, atenolol, nadolol, sotalol)

**Drug Interactions** CYP2D6 enzyme substrate

Alpha-blockers (prazosin, terazosin): Concurrent use of beta-blockers may increase risk of orthostasis

Clonidine: Hypertensive crisis after or during withdrawal of either agent

Drugs which slow AV conduction (digoxin): Effects may be additive with beta-blockers

Glucagon: Bisoprolol may blunt the hyperglycemic action of glucagon

Insulin: Bisoprolol may mask tachycardia from hypoglycemia

NSAIDs (ibuprofen, indomethacin, naproxen, piroxicam) may reduce the antihypertensive effects of beta-blockers

Salicylates may reduce the antihypertensive effects of beta-blockers

Sulfonylureas: Beta-blockers may alter response to hypoglycemic agents

**Usual Dosage** Oral:

Adults: 5 mg once daily, may be increased to 10 mg, and then up to 20 mg once daily, if necessary

Elderly: Initial dose: 2.5 mg/day; may be increased by 2.5-5 mg/day; maximum recommended dose: 20 mg/day

**Dosing adjustment in renal/hepatic impairment:** $Cl_{cr}$ <40 mL/minute: Initial: 2.5 mg/day; increase cautiously.

Hemodialysis: Not dialyzable

**Patient Information** Take exactly as directed. Do not increase, decrease, or adjust dosage without consulting prescriber. Do not take with antacids and do not use alcohol or OTC medications (eg, cold remedies) without consulting prescriber. If diabetic, monitor serum sugars closely (may alter glucose tolerance or mask signs of hypoglycemia). May cause fatigue, dizziness, or postural hypotension; use caution when changing position from lying or sitting to standing, or when driving or climbing stairs until response to medication is known. May cause alteration in sexual performance (reversible). Report palpitations, unresolved swelling of extremities, difficulty breathing or new cough, unresolved fatigue, unusual weight gain, unresolved constipation, or unusual muscle weakness.

**Dosage Forms** Tablet, as fumarate: 5 mg, 10 mg

## Bisoprolol and Hydrochlorothiazide

(bis OH proe lol & hye droe klor oh THYE a zide)

**U.S. Brand Names** Ziac™

**Pharmacologic Category** Antihypertensive Agent, Combination

**Use** Treatment of hypertension

**Effects on Mental Status** Fatigue is common; may cause insomnia, confusion, and depression

**Effects on Psychiatric Treatment** Barbiturates may decrease the effects of beta-blockers

**Usual Dosage** Adults: Oral: Dose is individualized, given once daily

**Dosage Forms** Tablet:

Bisoprolol fumarate 2.5 mg and hydrochlorothiazide 6.25 mg

Bisoprolol fumarate 5 mg and hydrochlorothiazide 6.25 mg

Bisoprolol fumarate 10 mg and hydrochlorothiazide 6.25 mg

## Bitolterol (bye TOLE ter ole)

**U.S. Brand Names** Tornalate®

**Pharmacologic Category** $Beta_2$ Agonist

**Use** Prevention and treatment of bronchial asthma and bronchospasm

**Effects on Mental Status** May cause nervousness and insomnia

**Effects on Psychiatric Treatment** Concurrent use with MAOIs or TCAs may result in increased toxicity

**Pregnancy Risk Factor** C

**Contraindications** Known hypersensitivity to bitolterol

**Warnings/Precautions** Use with caution in patients with unstable vasomotor symptoms, diabetes, hyperthyroidism, prostatic hypertrophy or a history of seizures; also use caution in the elderly and those patients with cardiovascular disorders such as coronary artery disease, arrhythmias, and hypertension; excessive use may result in cardiac arrest and death; do not use concurrently with other sympathomimetic bronchodilators

**Adverse Reactions**
>10%: Neuromuscular & skeletal: Trembling
1% to 10%:
Cardiovascular: Flushing of face, hypertension, pounding heartbeat
Central nervous system: Dizziness, lightheadedness, nervousness
Gastrointestinal: Xerostomia, nausea, unpleasant taste
Respiratory: Bronchial irritation, coughing
<1%: Arrhythmias, chest pain, insomnia, paradoxical bronchospasm, tachycardia

**Overdosage/Toxicology**
Signs and symptoms: Tremor, dizziness, nervousness, headache, nausea, coughing
Treatment: Symptomatic/supportive; in cases of severe overdose, supportive therapy should be instituted, and prudent use of a cardioselective beta-adrenergic blocker (eg, atenolol or metoprolol) should be considered, keeping in mind the potential for induction of bronchoconstriction in an asthmatic individual. Dialysis has not been shown to be of value in the treatment of an overdose with this agent.

**Drug Interactions**
Decreased effect: Beta-adrenergic blockers (eg, propranolol)
Increased effect: Inhaled ipratropium may increase duration of bronchodilation, nifedipine may increase FEV-1
Increased toxicity: MAO inhibitors, tricyclic antidepressants, sympathomimetic agents (eg, amphetamine, dopamine, dobutamine), inhaled anesthetics (eg, enflurane)

**Usual Dosage** Children >12 years and Adults:
Bronchospasm: 2 inhalations at an interval of at least 1-3 minutes, followed by a third inhalation if needed
Prevention of bronchospasm: 2 inhalations every 8 hours; do not exceed 3 inhalations every 6 hours or 2 inhalations every 4 hours

**Patient Information** Use exactly as directed. Do not use more often than recommended. Maintain adequate hydration (2-3 L/day of fluids unless instructed to restrict fluid intake). You may experience nervousness, dizziness, or fatigue (use caution when driving or engaging in tasks requiring alertness until response to drug is known); or dry mouth, stomach upset (frequent small meals, frequent mouth care, chewing gum, or sucking hard candy may help). Report unresolved GI upset; dizziness or fatigue; vision changes; chest pain, rapid heartbeat, or palpitations; nervousness or insomnia; muscle cramping or tremor; or unusual cough.

**Administration:** Self-administered inhalation: Store canister upside down; do not freeze. Shake canister before using. Sit when using medication. Close eyes when administering bitolterol to avoid spray getting into eyes. Exhale slowly and completely through nose; inhale deeply through mouth while administering aerosol. Hold breath for 1-3 seconds after inhalation. Wait at least 1 full minute between inhalations. Wash mouthpiece between use. If more than one inhalation medication is used, use bitolterol first and wait 5 minutes between medications.

Self-administered nebulizer: Wash hands before and after treatment. Wash and dry nebulizer after each treatment. Twist open the top of one unit dose vial and squeeze contents into nebulizer reservoir. Connect nebulizer reservoir to the mouthpiece or face-mask. Connect nebulizer to compressor. Sit in comfortable, upright position. Place mouthpiece in your mouth or put on face-mask and turn on compressor. If face-mask is used, avoid leakage around the mask to avoid mist getting into eyes which may cause vision problems. Breath calmly and deeply until no more mist is formed in nebulizer (about 5 minutes). At this point treatment is finished.

**Nursing Implications** Before using, the inhaler must be shaken well

**Dosage Forms**
Aerosol, oral, as mesylate: 0.8% [370 mcg/metered spray, 300 inhalations] (15 mL)
Solution, inhalation, as mesylate: 0.2% (10 mL, 30 mL, 60 mL)


- ♦ **Black Draught® [OTC]** *see* Senna *on page 509*
- ♦ **Black Susans** *see* Echinacea *on page 189*
- ♦ **BlemErase® Lotion [OTC]** *see* Benzoyl Peroxide *on page 62*
- ♦ **Blenoxane®** *see* Bleomycin *on page 71*


## Bleomycin (blee oh MYE sin)

**U.S. Brand Names** Blenoxane®
**Pharmacologic Category** Antineoplastic Agent, Antibiotic
**Use** Treatment of squamous cell carcinomas, melanomas, sarcomas, testicular carcinoma, Hodgkin's lymphoma, and non-Hodgkin's lymphoma; may also be used as a sclerosing agent for malignant pleural effusion
**Effects on Mental Status** None reported
**Effects on Psychiatric Treatment** May rarely produce myelosuppression; use caution with clozapine and carbamazepine
**Usual Dosage** Refer to individual protocols; 1 unit = 1 mg
May be administered I.M., I.V., S.C., or intracavitary
Children and Adults:
Test dose for lymphoma patients: I.M., I.V., S.C.: Because of the possibility of an anaphylactoid reaction, ≤2 units of bleomycin for the first 2 doses; monitor vital signs every 15 minutes; wait a minimum of 1 hour before administering remainder of dose; if no acute reaction occurs, then the regular dosage schedule may be followed
**Single-agent therapy:**
I.M./I.V./S.C.: Squamous cell carcinoma, lymphoma, testicular carcinoma: 0.25-0.5 units/kg (10-20 units/m$^2$) 1-2 times/week
CIV: 15 units/m$^2$ over 24 hours daily for 4 days
**Combination-agent therapy:**
I.M./I.V.: 3-4 units/m$^2$
I.V.: ABVD: 10 units/m$^2$ on days 1 and 15
Maximum cumulative lifetime dose: 400 units
**Dosing adjustment in renal impairment:**
$Cl_{cr}$ 10-50 mL/minute: Administer 75% of normal dose
$Cl_{cr}$ <10 mL/minute: Administer 50% of normal dose
Hemodialysis: None
CAPD effects: None
CAVH effects: None
Adults: Intracavitary injection for malignant pleural effusion: 60 international units (range of 15-120 units; dose generally does not exceed 1 unit/kg) in 50-100 mL SWI

**Dosage Forms** Powder for injection, as sulfate: 15 units


- ♦ **Bleph®-10 Ophthalmic** *see* Sulfacetamide *on page 522*
- ♦ **Blephamide® Ophthalmic** *see* Sulfacetamide Sodium and Prednisolone *on page 523*
- ♦ **Blis-To-Sol® [OTC]** *see* Tolnaftate *on page 555*
- ♦ **Blocadren® Oral** *see* Timolol *on page 549*
- ♦ **Bluboro® [OTC]** *see* Aluminum Sulfate and Calcium Acetate *on page 28*
- ♦ **Bonine® [OTC]** *see* Meclizine *on page 335*
- ♦ **Boropak® [OTC]** *see* Aluminum Sulfate and Calcium Acetate *on page 28*
- ♦ **B&O Supprettes®** *see* Belladonna and Opium *on page 60*
- ♦ **Botox®** *see* Botulinum Toxin Type A *on page 71*


## Botulinum Toxin Type A (BOT yoo lin num TOKS in type aye)

**U.S. Brand Names** Botox®
**Pharmacologic Category** Ophthalmic Agent, Toxin
**Use** Treatment of strabismus and blepharospasm associated with dystonia (including benign essential blepharospasm or VII nerve disorders in patients ≥12 years of age)
**Unlabeled use:** Treatment of hemifacial spasms, spasmodic torticollis (ie, cervical dystonia, clonic twisting of the head), oromandibular dystonia, spasmodic dysphonia (laryngeal dystonia) and other dystonias (ie, writer's cramp, focal task-specific dystonias)
**Orphan drug:** Treatment of dynamic muscle contracture in pediatric cerebral palsy patients
**Effects on Mental Status** None reported
**Effects on Psychiatric Treatment** None reported
**Pregnancy Risk Factor** C
**Contraindications** Hypersensitivity to botulinum A toxin; relative contraindications to botulinum toxin therapy include diseases of neuromuscular transmission and coagulopathy, including anticoagulant therapy; injections into the central area of the upper eyelid (rapid diffusion of toxin into the levator can occur resulting in a marked ptosis).
**Warnings/Precautions** Use with caution in patients taking aminoglycosides or any other antibiotic or other drugs that interfere with neuromuscular transmission; do not exceed recommended dose
**Adverse Reactions**
>10%: Ocular: Dry eyes, lagophthalmos, ptosis, photophobia, vertical deviation
1% to 10%:
Dermatologic: Diffuse rash
Ocular: Eyelid edema, blepharospasm
<1%: Diplopia, ectropion, entropion, keratitis
**Overdosage/Toxicology** In the event of an overdosage or injection into the wrong muscle, additional information may be obtained by contacting Allergan Pharmaceuticals at (800)-347-5063 from 8 AM to 4 PM Pacific time, or at (714)-724-5954 at other times
**Drug Interactions** Increased effect: Botulinum toxin may be potentiated by aminoglycosides
**Usual Dosage**
Strabismus: 1.25-5 units (0.05-0.15 mL) injected into any one muscle
Subsequent doses for residual/recurrent strabismus: Re-examine patients 7-14 days after each injection to assess the effect of that dose. Subsequent doses for patients experiencing incomplete paralysis of the target may be increased up to two fold the previously administered dose. Maximum recommended dose as a single injection for any one muscle is 25 units.
Blepharospasm: 1.25-2.5 units (0.05-0.10 mL) injected into the orbicularis oculi muscle
(Continued)

## Botulinum Toxin Type A *(Continued)*

Subsequent doses: Each treatment lasts approximately 3 months. At repeat treatment sessions, the dose may be increased up to twofold if the response from the initial treatment is considered insufficient (usually defined as an effect that does not last >2 months). There appears to be little benefit obtainable from injecting >5 units per site. Some tolerance may be found if treatments are given any more frequently than every 3 months.

The cumulative dose should not exceed 200 units in a 30-day period

**Patient Information** Patients with blepharospasm may have been extremely sedentary for a long time; caution these patients to resume activity slowly and carefully following administration

**Nursing Implications** To alleviate spatial disorientation or double vision in strabismic patients, cover the affected eye; have epinephrine ready for hypersensitivity reactions

**Dosage Forms** Injection: 100 units *Clostridium botulinum* toxin type A


- **Breezee® Mist Antifungal [OTC]** *see* Tolnaftate *on page 555*
- **Breezee® Mist Antifungal [OTC]** *see* Miconazole *on page 364*
- **Breonesin® [OTC]** *see* Guaifenesin *on page 256*
- **Brethaire®** *see* Terbutaline *on page 535*
- **Brethine®** *see* Terbutaline *on page 535*


## Bretylium (bre TIL ee um)

**U.S. Brand Names** Bretylol®

**Canadian Brand Names** Bretylate®

**Pharmacologic Category** Antiarrhythmic Agent, Class III

**Use** Treatment of ventricular tachycardia and fibrillation; treatment of other serious ventricular arrhythmias resistant to lidocaine

**Effects on Mental Status** May cause confusion

**Effects on Psychiatric Treatment** Hypotension is common; use caution with concurrent psychotropics

**Usual Dosage Note**: Patients should undergo defibrillation/cardioversion before and after bretylium doses as necessary.

Children (**Note:** Not well established, although the following dosing has been suggested):

I.M.: 2-5 mg/kg as a single dose

I.V.: Acute ventricular fibrillation: Initial: 5 mg/kg, then attempt electrical defibrillation; repeat with 10 mg/kg if ventricular fibrillation persists at 15- to 30-minute intervals to maximum total of 30 mg/kg.

Maintenance dose: I.M., I.V.: 5 mg/kg every 6 hours

Adults:

Immediate life-threatening ventricular arrhythmias (ventricular fibrillation, unstable ventricular tachycardia): Initial dose: I.V.: 5 mg/kg (undiluted) over 1 minute; if arrhythmia persists, administer 10 mg/kg (undiluted) over 1 minute and repeat as necessary (usually at 15- to 30-minute intervals) up to a total dose of 30-35 mg/kg.

Other life-threatening ventricular arrhythmias:

Initial dose: I.M., I.V.: 5-10 mg/kg, may repeat every 1-2 hours if arrhythmia persists; administer I.V. dose (diluted) over 8-10 minutes.

Maintenance dose: I.M.: 5-10 mg/kg every 6-8 hours; I.V. (diluted): 5-10 mg/kg every 6 hours; I.V. infusion (diluted): 1-2 mg/minute (little experience with doses >40 mg/kg/day)

Example dilution: 2 g/250 mL $D_5W$ (infusion pump should be used for I.V. infusion administration)

Rate of I.V. infusion: 1-4 mg/minute

1 mg/minute = 7 mL/hour
2 mg/minute = 15 mL/hour
3 mg/minute = 22 mL/hour
4 mg/minute = 30 mL/hour

**Dosing adjustment in renal impairment:**

$Cl_{cr}$ 10-50 mL/minute: Administer 25% to 50% of dose.

$Cl_{cr}$ <10 mL/minute: Administer 25% of dose.

Dialysis: Not dialyzable (0% to 5%) via hemo- or peritoneal dialysis; supplemental doses are not needed.

**Dosage Forms**

Injection, as tosylate: 50 mg/mL (10 mL, 20 mL)

Injection, as tosylate, premixed in $D_5W$: 1 mg/mL (500 mL); 2 mg/mL (250 mL); 4 mg/mL (250 mL, 500 mL)


- **Bretylol®** *see* Bretylium *on page 72*
- **Brevibloc® Injection** *see* Esmolol *on page 202*
- **Brevicon®** *see* Ethinyl Estradiol and Norethindrone *on page 212*
- **Brevital® Sodium** *see* Methohexital *on page 353*
- **Brevoxyl® Gel** *see* Benzoyl Peroxide *on page 62*
- **Bricanyl®** *see* Terbutaline *on page 535*


## Brimonidine (bri MOE ni deen)

**U.S. Brand Names** Alphagan®

**Pharmacologic Category** $Alpha_2$ Agonist, Ophthalmic; Ophthalmic Agent, Antiglaucoma

**Use** Lowering of intraocular pressure in patients with open-angle glaucoma or ocular hypertension

**Effects on Mental Status** Drowsiness is common

**Effects on Psychiatric Treatment** Contraindicated with MAOIs; concurrent use with psychotropics may produce additive sedation

**Usual Dosage** Adults: Ophthalmic: Instill 1 drop in affected eye(s) 3 times/day (approximately every 8 hours)

**Dosage Forms** Solution, ophthalmic, as tartrate: 0.2% (5 mL, 10 mL)

## Brinzolamide (brin ZOH la mide)

**Related Information**

Glaucoma Drug Therapy *on page 712*

**U.S. Brand Names** Azopt™

**Pharmacologic Category** Carbonic Anhydrase Inhibitor; Ophthalmic Agent, Antiglaucoma

**Use** Lowers intraocular pressure to treat glaucoma in patients with ocular hypertension or open-angle glaucoma

**Effects on Mental Status** May rarely cause dizziness

**Effects on Psychiatric Treatment** None reported

**Usual Dosage** Adults: Ophthalmic: Instill 1 drop in affected eye(s) 3 times/day

**Dosage Forms** Suspension, ophthalmic: 1% (2.5 mL, 5 mL, 10 mL, 15 mL)


- **BRL 43694** *see* Granisetron *on page 254*
- **Brofed® Elixir [OTC]** *see* Brompheniramine and Pseudoephedrine *on page 74*
- **Bromaline® Elixir [OTC]** *see* Brompheniramine and Phenylpropanolamine *on page 74*
- **Bromanate® DC** *see* Brompheniramine, Phenylpropanolamine, and Codeine *on page 74*
- **Bromanate® Elixir [OTC]** *see* Brompheniramine and Phenylpropanolamine *on page 74*
- **Bromarest® [OTC]** *see* Brompheniramine *on page 73*
- **Bromatapp® [OTC]** *see* Brompheniramine and Phenylpropanolamine *on page 74*
- **Brombay® [OTC]** *see* Brompheniramine *on page 73*
- **Bromfed® Syrup [OTC]** *see* Brompheniramine and Pseudoephedrine *on page 74*
- **Bromfed® Tablet [OTC]** *see* Brompheniramine and Pseudoephedrine *on page 74*
- **Bromfenex®** *see* Brompheniramine and Pseudoephedrine *on page 74*
- **Bromfenex® PD** *see* Brompheniramine and Pseudoephedrine *on page 74*


## Bromocriptine (broe moe KRIP teen)

**Related Information**

Discontinuation of Psychotropic Drugs - Withdrawal Symptoms and Recommendations *on page 798*

**Generic Available** No

**U.S. Brand Names** Parlodel®

**Canadian Brand Names** Apo® Bromocriptine

**Synonyms** Bromocriptine Mesylate

**Pharmacologic Category** Anti-Parkinson's Agent (Dopamine Agonist); Ergot Derivative

**Use**

Amenorrhea with or without galactorrhea; infertility or hypogonadism; prolactin-secreting adenomas; acromegaly; Parkinson's disease

**The indication for prevention of postpartum lactation was withdrawn** voluntarily by Sandoz Pharmaceuticals Corporation

**Unlabeled use:** Neuroleptic malignant syndrome

**Effects on Mental Status** Drowsiness is common; may cause hallucinations

**Effects on Psychiatric Treatment** Used to treat neuroleptic malignant syndrome and cocaine abuse; fluvoxamine and nefazodone may increase bromocriptine concentrations; monitor for hypotension, headache, nausea

**Pregnancy Risk Factor** B

**Contraindications** Hypersensitivity to bromocriptine, ergot alkaloids, or any component; uncontrolled hypertension; severe ischemic heart disease or peripheral vascular disorders; pregnancy (risk to benefit evaluation must be performed in women who become pregnant during treatment for acromegaly, prolactinoma, or Parkinson's disease - hypertension during treatment should generally result in efforts to withdraw)

**Warnings/Precautions** Use with caution in patients with impaired renal or hepatic function, a history of psychosis, or cardiovascular disease (myocardial infarction, arrhythmia). Patients who receive bromocriptine during and immediately following pregnancy as a continuation of previous therapy (ie, acromegaly) should be closely monitored for cardiovascular effects. Discontinuation of bromocriptine in patients with macroadenomas has been associated with rapid regrowth of tumor and increased prolactin serum levels. Use with caution in patients with a history of peptic ulcer disease, dementia, or concurrent antihypertensive therapy. Safety and effectiveness in patients <15 years of age have not been established.

**Adverse Reactions**

>10%:

Central nervous system: Headache, dizziness

Gastrointestinal: Nausea

1% to 10%:

Cardiovascular: Orthostatic hypotension

Central nervous system: Fatigue, lightheadedness, drowsiness

Gastrointestinal: Anorexia, vomiting, abdominal cramps, constipation

Respiratory: Nasal congestion

<1%: Arrhythmias, hair loss, insomnia, paranoia, visual hallucinations

**Overdosage/Toxicology**

Signs and symptoms: Nausea, vomiting, hypotension

Treatment: Hypotension, when unresponsive to I.V. fluids or Trendelenburg positioning, often responds to norepinephrine infusions started at 0.1-0.2 mcg/kg/minute followed by a titrated infusion.

**Drug Interactions** CYP3A3/4 enzyme substrate

Antipsychotics: Antipsychotics may inhibit bromocriptine's therapeutic effects (diminished ability to lower prolactin)

CYP3A3/4 inhibitors: Serum level and/or toxicity of bromocriptine may be increased; inhibitors include amiodarone, cimetidine, clarithromycin, erythromycin, delavirdine, diltiazem, dirithromycin, disulfiram, fluoxetine, fluvoxamine, grapefruit juice, indinavir, itraconazole, ketoconazole, nevirapine, propoxyfene, quinupristin-dalfopristin, ritonavir, saquinavir, verapamil, zafirlukast, zileuton; monitor for altered effects; a decrease in bromocriptine dosage may be required

Entacapone: Fibrotic complications (retroperitoneal or pulmonary fibrosis) have been associated with combinations of entacapone and bromocriptine

Ethanol: May increase the sensitivity of receptors to bromocriptine; monitor for increase effect

Sympathomimetics: May increase risk of hypertension and seizure; isometheptene and phenylpropanolamine (and other sympathomimetics) should be avoided in patients receiving bromocriptine

**Mechanism of Action** Semisynthetic ergot alkaloid derivative and a dopamine receptor agonist which activates postsynaptic dopamine receptors in the tuberoinfundibular and nigrostriatal pathways

**Pharmacodynamics/kinetics**

Protein binding: 90% to 96%

Metabolism: Majority of drug metabolized in the liver

Half-life (biphasic):

Initial: 6-8 hours

Terminal: 50 hours

Time to peak serum concentration: Oral: Within 1-2 hours

Elimination: In bile; only 2% to 6% excreted unchanged in urine

**Usual Dosage** Adults: Oral:

Parkinsonism: 1.25 mg 2 times/day, increased by 2.5 mg/day in 2- to 4-week intervals (usual dose range is 30-90 mg/day in 3 divided doses), though elderly patients can usually be managed on lower doses

Neuroleptic malignant syndrome: 2.5-5 mg 3 times/day

Hyperprolactinemia: 2.5 mg 2-3 times/day

Acromegaly: Initial: 1.25-2.5 mg increasing as necessary every 3-7 days; usual dose: 20-30 mg/day

**Dosing adjustment in hepatic impairment:** No guidelines are available, however, may be necessary

**Monitoring Parameters** Monitor blood pressure closely as well as hepatic, hematopoietic, and cardiovascular function

**Reference Range** Peak plasma level of 24.6 ng/mL achieved after a dose of 100 mg

**Test Interactions** Bromocriptine may increase blood urea nitrogen, serum AST, serum ALT, serum CPK, alkaline phosphatase, and serum uric acid

**Patient Information** Take with food or milk; drowsiness commonly occurs upon initiation of therapy; limit use of alcohol; avoid exposure to cold; incidence of side effects is high (68%) with nausea the most common; hypotension occurs commonly with initiation of therapy, usually upon rising after prolonged sitting or lying; discontinue immediately if pregnant; may restore fertility; women desiring not to become pregnant should use mechanical contraceptive means

**Nursing Implications** Raise bed rails and institute safety measures; aid patient with ambulation; may cause postural hypotension and drowsiness

**Additional Information** Usually used with levodopa or levodopa/carbidopa to treat Parkinson's disease; when adding bromocriptine, the dose of levodopa/carbidopa can usually be decreased

**Dosage Forms**

Capsule, as mesylate: 5 mg

Tablet, as mesylate: 2.5 mg

- **Bromocriptine Mesylate** *see* Bromocriptine *on page 72*
- **Bromphen® [OTC]** *see* Brompheniramine *on page 73*
- **Bromphen® DC w/Codeine** *see* Brompheniramine, Phenylpropanolamine, and Codeine *on page 74*

## Brompheniramine (brome fen IR a meen)

**U.S. Brand Names** Bromarest® [OTC]; Brombay® [OTC]; Bromphen® [OTC]; Brotane® [OTC]; Chlorphed® [OTC]; Cophene-B®; Diamine T.D.® [OTC]; Dimetane® Extentabs® [OTC]; Nasahist B®; ND-Stat®

**Synonyms** Parabromdylamine

**Pharmacologic Category** Antihistamine

**Use** Perennial and seasonal allergic rhinitis and other allergic symptoms including urticaria

**Effects on Mental Status** Sedation is common

**Effects on Psychiatric Treatment** Concurrent use with psychotropics may produce additive sedation

**Pregnancy Risk Factor** C

**Contraindications** Narrow-angle glaucoma; bladder neck obstruction; symptomatic prostatic hypertrophy; asthmatic attacks; stenosing peptic ulcer; hypersensitivity to brompheniramine or any component

**Warnings/Precautions** Use with caution in patients with heart disease, hypertension, thyroid disease, and asthma; swallow whole, do not crush or chew; antihistamines are more likely to cause dizziness, excessive sedation, syncope, toxic confusional states, and hypotension in the elderly

**Adverse Reactions**

>10%:

Central nervous system: Slight to moderate drowsiness (compared with other first generation antihistamines, brompheniramine is relatively nonsedating)

Respiratory: Thickening of bronchial secretions

1% to 10%:

Central nervous system: Headache, fatigue, nervousness, dizziness

Gastrointestinal: Appetite increase, weight gain, nausea, diarrhea, abdominal pain, xerostomia

Neuromuscular & skeletal: Arthralgia

Respiratory: Pharyngitis

**Overdosage/Toxicology**

Signs and symptoms: Dry mouth, flushed skin, dilated pupils, CNS depression

Treatment: There is no specific treatment for an antihistamine overdose, however, most of its clinical toxicity is due to anticholinergic effects; anticholinesterase inhibitors including physostigmine, neostigmine, pyridostigmine, and edrophonium may be useful by reducing acetylcholinesterase; for anticholinergic overdose with severe life-threatening symptoms, physostigmine 1-2 mg (0.5 or 0.02 mg/kg for children) I.V., slowly may be given to reverse these effects

**Drug Interactions** Increased toxicity: CNS depressants, MAO inhibitors, alcohol, tricyclic antidepressants

**Usual Dosage**

Oral:

Children:

≤6 years: 0.125 mg/kg/dose given every 6 hours; maximum: 6-8 mg/day

6-12 years: 2-4 mg every 6-8 hours; maximum: 12-16 mg/day

Adults: 4 mg every 4-6 hours or 8 mg of sustained release form every 8-12 hours or 12 mg of sustained release every 12 hours; maximum: 24 mg/day

Elderly: Initial: 4 mg once or twice daily. **Note:** Duration of action may be 36 hours or more, even when serum concentrations are low.

I.M., I.V., S.C.:

Children ≤12 years: 0.5 mg/kg/24 hours divided every 6-8 hours

Adults: 10 mg every 6-12 hours, maximum: 40 mg/24 hours

**Patient Information** Avoid alcohol; take with food or milk; swallow whole, do not crush or chew extended release products; may cause drowsiness

**Dosage Forms**

Elixir, as maleate: 2 mg/5 mL with 3% alcohol (120 mL, 480 mL, 4000 mL)

Injection, as maleate: 10 mg/mL (10 mL)

Tablet, as maleate: 4 mg, 8 mg, 12 mg

Tablet, sustained release, as maleate: 8 mg, 12 mg

## Brompheniramine and Phenylephrine
(brome fen IR a meen & fen il EF rin)

**U.S. Brand Names** Dimetane® Decongestant Elixir [OTC]

**Pharmacologic Category** Antihistamine/Decongestant Combination

**Use** Temporary relief of symptoms of seasonal and perennial allergic rhinitis, and vasomotor rhinitis, including nasal obstruction

**Effects on Mental Status** Drowsiness, nervousness, insomnia, and slight stimulation are common; may cause fatigue or dizziness; may rarely cause depression or hallucinations

**Effects on Psychiatric Treatment** Concurrent use with psychotropics and other CNS depressants may produce additive adverse effects; tachycardia is common; use caution with clozapine and TCAs

(Continued)

## Brompheniramine and Phenylephrine *(Continued)*

**Usual Dosage** Children >12 years and Adults: Oral: 10 mL every 4 hours

**Dosage Forms** Elixir: Brompheniramine maleate 4 mg and phenylephrine hydrochloride 5 mg per 5 mL

## Brompheniramine and Phenylpropanolamine

(brome fen IR a meen & fen il proe pa NOLE a meen)

**U.S. Brand Names** Bromaline® Elixir [OTC]; Bromanate® Elixir [OTC]; Bromatapp® [OTC]; Bromphen® Tablet [OTC]; Cold & Allergy® Elixir [OTC]; Dimaphen® Elixir [OTC]; Dimaphen® Tablets [OTC]; Dimetapp® 4-Hour Liqui-Gel Capsule [OTC]; Dimetapp® Elixir [OTC]; Dimetapp® Extentabs® [OTC]; Dimetapp® Tablet [OTC]; Genatap® Elixir [OTC]; Tamine® [OTC]; Vicks® DayQuil® Allergy Relief 4 Hour Tablet [OTC]

**Pharmacologic Category** Antihistamine/Decongestant Combination

**Use** Temporary relief of nasal congestion, running nose, sneezing, and itchy, watery eyes

**Effects on Mental Status** Drowsiness, nervousness, insomnia, and slight stimulation are common; may cause fatigue or dizziness; may rarely cause depression or hallucinations

**Effects on Psychiatric Treatment** Concurrent use with psychotropics and other CNS depressants may produce additive adverse effects; tachycardia is common; use with caution with clozapine and TCAs

**Usual Dosage** Oral:

Children:
- 1-6 months: 1.25 mL 3-4 times/day
- 7-24 months: 2.5 mL 3-4 times/day
- 2-4 years: 3.75 mL 3-4 times/day
- 4-12 years: 5 mL 3-4 times/day

Adults: 5-10 mL 3-4 times/day or 1 regular tablet every 4 hours; sustained release: 1 tablet every 12 hours

**Dosage Forms**

Capsule (Dimetapp® 4-Hour Liqui-Gel): Brompheniramine maleate 4 mg and phenylpropanolamine hydrochloride 25 mg

Liquid (Bromaline®, Bromanate®, Cold & Allergy®, Dimaphen®, Dimetapp®, Genatap®): Brompheniramine maleate 2 mg and phenylpropanolamine hydrochloride 12.5 mg per 5 mL

Tablet (Dimaphen®, Dimetapp®, Vicks® DayQuil® Allergy Relief 4 Hour): Brompheniramine maleate 4 mg and phenylpropanolamine hydrochloride 25 mg

Tablet, sustained release: Brompheniramine maleate 12 mg and phenylpropanolamine hydrochloride 75 mg

## Brompheniramine and Pseudoephedrine

(brome fen IR a meen & soo doe e FED rin)

**U.S. Brand Names** Brofed® Elixir [OTC]; Bromfed® Syrup [OTC]; Bromfed® Tablet [OTC]; Bromfenex®; Bromfenex® PD; Drixoral® Syrup [OTC]; Iofed®; Iofed® PD

**Pharmacologic Category** Antihistamine/Decongestant Combination

**Use** Temporary relief of symptoms of seasonal and perennial allergic rhinitis, and vasomotor rhinitis, including nasal obstruction

**Effects on Mental Status** Drowsiness, nervousness, insomnia, and slight stimulation are common; may cause fatigue or dizziness; may rarely cause depression or hallucinations

**Effects on Psychiatric Treatment** Concurrent use with psychotropics and other CNS depressants may produce additive adverse effects; tachycardia is common; use caution with clozapine and TCAs

**Usual Dosage** Children >12 years and Adults: Oral: 10 mL every 4-6 hours, up to 40 mL/day

**Dosage Forms**

Capsule, extended release:
- Bromfenex® PD, Iofed® PD: Brompheniramine maleate 6 mg and pseudoephedrine hydrochloride 60 mg
- Bromfenex®, Iofed®: Brompheniramine maleate 12 mg and pseudoephedrine hydrochloride 120 mg

Elixir:
- Brofed®: Brompheniramine maleate 4 mg and pseudoephedrine hydrochloride 30 mg per 5 mL
- Bromfed®: Brompheniramine maleate 2 mg and pseudoephedrine hydrochloride 30 mg per 5 mL
- Drixoral®: Brompheniramine maleate 2 mg and pseudoephedrine sulfate 30 mg per 5 mL

Tablet (Bromfed®): Brompheniramine maleate 4 mg and pseudoephedrine hydrochloride 60 mg

## Brompheniramine, Phenylpropanolamine, and Codeine

(brome fen IR a meen, fen il proe pa NOLE a meen, & KOE deen)

**U.S. Brand Names** Bromanate® DC; Bromphen® DC w/Codeine; Dimetane®-DC; Myphetane DC®; Poly-Histine CS®

**Pharmacologic Category** Antihistamine/Decongestant/Antitussive

**Use** Relief of coughs and upper respiratory symptoms, including nasal congestion, associated with allergy or the common cold

**Effects on Mental Status** Drowsiness, nervousness, insomnia, and slight stimulation are common; may cause fatigue or dizziness; may rarely cause depression or hallucinations

**Effects on Psychiatric Treatment** Concurrent use with psychotropics and other CNS depressants may produce additive adverse effects; tachycardia is common; use caution with clozapine and TCAs

**Restrictions** C-V

**Usual Dosage** Oral:

Children:
- 2-6 years: 2.5 mL every 4 hours
- 6-12 years: 5 mL every 4 hours

Children >12 years and Adults: 10 mL every 4 hours

**Dosage Forms** Liquid: Brompheniramine maleate 2 mg, phenylpropanolamine hydrochloride 12.5 mg, and codeine phosphate 10 mg per 5 mL with alcohol 0.95% (480 mL)


- ♦ **Bromphen® Tablet [OTC]** *see* Brompheniramine and Phenylpropanolamine *on page 74*
- ♦ **Bronchial®** *see* Theophylline and Guaifenesin *on page 539*
- ♦ **Bronitin®** *see* Epinephrine *on page 195*
- ♦ **Bronkaid® Mist [OTC]** *see* Epinephrine *on page 195*
- ♦ **Bronkephrine® Injection** *see* Ethylnorepinephrine *on page 214*
- ♦ **Bronkodyl®** *see* Theophylline Salts *on page 539*
- ♦ **Bronkometer®** *see* Isoetharine *on page 294*
- ♦ **Bronkosol®** *see* Isoetharine *on page 294*
- ♦ **Brontex® Liquid** *see* Guaifenesin and Codeine *on page 256*
- ♦ **Brontex® Tablet** *see* Guaifenesin and Codeine *on page 256*
- ♦ **Brotane® [OTC]** *see* Brompheniramine *on page 73*


## Bucindolol (byoo SIN doe lole)

**U.S. Brand Names** Bextra®

**Synonyms** Bucindolol Hydrochloride; MJ-13105-1

**Pharmacologic Category** Beta Blocker, Nonselective

**Effects on Mental Status** Sedation is common

**Effects on Psychiatric Treatment** Concurrent use with psychotropics may produce additive sedation

**Contraindications** Hypersensitivity to bucindolol or other beta-adrenergic blockers; bronchospastic disease; bradycardia; cardiogenic shock; greater than first-degree A-V block (except in patients with a functioning artificial pacemaker)

**Warnings/Precautions** Use with caution in patients with multiple allergies, ventricular tachycardia, first-degree A-V block, hypotension, bradycardia, Raynaud's syndrome, peripheral vascular disease, hyperthyroidism, cardiac tamponade, diabetes mellitus, myasthenia gravis, liver or renal disease, or pregnancy. Bucindolol has not been demonstrated to be of benefit in patients with Class III-IV congestive heart failure (BEST study).

**Adverse Reactions**

Cardiovascular: Postural hypotension, facial flushing, sinus bradycardia
Central nervous system: Dizziness, headache, fatigue
Gastrointestinal: Nausea, vomiting, dyspepsia, abdominal cramps
Neuromuscular & skeletal: Myalgia
Respiratory: Bronchospasm

**Drug Interactions** Anticipated to be similar to other beta-blockers

Alpha-blockers (prazosin, terazosin): Concurrent use of beta-blockers may increase risk of orthostasis

Ampicillin, in single doses of 1 gram, decrease bucindolol's pharmacologic actions

Antacids (magnesium-aluminum, calcium antacids or salts) may reduce the bioavailability of bucindolol

Clonidine: Hypertensive crisis after or during withdrawal of either agent

Drugs which slow AV conduction (digoxin): Effects may be additive with beta-blockers

Glucagon: Bucindolol may blunt the hyperglycemic action of glucagon

Insulin and oral hypoglycemics: Bucindolol masks the tachycardia that usually accompanies hypoglycemia

NSAIDs (ibuprofen, indomethacin, naproxen, piroxicam) may reduce the antihypertensive effects of beta-blockers

Salicylates may reduce the antihypertensive effects of beta-blockers

Sulfonylureas: Beta-blockers may alter response to hypoglycemic agents

Verapamil or diltiazem may have synergistic or additive pharmacological effects when taken concurrently with beta-blockers

**Usual Dosage**

Congestive heart failure: 6.25 mg twice daily for 1 week followed by doubling of dose weekly, as tolerated, to a maximum dose of 100 mg twice daily. **Note: The BEST study, presented in November 1999 at the AHA Scientific sessions, showed no benefit of bucindolol in patients with Class III-IV CHF.**

Hypertension: 50 mg 3 times/day up to 200 mg 3 times/day

- **Bucindolol Hydrochloride** *see* Bucindolol *on page 74*
- **Bucladin®-S Softab®** *see* Buclizine *on page 75*

## Buclizine (BYOO kli zeen)

**U.S. Brand Names** Bucladin®-S Softab®

**Pharmacologic Category** Antihistamine

**Use** Prevention and treatment of motion sickness; symptomatic treatment of vertigo

**Effects on Mental Status** Drowsiness is common

**Effects on Psychiatric Treatment** Concurrent use with psychotropics may produce additive sedation

**Pregnancy Risk Factor** C

**Contraindications** Known hypersensitivity to buclizine

**Warnings/Precautions** Product contains tartrazine; use with caution in patients with angle-closure glaucoma, peptic ulcer, urinary tract obstruction, hyperthyroidism; some preparations contain sodium bisulfite; syrup contains alcohol

**Adverse Reactions**

>10%: Central nervous system: Drowsiness

<1%: Blurred vision, dizziness, fatigue, hypotension, insomnia, nausea, palpitations, paradoxical excitement, sedation, tremor, urinary retention, vomiting

**Overdosage/Toxicology**

Signs and symptoms: CNS stimulation or depression; overdose may result in death in infants and children

Treatment: There is no specific treatment for an antihistamine overdose, however, most of its clinical toxicity is due to anticholinergic effects; anticholinesterase inhibitors including physostigmine, neostigmine, pyridostigmine, and edrophonium may be useful by reducing acetylcholinesterase; for anticholinergic overdose with severe life-threatening symptoms, physostigmine 1-2 mg (0.5 or 0.02 mg/kg for children) I.V., slowly may be given to reverse these effects

**Drug Interactions** Increased toxicity: CNS depressants, MAO inhibitors, tricyclic antidepressants

**Usual Dosage** Adults: Oral:

Motion sickness (prophylaxis): 50 mg 30 minutes prior to traveling; may repeat 50 mg after 4-6 hours

Vertigo: 50 mg twice daily, up to 150 mg/day

**Patient Information** Take as directed. Do not increase dose or take more often than recommended. May cause drowsiness; use caution when driving or engaging in tasks that require alertness until response to drug is known. May cause dry mouth; lozenges, gum, or liquids may help. May cause headache or feelings of jitteriness or anxiety; these will go away when drug is discontinued.

**Nursing Implications** Bucladin®-S Softab® may be chewed, swallowed whole, or allowed to dissolve in mouth

**Dosage Forms** Tablet, chewable, as hydrochloride: 50 mg

## Budesonide (byoo DES oh nide)

**Related Information**

Asthma Guidelines *on page 773*

**U.S. Brand Names** Pulmicort® Turbuhaler®; Rhinocort®; Rhinocort® Aqua™

**Canadian Brand Names** Entocort®; Pulmicort®

**Pharmacologic Category** Corticosteroid, Oral Inhaler; Corticosteroid, Nasal

**Use**

Intranasal: Children and Adults: Management of symptoms of seasonal or perennial rhinitis

Oral inhalation: Maintenance and prophylactic treatment of asthma; includes patients who require corticosteroids and those who may benefit from systemic dose reduction/elimination

**Effects on Mental Status** May cause nervousness and insomnia

**Effects on Psychiatric Treatment** None reported

**Pregnancy Risk Factor** C

**Warnings/Precautions** Controlled clinical studies have shown that inhaled and intranasal corticosteroids may cause a reduction in growth velocity in pediatric patients. Growth velocity provides a means of comparing the rate of growth among children of the same age.

In studies involving inhaled corticosteroids, the average reduction in growth velocity was approximately 1 cm (about 1/3 of an inch) per year. It appears that the reduction is related to dose and how long the child takes the drug.

FDA's Pulmonary and Allergy Drugs and Metabolic and Endocrine Drugs advisory committees discussed this issue at a July 1998 meeting. They recommended that the agency develop class-wide labeling to inform healthcare providers so they would understand this potential side effect and monitor growth routinely in pediatric patients who are treated with inhaled corticosteroids, intranasal corticosteroids or both.

Long-term effects of this reduction in growth velocity on final adult height are unknown. Likewise, it also has not yet been determined whether patients' growth will "catch up" if treatment in discontinued. Drug manufacturers will continue to monitor these drugs to learn more about long-term effects. Children are prescribed inhaled corticosteroids to treat asthma. Intranasal corticosteroids are generally used to prevent and treat allergy-related nasal symptoms.

Patients are advised not to stop using their inhaled or intranasal corticosteroids without first speaking to their healthcare providers about the benefits of these drugs compared to their risks.

**Adverse Reactions**

>10%:

Cardiovascular: Pounding heartbeat

Central nervous system: Dizziness, headache, nervousness

Dermatologic: Itching, rash

Gastrointestinal: Bitter taste, GI irritation, oral candidiasis

Respiratory: Bronchitis, coughing, hoarseness, upper respiratory tract infection

Miscellaneous: Diaphoresis, increased susceptibility to infections

1% to 10%:

Central nervous system: Insomnia, psychic changes

Dermatologic: Acne, urticaria

Endocrine & metabolic: Menstrual problems

Gastrointestinal: Anorexia, Dry throat, increase in appetite, loss of taste perception, xerostomia

Ocular: Cataracts

Respiratory: Epistaxis

Miscellaneous: Loss of smell

<1%: Abdominal fullness, bronchospasm, shortness of breath

**Overdosage/Toxicology**

Signs and symptoms: Irritation and burning of the nasal mucosa, sneezing, intranasal and pharyngeal *Candida* infections, nasal ulceration, epistaxis, rhinorrhea, nasal stuffiness, headache. When consumed in excessive quantities, systemic hypercorticism and adrenal suppression may occur

Treatment: In those cases when systemic hypercorticism and adrenal suppression occur, discontinuation and withdrawal of the corticosteroid should be done judiciously

**Drug Interactions** CYP3A3/4 enzyme substrate

Although there have been no reported drug interactions to date, one would expect budesonide could potentially interact with drugs known to interact with other corticosteroids

**Usual Dosage**

Children <6 years: Not recommended

Aerosol inhalation: Children ≥6 years and Adults:

Rhinocort®: Nasal: Initial: 8 sprays (4 sprays/nostril) per day (256 mcg/day), given as either 2 sprays in each nostril in the morning and evening or as 4 sprays in each nostril in the morning; after symptoms decrease (usually by 3-7 days), reduce dose slowly every 2-4 weeks to the smallest amount needed to control symptoms

Rhinocort® Aqua™: 64 mcg/day as a single 32 mcg spray in each nostril. Some patients who do not achieve adequate control may benefit from increased dosage. A reduced dosage may be effective after initial control is achieved.

Maximum dose: Children <12 years: 129 mcg/day; Adults: 256 mcg/day

Oral inhalation:

Children ≥6 years:

Previous therapy of bronchodilators alone: 200 mcg twice initially which may be increased up to 400 mcg twice daily

Previous therapy of inhaled corticosteroids: 200 mcg twice initially which may be increased up to 400 mcg twice daily

Previous therapy of oral corticosteroids: The highest recommended dose in children is 400 mcg twice daily

Adults:

Previous therapy of bronchodilators alone: 200-400 mcg twice initially which may be increased up to 400 mcg twice daily

Previous therapy of inhaled corticosteroids: 200-400 mcg twice initially which may be increased up to 800 mcg twice daily

Previous therapy of oral corticosteroids: 400-800 mcg twice daily which may be increased up to 800 mcg twice daily

NIH Guidelines (NIH, 1997) (give in divided doses twice daily):

Children:

"Low" dose: 100-200 mcg/day

"Medium" dose: 200-400 mcg/day (1-2 inhalations/day)

"High" dose: >400 mcg/day (>2 inhalation/day)

Adults:

"Low" dose: 200-400 mcg/day (1-2 inhalations/day)

"Medium" dose: 400-600 mcg/day (2-3 inhalations/day)

"High" dose: >600 mcg/day (>3 inhalation/day)

**Patient Information** Use as directed; do not increase dosage or discontinue abruptly without consulting prescriber. It may take several days for you to realize full effects of treatment. If you are also using an inhaled bronchodilator, wait 10 minutes before using this steroid aerosol. You may experience dizziness, anxiety, or blurred vision (rise slowly from sitting or lying position and use caution when driving or engaging in tasks requiring

(Continued)

## Budesonide *(Continued)*

alertness until response to drug is known); or taste disturbance or aftertaste (frequent mouth care and mouth rinses may help). Report pounding heartbeat or chest pain; acute nervousness or inability to sleep; severe sneezing or nosebleed; difficulty breathing, sore throat, hoarseness, or bronchitis; respiratory difficulty or bronchospasms; disturbed menstrual pattern; vision changes; loss of taste or smell perception; or worsening of condition or lack of improvement.

**Administration:** Take 3-5 deep breaths. Use inhaler on inspiration. Allow 1 full minute between inhalations. Rinse mouth with water after use to reduce aftertaste and incidence of candidiasis.

**Dosage Forms**

Aerosol: 50 mcg released per actuation to deliver ~32 mcg to patient via nasal adapter [200 metered doses] (7 g)

Rhinocort® Aqua™: 32 mcg (60, 120 metered sprays); 64 mcg (120 metered sprays)

Turbuhaler: ~160 mcg delivered (200 mcg released) with each actuation (200 doses/inhaler)

♦ **Bufferin® [OTC]** *see* Aspirin *on page 49*

♦ **Buffex® [OTC]** *see* Aspirin *on page 49*

## Bumetanide (byoo MET a nide)

**U.S. Brand Names** Bumex®

**Canadian Brand Names** Burinex®

**Pharmacologic Category** Diuretic, Loop

**Use** Management of edema secondary to congestive heart failure or hepatic or renal disease including nephrotic syndrome; may be used alone or in combination with antihypertensives in the treatment of hypertension; can be used in furosemide-allergic patients

**Effects on Mental Status** May cause dizziness

**Effects on Psychiatric Treatment** Lithium excretion may be decreased; monitor serum lithium levels

**Pregnancy Risk Factor** C (per manufacturer); D (based on expert analysis)

**Contraindications** Hypersensitivity to bumetanide or sulfonylureas; anuria; patients with hepatic coma or in states of severe electrolyte depletion until the condition improves or is corrected; pregnancy (based on expert analysis)

**Warnings/Precautions** Adjust dose to avoid dehydration. In cirrhosis, avoid electrolyte and acid/base imbalances that might lead to hepatic encephalopathy. Ototoxicity is associated with I.V. rapid administration, renal impairment, excessive doses, and concurrent use of other ototoxins. Hypersensitivity reactions can rarely occur. Monitor fluid status and renal function in an attempt to prevent oliguria, azotemia, and reversible increases in BUN and creatinine. Close medical supervision of aggressive diuresis required. Watch for and correct electrolyte disturbances. Coadministration of antihypertensives may increase the risk of hypotension. Use caution in patients with known hypersensitivity to sulfonamides or thiazides (due to possible cross-sensitivity); avoid in patients with history of severe reactions.

**Adverse Reactions**

>10%:
- Endocrine & metabolic: Hyperuricemia (18.4%), hypochloremia, hypokalemia
- Renal: Azotemia

1% to 10%:
- Central nervous system: Dizziness, encephalopathy, headache
- Endocrine & metabolic: Hyponatremia
- Neuromuscular & skeletal: Muscle cramps, weakness

<1%: Altered LFTs, cramps, hearing loss, hyperglycemia, hypotension, increased serum creatinine, nausea, pruritus, rash, vomiting

**Overdosage/Toxicology**

Signs and symptoms: Electrolyte depletion, volume depletion

Treatment: Primarily symptomatic and supportive

**Drug Interactions**

ACE inhibitors: Hypotensive effects and/or renal effects are potentiated by hypovolemia

Antidiabetic agents: Glucose tolerance may be decreased

Antihypertensive agents: Hypotensive effects may be enhanced

Cholestyramine or colestipol may reduce bioavailability of bumetanide

Digoxin: Ethacrynic acid-induced hypokalemia may predispose to digoxin toxicity; monitor potassium

Indomethacin (and other NSAIDs) may reduce natriuretic and hypotensive effects of diuretics

Lithium: Renal clearance may be reduced. Isolated reports of lithium toxicity have occurred; monitor lithium levels

NSAIDs: Risk of renal impairment may increase when used in conjunction with diuretics

Ototoxic drugs (aminoglycosides, cis-platinum): Concomitant use of bumetanide may increase risk of ototoxicity, especially in patients with renal dysfunction

Peripheral adrenergic-blocking drugs or ganglionic blockers: Effects may be increased

Salicylates (high-dose) with diuretics may predispose patients to salicylate toxicity due to reduced renal excretion or alter renal function

Sparfloxacin, gatifloxacin, and moxifloxacin: Risk of hypokalemia and cardiotoxicity may be increased; avoid use

Thiazides: Synergistic diuretic effects occur

**Usual Dosage**

Children (not FDA-approved for use in children <18 years of age):
- <6 months: Dose not established
- >6 months:
  - Oral: Initial: 0.015 mg/kg/dose once daily or every other day; maximum dose: 0.1 mg/kg/day
  - I.M., I.V.: Dose not established

Adults:
- Oral: 0.5-2 mg/dose 1-2 times/day; maximum: 10 mg/day
- I.M., I.V.: 0.5-1 mg/dose; maximum: 10 mg/day
- Continuous I.V. infusions of 0.9-1 mg/hour may be more effective than bolus dosing

**Patient Information** May be taken with food to reduce GI effects. Take single dose early in day (single dose) or last dose early in afternoon (twice daily) to prevent sleep interruptions. Include orange juice or bananas (or other sources of potassium-rich foods) in your daily diet but do not take supplemental potassium without consulting prescriber. You may experience dizziness, hypotension, lightheadedness, or weakness; use caution when changing position (rising from sitting or lying position), when driving, exercising, climbing stairs, or performing hazardous tasks, and avoid excessive exercise in hot weather. Report swelling of ankles or feet, weight increase or decrease more than 3 pounds in any one day, increased fatigue, muscle cramps or trembling, and any changes in hearing.

**Nursing Implications** Be alert to complaints about hearing difficulty

**Dosage Forms**

Injection: 0.25 mg/mL (2 mL, 4 mL, 10 mL)

Tablet: 0.5 mg, 1 mg, 2 mg

♦ **Bumex®** *see* Bumetanide *on page 76*

♦ **Buminate®** *see* Albumin *on page 21*

♦ **Bupap®** *see* Butalbital Compound and Acetaminophen *on page 80*

## Bupivacaine (byoo PIV a kane)

**U.S. Brand Names** Marcaine®; Sensorcaine®; Sensorcaine®-MPF

**Pharmacologic Category** Local Anesthetic

**Use** Local anesthetic (injectable) for peripheral nerve block, infiltration, sympathetic block, caudal or epidural block, retrobulbar block

**Effects on Mental Status** May cause anxiety and restlessness

**Effects on Psychiatric Treatment** Use with caution in patients receiving phenothiazines, MAOIs, or TCAs; severe hypertension or hypotension may result

**Usual Dosage** Dose varies with procedure, depth of anesthesia, vascularity of tissues, duration of anesthesia and condition of patient. Metabisulfites (in epinephrine-containing injection); do not use solutions containing preservatives for caudal or epidural block.

Caudal block (with or without epinephrine):
- Children: 1-3.7 mg/kg
- Adults: 15-30 mL of 0.25% or 0.5%

Epidural block (other than caudal block):
- Children: 1.25 mg/kg/dose
- Adults: 10-20 mL of 0.25% or 0.5%

Peripheral nerve block: 5 mL dose of 0.25% or 0.5% (12.5-25 mg); maximum: 2.5 mg/kg (plain); 3 mg/kg (with epinephrine); up to a maximum of 400 mg/day

Sympathetic nerve block: 20-50 mL of 0.25% (no epinephrine) solution

**Dosage Forms**

Injection, as hydrochloride: 0.25% (10 mL, 20 mL, 30 mL, 50 mL); 0.5% (10 mL, 20 mL, 30 mL, 50 mL); 0.75% (2 mL, 10 mL, 20 mL, 30 mL)

Injection, as hydrochloride, with epinephrine (1:200,000): 0.25% (10 mL, 30 mL, 50 mL); 0.5% (1.8 mL, 3 mL, 5 mL, 10 mL, 30 mL, 50 mL); 0.75% (30 mL)

♦ **Buprenex®** *see* Buprenorphine *on page 76*

## Buprenorphine (byoo pre NOR feen)

**Related Information**

Narcotic Agonists Comparison Chart *on page 720*

Substance-Related Disorders *on page 609*

**Generic Available** Yes

**U.S. Brand Names** Buprenex®

**Synonyms** Buprenorphine Hydrochloride

**Pharmacologic Category** Analgesic, Narcotic

**Use** Management of moderate to severe pain

**Unlabeled use:** Heroin and opioid withdrawal

**Effects on Mental Status** Drowsiness is common; rare reports of euphoria

**Effects on Psychiatric Treatment** Concurrent use with benzodiazepines or barbiturates may result in CNS or respiratory depression

**Restrictions** C-V

**Pregnancy Risk Factor** C

**Contraindications** Hypersensitivity to buprenorphine or any component

**Warnings/Precautions** May cause respiratory depression - use caution in patients with respiratory disease or pre-existing respiratory depression. Potential for drug dependency exists, abrupt cessation may precipitate withdrawal. Use caution in elderly, debilitated, or pediatric patients. Use with caution in patients with depression or suicidal tendencies, or in patients with a history of drug abuse. Tolerance, psychological and physical dependence may occur with prolonged use. Use with caution in patients with hepatic, pulmonary, or renal function impairment. May cause CNS depression, which may impair physical or mental abilities. Patients must be cautioned about performing tasks which require mental alertness (ie, operating machinery or driving). Effects with other sedative drugs or ethanol may be potentiated. Elderly may be more sensitive to CNS depressant and constipating effects. Use with caution in patients with head injury or increased ICP, biliary tract dysfunction, pancreatitis, patients with history of ileus or bowel obstruction, glaucoma, hyperthyroidism, adrenal insufficiency, prostatic hypertrophy, urinary stricture, CNS depression, toxic psychosis, alcoholism, delirium tremens, or kyphoscoliosis. Partial antagonist activity may precipitate acute narcotic withdrawal in opioid-dependent individuals.

**Adverse Reactions**

>10%: Central nervous system: Sedation

1% to 10%:

Cardiovascular: Hypotension

Central nervous system: Respiratory depression, dizziness, headache

Gastrointestinal: Vomiting, nausea

Ocular: Miosis

Miscellaneous: Diaphoresis

<1%: Blurred vision, bradycardia, confusion, constipation, cyanosis, depression, diplopia, dyspnea, euphoria, hypertension, nervousness, paresthesia, pruritus, slurred speech, tachycardia, urinary retention, xerostomia

**Overdosage/Toxicology**

Signs and symptoms: CNS depression, pinpoint pupils, hypotension, bradycardia

Treatment: Support of the patient's airway, establishment of an I.V. line, and administration of naloxone 2 mg I.V. (0.01 mg/kg for children) with repeat administration as necessary up to a total of 10 mg

**Drug Interactions**

Cimetidine: May increase sedation from narcotic analgesics; however, histamine blockers may attenuate the cardiovascular response from histamine release associated with narcotic analgesics

CNS depressants: May produce additive respiratory and CNS depression; includes benzodiazepines, barbiturates, ethanol, and other sedatives. Respiratory and CV collapse was reported in a patient who received diazepam and buprenorphine.

Naltrexone: May antagonize the effect of narcotic analgesics; concurrent use or use within 7-10 days is contraindicated

**Stability** Protect from excessive heat (>40°C/104°F) and light

**Compatible** with 0.9% sodium chloride, lactated Ringer's solution, 5% dextrose in water, scopolamine, haloperidol, glycopyrrolate, droperidol, and hydroxyzine

**Incompatible** with diazepam, lorazepam

**Mechanism of Action** Buprenorphine exerts its analgesic effect via high affinity binding to μ opiate receptors in the CNS; displays both agonist and antagonist activity

**Pharmacodynamics/kinetics**

Onset of analgesia: Within 10-30 minutes

Absorption: I.M., S.C.: 30% to 40%

Distribution: $V_d$: 97-187 L/kg

Protein binding: High

Metabolism: Mainly in the liver; undergoes extensive first-pass metabolism

Half-life: 2.2-3 hours

Elimination: 70% excreted in feces via bile and 20% in urine as unchanged drug

**Usual Dosage** I.M., slow I.V.:

Children ≥13 years and Adults: 0.3-0.6 mg every 6 hours as needed

Elderly: 0.15 mg every 6 hours; elderly patients are more likely to suffer from confusion and drowsiness compared to younger patients

**Long-term use is not recommended**

**Monitoring Parameters** Pain relief, respiratory and mental status, CNS depression, blood pressure

**Reference Range** I.V. dose of 0.3 mg results in a plasma buprenorphine level of 0.5 μg/L

**Test Interactions** ↑ amylase, lipase

**Patient Information** May cause drowsiness; avoid alcoholic beverages; may be habit forming

**Nursing Implications** Gradual withdrawal of drug is necessary to avoid withdrawal symptoms

**Additional Information** 0.3 mg = 10 mg morphine or 75 mg meperidine, has longer duration of action than either agent

**Dosage Forms** Injection, as hydrochloride: 0.3 mg/mL (1 mL)

♦ **Buprenorphine Hydrochloride** *see* Buprenorphine *on page 76*

## Bupropion (byoo PROE pee on)

**Related Information**

Addiction Treatments *on page 772*
Antidepressant Agents Comparison Chart *on page 704*
Clinical Issues in the Use of Antidepressants *on page 627*
Mood Disorders *on page 600*
Patient Information - Antidepressants (Bupropion) *on page 641*
Special Populations - Elderly *on page 662*
Substance-Related Disorders *on page 609*

**Generic Available** Yes

**U.S. Brand Names** Wellbutrin®; Wellbutrin SR®; Zyban™

**Pharmacologic Category** Antidepressant, Dopamine-Reuptake Inhibitor

**Use** Treatment of depression; adjunct in smoking cessation

**Pregnancy Risk Factor** B

**Contraindications** Seizure disorder; anorexia/bulimia; use of monoamine oxidase inhibitors within 14 days; hypersensitivity to bupropion

**Warnings/Precautions** Seizure risk is increased at total daily dosage >450 mg, individual dosages >150 mg, or by sudden, large increments in dose. The risk of seizures is increased in patients with a history of seizures, head trauma, CNS tumor, abrupt discontinuation of sedative-hypnotics or alcohol, medications which lower seizure threshold, stimulants, or hypoglycemic agents. May cause CNS stimulation (restlessness, anxiety, insomnia) or anorexia. Use with caution in patients where weight loss is not desirable. The incidence of sexual dysfunction with bupropion is generally lower than with SSRIs.

Use with caution in patients with hepatic or renal dysfunction and in elderly patients. Elderly patients may be at greater risk of accumulation during chronic dosing. May cause motor or cognitive impairment in some patients, use with caution if tasks requiring alertness such as operating machinery or driving are undertaken. May worsen psychosis in some patients or precipitate a shift to mania or hypomania in patients with bipolar disease. Use caution in patients with depression, particularly if suicidal risk may be present.

Arthralgia, myalgia, and fever with rash and other symptoms suggestive of delayed hypersensitivity resembling serum sickness reported

**Adverse Reactions**

>10%:

Cardiovascular: Tachycardia

Central nervous system: Agitation, insomnia, headache, dizziness, sedation

Gastrointestinal: Nausea, vomiting, xerostomia, constipation

Neuromuscular & skeletal: Tremor

Ocular: Blurred vision

Respiratory: Rhinitis

Miscellaneous: Diaphoresis

1% to 10%:

Cardiovascular: Hypertension, palpitations

Central nervous system: Anxiety, nervousness, confusion, hostility, abnormal dreams

Dermatologic: Rash, acne, dry skin

Endocrine & metabolic: Hyper- or hypoglycemia

Gastrointestinal: Anorexia, diarrhea, dyspepsia

Neuromuscular & skeletal: Arthralgia, myalgia

Otic: Tinnitus

Post-introduction adverse reactions: Arthralgia, myalgia, and fever with rash and other symptoms suggestive of delayed hypersensitivity resembling serum sickness reported

Hypertension (in some cases severe) requiring acute treatment has been reported in patients receiving bupropion alone and in combination with nicotine replacement therapy, orthostatic hypotension, third degree heart block, extrasystoles, myocardial infarction, phlebitis, pulmonary embolism

**Overdosage/Toxicology**

Signs and symptoms: Labored breathing, salivation, arched back, ataxia, convulsions

Treatment: Supportive; I.V. diazepam is useful in treating seizures

**Drug Interactions** CYP2B6 enzyme substrate, CYP3A3/4 enzyme substrate (minor)

**Note:** Seizure threshold-lowering agents: Use with caution in individuals receiving other agents that may lower seizure threshold (antipsychotics, antidepressants, fluoroquinolones, theophylline, abrupt discontinuation of benzodiazepines, systemic steroids)

Levodopa: Toxicity of bupropion is enhanced by levodopa

MAOIs: Toxicity of bupropion is enhanced by MAOIs (phenelzine); concurrent use in contraindicated

Nicotine: Treatment-emergent hypertension may occur; monitor BP in patients treated with bupropion and nicotine patch

(Continued)

## Bupropion *(Continued)*

Selegiline: When used in low doses (<10 mg/day), risk of interaction is theoretically lower than with nonselective MAOIs

Tricyclic antidepressants: Serum levels may be increased by bupropion; in addition, these agents lower seizure threshold (see above)

**Mechanism of Action** Antidepressant structurally different from all other previously marketed antidepressants; like other antidepressants the mechanism of bupropion's activity is not fully understood; weak inhibitor of the neuronal uptake of serotonin, norepinephrine, and dopamine

**Pharmacodynamics/kinetics**

Absorption: Rapidly absorbed from GI tract

Distribution: $V_d$: 19-21 L/kg

Protein binding: 82% to 88%

Metabolism: Extensively in the liver to multiple metabolites

Half-life: 14 hours

Time to peak serum concentration: Oral: Within 3 hours

**Usual Dosage** Oral:

Adults:

Depression:

Immediate release: 100 mg 3 times/day; begin at 100 mg twice daily; may increase to a maximum dose of 450 mg/day

Sustained release: Initial: 150 mg/day in the morning; may increase to 150 mg twice daily by day 4 if tolerated; target dose: 300 mg/day given as 150 mg twice daily; maximum dose: 400 mg/day given as 200 mg twice daily

Smoking cessation: Initiate with 150 mg once daily for 3 days; increase to 150 mg twice daily; treatment should continue for 7-12 weeks

Elderly: Depression: 50-100 mg/day, increase by 50-100 mg every 3-4 days as tolerated; there is evidence that the elderly respond at 150 mg/day in divided doses, but some may require a higher dose

**Dosing adjustment/comments in renal or hepatic impairment:** Patients with renal or hepatic failure should receive a reduced dosage initially and be closely monitored

**Dietary Considerations** Alcohol: Additive CNS effects, avoid use

**Monitoring Parameters** Body weight

**Reference Range** Therapeutic levels (trough, 12 hours after last dose): 50-100 ng/mL

**Test Interactions** Decreased prolactin levels

**Patient Information** Take in equally divided doses 3-4 times/day to minimize the risk of seizures; avoid alcohol; do not take more than recommended dose or more than 150 mg in a single dose; do not discontinue abruptly, may take 3-4 weeks for full effect; may impair driving or other motor or cognitive skills and judgment

**Nursing Implications** Be aware that drug may cause seizures; dose should not be increased by more than 150 mg/day once weekly

**Dosage Forms**

Tablet (Wellbutrin®): 75 mg, 100 mg

Tablet, sustained release (Wellbutrin® SR, Zyban™): 100 mg, 150 mg

♦ **BuSpar®** *see* Buspirone *on page 78*

## Buspirone (byoo SPYE rone)

**Related Information**

Anxiety Disorders *on page 606*
Clinical Issues in the Use of Anxiolytics and Sedative/Hypnotics *on page 634*
Impulse Control Disorders *on page 622*
Nonbenzodiazepine Anxiolytics and Hypnotics *on page 721*
Patient Information - Anxiolytics & Sedative Hypnotics (Buspirone) *on page 655*
Secondary Mental Disorders *on page 616*
Special Populations - Elderly *on page 662*
Special Populations - Mentally Retarded Patients *on page 665*
Teratogenic Risks of Psychotropic Medications *on page 812*

**Generic Available** Yes

**U.S. Brand Names** BuSpar®

**Synonyms** Buspirone Hydrochloride

**Pharmacologic Category** Antianxiety Agent, Miscellaneous

**Use** Management of anxiety disorders (GAD)

**Unlabeled use:** Management of aggression in mental retardation and secondary mental disorders; major depression; potential augmenting agent for antidepressants; premenstrual syndrome

**Pregnancy Risk Factor** B

**Contraindications** Hypersensitivity to buspirone or any component

**Warnings/Precautions** Safety and efficacy not established in children <18 years of age; use in hepatic or renal impairment is not recommended; does not prevent or treat withdrawal from benzodiazepines. Low potential for cognitive or motor impairment. Use with monoamine oxidase inhibitors may result in hypertensive reactions.

**Adverse Reactions**

>10%: Central nervous system: Dizziness

1% to 10%:

Central nervous system: Drowsiness, EPS, serotonin syndrome, confusion, nervousness, lightheadedness, excitement, anger, hostility, headache

Dermatologic: Rash

Gastrointestinal: Diarrhea, nausea

Neuromuscular & skeletal: Muscle weakness, numbness, paresthesia, incoordination, tremor

Ocular: Blurred vision, tunnel vision

Miscellaneous: Diaphoresis, allergic reactions

**Overdosage/Toxicology**

Signs and symptoms: Dizziness, drowsiness, pinpoint pupils, nausea, vomiting

Treatment: There is no known antidote for buspirone and most therapies are supportive and symptomatic in nature

**Drug Interactions** CYP3A3/4 enzyme substrate

Calcium channel blockers: Diltiazem and verapamil may increase serum concentrations of buspirone; consider a dihydropyridine calcium channel blocker

CYP3A3/4 inhibitors: Serum level and/or toxicity of buspirone may be increased; inhibitors include amiodarone, cimetidine, clarithromycin, erythromycin, delavirdine, diltiazem, dirithromycin, disulfiram, fluoxetine, fluvoxamine, grapefruit juice, indinavir, itraconazole, ketoconazole, nefazodone, nevirapine, propoxyfene, quinupristin-dalfopristin, ritonavir, saquinavir, verapamil, zafirlukast, zileuton; monitor for altered effects; a decrease in buspirone dosage may be required

Enzyme inducers: May reduce serum concentrations of buspirone resulting in loss of efficacy; includes barbiturates, carbamazepine, phenytoin, rifabutin and rifampin

MAO inhibitors: Buspirone should not be used concurrently with an MAO inhibitor due to reports of increased blood pressure; includes classic MAO inhibitors and linezolid (due to ability to inhibit MAO)

Selegiline: Theoretically, risk of interaction with selective MAO-B inhibitor would be less than with nonselective inhibitors; however, this combination is generally best avoided

SSRIs: Concurrent use of buspirone with SSRIs may cause serotonin syndrome. Some SSRIs may increase buspirone serum concentrations (see CYP3A3/4 inhibitors). Buspirone may increase the efficacy of fluoxetine in some patients; however, the anxiolytic activity of buspirone may be lost when combined with SSRIs (fluoxetine).

Trazodone: Concurrent use of buspirone with trazodone may cause serotonin syndrome

**Mechanism of Action** The mechanism of action of buspirone is unknown. Buspirone has a high affinity for serotonin 5HT1a and 5HT2 receptors, without affecting benzodiazepine-GABA receptors; buspirone has moderate affinity for dopamine $D_2$ receptors

**Pharmacodynamics/kinetics**

Protein binding: 95%

Metabolism: In the liver by oxidation and undergoes extensive first-pass metabolism

Half-life: 2-3 hours

Time to peak serum concentration: Oral: Within 40-60 minutes

**Usual Dosage** Adults: Oral: 15 mg/day (7.5 mg twice daily); may increase in increments of 5 mg/day every 2-4 days to a maximum of 60 mg/day; target dose for most people is 30 mg/day (15 mg twice daily)

**Dosing adjustment in renal or hepatic impairment:** Buspirone is metabolized by the liver and excreted by the kidneys. Patients with impaired hepatic or renal function demonstrated increased plasma levels and a prolonged half-life of buspirone. Therefore, use in patients with severe hepatic or renal impairment cannot be recommended.

**Dietary Considerations** Give orally with food

**Monitoring Parameters** Mental status, symptoms of anxiety

**Reference Range** Peak plasma levels ≤6 ng/mL noted up to 90 minutes after a 20 mg dose

**Test Interactions** ↑ AST, ALT, growth hormone(s), prolactin (S)

**Patient Information** Take with food; report any change in senses (ie, smelling, hearing, vision); cautious use with alcohol is recommended; cannot be substituted for benzodiazepines unless directed by a physician; takes 2-3 weeks to see the full effect of this medication; if you miss a dose, do **not** double your next dose

**Additional Information** Has shown little potential for abuse; needs continuous use; because of slow onset, not appropriate for "as needed" (prn) use or for brief, situational anxiety; ineffective for benzodiazepine or alcohol withdrawal

**Dosage Forms** Tablet, as hydrochloride: 5 mg, 10 mg, 15 mg Dividose®, 30 mg Dividose®

## Busulfan (byoo SUL fan)

**U.S. Brand Names** Myleran®

**Pharmacologic Category** Antineoplastic Agent, Alkylating Agent

**Use**

Oral: Chronic myelogenous leukemia and bone marrow disorders, such as polycythemia vera and myeloid metaplasia, conditioning regimens for bone marrow transplantation

I.V.: Combination therapy with cyclophosphamide as a conditioning regimen prior to allogeneic hematopoietic progenitor cell transplantation for chronic myelogenous leukemia

**Effects on Mental Status** None reported

**Effects on Psychiatric Treatment** May cause severe pancytopenia; use caution with clozapine and carbamazepine

**Usual Dosage** Busulfan should be based on adjusted ideal body weight because actual body weight, ideal body weight, or other factors can produce significant differences in busulfan clearance among lean, normal, and obese patients

Oral (refer to individual protocols):

Children:

For remission induction of CML: 0.06-0.12 mg/kg/day **OR** 1.8-4.6 mg/$m^2$/day; titrate dosage to maintain leukocyte count above 40,000/$mm^3$; reduce dosage by 50% if the leukocyte count reaches 30,000-40,000/$mm^3$; discontinue drug if counts fall to ≤20,000/$mm^3$

BMT marrow-ablative conditioning regimen: 1 mg/kg/dose (ideal body weight) every 6 hours for 16 doses

Adults:

BMT marrow-ablative conditioning regimen: 1 mg/kg/dose (ideal body weight) every 6 hours for 16 doses

Remission: Induction of CML: 4-8 mg/day (may be as high as 12 mg/day); Maintenance doses: Controversial, range from 1-4 mg/day to 2 mg/week; treatment is continued until WBC reaches 10,000-20,000 cells/$mm^3$ at which time drug is discontinued; when WBC reaches 50,000/$mm^3$, maintenance dose is resumed

**Unapproved uses:**

Polycythemia vera: 2-6 mg/day

Thrombocytosis: 4-6 mg/day

I.V.: 0.8 mg/kg (ideal body weight or actual body weight, whichever is lower) every 6 hours for 4 days (a total of 16 doses)

I.V. dosing in morbidly obese patients: Dosing should be based on adjusted ideal body weight (AIBW) which should be calculated as ideal body weight (IBW) + 0.25 times (actual weight minus ideal body weight)

AIBW = IBW + 0.25 x (AW - IBW)

Cyclophosphamide, in combination with busulfan, is given on each of two days as a 1-hour infusion at a dose of 160 mg/$m^2$ beginning on day 3, 6 hours following the 16th dose of busulfan

**Dosage Forms**

Injection: 60 mg/10 mL ampuls

Tablet: 2 mg

## Butabarbital Sodium (byoo ta BAR bi tal SOW dee um)

**Related Information**

Anxiolytic/Hypnotic Use in Long-Term Care Facilities *on page 754*

Federal OBRA Regulations Recommended Maximum Doses *on page 756*

Patient Information - Anxiolytics & Sedative Hypnotics (Barbiturates) *on page 654*

**Generic Available** Yes

**U.S. Brand Names** Butalan®; Buticaps®; Butisol Sodium®

**Pharmacologic Category** Barbiturate

**Use** Sedative; hypnotic

**Effects on Mental Status** Drowsiness is common

**Effects on Psychiatric Treatment** Rare reports of agranulocytosis; use caution with clozapine and carbamazepine; enzyme induction effects of barbiturates may decrease effects of psychotropics; CNS depressant effects of psychotropics may be enhanced by barbiturates

**Restrictions** C-III

**Pregnancy Risk Factor** D

**Contraindications** Hypersensitivity to barbiturates or any component of the formulation; porphyria

**Warnings/Precautions** Potential for drug dependency exists; abrupt cessation may precipitate withdrawal, including status epilepticus in epileptic patients. Do not administer to patients in acute pain. Use caution in elderly, debilitated, renally impaired, hepatic impairment, or pediatric patients. May cause paradoxical responses, including agitation and hyperactivity, particularly in acute pain and pediatric patients. Use with caution in patients with depression or suicidal tendencies, or in patients with a history of drug abuse. Tolerance, psychological and physical dependence may occur with prolonged use. May cause CNS depression, which may impair physical or mental abilities. Patients must be cautioned about performing tasks which require mental alertness (ie, operating machinery or driving). Effects with other sedative drugs or ethanol may be potentiated. May cause respiratory depression or hypotension. Use with caution in hemodynamically unstable patients or patients with respiratory disease.

**Adverse Reactions**

>10%: Central nervous system: Dizziness, lightheadedness, drowsiness, "hangover" effect

1% to 10%:

Central nervous system: Confusion, mental depression, unusual excitement, nervousness, faint feeling, headache, insomnia, nightmares

Gastrointestinal: Constipation, nausea, vomiting

<1%: Agranulocytosis, angioedema, dependence, exfoliative dermatitis, hallucinations, hypotension, megaloblastic anemia, rash, respiratory depression, Stevens-Johnson syndrome, thrombocytopenia, thrombophlebitis

**Overdosage/Toxicology**

Signs and symptoms: Slurred speech, confusion, nystagmus, tachycardia, hypotension

Treatment: If hypotension occurs, administer I.V. fluids and place the patient in the Trendelenburg position; if unresponsive, an I.V. vasopressor (eg, dopamine, epinephrine) may be required. Forced alkaline diuresis is of no value in the treatment of intoxications with short-acting barbiturates. Charcoal hemoperfusion or hemodialysis may be useful in the harder to treat intoxications, especially in the presence of very high serum barbiturate levels.

**Drug Interactions Note:** Barbiturates are cytochrome P-450 enzyme inducers. Patients should be monitored when these drugs are started or stopped for a decreased or increased therapeutic effect respectively.

Acetaminophen: Barbiturates may enhance the hepatotoxic potential of acetaminophen overdoses

Antiarrhythmics: Barbiturates may increase the metabolism of antiarrhythmics, decreasing their clinical effect; includes disopyramide, propafenone, and quinidine

Anticonvulsants: Barbiturates may increase the metabolism of anticonvulsants; includes ethosuximide, felbamate (possibly), lamotrigine, phenytoin, tiagabine, topiramate, and zonisamide; does not appear to affect gabapentin, or levetiracetam

Antineoplastics: Limited evidence suggests that enzyme-inducing anticonvulsant therapy may reduce the effectiveness of some chemotherapy regimens (specifically in ALL); teniposide and methotrexate may be cleared more rapidly in these patients

Antipsychotics: Barbiturates may enhance the metabolism (decrease the efficacy) of antipsychotics; monitor for altered response; dose adjustment may be needed

Beta-blockers: Metabolism of beta-blockers may be increased and clinical effect decreased; atenolol and nadolol are unlikely to interact given their renal elimination

Calcium channel blockers: Barbiturates may enhance the metabolism of calcium channel blockers, decreasing their clinical effect

Chloramphenicol: Barbiturates may increase the metabolism of chloramphenicol and chloramphenicol may inhibit barbiturate metabolism; monitor for altered response

Cimetidine: Barbiturates may enhance the metabolism of cimetidine, decreasing its clinical effect

CNS depressants: Sedative effects and/or respiratory depression with barbiturates may be additive with other CNS depressants; monitor for increased effect; includes ethanol, sedatives, antidepressants, narcotic analgesics, and benzodiazepines

Corticosteroids: Barbiturates may enhance the metabolism of corticosteroids, decreasing their clinical effect

Cyclosporine: Levels may be decreased by barbiturates; monitor

Immunosuppressants: Barbiturates may enhance the metabolism of immunosuppressants, decreasing its clinical effect; includes both cyclosporine and tacrolimus

Doxycycline: Barbiturates may enhance the metabolism of doxycycline, decreasing its clinical effect; higher dosages may be required

Estrogens: Barbiturates may increase the metabolism of estrogens and reduce their efficacy

Felbamate may inhibit the metabolism of barbiturates and barbiturates may increase the metabolism of felbamate

Griseofulvin: Barbiturates may impair the absorption of griseofulvin, and griseofulvin metabolism may be increased by barbiturates, decreasing clinical effect

Guanfacine: Effect may be decreased by barbiturates

Loop diuretics: Metabolism may be increased and clinical effects decreased; established for furosemide, effect with other loop diuretics not established

MAOIs: Metabolism of barbiturates may be inhibited, increasing clinical effect or toxicity of the barbiturates

Methadone: Barbiturates may enhance the metabolism of methadone resulting in methadone withdrawal

Methoxyflurane: Barbiturates may enhance the nephrotoxic effects of methoxyflurane

Oral contraceptives: Barbiturates may enhance the metabolism of oral contraceptives, decreasing their clinical effect; an alternative method of contraception should be considered

Theophylline: Barbiturates may increase metabolism of theophylline derivatives and decrease their clinical effect

Tricyclic antidepressants: Barbiturates may increase metabolism of tricyclic antidepressants and decrease their clinical effect; sedative effects may be additive

Valproic acid: Metabolism of barbiturates may be inhibited by valproic acid; monitor for excessive sedation; a dose reduction may be needed

(Continued)

## Butabarbital Sodium *(Continued)*

Warfarin: Barbiturates inhibit the hypoprothrombinemic effects of oral anticoagulants via increased metabolism; this combination should generally be avoided

**Mechanism of Action** Interferes with transmission of impulses from the thalamus to the cortex of the brain resulting in an imbalance in central inhibitory and facilitatory mechanisms

**Pharmacodynamics/kinetics**

Distribution: $V_d$: 0.8 L/kg

Protein binding: 26%

Metabolism: In the liver

Half-life: 40-140 hours

Time to peak serum concentration: Oral: Within 40-60 minutes

Elimination: In urine as metabolites

**Usual Dosage** Oral:

Children: Preop: 2-6 mg/kg/dose; maximum: 100 mg

Adults:

Sedative: 15-30 mg 3-4 times/day

Hypnotic: 50-100 mg

Preop: 50-100 mg 1-1$^1/_2$ hours before surgery

**Dietary Considerations** Alcohol: Additive CNS effects, avoid use

**Reference Range** Therapeutic: Not established; Toxic: 28-73 µg/mL

**Test Interactions** ↑ ammonia (B); ↓ bilirubin (S)

**Patient Information** May cause drowsiness, avoid alcohol or other CNS depressants, may impair judgment and coordination; may cause physical and psychological dependence with prolonged use; do not exceed recommended dose

**Nursing Implications** Raise bed rails; initiate safety measures; aid with ambulation; monitor for CNS depression

**Dosage Forms**

Capsule: 15 mg, 30 mg

Elixir, with alcohol 7%: 30 mg/5 mL (480 mL, 3780 mL); 33.3 mg/5 mL (480 mL, 3780 mL)

Tablet: 15 mg, 30 mg, 50 mg, 100 mg

♦ **Butalan®** *see* Butabarbital Sodium *on page 79*

## Butalbital Compound and Acetaminophen

(byoo TAL bi tal KOM pound & a seet a MIN oh fen)

**U.S. Brand Names** Amaphen®; Anoquan®; Axocet®; Bupap®; Endolor®; Esgic®; Esgic-Plus®; Femcet®; Fioricet®; G-1®; Medigesic®; Phrenilin®; Phrenilin® Forte; Repan®; Sedapap-10®; Triapin®; Two-Dyne®

**Synonyms** Acetaminophen and Butalbital Compound

**Pharmacologic Category** Barbiturate

**Use** Relief of the symptomatic complex of tension or muscle contraction headache

**Effects on Mental Status** Drowsiness is common; may cause depression, nervousness, insomnia, and nightmares; rare reports of hallucinations

**Effects on Psychiatric Treatment** Rare reports of agranulocytosis; use caution with clozapine and carbamazepine; CNS depressant effects of psychotropics may be enhance by barbiturates; enzyme induction effects of barbiturates may decrease effects of psychotropics

**Restrictions** C-III

**Contraindications** Porphyria; hypersensitivity to butalbital or any component

**Warnings/Precautions** Administer with caution, if at all, to patients who are mentally depressed, have suicidal tendencies, or a history of drug abuse. May be habit-forming.

**Adverse Reactions**

>10%:

Central nervous system: Dizziness, lightheadedness, drowsiness, "hangover" effect

Gastrointestinal: Nausea, heartburn, stomach pains, dyspepsia, epigastric discomfort

1% to 10%:

Central nervous system: Confusion, mental depression, unusual excitement, nervousness, faint feeling, headache, insomnia, nightmares, fatigue

Dermatologic: Skin rash

Gastrointestinal: Constipation, vomiting, gastrointestinal ulceration

Hematologic: Hemolytic anemia

Neuromuscular & skeletal: Weakness

Respiratory: Troubled breathing

Miscellaneous: Anaphylactic shock

**Overdosage/Toxicology**

Signs and symptoms: Slurred speech, confusion, nystagmus, tachycardia, hypotension, tinnitus, headache, dizziness, confusion, metabolic acidosis, hyperpyrexia, hypoglycemia, coma, hepatic necrosis, blood dyscrasias, respiratory depression

Treatment: Forced alkaline diuresis is of no value in the treatment of intoxications with short-acting barbiturates; charcoal hemoperfusion or hemodialysis may be useful in the harder to treat intoxications, especially in the presence of very high serum barbiturate levels

**Drug Interactions** Barbiturates are enzyme inducers; patients should be monitored when these drugs are started or stopped for a decreased or increased therapeutic effect respectively

Antineoplastics: Limited evidence suggests that enzyme-inducing anticonvulsant therapy may reduce the effectiveness of some chemotherapy regimens (specifically in ALL); teniposide and methotrexate may be cleared more rapidly in these patients

Decreased effect: Butalbital compound may reduce the efficacy of beta-blockers, chloramphenicol, cimetidine, clozapine, corticosteroids, cyclosporine, disopyramide, doxycycline, ethosuximide, furosemide, griseofulvin, haloperidol, lamotrigine, methadone, nifedipine, oral contraceptives, phenothiazine, phenytoin, propafenone, quinidine, tacrolimus, TCAs, theophylline, **warfarin** , and verapamil

Increased toxicity when combined with other CNS depressants, benzodiazepine, valproic acid, chloramphenicol, or antidepressants; respiratory and CNS depression may be additive. MAOIs may prolong the effect of butalbital compound; barbiturates inhibit the hypoprothombinemic response to warfarin.

**Usual Dosage** Adults: Oral: 1-2 tablets or capsules every 4 hours; not to exceed 6/day

**Dosing interval in renal or hepatic impairment:** Should be reduced

**Patient Information** If self-administered, use exactly as directed (do not increase dose or frequency); may cause physical and/or psychological dependence. Take with food or milk. While using this medication, do not use alcohol and other prescription or OTC medications (especially sedatives, tranquilizers, antihistamines, or pain medications) without consulting prescriber. Maintain adequate hydration (2-3 L/day of fluids unless instructed to restrict fluid intake). May cause dizziness, lightheadedness, confusion, or drowsiness (use caution when driving, climbing stairs, or changing position - rising from sitting or lying to standing, or when engaging in tasks requiring alertness until response to drug is known); heartburn or epigastric discomfort (frequent mouth care, frequent sips of fluids, chewing gum, or sucking lozenges may help); constipation (increased exercise, fluids, or dietary fruit and fiber may help). Report chest pain or palpitations; persistent dizziness; confusion, nightmares, excitation, or changes in mentation; shortness of breath or difficulty breathing; skin rash; unusual bleeding or bruising; or unusual fatigue and weakness.

**Dosage Forms**

Capsule:

Amaphen®, Anoquan®, Butace®, Endolor®, Esgic®, Femcet®, G-1®, Medigesic®, Repan®, Two-Dyne®: Butalbital 50 mg, caffeine 40 mg, and acetaminophen 325 mg

Axocet®, Phrenilin Forte®: Butalbital 50 mg and acetaminophen 650 mg

Bancap®, Triapin®: Butalbital 50 mg and acetaminophen 325 mg

Tablet:

Bupap®: Butalbital 50 mg and acetaminophen 650 mg

Esgic®, Fioricet®, Repan®: Butalbital 50 mg, caffeine 40 mg, and acetaminophen 325 mg

Phrenilin®: Butalbital 50 mg and acetaminophen 325 mg

Sedapap-10®: Butalbital 50 mg and acetaminophen 650 mg

## Butalbital Compound and Aspirin

(byoo TAL bi tal KOM pound & AS pir in)

**U.S. Brand Names** Fiorgen PF®; Fiorinal®; Isollyl® Improved; Lanorinal®

**Canadian Brand Names** Tecnal

**Synonyms** Aspirin and Butalbital Compound

**Pharmacologic Category** Barbiturate

**Use** Relief of the symptomatic complex of tension or muscle contraction headache

**Effects on Mental Status** Drowsiness is common; may cause depression, nervousness, insomnia, and nightmares; rare reports of hallucinations

**Effects on Psychiatric Treatment** Rare reports of agranulocytosis; use caution with clozapine and carbamazepine; CNS depressant effects of psychotropics may be enhance by barbiturates; enzyme induction effects of barbiturates may decrease effects of psychotropics

**Restrictions** C-III

**Contraindications** Porphyria; hypersensitivity to butalbital or any component

**Warnings/Precautions** Use with extreme caution in the presence of peptic ulcer or coagulation abnormality - can produce psychological/physical drug dependence. Children and teenagers should not use this product.

**Adverse Reactions**

>10%:

Central nervous system: Dizziness, lightheadedness, drowsiness, "hangover" effect

Gastrointestinal: Heartburn, stomach pains, dyspepsia, epigastric discomfort, nausea

1% to 10%:
Central nervous system: Confusion, mental depression, unusual excitement, nervousness, faint feeling, headache, insomnia, nightmares, fatigue
Dermatologic: Skin rash
Gastrointestinal: Constipation, vomiting, gastrointestinal ulceration
Hematologic: Hemolytic anemia
Neuromuscular & skeletal: Weakness
Respiratory: Troubled breathing
Miscellaneous: Anaphylactic shock

**Overdosage/Toxicology**
Signs and symptoms: Slurred speech, confusion, nystagmus, tachycardia, hypotension, tinnitus, headache, dizziness, confusion, metabolic acidosis, hyperpyrexia, hypoglycemia, coma, hepatic necrosis, blood dyscrasias, respiratory depression
Treatment: Forced alkaline diuresis is of no value in the treatment of intoxications with short-acting barbiturates; charcoal hemoperfusion or hemodialysis may be useful in the harder to treat intoxications, especially in the presence of very high serum barbiturate levels

**Drug Interactions** Barbiturates are enzyme inducers; patients should be monitored when these drugs are started or stopped for a decreased or increased therapeutic effect respectively
Antineoplastics: Limited evidence suggests that enzyme-inducing anticonvulsant therapy may reduce the effectiveness of some chemotherapy regimens (specifically in ALL); teniposide and methotrexate may be cleared more rapidly in these patients
Decreased effect: Butalbital compound may reduce the efficacy of beta-blockers, chloramphenicol, cimetidine, clozapine, corticosteroids, cyclosporine, disopyramide, doxycycline, ethosuximide, furosemide, griseofulvin, haloperidol, lamotrigine, methadone, nifedipine, oral contraceptives, phenothiazine, phenytoin, propafenone, quinidine, tacrolimus, TCAs, theophylline, **warfarin** , and verapamil
Increased toxicity when combined with other CNS depressants, benzodiazepine, valproic acid, chloramphenicol, or antidepressants; respiratory and CNS depression may be additive. MAOIs may prolong the effect of butalbital compound; barbiturates inhibit the hypoprothombinemic response to warfarin.

**Usual Dosage** Adults: Oral: 1-2 tablets or capsules every 4 hours; not to exceed 6/day
**Dosing interval in renal or hepatic impairment:** Should be reduced

**Patient Information** Take as directed; do not exceed prescribed amount. Avoid alcohol, aspirin or aspirin-containing medications, or any OTC medications unless approved by prescriber. Maintain adequate hydration (2-3 L/day of fluids unless instructed to restrict fluid intake) to prevent constipation. You may experience drowsiness, impaired judgment or coordination; use caution when driving or engaging in tasks that require alertness until response to drug is known. Small frequent meals may help reduce GI upset. Report any ringing in ears; abdominal pain; easy bruising or bleeding; blood in urine; severe weakness; acute unresolved dizziness or confusion, nervousness, nightmares, insomnia; or skin rash.

**Dosage Forms**
Capsule: (Fiorgen PF®, Fiorinal®, Isollyl® Improved, Lanorinal®, Marnal®): Butalbital 50 mg, caffeine 40 mg, and aspirin 325 mg
Tablet:
Axotal®: Butalbital 50 mg and aspirin 650 mg
B-A-C®: Butalbital 50 mg, caffeine 40 mg, and aspirin 650 mg
Fiorinal®, Isollyl® Improved, Lanorinal®, Marnal®: Butalbital 50 mg, caffeine 40 mg, and aspirin 325 mg

## Butalbital Compound and Codeine
(byoo TAL bi tal KOM pound & KOE deen)

**U.S. Brand Names** Fiorinal® With Codeine
**Canadian Brand Names** Fiorinal®-C 1/4, 1/2; Tecnal C1/4, C1/2
**Pharmacologic Category** Analgesic, Narcotic; Barbiturate
**Use** Mild to moderate pain when sedation is needed
**Effects on Mental Status** Drowsiness is common; may cause depression, nervousness, insomnia, and nightmares; rare reports of hallucinations
**Effects on Psychiatric Treatment** Rare reports of agranulocytosis; use caution with clozapine and carbamazepine; CNS depressant effects of psychotropics may be enhance by barbiturates; enzyme induction effects of barbiturates may decrease effects of psychotropics
**Restrictions** C-III
**Usual Dosage** Adults: Oral: 1-2 capsules every 4 hours as needed for pain; up to 6/day
**Dosage Forms** Capsule: Butalbital 50 mg, caffeine 40 mg, aspirin 325 mg and codeine phosphate 30 mg

♦ **Butazolidin®** *see* Phenylbutazone *on page 439*

## Butenafine (byoo TEN a fine)

**U.S. Brand Names** Mentax®
**Pharmacologic Category** Antifungal Agent, Topical
**Use** Topical treatment of tinea pedis (athlete's foot) and tinea cruris (jock itch)
**Effects on Mental Status** None reported
**Effects on Psychiatric Treatment** None reported
**Usual Dosage** Children >12 years and Adults: Topical: Apply once daily for 4 weeks to the affected area and surrounding skin
**Dosage Forms** Cream, as hydrochloride: 1% (2 g, 15 g, 30 g)

♦ **Buticaps®** *see* Butabarbital Sodium *on page 79*

♦ **Butisol Sodium®** *see* Butabarbital Sodium *on page 79*

## Butoconazole (byoo toe KOE na zole)

**U.S. Brand Names** Femstat®
**Pharmacologic Category** Antifungal Agent, Vaginal
**Use** Local treatment of vulvovaginal candidiasis
**Effects on Mental Status** None reported
**Effects on Psychiatric Treatment** None reported
**Usual Dosage** Adults:
Nonpregnant: Insert 1 applicatorful (~5 g) intravaginally at bedtime as a single dose; therapy may extend for up to 6 days, if necessary, as directed by physician
Pregnant: **Use only during 2nd or 3rd trimester**
**Dosage Forms** Cream, vaginal, as nitrate: 2% with applicator (28 g)

## Butorphanol (byoo TOR fa nole)

**Related Information**
Narcotic Agonists Comparison Chart *on page 720*
**U.S. Brand Names** Stadol®; Stadol® NS
**Pharmacologic Category** Analgesic, Narcotic
**Use** Management of moderate to severe pain
**Effects on Mental Status** Drowsiness is common; may rarely produce CNS stimulation or depression, hallucinations, and confusion
**Effects on Psychiatric Treatment** Contraindicated in opiate dependent patients; may precipitate opiate withdrawal; concurrent use with psychotropic may produce additive sedation
**Restrictions** C-IV
**Pregnancy Risk Factor** B (D if used for prolonged periods or in high doses at term)
**Contraindications** Hypersensitivity to butorphanol or any component; avoid use in opiate-dependent patients who have not been detoxified, may precipitate opiate withdrawal
**Warnings/Precautions** Use with caution in patients with hepatic/renal dysfunction, may elevate CSF pressure, may increase cardiac workload; tolerance of drug dependence may result from extended use
**Adverse Reactions**
>10%: Central nervous system: Drowsiness
1% to 10%:
Cardiovascular: Flushing of the face, hypotension
Central nervous system: Dizziness, lightheadedness, headache
Gastrointestinal: Anorexia, nausea, vomiting
Genitourinary: Decreased urination
Miscellaneous: Diaphoresis (increased)
<1%: Blurred vision, bradycardia or tachycardia, CNS depression, confusion, constipation, dependence with prolonged use, dyspnea, false sense of well being, hallucinations, hypertension, malaise, mental depression, nightmares, painful urination, paradoxical CNS stimulation, rash, respiratory depression, restlessness, shortness of breath, stomach cramps, tinnitus, weakness, xerostomia
**Overdosage/Toxicology**
Signs and symptoms: Respiratory depression, cardiac and CNS depression
Treatment: Includes support of the patient's airway, establishment of an I.V. line and administration of naloxone 2 mg I.V. (0.01 mg/kg for children) with repeat administration as necessary up to a total of 10 mg
**Drug Interactions** Increased toxicity: CNS depressants, phenothiazines, barbiturates, skeletal muscle relaxants, alfentanil, guanabenz, MAO inhibitors
**Usual Dosage** Adults:
I.M.: 1-4 mg every 3-4 hours as needed
I.V.: 0.5-2 mg every 3-4 hours as needed
Nasal spray: Headache: 1 spray in 1 nostril; if adequate pain relief is not achieved within 60-90 minutes, an additional 1 spray in 1 nostril may be given (each spray gives ~1 mg of butorphanol); may repeat in 3-4 hours after the last dose as needed
**Dosing adjustment in renal impairment:**
$Cl_{cr}$ 10-50 mL/minute: Administer 75% of dose
$Cl_{cr}$ <10 mL/minute: Administer 50% of dose
**Dietary Considerations** Alcohol: Additive CNS effects, avoid or limit use; watch for sedation
**Patient Information** If self-administered, use exactly as directed (do not increase dose or frequency); may cause physical and/or psychological dependence. While using this medication, do not use alcohol and other
(Continued)

## Butorphanol *(Continued)*

prescription or OTC medications (especially sedatives, tranquilizers, antihistamines, or pain medications) without consulting prescriber. May cause dizziness, drowsiness, confusion, or blurred vision (use caution when driving, climbing stairs, or changing position - rising from sitting or lying to standing, or when engaging in tasks requiring alertness until response to drug is known); nausea or vomiting, or loss of appetite (frequent mouth care, small frequent meals, sucking lozenges, or chewing gum may help). Report unresolved nausea or vomiting; difficulty breathing or shortness of breath; restlessness, insomnia, euphoria, or nightmares; excessive sedation or unusual weakness; facial flushing, rapid heartbeat, or palpitations; urinary difficulty; or vision changes.

**Nursing Implications** Observe for excessive sedation or confusion, respiratory depression; raise bed rails; aid with ambulation

**Dosage Forms**

Injection, as tartrate: 1 mg/mL (1 mL); 2 mg/mL (1 mL, 2 mL, 10 mL)

Spray, nasal, as tartrate: 10 mg/mL [14-15 doses] (2.5 mL)

- **BW-430C** *see* Lamotrigine *on page 306*
- **Byclomine® Injection** *see* Dicyclomine *on page 165*
- **Bydramine® Cough Syrup [OTC]** *see* Diphenhydramine *on page 174*
- **C7E3** *see* Abciximab *on page 12*
- **C8-CCK** *see* Sincalide *on page 513*
- **311C90** *see* Zolmitriptan *on page 593*

## Cabergoline (ca BER go leen)

**U.S. Brand Names** Dostinex®

**Pharmacologic Category** Ergot Derivative

**Use** Treatment of hyperprolactinemic disorders, either idiopathic or due to pituitary adenomas

**Unlabeled use:** Adjunct for the treatment of Parkinson's disease

**Effects on Mental Status** Dizziness is common; may cause depression

**Effects on Psychiatric Treatment** Antipsychotics may decrease the therapeutic effects of cabergoline; avoid combination

**Pregnancy Risk Factor** B

**Contraindications** Patients with uncontrolled hypertension or hypersensitivity to ergot derivatives

**Warnings/Precautions** Initial doses >1 mg may cause orthostatic hypotension. Use caution when patients are receiving other medications which may reduce blood pressure. Not indicated for the inhibition or suppression of physiologic lactation since it has been associated with cases of hypertension, stroke, and seizures. Because cabergoline is extensively metabolized by the liver, careful monitoring in patients with hepatic impairment is warranted. Female patients should instruct the physician if they are pregnant, become pregnant, or intend to become pregnant. Should not be used in patients with pregnancy-induced hypertension unless benefit outweighs potential risk. Do not give to postpartum women who are breast-feeding or planning to breast-feed. In all patients, prolactin concentrations should be monitored monthly until normalized.

**Adverse Reactions**

>10%:

Central nervous system: Headache (26%), dizziness (17%)

Gastrointestinal: Nausea (29%)

1% to 10%:

Body as whole: Asthenia (6%), fatigue (5%), syncope (1%), influenza-like symptoms (1%), malaise (1%), periorbital edema (1%), peripheral edema (1%)

Cardiovascular: Hot flashes (3%), hypotension (1%), dependent edema (1%), palpitations (1%)

Central nervous system: Vertigo (4%), depression (3%), somnolence (2%), anxiety (1%), insomnia (1%), impaired concentration (1%), nervousness (1%)

Dermatologic: Acne (1%), pruritus (1%)

Endocrine: Breast pain (2%), dysmenorrhea (1%)

Gastrointestinal: Constipation (7%), abdominal pain (5%), dyspepsia (5%), vomiting (4%), xerostomia (2%), diarrhea (2%), flatulence (2%), throat irritation (1%), toothache (1%), anorexia (1%)

Neuromuscular & skeletal: Pain (2%), arthralgia (1%), paresthesias (2%)

Ocular: Abnormal vision (1%)

Respiratory: Rhinitis (1%)

**Overdosage/Toxicology**

Signs and symptoms; An overdose may produce nasal congestion, syncope, hallucinations, or hypotension

Treatment: Measures to support blood pressure should be taken if necessary

**Drug Interactions**

Additive hypotensive effects may occur when cabergoline is administered with antihypertensive medications; dosage adjustment of the antihypertensive medication may be required

Decreased effect: Dopamine antagonists (eg, phenothiazines, butyrophenones, thioxanthenes, or metoclopramide) may reduce the therapeutic effects of cabergoline and should not be used concomitantly

**Usual Dosage** Initial dose: Oral: 0.25 mg twice weekly; the dose may be increased by 0.25 mg twice weekly up to a maximum of 1 mg twice weekly according to the patient's serum prolactin level. Dosage increases should not occur more rapidly than every 4 weeks. Once a normal serum prolactin level is maintained for 6 months, the dose may be discontinued and prolactin levels monitored to determine if cabergoline is still required. The durability of efficacy beyond 24 months of therapy has not been established.

Elderly: No dosage recommendations suggested, but start at the low end of the dosage range

**Patient Information** Patient should be instructed to notify physician if she suspects she is pregnant, becomes pregnant, or intends to become pregnant during therapy with cabergoline. A pregnancy test should be done if there is any suspicion of pregnancy and continuation of treatment should be discussed with physician.

**Dosage Forms** Tablet: 0.5 mg

- **Cafatine®** *see* Ergotamine *on page 200*
- **Cafatine-PB®** *see* Ergotamine *on page 200*
- **Cafergot®** *see* Ergotamine *on page 200*
- **Cafetrate®** *see* Ergotamine *on page 200*

## Caffeine, Citrated (KAF een, SIT rated)

**Pharmacologic Category** Respiratory Stimulant; Stimulant

**Use** Central nervous system stimulant; used in the treatment of apnea of prematurity (28 to <33 weeks gestational age). Has several advantages over theophylline in the treatment of neonatal apnea, its half-life is about 3 times as long, allowing once daily dosing, drug levels do not need to be drawn at peak and trough; has a wider therapeutic window, allowing more room between an effective concentration and toxicity.

**Effects on Mental Status** May cause anxiety, restlessness, agitation, and insomnia

**Effects on Psychiatric Treatment** None reported

**Pregnancy Risk Factor** B

**Contraindications** Hypersensitivity to caffeine or any component

**Warnings/Precautions** Do not interchange the caffeine citrate salt formulation with the caffeine sodium benzoate formulation; the sodium benzoate salt has been reported to produce kernicterus (by displacement of bilirubin) and neonatal "gasping syndrome"; its use (sodium benzoate) should be avoided in neonates; during a Cafcit® double-blind, placebo-controlled study, 6 of 85 patients developed necrotizing enterocolitis (NEC); 5 of these 6 patients had received caffeine citrate; although no causal relationship has been established, neonates who receive caffeine citrate should be closely monitored for the development of NEC.

**Adverse Reactions** >10%:

Cardiovascular: Cardiac arrhythmias, tachycardia, extrasystoles

Central nervous system: Insomnia, restlessness, agitation, irritability,

Gastrointestinal: Nausea, vomiting, gastric irritation

**Overdosage/Toxicology** Signs and symptoms: GI pain, mild delirium, insomnia, diuresis, dehydration, fever, cardiac arrhythmias, tonic-clonic seizures

**Drug Interactions** CYP1A2, 2E1, and 3A3/4 enzyme substrate

Caffeine may antagonize the cardiovascular effects of adenosine

Increased effects/levels of caffeine: Cimetidine, oral contraceptives, disulfiram, phenylpropanolamine, quinolones

Increased effects/levels of theophylline, beta-agonists (increased positive inotropic and chronotropic effects)

**Usual Dosage** Apnea of prematurity: Neonates:

Loading dose (usually administered I.V.): 10-20 mg/kg as caffeine citrate (5-10 mg/kg as caffeine base). If theophylline has been administered to the patient within the previous 3 days, a full or modified loading dose (50% to 75% of a loading dose) may be given (caffeine is a significant metabolite of theophylline in the newborn).

Maintenance dose: Oral, I.V.: 5 mg/kg/day as caffeine citrate (2.5 mg/kg/day as caffeine base) once daily starting 24 hours after the loading dose. Maintenance dose is adjusted based on patient's response (efficacy and adverse effects), and serum caffeine concentrations.

**Dosage Forms**

Solution, oral: 20 mg/mL [anhydrous caffeine 10 mg/mL]

Tablet: 65 mg [anhydrous caffeine 32.5 mg]

- **Calan®** *see* Verapamil *on page 583*
- **Calan® SR** *see* Verapamil *on page 583*
- **Cal Carb-HD® [OTC]** *see* Calcium Carbonate *on page 84*
- **Calci-Chew™ [OTC]** *see* Calcium Carbonate *on page 84*
- **Calciday-667® [OTC]** *see* Calcium Carbonate *on page 84*

## Calcifediol (kal si fe DYE ole)

**U.S. Brand Names** Calderol®
**Synonyms** 25-HCC; 25-Hydroxycholecalciferol; 25-Hydroxyvitamin $D_3$
**Pharmacologic Category** Vitamin D Analog
**Use** Treatment and management of metabolic bone disease associated with chronic renal failure or hypocalcemia in patients on chronic renal dialysis
**Effects on Mental Status** May cause sedation or irritability
**Effects on Psychiatric Treatment** None reported
**Pregnancy Risk Factor** C (per manufacturer); A/D (if dosage exceeds RDA)(based on expert analysis)
**Contraindications** Hypercalcemia; known hypersensitivity to calcifediol; malabsorption syndrome; hypervitaminosis D; significantly decreased renal function
**Warnings/Precautions** Adequate (supplemental) dietary calcium is necessary for clinical response to vitamin D; calcium-phosphate product (serum calcium times phosphorus) must not exceed 70; avoid hypercalcemia
**Adverse Reactions** Percentage unknown: Anorexia, bone pain, cardiac arrhythmias, conjunctivitis, constipation, elevated LFTs, headache, hypercalcemia, hypermagnesemia, hypertension, hypotension, irritability, metallic taste, myalgia, nausea, pancreatitis, photophobia, polydipsia, polyuria, pruritus, seizures (rare), somnolence, vomiting, xerostomia
**Overdosage/Toxicology**
Signs and symptoms: Rarely toxicity occurs from acute overdose; symptoms of chronic overdose include hypercalcemia, hypercalciuria with weakness, altered mental status, GI upset, renal tubular injury, and occasionally cardiac arrhythmias
Treatment: Following withdrawal of the drug, treatment consists of bed rest, liberal intake of fluids, reduced calcium intake, and cathartic administration. Severe hypercalcemia requires I.V. hydration and forced diuresis. I.V. saline may increase excretion of calcium. Calcitonin, cholestyramine, prednisone, sodium EDTA, biphosphonates, and mithramycin have all been used successfully to treat the more resistant cases of vitamin D-induced hypercalcemia.
**Drug Interactions**
Decreased effect: Cholestyramine, colestipol
Increased effect: Thiazide diuretics
Additive effect: Antacids (magnesium)
**Usual Dosage** Oral: Hepatic osteodystrophy:
Infants: 5-7 mcg/kg/day
Children and Adults: Usual dose: 20-100 mcg/day or 20-200 mcg every other day; titrate to obtain normal serum calcium/phosphate levels; increase dose at 4-week intervals; initial dose: 300-350 mcg/week, administered daily or on alternate days
**Patient Information** Take exact dose as prescribed; do not increase dose. Maintain recommended diet and calcium supplementation. Avoid taking magnesium-containing antacids. You may experience nausea, vomiting, or metallic taste (frequent small meals, frequent mouth care, chewing gum, or sucking lozenges may help) or hypotension (use caution when rising from sitting or lying position or when climbing stairs or bending over). Report chest pain or palpitations, acute headache, skin rash, change in vision or eye irritation, CNS changes, weakness or lethargy.
**Dosage Forms** Capsule: 20 mcg, 50 mcg

♦ **Calciferol™ Injection** *see* Ergocalciferol *on page 198*

♦ **Calciferol™ Oral** *see* Ergocalciferol *on page 198*

♦ **Calcijex™** *see* Calcitriol *on page 83*

♦ **Calcimar® Injection** *see* Calcitonin *on page 83*

♦ **Calci-Mix™ [OTC]** *see* Calcium Carbonate *on page 84*

## Calcipotriene (kal si POE try een)

**U.S. Brand Names** Dovonex®
**Pharmacologic Category** Topical Skin Product; Vitamin, Fat Soluble
**Use** Treatment of moderate plaque psoriasis
**Effects on Mental Status** None reported
**Effects on Psychiatric Treatment** None reported
**Usual Dosage** Adults: Topical: Apply in a thin film to the affected skin twice daily and rub in gently and completely
**Dosage Forms**
Cream: 0.005% (30 g, 60 g, 100 g)
Ointment, topical: 0.005% (30 g, 60 g, 100 g)
Solution, topical: 0.005%

## Calcitonin (kal si TOE nin)

**U.S. Brand Names** Calcimar® Injection; Cibacalcin® Injection; Miacalcin® Injection; Miacalcin® Nasal Spray; Osteocalcin® Injection; Salmonine® Injection
**Canadian Brand Names** Caltine®
**Synonyms** Calcitonin (Human); Calcitonin (Salmon)
**Pharmacologic Category** Antidote
**Use**
Calcitonin (salmon): Treatment of Paget's disease of bone and as adjunctive therapy for hypercalcemia; also used in postmenopausal osteoporosis and osteogenesis imperfecta
Calcitonin (human): Treatment of Paget's disease of bone
**Effects on Mental Status** None reported
**Effects on Psychiatric Treatment** None reported
**Pregnancy Risk Factor** C
**Contraindications** Hypersensitivity to salmon protein or gelatin diluent
**Warnings/Precautions** A skin test should be performed prior to initiating therapy of calcitonin salmon; have epinephrine immediately available for a possible hypersensitivity reaction
**Adverse Reactions**
>10%:
Cardiovascular: Facial flushing
Gastrointestinal: Nausea, diarrhea, anorexia
Local: Edema at injection site
1% to 10%: Genitourinary: Polyuria
<1%: Chills, dizziness, edema, headache, nasal congestion, paresthesia, rash, shortness of breath, urticaria, weakness
**Overdosage/Toxicology** Signs and symptoms: Nausea, vomiting, hypocalcemia, hypocalcemic tetany
**Drug Interactions** Plicamycin may enhance hypocalcemic effect
**Usual Dosage**
Children: Dosage not established
Adults:
Paget's disease:
Salmon calcitonin: I.M., S.C.: 100 units/day to start, 50 units/day or 50-100 units every 1-3 days maintenance dose
Human calcitonin: S.C.: Initial: 0.5 mg/day (maximum: 0.5 mg twice daily); maintenance: 0.5 mg 2-3 times/week or 0.25 mg/day
Hypercalcemia: Initial: Salmon calcitonin: I.M., S.C.: 4 units/kg every 12 hours; may increase up to 8 units/kg every 12 hours to a maximum of every 6 hours
Osteogenesis imperfecta: Salmon calcitonin: I.M., S.C.: 2 units/kg 3 times/week
Postmenopausal osteoporosis: Salmon calcitonin:
I.M., S.C.: 100 units/day
Intranasal: 200 units (1 spray)/day
**Patient Information** When this drug is given subcutaneously or I.M. it will be necessary for you or a significant other to learn to prepare and give the injections (keep drug vials in a refrigerator - do not freeze). Report significant nasal irritation if using calcitonin nasal spray. Follow directions exactly. Increased warmth and flushing may be experienced with this drug and should only last about 1 hour after administration (taking drug in the evening may minimize these discomforts). Immediately report twitching, muscle spasm, dark colored urine, hives, significant skin rash, palpitations, or difficulty breathing.
**Nursing Implications** Skin test should be performed prior to administration of salmon calcitonin; refrigerate; I.M. administration is preferred if the volume to injection exceeds 2 mL
**Dosage Forms**
Injection:
**Human** (Cibacalcin®): 0.5 mg/vial
**Salmon:** 200 units/mL (2 mL)
Spray, nasal: **Salmon** (Miacalcin®): 200 units/activation (0.09 mL/dose) (2 mL glass bottle with pump)

♦ **Calcitonin (Human)** *see* Calcitonin *on page 83*

♦ **Calcitonin (Salmon)** *see* Calcitonin *on page 83*

## Calcitriol (kal si TRYE ole)

**U.S. Brand Names** Calcijex™; Rocaltrol®
**Synonyms** 1,25 Dihydroxycholecalciferol
**Pharmacologic Category** Vitamin D Analog
**Use** Management of hypocalcemia in patients on chronic renal dialysis; reduce elevated parathyroid hormone levels
**Unlabeled use:** Decrease severity of psoriatic lesions in psoriatic vulgaris; vitamin D resistant rickets
**Effects on Mental Status** May cause sedation or irritability
**Effects on Psychiatric Treatment** None reported
**Pregnancy Risk Factor** C (per manufacturer); A/D (if dosage exceeds RDA)(based on expert analysis)
**Contraindications** Hypercalcemia; vitamin D toxicity; abnormal sensitivity to the effects of vitamin D; malabsorption syndrome
**Warnings/Precautions** Adequate dietary (supplemental) calcium is necessary for clinical response to vitamin D; maintain adequate fluid intake; calcium-phosphate product (serum calcium times phosphorus) must not exceed 70; avoid hypercalcemia or use with renal function impairment and secondary hyperparathyroidism
**Adverse Reactions**
>10%: Endocrine & metabolic: Hypercalcemia (33%)
(Continued)

## Calcitriol *(Continued)*

Percentage unknown: Anorexia, bone pain, cardiac arrhythmias, conjunctivitis, constipation, elevated LFTs, headache, hypermagnesemia, hypertension, hypotension, irritability, metallic taste, myalgia, nausea, pancreatitis, photophobia, polydipsia, polyuria, pruritus, seizures (rare), somnolence, vomiting, xerostomia

**Overdosage/Toxicology**

Signs and symptoms: Rarely toxicity occurs from acute overdose; symptoms of chronic overdose include hypercalcemia, hypercalciuria with weakness, altered mental status, GI upset, renal tubular injury, and occasionally cardiac arrhythmias

Treatment: Following withdrawal of the drug, treatment consists of bed rest, liberal intake of fluids, reduced calcium intake, and cathartic administration. Severe hypercalcemia requires I.V. hydration and forced diuresis. I.V. saline may increase excretion of calcium. Calcitonin, cholestyramine, prednisone, sodium EDTA, biphosphonates, and mithramycin have all been used successfully to treat the more resistant cases of vitamin D-induced hypercalcemia.

**Drug Interactions**

Decreased effect/absorption: Cholestyramine, colestipol

Increased effect: Thiazide diuretics

Additive effect: Magnesium-containing antacids

**Usual Dosage** Individualize dosage to maintain calcium levels of 9-10 mg/dL

Renal failure:

Children:

Oral: 0.25-2 mcg/day have been used (with hemodialysis); 0.014-0.041 mcg/kg/day (not receiving hemodialysis); increases should be made at 4- to 8-week intervals

I.V.: 0.01-0.05 mcg/kg 3 times/week if undergoing hemodialysis

Adults:

Oral: 0.25 mcg/day or every other day (may require 0.5-1 mcg/day); increases should be made at 4- to 8-week intervals

I.V.: 0.5 mcg/day 3 times/week (may require from 0.5-3 mcg/day given 3 times/week) if undergoing hemodialysis

Hypoparathyroidism/pseudohypoparathyroidism: Oral (evaluate dosage at 2- to 4-week intervals):

Children:

<1 year: 0.04-0.08 mcg/kg once daily

1-5 years: 0.25-0.75 mcg once daily

Children >6 years and Adults: 0.5-2 mcg once daily

Vitamin D-dependent rickets: Children and Adults: Oral: 1 mcg once daily

Vitamin D-resistant rickets (familial hypophosphatemia): Children and Adults: Oral: Initial: 0.015-0.02 mcg/kg once daily; maintenance: 0.03-0.06 mcg/kg once daily; maximum dose: 2 mcg once daily

Hypocalcemia in premature infants: Oral: 1 mcg once daily for 5 days

Hypocalcemic tetany in premature infants: I.V.: 0.05 mcg/kg once daily for 5-12 days

Elderly: No dosage recommendations, but start at the lower end of the dosage range

**Patient Information** Take exact dose as prescribed; do not increase dose. Maintain recommended diet and calcium supplementation. Avoid taking magnesium-containing antacids. You may experience nausea, vomiting, loss of appetite, or metallic taste (frequent small meals, frequent mouth care, chewing gum, or sucking lozenges may help); or hypotension (use caution when rising from sitting or lying position or when climbing stairs or bending over). Report chest pain or palpitations; acute headache; skin rash; change in vision or eye irritation; CNS changes; unusual weakness or fatigue; persistent nausea, vomiting, cramps, or diarrhea; or muscle or bone pain.

**Dosage Forms**

Capsule: 0.25 mcg, 0.5 mcg

Injection: 1 mcg/mL (1 mL); 2 mcg/mL (1 mL)

Solution, oral: 1 mcg/mL

## Calcium Acetate (KAL see um AS e tate)

**U.S. Brand Names** Calphron®; PhosLo®

**Pharmacologic Category** Antidote; Calcium Salt; Electrolyte Supplement, Oral

**Use**

Oral: Control of hyperphosphatemia in end-stage renal failure; calcium acetate binds to phosphorus in the GI tract better than other calcium salts due to its lower solubility and subsequent reduced absorption and increased formation of calcium phosphate; calcium acetate does not promote aluminum absorption

I.V.: Calcium supplementation in parenteral nutrition therapy

**Effects on Mental Status** May cause confusion and delirium (as a consequence of hypercalcemia)

**Effects on Psychiatric Treatment** None reported

**Usual Dosage**

Oral: Adults, on dialysis: Initial: 2 tablets with each meal, can be increased gradually to 3-4 tablets with each meal to bring the serum phosphate value <6 mg/dL as long as hypercalcemia does not develop

I.V.: Dose is dependent on the requirements of the individual patient; in central venous total parental nutrition (TPN), calcium is administered at a concentration of 5 mEq (10 mL)/L of TPN solution; the additive maintenance dose in neonatal TPN is 0.5 mEq calcium/kg/day (1.0 mL/kg/day)

Neonates: 70-200 mg/kg/day

Infants and Children: 70-150 mg/kg/day

Adolescents: 18-35 mg/kg/day

**Dosage Forms** Elemental calcium listed in brackets

Capsule: Phos-Ex® 125: 500 mg (125 mg)

Injection, 0.5 mEq calcium/mL (39.55 mg calcium acetate/mL) 10 mL vial

Tablet:

Calphron®: 667 mg [169 mg]

PhosLo®: 667 mg [169 mg]

## Calcium Carbonate (KAL see um KAR bun ate)

**U.S. Brand Names** Alka-Mints® [OTC]; Amitone® [OTC]; Cal Carb-HD® [OTC]; Calci-Chew™ [OTC]; Calciday-667® [OTC]; Calci-Mix™ [OTC]; Cal-Plus® [OTC]; Caltrate® 600 [OTC]; Caltrate, Jr.® [OTC]; Chooz® [OTC]; Dicarbosil® [OTC]; Equilet® [OTC]; Florical® [OTC]; Gencalc® 600 [OTC]; Mallamint® [OTC]; Nephro-Calci® [OTC]; Os-Cal® 500 [OTC]; Oyst-Cal 500 [OTC]; Oystercal® 500; Rolaids® Calcium Rich [OTC]; Tums® [OTC]; Tums® E-X Extra Strength Tablet [OTC]; Tums® Extra Strength Liquid [OTC]

**Canadian Brand Names** Apo®-Cal; Calcite-500; Calsan®; Pharmacal®

**Pharmacologic Category** Antacid; Antidote; Calcium Salt; Electrolyte Supplement, Oral

**Use** As an antacid, and treatment and prevention of calcium deficiency or hyperphosphatemia (eg, osteoporosis, osteomalacia, mild/moderate renal insufficiency, hypoparathyroidism, postmenopausal osteoporosis, rickets); has been used to bind phosphate

**Effects on Mental Status** May rarely produce irritability

**Effects on Psychiatric Treatment** None reported

**Usual Dosage** Oral (dosage is in terms of elemental calcium):

**Adequate intakes:**

0-6 months: 210 mg/day

7-12 months: 270 mg/day

1-3 years: 500 mg/day

4-8 years: 800 mg/day

Adults, male/female:

9-18 years: 1300 mg/day

19-50 years: 1000 mg/day

>51 years: 1200 mg/day

Female: Pregnancy:

≤18 years: 1300 mg/day

>19 years: 1000 mg/day

Female: Lactating:

≤18 years: 1300 mg/day

>19 years: 1000 mg/day

Hypocalcemia (dose depends on clinical condition and serum calcium level): Dose expressed in mg of **elemental calcium**

Neonates: 50-150 mg/kg/day in 4-6 divided doses; not to exceed 1 g/day

Children: 45-65 mg/kg/day in 4 divided doses

Adults: 1-2 g or more/day in 3-4 divided doses

Adults:

Dietary supplementation: 500 mg to 2 g divided 2-4 times/day

Antacid: 2 tablets or 10 mL every 2 hours, up to 12 times/day

Adults >51 years of age: Osteoporosis: 1200 mg/day

**Dosing adjustment in renal impairment:** $Cl_{cr}$ <25 mL/minute: Dosage adjustments may be necessary depending on the serum calcium levels

**Dosage Forms** Elemental calcium listed in brackets

Capsule: 1500 mg [600 mg]

Calci-Mix™: 1250 mg [500 mg]

Florical®: 364 mg [145.6 mg] with sodium fluoride 8.3 mg

Liquid (Tums® Extra Strength): 1000 mg/5 mL (360 mL)

Lozenge (Mylanta® Soothing Antacids): 600 mg [240 mg]

Powder (Cal Carb-HD®): 6.5 g/packet [2.6 g]

Suspension, oral: 1250 mg/5 mL [500 mg]

Tablet: 650 mg [260 mg], 1500 mg [600 mg]

Calciday-667®: 667 mg [267 mg]

Os-Cal® 500, Oyst-Cal 500, Oystercal® 500: 1250 mg [500 mg]

Cal-Plus®, Caltrate® 600, Gencalc® 600, Nephro-Calci®: 1500 mg [600 mg]

Chewable:

Alka-Mints®: 850 mg [340 mg]

Amitone®: 350 mg [140 mg]

Caltrate, Jr.®: 750 mg [300 mg]

Calci-Chew™, Os-Cal®: 750 mg [300 mg]

Chooz®, Dicarbosil®, Equilet®, Tums®: 500 mg [200 mg]

Mallamint®: 420 mg [168 mg]

Rolaids® Calcium Rich: 550 mg [220 mg]

Tums® E-X Extra Strength: 750 mg [300 mg]

Tums® Ultra®: 1000 mg [400 mg]

Florical®: 364 mg [145.6 mg] with sodium fluoride 8.3 mg

## Calcium Carbonate and Magnesium Carbonate

(KAL see um KAR bun ate & mag NEE zhum KAR bun ate)

**U.S. Brand Names** Mylanta® Gelcaps®
**Pharmacologic Category** Antacid
**Use** Hyperacidity
**Effects on Mental Status** May rarely produce irritability
**Effects on Psychiatric Treatment** None reported
**Usual Dosage** Adults: Oral: 2-4 Gelcaps® as needed
**Dosage Forms** Capsule: Calcium carbonate 311 mg and magnesium carbonate 232 mg

## Calcium Carbonate and Simethicone

(KAL see um KAR bun ate & sye METH i kone)

**U.S. Brand Names** Titralac® Plus Liquid [OTC]
**Pharmacologic Category** Antacid; Antiflatulent
**Use** Relief of acid indigestion, heartburn, peptic esophagitis, hiatal hernia, and gas
**Effects on Mental Status** None reported
**Effects on Psychiatric Treatment** None reported
**Usual Dosage** Oral: 0.5-2 g 4-6 times/day
**Dosage Forms** Elemental calcium listed in brackets
Liquid: Calcium carbonate 500 mg [200 mg] and simethicone 20 mg per 5 mL

♦ **Calcium Channel Blocking Agents Comparison Chart** *see page 710*

## Calcium Chloride (KAL see um KLOR ide)

**Pharmacologic Category** Calcium Salt; Electrolyte Supplement, Parenteral
**Use** Cardiac resuscitation when epinephrine fails to improve myocardial contractions, cardiac disturbances of hyperkalemia, hypocalcemia, or calcium channel blocking agent toxicity; emergent treatment of hypocalcemic tetany, treatment of hypermagnesemia
**Effects on Mental Status** May cause drowsiness; rare reports of mania
**Effects on Psychiatric Treatment** None reported
**Usual Dosage Note:** Calcium chloride is 3 times as potent as calcium gluconate
Cardiac arrest in the presence of hyperkalemia or hypocalcemia, magnesium toxicity, or calcium antagonist toxicity: I.V.:
Infants and Children: 20 mg/kg; may repeat in 10 minutes if necessary
Adults: 2-4 mg/kg (10% solution), repeated every 10 minutes if necessary
Hypocalcemia: I.V.:
Infants and Children: 10-20 mg/kg/dose (infants <1 mEq; children 1-7 mEq), repeat every 4-6 hours if needed
Adults: 500 mg to 1 g (7-14 mEq)/dose repeated every 4-6 hours if needed
Hypocalcemic tetany: I.V.:
Infants and Children: 10 mg/kg (0.5-0.7 mEq/kg) over 5-10 minutes; may repeat after 6-8 hours or follow with an infusion with a maximum dose of 200 mg/kg/day
Adults: 1 g over 10-30 minutes; may repeat after 6 hours
Hypocalcemia secondary to citrated blood transfusion: I.V.:
Neonates: Give 0.45 mEq **elemental** calcium for each 100 mL citrated blood infused
Adults: 1.35 mEq calcium with each 100 mL of citrated blood infused
**Dosing adjustment in renal impairment:** $Cl_{cr}$ <25 mL/minute: Dosage adjustments may be necessary depending on the serum calcium levels
**Dosage Forms** Elemental calcium listed in brackets
Injection: 10% = 100 mg/mL [27.2 mg/mL, 1.36 mEq/mL] (10 mL)

## Calcium Citrate (KAL see um SIT rate)

**U.S. Brand Names** Citracal® [OTC]
**Pharmacologic Category** Calcium Salt
**Use** Antacid; treatment and prevention of calcium deficiency or hyperphosphatemia (eg, osteoporosis, osteomalacia, mild/moderate renal insufficiency, hypoparathyroidism, postmenopausal osteoporosis, rickets)
**Effects on Mental Status** May cause confusion and delirium (as a consequence of hypercalcemia)
**Effects on Psychiatric Treatment** None reported
**Usual Dosage** Oral: Dosage is in terms of elemental calcium
Recommended daily allowance (RDA):
<6 months: 360 mg/day
6-12 months: 540 mg/day
1-10 years: 800 mg/day
10-18 years: 1200 mg/day
Adults: 1-2 g/day
Dietary supplement: Usual dose: 500 mg to 2 g 2-4 times/day
**Dosage Forms** Elemental calcium listed in brackets
Tablet: 950 mg [200 mg]
Tablet, effervescent: 2376 mg [500 mg]

## Calcium Glubionate (KAL see um gloo BYE oh nate)

**U.S. Brand Names** Neo-Calglucon® [OTC]
**Pharmacologic Category** Calcium Salt
**Use** Adjunct in treatment and prevention of postmenopausal osteoporosis; treatment and prevention of calcium depletion or hyperphosphatemia (eg, osteoporosis, osteomalacia, mild/moderate renal insufficiency, hypoparathyroidism, rickets)
**Effects on Mental Status** May cause confusion and delirium (as a consequence of hypercalcemia)
**Effects on Psychiatric Treatment** None reported
**Usual Dosage** Dosage is in terms of **elemental** calcium
**Adequate intakes:**
0-6 months: 210 mg/day
7-12 months: 270 mg/day
1-3 years: 500 mg/day
4-8 years: 800 mg/day
Adults, male/female:
9-18 years: 1300 mg/day
19-50 years: 1000 mg/day
>51 years: 1200 mg/day
Female: Pregnancy:
≤18 years: 1300 mg/day
>19 years: 1000 mg/day
Female: Lactating:
≤18 years: 1300 mg/day
>19 years: 1000 mg/day
Syrup is a hyperosmolar solution; dosage is in terms of calcium glubionate, elemental calcium is in parentheses
Neonatal hypocalcemia: 1200 mg (77 mg $Ca^{++}$)/kg/day in 4-6 divided doses
Maintenance: Infants and Children: 600-2000 mg (38-128 mg $Ca^{++}$)/kg/day in 4 divided doses up to a maximum of 9 g (575 mg $Ca^{++}$)/day
Adults: 6-18 g (~0.5-1 g $Ca^{++}$)/day in divided doses
**Dosing adjustment in renal impairment:** $Cl_{cr}$ <25 mL/minute: Dosage adjustments may be necessary depending on the serum calcium levels
**Dosage Forms** Elemental calcium listed in brackets
Syrup: 1.8 g/5 mL [115 mg/5 mL] (480 mL)

## Calcium Gluceptate (KAL see um gloo SEP tate)

**Pharmacologic Category** Calcium Salt
**Use** Treatment of cardiac disturbances of hyperkalemia, hypocalcemia, or calcium channel blocker toxicity; cardiac resuscitation when epinephrine fails to improve myocardial contractions; treatment of hypermagnesemia and hypocalcemia
**Effects on Mental Status** May rarely cause lethargy or mania
**Effects on Psychiatric Treatment** None reported
**Usual Dosage** Dose expressed in mg of calcium gluceptate (elemental calcium is in parentheses)
Cardiac resuscitation in the presence of hypocalcemia, hyperkalemia, magnesium toxicity, or calcium channel blocker toxicity: I.V.:
Children: 110 mg (9 mg $Ca^{++}$)/kg/dose
Adults: 1.1-1.5 g (90-123 mg $Ca^{++}$)
Hypocalcemia:
I.M.:
Children: 200-500 mg (16.4-41 mg $Ca^{++}$)/kg/day divided every 6 hours
Adults: 500 mg to 1.1 g/dose as needed
I.V.: Adults: 1.1-4.4 g (90-360 mg $Ca^{++}$) administered slowly as needed (≤2 mL/minute)
After citrated blood administration: Children and Adults: I.V.: 0.45 mEq $Ca^{++}$/100 mL blood infused
**Dosing adjustment in renal impairment:** $Cl_{cr}$ <25 mL/minute: Dosage adjustments may be necessary depending on the serum calcium levels
**Dosage Forms** Elemental calcium listed in brackets
Injection: 220 mg/mL [18 mg/mL, 0.9 mEq/mL] (5 mL, 50 mL)

## Calcium Gluconate (KAL see um GLOO koe nate)

**U.S. Brand Names** Kalcinate®
**Pharmacologic Category** Calcium Salt; Electrolyte Supplement, Oral; Electrolyte Supplement, Parenteral
**Use** Treatment and prevention of hypocalcemia; treatment of tetany, cardiac disturbances of hyperkalemia, cardiac resuscitation when epinephrine fails to improve myocardial contractions, hypocalcemia, or calcium channel blocker toxicity; calcium supplementation
**Effects on Mental Status** May cause drowsiness; may cause confusion and delirium (as a consequence of hypercalcemia)
**Effects on Psychiatric Treatment** None reported
**Usual Dosage** Dosage is in terms of **elemental** calcium
(Continued)

## Calcium Gluconate *(Continued)*

**Adequate intakes:**
0-6 months: 210 mg/day
7-12 months: 270 mg/day
1-3 years: 500 mg/day
4-8 years: 800 mg/day
Adults, male/female:
9-18 years: 1300 mg/day
19-50 years: 1000 mg/day
>51 years: 1200 mg/day
Female: Pregnancy:
≤18 years: 1300 mg/day
>19 years: 1000 mg/day
Female: Lactating:
≤18 years: 1300 mg/day
>19 years: 1000 mg/day

Dosage expressed in terms of **calcium gluconate**
Hypocalcemia: I.V.:
Neonates: 200-800 mg/kg/day as a continuous infusion or in 4 divided doses
Infants and Children: 200-500 mg/kg/day as a continuous infusion or in 4 divided doses
Adults: 2-15 g/24 hours as a continuous infusion or in divided doses
Hypocalcemia: Oral:
Children: 200-500 mg/kg/day divided every 6 hours
Adults: 500 mg to 2 g 2-4 times/day
Osteoporosis/bone loss: Oral: 1000-1500 mg in divided doses/day
Hypocalcemia secondary to citrated blood infusion: I.V.: Give 0.45 mEq **elemental** calcium for each 100 mL citrated blood infused
Hypocalcemic tetany: I.V.:
Neonates: 100-200 mg/kg/dose, may follow with 500 mg/kg/day in 3-4 divided doses or as an infusion
Infants and Children: 100-200 mg/kg/dose (0.5-0.7 mEq/kg/dose) over 5-10 minutes; may repeat every 6-8 hours **or** follow with an infusion of 500 mg/kg/day
Adults: 1-3 g (4.5-16 mEq) may be administered until therapeutic response occurs
Calcium antagonist toxicity, magnesium intoxication or cardiac arrest in the presence of hyperkalemia or hypocalcemia: Calcium chloride is recommended calcium salt: I.V.:
Infants and Children: 100 mg/kg/dose (maximum: 3 g/dose)
Adults: 500-800 mg; maximum: 3 g/dose
Maintenance electrolyte requirements for total parenteral nutrition: I.V.: Daily requirements: Adults: 8-16 mEq/1000 kcal/24 hours
**Dosing adjustment in renal impairment:** $Cl_{cr}$ <25 mL/minute: Dosage adjustments may be necessary depending on the serum calcium levels

**Dosage Forms** Elemental calcium listed in brackets
Injection: 10% = 100 mg/mL [9 mg/mL] (10 mL, 50 mL, 100 mL, 200 mL)
Tablet: 500 mg [45 mg], 650 mg [58.5 mg], 975 mg [87.75 mg], 1 g [90 mg]

## Calcium Lactate (KAL see um LAK tate)

**Pharmacologic Category** Calcium Salt
**Use** Adjunct in prevention of postmenopausal osteoporosis; treatment and prevention of calcium depletion
**Effects on Mental Status** May rarely cause confusion or dizziness
**Effects on Psychiatric Treatment** None reported
**Usual Dosage** Oral (in terms of calcium lactate)
Recommended daily allowance (RDA) (in terms of elemental calcium):
<6 months: 360 mg/day
6-12 months: 540 mg/day
1-10 years: 800 mg/day
10-18 years: 1200 mg/day
Adults: 800 mg/day
Children: 500 mg/kg/day divided every 6-8 hours
Maximum daily dose: 9 g
Adults: 1.5-3 g divided every 8 hours
**Dosage Forms** Elemental calcium listed in brackets
Tablet: 325 mg [42.25 mg], 650 mg [84.5 mg]

♦ **Calcium Leucovorin** *see* Leucovorin *on page 309*

## Calcium Phosphate, Tribasic
(KAL see um FOS fate tri BAY sik)

**U.S. Brand Names** Posture® [OTC]
**Pharmacologic Category** Calcium Salt
**Use** Adjunct in prevention of postmenopausal osteoporosis; treatment and prevention of calcium depletion
**Effects on Mental Status** None reported
**Effects on Psychiatric Treatment** None reported
**Usual Dosage** Oral (all doses in terms of elemental calcium):
Recommended daily allowance (RDA) (elemental calcium):
<6 months: 360 mg/day
6-12 months: 540 mg/day
1-10 years: 800 mg/day
10-18 years: 1200 mg/day
Adults: 800 mg/day
Children: 45-65 mg/kg/day
Adults: 1-2 g/day
**Dosage Forms** Elemental calcium listed in brackets
Tablet, sugar free: 1565.2 mg [600 mg]

## Calcium Polycarbophil (KAL see um pol i KAR boe fil)

**U.S. Brand Names** Equalactin® Chewable Tablet [OTC]; Fiberall® Chewable Tablet [OTC]; FiberCon® Tablet [OTC]; Fiber-Lax® Tablet [OTC]; Mitrolan® Chewable Tablet [OTC]
**Pharmacologic Category** Antidiarrheal; Laxative, Bulk-Producing
**Use** Treatment of constipation or diarrhea by restoring a more normal moisture level and providing bulk in the patient's intestinal tract; calcium polycarbophil is supplied as the approved substitute whenever a bulk-forming laxative is ordered in a tablet, capsule, wafer, or other oral solid dosage form
**Effects on Mental Status** None reported
**Effects on Psychiatric Treatment** None reported
**Usual Dosage** Oral:
Children:
2-6 years: 500 mg (1 tablet) 1-2 times/day, up to 1.5 g/day
6-12 years: 500 mg (1 tablet) 1-3 times/day, up to 3 g/day
Adults: 1 g 4 times/day, up to 6 g/day
**Dosage Forms** Tablet:
Sodium free:
Fiber-Lax®: 625 mg
FiberCon®: 500 mg
Chewable:
Equalactin®, Mitrolan®: 500 mg
Fiberall®: 1250 mg

♦ **Caldecort®** *see* Hydrocortisone *on page 273*
♦ **Caldecort® Anti-Itch Spray** *see* Hydrocortisone *on page 273*
♦ **Calderol®** *see* Calcifediol *on page 83*

## Calfactant (cal FAC tant)

**U.S. Brand Names** Infasurf®
**Pharmacologic Category** Lung Surfactant
**Use** Prevention of respiratory distress syndrome (RDS) in premature infants at high risk for RDS and for the treatment ("rescue") of premature infants who develop RDS
Prophylaxis: Therapy at birth with calfactant is indicated for premature infants <29 weeks of gestational age at significant risk for RDS. Should be administered as soon as possible, preferably within 30 minutes after birth.
Treatment: For infants ≤72 hours of age with RDS (confirmed by clinical and radiologic findings) and requiring endotracheal intubation.
**Effects on Mental Status** None reported
**Effects on Psychiatric Treatment** None reported
**Usual Dosage** Intratracheal administration **only**: Each dose is 3 mL/kg body weight at birth; should be administered every 12 hours for a total of up to 3 doses
**Dosage Forms** Suspension, intratracheal: 6 mL

♦ **Calm-X® Oral [OTC]** *see* Dimenhydrinate *on page 173*
♦ **Calphron®** *see* Calcium Acetate *on page 84*
♦ **Cal-Plus® [OTC]** *see* Calcium Carbonate *on page 84*
♦ **Caltrate® 600 [OTC]** *see* Calcium Carbonate *on page 84*
♦ **Caltrate, Jr.® [OTC]** *see* Calcium Carbonate *on page 84*
♦ **Cama® Arthritis Pain Reliever [OTC]** *see* Aspirin *on page 49*
♦ **Campho-Phenique® [OTC]** *see* Camphor and Phenol *on page 86*

## Camphor and Phenol (KAM for & FEE nole)

**U.S. Brand Names** Campho-Phenique® [OTC]
**Pharmacologic Category** Topical Skin Product
**Use** Relief of pain and for minor infections
**Effects on Mental Status** None reported
**Effects on Psychiatric Treatment** None reported
**Usual Dosage** Apply as needed
**Dosage Forms** Liquid: Camphor 10.8% and phenol 4.7%

♦ **Camphorated Tincture of Opium** *see* Paregoric *on page 420*

## Camphor, Menthol, and Phenol
(KAM for, MEN thol, & FEE nole)

**U.S. Brand Names** Sarna [OTC]
**Pharmacologic Category** Topical Skin Product
**Use** Relief of dry, itching skin
**Effects on Mental Status** None reported
**Effects on Psychiatric Treatment** None reported
**Usual Dosage** Topical: Apply as needed for dry skin
**Dosage Forms** Lotion, topical: Camphor 0.5%, menthol 0.5%, and phenol 0.5% in emollient base (240 mL)

♦ **Camptosar®** *see* Irinotecan *on page 292*

## Candesartan (kan de SAR tan)

**Related Information**
Angiotensin-Related Agents Comparison Chart *on page 700*
**U.S. Brand Names** Atacand™
**Synonyms** Candesartan Cilexetil
**Pharmacologic Category** Angiotensin II Antagonists
**Use** Alone or in combination with other antihypertensive agents in treating essential hypertension; may have an advantage over losartan due to minimal metabolism requirements and consequent use in mild to moderate hepatic impairment
**Effects on Mental Status** May cause dizziness or drowsiness; may rarely cause anxiety or depression
**Effects on Psychiatric Treatment** None reported
**Pregnancy Risk Factor** C (1st trimester); D (2nd and 3rd trimester)
**Contraindications** Hypersensitivity to candesartan or any component; hypersensitivity to other A-II receptor antagonists; primary hyperaldosteronism; bilateral renal artery stenosis; pregnancy (2nd and 3rd trimesters)
**Warnings/Precautions** Avoid use or use a smaller dose in patients who are volume depleted; correct depletion first. Deterioration in renal function can occur with initiation. Use with caution in unilateral renal artery stenosis and pre-existing renal insufficiency; significant aortic/mitral stenosis.
**Adverse Reactions**
Cardiovascular: Flushing, chest pain, peripheral edema, tachycardia, palpitations, angina, myocardial infarction,
Central nervous system: Dizziness, lightheadedness, drowsiness, fatigue, headache, vertigo, anxiety, depression, somnolence, fever
Dermatologic: Angioedema, rash (>0.5%)
Endocrine & metabolic: Hyperglycemia, hypertriglyceridemia
Gastrointestinal: Nausea, diarrhea, vomiting, dyspepsia, gastroenteritis
Genitourinary: Hyperuricemia, hematuria
Neuromuscular & skeletal: Back pain, arthralgia, paresthesias, increased CPK, myalgia, weakness
Respiratory: Upper respiratory tract infection, pharyngitis, rhinitis, bronchitis, cough, sinusitis, epistaxis, dyspnea
Miscellaneous: Diaphoresis (increased)
**Overdosage/Toxicology**
Signs and symptoms: Hypotension, tachycardia
Treatment: Supportive
**Drug Interactions**
Lithium: Risk of toxicity may be increased by candesartan; monitor lithium levels
Potassium-sparing diuretics (amiloride, spironolactone, triamterene): Increased risk of hyperkalemia
Potassium supplements may increase the risk of hyperkalemia
Trimethoprim (high dose) may increase the risk of hyperkalemia
**Usual Dosage** Adults: Oral: Usual dose is 4-32 mg once daily; dosage must be individualized. Blood pressure response is dose-related over the range of 2-32 mg. The usual recommended starting dose of 16 mg once daily when it is used as monotherapy in patients who are not volume depleted. It can be administered once or twice daily with total daily doses ranging from 8-32 mg. Larger doses do not appear to have a greater effect and there is relatively little experience with such doses.

No initial dosage adjustment is necessary for elderly patients (although higher concentrations ($C_{max}$) and AUC were observed in these populations), for patients with mildly impaired renal function, or for patients with mildly impaired hepatic function.
**Dietary Considerations** Food reduces the time to maximal concentration and increases the $C_{max}$
**Patient Information** Take exactly as directed; do not miss doses, alter dosage, or discontinue without consulting prescriber. Do not alter salt or potassium intake without consulting prescriber. Change position slowly when rising from sitting or lying or when climbing stairs. May cause transient drowsiness, dizziness, or headache; avoid driving or engaging in tasks requiring alertness until response to drug is known. Small frequent meals may help reduce any nausea or vomiting. Report unusual weight gain or swelling of ankles and hands; persistent fatigue; unusual flu or cold symptoms or dry cough; difficulty breathing; chest pain or palpitations; swelling of eyes, face, or lips; skin rash; muscle pain or weakness; unusual bleeding (in urine, stool, or gums); or excessive sweating.
**Dosage Forms** Tablet, as cilexetil: 4 mg, 8 mg, 16 mg, 32 mg

♦ **Candesartan Cilexetil** *see* Candesartan *on page 87*

## *Candida albicans (Monilia)*
(KAN dee da AL bi kans mo NIL ya)

**U.S. Brand Names** Dermatophytin-O
**Pharmacologic Category** Diagnostic Agent
**Use** Screen for detection of nonresponsiveness to antigens in immunocompromised individuals
**Effects on Mental Status** None reported
**Effects on Psychiatric Treatment** None reported
**Usual Dosage** Intradermal: 0.1 mL, examine reaction site in 24-48 hours; induration of ≥5 mm in diameter is a positive reaction
**Dosage Forms** Injection:
Intradermal: 1:100 (5 mL)
Scratch: 1:10 (5 mL)

♦ ***C. angustifolia*** *see* Senna *on page 509*

## Cantharidin (kan THAR e din)

**U.S. Brand Names** Verr-Canth™
**Canadian Brand Names** Canthacur®; Catharone®
**Pharmacologic Category** Keratolytic Agent
**Use** Removal of ordinary and periungual warts
**Effects on Mental Status** May cause delirium
**Effects on Psychiatric Treatment** None reported
**Usual Dosage** Apply directly to lesion, cover with nonporous tape, remove tape in 24 hours, reapply if necessary
**Dosage Forms** Liquid: 0.7% in a film-forming vehicle containing acetone, pyroxylin, castor oil and camphor (7.5 mL)

♦ **Cantil®** *see* Mepenzolate *on page 340*

♦ **Capastat® Sulfate** *see* Capreomycin *on page 88*

## Capecitabine (ka pe SITE a been)

**U.S. Brand Names** Xeloda®
**Pharmacologic Category** Antineoplastic Agent, Antimetabolite
**Use** Treatment of patients with metastatic breast cancer resistant to both paclitaxel and an anthracycline-containing chemotherapy regimen or resistant to paclitaxel and for whom further anthracycline therapy is not indicated (eg, patients who have received cumulative doses of 400 mg/m² of doxorubicin or doxorubicin equivalents). Resistance is defined as progressive disease while on treatment, with or without an initial response, or relapse within 6 months of completing treatment with an anthracycline-containing adjuvant regimen.
**Effects on Mental Status** Sedation is common; may cause dizziness or insomnia
**Effects on Psychiatric Treatment** Neutropenia is common; use caution with clozapine and carbamazepine
**Pregnancy Risk Factor** D
**Contraindications** Hypersensitivity to capecitabine, fluorouracil, or any component
**Warnings/Precautions** The U.S. Food and Drug Administration (FDA) currently recommends that procedures for proper handling and disposal of antineoplastic agents be considered. Use with caution in patients with bone marrow suppression, poor nutritional status, or renal or hepatic dysfunction. The drug should be discontinued if intractable diarrhea, stomatitis, bone marrow suppression, or myocardial ischemia develop. Use with caution in patients who have received extensive pelvic radiation or alkylating therapy.

Capecitabine can cause severe diarrhea; median time to first occurrence is 31 days; subsequent doses should be reduced after grade 3 or 4 diarrhea

Hand-and-foot syndrome (palmar-plantar erythrodysesthesia or chemotherapy-induced acral erythema) is characterized by numbness, dysesthesia/paresthesia, tingling, painless or painful swelling, erythema, desquamation, blistering, and severe pain. If grade 2 or 3 hand-and-foot syndrome occurs, interrupt administration of capecitabine until the event resolves or decreases in intensity to grade 1. Following grade 3 hand-and-foot syndrome, decrease subsequent doses of capecitabine.

There has been cardiotoxicity associated with fluorinated pyrimidine therapy, including myocardial infarction, angina, dysrhythmias, cardiogenic shock, sudden death, and EKG changes. These adverse events may be more common in patients with a history of coronary artery disease.
**Adverse Reactions**
>10%:
Central nervous system: Fatigue (41%), fever (12%)
Gastrointestinal: Diarrhea (57%), may be dose limiting; mild to moderate nausea (53%), vomiting (37%), stomatitis (24%), anorexia (23%), abdominal pain (20%), constipation (15%)
(Continued)

## Capecitabine *(Continued)*

Dermatologic: Palmar-plantar erythrodysesthesia (hand-and-foot syndrome) (57%), may be dose limiting; dermatitis (37%)
Hematologic: Lymphopenia (94%), anemia (72%), neutropenia (26%), thrombocytopenia (24%)
Hepatic: Increased bilirubin (22%)
Neuromuscular & skeletal: Paresthesia (21%)
Ocular: Eye irritation (15%)

1% to 10%:
Central nervous system: Headache (9%), dizziness (8%), insomnia (8%)
Dermatologic: Nail disorders (7%)
Gastrointestinal: Intestinal obstruction (1.1%)
Endocrine & metabolic: Dehydration (7%)
Neuromuscular & skeletal: Myalgia (9%)

<1%: Alopecia, ataxia, bone pain, bronchospasm, cachexia, cardiomyopathy, cerebral vascular accident, change in consciousness, chest pain, cholestasis, colitis, confusion, deep vein thrombosis, duodenitis, dyspnea, encephalopathy, epistaxis, esophagitis, gastritis, GI hemorrhage, hematemesis, hepatic fibrosis, hepatitis, hypersensitivity, hypertriglyceridemia, hypotension, increased diaphoresis, infections, joint stiffness, lymphedema, necrotizing enterocolitis, nocturia, oral candidiasis, pancytopenia, photosensitization, pulmonary embolism, radiation recall, respiratory distress, thrombocytopenic purpura, thrombophlebitis

**Overdosage/Toxicology**
Signs and symptoms: Myelosuppression, nausea, vomiting, diarrhea, and alopecia
Treatment is supportive; no specific antidote exists; monitor hematologically for at least 4 weeks

**Drug Interactions**
Increased effect: Taking capecitabine immediately before an aluminum hydroxide/magnesium hydroxide antacid, or a meal, increases the absorption of capecitabine. Phenytoin levels may be increased by capecitabine.
Increased toxicity: The concentration of 5-fluorouracil is increased and its toxicity may be enhanced by leucovorin. Deaths from severe enterocolitis, diarrhea, and dehydration have been reported in elderly patients receiving weekly leucovorin and fluorouracil. Warfarin: Altered coagulation parameters have been noted in cancer patients receiving coumarin derivatives concomitantly with capecitabine.

**Usual Dosage** Oral:
Adults: 2500 mg/m²/day in 2 divided doses (~12 hours apart) at the end of a meal for 2 weeks followed by a 1-week rest period given as 3-week cycles

**Capecitabine dose calculation according to BSA table:** The following can be used to determine the total daily dose (mg) based on a dosing level of 2500 mg/m²/day. (The number of tablets per dose, given morning and evening, are also listed):
Surface area ≤1.24 m²:
Total daily dose is 3000 mg (3 x 500 mg tablets per dose)
Surface area 1.25-1.36 m²:
Total daily dose is 3300 mg (1 x 150 mg tablet plus 3 x 500 mg tablets per dose)
Surface area 1.37-1.51 m²:
Total daily dose is 3600 mg (2 x 150 mg tablets plus 3 x 500 mg tablets per dose)
Surface area 1.52-1.64 m²:
Total daily dose is 4000 mg (4 x 500 mg tablets per dose)
Surface area 1.65-1.76 m²:
Total daily dose is 4300 mg (1 x 150 mg tablet plus 4 x 500 mg tablets per dose)
Surface area 1.77-1.91 m²:
Total daily dose is 4600 mg (2 x 150 mg tablets plus 4 x 500 mg tablets per dose)
Surface area 1.92-2.04 m²:
Total daily dose is 5000 mg (5 x 500 mg tablets per dose)
Surface area 2.05-2.17 m²:
Total daily dose is 5300 mg (1 x 150 mg tablets plus 5 x 500 mg tablets per dose)
Surface area ≥2.18 m²:
Total daily dose is 5600 mg (2 x 150 mg tablets plus 5 x 500 mg tablets per dose)

**Dosing adjustment in renal impairment:** There is little experience in patients with renal impairment; use with caution. There is insufficient data to provide a dosage recommendation.

**Dosing adjustment in hepatic impairment:**
Mild to moderate impairment: No starting dose adjustment is necessary; however, carefully monitor patients
Severe hepatic impairment: Patients have not been studied

**Dosing adjustment in elderly patients:** The elderly may be pharmacodynamically more sensitive to the toxic effects of 5-fluorouracil. Use with caution in monitoring the effects of capecitabine. Insufficient data are available to provide dosage modifications.

**Dosage modification guidelines:** Carefully monitor patients for toxicity. Toxicity caused by capecitabine administration may be managed by symptomatic treatment, dose interruptions, and adjustment of dose. Once the dose has been reduced, it should not be increased at a later time.
**Dosage reduction for toxicity:** The starting dose may be reduced by 25% in patients experiencing significant adverse effects at the full starting dose if symptoms persist, a further reduction (to 50% of the starting dose) may be considered. These recommendations were based on clinical studies reported at the 36th Annual Meeting of the American Society of Clinical Oncology (ASCO).

**Manufacturer-recommended dosage adjustments for various nonhematologic toxicities:**

NCI Grade 1:
Maintain dose level during course of therapy and for next cycle.

NCI Grade 2:
1st appearance: Interrupt therapy until resolved to grade 0-1 during course of therapy; administer 100% of initial dose for next cycle
2nd appearance: Interrupt therapy until resolved to grade 0- 1 during course of therapy; administer 75% of initial dose for next cycle
3rd appearance: Interrupt therapy until resolved to grade 0-1 during course of therapy; administer 50% of initial dose for next cycle
4th appearance: Discontinue treatment permanently

NCI Grade 3:
1st appearance: Interrupt therapy until resolved to grade 0-1 during course of therapy; administer 75% of starting dose for next cycle
2nd appearance: Interrupt therapy until resolved to grade 0-1; administer 50% of initial dose for next cycle
3rd appearance: Discontinue treatment permanently

NCI Grade 4:
1st appearance: Discontinue permanently, **or**, if physician deems it to be in the patient's best interest to continue, interrupt until resolved to grade 0-1; administer 50% of initial dose for next cycle.

**Dietary Considerations** Food reduced the rate and extent of absorption of capecitabine. Because current safety and efficacy data are based upon administration with food, it is recommended that capecitabine be administered with food. In all clinical trials, patients were instructed to administer capecitabine within 30 minutes after a meal.

**Patient Information** Take with food or within 30 minutes after meal. Avoid use of antacids within 2 hours of taking capecitabine. Do not crush, chew, or dissolve tablets. You will need frequent blood tests while taking this medication. Maintain adequate hydration (2-3 L/day of fluids unless instructed to restrict fluid intake). You may experience lethargy, dizziness, visual changes, confusion, anxiety (avoid driving or engaging in tasks requiring alertness until response to drug is known). For nausea, vomiting, loss of appetite, or dry mouth small, frequent meals, chewing gum, or sucking lozenges may help. You may experience loss of hair (will grow back when treatment is discontinued). You may experience photosensitivity (use sunscreen, wear protective clothing and eyewear, and avoid direct sunlight). You may experience dry, itchy, skin, and dry or irritated eyes (avoid contact lenses). You will be more susceptible to infection; avoid crowds or infected persons. Report chills or fever, confusion, persistent or violent vomiting or stomach pain, persistent diarrhea, respiratory difficulty, chest pain or palpitations, unusual bleeding or bruising, bone pain, muscle spasms/tremors, or vision changes immediately.

**Dosage Forms** Tablet: 150 mg, 500 mg

♦ **Capital® and Codeine** *see* Acetaminophen and Codeine *on page 14*

♦ **Capoten®** *see* Captopril *on page 89*

♦ **Capozide®** *see* Captopril and Hydrochlorothiazide *on page 90*

## Capreomycin (kap ree oh MYE sin)

**U.S. Brand Names** Capastat® Sulfate

**Pharmacologic Category** Antibiotic, Miscellaneous; Antitubercular Agent

**Use** Treatment of tuberculosis in conjunction with at least one other antituberculosis agent

**Effects on Mental Status** May cause dizziness

**Effects on Psychiatric Treatment** None reported

**Pregnancy Risk Factor** C

**Contraindications** Known hypersensitivity to capreomycin sulfate

**Warnings/Precautions** Use in patients with renal insufficiency or preexisting auditory impairment must be undertaken with great caution, and the risk of additional eighth nerve impairment or renal injury should be weighed against the benefits to be derived from therapy. Since other parenteral antituberculous agents (eg, streptomycin) also have similar and sometimes irreversible toxic effects, particularly on eighth cranial nerve and renal function, simultaneous administration of these agents with capreomycin is not recommended. Use with nonantituberculous drugs (ie, aminoglycoside antibiotics) having ototoxic or nephrotoxic potential should be undertaken only with great caution.

**Adverse Reactions**
>10%:
Otic: Ototoxicity [subclinical hearing loss (11%), clinical loss (3%)], tinnitus

Renal: Nephrotoxicity (36%, increased BUN)
1% to 10%: Hematologic: Eosinophilia (dose-related, mild)
<1%: Hypersensitivity (urticaria, rash, fever), hypokalemia, leukocytosis, pain/induration/bleeding at injection site, thrombocytopenia (rare), vertigo

**Overdosage/Toxicology**
Signs and symptoms: Renal failure, ototoxicity, thrombocytopenia
Treatment: Supportive

**Drug Interactions**
Increased effect/duration of nondepolarizing neuromuscular blocking agents
Additive toxicity (nephro- and ototoxicity, respiratory paralysis): Aminoglycosides (eg, streptomycin)

**Usual Dosage** I.M.:
Infants and Children: 15 mg/kg/day, up to 1 g/day maximum
Adults: 15-20 mg/kg/day up to 1 g/day for 60-120 days, followed by 1 g 2-3 times/week
**Dosing interval in renal impairment:** Adults:
$Cl_{cr}$ >100 mL/minute: Administer 13-15 mg/kg every 24 hours
$Cl_{cr}$ 80-100 mL/minute: Administer 10-13 mg/kg every 24 hours
$Cl_{cr}$ 60-80 mL/minute: Administer 7-10 mg/kg every 24 hours
$Cl_{cr}$ 40-60 mL/minute: Administer 11-14 mg/kg every 48 hours
$Cl_{cr}$ 20-40 mL/minute: Administer 10-14 mg/kg every 72 hours
$Cl_{cr}$ <20 mL/minute: Administer 4-7 mg/kg every 72 hours

**Patient Information** Take as prescribed; do not discontinue without consulting prescriber. Maintain adequate hydration (2-3 L/day of fluids unless instructed to restrict fluid intake) to reduce incidence of nephrotoxicity. While taking this medication, routine blood tests and auditory tests will be necessary. Report any hearing loss, dizziness or vertigo, persistent nausea or vomiting, loss of appetite, or increased frequency of urination.

**Nursing Implications** The solution for injection may acquire a pale straw color and darken with time; this is not associated with a loss of potency or development of toxicity

**Dosage Forms** Injection, as sulfate: 100 mg/mL (10 mL)

## Capsaicin (kap SAY sin)

**U.S. Brand Names** Capsin® [OTC]; Capzasin-P® [OTC]; Dolorac™ [OTC]; No Pain-HP® [OTC]; R-Gel® [OTC]; Zostrix® [OTC]; Zostrix®-HP [OTC]

**Pharmacologic Category** Analgesic, Topical; Topical Skin Product

**Use** FDA approved for the topical treatment of pain associated with postherpetic neuralgia, rheumatoid arthritis, osteoarthritis, diabetic neuropathy, and postsurgical pain.
**Unlabeled use:** Treatment of pain associated with psoriasis, chronic neuralgias unresponsive to other forms of therapy, and intractable pruritus

**Effects on Mental Status** None reported

**Effects on Psychiatric Treatment** None reported

**Contraindications** Hypersensitivity to capsaicin or any component

**Drug Interactions** No data reported

**Usual Dosage** Children ≥2 years and Adults: Topical: Apply to affected area at least 3-4 times/day; application frequency less than 3-4 times/day prevents the total depletion, inhibition of synthesis, and transport of substance P resulting in decreased clinical efficacy and increased local discomfort

**Patient Information** For external use only; wash hands immediately after application; discontinue if severe burning or itching occurs; if symptoms persist longer than 14-28 days, contact physician

**Dosage Forms**
Cream:
Capzasin-P®, Zostrix®: 0.025% (45 g, 90 g)
Dolorac™: 0.25% (28 g)
Zostrix®-HP: 0.075% (30 g, 60 g)
Gel (R-Gel®): 0.025% (15 g, 30 g)
Lotion (Capsin®): 0.025% (59 mL); 0.075% (59 mL)
Roll-on (No Pain-HP®): 0.075% (60 mL)

♦ **Capsin® [OTC]** *see* Capsaicin *on page 89*

## Captopril (KAP toe pril)

**Related Information**
Angiotensin-Related Agents Comparison Chart *on page 700*

**U.S. Brand Names** Capoten®

**Canadian Brand Names** Apo®-Capto; Novo-Captopril; Nu-Capto; Syn-Captopril

**Synonyms** ACE

**Pharmacologic Category** Angiotensin-Converting Enzyme (ACE) Inhibitors

**Use** Management of hypertension; treatment of congestive heart failure, left ventricular dysfunction after myocardial infarction, diabetic nephropathy
**Unlabeled use:** Treatment of hypertensive crisis, rheumatoid arthritis; diagnosis of anatomic renal artery stenosis, hypertension secondary to scleroderma renal crisis; diagnosis of aldosteronism, idiopathic edema, Bartter's syndrome, postmyocardial infarction for prevention of ventricular failure; increase circulation in Raynaud's phenomenon, hypertension secondary to Takayasu's disease

**Effects on Mental Status** May cause drowsiness or insomnia

**Effects on Psychiatric Treatment** May rarely cause agranulocytosis; use caution with clozapine and carbamazepine; may decrease lithium clearance resulting in an increase in serum lithium levels and potential lithium toxicity; monitor serum lithium levels

**Pregnancy Risk Factor** C (1st trimester); D (2nd and 3rd trimesters)

**Contraindications** Hypersensitivity to captopril or any component; angioedema related to previous treatment with an ACE inhibitor; primary hyperaldosteronism; patients with idiopathic or hereditary angioedema; bilateral renal artery stenosis; pregnancy (2nd or 3rd trimester)

**Warnings/Precautions** Anaphylactic reactions can occur. Angioedema can occur at any time during treatment (especially following first dose). Careful blood pressure monitoring with first dose (hypotension can occur especially in volume depleted patients). Dosage adjustment needed in renal impairment. Use with caution in hypovolemia; collagen vascular diseases; valvular stenosis (particularly aortic stenosis); hyperkalemia; or before, during, or immediately after anesthesia. Avoid rapid dosage escalation which may lead to renal insufficiency. Neutropenia/agranulocytosis with myeloid hyperplasia can rarely occur. If patient has renal impairment then a baseline WBC with differential and serum creatinine should be evaluated and monitored closely during the first 3 months of therapy. Hypersensitivity reactions may be seen during hemodialysis with high-flux dialysis membranes (eg, AN69). Deterioration in renal function can occur with initiation. Use with caution in unilateral renal artery stenosis and pre-existing renal insufficiency.

**Adverse Reactions**
>1%:
Cardiovascular: Tachycardia, chest pain, palpitations
Central nervous system: Insomnia, headache, dizziness, fatigue, malaise
Dermatologic: Rash (4% to 7%), pruritus, alopecia
Gastrointestinal: Abdominal pain, vomiting, nausea, diarrhea, anorexia, constipation, abnormal taste (2% to 4%), xerostomia
Neuromuscular & skeletal: Paresthesias
Renal: Oliguria
Respiratory: Transient cough (0.5% to 2%)
<1%: Agranulocytosis, angioedema, hyperkalemia, hypotension, increased BUN/serum creatinine, neutropenia, proteinuria

**Overdosage/Toxicology**
Signs and symptoms: Mild hypotension has been the only toxic effect seen with acute overdose; bradycardia may also occur. Hyperkalemia occurs even with therapeutic doses, especially in patients with renal insufficiency and those taking NSAIDs.
Treatment: Following initiation of essential overdose management, toxic symptom treatment and supportive treatment should be initiated. Hypotension usually responds to I.V. fluids or Trendelenburg positioning.

**Drug Interactions** CYP2D6 enzyme substrate
Allopurinol: Case reports (rare) indicate a possible increased risk of Stevens-Johnson syndrome when combined with captopril
Alpha$_1$ blockers: Hypotensive effect increased
Aspirin: The effects of ACE inhibitors may be blunted by aspirin administration, particularly at higher dosages
Diuretics: Hypovolemia due to diuretics may precipitate acute hypotensive events or acute renal failure
Insulin: Risk of hypoglycemia may be increased
Lithium: Risk of lithium toxicity may be increased; monitor lithium levels, especially the first 4 weeks of therapy
Mercaptopurine: Risk of neutropenia may be increased
NSAIDs may decrease ACE inhibitor efficacy and/or increase adverse renal effects
Potassium-sparing diuretics (amiloride, potassium, spironolactone, triamterene): Increased risk of hyperkalemia
Potassium supplements may increase the risk of hyperkalemia
Trimethoprim (high dose) may increase the risk of hyperkalemia

**Usual Dosage Note:** Dosage must be titrated according to patient's response; use lowest effective dose. Oral:
Infants: Initial: 0.15-0.3 mg/kg/dose; titrate dose upward to maximum of 6 mg/kg/day in 1-4 divided doses; usual required dose: 2.5-6 mg/kg/day
Children: Initial: 0.5 mg/kg/dose; titrate upward to maximum of 6 mg/kg/day in 2-4 divided doses
Older Children: Initial: 6.25-12.5 mg/dose every 12-24 hours; titrate upward to maximum of 6 mg/kg/day
Adolescents: Initial: 12.5-25 mg/dose given every 8-12 hours; increase by 25 mg/dose to maximum of 450 mg/day
Adults:
Hypertension:
Initial dose: 12.5-25 mg 2-3 times/day; may increase by 12.5-25 mg/dose at 1- to 2-week intervals up to 50 mg 3 times/day; add diuretic before further dosage increases
Maximum dose: 150 mg 3 times/day
(Continued)

## Captopril *(Continued)*

Congestive heart failure:

Initial dose: 6.25-12.5 mg 3 times/day in conjunction with cardiac glycoside and diuretic therapy; initial dose depends upon patient's fluid/electrolyte status

Target dose: 50 mg 3 times/day

Maximum dose: 150 mg 3 times/day

LVD after MI: Initial dose: 6.25 mg followed by 12.5 mg 3 times/day; then increase to 25 mg 3 times/day during next several days and then over next several weeks to target dose of 50 mg 3 times/day

Diabetic nephropathy: 25 mg 3 times/day; other antihypertensives often given concurrently

**Dosing adjustment in renal impairment:**

$Cl_{cr}$ 10-50 mL/minute: Administer at 75% of normal dose.

$Cl_{cr}$ <10 mL/minute: Administer at 50% of normal dose.

**Note:** Smaller dosages given every 8-12 hours are indicated in patients with renal dysfunction; renal function and leukocyte count should be carefully monitored during therapy.

Hemodialysis: Moderately dialyzable (20% to 50%); administer dose postdialysis or administer 25% to 35% supplemental dose.

Peritoneal dialysis: Supplemental dose is not necessary.

**Patient Information** Take exactly as directed; do not discontinue without consulting prescriber. Take first dose at bedtime. Take all doses on an empty stomach (30 minutes before or 2 hours after meals). This drug does not eliminate need for diet or exercise regimen as recommended by prescriber. Do not use potassium supplements or salt substitutes containing potassium without consulting prescriber. May cause dizziness, fainting, lightheadedness (use caution when driving or engaging in tasks that require alertness until response to drug is known); postural hypotension (use caution when rising from lying or sitting position or climbing stairs); nausea, vomiting, abdominal pain, dry mouth, or transient loss of appetite (small frequent meals, frequent mouth care, sucking lozenges, or chewing gum may help) - report if these persist. Report chest pain or palpitations; mouth sores; fever or chills; swelling of extremities, face, mouth, or tongue; skin rash; numbness, tingling, or pain in muscles; difficulty in breathing or unusual cough; other persistent adverse reactions.

**Nursing Implications** Watch for hypotensive effect within 1-3 hours of first dose or new higher dose

**Dosage Forms** Tablet: 12.5 mg, 25 mg, 50 mg, 100 mg

## Captopril and Hydrochlorothiazide

(KAP toe pril & hye droe klor oh THYE a zide)

**U.S. Brand Names** Capozide®

**Pharmacologic Category** Antihypertensive Agent, Combination

**Use** Management of hypertension and treatment of congestive heart failure

**Effects on Mental Status** May cause drowsiness or insomnia

**Effects on Psychiatric Treatment** May rarely cause agranulocytosis; use caution with clozapine and carbamazepine; may decrease lithium clearance resulting in an increase in serum lithium levels and potential lithium toxicity; monitor serum lithium levels

**Usual Dosage** Adults: Oral: Hypertension: Initial: 25 mg 2-3 times/day (captopril dose)

**Dosage Forms** Tablet:

25/15: Captopril 25 mg and hydrochlorothiazide 15 mg

25/25: Captopril 25 mg and hydrochlorothiazide 25 mg

50/15: Captopril 50 mg and hydrochlorothiazide 15 mg

50/25: Captopril 50 mg and hydrochlorothiazide 25 mg

♦ **Capzasin-P® [OTC]** *see* Capsaicin *on page 89*

♦ **Carafate®** *see* Sucralfate *on page 521*

## Caramiphen and Phenylpropanolamine

(kar AM i fen & fen il proe pa NOLE a meen)

**U.S. Brand Names** Detuss®; Ordrine AT® Extended Release Capsule; Rescaps-D® S.R. Capsule; Tuss-Allergine® Modified T.D. Capsule; Tuss-Genade® Modified Capsule; Tussogest® Extended Release Capsule

**Pharmacologic Category** Antihistamine

**Use** Symptomatic relief of cough and nasal congestion associated with the common cold

**Effects on Mental Status** May cause restlessness or insomnia

**Effects on Psychiatric Treatment** Contraindicated with concurrent MAOI therapy

**Usual Dosage** Oral:

Children:

2-6 years: ½ teaspoonful every 4 hours

6-12 years: 1 teaspoonful every 4 hours

Children >12 years and Adults: 1 capsule every 12 hours or 2 teaspoonfuls every 4 hours

**Dosage Forms**

Capsule, timed release: Caramiphen edisylate 40 mg and phenylpropanolamine hydrochloride 75 mg

Liquid: Caramiphen edisylate 6.7 mg and phenylpropanolamine hydrochloride 12.5 mg per 5 mL

## Carbachol (KAR ba kole)

**Related Information**

Glaucoma Drug Therapy *on page 712*

**U.S. Brand Names** Carbastat® Ophthalmic; Carboptic® Ophthalmic; Isopto® Carbachol Ophthalmic; Miostat® Intraocular

**Pharmacologic Category** Cholinergic Agonist; Ophthalmic Agent, Antiglaucoma; Ophthalmic Agent, Miotic

**Use** Lowers intraocular pressure in the treatment of glaucoma; cause miosis during surgery

**Effects on Mental Status** None reported

**Effects on Psychiatric Treatment** None reported

**Usual Dosage** Adults:

Ophthalmic: Instill 1-2 drops up to 3 times/day

Intraocular: 0.5 mL instilled into anterior chamber before or after securing sutures

**Dosage Forms** Solution:

Intraocular (Carbastat®, Miostat®): 0.01% (1.5 mL)

Topical, ophthalmic:

Carboptic®: 3% (15 mL)

Isopto® Carbachol: 0.75% (15 mL, 30 mL); 1.5% (15 mL, 30 mL); 2.25% (15 mL); 3% (15 mL, 30 mL)

## Carbamazepine (kar ba MAZ e peen)

**Related Information**

Anticonvulsants by Seizures Type *on page 703*
Anxiety Disorders *on page 606*
Clinical Issues in the Use of Mood Stabilizers *on page 632*
Epilepsy Treatment *on page 783*
Impulse Control Disorders *on page 622*
Liquid Compatibility With Antipsychotics and Mood Stabilizers *on page 718*
Mood Disorders *on page 600*
Mood Stabilizers *on page 719*
Patient Information - Mood Stabilizers (Carbamazepine) *on page 651*
Personality Disorders *on page 625*
Secondary Mental Disorders *on page 616*
Serum Drug Concentrations Commonly Monitored: Guidelines *on page 759*
Special Populations - Children and Adolescents *on page 663*
Special Populations - Elderly *on page 662*
Special Populations - Mentally Retarded Patients *on page 665*
Special Populations - Pregnant and Breast-Feeding Patients *on page 668*
Teratogenic Risks of Psychotropic Medications *on page 812*

**Generic Available** Yes: Tablet

**U.S. Brand Names** Epitol®; Tegretol®; Tegretol®-XR

**Canadian Brand Names** Apo®-Carbamazepine; Mazepine®; Novo-Carbamaz; Nu-Carbamazepine; PMS-Carbamazepine

**Synonyms** CBZ

**Pharmacologic Category** Anticonvulsant, Miscellaneous

**Use**

Epilepsy:

Partial seizures with complex symptomatology (psychomotor, temporal lobe)

Generalized tonic-clonic seizures (grand mal)

Mixed seizure patterns

Pain relief of trigeminal neuralgia

**Unlabeled use:** Treat bipolar disorders and other affective disorders, resistant schizophrenia, alcohol withdrawal, restless leg syndrome, psychotic behavior associated with dementia, post-traumatic stress disorders

**Pregnancy Risk Factor** D

**Pregnancy/Breast-Feeding Implications**

Clinical effects on the fetus: Crosses the placenta. Dysmorphic facial features, cranial defects, cardiac defects, spina bifida, intrauterine growth retardation, and multiple other malformations reported. Epilepsy itself, number of medications, genetic factors, or a combination of these probably influence the teratogenicity of anticonvulsant therapy.

Breast-feeding/lactation: Crosses into breast milk. American Academy of Pediatrics considers **compatible** with breast-feeding.

**Contraindications** Hypersensitivity to carbamazepine or any component; may have cross-sensitivity with tricyclic antidepressants; marrow depression; MAO inhibitor use; pregnancy (may harm fetus)

**Warnings/Precautions** MAO inhibitors should be discontinued for a minimum of 14 days before carbamazepine is begun; administer with caution to patients with history of cardiac damage or hepatic disease; potentially fatal blood cell abnormalities have been reported following treatment; early detection of hematologic change is important; advise patients of early signs and symptoms including fever, sore throat, mouth ulcers, infections, easy bruising, petechial or purpuric hemorrhage; carbamazepine is not effective in absence, myoclonic or akinetic seizures; exacerbation of certain seizure types have been seen after initiation of carbamazepine therapy in children with mixed seizure disorders. Elderly may have increased risk of SIADH-like syndrome.

**Adverse Reactions**

Cardiovascular: Edema, congestive heart failure, syncope, bradycardia, hypertension or hypotension, A-V block, arrhythmias, thrombophlebitis, thromboembolism, lymphadenopathy

Central nervous system: Sedation, dizziness, fatigue, ataxia, confusion, headache, slurred speech

Dermatologic: Rash, urticaria, toxic epidermal necrolysis, Stevens-Johnson syndrome, photosensitivity reaction, alterations in skin pigmentation, exfoliative dermatitis, erythema multiforme, purpura, alopecia

Endocrine & metabolic: Hyponatremia, SIADH, fever, chills

Gastrointestinal: Nausea, vomiting, gastric distress, abdominal pain, diarrhea, constipation, anorexia, pancreatitis

Genitourinary: Urinary retention, urinary frequency, azotemia, renal failure, impotence

Hematologic: Aplastic anemia, agranulocytosis, eosinophilia, leukopenia, pancytopenia, thrombocytopenia, bone marrow suppression, acute intermittent porphyria, leukocytosis

Hepatic: Hepatitis, abnormal liver function tests, jaundice, hepatic failure

Neuromuscular & skeletal: Peripheral neuritis

Ocular: Blurred vision, nystagmus, lens opacities, conjunctivitis

Otic: Tinnitus, hyperacusis

Miscellaneous: Hypersensitivity, diaphoresis

**Overdosage/Toxicology** Lowest known lethal dose: Adults: 3.2 g; children: 4 g and 1.6 g

Signs and symptoms: Dizziness, ataxia, drowsiness, nausea, vomiting, tremor, agitation, nystagmus, urinary retention, dysrhythmias, coma

Treatment: Activated charcoal is effective at binding certain chemicals and this is especially true for carbamazepine; other treatment is supportive/symptomatic

**Drug Interactions** CYP2C8 and 3A3/4 enzyme substrate; CYP1A2, 2C, and 3A3/4 inducer

**Note:** Carbamazepine (CBZ) is a heteroinducer. It induces its own metabolism as well as the metabolism of other drugs. If CBZ is added to a drug regimen, serum concentrations may decrease. Conversely, if CBZ is part of an ongoing regimen and it is discontinued, elevated concentrations of the other drugs may result.

Acetaminophen: Carbamazepine may enhance hepatotoxic potential of acetaminophen; risk is greater in acetaminophen overdose

Antipsychotics: Carbamazepine may enhance the metabolism (decrease the efficacy) of antipsychotics; monitor for altered response; dose adjustment may be needed

Barbiturates: May reduce serum concentrations of carbamazepine; monitor

Benzodiazepines: Serum concentrations and effect of benzodiazepines may be reduced by carbamazepine; monitor for decreased effect

Calcium channel blockers: Diltiazem and verapamil may increase carbamazepine levels, due to enzyme inhibition (see below); other calcium channel blockers (felodipine) may be decreased by carbamazepine due to enzyme induction

Corticosteroids: Metabolism may be increased by carbamazepine

Cyclosporine (and other immunosuppressants): Carbamazepine may enhance the metabolism of immunosuppressants, decreasing its clinical effect; includes both cyclosporine and tacrolimus

CYP2C8/9 inhibitors: Serum levels and/or toxicity of carbamazepine may be increased; inhibitors include amiodarone, cimetidine, fluvoxamine, some NSAIDs, metronidazole, ritonavir, sulfonamides, troglitazone, valproic acid, and zafirlukast; monitor for increased effect/toxicity

CYP3A3/4 inhibitors: Serum level and/or toxicity of carbamazepine may be increased; inhibitors include amiodarone, cimetidine, clarithromycin, erythromycin, delavirdine, diltiazem, dirithromycin, disulfiram, fluoxetine, fluvoxamine, grapefruit juice, indinavir, itraconazole, ketoconazole, metronidazole, nefazodone, nevirapine, propoxyfene, quinine, quinupristin-dalfopristin, ritonavir, saquinavir, ticlopidine, verapamil, zafirlukast, zileuton; monitor for altered effects; a decrease in carbamazepine dosage may be required

Danazol: May increase serum concentrations of carbamazepine; monitor

Doxycycline: Carbamazepine may enhance the metabolism of doxycycline, decreasing its clinical effect

Ethosuximide: Serum levels may be reduced by carbamazepine

Felbamate: May increase carbamazepine levels and toxicity (increased epoxide metabolite concentrations); carbamazepine may decrease felbamate levels due to enzyme induction

Immunosuppressants: Carbamazepine may enhance the metabolism of immunosuppressants, decreasing its clinical effect; includes both cyclosporine and tacrolimus

Isoniazid: May increase the serum concentrations and toxicity of carbamazepine; in addition, carbamazepine may increase the hepatic toxicity of isoniazid (INH)

Isotretinoin: May decrease the effect of carbamazepine

Lamotrigine: Increases the epoxide metabolite of carbamazepine resulting in toxicity; carbamazepine increases the metabolism of lamotrigine

Lithium: Neurotoxicity may result in patients receiving concurrent carbamazepine

Loxapine: May increase concentrations of epoxide metabolite and toxicity of carbamazepine

Methadone: Carbamazepine may enhance the metabolism of methadone resulting in methadone withdrawal

Methylphenidate: concurrent use of carbamazepine may reduce the therapeutic effect of methylphenidate; limited documentation; monitor for decreased effect

Neuromuscular blocking agents, nondepolarizing: Effects may be of shorter duration when administered to patients receiving carbamazepine

Oral contraceptives: Metabolism may be increased by carbamazepine, resulting in a loss of efficacy

Phenytoin: Carbamazepine levels may be decreased by phenytoin; metabolism may be altered by carbamazepine

SSRIs: Metabolism may be increased by carbamazepine (due to enzyme induction)

Theophylline: Serum levels may be reduced by carbamazepine

Thioridazine: Note: Carbamazepine suspension is incompatible with chlorpromazine solution and thioridazine liquid. Schedule carbamazepine suspension at least 1-2 hours apart from other liquid medicinals.

Thyroid: Serum levels may be reduced by carbamazepine

Tricyclic antidepressants: May increase serum concentrations of carbamazepine; carbamazepine may decrease concentrations of tricyclics due to enzyme induction

Valproic acid: Serum levels may be reduced by carbamazepine; carbamazepine levels may also be altered by valproic acid

Warfarin: Carbamazepine may inhibit the hypoprothrombinemic effects of oral anticoagulants via increased metabolism; this combination should generally be avoided

**Mechanism of Action** In addition to anticonvulsant effects, carbamazepine has anticholinergic, antineuralgic, antidiuretic, muscle relaxant and antiarrhythmic properties; may depress activity in the nucleus ventralis of the thalamus or decrease synaptic transmission or decrease summation of temporal stimulation leading to neural discharge by limiting influx of sodium ions across cell membrane or other unknown mechanisms; stimulates the release of ADH and potentiates its action in promoting reabsorption of water; chemically related to tricyclic antidepressants

**Pharmacodynamics/kinetics**

Absorption: Slowly absorbed from GI tract

Distribution: $V_d$:
- Neonates: 1.5 L/kg
- Children: 1.9 L/kg
- Adults: 0.59-2 L/kg

Protein binding: 75% to 90%; may be decreased in newborns

Metabolism: In the liver to active epoxide metabolite; induces liver enzymes to increase metabolism and shorten half-life over time

Bioavailability, oral: 85%

Half-life:
- Initial: 18-55 hours
- Multiple dosing:
  - Children: 8-14 hours
  - Adults: 12-17 hours

Time to peak serum concentration: Unpredictable, within 4-8 hours

Elimination: 1% to 3% excreted unchanged in urine

**Usual Dosage** Oral (dosage must be adjusted according to patient's response and serum concentrations):

Children:
- <6 years: Initial: 5 mg/kg/day; dosage may be increased every 5-7 days to 10 mg/kg/day; then up to 20 mg/kg/day if necessary; administer in 2-4 divided doses/day
- 6-12 years: Initial: 100 mg twice daily or 10 mg/kg/day in 2 divided doses; increase by 100 mg/day at weekly intervals depending upon response; usual maintenance: 20-30 mg/kg/day in 2-4 divided doses/day; maximum dose: 1000 mg/day

Children >12 years and Adults: 200 mg twice daily to start, increase by 200 mg/day at weekly intervals until therapeutic levels achieved; usual dose: 800-1200 mg/day in 3-4 divided doses; some patients have required up to 1.6-2.4 g/day

Trigeminal or glossopharyngeal neuralgia: Initial: 100 mg twice daily with food, gradually increasing in increments of 100 mg twice daily as needed usual maintenance: 400-800 mg daily in 2 divided doses

**Dosing adjustment in renal impairment:** $Cl_{cr}$ <10 mL/minute: Administer 75% of dose

**Dietary Considerations**

Food: Drug may cause GI upset, take with large amount of water or food to decrease GI upset. May need to split doses to avoid GI upset.

Sodium: SIADH and water intoxication; monitor fluid status; may need to restrict fluid

**Administration** May administer the suspension rectally if patient is NPO. XR tablet coating is not absorbed and is excreted in the feces; these coatings may be noticeable in the stool

**Monitoring Parameters** CBC with platelet count, liver function tests, serum drug concentration; observe patient for excessive sedation especially when instituting or increasing therapy

(Continued)

## Carbamazepine *(Continued)*

**Reference Range** Therapeutic: 6-12 μg/mL (SI: 25-51 μmol/L). Patients who require higher levels (8-12 μg/mL (SI: 34-51 μmol/L)) should be watched closely. Side effects including CNS effects occur commonly at higher dosage levels. If other anticonvulsants are given, therapeutic range is 4-8 μg/mL (SI: 17-34 μmol/L).

**Test Interactions** ↑ BUN, AST, ALT, bilirubin, alkaline phosphatase (S); ↓ calcium, $T_3$, $T_4$, sodium (S)

**Patient Information** Take with food, may cause drowsiness, periodic blood test monitoring required; notify physician if you observe bleeding, bruising, jaundice, abdominal pain, pale stools, mental disturbances, fever, chills, sore throat, or mouth ulcers

**Nursing Implications** Observe patient for excessive sedation; suspension dosage form must be given on a 3-4 times/day schedule versus tablets which can be given 2-4 times/day

**Additional Information** Suspension dosage should be given on a 3-4 times/day schedule vs tablet which can be given 2-4 times/day; carbamazepine is not effective in absence, myoclonic or akinetic seizures; exacerbation of certain seizure types have been seen after initiation of carbamazepine therapy in children with mixed seizure disorders

Investigationally, loading doses of the suspension (10 mg/kg for children <12 years of age and 8 mg/kg for children >12 years of age) were given (via NG or ND tubes followed by 5-10 mL of water to flush through tube) to PICU patients with frequent seizures/status; 5 of 6 patients attained mean Cp of 4.3 mcg/mL and 7.3 mcg/mL at 1 and 2 hours postload; concurrent enteral feeding or ileus may delay absorption

**Dosage Forms**
- Suspension, oral (citrus-vanilla flavor): 100 mg/5 mL (450 mL)
- Tablet: 200 mg
- Tablet, chewable: 100 mg
- Tablet, extended release: 100 mg, 200 mg, 400 mg

♦ **Carbamide** *see* Urea *on page 576*

## Carbamide Peroxide (KAR ba mide per OKS ide)

**U.S. Brand Names** Auro® Ear Drops [OTC]; Debrox® Otic [OTC]; E•R•O Ear [OTC]; Gly-Oxide® Oral [OTC]; Mollifene® Ear Wax Removing Formula [OTC]; Murine® Ear Drops [OTC]; Orajel® Perioseptic [OTC]; Proxigel® Oral [OTC]

**Canadian Brand Names** Clamurid®

**Pharmacologic Category** Otic Agent, Cerumenolytic

**Use** Relief of minor inflammation of gums, oral mucosal surfaces and lips including canker sores and dental irritation; emulsify and disperse ear wax

**Effects on Mental Status** None reported

**Effects on Psychiatric Treatment** None reported

**Usual Dosage** Children and Adults:

Gel: Gently massage on affected area 4 times/day; do not drink or rinse mouth for 5 minutes after use

Oral solution (should not be used for >7 days): Oral preparation should not be used in children <3 years of age; apply several drops undiluted on affected area 4 times/day after meals and at bedtime; expectorate after 2-3 minutes **or** place 10 drops onto tongue, mix with saliva, swish for several minutes, expectorate

Otic:

Children <12 years: Tilt head sideways and individualize the dose according to patient size; 3 drops (range: 1-5 drops) twice daily for up to 4 days, tip of applicator should not enter ear canal; keep drops in ear for several minutes by keeping head tilted and placing cotton in ear

Children ≥12 years and Adults: Tilt head sideways and instill 5-10 drops twice daily up to 4 days, tip of applicator should not enter ear canal; keep drops in ear for several minutes by keeping head tilted and placing cotton in ear

**Dosage Forms**

Gel, oral (Proxigel®): 10% (34 g)

Solution:

Oral:
- Gly-Oxide®: 10% in glycerin (15 mL, 60 mL)
- Orajel® Perioseptic: 15% in glycerin (13.3 mL)

Otic (Auro® Ear Drops, Debrox®, Mollifene® Ear Wax Removing, Murine® Ear Drops): 6.5% in glycerin (15 mL, 30 mL)

♦ **Carbastat® Ophthalmic** *see* Carbachol *on page 90*

## Carbenicillin (kar ben i SIL in)

**U.S. Brand Names** Geocillin®

**Canadian Brand Names** Geopen®

**Pharmacologic Category** Antibiotic, Penicillin

**Use** Treatment of serious urinary tract infections and prostatitis caused by susceptible gram-negative aerobic bacilli

**Effects on Mental Status** Penicillins have been reported to cause apprehension, illusions, agitation, insomnia, depersonalization, and encephalopathy

**Effects on Psychiatric Treatment** Rare reports of leukopenia and neutropenia; use caution with clozapine and carbamazepine

**Usual Dosage** Oral:

Children: 30-50 mg/kg/day divided every 6 hours; maximum dose: 2-3 g/day

Adults: 1-2 tablets every 6 hours for urinary tract infections or 2 tablets every 6 hours for prostatitis

**Dosing interval in renal impairment:** Adults:
- $Cl_{cr}$ 10-50 mL/minute: Administer 382-764 mg every 12-24 hours
- $Cl_{cr}$ <10 mL/minute: Administer 382-764 mg every 24-48 hours

Moderately dialyzable (20% to 50%)

**Dosage Forms** Tablet, film coated: 382 mg

♦ **Carbidopa and Levodopa** *see* Levodopa and Carbidopa *on page 313*

## Carbinoxamine (kar bi NOKS a meen)

**U.S. Brand Names** Allergefon®; Andec®; Carbodec®; Chemdec®; Clistin®; Humex®; Lergefin®; Naldecol®; Polistine®; Rondec®; Toscal®; Tussafed®; Tylex; Ziriton®

**Pharmacologic Category** Antihistamine

**Use** Allergic rhinitis

**Effects on Mental Status** May cause drowsiness

**Effects on Psychiatric Treatment** Concurrent use with TCAs and barbiturates may produce additive sedation; concurrent use with MAOI may prolong anticholinergic effects of carbinoxamine

**Usual Dosage**
- Children: 0.2-0.4 mg/kg/day
- Adults: 4-8 mg given 3 or 4 times/day

**Dosage Forms**
- Syrup, as maleate: 2 mg/5 mL
- Tablet, as maleate: 4 mg, 8 mg, 12 mg

## Carbinoxamine and Pseudoephedrine
(kar bi NOKS a meen & soo doe e FED rin)

**U.S. Brand Names** Biohist-LA®; Carbiset® Tablet; Carbiset-TR® Tablet; Carbodec® Syrup; Carbodec® Tablet; Carbodec® TR Tablet; Cardec-S® Syrup; Rondec® Drops; Rondec® Filmtab®; Rondec® Syrup; Rondec-TR®

**Pharmacologic Category** Adrenergic Agonist Agent; Antihistamine, $H_1$ Blocker; Decongestant

**Use** Temporary relief of nasal congestion, running nose, sneezing, itching of nose or throat, and itchy, watery eyes due to the common cold, hay fever, or other respiratory allergies

**Effects on Mental Status** Drowsiness is common; may cause fatigue, nervousness, or dizziness; may rarely produce depression

**Effects on Psychiatric Treatment** Contraindicated with MAOIs; concurrent use with sedating psychotropics or CNS depressants may produce additive adverse effects

**Usual Dosage** Oral:

Children:

Drops: 1-18 months: 0.25-1 mL 4 times/day

Syrup:
- 18 months to 6 years: 2.5 mL 3-4 times/day
- >6 years: 5 mL 2-4 times/day

Adults:
- Liquid: 5 mL 4 times/day
- Tablets: 1 tablet 4 times/day

**Dosage Forms**

Drops: Carbinoxamine maleate 2 mg and pseudoephedrine hydrochloride 25 mg per mL (30 mL with dropper)

Syrup: Carbinoxamine maleate 4 mg and pseudoephedrine hydrochloride 60 mg per 5 mL (120 mL, 480 mL)

Tablet:
- Film-coated: Carbinoxamine maleate 4 mg and pseudoephedrine hydrochloride 60 mg
- Extended release: Carbinoxamine maleate 8 mg and pseudoephedrine hydrochloride 90 mg
- Sustained release: Carbinoxamine maleate 8 mg and pseudoephedrine hydrochloride 120 mg

## Carbinoxamine, Pseudoephedrine, and Dextromethorphan
(kar bi NOKS a meen, soo doe e FED rin, & deks troe meth OR fan)

**U.S. Brand Names** Carbodec DM®; Cardec DM®; Pseudo-Car® DM; Rondamine-DM® Drops; Rondec®-DM; Tussafed® Drops

**Pharmacologic Category** Antihistamine/Decongestant/Antitussive

**Use** Relief of coughs and upper respiratory symptoms, including nasal congestion, associated with allergy or the common cold

**Effects on Mental Status** Drowsiness is common; may cause fatigue, nervousness, or dizziness; may rarely produce depression

**Effects on Psychiatric Treatment** Contraindicated with MAOIs; concurrent use with sedating psychotropics or CNS depressants may produce additive adverse effects

**Usual Dosage**

Infants: Drops:

1-3 months: 1/4 mL 4 times/day

3-6 months: 1/2 mL 4 times/day

6-9 months: 3/4 mL 4 times/day

9-18 months: 1 mL 4 times/day

Children 1 1/2 to 6 years: Syrup: 2.5 mL 4 times/day

Children >6 years and Adults: Syrup: 5 mL 4 times/day

**Dosage Forms**

Drops: Carbinoxamine maleate 2 mg, pseudoephedrine hydrochloride 25 mg, and dextromethorphan hydrobromide 4 mg per mL (30 mL)

Syrup: Carbinoxamine maleate 4 mg, pseudoephedrine hydrochloride 60 mg, and dextromethorphan hydrobromide 15 mg per 5 mL (120 mL, 480 mL, 4000 mL)

- **Carbiset® Tablet** *see* Carbinoxamine and Pseudoephedrine *on page 92*
- **Carbiset-TR® Tablet** *see* Carbinoxamine and Pseudoephedrine *on page 92*
- **Carbocaine®** *see* Mepivacaine *on page 342*
- **Carbodec®** *see* Carbinoxamine *on page 92*
- **Carbodec DM®** *see* Carbinoxamine, Pseudoephedrine, and Dextromethorphan *on page 92*
- **Carbodec® Syrup** *see* Carbinoxamine and Pseudoephedrine *on page 92*
- **Carbodec® Tablet** *see* Carbinoxamine and Pseudoephedrine *on page 92*
- **Carbodec® TR Tablet** *see* Carbinoxamine and Pseudoephedrine *on page 92*

## Carbol-Fuchsin Solution (kar bol-FOOK sin soe LOO shun)

**Pharmacologic Category** Antifungal Agent, Topical

**Use** Treatment of superficial mycotic infections

**Effects on Mental Status** None reported

**Effects on Psychiatric Treatment** None reported

**Usual Dosage** Apply to affected area 2-4 times/day

**Dosage Forms** Solution: Basic fuchsin 0.3%, boric acid 1%, phenol 4.5%, resorcinol 10%, acetone 5%, and alcohol 10%

## Carboplatin (KAR boe pla tin)

**U.S. Brand Names** Paraplatin®

**Pharmacologic Category** Antineoplastic Agent, Alkylating Agent

**Use** Ovarian carcinoma, cervical, small cell lung carcinoma, esophageal, testicular, bladder cancer, mesothelioma, pediatric brain tumors, sarcoma, neuroblastoma, osteosarcoma

**Effects on Mental Status** None reported

**Effects on Psychiatric Treatment** May cause myelosuppression; use caution with clozapine and carbamazepine

**Usual Dosage** IVPB, I.V. infusion, intraperitoneal (refer to individual protocols):

Children:

Solid tumor: 300-600 mg/m² once every 4 weeks

Brain tumor: 175 mg/m² once weekly for 4 weeks with a 2-week recovery period between courses; dose is then adjusted on platelet count and neutrophil count values

Adults:

Ovarian cancer: Usual doses range from 360 mg/m² I.V. every 3 weeks single agent therapy to 300 mg/m² every 4 weeks as combination therapy

In general, however, single intermittent courses of carboplatin should not be repeated until the neutrophil count is at least 2000 and the platelet count is at least 100,000

The following dose adjustments are modified from a controlled trial in previously treated patients with ovarian carcinoma. Blood counts were done weekly, and the recommendations are based on the lowest post-treatment platelet or neutrophil value.

**Carboplatin dosage adjustment based on pretreatment platelet counts**

- Platelets >100,00 cells/mm³ and neutrophils >2000 cells/mm³: Adjust dose 125% from prior course
- Platelets 50-100,000 cells/mm³ and neutrophils 500-2000 cells/mm³: No dose adjustment
- Platelets <50,000 cells/mm³ and neutrophils <500 cells/mm³: Adjust dose 75% from prior course

**Carboplatin dosage adjustment based on the Egorin formula** (based on platelet counts):

Previously untreated patients:

$$\text{dosage (mg/m}^2\text{)} = (0.091)\frac{(Cl_{cr})}{(BSA)}\frac{(\text{Pretreat Plt count - Plt nadir count desired} \times 100)}{(\text{Pretreatment Plt count})} + 86$$

Previously treated patients with heavily myelosuppressive agents:

$$\text{dosage (mg/m}^2\text{)} = (0.091)\frac{(Cl_{cr})}{(BSA)}\frac{[(\text{Pretreat Plt count - Plt nadir count desired} \times 100) - 17]}{(\text{Pretreatment Plt count})} + 86$$

Autologous BMT: I.V.: 1600 mg/m² (total dose) divided over 4 days **requires BMT (ie, FATAL without BMT)**

**Dosing adjustment in hepatic impairment:** There are no published studies available on the dosing of carboplatin in patients with impaired liver function. Human data regarding the biliary elimination of carboplatin are not available; however, pharmacokinetic studies in rabbits and rats reflect a biliary excretion of 0.4% to 0.7% of the dose (ie, 0.05 mL/minute/kg biliary clearance).

**Dosing adjustment in renal impairment:** These dosing recommendations apply to the initial course of treatment. Subsequent dosages should be adjusted according to the patient's tolerance based on the degree of bone marrow suppression.

$Cl_{cr}$ <60 mL/minute: Increased risk of severe bone marrow suppression. In renally impaired patients who received single agent carboplatin therapy, the incidence of severe leukopenia, neutropenia, or thrombocytopenia has been about 25% when the following dosage modifications have been used:

$Cl_{cr}$ 41-59 mL/minute: Recommended dose on day 1 is 250 mg/m²

$Cl_{cr}$ 16-40 mL/minute: Recommended dose on day 1 is 200 mg/m²

$Cl_{cr}$ <15 mL/minute: The data available for patients with severely impaired kidney function are too limited to permit a recommendation for treatment

**or**

**Dosing adjustment in renal impairment: CALVERT FORMULA**

**Total dose (mg) = Target AUC (mg/mL/minute) x (GFR [mL/minute] + 25)**

**Note: The dose of carboplatin calculated is TOTAL mg DOSE not** mg/m². AUC is the area under the concentration versus time curve.

Target AUC value will vary depending upon:

Number of agents in the regimen

Treatment status (ie, previously untreated or treated)

For single agent carboplatin/no prior chemotherapy: Total dose (mg): 6-8 (GFR + 25)

For single agent carboplatin/prior chemotherapy: Total dose (mg): 4-6 (GFR + 25)

For combination chemotherapy/no prior chemotherapy: Total dose (mg): 4.5-6 (GFR + 25)

For combination chemotherapy/prior chemotherapy: A reasonable approach for these patients would be to use a target AUC value <5 for the initial cycle

**Note:** The Jelliffe formula (below) substantially underestimates the creatinine clearance in patients with a serum creatinine <1.5 mg/dL. However, the Jelliffe formula is more accurate in estimating creatinine clearance in patients with significant renal impairment than the Cockroft and Gault formula.

$Cl_{cr}$ (mL/minute/1.73 m²) for males = 98 - [(0.8) (Age - 20)]/$S_{cr}$

$Cl_{cr}$ (mL/minute/1.73 m²) for females = 98 - [(0.8) (Age - 20)]/$S_{cr}$ multiplied by 90%

Intraperitoneal: 200-650 mg/m² in 2 L of dialysis fluid have been administered into the peritoneum of ovarian cancer patients

**Dosage Forms** Powder for injection, lyophilized: 50 mg, 150 mg, 450 mg

## Carboprost Tromethamine (KAR boe prost tro METH a meen)

**U.S. Brand Names** Hemabate™

**Pharmacologic Category** Abortifacient; Prostaglandin

**Use** Termination of pregnancy and refractory postpartum uterine bleeding

**Unlabeled use:** Hemorrhagic cystitis

**Effects on Mental Status** May cause drowsiness or nervousness; rare reports of dystonia

**Effects on Psychiatric Treatment** None reported

**Pregnancy Risk Factor** X

**Contraindications** Hypersensitivity to carboprost tromethamine or any component; acute pelvic inflammatory disease; pregnancy

**Warnings/Precautions** Use with caution in patients with history of asthma, hypotension or hypertension, cardiovascular, adrenal, renal or hepatic disease, anemia, jaundice, diabetes, epilepsy or compromised uteri

**Adverse Reactions**

>10%: Gastrointestinal: Nausea (33%)

1% to 10%: Cardiovascular: Flushing (7%)

<1%: Abnormal taste, asthma, bladder spasms, blurred vision, breast tenderness, coughing, diarrhea, drowsiness, dystonia, fever, headache, (Continued)

## Carboprost Tromethamine *(Continued)*

hematemesis, hiccups, hypertension, hypotension, myalgia, nervousness, respiratory distress, septic shock, vasovagal syndrome, vertigo, vomiting, xerostomia

**Drug Interactions** Increased toxicity: Oxytocic agents

**Usual Dosage** Adults: I.M.:

Abortion: Initial: 250 mcg, then 250 mcg at 1½-hour to 3½-hour intervals depending on uterine response; a 500 mcg dose may be given if uterine response is not adequate after several 250 mcg doses; do not exceed 12 mg total dose or continuous administration for >2 days

Refractory postpartum uterine bleeding: Initial: 250 mcg; may repeat at 15- to 90-minute intervals to a total dose of 2 mg

Bladder irrigation for hemorrhagic cystitis (refer to individual protocols): [0.4-1.0 mg/dL as solution] 50 mL instilled into bladder 4 times/day for 1 hour

**Patient Information** This medication is used to stimulate expulsion of uterine contents (fetal tissue) or stimulate uterine contractions to reduce uterine bleeding. Report increased blood loss, acute abdominal cramping, persistent elevation of temperature, foul-smelling vaginal discharge. Increased temperature (elevated temperature) may occur 1-16 hours after therapy and last for several hours.

**Dosage Forms** Injection: Carboprost 250 mcg and tromethamine 83 mcg per mL (1 mL)

♦ **Carboptic® Ophthalmic** *see* Carbachol *on page 90*

## Carboxymethylcellulose (kar boks ee meth il SEL yoo lose)

**U.S. Brand Names** Cellufresh™ [OTC]; Celluvisc® [OTC]

**Pharmacologic Category** Ophthalmic Agent, Miscellaneous

**Use** Preservative-free artificial tear substitute

**Effects on Mental Status** None reported

**Effects on Psychiatric Treatment** None reported

**Usual Dosage** Adults: Ophthalmic: Instill 1-2 drops into eye(s) 3-4 times/day

**Dosage Forms** Solution, ophthalmic, as sodium, preservative free: 0.5% (0.3 mL); 1% (0.3 mL)

♦ **Cardec DM®** *see* Carbinoxamine, Pseudoephedrine, and Dextromethorphan *on page 92*

♦ **Cardec-S® Syrup** *see* Carbinoxamine and Pseudoephedrine *on page 92*

♦ **Cardene®** *see* Nicardipine *on page 391*

♦ **Cardene® SR** *see* Nicardipine *on page 391*

♦ **Cardilate®** *see* Erythrityl Tetranitrate *on page 200*

♦ **Cardioquin®** *see* Quinidine *on page 485*

♦ **Cardizem® CD** *see* Diltiazem *on page 172*

♦ **Cardizem® Injectable** *see* Diltiazem *on page 172*

♦ **Cardizem® SR** *see* Diltiazem *on page 172*

♦ **Cardizem® Tablet** *see* Diltiazem *on page 172*

♦ **Cardura®** *see* Doxazosin *on page 183*

♦ **Carisoprodate** *see* Carisoprodol *on page 94*

## Carisoprodol (kar i soe PROE dole)

**U.S. Brand Names** Soma®

**Synonyms** Carisoprodate; Isobamate

**Pharmacologic Category** Skeletal Muscle Relaxant

**Use** Skeletal muscle relaxant

**Effects on Mental Status** Drowsiness is common; may produce depression or paradoxical CNS stimulation

**Effects on Psychiatric Treatment** Rarely may cause leukopenia or aplastic anemia; use caution with clozapine and carbamazepine; concurrent use with psychotropics may produce additive sedation

**Pregnancy Risk Factor** C

**Contraindications** Acute intermittent porphyria, hypersensitivity to carisoprodol, meprobamate or any component

**Warnings/Precautions** Use with caution in renal and hepatic dysfunction

**Adverse Reactions**

>10%: Central nervous system: Drowsiness

1% to 10%:

Cardiovascular: Tachycardia, tightness in chest, flushing of face, syncope

Central nervous system: Mental depression, allergic fever, dizziness, lightheadedness, headache, paradoxical CNS stimulation

Dermatologic: Angioedema

Gastrointestinal: Nausea, vomiting, stomach cramps

Neuromuscular & skeletal: Trembling

Ocular: Burning eyes

Respiratory: Shortness of breath

Miscellaneous: Hiccups

<1%: Aplastic anemia, ataxia, blurred vision, eosinophilia, erythema multiforme, leukopenia, rash, urticaria

**Overdosage/Toxicology**

Signs and symptoms: CNS depression, stupor, coma, shock, respiratory depression

Treatment: Supportive following attempts to enhance drug elimination. Hypotension should be treated with I.V. fluids and/or Trendelenburg positioning.

**Drug Interactions** CYP2C19 enzyme substrate

Increased toxicity: Alcohol, CNS depressants, phenothiazines

**Usual Dosage** Adults: Oral: 350 mg 3-4 times/day; take last dose at bedtime; compound: 1-2 tablets 4 times/day

**Dietary Considerations** Alcohol: Additive CNS effects, avoid use

**Patient Information** Take exactly as directed with food. Do not increase dose or discontinue without consulting prescriber. Do not use alcohol, prescriptive or OTC antidepressants, sedatives, and pain medications without consulting prescriber. You may experience drowsiness, dizziness, lightheadedness (avoid driving or engaging in tasks requiring alertness until response to drug is known); nausea, vomiting, or cramping (small, frequent meals, frequent mouth care, or sucking hard candy may help); or postural hypotension (change position slowly when rising from sitting or lying or when climbing stairs). Report excessive drowsiness or mental agitation; palpitations, rapid heartbeat, or chest pain; skin rash; muscle cramping or tremors; or respiratory difficulty.

**Nursing Implications** Raise bed rails; institute safety measures; assist with ambulation

**Dosage Forms** Tablet: 350 mg

## Carisoprodol and Aspirin (kar i soe PROE dole & AS pir in)

**U.S. Brand Names** Soma® Compound

**Pharmacologic Category** Skeletal Muscle Relaxant

**Use** Skeletal muscle relaxant

**Effects on Mental Status** Drowsiness is common; may produce depression or paradoxical CNS stimulation

**Effects on Psychiatric Treatment** Rarely may cause leukopenia or aplastic anemia; use caution with clozapine and carbamazepine; concurrent use with psychotropics may produce additive sedation

**Usual Dosage** Adults: Oral: 1-2 tablets 4 times/day

**Dosage Forms** Tablet: Carisoprodol 200 mg and aspirin 325 mg

## Carisoprodol, Aspirin, and Codeine
(kar i soe PROE dole, AS pir in, and KOE deen)

**U.S. Brand Names** Soma® Compound w/Codeine

**Pharmacologic Category** Skeletal Muscle Relaxant

**Use** Skeletal muscle relaxant

**Effects on Mental Status** Drowsiness is common; may produce depression or paradoxical CNS stimulation

**Effects on Psychiatric Treatment** Rarely may cause leukopenia or aplastic anemia; use caution with clozapine and carbamazepine; concurrent use with psychotropics may produce additive sedation

**Restrictions** C-III

**Usual Dosage** Adults: Oral: 1 or 2 tablets 4 times/day

**Dosage Forms** Tablet: Carisoprodol 200 mg, aspirin 325 mg, and codeine phosphate 16 mg

♦ **Carmol® Topical [OTC]** *see* Urea *on page 576*

## Carmustine (kar MUS teen)

**U.S. Brand Names** BiCNU®

**Pharmacologic Category** Antineoplastic Agent, Alkylating Agent

**Use** Treatment of brain tumors (glioblastoma, brainstem glioma, medulloblastoma, astrocytoma, ependymoma, and metastatic brain tumors), multiple myeloma, Hodgkin's disease (secondary therapy in combination with other approved drugs in patients who relapse while being treated with primary therapy or who fail to respond to primary therapy) and non-Hodgkin's lymphomas (secondary therapy in combination with other approved drugs in patients who relapse while being treated with primary therapy or who fail to respond to primary therapy), melanoma, lung cancer, colon cancer

**Effects on Mental Status** Dizziness is common

**Effects on Psychiatric Treatment** May cause myelosuppression; use caution with clozapine and carbamazepine

**Usual Dosage** I.V. (refer to individual protocols):

Children: 200-250 mg/m$^2$ every 4-6 weeks as a single dose

Adults: 150-200 mg/m$^2$ every 6 weeks as a single dose or divided into daily injections on 2 successive days; next dose is to be determined based on hematologic response to the previous dose. Listed are the suggested carmustine doses, based upon the nadir after the prior dose.

- Leukocytes >4000 $mm^3$ and platelets >100,000 $mm^3$: Give 100% of prior dose
- Leukocytes 3000-3999 $mm^3$ and platelets 75,000-99,999 $mm^3$: Give 100% of prior dose
- Leukocytes 2000-2999 $mm^3$ and platelets 25,000-74,999 $mm^3$: Give 70% of prior dose
- Leukocytes <2000 $mm^3$ and platelets <25,000 $mm^3$: Give 50% of prior dose

Primary brain cancer: 150-200 mg/$m^2$ every 6-8 weeks

Autologous BMT: ALL OF THE FOLLOWING DOSES ARE FATAL WITHOUT BMT

Combination therapy: Up to 300-900 mg/$m^2$

Single agent therapy: Up to 1200 mg/$m^2$ (fatal necrosis is associated with doses >2 g/$m^2$)

Hemodialysis: Supplemental dosing is not required

**Dosing adjustment in hepatic impairment**: Dosage adjustment may be necessary; however, no specific guidelines are available

**Dosage Forms** Powder for injection: 100 mg/vial packaged with 3 mL of absolute alcohol for use as a sterile diluent

♦ **Carnitor® Injection** *see* Levocarnitine *on page 312*

♦ **Carnitor® Oral** *see* Levocarnitine *on page 312*

## Carteolol (KAR tee oh lole)

**Related Information**

Beta-Blockers Comparison Chart *on page 709*

Glaucoma Drug Therapy *on page 712*

**U.S. Brand Names** Cartrol® Oral; Ocupress® Ophthalmic

**Pharmacologic Category** Beta Blocker (with Intrinsic Sympathomimetic Activity); Ophthalmic Agent, Antiglaucoma

**Use** Management of hypertension; treatment of chronic open-angle glaucoma and intraocular hypertension

**Effects on Mental Status** May cause fatigue, insomnia, confusion, and nightmares and clinically look like a major depression

**Effects on Psychiatric Treatment** Antipsychotics and MAOIs may increase the effects of beta-blockers; conversely beta-blockers may increase the effects of antipsychotics and benzodiazepines

**Pregnancy Risk Factor** C (per manufacturer); D (in second and third trimester, based on expert analysis)

**Contraindications** Hypersensitivity to carteolol or any component; sinus bradycardia; heart block greater than first-degree (except in patients with a functioning artificial pacemaker); cardiogenic shock; bronchial asthma, bronchospasm, or COPD; uncompensated cardiac failure; pulmonary edema; pregnancy (2nd and 3rd trimesters)

**Warnings/Precautions** Avoid abrupt discontinuation in patients with a history of CAD; slowly wean while monitoring for signs and symptoms of ischemia. Use caution in patients with PVD (can aggravate arterial insufficiency). Use caution with concurrent use of beta-blockers and either verapamil or diltiazem; bradycardia or heart block can occur. Patients with bronchospastic disease should not receive beta-blockers. Use cautiously in diabetics because it can mask prominent hypoglycemic symptoms. Can mask signs of thyrotoxicosis. Can cause fetal harm when administered in pregnancy. Dosage adjustment is required in patients with renal dysfunction. Use care with anesthetic agents that decrease myocardial function. Beta-blockers with intrinsic sympathomimetic activity have not been demonstrated to be of value in congestive heart failure.

**Adverse Reactions**

1% to 10%:

Cardiovascular: Congestive heart failure, arrhythmia

Central nervous system: Mental depression, headache, dizziness

Neuromuscular & skeletal: Back pain, arthralgia

<1%: A-V block, bradycardia, bronchospasm, chest pain, cold extremities, confusion, constipation, diarrhea, edema, fatigue, hyperglycemia, hypotension, impotence, insomnia, ischemic colitis, lethargy, mesenteric arterial thrombosis, nausea, nightmares, persistent bradycardia, purpura, Raynaud's phenomenon, thrombocytopenia

**Overdosage/Toxicology**

Signs and symptoms: Cardiac disturbances, CNS toxicity, bronchospasm, hypoglycemia, and hyperkalemia. The most common cardiac symptoms include hypotension and bradycardia; atrioventricular block, intraventricular conduction disturbances, cardiogenic shock, and asystole may occur with severe overdose, especially with membrane-depressant drugs (eg, propranolol); CNS effects include convulsions, coma, and respiratory arrest (commonly seen with propranolol and other membrane-depressant and lipid-soluble drugs).

Treatment: Symptomatic treatment of seizures, hypotension, hyperkalemia, and hypoglycemia; bradycardia and hypotension resistant to atropine, isoproterenol, or pacing may respond to glucagon; wide QRS defects caused by the membrane-depressant poisoning may respond to hypertonic sodium bicarbonate; repeat-dose charcoal, hemoperfusion, or hemodialysis may be helpful in removal of only those beta-blockers with a small $V_d$, long half-life, or low intrinsic clearance (acebutolol, atenolol, nadolol, sotalol).

**Drug Interactions**

Albuterol (and other $beta_2$ agonists): Effects may be blunted by nonspecific beta-blockers

Alpha-blockers (prazosin, terazosin): Concurrent use of beta-blockers may increase risk of orthostasis

Carteolol causes hypertension when used with local anesthetics (tetracaine, lidocaine, or bupivacaine) containing epinephrine

Clonidine: Hypertensive crisis after or during withdrawal of either agent

Drugs which slow AV conduction (digoxin): Effects may be additive with beta-blockers

Glucagon: Carteolol may blunt the hyperglycemic action of glucagon

Insulin: Carteolol may mask tachycardia from hypoglycemia

NSAIDs (ibuprofen, indomethacin, naproxen, piroxicam) may reduce the antihypertensive effects of beta-blockers

Salicylates may reduce the antihypertensive effects of beta-blockers

Sulfonylureas: Beta-blockers may alter response to hypoglycemic agents

Verapamil or diltiazem may have synergistic or additive pharmacological effects when taken concurrently with beta-blockers

**Usual Dosage** Adults:

Oral: 2.5 mg as a single daily dose, with a maintenance dose normally 2.5-5 mg once daily; doses >10 mg do not increase response and may in fact decrease effect.

Ophthalmic: Instill 1 drop in affected eye(s) twice daily.

**Dosing interval in renal impairment:**

$Cl_{cr}$ >60 mL/minute/1.73 $m^2$: Administer every 24 hours.

$Cl_{cr}$ 20-60 mL/minute/1.73 $m^2$: Administer every 48 hours.

$Cl_{cr}$ <20 mL/minute/1.73 $m^2$: Administer every 72 hours.

**Patient Information**

Oral: Take exactly as directed. Do not increase, decrease, or adjust dosage without consulting prescriber. Take pulse daily, prior to medication; follow prescriber's instruction about holding medication. Do not take with antacids and avoid alcohol or OTC medications (eg, cold remedies) without consulting prescriber. If diabetic, monitor serum blood glucose closely (may alter glucose tolerance or mask signs of hypoglycemia). May cause fatigue, dizziness, or postural hypotension; use caution when changing position from lying or sitting to standing, when driving, or climbing stairs until response to medication is known. May cause alteration in sexual performance (reversible). Report unresolved swelling of extremities, difficulty breathing or new cough, unresolved fatigue, unusual weight gain, unresolved constipation, or unusual muscle weakness.

Ophthalmic: Wash hands before instilling. Sit or lie down to instill. Open eye, look at ceiling, and instill prescribed amount of medication. Close eye and apply gentle pressure to inner corner of eye. Do not let tip of applicator touch eye or contaminate tip of applicator. Temporary stinging or burning may occur. Report persistent pain, burning, vision disturbances, swelling, itching, or worsening of condition.

**Nursing Implications** Advise against abrupt withdrawal; monitor orthostatic blood pressures, apical and peripheral pulse, and mental status changes (ie, confusion, depression)

**Dosage Forms**

Solution, ophthalmic, as hydrochloride (Ocupress®): 1% (5 mL, 10 mL)

Tablet, as hydrochloride (Cartrol®): 2.5 mg, 5 mg

♦ **Carter's Little Pills® [OTC]** *see* Bisacodyl *on page 69*

♦ **Cartrol® Oral** *see* Carteolol *on page 95*

## Carvedilol (KAR ve dil ole)

**U.S. Brand Names** Coreg®

**Pharmacologic Category** Alpha-/Beta- Blocker

**Use** Management of hypertension; can be used alone or in combination with other agents, especially thiazide-type diuretics; mild to moderate heart failure (NYHA Class II-III) following standardized therapy.

**Effects on Mental Status** May cause fatigue, insomnia, confusion, and nightmare and clinically look like a major depression

**Effects on Psychiatric Treatment** Fluoxetine and paroxetine may increase carvedilol's (a CYP2D6 substrate) serum levels

**Pregnancy Risk Factor** C (per manufacturer); D (in second and third trimester, based on expert analysis)

**Contraindications** Hypersensitivity to carvedilol or any component; patients with NYHA Class IV decompensated cardiac failure requiring intravenous therapy; bronchial asthma or related bronchospastic conditions; second- or third-degree AV block (except in patients with a functioning artificial pacemaker); sick sinus syndrome (except in patients with a functioning artificial pacemaker); cardiogenic shock; severe bradycardia; severe hepatic impairment; pregnancy (2nd and 3rd trimesters)

**Warnings/Precautions** Initiate cautiously and monitor for possible deterioration in CHF. Adjustment of other medications (ACE inhibitors and/or diuretics) may be required. Discontinue therapy if any evidence of liver injury occurs. Use caution in patients with PVD (can aggravate arterial insufficiency). Use caution with concurrent use of beta-blockers and either verapamil or diltiazem; bradycardia or heart block can occur. Patients with bronchospastic disease should not receive beta-blockers. Use cautiously in diabetics because it can mask prominent hypoglycemic symptoms. Can

(Continued)

## Carvedilol *(Continued)*

mask signs of thyrotoxicosis. Use care with anesthetic agents that decrease myocardial function.

**Adverse Reactions**

>1%:

Cardiovascular: Bradycardia, postural hypotension, edema
Central nervous system: Dizziness, somnolence, insomnia, fatigue
Gastrointestinal: Diarrhea, abdominal pain
Neuromuscular & skeletal: Back pain
Respiratory: Rhinitis, pharyngitis, dyspnea

<1%: Abnormal vision, anemia, asthma, ataxia, A-V block, constipation, cough, decreased male libido, depression, diaphoresis (increased), extrasystoles, flatulence, hyperbilirubinemia, hypercholesterolemia, hyperglycemia, hypertension, hyperuricemia, hypotension, impotence, increased LFTs, leukopenia, malaise, myalgia, nervousness, palpitations, paresthesia, peripheral ischemia, pruritus, rash, syncope, tinnitus, vertigo, weakness, xerostomia

**Overdosage/Toxicology**

Signs and symptoms: Cardiac disturbances, CNS toxicity, bronchospasm, hypoglycemia, and hyperkalemia. The most common cardiac symptoms include hypotension and bradycardia; atrioventricular block, intraventricular conduction disturbances, cardiogenic shock, and asystole may occur with severe overdose, especially with membrane-depressant drugs (eg, propranolol); CNS effects include convulsions, coma, and respiratory arrest which are commonly seen with propranolol and other membrane-depressant and lipid-soluble drugs.

Treatment: Symptomatic treatment of seizures, hypotension, hyperkalemia, and hypoglycemia; bradycardia and hypotension resistant to atropine, isoproterenol, or pacing may respond to glucagon; wide QRS defects caused by the membrane-depressant poisoning may respond to hypertonic sodium bicarbonate; repeat-dose charcoal, hemoperfusion, or hemodialysis may be helpful in removal of only those beta-blockers with a small $V_d$, long half-life, or low intrinsic clearance (acebutolol, atenolol, nadolol, sotalol)

**Drug Interactions** CYP2C, 2C9, 2D6 substrate

Inhibitors of CYP2D6 including quinidine, paroxetine, and propafenone are likely to increase blood levels of carvedilol
Alpha-blockers (prazosin, terazosin): Concurrent use of beta-blockers may increase risk of orthostasis
Clonidine: Hypertensive crisis after or during withdrawal of either agent
Cyclosporine blood levels may be increased by carvedilol
Digoxin blood levels may be increased
Drugs which slow AV conduction (digoxin): Effects may be additive with beta-blockers
Fluoxetine may increase carvedilol blood levels
Glucagon: Carvedilol may blunt the hyperglycemic action of glucagon
Insulin and oral hypoglycemics: Carvedilol may masks symptoms of hypoglycemia
NSAIDs (ibuprofen, indomethacin, naproxen, piroxicam) may reduce the antihypertensive effects of beta-blockers
Paroxetine may increase carvedilol blood levels
Rifampin may decrease in carvedilol blood concentration
Salicylates may reduce the antihypertensive effects of beta-blockers
Sulfonylureas: Beta-blockers may alter response to hypoglycemic agents
Verapamil or diltiazem may have synergistic or additive pharmacological effects when taken concurrently with beta-blockers

**Usual Dosage** Adults: Oral:

Hypertension: 6.25 mg twice daily; if tolerated, dose should be maintained for 1-2 weeks, then increased to 12.5 mg twice daily. Dosage may be increased to a maximum of 25 mg twice daily after 1-2 weeks. Reduce dosage if heart rate drops to <55 beats/minute.

Congestive heart failure: 3.125 mg twice daily for 2 weeks; if this dose is tolerated, may increase to 6.25 mg twice daily. Double the dose every 2 weeks to the highest dose tolerated by patient. (Prior to initiating therapy, other heart failure medications should be stabilized.)

Maximum recommended dose:
<85 kg: 25 mg twice daily
>85 kg: 50 mg twice daily

Angina pectoris (unlabeled use): 25-50 mg twice daily
Idiopathic cardiomyopathy (unlabeled use): 6.25-25 mg twice daily

**Dosing adjustment in renal impairment:** None necessary

**Dosing adjustment in hepatic impairment:** Use is contraindicated in liver dysfunction.

**Patient Information** Take exactly as directed. Do not increase, decrease, or adjust dosage without consulting prescriber. Take pulse daily, prior to medication; follow prescriber's instruction about holding medication. Do not take with antacids and avoid alcohol or OTC medications (eg, cold remedies) without consulting prescriber. If diabetic, monitor serum glucose closely (may alter glucose tolerance or mask signs of hypoglycemia). May cause fatigue, dizziness, or postural hypotension; use caution when changing position from lying or sitting to standing, when driving, or climbing stairs until response to medication is known. May cause alteration in sexual performance (reversible). Report unresolved swelling of extremities, difficulty breathing or new cough, unresolved fatigue, unusual weight gain, unresolved constipation, or unusual muscle weakness.

**Nursing Implications** Minimize risk of bradycardia with initiation of treatment with a low dose, slow upward titration, and administration with food; decrease dose if pulse rate drops <55 beats per minute

**Dosage Forms** Tablet: 3.125 mg, 6.25 mg, 12.5 mg, 25 mg


- **Casodex®** *see* Bicalutamide *on page 68*
- ***Cassia acutifolia*** *see* Senna *on page 509*
- **Cataflam® Oral** *see* Diclofenac *on page 163*
- **Catapres® Oral** *see* Clonidine *on page 133*
- **Catapres-TTS® Transdermal** *see* Clonidine *on page 133*
- **Caverject® Injection** *see* Alprostadil *on page 27*
- **CBZ** *see* Carbamazepine *on page 90*
- **CCNU** *see* Lomustine *on page 323*
- **C-Crystals® [OTC]** *see* Ascorbic Acid *on page 48*
- **Cebid® Timecelles® [OTC]** *see* Ascorbic Acid *on page 48*
- **Ceclor®** *see* Cefaclor *on page 96*
- **Ceclor® CD** *see* Cefaclor *on page 96*
- **Cecon® [OTC]** *see* Ascorbic Acid *on page 48*
- **Cedax®** *see* Ceftibuten *on page 101*
- **Cedilanid-D®** *see* Deslanoside *on page 156*
- **CeeNU®** *see* Lomustine *on page 323*
- **Ceepryn® [OTC]** *see* Cetylpyridinium *on page 106*


## Cefaclor (SEF a klor)

**U.S. Brand Names** Ceclor®; Ceclor® CD

**Canadian Brand Names** Apo®-Cefaclor

**Pharmacologic Category** Antibiotic, Cephalosporin (Second Generation)

**Use** Infections caused by susceptible organisms including *Staphylococcus aureus* and *H. influenzae*; treatment of otitis media, sinusitis, and infections involving the respiratory tract, skin and skin structure, bone and joint, and urinary tract

**Effects on Mental Status** May cause nervousness; case reports of euphoria, delusion, illusions, and depersonalization with cephalosporins

**Effects on Psychiatric Treatment** May rarely cause neutropenia; use caution with clozapine and carbamazepine

**Pregnancy Risk Factor** B

**Contraindications** Hypersensitivity to cefaclor, any component, or cephalosporins

**Warnings/Precautions** Modify dosage in patients with severe renal impairment; prolonged use may result in superinfection; a low incidence of cross-hypersensitivity to penicillins exists

**Adverse Reactions**

1% to 10%:

Gastrointestinal: Diarrhea (1.5%)
Hematologic: Eosinophilia (2%)
Hepatic: Elevated transaminases (2.5%)
Dermatologic: Rash (maculopapular, erythematous, or morbilliform) (1% to 1.5%)

<1%: Agitation, anaphylaxis, angioedema, arthralgia, cholestatic jaundice, CNS irritability, confusion, dizziness, hallucinations, hemolytic anemia, hepatitis, hyperactivity, insomnia, interstitial nephritis, nausea, nervousness, neutropenia, prolonged PT, pruritus, pseudomembranous colitis, seizures, serum-sickness, somnolence, Stevens-Johnson syndrome, urticaria, vaginitis, vomiting

Reactions reported with other cephalosporins include abdominal pain, cholestasis, fever, hemorrhage, renal dysfunction, superinfection, toxic nephropathy

**Overdosage/Toxicology**

Signs and symptoms: After acute overdose, most agents cause only nausea, vomiting, and diarrhea, although neuromuscular hypersensitivity and seizures are possible, especially in patients with renal insufficiency

Treatment: Hemodialysis may be helpful to aid in the removal of the drug from the blood but not usually indicated, otherwise most treatment is supportive or symptom directed following GI decontamination

**Drug Interactions**

Increased effect: Probenecid may decrease cephalosporin elimination
Increased toxicity: Furosemide, aminoglycosides may be a possible additive to nephrotoxicity

**Usual Dosage** Oral:

Children >1 month: 20-40 mg/kg/day divided every 8-12 hours; maximum dose: 2 g/day (total daily dose may be divided into two doses for treatment of otitis media or pharyngitis)
Adults: 250-500 mg every 8 hours

Extended release tablets: 500 mg every 12 hours for 7 days for acute bacterial exacerbations of or secondary infections with chronic bronchitis or 375 mg every 12 hour for 10 days for pharyngitis or tonsillitis or for uncomplicated skin and skin structure infections

**Dosing adjustment in renal impairment:** $Cl_{cr}$ <50 mL/minute: Administer 50% of dose

Hemodialysis: Moderately dialyzable (20% to 50%)

**Patient Information** Take as directed, at regular intervals around-the-clock (with or without food). Chilling oral suspension improves flavor (do not freeze). Do not chew or crush extended release tablets. Complete full course of medication, even if you feel better. Drink 2-3 L fluid/day. Small frequent meals, frequent mouth care, sucking lozenges, or chewing gum may reduce nausea or vomiting. If diarrhea occurs, yogurt or buttermilk may help. May cause false-positive test with Clinitest®; use another form of testing. May interfere with oral contraceptives; additional contraceptive measures are necessary. Report severe, unresolved diarrhea; vaginal itching or drainage; sores in mouth; blood, pus, or mucus in stool or urine; easy bleeding or bruising; unusual fever or chills; rash; or respiratory difficulty.

**Dosage Forms**

Capsule: 250 mg, 500 mg

Powder for oral suspension (strawberry flavor): 125 mg/5 mL (75 mL, 150 mL); 187 mg/5 mL (50 mL, 100 mL); 250 mg/5 mL (75 mL, 150 mL); 375 mg/5 mL (50 mL, 100 mL)

Tablet, extended release: 375 mg, 500 mg

## Cefadroxil (sef a DROKS il)

**U.S. Brand Names** Duricef®

**Pharmacologic Category** Antibiotic, Cephalosporin (First Generation)

**Use** Treatment of susceptible bacterial infections, including those caused by group A beta-hemolytic *Streptococcus*; prophylaxis against bacterial endocarditis in patients who are allergic to penicillin and undergoing surgical or dermal procedures

**Effects on Mental Status** May cause nervousness; case reports of euphoria, delusion, illusions, and depersonalization with cephalosporins

**Effects on Psychiatric Treatment** May rarely cause neutropenia; use caution with clozapine and carbamazepine

**Pregnancy Risk Factor** B

**Contraindications** Hypersensitivity to cefadroxil or other cephalosporins

**Warnings/Precautions** Modify dosage in patients with severe renal impairment; prolonged use may result in superinfection; use with caution in patients with a history of penicillin allergy especially IgE-mediated reactions (eg, anaphylaxis, urticaria); may cause antibiotic-associated colitis or colitis secondary to *C. difficile*

**Adverse Reactions**

1% to 10%: Gastrointestinal: Diarrhea

<1%: Abdominal pain, agranulocytosis, anaphylaxis, angioedema, arthralgia, cholestasis, dyspepsia, elevated transaminases, erythema multiforme, fever, nausea, neutropenia, pruritus, pseudomembranous colitis, rash (maculopapular and erythematous), serum sickness, Stevens-Johnson syndrome, thrombocytopenia, urticaria, vaginitis, vomiting

Reactions reported with other cephalosporins include abdominal pain, aplastic anemia, eosinophilia, hemolytic anemia, hemorrhage, increased BUN, increased creatinine, pancytopenia, prolonged prothrombin time, renal dysfunction, seizures, superinfection, toxic epidermal necrolysis, toxic nephropathy

**Overdosage/Toxicology**

Signs and symptoms: After acute overdose, most agents cause only nausea, vomiting, and diarrhea, although neuromuscular hypersensitivity and seizures are possible, especially in patients with renal insufficiency

Treatment: Hemodialysis may be helpful to aid in the removal of the drug from the blood but not usually indicated, otherwise most treatment is supportive or symptom directed following GI decontamination

**Drug Interactions**

Increased effect: Probenecid may decrease cephalosporin elimination

Increased toxicity: Furosemide, aminoglycosides may be a possible additive to nephrotoxicity

**Usual Dosage** Oral:

Children: 30 mg/kg/day divided twice daily up to a maximum of 2 g/day

Adults: 1-2 g/day in 2 divided doses

Prophylaxis against bacterial endocarditis: 2 g 1 hour prior to the procedure

**Dosing interval in renal impairment:**

$Cl_{cr}$ 10-25 mL/minute: Administer every 24 hours

$Cl_{cr}$ <10 mL/minute: Administer every 36 hours

**Patient Information** Take as directed, at regular intervals around-the-clock (with or without food). Chilling oral suspension improves flavor (do not freeze). Complete full course of medication, even if you feel better. Drink 2-3 L fluid/day. If diarrhea occurs, yogurt or buttermilk may help. May cause false-positive test with Clinitest®; use another form of testing. May interfere with oral contraceptives; additional contraceptive measures are necessary. Report severe, unresolved diarrhea; vaginal itching or drainage; sores in mouth; blood, pus, or mucus in stool or urine; easy bleeding or bruising; unusual fever or chills; rash; or respiratory difficulty.

**Dosage Forms**

Capsule, as monohydrate: 500 mg

Suspension, oral, as monohydrate: 125 mg/5 mL, 250 mg/5 mL, 500 mg/5 mL (50 mL, 100 mL)

Tablet, as monohydrate: 1 g

♦ **Cefadyl®** *see* Cephapirin *on page 104*

## Cefamandole (sef a MAN dole)

**U.S. Brand Names** Mandol®

**Pharmacologic Category** Antibiotic, Cephalosporin (Second Generation)

**Use** Treatment of susceptible bacterial infection; mainly respiratory tract, skin and skin structure, bone and joint, urinary tract and gynecologic, septicemia; surgical prophylaxis. Active against methicillin-sensitive staphylococci, many streptococci, and various gram-negative bacilli including *E. coli*, some *Klebsiella*, *P. mirabilis*, *H. influenzae*, and *Moraxella*.

**Effects on Mental Status** May cause nervousness; case reports of euphoria, delusion, illusions, and depersonalization with cephalosporins

**Effects on Psychiatric Treatment** May rarely cause neutropenia; use caution with clozapine and carbamazepine

**Usual Dosage** I.M., I.V.:

Children: 50-150 mg/kg/day in divided doses every 4-8 hours

Adults: Usual dose: 500-1000 mg every 4-8 hours; in life-threatening infections: 2 g every 4 hours may be needed

**Dosing interval in renal impairment:**

$Cl_{cr}$ 25-50 mL/minute: 1-2 g every 8 hours

$Cl_{cr}$ 10-25 mL/minute: 1 g every 8 hours

$Cl_{cr}$ <10 mL/minute: 1 g every 12 hours

Hemodialysis: Moderately dialyzable (20% to 50%)

**Dosage Forms** Powder for injection, as nafate: 500 mg (10 mL); 1 g (10 mL, 100 mL); 2 g (20 mL, 100 mL); 10 g (100 mL)

## Cefazolin (sef A zoe lin)

**U.S. Brand Names** Ancef®; Kefzol®; Zolicef®

**Pharmacologic Category** Antibiotic, Cephalosporin (First Generation)

**Use** Treatment of gram-positive bacilli and cocci (except enterococcus); some gram-negative bacilli including *E. coli*, *Proteus*, and *Klebsiella* may be susceptible

**Effects on Mental Status** May cause nervousness; case reports of euphoria, delusion, illusions, and depersonalization with cephalosporins

**Effects on Psychiatric Treatment** May rarely cause neutropenia; use caution with clozapine and carbamazepine

**Usual Dosage** I.M., I.V.:

Children >1 month: 25-100 mg/kg/day divided every 6-8 hours; maximum: 6 g/day

Adults: 250 mg to 2 g every 6-12 (usually 8) hours, depending on severity of infection; maximum dose: 12 g/day

**Dosing adjustment in renal impairment:**

$Cl_{cr}$ 10-30 mL/minute: Administer every 12 hours

$Cl_{cr}$ <10 mL/minute: Administer every 24 hours

Hemodialysis: Moderately dialyzable (20% to 50%); administer dose postdialysis or administer supplemental dose of 0.5-1 g after dialysis

Peritoneal dialysis: Administer 0.5 g every 12 hours

Continuous arteriovenous or venovenous hemofiltration (CAVH/CAVHD): Dose as for $Cl_{cr}$ 10-30 mL/minute; removes 30 mg of cefazolin per liter of filtrate per day

**Dosage Forms**

Infusion, premixed, as sodium, in $D_5W$ (frozen) (Ancef®): 500 mg (50 mL); 1 g (50 mL)

Injection, as sodium (Kefzol®): 500 mg, 1 g

Powder for injection, as sodium (Ancef®, Zolicef®): 250 mg, 500 mg, 1 g, 5 g, 10 g, 20 g

## Cefdinir (SEF di ner)

**U.S. Brand Names** Omnicef®

**Synonyms** CFDN

**Pharmacologic Category** Antibiotic, Cephalosporin (Third Generation)

**Use** Treatment of community-acquired pneumonia, acute exacerbations of chronic bronchitis, acute bacterial otitis media, acute maxillary sinusitis, pharyngitis/tonsillitis, and uncomplicated skin and skin structure infections.

**Effects on Mental Status** May cause nervousness; case reports of euphoria, delusion, illusions, and depersonalization with cephalosporins

**Effects on Psychiatric Treatment** May rarely cause neutropenia; use caution with clozapine and carbamazepine

**Pregnancy Risk Factor** B

**Contraindications** Hypersensitivity to cephalosporins or related antibiotics

**Warnings/Precautions** Administer cautiously to penicillin-sensitive patients. There is evidence of partial cross-allergenicity and

(Continued)

## Cefdinir *(Continued)*

cephalosporins cannot be assumed to be an absolutely safe alternative to penicillin in the penicillin-allergic patient. Serum sickness-like reactions have been reported. Signs and symptoms occur after a few days of therapy and resolve a few days after drug discontinuation with no serious sequelae. Pseudomembranous colitis occurs; consider its diagnosis in patients who develop diarrhea with antibiotic use.

**Adverse Reactions**

>1%: Gastrointestinal: Diarrhea

<1%: Arthralgia, candidiasis, cholestatic jaundice, eosinophilia, headache, hemolytic anemia, interstitial nephritis, nausea, nephrotoxicity with transient elevations of BUN/creatinine, nervousness, neutropenia, positive Coombs' test, pruritus, pseudomembranous colitis, rash, seizures (with high doses and renal dysfunction), serum sickness, slightly increased AST/ALT, Stevens-Johnson syndrome, thrombocytopenia, urticaria, vomiting

**Overdosage/Toxicology**

Signs and symptoms: After acute overdose, most agents cause only nausea, vomiting, and diarrhea, although neuromuscular hypersensitivity and seizures are possible, especially in patients with renal insufficiency

Treatment: Hemodialysis may be helpful to aid in the removal of the drug from the blood but not usually indicated, otherwise most treatment is supportive or symptom directed following GI decontamination

**Drug Interactions**

Decreased effect: Coadministration with iron or antacids reduces the rate and extent of cefdinir absorption

Increased effect: Probenecid increases the effects of cephalosporins by decreasing the renal elimination in those which are secreted by tubular secretion

Increased toxicity: Anticoagulant effects may be increased when administered with cephalosporins

**Usual Dosage** Oral:

Children: 7 mg/kg/dose twice daily or 14 mg/kg/dose once daily for 10 days (maximum: 600 mg/day)

Adolescents and Adults: 300 mg twice daily or 600 mg once daily for 10 days

**Dosing adjustment in renal impairment:** $Cl_{cr}$ <30 mL/minute: 300 mg once daily

Hemodialysis removes cefdinir; recommended initial dose: 300 mg (or 7 mg/kg/dose) every other day. At the conclusion of each hemodialysis session, 300 mg (or 7 mg/kg/dose) should be given. Subsequent doses (300 mg or 7 mg/kg/dose) should be administered every other day.

**Dosage Forms**

Capsule: 300 mg

Suspension, oral: 125 mg/5 mL (60 mL, 100 mL)

---

## Cefepime (SEF e pim)

**U.S. Brand Names** Maxipime®

**Pharmacologic Category** Antibiotic, Cephalosporin (Fourth Generation)

**Use** Treatment of uncomplicated and complicated urinary tract infections, including pyelonephritis caused by typical urinary tract pathogens; monotherapy for febrile neutropenia; uncomplicated skin and skin structure infections caused by *Streptococcus pyogenes*; moderate to severe pneumonia caused by pneumococcus, *Pseudomonas aeruginosa*, and other gram-negative organisms; complicated intra-abdominal infections (in combination with metronidazole). Also active against methicillin-susceptible staphylococci, *Enterobacter* sp, and many other gram-negative bacilli.

Pediatrics (2 months to 16 years of age): Empiric therapy of febrile neutropenia patients, uncomplicated skin/soft tissue infections, pneumonia, and uncomplicated/complicated urinary tract infections.

**Effects on Mental Status** May cause nervousness; case reports of euphoria, delusion, illusions, and depersonalization with cephalosporins

**Effects on Psychiatric Treatment** May rarely cause neutropenia; use caution with clozapine and carbamazepine

**Usual Dosage** I.V.:

Children:

Febrile neutropenia: 50 mg/kg every 8 hours for 7-10 days

Uncomplicated skin/soft tissue infections, pneumonia, and complicated/uncomplicated UTI: 50 mg/kg twice daily

Adults:

Most infections: 1-2 g every 12 hours for 5-10 days; higher doses or more frequent administration may be required in pseudomonal infections

Urinary tract infections, uncomplicated: 500 mg every 12 hours

Monotherapy for febrile neutropenic patients: 2 g every 8 hours for 7 days or until the neutropenia resolves

**Dosing adjustment in renal impairment:** Recommended maintenance schedule based on creatinine clearance (mL/minute), compared to normal dosing schedule:

When normal ($Cl_{cr}$ >60) dosing schedule is 500 mg every 12 hours

Adjust dose as follows:

$Cl_{cr}$ 30-60: 500 mg every 24 hours

$Cl_{cr}$ 11-29: 500 mg every 24 hours

$Cl_{cr}$ <10: 250 mg every 24 hours

When normal ($Cl_{cr}$ >60) dosing schedule is 1 g every 12 hours

Adjust dose as follows:

$Cl_{cr}$ 30-60: 1 g every 24 hours

$Cl_{cr}$ 11-29: 500 g every 24 hours

$Cl_{cr}$ <10: 250 mg every 24 hours

When normal ($Cl_{cr}$ >60) dosing schedule is 2 g every 12 hours

Adjust dose as follows:

$Cl_{cr}$ 30-60: 1 g every 24 hours

$Cl_{cr}$ 11-29: 1 mg every 24 hours

$Cl_{cr}$ <10: 500 mg every 24 hours

Hemodialysis: Removed by dialysis; administer supplemental dose of 250 mg after each dialysis session

Peritoneal dialysis: Removed to a lesser extent than hemodialysis; administer 250 mg every 48 hours

Continuous arteriovenous or venovenous hemofiltration (CAVH/CAVHD): Dose as normal $Cl_{cr}$ (eg, >30 mL/minute)

**Dosage Forms**

Infusion, piggy-back: 1 g (100 mL); 2 g (100 mL)

Infusion (ADD-Vantage®): 1 g

Injection: 500 mg, 1 g, 2 g

---

## Cefixime (sef IKS eem)

**U.S. Brand Names** Suprax®

**Pharmacologic Category** Antibiotic, Cephalosporin (Third Generation)

**Use** Treatment of urinary tract infections, otitis media, respiratory infections due to susceptible organisms including *S. pneumoniae* and *S. pyogenes*, *H. influenzae* and many Enterobacteriaceae; documented poor compliance with other oral antimicrobials; outpatient therapy of serious soft tissue or skeletal infections due to susceptible organisms; single-dose oral treatment of uncomplicated cervical/urethral gonorrhea due to *N. gonorrhoeae*

**Effects on Mental Status** May cause nervousness; case reports of euphoria, delusion, illusions, and depersonalization with cephalosporins

**Effects on Psychiatric Treatment** May rarely cause neutropenia; use caution with clozapine and carbamazepine

**Pregnancy Risk Factor** B

**Contraindications** Hypersensitivity to cefixime or cephalosporins

**Warnings/Precautions** Prolonged use may result in superinfection; modify dosage in patients with renal impairment; use with caution in patients with a history of penicillin allergy especially IgE-mediated reactions (eg, anaphylaxis, urticaria); may cause antibiotic-associated colitis or colitis secondary to *C. difficile*

**Adverse Reactions**

>10%: Gastrointestinal: Diarrhea (16%)

1% to 10%: Gastrointestinal: Abdominal pain, nausea, dyspepsia, flatulence

<1%: candidiasis, dizziness, eosinophilia, erythema multiforme, fever, headache, increased BUN, increased creatinine, leukopenia, prolonged PT, pruritus, pseudomembranous colitis, rash, serum sickness-like reaction, Stevens-Johnson syndrome, thrombocytopenia, transaminase elevations, urticaria, vaginitis, vomiting

Other reactions with cephalosporins include agranulocytosis, anaphylaxis, aplastic anemia, cholestasis, colitis, hemolytic anemia, hemorrhage, interstitial nephritis, neutropenia, pancytopenia, renal dysfunction, seizures, superinfection, toxic epidermal necrolysis, toxic nephropathy

**Drug Interactions**

Increased effect: Probenecid may decrease cephalosporin elimination

Increased toxicity: Furosemide, aminoglycosides may be a possible additive to nephrotoxicity

**Usual Dosage** Oral:

Children: 8 mg/kg/day divided every 12-24 hours

Adolescents and Adults: 400 mg/day divided every 12-24 hours

Uncomplicated cervical/urethral gonorrhea due to *N. gonorrhoeae*: 400 mg as a single dose

For *S. pyogenes* infections, treat for 10 days; use suspension for otitis media due to increased peak serum levels as compared to tablet form

**Dosing adjustment in renal impairment:**

$Cl_{cr}$ 21-60 mL/minute or with renal hemodialysis: Administer 75% of the standard dose

$Cl_{cr}$ <20 mL/minute or with CAPD: Administer 50% of the standard dose

Moderately dialyzable (10%)

**Patient Information** Take as directed, at regular intervals around-the-clock (with or without food). Chilling oral suspension improves flavor (do not freeze). Complete full course of medication, even if you feel better. Drink 2-3 L fluid/day. If diarrhea occurs, yogurt or buttermilk may help. May cause false-positive test with Clinitest®; use another form of testing. May interfere with oral contraceptives; additional contraceptive measures are necessary. Report severe, unresolved diarrhea; vaginal itching or drainage; sores in mouth; blood, pus, or mucus in stool or urine; easy bleeding or bruising; unusual fever or chills,; rash; or respiratory difficulty.

**Dosage Forms**

Powder for oral suspension (strawberry flavor): 100 mg/5 mL (50 mL, 100 mL)

Tablet, film coated: 200 mg, 400 mg

- **Cefizox®** *see* Ceftizoxime *on page 101*

## Cefmetazole (sef MET a zole)

**U.S. Brand Names** Zefazone®

**Pharmacologic Category** Antibiotic, Cephalosporin (Second Generation)

**Use** Second generation cephalosporin, useful for susceptible aerobic and anaerobic gram-positive and gram-negative bacteria; surgical prophylaxis, specifically colorectal and OB-GYN

**Effects on Mental Status** May cause nervousness; case reports of euphoria, delusion, illusions, and depersonalization with cephalosporins

**Effects on Psychiatric Treatment** May rarely cause neutropenia; use caution with clozapine and carbamazepine

**Usual Dosage** Adults: I.V.:

Infections: 2 g every 6-12 hours for 5-14 days

Prophylaxis: 2 g 30-90 minutes before surgery **or** 1 g 30-90 minutes before surgery; repeat 8 and 16 hours later

**Dosing interval in renal impairment:**

$Cl_{cr}$ 50-90 mL/minute: Administer every 12 hours

$Cl_{cr}$ 10-50 mL/minute: Administer every 16-24 hours

$Cl_{cr}$ <10 mL/minute: Administer every 48 hours

**Dosage Forms** Powder for injection, as sodium: 1 g, 2 g

- **Cefobid®** *see* Cefoperazone *on page 99*
- **Cefol® Filmtab®** *see* Vitamins, Multiple *on page 587*

## Cefonicid (se FON i sid)

**U.S. Brand Names** Monocid®

**Pharmacologic Category** Antibiotic, Cephalosporin (Second Generation)

**Use** Treatment of susceptible bacterial infection; mainly respiratory tract, skin and skin structure, bone and joint, urinary tract and gynecologic, septicemia; active against methicillin-sensitive staphylococci, many streptococci, and various gram-negative bacilli including *E. coli*, some *Klebsiella*, *P. mirabilis*, *H. influenzae*, and *Moraxella*.

**Effects on Mental Status** May cause nervousness; case reports of euphoria, delusion, illusions, and depersonalization with cephalosporins

**Effects on Psychiatric Treatment** May rarely cause neutropenia; use caution with clozapine and carbamazepine

**Usual Dosage** Adults: I.M., I.V.: 0.5-2 g every 24 hours

Prophylaxis: Preop: 1 g/hour

**Dosing interval in renal impairment:** Dosing based on $Cl_{cr}$ (mL/minute/1.73 $m^2$)

$Cl_{cr}$ 60-79: 10-24 mg/kg every 24 hours

$Cl_{cr}$ 40-59: 8-20 mg/kg every 24 ours

$Cl_{cr}$ 20-39: 4-15 mg/kg every 24 hours

$Cl_{cr}$ 10-19: 4-15 mg/kg every 48 hours

$Cl_{cr}$ 5-9: 4-15 mg/kg every 3-5 days

$Cl_{cr}$ <5: 3-4 mg/kg every 3-5 days

**Dosage Forms** Powder for injection, as sodium: 500 mg, 1 g, 10 g

## Cefoperazone (sef oh PER a zone)

**U.S. Brand Names** Cefobid®

**Pharmacologic Category** Antibiotic, Cephalosporin (Third Generation)

**Use** Treatment of susceptible bacterial infection; mainly respiratory tract, skin and skin structure, bone and joint, urinary tract and gynecologic as well as septicemia. Active against a variety of gram-negative bacilli, some gram-positive cocci, and has some activity against *Pseudomonas aeruginosa*.

**Effects on Mental Status** May cause nervousness; case reports of euphoria, delusion, illusions, and depersonalization with cephalosporins

**Effects on Psychiatric Treatment** May rarely cause neutropenia; use caution with clozapine and carbamazepine

**Usual Dosage** I.M., I.V.:

Children (not approved): 100-150 mg/kg/day divided every 8-12 hours; up to 12 g/day

Adults: 2-4 g/day in divided doses every 12 hours; up to 12 g/day

**Dosing adjustment in hepatic impairment:** Reduce dose 50% in patients with advanced liver cirrhosis; maximum daily dose: 4 g

**Dosage Forms**

Injection, as sodium, premixed (frozen): 1 g (50 mL); 2 g (50 mL)

Powder for injection, as sodium: 1 g, 2 g

- **Cefotan®** *see* Cefotetan *on page 99*

## Cefotaxime (sef oh TAKS eem)

**U.S. Brand Names** Claforan®

**Pharmacologic Category** Antibiotic, Cephalosporin (Third Generation)

**Use** Treatment of susceptible infection in respiratory tract, skin and skin structure, bone and joint, urinary tract, gynecologic as well as septicemia, and documented or suspected meningitis. Active against most gram-negative bacilli (not *Pseudomonas*) and gram-positive cocci (not enterococcus). Active against many penicillin-resistant pneumococci.

**Effects on Mental Status** May cause nervousness; case reports of euphoria, delusion, illusions, and depersonalization with cephalosporins

**Effects on Psychiatric Treatment** May rarely cause neutropenia; use caution with clozapine and carbamazepine

**Usual Dosage**

Neonates: I.V.:

0-1 week: 50 mg/kg every 12 hours

1-4 weeks: 50 mg/kg every 8 hours

Infants and Children 1 month to 12 years: I.M., I.V.: <50 kg: 50-180 mg/kg/day in divided doses every 4-6 hours

Meningitis: 200 mg/kg/day in divided doses every 6 hours

Children >12 years and Adults:

Gonorrhea: I.M.: 1 g as a single dose

Uncomplicated infections: I.M., I.V.: 1 g every 12 hours

Moderate/severe infections: I.M., I.V.: 1-2 g every 8 hours

Infections commonly needing higher doses (eg, septicemia): I.V.: 2 g every 6-8 hours

Life-threatening infections: I.V.: 2 g every 4 hours

Preop: I.M., I.V.: 1 g 30-90 minutes before surgery

C-section: 1 g as soon as the umbilical cord is clamped, then 1 g I.M., I.V. at 6- and 12-hours intervals

**Dosing interval in renal impairment:**

$Cl_{cr}$ 10-50 mL/minute: Administer every 8-12 hours

$Cl_{cr}$ <10 mL/minute: Administer every 24 hours

Hemodialysis: Moderately dialyzable

**Dosing adjustment in hepatic impairment:** Moderate dosage reduction is recommended in severe liver disease

Continuous arteriovenous or venovenous hemodiafiltration (CAVH) effects: Administer 1 g every 12 hour

**Dosage Forms**

Infusion, as sodium, premixed, in $D_5W$ (frozen): 1 g (50 mL); 2 g (50 mL)

Powder for injection, as sodium: 500 mg, 1 g, 2 g, 10 g

## Cefotetan (SEF oh tee tan)

**U.S. Brand Names** Cefotan®

**Pharmacologic Category** Antibiotic, Cephalosporin (Second Generation)

**Use** Less active against staphylococci and streptococci than first generation cephalosporins, but active against anaerobes including *Bacteroides fragilis*; active against gram-negative enteric bacilli including *E. coli*, *Klebsiella*, and *Proteus*; used predominantly for respiratory tract, skin and skin structure, bone and joint, urinary tract and gynecologic as well as septicemia; surgical prophylaxis; intra-abdominal infections and other mixed infections

**Effects on Mental Status** May cause nervousness; case reports of euphoria, delusion, illusions, and depersonalization with cephalosporins

**Effects on Psychiatric Treatment** May rarely cause neutropenia; use caution with clozapine and carbamazepine

**Usual Dosage** I.M., I.V.:

Children: 20-40 mg/kg/dose every 12 hours

Adults: 1-6 g/day in divided doses every 12 hours; usual dose: 1-2 g every 12 hours for 5-10 days; 1-2 g may be given every 24 hours for urinary tract infection

**Dosing interval in renal impairment:**

$Cl_{cr}$ 10-30 mL/minute: Administer every 24 hours

$Cl_{cr}$ <10 mL/minute: Administer every 48 hours

Hemodialysis: Slightly dialyzable (5% to 20%)

Continuous arteriovenous or venovenous hemodiafiltration (CAVH) effects: Administer 750 mg every 12 hours

**Dosage Forms** Powder for injection, as disodium: 1 g (10 mL, 100 mL); 2 g (20 mL, 100 mL); 10 g (100 mL)

## Cefoxitin (se FOKS i tin)

**U.S. Brand Names** Mefoxin®

**Pharmacologic Category** Antibiotic, Cephalosporin (Second Generation)

**Use** Less active against staphylococci and streptococci than first generation cephalosporins, but active against anaerobes including *Bacteroides fragilis*; active against gram-negative enteric bacilli including *E. coli*, *Klebsiella*, and *Proteus*; used predominantly for respiratory tract, skin and skin structure, bone and joint, urinary tract and gynecologic as well as septicemia; surgical prophylaxis; intra-abdominal infections and other mixed infections; indicated for bacterial *Eikenella corrodens* infections

**Effects on Mental Status** May cause nervousness; case reports of euphoria, delusion, illusions, and depersonalization with cephalosporins

**Effects on Psychiatric Treatment** May rarely cause neutropenia; use caution with clozapine and carbamazepine

**Usual Dosage** I.M., I.V.:

Infants >3 months and Children:

Mild to moderate infection: 80-100 mg/kg/day in divided doses every 4-6 hours

(Continued)

## Cefoxitin *(Continued)*

Severe infection: 100-160 mg/kg/day in divided doses every 4-6 hours
Maximum dose: 12 g/day

Adults: 1-2 g every 6-8 hours (I.M. injection is painful); up to 12 g/day

**Dosing interval in renal impairment:**

$Cl_{cr}$ 30-50 mL/minute: Administer every 8-12 hours
$Cl_{cr}$ 10-30 mL/minute: Administer every 12-24 hours
$Cl_{cr}$ <10 mL/minute: Administer every 24-48 hours

Hemodialysis: Moderately dialyzable (20% to 50%)

Continuous arteriovenous or venovenous hemodiafiltration (CAVH) effects: Dose as for $Cl_{cr}$ 10-50 mL/minute

**Dosage Forms**

Infusion, as sodium, premixed, in $D_5W$ (frozen): 1 g (50 mL); 2 g (50 mL)
Powder for injection, as sodium: 1 g, 2 g, 10 g

## Cefpodoxime (sef pode OKS eem)

**U.S. Brand Names** Vantin®

**Pharmacologic Category** Antibiotic, Cephalosporin (Third Generation)

**Use** Treatment of susceptible acute, community-acquired pneumonia caused by *S. pneumoniae* or nonbeta-lactamase producing *H. influenzae*; acute uncomplicated gonorrhea caused by *N. gonorrhoeae*; uncomplicated skin and skin structure infections caused by *S. aureus* or *S. pyogenes*; acute otitis media caused by *S. pneumoniae, H. influenzae*, or *M. catarrhalis*; pharyngitis or tonsillitis; and uncomplicated urinary tract infections caused by *E. coli, Klebsiella*, and *Proteus*

**Effects on Mental Status** May cause nervousness; case reports of euphoria, delusion, illusions, and depersonalization with cephalosporins

**Effects on Psychiatric Treatment** May rarely cause neutropenia; use caution with clozapine and carbamazepine

**Pregnancy Risk Factor** B

**Contraindications** Hypersensitivity to cefpodoxime or cephalosporins

**Warnings/Precautions** Modify dosage in patients with severe renal impairment; prolonged use may result in superinfection; a low incidence of cross-hypersensitivity to penicillins exists

**Adverse Reactions**

>10%:
Dermatologic: Diaper rash (12.1%)
Gastrointestinal: Diarrhea in infants and toddlers (15.4%)

1% to 10%:
Central nervous system: Headache (1.1%)
Dermatologic: Rash (1.4%)
Gastrointestinal: Diarrhea (7.2%), nausea (3.8%), abdominal pain (1.6%), vomiting (1.1% to 2.1%)
Genitourinary: Vaginal infections (3.1%)

<1%: Anaphylaxis, anxiety, chest pain, cough, decreased appetite, decreased salivation, dizziness, epistaxis, eye itching, fatigue, fever, flatulence, flushing, fungal skin infection, hypotension, insomnia, malaise, nightmares, pruritus, pseudomembranous colitis, purpuric nephritis, taste alteration, tinnitus, vaginal candidiasis, weakness

Other reactions with cephalosporins include agranulocytosis, aplastic anemia, cholestasis, colitis, erythema multiforme, hemolytic anemia, hemorrhage, interstitial nephritis, pancytopenia, renal dysfunction, seizures, serum-sickness reactions, Stevens-Johnson syndrome, superinfection, toxic epidermal necrolysis, toxic nephropathy, urticaria, vaginitis

**Overdosage/Toxicology**

Signs and symptoms: After acute overdose, most agents cause only nausea, vomiting, and diarrhea, although neuromuscular hypersensitivity and seizures are possible, especially in patients with renal insufficiency

Treatment: Hemodialysis may be helpful to aid in the removal of the drug from the blood but not usually indicated, otherwise most treatment is supportive or symptom directed following GI decontamination

**Drug Interactions**

Decreased effect: Antacids and $H_2$-receptor antagonists (reduce absorption and serum concentration of cefpodoxime)

Increased effect: Probenecid may decrease cephalosporin elimination

Increased toxicity: Furosemide, aminoglycosides may be a possible additive to nephrotoxicity

**Usual Dosage** Oral:

Children >5 months to 12 years:
Acute otitis media: 10 mg/kg/day as a single dose or divided every 12 hours (400 mg/day)
Pharyngitis/tonsillitis: 10 mg/kg/day in 2 divided doses (maximum: 200 mg/day)

Children ≥13 years and Adults:
Acute community-acquired pneumonia and bacterial exacerbations of chronic bronchitis: 200 mg every 12 hours for 14 days and 10 days, respectively
Skin and skin structure: 400 mg every 12 hours for 7-14 days
Uncomplicated gonorrhea (male and female) and rectal gonococcal infections (female): 200 mg as a single dose
Pharyngitis/tonsillitis: 100 mg every 12 hours for 10 days
Uncomplicated urinary tract infection: 100 mg every 12 hours for 7 days

**Dosing adjustment in renal impairment:** $Cl_{cr}$ <30 mL/minute: Administer every 24 hours

**Patient Information** Take as directed, at regular intervals around-the-clock (with or without food). Chilling oral suspension improves flavor (do not freeze). Complete full course of medication, even if you feel better. Drink 2-3 L fluid/day. If diarrhea occurs, yogurt or buttermilk may help. May cause false-positive test with Clinitest®; use another form of testing. May interfere with oral contraceptives; additional contraceptive measures are necessary. Report severe, unresolved diarrhea; vaginal itching or drainage; sores in mouth; blood, pus, or mucus in stool or urine; easy bleeding or bruising; unusual fever or chills; rash; or respiratory difficulty.

**Dosage Forms**

Granules for oral suspension, as proxetil (lemon creme flavor): 50 mg/5 mL (100 mL); 100 mg/5 mL (100 mL)
Tablet, film coated, as proxetil: 100 mg, 200 mg

## Cefprozil (sef PROE zil)

**U.S. Brand Names** Cefzil®

**Pharmacologic Category** Antibiotic, Cephalosporin (Second Generation)

**Use** Treatment of otitis media and infections involving the respiratory tract and skin and skin structure; Active against methicillin-sensitive staphylococci, many streptococci, and various gram-negative bacilli including *E. coli*, some *Klebsiella, P. mirabilis, H. influenzae*, and *Moraxella*.

**Effects on Mental Status** May cause nervousness; case reports of euphoria, delusion, illusions, and depersonalization with cephalosporins

**Effects on Psychiatric Treatment** May rarely cause neutropenia; use caution with clozapine and carbamazepine

**Pregnancy Risk Factor** B

**Contraindications** Hypersensitivity to cefprozil or any component or cephalosporins

**Warnings/Precautions** Modify dosage in patients with severe renal impairment; prolonged use may result in superinfection; use with caution in patients with a history of penicillin allergy especially IgE-mediated reactions (eg, anaphylaxis, urticaria); may cause antibiotic-associated colitis or colitis secondary to *C. difficile*

**Adverse Reactions**

1% to 10%:
Central nervous system: Dizziness (1%)
Dermatologic: Diaper rash (1.5%)
Gastrointestinal: Diarrhea (2.9%), nausea (3.5%), vomiting (1%), abdominal pain (1%)
Genitourinary: Vaginitis, genital pruritus (1.6%)
Hepatic: Increased transaminases (2%)
Miscellaneous: Superinfection

<1%: Anaphylaxis, angioedema, arthralgia, cholestatic jaundice, confusion, elevated BUN, elevated creatinine, eosinophilia, erythema multiforme, fever, headache, hyperactivity, insomnia, leukopenia, pseudomembranous colitis, rash, serum sickness, somnolence, Stevens-Johnson syndrome, thrombocytopenia, urticaria

Other reactions with cephalosporins include agranulocytosis, aplastic anemia, cholestasis, colitis, erythema multiforme, hemolytic anemia, hemorrhage, interstitial nephritis, pancytopenia, renal dysfunction, seizures, serum-sickness reactions, Stevens-Johnson syndrome, superinfection, toxic epidermal necrolysis, toxic nephropathy, urticaria, vaginitis

**Overdosage/Toxicology**

Signs and symptoms: After acute overdose, most agents cause only nausea, vomiting, and diarrhea, although neuromuscular hypersensitivity and seizures are possible, especially in patients with renal insufficiency

Treatment: Hemodialysis may be helpful to aid in the removal of the drug from the blood but not usually indicated, otherwise most treatment is supportive or symptom directed following GI decontamination

**Drug Interactions**

Increased effect: Probenecid may decrease cephalosporin elimination

Increased toxicity: Furosemide, aminoglycosides may be a possible additive to nephrotoxicity

**Usual Dosage** Oral:

Infants and Children >6 months to 12 years: Otitis media: 15 mg/kg every 12 hours for 10 days

Pharyngitis/tonsillitis:
Children 2-12 years: 7.5 -15 mg/kg/day divided every 12 hours for 10 days (administer for >10 days if due to *S. pyogenes*); maximum: 1 g/day
Children >13 years and Adults: 500 mg every 24 hours for 10 days

Uncomplicated skin and skin structure infections:
Children 2-12 years: 20 mg/kg every 24 hours for 10 days; maximum: 1 g/day
Children >13 years and Adults: 250 mg every 12 hours, or 500 mg every 12-24 hours for 10 days

Secondary bacterial infection of acute bronchitis or acute bacterial exacerbation of chronic bronchitis: 500 mg every 12 hours for 10 days

**Dosing adjustment in renal impairment:** $Cl_{cr}$ <30 mL/minute: Reduce dose by 50%

Hemodialysis: Reduced by hemodialysis; administer dose after the completion of hemodialysis

**Patient Information** Take as directed, at regular intervals around-the-clock (with or without food). Chilling oral suspension improves flavor (do not freeze). Complete full course of medication, even if you feel better. Drink 2-3 L fluid/day. If diarrhea occurs, yogurt or buttermilk may help. May cause false-positive test with Clinitest®; use another form of testing. May interfere with oral contraceptives; additional contraceptive measures are necessary. Report severe, unresolved diarrhea; vaginal itching or drainage; sores in mouth; blood, pus, or mucus in stool or urine; easy bleeding or bruising; unusual fever or chills; rash; or respiratory difficulty.

**Dosage Forms**

Powder for oral suspension, as anhydrous: 125 mg/5 mL (50 mL, 75 mL, 100 mL); 250 mg/5 mL (50 mL, 75 mL, 100 mL)

Tablet, as anhydrous: 250 mg, 500 mg

## Ceftazidime (SEF tay zi deem)

**U.S. Brand Names** Ceptaz™; Fortaz®; Tazicef®; Tazidime®

**Canadian Brand Names** Ceptaz™

**Pharmacologic Category** Antibiotic, Cephalosporin (Third Generation)

**Use** Treatment of documented susceptible *Pseudomonas aeruginosa* infection and infections due to other susceptible aerobic gram-negative organisms; empiric therapy of a febrile, granulocytopenic patient

**Effects on Mental Status** May cause nervousness; case reports of euphoria, delusion, illusions, and depersonalization with cephalosporins

**Effects on Psychiatric Treatment** May rarely cause neutropenia; use caution with clozapine and carbamazepine

**Usual Dosage**

Neonates 0-4 weeks: I.V.: 30 mg/kg every 12 hours

Infants and Children 1 month to 12 years: I.V.: 30-50 mg/kg/dose every 8 hours; maximum dose: 6 g/day

Adults: I.M., I.V.: 500 mg to 2 g every 8-12 hours

Urinary tract infections: 250-500 mg every 12 hours

**Dosing interval in renal impairment:**

$Cl_{cr}$ 30-50 mL/minute: Administer every 12 hours

$Cl_{cr}$ 10-30 mL/minute: Administer every 24 hours

$Cl_{cr}$ <10 mL/minute: Administer every 48-72 hours

Hemodialysis: Dialyzable (50% to 100%)

Continuous arteriovenous or venovenous hemodiafiltration (CAVH) effects: Dose as for $Cl_{cr}$ 30-50 mL/minute

**Dosage Forms**

Infusion, premixed (frozen) (Fortaz®): 1 g (50 mL); 2 g (50 mL)

Powder for injection: 500 mg, 1 g, 2 g, 6 g

## Ceftibuten (sef TYE byoo ten)

**U.S. Brand Names** Cedax®

**Pharmacologic Category** Antibiotic, Cephalosporin (Third Generation)

**Use** Oral cephalosporin for bronchitis, otitis media, and pharyngitis/tonsillitis due to *H. influenzae* and *M. catarrhalis*, both beta-lactamase-producing and nonproducing strains, as well as *S. pneumoniae* (weak) and *S. pyogenes*

**Effects on Mental Status** May cause nervousness; case reports of euphoria, delusion, illusions, and depersonalization with cephalosporins

**Effects on Psychiatric Treatment** May rarely cause neutropenia; use caution with clozapine and carbamazepine

**Pregnancy Risk Factor** B

**Contraindications** In patients with known allergy to the cephalosporin group of antibiotics

**Warnings/Precautions** Modify dosage in patients with severe renal impairment, prolonged use may result in superinfection; use with caution in patients with a history of penicillin allergy, especially IgE-mediated reactions (eg, anaphylaxis, urticaria); may cause antibiotic-associated colitis or colitis secondary to *C. difficile*

**Adverse Reactions**

1% to 10%:

Central nervous system: Headache (3%), dizziness (1%)

Gastrointestinal: Nausea (4%), diarrhea (3%), dyspepsia (2%), vomiting (1%), abdominal pain (1%)

Hematologic: Increased eosinophils (3%), decreased hemoglobin (2%), thrombocytosis

Hepatic: Increased ALT (1%), increased bilirubin (1%)

Renal: Increased BUN (4%)

<1%: Agitation, anorexia, candidiasis, constipation, fatigue, diaper rash, dyspnea, dysuria, increased creatinine, increased transaminases, insomnia, irritability, leukopenia, nasal congestion, paresthesia, rash, rigors, urticaria, xerostomia

Other reactions with cephalosporins include agranulocytosis, anaphylaxis, angioedema, aplastic anemia, asterixis, candidiasis, cholestasis, colitis, encephalopathy, erythema multiforme, fever, hemolytic anemia, hemorrhage, interstitial nephritis, neuromuscular excitability, pancytopenia, paresthesia, prolonged PT, pruritus, pseudomembranous colitis, renal dysfunction, seizures, serum-sickness reactions, Stevens-Johnson syndrome, superinfection, toxic epidermal necrolysis, toxic nephropathy, vaginitis

**Overdosage/Toxicology**

Signs and symptoms: After acute overdose, most agents cause only nausea, vomiting, and diarrhea, although neuromuscular hypersensitivity and seizures are possible, especially in patients with renal insufficiency

Treatment: Hemodialysis may be helpful to aid in the removal of the drug from the blood but not usually indicated, otherwise most treatment is supportive or symptom directed following GI decontamination

**Drug Interactions**

Increased effect: High-dose probenecid decreases clearance

Increased toxicity: Aminoglycosides increase nephrotoxic potential

**Usual Dosage** Oral:

Children <12 years: 9 mg/kg/day for 10 days; maximum daily dose: 400 mg

Children ≥12 years and Adults: 400 mg once daily for 10 days; maximum: 400 mg

**Dosage adjustment in renal impairment:**

$Cl_{cr}$ 30-49 mL//minute: Administer 4.5 mg/kg or 200 mg every 24 hours

$Cl_{cr}$ <29 mL/minute: Administer 2.25 mg/kg or 100 mg every 24 hours

**Patient Information** Take as directed, at regular intervals around-the-clock (with or without food). Chilling oral suspension improves flavor (do not freeze). Complete full course of medication, even if you feel better. Drink 2-3 L fluid/day. If diarrhea occurs, yogurt or buttermilk may help. May cause false-positive test with Clinitest®; use another form of testing. May interfere with oral contraceptives; additional contraceptive measures are necessary. Report severe, unresolved diarrhea; vaginal itching or drainage; sores in mouth; blood, pus, or mucus in stool or urine; easy bleeding or bruising; unusual fever or chills; rash; or respiratory difficulty.

**Dosage Forms**

Capsule: 400 mg

Powder for oral suspension (cherry flavor): 90 mg/5 mL (30 mL, 60 mL, 120 mL); 180 mg/5 mL (30 mL, 60 mL, 120 mL)

♦ **Ceftin® Oral** *see* Cefuroxime *on page 102*

## Ceftizoxime (sef ti ZOKS eem)

**U.S. Brand Names** Cefizox®

**Pharmacologic Category** Antibiotic, Cephalosporin (Third Generation)

**Use** Treatment of susceptible bacterial infection, mainly respiratory tract, skin and skin structure, bone and joint, urinary tract and gynecologic, as well as septicemia; active against many gram-negative bacilli (not *Pseudomonas*), some gram-positive cocci (not *Enterococcus*), and some anaerobes

**Effects on Mental Status** May cause nervousness; case reports of euphoria, delusion, illusions, and depersonalization with cephalosporins

**Effects on Psychiatric Treatment** May rarely cause neutropenia; use caution with clozapine and carbamazepine

**Usual Dosage** I.M., I.V.:

Children ≥6 months: 150-200 mg/kg/day divided every 6-8 hours (maximum of 12 g/24 hours)

Adults: 1-2 g every 8-12 hours, up to 2 g every 4 hours or 4 g every 8 hours for life-threatening infections

**Dosing adjustment in renal impairment:** Adults:

$Cl_{cr}$ 10-30 mL/minute: Administer 1 g every 12 hours

$Cl_{cr}$ <10 mL/minute: Administer 1 g every 24 hours

Moderately dialyzable (20% to 50%)

Continuous arteriovenous or venovenous hemodiafiltration (CAVH) effects: Dose as for $Cl_{cr}$ 10-50 mL/minute

**Dosage Forms**

Injection, as sodium, in $D_5W$ (frozen): 1 g (50 mL); 2 g (50 mL)

Powder for injection, as sodium: 500 mg, 1 g, 2 g, 10 g

## Ceftriaxone (sef trye AKS one)

**U.S. Brand Names** Rocephin®

**Pharmacologic Category** Antibiotic, Cephalosporin (Third Generation)

**Use** Treatment of lower respiratory tract infections, skin and skin structure infections, bone and joint infections, intra-abdominal and urinary tract infections, sepsis and meningitis due to susceptible organisms; documented or suspected infection due to susceptible organisms in home care patients and patients without I.V. line access; treatment of documented or suspected gonococcal infection or chancroid; emergency room management of patients at high risk for bacteremia, periorbital or buccal cellulitis, salmonellosis or shigellosis, and pneumonia of unestablished etiology (<5 years of age); treatment of Lyme disease, depends on the stage of the disease (used in Stage II and Stage III, but not stage I; doxycycline is the drug of choice for Stage I)

**Effects on Mental Status** Case reports of euphoria, delusion, illusions, and depersonalization with cephalosporins

**Effects on Psychiatric Treatment** May rarely cause neutropenia; use caution with clozapine and carbamazepine

**Usual Dosage** I.M., I.V.:

Neonates:

Postnatal age ≤7 days: 50 mg/kg/day given every 24 hours

(Continued)

## Ceftriaxone *(Continued)*

Postnatal age >7 days:
≤2000 g: 50 mg/kg/day given every 24 hours
>2000 g: 50-75 mg/kg/day given every 24 hours
Gonococcal prophylaxis: 25-50 mg/kg as a single dose (dose not to exceed 125 mg)
Gonococcal infection: 25-50 mg/kg/day (maximum dose: 125 mg) given every 24 hours for 10-14 days
Infants and Children: 50-75 mg/kg/day in 1-2 divided doses every 12-24 hours; maximum: 2 g/24 hours
Meningitis: 100 mg/kg/day divided every 12-24 hours, up to a maximum of 4 g/24 hours; loading dose of 75 mg/kg/dose may be given at start of therapy
Otitis media: Single I.M. injection
Uncomplicated gonococcal infections, sexual assault, and STD prophylaxis: I.M.: 125 mg as a single dose plus doxycycline
Complicated gonococcal infections:
Infants: I.M., I.V.: 25-50 mg/kg/day in a single dose (maximum: 125 mg/dose); treat for 7 days for disseminated infection and 7-14 days for documented meningitis
<45 kg: 50 mg/kg/day once daily; maximum: 1 g/day; for ophthalmia, peritonitis, arthritis, or bacteremia: 50-100 mg/kg/day divided every 12-24 hours; maximum: 2 g/day for meningitis or endocarditis
>45 kg: 1 g/day once daily for disseminated gonococcal infections; 1-2 g dose every 12 hours for meningitis or endocarditis
Acute epididymitis: I.M.: 250 mg in a single dose
Adults: 1-2 g every 12-24 hours (depending on the type and severity of infection); maximum dose: 2 g every 12 hours for treatment of meningitis
Uncomplicated gonorrhea: I.M.: 250 mg as a single dose
Surgical prophylaxis: 1 g 30 minutes to 2 hours before surgery
**Dosing adjustment in renal or hepatic impairment:** No change necessary
Hemodialysis: Not dialyzable (0% to 5%); administer dose postdialysis
Peritoneal dialysis: Administer 750 mg every 12 hours
Continuous arteriovenous or venovenous hemofiltration (CAVH/CAVHD): Removes 10 mg of ceftriaxone per liter of filtrate per day

**Dosage Forms**
Infusion, as sodium, premixed (frozen): 1 g in $D_{3.8}W$ (50 mL); 2 g in $D_{2.4}W$ (50 mL)
Powder for injection, as sodium: 250 mg, 500 mg, 1 g, 2 g, 10 g

## Cefuroxime (se fyoor OKS eem)

**U.S. Brand Names** Ceftin® Oral; Kefurox® Injection; Zinacef® Injection

**Pharmacologic Category** Antibiotic, Cephalosporin (Second Generation)

**Use** Treatment of infections caused by staphylococci, group B streptococci, *H. influenzae* (type A and B), *E. coli*, *Enterobacter*, *Salmonella*, and *Klebsiella*; treatment of susceptible infections of the lower respiratory tract, otitis media, urinary tract, skin and soft tissue, bone and joint, sepsis and gonorrhea

**Effects on Mental Status** May cause nervousness; case reports of euphoria, delusion, illusions, and depersonalization with cephalosporins

**Effects on Psychiatric Treatment** May rarely cause neutropenia; use caution with clozapine and carbamazepine

**Pregnancy Risk Factor** B

**Contraindications** Hypersensitivity to cefuroxime, any component, or cephalosporins

**Warnings/Precautions** Modify dosage in patients with severe renal impairment, prolonged use may result in superinfection; use with caution in patients with a history of penicillin allergy, especially IgE-mediated reactions (eg, anaphylaxis, urticaria); may cause antibiotic-associated colitis or colitis secondary to *C. difficile*

**Adverse Reactions**
1% to 10%:
Hematologic: Eosinophilia (7%), decreased hemoglobin and hematocrit (10%)
Hepatic: Increased transaminases (4%), increased alkaline phosphatase (2%)
Local: Thrombophlebitis (1.7%)
<1%: Anaphylaxis, angioedema, colitis, diarrhea, dizziness, erythema multiforme, fever, GI bleeding, headache, increased BUN, increased creatinine, interstitial nephritis, leukopenia, nausea, neutropenia, pain at injection site, pseudomembranous colitis, rash, seizures, Stevens-Johnson syndrome, stomach cramps, toxic epidermal necrolysis, vaginitis, vomiting
Other reactions with cephalosporins include agranulocytosis, aplastic anemia, asterixis, cholestasis, colitis, encephalopathy, hemolytic anemia, hemorrhage, neuromuscular excitability, pancytopenia, prolonged PT, serum-sickness reactions, superinfection, toxic nephropathy

**Overdosage/Toxicology**
Signs and symptoms: After acute overdose, most agents cause only nausea, vomiting, and diarrhea, although neuromuscular hypersensitivity and seizures are possible, especially in patients with renal insufficiency
Treatment: Hemodialysis may be helpful to aid in the removal of the drug from the blood but not usually indicated, otherwise most treatment is supportive or symptom directed following GI decontamination

**Drug Interactions**
Increased effect: High-dose probenecid decreases clearance
Increased toxicity: Aminoglycosides increase nephrotoxic potential

**Usual Dosage**
Children:
Pharyngitis, tonsillitis: Oral:
Suspension: 20 mg/kg/day (maximum: 500 mg/day) in 2 divided doses
Tablet: 125 mg every 12 hours
Acute otitis media, impetigo: Oral:
Suspension: 30 mg/kg/day (maximum: 1 g/day) in 2 divided doses
Tablet: 250 mg every 12 hours
I.M., I.V.: 75-150 mg/kg/day divided every 8 hours; maximum dose: 6 g/day
Meningitis: Not recommended (doses of 200-240 mg/kg/day divided every 6-8 hours have been used); maximum dose: 9 g/day
Adults:
Oral: 250-500 mg twice daily; uncomplicated urinary tract infection: 125-250 mg every 12 hours
I.M., I.V.: 750 mg to 1.5 g/dose every 8 hours or 100-150 mg/kg/day in divided doses every 6-8 hours; maximum: 6 g/24 hours
**Dosing adjustment in renal impairment:**
$Cl_{cr}$ 10-20 mL/minute: Administer every 12 hours
$Cl_{cr}$ <10 mL/minute: Administer every 24 hours
Hemodialysis: Dialyzable (25%)
**Note:** Cefuroxime axetil film-coated tablets and oral suspension are not bioequivalent and are not substitutable on a mg/mg basis
Continuous arteriovenous or venovenous hemodiafiltration (CAVH) effects: Dose as for $Cl_{cr}$ 10-20 mL/minute

**Patient Information** Take as directed, at regular intervals around-the-clock (with or without food). Chilling oral suspension improves flavor (do not freeze). Complete full course of medication, even if you feel better. Drink 2-3 L fluid/day. If diarrhea occurs, yogurt or buttermilk may help. May cause false-positive test with Clinitest®; use another form of testing. May interfere with oral contraceptives; additional contraceptive measures are necessary. Report severe, unresolved diarrhea; vaginal itching or drainage; sores in mouth; blood, pus, or mucus in stool or urine; easy bleeding or bruising; unusual fever or chills; rash; or respiratory difficulty.

**Nursing Implications** Do not admix with aminoglycosides in same bottle/bag; obtain specimens for culture and sensitivity prior to the first dose

**Dosage Forms**
Infusion, as sodium, premixed (frozen) (Zinacef®): 750 mg (50 mL); 1.5 g (50 mL)
Powder for injection, as sodium: 750 mg, 1.5 g, 7.5 g
Powder for injection, as sodium (Kefurox®, Zinacef®): 750 mg, 1.5 g, 7.5 g
Powder for oral suspension, as axetil (tutti-frutti flavor) (Ceftin®): 125 mg/5 mL (50 mL, 100 mL, 200 mL)
Tablet, as axetil (Ceftin®): 125 mg, 250 mg, 500 mg

♦ **Cefzil®** *see* Cefprozil *on page 100*

♦ **Celebrex™** *see* Celecoxib *on page 102*

## Celecoxib (ce le COX ib)

**Related Information**
Nonsteroidal Anti-inflammatory Agents Comparison Chart *on page 722*

**U.S. Brand Names** Celebrex™

**Pharmacologic Category** Nonsteroidal Anti-Inflammatory Agent (NSAID)

**Use** Relief of the signs and symptoms of osteoarthritis; relief of the signs and symptoms of rheumatoid arthritis in adults

**Effects on Mental Status** May cause dizziness and insomnia; may rarely, cause anxiety, depression, nervousness, or somnolence

**Effects on Psychiatric Treatment** Effects of benzodiazepines and antidepressants may be altered. Lithium concentrations may be increased by celecoxib via decreased renal lithium clearance; dose adjustment may be needed.

**Pregnancy Risk Factor** C (D after 34 weeks gestation or close to delivery)

**Contraindications** Hypersensitivity to celecoxib or any component, sulfonamides, aspirin, or other nonsteroidal anti-inflammatory drugs (NSAIDs)

**Warnings/Precautions** Gastrointestinal irritation, ulceration, bleeding, and perforation may occur with NSAIDs (it is unclear whether celecoxib is associated with rates of these events which are similar to nonselective NSAIDs). Use with caution in patients with a history of GI disease (bleeding or ulcers), decreased renal function, hepatic disease, congestive heart failure, hypertension, or asthma. Anaphylactoid reactions may occur, even with no prior exposure to celecoxib. Use caution in patients with known or suspected deficiency of cytochrome P-450 isoenzyme 2C9.

**Adverse Reactions**
>10%: Central nervous system: Headache (15.8%)
2% to 10%:
Cardiovascular: Peripheral edema (2.1%)

Central nervous system: Insomnia (2.3%), dizziness (2%)
Dermatologic: Skin rash (2.2%)
Gastrointestinal: Dyspepsia (8.8%), diarrhea (5.6%), abdominal pain (4.1%), nausea (3.5%), flatulence (2.2%)
Neuromuscular & skeletal: Back pain (2.8%)
Respiratory: Upper respiratory tract infection (8.1%), sinusitis (5%), pharyngitis (2.3%), rhinitis (2%)
Miscellaneous: Accidental injury (2.9%)

0.1% to 2%:
Cardiovascular: Hypertension (aggravated), chest pain, myocardial infarction, palpitation, tachycardia, facial edema, peripheral edema
Central nervous system: Migraine, vertigo, hypoesthesia, fatigue, fever, pain, hypotonia, anxiety, depression, nervousness, somnolence
Dermatologic: Alopecia, dermatitis, photosensitivity, pruritus, rash (maculopapular), rash (erythematous), dry skin, urticaria
Endocrine & metabolic: Hot flashes, diabetes mellitus, hyperglycemia, hypercholesterolemia, breast pain, dysmenorrhea, menstrual disturbances, hypokalemia
Gastrointestinal: Constipation, tenesmus, diverticulitis, eructation, esophagitis, gastroenteritis, vomiting, gastroesophageal reflux, hemorrhoids, hiatal hernia, melena, stomatitis, anorexia, increased appetite, taste disturbance, xerostomia, tooth disorder, weight gain
Genitourinary: Prostate disorder, vaginal bleeding, vaginitis, monilial vaginitis, dysuria, cystitis, urinary frequency, incontinence, urinary tract infection,
Hepatic: Elevated transaminases, increased alkaline phosphatase
Hematologic: Anemia, thrombocytopenia, ecchymosis
Neuromuscular & skeletal: Leg cramps, increased CPK, neck stiffness, arthralgia, myalgia, bone disorder, fracture, synovitis, tendonitis, neuralgia, paresthesia, neuropathy, weakness
Ocular: Glaucoma, blurred vision, cataract, conjunctivitis, eye pain
Otic: Deafness, tinnitus, earache, otitis media
Renal: Increased BUN, increased creatinine, albuminuria, hematuria, renal calculi
Respiratory: Bronchitis, bronchospasm, cough, dyspnea, laryngitis, pneumonia, epistaxis
Miscellaneous: Allergic reactions, flu-like syndrome, breast cancer, herpes infection, bacterial infection, moniliasis, viral infection, increased diaphoresis

<0.1% (limited to severe): Acute renal failure, ataxia, cerebrovascular accident, colitis, congestive heart failure, esophageal perforation, gangrene, gastrointestinal bleeding, intestinal obstruction, intestinal perforation, pancreatitis, pulmonary embolism, sepsis, sudden death, syncope, thrombocytopenia, thrombophlebitis, ventricular fibrillation

**Overdosage/Toxicology**
Symptoms may include epigastric pain, drowsiness, lethargy, nausea, and vomiting; gastrointestinal bleeding may occur. Rare manifestations include hypertension, respiratory depression, coma, and acute renal failure.
Treatment is symptomatic and supportive; forced diuresis, hemodialysis and/or urinary alkalinization may not be useful

**Drug Interactions** Celecoxib may be a cytochrome oxidase P-450 isoenzyme 2C9 substrate and an inhibitor of isoenzyme 2D6
ACE inhibitors: Effects may be reduced by celecoxib (limited information on effects with COX-2 inhibitors as compared to nonselective NSAIDs); monitor
Antacids (aluminum and magnesium containing): May reduce AUC by 10% ($C_{max}$ reduced by 37%)
Aspirin: Celecoxib may be used with low-dose aspirin; however, rates of gastrointestinal bleeding may be increased with coadministration
Corticosteroids: May increase the risk of GI ulceration (limited information on risk with selective COX-2 inhibitors); use caution
CYP2C9 inhibitors: May result in significant increases in celecoxib concentrations; inhibitors include amiodarone, cimetidine, fluvoxamine, metronidazole, omeprazole, sulfonamides, valproic acid, and zafirlukast
CYP2D6 substrates: Coadministration of drugs metabolized by CYP2D6 may result in increased serum concentrations of these agents; includes many psychotherapeutic agents
Fluconazole: Increases celecoxib concentrations two-fold
Hydralazine: Antihypertensive effect may be decreased; avoid concurrent use
Lithium: Serum levels can be increased; avoid concurrent use if possible or monitor lithium levels and adjust dose. Limited information with COX-2 selective agents as compared to NSAIDs. When NSAID is stopped, lithium may need adjustment again.
Loop diuretics: Therapeutic effects may be reduced by celecoxib; avoid
Thiazide diuretics: Antihypertensive effects are decreased; avoid
Warfarin: INRs may be increased by some NSAIDs. Individual cases have been reported with celecoxib. This may depend, in part, on dose and duration; monitor INR closely. Use the lowest dose of NSAIDs possible and for the briefest duration.

**Usual Dosage** Adults: Oral:
Osteoarthritis: 200 mg/day as a single dose or in divided dose twice daily
Rheumatoid arthritis: 100-200 mg twice daily
**Dosing adjustment in renal impairment:** No specific dosage adjustment is recommended
**Dosing adjustment in hepatic impairment:** Reduced dosage is recommended (AUC may be increased by 40% to 180%)
Dosing adjustment for elderly: No specific adjustment is recommended. However, the AUC in elderly patients may be increased by 50% as compared to younger subjects. Use the lowest recommended dose in patients weighing <50 kg.

**Dietary Considerations** Peak concentrations are delayed and AUC is increased by 10% to 20% when taken with a high-fat meal; celecoxib may be taken without regard to meals

**Patient Information** Do not take more than recommended dose. May be taken with food to reduce GI upset. Do not take with antacids. Avoid alcohol, aspirin, and OTC medication unless approved by prescriber. You may experience dizziness, confusion, or blurred vision (avoid driving or engaging in tasks requiring alertness until response to drug is known); anorexia, nausea, vomiting, taste disturbance, gastric distress (small frequent meals, frequent mouth care, sucking lozenges, or chewing gum may help). GI bleeding, ulceration, or perforation can occur with or without pain; it is unclear whether celecoxib has rates of these events which are similar to nonselective NSAIDs. Stop taking medication and report immediately stomach pain or cramping, unusual bleeding or bruising, or blood in vomitus, stool, or urine. Report persistent insomnia; skin rash; unusual fatigue or easy bruising or bleeding; muscle pain, tremors, or weakness; sudden weight gain; changes in hearing (ringing in ears); changes in vision; changes in urination pattern; or respiratory difficulty.

**Dosage Forms** Capsule: 100 mg, 200 mg


- **Celestone®** *see* Betamethasone *on page 65*
- **Celestone® Soluspan®** *see* Betamethasone *on page 65*
- **Celexa™** *see* Citalopram *on page 126*
- **CellCept®** *see* Mycophenolate *on page 377*
- **Cellufresh™ [OTC]** *see* Carboxymethylcellulose *on page 94*
- **Celluvisc® [OTC]** *see* Carboxymethylcellulose *on page 94*
- **Celontin®** *see* Methsuximide *on page 356*
- **Cel-U-Jec®** *see* Betamethasone *on page 65*
- **Cenafed® [OTC]** *see* Pseudoephedrine *on page 478*
- **Cenafed® Plus Tablet [OTC]** *see* Triprolidine and Pseudoephedrine *on page 572*
- **Cena-K®** *see* Potassium Chloride *on page 453*
- **Cenestin™** *see* Estrogens, Conjugated (Synthetic) *on page 207*
- **Centrax®** *see* Prazepam *on page 458*
- **Cēpacol® Anesthetic Troches [OTC]** *see* Cetylpyridinium and Benzocaine *on page 106*
- **Cēpacol® Troches [OTC]** *see* Cetylpyridinium *on page 106*


## Cephalexin (sef a LEKS in)

**U.S. Brand Names** Biocef; Keflex®; Keftab®

**Canadian Brand Names** Apo®-Cephalex; Novo-Lexin; Nu-Cephalex

**Pharmacologic Category** Antibiotic, Cephalosporin (First Generation)

**Use** Treatment of susceptible bacterial infections, including those caused by group A beta-hemolytic *Streptococcus, Staphylococcus, Klebsiella pneumoniae, E. coli, Proteus mirabilis,* and *Shigella*; predominantly used for lower respiratory tract, urinary tract, skin and soft tissue, and bone and joint; prophylaxis against bacterial endocarditis in high-risk patients undergoing surgical or dental procedures who are allergic to penicillin

**Effects on Mental Status** May cause nervousness; case reports of euphoria, delusion, illusions, and depersonalization with cephalosporins

**Effects on Psychiatric Treatment** May rarely cause neutropenia; use caution with clozapine and carbamazepine

**Pregnancy Risk Factor** B

**Contraindications** Hypersensitivity to cephalexin, any component, or cephalosporins

**Warnings/Precautions** Modify dosage in patients with severe renal impairment, prolonged use may result in superinfection; use with caution in patients with a history of penicillin allergy, especially IgE-mediated reactions (eg, anaphylaxis, urticaria); may cause antibiotic-associated colitis or colitis secondary to *C. difficile*

**Adverse Reactions**
1% to 10%: Gastrointestinal: Diarrhea
<1%: Abdominal pain, agitation, anaphylaxis, anemia, angioedema, arthralgia, cholestasis, confusion, dizziness, dyspepsia, eosinophilia, erythema multiforme, fatigue, gastritis, hallucinations, headache, hepatitis, increased transaminases, interstitial nephritis, nausea, neutropenia, pseudomembranous colitis, rash, serum-sickness reaction, Stevens-Johnson syndrome, thrombocytopenia, toxic epidermal necrolysis, urticaria, vomiting
Other reactions with cephalosporins include agranulocytosis, anaphylaxis, aplastic anemia, asterixis, colitis, encephalopathy, hemolytic anemia,
(Continued)

## Cephalexin *(Continued)*

hemorrhage, neuromuscular excitability, pancytopenia, prolonged PT, seizures, superinfection, vomiting

**Overdosage/Toxicology**

Signs and symptoms: After acute overdose, most agents cause only nausea, vomiting, and diarrhea, although neuromuscular hypersensitivity and seizures are possible, especially in patients with renal insufficiency

Treatment: Hemodialysis may be helpful to aid in the removal of the drug from the blood but not usually indicated, otherwise most treatment is supportive or symptom directed following GI decontamination

**Drug Interactions**

Increased effect: High-dose probenecid decreases clearance

Increased toxicity: Aminoglycosides increase nephrotoxic potential

**Usual Dosage** Oral:

Children: 25-50 mg/kg/day every 6 hours; severe infections: 50-100 mg/kg/day in divided doses every 6 hours; maximum: 3 g/24 hours

Adults: 250-1000 mg every 6 hours; maximum: 4 g/day

Prophylaxis of bacterial endocarditis: 2 g 1 hour prior to the procedure

**Dosing adjustment in renal impairment:** Adults:

$Cl_{cr}$ 10-40 mL/minute: 250-500 mg every 8-12 hours

$Cl_{cr}$ <10 mL/minute: 250 mg every 12-24 hours

Hemodialysis: Moderately dialyzable (20% to 50%)

**Dietary Considerations** Food: Peak antibiotic serum concentration is lowered and delayed, but total drug absorbed is not affected; take on an empty stomach. If GI distress, take with food.

**Patient Information** Take as directed, at regular intervals around-the-clock (with or without food). Chilling oral suspension improves flavor (do not freeze). Complete full course of medication, even if you feel better. Drink 2-3 L fluid/day. If diarrhea occurs, yogurt or buttermilk may help. May cause false-positive test with Clinitest®; use another form of testing. May interfere with oral contraceptives; additional contraceptive measures are necessary. Report severe, unresolved diarrhea; vaginal itching or drainage; sores in mouth; blood, pus, or mucus in stool or urine; easy bleeding or bruising; unusual fever or chills; rash; or respiratory difficulty.

**Dosage Forms**

Capsule, as monohydrate: 250 mg, 500 mg

Powder for oral suspension, as monohydrate: 125 mg/5 mL (5 mL unit dose, 60 mL, 100 mL, 200 mL); 250 mg/5 mL (5 mL unit dose, 100 mL, 200 mL)

Suspension, oral, as monohydrate, pediatric: 100 mg/mL [5 mg/drop] (10 mL)

Tablet, as monohydrate: 250 mg, 500 mg, 1 g

Tablet, as hydrochloride: 500 mg

## Cephalothin (sef A loe thin)

**Canadian Brand Names** Ceporacin®

**Pharmacologic Category** Antibiotic, Cephalosporin (First Generation)

**Use** Treatment of infections when caused by susceptible strains in respiratory, genitourinary, gastrointestinal, skin and soft tissue, bone and joint infections; septicemia; treatment of susceptible gram-positive bacilli and cocci (never enterococcus); some gram-negative bacilli including *E. coli*, *Proteus*, and *Klebsiella* may be susceptible

**Effects on Mental Status** May cause nervousness; case reports of euphoria, delusion, illusions, and depersonalization with cephalosporins

**Effects on Psychiatric Treatment** May rarely cause neutropenia; use caution with clozapine and carbamazepine

**Usual Dosage** I.M., I.V.:

Neonates:

Postnatal age <7 days:

<2000 g: 20 mg every 12 hours

>2000 g: 20 mg every 8 hours

Postnatal age >7 days:

<2000 g: 20 mg every 8 hours

>2000 g: 20 mg every 6 hours

Children: 75-125 mg/kg/day divided every 4-6 hours; maximum dose: 10 g in a 24-hour period

Adults: 500 mg to 2 g every 4-6 hours

**Dosing interval in renal impairment:**

$Cl_{cr}$ 10-50 mL/minute: Administer every 6-8 hours

$Cl_{cr}$ <10 mL/minute: Administer every 12 hours

Continuous arteriovenous or venovenous hemodiafiltration (CAVH) effects: Administer 1 g every 8 hours

**Dosage Forms** Powder for injection, as sodium: 1 g, 2 g (50 mL)

## Cephapirin (sef a PYE rin)

**U.S. Brand Names** Cefadyl®

**Pharmacologic Category** Antibiotic, Cephalosporin (First Generation)

**Use** Treatment of infections when caused by susceptible strains in respiratory, genitourinary, gastrointestinal, skin and soft tissue, bone and joint infections, septicemia; treatment of susceptible gram-positive bacilli and cocci (never enterococcus); some gram-negative bacilli including *E. coli*, *Proteus*, and *Klebsiella* may be susceptible

**Effects on Mental Status** May cause nervousness; case reports of euphoria, delusion, illusions, and depersonalization with cephalosporins

**Effects on Psychiatric Treatment** May rarely cause neutropenia; use caution with clozapine and carbamazepine

**Pregnancy Risk Factor** B

**Contraindications** Hypersensitivity to cephapirin sodium, any component, or cephalosporins

**Warnings/Precautions** Modify dosage in patients with severe renal impairment, prolonged use may result in superinfection; use with caution in patients with a history of penicillin allergy, especially IgE-mediated reactions (eg, anaphylaxis, urticaria); may cause antibiotic-associated colitis or colitis secondary to *C. difficile*

**Adverse Reactions**

1% to 10%: Gastrointestinal: Diarrhea

<1%: CNS irritation, fever, increased transaminases, leukopenia, rash, seizures, thrombocytopenia, urticaria

Other reactions with cephalosporins include agranulocytosis, anaphylaxis, angioedema, aplastic anemia, asterixis, cholestasis, decreased hemoglobin, dizziness, encephalopathy, erythema multiforme, fever, headache, hemolytic anemia, hemorrhage, interstitial nephritis, nausea, neuromuscular excitability, pain at injection site, pancytopenia, prolonged PT, pseudomembranous colitis, seizures, serum-sickness reactions, Stevens-Johnson syndrome, superinfection, toxic epidermal necrolysis, toxic nephropathy, vaginitis, vomiting

**Overdosage/Toxicology**

Signs and symptoms: Neuromuscular hypersensitivity, convulsions especially with renal insufficiency

Treatment: Hemodialysis may be helpful to aid in the removal of the drug from the blood, otherwise most treatment is supportive or symptom directed

**Drug Interactions**

Increased effect: High-dose probenecid decreases clearance

Increased toxicity: Aminoglycosides increase nephrotoxic potential

**Usual Dosage** I.M., I.V.:

Children: 10-20 mg/kg/dose every 6 hours up to 4 g/24 hours

Adults: 500 mg to 1 g every 6 hours up to 12 g/day

Perioperative prophylaxis: 1-2 g 30 minutes to 1 hour prior to surgery and every 6 hours as needed for 24 hours following

**Dosing interval in renal impairment:**

$Cl_{cr}$ 10-50 mL/minute: Administer every 6-8 hours

$Cl_{cr}$ <10 mL/minute: Administer every 12 hours

Continuous arteriovenous or venovenous hemodiafiltration (CAVH) effects: Administer 1 g every 8 hours

**Patient Information** This drug is administered I.M. or I.V. Drink 2-3 L fluid/day. If diarrhea occurs, yogurt or buttermilk may help. May cause false-positive test with Clinitest®; use another form of testing. May interfere with oral contraceptives; additional contraceptive measures are necessary. Report severe, unresolved diarrhea; vaginal itching or drainage; sores in mouth; blood, pus, or mucus in stool or urine; easy bleeding or bruising; unusual fever or chills; rash; or respiratory difficulty.

**Nursing Implications** Do not admix with aminoglycosides in same bottle/bag; obtain specimens for culture and sensitivity prior to administration of first dose

**Dosage Forms** Powder for injection, as sodium: 500 mg, 1 g, 2 g, 4 g, 20 g

## Cephradine (SEF ra deen)

**U.S. Brand Names** Velosef®

**Pharmacologic Category** Antibiotic, Cephalosporin (First Generation)

**Use** Treatment of infections when caused by susceptible strains in respiratory, genitourinary, gastrointestinal, skin and soft tissue, bone and joint infections; treatment of susceptible gram-positive bacilli and cocci (never enterococcus); some gram-negative bacilli including *E. coli*, *Proteus*, and *Klebsiella* may be susceptible

**Effects on Mental Status** May cause nervousness; case reports of euphoria, delusion, illusions, and depersonalization with cephalosporins

**Effects on Psychiatric Treatment** May rarely cause neutropenia; use caution with clozapine and carbamazepine

**Pregnancy Risk Factor** B

**Contraindications** Hypersensitivity to cephradine, any component, or cephalosporins

**Warnings/Precautions** Modify dosage in patients with severe renal impairment, prolonged use may result in superinfection; use with caution in patients with a history of penicillin allergy, especially IgE-mediated reactions (eg, anaphylaxis, urticaria); may cause antibiotic-associated colitis or colitis secondary to *C. difficile*

**Adverse Reactions**

1% to 10%: Gastrointestinal: Diarrhea

<1%: Increased BUN, increased creatinine, nausea, pseudomembranous colitis, rash, vomiting

Other reactions with cephalosporins include agranulocytosis, anaphylaxis, angioedema, aplastic anemia, asterixis, cholestasis, dizziness, encephalopathy, erythema multiforme, fever, headache, hemolytic anemia, hemorrhage, interstitial nephritis, leukopenia, neuromuscular excitability, neutropenia, pancytopenia, prolonged PT, seizures, serum-sickness reactions, Stevens-Johnson syndrome, superinfection, toxic epidermal necrolysis, toxic nephropathy, vaginitis

**Overdosage/Toxicology**

Signs and symptoms: Neuromuscular hypersensitivity, convulsions especially with renal insufficiency

Treatment: Hemodialysis may be helpful to aid in the removal of the drug from the blood, otherwise most treatment is supportive or symptom directed.

**Drug Interactions**

Increased effect: High-dose probenecid decreases clearance

Increased toxicity: Aminoglycosides increase nephrotoxic potential

**Usual Dosage** Oral:

Children ≥9 months: 25-50 mg/kg/day in divided doses every 6 hours

Adults: 250-500 mg every 6-12 hours

**Dosing adjustment in renal impairment:** Adults:

$Cl_{cr}$ 10-50 mL/minute: 250 mg every 6 hours

$Cl_{cr}$ <10 mL/minute: 125 mg every 6 hours

**Patient Information** Oral: Take as directed, at regular intervals around-the-clock (with or without food). Chilling oral suspension improves flavor (do not freeze). Complete full course of medication, even if you feel better. Drink 2-3 L fluid/day. If diarrhea occurs, yogurt or buttermilk may help. May cause false-positive test with Clinitest®; use another form of testing. May interfere with oral contraceptives; additional contraceptive measures are necessary. Report severe, unresolved diarrhea; vaginal itching or drainage; sores in mouth; blood, pus, or mucus in stool or urine; easy bleeding or bruising; unusual fever or chills; rash; or respiratory difficulty.

**Dosage Forms**

Capsule: 250 mg, 500 mg

Powder for injection: 250 mg, 500 mg, 1 g, 2 g, (in ready-to-use infusion bottles)

Powder for oral suspension: 125 mg/5 mL (5 mL, 100 mL, 200 mL); 250 mg/5 mL (5 mL, 100 mL, 200 mL)

- **Cephulac®** *see* Lactulose *on page 306*
- **Ceptaz™** *see* Ceftazidime *on page 101*
- **Cerebyx®** *see* Fosphenytoin *on page 242*
- **Ceredase®** *see* Alglucerase *on page 23*
- **Cerezyme®** *see* Imiglucerase *on page 282*

## Cerivastatin (se ree va STAT in)

**Related Information**

Lipid-Lowering Agents Comparison Chart *on page 717*

**U.S. Brand Names** Baycol™

**Pharmacologic Category** Antilipemic Agent (HMG-CoA Reductase Inhibitor)

**Use** In conjunction with diet, reduces total LDL serum cholesterol and increases HDL-C concentrations in patients with primary hypercholesterolemia and mixed dyslipidemia (Fredrickson types IIa and IIb)

**Effects on Mental Status** May cause insomnia

**Effects on Psychiatric Treatment** None reported

**Pregnancy Risk Factor** X

**Contraindications** Hypersensitivity to cerivastatin or any component; active liver disease; unexplained persistent elevations of serum transaminases; pregnancy

**Warnings/Precautions** Liver function must be monitored by periodic laboratory assessment. Rhabdomyolysis with acute renal failure has occurred. Risk is increased with concurrent use of clarithromycin, danazol, diltiazem, fluvoxamine, indinavir, nefazodone, nelfinavir, ritonavir, verapamil, troleandomycin, cyclosporine, fibric acid derivatives, erythromycin, niacin, or azole antifungals. Weigh the risk versus benefit when combining any of these drugs with cerivastatin. Use with caution in patients who have a history of liver disease and/or consume substantial quantities of alcohol. Temporarily discontinue in any patient experiencing an acute or serious condition predisposing to renal failure secondary to rhabdomyolysis. Has not been evaluated in homozygous familial hypercholesterolemia.

**Adverse Reactions**

1% to 10%:

Cardiovascular: Chest pain, peripheral edema (2%)

Central nervous system: Headache, dizziness, insomnia

Gastrointestinal: Pain (3%), diarrhea (4%), dyspepsia (6%), nausea (3%), constipation (2%)

Neuromuscular & skeletal: Myalgia (3%), arthralgia (7%), leg pain (2%), weakness (2%)

<1%: Cough, increased LFTs, myopathy, possible rhabdomyolysis with renal failure, rhinitis, sinusitis

**Drug Interactions** CYP3A3/4 enzyme substrate

Inhibitors of CYP3A3/4 (clarithromycin, cyclosporine, danazol, diltiazem, fluvoxamine, erythromycin, fluconazole, itraconazole, ketoconazole, miconazole, nefazodone,amprenavir, indinavir, nelfinavir, ritonavir, saquinavir troleandomycin, and verapamil) increase cerivastatin blood levels; may increase the risk of cerivastatin-induced myopathy and rhabdomyolysis.

Cholestyramine reduces cerivastatin absorption. Separate administration times by at least 4 hours

Cholestyramine and colestipol (bile acid sequestrants): Cholesterol-lowering effects are additive

Clofibrate and fenofibrate may increase the risk of myopathy and rhabdomyolysis

Gemfibrozil: Increased risk of myopathy and rhabdomyolysis

Grapefruit juice may inhibit metabolism of cerivastatin via CYP3A3/4; avoid high dietary intakes of grapefruit juice

Niacin may increase the risk of myopathy and rhabdomyolysis

**Usual Dosage** Adults: Oral: 0.4 mg once daily in the evening; may be taken with or without food; maximum effect of a given dose will be seen in 4 weeks; monitor lipid levels and adjust dose at that time; dosing range: 0.2-0.8 mg/day

**Dosing adjustment with renal impairment:** Moderate to severe impairment (<60 mL/minute): Starting dose: 0.2 mg

**Dosing adjustment in hepatic impairment:** Avoidance suggested; no guidelines for dosage reduction available.

**Patient Information** Take prescribed dose in the evening (with or without food). You will need laboratory evaluation during therapy. Maintain adequate hydration (2-3 L/day of fluids unless instructed to restrict fluid intake). May cause headache (mild analgesic may help); drowsiness, dizziness, or blurred vision (use caution when driving or engaging in tasks that require alertness until response to medication is known). Report chest pain; swelling of extremities; weight gain (>5 lb/week); respiratory difficulty; persistent vomiting or abdominal pain; muscle weakness or pain; persistent cough; swelling of mouth, lips, or face; unusual bruising or bleeding; or skin rash.

**Dosage Forms** Tablet, as sodium: 0.2 mg, 0.3 mg, 0.8 mg

- **Cerose-DM® [OTC]** *see* Chlorpheniramine, Phenylephrine, and Dextromethorphan *on page 115*
- **Cerubidine®** *see* Daunorubicin Hydrochloride *on page 152*
- **Cerumenex® Otic** *see* Triethanolamine Polypeptide Oleate-Condensate *on page 566*
- **Cervidil® Vaginal Insert** *see* Dinoprostone *on page 173*
- **C.E.S.** *see* Estrogens, Conjugated *on page 206*
- **Cesamet®** *see* Nabilone *on page 378*
- **Cetacaine®** *see* Benzocaine, Butyl Aminobenzoate, Tetracaine, and Benzalkonium Chloride *on page 62*
- **Cetamide® Ophthalmic** *see* Sulfacetamide *on page 522*
- **Cetapred® Ophthalmic** *see* Sulfacetamide Sodium and Prednisolone *on page 523*

## Cetirizine (se TI ra zeen)

**U.S. Brand Names** Zyrtec®

**Canadian Brand Names** Reactine™

**Synonyms** P-071; UCB-P071

**Pharmacologic Category** Antihistamine

**Use** Perennial and seasonal allergic rhinitis and other allergic symptoms including urticaria

**Effects on Mental Status** Drowsiness is common

**Effects on Psychiatric Treatment** Concurrent use with psychotropics may produce additive sedation

**Pregnancy Risk Factor** B

**Contraindications** Hypersensitivity to cetirizine, hydroxyzine, or any component

**Warnings/Precautions** Cetirizine should be used cautiously in patients with hepatic or renal dysfunction and the elderly. Use in breast-feeding women is not recommended. Doses >10 mg/day may cause significant drowsiness

**Adverse Reactions**

>10%: Central nervous system: Headache has been reported to occur in 10% to 12% of patients, drowsiness has been reported in as much as 26% of patients on high doses

1% to 10%:

Central nervous system: Somnolence, fatigue, dizziness

Gastrointestinal: Xerostomia

<1%: Depression

**Overdosage/Toxicology**

Signs and symptoms: Seizures, sedation, hypotension

Treatment: There is no specific treatment for an antihistamine overdose; however, most of its clinical toxicity is due to anticholinergic effects. Anticholinesterase inhibitors may be useful by reducing acetylcholinesterase. For anticholinergic overdose with severe life-threatening symptoms, physostigmine 1-2 mg (0.5 or 0.02 mg/kg for children) I.V., slowly may be given to reverse these effects.

**Drug Interactions** Increased toxicity: CNS depressants, anticholinergics

**Usual Dosage** Children ≥6 years and Adults: Oral: 5-10 mg once daily, depending upon symptom severity

(Continued)

## Cetirizine *(Continued)*

**Dosing interval in renal/hepatic impairment:** $Cl_{cr}$ ≤31 mL/minute: Administer 5 mg once daily

**Patient Information** Take as directed; do not exceed recommended dose. Avoid use of other depressants, alcohol, or sleep-inducing medications unless approved by prescriber. You may experience drowsiness or dizziness (use caution when driving or engaging in tasks requiring alertness until response to drug is known); or dry mouth, (frequent small meals, frequent mouth care, chewing gum, or sucking hard candy may help). Report persistent sedation, confusion, or agitation; persistent nausea or vomiting; changes in urinary pattern; blurred vision; chest pain or palpitations; or lack of improvement or worsening or condition.

**Dosage Forms**

Syrup, as hydrochloride: 5 mg/5 mL (120 mL)

Tablet, as hydrochloride: 5 mg, 10 mg

♦ **Cetobemidone** *see* Ketobemidone *on page 301*

## Cetylpyridinium (SEE til peer i DI nee um)

**U.S. Brand Names** Ceepryn® [OTC]; Cēpacol® Troches [OTC]

**Pharmacologic Category** Local Anesthetic

**Use** Temporary relief of sore throat

**Effects on Mental Status** None reported

**Effects on Psychiatric Treatment** None reported

**Usual Dosage** Children >6 years and Adults: Oral: Dissolve 1 lozenge in the mouth every 2 hours as needed

**Dosage Forms**

Troches, as chloride: 1:1500 (24s)

Mouthwash, as chloride: 0.05% and alcohol 14% (180 mL)

## Cetylpyridinium and Benzocaine
(SEE til peer i DI nee um & BEN zoe kane)

**U.S. Brand Names** Cēpacol® Anesthetic Troches [OTC]

**Pharmacologic Category** Local Anesthetic

**Use** Symptomatic relief of sore throat

**Effects on Mental Status** None reported

**Effects on Psychiatric Treatment** None reported

**Usual Dosage** Use as needed for sore throat

**Dosage Forms** Troche: Cetylpyridinium chloride 1:1500 and benzocaine 10 mg per troche (18s)

♦ **Cevalin® [OTC]** *see* Ascorbic Acid *on page 48*

♦ **Cevi-Bid® [OTC]** *see* Ascorbic Acid *on page 48*

♦ **Ce-Vi-Sol® [OTC]** *see* Ascorbic Acid *on page 48*

♦ **CF100** *see* Ginkgo Biloba *on page 249*

♦ **CFDN** *see* Cefdinir *on page 97*

♦ **CG** *see* Chorionic Gonadotropin *on page 122*

## Chamomile

**Related Information**

Natural/Herbal Products *on page 746*

Natural Products, Herbals, and Dietary Supplements *on page 742*

**Synonyms** *Matricaria chamomilla*; *Matricarta recutita*

**Pharmacologic Category** Herb

**Use** Has been used for indigestion and its hypnotic properties; topical anti-inflammatory agent; used for hemorrhoids, irritable bowel, eczema, mastitis and leg ulcers; used to flavor cigarette tobacco

**Contraindications** Known hypersensitivity to *Asteraceae/Compositae* family

**Warnings/Precautions** Use with caution in asthmatics; cross sensitivity may occur in individuals allergic to ragweed pollens, asters, or chrysanthemums

**Adverse Reactions** Associated with those with severe ragweed allergies

Dermatologic: Contact dermatitis, immunologic contact urticaria

Gastrointestinal: Emesis (from dried flowering heads)

Miscellaneous: Anaphylaxis

While the toxicity of its main chemical constituent (Bisabolol) is low, the tea is essentially prepared from various allergens (ie, pollen-laden flower heads) which can cause hypersensitivity reactions especially in atopic individuals; contains various flavonoids (apigenin, herniarin)

**Overdosage/Toxicology** Treatment: Supportive therapy; treat allergic reactions with standard therapy (ie, epinephrine, antihistamines, vasopressors, if required)

**Drug Interactions**

CNS depressants: Sedative effects may be additive with other CNS depressants; includes ethanol, barbiturates, narcotic analgesics, and other sedative agents; monitor for increased effect

Warfarin: Anticoagulant effects may be potentiated (only at very high dosages of chamomile)

**Usual Dosage**

Tea: ±150 mL $H_2O$ poured over heaping tablespoon (±3 g) of chamomile, covered and steeped 5-10 minutes; tea used 3-4 times/day for G.I. upset

Liquid extract: 1-4 mL 3 times/day

**Additional Information** Cross-sensitivity may occur in individuals allergic to ragweed pollens, asters, or chrysanthemums

## Chaparral

**Synonyms** *Larrea tridentata*

**Pharmacologic Category** Herb

**Use** Herbal medicine to treat acne, bowel cramps, analgesic agent and to "retard aging" (not substantiated)

**Adverse Reactions**

Dermatologic: Contact dermatitis

Gastrointestinal: Anorexia

Hematologic: Coagulopathy

Hepatic: Lobular necrosis, jaundice

Miscellaneous: Necrosis

**Overdosage/Toxicology**

Decontamination: Ipecac within 30 minutes or lavage (within 1 hour)/activated charcoal with cathartic

Treatment: Supportive therapy; orthotopic liver transplantation may be required to treat liver failure

**Patient Information** Considered unsafe by the FDA; large doses and/or prolonged use can cause liver damage

**Additional Information** A branched bush or shrub that is olive green and can grow to a height of 9 feet in the desert regions of Southwestern U.S. and Mexico. Approximately 200 tons of chaparral were sold in the U.S. for use as teas and herbal dietary supplements in the 20 years from 1973-1993, according to informal herb industry estimates. Few adverse reactions were reported during this period. A medical review by three physicians of patient records obtained from FDA regarding hepatitis associated with chaparral ingestion could not definitively conclude that chaparral was the causative agent. Idiosyncratic reactions were suggested.

♦ **CharcoAid® [OTC]** *see* Charcoal *on page 106*

## Charcoal (CHAR kole)

**U.S. Brand Names** Actidose-Aqua® [OTC]; Actidose® With Sorbitol [OTC]; CharcoAid® [OTC]; Charcocaps® [OTC]; Insta-Char® [OTC]; Liqui-Char® [OTC]

**Synonyms** Activated Carbon; Activated Charcoal; Adsorbent Charcoal; Liquid Antidote; Medicinal Carbon; Medicinal Charcoal

**Pharmacologic Category** Antidiarrheal; Antidote; Antiflatulent

**Use** Emergency treatment in poisoning by drugs and chemicals; repetitive doses for gastric dialysis in uremia to adsorb various waste products, and repetitive doses have proven useful to enhance the elimination of certain drugs (eg, theophylline, phenobarbital, and aspirin)

**Effects on Mental Status** None reported

**Effects on Psychiatric Treatment** Does not effectively remove lithium

**Pregnancy Risk Factor** C

**Contraindications** Not effective for cyanide, mineral acids, caustic alkalis, organic solvents, iron, ethanol, methanol poisoning, lithium; do not use charcoal with sorbitol in patients with fructose intolerance; charcoal with sorbitol is not recommended in children <1 year.

**Warnings/Precautions** When using ipecac with charcoal, induce vomiting with ipecac before administering activated charcoal since charcoal adsorbs ipecac syrup; charcoal may cause vomiting which is hazardous in petroleum distillate and caustic ingestions; if charcoal in sorbitol is administered, doses should be limited to prevent excessive fluid and electrolyte losses; do not mix charcoal with milk, ice cream, or sherbet

**Adverse Reactions**

>10%:

Gastrointestinal: Vomiting, diarrhea with sorbitol, constipation

Miscellaneous: Stools will turn black

<1%: Swelling of abdomen

**Drug Interactions** Do not administer concomitantly with syrup of ipecac; do not mix with milk, ice cream, or sherbet

**Usual Dosage** Oral:

Acute poisoning:

Charcoal with sorbitol: Single-dose:

Children 1-12 years: 1-2 g/kg/dose or 15-30 g or approximately 5-10 times the weight of the ingested poison; 1 g adsorbs 100-1000 mg of poison; the use of repeat oral charcoal with sorbitol doses is not recommended. In young children, sorbitol should be repeated no more than 1-2 times/day.

Adults: 30-100 g

Charcoal in water:

Single-dose:

Infants <1 year: 1 g/kg

Children 1-12 years: 15-30 g or 1-2 g/kg

Adults: 30-100 g or 1-2 g/kg
Multiple-dose:
Infants <1 year: 0.5 g/kg every 4-6 hours
Children 1-12 years: 20-60 g or 0.5-1 g/kg every 2-6 hours until clinical observations, serum drug concentration have returned to a subtherapeutic range, or charcoal stool apparent
Adults: 20-60 g or 0.5-1 g/kg every 2-6 hours
Gastric dialysis: Adults: 20-50 g every 6 hours for 1-2 days
Intestinal gas, diarrhea, GI distress: Adults: 520-975 mg after meals or at first sign of discomfort; repeat as needed to a maximum dose of 4.16 g/day

**Dietary Considerations** Milk, ice cream, sherbet, or marmalade may reduce charcoal's effectiveness

**Patient Information** Charcoal will cause your stools to turn black. Do not self-administer as an antidote before calling the poison control center, hospital emergency room, or physician for instructions (charcoal is not the antidote for all poisons).

**Nursing Implications** Too concentrated of slurries may clog airway; often given with a laxative or cathartic; check for presence of bowel sounds before administration

**Dosage Forms**
Capsule (Charcocaps®): 260 mg
Liquid, activated:
Actidose-Aqua®: 12.5 g (60 mL); 25 g (120 mL)
Liqui-Char®: 12.5 g (60 mL); 15 g (75 mL); 25 g (120 mL); 30 g (120 mL); 50 g (240 mL)
SuperChar®: 30 g (240 mL)
Liquid, activated, with propylene glycol: 12.5 g (60 mL); 25 g (120 mL)
Liquid, activated, with sorbitol:
Actidose® With Sorbitol: 25 g (120 mL); 50 g (240 mL)
Charcoaid®: 30 g (150 mL)
SuperChar®: 30 g (240 mL)
Powder for suspension, activated:
15 g, 30 g, 40 g, 120 g, 240 g
SuperChar®: 30 g

- **Charcocaps® [OTC]** *see* Charcoal *on page 106*

## Chaste Tree

**Synonyms** *Vitex agnus-castus*

**Pharmacologic Category** Herb

**Use** In herbal medicine, it is used in treatment of menstrual disorders, premenstrual syndrome and mastodynia

**Adverse Reactions** Dermatologic: Pruritus, rash

**Overdosage/Toxicology**
Decontamination: Lavage (within 1 hour)/activated charcoal with cathartic
Treatment: Supportive therapy; antihistamines can be used to treat pruritus although there is no data on this modality

**Drug Interactions** None known per Commission E but may counteract the effectiveness of birth control pills

**Usual Dosage**
As a concentrated alcoholic extract: ~20 mg/day
Per Commission E: Average daily dose: 3 g herb or equivalent preparations

**Additional Information** A small deciduous multi-trunk tree which can grow up to 25 feet; native to Mediterranean region with flowers blooming in summer; the dried ripe fruit (which is brown/black with a pepperish flavor or aroma) contains the active chemical ingredients; dried leaves contain some of the active ingredients

- **Chemdec®** *see* Carbinoxamine *on page 92*
- **Chemet®** *see* Succimer *on page 521*
- **Chenix®** *see* Chenodiol *on page 107*
- **Chenodeoxycholic Acid** *see* Chenodiol *on page 107*

## Chenodiol (kee noe DYE ole)

**U.S. Brand Names** Chenix®

**Synonyms** Chenodeoxycholic Acid

**Pharmacologic Category** Bile Acid

**Use** Oral dissolution of cholesterol gallstones in selected patients

**Effects on Mental Status** None reported

**Effects on Psychiatric Treatment** May rarely produce leukopenia; use caution with clozapine and carbamazepine

**Pregnancy Risk Factor** X

**Contraindications** Presence of known hepatocyte dysfunction or bile ductal abnormalities; a gallbladder confirmed as nonvisualizing after two consecutive single doses of dye; radiopaque stones; gallstone complications or compelling reasons for gallbladder surgery; inflammatory bowel disease or active gastric or duodenal ulcer; pregnancy

**Warnings/Precautions** Chenodiol is hepatotoxic in animal models including subhuman Primates; chenodiol should be discontinued if aminotransferases exceed 3 times the upper normal limit; chenodiol may contribute to colon cancer in otherwise susceptible individuals

**Adverse Reactions**
>10%:
Gastrointestinal: Diarrhea (mild), biliary pain
Miscellaneous: Aminotransferase increases
1% to 10%:
Endocrine & metabolic: Increases in cholesterol and LDL cholesterol
Gastrointestinal: Dyspepsia
<1%: Constipation, cramps, diarrhea (severe), flatulence, higher cholecystectomy rates intrahepatic cholestasis, leukopenia, nausea, vomiting

**Overdosage/Toxicology**
Signs and symptoms: Diarrhea and a rise in liver function tests have been observed
Treatment: No specific antidote, institute supportive therapy

**Drug Interactions** Decreased effect: Antacids, cholestyramine, colestipol, oral contraceptives

**Usual Dosage** Adults: Oral: 13-16 mg/kg/day in 2 divided doses, starting with 250 mg twice daily the first 2 weeks and increasing by 250 mg/day each week thereafter until the recommended or maximum tolerated dose is achieved

**Dosing comments in hepatic impairment:** Contraindicated for use in presence of known hepatocyte dysfunction or bile ductal abnormalities

**Patient Information** Take as directed, for entire length of therapy. Medication may need to be taken for 24 months before dissolution will occur. Avoid aluminum-based antacids during entire course of therapy. Blood studies and x-rays studies will be necessary during therapy. Report persistent diarrhea and gallstone attacks (abdominal pain, nausea and vomiting, yellowing of skin or eyes).

**Dosage Forms** Tablet, film coated: 250 mg

- **Cheracol®** *see* Guaifenesin and Codeine *on page 256*
- **Cheracol® D [OTC]** *see* Guaifenesin and Dextromethorphan *on page 257*
- **Chibroxin™ Ophthalmic** *see* Norfloxacin *on page 399*
- **Chiggertox® [OTC]** *see* Benzocaine *on page 61*
- **Children's Advil® Oral Suspension [OTC]** *see* Ibuprofen *on page 280*
- **Children's Dynafed® Jr [OTC]** *see* Acetaminophen *on page 14*
- **Children's Hold® [OTC]** *see* Dextromethorphan *on page 160*
- **Children's Kaopectate® [OTC]** *see* Attapulgite *on page 53*
- **Children's Motrin® Oral Suspension [OTC]** *see* Ibuprofen *on page 280*
- **Children's Silapap® [OTC]** *see* Acetaminophen *on page 14*
- **Children's Silfedrine® [OTC]** *see* Pseudoephedrine *on page 478*
- **Chirocaine®** *see* Levobupivacaine *on page 311*
- **Chlo-Amine® [OTC]** *see* Chlorpheniramine *on page 113*
- **Chlorafed® Liquid [OTC]** *see* Chlorpheniramine and Pseudoephedrine *on page 114*
- **Chloral** *see* Chloral Hydrate *on page 107*

## Chloral Hydrate (KLOR al HYE drate)

**Related Information**
Anxiolytic/Hypnotic Use in Long-Term Care Facilities *on page 754*
Clinical Issues in the Use of Anxiolytics and Sedative/Hypnotics *on page 634*
Federal OBRA Regulations Recommended Maximum Doses *on page 756*
Nonbenzodiazepine Anxiolytics and Hypnotics *on page 721*

**Generic Available** Yes

**U.S. Brand Names** Aquachloral® Supprettes®

**Canadian Brand Names** Novo-Chlorhydrate; PMS-Chloral Hydrate

**Synonyms** Chloral; Hydrated Chloral; Trichloroacetaldehyde Monohydrate

**Pharmacologic Category** Hypnotic, Miscellaneous

**Use** Short-term sedative and hypnotic (<2 weeks); sedative/hypnotic for dental and diagnostic procedures; sedative prior to EEG evaluations

**Restrictions** C-IV

**Pregnancy Risk Factor** C

**Contraindications** Hypersensitivity to chloral hydrate or any component; hepatic or renal impairment; gastritis or ulcers; severe cardiac disease

**Warnings/Precautions** Use with caution in patients with porphyria; use with caution in neonates, drug may accumulate with repeated use, prolonged use in neonates associated with hyperbilirubinemia; tolerance to hypnotic effect develops, therefore, not recommended for use >2 weeks; taper dosage to avoid withdrawal with prolonged use; trichloroethanol (TCE), a metabolite of chloral hydrate, is a carcinogen in mice; there is no data in humans. Chloral hydrate is considered a second line hypnotic

(Continued)

## Chloral Hydrate *(Continued)*

agent in the elderly. Recent interpretive guidelines from the Health Care Financing Administration (HCFA) discourage the use of chloral hydrate in residents of long-term care facilities.

**Adverse Reactions**

Central nervous system: Ataxia, disorientation, sedation, excitement (paradoxical), dizziness, fever, headache, confusion, lightheadedness, nightmares, hallucinations, drowsiness, "hangover" effect

Dermatologic: Rash, urticaria

Gastrointestinal: Gastric irritation, nausea, vomiting, diarrhea, flatulence

Hematologic: Leukopenia, eosinophilia, acute intermittent porphyria

Miscellaneous: Physical and psychological dependence may occur with prolonged use of large doses

**Overdosage/Toxicology** Doses >2 g may produce symptoms of toxicity

Signs and symptoms: Hypotension, respiratory depression, coma, hypothermia, cardiac arrhythmias

Treatment: Supportive and symptomatic; lidocaine or propranolol may be used for ventricular dysrhythmias, while isoproterenol or atropine may be required for torsade de pointes

**Drug Interactions**

CNS depressants: Sedative effects and/or respiratory depression with chloral hydrate may be additive with other CNS depressants; monitor for increased effect; includes ethanol, sedatives, antidepressants, narcotic analgesics, and benzodiazepines

Furosemide: Diaphoresis, flushing, and hypertension have occurred in patients who received I.V. furosemide within 24 hours after administration of chloral hydrate; consider using a benzodiazepine

Phenytoin: Half-life may be decreased by chloral hydrate; limited documentation (small, single-dose study); monitor

Warfarin: Effect of oral anticoagulants may be increased by chloral hydrate; monitor INR; warfarin dosage may require adjustment. Chloral hydrate's metabolite may displace warfarin from its protein binding sites resulting in an increase in the hypoprothrombinemic response to warfarin.

**Stability** Sensitive to light; exposure to air causes volatilization; store in light-resistant, airtight container

**Mechanism of Action** Central nervous system depressant effects are due to its active metabolite trichloroethanol, mechanism unknown

**Pharmacodynamics/kinetics**

Peak effect: Within 0.5-1 hour

Duration: 4-8 hours

Absorption: Oral, rectal: Well absorbed

Distribution: Crosses the placenta; negligible amounts appear in breast milk

Metabolism: Rapidly to trichloroethanol (active metabolite); variable amounts metabolized in liver and kidney to trichloroacetic acid (inactive)

Half-life: Active metabolite: 8-11 hours

Elimination: Metabolites excreted in urine, small amounts excreted in feces via bile

**Usual Dosage**

Children:

- Sedation, anxiety: Oral, rectal: 5-15 mg/kg/dose every 8 hours, maximum: 500 mg/dose
- Prior to EEG: Oral, rectal: 20-25 mg/kg/dose, 30-60 minutes prior to EEG; may repeat in 30 minutes to maximum of 100 mg/kg or 2 g total
- Hypnotic: Oral, rectal: 20-40 mg/kg/dose up to a maximum of 50 mg/kg/24 hours or 1 g/dose or 2 g/24 hours
- Sedation, nonpainful procedure: Oral: 50-75 mg/kg/dose 30-60 minutes prior to procedure; may repeat 30 minutes after initial dose if needed, to a total maximum dose of 120 mg/kg or 1 g total

Adults: Oral, rectal:

- Sedation, anxiety: 250 mg 3 times/day
- Hypnotic: 500-1000 mg at bedtime or 30 minutes prior to procedure, not to exceed 2 g/24 hours

**Dosing adjustment/comments in renal impairment:** $Cl_{cr}$ <50 mL/minute: Avoid use

Hemodialysis: Dialyzable (50% to 100%); supplemental dose is not necessary

**Dosing adjustment/comments in hepatic impairment:** Avoid use in patients with severe hepatic impairment

**Dietary Considerations** Alcohol: Additive CNS effects, avoid use

**Administration** Do not crush capsule, contains drug in liquid form

**Monitoring Parameters** Vital signs, $O_2$ saturation and blood pressure with doses used for conscious sedation

**Reference Range** Therapeutic: 2-12 µg/mL of trichloroethanol; 25 µg/mL of trichloroethanol correlated with fatalities

**Test Interactions** False-positive urine glucose using Clinitest® method; may interfere with fluorometric urine catecholamine and urinary 17-hydroxycorticosteroid tests

**Patient Information** Take a capsule with a full glass of water or fruit juice; swallow capsules whole, do not chew; avoid alcohol and other CNS depressants; avoid activities needing good psychomotor coordination until CNS effects are known; drug may cause physical or psychological dependence; avoid abrupt discontinuation after prolonged use; if taking at home prior to a diagnostic procedure, have someone else transport

**Nursing Implications** Gastric irritation may be minimized by diluting dose in water or other oral liquid

**Additional Information** Not an analgesic

**Dosage Forms**

Capsule: 250 mg, 500 mg

Suppository, rectal: 324 mg, 500 mg, 648 mg

Syrup: 250 mg/5 mL (10 mL); 500 mg/5 mL (5 mL, 10 mL, 480 mL)

## Chlorambucil (klor AM byoo sil)

**U.S. Brand Names** Leukeran®

**Pharmacologic Category** Antineoplastic Agent, Alkylating Agent

**Use** Management of chronic lymphocytic leukemia, Hodgkin's and non-Hodgkin's lymphoma; breast and ovarian carcinoma; Waldenström's macroglobulinemia, testicular carcinoma, thrombocythemia, choriocarcinoma

**Effects on Mental Status** May rarely produce agitation, confusion, and hallucinations

**Effects on Psychiatric Treatment** Myelosuppression is common; use caution with clozapine and carbamazepine

**Pregnancy Risk Factor** D

**Contraindications** Previous resistance; hypersensitivity to chlorambucil or any component or other alkylating agents

**Warnings/Precautions** The U.S. Food and Drug Administration (FDA) currently recommends that procedures for proper handling and disposal of antineoplastic agents be considered. Use with caution in patients with seizure disorder and bone marrow suppression; reduce initial dosage if patient has received radiation therapy, myelosuppressive drugs or has a depressed baseline leukocyte or platelet count within the previous 4 weeks. Can severely suppress bone marrow function; affects human fertility; carcinogenic in humans and probably mutagenic and teratogenic as well; chromosomal damage has been documented; secondary AML may be associated with chronic therapy.

**Adverse Reactions**

>10%:

Hematologic: Myelosuppressive: Use with caution when receiving radiation; bone marrow suppression frequently occurs and occasionally bone marrow failure has occurred; blood counts should be monitored closely while undergoing treatment; leukopenia, thrombocytopenia, anemia

WBC: Moderate

Platelets: Moderate

Onset (days): 7

Nadir (days): 10-14

Recovery (days): 28

1% to 10%:

Dermatologic: Skin rashes

Endocrine & metabolic: Hyperuricemia, menstrual changes

Gastrointestinal: Nausea, vomiting, diarrhea, oral ulceration are all infrequent

Emetic potential: Low (<10%)

<1%: Agitation, ataxia, confusion, drug fever, hallucination; rarely generalized or focal seizures, rash, fertility impairment: Has caused chromosomal damage in men, both reversible and permanent sterility have occurred in both sexes; can produce amenorrhea in females, oral ulceration, oligospermia, hepatotoxicity, hepatic necrosis, weakness, tremors, muscular twitching, peripheral neuropathy, pulmonary fibrosis, secondary malignancies; Increased incidence of AML; skin hypersensitivity

**Overdosage/Toxicology**

Signs and symptoms: Vomiting, ataxia, coma, seizures, pancytopenia

Treatment: There are no known antidotes for chlorambucil intoxication, and treatment is mainly supportive, directed at decontaminating the GI tract and controlling symptoms; blood products may be used to treat the hematologic toxicity

**Drug Interactions** Patients may experience impaired immune response to vaccines; possible infection after administration of live vaccines in patients receiving immunosuppressants

**Usual Dosage** Oral (refer to individual protocols):

Children:

- General short courses: 0.1-0.2 mg/kg/day **OR** 4.5 mg/m²/day for 3-6 weeks for remission induction (usual: 4-10 mg/day); maintenance therapy: 0.03-0.1 mg/kg/day (usual: 2-4 mg/day)
- Nephrotic syndrome: 0.1-0.2 mg/kg/day every day for 5-15 weeks with low-dose prednisone
- Chronic lymphocytic leukemia (CLL):
  - Biweekly regimen: Initial: 0.4 mg/kg/dose every 2 weeks; increase dose by 0.1 mg/kg every 2 weeks until a response occurs and/or myelosuppression occurs
  - Monthly regimen: Initial: 0.4 mg/kg, increase dose by 0.2 mg/kg every 4 weeks until a response occurs and/or myelosuppression occurs
- Malignant lymphomas:
  - Non-Hodgkin's lymphoma: 0.1 mg/kg/day
  - Hodgkin's lymphoma: 0.2 mg/kg/day

Adults: 0.1-0.2 mg/kg/day **OR** 3-6 mg/m²/day for 3-6 weeks, then adjust dose on basis of blood counts. Pulse dosing has been used in CLL as intermittent, biweekly, or monthly doses of 0.4 mg/kg and increased by 0.1 mg/kg until the disease is under control or toxicity ensues. An alternate regimen is 14 mg/m²/day for 5 days, repeated every 21-28 days.

Hemodialysis: Supplemental dosing is not necessary

Peritoneal dialysis: Supplemental dosing is not necessary

**Patient Information** Take exactly as directed (may be taken with chilled liquids). Maintain adequate hydration (2-3 L/day of fluids unless instructed to restrict fluid intake). Avoid alcohol, acidic, spicy, or hot foods, aspirin, or OTC medications unless approved by prescriber. Hair may be lost during treatment (reversible). You may experience menstrual irregularities and/or sterility. You will be more susceptible to infection; avoid crowds and exposure to infection. Frequent mouth care with soft toothbrush or cotton swab may reduce occurrence of mouth sores. Report easy bruising or bleeding; fever or chills; numbness, pain, or tingling of extremities; muscle cramping or weakness; unusual swelling of extremities; menstrual irregularities; or any difficulty breathing.

**Dosage Forms** Tablet, sugar coated: 2 mg

## Chloramphenicol (klor am FEN i kole)

**U.S. Brand Names** AK-Chlor® Ophthalmic; Chloromycetin®; Chloroptic® Ophthalmic

**Canadian Brand Names** Diochloram; Pentamycetin®; Sopamycetin

**Synonyms** Cloranfenicol

**Pharmacologic Category** Antibiotic, Ophthalmic; Antibiotic, Otic; Antibiotic, Miscellaneous

**Use** Treatment of serious infections due to organisms resistant to other less toxic antibiotics or when its penetrability into the site of infection is clinically superior to other antibiotics to which the organism is sensitive; useful in infections caused by *Bacteroides, H. influenzae, Neisseria meningitidis, Salmonella*, and *Rickettsia*; active against many vancomycin-resistant enterococci

**Effects on Mental Status** May rarely cause nightmares

**Effects on Psychiatric Treatment** May cause bone marrow suppression; use caution with clozapine and carbamazepine

**Pregnancy Risk Factor** C

**Contraindications** Hypersensitivity to chloramphenicol or any component

**Warnings/Precautions** Use with caution in patients with impaired renal or hepatic function and in neonates; reduce dose with impaired liver function; use with care in patients with glucose 6-phosphate dehydrogenase deficiency. Serious and fatal blood dyscrasias have occurred after both short-term and prolonged therapy; should not be used when less potentially toxic agents are effective; prolonged use may result in superinfection.

**Adverse Reactions** <1%: Nightmares, headache, rash, diarrhea, stomatitis, enterocolitis, nausea, vomiting, bone marrow suppression, aplastic anemia, peripheral neuropathy, optic neuritis, gray syndrome

**Three (3) major toxicities associated with chloramphenicol include:**

Aplastic anemia, an idiosyncratic reaction which can occur with any route of administration; usually occurs 3 weeks to 12 months after initial exposure to chloramphenicol

Bone marrow suppression is thought to be dose-related with serum concentrations >25 μg/mL and reversible once chloramphenicol is discontinued; anemia and neutropenia may occur during the first week of therapy

Gray syndrome is characterized by circulatory collapse, cyanosis, acidosis, abdominal distention, myocardial depression, coma, and death; reaction appears to be associated with serum levels ≥50 μg/mL; may result from drug accumulation in patients with impaired hepatic or renal function

**Overdosage/Toxicology**

Signs and symptoms: Anemia, metabolic acidosis, hypotension, hypothermia

Treatment: Supportive following GI decontamination

**Drug Interactions** CYP2C9 enzyme inhibitor

Decreased effect: Phenobarbital and rifampin may decrease concentration of chloramphenicol

Increased toxicity: Chloramphenicol inhibits the metabolism of chlorpropamide, phenytoin, oral anticoagulants

**Usual Dosage**

Meningitis: I.V.: Infants >30 days and Children: 50-100 mg/kg/day divided every 6 hours

Other infections: I.V.:

Infants >30 days and Children: 50-75 mg/kg/day divided every 6 hours; maximum daily dose: 4 g/day

Adults: 50-100 mg/kg/day in divided doses every 6 hours; maximum daily dose: 4 g/day

Ophthalmic: Children and Adults: Instill 1-2 drops or 1.25 cm (½" of ointment every 3-4 hours); increase interval between applications after 48 hours to 2-3 times/day

Otic solution: Instill 2-3 drops into ear 3 times/day

Topical: Gently rub into the affected area 1-4 times/day

**Dosing adjustment/comments in hepatic impairment:** Avoid use in severe liver impairment as increased toxicity may occur

Hemodialysis: Slightly dialyzable (5% to 20%) via hemo- and peritoneal dialysis; no supplemental doses needed in dialysis or continuous arterio-venous or veno-venous hemofiltration (CAVH/CAVHD)

**Dietary Considerations** Folic acid, iron salts, vitamin $B_{12}$: May decrease intestinal absorption of vitamin $B_{12}$; may have increased dietary need for riboflavin, pyridoxine, and vitamin $B_{12}$; monitor hematological status

**Patient Information**

Oral: Take as directed, at regular intervals around-the-clock, with a large glass of water. Maintain adequate hydration (2-3 L/day of fluids unless instructed to restrict fluid intake). During I.V. administration, a bitter taste may occur; this will pass. Diabetics: Drug may cause false-positive test with Clinitest® glucose monitoring; use alternative glucose monitoring. This drug may interfere with effectiveness of oral contraceptives. You may experience nausea, vomiting (frequent small meals, frequent mouth care, sucking lozenges, or chewing gum may help). Report persistent rash, diarrhea; pain, burning, or numbness of extremities; petechiae; sore throat; fatigue; unusual bleeding or bruising; vaginal itching or discharge; mouth sores; yellowing of skin or eyes; dark urine or stool discoloration (blue); CNS disturbances (nightmares acute headache); or lack or improvement or worsening of condition.

Ophthalmic: Wash hands before instilling. Sit or lie down to instill. Open eye, look at ceiling, and instill prescribed amount of medication. Close eye and apply gentle pressure to inner corner of eye. Do not let tip of applicator touch eye or contaminate tip of applicator. Temporary stinging or burning may occur. Report persistent pain, burning, vision disturbances, swelling, itching, rash, or worsening of condition.

Otic: Wash hands before instilling. Tilt head with affected ear upward. Gently grasp ear lobe and lift back and upward. Instill prescribed drops into ear canal. Do not push dropper into ear. Remain with head tilted for 2 minutes. Report ringing in ears, discharge, or worsening of condition.

Topical: Wash hands before applying or wear gloves. Apply thin film to affected area. May apply porous dressing. Report persistent burning, swelling, itching, or worsening of condition.

**Dosage Forms**

Capsule: 250 mg

Ointment, ophthalmic: 1% [10 mg/g] (3.5 g)

AK-Chlor®, Chloromycetin®, Chloroptic® S.O.P.: 1% [10 mg/g] (3.5 g)

Powder for injection, as sodium succinate: 1 g

Powder for ophthalmic solution (Chloromycetin®): 25 mg/vial (15 mL)

Solution: 0.5% [5 mg/mL] (7.5 mL, 15 mL)

Ophthalmic (AK-Chlor®, Chloroptic®): 0.5% [5 mg/mL] (2.5 mL, 7.5 mL, 15 mL)

Otic (Chloromycetin®): 0.5% (15 mL)

## Chloramphenicol and Prednisolone
(klor am FEN i kole & pred NIS oh lone)

**U.S. Brand Names** Chloroptic-P® Ophthalmic

**Pharmacologic Category** Antibiotic, Ophthalmic; Corticosteroid, Ophthalmic

**Use** Topical anti-infective and corticosteroid for treatment of ocular infections

**Effects on Mental Status** None reported

**Effects on Psychiatric Treatment** None reported

**Usual Dosage** Ophthalmic: Instill 1-2 drops in eye(s) 2-4 times/day

**Dosage Forms** Ointment, ophthalmic: Chloramphenicol 1% and prednisolone 0.5% (3.5 g)

## Chloramphenicol, Polymyxin B, and Hydrocortisone
(klor am FEN i kole, pol i MIKS in bee, & hye droe KOR ti sone)

**Pharmacologic Category** Antibiotic, Ophthalmic; Corticosteroid, Ophthalmic

**Use** Topical anti-infective and corticosteroid for treatment of ocular infections

**Effects on Mental Status** None reported

**Effects on Psychiatric Treatment** None reported

**Usual Dosage** Apply ½" ribbon every 3-4 hours until improvement occurs

**Dosage Forms** Solution, ophthalmic: Chloramphenicol 1%, polymyxin B sulfate 10,000 units, and hydrocortisone acetate 0.5% per g (3.75 g)

♦ **Chlorate® [OTC]** *see* Chlorpheniramine *on page 113*

## Chlordiazepoxide (klor dye az e POKS ide)

**Related Information**

Anxiolytic/Hypnotic Use in Long-Term Care Facilities *on page 754*
Benzodiazepines Comparison Chart *on page 708*
Clinical Issues in the Use of Anxiolytics and Sedative/Hypnotics *on page 634*
Federal OBRA Regulations Recommended Maximum Doses *on page 756*
Patient Information - Anxiolytics & Sedative Hypnotics (Benzodiazepines) *on page 653*

(Continued)

## Chlordiazepoxide *(Continued)*

**Generic Available** Yes

**U.S. Brand Names** Libritabs®; Librium®; Mitran® Oral; Reposans-10® Oral

**Canadian Brand Names** Apo®-Chlordiazepoxide; Corax®; Medilium®; Novo-Poxide; Solium®

**Synonyms** Methaminodiazepoxide Hydrochloride

**Pharmacologic Category** Benzodiazepine

**Use** Management of anxiety disorder or for the short-term relief of symptoms of anxiety; withdrawal symptoms of acute alcoholism; and preoperative apprehension and anxiety

**Restrictions** C-IV

**Pregnancy Risk Factor** D

**Contraindications** Hypersensitivity to this drug or any component of its formulation (cross-sensitivity with other benzodiazepines may exist); narrow angle glaucoma (not in product labeling: however, benzodiazepines are contraindicated); pregnancy

**Warnings/Precautions** Active metabolites with extended half-lives may lead to delayed accumulation and adverse effects. Use with caution in elderly or debilitated patients, pediatric patients, patients with hepatic disease (including alcoholics) or renal impairment. Use with caution in patients with respiratory disease or impaired gag reflex. Use with caution in patients with porphyria.

Parenteral administration should be avoided in comatose patients or shock. Adequate resuscitative equipment/personnel should be available, and appropriate monitoring should be conducted at the time of injection and for several hours following administration. The parenteral formulation should be diluted for I.M. administration with the supplied diluent only. This diluent should not be used when preparing the drug for intravenous administration.

Causes CNS depression (dose-related) resulting in sedation, dizziness, confusion, or ataxia which may impair physical and mental capabilities. Patients must be cautioned about performing tasks which require mental alertness (ie, operating machinery or driving). Use with caution in patients receiving other CNS depressants or psychoactive agents (lithium, phenothiazines). Effects with other sedative drugs or ethanol may be potentiated. Benzodiazepines have been associated with falls and traumatic injury and should be used with extreme caution in patients who are at risk of these events (especially the elderly).

Use caution in patients with depression, particularly if suicidal risk may be present. Use with caution in patients with a history of drug dependence. Benzodiazepines have been associated with dependence and acute withdrawal symptoms on discontinuation or reduction in dose. Acute withdrawal, including seizures, may be precipitated in patients after administration of flumazenil to patients receiving long-term benzodiazepine therapy.

Benzodiazepines have been associated with anterograde amnesia. Paradoxical reactions, including hyperactive or aggressive behavior have been reported with benzodiazepines, particularly in adolescent/pediatric or psychiatric patients. Does not have analgesic, antidepressant, or antipsychotic properties.

**Adverse Reactions**

>10%:
- Central nervous system: Drowsiness, fatigue, ataxia, lightheadedness, memory impairment, dysarthria, irritability
- Dermatologic: Rash
- Endocrine & metabolic: Decreased libido, menstrual disorders
- Gastrointestinal: Xerostomia, decreased salivation, increased or decreased appetite, weight gain or loss
- Genitourinary: Micturition difficulties

1% to 10%:
- Cardiovascular: Hypotension
- Central nervous system: Confusion, dizziness, disinhibition, akathisia, increased libido
- Dermatologic: Dermatitis
- Gastrointestinal: Increased salivation
- Genitourinary: Sexual dysfunction, incontinence
- Neuromuscular & skeletal: Rigidity, tremor, muscle cramps
- Otic: Tinnitus
- Respiratory: Nasal congestion

**Overdosage/Toxicology**

Signs and symptoms: Hypotension, respiratory depression, coma, hypothermia, cardiac arrhythmias

Treatment: Supportive, rarely is mechanical ventilation required, flumazenil has been shown to selectively block the binding of benzodiazepines to CNS receptors, resulting in a reversal of benzodiazepine- induced CNS depression. Respiratory depression may not be reversed.

**Drug Interactions** CYP3A3/4 enzyme substrate

CNS depressants: Sedative effects and/or respiratory depression may be additive with CNS depressants; includes ethanol, barbiturates, narcotic analgesics, and other sedative agents; monitor for increased effect

CYP enzyme inducers: Metabolism of some benzodiazepines may be increased, decreasing their therapeutic effect; consider using an alternative sedative/hypnotic agent; potential inducers include phenobarbital, phenytoin, carbamazepine, rifampin, and rifabutin

CYP3A3/4 inhibitors: Serum level and/or toxicity of some benzodiazepines may be increased; inhibitors include amiodarone, cimetidine, clarithromycin, erythromycin, delavirdine, diltiazem, dirithromycin, disulfiram, fluoxetine, fluvoxamine, grapefruit juice, indinavir, itraconazole, ketoconazole, nevirapine, propoxyfene, quinupristin-dalfopristin, ritonavir, saquinavir, verapamil, zafirlukast, zileuton; monitor for altered benzodiazepine response

Oral contraceptives: May decrease the clearance of some benzodiazepines (those which undergo oxidative metabolism); monitor for increased benzodiazepine effect

Theophylline: May partially antagonize some of the effects of benzodiazepines; monitor for decreased response; may require higher doses for sedation

**Stability** Refrigerate injection; protect from light; **incompatible** when mixed with Ringer's solution, ascorbic acid, benzquinamide, heparin, phenytoin, promethazine, secobarbital

**Mechanism of Action** Binds to stereospecific benzodiazepine receptors on the postsynaptic GABA neuron at several sites within the central nervous system, including the limbic system, reticular formation. Enhancement of the inhibitory effect of GABA on neuronal excitability results by increased neuronal membrane permeability to chloride ions. This shift in chloride ions results in hyperpolarization (a less excitable state) and stabilization.

**Pharmacodynamics/kinetics**

Distribution: $V_d$: 3.3 L/kg; crosses the placenta; appears in breast milk

Protein binding: 90% to 98%

Metabolism: Extensive in the liver to desmethyldiazepam (active and long-acting)

Half-life: 6.6-25 hours
- End-stage renal disease: 5-30 hours
- Cirrhosis: 30-63 hours

Time to peak serum concentration:
- Oral: Within 2 hours
- I.M.: Results in lower peak plasma levels than oral

Elimination: Very little excretion in urine as unchanged drug

**Usual Dosage**

Children:
- <6 years: Not recommended
- >6 years: Anxiety: Oral, I.M.: 0.5 mg/kg/24 hours divided every 6-8 hours

Adults:
- Anxiety:
  - Oral: 15-100 mg divided 3-4 times/day
  - I.M., I.V.: Initial: 50-100 mg followed by 25-50 mg 3-4 times/day as needed
- Preoperative anxiety: I.M.: 50-100 mg prior to surgery
- Alcohol withdrawal symptoms: Oral, I.V.: 50-100 mg to start, dose may be repeated in 2-4 hours as necessary to a maximum of 300 mg/24 hours

**Dosing adjustment in renal impairment:** $Cl_{cr}$ <10 mL/minute: Administer 50% of dose

Hemodialysis: Not dialyzable (0% to 5%)

**Dosing adjustment/comments in hepatic impairment:** Avoid use

**Dietary Considerations** Alcohol: Additive CNS effects, avoid use

**Administration** Up to 300 mg may be given I.M. or I.V. during a 6-hour period, but not more than this in any 24-hour period; do not use diluent provided with parenteral form for I.V. administration; dissolve with normal saline instead; I.V. form is a powder and should be reconstituted with 5 mL of sterile water or saline prior to administration. I.M. dosage form is poorly and erratically absorbed. If an I.M. benzodiazepine is necessary, lorazepam is preferred.

**Monitoring Parameters** Respiratory and cardiovascular status, mental status, check for orthostasis

**Reference Range** Therapeutic: 0.1-3 µg/mL (SI: 0-10 µmol/L); Toxic: >23 µg/mL (SI: >77 µmol/L)

**Test Interactions** ↑ triglycerides (S); ↓ HDL

**Patient Information** Avoid alcohol and other CNS depressants; avoid activities needing good psychomotor coordination until CNS effects are known; drug may cause physical or psychological dependence; avoid abrupt discontinuation after prolonged use, may cause drowsiness, poor balance

**Nursing Implications** Up to 300 mg may be given I.M. or I.V. during a 6-hour period, but not more than this in any 24-hour period; do not use diluent provided with parenteral form for I.V. administration; dissolve with normal saline instead; raise bed rails; initiate safety measures; aid with ambulation

**Additional Information** The I.V. formulation is a powder and should be reconstituted with 5 mL of sterile water or saline prior to administration, do not use diluent provided with ampul for I.V. administration

**Dosage Forms**

Capsule, as hydrochloride: 5 mg, 10 mg, 25 mg

Powder for injection, as hydrochloride: 100 mg

Tablet: 10 mg, 25 mg

♦ **Chlordiazepoxide and Amitriptyline** *see* Amitriptyline and Chlordiazepoxide *on page 34*

- **Chlordiazepoxide and Clidinium** *see* Clidinium and Chlordiazepoxide *on page 128*

## Chlorhexidine Gluconate (klor HEKS i deen GLOO koe nate)

**U.S. Brand Names** BactoShield® Topical [OTC]; Betasept® [OTC]; Dyna-Hex® Topical [OTC]; Exidine® Scrub [OTC]; Hibiclens® Topical [OTC]; Hibistat® Topical [OTC]; Peridex® Oral Rinse; PerioChip®; PerioGard®

**Pharmacologic Category** Antibiotic, Oral Rinse; Antibiotic, Topical

**Use** Skin cleanser for surgical scrub, cleanser for skin wounds, germicidal hand rinse, and an antibacterial dental rinse. Chlorhexidine is active against gram-positive and gram-negative organisms, facultative anaerobes, aerobes, and yeast.

**Effects on Mental Status** None reported

**Effects on Psychiatric Treatment** None reported

**Usual Dosage** Adults:

Oral rinse (Peridex®):

Precede use of solution by flossing and brushing teeth; completely rinse toothpaste from mouth. Swish 15 mL undiluted oral rinse around in mouth for 30 seconds, then expectorate. Caution patient not to swallow the medicine. Avoid eating for 2-3 hours after treatment. (The cap on bottle of oral rinse is a measure for 15 mL.)

When used as a treatment of gingivitis, the regimen begins with oral prophylaxis. Patient treats mouth with 15 mL chlorhexidine, swishes for 30 seconds, then expectorates. This is repeated twice daily (morning and evening). Patient should have a re-evaluation followed by a dental prophylaxis every 6 months.

Cleanser:

Surgical scrub: Scrub 3 minutes and rinse thoroughly, wash for an additional 3 minutes

Hand wash: Wash for 15 seconds and rinse

Hand rinse: Rub 15 seconds and rinse

Periodontal chip: Adults: One chip is inserted into a periodontal pocket with a probing pocket depth ≥5 mm. Up to 8 chips may be inserted in a single visit. Treatment is recommended every 3 months in pockets with a remaining depth ≥5 mm. If dislodgment occurs 7 days or more after placement, the subject is considered to have had the full course of treatment. If dislodgment occurs within 48 hours, a new chip should be inserted.

Insertion of periodontal chip: Pocket should be isolated and surrounding area dried prior to chip insertion. The chip should be grasped using forceps with the rounded edges away from the forceps. The chip should be inserted into the periodontal pocket to its maximum depth. It may be maneuvered into position using the tips of the forceps or a flat instrument. The chip biodegrades completely and does not need to be removed. Patients should avoid dental floss at the site of PerioChip® insertion for 10 days after placement because flossing might dislodge the chip.

**Dosage Forms**

Chip, for periodontal pocket insertion (PerioChip®): 2.5 mg

Foam, topical, with isopropyl alcohol 4% (BactoShield®): 4% (180 mL)

Liquid, topical, with isopropyl alcohol 4%:

Dyna-Hex® Skin Cleanser: 2% (120 mL, 240 mL, 480 mL, 960 mL, 4000 mL); 4% (120 mL, 240 mL, 480 mL, 4000 mL)

BactoShield® 2: 2% (960 mL)

BactoShield®, Betasept®, Exidine® Skin Cleanser, Hibiclens® Skin Cleanser: 4% (15 mL, 120 mL, 240 mL, 480 mL, 960 mL, 4000 mL)

Rinse:

Oral (mint flavor) (Peridex®, PerioGard®): 0.12% with alcohol 11.6% (480 mL)

Topical (Hibistat® Hand Rinse): 0.5% with isopropyl alcohol 70% (120 mL, 240 mL)

Sponge/Brush (Hibiclens®): 4% with isopropyl alcohol 4% (22 mL)

Wipes (Hibistat®): 0.5% (50s)

## Chlormezanone (klor me ZA none)

**U.S. Brand Names** Alinam®; Muskel Trancopal®; Trancopal®

**Pharmacologic Category** Antianxiety Agent, Miscellaneous

**Use** Anxiety; insomnia; muscle spasm

**Effects on Mental Status** May cause drowsiness

**Effects on Psychiatric Treatment** Concurrent use with other psychotropics may produce additive sedation

**Contraindications** Hypersensitivity to chlormezanone

**Adverse Reactions**

Cardiovascular: Flushing, toxic epidermal necrosis

Central nervous system: Drowsiness, confusion, headache

Gastrointestinal: Nausea, xerostomia

Hematologic: Porphyrinogenic

Hepatic: Reversible jaundice, hepatitis

Neuromuscular & skeletal: Tremor, muscle weakness

Respiratory: Hyposmia

**Drug Interactions** Increased effect with use of alcohol or other central nervous system depressants

**Usual Dosage** Oral:

Children >5 years: 50-100 mg 3-4 times/day

Adults:

Anxiety: 100-200 mg 3-4 times/day

Insomnia: 400 mg at bedtime (200 mg in elderly patients)

Muscle spasm: 200-400 mg 3-4 times/day

**Dosage Forms** Caplet: 100 mg, 200 mg

- **Chloromycetin®** *see* Chloramphenicol *on page 109*
- **Chloroptic® Ophthalmic** *see* Chloramphenicol *on page 109*
- **Chloroptic-P® Ophthalmic** *see* Chloramphenicol and Prednisolone *on page 109*

## Chloroquine and Primaquine
(KLOR oh kwin & PRIM a kween)

**U.S. Brand Names** Aralen® Phosphate With Primaquine Phosphate

**Synonyms** Primaquine and Chloroquine

**Pharmacologic Category** Antimalarial Agent

**Use** Prophylaxis of malaria, regardless of species, in all areas where the disease is endemic

**Effects on Mental Status** May rarely cause fatigue or personality changes

**Effects on Psychiatric Treatment** May cause blood dyscrasias; use caution with clozapine and carbamazepine

**Pregnancy Risk Factor** C

**Contraindications** Retinal or visual field changes, known hypersensitivity to chloroquine or primaquine

**Warnings/Precautions** Use with caution in patients with psoriasis, porphyria, hepatic dysfunction, G-6-PD deficiency

**Adverse Reactions**

1% to 10%: Gastrointestinal: Diarrhea, nausea

<1%: Anorexia, blood dyscrasias, blurred vision, EKG changes, fatigue, hair bleaching, headache, hypotension, personality changes, pruritus, retinopathy, stomatitis, vomiting

**Overdosage/Toxicology**

Signs and symptoms: Headache, visual changes, cardiovascular collapse, seizures, abdominal cramps, vomiting, cyanosis, methemoglobinemia, leukopenia, respiratory and cardiac arrest

Treatment: Following initial measures (immediate GI decontamination), treatment is supportive and symptomatic

**Drug Interactions**

Decreased absorption if administered concomitantly with kaolin and magnesium trisilicate

Increased toxicity/levels with cimetidine

**Usual Dosage** Oral: Start at least 1 day before entering the endemic area; continue for 8 weeks after leaving the endemic area

Children: Suggested weekly dosage based on body weight:

**Note:** Liquid doses contain approximately 40 mg of chloroquine base and 6 mg primaquine base per 5 mL, prepared from chloroquine phosphate with primaquine phosphate tablets

10-15 lb (4.5-6.8 kg): 20 mg chloroquine base and 3 mg primaquine base (2.5 mL)

16-25 lb (7.3-11.4 kg): 40 mg chloroquine base and 6 mg primaquine base (5 mL)

26-35 lb (11.8-15.9 kg): 60 mg chloroquine base and 9 mg primaquine base (7.5 mL)

36-45 lb (16.4-20.5 kg): 80 mg chloroquine base and 12 mg primaquine base (10 mL)

46-55 lb (20.9-25 kg): 100 mg chloroquine base and 15 mg primaquine base (12.5 mL)

56-100 lb (25.4-45.4 kg): 150 mg chloroquine base and 22.5 mg primaquine base (1/2 tablet)

>100 lb (>45.4 kg): 300 mg chloroquine base and 45 mg primaquine base (1 tablet)

Adults: 1 tablet/week on the same day each week

**Patient Information** See individual agents

**Dosage Forms** Tablet: Chloroquine phosphate 500 mg [base 300 mg] and primaquine phosphate 79 mg [base 45 mg]

## Chloroquine Phosphate (KLOR oh kwin FOS fate)

**U.S. Brand Names** Aralen® Phosphate

**Pharmacologic Category** Aminoquinoline (Antimalarial)

**Use** Suppression or chemoprophylaxis of malaria; treatment of uncomplicated or mild to moderate malaria; extraintestinal amebiasis

**Unlabeled use:** Rheumatoid arthritis; discoid lupus erythematosus, scleroderma, pemphigus

**Effects on Mental Status** May rarely cause fatigue or personality changes

**Effects on Psychiatric Treatment** May cause blood dyscrasias; use caution with clozapine and carbamazepine

**Pregnancy Risk Factor** C

(Continued)

## Chloroquine Phosphate *(Continued)*

**Contraindications** Retinal or visual field changes; patients with psoriasis; known hypersensitivity to chloroquine

**Warnings/Precautions** Use with caution in patients with liver disease, G-6-PD deficiency, alcoholism or in conjunction with hepatotoxic drugs, psoriasis, porphyria may be exacerbated; retinopathy (irreversible) has occurred with long or high-dose therapy; discontinue drug if any abnormality in the visual field or if muscular weakness develops during treatment

**Adverse Reactions**

>1%: Gastrointestinal: Nausea, diarrhea

<1%: Anorexia, blood dyscrasias, blurred vision, EKG changes, fatigue, hair bleaching, headache, hypotension, personality changes, pruritus, retinopathy, stomatitis, vomiting

**Overdosage/Toxicology**

Signs and symptoms: Headache, visual changes, cardiovascular collapse, seizures, abdominal cramps, vomiting, cyanosis, methemoglobinemia, leukopenia, respiratory and cardiac arrest

Treatment: Following initial measures (immediate GI decontamination), treatment is supportive and symptomatic

**Drug Interactions**

Chloroquine and other 4-aminoquinolones may be decreased due to GI binding with kaolin or magnesium trisilicate

Increased effect: Cimetidine increases levels of chloroquine and probably other 4-aminoquinolones

**Usual Dosage** Oral (**dosage expressed in terms of mg of base**):

Suppression or prophylaxis of malaria:

Children: Administer 5 mg base/kg/week on the same day each week (not to exceed 300 mg base/dose); begin 1-2 weeks prior to exposure; continue for 4-6 weeks after leaving endemic area; if suppressive therapy is not begun prior to exposure, double the initial loading dose to 10 mg base/kg and administer in 2 divided doses 6 hours apart, followed by the usual dosage regimen

Adults: 300 mg/week (base) on the same day each week; begin 1-2 weeks prior to exposure; continue for 4-6 weeks after leaving endemic area; if suppressive therapy is not begun prior to exposure, double the initial loading dose to 600 mg base and administer in 2 divided doses 6 hours apart, followed by the usual dosage regimen

Acute attack:

Oral:

Children: 10 mg/kg on day 1, followed by 5 mg/kg 6 hours later and 5 mg/kg on days 2 and 3

Adults: 600 mg on day 1, followed by 300 mg 6 hours later, followed by 300 mg on days 2 and 3

I.M. (as hydrochloride):

Children: 5 mg/kg, repeat in 6 hours

Adults: Initial: 160-200 mg, repeat in 6 hours if needed; maximum: 800 mg first 24 hours; begin oral dosage as soon as possible and continue for 3 days until 1.5 g has been given

Extraintestinal amebiasis:

Children: Oral: 10 mg/kg once daily for 2-3 weeks (up to 300 mg base/day)

Adults:

Oral: 600 mg base/day for 2 days followed by 300 mg base/day for at least 2-3 weeks

I.M., as hydrochloride: 160-200 mg/day for 10 days; resume oral therapy as soon as possible

**Dosing adjustment in renal impairment:** $Cl_{cr}$ <10 mL/minute: Administer 50% of dose

Hemodialysis: Minimally removed by hemodialysis

**Patient Information** It is important to complete full course of therapy which may take up to 6 months for full effect. May be taken with meals to decrease GI upset and bitter aftertaste. Avoid alcohol. You should have regular ophthalmic exams (every 4-6 months) if using this medication over extended periods. You may experience skin discoloration (blue/black), hair bleaching, or skin rash. If you have psoriasis, you may experience exacerbation. May turn urine black/brown (normal). You may experience nausea, vomiting, or loss of appetite (small frequent meals, frequent mouth care, sucking lozenges, or chewing gum may help) or increased sensitivity to sunlight (wear dark glasses and protective clothing, use sunblock, and avoid direct exposure to sunlight). Report vision changes, rash or itching, persistent diarrhea or GI disturbances, change in hearing acuity or ringing in the ears, chest pain or palpitation, CNS changes, unusual fatigue, easy bruising or bleeding, or any other persistent adverse reactions.

**Dosage Forms**

Injection: 50 mg [40 mg base]/mL (5 mL)

Tablet: 250 mg [150 mg base]; 500 mg [300 mg base]

## Chlorothiazide (klor oh THYE a zide)

**U.S. Brand Names** Diurigen®; Diuril®

**Pharmacologic Category** Diuretic, Thiazide

**Use** Management of mild to moderate hypertension, or edema associated with congestive heart failure, pregnancy, or nephrotic syndrome in patients unable to take oral hydrochlorothiazide; when a thiazide is the diuretic of choice

**Effects on Mental Status** May cause dizziness

**Effects on Psychiatric Treatment** Rare reports of agranulocytosis; use caution with clozapine and carbamazepine; thiazides decrease lithium clearance resulting in elevated serum lithium levels and potential toxicity; monitor serum lithium levels

**Pregnancy Risk Factor** C (per manufacturer); D (based on expert analysis)

**Contraindications** Hypersensitivity to chlorothiazide or any component, thiazides, or sulfonamide-derived drugs; anuria; renal decompensation; pregnancy

**Warnings/Precautions** Use with caution in severe renal disease. Electrolyte disturbances (hypokalemia, hypochloremic alkalosis, hyponatremia) can occur. Use with caution in severe hepatic dysfunction; hepatic encephalopathy can be caused by electrolyte disturbances. Gout can be precipitate in certain patients with a history of gout, a familial predisposition to gout, or chronic renal failure. Cautious use in diabetics; may see a change in glucose control. I.V. use is generally not recommended (but is available). Hypersensitivity reactions can occur. Can cause SLE exacerbation or activation. Use with caution in patients with moderate or high cholesterol concentrations. Photosensitization may occur. Correct hypokalemia before initiating therapy.

**Adverse Reactions**

1% to 10%: Endocrine & metabolic: Hypokalemia, hyponatremia

<1%: Agranulocytosis, aplastic anemia, arrhythmia, dizziness, fever, headache, hyperglycemia, hyperlipidemia, hyperuricemia, hypochloremic alkalosis, leukopenia, orthostatic hypotension, paresthesias, prerenal azotemia, photosensitivity, rarely blood dyscrasias, rash, vertigo, weak pulse

**Overdosage/Toxicology**

Signs and symptoms: Hypermotility, diuresis, lethargy, confusion, muscle weakness, coma

Treatment: Following GI decontamination, therapy is supportive with I.V. fluids, electrolytes, and I.V. pressors if needed

**Drug Interactions**

Angiotensin-converting enzyme inhibitors: Increased hypotension if aggressively diuresed with a thiazide diuretic

Beta-blockers increase hyperglycemic effects in Type 2 diabetes mellitus

Cyclosporine and thiazides can increase the risk of gout or renal toxicity; avoid concurrent use

Digoxin toxicity can be exacerbated if a thiazide induces hypokalemia or hypomagnesemia

Lithium toxicity can occur by reducing renal excretion of lithium; monitor lithium concentration and adjust as needed

Neuromuscular-blocking agents can prolong blockade; monitor serum potassium and neuromuscular status

NSAIDs can decrease the efficacy of thiazides reducing the diuretic and antihypertensive effects

**Usual Dosage**

Infants <6 months:

Oral: 20-40 mg/kg/day in 2 divided doses

I.V.: 2-8 mg/kg/day in 2 divided doses

Infants >6 months and Children:

Oral: 20 mg/kg/day in 2 divided doses

I.V.: 4 mg/kg/day

Adults:

Oral: 500 mg to 2 g/day divided in 1-2 doses

I.V.: 100-500 mg/day (for edema only)

Elderly: Oral: 500 mg once daily **or** 1 g 3 times/week

**Patient Information** Take once daily dose of chlorothiazide in morning or last of daily doses in early evening to avoid night-time disturbances. Additional potassium may be recommended; follow dietary suggestions of prescriber. You will be more sensitive to sunlight; use sunblock, wear protective clothing, or avoid direct sunlight. You may experience dizziness, weakness, or drowsiness; use caution when driving or engaging in tasks that require alertness until response to drug is known. You may experience postural hypotension; use caution when rising from sitting or lying position or when climbing stairs. Report muscle twitching or cramps; acute loss of appetite; GI distress; severe rash, redness, or itching of skin; sexual dysfunction; palpitations; or respiratory difficulty.

**Nursing Implications** Take blood pressure with patient lying down and standing; avoid extravasation of parenteral solution since it is extremely irritating to tissues

**Dosage Forms**

Powder for injection, lyophilized, as sodium: 500 mg

Suspension, oral: 250 mg/5 mL (237 mL)

Tablet: 250 mg, 500 mg

## Chlorothiazide and Methyldopa
(klor oh THYE a zide & meth il DOE pa)

**U.S. Brand Names** Aldoclor®

**Pharmacologic Category** Antihypertensive Agent, Combination

**Use** Treatment of hypertension

**Effects on Mental Status** May cause dizziness, drowsiness, anxiety, nightmares, or depression

**Effects on Psychiatric Treatment** Rare reports of agranulocytosis; use caution with clozapine and carbamazepine; thiazides decrease lithium clearance resulting in elevated serum lithium levels and potential toxicity; monitor serum lithium levels. Contraindicated with MAOIs; associated with lithium toxicity; use alternative antihypertensive agent; methyldopa may interact with psychotropics; monitor blood pressure and clinical status.

**Usual Dosage** Oral: 1 tablet 2-3 times/day for first 48 hours, then adjust

**Dosage Forms** Tablet:

150: Chlorothiazide 150 mg and methyldopa 250 mg
250: Chlorothiazide 250 mg and methyldopa 250 mg

## Chlorothiazide and Reserpine

(klor oh THYE a zide & re SER peen)

**Pharmacologic Category** Antihypertensive Agent, Combination

**Use** Management of hypertension

**Effects on Mental Status** May cause dizziness

**Effects on Psychiatric Treatment** Rare reports of agranulocytosis; use caution with clozapine and carbamazepine; thiazides decrease lithium clearance resulting in elevated serum lithium levels and potential toxicity; monitor serum lithium levels

**Usual Dosage** Oral: 1-2 tablets 1-2 times/day

**Dosage Forms** Tablet:

250: Chlorothiazide 250 mg and reserpine 0.125 mg
500: Chlorothiazide 500 mg and reserpine 0.125 mg

## Chlorotrianisene (klor oh trye AN i seen)

**U.S. Brand Names** TACE®

**Pharmacologic Category** Estrogen Derivative

**Use** Treat inoperable prostatic cancer; management of atrophic vaginitis, female hypogonadism, vasomotor symptoms of menopause

**Effects on Mental Status** May cause depression or anxiety

**Effects on Psychiatric Treatment** Barbiturates may increase the metabolism of estrogen resulting in lower levels

**Pregnancy Risk Factor** X

**Contraindications** Thrombophlebitis, breast cancer, undiagnosed abnormal vaginal bleeding, known or suspected pregnancy

**Warnings/Precautions** Estrogens have been reported to increase the risk of endometrial carcinoma; do not use estrogens during pregnancy

**Adverse Reactions**

>10%:
- Cardiovascular: Peripheral edema
- Endocrine & metabolic: Enlargement of breasts (female and male), breast tenderness
- Gastrointestinal: Nausea, anorexia, bloating

1% to 10%:
- Central nervous system: Headache
- Endocrine & metabolic: Increased libido (female), decreased libido (male)
- Gastrointestinal: Vomiting, diarrhea

<1%: Alterations in frequency and flow of menses, amenorrhea, anxiety, breast tumors, chloasma, cholestatic jaundice, decreased glucose tolerance, depression, dizziness, edema, GI distress, hypertension, increased susceptibility to *Candida* infection, increased triglycerides and LDL, intolerance to contact lenses, melasma, myocardial infarction, nausea, rash, stroke, thromboembolism

**Overdosage/Toxicology** Signs and symptoms: Serious adverse effects have not been reported following ingestion of large doses of estrogen-containing oral contraceptives; overdosage of estrogen may cause nausea; withdrawal bleeding may occur in females

**Drug Interactions** Barbiturates may produce lower estrogen levels due to increased hepatic metabolism; may result in an increase in the pharmacologic and toxicologic effect of corticosteroids; hydantoins and rifamycins may cause an increase in metabolism of estrogen compounds

**Usual Dosage** Adults: Oral:

- Atrophic vaginitis: 12-25 mg/day in 28-day cycles (21 days on and 7 days off)
- Female hypogonadism: 12-25 mg cyclically for 21 days. May be followed by I.M. progesterone 100 mg or 5 days of oral progestin; next course may begin on day 5 of induced uterine bleeding.
- Postpartum breast engorgement: 12 mg 4 times/day for 7 days or 50 mg every 6 hours for 6 doses; administer first dose within 8 hours after delivery
- Vasomotor symptoms associated with menopause: 12-25 mg cyclically for 30 days; one or more courses may be prescribed
- Prostatic cancer (inoperable/progressing): 12-25 mg/day

**Patient Information** Take as directed. May cause enlargement of breast (male/female), menstrual irregularity, increased libido (female), decreased libido (male), nausea or vomiting (small frequent meals, frequent mouth care, sucking lozenges, or chewing gum may help), or acute headache (mild analgesic may help). Report persistent diarrhea; swelling of feet, hands, or legs; sudden severe headache; disturbance of speech or vision; warmth, swelling, or pain in calves; severe abdominal pain; rash; emotional lability; chest pain or palpitations; or signs of vaginal infection.

**Dosage Forms** Capsule: 12 mg, 25 mg

- **Chlorphed® [OTC]** *see* Brompheniramine *on page 73*
- **Chlorphed®-LA Nasal Solution [OTC]** *see* Oxymetazoline *on page 415*

## Chlorphenesin (klor FEN e sin)

**U.S. Brand Names** Maolate®

**Pharmacologic Category** Skeletal Muscle Relaxant

**Use** Adjunctive treatment of discomfort in short-term, acute, painful musculoskeletal conditions

**Effects on Mental Status** Drowsiness is common; may cause depression or paradoxical stimulation

**Effects on Psychiatric Treatment** May rarely produce aplastic anemia or leukopenia; use caution with clozapine and carbamazepine

**Contraindications** Hypersensitivity to chlorphenesin

**Warnings/Precautions** Safe use for periods >8 weeks has not been established, use with caution in patients with impaired renal or hepatic function; product contains tartrazine

**Adverse Reactions**

>10%:
- Central nervous system: Drowsiness

1% to 10%:
- Cardiovascular: Tachycardia, tightness in chest, flushing of face
- Central nervous system: Syncope, mental depression, dizziness lightheadedness, headache, paradoxical stimulation
- Dermatologic: Angioedema
- Gastrointestinal: Stomach cramps, hiccups, nausea, vomiting
- Neuromuscular & skeletal: Trembling
- Ocular: Burning of eyes
- Respiratory: Shortness of breath
- Miscellaneous: Allergic fever

**Overdosage/Toxicology** Signs and symptoms: Drowsiness, respiratory depression, nausea, coma

**Usual Dosage** Adults: Oral: 800 mg 3 times/day, then adjusted to lowest effective dosage, usually 400 mg 4 times/day for up to a maximum of 2 months

**Patient Information** May cause drowsiness, may impair judgment and coordination; avoid alcohol and other CNS depressants

**Dosage Forms** Tablet, as carbamate: 400 mg

## Chlorpheniramine (klor fen IR a meen)

**U.S. Brand Names** Aller-Chlor® [OTC]; AL-R® [OTC]; Chlo-Amine® [OTC]; Chlorate® [OTC]; Chlor-Pro® [OTC]; Chlor-Trimeton® [OTC]; Telachlor®; Teldrin® [OTC]

**Canadian Brand Names** Chlor-Tripolon®

**Synonyms** CTM

**Pharmacologic Category** Antihistamine

**Use** Perennial and seasonal allergic rhinitis and other allergic symptoms including urticaria

**Effects on Mental Status** Drowsiness is common; may cause excitability, nervousness, fatigue, or depression

**Effects on Psychiatric Treatment** Dry mouth and sedation may be exacerbated by concurrent psychotropic use

**Contraindications** Hypersensitivity to chlorpheniramine maleate or any component; narrow-angle glaucoma; bladder neck obstruction; symptomatic prostate hypertrophy; during acute asthmatic attacks; stenosing peptic ulcer; pyloroduodenal obstruction. Avoid use in premature and term newborns due to possible association with SIDS.

**Warnings/Precautions** Do not administer to premature or full-term neonates; young children may be more susceptible to side effects and CNS stimulation; bladder neck obstruction, symptomatic prostate hypertrophy, asthmatic attacks, and stenosing peptic ulcer; swallow whole, do not crush or chew sustained release tablets. Anticholinergic action may cause significant confusional symptoms.

**Adverse Reactions**
- Genitourinary: Urinary retention
- Ocular: Diplopia
- Renal: Polyuria

>10%:
- Central nervous system: Slight to moderate drowsiness
- Respiratory: Thickening of bronchial secretions

1% to 10%:
- Central nervous system: Headache, excitability, fatigue, nervousness, dizziness
- Gastrointestinal: Nausea, xerostomia, diarrhea, abdominal pain, appetite increase, weight increase
- Neuromuscular & skeletal: Arthralgia, weakness
- Respiratory: Pharyngitis

(Continued)

## Chlorpheniramine *(Continued)*

**Overdosage/Toxicology**

Signs and symptoms: Dry mouth, flushed skin, dilated pupils, CNS depression

Treatment: There is no specific treatment for an antihistamine overdose, however, most of its clinical toxicity is due to anticholinergic effects. For anticholinergic overdose with severe life-threatening symptoms, physostigmine 1-2 mg (0.5 or 0.02 mg/kg for children) I.V., slowly may be given to reverse these effects.

**Drug Interactions** CYP2D6 enzyme substrate

Increased toxicity (CNS depression): CNS depressants, MAO inhibitors, tricyclic antidepressants, phenothiazines

**Usual Dosage**

Children: Oral: 0.35 mg/kg/day in divided doses every 4-6 hours
- 2-6 years: 1 mg every 4-6 hours, not to exceed 6 mg in 24 hours
- 6-12 years: 2 mg every 4-6 hours, not to exceed 12 mg/day or sustained release 8 mg at bedtime

Children >12 years and Adults: Oral: 4 mg every 4-6 hours, not to exceed 24 mg/day or sustained release 8-12 mg every 8-12 hours, not to exceed 24 mg/day

Adults: Allergic reactions: I.M., I.V., S.C.: 10-20 mg as a single dose; maximum recommended dose: 40 mg/24 hours

Elderly: 4 mg once or twice daily. **Note:** Duration of action may be 36 hours or more when serum concentrations are low.

Hemodialysis: Supplemental dose is not necessary

**Patient Information** May cause drowsiness; swallow whole, do not crush or chew sustained release product; avoid alcohol, may impair coordination and judgment

**Dosage Forms**

Capsule, as maleate: 12 mg

Capsule, as maleate, timed release: 8 mg, 12 mg

Injection, as maleate: 10 mg/mL (1 mL, 30 mL); 100 mg/mL (2 mL)

Syrup, as maleate: 2 mg/5 mL (120 mL, 473 mL)

Tablet, as maleate: 4 mg, 8 mg, 12 mg

Tablet, as maleate:
- Chewable: 2 mg
- Timed release: 8 mg, 12 mg

## Chlorpheniramine and Acetaminophen

(klor fen IR a meen & a seet a MIN oh fen)

**U.S. Brand Names** Coricidin® [OTC]

**Pharmacologic Category** Antihistamine/Analgesic

**Use** Symptomatic relief of congestion, headache, aches and pains of colds and flu

**Effects on Mental Status** Drowsiness is common; may cause excitability, nervousness, fatigue, or depression

**Effects on Psychiatric Treatment** Dry mouth and sedation may be exacerbated by concurrent psychotropic use

**Usual Dosage** Adults: Oral: 2 tablets every 4 hours, up to 20/day

**Dosage Forms** Tablet: Chlorpheniramine maleate 2 mg and acetaminophen 325 mg

## Chlorpheniramine and Phenylephrine

(klor fen IR a meen & fen il EF rin)

**U.S. Brand Names** Dallergy-D® Syrup; Ed A-Hist® Liquid; Histatab® Plus Tablet [OTC]; Histor-D® Syrup; Rolatuss® Plain Liquid; Ru-Tuss® Liquid

**Pharmacologic Category** Antihistamine/Decongestant Combination

**Use** Temporary relief of nasal congestion and eustachian tube congestion as well as runny nose, sneezing, itching of nose or throat, itchy and watery eyes

**Effects on Mental Status** Drowsiness is common; may cause excitability, nervousness, fatigue, or depression

**Effects on Psychiatric Treatment** Dry mouth and sedation may be exacerbated by concurrent psychotropic use

**Usual Dosage** Oral:

Children:
- 2-5 years: 2.5 mL every 4 hours
- 6-12 years: 5 mL every 4 hours

Adults: 10 mL every 4 hours

**Dosage Forms**

Capsule, sustained release: Chlorpheniramine maleate 8 mg and phenylephrine hydrochloride 20 mg

Liquid:
- Dallergy-D®, Histor-D®, Rolatuss® Plain, Ru-Tuss®: Chlorpheniramine maleate 2 mg and phenylephrine hydrochloride 5 mg per 5 mL
- Ed A-Hist® Liquid: Chlorpheniramine maleate 4 mg and phenylephrine hydrochloride 10 mg per 5 mL

Tablet (Histatab® Plus): Chlorpheniramine maleate 2 mg and phenylephrine hydrochloride 5 mg

## Chlorpheniramine and Phenylpropanolamine

(klor fen IR a meen & fen il proe pa NOLE a meen)

**U.S. Brand Names** Allerest® 12 Hour Capsule [OTC]; A.R.M.® Caplet [OTC]; Chlor-Rest® Tablet [OTC]; Demazin® Syrup [OTC]; Genamin® Cold Syrup [OTC]; Ornade® Spansule®; Resaid®; Rescon Liquid [OTC]; Silaminic® Cold Syrup [OTC]; Temazin® Cold Syrup [OTC]; Thera-Hist® Syrup [OTC]; Triaminic® Allergy Tablet [OTC]; Triaminic® Cold Tablet [OTC]; Triaminic® Syrup [OTC]; Tri-Nefrin® Extra Strength Tablet [OTC]; Triphenyl® Syrup [OTC]

**Pharmacologic Category** Antihistamine/Decongestant Combination

**Use** Symptomatic relief of nasal congestion, runny nose, sneezing, itchy nose or throat, and itchy or watery eyes due to the common cold or allergic rhinitis

**Effects on Mental Status** Drowsiness is common; may cause excitability, nervousness, fatigue, or depression

**Effects on Psychiatric Treatment** Dry mouth and sedation may be exacerbated by concurrent psychotropic use

**Usual Dosage**

Children <12 years: 5 mL every 3-4 hours

Children >12 years and Adults: 1 capsule every 12 hours or 5-10 mL every 3-4 hours

**Dosage Forms**

Capsule, sustained release: Chlorpheniramine maleate 12 mg and phenylpropanolamine hydrochloride 75 mg

Liquid:
- Triphenyl®, Genamin®: Chlorpheniramine maleate 1 mg and phenylpropanolamine hydrochloride 6.25 mg per 5 mL
- Demazin®, Rescon®, Silaminic®, Temazin®, Thera-Hist®: Chlorpheniramine maleate 2 mg and phenylpropanolamine hydrochloride 12.5 mg per 5 mL

Syrup: Chlorpheniramine maleate 2 mg and phenylpropanolamine hydrochloride 12.5 mg per 5 mL

Tablet:
- Triaminic® Cold: Chlorpheniramine maleate 2 mg and phenylpropanolamine hydrochloride 12.5 mg
- Chlor-Rest®: Chlorpheniramine maleate 2 mg and phenylpropanolamine hydrochloride 18.7 mg
- A.R.M.®, Triaminic® Allergy, Tri-Nefrin® Extra Strength: Chlorpheniramine maleate 4 mg and phenylpropanolamine hydrochloride 25 mg

Tablet, sustained release: Chlorpheniramine maleate 12 mg and phenylpropanolamine hydrochloride 75 mg

## Chlorpheniramine and Pseudoephedrine

(klor fen IR a meen & soo doe e FED rin)

**U.S. Brand Names** Allerest® Maximum Strength [OTC]; Anamine® Syrup [OTC]; Anaplex® Liquid [OTC]; Chlorafed® Liquid [OTC]; Chlor-Trimeton® 4 Hour Relief Tablet [OTC]; Co-Pyronil® 2 Pulvules® [OTC]; Deconamine® SR; Deconamine® Syrup [OTC]; Deconamine® Tablet [OTC]; Fedahist® Tablet [OTC]; Hayfebrol® Liquid [OTC]; Histalet® Syrup [OTC]; Klerist-D® Tablet [OTC]; Pseudo-Gest Plus® Tablet [OTC]; Rhinosyn® Liquid [OTC]; Rhinosyn-PD® Liquid [OTC]; Ryna® Liquid [OTC]; Sudafed® Plus Tablet [OTC]

**Pharmacologic Category** Antihistamine/Decongestant Combination

**Use** Relief of nasal congestion associated with the common cold, hay fever, and other allergies, sinusitis, eustachian tube blockage, and vasomotor and allergic rhinitis

**Effects on Mental Status** Drowsiness is common; may cause excitability, nervousness, fatigue, or depression

**Effects on Psychiatric Treatment** Dry mouth and sedation may be exacerbated by concurrent psychotropic use

**Usual Dosage** Oral:

Capsule: One every 12 hours

Tablet: One 3-4 times/day

**Dosage Forms**

Capsule:
- Co-Pyronil® 2 Pulvules®: Chlorpheniramine maleate 4 mg and pseudoephedrine hydrochloride 60 mg

Capsule, sustained release: Chlorpheniramine maleate 4 mg and pseudoephedrine hydrochloride 60 mg; chlorpheniramine maleate 8 mg and pseudoephedrine hydrochloride 120 mg

Liquid:
- Anamine®, Anaplex®, Chlorafed®, Deconamine®, Hayfebrol®, Rhinosyn-PD®, Ryna®: Chlorpheniramine maleate 2 mg and pseudoephedrine sulfate 30 mg per 5 mL
- Rhinosyn®: Chlorpheniramine maleate 2 mg and pseudoephedrine sulfate 60 mg per 5 mL

Histalet®: Chlorpheniramine maleate 3 mg and pseudoephedrine sulfate 45 mg per 5 mL

Tablet:
- Allerest® Maximum Strength: Chlorpheniramine maleate 2 mg and pseudoephedrine hydrochloride 30 mg

Deconamine®, Fedahist®, Klerist-D®, Pseudo-Gest Plus®, Sudafed® Plus: Chlorpheniramine maleate 4 mg and pseudoephedrine hydrochloride 60 mg

Chlor-Trimeton® 4 Hour Relief: Chlorpheniramine maleate 4 mg and pseudoephedrine sulfate 60 mg

## Chlorpheniramine, Ephedrine, Phenylephrine, and Carbetapentane

(klor fen IR a meen, e FED rin, fen il EF rin, & kar bay ta PEN tane)

**U.S. Brand Names** Rentamine®; Rynatuss® Pediatric Suspension; Tri-Tannate Plus®

**Pharmacologic Category** Antihistamine/Decongestant/Antitussive

**Use** Symptomatic relief of cough

**Effects on Mental Status** Drowsiness is common; may cause excitability, nervousness, fatigue, or depression

**Effects on Psychiatric Treatment** Dry mouth and sedation may be exacerbated by concurrent psychotropic use

**Usual Dosage** Children:

<2 years: Titrate dose individually

2-6 years: 2.5-5 mL every 12 hours

>6 years: 5-10 mL every 12 hours

**Dosage Forms** Liquid: Carbetapentane tannate 30 mg, ephedrine tannate 5 mg, phenylephrine tannate 5 mg, and chlorpheniramine tannate 4 mg per 5 mL

## Chlorpheniramine, Phenindamine, and Phenylpropanolamine

(klor fen IR a meen, fen IN dah meen, & fen il proe pa NOLE a meen)

**U.S. Brand Names** Nolamine®

**Pharmacologic Category** Antihistamine/Decongestant Combination

**Use** Upper respiratory and nasal congestion

**Effects on Mental Status** Drowsiness is common; may cause excitability, nervousness, fatigue, or depression

**Effects on Psychiatric Treatment** Dry mouth and sedation may be exacerbated by concurrent psychotropic use

**Usual Dosage** Adults: Oral: 1 tablet every 8-12 hours

**Dosage Forms** Tablet, timed release: Chlorpheniramine maleate 4 mg, phenindamine tartrate 24 mg, and phenylpropanolamine hydrochloride 50 mg

## Chlorpheniramine, Phenylephrine, and Codeine

(klor fen IR a meen, fen il EF rin, & KOE deen)

**U.S. Brand Names** Pediacof®; Pedituss®

**Pharmacologic Category** Antihistamine/Decongestant/Antitussive

**Use** Symptomatic relief of rhinitis, nasal congestion and cough due to colds or allergy

**Effects on Mental Status** Drowsiness is common; may cause excitability, nervousness, fatigue, or depression

**Effects on Psychiatric Treatment** Dry mouth and sedation may be exacerbated by concurrent psychotropic use

**Restrictions** C-IV

**Usual Dosage** Children 6 months to 12 years: 1.25-10 mL every 4-6 hours

**Dosage Forms** Liquid: Chlorpheniramine maleate 0.75 mg, phenylephrine hydrochloride 2.5 mg, and codeine phosphate 5 mg with potassium iodide 75 mg per 5 mL

## Chlorpheniramine, Phenylephrine, and Dextromethorphan

(klor fen IR a meen, fen il EF rin, & deks troe meth OR fan)

**U.S. Brand Names** Cerose-DM® [OTC]

**Pharmacologic Category** Antihistamine/Decongestant/Antitussive

**Use** Temporary relief of cough due to minor throat and bronchial irritation; relieves nasal congestion, runny nose and sneezing

**Effects on Mental Status** Drowsiness is common; may cause excitability, nervousness, fatigue, or depression

**Effects on Psychiatric Treatment** Dry mouth and sedation may be exacerbated by concurrent psychotropic use

**Usual Dosage** Adults: Oral: 5-10 mL 4 times/day

**Dosage Forms** Liquid: Chlorpheniramine maleate 4 mg, phenylephrine hydrochloride 10 mg, and dextromethorphan hydrobromide 15 mg per 5 mL

## Chlorpheniramine, Phenylephrine, and Methscopolamine

(klor fen IR a meen, fen il EF rin, & meth skoe POL a meen)

**U.S. Brand Names** D.A.II® Tablet; Dallergy®; Dura-Vent/DA®; Extendryl® SR; Histor-D® Timecelles®

**Pharmacologic Category** Antihistamine/Decongestant/Anticholinergic

**Use** Relieves nasal congestion, runny nose and sneezing

**Effects on Mental Status** Drowsiness is common; may cause excitability, nervousness, fatigue, or depression

**Effects on Psychiatric Treatment** Dry mouth and sedation may be exacerbated by concurrent psychotropic use

**Usual Dosage** Adults: Oral: 1 capsule every 12 hours

**Dosage Forms**

Caplet, sustained release: Chlorpheniramine maleate 8 mg, phenylephrine hydrochloride 20 mg, and methscopolamine nitrate 2.5 mg

Capsule, sustained release: Chlorpheniramine maleate 8 mg, phenylephrine hydrochloride 10 mg, and methscopolamine nitrate 2.5 mg

Syrup: Chlorpheniramine maleate 2 mg, phenylephrine hydrochloride 10 mg, and methscopolamine nitrate 0.625 mg per 5 mL

Tablet: Chlorpheniramine maleate 4 mg, phenylephrine hydrochloride 10 mg, and methscopolamine nitrate 1.25 mg

## Chlorpheniramine, Phenylephrine, and Phenylpropanolamine

(klor fen IR a meen, fen il EF rin, & fen il proe pa NOLE a meen)

**U.S. Brand Names** Hista-Vadrin® Tablet

**Pharmacologic Category** Antihistamine/Decongestant Combination

**Use** Symptomatic relief of rhinitis and nasal congestion due to colds or allergy

**Effects on Mental Status** Drowsiness is common; may cause excitability, nervousness, fatigue, or depression

**Effects on Psychiatric Treatment** Dry mouth and sedation may be exacerbated by concurrent psychotropic use

**Usual Dosage** Adults: Oral: 1 tablet every 6 hours

**Dosage Forms** Tablet: Chlorpheniramine maleate 6 mg, phenylephrine hydrochloride 5 mg, and phenylpropanolamine hydrochloride 40 mg

## Chlorpheniramine, Phenylephrine, and Phenyltoloxamine

(klor fen IR a meen, fen il EF rin, & fen il tole LOKS a meen)

**U.S. Brand Names** Comhist®; Comhist® LA

**Pharmacologic Category** Antihistamine/Decongestant Combination

**Use** Symptomatic relief of rhinitis and nasal congestion due to colds or allergy

**Effects on Mental Status** Drowsiness is common; may cause excitability, nervousness, fatigue, or depression

**Effects on Psychiatric Treatment** Dry mouth and sedation may be exacerbated by concurrent psychotropic use

**Usual Dosage** Oral: 1 capsule every 8-12 hours or 1-2 tablets 3 times/day

**Dosage Forms**

Capsule, sustained release (Comhist® LA): Chlorpheniramine maleate 4 mg, phenylephrine hydrochloride 20 mg, and phenyltoloxamine citrate 50 mg

Tablet (Comhist®): Chlorpheniramine maleate 2 mg, phenylephrine hydrochloride 10 mg, and phenyltoloxamine citrate 25 mg

## Chlorpheniramine, Phenylephrine, Phenylpropanolamine, and Belladonna Alkaloids

(klor fen IR a meen, fen il EF rin, fen il proe pa NOLE a meen, & bel a DON a AL ka loydz)

**U.S. Brand Names** Atrohist® Plus; Phenahist-TR®; Phenchlor® S.H.A.; Ru-Tuss®; Stahist®

**Pharmacologic Category** Cold Preparation

**Use** Relief of symptoms resulting from irritation of sinus, nasal, and upper respiratory tract tissues, including nasal congestion, watering eyes, and postnasal drip; this product contains anticholinergic agents and should be reserved for patients who do not respond to other antihistamine/decongestants

**Effects on Mental Status** Drowsiness is common; may cause excitability, nervousness, fatigue, or depression

**Effects on Psychiatric Treatment** Dry mouth and sedation may be exacerbated by concurrent psychotropic use

**Usual Dosage** Children ≥12 years and Adults: Oral: 1 tablet morning and evening, swallowed whole

**Dosage Forms** Tablet, sustained release: Chlorpheniramine 8 mg, phenylephrine 25 mg, phenylpropanolamine 50 mg, hyoscyamine 0.19 mg, atropine 0.04 mg, and scopolamine 0.01 mg

## Chlorpheniramine, Phenylpropanolamine, and Acetaminophen

(klor fen IR a meen, fen il proe pa NOLE a meen, & a seet a MIN oh fen)

**U.S. Brand Names** Congestant D® [OTC]; Coricidin D® [OTC]; Dapacin® Cold Capsule [OTC]; Duadacin® Capsule [OTC]; Tylenol® Cold Effervescent Medication Tablet [OTC]

**Pharmacologic Category** Antihistamine/Decongestant/Analgesic

**Use** Symptomatic relief of nasal congestion and headache from colds/sinus congestion

**Effects on Mental Status** Drowsiness is common; may cause excitability, nervousness, fatigue, or depression

**Effects on Psychiatric Treatment** Dry mouth and sedation may be exacerbated by concurrent psychotropic use

**Usual Dosage** Adults: Oral: 2 tablets every 4 hours, up to 12 tablets/day

**Dosage Forms**

Capsule: Chlorpheniramine maleate 2 mg, phenylpropanolamine hydrochloride 12.5 mg, and acetaminophen 325 mg

Tablet: Chlorpheniramine maleate 2 mg, phenylpropanolamine hydrochloride 12.5 mg, and acetaminophen 325 mg

## Chlorpheniramine, Phenylpropanolamine, and Dextromethorphan

(klor fen IR a meen, fen il proe pa NOLE a meen, & deks troe meth OR fan)

**U.S. Brand Names** Triaminicol® Multi-Symptom Cold Syrup [OTC]

**Pharmacologic Category** Antihistamine/Decongestant/Antitussive

**Use** Provides relief of runny nose, sneezing, suppresses cough, promotes nasal and sinus drainage

**Effects on Mental Status** Drowsiness is common; may cause excitability, nervousness, fatigue, or depression

**Effects on Psychiatric Treatment** Dry mouth and sedation may be exacerbated by concurrent psychotropic use

**Usual Dosage** Oral:

Children 6-12 years: 5 mL every 4 hours

Adults: 10 mL every 4 hours

**Dosage Forms** Liquid: Chlorpheniramine maleate 2 mg, phenylpropanolamine hydrochloride 12.5 mg, and dextromethorphan hydrobromide 10 mg per 5 mL

## Chlorpheniramine, Phenyltoloxamine, Phenylpropanolamine, and Phenylephrine

(klor fen IR a meen, fen il tole LOKS a meen, fen il proe pa NOLE a meen & fen il EF rin)

**U.S. Brand Names** Naldecon®; Naldelate®; Nalgest®; Nalspan®; New Decongestant®; Par Decon®; Tri-Phen-Chlor®; Uni-Decon®

**Pharmacologic Category** Antihistamine/Decongestant Combination

**Use** Symptomatic treatment of nasal and eustachian tube congestion associated with sinusitis and acute upper respiratory infection; symptomatic relief of perennial and allergic rhinitis

**Effects on Mental Status** Drowsiness is common; may cause excitability, nervousness, fatigue, or depression

**Effects on Psychiatric Treatment** Dry mouth and sedation may be exacerbated by concurrent psychotropic use

**Usual Dosage** Oral:

Children:

3-6 months: 1/4 mL (pediatric drops) every 3-4 hours

6-12 months: 2.5 mL (pediatric syrup) or 1/2 mL (pediatric drops) every 3-4 hours

1-6 years: 5 mL (pediatric syrup) or 1 mL (pediatric drops) every 3-4 hours

6-12 years: 2.5 mL (syrup) or 10 mL (pediatric syrup) or 1/2 tablet every 3-4 hours

Children >12 years and Adults: 5 mL (syrup) or 1 tablet every 3-4 hours

**Dosage Forms**

Drops, pediatric: Chlorpheniramine maleate 0.5 mg, phenyltoloxamine citrate 2 mg, phenylpropanolamine hydrochloride 5 mg, and phenylephrine hydrochloride 1.25 mg per mL

Syrup: Chlorpheniramine maleate 2.5 mg, phenyltoloxamine citrate 7.5 mg, phenylpropanolamine hydrochloride 20 mg, and phenylephrine hydrochloride 5 mg per 5 mL

Syrup, pediatric: Chlorpheniramine maleate 0.5 mg, phenyltoloxamine citrate 2 mg, phenylpropanolamine hydrochloride 5 mg, and phenylephrine hydrochloride 1.25 mg per 5 mL

Tablet, sustained release: Chlorpheniramine maleate 5 mg, phenyltoloxamine citrate 15 mg, phenylpropanolamine hydrochloride 40 mg, and phenylephrine hydrochloride 10 mg

## Chlorpheniramine, Pseudoephedrine, and Codeine

(klor fen IR a meen, soo doe e FED rin, & KOE deen)

**U.S. Brand Names** Codehist® DH; Decohistine® DH; Dihistine® DH; Ryna-C® Liquid

**Pharmacologic Category** Antihistamine/Decongestant/Antitussive

**Use** Temporary relief of cough associated with minor throat or bronchial irritation or nasal congestion due to common cold, allergic rhinitis, or sinusitis

**Effects on Mental Status** Drowsiness is common; may cause excitability, nervousness, fatigue, or depression

**Effects on Psychiatric Treatment** Dry mouth and sedation may be exacerbated by concurrent psychotropic use

**Restrictions** C-V

**Usual Dosage** Oral:

Children:

25-50 lb: 1.25-2.50 mL every 4-6 hours, up to 4 doses in 24-hour period

50-90 lb: 2.5-5 mL every 4-6 hours, up to 4 doses in 24-hour period

Adults: 10 mL every 4-6 hours, up to 4 doses in 24-hour period

**Dosage Forms** Liquid: Chlorpheniramine maleate 2 mg, pseudoephedrine hydrochloride 30 mg, and codeine phosphate 10 mg (120 mL, 480 mL)

## Chlorpheniramine, Pyrilamine, and Phenylephrine

(klor fen IR a meen, pye RIL a meen, & fen il EF rin)

**U.S. Brand Names** Rhinatate® Tablet; R-Tannamine® Tablet; R-Tannate® Tablet; Rynatan® Pediatric Suspension; Rynatan® Tablet; Tanoral® Tablet; Triotann® Tablet; Tri-Tannate® Tablet

**Pharmacologic Category** Antihistamine/Decongestant Combination

**Use** Symptomatic relief of nasal congestion associated with upper respiratory tract condition

**Effects on Mental Status** Drowsiness is common; may cause excitability, nervousness, fatigue, or depression

**Effects on Psychiatric Treatment** Dry mouth and sedation may be exacerbated by concurrent psychotropic use

**Usual Dosage** Children:

<2 years: Titrate dose individually

2-6 years: 2.5-5 mL every 12 hours

>6 years: 5-10 mL every 12 hours

**Dosage Forms**

Liquid: Chlorpheniramine tannate 2 mg, pyrilamine tannate 12.5 mg, and phenylephrine tannate 5 mg per 5 mL

Tablet: Chlorpheniramine tannate 8 mg, pyrilamine maleate 12.5 mg, and phenylephrine tannate 25 mg

## Chlorpheniramine, Pyrilamine, Phenylephrine, and Phenylpropanolamine

(klor fen IR a meen, pye RIL a meen, fen il EF rin, & fen il proe pa NOLE a meen)

**U.S. Brand Names** Histalet Forte® Tablet

**Pharmacologic Category** Antihistamine/Decongestant Combination

**Use** Symptomatic relief of rhinitis and nasal congestion due to colds or allergy

**Effects on Mental Status** Drowsiness is common; may cause excitability, nervousness, fatigue, or depression

**Effects on Psychiatric Treatment** Dry mouth and sedation may be exacerbated by concurrent psychotropic use

**Usual Dosage** Adults: Oral: 1 tablet 2-3 times/day

**Dosage Forms** Tablet: Chlorpheniramine maleate 4 mg, pyrilamine maleate 25 mg, phenylephrine hydrochloride 10 mg, and phenylpropanolamine hydrochloride 50 mg

♦ **Chlor-Pro® [OTC]** *see* Chlorpheniramine *on page 113*

## Chlorpromazine (klor PROE ma zeen)

**Related Information**

Antipsychotic Agents Comparison Chart *on page 706*

Antipsychotic Medication Guidelines *on page 751*

Clinical Issues in the Use of Antipsychotics *on page 630*

Discontinuation of Psychotropic Drugs - Withdrawal Symptoms and Recommendations *on page 798*

Federal OBRA Regulations Recommended Maximum Doses *on page 756*

Liquid Compatibility With Antipsychotics and Mood Stabilizers *on page 718*

Patient Information - Antipsychotics (General) *on page 646*

Schizophrenia *on page 604*

Special Populations - Pregnant and Breast-Feeding Patients *on page 668*

**Generic Available** Yes

**U.S. Brand Names** Ormazine; Thorazine®

**Canadian Brand Names** Apo®-Chlorpromazine; Chlorprom®; Chlorpromanyl®; Largactil®; Novo-Chlorpromazine

**Synonyms** Chlorpromazine Hydrochloride

**Pharmacologic Category** Antipsychotic Agent, Phenothiazine, Aliphatic

**Use** Psychoses and mania; to control nausea and vomiting; relief of restlessness and apprehension before surgery; acute intermittent porphyria; adjunct in the treatment of tetanus; intractable hiccups; combativeness and/or explosive hyperexcitable behavior in children 1-12 years of age and in short-term treatment of hyperactive children

**Pregnancy Risk Factor** C

**Contraindications** Hypersensitivity to chlorpromazine or any component (cross reactivity between phenothiazines may occur); severe CNS depression, coma

**Warnings/Precautions** Highly sedating, use with caution in disorders where CNS depression is a feature. Use with caution in Parkinson's disease. Caution in patients with hemodynamic instability; bone marrow suppression; predisposition to seizures, subcortical brain damage, severe cardiac, hepatic, renal, or respiratory disease. Esophageal dysmotility and aspiration have been associated with antipsychotic use - use with caution in patients at risk of pneumonia (ie, Alzheimer's disease). Caution in breast cancer or other prolactin-dependent tumors (may elevate prolactin levels). May alter temperature regulation or mask toxicity of other drugs due to antiemetic effects. May alter cardiac conduction - life-threatening arrhythmias have occurred with therapeutic doses of neuroleptics. May cause orthostatic hypotension - use with caution in patients at risk of this effect or those who would tolerate transient hypotensive episodes (cerebrovascular disease, cardiovascular disease, or other medications which may predispose). Significant hypotension may occur, particularly with parenteral administration. Injection contains sulfites and benzyl alcohol.

Phenothiazines may cause anticholinergic effects (confusion, agitation, constipation, dry mouth, blurred vision, urinary retention). Therefore, they should be used with caution in patients with decreased gastrointestinal motility, urinary retention, BPH, xerostomia, or visual problems. Conditions which also may be exacerbated by cholinergic blockade include narrow-angle glaucoma (screening is recommended) and worsening of myasthenia gravis. Relative to other neuroleptics, chlorpromazine has a moderate potency of cholinergic blockade.

May cause extrapyramidal reactions, including pseudoparkinsonism, acute dystonic reactions, akathisia, and tardive dyskinesia (risk of these reactions is low-moderate relative to other neuroleptics). May be associated with neuroleptic malignant syndrome (NMS) or pigmentary retinopathy.

**Adverse Reactions**

Cardiovascular: Postural hypotension, tachycardia, dizziness, nonspecific Q-T changes

Central nervous system: Drowsiness, dystonias, akathisia, pseudoparkinsonism, tardive dyskinesia, neuroleptic malignant syndrome, seizures

Dermatologic: Photosensitivity, dermatitis, skin pigmentation (slate gray)

Endocrine & metabolic: Lactation, breast engorgement, false-positive pregnancy test, amenorrhea, gynecomastia, hyper- or hypoglycemia

Gastrointestinal: Xerostomia, constipation, nausea

Genitourinary: Urinary retention, ejaculatory disorder, impotence

Hematologic: Agranulocytosis, eosinophilia, leukopenia, hemolytic anemia, aplastic anemia, thrombocytopenic purpura

Hepatic: Jaundice

Ocular: Blurred vision, corneal and lenticular changes, epithelial keratopathy, pigmentary retinopathy

**Overdosage/Toxicology**

Signs and symptoms: Deep sleep, coma, extrapyramidal symptoms, abnormal involuntary muscle movements, hypotension

Treatment:

Following initiation of essential overdose management, toxic symptom treatment and supportive treatment should be initiated

Hypotension usually responds to I.V. fluids or Trendelenburg positioning. If unresponsive to these measures, the use of a parenteral inotrope may be required

Seizures commonly respond to diazepam (I.V. 5-10 mg bolus in adults every 15 minutes if needed up to a total of 30 mg; I.V. 0.25-0.4 mg/kg/dose up to a total of 10 mg in children) or to phenytoin or phenobarbital

Also critical cardiac arrhythmias often respond to I.V. phenytoin (15 mg/kg up to 1 g), while other antiarrhythmics can be used

Neuroleptics often cause extrapyramidal symptoms (eg, dystonic reactions) requiring management with benztropine mesylate I.V. 1-2 mg (adults) may be effective. These agents are generally effective within 2-5 minutes.

**Drug Interactions** CYP1A2, 2D6, and 3A3/4 enzyme substrate; CYP2D6 enzyme inhibitor

Aluminum salts: May decrease the absorption of phenothiazines; monitor

Amphetamines: Efficacy may be diminished by antipsychotics; in addition, amphetamines may increase psychotic symptoms; avoid concurrent use

Anticholinergics: May inhibit the therapeutic response to phenothiazines and excess anticholinergic effects may occur; includes benztropine, trihexyphenidyl, biperiden, and drugs with significant anticholinergic activity (TCAs, antihistamines, disopyramide)

Antihypertensives: Concurrent use of phenothiazines with an antihypertensive may produce additive hypotensive effects (particularly orthostasis)

Bromocriptine: Phenothiazines inhibit the ability of bromocriptine to lower serum prolactin concentrations

CNS depressants: Sedative effects may be additive with phenothiazines; monitor for increased effect; includes barbiturates, benzodiazepines, narcotic analgesics, ethanol and other sedative agents

CYP1A2 inhibitors: Metabolism of phenothiazines may be decreased; increasing clinical effect or toxicity. Inhibitors include cimetidine, ciprofloxacin, fluvoxamine, isoniazid, ritonavir, and zileutin

CYP2D6 inhibitors: Metabolism of phenothiazines may be decreased; increasing clinical effect or toxicity; inhibitors include amiodarone, cimetidine, delavirdine, fluoxetine, paroxetine, propafenone, quinidine, and ritonavir; monitor for increased effect/toxicity

CYP3A3/4 inhibitors: Serum level and/or toxicity of chlorpromazine may be increased; inhibitors include amiodarone, cimetidine, clarithromycin, erythromycin, delavirdine, diltiazem, dirithromycin, disulfiram, fluoxetine, fluvoxamine, grapefruit juice, indinavir, itraconazole, ketoconazole, metronidazole, nefazodone, nevirapine, propoxyfene, quinupristin-dalfopristin, ritonavir, saquinavir, verapamil, zafirlukast, zileuton; monitor for increased response

CYP2D6 substrates: Chlorpromazine may decrease the metabolism of drugs metabolized by CYP2D6 (in addition to drugs specifically mentioned in this listing)

Enzyme inducers: May enhance the hepatic metabolism of phenothiazines; larger doses may be required; includes rifampin, rifabutin, barbiturates, phenytoin, and cigarette smoking

Epinephrine: Chlorpromazine (and possibly other low potency antipsychotics) may diminish the pressor effects of epinephrine

Guanethidine and guanadrel: Antihypertensive effects may be inhibited by chlorpromazine

Levodopa: Chlorpromazine may inhibit the antiparkinsonian effect of levodopa; avoid this combination

Lithium: Chlorpromazine may produce neurotoxicity with lithium; this is a rare effect

Phenytoin: May reduce serum levels of phenothiazines; phenothiazines may increase phenytoin serum levels

Propranolol: Serum concentrations of phenothiazines may be increased; propranolol also increases phenothiazine concentrations

Polypeptide antibiotics: Rare cases of respiratory paralysis have been reported with concurrent use of phenothiazines

QTc prolonging agents: Effects on QTc interval may be additive with phenothiazines, increasing the risk of malignant arrhythmias; includes type Ia antiarrhythmics, TCAs, and some quinolone antibiotics (sparfloxacin, moxifloxacin and gatifloxacin)

Sulfadoxine-pyrimethamine: May increase phenothiazine concentrations

Tricyclic antidepressants: Concurrent use may produce increased toxicity or altered therapeutic response

Trazodone: Phenothiazines and trazodone may produce additive hypotensive effects

Valproic acid: Serum levels may be increased by phenothiazines

**Stability** Protect oral dosage forms from light; a slightly yellowed solution does not indicate potency loss, but a markedly discolored solution should be discarded; diluted injection (1 mg/mL) with normal saline and stored in 5 mL vials remains stable for 30 days

**Mechanism of Action** Blocks postsynaptic mesolimbic dopaminergic receptors in the brain; exhibits a strong alpha-adrenergic blocking effect and depresses the release of hypothalamic and hypophyseal hormones; believed to depress the reticular activating system, thus affecting basal metabolism, body temperature, wakefulness, vasomotor tone, and emesis

**Pharmacodynamics/kinetics**

Distribution: Crosses the placenta; appears in breast milk

Metabolism: Extensively in the liver to active and inactive metabolites

Half-life, biphasic:

Initial: 2 hours

Terminal: 30 hours

Elimination: <1% excreted in urine as unchanged drug within 24 hours

Hemodialysis: Not dialyzable (0% to 5%)

**Usual Dosage**

Children >6 months:

Psychosis:

Oral: 0.5-1 mg/kg/dose every 4-6 hours; older children may require 200 mg/day or higher

I.M., I.V.: 0.5-1 mg/kg/dose every 6-8 hours; maximum dose for <5 years (22.7 kg): 40 mg/day; maximum for 5-12 years (22.7-45.5 kg): 75 mg/day

Nausea and vomiting:

Oral: 0.5-1 mg/kg/dose every 4-6 hours as needed

I.M., I.V.: 0.5-1 mg/kg/dose every 6-8 hours; maximum dose for <5 years (22.7 kg): 40 mg/day; maximum for 5-12 years (22.7-45.5 kg): 75 mg/day

Rectal: 1 mg/kg/dose every 6-8 hours as needed

Adults:

Psychosis:

Oral: Range: 30-2000 mg/day in 1-4 divided doses, initiate at lower doses and titrate as needed; usual dose: 400-600 mg/day; some patients may require 1-2 g/day

(Continued)

## Chlorpromazine *(Continued)*

I.M., I.V.: Initial: 25 mg, may repeat (25-50 mg) in 1-4 hours, gradually increase to a maximum of 400 mg/dose every 4-6 hours until patient is controlled; usual dose: 300-800 mg/day

Intractable hiccups: Oral, I.M.: 25-50 mg 3-4 times/day

Nausea and vomiting:

Oral: 10-25 mg every 4-6 hours

I.M., I.V.: 25-50 mg every 4-6 hours

Rectal: 50-100 mg every 6-8 hours

Elderly (nonpsychotic patient; dementia behavior): Initial: 10-25 mg 1-2 times/day; increase at 4- to 7-day intervals by 10-25 mg/day. Increase dose intervals (bid, tid, etc) as necessary to control behavior response or side effects; maximum daily dose: 800 mg; gradual increases (titration) may prevent some side effects or decrease their severity.

**Dosing adjustment/comments in hepatic impairment:** Avoid use in severe hepatic dysfunction

**Dietary Considerations** Alcohol: Additive CNS effects, avoid use

**Administration** Dilute oral concentrate solution in juice before administration

**Monitoring Parameters** Orthostatic blood pressures; tremors, gait changes, abnormal movement in trunk, neck, buccal area, or extremities; monitor target behaviors for which the agent is given; watch for hypotension when administering I.M. or I.V.

**Reference Range** Therapeutic: 50-300 ng/mL (SI: 157-942 nmol/L); Toxic: >750 ng/mL (SI: >2355 nmol/L)

**Test Interactions** False-positives for phenylketonuria, amylase, uroporphyrins, urobilinogen; may cause photosensitivity; avoid excessive sunlight; do not stop taking without consulting physician

**Patient Information** Do not stop taking unless informed by your physician; oral concentrate must be diluted in 2-4 oz of liquid (water, fruit juice, carbonated drinks, milk, or pudding); do not take antacid within 1 hour of taking drug; avoid alcohol; avoid excess sun exposure (use sun block); may cause drowsiness, rise slowly from recumbent position; use of supportive stockings may help prevent orthostatic hypotension

**Nursing Implications** Dilute oral concentrate solution in juice before administration; avoid contact of oral solution or injection with skin (contact dermatitis); watch for hypotension when administering I.M. or I.V.

**Additional Information** Avoid rectal administration in immunocompromised patients

**Dosage Forms**

Capsule, as hydrochloride, sustained action: 30 mg, 75 mg, 150 mg, 200 mg, 300 mg

Concentrate, oral, as hydrochloride: 30 mg/mL (120 mL); 100 mg/mL (60 mL, 240 mL)

Injection, as hydrochloride: 25 mg/mL (1 mL, 2 mL, 10 mL)

Suppository, rectal, as base: 25 mg, 100 mg

Syrup, as hydrochloride: 10 mg/5 mL (120 mL)

Tablet, as hydrochloride: 10 mg, 25 mg, 50 mg, 100 mg, 200 mg

♦ **Chlorpromazine Hydrochloride** *see* Chlorpromazine *on page 116*

## Chlorpropamide (klor PROE pa mide)

**Related Information**

Hypoglycemic Drugs and Thiazolidinedione Information *on page 714*

**U.S. Brand Names** Diabinese®

**Canadian Brand Names** Apo®-Chlorpropamide; Novo-Propamide

**Pharmacologic Category** Antidiabetic Agent (Sulfonylurea)

**Use** Control blood sugar in adult onset, noninsulin-dependent diabetes (type 2)

**Unlabeled use:** Neurogenic diabetes insipidus

**Effects on Mental Status** Dizziness is common

**Effects on Psychiatric Treatment** Rare reports of agranulocytosis; use caution with clozapine and carbamazepine

**Pregnancy Risk Factor** C

**Contraindications** Cross-sensitivity may exist with other hypoglycemics or sulfonamides; do not use with type 1 diabetes or with severe renal, hepatic, thyroid, or other endocrine disease

**Warnings/Precautions** Patients should be properly instructed in the early detection and treatment of hypoglycemia; long half-life may complicate recovery from excess effects. Because of chlorpropamide's long half-life, duration of action, and the increased risk for hypoglycemia, it is not considered a hypoglycemic agent of choice in the elderly

Product labeling states oral hypoglycemic drugs may be associated with an increased cardiovascular mortality as compared to treatment with diet alone or diet plus insulin. Data to support this association are limited, and several studies, including a large prospective trial (UKPDS) have not supported an association.

**Adverse Reactions**

>10%:

Central nervous system: Headache, dizziness

Gastrointestinal: Anorexia, constipation, heartburn, epigastric fullness, nausea, vomiting, diarrhea

1% to 10%: Dermatologic: Skin rash, urticaria, photosensitivity

<1%: Agranulocytosis, aplastic anemia, blood dyscrasias, bone marrow suppression, cholestatic jaundice, edema, hemolytic anemia, hypoglycemia, hyponatremia, SIADH, thrombocytopenia

**Overdosage/Toxicology**

Signs and symptoms: Low blood glucose levels, tingling of lips and tongue, tachycardia, convulsions, stupor, coma

Treatment: Antidote is glucose; intoxications with sulfonylureas can cause hypoglycemia and are best managed with glucose administration (oral for milder hypoglycemia or by injection in more severe forms); prolonged effects lasting up to 1 week may occur with this agent

**Drug Interactions**

Decreased effect: Thiazides and hydantoins (eg, phenytoin) decrease chlorpropamide effectiveness may increase blood glucose

Increased toxicity:

Increases alcohol-associated disulfiram reactions

Increases oral anticoagulant effects

Salicylates may increase chlorpropamide effects may decrease blood glucose

Sulfonamides may decrease sulfonylureas clearance

**Usual Dosage** Oral: The dosage of chlorpropamide is variable and should be individualized based upon the patient's response

Initial dose:

Adults: 250 mg/day in mild to moderate diabetes in middle-aged, stable diabetic

Elderly: 100-125 mg/day in older patients

Subsequent dosages may be increased or decreased by 50-125 mg/day at 3- to 5-day intervals

Maintenance dose: 100-250 mg/day; severe diabetics may require 500 mg/day; avoid doses >750 mg/day

**Dosing adjustment/comments in renal impairment:** $Cl_{cr}$ <50 mL/minute: Avoid use

Hemodialysis: Removed with hemoperfusion

Peritoneal dialysis: Supplemental dose is not necessary

**Dosing adjustment in hepatic impairment:** Dosage reduction is recommended. Conservative initial and maintenance doses are recommended in patients with liver impairment because chlorpropamide undergoes extensive hepatic metabolism.

**Dietary Considerations**

Alcohol: A disulfiram-like reaction characterized by flushing, headache, nausea, vomiting, sweating or tachycardia; avoid use. Inform patient of chlorpropamide-alcohol flush (facial reddening and an increase in facial temperature).

Food: Chlorpropamide may cause GI upset; take with food. Take at the same time each day; eat regularly and do not skip meals.

Glucose: Decreases blood glucose concentration; hypoglycemia may occur. Educate patients how to detect and treat hypoglycemia. Monitor for signs and symptoms of hypoglycemia. Administer glucose if necessary. Evaluate patient's diet and exercise regimen. May need to decrease or discontinue dose of sulfonylurea.

Sodium: Reports of hyponatremia and SIADH. Those at increased risk include patients on medications or who have medical conditions that predispose them to hyponatremia. Monitor sodium serum concentration and fluid status. May need to restrict water intake.

**Patient Information** This medication is used to control diabetes; it is not a cure. Other components of treatment plan are important: follow prescribed diet, medication, and exercise regimen. Take exactly as directed, at the same time each day. Do not change dose or discontinue without consulting prescriber. Avoid alcohol while taking this medication; could cause severe reaction. Inform prescriber of all other prescription or OTC medications you are taking; do not introduce new medication without consulting prescriber. If you experience hypoglycemic reaction, contact prescriber immediately. Maintain regular dietary intake and exercise routine and always carry quick source of sugar with you. You may experience side effects during first weeks of therapy (headache, constipation or diarrhea, bloating or loss of appetite); consult prescriber if these persist. Report severe or persistent side effects, including fever, extended vomiting or flu-like symptoms, skin rash, easy bruising or bleeding, or change in color of urine or stool.

**Dosage Forms** Tablet: 100 mg, 250 mg

## Chlorprothixene (klor proe THIKS een)

**Related Information**

Antipsychotic Agents Comparison Chart *on page 706*

Antipsychotic Medication Guidelines *on page 751*

Clinical Issues in the Use of Antipsychotics *on page 630*

Patient Information - Antipsychotics (General) *on page 646*

**Generic Available** No

**Pharmacologic Category** Antipsychotic Agent, Thioxanthene Derivative

**Use** Management of psychotic disorders

**Pregnancy Risk Factor** C

**Adverse Reactions**

>10%:

Cardiovascular: Hypotension, orthostatic hypotension

Central nervous system: Pseudoparkinsonism, akathisia, dystonias, tardive dyskinesia (persistent), dizziness

Gastrointestinal: Constipation
Ocular: Pigmentary retinopathy
Respiratory: Nasal congestion
Miscellaneous: Decreased sweating
1% to 10%:
Dermatologic: Photosensitivity, skin rash
Endocrine & metabolic: Changes in menstrual cycle, changes in libido, pain in breasts
Gastrointestinal: Weight gain, nausea, vomiting, stomach pain
Genitourinary: Dysuria, ejaculatory disturbances
Neuromuscular & skeletal: Trembling of fingers
<1%:
Central nervous system: Neuroleptic malignant syndrome (NMS)
Dermatologic: discoloration of skin (blue-gray)
Endocrine & metabolic: Galactorrhea
Genitourinary: Priapism
Hematologic: Agranulocytosis, leukopenia
Hepatic: Cholestatic jaundice, hepatotoxicity
Ocular: Cornea and lens changes, pigmentary retinopathy
Miscellaneous: Impairment of temperature regulation lowering of seizures threshold

**Drug Interactions**
Aluminum salts: May decrease the absorption of antipsychotics; monitor
Amphetamines: Efficacy may be diminished by antipsychotics; in addition, amphetamines may increase psychotic symptoms; avoid concurrent use
Anticholinergics: May inhibit the therapeutic response to antipsychotics and excess anticholinergic effects may occur; includes benztropine, trihexyphenidyl, biperiden, and drugs with significant anticholinergic activity (TCAs, antihistamines, disopyramide)
Antihypertensives: Concurrent use of antipsychotics with an antihypertensive may produce additive hypotensive effects (particularly orthostasis)
Bromocriptine: Antipsychotics inhibit the ability of bromocriptine to lower serum prolactin concentrations
CNS depressants: Sedative effects may be additive with antipsychotics; monitor for increased effect; includes barbiturates, benzodiazepines, narcotic analgesics, ethanol, and other sedative agents
CYP inhibitors: Serum levels may be increased; monitor for increased effect
Enzyme inducers: May enhance the hepatic metabolism of antipsychotics; larger doses may be required; includes rifampin, rifabutin, barbiturates, phenytoin, and cigarette smoking
Epinephrine: Chlorpromazine (and possibly other low-potency antipsychotics) may diminish the pressor effects of epinephrine
Guanethidine and guanadrel: Antihypertensive effects may be inhibited by antipsychotics
Levodopa: Antipsychotics may inhibit the antiparkinsonian effect of levodopa; avoid this combination
Lithium: Antipsychotics may produce neurotoxicity with lithium; this is a rare effect
Phenytoin: May reduce serum levels of antipsychotics; antipsychotics may increase phenytoin serum levels
Propranolol: Serum concentrations of antipsychotics may be increased; propranolol also increases antipsychotics concentrations
QTc prolonging agents: Effects on QTc interval may be additive with antipsychotics, increasing the risk of malignant arrhythmias; includes type Ia antiarrhythmics, TCAs, and some quinolone antibiotics (sparfloxacin, moxifloxacin, and gatifloxacin)
Sulfadoxine-pyrimethamine: May increase antipsychotic concentrations
Tricyclic antidepressants: Concurrent use may produce increased toxicity or altered therapeutic response
Trazodone: Antipsychotics and trazodone may produce additive hypotensive effects
Valproic acid: Serum levels may be increased by antipsychotics

**Stability** Protect all dosage forms from light, clear or slightly yellow solutions may be used; should be dispensed in amber or opaque vials/bottles. Solutions may be diluted or mixed with fruit juices or other liquids but must be administered immediately after mixing; do not prepare bulk dilutions or store bulk dilutions.

**Mechanism of Action** The mechanism of action for chlorprothixene, like other thioxanthenes and phenothiazines, is not fully understood. The sites of action appear to be the reticular activating system of the midbrain, the limbic system, the hypothalamus, and the globus pallidus and corpus striatum. The mechanism appears to be one or more of a combination of postsynaptic blockade of adrenergic, dopaminergic, or serotonergic receptor sites, metabolic inhibition of oxidative phosphorylation, or decrease in the excitability of neuronal membranes.

**Usual Dosage**
Children >6 years: Oral: 10-25 mg 3-4 times/day
Adults:
Oral: 25-50 mg 3-4 times/day, to be increased as needed; doses exceeding 600 mg/day are rarely required
I.M.: 25-50 mg up to 3-4 times/day

**Administration** I.M. dose is 4-10 times the activity of oral dose

**Patient Information** May cause drowsiness; avoid alcohol

**Dosage Forms**
Concentrate, oral, as lactate and hydrochloride (fruit flavor): 100 mg/5 mL (480 mL)
Injection, as hydrochloride: 12.5 mg/mL (2 mL)
Tablet: 10 mg, 25 mg, 50 mg, 100 mg

♦ **Chlor-Rest® Tablet [OTC]** *see* Chlorpheniramine and Phenylpropanolamine *on page 114*

## Chlortetracycline (klor tet ra SYE kleen)

**U.S. Brand Names** Aureomycin®
**Pharmacologic Category** Antibiotic, Ophthalmic; Antibiotic, Tetracycline Derivative; Antibiotic, Topical
**Use**
Ophthalmic: Treatment of superficial ocular infections involving the conjunctiva or cornea due to strains of susceptible microorganisms
Topical: Treatment of superficial infections of the skin due to susceptible organisms, also infection prophylaxis in minor skin abrasions
**Effects on Mental Status** None reported
**Effects on Psychiatric Treatment** None reported
**Usual Dosage**
Ophthalmic:
Acute infections: Instill ½" (1.25 cm) every 3-4 hours until improvement
Mild to moderate infections: Instill ½" (1.25 cm) 2-3 times/day
Topical: Apply 1-4 times/day, cover with sterile bandage if needed
**Dosage Forms** Ointment, as hydrochloride:
Ophthalmic: 1% [10 mg/g] (3.5 g)
Topical: 3% (14.2 g, 30 g)

## Chlorthalidone (klor THAL i done)

**U.S. Brand Names** Hygroton®; Thalitone®
**Canadian Brand Names** Apo®-Chlorthalidone; Novo-Thalidone; Uridon®
**Pharmacologic Category** Diuretic, Thiazide
**Use** Management of mild to moderate hypertension when used alone or in combination with other agents; treatment of edema associated with congestive heart failure, nephrotic syndrome, or pregnancy. Recent studies have found chlorthalidone effective in the treatment of isolated systolic hypertension in the elderly.
**Effects on Mental Status** None reported
**Effects on Psychiatric Treatment** Rare reports of blood dyscrasias; use caution with clozapine and carbamazepine; thiazides decrease lithium clearance resulting in elevated serum lithium levels and potential toxicity; monitor serum lithium levels
**Pregnancy Risk Factor** B (per manufacturer); D (based on expert analysis)
**Contraindications** Hypersensitivity to chlorthalidone or any component; cross-sensitivity with other thiazides or sulfonamides; anuria; renal decompensation; pregnancy
**Warnings/Precautions** Use with caution in patients with hypokalemia, renal disease, hepatic disease, gout, lupus erythematosus, or diabetes mellitus. Use with caution in severe renal diseases. Correct hypokalemia before initiating therapy.
**Adverse Reactions**
1% to 10%: Endocrine & metabolic: Hypokalemia
<1%: Fluid and electrolyte imbalances (hypocalcemia, hypomagnesemia, hyponatremia), hyperglycemia, hypotension, photosensitivity, prerenal azotemia, rarely blood dyscrasias
**Overdosage/Toxicology**
Signs and symptoms: Hypermotility, diuresis, lethargy, confusion, muscle weakness, coma
Treatment: Following GI decontamination, therapy is supportive with I.V. fluids, electrolytes, and I.V. pressors if needed
**Drug Interactions**
Angiotensin-converting enzyme inhibitors: Increased hypotension if aggressively diuresed with a thiazide diuretic
Beta-blockers increase hyperglycemic effects in Type 2 diabetes mellitus
Cyclosporine and thiazides can increase the risk of gout or renal toxicity; avoid concurrent use
Digoxin toxicity can be exacerbated if a thiazide induces hypokalemia or hypomagnesemia
Lithium toxicity can occur by reducing renal excretion of lithium; monitor lithium concentration and adjust as needed
Neuromuscular blocking agents can prolong blockade; monitor serum potassium and neuromuscular status
NSAIDs can decrease the efficacy of thiazides reducing the diuretic and antihypertensive effects
**Usual Dosage** Oral:
Children (nonapproved): 2 mg/kg/dose 3 times/week or 1-2 mg/kg/day
Adults: 25-100 mg/day or 100 mg 3 times/week
Elderly: Initial: 12.5-25 mg/day or every other day; there is little advantage to using doses >25 mg/day
**Dosage adjustment in renal impairment:** $Cl_{cr}$ <10 mL/minute: Administer every 48 hours
(Continued)

## Chlorthalidone *(Continued)*

**Patient Information** Take prescribed dose with food early in the day. Include orange juice or bananas in your diet, but do not take potassium supplements without consulting prescriber. You may experience postural hypotension (use caution when rising from lying or sitting position, when climbing stairs, or when driving); photosensitivity (use sunblock, wear protective clothing and eyewear, and avoid direct sunlight); decreased accommodation to heat (avoid excessive exercise in hot weather). Report muscle weakness, tremors, or cramping; persistent nausea or vomiting; swelling of extremities; significant increase in weight; respiratory difficulty; rash; unusual weakness or fatigue; or easy bruising or bleeding.

**Nursing Implications** Take blood pressure with patient lying down and standing

**Dosage Forms**

Tablet: 25 mg, 50 mg, 100 mg
- Hygroton®: 25 mg, 50 mg, 100 mg
- Thalitone®: 15 mg, 25 mg

♦ **Chlor-Trimeton® [OTC]** *see* Chlorpheniramine *on page 113*

♦ **Chlor-Trimeton® 4 Hour Relief Tablet [OTC]** *see* Chlorpheniramine and Pseudoephedrine *on page 114*

## Chlorzoxazone (klor ZOKS a zone)

**U.S. Brand Names** Flexaphen®; Paraflex®; Parafon Forte™ DSC

**Pharmacologic Category** Skeletal Muscle Relaxant

**Use** Symptomatic treatment of muscle spasm and pain associated with acute musculoskeletal conditions

**Effects on Mental Status** Drowsiness is common; may produce depression or paradoxical stimulation

**Effects on Psychiatric Treatment** May produce aplastic anemia and leukopenia; use caution with clozapine and carbamazepine

**Pregnancy Risk Factor** C

**Contraindications** Known hypersensitivity to chlorzoxazone; impaired liver function

**Warnings/Precautions** Use with caution in patients with liver dysfunction

**Adverse Reactions**

>10%: Central nervous system: Drowsiness

1% to 10%:
- Cardiovascular: Tachycardia, tightness in chest, flushing of face, syncope
- Central nervous system: Mental depression, allergic fever, dizziness, lightheadedness, headache, paradoxical stimulation
- Dermatologic: Angioedema
- Gastrointestinal: Nausea, vomiting, stomach cramps
- Neuromuscular & skeletal: Trembling
- Ocular: Burning of eyes
- Respiratory: Shortness of breath
- Miscellaneous: Hiccups

<1%: Aplastic anemia, ataxia, blurred vision, eosinophilia, erythema multiforme, leukopenia, rash, urticaria

**Overdosage/Toxicology**

Signs and symptoms: Nausea, vomiting, diarrhea, drowsiness, dizziness, headache, absent tendon reflexes, hypotension

Treatment: Supportive following attempts to enhance drug elimination. Hypotension should be treated with I.V. fluids and/or Trendelenburg positioning. Dialysis and hemoperfusion and osmotic diuresis have all been useful in reducing serum drug concentrations; patient should be observed for possible relapses due to incomplete gastric emptying.

**Drug Interactions** CYP2E1 enzyme substrate

Increased effect/toxicity: Alcohol, CNS depressants

**Usual Dosage** Oral:

Children: 20 mg/kg/day or 600 mg/m$^2$/day in 3-4 divided doses

Adults: 250-500 mg 3-4 times/day up to 750 mg 3-4 times/day

**Dietary Considerations** Alcohol: Additive CNS effects, avoid use

**Patient Information** Take exactly as directed, with food. Do not increase dose or discontinue without consulting prescriber. Do not use alcohol, prescriptive or OTC antidepressants, sedatives, or pain medications without consulting prescriber. May turn urine orange or red (normal). You may experience drowsiness, dizziness, lightheadedness (avoid driving or engaging in tasks that require alertness until response to drug is known); nausea, vomiting, or cramping (small, frequent meals, frequent mouth care, or sucking hard candy may help); postural hypotension (change position slowly when rising from sitting or lying or when climbing stairs); or constipation (increased dietary fluids and fibers or increased exercise may help). Report excessive drowsiness or mental agitation; palpitations, rapid heartbeat, or chest pain; skin rash or swelling of mouth or face; persistent diarrhea or constipation; or unusual weakness or bleeding.

**Nursing Implications** Raise bed rails; institute safety measures; assist with ambulation

**Dosage Forms**

Caplet (Parafon Forte™ DSC): 500 mg

Capsule (Flexaphen®, Mus-Lax®): 250 mg with acetaminophen 300 mg

Tablet: Paraflex®: 250 mg

♦ **Cholac®** *see* Lactulose *on page 306*

♦ **Cholan-HMB®** *see* Dehydrocholic Acid *on page 153*

## Cholecalciferol (kole e kal SI fer ole)

**U.S. Brand Names** Delta-D®

**Synonyms** $D_3$

**Pharmacologic Category** Vitamin D Analog

**Use** Dietary supplement, treatment of vitamin D deficiency or prophylaxis of deficiency

**Effects on Mental Status** May cause irritability; rare reports of psychosis

**Effects on Psychiatric Treatment** None reported

**Contraindications** Hypercalcemia; hypersensitivity to cholecalciferol or any component; malabsorption syndrome; evidence of vitamin D toxicity

**Warnings/Precautions** Administer with extreme caution in patients with impaired renal function, heart disease, renal stones, or arteriosclerosis

**Adverse Reactions** 1% to 10%:
- Cardiovascular: Hypotension, cardiac arrhythmias, hypertension, arrhythmia
- Central nervous system: Irritability, headache
- Dermatologic: Pruritus
- Endocrine & metabolic: Polydipsia
- Gastrointestinal: Nausea, vomiting, anorexia, pancreatitis, metallic taste
- Neuromuscular & skeletal: Bone pain, myalgia
- Ocular: Conjunctivitis, photophobia
- Renal: Polyuria

**Overdosage/Toxicology** Treatment: Following withdrawal of the drug, treatment consists of bed rest, liberal intake of fluids, reduced calcium intake, and cathartic administration. Severe hypercalcemia requires I.V. hydration and forced diuresis with I.V. furosemide (20-40 mg I.V. every 4-6 hours for adults). Urine output should be monitored and maintained at >3 mL/kg/hour. I.V. saline can quickly and significantly increase excretion of calcium into the urine. Calcitonin, cholestyramine, prednisone, sodium EDTA, and mithramycin have all been used successfully to treat the more resistant cases of vitamin D-induced hypercalcemia.

**Drug Interactions** Thiazide diuretics, cholestyramine, colestipol, corticosteroids, mineral oil, phenytoin, barbiturates, digitalis glycosides, antacids (magnesium)

**Usual Dosage** Adults: Oral: 400-1000 units/day

**Patient Information** Do not take more than the recommended amount. While taking this medication, your physician may want you to follow a special diet or take a calcium supplement. Follow this diet closely. Avoid taking magnesium supplements or magnesium containing antacids. Early symptoms of hypercalcemia include weakness, fatigue, somnolence, headache, anorexia, dry mouth, metallic taste, nausea, vomiting, cramps, diarrhea, muscle pain, bone pain, and irritability.

**Dosage Forms** Tablet: 400 units, 1000 units

♦ **Choledyl®** *see* Theophylline Salts *on page 539*

## Cholera Vaccine (KOL er a vak SEEN)

**Pharmacologic Category** Vaccine

**Use** The World Health Organization no longer recommends cholera vaccination for travel to or from cholera-endemic areas. Some countries may still require evidence of a complete primary series or a booster dose given within 6 months of arrival. Vaccination should not be considered as an alternative to continued careful selection of foods and water. Ideally, cholera and yellow fever vaccines should be administered at least 3 weeks apart.

**Effects on Mental Status** May cause malaise

**Effects on Psychiatric Treatment** None reported

**Usual Dosage**

Children:
- 6 months to 4 years: Two 0.2 mL doses I.M./S.C. 1 week to 1 month apart; booster doses (0.2 mL I.M./S.C.) every 6 months
- 5-10 years: Two 0.3 mL doses I.M./S.C. or two 0.2 mL intradermal doses 1 week to 1 month apart; booster doses (0.3 mL I.M./S.C. or 0.2 mL I.D.) every 6 months

Children ≥10 years and Adults: Two 0.5 mL doses given I.M./S.C. or two 0.2 mL doses I.D. 1 week to 1 month apart; booster doses (0.5 mL I.M. or S.C. or 0.2 mL I.D.) every 6 months

**Dosage Forms** Injection: Suspension of killed *Vibrio cholerae* (Inaba and Ogawa types) 8 units of each serotype per mL (1.5 mL, 20 mL)

## Cholestyramine Resin (koe LES tir a meen REZ in)

**Related Information**

Lipid-Lowering Agents Comparison Chart *on page 717*

**U.S. Brand Names** LoCHOLEST®; LoCHOLEST® Light; Prevalite®; Questran®; Questran® Light

**Canadian Brand Names** PMS-Cholestyramine

**Pharmacologic Category** Antilipemic Agent (Bile Acid Seqestrant)

**Use** Adjunct in the management of primary hypercholesterolemia; pruritus associated with elevated levels of bile acids; diarrhea associated with excess fecal bile acids; binding toxicologic agents; pseudomembraneous colitis

**Effects on Mental Status** None reported

**Effects on Psychiatric Treatment** May decrease the absorption of psychotropics including TCAs, beta-blockers, valproic acid, barbiturates

**Pregnancy Risk Factor** C

**Contraindications** Hypersensitivity of bile acid sequestering resins or any component of the products; complete biliary obstruction; bowel obstruction

**Warnings/Precautions** Not to be taken simultaneously with many other medicines (decreased absorption). Treat any diseases contributing to hypercholesterolemia first. May interfere with fat-soluble vitamins (A, D, E, K) and folic acid. Chronic use may be associated with bleeding problems (especially in high doses). May produce or exacerbate constipation problems. Fecal impaction may occur. Hemorrhoids may be worsened.

**Adverse Reactions**

1% to 10%: Gastrointestinal: Constipation

<1%: Abdominal distention and pain, hyperchloremic acidosis, hypoprothrombinemia (secondary to vitamin K deficiency), increased urinary calcium excretion, intestinal obstruction, irritation of perianal area or skin, malabsorption of fat-soluble vitamins, nausea, rash, steatorrhea, tongue irritation, vomiting

**Overdosage/Toxicology**

Signs and symptoms: GI obstruction

Treatment: Supportive

**Drug Interactions**

Cholestyramine can reduce the absorption of numerous medications when used concurrently. Give other medications 1 hour before or 4 hours after giving cholestyramine. Medications which may be affected include HMG-CoA reductase inhibitors, thiazide diuretics, propranolol (and potentially other beta-blockers), corticosteroids, thyroid hormones, digoxin, valproic acid, NSAIDs, loop diuretics, sulfonylureas, troglitazone (and potentially other agents in this class).

Warfarin and other oral anticoagulants: Hypoprothrombinemic effects may be reduced by cholestyramine. Separate administration times (as detailed above) and monitor INR closely when initiating or discontinuing.

**Usual Dosage** Oral (dosages are expressed in terms of anhydrous resin):

Powder:

Children: 240 mg/kg/day in 3 divided doses; need to titrate dose depending on indication

Adults: 4 g 1-2 times/day to a maximum of 24 g/day and 6 doses/day

Tablet: Adults: Initial: 4 g once or twice daily; maintenance: 8-16 g/day in 2 divided doses

Dialysis: Not removed by hemo- or peritoneal dialysis; supplemental doses not necessary with dialysis or continuous arteriovenous or venovenous hemofiltration effects

**Patient Information** Take once or twice a day as directed. Do not take the powder in its dry form; mix with fluid, applesauce, pudding, or jello. Chew bars thoroughly. Take other medications 2 hours before or 4 hours after cholestyramine. Ongoing medical follow-up and laboratory tests may be required. You may experience GI effects (these should resolve after continued use); nausea and vomiting (small frequent meals, frequent mouth care, sucking lozenges, or chewing gum may help); constipation (increased exercise, dietary fluid, fiber, or fruit may help - consult prescriber about use of stool softener or laxative). Report unusual stomach cramping, pain or blood in stool; unresolved nausea, vomiting, or constipation.

**Nursing Implications** Administer warfarin and other drugs at least 1-2 hours prior to, or 6 hours after cholestyramine because cholestyramine may bind to them, decreasing their total absorption. (**Note:** Cholestyramine itself may cause hypoprothrombinemia in patients with impaired enterohepatic circulation.)

**Dosage Forms**

Powder: 4 g of resin/9 g of powder (9 g, 378 g)

Powder, for oral suspension, with aspartame: 4 g of resin/5 g of powder (5 g, 210 g)

Powder, for oral suspension, with phenylalanine: 4 g of resin/5.5 g of powder (60s)

## Choline Magnesium Trisalicylate

(KOE leen mag NEE zhum trye sa LIS i late)

**U.S. Brand Names** Trilisate®

**Pharmacologic Category** Salicylate

**Use** Management of osteoarthritis, rheumatoid arthritis, and other arthritis; salicylate salts may not inhibit platelet aggregation and, therefore, should not be substituted for aspirin in the prophylaxis of thrombosis

**Effects on Mental Status** May cause sedation; may rarely cause nervousness or insomnia

**Effects on Psychiatric Treatment** May rarely cause leukopenia; use caution with clozapine and carbamazepine

**Pregnancy Risk Factor** C (D if used in third trimester)

**Contraindications** Bleeding disorders; hypersensitivity to salicylates or other nonacetylated salicylates or other NSAIDs; tartrazine dye hypersensitivity, asthma

**Warnings/Precautions** Use with caution in patients with impaired renal function, dehydration, erosive gastritis, or peptic ulcer; avoid use in patients with suspected varicella or influenza (salicylates have been associated with Reye's syndrome in children <16 years of age when used to treat symptoms of chickenpox or the flu). Tinnitus or impaired hearing may indicate toxicity; discontinue use 1 week prior to surgical procedures.

Elderly are a high-risk population for adverse effects from nonsteroidal anti-inflammatory agents. As much as 60% of elderly can develop peptic ulceration and/or hemorrhage asymptomatically. Use lowest effective dose for shortest period possible. Tinnitus may be a difficult and unreliable indication of toxicity due to age-related hearing loss or eighth cranial nerve damage. CNS adverse effects may be observed in the elderly at lower doses than younger adults.

**Adverse Reactions**

>10%: Gastrointestinal: Nausea, heartburn, stomach pains, dyspepsia, epigastric discomfort

1% to 10%:

Central nervous system: Fatigue

Dermatologic: Rash

Gastrointestinal: Gastrointestinal ulceration

Hematologic: Hemolytic anemia

Neuromuscular & skeletal: Weakness

Respiratory: Dyspnea

Miscellaneous: Anaphylactic shock

<1%: Bronchospasm, hepatotoxicity, impaired renal function, increased uric acid, insomnia, iron deficiency anemia, jitters, leukopenia, nervousness, occult bleeding, prolongation of bleeding time, thrombocytopenia

**Overdosage/Toxicology**

Signs and symptoms: Tinnitus, vomiting, acute renal failure, hyperthermia, irritability, seizures, coma, metabolic acidosis

Treatment: For acute ingestions, determine serum salicylate levels 6 hours after ingestion; the "Done" nomogram may be helpful for estimating the severity of aspirin poisoning and directing treatment using serum salicylate levels. Treatment can also be based upon symptomatology.

**Salicylates**

| Toxic Symptoms | Treatment |
|---|---|
| Overdose | Induce emesis with ipecac, and/or lavage with saline, followed with activated charcoal |
| Dehydration | I.V. fluids with KCl (no $D_5W$ only) |
| Metabolic acidosis (must be treated) | Sodium bicarbonate |
| Hyperthermia | Cooling blankets or sponge baths |
| Coagulopathy/hemorrhage | Vitamin K I.V. |
| Hypoglycemia (with coma, seizures, or change in mental status) | Dextrose 25 g I.V. |
| Seizures | Diazepam 5-10 mg I.V. |

**Drug Interactions**

Decreased effect: Antacids + Trilisate® → decreased salicylate concentration; ACE inhibitor effects may be decreased by concurrent therapy with NSAIDs

Increased toxicity: Warfarin + Trilisate® → possible increased hypoprothrombinemic effect

**Usual Dosage** Oral (based on total salicylate content):

Children <37 kg: 50 mg/kg/day given in 2 divided doses

Adults: 500 mg to 1.5 g 2-3 times/day; usual maintenance dose: 1-4.5 g/day

**Dosing adjustment/comments in renal impairment:** Avoid use in severe renal impairment

**Dietary Considerations**

Alcohol: Combination causes GI irritation, possible bleeding; avoid or limit alcohol. Patients at increased risk include those prone to hypoprothrombinemia, vitamin K deficiency, thrombocytopenia, thrombotic thrombocytopenia purpura, severe hepatic impairment, and those receiving anticoagulants.

Food: May decrease the rate but not the extent of oral absorption. Drug may cause GI upset, bleeding, ulceration, perforation. Take with food or or large volume of water or milk to minimize GI upset.

Folic acid: Hyperexcretion of folate; folic acid deficiency may result, leading to macrocytic anemia. Supplement with folic acid if necessary.

Iron: With chronic use and at doses of 3-4 g/day, iron deficiency anemia may result; supplement with iron if necessary

Magnesium: Hypermagnesemia resulting from magnesium salicylate; avoid or use with caution in renal insufficiency

Sodium: Hypernatremia resulting from buffered aspirin solutions or sodium salicylate containing high sodium content. Avoid or use with caution in CHF or any condition where hypernatremia would be detrimental.

Curry powder, paprika, licorice, Benedictine liqueur, prunes, raisins, tea and gherkins: Potential salicylate accumulation. These foods contain 6 mg salicylate/100 g. An ordinary American diet contains 10-200 mg/day of salicylate. Foods containing salicylates may contribute to aspirin

(Continued)

## Choline Magnesium Trisalicylate *(Continued)*

hypersensitivity. Patients at greatest risk for aspirin hypersensitivity include those with asthma, nasal polyposis, or chronic urticaria.

**Patient Information** If self-administered, use exactly as directed (do not increase dose or frequency); adverse reactions can occur with overuse. Take with food or milk. While using this medication, do not use alcohol, excessive amounts of vitamin C, or salicylate-containing foods (curry powder, prunes, raisins, tea, or licorice), other prescription or OTC medications containing aspirin or salicylate, or other NSAIDs without consulting prescriber. Maintain adequate hydration (2-3 L/day of fluids unless instructed to restrict fluid intake). You may experience nausea, vomiting, gastric discomfort (frequent mouth care, small frequent meals, sucking lozenges, or chewing gum may help). GI bleeding, ulceration, or perforation can occur with or without pain. Stop taking medication and report ringing in ears; persistent pain in stomach; unresolved nausea or vomiting; difficulty breathing or shortness of breath; unusual bruising or bleeding (mouth, urine, stool); or skin rash.

**Nursing Implications** Liquid may be mixed with fruit juice just before drinking; do not administer with antacids

**Dosage Forms** See table.

**Choline Magnesium Trisalicylate**

| Brand Name | Dosage Form | Total Salicylate | Choline Salicylate | Magnesium Salicylate |
|---|---|---|---|---|
| Trilisate® | Liquid | 500 mg/5 mL | 293 mg/5 mL | 362 mg/5 mL |
| Trilisate 500® | Tablet | 500 mg | 293 mg | 362 mg |
| Trilisate 750® | Tablet | 750 mg | 440 mg | 544 mg |
| Trilisate 1000® | Tablet | 1000 mg | 587 mg | 725 mg |

♦ **Choline Theophyllinate** *see* Theophylline Salts *on page 539*

♦ **Choloxin®** *see* Dextrothyroxine *on page 161*

## Chondroitin Sulfate-Sodium Hyaluronate

(kon DROY tin SUL fate-SOW de um hye al yoor ON ate)

**U.S. Brand Names** Viscoat®

**Pharmacologic Category** Ophthalmic Agent, Viscoelastic

**Use** Surgical aid in anterior segment procedures, protects corneal endothelium and coats intraocular lens thus protecting it

**Effects on Mental Status** None reported

**Effects on Psychiatric Treatment** None reported

**Usual Dosage** Carefully introduce (using a 27-gauge needle or cannula) into anterior chamber after thoroughly cleaning the chamber with a balanced salt solution

**Dosage Forms** Solution: Sodium chondroitin 40 mg and sodium hyaluronate 30 mg (0.25 mL, 0.5 mL)

♦ **Chooz® [OTC]** *see* Calcium Carbonate *on page 84*

♦ **Chorex®** *see* Chorionic Gonadotropin *on page 122*

## Chorionic Gonadotropin (kor ee ON ik goe NAD oh troe pin)

**U.S. Brand Names** A.P.L.®; Chorex®; Choron®; Gonic®; Pregnyl®; Profasi® HP

**Synonyms** CG; hCG

**Pharmacologic Category** Ovulation Stimulator

**Use** Induces ovulation and pregnancy in anovulatory, infertile females; treatment of hypogonadotropic hypogonadism, prepubertal cryptorchidism

**Effects on Mental Status** May cause drowsiness or depression; rarely may cause restlessness or irritability

**Effects on Psychiatric Treatment** None reported

**Pregnancy Risk Factor** C

**Contraindications** Hypersensitivity to chorionic gonadotropin or any component; precocious puberty, prostatic carcinoma or similar neoplasms

**Warnings/Precautions** Use with caution in asthma, seizure disorders, migraine, cardiac or renal disease; **not** effective in the treatment of obesity

**Adverse Reactions**

1% to 10%:

Central nervous system: Mental depression, fatigue

Endocrine & metabolic: Pelvic pain, ovarian cysts, enlargement of breasts, precocious puberty

Local: Pain at the injection site

Neuromuscular & skeletal: Premature closure of epiphyses

<1%: Gynecomastia, headache, irritability, ovarian hyperstimulation syndrome, peripheral edema, restlessness

**Drug Interactions** No data reported

**Usual Dosage** I.M.:

Children:

Prepubertal cryptorchidism: 1000-2000 units/m$^2$/dose 3 times/week for 3 weeks **OR** 4000 units 3 times/week for 3 weeks **OR** 5000 units every second day for 4 injections **OR** 500 units 3 times/week for 4-6 weeks

Hypogonadotropic hypogonadism: 500-1000 units 3 times/week for 3 weeks, followed by the same dose twice weekly for 3 weeks **OR** 1000-2000 units 3 times/week **OR** 4000 units 3 times/week for 6-9 months; reduce dosage to 2000 units 3 times/week for additional 3 months

Adults: Induction of ovulation: 5000-10,000 units one day following last dose of menotropins

**Patient Information** Discontinue immediately if possibility of pregnancy

**Dosage Forms** Powder for injection (human origin): 200 units/mL (10 mL, 25 mL); 500 units/mL (10 mL); 1000 units/mL (10 mL); 2000 units/mL (10 mL)

♦ **Choron®** *see* Chorionic Gonadotropin *on page 122*

## Chromium

**Pharmacologic Category** Nutritional Supplement

**Use** Improves glycemic control; increases lean body mass; reduces obesity; improves lipid profile by decreasing total cholesterol and triglycerides, increasing HDL

**Adverse Reactions** Gastrointestinal: Nausea, loose stools, flatulence, changes in appetite

Isolated reports of anemia, cognitive impairment, renal failure

**Drug Interactions** Any medications that may also affect blood sugars; (eg, beta-blockers, thiazides, any medications prescribed to treat diabetes); discuss chromium use prior to initiating

**Usual Dosage** 50-600 mcg/day

♦ **Chronulac®** *see* Lactulose *on page 306*

♦ **Chymodiactin®** *see* Chymopapain *on page 122*

## Chymopapain (KYE moe pa pane)

**U.S. Brand Names** Chymodiactin®

**Pharmacologic Category** Enzyme

**Use** Alternative to surgery in patients with herniated lumbar intervertebral discs

**Effects on Mental Status** May cause dizziness

**Effects on Psychiatric Treatment** None reported

**Usual Dosage** Adults: 2000-4000 units/disc with a maximum cumulative dose not to exceed 8000 units for patients with multiple disc herniations

**Dosage Forms** Injection: 4000 units [4 nKat]; 10,000 units [10 nKat]

♦ **Cibacalcin® Injection** *see* Calcitonin *on page 83*

## Ciclopirox (sye kloe PEER oks)

**U.S. Brand Names** Loprox®

**Pharmacologic Category** Antifungal Agent, Topical

**Use** Treatment of tinea pedis (athlete's foot), tinea cruris (jock itch), tinea corporis (ringworm), cutaneous candidiasis, and tinea versicolor (pityriasis)

**Effects on Mental Status** None reported

**Effects on Psychiatric Treatment** None reported

**Usual Dosage** Children >10 years and Adults: Apply twice daily, gently massage into affected areas; if no improvement after 4 weeks of treatment, re-evaluate the diagnosis

**Dosage Forms**

Cream, topical, as olamine: 1% (15 g, 30 g, 90 g)

Lotion, as olamine: 1% (30 mL, 60 mL)

## Cidofovir (si DOF o veer)

**U.S. Brand Names** Vistide®

**Pharmacologic Category** Antiviral Agent

**Use** Treatment of cytomegalovirus (CMV) retinitis in patients with acquired immunodeficiency syndrome (AIDS). **Note:** Should be administered with probenecid.

**Effects on Mental Status** Anxiety, confusion, amnesia, and insomnia are common; may cause depression or hallucinations

**Effects on Psychiatric Treatment** Anemia and neutropenia are common; use caution with clozapine and carbamazepine

**Usual Dosage**

Induction: 5 mg/kg I.V. over 1 hour once weekly for 2 consecutive weeks

Maintenance: 5 mg/kg over 1 hour once every other week

**Administer with probenecid - 2 g orally 3 hours prior to each cidofovir dose and 1 g at 2 and 8 hours after completion of the infusion (total: 4 g)**

Hydrate with 1 L of 0.9% NS I.V. prior to cidofovir infusion; a second liter may be administered over a 1- to 3-hour period immediately following infusion, if tolerated

**Dosing adjustment in renal impairment:**

$Cl_{cr}$ 41-55 mL/minute: 2 mg/kg

$Cl_{cr}$ 30-40 mL/minute: 1.5 mg/kg

$Cl_{cr}$ 20-29 mL/minute: 1 mg/kg

$Cl_{cr}$ <19 mL/minute: 0.5 mg/kg

If the creatinine increases by 0.3-0.4 mg/dL, reduce the cidofovir dose to 3 mg/kg; discontinue therapy for increases ≥0.5 mg/dL or development of ≥3+ proteinuria

**Dosage Forms** Injection: 75 mg/mL (5 mL)

## Cilostazol (sil OH sta zol)

**U.S. Brand Names** Pletal®

**Pharmacologic Category** Phosphodiesterase Enzyme Inhibitor; Platelet Aggregation Inhibitor

**Use** Symptomatic management of peripheral vascular disease, primarily intermittent claudication; currently being investigated for the treatment of acute coronary syndromes

**Effects on Mental Status** Headache and dizziness are common; may rarely cause anxiety or insomnia

**Effects on Psychiatric Treatment** CYP3A4 inhibitors (fluvoxamine, fluoxetine, nefazodone, sertraline) may increase the concentrations of cilostazol

**Usual Dosage** Adults: Oral: 100 mg twice daily taken at least one-half hour before or 2 hours after breakfast and dinner; dosage should be reduced to 50 mg twice daily during concurrent therapy with inhibitors of CYP3A4 or CYP2C19

**Dosage Forms** Tablet: 50 mg, 100 mg

♦ **Ciloxan™ Ophthalmic** *see* Ciprofloxacin *on page 123*

## Cimetidine (sye MET i deen)

**U.S. Brand Names** Tagamet®; Tagamet® HB [OTC]

**Canadian Brand Names** Apo®-Cimetidine; Novo-Cimetine; Nu-Cimet; Peptol®

**Pharmacologic Category** Histamine $H_2$ Antagonist

**Use** Short-term treatment of active duodenal ulcers and benign gastric ulcers; long-term prophylaxis of duodenal ulcer; gastric hypersecretory states; gastroesophageal reflux; prevention of upper GI bleeding in critically ill patients.

**Effects on Mental Status** May cause agitation or drowsiness; rare reports of confusion

**Effects on Psychiatric Treatment** Rare reports of agranulocytosis; use caution with clozapine and carbamazepine; may inhibit the metabolism of TCAs and benzodiazepines; monitor for adverse effects

**Pregnancy Risk Factor** B

**Contraindications** Hypersensitivity to cimetidine, other component, or other $H_2$-antagonists

**Warnings/Precautions** Adjust dosages in renal/hepatic impairment or patients receiving drugs metabolized through the P-450 system

**Adverse Reactions**

1% to 10%:

Central nervous system: Dizziness, agitation, headache, drowsiness

Gastrointestinal: Diarrhea, nausea, vomiting

<1%: Agranulocytosis, bradycardia, confusion, decreased sexual ability, edema of the breasts, elevated creatinine fever, gynecomastia, hypotension, increased AST/ALT, myalgia, neutropenia, rash, tachycardia, thrombocytopenia

**Overdosage/Toxicology**

Signs and symptoms: Animal data have shown respiratory failure, tachycardia, muscle tremors, vomiting, restlessness, hypotension, salivation, emesis, and diarrhea.

Treatment: Primarily symptomatic and supportive. No experience with intentional overdose; reported ingestions of 20 g have had transient side effects seen with recommended doses

**Drug Interactions** CYP3A3/4 enzyme substrate; CYP1A2, 2C9, 2C18, 2C19, 2D6, and 3A3/4 enzyme inhibitor

Increased toxicity: Decreased elimination of lidocaine, theophylline, phenytoin, metronidazole, triamterene, procainamide, quinidine, and propranolol

Inhibition of warfarin metabolism, tricyclic antidepressant metabolism, diazepam elimination and cyclosporine elimination

**Usual Dosage**

Children: Oral, I.M., I.V.: 20-40 mg/kg/day in divided doses every 6 hours

Adults: Short-term treatment of active ulcers:

Oral: 300 mg 4 times/day or 800 mg at bedtime or 400 mg twice daily for up to 8 weeks

I.M., I.V.: 300 mg every 6 hours or 37.5 mg/hour by continuous infusion; I.V. dosage should be adjusted to maintain an intragastric pH ≥5

Patients with an active bleed: Administer cimetidine as a continuous infusion (see above)

Duodenal ulcer prophylaxis: Oral: 400-800 mg at bedtime

Gastric hypersecretory conditions: Oral, I.M., I.V.: 300-600 mg every 6 hours; dosage not to exceed 2.4 g/day

**Dosing adjustment/interval in renal impairment**: Children and Adults:

$Cl_{cr}$ 20-40 mL/minute: Administer every 8 hours or 75% of normal dose

$Cl_{cr}$ 0-20 mL/minute: Administer every 12 hours or 50% of normal dose

Hemodialysis: Slightly dialyzable (5% to 20%)

**Dosing adjustment/comments in hepatic impairment:** Usual dose is safe in mild liver disease but use with caution and in reduced dosage in severe liver disease; increased risk of CNS toxicity in cirrhosis suggested by enhanced penetration of CNS

**Dietary Considerations** Alcohol: Additive CNS effects, avoid or limit use

**Patient Information** Take with meals. Limit xanthine-containing foods and beverages which may decrease iron absorption. To be effective, continue to take for the prescribed time (possibly 4-8 weeks) even though symptoms may have improved. Smoking decreases the effectiveness of cimetidine; stop smoking if possible. Avoid use of caffeine or aspirin products. Report diarrhea, black tarry stools, coffee ground like emesis, dizziness, confusion, rash, unusual bleeding or bruising, sore throat, and fever.

**Dosage Forms**

Infusion, as hydrochloride, in NS: 300 mg (50 mL)

Injection, as hydrochloride: 150 mg/mL (2 mL, 8 mL)

Liquid, oral, as hydrochloride (mint-peach flavor): 300 mg/5 mL with alcohol 2.8% (5 mL, 240 mL)

Tablet: 200 mg, 300 mg, 400 mg, 800 mg

♦ **Cinobac® Pulvules®** *see* Cinoxacin *on page 123*

## Cinoxacin (sin OKS a sin)

**U.S. Brand Names** Cinobac® Pulvules®

**Pharmacologic Category** Antibiotic, Quinolone

**Use** Treatment of urinary tract infections

**Effects on Mental Status** May cause dizziness, insomnia or confusion; quinolones reported to cause restlessness, hallucinations, euphoria, depression, panic, and paranoia

**Effects on Psychiatric Treatment** None reported

**Pregnancy Risk Factor** B

**Contraindications** History of convulsive disorders, hypersensitivity to cinoxacin or any component or other quinolones

**Warnings/Precautions** CNS stimulation may occur (tremor, restlessness, confusion, and very rarely hallucinations or seizures). Use with caution in patients with known or suspected CNS disorders or renal impairment. Not recommended in children <18 years of age, ciprofloxacin (a related compound), has caused a transient arthropathy in children; prolonged use may result in superinfection; modify dosage in patients with renal impairment.

**Adverse Reactions** Generally well tolerated

1% to 10%:

Central nervous system: Headache, dizziness

Gastrointestinal: Heartburn, abdominal pain, GI bleeding, belching, flatulence, anorexia, nausea

<1%: Confusion, diarrhea, insomnia, photophobia, seizures (rare), thrombocytopenia, tinnitus

**Overdosage/Toxicology**

Signs and symptoms: Acute renal failure, seizures

Treatment: GI decontamination and supportive care; not removed by peritoneal or hemodialysis

**Drug Interactions**

Decreased effect: Decreased urine levels with probenecid; decreased absorption with aluminum-, magnesium-, calcium-containing antacids

Increased serum levels: Probenecid

**Usual Dosage** Children >12 years and Adults: Oral: 1 g/day in 2-4 doses for 7-14 days

**Dosing interval in renal impairment:**

$Cl_{cr}$ 20-50 mL/minute: 250 mg twice daily

$Cl_{cr}$ <20 mL/minute: 250 mg/day

**Patient Information** Take prescribed dose with food. Maintain adequate hydration (2-3 L/day of fluids unless instructed to restrict fluid intake). Avoid antacid use. May cause dizziness; avoid driving or engaging in tasks that require alertness until response to drug is known. Small frequent meals, frequent mouth care, sucking lozenges, or chewing gum may reduce nausea or vomiting. Report skin rash, itching, redness, or swelling; pain, inflammation, or rupture of tendon; pain or burning on urination; or persistent diarrhea or vomiting.

**Nursing Implications** Hold antacids for 3-4 hours after giving

**Dosage Forms** Capsule: 250 mg, 500 mg

## Ciprofloxacin (sip roe FLOKS a sin)

**U.S. Brand Names** Ciloxan™ Ophthalmic; Cipro® Injection; Cipro® Oral

**Pharmacologic Category** Antibiotic, Ophthalmic; Antibiotic, Quinolone

**Use** Treatment of documented or suspected infections of the lower respiratory tract, sinuses, skin and skin structure, bone/joints, and urinary tract including prostatitis, due to susceptible bacterial strains; especially indicated for *Pseudomonal* infections and those due to multidrug resistant gram-negative organisms, chronic bacterial prostatitis, infectious diarrhea, complicated gram-negative and anaerobic intra-abdominal infections (with metronidazole) due to *E. coli* (enteropathic strains), *B. fragilis, P. mirabilis, K. pneumoniae, P. aeruginosa, Campylobacter jejuni* or *Shigella*; approved for acute sinusitis caused by *H. influenzae* or *M. catarrhalis*; also used to treat typhoid fever due to *Salmonella typhi* (although eradication of the

(Continued)

## Ciprofloxacin *(Continued)*

chronic typhoid carrier state has not been proven), osteomyelitis when parenteral therapy is not feasible, and sexually transmitted diseases such as uncomplicated cervical and urethral gonorrhea due to *Neisseria gonorrhoeae*; used ophthalmologically for superficial ocular infections (corneal ulcers, conjunctivitis) due to susceptible strains

**Effects on Mental Status** May cause dizziness, insomnia, or confusion; quinolones reported to cause restlessness, hallucinations, euphoria, depression, panic, and paranoia

**Effects on Psychiatric Treatment** Inhibits CYP1A2 isoenzyme; use caution with clozapine and other psychotropics; monitor for adverse effects

**Pregnancy Risk Factor** C

**Contraindications** Hypersensitivity to ciprofloxacin, any component or other quinolones

**Warnings/Precautions** Not recommended in children <18 years of age; has caused transient arthropathy in children; CNS stimulation may occur (tremor, restlessness, confusion, and very rarely hallucinations or seizures); use with caution in patients with known or suspected CNS disorder; green discoloration of teeth in newborns has been reported; prolonged use may result in superinfection; may rarely cause inflamed or ruptured tendons (discontinue use immediately with signs of inflammation or tendon pain)

**Adverse Reactions**

1% to 10%:
- Central nervous system: Headache, restlessness
- Gastrointestinal: Nausea, diarrhea, vomiting, abdominal pain
- Dermatologic: Rash

<1%: Acute renal failure, anemia, arthralgia, confusion, dizziness, increased liver enzymes, ruptured tendons, seizures, tremor

**Overdosage/Toxicology**

Signs and symptoms: Acute renal failure, seizures

Treatment: GI decontamination and supportive care; not removed by peritoneal or hemodialysis

**Drug Interactions** CYP1A2 enzyme inhibitor

Decreased effect:

Enteral feedings may decrease plasma concentrations of ciprofloxacin probably by >30% inhibition of absorption. Ciprofloxacin should not be administered with enteral feedings. The feeding would need to be discontinued for 1-2 hours prior to and after ciprofloxacin administration. Nasogastric administration produces a greater loss of ciprofloxacin bioavailability than does nasoduodenal administration.

Aluminum/magnesium products, didanosine, and sucralfate may decrease absorption of ciprofloxacin by ≥90% if administered concurrently

RECOMMENDATION: Administer ciprofloxacin 2 hours before dose OR administer ciprofloxacin at least 4 hours and preferably 6 hours after the dose of these agents OR change to an $H_2$-antagonist or omeprazole

Calcium, iron, zinc, and multivitamins with minerals products may decrease absorption of ciprofloxacin significantly if administered concurrently

RECOMMENDATION: Administer ciprofloxacin 2 hours before dose OR administer ciprofloxacin at least 2 hours after the dose of these agents

Increased toxicity:

Caffeine and theophylline → CNS stimulation when concurrent with ciprofloxacin

Cyclosporine may increase serum creatinine levels

**Usual Dosage**

Children:

Oral: 20-30 mg/kg/day in 2 divided doses; maximum: 1.5 g/day

Cystic fibrosis: 20-40 mg/kg/day divided every 12 hours

I.V.: 15-20 mg/kg/day divided every 12 hours

Cystic fibrosis: 15-30 mg/kg/day divided every 8-12 hours

Adults: Oral:

Urinary tract infection: 250-500 mg every 12 hours for 7-10 days, depending on severity of infection and susceptibility; (3 investigations (n=975) indicate the minimum effective dose for women with acute, uncomplicated urinary tract infection may be 100 mg twice daily for 3 days)

Lower respiratory tract, skin/skin structure infections: 500-750 mg twice daily for 7-14 days depending on severity and susceptibility

Bone/joint infections: 500-750 mg twice daily for 4-6 weeks, depending on severity and susceptibility

Infectious diarrhea: 500 mg every 12 hours for 5-7 days

Typhoid fever: 500 mg every 12 hours for 10 days

Urethral/cervical gonococcal infections: 250-500 mg as a single dose (CDC recommends concomitant doxycycline or azithromycin due to developing resistance; avoid use in Asian or Western Pacific travelers)

Disseminated gonococcal infection: 500 mg twice daily to complete 7 days of therapy (initial treatment with ceftriaxone 1 g I.M./I.V. daily for 24-48 hours after improvement begins)

Chancroid: 500 mg twice daily for 3 days

Mild to moderate sinusitis: 500 mg every 12 hours for 10 days

Adults: I.V.

Urinary tract infection: 200-400 mg every 12 hours for 7-10 days

Lower respiratory tract, skin/skin structure infection (mild to moderate): 400 mg every 12 hours for 7-14 days

Ophthalmic: Instill 1-2 drops in eye(s) every 2 hours while awake for 2 days and 1-2 drops every 4 hours while awake for the next 5 days

**Dosing adjustment in renal impairment:**

$Cl_{cr}$ <30 mL/minute:

500 mg every 24 hours or

750 mg every 24 hours

Dialysis: Only small amounts of ciprofloxacin are removed by hemo- or peritoneal dialysis (<10%); usual dose: 250-500 mg every 24 hours following dialysis

Continuous arteriovenous or venovenous hemodiafiltration (CAVH) effects: Administer 200-400 mg I.V. every 12 hours

**Dietary Considerations**

Food: Decreases rate, but not extent, of absorption. Drug may cause GI upset; take without regard to meals (manufacturer prefers that drug is taken 2 hours after meals)

Dairy products, oral multivitamins, and mineral supplements: Absorption decreased by divalent and trivalent cations. These cations bind to and form insoluble complexes with quinolones. Avoid taking these substrates with ciprofloxacin. The manufacturer states that the usual dietary intake of calcium has not been shown to interfere with ciprofloxacin absorption.

Caffeine: Possible exaggerated or prolonged effects of caffeine. Ciprofloxacin reduces total body clearance of caffeine. Patients consuming regular large quantities of caffeinated beverages may need to restrict caffeine intake if excessive cardiac or CNS stimulation occurs.

**Patient Information** Take as directed, preferably on an empty stomach (30 minutes before or 2 hours after meals). Take entire prescription even if feeling better. Maintain adequate hydration (2-3 L/day of fluids unless instructed to restrict fluid intake) to avoid concentrated urine and crystal formation. You may experience nausea, vomiting, or anorexia (small frequent meals, frequent mouth care, sucking lozenges, or chewing gum may help). Report immediately any signs of skin rash, joint or back pain, or difficulty breathing. Report unusual fever or chills; vaginal itching or foul-smelling vaginal discharge; easy bruising or bleeding; or pain, inflammation, or rupture of a tendon.

**Nursing Implications** Hold antacids for 2 hours after giving

**Dosage Forms**

Infusion, as hydrochloride, in $D_5W$: 400 mg (200 mL)

Infusion, as hydrochloride, in NS or $D_5W$: 200 mg (100 mL)

Injection, as hydrochloride: 200 mg (20 mL); 400 mg (40 mL)

Solution, ophthalmic, as hydrochloride: 3.5 mg/mL (2.5 mL, 5 mL)

Suspension, oral, as hydrochloride: 250 mg/5 mL (100 mL); 500 mg/5 mL (100 mL)

Tablet, as hydrochloride: 100 mg, 250 mg, 500 mg, 750 mg

## Ciprofloxacin and Hydrocortisone

(sip roe FLOKS a sin & hye droe KOR ti sone)

**U.S. Brand Names** Cipro® HC Otic

**Pharmacologic Category** Antibiotic/Corticosteroid, Otic

**Use** Treatment of acute otitis externa, sometimes known as "swimmer's ear"

**Effects on Mental Status** None reported

**Effects on Psychiatric Treatment** None reported

**Usual Dosage** Children >1 year of age and Adults: Otic: The recommended dosage for all patients is three drops of the suspension in the affected ear twice daily for seven day; twice-daily dosing schedule is more convenient for patients than that of existing treatments with hydrocortisone, which are typically administered three or four times a day; a twice-daily dosage schedule may be especially helpful for parents and caregivers of young children

**Dosage Forms** Suspension, otic: Ciprofloxacin hydrochloride 0.2% and hydrocortisone 1%

♦ **Cipro® HC Otic** *see* Ciprofloxacin and Hydrocortisone *on page 124*

♦ **Cipro® Injection** *see* Ciprofloxacin *on page 123*

♦ **Cipro® Oral** *see* Ciprofloxacin *on page 123*

♦ **Circo-Maren®** *see* Nicergoline *on page 392*

## Cisapride (SIS a pride)

**U.S. Brand Names** Propulsid®

**Canadian Brand Names** Prepulsid®

**Synonyms** R-51619

**Pharmacologic Category** Gastrointestinal Agent, Prokinetic

**Use** Treatment of nocturnal symptoms of gastroesophageal reflux disease (GERD), also demonstrated effectiveness for gastroparesis, refractory constipation, and nonulcer dyspepsia

**Effects on Mental Status** May cause sedation, insomnia, anxiety, or extrapyramidal effects

**Effects on Psychiatric Treatment** Contraindicated with nefazodone; may increase cisapride levels which have been associated with Q-T prolongation and torsade de pointes

**Pregnancy Risk Factor** C

**Contraindications** Hypersensitivity to cisapride or any of its components; GI hemorrhage, mechanical obstruction, GI perforation, or other situations when GI motility stimulation is dangerous

Serious cardiac arrhythmias including ventricular tachycardia, ventricular fibrillation, torsade de pointes, and Q-T prolongation have been reported in patients taking cisapride with other drugs that inhibit CYP3A4. Some of these events have been fatal. Concomitant oral or intravenous administration of the following drugs with cisapride may lead to elevated cisapride blood levels and is contraindicated:

- Antibiotics: Oral or I.V. erythromycin, clarithromycin, troleandomycin
- Antidepressants: Nefazodone
- Antifungals: Oral or I.V. fluconazole, itraconazole, miconazole, oral ketoconazole
- Protease inhibitors: Indinavir, ritonavir, amprenavir

Cisapride is also contraindicated for patients with a prolonged electrocardiographic Q-T intervals (QTc >450 milliseconds), a history of QTc prolongation, or known family history of congenital long Q-T syndrome; clinically significant bradycardia, renal failure, history of ventricular arrhythmias, ischemic heart disease, and congestive heart failure; uncorrected electrolyte disorders (hypokalemia, hypomagnesemia); respiratory failure; and concomitant medications known to prolong the Q-T interval and increase the risk of arrhythmia, such as certain antiarrhythmics, certain antipsychotics, certain antidepressants, astemizole, bepridil, sparfloxacin, and terodiline. The preceding lists of drugs are not comprehensive. Cisapride should not be used in patients with uncorrected hypokalemia or hypomagnesemia or who might experience rapid reduction of plasma potassium such as those administered potassium-wasting diuretics and/or insulin in acute settings.

**Warnings/Precautions On March 24, 2000 the FDA announced that the manufacturer of cisapride would voluntarily withdraw its product from the U.S. market on July 14, 2000. This decision was based on 341 reports of heart rhythm abnormalities including 80 reports of deaths. The company will continue to make the drug available to patients who meet specific clinical eligibility criteria for a limited-access protocol (Contact 1-800-JANSSEN). Serious cardiac arrhythmias including ventricular tachycardia, ventricular fibrillation, torsade de pointes, and Q-T prolongation have been reported in patients taking this drug.**

Many of these patients also took drugs expected to increase cisapride blood levels by inhibiting the CYP3A4 enzymes that metabolize cisapride. These drugs include clarithromycin, erythromycin, troleandomycin, nefazodone, fluconazole, itraconazole, ketoconazole, indinavir and ritonavir. Some of these events have been fatal. Cisapride is contraindicated in patients taking any of these drugs. **Q-T prolongation, torsade de pointes (sometimes with syncope), cardiac arrest and sudden death have been reported in patients taking cisapride without the above-mentioned contraindicated drugs.** Most patients had disorders that may have predisposed them to arrhythmias with cisapride. Cisapride is contraindicated for those patients with: history of prolonged electrocardiographic Q-T intervals; renal failure; history of ventricular arrhythmias, ischemic heart disease, and congestive heart failure; uncorrected electrolyte disorders (hypokalemia, hypomagnesemia); respiratory failure; and concomitant medications known to prolong the Q-T interval and increase the risk of arrhythmia, such as certain antiarrhythmics, including those of Class 1A (such as quinidine and procainamide) and Class III (such as sotalol); tricyclic antidepressants (such as amitriptyline); certain tetracyclic antidepressants (such as maprotiline); certain antipsychotic medications (such as certain phenothiazines and sertindole),protease inhibitors, astemizole, bepridil, sparfloxacin and terodiline. (The preceding lists of drugs are not comprehensive.) Recommended doses of cisapride should not be exceeded.

Patients should have a baseline EKG and an electrolyte panel (magnesium, calcium, potassium) prior to initiating cisapride. Potential benefits should be weighed against risks prior administration of cisapride to patients who have or may develop prolongation of cardiac conduction intervals, particularly $QT_c$. These include patients with conditions that could predispose them to the development of serious arrhythmias, such as multiple organ failure, COPD, apnea and advanced cancer. Cisapride should not be used in patients with uncorrected hypokalemia or hypomagnesemia, such as those with severe dehydration, vomiting or malnutrition, or those taking potassium-wasting diuretics. Cisapride should not be used in patients who might experience rapid reduction of plasma potassium, such as those administered potassium-wasting diuretics and/or insulin in acute settings.

**Adverse Reactions**

>5%:

- Central nervous system: Headache
- Dermatologic: Rash
- Gastrointestinal: Diarrhea, GI cramping, dyspepsia, flatulence, nausea, xerostomia
- Respiratory: Rhinitis

<5%:

- Cardiovascular: Tachycardia
- Central nervous system: Extrapyramidal effects, somnolence, fatigue, seizures, insomnia, anxiety
- Hematologic: Thrombocytopenia, increased LFTs, pancytopenia, leukopenia, granulocytopenia, aplastic anemia
- Respiratory: Sinusitis, coughing, upper respiratory tract infection, increased incidence of viral infection

**Drug Interactions** CYP3A3/4 enzyme substrate

- Azole antifungals (fluconazole, itraconazole, ketoconazole, miconazole) increase cisapride's concentration. Pre-existing cardiovascular disease or electrolyte imbalances increase the risk of malignant arrhythmias; concurrent use is contraindicated.
- Bepridil increases the risk of malignant arrhythmias; concurrent use is contraindicated
- Cimetidine increases the bioavailability of cisapride; use an alternative $H_2$ antagonist
- Class Ia (quinidine, procainamide) and Class III (amiodarone, sotalol) antiarrhythmics increase the risk of malignant arrhythmias; concurrent use is contraindicated
- Increased bioavailability of cisapride with grapefruit juice; concomitant use should be avoided
- Macrolides (clarithromycin, erythromycin, troleandomycin) increase cisapride; risk of arrhythmias; concurrent use is contraindicated
- Nefazodone and maprotiline may increase the risk of malignant arrhythmias; concurrent use is contraindicated
- Phenothiazines (prochlorperazine, promethazine) may increase the risk of malignant arrhythmias; concurrent use is contraindicated
- Protease inhibitors (amprenavir, indinavir, nelfinavir, ritonavir) increase cisapride's concentration; increased risk of malignant arrhythmias; concurrent use is contraindicated
- Quinolone antibiotics: Sparfloxacin, gatifloxacin, moxifloxacin increase the risk of malignant arrhythmias; concurrent use is contraindicated
- Sertindole may increase the risk of malignant arrhythmias; concurrent use is contraindicated
- TCAs increase the risk of malignant arrhythmias; concurrent use is contraindicated
- Warfarin: Isolated cases of increased INR; monitor closely

**Usual Dosage** Oral:

- Children: 0.15-0.3 mg/kg/dose 3-4 times/day; maximum: 10 mg/dose
- Adults: Initial: 10 mg 4 times/day at least 15 minutes before meals and at bedtime; in some patients the dosage will need to be increased to 20 mg to obtain a satisfactory result

**Dietary Considerations** Concomitant use with grapefruit juice should be avoided as it increases the bioavailability of cisapride

**Patient Information** Take before meals. Avoid alcohol and other CNS depressants. May cause increased sedation. Report severe abdominal pain, prolonged diarrhea, weight loss, or extreme fatigue.

**Dosage Forms**

- Suspension, oral (cherry cream flavor): 1 mg/mL (450 mL)
- Tablet, scored: 10 mg, 20 mg

## Cisatracurium (sis a tra KYOO ree um)

**U.S. Brand Names** Nimbex®

**Pharmacologic Category** Neuromuscular Blocker Agent, Nondepolarizing

**Use** Drug for neuromuscular blockade in patients with renal and/or hepatic failure; eases endotracheal intubation as an adjunct to general anesthesia and relaxes skeletal muscle during surgery or mechanical ventilation; does not relieve pain

**Effects on Mental Status** None reported

**Effects on Psychiatric Treatment** Concurrent use with lithium may prolong neuromuscular blockade; conversely, neuromuscular blockade may be diminished if used with carbamazepine

**Usual Dosage** I.V. (not to be used I.M.):

**Operating room administration:**

- Children 2-12 years: Intubating doses: 0.1 mg over 5-15 seconds during either halothane or opioid anesthesia. (**Note**: When given during stable opioid nitrous oxide/oxygen anesthesia, 0.1 mg/kg produces maximum neuromuscular block in an average of 2.8 minutes and clinically effective block for 28 minutes.)
- Adults: Intubating doses: 0.15-0.2 mg/kg as components of propofol/nitrous oxide/oxygen induction-intubation technique. (**Note**: May produce generally good or excellent conditions for tracheal intubation in 1.5-2 minutes with clinically effective duration of action during propofol anesthesia of 55-61 minutes.)
- Children ≥2 years and Adults: Continuous infusion: After an initial bolus, a diluted solution can be given by continuous infusion for maintenance of neuromuscular blockade during extended surgery; adjust the rate of administration according to the patient's response as determined by peripheral nerve stimulation. An initial infusion rate of 3 mcg/kg/minute may be required to rapidly counteract the spontaneous recovery of neuromuscular function; thereafter, a rate of 1-2 mcg/kg/minute should be adequate to maintain continuous neuromuscular block in the 89% to

(Continued)

## Cisatracurium *(Continued)*

99% range in most pediatric and adult patients. Consider reduction of the infusion rate by 30% to 40% when administering during stable isoflurane or enflurane anesthesia. Spontaneous recovery from neuromuscular blockade following discontinuation of infusion of cisatracurium may be expected to proceed at a rate comparable to that following single bolus administration.

**Intensive care unit administration:** Follow the principles for infusion in the operating rooms. An infusion rate of ~3 mcg/kg/minute should provide adequate neuromuscular blockade in adult patients. Following recovery from neuromuscular block, readministration of a bolus dose may be necessary to quickly re-establish neuromuscular block prior to reinstituting the infusion; dosage ranges of 0.5-10 mcg/kg/minute have been reported.

**Dosing adjustment in renal impairment:** Because slower times to onset of complete neuromuscular block were observed in renal dysfunction patients, extending the interval between the administration of cisatracurium and intubation attempt may be required to achieve adequate intubation conditions.

**Dosage Forms** Injection, as besylate: 2 mg/mL (5 mL, 10 mL); 10 mg/mL (20 mL)

## Cisplatin (SIS pla tin)

**U.S. Brand Names** Platinol®; Platinol®-AQ

**Pharmacologic Category** Antineoplastic Agent, Alkylating Agent

**Use** Treatment of head and neck, breast, testicular, and ovarian cancer; Hodgkin's and non-Hodgkin's lymphoma; neuroblastoma; sarcomas, bladder, gastric, lung, esophageal, cervical, and prostate cancer; myeloma, melanoma, mesothelioma, small cell lung cancer, and osteosarcoma

**Effects on Mental Status** None reported

**Effects on Psychiatric Treatment** May cause myelosuppression; use caution with clozapine and carbamazepine

**Usual Dosage** I.V. (refer to individual protocols):

An estimated $Cl_{cr}$ should be on all cisplatin chemotherapy orders along with other patient parameters (ie, patient's height, weight, and body surface area). Pharmacy and nursing staff should check the $Cl_{cr}$ on the order and determine the appropriateness of cisplatin dosing.

The manufacturer recommends that subsequent cycles should only be given when serum creatinine <1.5 mg%, WBC ≥4,000/mm³, platelets ≥ 100,000/mm³, and BUN <25.

It is recommended that a 24-hour urine creatinine clearance be checked prior to a patient's first dose of cisplatin and periodically thereafter (ie, after every 2-3 cycles of cisplatin)

Pretreatment hydration with 1-2 L of chloride-containing fluid is recommended prior to cisplatin administration; adequate hydration and urinary output (>100 mL/hour) should be maintained for 24 hours after administration

**If the dose prescribed is a reduced dose, then this should be indicated on the chemotherapy order**

Children: Various dosage schedules range from 30-100 mg/m² once every 2-3 weeks; may also dose similar to adult dosing

Recurrent brain tumors: 60 mg/m² once daily for 2 consecutive days every 3-4 weeks

Adults:

Advanced bladder cancer: 50-70 mg/m² every 3-4 weeks

Head and neck cancer: 100-120 mg/m² every 3-4 weeks

Testicular cancer: 10-20 mg/m²/day for 5 days repeated every 3-4 weeks

Metastatic ovarian cancer: 75-100 mg/m² every 3 weeks

Intraperitoneal: cisplatin has been administered intraperitoneal with systemic sodium thiosulfate for ovarian cancer; doses up to 90-270 mg/m² have been administered and retained for 4 hours before draining

**Dosing adjustment in renal impairment:**

$Cl_{cr}$ 10-50 mL/minute: Administer 50% of normal dose

$Cl_{cr}$ <10 mL/minute: Do not administer

Hemodialysis: Partially cleared by hemodialysis; administer dose posthemodialysis

CAPD effects: Unknown

CAVH effects: Unknown

**Dosage Forms**

Injection, aqueous: 1 mg/mL (50 mL, 100 mL)

Powder for injection: 10 mg, 50 mg

♦ **13-*cis*-Retinoic Acid** *see* Isotretinoin *on page 297*

## Citalopram (sye TAL oh pram)

**Related Information**

Antidepressant Agents Comparison Chart *on page 704*

Clinical Issues in the Use of Antidepressants *on page 627*

Discontinuation of Psychotropic Drugs - Withdrawal Symptoms and Recommendations *on page 798*

Patient Information - Antidepressants (SSRIs) *on page 639*

Pharmacokinetics of Selective Serotonin-Reuptake Inhibitors (SSRIs) *on page 723*

Teratogenic Risks of Psychotropic Medications *on page 812*

**U.S. Brand Names** Celexa™

**Synonyms** Citalopram Hydrobromide; Nitalapram

**Pharmacologic Category** Antidepressant, Selective Serotonin Reuptake Inhibitor

**Use** Depression

**Pregnancy Risk Factor** C

**Contraindications** Hypersensitivity to citalopram; use of MAO inhibitors within 14 days

**Warnings/Precautions** Potential for severe reaction when used with MAO inhibitors - serotonin syndrome (hyperthermia, muscular rigidity, mental status changes/agitation, autonomic instability) may occur. May precipitate a shift to mania or hypomania in patients with bipolar disease. Has a low potential to impair cognitive or motor performance - caution operating hazardous machinery or driving. Use caution in patients with depression, particularly if suicidal risk may be present. Use caution in patients with a previous seizure disorder or condition predisposing to seizures such as brain damage, alcoholism, or concurrent therapy with other drugs which lower the seizure threshold. Use with caution in patients with hepatic or renal dysfunction and in elderly patients. May cause hyponatremia/SIADH. Use with caution in patients with other concurrent illness (due to limited experience). May cause or exacerbate sexual dysfunction.

**Adverse Reactions**

>10%:

Central nervous system: Somnolence, insomnia

Gastrointestinal: Nausea, xerostomia

Miscellaneous: Diaphoresis

<10%:

Central nervous system: Anxiety, anorexia, agitation, yawning

Dermatologic: Rash, pruritus

Gastrointestinal: Diarrhea, dyspepsia, vomiting, abdominal pain

Endocrine & metabolic: Sexual dysfunction

Neuromuscular & skeletal: Tremor, arthralgia, myalgia

Respiratory: Cough, rhinitis, sinusitis

**Overdosage/Toxicology** Signs and symptoms: Dizziness, sweating, nausea, vomiting, tremor, somnolence, tachycardia, EKG changes

**Drug Interactions** CYP3A3/4 and CYP2C19 enzyme substrate; CYP2D6, 1A2, and 2C19 enzyme inhibitor (weak)

Beta-blockers: Citalopram may increase levels of some beta-blockers (see carvedilol and metoprolol); monitor carefully

Buspirone: Concurrent use of citalopram with buspirone may cause serotonin syndrome; avoid concurrent use

Carbamazepine: May enhance the metabolism of citalopram

Carvedilol: Serum concentrations may be increased; monitor carefully for increased carvedilol effect (hypotension and bradycardia)

Cimetidine: May inhibit the metabolism of citalopram

CYP3A3/4 inhibitors: Serum level and/or toxicity of citalopram may be increased; inhibitors include amiodarone, cimetidine, clarithromycin, erythromycin, delavirdine, diltiazem, dirithromycin, disulfiram, fluoxetine, fluvoxamine, grapefruit juice, indinavir, itraconazole, ketoconazole, metronidazole, nefazodone, nevirapine, propoxyfene, quinupristin-dalfopristin, ritonavir, saquinavir, verapamil, zafirlukast, zileuton; monitor for increased response

CYP2C19 inhibitors: Serum levels of citalopram may be increased; inhibitors include cimetidine, felbamate, fluconazole, fluoxetine, fluvoxamine, omeprazole, teniposide, tolbutamide, and troglitazone

Linezolid: Hyperpyrexia, hypertension, tachycardia, confusion, seizures, and **deaths have been reported** with agents which inhibit MAO (serotonin syndrome); this combination should be avoided

MAO inhibitors: Hyperpyrexia, hypertension, tachycardia, confusion, seizures, and **deaths have been reported** with MAO inhibitors (serotonin syndrome); this combination should be avoided

Meperidine: Combined use theoretically may increase the risk of serotonin syndrome

Metoprolol: Citalopram may increase plasma levels of metoprolol; monitor for increased effect

Moclobemide: Concurrent use of citalopram with moclobemide may cause serotonin syndrome; avoid concurrent use

Nefazodone: Concurrent use of citalopram with nefazodone may cause serotonin syndrome

Selegiline: Concurrent use with citalopram has been reported to cause serotonin syndrome; as a MAO-B inhibitor, the risk of serotonin syndrome may be less than with nonselective MAO inhibitors, and reports indicate that this combination has been well tolerated in Parkinson's patients

Serotonin agonists: Theoretically may increase the risk of serotonin syndrome; includes sumatriptan, naratriptan, rizatriptan, and zolmitriptan

Serotonin reuptake inhibitors: Concurrent use with other reuptake inhibitors may increase the risk of serotonin syndrome

Sibutramine: May increase the risk of serotonin syndrome with SSRIs

Tramadol: Concurrent use of citalopram with tramadol may cause serotonin syndrome; avoid concurrent use

Trazodone: Concurrent use of citalopram with trazodone may cause serotonin syndrome

Venlafaxine: Sertraline may increase the risk of serotonin syndrome

**Mechanism of Action** A bicyclic phthalane derivative, citalopram selectively inhibits serotonin reuptake in the presynaptic neurons

**Pharmacodynamics/kinetics**

Peak plasma level: 4 hours

Distribution: $V_d$: 12 L/kg

Protein binding: 80%

Metabolism: Hepatic desmethylcitalopram, didemethylcitalopram, citalopram-N-oxide, and a deaminated propionic acid derivative

Bioavailability: 80%

Half-life: 35 hours

Elimination:

Fecal: 80%

Renal: 20%

**Usual Dosage** Oral: Initial: 20 mg/day, generally with an increase to 40 mg/day; doses of more than 40 mg are not usually necessary. Should a dose increase be necessary, it should occur in 20 mg increments at intervals of no less than 1 week. Maximum dose: 60 mg/day; reduce dosage in elderly or those with hepatic impairment.

**Dietary Considerations** May be taken without regard to food

**Monitoring Parameters** Signs and symptoms of depression, anxiety, sleep

**Reference Range** Following a 50 mg oral dose, peak serum citalopram levels range from 120-160 nmol/L

**Patient Information** Use caution when operating hazardous machinery, including automobiles, until certain how citalopram affects; avoid alcohol

**Dosage Forms**

Solution, oral, peppermint, sugar free, alcohol free: 10 mg/5 mL

Tablet, as hydrobromide: 20 mg, 40 mg, 60 mg

♦ **Citalopram Hydrobromide** *see* Citalopram *on page 126*

♦ **Citracal® [OTC]** *see* Calcium Citrate *on page 85*

♦ **Citrovorum Factor** *see* Leucovorin *on page 309*

♦ **CI-719** *see* Gemfibrozil *on page 247*

♦ **Cla** *see* Clarithromycin *on page 127*

## Cladribine (KLA dri been)

**U.S. Brand Names** Leustatin™

**Pharmacologic Category** Antineoplastic Agent, Antimetabolite

**Use** Treatment of hairy cell leukemia (HCL) and chronic lymphocytic leukemias

**Effects on Mental Status** May cause drowsiness, dizziness, or insomnia

**Effects on Psychiatric Treatment** May cause bone marrow suppression; use caution with clozapine and carbamazepine

**Usual Dosage** I.V.:

Children:

Acute leukemia: The safety and effectiveness of cladribine in children have not been established; in a phase I study involving patients 1-21 years of age with relapsed acute leukemia, cladribine was administered by CIV at doses ranging from 3-10.7 mg/m²/day for 5 days (0.5-2 times the dose recommended in HCL). Investigators reported beneficial responses in this study; the dose-limiting toxicity was severe myelosuppression with profound neutropenia and thrombocytopenia.

CIV: 15-18 mg/m²/day for 5 days

Adults:

Hairy cell leukemia:

CIV: 0.09-0.1 mg/kg/day continuous infusion for 7 consecutive days

CIV: 4 mg/m²/day for 7 days

Non-Hodgkin's lymphoma: CIV: 0.1 mg/kg/day for 7 days

**Dosage Forms** Injection, preservative free: 1 mg/mL (10 mL)

♦ **Claforan®** *see* Cefotaxime *on page 99*

## Clarithromycin (kla RITH roe mye sin)

**U.S. Brand Names** Biaxin™; Biaxin™ XL

**Synonyms** Cla

**Pharmacologic Category** Antibiotic, Macrolide

**Use** In adults, for treatment of pharyngitis/tonsillitis, acute maxillary sinusitis, acute exacerbation of chronic bronchitis, pneumonia, uncomplicated skin/skin structure infections due to susceptible *S. pyogenes, S. pneumoniae, S. agalactiae*, viridans *Streptococcus, M. catarrhalis, C. trachomatis, Legionella* sp, *Mycoplasma pneumoniae, S. aureus, H. influenzae*; has activity against *M. avium* and *M. intracellulare* infection and is indicated for treatment of and prevention of disseminated mycobacterial infections due to *M. avium* complex disease (eg, patients with advanced HIV infection); indicated for the treatment of duodenal ulcer disease due to *H. pylori* in regimens with other drugs including amoxicillin and lansoprazole or omeprazole, ranitidine, bismuth citrate, bismuth subsalicylate, tetracycline and/or an $H_2$-antagonist; also indicated for prophylaxis of bacterial endocarditis in patients who are allergic to penicillin and undergoing surgical or dental procedures

In children, for treatment of pharyngitis/tonsillitis, acute maxillary sinusitis, acute otitis media, uncomplicated skin/skin structure infections due to the above organisms; treatment of and prevention of disseminated mycobacterial infections due to *M. avium* complex disease (eg, patients with advanced HIV infection)

Exhibits the same spectrum of *in vitro* activity as erythromycin, but with significantly increased potency against those organisms

**Effects on Mental Status** Macrolides have been reported to cause nightmares, confusion, anxiety, and mood lability

**Effects on Psychiatric Treatment** Contraindicated with pimozide; increases carbamazepine and triazolam levels; monitor for signs of toxicity

**Pregnancy Risk Factor** C

**Contraindications** Hypersensitivity to clarithromycin, erythromycin, or any macrolide antibiotic; use with pimozide, astemizole, cisapride, terfenadine

**Warnings/Precautions** In presence of severe renal impairment with or without coexisting hepatic impairment, decreased dosage or prolonged dosing interval may be appropriate; antibiotic-associated colitis has been reported with use of clarithromycin; elderly patients have experienced increased incidents of adverse effects due to known age-related decreases in renal function

**Adverse Reactions**

1% to 10%:

Central nervous system: Headache

Gastrointestinal: Diarrhea, nausea, abnormal taste, dyspepsia, abdominal pain

<1%: Elevated BUN/serum creatinine, hypoglycemia, increased AST/alkaline phosphatase/bilirubin, leukopenia, manic behavior, neutropenia, prolonged PT, torsade de pointes, tremor, ventricular tachycardia

**Overdosage/Toxicology**

Signs and symptoms: Nausea, vomiting, diarrhea, prostration, reversible pancreatitis, hearing loss with or without tinnitus or vertigo

Treatment: Symptomatic and supportive care

**Drug Interactions** CYP3A3/4 enzyme substrate; CYP1A2 and 3A3/4 enzyme inhibitor

Increased levels:

Clarithromycin increases serum theophylline levels by as much as 20%

Increased concentration of HMG CoA-reductase inhibitors (lovastatin and simvastatin)

Amprenavir's serum concentration may be increased.

Significantly increases carbamazepine levels and those of cyclosporine, digoxin, ergot alkaloid, tacrolimus, omeprazole and triazolam

Peak levels (but not AUC) of zidovudine are often increased; terfenadine and astemizole should be avoided with use of clarithromycin since plasma levels may be increased by >3 times; serious arrhythmias have occurred with cisapride and other drugs which inhibit cytochrome P-450 3A4 (eg, clarithromycin)

Fluconazole increases clarithromycin levels and AUC by ~25%; death has been reported with administration of pimozide and clarithromycin. Concurrent use is contraindicated.

**Note:** While other drug interactions (bromocriptine, disopyramide, lovastatin, phenytoin, and valproate) known to occur with erythromycin have not been reported in clinical trials with clarithromycin, concurrent use of these drugs should be monitored closely

**Usual Dosage** Safe use in children has not been established

Children ≥6 months: 15 mg/kg/day divided every 12 hours; dosages of 7.5 mg/kg twice daily up to 500 mg twice daily children with AIDS and disseminated MAC infection

Adults: Oral:

Usual dose: 250-500 mg every 12 hours **or** 1000 mg (2 x 500 mg extended release tablets) once daily for for 7-14 days

Upper respiratory tract: 250-500 mg every 12 hours for 10-14 days

Pharyngitis/tonsillitis: 250 mg every 12 hours for 10 days

Acute maxillary sinusitis: 500 mg every 12 hours **or** 1000 mg (2 x 500 mg extended release tablets) once daily for 14 days

Lower respiratory tract: 250-500 mg every 12 hours for 7-14 days

Acute exacerbation of chronic bronchitis due to:

*M. catarrhalis* and *S. pneumoniae*: 250 mg every 12 hours **or** 1000 mg (2 x 500 mg extended release tablets) once daily for 7-14 days

*H. influenzae*: 500 mg every 12 hours for 7-14 days

Pneumonia due to *M. pneumoniae* and *S. pneumoniae*: 250 mg every 12 hours for 7-14 days

Mycobacterial infection (prevention and treatment): 500 mg twice daily (use with other antimycobacterial drugs, eg, ethambutol, clofazimine, or rifampin)

Prophylaxis of bacterial endocarditis: 500 mg 1 hour prior to procedure

Uncomplicated skin and skin structure: 250 mg every 12 hours for 7-14 days

*Helicobacter pylori*: Combination regimen with bismuth subsalicylate, tetracycline, clarithromycin, and an $H_2$-receptor antagonist; or combination of omeprazole and clarithromycin; 250 mg twice daily to 500 mg 3 times/day

**Dosing adjustment in renal impairment:** Adults: Oral:

$Cl_{cr}$ <30 mL/minute: 500 mg loading dose, then 250 mg once or twice daily

(Continued)

## Clarithromycin *(Continued)*

**Dosing adjustment in severe renal impairment:** Decreased doses or prolonged dosing intervals are recommended

**Patient Information** Take full course of therapy; do not discontinue without consulting prescriber. Maintain adequate hydration (2-3 L/day of fluids unless instructed to restrict fluid intake). You may experience nausea (small frequent meals, or sucking lozenges may help); abnormal taste (frequent mouth care or chewing gum may help); diarrhea, headache, or abdominal cramps (medication may be ordered). Report persistent fever or chills, easy bruising or bleeding, or joint pain. Report severe persistent diarrhea, skin rash, sores in mouth, foul-smelling urine, rapid heartbeat or palpitations, or difficulty breathing. Do not refrigerate oral suspension (more palatable at room temperature).

**Dosage Forms**

Granules for oral suspension: 125 mg/5 mL (50 mL, 100 mL); 250 mg/5 mL (50 mL, 100 mL)

Tablet, film coated: 250 mg, 500 mg

Tablet, film coated, extended release: 500 mg


- **Claritin-D® 12-Hour** *see* Loratadine and Pseudoephedrine *on page 325*
- **Claritin-D® 24-Hour** *see* Loratadine and Pseudoephedrine *on page 325*
- **Claritin® RediTabs®** *see* Loratadine *on page 324*
- **Claritin® Syrup** *see* Loratadine *on page 324*
- **Claritin® Tablets** *see* Loratadine *on page 324*
- **Clear By Design® Gel [OTC]** *see* Benzoyl Peroxide *on page 62*
- **Clear Eyes® [OTC]** *see* Naphazoline *on page 383*
- **Clearsil® Maximum Strength [OTC]** *see* Benzoyl Peroxide *on page 62*
- **Clear Tussin® 30** *see* Guaifenesin and Dextromethorphan *on page 257*


## Clemastine (KLEM as teen)

**U.S. Brand Names** Antihist-1® [OTC]; Tavist®; Tavist®-1 [OTC]

**Pharmacologic Category** Antihistamine

**Use** Perennial and seasonal allergic rhinitis and other allergic symptoms including urticaria

**Effects on Mental Status** Drowsiness is common; may cause nervousness; rare reports of depression

**Effects on Psychiatric Treatment** Concurrent use with psychotropics may result in additive sedation

**Pregnancy Risk Factor** C

**Contraindications** Narrow-angle glaucoma, hypersensitivity to clemastine or any component

**Warnings/Precautions** Safety and efficacy have not been established in children <6 years of age; bladder neck obstruction, symptomatic prostate hypertrophy, asthmatic attacks, and stenosing peptic ulcer

**Adverse Reactions**

>10%:

Central nervous system: Slight to moderate drowsiness

Respiratory: Thickening of bronchial secretions

1% to 10%:

Central nervous system: Headache, fatigue, nervousness, increased dizziness

Gastrointestinal: Appetite increase, weight gain, nausea, diarrhea, abdominal pain, xerostomia

Neuromuscular & skeletal: Arthralgia

Respiratory: Pharyngitis

<1%: Angioedema, bronchospasm, depression, edema, epistaxis, hepatitis, myalgia, palpitations, paresthesia, photosensitivity, rash

**Overdosage/Toxicology**

Signs and symptoms: Anemia, metabolic acidosis, hypotension, hypothermia

Treatment: There is no specific treatment for an antihistamine overdose, however, most of its clinical toxicity is due to anticholinergic effects. For anticholinergic overdose with severe life-threatening symptoms, physostigmine 1-2 mg (0.5 or 0.02 mg/kg for children) I.V., slowly may be given to reverse these effects.

**Drug Interactions** Increased toxicity (CNS depression): CNS depressants, MAO inhibitors, tricyclic antidepressants, phenothiazines

**Usual Dosage** Oral:

Children: <12 years: 0.4-1 mg twice daily

Children >12 years and Adults: 1.34 mg twice daily to 2.68 mg 3 times/day; do not exceed 8.04 mg/day; lower doses should be considered in patients >60 years

**Dietary Considerations** Alcohol: Additive CNS effects, avoid use

**Patient Information** Avoid alcohol; may cause drowsiness, may impair coordination or judgment

**Nursing Implications** Raise bed rails, institute safety measures, assist with ambulation

**Dosage Forms**

Syrup, as fumarate (citrus flavor): 0.67 mg/5 mL with alcohol 5.5% (120 mL)

Tablet, as fumarate: 1.34 mg, 2.68 mg

## Clemastine and Phenylpropanolamine

(KLEM as teen & fen il proe pa NOLE a meen)

**U.S. Brand Names** Antihist-D®; Tavist-D®

**Pharmacologic Category** Antihistamine/Decongestant Combination

**Use** Symptomatic relief of allergic rhinitis; pruritus of the eyes, nose or throat, lacrimation and nasal congestion

**Effects on Mental Status** Drowsiness is common; may case nervousness; rare reports of depression

**Effects on Psychiatric Treatment** Concurrent use with psychotropics may result in additive sedation

**Usual Dosage** Children >12 years and Adults: Oral: 1 tablet every 12 hours

**Dosage Forms** Tablet: Clemastine fumarate 1.34 mg and phenylpropanolamine hydrochloride 75 mg


- **Cleocin-3®** *see* Clindamycin *on page 128*
- **Cleocin HCl®** *see* Clindamycin *on page 128*
- **Cleocin Pediatric®** *see* Clindamycin *on page 128*
- **Cleocin Phosphate®** *see* Clindamycin *on page 128*
- **Cleocin T®** *see* Clindamycin *on page 128*


## Clidinium and Chlordiazepoxide

(kli DI nee um & klor dye az e POKS ide)

**U.S. Brand Names** Clindex®; Librax®

**Canadian Brand Names** Apo®-Chlorax; Corium®; ProChlorax

**Synonyms** Chlordiazepoxide and Clidinium

**Pharmacologic Category** Antispasmodic Agent, Gastrointestinal

**Use** Adjunct treatment of peptic ulcer; treatment of irritable bowel syndrome

**Effects on Mental Status** Drowsiness is common; may cause confusion

**Effects on Psychiatric Treatment** Concurrent use with psychotropics may result in additive sedation

**Pregnancy Risk Factor** D

**Contraindications** Glaucoma; prostatic hypertrophy; benign bladder neck obstruction; hypersensitivity to clidinium, chlordiazepoxide, or any component

**Warnings/Precautions** Use with caution with alcohol or other CNS depressants because of possible combined effects. Do not abruptly discontinue this medication after prolonged use; taper dose gradually.

**Adverse Reactions** 1% to 10%: Drowsiness ataxia, confusion, anticholinergic side effects

**Drug Interactions** Additive effects may result from concomitant benzodiazepine and/or anticholinergic therapy

**Usual Dosage** Oral: 1-2 capsules 3-4 times/day, before meals or food and at bedtime

**Patient Information** Take as directed before meals; do not increase dose and do not discontinue without consulting prescriber first. Avoid alcohol and other CNS depressant medications (antihistamines, sleeping aids, antidepressants) unless approved by prescriber. Void before taking medication. This drug may impair mental alertness (use caution when driving or engaging in tasks that require alertness until response to drug is known). Report excessive and persistent anticholinergic effects (blurred vision, headache, flushing, tachycardia, nervousness, constipation, dizziness, insomnia, mental confusion or excitement, dry mouth, altered taste perception, dysphagia, palpitations, bradycardia, urinary hesitancy or retention, impotence, decreased sweating), or change in color of urine or stools.

**Dosage Forms** Capsule: Clidinium bromide 2.5 mg and chlordiazepoxide hydrochloride 5 mg


- **Climara® Transdermal** *see* Estradiol *on page 203*
- **Clinda-Derm® Topical Solution** *see* Clindamycin *on page 128*


## Clindamycin (klin da MYE sin)

**U.S. Brand Names** Cleocin-3®; Cleocin HCl®; Cleocin Pediatric®; Cleocin Phosphate®; Cleocin T®; Clinda-Derm® Topical Solution; Clindets® Pledgets; C/T/S® Topical Solution

**Canadian Brand Names** Dalacin® C [Hydrochloride]

**Pharmacologic Category** Antibiotic, Miscellaneous

**Use** Treatment against aerobic and anaerobic streptococci (except enterococci), most staphylococci, *Bacteroides* sp and *Actinomyces*; used topically in treatment of severe acne, vaginally for *Gardnerella vaginalis* or bacterial vaginosis; alternate treatment for toxoplasmosis; prophylaxis in the prevention of bacterial endocarditis in high-risk patients undergoing surgical or dental procedures in patients allergic to penicillin; may be useful in PCP

**Effects on Mental Status** None reported

**Effects on Psychiatric Treatment** May cause neutropenia; use caution with clozapine and carbamazepine

**Pregnancy Risk Factor** B

**Contraindications** Hypersensitivity to clindamycin or any component; previous pseudomembranous colitis, hepatic impairment

**Warnings/Precautions** Dosage adjustment may be necessary in patients with severe hepatic dysfunction; can cause severe and possibly fatal colitis; use with caution in patients with a history of pseudomembranous colitis; discontinue drug if significant diarrhea, abdominal cramps, or passage of blood and mucus occurs

**Adverse Reactions**

>10%: Gastrointestinal: Diarrhea

1% to 10%:

Dermatologic: Rashes

Gastrointestinal: Pseudomembranous colitis (more common with oral form), nausea, vomiting

<1%: Elevated liver enzymes, eosinophilia, granulocytopenia, hypotension, neutropenia, polyarthritis, rare renal dysfunction, sterile abscess at I.M. injection site, Stevens-Johnson syndrome, thrombocytopenia, thrombophlebitis, urticaria

**Overdosage/Toxicology**

Signs and symptoms: Diarrhea, nausea, vomiting

Treatment: Following GI decontamination, treatment is supportive

**Drug Interactions** CYP3A3/4 enzyme substrate

Increased duration of neuromuscular blockade from tubocurarine, pancuronium

**Usual Dosage** Avoid in neonates (contains benzyl alcohol)

Infants and Children:

Oral: 8-20 mg/kg/day as hydrochloride; 8-25 mg/kg/day as palmitate in 3-4 divided doses; minimum dose of palmitate: 37.5 mg 3 times/day

I.M., I.V.:

<1 month: 15-20 mg/kg/day

>1 month: 20-40 mg/kg/day in 3-4 divided doses

Children and Adults: Topical: Apply a thin film twice daily

Adults:

Oral: 150-450 mg/dose every 6-8 hours; maximum dose: 1.8 g/day

I.M., I.V.: 1.2-1.8 g/day in 2-4 divided doses; maximum dose: 4.8 g/day

Bacterial endocarditis prophylaxis: 600 mg 1 hour prior to the procedure

Pelvic inflammatory disease: I.V.: 900 mg every 8 hours with gentamicin 2 mg/kg, then 1.5 mg/kg every 8 hours; continue after discharge with doxycycline 100 mg twice daily or oral clindamycin 450 mg 5 times/day for 10-14 days

*Pneumocystis carinii* pneumonia:

Oral: 300-450 mg 4 times/day with primaquine

I.M., I.V.: 1200-2400 mg/day with pyrimethamine

I.V.: 600 mg 4 times/day with primaquine

Vaginal: One full applicator (100 mg) inserted intravaginally once daily before bedtime for 3 or 7 consecutive days

Intravaginal suppositories: Insert one ovule (100 mg clindamycin) daily into vagina at bedtime for 3 days

**Dosing adjustment in hepatic impairment:** Adjustment recommended in patients with severe hepatic disease

**Patient Information**

Oral: Take each dose with a full glass of water. Complete full prescription, even if feeling better. You may experience nausea or vomiting (small frequent meals, frequent mouth care, chewing gum, or sucking lozenges may help). Report dizziness; persistent gastrointestinal effects (pain, diarrhea, vomiting); skin redness, rash, or burning; fever; chills; unusual bruising or bleeding; signs of infection; excessive fatigue; yellowing of eyes or skin; change in color of urine or blackened stool; swelling, warmth, or pain in extremities; difficult respirations; bloody or fatty stool (do not take antidiarrheal without consulting prescriber); or lack or improvement or worsening of condition.

Topical: Wash hands before applying or wear gloves. Apply thin film of gel, lotion, or solution to affected area. May apply porous dressing. Report persistent burning, swelling, itching, or worsening of condition.

Vaginal: Wash hands before using. At bedtime, gently insert full applicator into vagina and expel cream. Wash applicator with soap and water following use. Remain lying down for 30 minutes following administration. Avoid intercourse during 7 days of therapy. Report adverse reactions (dizziness, nausea, vomiting, stomach cramps, or headache) or lack of improvement or worsening of condition.

**Dosage Forms**

Capsule, as hydrochloride: 75 mg, 150 mg, 300 mg

Cream, vaginal: 2% (40 g)

Gel, topical, as phosphate: 1% [10 mg/g] (7.5 g, 30 g)

Granules for oral solution, as palmitate: 75 mg/5 mL (100 mL)

Infusion, as phosphate, in $D_5W$: 300 mg (50 mL); 600 mg (50 mL)

Injection, as phosphate: 150 mg/mL (2 mL, 4 mL, 6 mL, 50 mL, 60 mL)

Lotion: 1% [10 mg/mL] (60 mL)

Pledgets: 1%

Solution, topical, as phosphate: 1% [10 mg/mL] (30 mL, 60 mL, 480 mL)

♦ **Clindets® Pledgets** *see* Clindamycin *on page 128*

♦ **Clindex®** *see* Clidinium and Chlordiazepoxide *on page 128*

♦ **Clinical Issues in the Use of Antidepressants** *see page 627*

♦ **Clinical Issues in the Use of Antipsychotics** *see page 630*

♦ **Clinical Issues in the Use of Anxiolytics and Sedative/Hypnotics** *see page 634*

♦ **Clinical Issues in the Use of Mood Stabilizers** *see page 632*

♦ **Clinical Issues in the Use of Stimulants** *see page 637*

♦ **Clinoril®** *see* Sulindac *on page 527*

## Clioquinol (klye oh KWIN ole)

**U.S. Brand Names** Vioform® [OTC]

**Pharmacologic Category** Antifungal Agent, Topical

**Use** Topically in the treatment of tinea pedis, tinea cruris, and skin infections caused by dermatophytic fungi (ringworm)

**Effects on Mental Status** None reported

**Effects on Psychiatric Treatment** May interfere with thyroid function tests

**Usual Dosage** Children and Adults: Topical: Apply 2-3 times/day; do not use for longer than 7 days

**Dosage Forms**

Cream: 3% (30 g)

Ointment, topical: 3% (30 g)

## Clioquinol and Hydrocortisone

(klye oh KWIN ole & hye droe KOR ti sone)

**U.S. Brand Names** Corque® Topical; Pedi-Cort V® Creme

**Pharmacologic Category** Antifungal Agent, Topical

**Use** Treatment of contact or atopic dermatitis, eczema, neurodermatitis, anogenital pruritus, mycotic dermatoses, moniliasis

**Effects on Mental Status** None reported

**Effects on Psychiatric Treatment** None reported

**Usual Dosage** Apply in a thin film 3-4 times/day

**Dosage Forms** Cream: Clioquinol 3% and hydrocortisone 1% (20 g)

♦ **Cliradon®** *see* Ketobemidone *on page 301*

♦ **Clistin®** *see* Carbinoxamine *on page 92*

## Clobetasol (kloe BAY ta sol)

**Related Information**

Corticosteroids Comparison Chart *on page 711*

**U.S. Brand Names** Temovate® Topical

**Canadian Brand Names** Dermasone; Dermovate®; Gen-Clobetasol; Novo-Clobetasol

**Pharmacologic Category** Corticosteroid, Topical

**Use Short-term** relief of inflammation of moderate to severe corticosteroid-responsive dermatosis (very high potency topical corticosteroid)

**Effects on Mental Status** None reported

**Effects on Psychiatric Treatment** None reported

**Usual Dosage** Adults: Topical: Apply twice daily for up to 2 weeks with no more than 50 g/week. Therapy should be discontinued when control is achieved; if no improvement is seen, reassessment of diagnosis may be necessary.

**Dosage Forms**

Cream, as propionate: 0.05% (15 g, 30 g, 45 g)

Cream, as propionate, in emollient base: 0.05% (15 g, 30 g, 60 g)

Gel, as propionate: 0.05% (15 g, 30 g, 45 g)

Ointment, topical, as propionate: 0.05% (15 g, 30 g, 45 g)

Scalp application, as propionate: 0.05% (25 mL, 50 mL)

♦ **Clocort® Maximum Strength** *see* Hydrocortisone *on page 273*

## Clocortolone (kloe KOR toe lone)

**Related Information**

Corticosteroids Comparison Chart *on page 711*

**U.S. Brand Names** Cloderm® Topical

**Pharmacologic Category** Corticosteroid, Topical

**Use** Inflammation of corticosteroid-responsive dermatoses (medium potency topical corticosteroid)

**Effects on Mental Status** None reported

**Effects on Psychiatric Treatment** None reported

**Usual Dosage** Adults: Apply sparingly and gently; rub into affected area from 1-4 times/day. Therapy should be discontinued when control is achieved; if no improvement is seen, reassessment of diagnosis may be necessary.

**Dosage Forms** Cream, as pivalate: 0.1% (15 g, 45 g)

♦ **Cloderm® Topical** *see* Clocortolone *on page 129*

## Clofazimine (kloe FA zi meen)

**U.S. Brand Names** Lamprene®
**Pharmacologic Category** Leprostatic Agent
**Use Orphan drug:** Treatment of dapsone-resistant leprosy; multibacillary dapsone-sensitive leprosy; erythema nodosum leprosum; *Mycobacterium avium-intracellulare* (MAI) infections
**Effects on Mental Status** May cause drowsiness or giddiness
**Effects on Psychiatric Treatment** None reported
**Pregnancy Risk Factor** C
**Contraindications** Hypersensitivity to clofazimine or any component
**Warnings/Precautions** Use with caution in patients with GI problems; dosages >100 mg/day should be used for as short a duration as possible; skin discoloration may lead to depression
**Adverse Reactions**
>10%:
Dermatologic: Dry skin
Gastrointestinal: Abdominal pain, nausea, vomiting, diarrhea
Miscellaneous: Pink to brownish-black discoloration of the skin and conjunctiva
1% to 10%:
Dermatologic: Rash, pruritus
Endocrine & metabolic: Elevated blood sugar
Gastrointestinal: Fecal discoloration
Genitourinary: Discoloration of urine
Ocular: Irritation of the eyes
Miscellaneous: Discoloration of sputum, sweat
<1%: Acneiform eruptions, anemia, anorexia, bone pain, bowel obstruction, constipation, cystitis, diminished vision, dizziness, drowsiness, edema, enlarged liver, eosinophilia, eosinophilic enteritis, erythroderma, fatigue, fever, GI bleeding, giddiness, headache, hepatitis, hypokalemia, increased albumin/serum bilirubin/AST, jaundice, lymphadenopathy, monilial cheilosis, neuralgia, phototoxicity, taste disorder, vascular pain, weight loss
**Overdosage/Toxicology** Treatment: Following GI decontamination, treatment is supportive
**Drug Interactions** Decreased effect with dapsone (unconfirmed)
**Usual Dosage** Oral:
Children: Leprosy: 1 mg/kg/day every 24 hours in combination with dapsone and rifampin
Adults:
Dapsone-resistant leprosy: 100 mg/day in combination with one or more antileprosy drugs for 3 years; then alone 100 mg/day
Dapsone-sensitive multibacillary leprosy: 100 mg/day in combination with two or more antileprosy drugs for at least 2 years and continue until negative skin smears are obtained, then institute single drug therapy with appropriate agent
Erythema nodosum leprosum: 100-200 mg/day for up to 3 months or longer then taper dose to 100 mg/day when possible
Pyoderma gangrenosum: 300-400 mg/day for up to 12 months
**Dosing adjustment in hepatic impairment:** Should be considered in severe hepatic dysfunction
**Patient Information** May be taken with meals. Drug may cause a pink to brownish-black discoloration of the skin, conjunctiva, tears, sweat, urine, feces, and nasal secretions. Although reversible, it may take months to years for skin discoloration to disappear after therapy is complete. Report promptly bone or joint pain, GI disturbance, or vision disturbances.
**Dosage Forms** Capsule, as palmitate: 50 mg

## Clofibrate (kloe FYE brate)

**Related Information**
Lipid-Lowering Agents Comparison Chart *on page 717*
**U.S. Brand Names** Atromid-S®
**Canadian Brand Names** Abitrate®; Claripex®; Novo-Fibrate
**Pharmacologic Category** Antilipemic Agent (Fibric Acid)
**Use** Adjunct to dietary therapy in the management of hyperlipidemias associated with high triglyceride levels (Types III, IV, V); primarily lowers triglycerides and very low density lipoprotein
**Effects on Mental Status** May cause sedation or dizziness
**Effects on Psychiatric Treatment** Rare reports of agranulocytosis; use caution with clozapine and carbamazepine
**Pregnancy Risk Factor** C
**Contraindications** Hypersensitivity to clofibrate or any component; significant hepatic or renal dysfunction; primary biliary cirrhosis
**Warnings/Precautions** Possible increased risk of malignancy and cholelithiasis. No evidence of cardiovascular mortality benefit. Anemia and leukopenia have been reported. Elevations in serum transaminases can be seen. Discontinue if lipid response is not seen. Use with caution in peptic ulcer disease. Flu-like symptoms may occur. Be careful in patient selection; this is not a first- or second-line choice. Other agents may be more suitable.
**Adverse Reactions** Percentage unknown: Abdominal distress, aching, agranulocytosis, alopecia, anemia, angina, cardiac arrhythmias, diarrhea, dizziness, dry/brittle hair, dyspepsia, eosinophilia, fatigue, flatulence, gallstones, headache, impotence, increased LFTs, leukopenia, muscle cramping, myalgia, nausea, pruritus, rash, renal toxicity, rhabdomyolysis-induced renal failure, urticaria, vomiting, weakness
**Overdosage/Toxicology**
Signs and symptoms: Nausea, vomiting, diarrhea, GI distress
Treatment: Following GI decontamination, treatment is supportive
**Drug Interactions**
Chlorpropamide: May increase risk of hypoglycemia.
Furosemide: Blood levels of furosemide and fibric acid derivatives (ie, clofibrate and fenofibrate) may be increased during concurrent dosing (particularly in hypoalbuminemia). Limited documentation; monitor for increased effect/toxicity.
HMG-CoA reductase inhibitors (atorvastatin, cerivastatin, fluvastatin, lovastatin, pravastatin, simvastatin) may increase the risk of myopathy and rhabdomyolysis. The manufacturer warns against the concomitant use. However, combination therapy with statins has been used in some patients with resistant hyperlipidemias (with great caution).
Insulin: Hypoglycemic effects may be potentiated by an unknown mechanism.
Probenecid may decrease the clearance of clofibrate.
Rifampin: Decreased clofibrate blood levels.
Sulfonylureas (including glyburide, glipizide): Hypoglycemic effects may be potentiated by an unknown mechanism.
Warfarin: Increased hypoprothrombinemic response; monitor INRs closely when clofibrate is initiated or discontinued.
**Usual Dosage** Adults: Oral: 500 mg 4 times/day; some patients may respond to lower doses
**Dosing interval in renal impairment:**
$Cl_{cr}$ >50 mL/minute: Administer every 6-12 hours
$Cl_{cr}$ 10-50 mL/minute: Administer every 12-18 hours
$Cl_{cr}$ <10 mL/minute: Avoid use
Hemodialysis: Elimination is not enhanced via hemodialysis; supplemental dose is not necessary
**Patient Information** This drug will have to be taken long-term and ongoing follow-up is essential. Adherence to a cardiac risk reduction program, including adherence to prescribed diet, is of major importance. This drug may cause stomach upset; if this occurs, take medication with food or milk. Report chest pain, shortness of breath, irregular heartbeat, palpitations, severe stomach pain with nausea and vomiting, persistent fever, sore throat, or unusual bleeding or bruising.
**Dosage Forms** Capsule: 500 mg

◆ **Clomid®** *see* Clomiphene *on page 130*

## Clomiphene (KLOE mi feen)

**U.S. Brand Names** Clomid®; Milophene®; Serophene®
**Pharmacologic Category** Ovulation Stimulator
**Use** Treatment of ovulatory failure in patients desiring pregnancy
**Unlabeled use:** Male infertility
**Effects on Mental Status** May cause insomnia, fatigue, or depression
**Effects on Psychiatric Treatment** None reported
**Pregnancy Risk Factor** X
**Contraindications** Hypersensitivity or allergy to clomiphene citrate or any of its components; liver disease, abnormal uterine bleeding, suspected pregnancy, enlargement or development of ovarian cyst, uncontrolled thyroid or adrenal dysfunction in the presence of an organic intracranial lesion such as pituitary tumor
**Warnings/Precautions** Patients unusually sensitive to pituitary gonadotropins (eg, polycystic ovary disease); multiple pregnancies, blurring or other visual symptoms can occur, ovarian hyperstimulation syndrome, and abdominal pain
**Adverse Reactions**
>10%: Endocrine & metabolic: Hot flashes, ovarian enlargement
1% to 10%:
Cardiovascular: Thromboembolism
Central nervous system: Mental depression, headache
Endocrine & metabolic: Breast enlargement (males), breast discomfort (females), abnormal menstrual flow
Gastrointestinal: Distention, bloating, nausea, vomiting, hepatotoxicity
Ocular: Blurring of vision, diplopia, floaters, after-images, phosphenes, photophobia
<1%: Alopecia (reversible), fatigue, insomnia, polyuria, weight gain
**Drug Interactions** Decreased response when used with danazol; decreased estradiol response when used with clomiphene
**Usual Dosage** Adults: Oral:
Male (infertility): 25 mg/day for 25 days with 5 days rest, or 100 mg every Monday, Wednesday, Friday
Female (ovulatory failure): 50 mg/day for 5 days (first course); start the regimen on or about the fifth day of cycle. The dose should be increased only in those patients who do not ovulate in response to cyclic 50 mg Clomid®. A low dosage or duration of treatment course is particularly recommended if unusual sensitivity to pituitary gonadotropin is suspected, such as in patients with polycystic ovary syndrome.

If ovulation does not appear to occur after the first course of therapy, a second course of 100 mg/day (two 50 mg tablets given as a single daily dose) for 5 days should be given. This course may be started as early as 30 days after the previous one after precautions are taken to exclude the presence of pregnancy. Increasing the dosage or duration of therapy beyond 100 mg/day for 5 days is not recommended. The majority of patients who are going to ovulate will do so after the first course of therapy. If ovulation does not occur after 3 courses of therapy, further treatment is not recommended and the patient should be re-evaluated. If 3 ovulatory responses occur, but pregnancy has not been achieved, further treatment is not recommended. If menses does not occur after an ovulatory response, the patient should be re-evaluated. Long-term cyclic therapy is not recommended beyond a total of about 6 cycles.

**Patient Information** Follow recommended schedule of dosing. You may experience hot flashes (cool clothes and cool environment may help). Report acute sudden headache; difficulty breathing; warmth, pain, redness, or swelling in calves; breast enlargement (male) or breast discomfort (female); abnormal menstrual bleeding; vision changes (blurring, diplopia, photophobia, floaters); acute abdominal discomfort; or fever.

**Dosage Forms** Tablet, as citrate: 50 mg

## Clomipramine (kloe MI pra meen)

**Related Information**

Antidepressant Agents Comparison Chart *on page 704*
Anxiety Disorders *on page 606*
Clinical Issues in the Use of Antidepressants *on page 627*
Clinical Issues in the Use of Anxiolytics and Sedative/Hypnotics *on page 634*
Discontinuation of Psychotropic Drugs - Withdrawal Symptoms and Recommendations *on page 798*
Patient Information - Antidepressants (TCAs) *on page 640*
Personality Disorders *on page 625*
Special Populations - Pregnant and Breast-Feeding Patients *on page 668*
Substance-Related Disorders *on page 609*
Teratogenic Risks of Psychotropic Medications *on page 812*

**Generic Available** Yes

**U.S. Brand Names** Anafranil®

**Canadian Brand Names** Apo®-Clomipramine

**Synonyms** Clomipramine Hydrochloride

**Pharmacologic Category** Antidepressant, Tricyclic (Tertiary Amine)

**Use** Treatment of obsessive-compulsive disorder (OCD)

**Unlabeled use:** May also relieve depression, panic attacks, and chronic pain

**Pregnancy Risk Factor** C

**Contraindications** Hypersensitivity to this drug or other tricyclic agents; use of monoamine oxidase inhibitors within 14 days; use in a patient during the acute recovery phase of MI

**Warnings/Precautions** May cause seizures (relationship to dose and/or duration of therapy) - do not exceed maximum doses. Use caution in patients with a previous seizure disorder or condition predisposing to seizures such as brain damage, alcoholism, or concurrent therapy with other drugs which lower the seizure threshold. Has been associated with a high incidence of sexual dysfunction. Weight gain may occur. May cause sedation, resulting in impaired performance of tasks requiring alertness (ie, operating machinery or driving). Sedative effects may be additive with other CNS depressants and/or ethanol. The degree of sedation is very high relative to other antidepressants. May worsen psychosis in some patients or precipitate a shift to mania or hypomania in patients with bipolar disease. May increase the risks associated with electroconvulsive therapy. This agent should be discontinued, when possible, prior to elective surgery. Therapy should not be abruptly discontinued in patients receiving high doses for prolonged periods.

May cause orthostatic hypotension (risk is moderate relative to other antidepressants) - use with caution in patients at risk of hypotension or in patients where transient hypotensive episodes would be poorly tolerated (cardiovascular disease or cerebrovascular disease). The degree of anticholinergic blockade produced by this agent is very high relative to other cyclic antidepressants - use caution in patients with urinary retention, benign prostatic hypertrophy, narrow-angle glaucoma, xerostomia, visual problems, constipation, or history of bowel obstruction.

Use caution in patients with depression, particularly if suicidal risk may be present. Use with caution in patients with a history of cardiovascular disease (including previous MI, stroke, tachycardia, or conduction abnormalities). The risk conduction abnormalities with this agent is high relative to other antidepressants. Use with caution in hyperthyroid patients or those receiving thyroid supplementation. Use with caution in patients with hepatic or renal dysfunction and in elderly patients.

**Adverse Reactions**

>10%:

Central nervous system: Dizziness, drowsiness, headache, insomnia, nervousness
Endocrine & metabolic: Libido changes
Gastrointestinal: Xerostomia, constipation, increased appetite, nausea, weight gain, dyspepsia, anorexia, abdominal pain
Neuromuscular & skeletal: Fatigue, tremor, myoclonus
Miscellaneous: Increased diaphoresis

1% to 10%:

Cardiovascular: Hypotension, palpitations, tachycardia
Central nervous system: Confusion, hypertonia, sleep disorder, yawning, speech disorder, abnormal dreaming, paresthesia, memory impairment, anxiety, twitching, impaired coordination, agitation, migraine, depersonalization, emotional lability, flushing, fever
Dermatologic: Rash, pruritus, dermatitis
Gastrointestinal: Diarrhea, vomiting
Genitourinary: Difficult urination
Ocular: Blurred vision, eye pain

<1%: Abnormal accommodation, alopecia, breast enlargement, decreased lower esophageal sphincter tone may cause GE reflux, galactorrhea, hyperacusis, increased liver enzymes, marrow depression, photosensitivity, prostatic disorder, seizures, SIADH, trouble with gums

**Overdosage/Toxicology**

Signs and symptoms: Agitation, confusion, hallucinations, urinary retention, hypothermia, hypotension, tachycardia, ventricular tachycardia, seizures, coma

Treatment: Following initiation of essential overdose management, toxic symptoms should be treated; ventricular arrhythmias often respond to systemic alkalinization (sodium bicarbonate 0.5-2 mEq/kg I.V.) and/or phenytoin 15-20 mg/kg (adults). Arrhythmias unresponsive to this therapy may respond to lidocaine 1 mg/kg I.V. followed by a titrated infusion. Physostigmine (1-2 mg I.V. slowly for adults or 0.5 mg I.V. slowly for children) may be indicated in reversing cardiac arrhythmias that are life-threatening. Seizures usually respond to diazepam I.V. boluses (5-10 mg for adults up to 30 mg or 0.25-0.4 mg/kg/dose for children up to 10 mg/dose). If seizures are unresponsive or recur, phenytoin or phenobarbital may be required.

**Drug Interactions** CYP1A2, 2C19, 2D6, and 3A3/4 enzyme substrate; CYP2D6 enzyme inhibitor

Altretamine: Concurrent use may cause orthostatic hypertension
Amphetamines: TCAs may enhance the effect of amphetamines; monitor for adverse CV effects
Anticholinergics: Combined use with TCAs may produce additive anticholinergic effects
Antihypertensives: TCAs inhibit the antihypertensive response to bethanidine, clonidine, debrisoquin, guanadrel, guanethidine, guanabenz, guanfacine; monitor BP; consider alternate antihypertensive agent
Beta-agonists: When combined with TCAs may predispose patients to cardiac arrhythmias
Bupropion: May increase the levels of tricyclic antidepressants; based on limited information; monitor response
Carbamazepine: Tricyclic antidepressants may increase carbamazepine levels; monitor
Cholestyramine and colestipol: May bind TCAs and reduce their absorption; monitor for altered response
Clonidine: Abrupt discontinuation of clonidine may cause hypertensive crisis, amitriptyline may enhance the response
CNS depressants: Sedative effects may be additive with TCAs; monitor for increased effect; includes benzodiazepines, barbiturates, antipsychotics, ethanol, and other sedative medications
CYP2C8/9 inhibitors: Serum levels and/or toxicity of some tricyclic antidepressants may be increased; inhibitors include amiodarone, cimetidine, fluvoxamine, some NSAIDs, metronidazole, ritonavir, sulfonamides, troglitazone, valproic acid, and zafirlukast; monitor for increased effect/toxicity
CYP2D6 inhibitors: Serum levels and/or toxicity of some tricyclic antidepressants may be increased; inhibitors include amiodarone, cimetidine, delavirdine, fluoxetine, paroxetine, propafenone, quinidine, and ritonavir; monitor for increased effect/toxicity
CYP3A3/4 inhibitors: Serum level and/or toxicity of some tricyclic antidepressants may be increased; inhibitors include amiodarone, cimetidine, clarithromycin, erythromycin, delavirdine, diltiazem, dirithromycin, disulfiram, fluoxetine, fluvoxamine, grapefruit juice, indinavir, itraconazole, ketoconazole, nefazodone, nevirapine, propoxyfene, quinupristin-dalfopristin, ritonavir, saquinavir, verapamil, zafirlukast, zileuton; monitor for altered effects; a decrease in TCA dosage may be required
Enzyme inducers: May increase the metabolism of TCAs resulting in decreased effect; includes carbamazepine, phenobarbital, phenytoin, and rifampin; monitor for decreased response
Epinephrine (and other direct alpha-agonists): The pressor response to I.V. epinephrine, norepinephrine, and phenylephrine may be enhanced in patients receiving TCAs; this combination is best avoided
Fenfluramine: May increase tricyclic antidepressant levels/effects
Hypoglycemic agents (including insulin): TCAs may enhance the hypoglycemic effects of tolazamide, chlorpropamide, or insulin; monitor for changes in blood glucose levels; reported with chlorpropamide, tolazamide, and insulin
Levodopa: Tricyclic antidepressants may decrease the absorption (bioavailability) of levodopa; rare hypertensive episodes have also been attributed to this combination

(Continued)

## Clomipramine *(Continued)*

Linezolid: Hyperpyrexia, hypertension, tachycardia, confusion, seizures, and **deaths have been reported** with agents which inhibit MAO (serotonin syndrome); this combination should be avoided

Lithium: Concurrent use with a TCA may increase the risk for neurotoxicity

MAO inhibitors: Hyperpyrexia, hypertension, tachycardia, confusion, seizures, and **deaths have been reported** (serotonin syndrome); this combination should be avoided

Methylphenidate: Metabolism of some TCAs may be decreased

Olanzapine: When used in combination, clomipramine and olanzapine have been reported to be associated with the development of seizures; limited documentation (case report)

Phenothiazines: Serum concentrations of some TCAs may be increased; in addition, TCAs may increase concentration of phenothiazines; monitor for altered clinical response

QTc prolonging agents: Concurrent use of tricyclic agents with other drugs which may prolong QTc interval may increase the risk of potentially fatal arrhythmias; includes type Ia and type III antiarrhythmics agents, selected quinolones (sparfloxacin, gatifloxacin, moxifloxacin, grepafloxacin), cisapride, and other agents

Sucralfate: Absorption of tricyclic antidepressants may be reduced with coadministration

Sympathomimetics, indirect-acting: Tricyclic antidepressants may result in a decreased sensitivity to indirect-acting sympathomimetics; includes dopamine and ephedrine; also see interaction with epinephrine (and direct-acting sympathomimetics)

Valproic acid: May increase serum concentrations/adverse effects of some tricyclic antidepressants

Warfarin (and other oral anticoagulants): TCAs may increase the anticoagulant effect in patients stabilized on warfarin; monitor INR

**Mechanism of Action** Clomipramine appears to affect serotonin uptake while its active metabolite, desmethylclomipramine, affects norepinephrine uptake

**Pharmacodynamics/kinetics**

Absorption: Oral: Rapid

Metabolism: Extensive first-pass metabolism; metabolized to desmethylclomipramine (active) in the liver

Half-life: 20-30 hours

**Usual Dosage** Oral: Initial:

Children: 25 mg/day and gradually increase, as tolerated, to a maximum of 3 mg/kg/day or 200 mg/day, whichever is smaller

Adults: 25 mg/day and gradually increase, as tolerated, to 100 mg/day the first 2 weeks, may then be increased to a total of 250 mg/day maximum

**Administration** Administer initially in divided doses with meals to avoid GI side effects

**Monitoring Parameters** Pulse rate and blood pressure prior to and during therapy; EKG/cardiac status in older adults

**Reference Range** 80-100 ng/mL, 7-14 days to steady-state

**Test Interactions** ↑ glucose

**Patient Information** May cause seizures; caution should be used in activities that require alertness like driving, operating machinery, or swimming; effect of drug may take several weeks to appear

**Nursing Implications** Evaluate mental status

**Additional Information** May also relieve depression, panic attacks and chronic pain

**Dosage Forms** Capsule, as hydrochloride: 25 mg, 50 mg, 75 mg

♦ **Clomipramine Hydrochloride** *see* Clomipramine *on page 131*

♦ **Clomycin® [OTC]** *see* Bacitracin, Neomycin, Polymyxin B, and Lidocaine *on page 57*

## Clonazepam (kloe NA ze pam)

**Related Information**

Agents for Treatment of Extrapyramidal Symptoms *on page 638*
Anticonvulsants by Seizures Type *on page 703*
Anxiety Disorders *on page 606*
Anxiolytic/Hypnotic Use in Long-Term Care Facilities *on page 754*
Benzodiazepines Comparison Chart *on page 708*
Mood Disorders *on page 600*
Patient Information - Anxiolytics & Sedative Hypnotics (Benzodiazepines) *on page 653*
Special Populations - Children and Adolescents *on page 663*
Substance-Related Disorders *on page 609*

**Generic Available** Yes

**U.S. Brand Names** Klonopin™

**Canadian Brand Names** PMS-Clonazepam; Rivotril®

**Pharmacologic Category** Benzodiazepine

**Use** Seizure disorder: Alone or as an adjunct in the treatment of petit mal variant (Lennox-Gastaut), akinetic, and myoclonic seizures; petit mal (absence) seizures unresponsive to succimides; panic disorder with or without agoraphobia

**Unlabeled use:** Restless legs syndrome; neuralgia; multifocal tic disorder; parkinsonian dysarthria; acute manic episodes; adjunct therapy for schizophrenia

**Restrictions** C-IV

**Pregnancy Risk Factor** D

**Pregnancy/Breast-Feeding Implications**

Clinical effects on the fetus: Crosses into breast milk. Two reports of cardiac defects; respiratory depression, lethargy, hypotonia may be observed in newborns exposed near time of delivery. Epilepsy itself, number of medications, genetic factors, or a combination of these probably influence the teratogenicity of anticonvulsant therapy.

Breast-feeding/lactation: Crosses into breast milk

Clinical effects on the infant: CNS depression, respiratory depression reported. The American Academy of Pediatrics has **no recommendation.**

**Contraindications** Hypersensitivity to clonazepam or any component of its formulation (cross-sensitivity with other benzodiazepines may exist); significant liver disease; narrow angle glaucoma; pregnancy

**Warnings/Precautions** Use with caution in elderly or debilitated patients, patients with hepatic disease (including alcoholics), or renal impairment. Use with caution in patients with respiratory disease or impaired gag reflex or ability to protect the airway from secretions (salivation may be increased). Worsening of seizures may occur when added to patients with multiple seizure types. Concurrent use with valproic acid may result in absence status. Monitoring of CBC and liver function tests has been recommended during prolonged therapy.

Causes CNS depression (dose-related) resulting in sedation, dizziness, confusion, or ataxia which may impair physical and mental capabilities. Patients must be cautioned about performing tasks which require mental alertness (ie, operating machinery or driving). Use with caution in patients receiving other CNS depressants or psychoactive agents. Effects with other sedative drugs or ethanol may be potentiated. Benzodiazepines have been associated with falls and traumatic injury and should be used with extreme caution in patients who are at risk of these events (especially the elderly).

Use caution in patients with depression, particularly if suicidal risk may be present. Use with caution in patients with a history of drug dependence. Benzodiazepines have been associated with dependence and acute withdrawal symptoms, including seizures, on discontinuation or reduction in dose. Acute withdrawal, including seizures, may be precipitated in patients after administration of flumazenil to patients receiving long-term benzodiazepine therapy.

Benzodiazepines have been associated with anterograde amnesia. Paradoxical reactions, including hyperactive or aggressive behavior, have been reported with benzodiazepines, particularly in adolescent/pediatric or psychiatric patients. Does not have analgesic, antidepressant, or antipsychotic properties.

**Adverse Reactions**

>10%: Central nervous system: Drowsiness

1% to 10%:

Central nervous system: Dizziness, abnormal coordination, ataxia, dysarthria, depression, memory disturbance, fatigue

Dermatologic: Dermatitis, allergic reactions

Endocrine & metabolic: Decreased libido

Gastrointestinal: Anorexia, constipation, diarrhea, xerostomia

Respiratory: Upper respiratory tract infection, sinusitis, rhinitis, coughing

<1%: Blood dyscrasias, menstrual irregularities

**Overdosage/Toxicology**

Signs and symptoms: Somnolence, confusion, ataxia, diminished reflexes, or coma

Treatment: Supportive. Rarely is mechanical ventilation required.

Flumazenil has been shown to selectively block the binding of benzodiazepines to CNS receptors, resulting in a reversal of benzodiazepine-induced CNS depression, but not respiratory depression

**Drug Interactions** CYP3A3/4 enzyme substrate

CNS depressants: Sedative effects and/or respiratory depression may be additive with CNS depressants; includes ethanol, barbiturates, narcotic analgesics, and other sedative agents; monitor for increased effect

Enzyme inducers: Metabolism of some benzodiazepines may be increased, decreasing their therapeutic effect; consider using an alternative sedative/hypnotic agent; potential inducers include phenobarbital, phenytoin, carbamazepine, rifampin, and rifabutin

CYP3A3/4 inhibitors: Serum level and/or toxicity of some benzodiazepines may be increased; inhibitors include amiodarone, cimetidine, clarithromycin, erythromycin, delavirdine, diltiazem, dirithromycin, disulfiram, fluoxetine, fluvoxamine, grapefruit juice, indinavir, itraconazole, ketoconazole, nevirapine, propoxyfene, quinupristin-dalfopristin, ritonavir, saquinavir, verapamil, zafirlukast, zileuton; monitor for altered benzodiazepine response

Disulfiram: Disulfiram may inhibit the metabolism of clonazepam; monitor for increased benzodiazepine effect

Oral contraceptives: May decrease the clearance of some benzodiazepines (those which undergo oxidative metabolism); monitor for increased benzodiazepine effect

Theophylline: May partially antagonize some of the effects of benzodiazepines; monitor for decreased response; may require higher doses for sedation

Valproic acid: The combined use of clonazepam and valproic acid has been associated with absence seizures

**Mechanism of Action** The exact mechanism is unknown, but believed to be related to its ability to enhance the activity of GABA; suppresses the spike-and-wave discharge in absence seizures by depressing nerve transmission in the motor cortex

**Pharmacodynamics/kinetics**

Onset of effect: 20-60 minutes

Duration: Up to 6-8 hours in infants and young children, up to 12 hours in adults

Absorption: Oral: Well absorbed

Distribution: Adults: $V_d$: 1.5-4.4 L/kg

Protein binding: 85%

Metabolism: Extensive; glucuronide and sulfate conjugation

Half-life:

Children: 22-33 hours

Adults: 19-50 hours

Time to peak serum concentration: Oral: 1-3 hours

Steady-state: 5-7 days

Elimination: <2% excreted unchanged in urine; metabolites excreted as glucuronide or sulfate conjugates

**Usual Dosage** Oral:

Children <10 years or 30 kg:

Initial daily dose: 0.01-0.03 mg/kg/day (maximum: 0.05 mg/kg/day) given in 2-3 divided doses; increase by no more than 0.5 mg every third day until seizures are controlled or adverse effects seen

Usual maintenance dose: 0.1-0.2 mg/kg/day divided 3 times/day; not to exceed 0.2 mg/kg/day

Adults:

Initial daily dose not to exceed 1.5 mg given in 3 divided doses; may increase by 0.5-1 mg every third day until seizures are controlled or adverse effects seen

Usual maintenance dose: 0.05-0.2 mg/kg; do not exceed 20 mg/day

Hemodialysis: Supplemental dose is not necessary

**Dietary Considerations** Alcohol: Additive CNS depression has been reported with benzodiazepines; avoid or limit alcohol

**Monitoring Parameters** CBC, liver function tests

**Reference Range** Therapeutic: 5-70 ng/mL; Toxic: >80 ng/mL; Timing of serum sample: Peak serum levels occur 1-3 hours after oral ingestion; steady-state occurs in 5-7 days

**Patient Information** Avoid alcohol and other CNS depressants; avoid activities needing good psychomotor coordination until CNS effects are known; drug may cause physical or psychological dependence; avoid abrupt discontinuation after prolonged use

**Nursing Implications** Observe patient for excess sedation, respiratory depression; raise bed rails, initiate safety measures, assist with ambulation

**Additional Information** Ethosuximide or valproic acid may be preferred for treatment of absence (petit mal) seizures; clonazepam-induced behavioral disturbances may be more frequent in mentally handicapped patients

**Dosage Forms** Tablet: 0.5 mg, 1 mg, 2 mg

## Clonidine (KLOE ni deen)

**Related Information**

Addiction Treatments *on page 772*
Agents for Treatment of Extrapyramidal Symptoms *on page 638*
Clozapine-Induced Side Effects *on page 780*
Special Populations - Children and Adolescents *on page 663*
Substance-Related Disorders *on page 609*

**Generic Available** Yes: Tablet

**U.S. Brand Names** Catapres® Oral; Catapres-TTS® Transdermal; Duraclon®

**Canadian Brand Names** Apo®-Clonidine; Dixarit®; Novo-Clonidine; Nu-Clonidine

**Synonyms** Clonidine Hydrochloride

**Pharmacologic Category** $Alpha_2$ Agonist

**Use** Management of mild to moderate hypertension; either used alone or in combination with other antihypertensives

**Unlabeled use:** Heroin or nicotine withdrawal; severe pain; prophylaxis of migraines, glaucoma, and diabetes-associated diarrhea, impulse control disorder, ADHD, clozapine-induced diarrhea

**Effects on Mental Status** Drowsiness is common

**Effects on Psychiatric Treatment** Dry mouth, orthostatic hypotension, and sedation may be increased with concurrent psychotropic use; used to treat clozapine-induced sialorrhea; TCAs may antagonize clonidine's hypotensive effect

**Pregnancy Risk Factor** C

**Pregnancy/Breast-Feeding Implications**

Clinical effects on the fetus: Crosses the placenta. Caution should be used with this drug due to the potential of rebound hypertension with abrupt discontinuation.

Breast-feeding/lactation: Crosses into breast milk. American Academy of Pediatrics has **no recommendation.**

**Contraindications** Hypersensitivity to clonidine hydrochloride or any component

**Warnings/Precautions** Use with caution in cerebrovascular disease, coronary insufficiency, renal impairment, sinus node dysfunction; do not abruptly discontinue (rapid increase in blood pressure, and symptoms of sympathetic overactivity, ie, increased heart rate, tremor, agitation, anxiety, insomnia, sweating, palpitations) may occur; **if need to discontinue, taper dose gradually over 1 week or more (2-4 days with epidural product)**; adjust dosage in patients with renal dysfunction (especially the elderly); not recommended for obstetrical, postpartum or perioperative pain management or in those with severe hemodynamic instability due to unacceptable risk of hypotension and bradycardia; clonidine injection should be administered via a continuous epidural infusion device

**Adverse Reactions**

>10%:

Central nervous system: Drowsiness, dizziness

Gastrointestinal: Xerostomia

1% to 10%:

Cardiovascular: Chest pain, orthostatic hypotension, palpitations, tachycardia, bradycardia, EKG abnormalities

Central nervous system: Mental depression, headache, fatigue, nervousness, agitation, insomnia

Dermatologic: Rash

Endocrine & metabolic: Decreased sexual activity, loss of libido

Gastrointestinal: vomiting, constipation, nausea, anorexia, malaise, weight gain

Genitourinary: Nocturia, impotence

Neuromuscular & skeletal: Weakness

<1%: Abdominal pain, abnormal liver function tests, alopecia, anxiety, blurred vision, burning eyes, congestive heart failure, constipation, delirium, micturition difficulty, nightmares, pruritus, Raynaud's phenomenon, restlessness, syncope, thrombocytopenia, urinary retention, urticaria, visual and auditory hallucinations, vivid dreams

**Overdosage/Toxicology**

Signs and symptoms: Bradycardia, CNS depression, hypothermia, diarrhea, respiratory depression, apnea

Treatment: Primarily supportive and symptomatic. Hypotension usually responds to I.V. fluids or Trendelenburg positioning. If unresponsive to these measures, the use of a parenteral vasoconstrictor may be required (eg, norepinephrine 0.1-0.2 mcg/kg/minute titrated to response). Naloxone may be utilized in treating the CNS depression and/or apnea and should be given I.V. 0.4-2 mg, with repeats as needed. Atropine 15 mcg/kg I.V. or may be needed for symptomatic bradycardia.

**Drug Interactions**

Antipsychotics: Concurrent use with antipsychotics (especially low potency) or nitroprusside may produce additive hypotensive effects

Beta-blockers: May potentiate bradycardia in patients receiving clonidine and may increase the rebound hypertension of withdrawal; discontinue beta-blocker several days before clonidine is tapered

CNS depressants: Sedative effects may be additive; monitor for increased effect; includes barbiturates, benzodiazepines, narcotic analgesics, ethanol, and other sedative agents

Cyclosporine: Clonidine may increase cyclosporine (and perhaps tacrolimus) serum concentrations; cyclosporine dosage adjustment may be needed

Hypoglycemic agents: Clonidine may decrease the symptoms of hypoglycemia; monitor patients receiving antidiabetic agents

Levodopa: Effects may be reduced by clonidine in some patients with Parkinson's disease (limited documentation); monitor

Local anesthetics: Epidural clonidine may prolong the sensory and motor blockade of local anesthetics

Mirtazapine: Antihypertensive effects of clonidine may be antagonized by mirtazapine (hypertensive urgency has been reported following addition of mirtazapine to clonidine); in addition, mirtazapine may potentially enhance the hypertensive response associated with abrupt clonidine withdrawal. Avoid this combination; consider an alternative agent.

Narcotic analgesics: May potentiate hypotensive effects of clonidine

Tricyclic antidepressants: Antihypertensive effects of clonidine may be antagonized by tricyclic antidepressants; in addition, tricyclic antidepressants may enhance the hypertensive response associated with abrupt clonidine withdrawal; avoid this combination; consider an alternative agent

Verapamil: Concurrent administration may be associated with hypotension and AV block in some patients (limited documentation); monitor

**Mechanism of Action** Stimulates $alpha_2$-adrenoceptors in the brain stem, thus activating an inhibitory neuron, resulting in reduced sympathetic outflow from the CNS, producing a decrease in peripheral resistance, renal vascular resistance, heart rate, and blood pressure; epidural clonidine may produce pain relief at spinal presynaptic and postjunctional $alpha_2$-adrenoceptors by preventing pain signal transmission; pain relief occurs only for the body regions innervated by the spinal segments where analgesic concentrations of clonidine exist

**Pharmacodynamics/kinetics**

Onset of effect: Oral: 0.5-1 hour; $T_{max}$: 2-4 hours

(Continued)

## Clonidine *(Continued)*

Duration: 6-10 hours

Distribution: $V_d$: 2.1 L/kg (adults); highly lipid soluble; distributes readily into extravascular sites; protein binding: 20% to 40%

Metabolism: Hepatic (enterohepatic recirculation); extensively metabolized to inactive metabolites

Bioavailability: 75% to 95%

Half-life: Adults:

Normal renal function: 6-20 hours

Renal impairment: 18-41 hours

Elimination: 65% excreted in urine, 32% unchanged, and 22% excreted in feces; not removed significantly by hemodialysis

**Usual Dosage**

Oral:

Children: Initial: 5-10 mcg/kg/day in divided doses every 8-12 hours; increase gradually at 5- to 7-day intervals to 25 mcg/kg/day in divided doses every 6 hours; maximum: 0.9 mg/day

Clonidine tolerance test (test of growth hormone release from pituitary): 0.15 mg/m² or 4 mcg/kg as single dose

Adults: Initial dose: 0.1 mg twice daily, usual maintenance dose: 0.2-1.2 mg/day in 2-4 divided doses; maximum recommended dose: 2.4 mg/day

Nicotine withdrawal symptoms: 0.1 mg twice daily to maximum of 0.4 mg/day for 3-4 weeks

Elderly: Initial: 0.1 mg once daily at bedtime, increase gradually as needed

Transdermal: Apply once every 7 days; for initial therapy start with 0.1 mg and increase by 0.1 mg at 1- to 2-week intervals; dosages >0.6 mg do not improve efficacy

Epidural infusion: Starting dose: 30 mcg/hour; titrate as required for relief of pain or presence of side effects; minimal experience with doses >40 mcg/hour; should be considered an adjunct to intraspinal opiate therapy

**Dosing adjustment in renal impairment:** $Cl_{cr}$ <10 mL/minute: Administer 50% to 75% of normal dose initially

Dialysis: Not dialyzable (0% to 5%) via hemo- or peritoneal dialysis; supplemental dose not necessary

**Administration** Catapres-TTS® comes in two parts - the small patch containing the drug and an overlay to keep the patch in place for 1 week; both parts should be used for maximum efficacy; it may be useful to note on the patch which day it should be changed

**Monitoring Parameters** Blood pressure, standing and sitting/supine, mental status, heart rate

**Reference Range** Therapeutic: 1-2 ng/mL (SI: 4.4-8.7 nmol/L)

**Test Interactions** ↑ sodium (S); ↓ catecholamines (U)

**Patient Information** Do not discontinue drug except on instruction of physician; check daily to be sure patch is present; may cause drowsiness, impaired coordination, and judgment

**Nursing Implications** Patches should be applied weekly at bedtime to a clean, hairless area of the upper outer arm or chest; rotate patch sites weekly; redness under patch may be reduced if a topical corticosteroid spray is applied to the area before placement of the patch; if needed, gradually reduce dose over 2-4 days to avoid rebound hypertension

**Additional Information** Transdermal clonidine should only be used in patients unable to take oral medication; the transdermal product is much more expensive than oral clonidine and produces no better therapeutic effects

**Dosage Forms**

Injection, preservative free, as hydrochloride: 100 mcg/mL (10 mL); 500 mcg/mL (10 mL)

Patch, transdermal, as hydrochloride: 1, 2, and 3 (0.1, 0.2, 0.3 mg/day, 7-day duration)

Tablet, as hydrochloride: 0.1 mg, 0.2 mg, 0.3 mg

## Clonidine and Chlorthalidone

(KLOE ni deen & klor THAL i done)

**U.S. Brand Names** Combipres®

**Pharmacologic Category** Antihypertensive Agent, Combination

**Use** Management of mild to moderate hypertension

**Effects on Mental Status** Drowsiness is common

**Effects on Psychiatric Treatment** Dry mouth, orthostatic hypotension, and sedation may be increased with concurrent psychotropic use; TCAs may antagonize clonidine's hypotensive effect; rare reports of blood dyscrasias; use caution with clozapine and carbamazepine; thiazides decrease lithium clearance resulting in elevated serum lithium levels and potential toxicity; monitor serum lithium levels

**Usual Dosage** Oral: 1 tablet 1-2 times/day

**Dosage Forms** Tablet:

0.1: Clonidine 0.1 mg and chlorthalidone 15 mg

0.2: Clonidine 0.2 mg and chlorthalidone 15 mg

0.3: Clonidine 0.3 mg and chlorthalidone 15 mg

♦ **Clonidine Hydrochloride** *see* Clonidine *on page 133*

## Clopidogrel (kloh PID oh grel)

**U.S. Brand Names** Plavix®

**Pharmacologic Category** Antiplatelet Agent

**Use** Reduce atherosclerotic events (myocardial infarction, stroke, vascular deaths) in patients with atherosclerosis documented by recent myocardial infarction, recent stroke, or established peripheral arterial disease; prevention of thrombotic complications after coronary stenting

**Effects on Mental Status** None reported

**Effects on Psychiatric Treatment** Rarely may produce neutropenia; use caution with clozapine and carbamazepine

**Pregnancy Risk Factor** B

**Contraindications** Hypersensitivity to clopidogrel or any component; active pathological bleeding such as PUD or intracranial hemorrhage; coagulation disorders

**Warnings/Precautions** Use with caution in patients who may be at risk of increased bleeding. Consider discontinuing 7 days before elective surgery. Use caution in mixing with other antiplatelet drugs. Use with caution in patients with severe liver disease (experience is limited). Cases of thrombotic thrombocytopenic purpura (usually occurring within the first 2 weeks of therapy) have been reported.

**Adverse Reactions**

>10%: Gastrointestinal: Indigestion, nausea, vomiting (15%)

1% to 10%:

Dermatologic: Rash (4.2%), pruritus (3.3%)

Gastrointestinal: Diarrhea (4.5%), GI hemorrhage (2%)

Hepatic: Liver function test abnormalities (<3%) (0.11% discontinued)

<1%: Intracranial bleeding (0.35%), neutropenia (0.1%), prolonged bleeding time

**Overdosage/Toxicology**

Signs and symptoms: Vomiting, prostration, difficulty breathing, and gastrointestinal hemorrhage. Only one case of overdose with clopidogrel has been reported to date, no symptoms were reported with this case and no specific treatments were required.

Treatment: Based on its pharmacology, platelet transfusions may be an appropriate treatment when attempting to reverse the effects of clopidogrel. After decontamination, treatment is symptomatic and supportive.

**Drug Interactions** CYP2C9 inhibitor

Substrates of CYP2C9 (including phenytoin, tamoxifen, tolbutamide, torsemide, fluvastatin, losartan, irbesartan, valsartan, and many NSAIDs) may have increased blood levels during concomitant therapy with clopidogrel. However, these combinations have not been investigated. Use caution during concomitant administration.

Anticoagulants or other antiplatelet agents may increase the risk of bleeding

Warfarin metabolism may be decreased due to clopidogrel inhibition of CYP2C9. Hypoprothrombinemic effects may be increased; monitor INR carefully during initiation or withdrawal.

**Usual Dosage** Adults: Oral: 75 mg once daily

**Dosing adjustment in renal impairment and elderly:** None necessary

**Dietary Considerations** Food: May be taken without regard to meals

**Patient Information** Take as directed. May cause headache or dizziness; use caution when driving or engaging in tasks that require alertness until response to drug is known. Small frequent meals, frequent mouth care, sucking lozenges, or chewing gum may reduce nausea or vomiting. Mild analgesics may reduce arthralgia or back pain. Report immediately unusual or acute chest pain or respiratory difficulties, skin rash, unresolved diarrhea or gastrointestinal distress, nosebleed, or acute headache.

**Dosage Forms** Tablet, as bisulfate: 75 mg

♦ **Cloranfenicol** *see* Chloramphenicol *on page 109*

## Clorazepate (klor AZ e pate)

**Related Information**

Anxiolytic/Hypnotic Use in Long-Term Care Facilities *on page 754*

Benzodiazepines Comparison Chart *on page 708*

Federal OBRA Regulations Recommended Maximum Doses *on page 756*

Patient Information - Anxiolytics & Sedative Hypnotics (Benzodiazepines) *on page 653*

**Generic Available** Yes

**U.S. Brand Names** Gen-XENE®; Tranxene®

**Canadian Brand Names** Apo®-Clorazepate; Novo-Clopate

**Synonyms** Clorazepate Dipotassium

**Pharmacologic Category** Benzodiazepine

**Use** Treatment of generalized anxiety disorder; management of alcohol withdrawal; adjunct anticonvulsant in management of partial seizures

**Restrictions** C-IV

**Pregnancy Risk Factor** D

**Contraindications** Hypersensitivity to this drug or any component of its formulation (cross-sensitivity with other benzodiazepines may exist); narrow angle glaucoma; lactation; pregnancy

**Warnings/Precautions** Not recommended for use in patients <9 years of age or patients with depressive or psychotic disorders. Use with caution in elderly or debilitated patients, patients with hepatic disease (including alcoholics), or renal impairment. Active metabolites with extended half-lives may lead to delayed accumulation and adverse effects. Use with caution in patients with respiratory disease or impaired gag reflex. Use is not recommended in patients with depressive disorders or psychoses. Avoid use in patients with sleep apnea.

Causes CNS depression (dose-related) resulting in sedation, dizziness, confusion, or ataxia which may impair physical and mental capabilities. Patients must be cautioned about performing tasks which require mental alertness (ie, operating machinery or driving). Use with caution in patients receiving other CNS depressants or psychoactive agents. Effects with other sedative drugs or ethanol may be potentiated. Benzodiazepines have been associated with falls and traumatic injury and should be used with extreme caution in patients who are at risk of these events (especially the elderly).

Use caution in patients with depression, particularly if suicidal risk may be present. Use with caution in patients with a history of drug dependence. Benzodiazepines have been associated with dependence and acute withdrawal symptoms on discontinuation or reduction in dose. Acute withdrawal, including seizures, may be precipitated in patients after administration of flumazenil to patients receiving long-term benzodiazepine therapy.

Benzodiazepines have been associated with anterograde amnesia. Paradoxical reactions, including hyperactive or aggressive behavior, have been reported with benzodiazepines, particularly in adolescent/pediatric or psychiatric patients. Does not have analgesic, antidepressant, or antipsychotic properties.

**Adverse Reactions**

Cardiovascular: Hypotension

Central nervous system: Drowsiness, fatigue, ataxia, lightheadedness, memory impairment, insomnia, anxiety, headache, depression, slurred speech, confusion, nervousness, dizziness, irritability

Dermatologic: Rash

Endocrine & metabolic: Decreased libido

Gastrointestinal: Xerostomia, constipation, diarrhea, decreased salivation, nausea, vomiting, increased or decreased appetite

Neuromuscular & skeletal: Dysarthria, tremor

Ocular: Blurred vision, diplopia

**Overdosage/Toxicology**

Signs and symptoms: Somnolence, confusion, ataxia, diminished reflexes, coma

Treatment: Supportive; rarely is mechanical ventilation required

Flumazenil has been shown to selectively block the binding of benzodiazepines to CNS receptors, resulting in a reversal of benzodiazepine-induced CNS depression, but not respiratory depression

**Drug Interactions** CYP3A3/4 enzyme substrate

CNS depressants: Sedative effects and/or respiratory depression may be additive with CNS depressants; includes ethanol, barbiturates, narcotic analgesics, and other sedative agents; monitor for increased effect

Enzyme inducers: Metabolism of some benzodiazepines may be increased, decreasing their therapeutic effect; consider using an alternative sedative/hypnotic agent; potential inducers include phenobarbital, phenytoin, carbamazepine, rifampin, and rifabutin

CYP3A3/4 inhibitors: Serum level and/or toxicity of some benzodiazepines may be increased; inhibitors include amiodarone, cimetidine, clarithromycin, erythromycin, delavirdine, diltiazem, dirithromycin, disulfiram, fluoxetine, fluvoxamine, grapefruit juice, indinavir, itraconazole, ketoconazole, nefazodone, nevirapine, propoxyfene, quinupristin-dalfopristin, ritonavir, saquinavir, verapamil, zafirlukast, zileuton; monitor for altered benzodiazepine response

Oral contraceptives: May decrease the clearance of some benzodiazepines (those which undergo oxidative metabolism); monitor for increased benzodiazepine effect

Theophylline: May partially antagonize some of the effects of benzodiazepines; monitor for decreased response; may require higher doses for sedation

**Stability** Unstable in water

**Mechanism of Action** Binds to stereospecific benzodiazepine receptors on the postsynaptic GABA neuron at several sites within the central nervous system, including the limbic system, reticular formation. Enhancement of the inhibitory effect of GABA on neuronal excitability results by increased neuronal membrane permeability to chloride ions. This shift in chloride ions results in hyperpolarization (a less excitable state) and stabilization.

**Pharmacodynamics/kinetics**

Distribution: Crosses the placenta; appears in urine

Metabolism: Rapidly decarboxylated to desmethyldiazepam (active) in acidic stomach prior to absorption; metabolized in the liver to oxazepam (active)

Half-life: Adults:

Desmethyldiazepam: 48-96 hours

Oxazepam: 6-8 hours

Time to peak serum concentration: Oral: Within 1 hour

Elimination: Primarily in urine

**Usual Dosage** Oral:

Children 9-12 years: Anticonvulsant: Initial: 3.75-7.5 mg/dose twice daily; increase dose by 3.75 mg at weekly intervals, not to exceed 60 mg/day in 2-3 divided doses

Children >12 years and Adults: Anticonvulsant: Initial: Up to 7.5 mg/dose 2-3 times/day; increase dose by 7.5 mg at weekly intervals; not to exceed 90 mg/day

Adults:

Anxiety: 7.5-15 mg 2-4 times/day, or given as single dose of 11.25 or 22.5 mg at bedtime

Alcohol withdrawal: Initial: 30 mg, then 15 mg 2-4 times/day on first day; maximum daily dose: 90 mg; gradually decrease dose over subsequent days

**Dietary Considerations** Alcohol: Additive CNS effects, avoid use

**Monitoring Parameters** Respiratory and cardiovascular status, excess CNS depression

**Reference Range** Therapeutic: 0.12-1 μg/mL (SI: 0.36-3.01 μmol/L)

**Test Interactions** ↓ hematocrit, abnormal liver and renal function tests

**Patient Information** Avoid alcohol and other CNS depressants; avoid activities needing good psychomotor coordination until CNS effects are known; drug may cause physical or psychological dependence; avoid abrupt discontinuation after prolonged use

**Nursing Implications** Observe patient for excess sedation, respiratory depression; raise bed rails, initiate safety measures, assist with ambulation

**Additional Information** Abrupt discontinuation after sustained use (generally >10 days) may cause withdrawal symptoms

**Dosage Forms**

Capsule, as dipotassium: 3.75 mg, 7.5 mg, 15 mg

Tablet, as dipotassium: 3.75 mg, 7.5 mg, 15 mg

Tablet, as dipotassium, single dose: 11.25 mg, 22.5 mg

♦ **Clorazepate Dipotassium** *see* Clorazepate *on page 134*

♦ **Clorpactin® WCS-90** *see* Oxychlorosene *on page 413*

## Clotrimazole (kloe TRIM a zole)

**U.S. Brand Names** Femizole-7® [OTC]; Gyne-Lotrimin® [OTC]; Lotrimin®; Lotrimin® AF Cream [OTC]; Lotrimin® AF Lotion [OTC]; Lotrimin® AF Solution [OTC]; Mycelex®; Mycelex®-7; Mycelex®-G

**Canadian Brand Names** Canesten®; Clotrimaderm®; Myclo-Derm®; Myclo-Gyne®

**Pharmacologic Category** Antifungal Agent, Oral Nonabsorbed; Antifungal Agent, Topical; Antifungal Agent, Vaginal

**Use** Treatment of susceptible fungal infections, including oropharyngeal, candidiasis, dermatophytoses, superficial mycoses, and cutaneous candidiasis, as well as vulvovaginal candidiasis; limited data suggest that clotrimazole troches may be effective for prophylaxis against oropharyngeal candidiasis in neutropenic patients

**Effects on Mental Status** None reported

**Effects on Psychiatric Treatment** None reported

**Usual Dosage**

Children >3 years and Adults:

Oral:

Prophylaxis: 10 mg troche dissolved 3 times/day for the duration of chemotherapy or until steroids are reduced to maintenance levels

Treatment: 10 mg troche dissolved slowly 5 times/day for 14 consecutive days

Topical: Apply twice daily; if no improvement occurs after 4 weeks of therapy, re-evaluate diagnosis

Children >12 years and Adults:

Vaginal:

Cream: Insert 1 applicatorful of 1% vaginal cream daily (preferably at bedtime) for 7 consecutive days

Tablet: Insert 100 mg/day for 7 days or 500 mg single dose

Topical: Apply to affected area twice daily (morning and evening) for 7 consecutive days

**Dosage Forms**

Combination pack (Mycelex®-7): Vaginal tablet 100 mg (7s) and vaginal cream 1% (7 g)

Cream:

Topical (Lotrimin®, Lotrimin® AF, Mycelex®, Mycelex® OTC) : 1% (15 g, 30 g, 45 g, 90 g)

Vaginal (Femizole-7®, Gyne-Lotrimin®, Mycelex®-G): 1% (45 g, 90 g)

Lotion (Lotrimin®): 1% (30 mL)

Solution, topical (Fungoid®, Lotrimin®, Lotrimin® AF, Mycelex®, Mycelex® OTC): 1% (10 mL, 30 mL)

Tablet, vaginal (Gyne-Lotrimin®, Gynix®, Mycelex®-G): 100 mg (7s); 500 mg (1s)

Troche (Mycelex®): 10 mg

Twin pack (Mycelex®): Vaginal tablet 500 mg (1s) and vaginal cream 1% (7 g)

## Cloxacillin (kloks a SIL in)

**U.S. Brand Names** Cloxapen®; Tegopen®

**Canadian Brand Names** Apo®-Cloxi; Novo-Cloxin; Nu-Cloxi; Orbenin®; Taro-Cloxacillin®

**Pharmacologic Category** Antibiotic, Penicillin

**Use** Treatment of susceptible bacterial infections, notably penicillinase-producing staphylococci causing respiratory tract, skin and skin structure, bone and joint, urinary tract infections

**Effects on Mental Status** Penicillins have been reported to cause apprehension, illusions, agitation, insomnia, depersonalization, and encephalopathy

**Effects on Psychiatric Treatment** Rare reports of agranulocytosis; use caution with clozapine and carbamazepine

**Usual Dosage** Oral:

Children >1 month (<20 kg): 50-100 mg/kg/day in divided doses every 6 hours; up to a maximum of 4 g/day

Children (>20 kg) and Adults: 250-500 mg every 6 hours

Hemodialysis: Not dialyzable (0% to 5%)

**Dosage Forms**

Capsule, as sodium: 250 mg, 500 mg

Powder for oral suspension, as sodium: 125 mg/5 mL (100 mL, 200 mL)

♦ **Cloxapen®** *see* Cloxacillin *on page 136*

## Clozapine (KLOE za peen)

**Related Information**

Antipsychotic Agents Comparison Chart *on page 706*
Antipsychotic Medication Guidelines *on page 751*
Atypical Antipsychotics *on page 707*
Clinical Issues in the Use of Antipsychotics *on page 630*
Clozapine-Induced Side Effects *on page 780*
Discontinuation of Psychotropic Drugs - Withdrawal Symptoms and Recommendations *on page 798*
Federal OBRA Regulations Recommended Maximum Doses *on page 756*
Patient Information - Antipsychotics (Clozapine) *on page 648*
Schizophrenia *on page 604*
Special Populations - Children and Adolescents *on page 663*
Substance-Related Disorders *on page 609*
Teratogenic Risks of Psychotropic Medications *on page 812*

**Generic Available** Yes: Capsule

**U.S. Brand Names** Clozaril®

**Pharmacologic Category** Antipsychotic Agent, Dibenzodiazepine

**Use** Management of treatment of refractory schizophrenia

**Unlabeled uses:** Schizoaffective disorder; bipolar disorder; psychosis

**Pregnancy Risk Factor** B

**Contraindications** Hypersensitivity to clozapine or any component of the formulation; history of agranulocytosis or granulocytopenia with clozapine; uncontrolled epilepsy; severe central nervous system depression or comatose state; myeloproliferative disorders or use with other agents which have a well-known risk of agranulocytosis or bone marrow suppression

In patients with WBC ≤3500 cells/mm³ before therapy; if WBC falls to <3000 cells/mm³ during therapy the drug should be withheld until signs and symptoms of infection disappear and WBC rises to >3000 cells/mm³

**Warnings/Precautions** Medication should not be stopped abruptly; taper off over 1-2 weeks. WBC testing should occur weekly for the first 6 months of therapy; thereafter, if acceptable, WBC counts are maintained (WBC >3000/mm³, ANC >1500/mm³) then WBC counts can be monitored every other week. WBCs must be monitored weekly for the first 4 weeks after therapy discontinuation. Significant risk of agranulocytosis, potentially life-threatening. Use with caution in patients receiving other marrow suppressive agents. Elderly patients are more susceptible to adverse effects (including cardiovascular, anticholinergic, and tardive dyskinesia).

Cognitive and/or motor impairment (sedation) is common with clozapine, resulting in impaired performance of tasks requiring alertness (ie, operating machinery or driving).

May cause orthostatic hypotension and tachycardia; use with caution in patients at risk of hypotension or in patients where transient hypotensive episodes would be poorly tolerated (cardiovascular disease or cerebrovascular disease). Concurrent use of psychotropics and benzodiazepines may increase the risk of severe cardiopulmonary reactions. Use with caution in patients at risk of seizures, including those with a history of seizures, head trauma, brain damage, alcoholism, or concurrent therapy with medications which may lower seizure threshold.

Has been associated with benign, self-limiting fever (<100.4 F, usually within first three weeks). However, clozapine may also be associated with severe febrile reactions, including neuroleptic malignant syndrome (NMS). Clozapine's potential for extrapyramidal reactions appears to be extremely low.

May cause anticholinergic effects; use with caution in patients with urinary retention, benign prostatic hypertrophy, narrow-angle glaucoma, xerostomia, visual problems, constipation, or history of bowel obstruction.

Eosinophilia has been reported to occur with clozapine and may require temporary or permanent interruption of therapy. Pulmonary embolism has been associated with clozapine therapy. May cause hyperglycemia - use with caution in patients with diabetes or other disorders of glucose regulation. Use with caution in patients with hepatic disease or impairment - hepatitis has been reported as a consequence of therapy.

Rare cases of thromboembolism, including pulmonary embolism and stroke resulting in fatalities, have been associated with clozapine.

**Adverse Reactions**

>10%:

Cardiovascular: Tachycardia

Central nervous system: Drowsiness, dizziness

Gastrointestinal: Constipation, unusual weight gain, diarrhea, sialorrhea

Genitourinary: Urinary incontinence

1% to 10%:

Cardiovascular: EKG changes, hypertension, hypotension, syncope

Central nervous system: Akathisia, seizures, headache, nightmares, akinesia, confusion, insomnia, fatigue, myoclonic jerks

Dermatologic: Rash

Gastrointestinal: Abdominal discomfort, heartburn, xerostomia, nausea, vomiting

Hematologic: Eosinophilia, leukopenia

Neuromuscular & skeletal: Tremor

Miscellaneous: Diaphoresis (increased), fever

<1%: Agranulocytosis, arrhythmias, blurred vision, congestive heart failure, difficult urination, granulocytopenia, impotence, myocardial infarction, myocarditis, neuroleptic malignant syndrome, pericardial effusion, pericarditis, rigidity, tardive dyskinesia, thrombocytopenia, thromboembolism, pulmonary embolism, stroke

**Overdosage/Toxicology**

Signs and symptoms: Altered states of consciousness, tachycardia, hypotension, hypersalivation, respiratory depression

Treatment:

Following initiation of essential overdose management, toxic symptom treatment and supportive treatment should be initiated

Hypotension usually responds to I.V. fluids or Trendelenburg positioning. If unresponsive to these measures, the use of a parenteral inotrope may be required

Seizures commonly respond to diazepam (I.V. 5-10 mg bolus in adults every 15 minutes if needed up to a total of 30 mg; I.V. 0.25-0.4 mg/kg/dose up to a total of 10 mg in children) or to phenytoin or phenobarbital; in situations where clozapine is to be continued, valproate is the anticonvulsant of choice

Also critical cardiac arrhythmias often respond to I.V. phenytoin (15 mg/kg up to 1 g), while other antiarrhythmics can be used

Neuroleptics often cause extrapyramidal symptoms (eg, dystonic reactions) requiring management with benztropine mesylate I.V. 1-2 mg (adults) may be effective. These agents are generally effective within 2-5 minutes.

**Drug Interactions** CYP1A2, 2C (minor), 2D6 (minor), 2E1, 3A3/4 enzyme substrate

Benzodiazepines: In combination with clozapine may produce respiratory depression and hypotension, especially during the first few weeks of therapy; monitor for altered response

Carbamazepine: A case of neuroleptic malignant syndrome has been reported in combination with clozapine; in addition, carbamazepine may alter clozapine levels (see enzyme inducers); monitor

CYP enzyme inducers: Metabolism of clozapine may be increased, decreasing its therapeutic effect; potential inducers include phenobarbital, phenytoin, carbamazepine, rifampin, rifabutin, and cigarette smoking

CYP1A2 inhibitors: Serum level and/or toxicity of clozapine may be increased; inhibitors include cimetidine, ciprofloxacin, fluvoxamine, isoniazid, ritonavir, and zileutin; monitor for altered effects; a decrease in clozapine dosage may be required

CYP2E1 inhibitors: Serum level and/or toxicity of clozapine may be increased; inhibitors include disulfiram and ritonavir; monitor for altered effects; a decrease in clozapine dosage may be required

CYP3A3/4 inhibitors: Serum level and/or toxicity of clozapine may be increased; inhibitors include amiodarone, cimetidine, clarithromycin, erythromycin, delavirdine, diltiazem, dirithromycin, disulfiram, fluoxetine, fluvoxamine, grapefruit juice, indinavir, itraconazole, ketoconazole, metronidazole, nefazodone, nevirapine, propoxyfene, quinupristin-dalfopristin, ritonavir, saquinavir, verapamil, zafirlukast, zileuton; monitor for altered effects; a decrease in clozapine dosage may be required

Epinephrine: Clozapine may reverse the pressor effect of epinephrine

Risperidone: Effects and/or toxicity may be increased when combined with clozapine; monitor

Valproic acid: May cause reductions in clozapine concentrations; monitor for altered response

**Mechanism of Action** Clozapine is a weak dopamine$_1$ and dopamine$_2$ receptor blocker, but blocks $D_1$-$D_5$ receptors; in addition, it blocks the serotonin$_2$, alpha-adrenergic, histamine $H_1$, and cholinergic receptors

**Pharmacodynamics/kinetics**

Protein binding: 95% bound to serum proteins

Metabolism: Undergoes extensive metabolism primarily to unconjugated forms

Half-life: 12 hours

Elimination: In urine

**Usual Dosage** Adults: Oral: 25 mg once or twice daily initially and increased, as tolerated to a target dose of 300-450 mg/day after 2-4 weeks, but may require doses as high as 600-900 mg/day

**Dietary Considerations** May be taken without regard to food

**Monitoring Parameters** White blood cell counts, EKG, liver function tests

**Reference Range** Not well established

**Patient Information** Report any lethargy, fever, sore throat, flu-like symptoms, or any other signs or symptoms of infection; may cause drowsiness; frequent blood samples must be taken; do not stop taking even if you think it is not working

**Nursing Implications** Benign, self-limiting temperature elevations sometimes occur during the first 3 weeks of treatment, weekly CBC mandatory

**Additional Information** Medication should not be stopped abruptly; taper off over 1-2 weeks

**Dosage Forms** Tablet: 25 mg, 100 mg

♦ **Clozapine-Induced Side Effects** *see page 780*

♦ **Clozaril®** *see* Clozapine *on page 136*

♦ **Clysodrast®** *see* Bisacodyl *on page 69*

## Cocaine (koe KANE)

**Related Information**

Hallucinogenic Drugs *on page 713*

Substance-Related Disorders *on page 609*

**Pharmacologic Category** Local Anesthetic

**Use** Topical anesthesia for mucous membranes

**Effects on Mental Status** CNS stimulation is common; may cause exacerbation of psychosis, nervousness, euphoria, restlessness, hallucinations, paranoia

**Effects on Psychiatric Treatment** Concurrent use with MAOIs may result in hypertensive crisis

**Restrictions** C-II

**Pregnancy Risk Factor** C (X if nonmedicinal use)

**Contraindications** Hypersensitivity to cocaine or to any components of the topical solution; ophthalmologic anesthesia (causing sloughing of the corneal epithelium); pregnancy (nonmedicinal use)

**Warnings/Precautions** For topical use only. Limit to office and surgical procedures only. Resuscitative equipment and drugs should be immediately available when any local anesthetic is used. Debilitated, elderly patients, acutely ill patients, and children should be given reduced doses consistent with their age and physical status. Use caution in patients with severely traumatized mucosa and sepsis in the region of the proposed application. Use with caution in patients with cardiovascular disease or a history of cocaine abuse. In patients being treated for cardiovascular complication of cocaine abuse, avoid beta-blockers for treatment.

**Adverse Reactions**

>10%:

- Central nervous system: CNS stimulation
- Gastrointestinal: Loss of taste perception
- Respiratory: Chronic rhinitis, nasal congestion
- Miscellaneous: Loss of smell

1% to 10%:

- Cardiovascular: Decreased heart rate with low doses, increased heart rate with moderate doses, hypertension, tachycardia, cardiac arrhythmias
- Central nervous system: Nervousness, restlessness, euphoria, excitement, hallucination, seizures
- Gastrointestinal: Vomiting
- Neuromuscular & skeletal: Tremors and clonic-tonic reactions
- Ocular: Sloughing of the corneal epithelium, ulceration of the cornea
- Respiratory: Tachypnea, respiratory failure

**Overdosage/Toxicology**

Signs and symptoms: Anxiety, excitement, confusion, nausea, vomiting, headache, rapid pulse, irregular respiration, delirium, fever, seizures, respiratory arrest, hallucinations, dilated pupils, muscle spasms, sensory aberrations, cardiac arrhythmias

Fatal dose: Oral: 500 mg to 1.2 g; severe toxic effects have occurred with doses as low as 20 mg

Treatment: Since no specific antidote for cocaine exists, serious toxic effects are treated symptomatically. Maintain airway and respiration. Attempt delay of absorption (if ingested) with activated charcoal, gastric lavage or emesis. Seizures are treated with diazepam while propranolol or labetalol may be useful for life-threatening arrhythmias, agitation, and/or hypertension.

**Drug Interactions** CYP3A3/4 enzyme substrate

Beta-blockers potentiate cocaine-induced coronary vasoconstriction (potentiate alpha-adrenergic effect of cocaine); avoid concurrent use

Sympathomimetic amines may cause malignant arrhythmias; avoid concurrent use

**Usual Dosage** Dosage depends on the area to be anesthetized, tissue vascularity, technique of anesthesia, and individual patient tolerance; use the lowest dose necessary to produce adequate anesthesia should be used, not to exceed 1 mg/kg. Use reduced dosages for children, elderly, or debilitated patients.

Topical application (ear, nose, throat, bronchoscopy): Concentrations of 1% to 4% are used. Concentrations >4% are not recommended because of potential for increased incidence and severity of systemic toxic reactions.

**Patient Information** When used orally, do not take anything by mouth until full sensation returns. Ocular: Use caution when driving or engaging in tasks that require alert vision (mydriasis may last for several hours). At time of use or immediately thereafter, report any unusual cardiovascular, CNS, or respiratory symptoms immediately. Following use, report skin irritation or eruption; alterations in vision, eye pain or irritation; persistent gastrointestinal effects; muscle or skeletal tremors, numbness, or rigidity; urinary or genital problems; or persistent fatigue. When used orally, do not take anything by mouth until full sensation returns.

**Nursing Implications** Use only on mucous membranes of the oral, laryngeal, and nasal cavities, do not use on extensive areas of broken skin

**Dosage Forms**

Powder, as hydrochloride: 5 g, 25 g

Solution, topical:

- As hydrochloride: 4% [40 mg/mL] (2 mL, 4 mL, 10 mL); 10% [100 mg/mL] (4 mL, 10 mL)
- Viscous, as hydrochloride: 4% [40 mg/mL] (4 mL, 10 mL); 10% [100 mg/mL] (4 mL, 10 mL)

Tablet, soluble, for topical solution, as hydrochloride: 135 mg

♦ **Codafed® Expectorant** *see* Guaifenesin, Pseudoephedrine, and Codeine *on page 258*

♦ **Codamine®** *see* Hydrocodone and Phenylpropanolamine *on page 273*

♦ **Codamine® Pediatric** *see* Hydrocodone and Phenylpropanolamine *on page 273*

♦ **Codehist® DH** *see* Chlorpheniramine, Pseudoephedrine, and Codeine *on page 116*

## Codeine (KOE deen)

**Related Information**

Narcotic Agonists Comparison Chart *on page 720*

**Canadian Brand Names** Codeine Contin®; Linctus Codeine Blac; Linctus With Codeine Phosphate; Paveral Stanley Syrup With Codeine Phosphate

**Synonyms** Methylmorphine

**Pharmacologic Category** Analgesic, Narcotic; Antitussive

**Use** Treatment of mild to moderate pain; antitussive in lower doses; dextromethorphan has equivalent antitussive activity but has much lower toxicity in accidental overdose

**Effects on Mental Status** Drowsiness is common; may cause euphoria, confusion, insomnia, hallucinations, or depression

**Effects on Psychiatric Treatment** Concurrent use with psychotropics may produce additive toxicity; concurrent use with fluoxetine or paroxetine may result in loss of pain control

**Restrictions** C-II

**Pregnancy Risk Factor** C (D if used for prolonged periods or in high doses at term)

**Contraindications** Hypersensitivity to codeine or any component

**Warnings/Precautions** Use with caution in patients with hypersensitivity reactions to other phenanthrene derivative opioid agonists (morphine, hydrocodone, hydromorphone, levorphanol, oxycodone, oxymorphone); respiratory diseases including asthma, emphysema, COPD, or severe liver or renal insufficiency; some preparations contain sulfites which may cause allergic reactions; tolerance or drug dependence may result from extended use

Not recommended for use for cough control in patients with a productive cough; not recommended as an antitussive for children <2 years of age; the elderly may be particularly susceptible to the CNS depressant and confusion as well as constipating effects of narcotics

**Adverse Reactions**

Percentage unknown: Increased AST, ALT

>10%:

- Central nervous system: Drowsiness
- Gastrointestinal: Constipation

1% to 10%:

- Cardiovascular: Tachycardia or bradycardia, hypotension
- Central nervous system: Dizziness, lightheadedness, false feeling of well being, malaise, headache, restlessness, paradoxical CNS stimulation, confusion

(Continued)

## Codeine *(Continued)*

Dermatologic: Rash, urticaria
Gastrointestinal: Xerostomia, anorexia, nausea, vomiting,
Genitourinary: Decreased urination, ureteral spasm
Hepatic: Increased LFTs
Local: Burning at injection site
Ocular: Blurred vision
Neuromuscular & skeletal: Weakness
Respiratory: Shortness of breath, dyspnea
Miscellaneous: Histamine release

<1%: Biliary spasm, convulsions, hallucinations, insomnia, mental depression, nightmares, paralytic ileus, muscle rigidity, stomach cramps, trembling

**Overdosage/Toxicology**

Signs and symptoms: CNS and respiratory depression, gastrointestinal cramping, constipation

Treatment: Naloxone 2 mg I.V. (0.01 mg/kg for children) with repeat administration as necessary up to a total of 10 mg

**Drug Interactions** CYP2D6 and 3A3/4 enzyme substrate; CYP2D6 enzyme inhibitor

Decreased effect with cigarette smoking

Increased toxicity: CNS depressants, phenothiazines, TCAs, other narcotic analgesics, guanabenz, MAO inhibitors, neuromuscular blockers

**Usual Dosage** Doses should be titrated to appropriate analgesic effect; when changing routes of administration, note that oral dose is $^2/_3$ as effective as parenteral dose

Analgesic:
- Children: Oral, I.M., S.C.: 0.5-1 mg/kg/dose every 4-6 hours as needed; maximum: 60 mg/dose
- Adults: Oral, I.M., I.V., S.C.: 30 mg/dose; range: 15-60 mg every 4-6 hours as needed

Antitussive: Oral (for nonproductive cough):
- Children: 1-1.5 mg/kg/day in divided doses every 4-6 hours as needed: Alternative dose according to age:
  - 2-6 years: 2.5-5 mg every 4-6 hours as needed; maximum: 30 mg/day
  - 6-12 years: 5-10 mg every 4-6 hours as needed; maximum: 60 mg/day
- Adults: 10-20 mg/dose every 4-6 hours as needed; maximum: 120 mg/day

**Dosing adjustment in renal impairment:**
- $Cl_{cr}$ 10-50 mL/minute: Administer 75% of dose
- $Cl_{cr}$ <10 mL/minute: Administer 50% of dose

**Dosing adjustment in hepatic impairment:** Probably necessary in hepatic insufficiency

**Dietary Considerations**

Alcohol: Additive CNS effects, avoid or limit alcohol; watch for sedation

Food: Glucose may cause hyperglycemia; monitor blood glucose concentrations

**Patient Information** If self-administered, use exactly as directed (do not increase dose or frequency); may cause physical and/or psychological dependence. While using this medication, do not use alcohol and other prescription or OTC medications (especially sedatives, tranquilizers, antihistamines, or pain medications) without consulting prescriber. Maintain adequate hydration (2-3 L/day of fluids unless instructed to restrict fluid intake). May cause dizziness, drowsiness, confusion, agitation, impaired coordination, or blurred vision (use caution when driving, climbing stairs, or changing position - rising from sitting or lying to standing, or when engaging in tasks requiring alertness until response to drug is known); nausea or vomiting, or loss of appetite (frequent mouth care, small frequent meals, sucking lozenges, or chewing gum may help); constipation (increased exercise, fluids, or dietary fruit and fiber may help - if constipation remains an unresolved problem, consult prescriber about use of stool softeners). Report confusion, insomnia, excessive nervousness, excessive sedation or drowsiness, or shakiness; acute GI upset; difficulty breathing or shortness of breath; facial flushing, rapid heartbeat or palpitations; urinary difficulty; unusual muscle weakness; or vision changes.

**Nursing Implications** Observe patient for excessive sedation, respiratory depression, implement safety measures, assist with ambulation

**Dosage Forms**

Injection, as phosphate: 30 mg (1 mL, 2 mL); 60 mg (1 mL, 2 mL)
Solution, oral: 15 mg/5 mL
Tablet, as phosphate, soluble: 30 mg, 60 mg
Tablet, as sulfate: 15 mg, 30 mg, 60 mg
Tablet, as sulfate, soluble: 15 mg, 30 mg, 60 mg


♦ **Codiclear® DH** *see* Hydrocodone and Guaifenesin *on page 272*

♦ **Codoxy®** *see* Oxycodone and Aspirin *on page 414*

♦ **Codroxomin®** *see* Hydroxocobalamin *on page 276*

♦ **Cogentin®** *see* Benztropine *on page 63*

♦ **Co-Gesic®** *see* Hydrocodone and Acetaminophen *on page 272*

♦ **Cognex®** *see* Tacrine *on page 529*

♦ **Co-Hist® [OTC]** *see* Acetaminophen, Chlorpheniramine, and Pseudoephedrine *on page 15*

♦ **Colace® [OTC]** *see* Docusate *on page 179*


## Colchicine (KOL chi seen)

**Synonyms** Vegetable arsenic

**Pharmacologic Category** Colchicine

**Use** Treat acute gouty arthritis attacks and prevent recurrences of such attacks, management of familial Mediterranean fever

**Effects on Mental Status** May cause drowsiness

**Effects on Psychiatric Treatment** Rare reports of agranulocytosis; use caution with clozapine and carbamazepine; CNS depressant effects may be enhanced

**Pregnancy Risk Factor** C (oral)/D (parenteral)

**Contraindications** Hypersensitivity to colchicine or any component; serious renal, gastrointestinal, hepatic, or cardiac disorders; blood dyscrasias

**Warnings/Precautions** Severe local irritation can occur following S.C. or I.M. administration; use with caution in debilitated patients or elderly patients or patients with severe GI, renal, or liver disease

**Adverse Reactions**

>10%: Gastrointestinal: Nausea, vomiting, diarrhea, abdominal pain

1% to 10%:
- Dermatologic: Alopecia
- Gastrointestinal: Anorexia

<1%: Agranulocytosis, aplastic anemia, azoospermia, bone marrow suppression, hepatotoxicity, myopathy, peripheral neuritis, rash

**Overdosage/Toxicology**

Signs and symptoms: Nausea, vomiting, abdominal pain, shock, kidney damage, muscle weakness, burning in throat, watery to bloody diarrhea, hypotension, anuria, cardiovascular collapse, delirium, convulsions

Treatment: Gastric lavage and measures to prevent shock, hemodialysis or peritoneal dialysis; atropine and morphine may relieve abdominal pain

**Drug Interactions**

Decreased effect: Vitamin $B_{12}$ absorption may be decreased

Increased toxicity:
- Sympathomimetic agents
- CNS depressant effects are enhanced

**Usual Dosage**

Prophylaxis of familial Mediterranean fever: Oral:
- Children:
  - ≤5 years: 0.5 mg/day
  - >5 years: 1-1.5 mg/day in 2-3 divided doses
- Adults: 1-2 mg/day in 2-3 divided doses

Gouty arthritis, acute attacks: Adults:
- Oral: Initial: 0.5-1.2 mg, then 0.5-0.6 mg every 1-2 hours or 1-1.2 mg every 2 hours until relief or GI side effects (nausea, vomiting, or diarrhea) occur to a maximum total dose of 8 mg; wait 3 days before initiating another course of therapy
- I.V.: Initial: 1-3 mg, then 0.5 mg every 6 hours until response, not to exceed 4 mg/day; if pain recurs, it may be necessary to administer a daily dose of 1-2 mg for several days, however, do not administer more colchicine by any route for at least 7 days after a full course of I.V. therapy (4 mg), transfer to oral colchicine in a dose similar to that being given I.V.

Gouty arthritis, prophylaxis of recurrent attacks: Adults: Oral: 0.5-0.6 mg/day or every other day

**Dosing adjustment in renal impairment:**
- $Cl_{cr}$ <50 mL/minute: Avoid chronic use or administration
- $Cl_{cr}$ <10 mL/minute: Decrease dose by 50% for treatment of acute attacks

Hemodialysis: Not dialyzable (0% to 5%); supplemental dose is not necessary

Peritoneal dialysis: Supplemental dose is not necessary

**Dietary Considerations**

Alcohol: Avoid use

Food: Cyanocobalamin (Vitamin $B_{12}$): Malabsorption of the substrate. May result in macrocytic anemia or neurologic dysfunction. May need to supplement with Vitamin $B_{12}$.

**Patient Information** Take as directed; do not exceed recommended dosage. Consult prescriber about a low-purine diet. Maintain adequate hydration (2-3 L/day of fluids unless instructed to restrict fluid intake). Do not use alcohol or aspirin-containing medication without consulting prescriber. You may experience nausea, vomiting, or anorexia (small frequent meals, frequent mouth care, chewing gum, or sucking lozenges may help); hair loss (reversible). Stop medication and report to prescriber if severe vomiting, watery or bloody diarrhea, or abdominal pain occurs. Report muscle tremors or weakness; fatigue; easy bruising or bleeding; yellowing of eyes or skin; or pale stool or dark urine.

**Dosage Forms**

Injection: 0.5 mg/mL (2 mL)
Tablet: 0.5 mg, 0.6 mg

## Colchicine and Probenecid (KOL chi seen & proe BEN e sid)

**Pharmacologic Category** Antigout Agent

**Use** Treatment of chronic gouty arthritis when complicated by frequent, recurrent acute attacks of gout

**Effects on Mental Status** May cause drowsiness or dizziness

**Effects on Psychiatric Treatment** Rare reports of agranulocytosis; use caution with clozapine and carbamazepine; CNS depressant effects may be enhanced

**Usual Dosage** Adults: Oral: 1 tablet daily for 1 week, then 1 tablet twice daily thereafter

**Dosage Forms** Tablet: Colchicine 0.5 mg and probenecid 0.5 g

♦ **Cold & Allergy® Elixir [OTC]** *see* Brompheniramine and Phenylpropanolamine *on page 74*

♦ **Coldlac-LA®** *see* Guaifenesin and Phenylpropanolamine *on page 257*

♦ **Coldloc®** *see* Guaifenesin, Phenylpropanolamine, and Phenylephrine *on page 258*

♦ **Coldrine® [OTC]** *see* Acetaminophen and Pseudoephedrine *on page 15*

## Colesevelam (koh le SEV a lam)

**U.S. Brand Names** Welchol™

**Pharmacologic Category** Antilipemic Agent (Bile Acid Seqestrant)

**Use** Adjunctive therapy to diet and exercise in the management of elevated LDL in primary hypercholesterolemia (Fredrickson type IIa) when used alone or in combination with an HMG-CoA reductase inhibitor

**Effects on Mental Status** None reported

**Effects on Psychiatric Treatment** Constipation is common, concurrent use with psychotropic agents may exacerbate this effect

**Pregnancy Risk Factor** B

**Contraindications** Hypersensitivity to colesevelam or any component; bowel obstruction

**Warnings/Precautions** Use caution in treating patients with serum triglyceride levels >300 mg/dL (excluded from trials). Safety and efficacy has not been established in pediatric patients. Use caution in dysphagia, swallowing disorders, severe GI motility disorders, major GI tract surgery, and in patients susceptible to fat-soluble vitamin deficiencies. Minimal effects are seen on HDL-C and triglyceride levels. Secondary causes of hypercholesterolemia should be excluded before initiation.

**Adverse Reactions**

>10%: Gastrointestinal: Constipation (11%)

2% to 10%:

Gastrointestinal: Dyspepsia (8%)

Neuromuscular & skeletal: Weakness (4%), myalgia (2%)

Respiratory: Pharyngitis (3%)

Incidence less than or equal to placebo: Infection, headache, pain, back pain, abdominal pain, flu syndrome, flatulence, diarrhea, nausea, sinusitis, rhinitis, cough

**Overdosage/Toxicology** Systemic toxicity is low since the drug is not absorbed.

**Drug Interactions**

Sustained-release verapamil AUC and $C_{max}$ were reduced; clinical significance unknown

Digoxin, lovastatin, metoprolol, quinidine, valproic acid, or warfarin absorption was not significantly affected with concurrent administration

Clinical effects of atorvastatin, lovastatin, and simvastatin were not changed by concurrent administration

**Usual Dosage** Adults: Oral:

Monotherapy: 3 tablets twice daily with meals or 6 tablets once daily with a meal; maximum dose: 7 tablets/day

Combination therapy with an HMG-CoA reductase inhibitor: 4-6 tablets daily; maximum dose: 6 tablets/day

**Dosage adjustment in renal impairment:** No recommendations made

**Dosage adjustment in hepatic impairment:** No recommendations made

Elderly: No recommendations made

**Dietary Considerations** Take with meal(s). Follow dietary guidelines.

**Patient Information** Take once or twice daily with meals. Follow diet and exercise plan as recommended by healthcare provider. Tell healthcare provider if you are pregnant, plan on getting pregnant, or are breast-feeding.

**Nursing Implications** Give with meal(s). Make sure patient understands dietary guidelines.

**Dosage Forms** Tablet: 625 mg

♦ **Colestid®** *see* Colestipol *on page 139*

## Colestipol (koe LES ti pole)

**Related Information**

Lipid-Lowering Agents Comparison Chart *on page 717*

**U.S. Brand Names** Colestid®

**Pharmacologic Category** Antilipemic Agent (Bile Acid Seqestrant)

**Use** Adjunct in management of primary hypercholesterolemia; regression of arteriolosclerosis; relief of pruritus associated with elevated levels of bile acids; possibly used to decrease plasma half-life of digoxin in toxicity

**Effects on Mental Status** May cause drowsiness or anxiety

**Effects on Psychiatric Treatment** Constipation is common; may be exacerbated by concurrent psychotropic use; may decrease the absorption of TCAs

**Pregnancy Risk Factor** C

**Contraindications** Hypersensitivity of bile acid sequestering resins or any components of the products; bowel obstruction

**Warnings/Precautions** Not to be taken simultaneously with many other medicines (decreased absorption). Treat any diseases contributing to hypercholesterolemia first. May interfere with fat soluble vitamins (A, D, E, K) and folic acid. Chronic use may be associated with bleeding problems. May produce or exacerbate constipation problems. Fecal impaction may occur. Hemorrhoids may be worsened.

**Adverse Reactions**

>10%: Gastrointestinal: Constipation

1% to 10%: Gastrointestinal: Abdominal pain and distention, belching, flatulence, nausea, vomiting, diarrhea

<1%: Anorexia, anxiety, arthralgia, arthritis, cholecystitis, cholelithiasis, dermatitis, dizziness, drowsiness, fatigue, GI irritation and bleeding, headache, increased serum phosphorous and chloride with decrease of sodium and potassium, peptic ulceration, shortness of breath, urticaria, vertigo, weakness

**Overdosage/Toxicology**

Signs and symptoms: GI obstruction, nausea, GI distress

Treatment: Supportive

**Drug Interactions**

Colestipol can reduce the absorption of numerous medications when used concurrently. Give other medications 1 hour before or 4 hours after giving colestipol. Medications which may be affected include HMG-CoA reductase inhibitors, thiazide diuretics, propranolol (and potentially other beta-blockers), corticosteroids, thyroid hormones, digoxin, valproic acid, NSAIDs, loop diuretics, sulfonylureas, troglitazone (and potentially other agents in this class).

Warfarin and other oral anticoagulants: Absorption is reduced by cholestyramine, may also be reduced by colestipol. Separate administration times (as detailed above) and monitor INR closely when initiating or discontinuing.

**Usual Dosage** Adults: Oral:

Granules: 5-30 g/day given once or in divided doses 2-4 times/day; initial dose: 5 g 1-2 times/day; increase by 5 g at 1- to 2-month intervals

Tablets: 2-16 g/day; initial dose: 2 g 1-2 times/day; increase by 2 g at 1- to 2-month intervals

**Patient Information** Take with 38-45 ounces of water or fruit juice. Rinse glass with small amount of water to ensure full dose is taken. Other medications should be taken 2 hours before or 2 hours after colestipol. You may experience constipation (increased exercise, increased dietary fluids, fruit, fiber, or stool softener may help) or drowsiness or dizziness (use caution when driving or engaging in tasks that require alertness until response to drug is known). Report acute gastric pain, tarry stools, or difficulty breathing.

**Dosage Forms**

Granules, as hydrochloride: 5 g packet, 300 g, 500 g

Tablet, as hydrochloride: 1 g

## Colistin (koe LIS tin)

**U.S. Brand Names** Coly-Mycin® S Oral

**Synonyms** Polymyxin E

**Pharmacologic Category** Antibiotic, Miscellaneous; Antidiarrheal

**Use** Treatment of diarrhea in infants and children caused by susceptible organisms, especially *E. coli* and *Shigella*, however, other agents are preferred; treatment of superficial infections of external ear canal and of mastoidectomy and fenestration cavities

**Effects on Mental Status** None reported

**Effects on Psychiatric Treatment** None reported

**Pregnancy Risk Factor** C

**Contraindications** Known hypersensitivity to colistin

**Warnings/Precautions** Use with caution in patients with impaired renal function; some systemic absorption may occur; potential for renal toxicity exists; prolonged use may lead to superinfection

**Adverse Reactions** <1%: Hypersensitivity reactions, nausea, nephrotoxicity, neuromuscular blockade, respiratory arrest, superinfections, vomiting

**Usual Dosage** Diarrhea: Children: Oral: 5-15 mg/kg/day in 3 divided doses given every 8 hours

**Patient Information** Keep refrigerated, shake well, discard after 14 days

**Dosage Forms** Powder for oral suspension: 25 mg/5 mL (60 mL)

## Colistin, Neomycin, and Hydrocortisone

(koe LIS tin, nee oh MYE sin & hye droe KOR ti sone)

**U.S. Brand Names** Coly-Mycin® S Otic Drops; Cortisporin-TC® Otic

**Pharmacologic Category** Antibiotic/Corticosteroid, Otic

(Continued)

## Colistin, Neomycin, and Hydrocortisone *(Continued)*

**Use** Treatment of superficial and susceptible bacterial infections of the external auditory canal; for treatment of susceptible bacterial infections of mastoidectomy and fenestration cavities

**Effects on Mental Status** None reported

**Effects on Psychiatric Treatment** None reported

**Usual Dosage**

Children: 3 drops in affected ear 3-4 times/day

Adults: 4 drops in affected ear 3-4 times/day

**Dosage Forms** Suspension, otic:

Coly-Mycin® S Otic Drops: Colistin sulfate 0.3%, neomycin sulfate 0.47%, and hydrocortisone acetate 1% (5 mL, 10 mL)

Cortisporin-TC®: Colistin sulfate 0.3%, neomycin sulfate 0.33%, and hydrocortisone acetate 1% (5 mL, 10 mL)


- ♦ **Collyrium Fresh® Ophthalmic [OTC]** *see* Tetrahydrozoline *on page 538*
- ♦ **Colovage®** *see* Polyethylene Glycol-Electrolyte Solution *on page 451*
- ♦ **Coly-Mycin® S Oral** *see* Colistin *on page 139*
- ♦ **Coly-Mycin® S Otic Drops** *see* Colistin, Neomycin, and Hydrocortisone *on page 139*
- ♦ **CoLyte®** *see* Polyethylene Glycol-Electrolyte Solution *on page 451*
- ♦ **Comb Flower** *see* Echinacea *on page 189*
- ♦ **CombiPatch™** *see* Estradiol and Norethindrone *on page 205*
- ♦ **Combipres®** *see* Clonidine and Chlorthalidone *on page 134*
- ♦ **Combivent®** *see* Ipratropium and Albuterol *on page 292*
- ♦ **Combivir™** *see* Zidovudine and Lamivudine *on page 592*
- ♦ **Comfort® Ophthalmic [OTC]** *see* Naphazoline *on page 383*
- ♦ **Comfort® Tears Solution [OTC]** *see* Artificial Tears *on page 48*
- ♦ **Comhist®** *see* Chlorpheniramine, Phenylephrine, and Phenyltoloxamine *on page 115*
- ♦ **Comhist® LA** *see* Chlorpheniramine, Phenylephrine, and Phenyltoloxamine *on page 115*
- ♦ **Compazine®** *see* Prochlorperazine *on page 465*
- ♦ **Comphor of the Poor** *see* Garlic *on page 246*
- ♦ **Compound E** *see* Cortisone *on page 141*
- ♦ **Compound S** *see* Zidovudine *on page 592*
- ♦ **Compoz® Gel Caps [OTC]** *see* Diphenhydramine *on page 174*
- ♦ **Compoz® Nighttime Sleep Aid [OTC]** *see* Diphenhydramine *on page 174*
- ♦ **Comtan®** *see* Entacapone *on page 194*
- ♦ **Comtrex® Maximum Strength Non-Drowsy [OTC]** *see* Acetaminophen, Dextromethorphan, and Pseudoephedrine *on page 16*
- ♦ **Comvax®** *see Haemophilus* b Conjugate and Hepatitis b Vaccine *on page 261*
- ♦ **Concerta™** *see* Methylphenidate *on page 357*
- ♦ **Conex® [OTC]** *see* Guaifenesin and Phenylpropanolamine *on page 257*
- ♦ **Congess® Jr** *see* Guaifenesin and Pseudoephedrine *on page 257*
- ♦ **Congess® Sr** *see* Guaifenesin and Pseudoephedrine *on page 257*
- ♦ **Congestac®** *see* Guaifenesin and Pseudoephedrine *on page 257*
- ♦ **Congestant D® [OTC]** *see* Chlorpheniramine, Phenylpropanolamine, and Acetaminophen *on page 116*
- ♦ **Conjugated Estrogen and Methyltestosterone** *see* Estrogens and Methyltestosterone *on page 206*
- ♦ **Constant-T®** *see* Theophylline Salts *on page 539*
- ♦ **Constilac®** *see* Lactulose *on page 306*
- ♦ **Constulose®** *see* Lactulose *on page 306*
- ♦ **Contac® Cough Formula Liquid [OTC]** *see* Guaifenesin and Dextromethorphan *on page 257*
- ♦ **Contergan®** *see* Thalidomide *on page 538*
- ♦ **Control® [OTC]** *see* Phenylpropanolamine *on page 440*
- ♦ **Controlled Substances - Uses and Effects** *see page 796*
- ♦ **Contuss®** *see* Guaifenesin, Phenylpropanolamine, and Phenylephrine *on page 258*
- ♦ **Contuss® XT** *see* Guaifenesin and Phenylpropanolamine *on page 257*
- ♦ **Copaxone®** *see* Glatiramer *on page 250*
- ♦ **Cophene-B®** *see* Brompheniramine *on page 73*
- ♦ **Cophene XP®** *see* Hydrocodone, Pseudoephedrine, and Guaifenesin *on page 273*
- ♦ **Copolymer-1** *see* Glatiramer *on page 250*
- ♦ **Co-Pyronil® 2 Pulvules® [OTC]** *see* Chlorpheniramine and Pseudoephedrine *on page 114*
- ♦ **Cordarone®** *see* Amiodarone *on page 32*
- ♦ **Coreg®** *see* Carvedilol *on page 95*
- ♦ **Corgard®** *see* Nadolol *on page 379*
- ♦ **Coricidin® [OTC]** *see* Chlorpheniramine and Acetaminophen *on page 114*
- ♦ **Coricidin D® [OTC]** *see* Chlorpheniramine, Phenylpropanolamine, and Acetaminophen *on page 116*
- ♦ **Corlopam®** *see* Fenoldopam *on page 221*
- ♦ **Corque® Topical** *see* Clioquinol and Hydrocortisone *on page 129*
- ♦ **CortaGel® [OTC]** *see* Hydrocortisone *on page 273*
- ♦ **Cortaid® Maximum Strength [OTC]** *see* Hydrocortisone *on page 273*
- ♦ **Cortaid® With Aloe [OTC]** *see* Hydrocortisone *on page 273*
- ♦ **Cortatrigen® Otic** *see* Neomycin, Polymyxin B, and Hydrocortisone *on page 389*
- ♦ **Cort-Dome®** *see* Hydrocortisone *on page 273*
- ♦ **Cortef®** *see* Hydrocortisone *on page 273*
- ♦ **Cortef® Feminine Itch** *see* Hydrocortisone *on page 273*
- ♦ **Cortenema®** *see* Hydrocortisone *on page 273*
- ♦ **Corticaine® Topical** *see* Dibucaine and Hydrocortisone *on page 163*
- ♦ **Corticosteroids Comparison Chart** *see page 711*


## Corticotropin (kor ti koe TROE pin)

**Related Information**

Anticonvulsants by Seizures Type *on page 703*

**U.S. Brand Names** Acthar®; H.P. Acthar® Gel

**Synonyms** ACTH; Adrenocorticotropic Hormone; Corticotropin, Repository

**Pharmacologic Category** Corticosteroid, Parenteral

**Use** Acute exacerbations of multiple sclerosis; diagnostic aid in adrenocortical insufficiency, severe muscle weakness in myasthenia gravis

Cosyntropin is preferred over corticotropin for diagnostic test of adrenocortical insufficiency (cosyntropin is less allergenic and test is shorter in duration)

**Effects on Mental Status** Insomnia and nervousness are common; may cause euphoria or hallucinations

**Effects on Psychiatric Treatment** Barbiturates may decrease the levels of corticotropin

**Contraindications** Scleroderma; osteoporosis; systemic fungal infections; ocular herpes simplex; peptic ulcer; hypersensitivity to corticotropin or any component

**Warnings/Precautions** Use with caution in patients with hypothyroidism, cirrhosis, thromboembolic disorders, seizure disorders or renal insufficiency, hypertension, congestive heart failure; may mask signs of infection; do not administer live vaccines

**Adverse Reactions**

>10%:

Central nervous system: Insomnia, nervousness

Gastrointestinal: Increased appetite, indigestion

1% to 10%:

Dermatologic: Hirsutism

Endocrine & metabolic: Diabetes mellitus

Neuromuscular & skeletal: Arthralgia

Ocular: Cataracts

Respiratory: Epistaxis

**Drug Interactions**

Decreased effect: Can antagonize the effect of anticholinesterases (eg, neostigmine) in patients with myasthenia gravis

Decreased corticotropin levels with barbiturates

**Usual Dosage** Injection has a rapid onset and duration of activity of approximately 2 hours; the repository injection has a slower onset, but may sustain effects for ≤3 days

Children:

Anti-inflammatory/immunosuppressant:

I.M., I.V., S.C. (aqueous): 1.6 units/kg/day or 50 units/m$^2$/day divided every 6-8 hours

I.M. (gel): 0.8 units/kg/day or 25 units/m$^2$/day divided every 12-24 hours

Infantile spasms: Various regimens have been used. Some neurologists recommend low-dose ACTH (5-40 units/day) for short periods (1-6

weeks), while others recommend larger doses of ACTH (40-160 units/day) for long periods of treatment (3-12 months). Well designed comparative dosing studies are needed. Example of low dose regimen:
Initial: I.M. (gel): 20 units/day for 2 weeks, if patient responds, taper and discontinue; if patient does not respond, increase dose to 30 units/day for 4 weeks then taper and discontinue
I.M. usual dose (gel): 20-40 units/day or 5-8 units/kg/day in 1-2 divided doses; range: 5-160 units/day
Oral prednisone (2 mg/kg/day) was as effective as I.M. ACTH gel (20 units/day) in controlling infantile spasms
Adults: Acute exacerbation of multiple sclerosis: I.M.: 80-120 units/day for 2-3 weeks
Diagnostic purposes: I.V.: 10-25 units in 500 mL 5% dextrose in water infused over 8 hours
Repository injection: I.M., S.C.: 40-80 units every 24-72 hours

**Patient Information** Do not abruptly discontinue the medication; your physician may want you to follow a low salt/potassium rich diet; tell physician you are using this drug before having skin tests, before surgery, or emergency treatment if you get a serious infection or injury

**Dosage Forms**
Injection, repository (H.P. Acthar® Gel): 40 units/mL (1 mL, 5 mL); 80 units/mL (1 mL, 5 mL)
Powder for injection (Acthar®): 25 units, 40 units

- **Corticotropin, Repository** *see* Corticotropin *on page 140*
- **Cortifoam®** *see* Hydrocortisone *on page 273*

## Cortisone (KOR ti sone AS e tate)

**Related Information**
Corticosteroids Comparison Chart *on page 711*

**U.S. Brand Names** Cortone® Acetate

**Synonyms** Compound E

**Pharmacologic Category** Corticosteroid, Oral; Corticosteroid, Parenteral

**Use** Management of adrenocortical insufficiency

**Effects on Mental Status** Insomnia and nervousness are common; may cause euphoria or hallucinations

**Effects on Psychiatric Treatment** Barbiturates may decrease the levels of cortisone

**Pregnancy Risk Factor** D

**Contraindications** Serious infections, except septic shock or tuberculous meningitis; administration of live virus vaccines

**Warnings/Precautions** Use with caution in patients with hypothyroidism, cirrhosis, hypertension, congestive heart failure, ulcerative colitis, thromboembolic disorders, osteoporosis, convulsive disorders, peptic ulcer, diabetes mellitus, myasthenia gravis; prolonged therapy (>5 days) of pharmacologic doses of corticosteroids may lead to hypothalamic-pituitary-adrenal suppression, the degree of adrenal suppression varies with the degree and duration of glucocorticoid therapy; this must be taken into consideration when taking patients off steroids

**Adverse Reactions**
>10%:
Central nervous system: Insomnia, nervousness
Gastrointestinal: Increased appetite, indigestion
1% to 10%:
Dermatologic: Hirsutism
Endocrine & metabolic: Diabetes mellitus
Neuromuscular & skeletal: Arthralgia
Ocular: Cataracts, glaucoma
Respiratory: Epistaxis
<1%: Abdominal distention, acne, alkalosis, amenorrhea, bruising, Cushing's syndrome, delirium, edema, euphoria, fractures, glucose intolerance, growth suppression, hallucinations, headache, hyperglycemia, hyperpigmentation, hypersensitivity reactions, hypertension, hypokalemia, mood swings, muscle wasting, myalgia, nausea, osteoporosis, pancreatitis, peptic ulcer, pituitary-adrenal axis suppression, pseudotumor cerebri, psychoses, seizures, skin atrophy, sodium and water retention, ulcerative esophagitis, vertigo, vomiting

**Overdosage/Toxicology** Signs and symptoms: When consumed in excessive quantities for prolonged periods, systemic hypercorticism and adrenal suppression may occur; in those cases, discontinuation and withdrawal of the corticosteroid should be done judiciously. Cushingoid changes from continued administration of large doses results in moon face, central obesity, striae, hirsutism, acne, ecchymoses, hypertension, osteoporosis, myopathy, sexual dysfunction, diabetes, hyperlipidemia, peptic ulcer, increased susceptibility to infection, and electrolyte and fluid imbalance.

**Drug Interactions** CYP3A3/4 enzyme substrate
Decreased effect:
Barbiturates, phenytoin, rifampin may decrease cortisone effects
Live virus vaccines
Anticholinesterase agents may decrease effect
Cortisone may decrease warfarin effects
Cortisone may decrease effects of salicylates
Increased effect: Estrogens (increase cortisone effects)
Increased toxicity:
Cortisone + NSAIDs may increase ulcerogenic potential
Cortisone may increase potassium deletion due to diuretics

**Usual Dosage** If possible, administer glucocorticoids before 9 AM to minimize adrenocortical suppression; dosing depends upon the condition being treated and the response of the patient; supplemental doses may be warranted during times of stress in the course of withdrawing therapy
Children:
Anti-inflammatory or immunosuppressive: Oral: 2.5-10 mg/kg/day **or** 20-300 mg/m$^2$/day in divided doses every 6-8 hours
Physiologic replacement: Oral: 0.5-0.75 mg/kg/day **or** 20-25 mg/m$^2$/day in divided doses every 8 hours
Adults: Oral: 25-300 mg/day in divided doses every 12-24 hours
Hemodialysis: Supplemental dose is not necessary
Peritoneal dialysis: Supplemental dose is not necessary

**Patient Information** Take oral formulation as directed, with food or milk in the morning. Do not take more than prescribed or discontinue without consulting prescriber. Maintain adequate nutritional intake; consult prescriber for possibility of special dietary instructions. If diabetic, monitor serum glucose closely and notify prescriber of any changes; this medication can alter hypoglycemic requirements. Inform prescriber if you are experiencing unusual stress; dosage may need to be adjusted. You will be susceptible to infection; avoid crowds or infected persons or persons with contagious diseases. You may experience insomnia or nervousness; use caution when driving or engaging in tasks requiring alertness until response to drug is known. Report excessive or sudden weight gain, swelling of extremities, difficulty breathing, muscle pain or weakness, change in menstrual pattern, vision changes, signs of hyperglycemia, signs of infection (eg, fever, chills, mouth sores, perianal itching, vaginal discharge), other persistent side effects, or worsening of condition.

**Nursing Implications** Withdraw gradually following long-term therapy

**Dosage Forms** Tablet: 5 mg, 10 mg, 25 mg

- **Cortisporin® Ophthalmic Ointment** *see* Bacitracin, Neomycin, Polymyxin B, and Hydrocortisone *on page 57*
- **Cortisporin® Ophthalmic Suspension** *see* Neomycin, Polymyxin B, and Hydrocortisone *on page 389*
- **Cortisporin® Otic** *see* Neomycin, Polymyxin B, and Hydrocortisone *on page 389*
- **Cortisporin-TC® Otic** *see* Colistin, Neomycin, and Hydrocortisone *on page 139*
- **Cortisporin®-TC Otic Suspension** *see* Neomycin, Colistin, Hydrocortisone, and Thonzonium *on page 389*
- **Cortisporin® Topical Cream** *see* Neomycin, Polymyxin B, and Hydrocortisone *on page 389*
- **Cortisporin® Topical Ointment** *see* Bacitracin, Neomycin, Polymyxin B, and Hydrocortisone *on page 57*
- **Cortizone®-5 [OTC]** *see* Hydrocortisone *on page 273*
- **Cortizone®-10 [OTC]** *see* Hydrocortisone *on page 273*
- **Cortone® Acetate** *see* Cortisone *on page 141*
- **Cortrosyn®** *see* Cosyntropin *on page 141*
- **Corvert®** *see* Ibutilide *on page 281*
- ***Corynanthe yohimbe*** *see* Yohimbine *on page 589*
- **Cosmegen®** *see* Dactinomycin *on page 149*
- **Cosopt™** *see* Dorzolamide and Timolol *on page 182*

## Cosyntropin (koe sin TROE pin)

**U.S. Brand Names** Cortrosyn®

**Canadian Brand Names** Synacthen® Depot

**Pharmacologic Category** Diagnostic Agent, Adrenocortical Insufficiency

**Use** Diagnostic test to differentiate primary adrenal from secondary (pituitary) adrenocortical insufficiency

**Effects on Mental Status** None reported

**Effects on Psychiatric Treatment** Barbiturates may decrease the levels of cosyntropin

**Usual Dosage**
Adrenocortical insufficiency: I.M., I.V. (over 2 minutes): Peak plasma cortisol concentrations usually occur 45-60 minutes after cosyntropin administration
Neonates: 0.015 mg/kg/dose
Children <2 years: 0.125 mg
Children >2 years and Adults: 0.25-0.75 mg
When greater cortisol stimulation is needed, an I.V. infusion may be used:
Children >2 years and Adults: 0.25 mg administered at 0.04 mg/hour over 6 hours
(Continued)

## Cosyntropin *(Continued)*

Congenital adrenal hyperplasia evaluation: 1 mg/m²/dose up to a maximum of 1 mg

**Dosage Forms** Powder for injection: 0.25 mg


- **Cotazym®** *see* Pancrelipase *on page 418*
- **Cotazym-S®** *see* Pancrelipase *on page 418*
- **Cotrim®** *see* Co-Trimoxazole *on page 142*
- **Cotrim® DS** *see* Co-Trimoxazole *on page 142*


## Co-Trimoxazole (koe trye MOKS a zole)

**U.S. Brand Names** Bactrim™; Bactrim™ DS; Cotrim®; Cotrim® DS; Septra®; Septra® DS; Sulfatrim®

**Canadian Brand Names** Apo®-Sulfatrim; Novo-Trimel; Nu-Cotrimox; Pro-Trin®; Roubac®; Trisulfa®; Trisulfa-S®

**Synonyms** SMZ-TMP; Sulfamethoxazole and Trimethoprim; TMP-SMZ; Trimethoprim and Sulfamethoxazole

**Pharmacologic Category** Antibiotic, Sulfonamide Derivative

**Use**

Oral treatment of urinary tract infections due to *E. coli, Klebsiella* and *Enterobacter* sp, *M. morganii, P. mirabilis* and *P. vulgaris*; acute otitis media in children and acute exacerbations of chronic bronchitis in adults due to susceptible strains of *H. influenzae* or *S. pneumoniae*; prophylaxis of *Pneumocystis carinii* pneumonitis (PCP), traveler's diarrhea due to enterotoxigenic *E. coli* or *Cyclospora*

I.V. treatment or severe or complicated infections when oral therapy is not feasible, for documented PCP, empiric treatment of PCP in immune compromised patients; treatment of documented or suspected shigellosis, typhoid fever, *Nocardia asteroides* infection, or other infections caused by susceptible bacteria

**Unlabeled use:** Cholera and salmonella-type infections and nocardiosis; chronic prostatitis; as prophylaxis in neutropenic patients with *P. carinii* infections, in leukemics, and in patients following renal transplantation, to decrease incidence of gram-negative rod infections

**Effects on Mental Status** Rarely may cause depression, hallucination, or confusion; sulfonamides may cause euphoria, restlessness, irritability, disorientation, panic, and delusions

**Effects on Psychiatric Treatment** May rarely cause granulocytopenia; use caution with clozapine and carbamazepine

**Pregnancy Risk Factor** C (per manufacturer); D (if near term, based on expert analysis)

**Contraindications** Hypersensitivity to any sulfa drug or any component; porphyria; megaloblastic anemia due to folate deficiency; infants <2 months of age; marked hepatic damage

**Warnings/Precautions** Use with caution in patients with G-6-PD deficiency, impaired renal or hepatic function; maintain adequate hydration to prevent crystalluria; adjust dosage in patients with renal impairment. Injection vehicle contains benzyl alcohol and sodium metabisulfite. Fatalities associated with severe reactions including Stevens-Johnson syndrome, toxic epidermal necrolysis, hepatic necrosis, agranulocytosis, aplastic anemia and other blood dyscrasias; discontinue use at first sign of rash. Elderly patients appear at greater risk for more severe adverse reactions. May cause hypoglycemia, particularly in malnourished, or patients with renal or hepatic impairment. Use with caution in patients with porphyria or thyroid dysfunction. Slow acetylators may be more prone to adverse reactions.

**Adverse Reactions**

>10%:

Dermatologic: Allergic skin reactions including rashes and urticaria, photosensitivity

Gastrointestinal: Nausea, vomiting, anorexia

1% to 10%:

Dermatologic: Stevens-Johnson syndrome, toxic epidermal necrolysis (rare)

Hematologic: Blood dyscrasias

Hepatic: Hepatitis

<1%: Aplastic anemia, ataxia, cholestatic jaundice, confusion, depression, diarrhea, erythema multiforme, fever, granulocytopenia, hallucinations, hemolysis (with G-6-PD deficiency), interstitial nephritis, kernicterus in neonates, megaloblastic anemia, pancreatitis, pancytopenia, pseudomembranous colitis, rhabdomyolysis, seizures, serum sickness, stomatitis, thrombocytopenia

**Overdosage/Toxicology**

Signs and symptoms: Nausea, vomiting, GI distress, hematuria, crystalluria

Treatment: Following GI decontamination, treatment is supportive; adequate fluid intake is essential; peritoneal dialysis is not effective and hemodialysis only moderately effective in removing co-trimoxazole

**Drug Interactions** CYP2C9 enzyme inhibitor

Decreased effect: Cyclosporines

Increased effect/toxicity: Phenytoin, cyclosporines (nephrotoxicity), methotrexate (displaced from binding sites), dapsone, sulfonylureas, and oral anticoagulants; may compete for renal secretion of methotrexate; digoxin concentrations increased

**Usual Dosage** Dosage recommendations are based on the trimethoprim component

Children >2 months:

Mild to moderate infections: Oral, I.V.: 8 mg TMP/kg/day in divided doses every 12 hours

Serious infection/*Pneumocystis*: I.V.: 20 mg TMP/kg/day in divided doses every 6 hours

Urinary tract infection prophylaxis: Oral: 2 mg TMP/kg/dose daily

Prophylaxis of *Pneumocystis*: Oral, I.V.: 10 mg TMP/kg/day or 150 mg TMP/m²/day in divided doses every 12 hours for 3 days/week; dose should not exceed 320 mg trimethoprim and 1600 mg sulfamethoxazole 3 days/week

Adults:

Urinary tract infection/chronic bronchitis: Oral: 1 double strength tablet every 12 hours for 10-14 days

Sepsis: I.V.: 20 TMP/kg/day divided every 6 hours

*Pneumocystis carinii*:

Prophylaxis: Oral: 1 double strength tablet daily or 3 times/week

Treatment: Oral, I.V.: 15-20 mg TMP/kg/day in 3-4 divided doses

**Dosing adjustment in renal impairment:** Adults:

I.V.:

$Cl_{cr}$ 15-30 mL/minute: Administer 2.5-5 mg/kg every 12 hours

$Cl_{cr}$ <15 mL/minute: Administer 2.5-5 mg/kg every 24 hours

Oral:

$Cl_{cr}$ 15-30 mL/minute: Administer 1 double strength tablet every 24 hours or 1 single strength tablet every 12 hours

$Cl_{cr}$ <15 mL/minute: Not recommended

**Patient Information** Take oral medication with 8 oz of water on an empty stomach (1 hour before or 2 hours after meals) for best absorption. Finish all medication; do not skip doses. You may experience increased sensitivity to sunlight; use sunblock, wear protective clothing and dark glasses, or avoid direct exposure to sunlight. Small frequent meals, frequent mouth care, sucking lozenges, or chewing gum may reduce nausea or vomiting. Report skin rash, sore throat, blackened stool, or unusual bruising or bleeding immediately.

**Dosage Forms** The 5:1 ratio (SMX to TMP) remains constant in all dosage forms:

Injection: Sulfamethoxazole 80 mg and trimethoprim 16 mg per mL (5 mL, 10 mL, 20 mL, 30 mL, 50 mL)

Suspension, oral: Sulfamethoxazole 200 mg and trimethoprim 40 mg per 5 mL (20 mL, 100 mL, 150 mL, 200 mL, 480 mL)

Tablet: Sulfamethoxazole 400 mg and trimethoprim 80 mg

Tablet, double strength: Sulfamethoxazole 800 mg and trimethoprim 160 mg


- **Coumadin®** *see* Warfarin *on page 587*
- **Covera-HS®** *see* Verapamil *on page 583*
- **Cozaar®** *see* Losartan *on page 326*
- **CP-99,219-27** *see* Trovafloxacin *on page 574*
- **CPM** *see* Cyclophosphamide *on page 145*
- ***Crataegus laevigata*** *see* Hawthorn *on page 264*
- ***Crataegus monogyna*** *see* Hawthorn *on page 264*
- ***Crataegus oxyacantha*** *see* Hawthorn *on page 264*
- ***Crataegus pinnatifida*** *see* Hawthorn *on page 264*
- **Creon® 10** *see* Pancrelipase *on page 418*
- **Creon® 20** *see* Pancrelipase *on page 418*
- **Creo-Terpin® [OTC]** *see* Dextromethorphan *on page 160*
- **Crinone™** *see* Progesterone *on page 468*
- **Crixivan®** *see* Indinavir *on page 285*
- **Crolom® Ophthalmic Solution** *see* Cromolyn Sodium *on page 142*
- **Cromoglycic Acid** *see* Cromolyn Sodium *on page 142*


## Cromolyn Sodium (KROE moe lin SOW dee um)

**Related Information**

Asthma Guidelines *on page 773*

**U.S. Brand Names** Crolom® Ophthalmic Solution; Gastrocrom® Oral; Intal® Nebulizer Solution; Intal® Oral Inhaler; Nasalcrom® Nasal Solution [OTC]

**Canadian Brand Names** Novo-Cromolyn; Opticrom®; PMS-Sodium Cromoglycate; Rynacrom®

**Synonyms** Cromoglycic Acid; Disodium Cromoglycate; DSCG

**Pharmacologic Category** Antihistamine, Inhalation; Mast Cell Stabilizer

**Use** Adjunct in the prophylaxis of allergic disorders, including rhinitis, giant papillary conjunctivitis, and asthma; inhalation product may be used for prevention of exercise-induced bronchospasm; systemic mastocytosis, food allergy, and treatment of inflammatory bowel disease; **cromolyn is a prophylactic drug with no benefit for acute situations**

**Effects on Mental Status** May cause dizziness

**Effects on Psychiatric Treatment** None reported

**Pregnancy Risk Factor** B

**Contraindications** Hypersensitivity to cromolyn or any component; acute asthma attacks

**Warnings/Precautions** Severe anaphylactic reactions may occur rarely; cromolyn is a prophylactic drug with no benefit for acute situations; do not use in patients with severe renal or hepatic impairment; caution should be used when withdrawing the drug or tapering the dose as symptoms may reoccur; use with caution in patients with a history of cardiac arrhythmias

**Adverse Reactions**

>10%:

Gastrointestinal: Unpleasant taste (inhalation aerosol)
Respiratory: Hoarseness, coughing

1% to 10%:

Dermatologic: Angioedema
Gastrointestinal: Xerostomia
Genitourinary: Dysuria
Respiratory: Sneezing, nasal congestion

<1%: Anaphylactic reactions, arthralgia, diarrhea, dizziness, eosinophilic pneumonia, headache, lacrimation, nasal burning, nausea, ocular stinging, pulmonary infiltrates, rash, throat irritation, urticaria, vomiting, wheezing

**Overdosage/Toxicology** Signs and symptoms: Bronchospasm, laryngeal edema, dysuria

**Drug Interactions** Isoproterenol

**Usual Dosage**

Oral:

Systemic mastocytosis:

Neonates and preterm Infants: Not recommended
Infants and Children <2 years: 20 mg/kg/day in 4 divided doses; may increase in patients 6 months to 2 years of age if benefits not seen after 2-3 weeks; do not exceed 30 mg/kg/day
Children 2-12 years: 100 mg 4 times/day; not to exceed 40 mg/kg/day
Children >12 years and Adults: 200 mg 4 times/day

Food allergy and inflammatory bowel disease:

Children <2 years: Not recommended
Children 2-12 years: Initial dose: 100 mg 4 times/day; may double the dose if effect is not satisfactory within 2-3 weeks; not to exceed 40 mg/kg/day
Children >12 years and Adults: Initial dose: 200 mg 4 times/day; may double the dose if effect is not satisfactory within 2-3 weeks; up to 400 mg 4 times/day
Once desired effect is achieved, dose may be tapered to lowest effective dose

Inhalation:

For chronic control of asthma, taper frequency to the lowest effective dose (ie, 4 times/day to 3 times/day to twice daily):

Nebulization solution: Children >2 years and Adults: Initial: 20 mg 4 times/day; usual dose: 20 mg 3-4 times/day

Metered spray:

Children 5-12 years: Initial: 2 inhalations 4 times/day; usual dose: 1-2 inhalations 3-4 times/day
Children ≥12 years and Adults: Initial: 2 inhalations 4 times/day; usual dose: 2-4 inhalations 3-4 times/day

Prevention of allergen- or exercise-induced bronchospasm: Administer 10-15 minutes prior to exercise or allergen exposure but no longer than 1 hour before:

Nebulization solution: Children >2 years and Adults: Single dose of 20 mg
Metered spray: Children >5 years and Adults: Single dose of 2 inhalations

**Patient Information** Oral: Use as directed; do not increase dosage or discontinue abruptly without consulting prescriber. You may experience dizziness or nervousness (use caution when driving or engaging in tasks requiring alertness until response to drug is known); diarrhea (boiled milk, yogurt, or buttermilk may help); or headache or muscle pain (mild analgesic may offer relief). Report persistent insomnia; skin rash or irritation; abdominal pain or difficulty swallowing; unusual cough, bronchospasm, or difficulty breathing; decreased urination; or if condition worsens or fails to improve.

Nebulizer: Store nebulizer solution away from light. Prepare nebulizer according to package instructions. Clear as much mucus as possible before use. Rinse mouth following each use to prevent opportunistic infection and reduce unpleasant aftertaste. Report if symptoms worsen or condition fails to improve.

Nasal: Instill 1 spray into each nostril 3-4 times a day. You may experience unpleasant taste (rinsing mouth and frequent oral care may help); or headache (mild analgesic may help). Report increased sneezing, burning, stinging, or irritation inside of nose; sore throat, hoarseness, nosebleed; anaphylactic reaction (skin rash, fever, chills, backache, difficulty breathing, chest pain); or worsening of condition or lack of improvement.

Ophthalmic: For ophthalmic use only. Wash hands before using. Tilt head back and look upward. Put drops of suspension or apply thin ribbon of ointment inside lower eyelid. Close eye and roll eyeball in all directions. Do not blink for ½ minute. apply gentle pressure to inner corner of eye for 30 seconds. Do not use any other eye preparation for at least 10 minutes. Do not let tip of applicator touch eye or contaminate tip of applicator. Do not share medication with anyone else. Temporary stinging or blurred vision may occur. Inform prescriber if condition worsens or fails to improve or if you experience eye pain, redness, burning, watering, dryness, double vision, puffiness around eye, vision disturbances, or other adverse eye response; or worsening of condition or lack of improvement.

**Nursing Implications** Advise patient to clear as much mucus as possible before inhalation treatments

**Dosage Forms**

Inhalation, oral (Intal®): 800 mcg/spray (8.1 g)
Solution, for nebulization:
10 mg/mL (2 mL)
Intal®: 10 mg/mL (2 mL)
Solution, as sodium (Gastrocrom®): 100 mg/5 mL
Solution, nasal (Nasalcrom®): 40 mg/mL (13 mL)
Solution, ophthalmic (Crolom®): 4% (2.5 mL, 10 mL)


- **Crystamine®** *see* Cyanocobalamin *on page 143*
- **Crysti 1000®** *see* Cyanocobalamin *on page 143*
- **Crysticillin® A.S.** *see* Penicillin G Procaine *on page 425*
- **CS-045** *see* Troglitazone *on page 573*
- **CSA** *see* Cyclosporine *on page 146*
- **CTM** *see* Chlorpheniramine *on page 113*
- **C/T/S® Topical Solution** *see* Clindamycin *on page 128*
- **CTX** *see* Cyclophosphamide *on page 145*
- **Cuprimine®** *see* Penicillamine *on page 424*
- **Curretab® Oral** *see* Medroxyprogesterone *on page 336*
- **Cutivate™** *see* Fluticasone *on page 237*
- **CyA** *see* Cyclosporine *on page 146*


## Cyanocobalamin (sye an oh koe BAL a min)

**U.S. Brand Names** Crystamine®; Crysti 1000®; Cyanoject®; Cyomin®; Ener-B®; Nascobal®

**Canadian Brand Names** Rubramin®

**Synonyms** Vitamin $B_{12}$

**Pharmacologic Category** Vitamin, Water Soluble

**Use** Treatment of pernicious anemia; vitamin $B_{12}$ deficiency; increased $B_{12}$ requirements due to pregnancy, thyrotoxicosis, hemorrhage, malignancy, liver or kidney disease

**Effects on Mental Status** None reported

**Effects on Psychiatric Treatment** Anticonvulsants may decrease the absorption of cyanocobalamin

**Pregnancy Risk Factor** A (C if dose exceeds RDA recommendation)

**Contraindications** Hypersensitivity to cyanocobalamin or any component, cobalt; patients with hereditary optic nerve atrophy

**Warnings/Precautions** I.M. route used to treat pernicious anemia; vitamin $B_{12}$ deficiency for >3 months results in irreversible degenerative CNS lesions; treatment of vitamin $B_{12}$ megaloblastic anemia may result in severe hypokalemia, sometimes, fatal, when anemia corrects due to cellular potassium requirements. $B_{12}$ deficiency masks signs of polycythemia vera; vegetarian diets may result in $B_{12}$ deficiency; pernicious anemia occurs more often in gastric carcinoma than in general population.

**Adverse Reactions**

1% to 10%:

Dermatologic: Itching
Gastrointestinal: Diarrhea

<1%: Anaphylaxis, peripheral vascular thrombosis, urticaria

**Drug Interactions** Neomycin, colchicine, anticonvulsants may decrease absorption, chloramphenicol may decrease $B_{12}$ effects

**Usual Dosage**

Recommended daily allowance (RDA):

Children: 0.3-2 mcg
Adults: 2 mcg

Nutritional deficiency: Oral: 25-250 mcg/day

Anemias: I.M. or deep S.C. (oral is not generally recommended due to poor absorption and I.V. is not recommended due to more rapid elimination):

Pernicious anemia, congenital (if evidence of neurologic involvement): 1000 mcg/day for at least 2 weeks; maintenance: 50-100 mcg/month or 100 mcg for 6-7 days; if there is clinical improvement, give 100 mcg every other day for 7 doses, then every 3-4 days for 2-3 weeks; follow with 100 mcg/month for life. Administer with folic acid if needed.

Children: 30-50 mcg/day for 2 or more weeks (to a total dose of 1000-5000 mcg), then follow with 100 mcg/month as maintenance dosage

(Continued)

## Cyanocobalamin *(Continued)*

Adults: 100 mcg/day for 6-7 days; if improvement, administer same dose on alternate days for 7 doses; then every 3-4 days for 2-3 weeks; once hematologic values have returned to normal, maintenance dosage: 100 mcg/month. **Note:** Use only parenteral therapy as oral therapy is not dependable.

Vitamin $B_{12}$ deficiency:

Children:

Neurologic signs: 100 mcg/day for 10-15 days (total dose of 1-1.5 mg), then once or twice weekly for several months; may taper to 60 mcg every month

Hematologic signs: 10-50 mcg/day for 5-10 days, followed by 100-250 mcg/dose every 2-4 weeks

Adults: Initial: 30 mcg/day for 5-10 days; maintenance: 100-200 mcg/month

Schilling test: I.M.: 1000 mcg

**Patient Information** Use exactly as directed. Pernicious anemia may require monthly injections for life. Report skin rash; swelling, pain, or redness of extremities; or acute persistent diarrhea.

**Nursing Implications** Oral therapy is markedly inferior to parenteral therapy; monitor potassium concentrations during early therapy

**Dosage Forms**

Gel, nasal:

Ener-B®: 400 mcg/0.1 mL

Nascobal™: 500 mcg/0.1 mL (5 mL)

Injection: 30 mcg/mL (30 mL); 100 mcg/mL (1 mL, 10 mL, 30 mL); 1000 mcg/mL (1 mL, 10 mL, 30 mL)

Tablet [OTC]: 25 mcg, 50 mcg, 100 mcg, 250 mcg, 500 mcg, 1000 mcg

♦ **Cyanoject®** *see* Cyanocobalamin *on page 143*

♦ **Cyclan®** *see* Cyclandelate *on page 144*

## Cyclandelate (sye KLAN de late)

**U.S. Brand Names** Cyclan®; Cyclospasmol®

**Pharmacologic Category** Vasodilator

**Use** Considered as "possibly effective" for adjunctive therapy in peripheral vascular disease and possibly senility due to cerebrovascular disease or multi-infarct dementia; migraine prophylaxis, vertigo, tinnitus, and visual disturbances secondary to cerebrovascular insufficiency and diabetic peripheral polyneuropathy

**Effects on Mental Status** May cause dizziness

**Effects on Psychiatric Treatment** None reported

**Contraindications** Hypersensitivity to cyclandelate or any component

**Warnings/Precautions** Use with caution in patients with severe obliterative coronary artery or cerebral vascular disease, in patients with active bleeding or a bleeding tendency, and patients with glaucoma

**Adverse Reactions** <1%: Belching, dizziness, flushing of face, headache, heartburn, pain, tachycardia, tingling sensation in face/fingers/toes, weakness

**Overdosage/Toxicology**

Signs and symptoms: Drowsiness, weakness, respiratory depression, hypotension

Treatment: Following decontamination, supportive; fluids followed by vasopressors are most helpful

**Drug Interactions** May enhance action of drugs causing vasodilation/hypotension

**Usual Dosage** Adults: Oral: Initial: 1.2-1.6 g/day in divided doses before meals and at bedtime until response; maintenance therapy: 400-800 mg/day in 2-4 divided doses; start with lowest dose in elderly due to hypotensive potential; decrease dose by 200 mg decrements to achieve minimal maintenance dose; improvement can usually be seen over weeks of therapy and prolonged use; short courses of therapy are usually ineffective and not recommended

**Patient Information** Take with meals or antacids to reduce GI distress

**Dosage Forms**

Capsule: 200 mg, 400 mg

Tablet: 200 mg, 400 mg

## Cyclizine (SYE kli zeen)

**U.S. Brand Names** Marezine® [OTC]

**Synonyms** Cyclizine Hydrochloride; Cyclizine Lactate

**Pharmacologic Category** Antihistamine

**Use** Prevention and treatment of nausea, vomiting, and vertigo associated with motion sickness; control of postoperative nausea and vomiting

**Effects on Mental Status** Drowsiness is common

**Effects on Psychiatric Treatment** Concurrent use with psychotropics may exacerbate the dry mouth and sedation commonly seen with cyclizine

**Contraindications** Hypersensitivity to cyclizine or any component

**Warnings/Precautions** Do not administer to premature or full-term neonates; young children may be more susceptible to side effects and CNS stimulation; bladder neck obstruction, symptomatic prostate hypertrophy, asthmatic attacks, and stenosing peptic ulcer

**Adverse Reactions**

>10%:

Central nervous system: Drowsiness

Gastrointestinal: Xerostomia

1% to 10%:

Central nervous system: Headache

Dermatologic: Dermatitis

Gastrointestinal: Nausea

Genitourinary: Urinary retention

Ocular: Diplopia

Renal: Polyuria

**Overdosage/Toxicology**

Signs and symptoms: Dry mouth, flushed skin, dilated pupils, CNS depression

Treatment: There is no specific treatment for an antihistamine overdose, however, most of its clinical toxicity is due to anticholinergic effects. For anticholinergic overdose with severe life-threatening symptoms, physostigmine 1-2 mg (0.5 or 0.02 mg/kg for children) I.V., slowly may be given to reverse these effects.

**Drug Interactions** Increased effect/toxicity with CNS depressants, alcohol

**Usual Dosage** Oral:

Children 6-12 years: 25 mg up to 3 times/day

Adults: 50 mg taken 30 minutes before departure, may repeat in 4-6 hours if needed, up to 200 mg/day

**Patient Information** May cause drowsiness, may impair judgment and coordination; avoid alcohol; drink plenty of fluids for dry mouth and to prevent constipation

**Dosage Forms**

Injection, as lactate: 50 mg/mL (1 mL)

Tablet, as hydrochloride: 50 mg

♦ **Cyclizine Hydrochloride** *see* Cyclizine *on page 144*

♦ **Cyclizine Lactate** *see* Cyclizine *on page 144*

## Cyclobenzaprine (sye kloe BEN za preen)

**U.S. Brand Names** Flexeril®

**Canadian Brand Names** Novo-Cycloprine

**Pharmacologic Category** Skeletal Muscle Relaxant

**Use** Treatment of muscle spasm associated with acute painful musculoskeletal conditions; supportive therapy in tetanus

**Effects on Mental Status** Drowsiness and dizziness are common; may cause nervousness or confusion

**Effects on Psychiatric Treatment** Contraindicated with MAOIs or within 14 days of MAOI; concurrent use with psychotropics may exacerbate the dry mouth and sedation commonly seen with cyclobenzaprine

**Pregnancy Risk Factor** B

**Contraindications** Hypersensitivity to cyclobenzaprine or any component; do not use concomitantly or within 14 days of MAO inhibitors; hyperthyroidism, congestive heart failure, arrhythmias

**Warnings/Precautions** Cyclobenzaprine shares the toxic potentials of the tricyclic antidepressants and the usual precautions of tricyclic antidepressant therapy should be observed; use with caution in patients with urinary hesitancy or angle-closure glaucoma

**Adverse Reactions**

>10%:

Central nervous system: Drowsiness, dizziness, lightheadedness

Gastrointestinal: Xerostomia

1% to 10%:

Cardiovascular: Edema of the face/lips, syncope

Gastrointestinal: Bloated feeling

Genitourinary: Problems in urinating, polyuria

Hepatic: Hepatitis

Neuromuscular & skeletal: Problems in speaking, muscle weakness

Ocular: Blurred vision

Otic: Tinnitus

<1%: Arrhythmia, ataxia, confusion, constipation, dermatitis, dyspepsia, fatigue, headache, hypotension, nausea, nervousness, rash, stomach cramps, tachycardia, unpleasant taste

**Overdosage/Toxicology**

Signs and symptoms: Troubled breathing, drowsiness, syncope, seizures, tachycardia, hallucinations, vomiting

Treatment: Following initiation of essential overdose management, toxic symptoms should be treated. Ventricular arrhythmias often respond to systemic alkalinization (sodium bicarbonate 0.5-2 mEq/kg I.V.) and/or phenytoin 15-20 mg/kg (adults). Arrhythmias unresponsive to this therapy may respond to lidocaine 1 mg/kg I.V. followed by a titrated infusion. Physostigmine (1-2 mg I.V. slowly for adults or 0.5 mg I.V. slowly for children) may be indicated in reversing cardiac arrhythmias that are life-threatening. Seizures usually respond to diazepam I.V. boluses (5-10 mg for adults up to 30 mg or 0.25-0.4 mg/kg/dose for children up to 10 mg/dose). If seizures are unresponsive or recur, phenytoin or phenobarbital may be required.

**Drug Interactions** CYP1A2, 2D6 and 3A3/4 enzyme substrate

Increased toxicity:

Do not use concomitantly or within 14 days after MAO inhibitors

Because of similarities to the tricyclic antidepressants, may have additive toxicities

Anticholinergics: Because of cyclobenzaprine's anticholinergic action, use with caution in patients receiving these agents

Alcohol, barbiturates, and other CNS depressants: Effects may be enhanced by cyclobenzaprine

**Usual Dosage** Oral: **Note:** Do not use longer than 2-3 weeks

Children: Dosage has not been established

Adults: 20-40 mg/day in 2-4 divided doses; maximum dose: 60 mg/day

**Patient Information** Take exactly as directed. Do not increase dose or discontinue without consulting prescriber. Do not use alcohol, prescriptive or OTC antidepressants, sedatives, or pain medications without consulting prescriber. You may experience drowsiness, dizziness, lightheadedness (avoid driving or engaging in tasks that require alertness until response to drug is known); or urinary retention (void before taking medication). Report excessive drowsiness or mental agitation, chest pain, skin rash, swelling of mouth/face, difficulty speaking, ringing in ears, or blurred vision.

**Nursing Implications** Raise bed rails, institute safety measures, assist with ambulation

**Dosage Forms** Tablet, as hydrochloride: 10 mg

♦ **Cyclocort®** *see* Amcinonide *on page 29*

♦ **Cyclogyl®** *see* Cyclopentolate *on page 145*

♦ **Cyclomydril® Ophthalmic** *see* Cyclopentolate and Phenylephrine *on page 145*

## Cyclopentolate (sye kloe PEN toe late)

**U.S. Brand Names** AK-Pentolate®; Cyclogyl®; I-Pentolate®

**Pharmacologic Category** Anticholinergic Agent, Ophthalmic

**Use** Diagnostic procedures requiring mydriasis and cycloplegia

**Effects on Mental Status** Cyclopentolate may cause restlessness, hallucinations, psychosis, hyperactivity, seizures, incoherent speech, or ataxia. The 2% solution may result in psychotic reactions and behavioral disturbances in children, usually occurring approximately 30-45 minutes after instillation.

**Effects on Psychiatric Treatment** None reported; may counteract the effects of antipsychotics, especially in children; monitor

**Usual Dosage** Ophthalmic:

Neonates and Infants: See Cyclopentolate and Phenylephrine (preferred agent for use in neonates and infants due to lower cyclopentolate concentration and reduced risk for systemic reactions)

Children: Instill 1 drop of 0.5%, 1%, or 2% in eye followed by 1 drop of 0.5% or 1% in 5 minutes, if necessary

Adults: Instill 1 drop of 1% followed by another drop in 5 minutes; 2% solution in heavily pigmented iris

**Dosage Forms** Solution, ophthalmic, as hydrochloride: 0.5% (2 mL, 5 mL, 15 mL); 1% (2 mL, 5 mL, 15 mL); 2% (2 mL, 5 mL, 15 mL)

## Cyclopentolate and Phenylephrine
(sye kloe PEN toe late & fen il EF rin)

**U.S. Brand Names** Cyclomydril® Ophthalmic

**Pharmacologic Category** Ophthalmic Agent, Antiglaucoma

**Use** Induce mydriasis greater than that produced with cyclopentolate HCl alone

**Effects on Mental Status** Cyclopentolate may cause restlessness, hallucinations, psychosis, hyperactivity, seizures, incoherent speech, or ataxia. The 2% solution may result in psychotic reactions and behavioral disturbances in children, usually occurring approximately 30-45 minutes after instillation.

**Effects on Psychiatric Treatment** None reported; may counteract the effects of antipsychotics, especially in children; monitor

**Usual Dosage** Ophthalmic: Neonates, Infants, Children, and Adults: Instill 1 drop into the eye every 5-10 minutes, for up to 3 doses, approximately 40-50 minutes before the examination

**Dosage Forms** Solution, ophthalmic: Cyclopentolate hydrochloride 0.2% and phenylephrine hydrochloride 1% (2 mL, 5 mL)

## Cyclophosphamide (sye kloe FOS fa mide)

**U.S. Brand Names** Cytoxan® Injection; Cytoxan® Oral; Neosar® Injection

**Canadian Brand Names** Procytox®

**Synonyms** CPM; CTX; CYT; NSC 26271

**Pharmacologic Category** Antineoplastic Agent, Alkylating Agent

**Use** Treatment of Hodgkin's and non-Hodgkin's lymphoma, Burkitt's lymphoma, chronic lymphocytic leukemia, chronic granulocytic leukemia, AML, ALL, mycosis fungoides, breast cancer, multiple myeloma, neuroblastoma, retinoblastoma, rhabdomyosarcoma, Ewing's sarcoma; testicular, endometrium and ovarian, and lung cancer, and as a conditioning regimen for BMT; prophylaxis of rejection for kidney, heart, liver, and BMT transplants, severe rheumatoid disorders, nephrotic syndrome, Wegener's granulomatosis, idiopathic pulmonary hemosideroses, myasthenia gravis, multiple sclerosis, systemic lupus erythematosus, lupus nephritis, autoimmune hemolytic anemia, idiopathic thrombocytic purpura, macroglobulinemia, and antibody-induced pure red cell aplasia

**Effects on Mental Status** May cause dizziness

**Effects on Psychiatric Treatment** May cause myelosuppression; use caution with clozapine and carbamazepine

**Pregnancy Risk Factor** D

**Contraindications** Hypersensitivity to cyclophosphamide or any component

**Warnings/Precautions** The U.S. Food and Drug Administration (FDA) currently recommends that procedures for proper handling and disposal of antineoplastic agents be considered. Possible dosage adjustment needed for renal or hepatic failure; use with caution in patients with bone marrow suppression.

**Adverse Reactions**

>10%:

Dermatologic: Alopecia is frequent, but hair will regrow although it may be of a different color or texture; alopecia usually occurs 3 weeks after therapy

Endocrine & metabolic: Fertility: May cause sterility; interferes with oogenesis and spermatogenesis; may be irreversible in some patients; gonadal suppression (amenorrhea)

Gastrointestinal: Nausea and vomiting occur more frequently with larger doses, usually beginning 6-10 hours after administration; also seen are anorexia, diarrhea, stomatitis; mucositis

Emetic potential:

Oral: Low (<10%)

<1 g: Moderate (30% to 60%)

≥1 g: High (>90%)

Time course of nausea/vomiting: Onset: 6-8 hours; Duration: 8-24 hours

Hepatic: Jaundice seen occasionally

1% to 10%:

Central nervous system: Headache

Dermatologic: Skin rash, facial flushing

Hematologic: Myelosuppressive: Thrombocytopenia occurs less frequently than with mechlorethamine, anemia

WBC: Moderate

Platelets: Moderate

Onset (days): 7

Nadir (days): 10-14

Recovery (days): 21

<1%: High-dose therapy may cause cardiac dysfunction manifested as congestive heart failure; cardiac necrosis or hemorrhagic myocarditis has occurred rarely, but is fatal. Cyclophosphamide may also potentiate the cardiac toxicity of anthracyclines.

Dizziness, darkening of skin/fingernails, hyperglycemia, hypokalemia, distortion, hyperuricemia, SIADH has occurred with I.V. doses >50 mg/kg, stomatitis, acute hemorrhagic cystitis is believed to be a result of chemical irritation of the bladder by acrolein, a cyclophosphamide metabolite. Acute hemorrhagic cystitis occurs in 7% to 12% of patients, and has been reported in up to 40% of patients. Hemorrhagic cystitis can be severe and even fatal. Patients should be encouraged to drink plenty of fluids (3-4 L/day) during therapy, void frequently, and avoid taking the drug at nighttime. If large I.V. doses are being administered, I.V. hydration should be given during therapy. The administration of mesna or continuous bladder irrigation may also be warranted.

Hepatic toxicity, renal tubular necrosis has occurred, but usually resolves after the discontinuation of therapy, nasal congestion occurs when given in large I.V. doses via 30-60 minute infusion; patients experience runny eyes, nasal burning, rhinorrhea, sinus congestion, and sneezing during or immediately after the infusion; interstitial pulmonary fibrosis with prolonged high dosage has occurred; secondary malignancy has developed with cyclophosphamide alone or in combination with other antineoplastics; both bladder carcinoma and acute leukemia are well documented; rare instances of anaphylaxis have been reported

**Overdosage/Toxicology**

Signs and symptoms: Myelosuppression, alopecia, nausea, vomiting

Treatment: Supportive; cyclophosphamide is moderately dialyzable (20% to 50%)

**Drug Interactions** CYP2B6, 2D6, and 3A3/4 enzyme substrate

Allopurinol may cause increase in bone marrow depression and may result in significant elevations of cyclophosphamide cytotoxic metabolites

Anesthetic agents: Cyclophosphamide reduces serum pseudocholinesterase concentrations and may prolong the neuromuscular blocking activity of succinylcholine; use with caution with halothane, nitrous oxide, and succinylcholine

Chloramphenicol results in prolonged cyclophosphamide half-life to increase toxicity

Cimetidine inhibits hepatic metabolism of drugs and may decrease or increase the activation of cyclophosphamide

Digoxin: Cyclophosphamide may decrease digoxin serum levels

(Continued)

## Cyclophosphamide *(Continued)*

Doxorubicin: Cyclophosphamide may enhance cardiac toxicity of anthracyclines

Phenobarbital and phenytoin induce hepatic enzymes and cause a more rapid production of cyclophosphamide metabolites with a concurrent decrease in the serum half-life of the parent compound

Tetrahydrocannabinol results in enhanced immunosuppression in animal studies

Thiazide diuretics: Leukopenia may be prolonged

**Usual Dosage** Refer to individual protocols

Patients with compromised bone marrow function may require a 33% to 50% reduction in initial loading dose

Children:

SLE: I.V.: 500-750 mg/m$^2$ every month; maximum dose: 1 g/m$^2$

JRA/vasculitis: I.V.: 10 mg/kg every 2 weeks

Children and Adults:

Oral: 50-100 mg/m$^2$/day as continuous therapy or 400-1000 mg/m$^2$ in divided doses over 4-5 days as intermittent therapy

I.V.:

Single doses: 400-1800 mg/m$^2$ (30-50 mg/kg) per treatment course (1-5 days) which can be repeated at 2- to 4-week intervals

**MAXIMUM SINGLE DOSE WITHOUT BMT is 7 g/m$^2$ (190 mg/kg) SINGLE AGENT THERAPY**

Continuous daily doses: 60-120 mg/m$^2$ (1-2.5 mg/kg) per day

Autologous BMT: IVPB: 50 mg/kg/dose x 4 days or 60 mg/kg/dose for 2 days; total dose is usually divided over 2-4 days

Nephrotic syndrome: Oral: 2-3 mg/kg/day every day for up to 12 weeks when corticosteroids are unsuccessful

**Dosing adjustment in renal impairment:** A large fraction of cyclophosphamide is eliminated by hepatic metabolism

Some authors recommend no dose adjustment unless severe renal insufficiency ($Cl_{cr}$ <20 mL/minute)

$Cl_{cr}$ >10 mL/minute: Administer 100% of normal dose

$Cl_{cr}$ <10 mL/minute: Administer 75% of normal dose

Hemodialysis: Moderately dialyzable (20% to 50%); administer dose posthemodialysis or administer supplemental 50% dose

CAPD effects: Unknown

CAVH effects: Unknown

**Dosing adjustment in hepatic impairment:** Some authors recommend dosage reductions (of up to 30%); however, the pharmacokinetics of cyclophosphamide are not significantly altered in the presence of hepatic insufficiency. Cyclophosphamide undergoes hepatic transformation in the liver to its 4-hydroxycyclophosphamide, which breaks down to its active form, phosphoramide mustard.

**Patient Information** Tablets may be taken during or after meals to reduce GI effects. Maintain adequate fluid balance (2-3 L/day of fluids unless instructed to restrict fluid intake). Void frequently and report any difficulty or pain with urination. May cause hair loss (reversible after treatment) or sterility or amenorrhea (sometimes reversible). If you are diabetic, you will need to monitor serum glucose closely to avoid hypoglycemia. You may be more susceptible to infection; avoid crowds and unnecessary exposure to infection. Report unusual bleeding or bruising; persistent fever or sore throat; blood in urine, stool (black stool), or vomitus; delayed healing of any wounds; skin rash; yellowing of skin or eyes; or changes in color of urine or stool.

**Nursing Implications** Encourage adequate hydration and frequent voiding to help prevent hemorrhagic cystitis

**Dosage Forms**

Powder for injection: 100 mg, 200 mg, 500 mg, 1 g, 2 g

Powder for injection, lyophilized: 100 mg, 200 mg, 500 mg, 1 g, 2 g

Tablet: 25 mg, 50 mg

## Cycloserine (sye kloe SER een)

**U.S. Brand Names** Seromycin® Pulvules®

**Pharmacologic Category** Antibiotic, Miscellaneous; Antitubercular Agent

**Use** Adjunctive treatment in pulmonary or extrapulmonary tuberculosis; has been studied for use in Gaucher's disease

**Effects on Mental Status** May cause drowsiness, confusion, depression, and psychosis

**Effects on Psychiatric Treatment** Low doses (50 mg) have been used to treat negative symptoms of schizophrenia

**Pregnancy Risk Factor** C

**Contraindications** Known hypersensitivity to cycloserine

**Warnings/Precautions** Epilepsy, depression, severe anxiety, psychosis, severe renal insufficiency, chronic alcoholism

**Adverse Reactions** Percentage unknown: Cardiac arrhythmias, coma, confusion, dizziness, drowsiness, elevated liver enzymes, folate deficiency, headache, paresis, psychosis, rash, seizures, tremor, vertigo, vitamin $B_{12}$ deficiency

**Overdosage/Toxicology**

Signs and symptoms: Confusion, agitation, CNS depression, psychosis, coma, seizures

Treatment: Decontaminate with activated charcoal; can be hemodialyzed; management is supportive; administer 100-300 mg/day of pyridoxine to reduce neurotoxic effects; acute toxicity can occur with ingestions >1 g; chronic toxicity: >500 mg/day

**Drug Interactions** Increased toxicity: Alcohol, isoniazid, ethionamide increase toxicity of cycloserine; cycloserine inhibits the hepatic metabolism of phenytoin

**Usual Dosage** Some of the neurotoxic effects may be relieved or prevented by the concomitant administration of pyridoxine

Tuberculosis: Oral:

Children: 10-20 mg/kg/day in 2 divided doses up to 1000 mg/day for 18-24 months

Adults: Initial: 250 mg every 12 hours for 14 days, then administer 500 mg to 1 g/day in 2 divided doses for 18-24 months (maximum daily dose: 1 g)

**Dosing interval in renal impairment:**

$Cl_{cr}$ 10-50 mL/minute: Administer every 24 hours

$Cl_{cr}$ <10 mL/minute: Administer every 36-48 hours

**Patient Information** Take as prescribed; do not discontinue without consulting prescriber. Avoid alcohol. Maintain recommended diet and adequate hydration (2-3 L/day of fluids unless instructed to restrict fluid intake). You may experience drowsiness or restlessness (use caution when driving or engaging in tasks that require alertness until response to drug is known). Report skin rash, acute headache, tremors or changes in mentation (confusion, nightmares, depression, or suicide ideation), or fluid retention (respiratory difficulty, swelling of extremities, unusual weight gain).

**Dosage Forms** Capsule: 250 mg

♦ **Cyclospasmol®** *see* Cyclandelate *on page 144*

♦ **Cyclosporin A** *see* Cyclosporine *on page 146*

## Cyclosporine (SYE kloe spor een)

**Related Information**

Serum Drug Concentrations Commonly Monitored: Guidelines *on page 759*

**U.S. Brand Names** Neoral® Oral; Sandimmune® Injection; Sandimmune® Oral

**Synonyms** CSA; CyA; Cyclosporin A

**Pharmacologic Category** Immunosuppressant Agent

**Use** Immunosuppressant which may be used with azathioprine and/or corticosteroids to prolong organ and patient survival in kidney, liver, and heart transplants; used in allogeneic bone marrow transplants for prevention and treatment of graft-versus-host disease; also used in some cases of severe autoimmune disease that are resistant to corticosteroids and other therapy.

**Unlabeled use:** Short-term high-dose cyclosporine as a modulator of multidrug resistance in cancer treatment

**Effects on Mental Status** None reported

**Effects on Psychiatric Treatment** Carbamazepine and phenobarbital may increase the clearance of cyclosporine resulting in decreased levels; nefazodone may inhibit the clearance of cyclosporine resulting in increased levels of cyclosporine

**Pregnancy Risk Factor** C

**Contraindications** Hypersensitivity to cyclosporine, Cremophor® EL (I.V. solution), or any other I.V. component (ie, polyoxyl 35 castor oil is an ingredient of the parenteral formulation, and polyoxyl 40 hydrogenated castor oil is an ingredient of cyclosporine capsules and solution for microemulsion)

**Warnings/Precautions** Infection and possible development of lymphoma may result. Make dose adjustments to avoid toxicity or possible organ rejection using cyclosporine blood levels because absorption is erratic and elimination is highly variable. Administer with adrenal corticosteroids but not with other immunosuppressive agents. Adjustment of dose should only be made under the direct supervision of an experienced physician. Reserve I.V. use for patients who cannot take oral form. Maintain patent airway; other supportive measures and agents for treating anaphylaxis should be present when I.V. drug is given. Nephrotoxic: If possible avoid concomitant use of other potentially nephrotoxic drugs (eg, acyclovir, aminoglycoside antibiotics, amphotericin B, ciprofloxacin). Injectable form contains ethanol.

**Adverse Reactions**

>10%:

Cardiovascular: Hypertension

Dermatologic: Hirsutism

Endocrine & metabolic: Hypomagnesemia, hypokalemia

Gastrointestinal: Gingival hypertrophy

Neuromuscular & skeletal: Tremor

Renal: Nephrotoxicity

1% to 10%:

Central nervous system: Seizure, headache

Dermatologic: Acne

Gastrointestinal: Abdominal discomfort, nausea, vomiting

Neuromuscular & skeletal: Leg cramps

<1%: Anaphylaxis, flushing, hepatotoxicity, hyperkalemia, hyperuricemia, hypomagnesemia, hypotension, increased susceptibility to infection, myositis, pancreatitis, paresthesias, respiratory distress, sensitivity to temperature extremes, sinusitis, tachycardia, warmth

**Overdosage/Toxicology** Signs and symptoms: Hepatotoxicity, nephrotoxicity, nausea, vomiting, tremor. CNS secondary to direct action of the drug may not be reflected in serum concentrations, may be more predictable by renal magnesium loss.

**Drug Interactions** CYP3A3/4 enzyme substrate

Decreased effect: Drugs that decrease cyclosporine concentrations: Carbamazepine, phenobarbital, phenytoin, rifampin, isoniazid

Increased toxicity:

Drugs that increase cyclosporine concentrations: Azithromycin, clarithromycin, diltiazem, erythromycin, fluconazole, itraconazole, ketoconazole, nicardipine, verapamil, grapefruit juice

Drugs that enhance nephrotoxicity of cyclosporine: Aminoglycosides, amphotericin B, acyclovir

Lovastatin - myositis, myalgias, rhabdomyolysis, acute renal failure

Nifedipine - increases risk of gingival hyperplasia

**Usual Dosage** Children and Adults (oral dosage is ~3 times the I.V. dosage); dosage should be based on ideal body weight:

I.V.:

Initial: 5-6 mg/kg/day beginning 4-12 hours prior to organ transplantation. Patients should be switched to oral cyclosporine as soon as possible; dose should be infused over 2-24 hours.

Maintenance: 2-10 mg/kg/day in divided doses every 8-12 hours; dose should be adjusted to maintain whole blood FPIA trough concentrations in the reference range

Oral: Solution or soft gelatin capsule (Sandimmune®):

Initial: 14-18 mg/kg/day, beginning 4-12 hours prior to organ transplantation

Maintenance: 5-15 mg/kg/day divided every 12-24 hours; maintenance dose is usually tapered to 3-10 mg/kg/day.

Focal segmental glomerulosclerosis: Initial: 3 mg/kg/day divided every 12 hours

Autoimmune diseases: 1-3 mg/kg/day

**Dosing considerations of cyclosporine:**

Switch from I.V. to oral therapy:

Threefold increase in dose

T-tube clamping:

Decrease dose; increased availability of bile facilitates absorption of CsA

Pediatric patients:

About 2-3 times higher dose compared to adults

Liver dysfunction:

Decrease I.V. dose; increase oral dose

Renal dysfunction:

Decrease dose to decrease levels if renal dysfunction is related to the drug.

Dialysis:

Not removed

Inhibitors of hepatic metabolism:

Decrease dose

Inducers of hepatic metabolism:

Monitor drug level; may need to increase dose

Oral: **Solution or soft gelatin capsule in a microemulsion (Neoral®):**

Based on the organ transplant population:

Initial: Same as the initial dose for solution or soft gelatin capsule (listed above) **or**

Renal: 9 mg/kg/day (range: 6-12 mg/kg/day)

Liver: 8 mg/kg/day (range: 4-12 mg/kg/day)

Heart: 7 mg/kg/day (range: 4-10 mg/kg/day)

**Note:** A 1:1 ratio conversion from Sandimmune® to Neoral® has been recommended initially; however, lower doses of Neoral® may be required after conversion to prevent overdose. Total daily doses should be adjusted based on the cyclosporine trough blood concentration and clinical assessment of organ rejection. CsA blood trough levels should be determined prior to conversion. After conversion to Neoral®, CsA trough levels should be monitored every 4-7 days. **Neoral® and Sandimmune® are not bioequivalent and cannot be used interchangeably.**

Hemodialysis: Supplemental dose is not necessary.

Peritoneal dialysis: Supplemental dose is not necessary.

**Dosing adjustment in hepatic impairment:** Probably necessary, monitor levels closely.

**Dosing adjustment recommendations for renal impairment during cyclosporine therapy for severe psoriasis:**

**Serum creatinine levels ≥25% above pretreatment levels:** Take another sample within 2 weeks. If the level remains ≥25% above pretreatment levels, decrease dosage of cyclosporine microemulsion by 25% to 50%. If 2 dosage adjustments do not reverse the increase in serum creatinine levels, treatment should be discontinued.

**Serum creatinine ≥50% above pretreatment levels:** Decrease cyclosporine dosage by 25% to 50%. If 2 dosage adjustments do not reverse the increase in serum creatinine levels, treatment should be discontinued.

**Note:** Increase the frequency of blood pressure monitoring after each alteration in dosage of cyclosporine. Cyclosporine dosage should be decreased by 25% to 50% in patients with no history of hypertension who develop sustained hypertension during therapy and, if hypertension persists, treatment with cyclosporine should be discontinued.

**Dietary Considerations** Grapefruit juice will increase absorption, avoid use; mix with diluent at room temperature. May dilute Neoral® oral solution with orange juice or apple juice. May dilute Sandimmune® oral solution with milk, chocolate milk, or orange juice. Avoid changing diluents frequently.

**Patient Information** Use glass container for liquid solution (do not use plastic or styrofoam cup). Diluting oral solution improves flavor. May dilute Neoral® oral solution with orange juice or apple juice. May dilute Sandimmune® oral solution with milk, chocolate milk, or orange juice. Avoid changing diluents frequently. Mix thoroughly and drink at once. Take dose at the same time each day. You will be susceptible to infection; avoid crowds and exposure to any infectious diseases. Do not have any vaccinations without consulting prescriber. Practice good oral hygiene to reduce gum inflammation; see dentist regularly during treatment. Report acute headache; unusual hair growth or deepening of voice; mouth sores or swollen gums; persistent nausea, vomiting, or abdominal pain; muscle pain or cramping; unusual swelling of extremities, weight gain, or change in urination; or chest pain or rapid heartbeat.

**Nursing Implications** Do not administer liquid from plastic or styrofoam cup. Diluting oral solution improves flavor. May dilute Neoral® oral solution with orange juice or apple juice. May dilute Sandimmune® oral solution with milk, chocolate milk, or orange juice. Stir well; do not allow to stand before drinking; rinse with more diluent to ensure that the total dose is taken; after use, dry outside of pipette; do not rinse with water or other cleaning agents; may cause inflamed gums

**Additional Information** In July, 2000, the SangCya™ brand of cyclosporine was voluntarily recalled due to lack of bioequivalency with Neoral® oral solution when mixed in apple juice. The product was allowed to remain in pharmacies to provide a transition time for changing patients to another cyclosporine product. Patients who were previously stabilized on this product should be instructed not to change how they mix their medication until they can be switched to another product.

**Dosage Forms**

Capsule, microemulsion (Neoral®): 25 mg; 100 mg

Capsule, soft gelatin (Sandimmune®): 25 mg; 50 mg; 100 mg

Injection: 50 mg/mL (5 mL)

Solution, oral (Sandimmune®): 100 mg/mL (50 mL)

Solution, oral, microemulsion (Neoral®): 100 mg/mL (50 mL)

## Cyclothiazide (sye kloe THYE a zide)

**U.S. Brand Names** Anhydron®

**Pharmacologic Category** Diuretic, Thiazide

**Use** Management of mild to moderate hypertension; treatment of edema in congestive heart failure and nephrotic syndrome

**Effects on Mental Status** None reported

**Effects on Psychiatric Treatment** Thiazides decrease lithium clearance resulting in elevated serum lithium levels and potential toxicity; monitor serum lithium levels

**Pregnancy Risk Factor** C

**Contraindications** Hypersensitivity to cyclothiazide or any component; cross-sensitivity with other thiazides or sulfonamides; anuria; renal decompensation

**Warnings/Precautions** Use with caution in severe renal disease. Electrolyte disturbances (hypokalemia, hypochloremic alkalosis, hyponatremia) can occur. Use with caution in severe hepatic dysfunction; hepatic encephalopathy can be caused by electrolyte disturbances. Gout can be precipitate in certain patients with a history of gout, a familial predisposition to gout, or chronic renal failure. Cautious use in diabetics; may see a change in glucose control. I.V. use is generally not recommended (but is available). Hypersensitivity reactions can occur. Can cause SLE exacerbation or activation. Use with caution in patients with moderate or high cholesterol concentrations. Photosensitization may occur. Correct hypokalemia before initiating therapy.

**Adverse Reactions** 1% to 10%: Hypokalemia

**Drug Interactions**

Angiotensin-converting enzyme inhibitors: Increased hypotension if aggressively diuresed with a thiazide diuretic

Beta-blockers increase hyperglycemic effects in Type 2 diabetes mellitus

Cyclosporine and thiazides can increase the risk of gout or renal toxicity; avoid concurrent use

Digoxin toxicity can be exacerbated if a thiazide induces hypokalemia or hypomagnesemia

Lithium toxicity can occur by reducing renal excretion of lithium; monitor lithium concentration and adjust as needed

Neuromuscular blocking agents can prolong blockade; monitor serum potassium and neuromuscular status

NSAIDs can decrease the efficacy of thiazides reducing the diuretic and antihypertensive effects

**Usual Dosage** Adults: Oral: 2 mg/day; up to 2 mg 2-3 times/day

(Continued)

## Cyclothiazide *(Continued)*

**Dosage Forms** Tablet: 2 mg

♦ **Cycofed® Pediatric** *see* Guaifenesin, Pseudoephedrine, and Codeine *on page 258*

♦ **Cycrin® Oral** *see* Medroxyprogesterone *on page 336*

♦ **Cyklokapron®** *see* Tranexamic Acid *on page 559*

♦ **Cylert®** *see* Pemoline *on page 423*

♦ **Cylex® [OTC]** *see* Benzocaine *on page 61*

♦ **Cyomin®** *see* Cyanocobalamin *on page 143*

## Cyproheptadine (si proe HEP ta deen)

**U.S. Brand Names** Periactin®
**Canadian Brand Names** PMS-Cyproheptadine
**Pharmacologic Category** Antihistamine
**Use** Perennial and seasonal allergic rhinitis and other allergic symptoms including urticaria

**Unlabeled use:** Appetite stimulation, blepharospasm, cluster headaches, migraine headaches, Nelson's syndrome, pruritus, schizophrenia, spinal cord damage associated spasticity, and tardive dyskinesia

**Effects on Mental Status** Drowsiness is common; may cause nervousness or depression

**Effects on Psychiatric Treatment** Contraindicated with MAOIs; concurrent use with psychotropic may produce additive sedation

**Pregnancy Risk Factor** B

**Contraindications** Hypersensitivity to cyproheptadine or any component; narrow-angle glaucoma, bladder neck obstruction, acute asthmatic attack, stenosing peptic ulcer, GI tract obstruction, those on MAO inhibitors; avoid use in premature and term newborns due to potential association with SIDS

**Warnings/Precautions** Do not use in neonates, safety and efficacy have not been established in children <2 years of age; symptomatic prostate hypertrophy; antihistamines are more likely to cause dizziness, excessive sedation, syncope, toxic confusion states, and hypotension in the elderly. In case reports, cyproheptadine has promoted weight gain in anorexic adults, though it has not been specifically studied in the elderly. All cases of weight loss or decreased appetite should be adequately assessed.

**Adverse Reactions**

>10%:
- Central nervous system: Slight to moderate drowsiness
- Respiratory: Thickening of bronchial secretions

1% to 10%:
- Central nervous system: Headache, fatigue, nervousness, dizziness
- Gastrointestinal: Appetite stimulation, nausea, diarrhea, abdominal pain, xerostomia
- Neuromuscular & skeletal: Arthralgia
- Respiratory: Pharyngitis

<1%: Allergic reactions, angioedema, bronchospasm, CNS stimulation, depression, edema, epistaxis, hemolytic anemia, hepatitis, leukopenia, myalgia, palpitations, paresthesia, photosensitivity, rash, sedation, seizures, tachycardia, thrombocytopenia

**Overdosage/Toxicology**

Signs and symptoms: CNS depression or stimulation, dry mouth, flushed skin, fixed and dilated pupils, apnea

Treatment: There is no specific treatment for an antihistamine overdose, however, most of its clinical toxicity is due to anticholinergic effects. Anticholinesterase inhibitors may be useful by reducing acetylcholinesterase. Anticholinesterase inhibitors include physostigmine, neostigmine, pyridostigmine, and edrophonium. For anticholinergic overdose with severe life-threatening symptoms, physostigmine 1-2 mg (0.5 or 0.02 mg/kg for children) I.V., slowly may be given to reverse these effects.

**Drug Interactions** Increased toxicity: MAO inhibitors → hallucinations

**Usual Dosage** Oral:

Children: 0.25 mg/kg/day in 2-3 divided doses or 8 mg/m²/day in 2-3 divided doses
- 2-6 years: 2 mg every 8-12 hours (not to exceed 12 mg/day)
- 7-14 years: 4 mg every 8-12 hours (not to exceed 16 mg/day)

Adults: 4-20 mg/day divided every 8 hours (not to exceed 0.5 mg/kg/day)

**Dosing adjustment in hepatic impairment:** Dosage should be reduced in patients with significant hepatic dysfunction

**Dietary Considerations** Alcohol: Additive CNS effects, avoid use

**Patient Information** Take as directed; do not exceed recommended dose. Avoid use of other depressants, alcohol, or sleep-inducing medications unless approved by prescriber. You may experience drowsiness or dizziness (use caution when driving or engaging in tasks requiring alertness until response to drug is known); or dry mouth, nausea, or abdominal pain (frequent small meals, frequent mouth care, chewing gum, or sucking hard candy may help). Report persistent sedation, confusion, or agitation; changes in urinary pattern; blurred vision; chest pain or palpitations; sore throat difficulty breathing or expectorating (thick secretions); or lack of improvement or worsening or condition.

**Nursing Implications** Raise bed rails, institute safety measures, assist with ambulation

**Dosage Forms**
- Syrup, as hydrochloride: 2 mg/5 mL with alcohol 5% (473 mL)
- Tablet, as hydrochloride: 4 mg

♦ **Cystadane®** *see* Betaine Anhydrous *on page 65*

♦ **Cystagon®** *see* Cysteamine *on page 148*

## Cysteamine (sis TEE a meen)

**U.S. Brand Names** Cystagon®
**Pharmacologic Category** Anticystine Agent; Urinary Tract Product
**Use Orphan drug:** Management of nephropathic cystinosis
**Effects on Mental Status** Sedation is common; may cause confusion, nervousness, impaired cognition, and hallucinations
**Effects on Psychiatric Treatment** Concurrent use with psychotropic may produce additive sedation
**Usual Dosage** Initiate therapy with 1/4 to 1/8 of maintenance dose; titrate slowly upward over 4-6 weeks

Children <12 years: Oral: Maintenance: 1.3 g/m²/day divided into 4 doses

Children >12 years and Adults (>110 lbs): 2 g/day in 4 divided doses; dosage may be increased to 1.95 g/m²/day if cystine levels are <1 nmol/1/2 cystine/mg protein, although intolerance and incidence of adverse events may be increased

**Dosage Forms** Capsule, as bitartrate: 50 mg, 150 mg

♦ **Cystospaz®** *see* Hyoscyamine *on page 279*

♦ **Cystospaz-M®** *see* Hyoscyamine *on page 279*

♦ **CYT** *see* Cyclophosphamide *on page 145*

♦ **Cytadren®** *see* Aminoglutethimide *on page 31*

## Cytarabine (sye TARE a been)

**U.S. Brand Names** Cytosar-U®
**Pharmacologic Category** Antineoplastic Agent, Antimetabolite
**Use** Ara-C is one of the most active agents in leukemia; also active against lymphoma, meningeal leukemia, and meningeal lymphoma; has little use in the treatment of solid tumors
**Effects on Mental Status** May cause sedation or confusion
**Effects on Psychiatric Treatment** May cause myelosuppression; use caution with clozapine and carbamazepine
**Usual Dosage I.V. bolus, IVPB, and CIV doses of cytarabine are very different.** Bolus doses are relatively well tolerated since the drug is rapidly metabolized; bolus doses are associated with greater gastrointestinal and neurotoxicity; continuous infusion uniformly results in myelosuppression. Refer to individual protocols.

Children and Adults:

Induction remission:
- I.V.: 200 mg/m²/day for 5 days at 2-week intervals
- 100-200 mg/m²/day for 5- to 10-day therapy course or every day until remission
- I.T.: 5-75 mg/m² every 4 days until CNS findings normalize

**or**
- <1 year: 20 mg
- 1-2 years: 30 mg
- 2-3 years: 50 mg
- >3 years: 70 mg

Maintenance remission:
- I.V.: 70-200 mg/m²/day for 2-5 days at monthly intervals
- I.M., S.C.: 1-1.5 mg/kg single dose for maintenance at 1- to 4-week intervals

High-dose therapies:
- Doses as high as 1-3 g/m² have been used for refractory or secondary leukemias or refractory non-Hodgkin's lymphoma
- Doses of 3 g/m² every 12 hours for up to 12 doses have been used

Bone marrow transplant: 1.5 g/m² continuous infusion over 48 hours

**Dosage adjustment of high-dose therapy in patients with renal insufficiency:** In one study, 76% of patients with a $Cl_{cr}$ <60 mL/minute experienced neurotoxicity; dosage adjustment should be considered in these patients

Hemodialysis: Supplemental dose is not necessary

Peritoneal dialysis: Supplemental dose is not necessary

**Dose may need to be adjusted in patients with liver failure** since cytarabine is partially detoxified in the liver

**Dosage Forms**
- Powder for injection, as hydrochloride: 100 mg, 500 mg, 1 g, 2 g
- Powder for injection, as hydrochloride (Cytosar-U®): 100 mg, 500 mg, 1 g, 2 g

## Cytarabine (Liposomal) (sye TARE a been lip po SOE mal)

**U.S. Brand Names** DepoCyt™

**Pharmacologic Category** Antineoplastic Agent, Antimetabolite

**Use** Intrathecal treatment of lymphomatous meningitis

**Effects on Mental Status** Cerebellar syndrome is common; may cause dizziness, confusion, or sedation

**Effects on Psychiatric Treatment** Myelosuppression is common; use caution with clozapine and carbamazepine. GI side effects are common and dose related; use caution with SSRIs.

**Usual Dosage** Adults:

Induction: 50 mg intrathecally every 14 days for a total of 2 doses (weeks 1 and 3)

Consolidation: 50 mg intrathecally every 14 days for 3 doses (weeks 5, 7, and 9), followed by an additional dose at week 13

Maintenance: 50 mg intrathecally every 28 days for 4 doses (weeks 17, 21, 25, and 29)

If drug-related neurotoxicity develops, the dose should be reduced to 25 mg; if toxicity persists, treatment with liposomal cytarabine should be discontinued

**Note:** Patients should be started on dexamethasone 4 mg twice daily (oral or I.V.) for 5 days, beginning on the day of liposomal cytarabine injection

**Dosage Forms** Injection: 50 mg per 5 mL

- **Cytochrome P-450 Enzymes and Drug Metabolism** *see page 730*
- **Cytochrome P-450 Enzymes and Respective Metabolized Drugs** *see page 731*
- **CytoGam™** *see* Cytomegalovirus Immune Globulin (Intravenous-Human) *on page 149*

## Cytomegalovirus Immune Globulin (Intravenous-Human)

(sye toe meg a low VYE rus i MYUN GLOB yoo lin in tra VEE nus HYU man)

**U.S. Brand Names** CytoGam™

**Pharmacologic Category** Immune Globulin

**Use** Attenuation of primary CMV disease associated with immunosuppressed recipients of kidney transplantation; especially indicated for CMV-negative recipients of CMV-positive donor; has been used as adjunct therapy in the treatment of CMV disease in immunocompromised patients

**Effects on Mental Status** None reported

**Effects on Psychiatric Treatment** None reported

**Usual Dosage** I.V.:

Dosing schedule:

Initial dose (within 72 hours after transplant): 150 mg/kg/dose

2, 4, 6, 8 weeks after transplant: 100 mg/kg/dose

12 and 16 weeks after transplant: 50 mg/kg/dose

Severe CMV pneumonia: Regimens of 400 mg/kg on days 1, 2, 7 or 8, followed by 200 mg/kg have been used

Administration rate: Administer at 15 mg/kg/hour initially, then increase to 30 mg/kg/hour after 30 minutes if no untoward reactions, then increase to 60 mg/kg/hour after another 30 minutes; volume not to exceed 75 mL/hour

**Dosage Forms** Powder for injection, lyophilized, detergent treated: 2500 mg ± 250 mg (50 mL)

- **Cytomel® Oral** *see* Liothyronine *on page 319*
- **Cytosar-U®** *see* Cytarabine *on page 148*
- **Cytotec®** *see* Misoprostol *on page 369*
- **Cytovene®** *see* Ganciclovir *on page 245*
- **Cytoxan® Injection** *see* Cyclophosphamide *on page 145*
- **Cytoxan® Oral** *see* Cyclophosphamide *on page 145*
- **$D_3$** *see* Cholecalciferol *on page 120*
- **D-3-Mercaptovaline** *see* Penicillamine *on page 424*
- **d4T** *see* Stavudine *on page 519*

## Dacarbazine (da KAR ba zeen)

**U.S. Brand Names** DTIC-Dome®

**Pharmacologic Category** Antineoplastic Agent, Alkylating Agent

**Use** Treatment of malignant melanoma, Hodgkin's disease, soft-tissue sarcomas, fibrosarcomas, rhabdomyosarcoma, islet cell carcinoma, medullary carcinoma of the thyroid, and neuroblastoma

**Effects on Mental Status** May cause headache

**Effects on Psychiatric Treatment** May cause myelosuppression; use caution with clozapine and carbamazepine

**Usual Dosage** I.V. (refer to individual protocols):

Children:

Pediatric solid tumors: 200-470 mg/m²/day over 5 days every 21-28 days

Pediatric neuroblastoma: 800-900 mg/m² as a single dose on day 1 of therapy every 3-4 weeks in combination therapy

Hodgkin's disease: 375 mg/m² on days 1 and 15 of treatment course, repeat every 28 days

Adults:

Malignant melanoma: 2-4.5 mg/kg/day for 10 days, repeat in 4 weeks **OR** may use 250 mg/m²/day for 5 days, repeat in 3 weeks

Hodgkin's disease: 150 mg/m²/day for 5 days, repeat every 4 weeks **OR** 375 mg/m² on day 1, repeat in 15 days of each 28-day cycle in combination with other agents **OR** 375 mg/m² repeated in 15 days of each 28-day cycle

**Dosing adjustment in renal impairment:** Adjustment is warranted

**Dosing adjustment/comments in hepatic impairment:** Monitor closely for signs of toxicity

**Dosage Forms** Injection: 100 mg (10 mL, 20 mL); 200 mg (20 mL, 30 mL); 500 mg (50 mL)

## Daclizumab (da KLIK si mab)

**U.S. Brand Names** Zenapax®

**Pharmacologic Category** Immunosuppressant Agent

**Use** Prophylaxis of acute organ rejection in patients receiving renal transplants; used as part of an immunosuppressive regimen that includes cyclosporine and corticosteroids

**Effects on Mental Status** May cause depression, anxiety, or insomnia

**Effects on Psychiatric Treatment** None reported

**Usual Dosage** Children and Adults: IVPB: 1 mg/kg, used as part of an immunosuppressive regimen that includes cyclosporine and corticosteroids for a total of 5 doses; give the first dose ≤24 hours before transplantation. The 4 remaining doses should be administered at intervals of 14 days.

**Dosing adjustment in renal impairment:** None necessary

**Dosage Forms** Injection: 5 mg/mL (5 mL)

- **Dacodyl® [OTC]** *see* Bisacodyl *on page 69*

## Dactinomycin (dak ti noe MYE sin)

**U.S. Brand Names** Cosmegen®

**Pharmacologic Category** Antineoplastic Agent, Antibiotic

**Use** Treatment of testicular tumors, melanoma, choriocarcinoma, Wilms' tumor, neuroblastoma, retinoblastoma, rhabdomyosarcoma, uterine sarcomas, Ewing's sarcoma, Kaposi's sarcoma, and soft tissue sarcoma

**Effects on Mental Status** Sedation is common

**Effects on Psychiatric Treatment** May cause myelosuppression; use caution with clozapine and carbamazepine

**Usual Dosage** Refer to individual protocols

**Calculation of the dosage for obese or edematous patients should be on the basis of surface area in an effort to relate dosage to lean body mass**

Children >6 months and Adults: I.V.:

15 mcg/kg/day **or** 400-600 mcg/m²/day (maximum: 500 mcg) for 5 days, may repeat every 3-6 weeks **or**

2.5 mg/m² given in divided doses over 1-week period and repeated at 2-week intervals **or**

0.75-2 mg/m² as a single dose given at intervals of 1-4 weeks have been used

**Dosing in renal impairment:** No adjustment necessary

**Dosage Forms** Powder for injection, lyophilized: 0.5 mg

- **D.A.II® Tablet** *see* Chlorpheniramine, Phenylephrine, and Methscopolamine *on page 115*
- **Dairy Ease® [OTC]** *see* Lactase *on page 305*
- **Dakrina® Ophthalmic Solution [OTC]** *see* Artificial Tears *on page 48*
- **Dalalone®** *see* Dexamethasone *on page 157*
- **Dalalone D.P.®** *see* Dexamethasone *on page 157*
- **Dalalone L.A.®** *see* Dexamethasone *on page 157*
- **Dalgan®** *see* Dezocine *on page 161*
- **Dallergy®** *see* Chlorpheniramine, Phenylephrine, and Methscopolamine *on page 115*
- **Dallergy-D® Syrup** *see* Chlorpheniramine and Phenylephrine *on page 114*
- **Dalmane®** *see* Flurazepam *on page 235*
- ***d*-Alpha Tocopherol** *see* Vitamin E *on page 586*

## Dalteparin (dal TE pa rin)

**U.S. Brand Names** Fragmin®

**Pharmacologic Category** Low Molecular Weight Heparin

**Use** Prevention of deep vein thrombosis which may lead to pulmonary embolism, in patients requiring abdominal surgery who are at risk for thromboembolism complications (ie, patients >40 years of age, obese, patients with malignancy, history of deep vein thrombosis or pulmonary embolism, and surgical procedures requiring general anesthesia and lasting longer than 30 minutes); prevention of DVT in patients undergoing hip surgery; acute treatment of unstable angina or non-Q-wave myocardial infarction

**Effects on Mental Status** None reported

**Effects on Psychiatric Treatment** None reported

**Usual Dosage** Adults: S.C.:

Low-moderate risk patients undergoing abdominal surgery: 2500 units 1-2 hours prior to surgery, then once daily for 5-10 days postoperatively

High-risk patients undergoing abdominal surgery: 5000 units 1-2 hours prior to surgery and then once daily for 5-10 days postoperatively

Patients undergoing total hip surgery: 2500 units 1-2 hours prior to surgery, then 2500 units 6 hours after surgery (evening of the day of surgery), followed by 5000 units once daily for 7-10 days

Patients with unstable angina or non-Q-wave myocardial infarction: 120 IU/kg body weight (maximum dose: 10,000 IU) every 12 hours for 5-8 days with concurrent aspirin therapy. Discontinue dalteparin once patient is clinically stable.

**Dosage Forms** Injection:

Prefilled syringe: Antifactor Xa 2500 units per 0.2 mL; antifactor Xa 5000 units per 0.2 mL

Multidose vial: 95,000 international units

♦ **Damason-P®** *see* Hydrocodone and Aspirin *on page 272*

## Danaparoid (da NAP a roid)

**U.S. Brand Names** Orgaran®

**Pharmacologic Category** Anticoagulant

**Use** Prevention of postoperative deep vein thrombosis following elective hip replacement surgery

**Unlabeled use:** Systemic anticoagulation for patients with heparin-induced thrombocytopenia: Factor Xa inhibition is used to monitor degree of anticoagulation if necessary

**Adult Danaparoid Treatment Dosing Regimens**

| | Body Weight (kg) | I.V. Bolus aFXaU | Long-Term Infusion aFXaU | Level of aFXaU/mL | Monitoring |
|---|---|---|---|---|---|
| **Deep Vein Thrombosis OR Acute Pulmonary Embolism** | <55<br>55-90<br>>90 | 1250<br>2500<br>3750 | 400 units/h over 4 h then 300 units/h over 4 h, then 150-200 units/h maintenance dose | 0.5-0.8 | Days 1-3 daily, then every alternate day |
| **Deep Vein Thrombosis OR Pulmonary Embolism >5 d old** | <90<br>>90 | 1250<br>1250 | S.C.: 3 x 750/d<br>S.C.: 3 x 1250/d | <0.5 | Not necessary |
| **Embolectomy** | <90<br>>90 and high risk | 2500 preoperatively<br>2500 preoperatively | S.C.: 2 x 1250/d postoperatively<br>150-200 units/hour I.V.; perioperative arterial irrigation, if necessary: 750 units/20 mL NaCl | <0.4<br>0.5-0.8 | Not necessary<br>Days 1-3 daily, then every alternate day |
| **Peripheral Arterial Bypass** | | 2500 preoperatively | 150-200 units/h | 0.5-0.8 | Days 1-3 daily, then every alternate day |
| **Cardiac Catheter** | <90<br>>90 | 2500 preoperatively<br>3750 preoperatively | | | |
| **Surgery (excluding vascular)** | | | S.C.: 750, 1-4 h preoperatively<br>S.C.: 750, 2-5 h postoperatively, then 2 x 750/d | <0.35 | Not necessary |

**Effects on Mental Status** May cause insomnia

**Effects on Psychiatric Treatment** None reported

**Usual Dosage** S.C.:

Children: Safety and effectiveness have not been established

Adults: 750 anti-Xa units twice daily; beginning 1-4 hours before surgery and then not sooner than 2 hours after surgery and every 12 hours until the risk of DVT has diminished, the average duration of therapy is 7-10 days

Treatment: See table.

**Dosing adjustment in elderly and severe renal impairment:** Adjustment may be necessary; patients with serum creatinine levels ≥2.0 mg/dL should be carefully monitored

**Dosage Forms** Injection, as sodium: 750 anti-Xa units/0.6 mL

## Danazol (DA na zole)

**U.S. Brand Names** Danocrine®

**Canadian Brand Names** Cyclomen®

**Pharmacologic Category** Androgen

**Use** Treatment of endometriosis, fibrocystic breast disease, and hereditary angioedema

**Effects on Mental Status** May cause dizziness

**Effects on Psychiatric Treatment** None reported

**Pregnancy Risk Factor** X

**Contraindications** Undiagnosed genital bleeding, hypersensitivity to danazol or any component; pregnancy

**Warnings/Precautions** Use with caution in patients with seizure disorders, migraine, or conditions influenced by edema; impaired hepatic, renal, or cardiac disease, pregnancy, lactation

**Adverse Reactions**

>10%:

- Cardiovascular: Edema
- Dermatologic: Oily skin, acne, hirsutism
- Endocrine & metabolic: Fluid retention, breakthrough bleeding, irregular menstrual periods, decreased breast size
- Gastrointestinal: Weight gain
- Hepatic: Hepatic impairment
- Miscellaneous: Voice deepening

1% to 10%:

- Endocrine & metabolic: Virilization, androgenic effects, amenorrhea, hypoestrogenism
- Neuromuscular & skeletal: Weakness

<1%: Benign intracranial hypertension, bleeding gums, carpal tunnel syndrome, cholestatic jaundice, dizziness, enlarged clitoris, headache, pancreatitis, photosensitivity, monilial vaginitis, skin rashes, testicular atrophy

**Drug Interactions** CYP3A3/4 enzyme inhibitor

Increased toxicity: Decreased insulin requirements; warfarin may increase anticoagulant effects

**Usual Dosage** Adults: Oral:

Female: Endometriosis: Initial: 200-400 mg/day in 2 divided doses for mild disease; individualize dosage. Usual maintenance dose: 800 mg/day in 2 divided doses to achieve amenorrhea and rapid response to painful symptoms. Continue therapy uninterrupted for 3-6 months (up to 9 months).

Female: Fibrocystic breast disease: Range: 10-400 mg/day in 2 divided doses

Male/Female: Hereditary angioedema: Initial: 200 mg 2-3 times/day; after favorable response, decrease the dosage by 50% or less at intervals of 1-3 months or longer if the frequency of attacks dictates. If an attack occurs, increase the dosage by up to 200 mg/day.

**Patient Information** Take as directed; do not discontinue without consulting prescriber. Therapy may take up to several months depending on purpose for therapy. Diabetics should monitor serum glucose closely and notify prescriber of changes; this medication can alter hypoglycemic requirements. You may experience acne, growth of body hair, deepening of voice, loss of libido, impotence, or menstrual irregularity (usually reversible). Report changes in menstrual pattern; deepening of voice or unusual growth of body hair; persistent penile erections; fluid retention (swelling of ankles, feet, or hands, difficulty breathing, or sudden weight gain); change in color of urine or stool; yellowing of eyes or skin; unusual bruising or bleeding; or other adverse reactions.

**Dosage Forms** Capsule: 50 mg, 100 mg, 200 mg

♦ **Danocrine®** *see* Danazol *on page 150*

♦ **Dantrium®** *see* Dantrolene *on page 150*

## Dantrolene (DAN troe leen)

**Related Information**

Psychiatric Emergencies - Neuroleptic Malignant Syndrome *on page 660*

Special Populations - Elderly *on page 662*

**U.S. Brand Names** Dantrium®

**Pharmacologic Category** Skeletal Muscle Relaxant

**Use** Treatment of spasticity associated with spinal cord injury, stroke, cerebral palsy, or multiple sclerosis; also used as treatment of malignant hyperthermia

**Effects on Mental Status** Drowsiness is common; may cause insomnia, nervousness, confusion, or depression

**Effects on Psychiatric Treatment** Concurrent use with psychotropic may result in additive sedation; use to treat neuroleptic malignant syndrome

**Pregnancy Risk Factor** C

**Contraindications** Active hepatic disease; should not be used where spasticity is used to maintain posture or balance

**Warnings/Precautions** Use with caution in patients with impaired cardiac function or impaired pulmonary function; has potential for hepatotoxicity; overt hepatitis has been most frequently observed between the third and twelfth month of therapy; hepatic injury appears to be greater in females and in patients >35 years of age

**Adverse Reactions**

>10%:

Central nervous system: Drowsiness, dizziness, lightheadedness, fatigue

Dermatologic: Rash

Gastrointestinal: Diarrhea (mild), nausea, vomiting

Neuromuscular & skeletal: Muscle weakness

1% to 10%:

Cardiovascular: Pleural effusion with pericarditis

Central nervous system: Chills, fever, headache, insomnia, nervousness, mental depression

Gastrointestinal: Diarrhea (severe), constipation, anorexia, stomach cramps

Ocular: Blurred vision

Respiratory: Respiratory depression

<1%: Confusion, hepatitis, seizures

**Overdosage/Toxicology**

Signs and symptoms: CNS depression, hypotension, nausea, vomiting

Treatment: For decontamination, lavage/activated charcoal with cathartic; do not use ipecac; hypotension can be treated with isotonic I.V. fluids with the patient placed in the Trendelenburg position; dopamine or norepinephrine can be given if hypotension is refractory to above therapy

**Drug Interactions** Increased toxicity: Estrogens (hepatotoxicity), CNS depressants (sedation), MAO inhibitors, phenothiazines, clindamycin (increased neuromuscular blockade), verapamil (hyperkalemia and cardiac depression), warfarin, clofibrate and tolbutamide

**Usual Dosage**

Spasticity: Oral:

Children: Initial: 0.5 mg/kg/dose twice daily, increase frequency to 3-4 times/day at 4- to 7-day intervals, then increase dose by 0.5 mg/kg to a maximum of 3 mg/kg/dose 2-4 times/day up to 400 mg/day

Adults: 25 mg/day to start, increase frequency to 2-4 times/day, then increase dose by 25 mg every 4-7 days to a maximum of 100 mg 2-4 times/day or 400 mg/day

Malignant hyperthermia: Children and Adults:

Oral: 4-8 mg/kg/day in 4 divided doses

Preoperative prophylaxis: Begin 1-2 days prior to surgery with last dose 3-4 hours prior to surgery

I.V.: 1 mg/kg; may repeat dose up to cumulative dose of 10 mg/kg (mean effective dose is 2.5 mg/kg), then switch to oral dosage

Preoperative: 2.5 mg/kg ~1¼ hours prior to anesthesia and infused over 1 hour with additional doses as needed and individualized

**Dietary Considerations** Alcohol: Additive CNS effects, avoid use

**Patient Information** Take exactly as directed. Do not increase dose or discontinue without consulting prescriber. Do not use alcohol, prescriptive or OTC antidepressants, sedatives, or pain medications without consulting prescriber. You may experience drowsiness, dizziness, lightheadedness (avoid driving or engaging in tasks that require alertness until response to drug is known); nausea or vomiting (small, frequent meals, frequent mouth care, or sucking hard candy may help); or diarrhea (buttermilk, boiled milk, or yogurt may help). Report excessive confusion; drowsiness or mental agitation; chest pain, palpitations, or difficulty breathing; skin rash; or vision disturbances.

**Nursing Implications** 36 vials needed for adequate hyperthermia therapy; exercise caution at meals on the day of administration because difficulty swallowing and choking has been reported; avoid extravasation as is a tissue irritant

**Dosage Forms**

Capsule, as sodium: 25 mg, 50 mg, 100 mg

Powder for injection, as sodium: 20 mg

♦ **Dapacin® Cold Capsule [OTC]** *see* Chlorpheniramine, Phenylpropanolamine, and Acetaminophen *on page 116*

## Dapiprazole (DA pi pray zole)

**U.S. Brand Names** Rēv-Eyes™

**Pharmacologic Category** Alpha$_1$ Blocker, Ophthalmic

**Use** Reverse dilation due to drugs (adrenergic or parasympathomimetic) after eye exams

**Effects on Mental Status** None reported

**Effects on Psychiatric Treatment** None reported

**Usual Dosage** Adults: Administer 2 drops followed 5 minutes later by an additional 2 drops applied to the conjunctiva of each eye; should not be used more frequently than once a week in the same patient

**Dosage Forms** Powder, lyophilized, as hydrochloride: 25 mg [0.5% solution when mixed with supplied diluent]

## Dapsone (DAP sone)

**U.S. Brand Names** Avlosulfon®

**Synonyms** Diaminodiphenylsulfone

**Pharmacologic Category** Antibiotic, Miscellaneous

**Use** Treatment of leprosy and dermatitis herpetiformis (infections caused by *Mycobacterium leprae*)

Prophylaxis of toxoplasmosis in severely immunocompromised patients; alternative agent for *Pneumocystis carinii* pneumonia prophylaxis (given alone) and treatment (given with trimethoprim)

May be useful in relapsing polychondritis, prophylaxis of malaria, inflammatory bowel disorders, *Leishmaniasis*, rheumatic/connective tissue disorders, brown recluse spider bites

**Effects on Mental Status** May cause insomnia

**Effects on Psychiatric Treatment** None reported

**Pregnancy Risk Factor** C

**Contraindications** Hypersensitivity to dapsone or any component

**Warnings/Precautions** Use with caution in patients with severe anemia, G-6-PD, methemoglobin reductase or hemoglobin M deficiency; hypersensitivity to other sulfonamides; aplastic anemia, agranulocytosis and other severe blood dyscrasias have resulted in death; monitor carefully; treat severe anemia prior to therapy; serious dermatologic reactions (including toxic epidermal necrolysis) are rare but potential occurrences; sulfone reactions may also occur as potentially fatal hypersensitivity reactions; these, but not leprosy reactional states, require drug discontinuation; dapsone is carcinogenic in small animals

**Adverse Reactions**

1% to 10%: Hematologic: Hemolysis, methemoglobinemia

<1%: Agranulocytosis, anemia, blurred vision, cholestatic jaundice, exfoliative dermatitis, headache, hepatitis, insomnia, leukopenia, nausea, peripheral neuropathy (usually in nonleprosy patients), photosensitivity, reactional states (ie, abrupt changes in clinical activity occurring during any leprosy treatment; classified as reversal of erythema nodosum leprosum reactions); SLE, tinnitus, vomiting

**Overdosage/Toxicology**

Signs and symptoms: Nausea, vomiting, confusion, hyperexcitability, seizures, cyanosis, hemolysis, methemoglobinemia, sulfhemoglobinemia, metabolic acidosis, hallucinations, hepatitis

Treatment: Following decontamination, methylene blue 1-2 mg/kg I.V. is treatment of choice if MHb level is >15%; may repeat every 6-8 hours for 2-3 days if needed; if hemolysis is present, give I.V. fluids and alkalinize urine to prevent acute tubular necrosis

**Drug Interactions** CYP2C9, 2E1, and 3A3/4 enzyme substrate

Decreased effect/levels: Para-aminobenzoic acid, didanosine, and rifampin decrease dapsone effects

Increased toxicity: Folic acid antagonists may increase the risk of hematologic reactions of dapsone; probenecid decreases dapsone excretion; trimethoprim with dapsone may increase toxic effects of both drugs; Protease inhibitor like amprenavir and ritonavir may increase dapsone's serum concentration.

**Usual Dosage** Oral:

Leprosy:

Children: 1-2 mg/kg/24 hours, up to a maximum of 100 mg/day

Adults: 50-100 mg/day for 3-10 years

Dermatitis herpetiformis: Adults: Start at 50 mg/day, increase to 300 mg/day, or higher to achieve full control, reduce dosage to minimum level as soon as possible

Prophylaxis of *Pneumocystis carinii* pneumonia:

Children >1 month: 1 mg/kg/day; maximum: 100 mg

Adults: 100 mg/day

Treatment of *Pneumocystis carinii* pneumonia: Adults: 100 mg/day in combination with trimethoprim (15-20 mg/kg/day) for 21 days

**Dosing in renal impairment:** No specific guidelines are available

**Patient Information** Take as directed, for full term of therapy (treatment for leprosy may take 3-10 years). Do not take with antacids, alkaline foods, or drugs (may decrease dapsone absorption). Frequent blood tests may be required during therapy. Discontinue if rash develops and notify prescriber. Report persistent sore throat, fever, chills; constant fatigue; yellowing of skin or eyes; or easy bruising or bleeding.

**Dosage Forms** Tablet: 25 mg, 100 mg

♦ **Daranide®** *see* Dichlorphenamide *on page 163*

♦ **Daraprim®** *see* Pyrimethamine *on page 481*

♦ **Darbid®** *see* Isopropamide *on page 295*

- **Daricon®** *see* Oxyphencyclimine *on page 416*
- **Darvocet-N®** *see* Propoxyphene and Acetaminophen *on page 474*
- **Darvocet-N® 100** *see* Propoxyphene and Acetaminophen *on page 474*
- **Darvon®** *see* Propoxyphene *on page 474*
- **Darvon® Compound-65 Pulvules®** *see* Propoxyphene and Aspirin *on page 475*
- **Darvon-N®** *see* Propoxyphene *on page 474*

## Daunorubicin Citrate (Liposomal)

(daw noe ROO bi sin SI trate lip po SOE mal)

**Related Information**
Daunorubicin Hydrochloride *on page 152*
**U.S. Brand Names** DaunoXome®
**Pharmacologic Category** Antineoplastic Agent, Antibiotic
**Use** Advanced HIV-associated Kaposi's sarcoma; first-line cytotoxic therapy for advanced HIV-associated Kaposi's sarcoma
**Effects on Mental Status** May produce myelosuppression; caution with clozapine and carbamazepine
**Effects on Psychiatric Treatment** None reported
**Usual Dosage** Adults: I.V.: 40 mg/m$^2$ over 1 hour; repeat every 2 weeks; continue treatment until there is evidence of progressive disease
**Dosing adjustment in renal/hepatic impairment:**
Serum bilirubin 1.2-3 mg/dL: $^3/_4$ normal dose recommended
Serum bilirubin >3 mg/dL; serum creatinine >3 mg/dL: $^1/_2$ normal dose recommended
**Dosage Forms** Injection: 2 mg/mL (equivalent to 50 mg daunorubicin base) (1 mL, 4 mL, 10 mL unit packs)

## Daunorubicin Hydrochloride

(daw noe ROO bi sin hye droe KLOR ide)

**U.S. Brand Names** Cerubidine®
**Pharmacologic Category** Antineoplastic Agent, Antibiotic
**Use** Treatment of ANLL and myeloblastic leukemia; lymphoma
**Effects on Mental Status** None reported
**Effects on Psychiatric Treatment** May produce myelosuppression; use caution with clozapine and carbamazepine
**Usual Dosage** I.V. (refer to individual protocols):
Children:
ALL combination therapy: Remission induction: 25-45 mg/m$^2$ on day 1 every week for 4 cycles **or** 30-45 mg/m$^2$/day for 3 days
AML combination therapy: Induction: I.V. continuous infusion: 30-60 mg/m$^2$/day on days 1-3 of cycle
**Note:** In children <2 years or <0.5 m$^2$, daunorubicin should be based on weight - mg/kg: 1 mg/kg per protocol with frequency dependent on regimen employed
Cumulative dose should not exceed 300 mg/m$^2$ in children >2 years or 10 mg/kg in children <2 years
Adults:
30-60 mg/m$^2$/day for 3-5 days, repeat dose in 3-4 weeks
AML: Single agent induction: 60 mg/m$^2$/day for 3 days; repeat every 3-4 weeks
AML: Combination therapy induction: 45 mg/m$^2$/day for 3 days of the first course of induction therapy; subsequent courses: Every day for 2 days
ALL combination therapy: 45 mg/m$^2$/day for 3 days
Cumulative dose should not exceed 400-600 mg/m$^2$
**Dosing adjustment in renal impairment:**
$Cl_{cr}$ <10 mL/minute: Administer 75% of normal dose
$S_{cr}$ >3 mg/dL: Administer 50% of normal dose
**Dosing adjustment in hepatic impairment:**
Serum bilirubin 1.2-3 mg/dL or AST 60-180 int. units: Reduce dose to 75%
Serum bilirubin 3.1-5 mg/dL or AST >180 int. units: Reduce dose to 50%
Serum bilirubin >5 mg/dL: Omit use
**Dosage Forms** Powder for injection, lyophilized: 20 mg

- **DaunoXome®** *see* Daunorubicin Citrate (Liposomal) *on page 152*
- **Daypro™** *see* Oxaprozin *on page 409*
- **Dayto Himbin®** *see* Yohimbine *on page 589*
- **DC 240® Softgels® [OTC]** *see* Docusate *on page 179*
- **DCF** *see* Pentostatin *on page 430*
- **DDAVP®** *see* Desmopressin *on page 156*
- **ddC** *see* Zalcitabine *on page 590*
- **ddI** *see* Didanosine *on page 166*
- **1-Deamino-8-D-Arginine Vasopressin** *see* Desmopressin *on page 156*
- **Deaner®** *see* Deanol *on page 152*

## Deanol (DE ah nol)

**U.S. Brand Names** Acumen®; Atrol®; Deaner®; Elevan®; Panclar®
**Synonyms** Demanol; 2-Dimethylaminoethanol
**Pharmacologic Category** Stimulant
**Use** Psychostimulant, antispasmodic; not available in U.S. since 1983; has been used to reverse levodopa-induced dyskinesias; used for hyperkinetic children
**Effects on Mental Status** May cause insomnia
**Effects on Psychiatric Treatment** Do not use with other stimulants
**Contraindications** Seizure disorders
**Adverse Reactions**
Cardiovascular: Hypotension (orthostatic) rare
Central nervous system: Headache, insomnia, trismus
Dermatologic: Pruritus, rash
Gastrointestinal: Constipation
**Drug Interactions** Avoid concomitant use of amphetamines
**Usual Dosage**
Reduce levodopa dyskinesias: Initial: 100 mg 3 times/day for 5 days; can increase dosage from 500-900 mg/day; improvement noted in 10-94 days
Hyperactivity syndrome: Children: Recommended daily dosage: 300 mg
**Dosage Forms**
Injection: 1.5 g (15 mL), 3 g (15 mL)
Tablet:
Deanol: 100 mg
Deanol acetamidobenzoate: 100 mg
Deanol benzilate: 0.3 mg

- **Debrox® Otic [OTC]** *see* Carbamide Peroxide *on page 92*
- **Decadron®** *see* Dexamethasone *on page 157*
- **Decadron®-LA** *see* Dexamethasone *on page 157*
- **Decadron® Phosphate** *see* Dexamethasone *on page 157*
- **Deca-Durabolin® Injection** *see* Nandrolone *on page 383*
- **Decaject®** *see* Dexamethasone *on page 157*
- **Decaject-LA®** *see* Dexamethasone *on page 157*
- **Decholin®** *see* Dehydrocholic Acid *on page 153*
- **Declomycin®** *see* Demeclocycline *on page 153*
- **Decofed® Syrup [OTC]** *see* Pseudoephedrine *on page 478*
- **Decohistine® DH** *see* Chlorpheniramine, Pseudoephedrine, and Codeine *on page 116*
- **Decohistine® Expectorant** *see* Guaifenesin, Pseudoephedrine, and Codeine *on page 258*
- **Deconamine® SR** *see* Chlorpheniramine and Pseudoephedrine *on page 114*
- **Deconamine® Syrup [OTC]** *see* Chlorpheniramine and Pseudoephedrine *on page 114*
- **Deconamine® Tablet [OTC]** *see* Chlorpheniramine and Pseudoephedrine *on page 114*
- **Deconsal® II** *see* Guaifenesin and Pseudoephedrine *on page 257*
- **Deconsal® Sprinkle®** *see* Guaifenesin and Phenylephrine *on page 257*
- **Defen®-LA** *see* Guaifenesin and Pseudoephedrine *on page 257*

## Deferoxamine (de fer OKS a meen)

**U.S. Brand Names** Desferal® Mesylate
**Pharmacologic Category** Antidote
**Use** Acute iron intoxication when serum iron is >450-500 mcg/dL or when clinical signs of significant iron toxicity exist; chronic iron overload secondary to multiple transfusions; diagnostic test for iron overload; iron overload secondary to congenital anemias; hemochromatosis; removal of corneal rust rings following surgical removal of foreign bodies
**Unlabeled use:** Treatment of aluminum accumulation in renal failure
**Effects on Mental Status** None reported
**Effects on Psychiatric Treatment** Loss of consciousness has been reported with concurrent use of prochlorperazine
**Usual Dosage**
Children and Adults:
Acute iron toxicity: I.V. route is used when severe toxicity is evidenced by systemic symptoms (coma, shock, metabolic acidosis, or severe gastrointestinal bleeding) or potentially severe intoxications (serum iron level >500 μg/dL). When severe symptoms are not present, the I.M. route may be preferred, however the use of deferoxamine in situations where the serum iron concentration is <500 μg/dL or when severe toxicity is not evident is a subject of some clinical debate.
Dose: 15 mg/kg/hour (although rates up to 40-50 mg/kg/hour have been given in patients with massive iron intoxication); maximum

recommended dose: 6 g/day (however, doses as high as 16-37 g have been administered)

Children:

Chronic iron overload: S.C.: 20-40 mg/kg/day over 8-12 hours (via a portable, controlled infusion device)

Aluminum-induced bone disease: 20-40 mg/kg every hemodialysis treatment, frequency dependent on clinical status of the patient

Adults: Chronic iron overload:

I.V.: 2 g after each unit of blood infusion at 15 mg/kg/hour

S.C.: 1-2 g every day over 8-24 hours

**Dosing adjustment in renal impairment:** $Cl_{cr}$ <10 mL/minute: Administer 50% of dose

Has been used investigationally as a single 40 mg/kg I.V. dose over 2 hours, to promote mobilization of aluminum from tissue stores as an aid in the diagnosis of aluminum-associated osteodystrophy

**Dosage Forms** Powder for injection, as mesylate: 500 mg


- ♦ **Deficol® [OTC]** *see* Bisacodyl *on page 69*
- ♦ **Degas® [OTC]** *see* Simethicone *on page 512*
- ♦ **Degest® 2 Ophthalmic [OTC]** *see* Naphazoline *on page 383*


## Dehydrocholic Acid (dee hye droe KOE lik AS id)

**U.S. Brand Names** Cholan-HMB®; Decholin®

**Canadian Brand Names** Dycholium®

**Pharmacologic Category** Bile Acid; Laxative, Hydrocholeretic

**Use** Relief of constipation; adjunct to various biliary tract conditions

**Effects on Mental Status** None reported

**Effects on Psychiatric Treatment** None reported

**Usual Dosage** Children >12 years and Adults: 250-500 mg 2-3 times/day after meals up to 1.5 g/day

**Dosage Forms** Tablet: 250 mg


- ♦ **Deiten®** *see* Nitrendipine *on page 396*
- ♦ **Deladumone® Injection** *see* Estradiol and Testosterone *on page 205*
- ♦ **Del Aqua-5® Gel** *see* Benzoyl Peroxide *on page 62*
- ♦ **Del Aqua-10® Gel** *see* Benzoyl Peroxide *on page 62*
- ♦ **Delatest® Injection** *see* Testosterone *on page 536*
- ♦ **Delatestryl® Injection** *see* Testosterone *on page 536*


## Delavirdine (de la VIR deen)

**U.S. Brand Names** Rescriptor®

**Synonyms** U-90152S

**Pharmacologic Category** Antiretroviral Agent, Reverse Transcriptase Inhibitor (Non-Nucleoside)

**Use** Treatment of HIV-1 infection in combination with at least two additional antiretroviral agents

**Effects on Mental Status** May cause sedation

**Effects on Psychiatric Treatment** Fluoxetine may increase plasma concentrations of delavirdine; carbamazepine and phenobarbital may decrease plasma concentrations of delavirdine; delavirdine may increase concentrations of alprazolam, midazolam, and triazolam

**Pregnancy Risk Factor** C

**Contraindications** Known hypersensitivity to delavirdine or any components

**Warnings/Precautions** Avoid use with terfenadine, astemizole, benzodiazepines, clarithromycin, dapsone, cisapride, rifabutin, rifampin; use with caution in patients with hepatic or renal dysfunction; due to rapid emergence of resistance, delavirdine should not be used as monotherapy; cross-resistance may be conferred to other non-nucleoside reverse transcriptase inhibitors, although potential for cross-resistance with protease inhibitors is low. Long-term effects of delavirdine are not known. Safety and efficacy have not been established in children. Rash, which occurs frequently, may require discontinuation of therapy; usually occurs within 1-3 weeks and lasts <2 weeks. Most patients may resume therapy following a treatment interruption.

**Adverse Reactions** >2%:

Central nervous system: Headache, fatigue

Dermatologic: Rash, pruritus

Gastrointestinal: Nausea, diarrhea, vomiting

Metabolic: Increased ALT/AST

**Overdosage/Toxicology**

Human reports of overdose with delavirdine are not available

Treatment: GI decontamination and supportive measures are recommended, dialysis unlikely to be of benefit in removing drug since it is extensively metabolized by the liver and is highly protein bound

**Drug Interactions** CYP2D6 and 3A3/4 enzyme substrate; CYP2D6 and 3A3/4 enzyme inhibitor

Increased plasma concentrations of delavirdine: Clarithromycin, ketoconazole, fluoxetine

Decreased plasma concentrations of delavirdine: Carbamazepine, phenobarbital, phenytoin, rifabutin, rifampin, didanosine, saquinavir

Decreased absorption of delavirdine: Antacids, histamine-2 receptor antagonists, didanosine

Delavirdine increases plasma concentrations of: Indinavir, saquinavir, terfenadine, astemizole, clarithromycin, dapsone, rifabutin, ergot derivatives, alprazolam, midazolam, triazolam, dihydropyridines, cisapride, quinidine, warfarin, antiarrhythmics, nonsedating antihistamines, sedative-hypnotics, calcium channel blockers, amprenavir

Delavirdine decreases plasma concentrations of: Didanosine

**Usual Dosage** Adults: Oral: 400 mg 3 times/day

**Dietary Considerations** Delavirdine may be taken without regard to food

**Patient Information** Delavirdine is not a cure for HIV nor has it been found to reduce transmission of HIV. Take as directed, with food. Do not take antacids within 1 hour of delavirdine. Mix 4 tablets in 3-5 ounces of water, allow to stand a few minutes, and stir; drink immediately. You may experience nausea or vomiting (small frequent meals, frequent mouth care, sucking lozenges, or chewing gum may help - consult prescriber if nausea or vomiting persists). Report mouth sores; skin rash or irritation; muscle weakness or tremors; easy bruising or bleeding, fever or chills; CNS changes (eg, hallucinations, confusion, dizziness, altered coordination); swelling of face, lips, or tongue; yellowing of eyes or skin; or dark urine or pale stools.

**Dosage Forms**

Capsule: 200 mg

Tablet: 100 mg


- ♦ **Delcort®** *see* Hydrocortisone *on page 273*
- ♦ **Delestrogen® Injection** *see* Estradiol *on page 203*
- ♦ **Delfen® [OTC]** *see* Nonoxynol 9 *on page 398*
- ♦ **Del-Mycin® Topical** *see* Erythromycin, Ophthalmic/Topical *on page 202*
- ♦ **Delsym® [OTC]** *see* Dextromethorphan *on page 160*
- ♦ **Delta-Cortef® Oral** *see* Prednisolone *on page 459*
- ♦ **Deltacortisone** *see* Prednisone *on page 461*
- ♦ **Delta-D®** *see* Cholecalciferol *on page 120*
- ♦ **Deltadehydrocortisone** *see* Prednisone *on page 461*
- ♦ **Deltasone®** *see* Prednisone *on page 461*
- ♦ **Delta-Tritex®** *see* Triamcinolone *on page 563*
- ♦ **Del-Vi-A®** *see* Vitamin A *on page 585*
- ♦ **Demadex®** *see* Torsemide *on page 557*
- ♦ **Demanol** *see* Deanol *on page 152*
- ♦ **Demazin® Syrup [OTC]** *see* Chlorpheniramine and Phenylpropanolamine *on page 114*


## Demecarium (dem e KARE ee um)

**Related Information**

Glaucoma Drug Therapy *on page 712*

**U.S. Brand Names** Humorsol® Ophthalmic

**Pharmacologic Category** Cholinergic Agonist; Ophthalmic Agent, Antiglaucoma; Ophthalmic Agent, Miotic

**Use** Management of chronic simple glaucoma, chronic and acute angle-closure glaucoma; strabismus

**Effects on Mental Status** None reported

**Effects on Psychiatric Treatment** None reported

**Usual Dosage** Children/Adults: Ophthalmic:

Glaucoma: Instill 1 drop into eyes twice weekly to a maximum dosage of 1 or 2 drops twice daily for up to 4 months

Strabismus:

Diagnosis: Instill 1 drop daily for 2 weeks, then 1 drop every 2 days for 2-3 weeks. If eyes become straighter, an accommodative factor is demonstrated.

Therapy: Instill not more than 1 drop at a time in both eyes every day for 2-3 weeks. Then reduce dosage to 1 drop every other day for 3-4 weeks and re-evaluate. Continue at 1 drop every 2 days to 1 drop twice a week and evaluate the patient's condition every 4-12 weeks. If improvement continues, reduce dose to 1 drop once a week and eventually off of medication. Discontinue therapy after 4 months if control of the condition still requires 1 drop every 2 days.

**Dosage Forms** Solution, ophthalmic, as bromide: 0.125% (5 mL); 0.25% (5 mL)

## Demeclocycline (dem e kloe SYE kleen)

**U.S. Brand Names** Declomycin®

**Synonyms** Demethylchlortetracycline

**Pharmacologic Category** Antibiotic, Tetracycline Derivative

(Continued)

## Demeclocycline *(Continued)*

**Use** Treatment of susceptible bacterial infections (acne, gonorrhea, pertussis and urinary tract infections) caused by both gram-negative and gram-positive organisms; used when penicillin is contraindicated (other agents are preferred); treatment of chronic syndrome of inappropriate secretion of antidiuretic hormone (SIADH)

**Effects on Mental Status** Tetracyclines reported to cause memory disturbances, mood stabilizing and antidepressant effects

**Effects on Psychiatric Treatment** Barbiturates and carbamazepine may decrease the effects of demeclocycline

**Pregnancy Risk Factor** D

**Contraindications** Hypersensitivity to demeclocycline, tetracyclines, or any component

**Warnings/Precautions** Do not administer to children <9 years of age; photosensitivity reactions occur frequently with this drug, avoid prolonged exposure to sunlight, do not use tanning equipment

**Adverse Reactions**

1% to 10%:

Dermatologic: Photosensitivity

Gastrointestinal: Nausea, diarrhea

<1%: Abdominal cramps, acute renal failure, anaphylaxis, anorexia, azotemia, bulging fontanels in infants, dermatologic effects, diabetes insipidus syndrome, esophagitis, exfoliative dermatitis, increased intracranial pressure, paresthesia, pericarditis, pigmentation of nails, pruritus, superinfections, vomiting

**Overdosage/Toxicology**

Signs and symptoms: Diabetes insipidus, nausea, anorexia, diarrhea

Treatment: Following GI decontamination, treatment is supportive

**Drug Interactions**

Decreased effect with antacids (aluminum, calcium, zinc, or magnesium), bismuth salts, sodium bicarbonate, barbiturates, carbamazepine, hydantoins

Decreased effect of oral contraceptives

Increased effect of warfarin

**Usual Dosage** Oral:

Children ≥8 years: 8-12 mg/kg/day divided every 6-12 hours

Adults: 150 mg 4 times/day or 300 mg twice daily

Uncomplicated gonorrhea (penicillin sensitive): 600 mg stat, 300 mg every 12 hours for 4 days (3 g total)

SIADH: 900-1200 mg/day or 13-15 mg/kg/day divided every 6-8 hours initially, then decrease to 600-900 mg/day

**Dosing adjustment/comments in renal/hepatic impairment:** Should be avoided in patients with renal/hepatic dysfunction

**Patient Information** Preferable to take on an empty stomach (1 hour before or 2 hours after meals). Take at regularly scheduled times around-the-clock. Avoid antacids, iron, or dairy products within 2 hours of taking demeclocycline. You may experience photosensitivity (use sunscreen, wear protective clothing and eyewear, and avoid direct sunlight); dizziness or lightheadedness (use caution when driving or engaging in tasks that require alertness until response to drug is known); nausea/vomiting (frequent small meals, frequent mouth care, sucking lozenges, or chewing gum may help); or diarrhea (buttermilk, yogurt, or boiled milk may help). If diabetic, drug may cause false tests with Clinitest® urine glucose monitoring; use of glucose oxidase methods (Clinistix®) or serum glucose monitoring is preferable. Report rash or intense itching; yellowing of skin or eyes; change in color of urine or stools; fever or chills; dark urine or pale stools; vaginal itching or discharge; foul-smelling stools; excessive thirst or urination; acute headache; unresolved diarrhea; or difficulty breathing.

**Dosage Forms**

Capsule, as hydrochloride: 150 mg

Tablet, as hydrochloride: 150 mg, 300 mg


♦ **Demerol®** *see* Meperidine *on page 341*

♦ **Demethylchlortetracycline** *see* Demeclocycline *on page 153*

♦ **Demorphan** *see* Dextromethorphan *on page 160*

♦ **Demser®** *see* Metyrosine *on page 363*

♦ **Demulen®** *see* Estradiol and Ethynodiol Diacetate *on page 204*

♦ **Denavir™** *see* Penciclovir *on page 424*


## Denileukin Diftitox (de ne LU kin DEFT e tox)

**U.S. Brand Names** Ontak™

**Pharmacologic Category** Antineoplastic Agent, Miscellaneous

**Use** Treatment of patients with persistent or recurrent cutaneous T-cell lymphoma whose malignant cells express the CD25 component of the IL-2 receptor

**Effects on Mental Status** Dizziness and nervousness are common; may cause insomnia or confusion

**Effects on Psychiatric Treatment** Hypotension and tachycardia are common; use caution with low potency antipsychotics and other psychotropics. Nausea and vomiting are common; use caution with SSRIs.

**Usual Dosage** Adults: I.V.: A treatment cycle consists of 9 or 18 mcg/kg/day for 5 consecutive days administered every 21 days. The optimal duration of therapy has not been determined. Only 2% of patients who failed to demonstrate a response (at least a 25% decrease in tumor burden) prior to the fourth cycle responded to subsequent treatment.

**Dosage Forms** Injection: 150 mcg/mL (2 mL)


♦ **Deodorized Opium Tincture** *see* Opium Tincture *on page 406*

♦ **Deoxycoformycin** *see* Pentostatin *on page 430*

♦ **2′-deoxycoformycin** *see* Pentostatin *on page 430*

♦ **Depacon™** *see* Valproic Acid and Derivatives *on page 578*

♦ **Depakene®** *see* Valproic Acid and Derivatives *on page 578*

♦ **Depakote® Delayed Release** *see* Valproic Acid and Derivatives *on page 578*

♦ **Depakote® ER** *see* Valproic Acid and Derivatives *on page 578*

♦ **depAndrogyn® Injection** *see* Estradiol and Testosterone *on page 205*

♦ **depAndro® Injection** *see* Testosterone *on page 536*

♦ **Depen®** *see* Penicillamine *on page 424*

♦ **depGynogen® Injection** *see* Estradiol *on page 203*

♦ **depMedalone® Injection** *see* Methylprednisolone *on page 359*

♦ **DepoCyt™** *see* Cytarabine (Liposomal) *on page 149*

♦ **Depo®-Estradiol Injection** *see* Estradiol *on page 203*

♦ **Depogen® Injection** *see* Estradiol *on page 203*

♦ **Depoject® Injection** *see* Methylprednisolone *on page 359*

♦ **Depo-Medrol® Injection** *see* Methylprednisolone *on page 359*

♦ **Deponit® Patch** *see* Nitroglycerin *on page 397*

♦ **Depopred® Injection** *see* Methylprednisolone *on page 359*

♦ **Depo-Provera® Injection** *see* Medroxyprogesterone *on page 336*

♦ **Depo-Testadiol® Injection** *see* Estradiol and Testosterone *on page 205*

♦ **Depotest® Injection** *see* Testosterone *on page 536*

♦ **Depotestogen® Injection** *see* Estradiol and Testosterone *on page 205*

♦ **Depo®-Testosterone Injection** *see* Testosterone *on page 536*

♦ **Deprenyl** *see* Selegiline *on page 508*

♦ **Depression Treatment** *see page 781*

♦ **Deproist® Expectorant With Codeine** *see* Guaifenesin, Pseudoephedrine, and Codeine *on page 258*

♦ **Dermacort®** *see* Hydrocortisone *on page 273*

♦ **Dermaflex® Gel** *see* Lidocaine *on page 317*

♦ **Dermarest Dricort®** *see* Hydrocortisone *on page 273*

♦ **Derma-Smoothe/FS®** *see* Fluocinolone *on page 231*

♦ **Dermatop®** *see* Prednicarbate *on page 459*

♦ **Dermatophytin-O** *see Candida albicans* (*Monilia*) *on page 87*

♦ **DermiCort®** *see* Hydrocortisone *on page 273*

♦ **Dermolate® [OTC]** *see* Hydrocortisone *on page 273*

♦ **Dermoplast® [OTC]** *see* Benzocaine *on page 61*

♦ **Dermtex® HC With Aloe** *see* Hydrocortisone *on page 273*

♦ **DES** *see* Diethylstilbestrol *on page 168*

♦ **Desace®** *see* Deslanoside *on page 156*

♦ **Desaci®** *see* Deslanoside *on page 156*

♦ **Desferal® Mesylate** *see* Deferoxamine *on page 152*

♦ **Desiccated Thyroid** *see* Thyroid *on page 547*


## Desipramine (des IP ra meen)

**Related Information**


Antidepressant Agents Comparison Chart *on page 704*

Clinical Issues in the Use of Antidepressants *on page 627*

Discontinuation of Psychotropic Drugs - Withdrawal Symptoms and Recommendations *on page 798*

Federal OBRA Regulations Recommended Maximum Doses *on page 756*

Patient Information - Antidepressants (TCAs) *on page 640*

Pharmacotherapy of Urinary Incontinence *on page 758*

Serum Drug Concentrations Commonly Monitored: Guidelines *on page 759*

Special Populations - Elderly *on page 662*

Substance-Related Disorders *on page 609*

Teratogenic Risks of Psychotropic Medications *on page 812*

**Generic Available** Yes: Tablet

**U.S. Brand Names** Norpramin®

**Canadian Brand Names** PMS-Desipramine

**Synonyms** Desipramine Hydrochloride; Desmethylimipramine Hydrochloride

**Pharmacologic Category** Antidepressant, Tricyclic (Secondary Amine)

**Use** Treatment of depression

**Unlabeled uses:** Analgesic adjunct in chronic pain; peripheral neuropathies

**Pregnancy Risk Factor** C

**Contraindications** Hypersensitivity to this drug and similar chemical class; use of monoamine oxidase inhibitors within 14 days; use in a patient during the acute recovery phase of MI

**Warnings/Precautions** May cause sedation, resulting in impaired performance of tasks requiring alertness (ie, operating machinery or driving). Sedative effects may be additive with other CNS depressants and/or ethanol. The degree of sedation is low-moderate relative to other antidepressants. May worsen psychosis in some patients or precipitate a shift to mania or hypomania in patients with bipolar disease. May cause hyponatremia/SIADH. May increase the risks associated with electroconvulsive therapy. This agent should be discontinued, when possible, prior to elective surgery. Therapy should not be abruptly discontinued in patients receiving high doses for prolonged periods.

May cause orthostatic hypotension (risk is moderate relative to other antidepressants) - use with caution in patients at risk of hypotension or in patients where transient hypotensive episodes would be poorly tolerated (cardiovascular disease or cerebrovascular disease). The degree of anticholinergic blockade produced by this agent is low relative to other cyclic antidepressants - however, caution should be used in patients with urinary retention, benign prostatic hypertrophy, narrow-angle glaucoma, xerostomia, visual problems, constipation, or a history of bowel obstruction.

Use caution in patients with depression, particularly if suicidal risk may be present. Use with caution in patients with a history of cardiovascular disease (including previous MI, stroke, tachycardia, or conduction abnormalities). The risk conduction abnormalities with this agent is moderate relative to other antidepressants. Use caution in patients with a previous seizure disorder or condition predisposing to seizures such as brain damage, alcoholism, or concurrent therapy with other drugs which lower the seizure threshold. Use with caution in hyperthyroid patients or those receiving thyroid supplementation. Use with caution in patients with hepatic or renal dysfunction and in elderly patients.

**Adverse Reactions**

Cardiovascular: Arrhythmias, hypotension, hypertension, palpitations, heart block, tachycardia

Central nervous system: Dizziness, drowsiness, headache, confusion, delirium, hallucinations, nervousness, restlessness, parkinsonian syndrome, insomnia, disorientation, anxiety, agitation, hypomania, exacerbation of psychosis, incoordination, seizures, extrapyramidal symptoms

Dermatologic: Alopecia, photosensitivity, skin rash, urticaria

Endocrine & metabolic: Breast enlargement, galactorrhea, SIADH

Gastrointestinal: Xerostomia, decreased lower esophageal sphincter tone may cause GE reflux, constipation, nausea, unpleasant taste, weight gain, anorexia, abdominal cramps, weight loss, diarrhea, heartburn

Genitourinary: Difficult urination, sexual dysfunction, testicular edema

Hematologic: Agranulocytosis, eosinophilia, purpura, thrombocytopenia

Hepatic: Cholestatic jaundice, increased liver enzyme

Neuromuscular & skeletal: Fine muscle tremors, weakness, numbness, tingling, paresthesia of extremities, ataxia

Ocular: Blurred vision, disturbances of accommodation, mydriasis, increased intraocular pressure

Miscellaneous: Diaphoresis (excessive), allergic reactions

**Overdosage/Toxicology**

Signs and symptoms: Agitation, confusion, hallucinations, hyperthermia, urinary retention, CNS depression, cyanosis, dry mucous membranes, cardiac arrhythmias, seizures

Treatment:

Following initiation of essential overdose management, toxic symptoms should be treated

Ventricular arrhythmias often respond with concurrent systemic alkalinization (sodium bicarbonate 0.5-2 mEq/kg I.V.). Arrhythmias unresponsive to phenytoin 15-20 mg/kg (adults) may respond to lidocaine 1 mg/kg I.V. followed by a titrated infusion. Physostigmine (1-2 mg I.V. slowly for adults or 0.5 mg I.V. slowly for children) may be indicated in reversing cardiac arrhythmias that are life-threatening.

Seizures usually respond to diazepam I.V. boluses (5-10 mg for adults up to 30 mg or 0.25-0.4 mg/kg/dose for children up to 10 mg/dose). If seizures are unresponsive or recur, phenytoin or phenobarbital may be required.

**Drug Interactions** CYP1A2 and 2D6 enzyme substrate; CYP2D6 inhibitor

Altretamine: Concurrent use may cause orthostatic hypertension

Amphetamines: TCAs may enhance the effect of amphetamines; monitor for adverse CV effects

Anticholinergics: Combined use with TCAs may produce additive anticholinergic effects

Antihypertensives: TCAs inhibit the antihypertensive response to bethanidine, clonidine, debrisoquin, guanadrel, guanethidine, guanabenz, guanfacine; monitor BP; consider alternate antihypertensive agent

Beta-agonists: When combined with TCAs may predispose patients to cardiac arrhythmias

Bupropion: May increase the levels of tricyclic antidepressants; based on limited information; monitor response

Carbamazepine: Tricyclic antidepressants may increase carbamazepine levels; monitor

Cholestyramine and colestipol: May bind TCAs and reduce their absorption; monitor for altered response

Clonidine: Abrupt discontinuation of clonidine may cause hypertensive crisis; amitriptyline may enhance the response

CNS depressants: Sedative effects may be additive with TCAs; monitor for increased effect; includes benzodiazepines, barbiturates, antipsychotics, ethanol, and other sedative medications

CYP2C8/9 inhibitors: Serum levels and/or toxicity of some tricyclic antidepressants may be increased; inhibitors include amiodarone, cimetidine, fluvoxamine, some NSAIDs, metronidazole, ritonavir, sulfonamides, troglitazone, valproic acid, and zafirlukast; monitor for increased effect/toxicity

CYP2D6 inhibitors: Serum levels and/or toxicity of some tricyclic antidepressants may be increased; inhibitors include amiodarone, cimetidine, delavirdine, fluoxetine, paroxetine, propafenone, quinidine, and ritonavir; monitor for increased effect/toxicity

CYP3A3/4 inhibitors: Serum level and/or toxicity of some tricyclic antidepressants may be increased; inhibitors include amiodarone, cimetidine, clarithromycin, erythromycin, delavirdine, diltiazem, dirithromycin, disulfiram, fluoxetine, fluvoxamine, grapefruit juice, indinavir, itraconazole, ketoconazole, nevirapine, propoxyfene, quinupristin-dalfopristin, ritonavir, saquinavir, verapamil, zafirlukast, zileuton; monitor for altered effects; a decrease in TCA dosage may be required

Enzyme inducers: May increase the metabolism of TCAs resulting in decreased effect; includes carbamazepine, phenobarbital, phenytoin, and rifampin; monitor for decreased response

Epinephrine (and other direct alpha-agonists): The pressor response to I.V. epinephrine, norepinephrine, and phenylephrine may be enhanced in patients receiving TCAs; this combination is best avoided

Fenfluramine: May increase tricyclic antidepressant levels/effects

Hypoglycemic agents (including insulin): TCAs may enhance the hypoglycemic effects of tolazamide, chlorpropamide, or insulin; monitor for changes in blood glucose levels; reported with chlorpropamide, tolazamide, and insulin

Levodopa: Tricyclic antidepressants may decrease the absorption (bioavailability) of levodopa; rare hypertensive episodes have also been attributed to this combination

Linezolid: Hyperpyrexia, hypertension, tachycardia, confusion, seizures, and **deaths have been reported** with agents which inhibit MAO (serotonin syndrome); this combination should be avoided

Lithium: Concurrent use with a TCA may increase the risk for neurotoxicity

MAO inhibitors: Hyperpyrexia, hypertension, tachycardia, confusion, seizures, and **deaths have been reported** (serotonin syndrome); this combination should be avoided

Methylphenidate: Metabolism of TCAs may be decreased

Phenothiazines: Serum concentrations of some TCAs may be increased; in addition, TCAs may increase concentration of phenothiazines; monitor for altered clinical response

QTc prolonging agents: Concurrent use of tricyclic agents with other drugs which may prolong QTc interval may increase the risk of potentially fatal arrhythmias; includes type Ia and type III antiarrhythmics agents, selected quinolones (sparfloxacin, gatifloxacin, moxifloxacin, grepafloxacin), cisapride, and other agents

Sucralfate: Absorption of tricyclic antidepressants may be reduced with coadministration

Sympathomimetics, indirect-acting: Tricyclic antidepressants may result in a decreased sensitivity to indirect-acting sympathomimetics; includes dopamine and ephedrine; also see interaction with epinephrine (and direct-acting sympathomimetics)

Valproic acid: May increase serum concentrations/adverse effects of some tricyclic antidepressants

Warfarin (and other oral anticoagulants): TCAs may increase the anticoagulant effect in patients stabilized on warfarin; monitor INR

**Mechanism of Action** Traditionally believed to increase the synaptic concentration of norepinephrine (and to a lesser extent, serotonin) in the central nervous system by inhibition of its reuptake by the presynaptic neuronal membrane. However, additional receptor effects have been found including desensitization of adenyl cyclase, down regulation of beta-adrenergic receptors, and down regulation of serotonin receptors.

**Pharmacodynamics/kinetics**

Onset of action: 1-3 weeks

Absorption: Well absorbed from GI tract

Metabolism: In the liver

Half-life: Adults: 7-60 hours

Peak plasma levels occur within 4-6 hours

(Continued)

## Desipramine *(Continued)*

Elimination: 70% excreted in urine

**Usual Dosage** Oral:

Children 6-12 years: 10-30 mg/day or 1-5 mg/kg/day in divided doses; do not exceed 5 mg/kg/day

Adolescents: Initial: 25-50 mg/day; gradually increase to 100 mg/day in single or divided doses; maximum: 150 mg/day

Adults: Initial: 75 mg/day in divided doses; increase gradually to 150-200 mg/day in divided or single dose; maximum: 300 mg/day

Elderly: Initial dose: 10-25 mg/day; increase by 10-25 mg every 3 days for inpatients and every week for outpatients if tolerated; usual maintenance dose: 75-100 mg/day, but doses up to 150 mg/day may be necessary

Hemodialysis/peritoneal dialysis: Supplemental dose is not necessary

**Dietary Considerations** Alcohol: Additive CNS effects, avoid use

**Monitoring Parameters** Monitor blood pressure and pulse rate prior to and during initial therapy evaluate mental status; monitor weight; EKG in older adults

**Reference Range** Therapeutic: 150-300 ng/mL (SI: 560-1125 nmol/L); possible toxicity: >300 ng/mL (SI: >1070 nmol/L); Toxic: >1000 ng/mL (SI: >3750 nmol/L)

**Test Interactions** ↑ glucose

**Patient Information** Avoid alcohol ingestion; do not discontinue medication abruptly; may cause urine to turn blue-green; may cause drowsiness; avoid unnecessary exposure to sunlight; sugarless hard candy or gum can help with dry mouth; full effect may not occur for 4-6 weeks

**Nursing Implications** May increase appetite

**Additional Information** Less sedation and anticholinergic effects than with amitriptyline or imipramine

**Dosage Forms** Tablet, as hydrochloride: 10 mg, 25 mg, 50 mg, 75 mg, 100 mg, 150 mg

♦ **Desipramine Hydrochloride** *see* Desipramine *on page 154*

## Deslanoside (des LAN oh side)

**U.S. Brand Names** Cedilanid-D®; Desace®; Desaci®; Verdiana®

**Pharmacologic Category** Cardiac Glycoside

**Use** Rapid digitalizing effect in emergency treatment of congestive heart failure, paroxysmal atrial tachycardia, fibrillation (atrial) and flutter

**Effects on Mental Status** May cause drowsiness, hallucinations, or paranoia

**Effects on Psychiatric Treatment** None reported

**Usual Dosage** I.M., I.V.:

Children:

Neonates, premature and full-term: 22 mcg divided into 2-3 doses every 3-4 hours

2 weeks to 3 years: 25 mcg/kg divided into 2-3 doses every 3-4 hours

>3 years: 22.5 mcg/kg divided into 2-3 doses every 3-4 hours

Children and Adults: Highly individualized

Adults: Loading dose: 1.2-1.6 mg in 2 divided doses over 24 hours

**Dosage Forms** Injection: 0.2 mg/mL (2 mL)

♦ **Desmethylimipramine Hydrochloride** *see* Desipramine *on page 154*

## Desmopressin (des moe PRES in)

**Related Information**

Clozapine-Induced Side Effects *on page 780*

Special Populations - Children and Adolescents *on page 663*

**U.S. Brand Names** DDAVP®; Stimate™ Nasal

**Canadian Brand Names** Octostim®

**Synonyms** 1-Deamino-8-D-Arginine Vasopressin

**Pharmacologic Category** Vasopressin Analog, Synthetic

**Use** Treatment of diabetes insipidus and controlling bleeding in mild hemophilia, von Willebrand disease, and thrombocytopenia (eg, uremia), nocturnal enuresis

**Effects on Mental Status** May cause dizziness

**Effects on Psychiatric Treatment** May decrease lithium's effect on ADH, however, hydrochlorothiazide or amiloride are better choices

**Pregnancy Risk Factor** B

**Contraindications** Hypersensitivity to desmopressin or any component; avoid using in patients with type IIB or platelet-type von Willebrand disease, patients with <5% factor VIII activity level

**Warnings/Precautions** Avoid overhydration especially when drug is used for its hemostatic effect

**Adverse Reactions**

1% to 10%:

Cardiovascular: Facial flushing

Central nervous system: Headache, dizziness

Gastrointestinal: Nausea, abdominal cramps

Genitourinary: Vulval pain

Local: Pain at the injection site

Respiratory: Nasal congestion

<1%: Hyponatremia, increase in blood pressure, water intoxication

**Overdosage/Toxicology** Signs and symptoms: Drowsiness, headache, confusion, anuria, water intoxication

**Drug Interactions**

Decreased effect: Demeclocycline, lithium may decrease ADH effects

Increased effect: Chlorpropamide, fludrocortisone may increase ADH response

**Usual Dosage**

Children:

Diabetes insipidus: 3 months to 12 years: Intranasal (using 100 mcg/mL nasal solution): Initial: 5 mcg/day (0.05 mL/day) divided 1-2 times/day; range: 5-30 mcg/day (0.05-0.3 mL/day) divided 1-2 times/day; adjust morning and evening doses separately for an adequate diurnal rhythm of water turnover

Hemophilia: >3 months: I.V. 0.3 mcg/kg; may repeat dose if needed; begin 30 minutes before procedure; dilute I.V. dose in 50 mL 0.9% sodium chloride and infuse over 15-30 minutes

Nocturnal enuresis: ≥6 years: Intranasal (using 100 mcg/mL nasal solution): Initial: 20 mcg (0.2 mL) at bedtime; range: 10-40 mcg; it is recommended that $^1/_2$ of the dose be given in each nostril

Children 12 years and Adults:

Diabetes insipidus:

I.V., S.C.: 2-4 mcg/day in 2 divided doses or $^1/_{10}$ of the maintenance intranasal dose; dilute I.V. dose in 50 mL 0.9% sodium chloride and infuse over 15-30 minutes

Intranasal (using 100 mcg/mL nasal solution): 5-40 mcg/day (0.05-0.4 mL) divided 1-3 times/day; adjust morning and evening doses separately for an adequate diurnal rhythm of water turnover. **Note:** The nasal spray pump can only deliver doses of 10 mcg (0.1 mL) or multiples of 10 mcg (0.1 mL), if doses other than this are needed, the rhinal tube delivery system is preferred.

Hemophilia/uremic bleeding:

I.V.: 0.3 mcg/kg by slow infusion, begin 30 minutes before procedure; dilute I.V. dose in 50 mL 0.9% sodium chloride and infuse over 15-30 minutes

Nasal spray: Using high concentration spray: <50 kg: 150 mcg (1 spray); >50 kg: 300 mcg (1 spray each nostril); repeat use is determined by the patient's clinical condition and laboratory work; if using preoperatively, administer 2 hours before surgery

Oral: Begin therapy 12 hours after the last intranasal dose for patients previously on intranasal therapy

Children: Initial: 0.05 mg; fluid restrictions are required in children to prevent hyponatremia and water intoxication

Adults: 0.05 mg twice daily; adjust individually to optimal therapeutic dose. Total daily dose should be increased or decreased (range: 0.1-1.2 mg divided 2-3 times/day) as needed to obtain adequate antidiuresis.

**Patient Information** Use specific product as directed. Diabetes insipidus: Avoid overhydration. Weigh yourself daily at the same time in the same clothes. Report increased weight or swelling of extremities. If using intranasal product, inspect nasal membranes regularly. Report swelling or increased nasal congestion. All uses: Report unresolved headache, difficulty breathing, acute heartburn or nausea, abdominal cramping, or vulval pain.

**Dosage Forms**

Injection (DDAVP®): 4 mcg/mL (1 mL)

Solution, nasal:

DDAVP®: 100 mcg/mL (2.5 mL, 5 mL)

Stimate™: 1.5 mg/mL (2.5 mL)

Tablet (DDAVP®): 0.1 mg, 0.2 mg

♦ **Desogen®** *see* Ethinyl Estradiol and Desogestrel *on page 211*

## Desoximetasone (des oks i MET a sone)

**Related Information**

Corticosteroids Comparison Chart *on page 711*

**U.S. Brand Names** Topicort®; Topicort®-LP

**Pharmacologic Category** Corticosteroid, Topical

**Use** Relieves inflammation and pruritic symptoms of corticosteroid-responsive dermatosis [medium to high potency topical corticosteroid]

**Effects on Mental Status** None reported

**Effects on Psychiatric Treatment** None reported

**Usual Dosage** Desoximetasone is a potent fluorinated topical corticosteroid. All of the preparations are considered high potency. Therapy should be discontinued when control is achieved; if no improvement is seen, reassessment of diagnosis may be necessary.

Children: Apply sparingly in a very thin film to affected area 1-2 times/day

Adults: Apply sparingly in a thin film twice daily

**Dosage Forms** Topical:

Cream:

Topicort®: 0.25% (15 g, 60 g, 120 g)

Topicort®-LP: 0.05% (15 g, 60 g)

Gel, topical: 0.05% (15 g, 60 g)

Ointment (Topicort®): 0.25% (15 g, 60 g)

## Dexamethasone (deks a METH a sone)

**Related Information**

Corticosteroids Comparison Chart *on page 711*

**U.S. Brand Names** Aeroseb-Dex®; AK-Dex® Ophthalmic; Baldex®; Dalalone®; Dalalone D.P.®; Dalalone L.A.®; Decadron®; Decadron®-LA; Decadron® Phosphate; Decaject®; Decaject-LA®; Dexacort® Phosphate in Respihaler®; Dexacort® Phosphate Turbinaire®; Dexasone®; Dexasone® L.A.; Dexone®; Dexone® LA; Dexotic®; Hexadrol®; Hexadrol® Phosphate; Maxidex®; Solurex®; Solurex L.A.®

**Synonyms** Dexamethasone Acetate; Dexamethasone Sodium Phosphate

**Pharmacologic Category** Corticosteroid, Oral; Corticosteroid, Oral Inhaler; Corticosteroid, Nasal; Corticosteroid, Ophthalmic; Corticosteroid, Parenteral; Corticosteroid, Topical

**Use** Systemically and locally for chronic swelling, allergic, hematologic, neoplastic, and autoimmune diseases; may be used in management of cerebral edema, septic shock, as a diagnostic agent, antiemetic

**Effects on Mental Status** Insomnia and nervousness are common; may cause euphoria, confusion, or hallucinations

**Effects on Psychiatric Treatment** Barbiturates and carbamazepine may decrease dexamethasone effects

**Pregnancy Risk Factor** C

**Contraindications** Active untreated infections; use in ophthalmic viral, fungal, or tuberculosis diseases of the eye

**Warnings/Precautions** Fatalities have occurred due to adrenal insufficiency in asthmatic patients during and after transfer from systemic corticosteroids to aerosol steroids; aerosol steroids do **not** provide the systemic steroid needed to treat patients having trauma, surgery, or infections; use with caution in patients with hypothyroidism, cirrhosis, hypertension, congestive heart failure, ulcerative colitis, thromboembolic disorders. Because of the risk of adverse effects, systemic corticosteroids should be used cautiously in the elderly in the smallest possible dose and for the shortest possible time.

Controlled clinical studies have shown that inhaled and intranasal corticosteroids may cause a reduction in growth velocity in pediatric patients. Growth velocity provides a means of comparing the rate of growth among children of the same age.

In studies involving inhaled corticosteroids, the average reduction in growth velocity was approximately 1 cm (about 1/3 of an inch) per year. It appears that the reduction is related to dose and how long the child takes the drug.

FDA's Pulmonary and Allergy Drugs and Metabolic and Endocrine Drugs advisory committees discussed this issue at a July 1998 meeting. They recommended that the agency develop class-wide labeling to inform health care providers so they would understand this potential side effect and monitor growth routinely in pediatric patients who are treated with inhaled corticosteroids, intranasal corticosteroids or both.

Long-term effects of this reduction in growth velocity on final adult height are unknown. Likewise, it also has not yet been determined whether patients' growth will "catch up" if treatment in discontinued. Drug manufacturers will continue to monitor these drugs to learn more about long-term effects. Children are prescribed inhaled corticosteroids to treat asthma. Intranasal corticosteroids are generally used to prevent and treat allergy-related nasal symptoms.

Patients are advised not to stop using their inhaled or intranasal corticosteroids without first speaking to their health care providers about the benefits of these drugs compared to their risks.

**Adverse Reactions**

**Systemic:**

>10%:
- Central nervous system: Insomnia, nervousness
- Gastrointestinal: Increased appetite, indigestion

1% to 10%:
- Dermatologic: Hirsutism
- Endocrine & metabolic: Diabetes mellitus
- Neuromuscular & skeletal: Arthralgia
- Ocular: Cataracts
- Respiratory: Epistaxis

<1%: Abdominal distention, acne, amenorrhea, bone growth suppression, bruising, Cushing's syndrome, delirium, euphoria, hallucinations, headache, hyperglycemia, hyperpigmentation, hypersensitivity reactions, mood swings, muscle wasting, pancreatitis, seizures, skin atrophy, sodium and water retention, ulcerative esophagitis

**Topical:** <1%: Acneiform eruptions, allergic contact dermatitis, dryness, folliculitis, hypertrichosis, hypopigmentation, irritation, itching, local burning, miliaria, perioral dermatitis, secondary infection, skin atrophy, skin maceration, striae

**Overdosage/Toxicology** Signs and symptoms: Moon face, central obesity, hypertension, psychosis, hallucinations, diabetes, hyperlipidemia, peptic ulcer, increased susceptibility to infection, electrolyte and fluid imbalance. When consumed in excessive quantities, systemic hypercorticism and adrenal suppression may occur.

Treatment: In those cases when systemic hypercorticism and adrenal suppression occur, discontinuation and withdrawal of the corticosteroid should be done judiciously.

**Drug Interactions** CYP3A3/4 enzyme substrate; CYP3A3/4 enzyme inducer; CYP3A3/4 enzyme inhibitor

Decreased effect: Barbiturates, phenytoin, rifampin may decrease dexamethasone effects; dexamethasone decreases effect of salicylates, vaccines, toxoids

**Usual Dosage**

Neonates:
- Airway edema or extubation: I.V.: Usual: 0.25 mg/kg/dose given 4 hours prior to scheduled extubation and then every 8 hours for 3 doses total; range: 0.25-1 mg/kg/dose for 1-3 doses; maximum dose: 1 mg/kg/day. **Note:** A longer duration of therapy may be needed with more severe cases.
- Bronchopulmonary dysplasia (to facilitate ventilator weaning): Oral:, I.V.: Numerous dosing schedules have been proposed; range: 0.5-0.6 mg/kg/day given in divided doses every 12 hours for 3-7 days, then taper over 1-6 weeks

Children:
- Antiemetic (prior to chemotherapy): I.V. (should be given as sodium phosphate): 10 mg/m$^2$/dose (maximum: 20 mg) for first dose then 5 mg/m$^2$/dose every 6 hours as needed
- Anti-inflammatory immunosuppressant: Oral, I.M., I.V. (injections should be given as sodium phosphate): 0.08-0.3 mg/kg/day **or** 2.5-10 mg/m$^2$/day in divided doses every 6-12 hours
- Extubation or airway edema: Oral, I.M., I.V. (injections should be given as sodium phosphate): 0.5-2 mg/kg/day in divided doses every 6 hours beginning 24 hours prior to extubation and continuing for 4-6 doses afterwards
- Cerebral edema: I.V. (should be given as sodium phosphate): Loading dose: 1-2 mg/kg/dose as a single dose; maintenance: 1-1.5 mg/kg/day (maximum: 16 mg/day) in divided doses every 4-6 hours for 5 days then taper for 5 days, then discontinue
- Bacterial meningitis in infants and children >2 months: I.V. (should be given as sodium phosphate): 0.6 mg/kg/day in 4 divided doses every 6 hours for the first 4 days of antibiotic treatment; start dexamethasone at the time of the first dose of antibiotic
- Physiologic replacement: Oral, I.M., I.V.: 0.03-0.15 mg/kg/day or 0.6-0.75 mg/m$^2$/day in divided doses every 6-12 hours

Adults:
- Acute nonlymphoblastic leukemia (ANLL) protocol: I.V.: 2 mg/m$^2$/dose every 8 hours for 12 doses
- Antiemetic (prior to chemotherapy): Oral/I.V. (should be given as sodium phosphate): 10 mg/m$^2$/dose (usually 20 mg) for first dose then 5 mg/m$^2$/dose every 6 hours as needed
- Anti-inflammatory:
  - Oral, I.M., I.V. (injections should be given as sodium phosphate): 0.75-9 mg/day in divided doses every 6-12 hours
  - I.M. (as acetate): 8-16 mg; may repeat in 1-3 weeks
  - Intralesional (as acetate): 0.8-1.6 mg
  - Intra-articular/soft tissue (as acetate): 4-16 mg; may repeat in 1-3 weeks
  - Intra-articular, intralesional, or soft tissue (as sodium phosphate): 0.4-6 mg/day
- Cerebral edema: I.V. 10 mg stat, 4 mg I.M./I.V. (should be given as sodium phosphate) every 6 hours until response is maximized, then switch to oral regimen, then taper off if appropriate; dosage may be reduced after 24 days and gradually discontinued over 5-7 days
- Diagnosis for Cushing's syndrome: Oral: 1 mg at 11 PM, draw blood at 8 AM the following day for plasma cortisol determination

(Continued)

## Dexamethasone *(Continued)*

Physiological replacement: Oral, I.M., I.V. (should be given as sodium phosphate): 0.03-0.15 mg/kg/day **OR** 0.6-0.75 mg/m²/day in divided doses every 6-12 hours

Shock therapy:

Addisonian crisis/shock (ie, adrenal insufficiency/responsive to steroid therapy): I.V. (given as sodium phosphate): 4-10 mg as a single dose, which may be repeated if necessary

Unresponsive shock (ie, unresponsive to steroid therapy): I.V. (given as sodium phosphate): 1-6 mg/kg as a single I.V. dose or up to 40 mg initially followed by repeat doses every 2-6 hours while shock persists

Hemodialysis: Supplemental dose is not necessary

Peritoneal dialysis: Supplemental dose is not necessary

Ophthalmic:

Ointment: Apply thin coating into conjunctival sac 3-4 times/day; gradually taper dose to discontinue

Suspension: Instill 2 drops into conjunctival sac every hour during the day and every other hour during the night; gradually reduce dose to every 3-4 hours, then to 3-4 times/day

Topical: Apply 1-4 times/day. Therapy should be discontinued when control is achieved; if no improvement is seen, reassessment of diagnosis may be necessary.

**Patient Information** Take exactly as directed; do not increase dose or discontinue abruptly without consulting prescriber. Take oral medication with or after meals. Limit intake of caffeine or stimulants. Prescriber may recommend increased dietary vitamins, minerals, or iron. Diabetics should monitor glucose levels closely (antidiabetic medication may need to be adjusted). Inform prescriber if you are experiencing greater than normal levels of stress (medication may need adjustment). Some forms of this medication may cause GI upset (oral medication may be taken with meals to reduce GI upset; small frequent meals and frequent mouth care may reduce GI upset). You may be more susceptible to infection (avoid crowds and persons with contagious or infective conditions). Report promptly excessive nervousness or sleep disturbances; any signs of infection (sore throat, unhealed injuries); excessive growth of body hair or loss of skin color; changes in vision; excessive or sudden weight gain (>3 lb/week); swelling of face or extremities; difficulty breathing; muscle weakness; change in color of stools (tarry) or persistent abdominal pain; or worsening of condition or failure to improve.

Ophthalmic: For ophthalmic use only. Wash hands before using. Tilt head back and look upward. Put drops of suspension or apply thin ribbon of ointment inside lower eyelid. Close eye and roll eyeball in all directions. Do not blink for ½ minute. Apply gentle pressure to inner corner of eye for 30 seconds. Do not use any other eye preparation for at least 10 minutes. Do not touch tip of applicator to eye or contaminate tip of applicator. Do not share medication with anyone else. Wear sunglasses when in sunlight; you may be more sensitive to bright light. Inform prescriber if condition worsens or fails to improve or if you experience eye pain, disturbances of vision, or other adverse eye response.

Topical: For external use only. Not for eyes or mucous membranes or open wounds. Apply in very thin layer to occlusive dressing. Apply dressing to area being treated. Avoid prolonged or excessive use around sensitive tissues, genital, or rectal areas. Inform prescriber if condition worsens (swelling, redness, irritation, pain, open sores) or fails to improve.

Aerosol: Not for use during acute asthmatic attack. Follow directions that accompany product. Rinse mouth and throat after use to prevent candidiasis. Do not use intranasal product if you have a nasal infection, nasal injury, or recent nasal surgery. If using two products, consult prescriber in which order to use the two products. Inform prescriber if condition worsens or does not improve.

**Nursing Implications** Topical formation is for external use, do not use on open wounds; apply sparingly to occlusive dressings; should not be used in the presence of open or weeping lesions; **acetate injection is not for I.V. use**

**Dosage Forms**

Aerosol:

Oral, as sodium phosphate: 84 mcg dexamethasone per activation (12.6 g)

Nasal, as sodium phosphate: 84 mcg dexamethasone/spray (12.6 g)

Topical: 0.01% (58 g); 0.04% (25 g)

Cream, as sodium phosphate: 0.1% (15 g, 30 g)

Elixir: 0.5 mg/5 mL (5 mL, 20 mL, 100 mL, 120 mL, 237 mL, 240 mL, 500 mL)

Injection, as acetate suspension: 8 mg/mL (1 mL, 5 mL); 16 mg/mL (1 mL, 5 mL)

Injection, as sodium phosphate: 4 mg/mL (1 mL, 5 mL, 10 mL, 25 mL, 30 mL); 10 mg/mL (1 mL, 10 mL); 20 mg/mL (5 mL); 24 mg/mL (5 mL, 10 mL)

Ointment, ophthalmic, as sodium phosphate: 0.05% (3.5 g)

Solution, oral:

Concentrate: 0.5 mg/0.5 mL (30 mL) (30% alcohol)

Oral: 0.5 mg/5 mL (5 mL, 20 mL, 500 mL)

Suspension, ophthalmic, as sodium phosphate: 0.1% with methylcellulose 0.5% (5 mL, 15 mL)

Tablet: 0.25 mg, 0.5 mg, 0.75 mg, 1 mg, 1.5 mg, 2 mg, 4 mg, 6 mg

Tablet, therapeutic pack: 6 x 1.5 mg; 8 x 0.75 mg

- **Dexamethasone Acetate** *see* Dexamethasone *on page 157*
- **Dexamethasone Sodium Phosphate** *see* Dexamethasone *on page 157*
- **Dexasone®** *see* Dexamethasone *on page 157*
- **Dexasone® L.A.** *see* Dexamethasone *on page 157*
- **Dexasporin®** *see* Neomycin, Polymyxin B, and Dexamethasone *on page 389*
- **Dexatrim® Pre-Meal [OTC]** *see* Phenylpropanolamine *on page 440*

## Dexbrompheniramine and Pseudoephedrine

(deks brom fen EER a meen & soo doe e FED rin)

**U.S. Brand Names** Disobrom® [OTC]; Disophrol® Chronotabs® [OTC]; Disophrol® Tablet [OTC]; Drixomed®; Drixoral® [OTC]

**Pharmacologic Category** Antihistamine/Decongestant Combination

**Use** Relief of symptoms of upper respiratory mucosal congestion in seasonal and perennial nasal allergies, acute rhinitis, rhinosinusitis and eustachian tube blockage

**Effects on Mental Status** May cause drowsiness, anxiety, and nervousness

**Effects on Psychiatric Treatment** Dry mouth is common; this effect may be worsened by concurrent psychotropic use

**Usual Dosage** Children >12 years and Adults: Oral: 1 tablet every 12 hours, may require 1 tablet every 8 hours

**Dosage Forms**

Tablet (Disophrol®): Dexbrompheniramine maleate 2 mg and pseudoephedrine sulfate 60 mg

Timed release (Disobrom®, Disophrol® Chrontabs®, Drixomed®, Drixoral®, Histrodrix®, Resporal®): Dexbrompheniramine maleate 6 mg and pseudoephedrine sulfate 120 mg

- **Dexchlor®** *see* Dexchlorpheniramine *on page 158*

## Dexchlorpheniramine (deks klor fen EER a meen)

**U.S. Brand Names** Dexchlor®; Poladex®; Polaramine®

**Pharmacologic Category** Antihistamine

**Use** Perennial and seasonal allergic rhinitis and other allergic symptoms including urticaria

**Effects on Mental Status** Drowsiness is common; may cause nervousness and depression

**Effects on Psychiatric Treatment** Concurrent use with psychotropics may cause additive sedation

**Usual Dosage** Oral:

Children:

2-5 years: 0.5 mg every 4-6 hours (do not use timed release)

6-11 years: 1 mg every 4-6 hours or 4 mg timed release at bedtime

Adults: 2 mg every 4-6 hours or 4-6 mg timed release at bedtime or every 8-10 hours

**Dosage Forms**

Syrup, as maleate (orange flavor): 2 mg/5 mL with alcohol 6% (480 mL)

Tablet, as maleate: 2 mg

Tablet, as maleate, sustained action: 4 mg, 6 mg

- **Dexedrine®** *see* Dextroamphetamine *on page 159*
- **Dexferrum® Injection** *see* Iron Dextran Complex *on page 293*
- **Dexone®** *see* Dexamethasone *on page 157*
- **Dexone® LA** *see* Dexamethasone *on page 157*
- **Dexotic®** *see* Dexamethasone *on page 157*

## Dexpanthenol (deks PAN the nole)

**U.S. Brand Names** Ilopan-Choline® Oral; Ilopan® Injection; Panthoderm® Cream [OTC]

**Pharmacologic Category** Gastrointestinal Agent, Stimulant

**Use** Prophylactic use to minimize paralytic ileus, treatment of postoperative distention

**Effects on Mental Status** None reported

**Effects on Psychiatric Treatment** None reported

**Usual Dosage**

Children and Adults: Relief of itching and aid in skin healing: Topical: Apply to affected area 1-2 times/day

Adults:

Relief of gas retention: Oral: 2-3 tablets 3 times/day

Prevention of postoperative ileus: I.M.: 250-500 mg stat, repeat in 2 hours, followed by doses every 6 hours until danger passes

Paralyzed ileus: I.M.: 500 mg stat, repeat in 2 hours, followed by doses every 6 hours, if needed

**Dosage Forms**
Cream: 2% (30 g, 60 g)
Injection (Ilopan®): 250 mg/mL (2 mL, 10 mL, 30 mL)
Tablet (Ilopan-Choline®): 50 mg with choline bitartrate 25 mg

## Dexrazoxane (deks ray ZOKS ane)

**U.S. Brand Names** Zinecard®

**Pharmacologic Category** Cardioprotectant

**Use** Reduction of the incidence and severity of cardiomyopathy associated with doxorubicin administration in women with metastatic breast cancer who have received a cumulative doxorubicin dose of 300 mg/m$^2$ and who would benefit from continuing therapy with doxorubicin. It is not recommended for use with the initiation of doxorubicin therapy.

**Effects on Mental Status** None reported

**Effects on Psychiatric Treatment** May cause granulocytopenia; use caution with clozapine or carbamazepine

**Usual Dosage** Adults: I.V.: The recommended dosage ratio of dexrazoxane:doxorubicin is 10:1 (eg, 500 mg/m$^2$ dexrazoxane:50 mg/m$^2$ doxorubicin). Administer the reconstituted solution by slow I.V. push or rapid I.V. infusion from a bag. After completing the infusion, and prior to a total elapsed time of 30 minutes (from the beginning of the dexrazoxane infusion), administer the I.V. injection of doxorubicin.

**Dosage Forms** Powder for injection, lyophilized: 250 mg, 500 mg (10 mg/mL when reconstituted)

## Dextroamphetamine (deks troe am FET a meen)

**Related Information**
Clinical Issues in the Use of Stimulants *on page 637*
Patient Information - Stimulants *on page 652*
Special Populations - Children and Adolescents *on page 663*
Stimulant Agents Used for ADHD *on page 728*
Substance-Related Disorders *on page 609*

**Generic Available** Yes

**U.S. Brand Names** Dexedrine®; Oxydess® II; Spancap® No. 1

**Synonyms** Dextroamphetamine Sulfate

**Pharmacologic Category** Stimulant

**Use** Narcolepsy; attention deficit/hyperactivity disorder (ADHD)
**Unlabeled uses:** Exogenous obesity; depression; abnormal behavioral syndrome in children (minimal brain dysfunction)

**Restrictions** C-II

**Pregnancy Risk Factor** C

**Contraindications** Known hypersensitivity or idiosyncrasy to dextroamphetamine or other sympathomimetic amines. Patients with advanced arteriosclerosis, symptomatic cardiovascular disease, moderate to severe hypertension (stage II or III), hyperthyroidism, glaucoma, diabetes mellitus, agitated states, patients with a history of drug abuse, and during or within 14 days following MAO inhibitor therapy. Stimulant medications are contraindicated for use in children with attention deficit/hyperactivity disorders and concomitant Tourette's syndrome or tics.

**Warnings/Precautions** Use with caution in patients with bipolar disorder, cardiovascular disease, seizure disorders, insomnia, porphyria, mild hypertension (stage I), or history of substance abuse. May exacerbate symptoms of behavior and thought disorder in psychotic patients. Potential for drug dependency exists - avoid abrupt discontinuation in patients who have received for prolonged periods. Use in weight reduction programs only when alternative therapy has been ineffective. Products may contain tartrazine - use with caution in potentially sensitive individuals. Stimulant use in children has been associated with growth suppression.

**Adverse Reactions**
Cardiovascular: Palpitations, tachycardia, hypertension, cardiomyopathy
Central nervous system: Overstimulation, euphoria, dyskinesia, dysphoria, exacerbation of motor and phonic tics, restlessness, insomnia, dizziness, headache, psychosis, Tourette's syndrome
Dermatologic: Rash, urticaria
Endocrine & metabolic: Changes in libido
Gastrointestinal: Diarrhea, constipation, anorexia, weight loss, xerostomia, unpleasant taste
Genitourinary: Impotence
Neuromuscular & skeletal: Tremor

**Overdosage/Toxicology**
Signs and symptoms: Restlessness, tremor, confusion, hallucinations, panic, dysrhythmias, nausea, vomiting
Treatment:
There is no specific antidote for dextroamphetamine intoxication and the bulk of the treatment is supportive
Hyperactivity and agitation usually respond to reduced sensory input; however, with extreme agitation, haloperidol (2-5 mg I.M. for adults) may be required
Hyperthermia is best treated with external cooling measures, or when severe or unresponsive, muscle paralysis with pancuronium may be needed
Hypertension is usually transient and generally does not require treatment unless severe. For diastolic blood pressures >110 mm Hg, a nitroprusside infusion should be initiated.
Seizures usually respond to diazepam I.V. and/or phenytoin maintenance regimens

**Drug Interactions**
Acidifiers: Very large doses of potassium acid phosphate or ammonium chloride may increase the renal elimination of amphetamines due to urinary acidification
Alkalinizers: Large doses of sodium bicarbonate or other alkalinizers may increase renal tubular reabsorption (decreased elimination) and diminish the effect of amphetamine; includes potassium or sodium citrate and acetate
Antipsychotics: Efficacy of amphetamines may be decreased by antipsychotics; in addition, amphetamines may induce an increase in psychotic symptoms in some patients
CYP2D6 inhibitors: Serum levels and/or toxicity of amphetamine may be increased; inhibitors include amiodarone, cimetidine, delavirdine, fluoxetine, paroxetine, propafenone, quinidine, and ritonavir; monitor for increased effect/toxicity
Enzyme inducers: Metabolism of amphetamine may be increased; decreasing clinical effect; inducers include barbiturates, carbamazepine, phenytoin, and rifampin
Furazolidine: Amphetamines may induce hypertensive episodes in patients receiving furazolidone
Guanethidine: Amphetamines inhibit the antihypertensive response to guanethidine; probably also may occur with guanadrel
MAOIs: Severe hypertensive episodes have occurred with amphetamine when used in patients receiving MAOIs; concurrent use or use within 14 days is contraindicated.
Norepinephrine: Amphetamines enhance the pressor response to norepinephrine
Sibutramine: Concurrent use of sibutramine and amphetamines may cause severe hypertension and tachycardia; use is contraindicated with SSRIs; amphetamines may increase the potential for serotonin syndrome when used concurrently with selective serotonin re-uptake inhibitors (including fluoxetine, fluvoxamine, paroxetine, and sertraline)
Tricyclic antidepressants: Concurrent of amphetamines with TCAs may result in hypertension and CNS stimulation; avoid this combination

**Stability** Protect from light

**Mechanism of Action** Blocks reuptake of dopamine and norepinephrine from the synapse, thus increases the amount of circulating dopamine and norepinephrine in cerebral cortex to reticular activating system; inhibits the action of monoamine oxidase and causes catecholamines to be released. Peripheral actions include elevated blood pressure, weak bronchodilator, and respiratory stimulant action.

**Pharmacodynamics/kinetics**
Onset of action: 1-1.5 hours
Metabolism: In the liver
Half-life: Adults: 34 hours (pH dependent)
Time to peak serum concentration: Oral: Within 3 hours
Elimination: In urine as unchanged drug and inactive metabolites after oral dose

**Usual Dosage** Oral:
Children:
Narcolepsy: 6-12 years: Initial: 5 mg/day, may increase at 5 mg increments in weekly intervals until side effects appear; maximum dose: 60 mg/day
Attention deficit/hyperactivity disorder:
3-5 years: Initial: 2.5 mg/day given every morning; increase by 2.5 mg/day in weekly intervals until optimal response is obtained, usual range: 0.1-0.5 mg/kg/dose every morning with maximum of 40 mg/day
≥6 years: 5 mg once or twice daily; increase in increments of 5 mg/day at weekly intervals until optimal response is reached, usual range: 0.1-0.5 mg/kg/dose every morning (5-20 mg/day) with maximum of 40 mg/day
Children >12 years and Adults:
Narcolepsy: Initial: 10 mg/day, may increase at 10 mg increments in weekly intervals until side effects appear; maximum: 60 mg/day
Exogenous obesity: 5-30 mg/day in divided doses of 5-10 mg 30-60 minutes before meals

**Administration** Administer as single dose in morning or as divided doses with breakfast and lunch

**Monitoring Parameters** Growth in children and CNS activity in all

**Reference Range** Therapeutic: 20-30 ng/mL; Toxic: >200 ng/mL

**Test Interactions** False-positive amphetamine assays may occur from coadministration with ranitidine, phenylpropanolamine, brompheniramine, chlorpromazine, fluspirilene, or pipothiazine

**Patient Information** Take during day to avoid insomnia; do not discontinue abruptly, may cause physical and psychological dependence with prolonged use

**Nursing Implications** Last daily dose should be given 6 hours before retiring; do not crush sustained release drug product; dose should not be given in evening or at bedtime

**Additional Information** Tablets (5 mg) contain tartrazine

(Continued)

## Dextroamphetamine *(Continued)*

**Dosage Forms**
Capsule, as sulfate, sustained release: 5 mg, 10 mg, 15 mg
Elixir, as sulfate: 5 mg/5 mL (480 mL)
Tablet, as sulfate: 5 mg, 10 mg (5 mg tablets contain tartrazine)

## Dextroamphetamine and Amphetamine

(deks troe am FET a meen & am FET a meen)

**Related Information**
Patient Information - Stimulants *on page 652*
Stimulant Agents Used for ADHD *on page 728*
Substance-Related Disorders *on page 609*

**Generic Available** No

**U.S. Brand Names** Adderall®

**Pharmacologic Category** Stimulant

**Use** Attention-deficit disorder with hyperactivity; narcolepsy

**Restrictions** C-II

**Pregnancy Risk Factor** C

**Pregnancy/Breast-Feeding Implications** Amphetamines are embryotoxic and teratogenic in mice; report of severe congenital bony deformity, tracheoesophageal fistula, and anal atresia in a mother who took dextroamphetamine and lovastatin in first trimester; use if benefit outweighs risk to fetus. Excreted in human milk; advise against nursing.

Infants born to mothers dependent on amphetamines have an increased risk of premature delivery and low birth weight. Infants may experience symptoms withdrawal as demonstrated by dysphoria including agitation and significant lassitude.

**Contraindications** Advanced arteriosclerosis; symptomatic cardiovascular disease; moderate to severe hypertension; hyperthyroidism; hypersensitivity or idiosyncrasy to the sympathomimetic amines; glaucoma; agitated states; patients with a history of drug abuse; during or within 14 days following MAOI (hypertensive crisis)

**Warnings/Precautions** When tolerance to the anorectic effect develops, the recommended dose should not be exceeded in attempt to increase the effect; rather the drug should be discontinued. Use caution in mildly hypertensive patients; amphetamines may impair the ability to engage in potentially hazardous activities.

In psychotic children, amphetamines may exacerbate symptoms of behavior disturbance and thought disorder

**Adverse Reactions**
Cardiovascular: Palpitations, tachycardia, hypertension, cardiomyopathy
Central nervous system: Overstimulation, euphoria, dyskinesia, dysphoria, exacerbation of motor and phonic tics, restlessness, insomnia, dizziness, headache, psychosis, Tourette's syndrome
Dermatologic: Rash, urticaria
Endocrine & metabolic: Changes in libido
Gastrointestinal: Diarrhea, constipation, anorexia, weight loss, xerostomia, unpleasant taste
Genitourinary: Impotence
Neuromuscular & skeletal: Tremor

**Drug Interactions**
Acidifiers: Very large doses of potassium acid phosphate or ammonium chloride may increase the renal elimination of amphetamines due to urinary acidification
Alkalinizers: Large doses of sodium bicarbonate or other alkalinizers may increase renal tubular reabsorption (decreased elimination) and diminish the effect of amphetamine; includes potassium or sodium citrate and acetate
Antipsychotics: Efficacy of amphetamines may be decreased by antipsychotics; in addition, amphetamines may induce an increase in psychotic symptoms in some patients
CYP2D6 inhibitors: Serum levels and/or toxicity of amphetamine may be increased; inhibitors include amiodarone, cimetidine, delavirdine, fluoxetine, paroxetine, propafenone, quinidine, and ritonavir; monitor for increased effect/toxicity
Enzyme inducers: Metabolism of amphetamine may be increased; decreasing clinical effect; inducers include barbiturates, carbamazepine, phenytoin, and rifampin
Furazolidine: Amphetamines may induce hypertensive episodes in patients receiving furazolidone
Guanethidine: Amphetamines inhibit the antihypertensive response to guanethidine; probably also may occur with guanadrel
MAOIs: Severe hypertensive episodes have occurred with amphetamine when used in patients receiving MAOIs; concurrent use or use within 14 days is contraindicated
Norepinephrine: Amphetamines enhance the pressor response to norepinephrine
Sibutramine: Concurrent use of sibutramine and amphetamines may cause severe hypertension and tachycardia; use is contraindicated with SSRIs; amphetamines may increase the potential for serotonin syndrome when used concurrently with selective serotonin reuptake inhibitors (including fluoxetine, fluvoxamine, paroxetine, and sertraline)
Tricyclic antidepressants: Concurrent of amphetamines with TCAs may result in hypertension and CNS stimulation; avoid this combination

**Mechanism of Action** Blocks reuptake of dopamine and norepinephrine from the synapse, thus increases the amount of circulating dopamine and norepinephrine in cerebral cortex to reticular activating system; inhibits the action of monoamine oxidase and causes catecholamines to be released. Peripheral actions include elevated blood pressure, weak bronchodilator, and respiratory stimulant action.

**Dosage Forms** Tablet:
5 mg [dextroamphetamine sulfate 1.25 mg, dextroamphetamine saccharate 1.25 mg and amphetamine aspartate 1.25 mg, amphetamine sulfate 1.25 mg]
10 mg [dextroamphetamine sulfate 2.5 mg, dextroamphetamine saccharate 2.5 mg and amphetamine aspartate 2.5 mg, amphetamine sulfate 2.5 mg]
20 mg [dextroamphetamine sulfate 5 mg, dextroamphetamine saccharate 5 mg and amphetamine aspartate 5 mg, amphetamine sulfate 5 mg]
30 mg [dextroamphetamine sulfate 7.5 mg, dextroamphetamine saccharate 7.5 mg and amphetamine aspartate 7.5 mg, amphetamine sulfate 7.5 mg]

♦ **Dextroamphetamine Sulfate** *see* Dextroamphetamine *on page 159*

## Dextromethorphan (deks troe meth OR fan)

**U.S. Brand Names** Benylin DM® [OTC]; Benylin® Pediatric [OTC]; Children's Hold® [OTC]; Creo-Terpin® [OTC]; Delsym® [OTC]; Drixoral® Cough Liquid Caps [OTC]; Hold® DM [OTC]; Pertussin® CS [OTC]; Pertussin® ES [OTC]; Robitussin® Cough Calmers [OTC]; Robitussin® Pediatric [OTC]; Scot-Tussin DM® Cough Chasers [OTC]; Silphen DM® [OTC]; St. Joseph® Cough Suppressant [OTC]; Sucrets® Cough Calmers [OTC]; Suppress® [OTC]; Trocal® [OTC]; Vicks Formula 44® [OTC]; Vicks Formula 44® Pediatric Formula [OTC]

**Canadian Brand Names** Balminil®-DM, -DM Children; Koffex® DM, -DM Children; Triaminic DM

**Synonyms** Demorphan; d-Methorphan

**Pharmacologic Category** Antitussive

**Use** Symptomatic relief of coughs caused by minor viral upper respiratory tract infections or inhaled irritants; most effective for a chronic nonproductive cough

**Effects on Mental Status** May cause drowsiness or depression

**Effects on Psychiatric Treatment** Use with MAOIs may cause hypertensive crisis; avoid combination

**Contraindications** Hypersensitivity to dextromethorphan or any component

**Warnings/Precautions** Research on chicken embryos exposed to concentrations of dextromethorphan relative to those typically taken by humans has shown to cause birth defects and fetal death; more study is needed, but it is suggested that pregnant women should be advised not to use dextromethorphan-containing medications

**Adverse Reactions** <1%: Abdominal discomfort, coma, constipation, dizziness, drowsiness, GI upset, nausea, respiratory depression

**Overdosage/Toxicology**
Signs and symptoms: Nausea, vomiting, drowsiness, blurred vision, nystagmus, urinary retention, stupor, hallucinations, ataxia, respiratory depression, convulsions
Treatment: Supportive; naloxone 2 mg I.V. with repeat administration as necessary up to a total of 10 mg

**Drug Interactions** CYP2D6, 2E1, 3A3/4 enzyme substrate
MAO inhibitors

**Usual Dosage** Oral:
Children:
<2 years: Use only as directed by a physician
2-6 years (syrup): 2.5-7.5 mg every 4-8 hours; extended release is 15 mg twice daily (maximum: 30 mg/24 hours)
6-12 years: 5-10 mg every 4 hours or 15 mg every 6-8 hours; extended release is 30 mg twice daily (maximum: 60 mg/24 hours)
Children >12 years and Adults: 10-20 mg every 4 hours or 30 mg every 6-8 hours; extended release: 60 mg twice daily; maximum: 120 mg/day

**Patient Information** Shake well; do not exceed recommended dosage; take with a large glass of water; if cough lasts more than 1 week or is accompanied by a rash, fever, or headache, notify physician

**Dosage Forms**
Capsule (Drixoral® Cough Liquid Caps): 30 mg
Liquid:
Creo-Terpin®: 10 mg/15 mL (120 mL)
Pertussin® CS: 3.5 mg/5 mL (120 mL)
Robitussin® Pediatric, St. Joseph® Cough Suppressant: 7.5 mg/5 mL (60 mL, 120 mL, 240 mL)
Pertussin® ES, Vicks Formula 44®: 15 mg/5 mL (120 mL, 240 mL)
Liquid, sustained release, as polistirex (Delsym®): 30 mg/5 mL (89 mL)
Lozenges:
Scot-Tussin DM® Cough Chasers: 2.5 mg
Children's Hold®, Hold® DM, Robitussin® Cough Calmers, Sucrets® Cough Calmers: 5 mg

Suppress®, Trocal®: 7.5 mg
Syrup:
Benylin® Pediatric: 7.5 mg/mL (118 mL)
Benylin DM®, Silphen DM®: 10 mg/5 mL (120 mL, 3780 mL)
Vicks Formula 44® Pediatric Formula: 15 mg/15 mL (120 mL)

♦ **Dextropropoxyphene** *see* Propoxyphene *on page 474*

## Dextrothyroxine (deks troe thye ROKS een)

**U.S. Brand Names** Choloxin®

**Pharmacologic Category** Antilipemic Agent (Miscellaneous)

**Use** Reduction of elevated serum cholesterol

**Effects on Mental Status** May cause insomnia

**Effects on Psychiatric Treatment** Concurrent use with TCAs may increase their toxicity

**Pregnancy Risk Factor** C

**Contraindications** Euthyroid patients with one of the following: Organic heart disease (including ischemic); congestive heart failure, advanced renal or hepatic disease, history of myocardial infarction, cardiac arrhythmias, rheumatic heart disease, hypertension

**Warnings/Precautions** Use with caution in patients with a history of angina pectoris, severe hypertension, or myocardial infarction, Do not use for treatment of obesity due to risk of life-threatening toxicity. Discontinue 2 weeks prior to elective surgery. Increased serum thyroxine levels are to be expected; do not interpret as hypermetabolism.

**Adverse Reactions** <1%: Alopecia, angina, arrhythmias, diaphoresis, headache, insomnia, myocardial infarction, paresthesia, rash, tinnitus, tremor, visual disturbances, weight loss

**Overdosage/Toxicology**
Signs and symptoms: Palpitations, diarrhea, abdominal cramps, sweating, heat intolerance, congestive heart failure, tachycardia, hypertension, cardiac arrhythmias, angina, restlessness, tremor, seizures
Treatment: Propranolol can be used to treat adrenergic adverse effects, adults rarely have severe toxicity following a single overdose

**Drug Interactions**
Warfarin's effects are increased; avoid concurrent use or decrease warfarin's dose and monitor INR closely
Cholestyramine decreases the absorption of dextrothyroxine; separate administration
TCAs may increase nervousness, CNS stimulation, tachycardia, and other arrhythmias
Beta-blockers may decrease the pharmacologic effects of dextrothyroxine
Digoxin's efficacy may be reduced with exacerbation of arrhythmias or heart failure
Antidiabetic agents may need dose increased to combat hyperglycemia caused by dextrothyroxine

**Usual Dosage** Oral:
Children: 0.05 mg/kg/day, increase at 1-month intervals by 0.05 mg/kg/day to a maximum of 0.4 mg/kg/day or 4 mg/day
Adults: 1-2 mg/day, increase at 1-2 mg at intervals of 4 weeks, up to a maximum of 8 mg/day

**Patient Information** If chest pain, palpitations, sweating, diarrhea develop during therapy, discontinue drug

**Dosage Forms** Tablet, as sodium: 2 mg, 4 mg, 6 mg

♦ **Dey-Dose® Isoproterenol** *see* Isoproterenol *on page 295*

♦ **Dey-Dose® Metaproterenol** *see* Metaproterenol *on page 347*

♦ **Dey-Drop® Ophthalmic Solution** *see* Silver Nitrate *on page 512*

♦ **Dey-Lute® Isoetharine** *see* Isoetharine *on page 294*

## Dezocine (DEZ oh seen)

**Related Information**
Narcotic Agonists Comparison Chart *on page 720*

**U.S. Brand Names** Dalgan®

**Pharmacologic Category** Analgesic, Narcotic

**Use** Relief of moderate to severe postoperative, acute renal and ureteral colic, and cancer pain

**Effects on Mental Status** Sedation is common; may see depression

**Effects on Psychiatric Treatment** Contraindicated with other CNS depressants

**Pregnancy Risk Factor** C

**Contraindications** Patients experiencing immediate type hypersensitivity reactions (anaphylaxis) to dezocine or structurally related compounds should not receive this drug. Use of other central nervous system depressants concurrently to dezocine is contraindicated.

**Warnings/Precautions** Use with caution in patients with head injuries or increased intracranial pressure, respiratory depression, asthma, emphysema, COPD, renal or hepatic disease, labor and delivery, biliary surgery, or in patients with a history of drug abuse; abuse potential is apparent; may be better tolerated than other opioid agonist-antagonist; does not affect cardiac performance; contains bisulfites, avoid use in those sensitive to bisulfites

**Adverse Reactions**
1% to 10%:
Central nervous system: Sedation, dizziness, vertigo
Gastrointestinal: Nausea, vomiting
Local: Injection site reactions
<1%: Antidiuretic hormone release, biliary tract spasm, bradycardia, CNS depression, constipation, drowsiness, histamine release, hypotension, increased intracranial pressure, miosis, palpitations, peripheral vasodilation, physical and psychological dependence with prolonged use, respiratory depression, urinary tract spasm

**Overdosage/Toxicology**
Signs and symptoms: CNS and respiratory depression, gastrointestinal cramping, constipation
Treatment: Naloxone 2 mg I.V. (0.01 mg/kg for children) with repeat administration as necessary up to a total of 10 mg

**Drug Interactions** Increased effect with CNS depressants

**Usual Dosage** Adults (not recommended for patients <18 years):
I.M.: Initial: 5-20 mg; may be repeated every 3-6 hours as needed; maximum: 120 mg/day and 20 mg/dose
I.V.: Initial: 2.5-10 mg; may be repeated every 2-4 hours as needed
**Dosing adjustment in renal impairment:** Should be used cautiously at reduced doses

**Patient Information** Avoid driving or operating machinery until the effect of drug wears off; may cause physical and psychological dependence with prolonged use

**Nursing Implications** Watch closely for respiratory depression; induced respiratory depression is greater than that seen with morphine during the first hour after administration

**Dosage Forms** Injection, single-dose vial: 5 mg/mL (2 mL); 10 mg/mL (2 mL); 15 mg/mL (2 mL)

♦ **DHC Plus®** *see* Dihydrocodeine Compound *on page 170*

♦ **D.H.E. 45® Injection** *see* Dihydroergotamine *on page 171*

♦ **DHPG Sodium** *see* Ganciclovir *on page 245*

♦ **DHT™** *see* Dihydrotachysterol *on page 171*

♦ **Diaβeta®** *see* Glyburide *on page 252*

♦ **Diabetes Mellitus Treatment** *see page 782*

♦ **Diabetic Tussin DM® [OTC]** *see* Guaifenesin and Dextromethorphan *on page 257*

♦ **Diabetic Tussin® EX [OTC]** *see* Guaifenesin *on page 256*

♦ **Diabinese®** *see* Chlorpropamide *on page 118*

♦ **Diacetylmorphine** *see* Heroin *on page 267*

♦ **Diagnostic and Statistical Manual of Mental Disorders (DSM-IV)** *see page 671*

♦ **Dialose® [OTC]** *see* Docusate *on page 179*

♦ **Dialume® [OTC]** *see* Aluminum Hydroxide *on page 28*

♦ **Diamine T.D.® [OTC]** *see* Brompheniramine *on page 73*

♦ **Diaminodiphenylsulfone** *see* Dapsone *on page 151*

♦ **Diamorphine Hydrochloride** *see* Heroin *on page 267*

♦ **Diamox®** *see* Acetazolamide *on page 16*

♦ **Diamox Sequels®** *see* Acetazolamide *on page 16*

♦ **Diapid® Nasal Spray** *see* Lypressin *on page 329*

♦ **Diar-aid® [OTC]** *see* Loperamide *on page 324*

♦ **Diasorb® [OTC]** *see* Attapulgite *on page 53*

♦ **Diastat® Gel** *see* Diazepam *on page 161*

♦ **Diazemuls® Injection** *see* Diazepam *on page 161*

## Diazepam (dye AZ e pam)

**Related Information**
Agents for Treatment of Extrapyramidal Symptoms *on page 638*
Anxiolytic/Hypnotic Use in Long-Term Care Facilities *on page 754*
Benzodiazepines Comparison Chart *on page 708*
Federal OBRA Regulations Recommended Maximum Doses *on page 756*
Patient Information - Anxiolytics & Sedative Hypnotics (Benzodiazepines) *on page 653*
Schizophrenia *on page 604*
Special Populations - Elderly *on page 662*
Substance-Related Disorders *on page 609*

**Generic Available** Yes

**U.S. Brand Names** Diastat® Gel; Diazemuls® Injection; Emulsified Dizac® Injection; Emulsified Valium®
(Continued)

## Diazepam *(Continued)*

**Canadian Brand Names** Apo®-Diazepam; Diazemuls®; E Pam®; Meval®; Novo-Dipam; PMS-Diazepam; Vivol®

**Pharmacologic Category** Benzodiazepine

**Use** Management of anxiety disorders; alcohol withdrawal symptoms; skeletal muscle relaxant; convulsive disorders

**Unlabeled uses:** Panic disorders; provide preoperative sedation; light anesthesia; amnesia

**Restrictions** C-IV

**Pregnancy Risk Factor** D

**Pregnancy/Breast-Feeding Implications**

Clinical effects on the fetus: Crosses the placenta. Oral clefts reported, however, more recent data does not support an association between drug and oral clefts; inguinal hernia, cardiac defects, spina bifida, dysmorphic facial features, skeletal defects, multiple other malformations reported; hypotonia and withdrawal symptoms reported following use near time of delivery

Breast-feeding/lactation: Crosses into breast milk

Clinical effects on the infant: Sedation; American Academy of Pediatrics reports that **use may be of concern.**

**Contraindications** Hypersensitivity to this drug or any component of its formulation (cross-sensitivity with other benzodiazepines may exist); narrow angle glaucoma; pregnancy; not for use in children <6 months of age (oral) or <30 days of age (parenteral)

**Warnings/Precautions** Diazepam has been associated with increasing the frequency of grand mal seizures. Withdrawal has also been associated with an increase in the seizure frequency. Use with caution with drugs which may decrease diazepam metabolism. Use with caution in elderly or debilitated patients, patients with hepatic disease (including alcoholics), or renal impairment. Active metabolites with extended half-lives may lead to delayed accumulation and adverse effects. Use with caution in patients with respiratory disease or impaired gag reflex.

Acute hypotension, muscle weakness, apnea, and cardiac arrest have occurred with parenteral administration. Acute effects may be more prevalent in patients receiving concurrent barbiturates, narcotics, or ethanol. Appropriate resuscitative equipment and qualified personnel should be available during administration and monitoring. Avoid use of the injection in patients with shock, coma, or acute ethanol intoxication. Intra-arterial injection or extravasation of the parenteral formulation should be avoided. Parenteral formulation contains propylene glycol, which has been associated with toxicity when administered in high dosages.

Causes CNS depression (dose-related) resulting in sedation, dizziness, confusion, or ataxia which may impair physical and mental capabilities. Patients must be cautioned about performing tasks which require mental alertness (ie, operating machinery or driving). Use with caution in patients receiving other CNS depressants or psychoactive agents. Effects with other sedative drugs or ethanol may be potentiated. The dosage of narcotics should be reduced by approximately 1/3 when diazepam is added. Benzodiazepines have been associated with falls and traumatic injury and should be used with extreme caution in patients who are at risk of these events (especially the elderly).

Use caution in patients with depression, particularly if suicidal risk may be present. Use with caution in patients with a history of drug dependence. Benzodiazepines have been associated with dependence and acute withdrawal symptoms on discontinuation or reduction in dose. Acute withdrawal, including seizures, may be precipitated in patients after administration of flumazenil to patients receiving long-term benzodiazepine therapy.

Diazepam has been associated with anterograde amnesia. Paradoxical reactions, including hyperactive or aggressive behavior, have been reported with benzodiazepines, particularly in adolescent/pediatric or psychiatric patients. Does not have analgesic, antidepressant, or antipsychotic properties.

**Adverse Reactions**

Cardiovascular: Hypotension

Central nervous system: Drowsiness, ataxia, amnesia, slurred speech, paradoxical excitement or rage, fatigue, insomnia, memory impairment, headache, anxiety, depression, vertigo, confusion

Dermatologic: Rash

Endocrine & metabolic: Changes in libido

Gastrointestinal: Changes in salivation, constipation, nausea

Genitourinary: Incontinence, urinary retention

Hepatic: Jaundice

Local: Phlebitis, pain with injection

Neuromuscular & skeletal: Dysarthria, tremor

Ocular: Blurred vision, diplopia

Respiratory: Decrease in respiratory rate, apnea

**Overdosage/Toxicology**

Signs and symptoms: Somnolence, confusion, coma, hypoactive reflexes, dyspnea, hypotension, slurred speech, impaired coordination

Treatment: Treatment for benzodiazepine overdose is supportive. Rarely is mechanical ventilation required. Flumazenil has been shown to selectively block the binding of benzodiazepines to CNS receptors, resulting in a reversal of benzodiazepine-induced CNS depression, but not respiratory depression.

**Drug Interactions** CYP1A2 and 2C8/9 enzyme substrate; minor pathways include CYP2C19 and 3A3/4

CNS depressants: Sedative effects and/or respiratory depression may be additive with CNS depressants; includes ethanol, barbiturates, narcotic analgesics, and other sedative agents; monitor for increased effect

CYP1A2 inhibitors: Metabolism of diazepam may be decreased; increasing clinical effect or toxicity; inhibitors include cimetidine, ciprofloxacin, fluvoxamine, isoniazid, ritonavir, and zileutin

CYP2C8/9 inhibitors: Serum levels and/or toxicity of diazepam may be increased; inhibitors include amiodarone, cimetidine, fluvoxamine, some NSAIDs, metronidazole, ritonavir, sulfonamides, troglitazone, valproic acid, and zafirlukast; monitor for increased sedation

Enzyme inducers: Metabolism of some benzodiazepines may be increased, decreasing their therapeutic effect; consider using an alternative sedative/hypnotic agent; potential inducers include phenobarbital, phenytoin, carbamazepine, rifampin, and rifabutin

Oral contraceptives: May decrease the clearance of some benzodiazepines (those which undergo oxidative metabolism); monitor for increased benzodiazepine effect

Theophylline: May partially antagonize some of the effects of benzodiazepines; monitor for decreased response; may require higher doses for sedation

**Stability** Protect parenteral dosage form from light; potency is retained for up to 3 months when kept at room temperature; most stable at pH 4-8, hydrolysis occurs at pH <3; do not mix I.V. product with other medications

**Mechanism of Action** Binds to stereospecific benzodiazepine receptors on the postsynaptic GABA neuron at several sites within the central nervous system, including the limbic system, reticular formation. Enhancement of the inhibitory effect of GABA on neuronal excitability results by increased neuronal membrane permeability to chloride ions. This shift in chloride ions results in hyperpolarization (a less excitable state) and stabilization.

**Pharmacodynamics/kinetics**

I.V. for status epilepticus:
- Onset of action: Almost immediate
- Duration: Short, 20-30 minutes

Absorption: Oral: 85% to 100%, more reliable than I.M.

Protein binding: 98%

Metabolism: In the liver

Half-life:
- Parent drug: Adults: 20-50 hours, increased half-life in neonates, elderly, and those with severe hepatic disorders
- Active major metabolite (desmethyldiazepam): 50-100 hours, can be prolonged in neonates

**Usual Dosage**

Children:
- Conscious sedation for procedures: Oral: 0.2-0.3 mg/kg (maximum: 10 mg) 45-60 minutes prior to procedure
- Sedation or muscle relaxation or anxiety:
  - Oral: 0.12-0.8 mg/kg/day in divided doses every 6-8 hours
  - I.M., I.V.: 0.04-0.3 mg/kg/dose every 2-4 hours to a maximum of 0.6 mg/kg within an 8-hour period if needed
- Status epilepticus:
  - Infants 30 days to 5 years: I.V.: 0.05-0.3 mg/kg/dose given over 2-3 minutes, every 15-30 minutes to a maximum total dose of 5 mg; repeat in 2-4 hours as needed **or** 0.2-0.5 mg/dose every 2-5 minutes to a maximum total dose of 5 mg
  - >5 years: I.V.: 0.05-0.3 mg/kg/dose given over 2-3 minutes every 15-30 minutes to a maximum total dose of 10 mg; repeat in 2-4 hours as needed **or** 1 mg/dose given over 2-3 minutes, every 2-5 minutes to a maximum total dose of 10 mg
  - Rectal: 0.5 mg/kg, then 0.25 mg/kg in 10 minutes if needed

Adolescents: Conscious sedation for procedures:
- Oral: 10 mg
- I.V.: 5 mg, may repeat with ½ dose if needed

Adults:
- Anxiety/sedation/skeletal muscle relaxation:
  - Oral: 2-10 mg 2-4 times/day
  - I.M., I.V.: 2-10 mg, may repeat in 3-4 hours if needed
- Status epilepticus: I.V.: 5-10 mg every 10-20 minutes, up to 30 mg in an 8-hour period; may repeat in 2-4 hours if necessary
- Rapid tranquilization of agitated patient (administer every 30-60 minutes): Oral: 5-10 mg; average total dose for tranquilization: 20-60 mg

Elderly: Oral: Initial:
- Anxiety: 1-2 mg 1-2 times/day; increase gradually as needed, rarely need to use >10 mg/day (watch for hypotension and excessive sedation)
- Skeletal muscle relaxant: 2-5 mg 2-4 times/day

Hemodialysis: Not dialyzable (0% to 5%); supplemental dose is not necessary

**Dosing adjustment in hepatic impairment:** Reduce dose by 50% in cirrhosis and avoid in severe/acute liver disease

**Dietary Considerations** Alcohol: Additive CNS depression has been reported with benzodiazepines; avoid or limit alcohol

**Administration** In children, do not exceed 1-2 mg/minute IVP; adults 5 mg/minute; I.M. absorption may be erratic

**Monitoring Parameters** Respiratory, cardiovascular, and mental status; check for orthostasis

**Reference Range** Therapeutic: Diazepam: 0.2-1.5 μg/mL (SI: 0.7-5.3 μmol/L); N-desmethyldiazepam (nordiazepam): 0.1-0.5 μg/mL (SI: 0.35-1.8 μmol/L)

**Test Interactions** False-negative urinary glucose determinations when using Clinistix® or Diastix®

**Patient Information** Avoid alcohol and other CNS depressants; avoid activities needing good psychomotor coordination until CNS effects are known; drug may cause physical or psychological dependence; avoid abrupt discontinuation after prolonged use

**Nursing Implications** Provide safety measures (ie, side rails, night light, and call button); supervise ambulation

**Additional Information** Oral absorption more reliable than I.M.; Intensol® should be diluted before use; diazepam does not have any analgesic effects

**Dosage Forms**

Gel, rectal delivery system (Diastat®):
- Pediatric rectal tip (4.4 cm): 5 mg/mL (2.5 mg, 5 mg, 10 mg) [twin packs]
- Adult rectal tip (6 cm): 5 mg/mL (10 mg, 15 mg, 20 mg) [twin packs]

Injection: 5 mg/mL (1 mL, 2 mL, 5 mL, 10 mL)

Injection, emulsified:
- Dizac®: 5 mg/mL (3 mL)
- Diazemuls®: 5 mg/mL (2 mL)

Solution, oral (wintergreen-spice flavor): 5 mg/5 mL (5 mL, 10 mL, 500 mL)

Solution, oral concentrate (Diazepam Intensol®): 5 mg/mL (30 mL)

Tablet: 2 mg, 5 mg, 10 mg

## Diazoxide (dye az OKS ide)

**U.S. Brand Names** Hyperstat® I.V.; Proglycem® Oral

**Synonyms** Diazoxidum

**Pharmacologic Category** Antihypoglycemic Agent; Vasodilator

**Use**

Oral: Hypoglycemia related to islet cell adenoma, carcinoma, hyperplasia, or adenomatosis, nesidioblastosis, leucine sensitivity, or extrapancreatic malignancy

I.V.: Severe hypertension

**Effects on Mental Status** May cause dizziness; may rarely cause extrapyramidal symptoms

**Effects on Psychiatric Treatment** May cause leukopenia; use caution with clozapine and carbamazepine

**Pregnancy Risk Factor** C

**Contraindications** Hypersensitivity to diazoxide, thiazides, or other sulfonamide derivatives; hypertension associated with aortic coarctation, arteriovenous shunts, pheochromocytoma, dissecting aortic aneurysm

**Warnings/Precautions** Diabetes mellitus, renal or liver disease, coronary artery disease, or cerebral vascular insufficiency; patients may require a diuretic with repeated I.V. doses; use caution when reducing severely elevated blood pressure (use 150 mg minibolus only)

**Adverse Reactions**

1% to 10%:
- Cardiovascular: Hypotension
- Central nervous system: Dizziness
- Gastrointestinal: Nausea, vomiting
- Neuromuscular & skeletal: Weakness

<1%: Angina, anorexia, burning, cellulitis, cerebral infarction, chronic oral use, constipation, extrapyramidal symptoms and development of abnormal facies with flushing, headache, hirsutism, hyperglycemia, hyperuricemia, inhibition of labor, ketoacidosis, leukopenia, myocardial infarction, pain, phlebitis upon extravasation, rash, seizures, sodium and water retention, tachycardia, thrombocytopenia

**Overdosage/Toxicology**

Signs and symptoms: Hyperglycemia, ketoacidosis, hypotension

Treatment: Insulin, fluid, and electrolyte restoration; I.V. pressors may be needed to support blood pressure

**Drug Interactions**

Decreased effect: Diazoxide may increase phenytoin metabolism or free fraction

Increased toxicity:
- Diuretics and hypotensive agents may potentiate diazoxide adverse effects
- Diazoxide may decrease warfarin protein binding

**Usual Dosage**

Hypertension: Children and Adults: I.V.: 1-3 mg/kg up to a maximum of 150 mg in a single injection; repeat dose in 5-15 minutes until blood pressure adequately reduced; repeat administration at intervals of 4-24 hours; monitor the blood pressure closely; do not use longer than 10 days

Hyperinsulinemic hypoglycemia: Oral: **Note:** Use lower dose listed as initial dose
- Newborns and Infants: 8-15 mg/kg/day in divided doses every 8-12 hours
- Children and Adults: 3-8 mg/kg/day in divided doses every 8-12 hours

**Dosing adjustment in renal impairment:** None

Dialysis: Elimination is not enhanced via hemo- or peritoneal dialysis; supplemental dose is not necessary

**Patient Information**

I.V. emergency treatment of hypertension: Remain lying down for at least 1 hour following infusion. When up, change positions from sitting or lying to standing slowly.

Oral treatment of hypoglycemia: Monitor serum glucose as directed by prescriber. Report significant changes in serum glucose levels, increased swelling of extremities, increased weight, unresolved constipation, GI upset (eg, nausea, vomiting, constipation, anorexia), chest pain, or palpitations.

**Nursing Implications** Extravasation can be treated with warm compresses; monitor blood glucose daily in patients receiving I.V. therapy

**Dosage Forms**

Capsule (Proglycem®): 50 mg

Injection (Hyperstat®): 15 mg/mL (1 mL, 20 mL)

Suspension, oral (chocolate-mint flavor) (Proglycem®): 50 mg/mL (30 mL)

♦ **Diazoxidum** *see* Diazoxide *on page 163*

♦ **Dibent® Injection** *see* Dicyclomine *on page 165*

♦ **Dibenzyline®** *see* Phenoxybenzamine *on page 437*

## Dibucaine (DYE byoo kane)

**U.S. Brand Names** Nupercainal® [OTC]

**Pharmacologic Category** Local Anesthetic

**Use** Amide derivative local anesthetic for minor skin conditions; fast, temporary relief of pain and itching due to hemorrhoids; minor burns

**Effects on Mental Status** None reported

**Effects on Psychiatric Treatment** None reported

**Usual Dosage** Children and Adults: Topical: Apply gently to the affected areas; no more than 30 g for adults or 7.5 g for children should be used in any 24-hour period

**Dosage Forms**

Cream, topical: 0.5% (45 g)

Ointment, topical: 1% (30 g, 60 g, 454 g)

## Dibucaine and Hydrocortisone
(DYE byoo kane & hye droe KOR ti sone)

**U.S. Brand Names** Corticaine® Topical

**Pharmacologic Category** Local Anesthetic

**Use** Relief of the inflammatory and pruritic manifestations of corticosteroid-responsive dermatoses and for external anal itching

**Effects on Mental Status** None reported

**Effects on Psychiatric Treatment** None reported

**Usual Dosage** Topical: Apply to affected areas 2-4 times/day

**Dosage Forms** Cream: Dibucaine 5% and hydrocortisone 5%

♦ **Dicarbosil® [OTC]** *see* Calcium Carbonate *on page 84*

## Dichlorphenamide (dye klor FEN a mide)

**U.S. Brand Names** Daranide®

**Pharmacologic Category** Carbonic Anhydrase Inhibitor; Diuretic, Carbonic Anhydrase Inhibitor; Ophthalmic Agent, Antiglaucoma

**Use** Adjunct in treatment of open-angle glaucoma and perioperative treatment for angle-closure glaucoma

**Effects on Mental Status** Sedation is common; may cause depression

**Effects on Psychiatric Treatment** May rarely cause bone marrow suppression; use caution with clozapine and carbamazepine; may increase the excretion of lithium but should not be used to treat lithium toxicity

**Usual Dosage** Adults: Oral: 100-200 mg to start followed by 100 mg every 12 hours until desired response is obtained; maintenance dose: 25-50 mg 1-3 times/day

**Dosage Forms** Tablet: 50 mg

♦ **Dichysterol** *see* Dihydrotachysterol *on page 171*

## Diclofenac (dye KLOE fen ak)

**Related Information**

Nonsteroidal Anti-inflammatory Agents Comparison Chart *on page 722*

**U.S. Brand Names** Cataflam® Oral; Voltaren® Ophthalmic; Voltaren® Oral; Voltaren®-XR Oral

**Canadian Brand Names** Apo®-Diclo; Novo-Difenac®; Novo-Difenac®-SR; Nu-Diclo; Voltaren Rapide®

**Synonyms** Diclofenac Potassium; Diclofenac Sodium

(Continued)

## Diclofenac *(Continued)*

**Pharmacologic Category** Nonsteroidal Anti-Inflammatory Agent (NSAID)

**Use** Acute treatment of mild to moderate pain; acute and chronic treatment of rheumatoid arthritis, ankylosing spondylitis, and osteoarthritis; used for juvenile rheumatoid arthritis, gout, dysmenorrhea; ophthalmic solution for postoperative inflammation after cataract extraction

**Effects on Mental Status** May cause nervousness or dizziness; may rarely cause depression

**Effects on Psychiatric Treatment** May rarely cause agranulocytosis; use caution with clozapine and carbamazepine; may decrease the clearance of lithium resulting in elevated serum levels and potential toxicity; monitor serum lithium levels

**Pregnancy Risk Factor** B (D if used in third trimester)

**Contraindications** Known hypersensitivity to diclofenac, any component, aspirin or other nonsteroidal anti-inflammatory drugs (NSAIDs); porphyria

**Warnings/Precautions** Use with caution in patients with congestive heart failure, dehydration, hypertension, decreased renal or hepatic function, history of GI disease, or those receiving anticoagulants

**Adverse Reactions**

>10%:

Dermatologic: Rash

Gastrointestinal: Abdominal cramps, heartburn, indigestion, nausea

1% to 10%:

Cardiovascular: Angina pectoris, arrhythmias

Central nervous system: Dizziness, nervousness

Dermatologic: Itching

Gastrointestinal: GI ulceration, vomiting

Genitourinary: Vaginal bleeding

Otic: Tinnitus

<1%: Agranulocytosis, anaphylaxis, anemia, angioedema, blurred vision, change in vision, chest pain, congestive heart failure, convulsions, cystitis, decreased hearing, diaphoresis (increased), drowsiness, epistaxis, erythema multiforme, exfoliative dermatitis, forgetfulness, hepatitis, hypertension, insomnia, interstitial nephritis, laryngeal edema, leukopenia, mental depression, nephrotic syndrome, pancytopenia, peripheral neuropathy, renal impairment, shortness of breath, Stevens-Johnson syndrome, stomatitis, tachycardia, thrombocytopenia, trembling, urticaria, weakness, wheezing

**Overdosage/Toxicology**

Signs and symptoms: Acute renal failure, vomiting, drowsiness, leukocytosis

Treatment: Management of a nonsteroidal anti-inflammatory drug (NSAID) intoxication is primarily supportive and symptomatic. Fluid therapy is commonly effective in managing the hypotension that may occur following an acute NSAID overdose, except when this is due to an acute blood loss.

**Drug Interactions** CYP2C8 and 2C9 enzyme substrate; CYP2C9 enzyme inhibitor

ACE inhibitors: Effects may be reduced by NSAIDs; use lowest possible dose for shortest duration possible; monitor

Cholestyramine and colestipol: Absorption may be reduced by concurrent administration

Corticosteroids: May increase the risk of GI ulceration; use caution

Cyclosporine: Nephrotoxicity may be increased with concurrent NSAID use; monitor

CYP2C9 inhibitors: May increase in diclofenac concentrations; inhibitors include amiodarone, cimetidine, fluvoxamine, metronidazole, omeprazole, sulfonamides, valproic acid, and zafirlukast

CYP2C9 substrates: Coadministration of drugs metabolized by CYP2C9 may result in increased serum concentrations of these agents

Hydralazine: Antihypertensive effect may be decreased; avoid concurrent use

Lithium: Serum levels can be increased; avoid concurrent use if possible or monitor lithium levels and adjust dose. When NSAID is stopped, lithium may need adjustment again.

Loop diuretics: Therapeutic effects may be reduced by NSAIDs; avoid

Methotrexate: Toxicity may be increased by concurrent NSAID use; risk is limited in low-dose methotrexate regimens (such as for rheumatoid arthritis); prolonged leucovorin rescue may be required at antineoplastic doses; monitor

Thiazide diuretics: Antihypertensive effects are decreased; avoid concurrent use

Warfarin: INRs may be increased by some NSAIDs. This may depend, in part, on dose and duration; monitor INR closely. Use the lowest dose of NSAIDs possible and for the briefest duration.

**Usual Dosage** Adults:

Oral:

Analgesia: Starting dose: 50 mg 3 times/day

Rheumatoid arthritis: 150-200 mg/day in 2-4 divided doses (100 mg/day of sustained release product)

Osteoarthritis: 100-150 mg/day in 2-3 divided doses (100-200 mg/day of sustained release product)

Ankylosing spondylitis: 100-125 mg/day in 4-5 divided doses

Ophthalmic: Instill 1 drop into affected eye 4 times/day beginning 24 hours after cataract surgery and continuing for 2 weeks

**Patient Information**

Oral: Take this medication exactly as directed; do not increase dose without consulting prescriber. Do not crush or chew tablets. Take with 8 ounces of water, along with food or milk products to reduce GI distress. Maintain adequate fluid intake (2-3 L/day of fluids unless instructed to restrict fluid intake). Avoid excessive alcohol, aspirin and aspirin-containing medication, and all other anti-inflammatory medications unless consulting prescriber. You may experience dizziness, nervousness, or headache (use caution when driving or engaging in tasks requiring alertness until response to drug is known); nausea, vomiting, dry mouth, or heartburn (frequent small meals, frequent mouth care, sucking lozenges, or chewing gum may help); or constipation (increased exercise, fluids, or dietary fruit and fiber may help). GI bleeding, ulceration, or perforation can occur with or without pain; discontinue medication and contact prescriber if persistent abdominal pain or cramping, or blood in stool occurs. Report chest pain or palpitations; breathlessness or difficulty breathing; unusual bruising/bleeding or blood in urine, stool, mouth, or vomitus; unusual fatigue; skin rash or itching; unusual weight gain or swelling of extremities; change in urinary pattern; change in vision or hearing; or ringing in ears.

Ophthalmic: For ophthalmic use only. Apply prescribed amount as often as directed. Wash hands before using and do not let tip of applicator touch eye or contaminate tip of applicator. Tilt head back and look upward. Gently pull down lower lid and put drop(s) in inner corner of eye. Close eye and roll eyeball in all directions. Do not blink for ½ minute. Apply gentle pressure to inner corner of eye for 30 seconds. Wipe away excess from skin around eye. Do not use any other eye preparation for at least 10 minutes. Do not touch tip of applicator to eye or contaminate tip of applicator. Do not share medication with anyone else. May cause sensitivity to bright light (dark glasses may help); temporary stinging or blurred vision may occur. Inform prescriber if you experience eye pain, redness, burning, watering, dryness, double vision, puffiness around eye, vision disturbances, or other adverse eye response; worsening of condition or lack of improvement.

**Nursing Implications** Do not crush tablets

**Dosage Forms**

Solution, ophthalmic, as sodium (Voltaren®): 0.1% (2.5 mL, 5 mL)

Tablet, enteric coated, as sodium: 25 mg, 50 mg, 75 mg

Voltaren®: 25 mg, 50 mg, 75 mg

Tablet, extended release, as sodium (Voltaren®-XR): 100 mg

Tablet, as potassium (Cataflam®): 50 mg

## Diclofenac and Misoprostol

(dye KLOE fen ak & mye soe PROST ole)

**U.S. Brand Names** Arthrotec®

**Pharmacologic Category** Nonsteroidal Anti-Inflammatory Agent (NSAID); Prostaglandin

**Use** The diclofenac component is indicated for the treatment of osteoarthritis and rheumatoid arthritis; the misoprostol component is indicated for the prophylaxis of NSAID-induced gastric and duodenal ulceration

**Effects on Mental Status** May cause nervousness or dizziness; may rarely cause depression

**Effects on Psychiatric Treatment** May rarely cause may agranulocytosis; use caution with clozapine and carbamazepine; may decrease the clearance of lithium resulting in elevated serum levels and potential toxicity; monitor serum lithium levels

**Pregnancy Risk Factor** X

**Contraindications** Pregnancy; patients who have demonstrated hypersensitivity to diclofenac, aspirin, other NSAIDs, misoprostol, other prostaglandins, or any component of the drug product

**Warnings/Precautions** Use in premenopausal women; should not be used in premenopausal women unless they use effective contraception and have been advised of the risks of taking the product if pregnant

**Adverse Reactions**

>10%: Gastrointestinal: Abdominal pain (21%), diarrhea (19%), nausea (11%), dyspepsia (14%)

1% to 10%:

Endocrine & metabolic: Elevated transaminase levels

Gastrointestinal: Flatulence (9%)

Hematologic: Anemia

Miscellaneous: Anaphylactic reactions

**Overdosage/Toxicology**

Signs and symptoms: Clinical signs that may suggest NSAID overdose include GI complaints, confusion, drowsiness, or general hypotonia. Clinical signs that may indicate a misoprostol overdose are sedation, tremor, convulsions, dyspnea, abdominal pain, diarrhea, fever, palpitations, hypotension, or bradycardia. The toxic dose of misoprostol in humans has not been determined. In animals, the acute toxic effects are diarrhea, GI lesions, focal cardiac necrosis, hepatic necrosis, renal tubular necrosis, testicular atrophy, respiratory difficulties, and depression of the central nervous system.

Treatment: Supportive therapy. In the case of acute overdosage, gastric lavage is recommended. Induced diuresis may be beneficial because diclofenac and misoprostol metabolites are excreted in the urine. The effect of dialysis or hemoperfusion on the drug's elimination remains unproven. The use of oral activated charcoal may help to reduce its absorption.

**Drug Interactions**

Increased effect/toxicity: Aspirin (shared toxicity), digoxin (elevated digoxin levels), warfarin (synergistic bleeding potential), methotrexate (increased methotrexate levels), cyclosporine (increased nephrotoxicity), lithium (increased lithium levels)

Decreased effects: Aspirin (displaces diclofenac from binding sites), antihypertensive agents (decreased blood pressure control), antacids (may decrease absorption)

**Usual Dosage** Adults: Oral:

Arthrotec® 50:

Osteoarthritis: 1 tablet 2-3 times/day

Rheumatoid arthritis: 1 tablet 3-4 times/day

For both regimens, if not tolerated by patient, the dose may be reduced to 1 tablet twice daily

Arthrotec® 75:

Patients who cannot tolerate full daily Arthrotec® 50 regimens: 1 tablet twice daily

**Note:** The use of these tablets may not be as effective at preventing GI ulceration

**Patient Information** See individual agents

**Dosage Forms** Tablet: Diclofenac 50 mg and misoprostol 200 mcg; diclofenac 75 mg and misoprostol 200 mcg

♦ **Diclofenac Potassium** *see* Diclofenac *on page 163*

♦ **Diclofenac Sodium** *see* Diclofenac *on page 163*

## Dicloxacillin (dye kloks a SIL in)

**U.S. Brand Names** Dycill®; Dynapen®; Pathocil®

**Pharmacologic Category** Antibiotic, Penicillin

**Use** Treatment of systemic infections such as pneumonia, skin and soft tissue infections, and osteomyelitis caused by penicillinase-producing staphylococci

**Effects on Mental Status** Penicillins have been reported to cause apprehension, illusions, agitation, insomnia, depersonalization, and encephalopathy

**Effects on Psychiatric Treatment** Rarely may cause agranulocytosis; use caution with clozapine and carbamazepine

**Pregnancy Risk Factor** B

**Contraindications** Known hypersensitivity to dicloxacillin, penicillin, or any components

**Warnings/Precautions** Monitor PT if patient concurrently on warfarin; elimination of drug is slow in neonates; use with caution in patients allergic to cephalosporins; bad taste of suspension may make compliance difficult

**Adverse Reactions**

1% to 10%: Gastrointestinal: Nausea, diarrhea, abdominal pain

<1%: Agranulocytosis, anemia, eosinophilia, fever, hematuria, hemolytic anemia, hepatotoxicity, hypersensitivity, increased BUN/creatinine, interstitial nephritis, leukopenia, neutropenia, prolonged PT, pseudomembranous colitis, rash (maculopapular to exfoliative), seizures with extremely high doses and/or renal failure, serum sickness-like reactions, thrombocytopenia, transient elevated LFTs, vaginitis, vomiting

**Overdosage/Toxicology**

Signs and symptoms: Neuromuscular hypersensitivity (agitation, hallucinations, asterixis, encephalopathy, confusion, and seizures) and electrolyte imbalance with potassium or sodium salts, especially in renal failure

Treatment: Hemodialysis may be helpful to aid in the removal of the drug from the blood, otherwise most treatment is supportive or symptom directed

**Drug Interactions**

Decreased effect: Efficacy of oral contraceptives may be reduced; decreased effect of warfarin

Increased effect: Disulfiram, probenecid may increase penicillin levels

**Usual Dosage** Oral:

Use in newborns not recommended

Children <40 kg: 12.5-25 mg/kg/day divided every 6 hours; doses of 50-100 mg/kg/day in divided doses every 6 hours have been used for therapy of osteomyelitis

Children >40 kg and Adults: 125-250 mg every 6 hours

**Dosage adjustment in renal impairment:** Not necessary

Hemodialysis: Not dialyzable (0% to 5%); supplemental dosage not necessary

Peritoneal dialysis: Supplemental dosage not necessary

Continuous arteriovenous or venovenous hemofiltration (CAVH/CAVHD): Supplemental dosage not necessary

**Dietary Considerations** Food: Decreases drug absorption rate; decreases drug serum concentration. Administer on an empty stomach 1 hour before or 2 hours after meals.

**Patient Information** Take medication as directed, with a large glass of water 1 hour before or 2 hours after meals. Take at regular intervals around-the-clock and take for length of time prescribed. You may experience some gastric distress (small frequent meals may help) and diarrhea (if this persists, consult prescriber). If diabetic, drug may cause false tests with Clinitest® urine glucose monitoring; use of glucose oxidase methods (Clinistix®) or serum glucose monitoring is preferable. This drug may interfere with oral contraceptives; an alternate form of birth control should be used. Report fever, vaginal itching, sores in the mouth, loose foul-smelling stools, yellowing of skin or eyes, and change in color of urine or stool.

**Dosage Forms**

Capsule, as sodium: 125 mg, 250 mg, 500 mg

Powder for oral suspension, as sodium: 62.5 mg/5 mL (80 mL, 100 mL, 200 mL)

## Dicumarol (dye KOO ma role)

**Synonyms** Bishydroxycoumarin

**Pharmacologic Category** Anticoagulant, Coumarin Derivative

**Use** Prophylaxis and treatment of thromboembolic disorders

**Effects on Mental Status** None reported

**Effects on Psychiatric Treatment** May cause leukopenia and agranulocytosis; use caution with clozapine and carbamazepine; psychotropics may increase or decrease prothrombin times; monitor prothrombin times

**Pregnancy Risk Factor** D

**Contraindications** Severe liver or kidney disease; open wounds; uncontrolled bleeding; hypersensitivity to dicumarol or any component

**Warnings/Precautions** Concomitant use with vitamin K may decrease anticoagulant effect; monitor carefully; concomitant use with ethacrynic acid, indomethacin, mefenamic acid, phenylbutazone, or aspirin increases warfarin's anticoagulant effect and may cause severe GI bleeding; the plasma half-life of dicumarol is 1-2 days and its duration of action is 2-10 days; as this is considerably longer than warfarin, prescribers should be aware of this difference; peak levels should be expected 1-2 weeks after dose adjustment

**Adverse Reactions** 1% to 10%:

Dermatologic: Alopecia

Gastrointestinal: Stomach cramps, nausea, vomiting, diarrhea

Hematologic: Leukopenia

**Drug Interactions** May accentuate toxicities of oral hypoglycemics and anticonvulsants. The following will decrease prothrombin time - antacids, antihistamines, phenobarbital, carbamazepine, cholestyramine, meprobamate, glutethimide, ethchlorvynol, oral contraceptives, ranitidine, chloral hydrate, diuretics. Increased prothrombin time due to allopurinol, amiodarone, cimetidine, clofibrate, dextran, diazoxide, diflunisal, diuretics, disulfiram, fenoprofen, ibuprofen, indomethacin, influenza virus vaccine, methyldopa, methylphenidate, MAO inhibitors, naproxen, nortriptyline, phenytoin, propylthiouracil, salicylates, quinidine, quinine, ranitidine, tolbutamide, thyroid drugs, sulindac, co-trimoxazole

**Usual Dosage** Adults: Oral: 25-200 mg/day based on prothrombin time (PT) determinations

**Dosage Forms** Tablet: 25 mg, 50 mg, 100 mg

## Dicyclomine (dye SYE kloe meen)

**Related Information**

Pharmacotherapy of Urinary Incontinence *on page 758*

**U.S. Brand Names** Antispas® Injection; Bentyl® Hydrochloride Injection; Bentyl® Hydrochloride Oral; Byclomine® Injection; Dibent® Injection; Di-Spaz® Injection; Di-Spaz® Oral; Or-Tyl® Injection

**Canadian Brand Names** Bentylol®; Formulex®

**Synonyms** Dicyclomine Hydrochloride; Dicycloverine Hydrochloride

**Pharmacologic Category** Anticholinergic Agent

**Use** Treatment of functional disturbances of GI motility such as irritable bowel syndrome

**Unlabeled use:** Urinary incontinence

**Effects on Mental Status** May cause nervousness, excitement, insomnia, confusion, drowsiness, dyskinesia

**Effects on Psychiatric Treatment** Concurrent use with psychotropics may produce additive sedation and dry mouth

**Pregnancy Risk Factor** B

**Contraindications** Hypersensitivity to any anticholinergic drug; narrow-angle glaucoma, myasthenia gravis; should not be used in infants <6 months of age; nursing mothers

**Warnings/Precautions** Use with caution in patients with hepatic or renal disease, ulcerative colitis, hyperthyroidism, cardiovascular disease, hypertension, tachycardia, GI obstruction, obstruction of the urinary tract. The elderly are at increased risk for anticholinergic effects, confusion and hallucinations.

**Adverse Reactions** Adverse reactions are included here that have been reported for pharmacologically similar drugs with anticholinergic/antispasmodic action

Cardiovascular: Syncope, tachycardia, palpitations

(Continued)

## Dicyclomine *(Continued)*

Central nervous system: Dizziness, lightheadedness, tingling, headache, drowsiness, nervousness, numbness, mental confusion and/or excitement, dyskinesia, lethargy, speech disturbance, insomnia

Dermatologic: Rash, urticaria, itching, and other dermal manifestations; severe allergic reaction or drug idiosyncrasies including anaphylaxis

Endocrine & metabolic: Suppression of lactation

Gastrointestinal: Xerostomia, nausea, vomiting, constipation, bloated feeling, abdominal pain, taste loss, anorexia

Genitourinary: Urinary hesitancy, urinary retention, impotence

Neuromuscular & skeletal: Weakness

Ocular: Blurred vision, diplopia, mydriasis, cycloplegia, increased ocular tension

Respiratory: Dyspnea, apnea, asphyxia, nasal stuffiness or congestion, sneezing, throat congestion

Miscellaneous: Decreased diaphoresis

**Overdosage/Toxicology**

Signs and symptoms: CNS stimulation followed by depression, confusion, delusions, nonreactive pupils, tachycardia, hypertension

Treatment: Anticholinergic toxicity is caused by strong binding of the drug to cholinergic receptors. For anticholinergic overdose with severe life-threatening symptoms, physostigmine 1-2 mg (0.5 or 0.02 mg/kg for children) S.C. or I.V., slowly may be given to reverse these effects.

**Drug Interactions**

Decreased effect: Phenothiazines, anti-Parkinson's drugs, haloperidol, sustained release dosage forms; decreased effect with antacids

Increased toxicity: Anticholinergics, amantadine, narcotic analgesics, type I antiarrhythmics, antihistamines, phenothiazines, TCAs

**Usual Dosage**

Oral:

Infants >6 months: 5 mg/dose 3-4 times/day

Children: 10 mg/dose 3-4 times/day

Adults: Begin with 80 mg/day in 4 equally divided doses, then increase up to 160 mg/day

I.M. **(should not be used I.V.)**: Adults: 80 mg/day in 4 divided doses (20 mg/dose)

**Dietary Considerations** Alcohol: Additive CNS effects, avoid use

**Patient Information** Take as directed before meals; do not increase dose and do not discontinue without consulting prescriber. Avoid alcohol and other CNS depressant medications (antihistamines, sleeping aids, antidepressants) unless approved by prescriber. Void before taking medication. This drug may impair mental alertness (use caution when driving or engaging in tasks that require alertness until response to drug is known); constipation (increased dietary fluid, fruit, or fiber and increased exercise may help). Report excessive and persistent anticholinergic effects (blurred vision, headache, flushing, tachycardia, nervousness, dizziness, insomnia, mental confusion or excitement, dry mouth, altered taste perception, dysphagia, palpitations, bradycardia, urinary hesitancy or retention, impotence, decreased sweating), change in color of urine or stools, or irritation or redness at injection site.

**Nursing Implications** Raise bed rails, institute safety measures

**Dosage Forms**

Capsule, as hydrochloride: 10 mg, 20 mg

Injection, as hydrochloride: 10 mg/mL (2 mL, 10 mL)

Syrup, as hydrochloride: 10 mg/5 mL (118 mL, 473 mL, 946 mL)

Tablet, as hydrochloride: 20 mg

♦ **Dicyclomine Hydrochloride** *see* Dicyclomine *on page 165*

♦ **Dicycloverine Hydrochloride** *see* Dicyclomine *on page 165*

## Didanosine (dye DAN oh seen)

**U.S. Brand Names** Videx®

**Synonyms** ddI

**Pharmacologic Category** Antiretroviral Agent, Reverse Transcriptase Inhibitor (Nucleoside)

**Use** Treatment of HIV infection; always to be used in combination with at least two other antiretroviral agents

**Effects on Mental Status** Anxiety; irritability and insomnia are common; may produce depression

**Effects on Psychiatric Treatment** May cause granulocytopenia; use caution with clozapine and carbamazepine

**Pregnancy Risk Factor** B

**Contraindications** Hypersensitivity to any component

**Warnings/Precautions** Peripheral neuropathy occurs in ~35% of patients receiving the drug; pancreatitis (sometimes fatal) occurs in ~9%; risk factors for developing pancreatitis include a previous history of the condition, concurrent cytomegalovirus or *Mycobacterium avium-intracellulare* infection, and concomitant use of pentamidine or co-trimoxazole; discontinue didanosine if clinical signs of pancreatitis occur. Didanosine may cause retinal depigmentation in children receiving doses >300 mg/m²/day. Patients should undergo retinal examination every 6-12 months. Use with caution in patients with decreased renal or hepatic function, phenylketonuria, sodium-restricted diets, or with edema, congestive heart failure or hyperuricemia; in high concentrations, didanosine is mutagenic. Lactic acidosis and severe hepatomegaly have occurred with antiretroviral nucleoside analogues.

**Adverse Reactions**

>10%:

Central nervous system: Anxiety, headache, irritability, insomnia, restlessness

Gastrointestinal: Abdominal pain, nausea, diarrhea

Neuromuscular & skeletal: Peripheral neuropathy

1% to 10%:

Central nervous system: Depression

Dermatologic: Rash, pruritus

Gastrointestinal: Pancreatitis (2% to 3%)

<1%: Alopecia, anaphylactoid reaction, anemia, diabetes mellitus, granulocytopenia, hepatitis, hypersensitivity, lactic acidosis/hepatomegaly, leukopenia, optic neuritis, renal impairment, retinal depigmentation, seizures, thrombocytopenia

**Overdosage/Toxicology**

signs and symptoms: Chronic overdose may cause pancreatitis, peripheral neuropathy, diarrhea, hyperuricemia, and hepatic impairment

Treatment: There is no known antidote for didanosine overdose; treatment is asymptomatic

**Drug Interactions** Drugs whose absorption depends on the level of acidity in the stomach such as ketoconazole, itraconazole, and dapsone should be administered at least 2 hours prior to didanosine

Decreased effect: Didanosine may decrease absorption of quinolones or tetracyclines, didanosine should be held during PCP treatment with pentamidine; didanosine may decrease levels of indinavir

Increased toxicity: Concomitant administration of other drugs which have the potential to cause peripheral neuropathy or pancreatitis may increase the risk of these toxicities

**Usual Dosage** Oral (administer on an empty stomach):

Children: 180 mg/m²/day divided every 12 hours **or** dosing is based on body surface area (m²) as follows:

BSA ≤0.4 m²: 25 mg twice daily (tablets)

BSA 0.5-0.7 m²: 50 mg twice daily (tablets)

BSA 0.8-1.0 m²: 75 mg twice daily (tablets)

BSA 1.1-1.4 m² :100 mg twice daily (tablets)

Adults: Dosing based on patient weight:

**Note:** Preferred dosing is twice daily

Tablets:

<60 kg: 125 mg twice daily (tablets) or 250 mg once daily

≥60 kg: 200 mg twice daily (tablets) or 400 mg once daily

**Note:** Children >1 year and Adults should receive 2 tablets per dose and children <1 year should receive 1 tablet per dose for adequate buffering and absorption; tablets should be chewed; didanosine has also been used as 300 mg once daily

Buffered Powder:

<60 kg: 167 mg twice daily

≥60 kg; 250 mg twice daily

**Dosage adjustment in renal impairment:** Dosing based on patient weight, creatinine clearance, and dosage form (tablet*or buffered powder for oral solution**):

**Dosing for patients ≥60 kg:**

$Cl_{cr}$ ≥60 mL/minute:

Tablet*: 400 mg once daily or 200 mg twice daily

Solution**: 250 mg twice daily

$Cl_{cr}$ 30-59 mL/minute:

Tablet*: 200 mg once daily or 100 mg twice daily

Solution**: 100 mg twice daily

$Cl_{cr}$ 10-29 mL/minute:

Tablet*: 150 mg once daily

Solution**: 167 mg once daily

$Cl_{cr}$ <10 mL/minute:

Tablet*: 100 mg once daily

Solution**: 100 mg once daily

**Dosing for patients <60 kg:**

$Cl_{cr}$ ≥60 mL/minute:

Tablet*: 250 mg once daily or 125 mg twice daily

Solution**: 167 mg twice daily

$Cl_{cr}$ 30-59 mL/minute:

Tablet*: 150 mg once daily or 75 mg twice daily

Solution**: 100 mg twice daily

$Cl_{cr}$ 10-29 mL/minute:

Tablet*: 100 mg once daily

Solution**: 100 mg once daily

$Cl_{cr}$ <10 mL/minute:

Tablet*: 75 mg once daily

Solution**: 100 mg once daily

*Chewable/dispersible buffered tablet; 2 tablets must be taken with each dose; different strengths of tablets may be combined to yield the recommended dose.

**Buffered powder for oral solution

Hemodialysis: Removed by hemodialysis (40% to 60%)

**Dosing adjustment in hepatic impairment:** Should be considered

**Patient Information** Take as directed, 1 hour before or 2 hours after eating. Chew tablets thoroughly and/or dissolve in water. Pour powder into 4 oz of liquid, stir, and drink immediately. Do not mix with fruit juice or other acid-containing liquids. You may experience dizziness; use caution when driving or engaging in tasks that require alertness until response to drug is known. You will be susceptible to infection; avoid crowds. Report numbness or tingling of fingers, toes, or feet; abdominal pain; or persistent nausea or vomiting. Should have a retinal exam every 6-12 months.

**Nursing Implications** Administer liquified powder immediately after dissolving; avoid creating dust if powder spilled, use wet mop or damp sponge

**Dosage Forms**

Powder for oral solution:

Buffered (single dose packet): 100 mg, 167 mg, 250 mg, 375 mg

Pediatric: 2 g, 4 g

Tablet, buffered, chewable (mint flavor): 25 mg, 50 mg, 100 mg, 150 mg

♦ **Dideoxycytidine** *see* Zalcitabine *on page 590*

♦ **Didrex®** *see* Benzphetamine *on page 62*

♦ **Didronel®** *see* Etidronate Disodium *on page 215*

## Dienestrol (dye en ES trole)

**U.S. Brand Names** DV® Vaginal Cream; Ortho® Dienestrol Vaginal

**Pharmacologic Category** Estrogen Derivative

**Use** Symptomatic management of atrophic vaginitis or kraurosis vulvae in postmenopausal women

**Effects on Mental Status** May cause anxiety or depression

**Effects on Psychiatric Treatment** None reported

**Usual Dosage** Adults: Vaginal: Insert 1 applicatorful once or twice daily for 1-2 weeks and then 1/2 of that dose for 1-2 weeks; maintenance dose: 1 applicatorful 1-3 times/week for 3-6 months

**Dosage Forms** Cream, vaginal: 0.01% (30 g with applicator; 78 g with applicator)

## Diethylcarbamazine (dye eth il kar BAM a zeen)

**U.S. Brand Names** Banocide®; Hetrazan®; Notézine®, Filarcidan®

**Pharmacologic Category** Anthelmintic

**Use** An antihelmintic agent used to treat *Wuchereria bancrofti, Brugia malayi, Brugia timori*, or *Onchocerca volvulus*; has been used to treat dog heartworm

**Effects on Mental Status** May cause dizziness

**Effects on Psychiatric Treatment** None reported

**Usual Dosage**

Bancroftian filariasis: 6 mg/kg/day in 3 divided doses for 12 days

Brugian filariasis: 3-6 mg/kg/day in 3 divided doses for 6-12 days

In order to decrease severity of hypersensitivity reactions, initial dosage of 1 mg/kg/day can be increased to 6 mg/kg/day over 3 days; a corticosteroid agent can be added

Prophylaxis of Bancroftian/Malayan filariasis: 50 mg/month

Prophylaxis of loiasis: 4-5 mg/kg for 3 successive days each month

Onchocerciasis: 0.5-1 mg/kg for first 1-2 days, then 2 mg/kg twice daily for next 5-7 days

## Diethylpropion (dye eth il PROE pee on)

**Related Information**

Phentermine *on page 438*

**Generic Available** Yes

**U.S. Brand Names** Tenuate®; Tenuate® Dospan®

**Canadian Brand Names** Nobesine®

**Body Mass Index (BMI), kg/m²**
**Height (feet, inches)**

| Weight (lb) | 5'0" | 5'3" | 5'6" | 5'9" | 6'0" | 6'3" |
|---|---|---|---|---|---|---|
| 140 | 27 | 25 | 23 | 21 | 19 | 18 |
| 150 | 29 | 27 | 24 | 22 | 20 | 19 |
| 160 | 31 | 28 | 26 | 24 | 22 | 20 |
| 170 | 33 | 30 | 28 | 25 | 23 | 21 |
| 180 | 35 | 32 | 29 | 27 | 25 | 23 |
| 190 | 37 | 34 | 31 | 28 | 26 | 24 |
| 200 | 39 | 36 | 32 | 30 | 27 | 25 |
| 210 | 41 | 37 | 34 | 31 | 29 | 26 |
| 220 | 43 | 39 | 36 | 33 | 30 | 28 |
| 230 | 45 | 41 | 37 | 34 | 31 | 29 |
| 240 | 47 | 43 | 39 | 36 | 33 | 30 |
| 250 | 49 | 44 | 40 | 37 | 34 | 31 |

**Synonyms** Amfepramone; Diethylpropion Hydrochloride

**Pharmacologic Category** Anorexiant

**Use** Short-term adjunct in a regimen of weight reduction based on exercise, behavioral modification, and caloric reduction in the management of exogenous obesity for patients with an initial body mass index ≥30 kg/m² or ≥27 kg/m² in the presence of other risk factors (diabetes, hypertension); see table

**Unlabeled uses:** Migraine

**Effects on Mental Status** Insomnia, nervousness, and euphoria are common; may cause confusion, depression, or psychosis

**Effects on Psychiatric Treatment** Concurrent use with MAOIs may cause hypertensive crisis; avoid combination; antipsychotics may blunt effect of diethylpropion. May cause bone marrow depression; use caution with clozapine.

**Restrictions** C-IV

**Pregnancy Risk Factor** B

**Contraindications** Known hypersensitivity or idiosyncrasy to sympathomimetic amines. Patients with advanced arteriosclerosis, symptomatic cardiovascular disease, moderate to severe hypertension (stage II or III), hyperthyroidism, glaucoma, agitated states, patients with a history of drug abuse, and during or within 14 days following MAO inhibitor therapy. Concurrent use with other anorectic agents; stimulant medications are contraindicated for use in children with attention deficit/hyperactivity disorders and concomitant Tourette's syndrome or tics.

**Warnings/Precautions** Use with caution in patients with bipolar disorder, diabetes mellitus, cardiovascular disease, seizure disorders, insomnia, porphyria, or mild hypertension (stage I). May exacerbate symptoms of behavior and thought disorder in psychotic patients. Potential for drug dependency exists - avoid abrupt discontinuation in patients who have received for prolonged periods. Stimulant use in children has been associated with growth suppression. Not recommended for use in patients < 12 years of age.

**Adverse Reactions**

Cardiovascular: Hypertension, palpitations, tachycardia, chest pain, T-wave changes, arrhythmias, pulmonary hypertension, valvalopathy

Central nervous system: Euphoria, nervousness, insomnia, restlessness, dizziness, anxiety, headache, agitation, confusion, mental depression, psychosis, CVA, seizure

Dermatologic: Alopecia, urticaria, skin rash, ecchymosis, erythema

Endocrine & metabolic: Changes in libido, gynecomastia, menstrual irregularities, porphyria

Gastrointestinal: Nausea, vomiting, abdominal cramps, constipation, xerostomia, metallic taste

Genitourinary: Impotence

Hematologic: Bone marrow depression, agranulocytosis, leukopenia

Neuromuscular & skeletal: Tremor

Ocular: Blurred vision, mydriasis

**Overdosage/Toxicology** Treatment: There is no specific antidote for amphetamine intoxication and the bulk of the treatment is supportive. Hyperactivity and agitation usually respond to reduced sensory input; however, with extreme agitation, haloperidol (2-5 mg I.M. for adults) may be required. Hyperthermia is best treated with external cooling measures, or when severe or unresponsive, muscle paralysis with pancuronium may be needed. Hypertension is usually transient and generally does not require treatment unless severe. For diastolic blood pressures >110 mm Hg, a nitroprusside infusion should be initiated. Seizures usually respond to diazepam I.V. and/or phenytoin maintenance regimens.

**Drug Interactions**

Anorectic agents: Concurrent use with other anorectic agents may cause serious cardiac problems and is contraindicated

Furazolidine: May induce a hypertensive episode in patients receiving furazolidone

Guanethidine: Diethylpropion may inhibit the antihypertensive response to guanethidine; probably also may occur with guanadrel

MAOIs: Severe hypertensive episodes have occurred with amphetamine when used in patients receiving MAOIs; concurrent use or use within 14 days is contraindicated

Norepinephrine: Diethylpropion may enhance the pressor response to norepinephrine

Sibutramine: Concurrent use of sibutramine and diethylpropion may cause severe hypertension and tachycardia; use is contraindicated

Tricyclic antidepressants: Concurrent use with tricyclic antidepressants may result in hypertension and CNS stimulation; avoid this combination

**Mechanism of Action** Diethylpropion is used as an anorexiant agent possessing pharmacological and chemical properties similar to those of amphetamines. The mechanism of action of diethylpropion in reducing appetite appears to be secondary to CNS effects, specifically stimulation of the hypothalamus to release catecholamines into the central nervous system; anorexiant effects are mediated via norepinephrine and dopamine metabolism. An increase in physical activity and metabolic effects (inhibition of lipogenesis and enhancement of lipolysis) may also contribute to weight loss.

**Usual Dosage** Adults: Oral:

Tablet: 25 mg 3 times/day before meals or food

Tablet, controlled release: 75 mg at midmorning

(Continued)

## Diethylpropion *(Continued)*

**Dietary Considerations** Alcohol: Avoid use

**Monitoring Parameters** Monitor CNS

**Patient Information** Avoid alcoholic beverages; take during day to avoid insomnia; do not discontinue abruptly, may cause physical and psychological dependence with prolonged use

**Nursing Implications** Do not crush 75 mg controlled release tablets; dose should not be given in evening or at bedtime

**Dosage Forms**

Tablet, as hydrochloride: 25 mg

Tablet, as hydrochloride, controlled release: 75 mg

♦ **Diethylpropion Hydrochloride** *see* Diethylpropion *on page 167*

## Diethylstilbestrol (dye eth il stil BES trole)

**U.S. Brand Names** Stilphostrol®

**Canadian Brand Names** Honvol®

**Synonyms** DES; Diethylstilbestrol Diphosphate Sodium; Stilbestrol

**Pharmacologic Category** Estrogen Derivative

**Use** Palliative treatment of inoperable metastatic prostatic carcinoma and postmenopausal inoperable, progressing breast cancer

**Effects on Mental Status** May rarely cause anxiety or depression

**Effects on Psychiatric Treatment** Barbiturates may lower levels of diethylstilbestrol

**Pregnancy Risk Factor** X

**Contraindications** Undiagnosed vaginal bleeding, during pregnancy; breast cancer except in select patients with metastatic disease

**Warnings/Precautions** Use with caution in patients with a history of thromboembolism, stroke, myocardial infarction (especially >40 years of age who smoke), liver tumor, hypertension, cardiac, renal or hepatic insufficiency; estrogens have been reported to increase the risk of endometrial carcinoma; do not use estrogens during pregnancy

**Adverse Reactions**

>10%:

Cardiovascular: Peripheral edema

Endocrine & metabolic: Enlargement of breasts (female and male), breast tenderness

Gastrointestinal: Anorexia, bloating

1% to 10%:

Central nervous system: Headache

Endocrine & metabolic: Increased libido (female), decreased libido (male)

Gastrointestinal: Vomiting, diarrhea

<1%: Alterations in frequency and flow of menses, amenorrhea, anxiety, breast tumors, chloasma, cholestatic jaundice, decreased glucose tolerance, depression, dizziness, edema, GI distress, hypertension, increased LDL, increased susceptibility to *Candida* infection, increased triglycerides, intolerance to contact lenses, melasma, myocardial infarction, nausea, rash, stroke, thromboembolism

**Overdosage/Toxicology** Signs and symptoms: Nausea

**Drug Interactions**

Decreased effect of oral anticoagulants

Increased effect of corticosteroids, succinylcholine, TCAs

Decreased DES levels: Barbiturates, phenytoin, rifampin

**Usual Dosage** Adults:

Male:

Prostate carcinoma (inoperable, progressing): Oral: 1-3 mg/day

Diphosphate: (inoperable, progressing): Oral: 50 mg 3 times/day; increase up to 200 mg or more 3 times/day; maximum daily dose: 1 g

I.V.: Administer 0.5 g, dissolved in 250 mL of saline or $D_5W$, administer slowly the first 10-15 minutes then adjust rate so that the entire amount is given in 1 hour; repeat for ≥5 days depending on patient response, then repeat 0.25-0.5 g 1-2 times for one week or change to oral therapy

Female: Postmenopausal (inoperable, progressing) breast carcinoma: Oral: 15 mg/day

**Patient Information** Use as directed with or after meals (sustained release may be taken at midmorning - do not crush or chew). May cause breast tenderness or enlargement (consult prescriber for relief). You may be more sensitive to sunlight; use sunblock, wear protective clothing and dark glasses, or avoid direct exposure to sunlight. If you are diabetic, monitor serum glucose closely; antidiabetic agent may need to be adjusted. Discontinue use and report promptly any pain, redness, warmth, or swelling in calves; sudden onset difficulty breathing; headache; loss of vision; difficulty speaking; sharp or sudden chest pain; severe abdominal pain; or unusual bleeding or speech.

**Dosage Forms**

Injection, as diphosphate sodium (Stilphostrol®): 0.25 g (5 mL)

Tablet: 1 mg, 2.5 mg, 5 mg

Tablet (Stilphostrol®): 50 mg

♦ **Diethylstilbestrol Diphosphate Sodium** *see* Diethylstilbestrol *on page 168*

## Difenoxin and Atropine (dye fen OKS in & A troe peen)

**U.S. Brand Names** Motofen®

**Pharmacologic Category** Antidiarrheal

**Use** Treatment of diarrhea

**Effects on Mental Status** May cause drowsiness; confusion

**Effects on Psychiatric Treatment** Concurrent use with psychotropic may cause additive sedation or dry mouth

**Restrictions** C-IV

**Pregnancy Risk Factor** C

**Contraindications** Hypersensitivity to difenoxin, atropine, or any component; severe liver disease; jaundice; dehydrated patient; angle-closure glaucoma; children <2 years of age

**Warnings/Precautions** Dosage recommendations should be strictly adhered to. If severe dehydration or electrolyte imbalance is manifested, withhold until appropriate corrective therapy has been initiated. Patients with acute ulcerative colitis should be carefully observed. Use with caution in patients with advanced hepatorenal disease.

**Adverse Reactions** 1% to 10%:

Central nervous system: Dizziness, drowsiness, lightheadedness, headache

Gastrointestinal: Nausea, vomiting, xerostomia, epigastric distress

**Usual Dosage** Adults: Oral: Initial: 2 tablets, then 1 tablet after each loose stool; 1 tablet every 3-4 hours, up to 8 tablets in a 24-hour period; if no improvement after 48 hours, continued administration is not indicated

**Patient Information** Take as directed; do not exceed recommended dose. If no relief in 48 hours, contact prescriber. Avoid alcohol. Keep out of reach of children; can cause severe and fatal respiratory depression if accidentally ingested. You may experience lightheadedness, depression, dizziness, or weakness; use caution when driving or engaging in tasks that require alertness until response to drug is known. Report acute dizziness, headache, or gastrointestinal symptoms.

**Dosage Forms** Tablet: Difenoxin hydrochloride 1 mg and atropine sulfate 0.025 mg

♦ **Differin®** *see* Adapalene *on page 20*

## Diflorasone (dye FLOR a sone)

**Related Information**

Corticosteroids Comparison Chart *on page 711*

**U.S. Brand Names** Florone®; Florone E®; Maxiflor®; Psorcon™

**Pharmacologic Category** Corticosteroid, Topical

**Use** Relieves inflammation and pruritic symptoms of corticosteroid-responsive dermatosis (high to very high potency topical corticosteroid)

Maxiflor®: High potency topical corticosteroid

Psorcon™: Very high potency topical corticosteroid

**Effects on Mental Status** None reported

**Effects on Psychiatric Treatment** None reported

**Usual Dosage** Topical: Apply ointment sparingly 1-3 times/day; apply cream sparingly 2-4 times/day. Therapy should be discontinued when control is achieved; if no improvement is seen, reassessment of diagnosis may be necessary.

**Dosage Forms**

Cream, as diacetate: 0.05% (15 g, 30 g, 60 g)

Ointment, topical, as diacetate: 0.05% (15 g, 30 g, 60 g)

♦ **Diflucan®** *see* Fluconazole *on page 227*

## Diflunisal (dye FLOO ni sal)

**U.S. Brand Names** Dolobid®

**Canadian Brand Names** Apo®-Diflunisal; Novo-Diflunisal; Nu-Diflunisal

**Pharmacologic Category** Nonsteroidal Anti-Inflammatory Agent (NSAID)

**Use** Management of inflammatory disorders usually including rheumatoid arthritis and osteoarthritis; can be used as an analgesic for treatment of mild to moderate pain

**Effects on Mental Status** May cause dizziness; rarely may cause insomnia, nervousness, depression, and hallucinations

**Effects on Psychiatric Treatment** May rarely cause may agranulocytosis; use caution with clozapine and carbamazepine; may decrease the clearance of lithium resulting in elevated serum levels and potential toxicity; monitor serum lithium levels

**Pregnancy Risk Factor** C (D if used in the 3rd trimester)

**Contraindications** Hypersensitivity to diflunisal or any component, may be a cross-sensitivity with other nonsteroidal anti-inflammatory agents including aspirin; should not be used in patients with active GI bleeding

**Warnings/Precautions** Peptic ulceration and GI bleeding have been reported; platelet function and bleeding time are inhibited; ophthalmologic effects; impaired renal function, use lower dosage; dehydration; peripheral edema; possibility of Reye's syndrome; elevation in liver tests

**Adverse Reactions**

>10%:

Central nervous system: Headache

Endocrine & metabolic: Fluid retention

1% to 10%:

Cardiovascular: Angina pectoris, arrhythmias

Central nervous system: Dizziness

Dermatologic: Rash

Gastrointestinal: GI ulceration

Genitourinary: Vaginal bleeding

Otic: Tinnitus

<1%: Agranulocytosis, anaphylaxis, angioedema, blurred vision, change in vision, chest pain, convulsions, cystitis, decreased hearing, diaphoresis (increased), drowsiness, erythema multiforme, esophagitis or gastritis, exfoliative dermatitis, hallucinations, hemolytic anemia, hepatitis, insomnia, interstitial nephritis, itching, mental depression, nephrotic syndrome, nervousness, peripheral neuropathy, renal impairment, shortness of breath, Stevens-Johnson syndrome, stomatitis, tachycardia, thrombocytopenia, toxic epidermal necrolysis, trembling, urticaria, vasculitis, weakness, wheezing

**Overdosage/Toxicology**

Signs and symptoms: Drowsiness, nausea, vomiting, hyperventilation, tachycardia, tinnitus, stupor, coma, renal failure, leukocytosis

Treatment: Management of a nonsteroidal anti-inflammatory drug (NSAID) intoxication is primarily supportive and symptomatic. Fluid therapy is commonly effective in managing the hypotension that may occur following an acute NSAID overdose, except when this is due to an acute blood loss.

**Drug Interactions**

ACE inhibitors: Effects may be reduced by NSAIDs; use lowest possible dose for shortest duration possible; monitor

Antacids: Absorption may be reduced; monitor

Cholestyramine and colestipol: Absorption may be reduced by concurrent administration

Hydralazine: Antihypertensive effect may be decreased; avoid concurrent use

Lithium: Serum levels can be increased; avoid concurrent use if possible or monitor lithium levels and adjust dose. When NSAID is stopped, lithium may need adjustment again.

Loop diuretics: Therapeutic effects may be reduced by NSAIDs; avoid

Methotrexate: Toxicity may be increased by concurrent NSAID use; risk is limited in low-dose methotrexate regimens (such as for rheumatoid arthritis); prolonged leucovorin rescue may be required at antineoplastic doses; monitor

Probenecid: May increase the effect and/or toxicity of diflunisal

Thiazide diuretics: Antihypertensive effects may be decreased; avoid concurrent use

Warfarin: INRs may be increased by some NSAIDs. This may depend, in part, on dose and duration; monitor INR closely. Use the lowest dose of NSAIDs possible and for the briefest duration.

**Usual Dosage** Adults: Oral:

Pain: Initial: 500-1000 mg followed by 250-500 mg every 8-12 hours; maximum daily dose: 1.5 g

Inflammatory condition: 500-1000 mg/day in 2 divided doses; maximum daily dose: 1.5 g

**Dosing adjustment in renal impairment:** $Cl_{cr}$ <50 mL/minute: Administer 50% of normal dose

**Patient Information** If self-administered, use exactly as directed (do not increase dose or frequency); adverse reactions can occur with overuse. Do not take longer than 3 days for fever, or 10 days for pain without consulting medical advisor. Take with food or milk. While using this medication, do not use alcohol, excessive amounts of vitamin C, or salicylate-containing foods (curry powder, prunes, raisins, tea, or licorice), other prescription or OTC medications containing aspirin or salicylate, or other NSAIDs without consulting prescriber. Maintain adequate hydration (2-3 L/day of fluids unless instructed to restrict fluid intake). You may experience nausea, vomiting, gastric discomfort (frequent mouth care, small frequent meals, chewing gum, or sucking lozenges may help). GI bleeding, ulceration, or perforation can occur with or without pain. Stop taking medication and report ringing in ears; persistent pain in stomach; unresolved nausea or vomiting; difficulty breathing or shortness of breath; unusual bruising or bleeding (mouth, urine, stool); skin rash; unusual swelling of extremities; chest pain; or palpitations.

**Dosage Forms** Tablet: 250 mg, 500 mg

♦ **Digacin** *see* Digoxin *on page 169*

♦ **Digibind®** *see* Digoxin Immune Fab *on page 170*

## Digoxin (di JOKS in)

**Related Information**

Serum Drug Concentrations Commonly Monitored: Guidelines *on page 759*

**U.S. Brand Names** Lanoxicaps®; Lanoxin®

**Canadian Brand Names** Novo-Digoxin

**Synonyms** Digacin

**Pharmacologic Category** Antiarrhythmic Agent, Class IV; Cardiac Glycoside

**Use** Treatment of congestive heart failure and to slow the ventricular rate in tachyarrhythmias such as atrial fibrillation, atrial flutter, and supraventricular tachycardia (paroxysmal atrial tachycardia); cardiogenic shock

**Effects on Mental Status** May cause sedation

**Effects on Psychiatric Treatment** Phenytoin may decrease levels of digoxin; monitor levels

**Pregnancy Risk Factor** C

**Contraindications** Hypersensitivity to digoxin or any component; hypersensitivity to cardiac glycosides (another may be tried); history of toxicity; ventricular tachycardia or fibrillation; idiopathic hypertrophic subaortic stenosis; constrictive pericarditis; amyloid disease; second- or third-degree heart block (except in patients with a functioning artificial pacemaker); Wolff-Parkinson-White syndrome and atrial fibrillation concurrently

**Warnings/Precautions** Withdrawal in CHF patients may lead to recurrence of CHF symptoms. Some arrhythmias that digoxin is used to treat may be exacerbated in digoxin toxicity. Sinus nodal disease may be worsened. Adjust doses in renal impairment and when verapamil, quinidine or amiodarone are added to a patient on digoxin. Correct hypokalemia and hypomagnesemia before initiating therapy. Calcium, especially when administered rapidly I.V., can produce serious arrhythmias. Atrial arrhythmias associated with hypermetabolic states are very difficult to treat. Rate control in atrial fibrillation may be better in a sedentary patient than an active one. Use with caution in acute MI (within 6 months). Serum concentration monitoring should be done before the next dose (patient can hold AM dose for blood test) for an accurate assessment. Reduce or hold dose 1-2 days before elective electrical cardioversion.

**Adverse Reactions**

1% to 10%: Gastrointestinal: Anorexia, nausea, vomiting

<1%: Abdominal pain, atrial or nodal ectopic beats, atrial tachycardia with A-V block, A-V block, bigeminy, blurred vision, diarrhea, diplopia, disorientation, drowsiness, fatigue, feeding intolerance, flashing lights, halos, headache, hyperkalemia with acute toxicity, lethargy, neuralgia, photophobia, S-A block, sinus bradycardia, trigeminy, ventricular arrhythmias, vertigo, yellow or green vision

**Overdosage/Toxicology**

Signs and symptoms: Vomiting, hyperkalemia, sinus bradycardia, S-A arrest and A-V block are common, ventricular tachycardia, and fibrillation may occur

Chronic intoxication: Visual disturbances, weakness, sinus bradycardia, atrial fibrillation with slowed ventricular response, and ventricular arrhythmias

Treatment: After GI decontamination, treat hyperkalemia if >5.5 mEq/L with sodium bicarbonate and glucose with insulin or Kayexalate®. Treat bradycardia or heart block with atropine or pacemaker and other arrhythmias with conventional antiarrhythmics. Use Digibind® for severe hyperkalemia, symptomatic arrhythmias unresponsive to other drugs, and for prophylactic treatment in massive overdose.

**Drug Interactions**

Amiloride may reduce the inotropic response to digoxin

Amiodarone reduces renal and nonrenal clearance of digoxin and may have additive effects on heart rate; reduce digoxin dose by 50% with start of amiodarone

Benzodiazepines (alprazolam, diazepam) have been associated with isolated reports of digoxin toxicity

Beta-blocking agents (propranolol) may have additive effects on heart rate

Calcium preparations: Rare cases of acute digoxin toxicity have been associated with parenteral calcium (bolus) administration

Carvedilol may increase digoxin blood levels in addition to potentiating its effects on heart rate

Cholestyramine, colestipol, kaolin-pectin may reduce digoxin absorption; separate administration

Cyclosporine may increase digoxin levels, possibly due to reduced renal clearance

Erythromycin, clarithromycin, and tetracyclines may increase digoxin (not capsule form) blood levels in a subset of patients

Indomethacin has been associated with isolated reports of increased digoxin blood levels/toxicity

Itraconazole may increase digoxin blood levels in some patients; monitor

Levothyroxine (and other thyroid supplements) may decrease digoxin blood levels

Metoclopramide may reduce the absorption of digoxin tablets.

Moricizine may increase the toxicity of digoxin (mechanism undefined)

Penicillamine has been associated with reductions in digoxin blood levels

Propafenone increases digoxin blood levels; effects are highly variable; monitor closely

Propylthiouracil (and methimazole) may increase digoxin blood levels by reducing thyroid hormone

Quinidine increases digoxin blood levels substantially; effect is variable (33% to 50%). Monitor digoxin blood levels/effect closely; reduce digoxin dose by 50% with start of quinidine. Other related agents (hydroxychloroquine, quinine) should be used with caution.

(Continued)

## Digoxin *(Continued)*

Spironolactone may interfere with some digoxin assays, but may also increase blood levels directly; however, spironolactone may attenuate the inotropic effect of digoxin. Monitor effects of digoxin closely.

St John's wort may decrease trough concentrations (33%); monitor

Succinylcholine administration to patients on digoxin has been associated with an increased risk of arrhythmias

Verapamil diltiazem, bepridil, and nitrendipine increased serum digoxin concentrations. Other calcium channel blocking agents do not appear to share this effect. Reduce digoxin's dose with the start of verapamil.

Drugs which cause hypokalemia (thiazide and loop diuretics, amphotericin B): Hypokalemia may potentiate digoxin toxicity

These medications have been associated with reduced digoxin blood levels which appear to be of limited clinical significance: Aminoglutethimide, aminosalicylic acid, aluminum-containing antacids, sucralfate, sulfasalazine, neomycin, ticlopidine

These medications have been associated with increased digoxin blood levels which appear to be of limited clinical significance: Famciclovir, flecainide, ibuprofen, fluoxetine, nefazodone, cimetidine, famotidine, ranitidine, omeprazole, trimethoprim

**Usual Dosage** When changing from oral (tablets or liquid) or I.M. to I.V. therapy, dosage should be reduced by 20% to 25%

**Dosage recommendations for digoxin:**

Preterm infant*
- Total digitalizing dose **: Oral: 20-30 mcg/kg*; I.V. or I.M.: 15-25 mcg/kg*
- Daily maintenance dose***: Oral: 5-7.5 mcg/kg*; I.V. or I.M.: 4-6 mcg/kg* I.V. or I.M.

Full-term infant*
- Total digitalizing dose **: Oral: 25-35 mcg/kg*; I.V. or I.M.: 20-30 mcg/kg* I.V. or I.M.
- Daily maintenance dose***: Oral: 6-10 mcg/kg*; I.V. or I.M.: 5-8 mcg/kg* I.V. or I.M.

1 month to 2 years*
- Total digitalizing dose **: Oral: 35-60 mcg/kg*; I.V. or I.M.: 30-50 mcg/kg* I.V. or I.M.
- Daily maintenance dose***: Oral: 10-15 mcg/kg*; I.V. or I.M.: 7.5- 12 mcg/kg*

2-5 years*
- Total digitalizing dose **: Oral: 30-40 mcg/kg*; I.V. or I.M.: 25-35 mcg/kg*
- Daily maintenance dose***: Oral: 7.5-10 mcg/kg*; I.V. or I.M.: 6-9 mcg/kg*

5-10 years*
- Total digitalizing dose **: Oral: 20-35 mcg/kg*; I.V. or I.M.: 15-30 mcg/kg*
- Daily maintenance dose***: Oral: 5-10 mcg/kg*; I.V. or I.M.: 4-8 mcg/kg*

>10 years*
- Total digitalizing dose **: Oral: 10-15 mcg/kg*; I.V. or I.M.: 8-12 mcg/kg*
- Daily maintenance dose***: Oral: 2.5-5 mcg/kg*; I.V. or I.M.: 2-3 mcg/kg*

Adults
- Total digitalizing dose **: Oral: 0.75-1.5 mg; I.V. or I.M.: 0.5-1 mg
- Daily maintenance dose***: Oral: 0.125 mg- 0.5 mg; I.V. or I.M.: 0.1 mg- 0.4 mg

*Based on lean body weight and normal renal function for age. Decrease dose in patients with decreased renal function; digitalizing dose often not recommended in infants and children.

**Give one-half of the total digitalizing dose (TDD) in the initial dose, then give one-quarter of the TDD in each of two subsequent doses at 8- to 12-hour intervals. Obtain EKG 6 hours after each dose to assess potential toxicity.

***Divided every 12 hours in infants and children <10 years of age; given once daily to children >10 years of age and adults

**Dosing adjustment/interval in renal impairment:**

$Cl_{cr}$ 10-50 mL/minute: Administer 25% to 75% of dose or every 36 hours

$Cl_{cr}$ <10 mL/minute: Administer 10% to 25% of dose or every 48 hours

Reduce loading dose by 50% in ESRD

Hemodialysis: Not dialyzable (0% to 5%)

**Patient Information** Take as directed; do not discontinue without consulting prescriber. Maintain adequate dietary intake of potassium (do not increase without consulting prescriber). Adequate dietary potassium will reduce risk of digoxin toxicity. Take pulse at the same time each day; follow prescriber instructions for holding medication if pulse is below 50. Notify prescriber of acute changes in pulse. Report loss of appetite, nausea, vomiting, persistent diarrhea, swelling of extremities, palpitations, "yellowing" or blurred vision, mental confusion or depression, or unusual fatigue.

**Nursing Implications** Observe patients for noncardiac signs of toxicity, ie, anorexia, vision changes (blurred), confusion, and depression

**Dosage Forms**

Capsule: 50 mcg, 100 mcg, 200 mcg

Elixir, pediatric (lime flavor): 50 mcg/mL with alcohol 10% (60 mL)

Injection: 250 mcg/mL (1 mL, 2 mL)

Injection, pediatric: 100 mcg/mL (1 mL)

Tablet: 125 mcg, 250 mcg, 500 mcg

## Digoxin Immune Fab (di JOKS in i MYUN fab)

**U.S. Brand Names** Digibind®

**Pharmacologic Category** Antidote

**Use** Digoxin immune antigen-binding fragments (Fab) are specific antibodies for the treatment of digitalis intoxication in carefully selected patients; used in life-threatening ventricular arrhythmias secondary to digoxin, acute digoxin ingestion (ie, >10 mg in adults or >4 mg in children), hyperkalemia (serum potassium >5 mEq/L) in the setting of digoxin toxicity

**Effects on Mental Status** None reported

**Effects on Psychiatric Treatment** None reported

**Usual Dosage** Each vial of Digibind® 40 mg will bind ~0.6 mg of digoxin or digitoxin.

Estimation of the dose is based on the body burden of digitalis. This may be calculated if the amount ingested is known or the postdistribution serum drug level is known.

**Fab dose based on number of tablets (0.25 mg) ingested:**
- 5 tablets ingested: Fab dose 68 mg (1.7 vials)
- 10 tablets ingested: Fab dose 136 mg (3.4 vials)
- 25 tablets ingested: Fab dose 340 mg (8.5 vials)
- 50 tablets ingested: Fab dose 680 mg (17 vials)
- 75 tablets ingested: Fab dose 1000 mg (25 vials)
- 100 tablets ingested: Fab dose 1360 mg (34 vials)
- 150 tablets ingested: Fab dose 2000 mg (50 vials)

**Fab dose based on serum drug level postdistribution:**
- Digoxin: No. of vials = level (ng/mL) x body weight (kg) divided by 100
- Digitoxin: No. of vials = digitoxin (ng/mL) x body weight (kg) divided by 1000

If neither amount ingested nor drug level are known, dose empirically with 10 and 5 vials for acute and chronic toxicity, respectively

**Dosage Forms** Powder for injection, lyophilized: 38 mg


◆ **Dihistine® DH** *see* Chlorpheniramine, Pseudoephedrine, and Codeine *on page 116*

◆ **Dihistine® Expectorant** *see* Guaifenesin, Pseudoephedrine, and Codeine *on page 258*

◆ **Dihydrex® Injection** *see* Diphenhydramine *on page 174*


## Dihydrocodeine Compound

(dye hye droe KOE deen KOM pound)

**U.S. Brand Names** DHC Plus®; Synalgos®-DC

**Pharmacologic Category** Analgesic, Narcotic

**Use** Management of mild to moderate pain that requires relaxation

**Effects on Mental Status** Sedation is common

**Effects on Psychiatric Treatment** Concurrent use with MAOIs may produce additive side effects

**Restrictions** C-III

**Pregnancy Risk Factor** B (D if used for prolonged periods or in high doses at term)

**Contraindications** Hypersensitivity to dihydrocodeine or any component

**Warnings/Precautions** Use with caution in patients with hypersensitivity reactions to other phenanthrene derivative opioid agonists (morphine, hydrocodone, hydromorphone, levorphanol, oxycodone, oxymorphone); respiratory diseases including asthma, emphysema, COPD, or severe liver or renal insufficiency; some preparations contain sulfites which may cause allergic reactions; dextromethorphan has equivalent antitussive activity but has much lower toxicity in accidental overdose; tolerance of drug dependence may result from extended use

**Adverse Reactions**

>10%:
- Central nervous system: Lightheadedness, dizziness, drowsiness, sedation
- Dermatologic: Pruritus, skin reactions
- Gastrointestinal: Nausea, vomiting, constipation

1% to 10%:
- Cardiovascular: Hypotension, palpitations, bradycardia, peripheral vasodilation
- Central nervous system: Increased intracranial pressure
- Endocrine & metabolic: Antidiuretic hormone release
- Gastrointestinal: Biliary tract spasm
- Genitourinary: Urinary tract spasm
- Ocular: Miosis
- Respiratory: Respiratory depression
- Miscellaneous: Histamine release, physical and psychological dependence with prolonged use

**Overdosage/Toxicology** Treatment: Naloxone 2 mg I.V. (0.01 mg/kg for children) with repeat administration as necessary up to a total of 10 mg

**Drug Interactions** CYP2D6 enzyme substrate

MAO inhibitors may increase adverse symptoms

**Usual Dosage** Adults: Oral: 1-2 capsules every 4-6 hours as needed for pain

**Dietary Considerations** Alcohol: Additive CNS effects, avoid use

**Patient Information** If self-administered, use exactly as directed (do not increase dose or frequency); may cause physical and/or psychological dependence. While using this medication, do not use alcohol and other prescription or OTC medications (especially sedatives, tranquilizers, antihistamines, or pain medications) without consulting prescriber. Maintain adequate hydration (2-3 L/day of fluids unless instructed to restrict fluid intake). May cause dizziness, drowsiness, impaired coordination, or blurred vision (use caution when driving, climbing stairs, or changing position - rising from sitting or lying to standing or when engaging in tasks requiring alertness until response to drug is known); nausea or vomiting (frequent mouth care, small frequent meals, chewing gum, or sucking lozenges may help); constipation (increased exercise, fluids, or dietary fruit and fiber may help - if constipation remains an unresolved problem, consult prescriber about use of stool softeners). Report chest pain or rapid heartbeat; acute headache; swelling of extremities or unusual weight gain; changes in urinary elimination; acute headache; back or flank pain or spasms; or other adverse reactions.

**Nursing Implications** Observe patient for excessive sedation, respiratory depression; implement safety measures, assist with ambulation

**Dosage Forms** Capsule:

DHC Plus®: Dihydrocodeine bitartrate 16 mg, acetaminophen 356.4 mg, and caffeine 30 mg

Synalgos®-DC: Dihydrocodeine bitartrate 16 mg, aspirin 356.4 mg, and caffeine 30 mg

## Dihydroergotamine (dye hye droe er GOT a meen)

**U.S. Brand Names** D.H.E. 45® Injection; Migranal® Nasal Spray

**Pharmacologic Category** Ergot Derivative

**Use** Aborts or prevents vascular headaches; also as an adjunct for DVT prophylaxis for hip surgery, for orthostatic hypotension, xerostomia secondary to antidepressant use, and pelvic congestion with pain

**Effects on Mental Status** Drowsiness is common

**Effects on Psychiatric Treatment** None reported

**Pregnancy Risk Factor** X

**Contraindications** High-dose aspirin therapy, hypersensitivity to dihydroergotamine or any component. DHE should not be used within 24 hours of sumatriptan, zolmitriptan, other serotonin agonists or ergot-like agents. DHE should be avoided during or within 2 weeks of discontinuing MAO inhibitors. Pregnancy is contraindicated. Contraindicated with ritonavir, nelfinavir and amprenavir.

**Warnings/Precautions** Use with caution in hypertension, angina, peripheral vascular disease, impaired renal or hepatic function; avoid pregnancy

**Adverse Reactions**

>10%:

- Cardiovascular: Localized edema, peripheral vascular effects (numbness and tingling of fingers and toes)
- Central nervous system: Drowsiness, dizziness
- Gastrointestinal: Xerostomia, diarrhea, nausea, vomiting

1% to 10%:

- Cardiovascular: Precordial distress and pain, transient tachycardia or bradycardia
- Neuromuscular & skeletal: Muscle pain in the extremities, weakness in the legs

**Overdosage/Toxicology**

Signs and symptoms: Peripheral ischemia, paresthesia, headache, nausea, vomiting

Treatment: Activated charcoal is effective at binding certain chemicals; this is especially true for ergot alkaloids

**Drug Interactions**

Increased effect of heparin

Increased toxicity with erythromycin, clarithromycin, nitroglycerin, propranolol, troleandomycin, protease inhibitors. Ritonavir, amprenavir and nelfinavir increase blood levels of ergot alkaloids. Avoid concurrent use.

**Usual Dosage** Adults:

I.M.: 1 mg at first sign of headache; repeat hourly to a maximum dose of 3 mg total

I.V.: Up to 2 mg maximum dose for faster effects; maximum dose: 6 mg/week

Intranasal: 1 spray (0.5 mg) of nasal spray should be administered into each nostril; repeat as needed within 15 minutes, up to a total of 6 sprays in any 24-hour period and no more than 8 sprays in a week

**Dosing adjustment in hepatic impairment:** Dosage reductions are probably necessary but specific guidelines are not available

**Patient Information** Take this drug as rapidly as possible when first symptoms occur. Rare feelings of numbness or tingling of fingers, toes, or face may occur; use caution and avoid injury. May cause drowsiness; avoid activities requiring alertness until effects of medication are known. Report heart palpitations, severe nausea or vomiting, or severe numbness of fingers or toes.

**Dosage Forms**

Injection, as mesylate: 1 mg/mL (1 mL)

Spray, nasal: 4 mg/mL [0.5 mg/spray] (1 mL)

- **Dihydroergotoxine** *see* Ergoloid Mesylates *on page 199*
- **Dihydrogenated Ergot Alkaloids** *see* Ergoloid Mesylates *on page 199*
- **Dihydrohydroxycodeinone** *see* Oxycodone *on page 413*
- **Dihydromorphinone** *see* Hydromorphone *on page 275*

## Dihydrotachysterol (dye hye droe tak IS ter ole)

**U.S. Brand Names** DHT™; Hytakerol®

**Synonyms** Dichysterol

**Pharmacologic Category** Vitamin D Analog

**Use** Treatment of hypocalcemia associated with hypoparathyroidism; prophylaxis of hypocalcemic tetany following thyroid surgery

**Effects on Mental Status** None reported

**Effects on Psychiatric Treatment** Concurrent use with phenytoin or phenobarbital may decrease effectiveness

**Pregnancy Risk Factor** A (D if used in doses above the recommended daily allowance)

**Contraindications** Hypercalcemia, known hypersensitivity to dihydrotachysterol

**Warnings/Precautions** Calcium-phosphate product (serum calcium and phosphorus) must not exceed 70; avoid hypercalcemia; use with caution in coronary artery disease, decreased renal function (especially with secondary hyperparathyroidism), renal stones, and elderly

**Adverse Reactions**

>10%:

- Endocrine & metabolic: Hypercalcemia
- Renal: Elevated serum creatinine, hypercalciuria

<1%: Anemia, anorexia, convulsions, metastatic calcification, nausea, polydipsia, polyuria, renal damage, vomiting, weakness, weight loss

**Overdosage/Toxicology**

Signs and symptoms: Hypercalcemia, anorexia, nausea, weakness, constipation, diarrhea, vague aches, mental confusion, tinnitus, ataxia, depression, hallucinations, syncope, coma; polyuria, polydypsia, nocturia, hypercalciuria, irreversible renal insufficiency or proteinuria, azotemia; will spread tissue calcifications, hypertension

Treatment: Following withdrawal of the drug, treatment consists of bed rest, liberal intake of fluids, reduced calcium intake, and cathartic administration. Severe hypercalcemia requires I.V. hydration and forced diuresis. Urine output should be monitored and maintained at >3 mL/kg/hour. I.V. saline can quickly and significantly increase excretion of calcium into the urine. Calcitonin, cholestyramine, prednisone, sodium EDTA and mithramycin have all been used successfully to treat the more resistant cases of vitamin D-induced hypercalcemia.

**Drug Interactions**

Decreased effect/levels of vitamin D: Cholestyramine, colestipol, mineral oil; phenytoin and phenobarbital may inhibit activation may decrease effectiveness

Increased toxicity: Thiazide diuretics increase calcium

**Usual Dosage** Oral:

Hypoparathyroidism:

- Infants and young Children: Initial: 1-5 mg/day for 4 days, then 0.1-0.5 mg/day
- Older Children and Adults: Initial: 0.8-2.4 mg/day for several days followed by maintenance doses of 0.2-1 mg/day

Nutritional rickets: 0.5 mg as a single dose or 13-50 mcg/day until healing occurs

Renal osteodystrophy: Maintenance: 0.25-0.6 mg/24 hours adjusted as necessary to achieve normal serum calcium levels and promote bone healing

**Patient Information** Take exact dose prescribed; do not take more than recommended. Your prescriber may recommend a special diet. Do not increase calcium intake without consulting prescriber. Avoid magnesium supplements or magnesium-containing antacids. You may experience nausea, vomiting, or metallic taste (frequent small meals, frequent mouth care, or sucking hard candy may help); hypotension (use caution when rising from sitting or lying position or when climbing stairs or bending over). Report chest pain or palpitations; acute headache, dizziness, or feeling of weakness; unresolved nausea or vomiting; persistent metallic taste; unrelieved muscle or bone pain; or CNS irritability.

**Nursing Implications** Monitor symptoms of hypercalcemia (weakness, fatigue, somnolence, headache, anorexia, dry mouth, metallic taste, nausea, vomiting, cramps, diarrhea, muscle pain, bone pain, and irritability)

**Dosage Forms**

Capsule (Hytakerol®): 0.125 mg

Solution:

- Oral Concentrate (DHT™): 0.2 mg/mL (30 mL)
- Oral, in oil (Hytakerol®): 0.25 mg/mL (15 mL)

Tablet (DHT™): 0.125 mg, 0.2 mg, 0.4 mg

## Dihydroxyaluminum Sodium Carbonate

(dye hye DROKS i a LOO mi num SOW dee um KAR bun ate)

**U.S. Brand Names** Rolaids® [OTC]
**Pharmacologic Category** Antacid
**Use** Symptomatic relief of upset stomach associated with hyperacidity
**Effects on Mental Status** None reported
**Effects on Psychiatric Treatment** Concurrent use with psychotropic may produce additive constipation
**Usual Dosage** Oral: Chew 1-2 tablets as needed
**Dosage Forms** Tablet, chewable: 334 mg


- ♦ **1,25 Dihydroxycholecalciferol** *see* Calcitriol *on page 83*
- ♦ **Diiodohydroxyquin** *see* Iodoquinol *on page 291*
- ♦ **Dilacor™ XR** *see* Diltiazem *on page 172*
- ♦ **Dilantin®** *see* Phenytoin *on page 441*
- ♦ **Dilatrate®-SR** *see* Isosorbide Dinitrate *on page 296*
- ♦ **Dilaudid®** *see* Hydromorphone *on page 275*
- ♦ **Dilaudid-5®** *see* Hydromorphone *on page 275*
- ♦ **Dilaudid-HP®** *see* Hydromorphone *on page 275*
- ♦ **Dilocaine®** *see* Lidocaine *on page 317*
- ♦ **Dilor®** *see* Dyphylline *on page 189*


## Diltiazem (dil TYE a zem)

**Related Information**
Calcium Channel Blocking Agents Comparison Chart *on page 710*
**U.S. Brand Names** Cardizem® CD; Cardizem® Injectable; Cardizem® SR; Cardizem® Tablet; Dilacor™ XR; Tiamate®; Tiazac™
**Canadian Brand Names** Apo®-Diltiaz; Novo-Diltazem; Nu-Diltiaz; Syn-Diltiazem
**Pharmacologic Category** Calcium Channel Blocker
**Use**
Capsule: Essential hypertension (alone or in combination) - sustained release only; chronic stable angina or angina from coronary artery spasm
Injection: Atrial fibrillation or atrial flutter; paroxysmal supraventricular tachycardia (PSVT)
**Effects on Mental Status** May cause dizziness, insomnia, nervousness, or sedation
**Effects on Psychiatric Treatment** May produce leukopenia; use caution with clozapine and carbamazepine; lithium levels may be increased or decreased; monitor serum lithium levels; carbamazepine levels may be increased; monitor levels
**Pregnancy Risk Factor** C
**Contraindications** Hypersensitivity to diltiazem or any component; sick sinus syndrome; second- or third- degree AV block (except in patients with a functioning artificial pacemaker); hypotension (systolic <90 mm Hg); acute MI and pulmonary congestion by x-ray
**Warnings/Precautions** Concomitant use with beta-blockers or digoxin can result in conduction disturbances. Avoid concurrent I.V. use of diltiazem and a beta-blocker - monitor closely when I.V. diltiazem is used. Use caution in left ventricular dysfunction and CHF (can exacerbate condition). Symptomatic hypotension can occur. Use with caution in hepatic or renal dysfunction.
**Adverse Reactions**
1% to 10% (generally well tolerated):
Cardiovascular: Bradycardia, A-V block (0.6% to 7.6%), EKG abnormality, peripheral edema, flushing
Central nervous system: Dizziness, headache
Gastrointestinal: Nausea
Neuromuscular & skeletal: Weakness
<1%: Abdominal cramps, abnormal taste, alopecia, amblyopia, angina, anorexia, congestive heart failure, constipation, diarrhea, dyspepsia, ecchymosis, hypotension, insomnia, joint stiffness, leukopenia, micturition disorder, nasal or chest congestion, nervousness, palpitations, paresthesia, petechiae, photosensitivity, psychiatric disturbances, rash, retinopathy, sexual difficulties, shortness of breath, sleep disturbances, somnolence, tachycardia, tinnitus, tremor, urticaria, vomiting, xerostomia
**Overdosage/Toxicology**
Signs and symptoms: The primary cardiac symptoms of calcium blocker overdose includes hypotension and bradycardia. The hypotension is caused by peripheral vasodilation, myocardial depression, and bradycardia. Bradycardia results from sinus bradycardia, second- or third-degree atrioventricular block, or sinus arrest with junctional rhythm. Intraventricular conduction is usually not affected so QRS duration is normal (verapamil does prolong the P-R interval and bepridil prolongs the Q-T and may cause ventricular arrhythmias, including torsade de pointes).
The noncardiac symptoms include confusion, stupor, nausea, vomiting, metabolic acidosis and hyperglycemia
Treatment: Following initial gastric decontamination, if possible, repeated calcium administration may promptly reverse the depressed cardiac contractility (but not sinus node depression or peripheral vasodilation); glucagon, epinephrine, and inamrinone may treat refractory hypotension; glucagon and epinephrine also increase the heart rate (outside the U.S., 4-aminopyridine may be available as an antidote); dialysis and hemoperfusion are not effective in enhancing elimination although repeat-dose activated charcoal may serve as an adjunct with sustained-release preparations.
**Drug Interactions** CYP3A3/4 enzyme substrate; CYP3A3/4, 1A2, 2D6 enzyme inhibitor
Alfentanil's plasma concentration is increased. Fentanyl and sufentanil may be affected similarly
Amiodarone use may lead to bradycardia, other conduction delays, and decreased cardiac output; monitor closely if using together
Azole antifungals may inhibit the calcium channel blocker's metabolism; avoid this combination. Try an antifungal like terbinafine (if appropriate) or monitor closely for altered effect of the calcium channel blocker.
Benzodiazepines (midazolam, triazolam) plasma concentrations are increased by diltiazem; monitor for prolonged CNS depression
Beta-blockers may have increased pharmacodynamic interactions with diltiazem (see Warnings/Precautions)
Calcium may reduce the calcium channel blocker's effects, particularly hypotension
Carbamazepine's serum concentration is increased and toxicity may result; avoid this combination
Cimetidine reduced diltiazem's metabolism; consider an alternative $H_2$-antagonist
Cyclosporine's serum concentrations are increased by diltiazem; avoid the combination. Use another calcium channel blocker or monitor cyclosporine trough levels and renal function closely.
Digoxin's serum concentration can be increased in some patients; monitor for increased effects of digoxin
HMG-CoA reductase inhibitors (atorvastatin, cerivastatin, lovastatin, simvastatin): Serum concentration will likely be increased; consider pravastatin/fluvastatin or a dihydropyridine calcium channel blocker as an alternative
Lithium neurotoxicity may result when diltiazem is added; monitor lithium levels
Moricizine's serum concentration is increased; monitor clinical response closely
Nafcillin decreases plasma concentration of diltiazem; avoid this combination
Nitroprusside's dose required reduction in patients started on diltiazem; monitor blood pressure
Protease inhibitor like amprenavir and ritonavir may increase diltiazem's serum concentration
Rifampin increases the metabolism of calcium channel blockers; adjust the dose of the calcium channel blocker to maintain efficacy or consider an alternative to rifampin
Tacrolimus's serum concentrations are increased by diltiazem; avoid the combination. Use another calcium channel blocker or monitor tacrolimus trough levels and renal function closely.
**Usual Dosage** Adults:
Angina: Oral: Usual starting dose: 30 mg 4 times/day; sustained release: 120-180 mg once daily; dosage should be increased gradually at 1- to 2-day intervals until optimum response is obtained. Doses up to 360 mg/day have been effectively used. Hypertension is controllable with single daily doses of sustained release products, or divided daily doses of regular release products, in the range of 240-360 mg/day.
Sustained-release capsules:
**Cardizem® SR:** Initial: 60-120 mg twice daily; adjust to maximum antihypertensive effect (usually within 14 days); usual range: 240-360 mg/day
**Cardizem® CD, Tiazac™:** Hypertension: Total daily dose of short-acting administered once daily or initially 180 or 240 mg once daily; adjust to maximum effect (usually within 14 days); maximum: 480 mg/day; usual range: 240-360 mg/day
**Cardizem® CD:** Angina: Initial: 120-180 mg once daily; maximum: 480 mg once/day
**Dilacor™ XR:**
Hypertension: 180-240 mg once daily; maximum: 540 mg/day; usual range: 180-480 mg/day; use lower dose in elderly
Angina: Initial: 120 mg/day; titrate slowly over 7-14 days up to 480 mg/day, as needed
I.V. (requires an infusion pump):
- Initial bolus dose: 0.25 mg/kg actual body weight over 2 minutes (average adult dose: 20 mg)
- Repeat bolus dose (may be administered after 15 minutes if the response is inadequate.): 0.35 mg/kg actual body weight over 2 minutes (average adult dose: 25 mg)
- Continuous infusion (infusions >24 hours or infusion rates >15 mg/hour are not recommended.): Initial infusion rate of 10 mg/hour; rate may be increased in 5 mg/hour increments up to 15 mg/hour as needed; some patients may respond to an initial rate of 5 mg/hour.

If Cardizem® injectable is administered by continuous infusion for >24 hours, the possibility of decreased diltiazem clearance, prolonged elimination half-life, and increased diltiazem and/or diltiazem metabolite plasma concentrations should be considered.

**Conversion from I.V. diltiazem to oral diltiazem:** Start oral approximately 3 hours after bolus dose.

**Oral dose (mg/day) is approximately equal to [rate (mg/hour) x 3 + 3] x 10.**

3 mg/hour = 120 mg/day
5 mg/hour = 180 mg/day
7 mg/hour = 240 mg/day
11 mg/hour = 360 mg/day

**Dosing comments in renal/hepatic impairment:** Use with caution as extensively metabolized by the liver and excreted in the kidneys and bile.

Dialysis: Not removed by hemo- or peritoneal dialysis; supplemental dose is not necessary.

**Dietary Considerations** Alcohol: Avoid use

**Patient Information** Oral: Take as directed; do not alter dosage or discontinue therapy without consulting prescriber. Do not crush or chew extended release form. Avoid (or limit) alcohol and caffeine. You may experience dizziness or lightheadedness (use caution when driving or engaging in tasks requiring alertness until response to drug is known); nausea or vomiting (small frequent meals, frequent mouth care, chewing gum, or sucking lozenges may help); constipation (increased exercise, dietary fiber, fruit, or fluid may help); diarrhea (buttermilk, boiled milk, or yogurt may help). Report chest pain, palpitations, irregular heartbeat, unusual cough, difficulty breathing, swelling of extremities, muscle tremors or weakness, confusion or acute lethargy, or skin rash.

**Nursing Implications** Do not crush sustained release capsules

**Dosage Forms**

Capsule, sustained release, as hydrochloride:
- Cardizem® CD: 120 mg, 180 mg, 240 mg, 300 mg
- Cardizem® SR: 60 mg, 90 mg, 120 mg
- Dilacor™ XR: 180 mg, 240 mg
- Tiazac™: 120 mg, 180 mg, 240 mg, 300 mg, 360 mg

Injection, as hydrochloride: 5 mg/mL (5 mL, 10 mL)
- Cardizem®: 5 mg/mL (5 mL, 10 mL)

Tablet, as hydrochloride (Cardizem®): 30 mg, 60 mg, 90 mg, 120 mg

Tablet, extended release, as hydrochloride (Tiamate®): 120 mg, 180 mg, 240 mg

♦ **Dimacol® Caplets [OTC]** *see* Guaifenesin, Pseudoephedrine, and Dextromethorphan *on page 259*

♦ **Dimaphen® Elixir [OTC]** *see* Brompheniramine and Phenylpropanolamine *on page 74*

♦ **Dimaphen® Tablets [OTC]** *see* Brompheniramine and Phenylpropanolamine *on page 74*

## Dimenhydrinate (dye men HYE dri nate)

**U.S. Brand Names** Calm-X® Oral [OTC]; Dimetabs® Oral; Dinate® Injection; Dramamine® Oral [OTC]; Dymenate® Injection; Hydrate® Injection; TripTone® Caplets® [OTC]

**Canadian Brand Names** Apo®-Dimenhydrinate; Gravol®; PMS-Dimenhydrinate; Travel Aid®; Travel Tabs

**Pharmacologic Category** Antihistamine

**Use** Treatment and prevention of nausea, vertigo, and vomiting associated with motion sickness

**Effects on Mental Status** Drowsiness is common; may cause depression, nervousness, or paradoxical CNS stimulation

**Effects on Psychiatric Treatment** Concurrent use with psychotropic may result in additive sedation

**Usual Dosage**

Children:
- Oral:
  - 2-5 years: 12.5-25 mg every 6-8 hours, maximum: 75 mg/day
  - 6-12 years: 25-50 mg every 6-8 hours, maximum: 150 mg/day
- I.M.: 1.25 mg/kg or 37.5 mg/m$^2$ 4 times/day, not to exceed 300 mg/day

Adults: Oral, I.M., I.V.: 50-100 mg every 4-6 hours, not to exceed 400 mg/day

**Dosage Forms**

Capsule: 50 mg
Injection: 50 mg/mL (1 mL, 5 mL, 10 mL)
Liquid: 12.5 mg/4 mL (90 mL, 473 mL); 16.62 mg/5 mL (480 mL)
Tablet: 50 mg
Tablet, chewable: 50 mg

## Dimercaprol (dye mer KAP role)

**U.S. Brand Names** BAL in Oil®

**Pharmacologic Category** Antidote

**Use** Antidote to gold, arsenic (except arsine), and mercury poisoning (except nonalkyl mercury); adjunct to edetate calcium disodium in lead poisoning; possibly effective for antimony, bismuth, chromium, copper, nickel, tungsten, or zinc

**Effects on Mental Status** May cause nervousness

**Effects on Psychiatric Treatment** May produce neutropenia; use caution with clozapine and carbamazepine

**Usual Dosage** Children and Adults: Deep I.M.:

Arsenic, mercury, and gold poisoning: 3 mg/kg every 4-6 hours for 2 days, then every 12 hours for 7-10 days or until recovery (initial dose may be up to 5 mg if severe poisoning)

Lead poisoning (in conjunction with calcium EDTA): For symptomatic acute encephalopathy or blood level >100 mcg/dL: 4-5 mg/kg every 4 hours for 3-5 days

**Dosage Forms** Injection: 100 mg/mL (3 mL)

♦ **Dimetabs® Oral** *see* Dimenhydrinate *on page 173*

♦ **Dimetane®-DC** *see* Brompheniramine, Phenylpropanolamine, and Codeine *on page 74*

♦ **Dimetane® Decongestant Elixir [OTC]** *see* Brompheniramine and Phenylephrine *on page 73*

♦ **Dimetane® Extentabs® [OTC]** *see* Brompheniramine *on page 73*

♦ **Dimetapp® 4-Hour Liqui-Gel Capsule [OTC]** *see* Brompheniramine and Phenylpropanolamine *on page 74*

♦ **Dimetapp® Elixir [OTC]** *see* Brompheniramine and Phenylpropanolamine *on page 74*

♦ **Dimetapp® Extentabs® [OTC]** *see* Brompheniramine and Phenylpropanolamine *on page 74*

♦ **Dimetapp® Sinus Caplets [OTC]** *see* Pseudoephedrine and Ibuprofen *on page 479*

♦ **Dimetapp® Tablet [OTC]** *see* Brompheniramine and Phenylpropanolamine *on page 74*

♦ **2-Dimethylaminoethanol** *see* Deanol *on page 152*

♦ **β,β-Dimethylcysteine** *see* Penicillamine *on page 424*

## Dimethyl Sulfoxide (dye meth il sul FOKS ide)

**U.S. Brand Names** Rimso®-50

**Synonyms** DMSO

**Pharmacologic Category** Urinary Tract Product

**Use** Symptomatic relief of interstitial cystitis

**Effects on Mental Status** May cause sedation

**Effects on Psychiatric Treatment** None reported

**Pregnancy Risk Factor** C

**Warnings/Precautions** Use with caution in patients with urinary tract malignancies

**Adverse Reactions**

>10%: Gastrointestinal: Garlic-like breath

1% to 10%:
- Central nervous system: Headache, sedation
- Gastrointestinal: Nausea, vomiting
- Local: Local dermatitis
- Ocular: Burning eyes

**Drug Interactions** Increased toxicity with sulindac

**Usual Dosage** Instill 50 mL directly into bladder and allow to remain for 15 minutes; repeat every 2 weeks until maximum symptomatic relief is obtained

**Dosage Forms** Solution: 50% [500 mg/mL] (50 mL)

♦ **Dinate® Injection** *see* Dimenhydrinate *on page 173*

## Dinoprostone (dye noe PROST one)

**U.S. Brand Names** Cervidil® Vaginal Insert; Prepidil® Vaginal Gel; Prostin E$_2$® Vaginal Suppository

**Synonyms** PGE$_2$; Prostaglandin E$_2$

**Pharmacologic Category** Abortifacient; Prostaglandin

**Use**

Gel: Promote cervical ripening prior to labor induction; usage for gel include any patient undergoing induction of labor with an unripe cervix, most commonly for pre-eclampsia, eclampsia, postdates, diabetes, intrauterine growth retardation, and chronic hypertension

Suppositories: Terminate pregnancy from 12th through 28th week of gestation; evacuate uterus in cases of missed abortion or intrauterine fetal death; manage benign hydatidiform mole

Vaginal insert: Initiation and/or cervical ripening in patients at or near term in whom there is a medical or obstetrical indication for the induction of labor

**Effects on Mental Status** May cause dizziness

**Effects on Psychiatric Treatment** None reported

**Pregnancy Risk Factor** C

(Continued)

## Dinoprostone *(Continued)*

**Contraindications**

Vaginal insert: Known hypersensitivity to prostaglandins; fetal distress (suspicion or clinical evidence unless delivery is imminent); unexplained vaginal bleeding during this pregnancy; strong suspicion of marked cephalopelvic disproportion; patients in whom oxytoxic drugs are contraindicated or when prolonged contraction of the uterus may be detrimental to fetal safety or uterine integrity (including previous cesarean section or major uterine surgery); greater than 6 previous term pregnancies; patients already receiving oxytoxic drugs

Gel: Hypersensitivity to prostaglandins or any constituents of the cervical gel, history of asthma, contracted pelvis, malpresentation of the fetus

Gel: The following are "relative" contraindications and should only be considered by the physician under these circumstances: Patients in whom vaginal delivery is not indicated (ie, herpes genitalia with a lesion at the time of delivery), prior uterine surgery, breech presentation, multiple gestation, polyhydramnios, premature rupture of membranes

Suppository: Known hypersensitivity to dinoprostone, acute pelvic inflammatory disease, uterine fibroids, cervical stenosis

**Warnings/Precautions** Dinoprostone should be used only by medically trained personnel in a hospital; caution in patients with cervicitis, infected endocervical lesions, acute vaginitis, compromised (scarred) uterus or history of asthma, hypertension or hypotension, epilepsy, diabetes mellitus, anemia, jaundice, or cardiovascular, renal, or hepatic disease. Oxytocin should not be used simultaneously with Prepidil® (>6 hours of the last dose of Prepidil®).

**Adverse Reactions**

>10%:
- Central nervous system: Headache
- Gastrointestinal: Vomiting, diarrhea, nausea

1% to 10%:
- Cardiovascular: Bradycardia
- Central nervous system: Fever
- Neuromuscular & skeletal: Back pain

<1%: Bronchospasm, cardiac arrhythmias, chills, coughing, dizziness, dyspnea, flushing, hot flashes, hypotension, pain, shivering, syncope, tightness of the chest, vasomotor and vasovagal reactions, wheezing

**Overdosage/Toxicology**

Signs and symptoms: Vomiting, bronchospasm, hypotension, chest pain, abdominal cramps, uterine contractions

Treatment: Symptomatic

**Drug Interactions** Increased effect of oxytocics

**Usual Dosage**

Abortifacient: Insert 1 suppository high in vagina, repeat at 3- to 5-hour intervals until abortion occurs up to 240 mg (maximum dose); continued administration for longer than 2 days is not advisable

Cervical ripening:
- Gel:
  - Intracervical: 0.25-1 mg
  - Intravaginal: 2.5 mg
- Suppositories: Intracervical: 2-3 mg
- Vaginal Insert (Cervidil®): 10 mg (to be removed at the onset of active labor or after 12 hours)

**Patient Information** Nausea and vomiting, cramping or uterine pain, or fever may occur. Report acute pain, respiratory difficulty, or skin rash. Closely monitor for vaginal discharge for several days. Report vaginal bleeding, itching, malodorous or bloody discharge, or severe cramping.

**Nursing Implications** Bring suppository to room temperature just prior to use; patient should remain supine for 10 minutes following insertion; commercially available suppositories should not be used for extemporaneous preparation of any other dosage form of drug

**Dosage Forms**

Insert, vaginal (Cervidil®): 10 mg

Gel, endocervical: 0.5 mg in 3 g syringes [each package contains a 10-mm and 20-mm shielded catheter]

Suppository, vaginal: 20 mg

## Dinoprost Tromethamine (DYE noe prost tro METH a meen)

**U.S. Brand Names** Prostin $F_2$ Alpha®

**Synonyms** $PGF_{2\alpha}$; Prostaglandin $F_2$ Alpha

**Pharmacologic Category** Prostaglandin

**Use** Abort 2nd trimester pregnancy

**Effects on Mental Status** None reported

**Effects on Psychiatric Treatment** None reported

**Pregnancy Risk Factor** X

**Contraindications** Hypersensitivity to dinoprost tromethamine; acute pelvic inflammatory disease; uterine fibroids; cervical stenosis

**Adverse Reactions** 1% to 10%:
- Hematologic: Blood loss
- Miscellaneous: Uterine infection

**Usual Dosage** 40 mg (8 mL) via transabdominal tap, if abortion not completed in 24 hours, another 10-40 mg may be given

**Dosage Forms** Injection: 5 mg/mL (4 mL, 8 mL)


- ♦ **Diocto® [OTC]** *see* Docusate *on page 179*
- ♦ **Diocto-K® [OTC]** *see* Docusate *on page 179*
- ♦ **Dioeze® [OTC]** *see* Docusate *on page 179*
- ♦ **Dioval® Injection** *see* Estradiol *on page 203*
- ♦ **Diovan™** *see* Valsartan *on page 580*
- ♦ **Diovan HCTZ®** *see* Valsartan and Hydrochlorothiazide *on page 580*
- ♦ **Dipentum®** *see* Olsalazine *on page 404*
- ♦ **Diphenacen-50® Injection** *see* Diphenhydramine *on page 174*
- ♦ **Diphen® Cough [OTC]** *see* Diphenhydramine *on page 174*
- ♦ **Diphenhist [OTC]** *see* Diphenhydramine *on page 174*


## Diphenhydramine (dye fen HYE dra meen)

**Related Information**


Agents for Treatment of Extrapyramidal Symptoms *on page 638*
Antiparkinsonian Agents Comparison Chart *on page 705*
Anxiolytic/Hypnotic Use in Long-Term Care Facilities *on page 754*
Clinical Issues in the Use of Anxiolytics and Sedative/Hypnotics *on page 634*
Discontinuation of Psychotropic Drugs - Withdrawal Symptoms and Recommendations *on page 798*
Federal OBRA Regulations Recommended Maximum Doses *on page 756*
Nonbenzodiazepine Anxiolytics and Hypnotics *on page 721*
Patient Information - Agents for Treatment of Extrapyramidal Symptoms *on page 657*
Sleep Disorders *on page 620*
Special Populations - Elderly *on page 662*


**Generic Available** Yes

**U.S. Brand Names** AllerMax® Oral [OTC]; Banophen® Oral [OTC]; Belix® Oral [OTC]; Benadryl® Injection; Benadryl® Oral [OTC]; Benadryl® Topical; Ben-Allergin-50® Injection; Benylin® Cough Syrup [OTC]; Bydramine® Cough Syrup [OTC]; Compoz® Gel Caps [OTC]; Compoz® Nighttime Sleep Aid [OTC]; Dihydrex® Injection; Diphenacen-50® Injection; Diphen® Cough [OTC]; Diphenhist [OTC]; Dormarex® 2 Oral [OTC]; Dormin® Oral [OTC]; Genahist® Oral; Hydramyn® Syrup [OTC]; Hyrexin-50® Injection; Maximum Strength Nytol® [OTC]; Miles Nervine® Caplets [OTC]; Nordryl® Injection; Nordryl® Oral; Nytol® Oral [OTC]; Phendry® Oral [OTC]; Siladryl® Oral [OTC]; Silphen® Cough [OTC]; Sleep-eze 3® Oral [OTC]; Sleepinal® [OTC]; Sleepwell 2-nite® [OTC]; Sominex® Oral [OTC]; Tusstat® Syrup; Twilite® Oral [OTC]; Uni-Bent® Cough Syrup; 40 Winks® [OTC]

**Canadian Brand Names** Allerdryl®; Allernix®; Nytol® Extra Strength

**Synonyms** Diphenhydramine Hydrochloride

**Pharmacologic Category** Antihistamine

**Use** Symptomatic relief of allergic symptoms caused by histamine release which include nasal allergies and allergic dermatosis; can be used for mild nighttime sedation; prevention of motion sickness and as an antitussive; has antinauseant and topical anesthetic properties; treatment of antipsychotic-induced extrapyramidal reactions

**Pregnancy Risk Factor** B

**Contraindications** Hypersensitivity to diphenhydramine or any component; should not be used in acute attacks of asthma; use in neonates is contraindicated

**Warnings/Precautions** Causes sedation, caution must be used in performing tasks which require alertness (ie, operating machinery or driving). Sedative effects of CNS depressants or ethanol are potentiated. Use with caution in patients with angle-closure glaucoma, pyloroduodenal obstruction (including stenotic peptic ulcer), urinary tract obstruction (including bladder neck obstruction and symptomatic prostatic hypertrophy), hyperthyroidism, increased intraocular pressure, and cardiovascular disease (including hypertension and tachycardia). Diphenhydramine has high sedative and anticholinergic properties, so it may not be considered the antihistamine of choice for prolonged use in the elderly. May cause paradoxical excitation in pediatric patients, and can result in hallucinations, coma, and death in overdose. Some preparations contain sodium bisulfite; syrup formulations may contain alcohol.

**Adverse Reactions**
- Cardiovascular: Hypotension, palpitations, tachycardia
- Central nervous system: Sedation, sleepiness, dizziness, disturbed coordination, headache, fatigue, nervousness, paradoxical excitement, insomnia, euphoria, confusion
- Dermatologic: Photosensitivity, rash, angioedema, urticaria
- Gastrointestinal: Nausea, vomiting, diarrhea, abdominal pain, xerostomia, appetite increase, weight gain, dry mucous membranes, anorexia
- Genitourinary: Urinary retention, urinary frequency, difficult urination
- Hematologic: Hemolytic anemia, thrombocytopenia, agranulocytosis
- Neuromuscular & skeletal: Tremor, paresthesia
- Ocular: blurred vision
- Respiratory: Thickening of bronchial secretions

**Overdosage/Toxicology**
Signs and symptoms: CNS stimulation or depression; overdose may result in death in infants and children
Treatment: There is no specific treatment for an antihistamine overdose, however, most of its clinical toxicity is due to anticholinergic effects. Anticholinesterase inhibitors (eg, physostigmine, neostigmine, pyridostigmine, or edrophonium) may be useful by reducing acetylcholinesterase. For anticholinergic overdose with severe life-threatening symptoms, physostigmine 1-2 mg (0.5 or 0.02 mg/kg for children) I.V., slowly may be given to reverse these effects.

**Drug Interactions** CYP2D6 enzyme substrate
Amantadine, rimantadine: Central and/or peripheral anticholinergic syndrome can occur when administered with amantadine or rimantadine
Anticholinergic agents: Central and/or peripheral anticholinergic syndrome can occur when administered with narcotic analgesics, phenothiazines and other antipsychotics (especially with high anticholinergic activity), tricyclic antidepressants, quinidine and some other antiarrhythmics, and antihistamines
Atenolol: Drugs with high anticholinergic activity may increase the bioavailability of atenolol (and possibly other beta-blockers); monitor for increased effect
Cholinergic agents: Drugs with high anticholinergic activity may antagonize the therapeutic effect of cholinergic agents; includes donepezil, rivastigmine, and tacrine
CNS depressants: Sedative effects may be additive with CNS depressants; includes ethanol, benzodiazepines, barbiturates, narcotic analgesics, and other sedative agents; monitor for increased effect
Digoxin: Drugs with high anticholinergic activity may decrease gastric degradation and increase the amount of digoxin absorbed by delaying gastric emptying
Ethanol: Syrup should not be given to patients taking drugs that can cause disulfiram reactions (ie, metronidazole, chlorpropamide) due to high alcohol content
Levodopa: Drugs with high anticholinergic activity may increase gastric degradation and decrease the amount of levodopa absorbed by delaying gastric emptying
Neuroleptics: Drugs with high anticholinergic activity may antagonize the therapeutic effects of neuroleptics

**Stability** Protect from light; the following drugs are **incompatible** with diphenhydramine when mixed in the same syringe: Amobarbital, amphotericin B, cephalothin, diatrizoate, foscarnet, heparin, hydrocortisone, hydroxyzine, pentobarbital, phenobarbital, phenytoin, prochlorperazine, promazine, promethazine, tetracycline, thiopental

**Mechanism of Action** Competes with histamine for $H_1$-receptor sites on effector cells in the gastrointestinal tract, blood vessels, and respiratory tract; anticholinergic and sedative effects are also seen

**Pharmacodynamics/kinetics**
Maximum sedative effect: 1-3 hours
Duration of action: 4-7 hours
Absorption: Oral: 40% to 60% reaches systemic circulation due to first-pass metabolism
Metabolism: Extensive in the liver and, to smaller degrees, in the lung and kidney
Half-life: 2-8 hours; elderly: 13.5 hours
Protein binding: 78%
Time to peak serum concentration: 2-4 hours

**Usual Dosage**
Children:
Oral: (>10 kg): 12.5-25 mg 3-4 times/day; maximum daily dose: 300 mg
I.M., I.V.: 5 mg/kg/day or 150 mg/m$^2$/day in divided doses every 6-8 hours, not to exceed 300 mg/day
Adults:
Oral: 25-50 mg every 6-8 hours
Nighttime sleep aid: 50 mg at bedtime
I.M., I.V.: 10-50 mg in a single dose every 2-4 hours, not to exceed 400 mg/day
Topical: For external application, not longer than 7 days

**Dietary Considerations** Alcohol: Additive CNS effects, avoid use

**Administration** Dilute to a maximum concentration of 25 mg/mL and infuse over 10-15 minutes (maximum rate of infusion: 25 mg/minute)

**Monitoring Parameters** Relief of symptoms, mental alertness

**Reference Range** Antihistamine effects at levels >25 ng/mL; drowsiness at levels: 30-40 ng/mL; mental impairment at levels >60 ng/mL; Therapeutic: Not established; Toxic: >0.1 µg/mL

**Test Interactions** May suppress the wheal and flare reactions to skin test antigens

**Patient Information** May cause drowsiness; swallow whole, do not crush or chew sustained release product; avoid alcohol, may impair coordination and judgment

**Nursing Implications** Raise bed rails, institute safety measures, assist with ambulation

**Additional Information** Has antinauseant and topical anesthetic properties

**Dosage Forms**
Capsule, as hydrochloride: 25 mg, 50 mg
Cream, as hydrochloride: 1%, 2%
Elixir, as hydrochloride: 12.5 mg/5 mL (5 mL, 10 mL, 20 mL, 120 mL, 480 mL, 3780 mL)
Injection, as hydrochloride: 10 mg/mL (10 mL, 30 mL); 50 mg/mL (1 mL, 10 mL)
Lotion, as hydrochloride: 1% (75 mL)
Solution, topical spray, as hydrochloride: 1% (60 mL)
Syrup, as hydrochloride: 12.5 mg/5 mL (5 mL, 120 mL, 240 mL, 480 mL, 3780 mL)
Tablet, as hydrochloride: 25 mg, 50 mg

## Diphenhydramine and Pseudoephedrine
(dye fen HYE dra meen & soo doe e FED rin)

**U.S. Brand Names** Actifed® Allergy Tablet (Night) [OTC]; Banophen® Decongestant Capsule [OTC]; Benadryl® Decongestant Allergy Tablet [OTC]

**Pharmacologic Category** Antihistamine/Decongestant Combination

**Use** Relief of symptoms of upper respiratory mucosal congestion in seasonal and perennial nasal allergies, acute rhinitis, rhinosinusitis, and eustachian tube blockage

**Effects on Mental Status** Diphenhydramine may cause paradoxical excitation in pediatric patients, and can result in hallucinations, coma, and death in overdose. May cause sedation, sleepiness, dizziness, disturbed coordination, headache, fatigue, nervousness, paradoxical excitement, insomnia, euphoria, or confusion. Pseudoephedrine may cause dizziness, drowsiness, nervousness, and insomnia; may rarely cause hallucinations.

**Effects on Psychiatric Treatment** Rare reports of agranulocytosis and thrombocytopenia; use caution with clozapine, carbamazepine, and valproic acid; may increase gastric degradation of levodopa and decrease the amount of levodopa absorbed by delaying gastric emptying. Therapeutic effects of cholinergic agents (tacrine, donepezil,rivastigmine, galantamine) and neuroleptics may be antagonized. Central and/or peripheral anticholinergic syndrome can occur when administered with amantadine, rimantadine, narcotic analgesics, phenothiazines, and other antipsychotics (especially with high anticholinergic activity), tricyclic antidepressants and antihistamines. Pseudoephedrine is contraindicated with MAOIs.

**Usual Dosage** Adults: Oral: 1 capsule or tablet every 4-6 hours, up to 4/day

**Dosage Forms**
Capsule: Diphenhydramine hydrochloride 25 mg and pseudoephedrine hydrochloride 60 mg
Tablet:
Actifed® Allergy (Night): Diphenhydramine hydrochloride 25 mg and pseudoephedrine hydrochloride 30 mg
Benadryl® Decongestant Allergy: Diphenhydramine hydrochloride 25 mg and pseudoephedrine hydrochloride 60 mg

♦ **Diphenhydramine Hydrochloride** *see* Diphenhydramine *on page 174*

## Diphenidol (dye FEN i dole)

**U.S. Brand Names** Vontrol®

**Pharmacologic Category** Antiemetic

**Use** Control of nausea and vomiting; peripheral vertigo and associated nausea and vomiting, Ménière's disease and middle and inner ear surgery

**Effects on Mental Status** Drowsiness is common; may cause nervousness or insomnia

**Effects on Psychiatric Treatment** Concurrent use with psychotropics may produce additive sedation

**Adverse Reactions**
>10%: Central nervous system: Drowsiness
1% to 10%:
Central nervous system: Headache, dizziness, nervousness, insomnia
Gastrointestinal: Xerostomia, heartburn
Neuromuscular & skeletal: Weakness
Ocular: Blurred vision

**Usual Dosage** Oral:
Children: 0.88 mg/kg, children weighing 50-100 pounds the dose in 25 mg given no more often than every 4 hours; total dose in 24 hours should not exceed 5.5 mg/kg
Adults: 25 mg every 4 hours

**Patient Information** Take as directed; may be taken with food to reduce GI upset. You may experience drowsiness or nervousness; use caution when driving or engaging in tasks requiring alertness. Report excessive drowsiness or nervousness, rash, or muscle weakness. Inform prescriber if you are or intend to be pregnant. Consult prescriber if breast-feeding.

**Dosage Forms** Tablet, as hydrochloride: 25 mg

## Diphenoxylate and Atropine
(dye fen OKS i late & A troe peen)

**U.S. Brand Names** Logen®; Lomanate®; Lomotil®; Lonox®

**Synonyms** Atropine and Diphenoxylate

(Continued)

## Diphenoxylate and Atropine *(Continued)*

**Pharmacologic Category** Antidiarrheal

**Use** Treatment of diarrhea

**Effects on Mental Status** May cause nervousness, restlessness, drowsiness, or insomnia; rarely may produce euphoria

**Effects on Psychiatric Treatment** Concurrent use with MAOIs may result in hypertensive crisis; additive sedation and dry mouth with psychotropics; use with benztropine or other anticholinergic agents may result in ileus

**Restrictions** C-V

**Pregnancy Risk Factor** C

**Contraindications** Hypersensitivity to diphenoxylate, atropine or any component; severe liver disease, jaundice, dehydrated patient, and narrow-angle glaucoma; it should not be used for children <2 years of age

**Warnings/Precautions** High doses may cause physical and psychological dependence with prolonged use; use with caution in patients with ulcerative colitis, dehydration, and hepatic dysfunction; reduction of intestinal motility may be deleterious in diarrhea resulting from *Shigella*, *Salmonella*, toxigenic strains of *E. coli*, and from pseudomembranous enterocolitis associated with broad spectrum antibiotics; children may develop signs of atropinism (dryness of skin and mucous membranes, thirst, hyperthermia, tachycardia, urinary retention, flushing) even at the recommended dosages; if there is no response with 48 hours, the drug is unlikely to be effective and should be discontinued; if chronic diarrhea is not improved symptomatically within 10 days at maximum dosage of 20 mg/day, control is unlikely with further use.

**Adverse Reactions**

1% to 10%:

- Central nervous system: Nervousness, restlessness, dizziness, drowsiness, headache, mental depression
- Gastrointestinal: Paralytic ileus, xerostomia
- Genitourinary: Urinary retention and dysuria
- Ocular: Blurred vision
- Respiratory: Respiratory depression

<1%: Abdominal discomfort, diaphoresis (increased), euphoria, hyperthermia, muscle cramps, nausea, pancreatitis, pruritus, sedation, stomach cramps, tachycardia, urticaria, vomiting, weakness

**Overdosage/Toxicology**

Signs and symptoms: Drowsiness, hypotension, blurred vision, flushing, dry mouth, miosis

Treatment: Administration of activated charcoal will reduce bioavailability of diphenoxylate; naloxone 2 mg I.V. (0.01 mg/kg for children) with repeat administration as necessary up to a total of 10 mg; for anticholinergic overdose with severe life-threatening symptoms, physostigmine 1-2 mg (0.5 or 0.02 mg/kg for children) S.C. or I.V., slowly may be given to reverse these effects

**Drug Interactions** Increased toxicity: MAO inhibitors (hypertensive crisis), CNS depressants, antimuscarinics (paralytic ileus); may prolong half-life of drugs metabolized in liver

**Usual Dosage** Oral:

Children (use with caution in young children due to variable responses):

- Liquid: 0.3-0.4 mg of diphenoxylate/kg/day in 2-4 divided doses **or**
- <2 years: Not recommended
- 2-5 years: 2 mg of diphenoxylate 3 times/day
- 5-8 years: 2 mg of diphenoxylate 4 times/day
- 8-12 years: 2 mg of diphenoxylate 5 times/day

Adults: 15-20 mg/day of diphenoxylate in 3-4 divided doses; maintenance: 5-15 mg/day in 2-3 divided doses

**Dietary Considerations** Alcohol: Additive CNS effects, avoid use

**Patient Information** Take as directed; do not exceed recommended dosage. If no response within 48 hours, notify prescriber. Avoid alcohol or other prescriptive or OTC sedatives or depressants. You may experience drowsiness, blurred vision, impaired coordination; use caution when driving or engaging in tasks that require alertness until response to drug is known. Sucking on lozenges or chewing gum may reduce dry mouth. Report difficulty urinating, persistent diarrhea, respiratory difficulties, fever, or palpitations.

**Nursing Implications** Raise bed rails, institute safety measures

**Dosage Forms**

Solution, oral: Diphenoxylate hydrochloride 2.5 mg and atropine sulfate 0.025 mg per 5 mL (4 mL, 10 mL, 60 mL)

Tablet: Diphenoxylate hydrochloride 2.5 mg and atropine sulfate 0.025 mg

♦ **Diphenylan Sodium®** *see* Phenytoin *on page 441*

♦ **Diphenylhydantoin** *see* Phenytoin *on page 441*

♦ **Diphtheria $CRM_{197}$ Protein** *see* Pneumococcal Conjugate Vaccine, 7-Valent *on page 450*

## Dipivefrin (dye PI ve frin)

**Related Information**

Glaucoma Drug Therapy *on page 712*

**U.S. Brand Names** AKPro® Ophthalmic; Propine® Ophthalmic

**Pharmacologic Category** Alpha/Beta Agonist; Ophthalmic Agent, Antiglaucoma; Ophthalmic Agent, Vasoconstrictor

**Use** Reduces elevated intraocular pressure in chronic open-angle glaucoma; also used to treat ocular hypertension, low tension, and secondary glaucomas

**Effects on Mental Status** None reported

**Effects on Psychiatric Treatment** None reported

**Usual Dosage** Adults: Ophthalmic: Instill 1 drop every 12 hours into the eyes

**Dosage Forms** Solution, ophthalmic, as hydrochloride: 0.1% (5 mL, 10 mL, 15 mL)

♦ **Diprivan® Injection** *see* Propofol *on page 473*

♦ **Diprolene®** *see* Betamethasone *on page 65*

♦ **Diprolene® AF** *see* Betamethasone *on page 65*

♦ **Dipropylacetic Acid** *see* Valproic Acid and Derivatives *on page 578*

♦ **Diprosone®** *see* Betamethasone *on page 65*

## Dipyridamole (dye peer ID a mole)

**U.S. Brand Names** Persantine®

**Canadian Brand Names** Apo®-Dipyridamole FC; Apo®-Dipyridamole SC; Novo-Dipiradol

**Pharmacologic Category** Antiplatelet Agent; Vasodilator

**Use** Maintains patency after surgical grafting procedures including coronary artery bypass; used with warfarin to decrease thrombosis in patients after artificial heart valve replacement; used with aspirin to prevent coronary artery thrombosis; in combination with aspirin or warfarin to prevent other thromboembolic disorders. Dipyridamole may also be given 2 days prior to open heart surgery to prevent platelet activation by extracorporeal bypass pump and as a diagnostic agent in CAD.

**Effects on Mental Status** Dizziness is common

**Effects on Psychiatric Treatment** None reported

**Pregnancy Risk Factor** B

**Contraindications** Hypersensitivity to dipyridamole or any component

**Warnings/Precautions** Use caution in patients with hypotension. Use caution in patients on other antiplatelet agents or anticoagulation. Severe adverse reactions have occurred rarely with I.V. administration. Use the I.V. form with caution in patients with bronchospastic disease or unstable angina. Have aminophylline ready in case of urgency or emergency with I.V. use.

**Adverse Reactions**

>10%:

- Cardiovascular: Exacerbation of angina pectoris (I.V.), headache (I.V.)
- Central nervous system: Dizziness

1% to 10%:

- Cardiovascular: Hypotension, hypertension, tachycardia
- Central nervous system: Headache
- Dermatologic: Rash
- Gastrointestinal: Abdominal distress
- Respiratory: Dyspnea

<1%: Allergic reaction, angina, diarrhea, edema, flushing, hepatic dysfunction, hypertonia, hyperventilation, migraine, pleural pain, rhinitis, syncope, vasodilatation, vomiting, weakness

**Overdosage/Toxicology**

Signs and symptoms: Hypotension, peripheral vasodilation; dialysis is not effective

Treatment: Includes fluids and vasopressors although hypotension is often transient

**Drug Interactions**

Adenosine blood levels and pharmacologic effects are increased; consider reduced doses of adenosine

Theophylline may reduce the pharmacologic effects of dipyridamole; hold theophylline preparations for 36-48 hours before dipyridamole facilitated stress test

**Usual Dosage**

Children: Oral: 3-6 mg/kg/day in 3 divided doses

- Doses of 4-10 mg/kg/day have been used investigationally to treat proteinuria in pediatric renal disease
- Mechanical prosthetic heart valves: Oral: 2-5 mg/kg/day (used in combination with an oral anticoagulant in children who have systemic embolism despite adequate oral anticoagulant therapy, and used in combination with low-dose oral anticoagulation (INR 2-3) plus aspirin in children in whom full-dose oral anticoagulation is contraindicated)

Adults:

- Oral: 75-400 mg/day in 3-4 divided doses
- Evaluation of coronary artery disease: I.V.: 0.14 mg/kg/minute for 4 minutes; maximum dose: 60 mg

Hemodialysis: Significant drug removal is unlikely based on physiochemical characteristics

**Patient Information** Oral: Take exactly as directed, with or without food. You may experience mild headache, transient diarrhea, or temporary dizziness (sit or lie down when taking medication). You may have a tendency to bleed easy; use caution with sharps, needles, or razors. Report chest pain, redness around mouth, acute abdominal cramping or severe diarrhea, acute and persistent headache or dizziness, rash, difficulty breathing, or swelling of extremities.

**Dosage Forms**

Injection: 10 mg/2 mL

Tablet: 25 mg, 50 mg, 75 mg

♦ **Dipyridamole and Aspirin** *see* Aspirin and Extended-Release Dipyridamole *on page 50*

## Dirithromycin (dye RITH roe mye sin)

**U.S. Brand Names** Dynabac®

**Synonyms** ASE-136BS; LY-237216

**Pharmacologic Category** Antibiotic, Macrolide

**Use** Treatment of mild to moderate upper and lower respiratory tract infections due to *Moraxella catarrhalis, Streptococcus pneumoniae, Legionella pneumophila, H. influenzae*, or *S. pyogenes* ie, acute exacerbation of chronic bronchitis, secondary bacterial infection of acute bronchitis, community-acquired pneumonia, pharyngitis/tonsillitis, and uncomplicated infections of the skin and skin structure due to *Staphylococcus aureus*

**Effects on Mental Status** May cause insomnia; rarely may cause anxiety, drowsiness, or depression; macrolides have been reported to cause nightmares, confusion, and mood lability

**Effects on Psychiatric Treatment** Contraindicated with pimozide; may cause neutropenia; use caution with clozapine and carbamazepine; may increase carbamazepine and triazolam levels

**Pregnancy Risk Factor** C

**Contraindications** Hypersensitivity to any macrolide or component of dirithromycin; use with pimozide

**Warnings/Precautions** Contrary to potential serious consequences with other macrolides (eg, cardiac arrhythmias), the combination of terfenadine and dirithromycin has not shown alteration of terfenadine metabolism; however, caution should be taken during coadministration of dirithromycin and terfenadine; pseudomembranous colitis has been reported and should be considered in patients presenting with diarrhea subsequent to therapy with dirithromycin

**Adverse Reactions**

1% to 10%:

Central nervous system: Headache, dizziness, vertigo, insomnia

Dermatologic: Rash, pruritus, urticaria

Endocrine & metabolic: Hyperkalemia

Gastrointestinal: Abdominal pain, nausea, diarrhea, vomiting, dyspepsia, flatulence

Hematologic: Thrombocytosis, eosinophilia, segmented neutrophils

Neuromuscular & skeletal: Weakness, pain, increased CPK

Respiratory: Increased cough, dyspnea

<1%: Abdominal pain, abnormal stools, abnormal taste, amblyopia, anorexia, anxiety, constipation, decreased hemoglobin/hematocrit, dehydration, depression, diaphoresis, dysmenorrhea, edema, epistaxis, fever, flu-like syndrome, gastritis, hemoptysis, hyperbilirubinemia, hyperventilation, hypoalbuminemia, hypochloremia, hypophosphatemia, increased alkaline phosphatase/bands/basophils, increased ALT/AST/GGT, increased creatinine/phosphorus, increased uric acid, leukocytosis, malaise, monocytosis, mouth ulceration, myalgia, neutropenia, palpitations, paresthesia, polyuria, somnolence, syncope, thirst, thrombocytopenia, tinnitus, tremor, vaginitis, vasodilation, xerostomia

**Overdosage/Toxicology**

Signs and symptoms: Nausea, vomiting, abdominal pain, diarrhea

Treatment: Supportive; dialysis has not been found effective

**Drug Interactions** CYP3A3/4 enzyme inhibitor

Increased effect: Absorption of dirithromycin is slightly enhanced with concomitant antacids and $H_2$-antagonists; dirithromycin may, like erythromycin, increase the effect of alfentanil, anticoagulants, bromocriptine, carbamazepine, cyclosporine, digoxin, disopyramide, ergots, methylprednisolone, cisapride, astemizole

Increased toxicity: Avoid use with pimozide (due to risk of significant cardiotoxicity) and triazolam

**Note:** Interactions with nonsedating antihistamines (eg, terfenadine, astemizole), cisapride, and theophylline are not known to occur, however, caution is advised with coadministration.

**Usual Dosage** Adults: Oral: 500 mg once daily for 5-14 days (14 days required for treatment of community-acquired pneumonia due to *Legionella, Mycoplasma*, or *S. pneumoniae*; 10 days is recommended for treatment of *S. pyogenes* pharyngitis/tonsillitis)

**Dosing adjustment in renal impairment:** None necessary

**Dosing adjustment in hepatic impairment:** None needed in mild dysfunction; not studied in moderate to severe dysfunction

**Patient Information** Take with food or after meals around-the-clock. Do not chew, cut, or crush tablets. Take complete prescription even if you are feeling better. You may experience dizziness or drowsiness (use caution when driving or engaging in tasks that require alertness until response to drug is known); nausea or vomiting (small frequent meals, frequent mouth care, sucking lozenges, or chewing gum may help); constipation (increased exercise, dietary fiber, fruit, or fluid may help); or diarrhea (buttermilk, boiled milk, or yogurt may help). Report skin rash or itching, easy bruising or bleeding, unhealed sores of mouth, itching or vaginal discharge, fever or chills, unusual cough, muscle cramping or weakness, or palpitations or chest pain.

**Nursing Implications** Do not crush tablets

**Dosage Forms** Tablet, enteric coated: 250 mg

♦ **Disalcid®** *see* Salsalate *on page 503*

♦ **Disalicylic Acid** *see* Salsalate *on page 503*

♦ **Discontinuation of Psychotropic Drugs - Withdrawal Symptoms and Recommendations** *see page 798*

♦ **Disobrom® [OTC]** *see* Dexbrompheniramine and Pseudoephedrine *on page 158*

♦ **Disodium Cromoglycate** *see* Cromolyn Sodium *on page 142*

♦ ***d*-Isoephedrine Hydrochloride** *see* Pseudoephedrine *on page 478*

♦ **Disonate® [OTC]** *see* Docusate *on page 179*

♦ **Disophrol® Chronotabs® [OTC]** *see* Dexbrompheniramine and Pseudoephedrine *on page 158*

♦ **Disophrol® Tablet [OTC]** *see* Dexbrompheniramine and Pseudoephedrine *on page 158*

## Disopyramide (dye soe PEER a mide)

**U.S. Brand Names** Norpace®

**Pharmacologic Category** Antiarrhythmic Agent, Class I-A

**Use** Suppression and prevention of unifocal and multifocal atrial and premature, ventricular premature complexes, coupled ventricular tachycardia; effective in the conversion of atrial fibrillation, atrial flutter, and paroxysmal atrial tachycardia to normal sinus rhythm and prevention of the recurrence of these arrhythmias after conversion by other methods

**Effects on Mental Status** May cause drowsiness or nervousness; rare reports of depression and psychosis

**Effects on Psychiatric Treatment** Use cautiously with TCAs; may cause AV block or Q-T prolongation; phenobarbital and carbamazepine may decrease the effects of disopyramide via enzyme induction

**Pregnancy Risk Factor** C

**Contraindications** Hypersensitivity to disopyramide or any component; cardiogenic shock; pre-existing second- or third-degree heart block (except in patients with a functioning artificial pacemaker); congenital Q-T syndrome; sick sinus syndrome

**Warnings/Precautions** Monitor and adjust dose to prevent QTc prolongation. Watch for proarrhythmic effects. May precipitate or exacerbate CHF. Due to significant anticholinergic effects, do not use in patients with urinary retention, BPH, glaucoma, or myasthenia gravis. Reduce dosage in renal or hepatic impairment. The extended release form is not recommended for $Cl_{cr}$ <40 mL/minute. In patients with atrial fibrillation or flutter, block the AV node before initiating. Use caution in Wolff-Parkinson-White syndrome or bundle branch block. Correct hypokalemia before initiating therapy. Hypokalemia may worsen toxicity. Monitor closely for hypotension during the initiation of therapy. Avoid concurrent use with other medications with prolong Q-T interval or decrease myocardial contractility.

**Adverse Reactions**

>10%: Genitourinary: Urinary retention/hesitancy

1% to 10%:

Cardiovascular: Chest pains, congestive heart failure, hypotension

Endocrine & metabolic: Hypokalemia

Gastrointestinal: Stomach pain, bloating, xerostomia

Neuromuscular & skeletal: Muscle weakness

Ocular: Blurred vision

<1%: Acute psychosis, anorexia, constipation, depression, diarrhea, dizziness, dry eyes, dry nose, dry throat, dyspnea, elevated liver enzymes, fatigue, flatulence, generalized rashes, headache, hepatic cholestasis, hyperkalemia may enhance toxicities, hypoglycemia, increased cholesterol and triglycerides, malaise, may initiate contractions of pregnant uterus, nausea, nervousness, pain, syncope and conduction disturbances including A-V block, vomiting, weight gain, widening QRS complex and lengthening of Q-T interval

**Overdosage/Toxicology**

Signs and symptoms: Has a low toxic therapeutic ratio and may easily produce fatal intoxication (acute toxic dose: 1 g in adults); symptoms of overdose include sinus bradycardia, sinus node arrest or asystole, P-R, QRS or Q-T interval prolongation, torsade de pointes (polymorphous ventricular tachycardia) and depressed myocardial contractility, which along with alpha-adrenergic or ganglionic blockade, may result in hypotension and pulmonary edema; other effects are anticholinergic (dry mouth, dilated pupils, and delirium) as well as seizures, coma and respiratory arrest.

Treatment: Primarily symptomatic and effects usually respond to conventional therapies (fluids, positioning, vasopressors, anticonvulsants, antiarrhythmics). **Note:** Do not use other type Ia or Ic antiarrhythmic agents to treat ventricular tachycardia; sodium bicarbonate may treat

(Continued)

## Disopyramide *(Continued)*

wide QRS intervals or hypotension; markedly impaired conduction or high degree A-V block, unresponsive to bicarbonate, indicates consideration of a pacemaker.

**Drug Interactions** CYP3A3/4 enzyme substrate

Inhibitors of CYP3A3/4 may increase blood levels

Beta-blockers may cause additive/excessive negative inotropic activity

Drugs which may prolong the Q-T interval include amiodarone, amitriptyline, astemizole, bepridil, cisapride, disopyramide, erythromycin, haloperidol, imipramine, pimozide, quinidine, sotalol, and thioridazine may be additive with disopyramide; use with caution

Enzyme inducers (phenobarbital, phenytoin, rifampin) decrease disopyramide blood levels

Erythromycin and clarithromycin increase disopyramide blood levels; may cause QRS widening and/or Q-T interval prolongation

Procainamide, quinidine, propafenone, or flecainide can cause increased/excessive negative inotropic effects or prolonged conduction

Sparfloxacin, gatifloxacin, and moxifloxacin may result in additional prolongation of the Q-T interval; concurrent use is contraindicated

**Usual Dosage** Oral:

Children:

- <1 year: 10-30 mg/kg/24 hours in 4 divided doses
- 1-4 years: 10-20 mg/kg/24 hours in 4 divided doses
- 4-12 years: 10-15 mg/kg/24 hours in 4 divided doses
- 12-18 years: 6-15 mg/kg/24 hours in 4 divided doses

Adults:

- <50 kg: 100 mg every 6 hours or 200 mg every 12 hours (controlled release)
- >50 kg: 150 mg every 6 hours or 300 mg every 12 hours (controlled release); if no response, increase to 200 mg every 6 hours. Maximum dose required for patients with severe refractory ventricular tachycardia is 400 mg every 6 hours.

**Dosing adjustment in renal impairment:** 100 mg (nonsustained release) given at the following intervals, based on creatinine clearance (mL/minute):

- $Cl_{cr}$ 30-40 mL/minute: Administer every 8 hours
- $Cl_{cr}$ 15-30 mL/minute: Administer every 12 hours
- $Cl_{cr}$ <15 mL/minute: Administer every 24 hours

or alter the dose as follows:

- $Cl_{cr}$ 30-<40 mL/minute: Reduce dose 50%
- $Cl_{cr}$ 15-30 mL/minute: Reduce dose 75%

Dialysis: Not dialyzable (0% to 5%) by hemo- or peritoneal methods; supplemental dose is not necessary.

**Dosing interval in hepatic impairment:** 100 mg every 6 hours or 200 mg every 12 hours (controlled release)

**Patient Information** Take as directed, at regular intervals around-the-clock. Do not alter dosage or discontinue therapy without consulting prescriber. Do not crush or chew extended release form. Avoid (or limit) alcohol and caffeine. You may experience dizziness or blurred vision (use caution when driving or engaging in tasks requiring alertness until response to drug is known); or dry mouth (frequent mouth care or sucking on lozenges may help). Report any change in urinary pattern or difficulty urinating; chest pain, palpitations, irregular heartbeat; unusual cough, difficulty breathing, swelling of extremities; muscle tremors or weakness; confusion or acute lethargy; or skin rash.

**Nursing Implications** Do not crush controlled release capsules

**Dosage Forms**

Capsule, as phosphate: 100 mg, 150 mg

Capsule, sustained action, as phosphate: 100 mg, 150 mg

♦ **Di-Spaz® Injection** *see* Dicyclomine *on page 165*

♦ **Di-Spaz® Oral** *see* Dicyclomine *on page 165*

♦ **Distaval®** *see* Thalidomide *on page 538*

## Disulfiram (dye SUL fi ram)

**Related Information**

Addiction Treatments *on page 772*

Substance-Related Disorders *on page 609*

**Generic Available** Yes

**U.S. Brand Names** Antabuse®

**Pharmacologic Category** Aldehyde Dehydrogenase Inhibitor

**Use** Management of chronic alcoholism

**Effects on Mental Status** Psychotic reactions have been noted

**Pregnancy Risk Factor** C

**Contraindications** Severe myocardial disease and coronary occlusion; psychoses; hypersensitivity to disulfiram and related compounds or any component; patients receiving or using alcohol, metronidazole, paraldehyde, or alcohol-containing preparations like cough syrup or tonics

**Warnings/Precautions** Use with caution in patients with diabetes, hypothyroidism, seizure disorders, nephritis (acute or chronic); hepatic cirrhosis or insufficiency; should never be administered to a patient when he/she is in a state of alcohol intoxication, or without his/her knowledge. Patient must receive appropriate counseling, including information on "disguised" forms of alcohol (tonics, mouthwashes, etc) and the duration of the drug's activity (up to 14 days).

**Adverse Reactions**

Central nervous system: Drowsiness, headache, fatigue, psychosis

Dermatologic: Rash, acneiform eruptions, allergic dermatitis

Gastrointestinal: Metallic or garlic-like aftertaste

Genitourinary: Impotence

Hepatic: Hepatitis

Neuromuscular & skeletal: Peripheral neuritis, polyneuritis, peripheral neuropathy

Ocular: Optic neuritis

**Overdosage/Toxicology** Treatment: Management of disulfiram reaction: Institute support measures to restore blood pressure (pressors and fluids); monitor for hypokalemia

**Drug Interactions** CYP2C9 and 2E1 enzyme inhibitor, both disulfiram and diethyldithiocarbamate (disulfiram metabolite) are CYP3A3/4 inhibitors

Benzodiazepines: Disulfiram may increase serum concentrations of benzodiazepines; includes only benzodiazepines which undergo oxidative metabolism (all but oxazepam, lorazepam, temazepam)

Cocaine: Disulfiram may increase serum concentrations of cocaine; avoid concurrent use

Co-trimoxazole: Intravenous trimethoprim-sulfamethoxazole contains 10% ethanol as a solubilizing agent and may interact with disulfiram; monitor for Antabuse® reaction

CYP2C9 substrates: Potentially, disulfiram may inhibit the metabolism of drugs metabolized by this isoenzyme system, increasing the serum levels/effect; use caution

CYP3A3/4 substrates: Potentially, disulfiram may inhibit the metabolism of drugs metabolized by this isoenzyme system, increasing the serum levels/effect. Some drugs metabolized by this system have been associated with significant toxicity when dosed with inhibitors (including astemizole, benzodiazepines, cisapride, cyclosporine, erythromycin, and statins). Review potential for this interaction and avoid combination when significant toxicity may result from increased levels.

Diphenhydramine: Syrup contains ethanol, avoid use of syrup; monitor for Antabuse® reaction

Ethanol: Disulfiram results in severe ethanol intolerance (Antabuse® reaction) secondary to disulfiram's ability to inhibit aldehyde dehydrogenase; this combination should be avoided. Pharmaceutical products should be evaluated for possible inclusion of ethanol (ie, elixirs, etc).

Isoniazid: Concurrent use with disulfiram may result in adverse CNS effects; this combination should be avoided

MAOIs: Concurrent use with disulfiram may result in adverse CNS effects; this combination should be avoided

Metronidazole: Concurrent use with disulfiram may result in adverse CNS effects; this combination should be avoided

Omeprazole: May cause CNS adverse effects (limited documentation); monitor

Phenytoin: Disulfiram may increase theophylline serum concentrations; toxicity may occur

Theophylline: Disulfiram may increase theophylline serum concentrations; toxicity may occur

Tricyclic antidepressants: Disulfiram may increase adverse CNS effects; monitor for acute changes in mental status

Warfarin: Disulfiram inhibits the metabolism of warfarin resulting in an increased hypoprothombinemic response; avoid when possible or monitor INR closely and adjust warfarin dosage

**Mechanism of Action** Disulfiram is a thiuram derivative which interferes with aldehyde dehydrogenase. When taken concomitantly with alcohol, there is an increase in serum acetaldehyde levels. High acetaldehyde causes uncomfortable symptoms including flushing, nausea, thirst, palpitations, chest pain, vertigo, and hypotension. This reaction is the basis for disulfiram use in postwithdrawal long-term care of alcoholism.

**Pharmacodynamics/kinetics**

Absorption: Rapid from GI tract

Full effect: 12 hours

Metabolism: To diethylthiocarbamate

Duration: May persist for 1-2 weeks after last dose

**Usual Dosage** Adults: Oral: Do not administer until the patient has abstained from alcohol for at least 12 hours

Initial: 500 mg/day as a single dose for 1-2 weeks; maximum daily dose is 500 mg

Average maintenance dose: 250 mg/day; range: 125-500 mg; duration of therapy is to continue until the patient is fully recovered socially and a basis for permanent self control has been established; maintenance therapy may be required for months or even years

**Dietary Considerations** Alcohol: Avoid use, including alcohol-containing products

**Monitoring Parameters** Hypokalemia; liver function tests at baseline and after 10-14 days of treatment

**Reference Range** Peak blood disulfiram level after a 500 mg dose: 0.38 mg/L; peak DDC level is ~1.2 mg/L; peak carbon disulfide level is 14 mg/L; concomitant ethanol levels >0.12 g/dL associated with unconsciousness when ethanol is used with disulfiram

**Test Interactions** Decreases catecholamines (U)

**Patient Information** Do not drink any alcohol, including products containing alcohol (cough and cold syrups), or use alcohol-containing skin products for at least 3 days and preferably 14 days after stopping this medication or while taking this medication; not for treatment of alcohol intoxication; may cause drowsiness; tablets can be crushed or mixed with water

**Nursing Implications** Administration of any medications containing alcohol including topicals is contraindicated

**Dosage Forms** Tablet: 250 mg, 500 mg


- ♦ **Ditropan®** *see* Oxybutynin *on page 412*
- ♦ **Diucardin®** *see* Hydroflumethiazide *on page 275*
- ♦ **Diurigen®** *see* Chlorothiazide *on page 112*
- ♦ **Diuril®** *see* Chlorothiazide *on page 112*
- ♦ **Divalproex Sodium** *see* Valproic Acid and Derivatives *on page 578*
- ♦ **Dizmiss® [OTC]** *see* Meclizine *on page 335*
- ♦ ***dl*-Alpha Tocopherol** *see* Vitamin E *on page 586*
- ♦ ***dl*-Norephedrine Hydrochloride** *see* Phenylpropanolamine *on page 440*
- ♦ ***D*-Mannitol** *see* Mannitol *on page 331*
- ♦ **D-Med® Injection** *see* Methylprednisolone *on page 359*
- ♦ **d-Methorphan** *see* Dextromethorphan *on page 160*
- ♦ **DMSO** *see* Dimethyl Sulfoxide *on page 173*
- ♦ **D-Norgestrel** *see* Levonorgestrel *on page 315*
- ♦ **Doan's®, Original [OTC]** *see* Magnesium Salicylate *on page 331*


## Dobutamine (doe BYOO ta meen)

**U.S. Brand Names** Dobutrex® Injection

**Pharmacologic Category** Adrenergic Agonist Agent

**Use** Short-term management of patients with cardiac decompensation

**Effects on Mental Status** None reported

**Effects on Psychiatric Treatment** None reported

**Usual Dosage** Administration requires the use of an infusion pump; I.V. infusion: See table.

**Infusion Rates of Various Dilutions of Dobutamine**

| Desired Delivery Rate (mcg/kg/min) | Infusion Rate (mL/kg/min) | |
|---|---|---|
| | 250 mg/500 mL diluent (500 mcg/mL) | 500 mg/500 mL diluent (1 mg/mL) |
| 2.5 | 0.005 | 0.0025 |
| 5 | 0.01 | 0.005 |
| 7.5 | 0.015 | 0.0075 |
| 10 | 0.02 | 0.01 |
| 12.5 | 0.025 | 0.0125 |
| 15 | 0.03 | 0.015 |
| 20 | 0.04 | 0.02 |

Neonates: 2-15 mcg/kg/minute, titrate to desired response

Children and Adults: 2.5-20 mcg/kg/minute; maximum: 40 mcg/kg/minute, titrate to desired response

**Dosage Forms** Infusion, as hydrochloride: 12.5 mg/mL (20 mL)


- ♦ **Dobutrex® Injection** *see* Dobutamine *on page 179*


## Docetaxel (doe se TAKS el)

**U.S. Brand Names** Taxotere®

**Pharmacologic Category** Antineoplastic Agent, Natural Source (Plant) Derivative

**Use** Treatment of patients with locally advanced or metastatic breast cancer who have progressed during anthracycline-based therapy or have relapsed during anthracycline-based adjuvant therapy; treatment of patients with locally advanced or metastatic nonsmall cell lung cancer after failure of prior platinum-based chemotherapy

**Unlabeled use:** Treatment of gastric, pancreatic, head and neck, ovarian, soft tissue sarcoma, and melanoma

**Effects on Mental Status** None reported

**Effects on Psychiatric Treatment** May cause leukopenia; use caution with clozapine and carbamazepine

**Usual Dosage** Corticosteroids (oral dexamethasone 8 mg twice daily for 3 days or 5 days starting 1 day prior to docetaxel administration) are necessary to reduce the potential for hypersensitivity and severe fluid retention

Adults: I.V. infusion: Refer to individual protocols:

Locally advanced or metastatic carcinoma of the breast: 60-100 mg/m² over 1 hour every 3 weeks

Dosage adjustment in patients who are initially started at 100 mg/m² (>1 week), cumulative cutaneous reactions, or severe peripheral neuropathy: 75 mg/m²

**Note:** If the patient continues to experience these adverse reactions, the dosage should be reduced to 55 mg/m² or therapy should be discontinued

**Dosing adjustment in hepatic impairment:**

Total bilirubin ≥ the upper limit of normal (ULN), or AST/ALT >1.5 times the ULN concomitant with alkaline phosphatase >2.5 times the ULN: Docetaxel **should not be administered** secondary to increased incidence of treatment-related mortality

**Dosage Forms** Injection: 40 mg/mL (0.5 mL, 2 mL)

## Docusate (DOK yoo sate)

**Related Information**

Laxatives, Classification and Properties *on page 716*

**U.S. Brand Names** Colace® [OTC]; DC 240® Softgels® [OTC]; Dialose® [OTC]; Diocto® [OTC]; Diocto-K® [OTC]; Dioeze® [OTC]; Disonate® [OTC]; DOK® [OTC]; DOS® Softgel® [OTC]; D-S-S® [OTC]; Kasof® [OTC]; Modane® Soft [OTC]; Pro-Cal-Sof® [OTC]; Regulax SS® [OTC]; Sulfalax® [OTC]; Surfak® [OTC]

**Canadian Brand Names** Albert® Docusate; Colax-C®; PMS-Docusate Calcium; Regulex®; Selax®; SoFlax™

**Pharmacologic Category** Stool Softener

**Use** Stool softener in patients who should avoid straining during defecation and constipation associated with hard, dry stools; prophylaxis for straining (Valsalva) following myocardial infarction. A safe agent to be used in elderly; some evidence that doses <200 mg are ineffective; stool softeners are unnecessary if stool is well hydrated or "mushy" and soft; shown to be ineffective used long-term.

**Effects on Mental Status** None reported

**Effects on Psychiatric Treatment** None reported

**Pregnancy Risk Factor** C

**Contraindications** Concomitant use of mineral oil; intestinal obstruction, acute abdominal pain, nausea, vomiting; hypersensitivity to docusate or any component

**Warnings/Precautions** Prolonged, frequent or excessive use may result in dependence or electrolyte imbalance

**Adverse Reactions** 1% to 10%:

Gastrointestinal: Intestinal obstruction, diarrhea, abdominal cramping

Miscellaneous: Throat irritation

**Overdosage/Toxicology**

Signs and symptoms: Abdominal cramps, diarrhea, fluid loss, hypokalemia

Treatment: Symptomatic

**Drug Interactions** Increased toxicity with mineral oil, phenolphthalein

**Usual Dosage** Docusate salts are interchangeable; the amount of sodium, calcium, or potassium per dosage unit is clinically insignificant

Infants and Children <3 years: Oral: 10-40 mg/day in 1-4 divided doses

Children: Oral:

- 3-6 years: 20-60 mg/day in 1-4 divided doses
- 6-12 years: 40-150 mg/day in 1-4 divided doses

Adolescents and Adults: Oral: 50-500 mg/day in 1-4 divided doses

Older Children and Adults: Rectal: Add 50-100 mg of docusate liquid to enema fluid (saline or water); administer as retention or flushing enema

**Patient Information** Docusate should be taken with a full glass of water, milk, or fruit juice. Do not use if abdominal pain, nausea, or vomiting are present. Laxative use should be used for a short period of time (<1 week). Prolonged use may result in abuse, dependence, as well as fluid and electrolyte loss. Report bleeding or if constipation occurs.

**Nursing Implications** Docusate liquid should be given with milk, fruit juice, or infant formula to mask the bitter taste

**Dosage Forms**

Capsule, as calcium:

- DC 240® Softgels®, Pro-Cal-Sof®, Sulfalax®: 240 mg
- Surfak®: 50 mg, 240 mg

Capsule, as potassium:

- Diocto-K®: 100 mg
- Kasof®: 240 mg

Capsule, as sodium:

- Colace®: 50 mg, 100 mg
- Dioeze®: 250 mg
- Disonate®: 100 mg, 240 mg
- DOK®: 100 mg, 250 mg
- DOS® Softgel®: 100 mg, 250 mg
- D-S-S®: 100 mg
- Modane® Soft: 100 mg
- Regulax SS®: 100 mg, 250 mg

Liquid, as sodium (Diocto®, Colace®, Disonate®, DOK®): 150 mg/15 mL (30 mL, 60 mL, 480 mL)

Solution, oral, as sodium (Doxinate®): 50 mg/mL with alcohol 5% (60 mL, 3780 mL)

Syrup, as sodium:

- 50 mg/15 mL (15 mL, 30 mL)

(Continued)

## Docusate *(Continued)*

Colace®, Diocto®, Disonate®, DOK®: 60 mg/15 mL (240 mL, 480 mL, 3780 mL)
Tablet, as sodium (Dialose®): 100 mg

## Dofetilide doe FET il ide

**U.S. Brand Names** Tikosyn™

**Pharmacologic Category** Antiarrhythmic Agent, Class III

**Use** Maintenance of normal sinus rhythm in patients with atrial fibrillation/atrial flutter of longer than 1-week duration who have been converted to normal sinus rhythm; conversion of atrial fibrillation and atrial flutter to normal sinus rhythm

**Effects on Mental Status** Insomnia is common

**Effects on Psychiatric Treatment** Contraindicated with drugs that prolong QTc (phenothiazines, TCAs)

**Pregnancy Risk Factor** C

**Contraindications** Patients with paroxysmal atrial fibrillation; patients with congenital or acquired long Q-T syndromes, do not use if a baseline Q-T interval or QTc is >440 msec (500 msec in patients with ventricular conduction abnormalities); severe renal impairment (estimated $Cl_{cr}$ <20 mL/minute); concurrent use with verapamil, cimetidine, trimethoprim (alone or in combination with sulfamethoxazole), ketoconazole, prochlorperazine, or megestrol; known hypersensitivity to dofetilide, baseline heart rate <50 beats/minute; other drugs that prolong Q-T intervals (phenothiazines, cisapride, bepridil, tricyclic antidepressants, certain oral macrolides: sparfloxacin, gatifloxacin, moxifloxacin); hypokalemia or hypomagnesemia; concurrent amiodarone

**Warnings/Precautions Note: Must be initiated (or reinitiated) in a setting with continuous monitoring and staff familiar with the recognition and treatment of life-threatening arrhythmias. Patients must be monitored with continuous EKG for a minimum of 3 days, or for a minimum of 12 hours after electrical or pharmacological cardioversion to normal sinus rhythm, whichever is greater. Patients should be readmitted for continuous monitoring if dosage is later increased.**

Reserve for patients who are highly symptomatic with atrial fibrillation/atrial flutter; torsade de pointes significantly increases with doses >500 mcg twice daily; hold Class Ia or Class II antiarrhythmics for at least three half-lives prior to starting dofetilide; use in patients on amiodarone therapy only if serum amiodarone level is <0.3 mg/L or if amiodarone was stopped for >3 months previously; correct hypokalemia or hypomagnesemia before initiating dofetilide and maintain within normal limits during treatment.

Patients with sick sinus syndrome or with second or third-degree heart block should not receive dofetilide unless a functional pacemaker is in place. Defibrillation threshold is reduced in patients with ventricular tachycardia or ventricular fibrillation undergoing implantation of a cardioverter-defibrillator device. Safety and efficacy in children (<18 years old) have not been established. Use with caution in renal impairment; not recommended in patients receiving drugs which may compete for renal secretion via cationic transport. Use with caution in patients with severe hepatic impairment.

**Adverse Reactions**

**Supraventricular arrhythmia patients** (incidence > placebo)

>10%: Central nervous system: Headache (11%)

2% to 10%:
- Central nervous system: Dizziness (8%), insomnia (4%)
- Cardiovascular: Ventricular tachycardia (2.6% to 3.7%), chest pain (10%), torsade de pointes (3.3% in CHF patients and 0.9% in patients with a recent MI; up to 10.5% in patients receiving doses in excess of those recommended). Torsade de pointes occurs most frequently within the first 3 days of therapy.
- Dermatologic: Rash (3%)
- Gastrointestinal: Nausea (5%), diarrhea (3%), abdominal pain (3%)
- Neuromuscular & skeletal: Back pain (3%)
- Respiratory: Dyspnea (6%), respiratory tract infection (7%)
- Miscellaneous: Flu syndrome (4%)

<2%:
- Central nervous system: CVA, facial paralysis, flaccid paralysis, migraine, paralysis
- Cardiovascular: AV block (0.4% to 1.5%), ventricular fibrillation (0% to 0.4%), bundle branch block, heart block, edema, heart arrest, myocardial infarct, sudden death, syncope
- Dermatologic: Angioedema
- Gastrointestinal: Liver damage
- Neuromuscular & skeletal: Paresthesia
- Respiratory: Cough

>2% (incidence ≤ placebo): Anxiety, pain, angina, atrial fibrillation, hypertension, palpitation, supraventricular tachycardia, peripheral edema, urinary tract infection, weakness, arthralgia, sweating

**Overdosage/Toxicology** The major dose-related toxicity is torsade de pointes. Treatment should be symptomatic and supportive. Watch for excessive prolongation of the Q-T interval in overdose situations. Continuous cardiac monitoring is necessary. A charcoal slurry is helpful when given early (15 minutes) after the overdose. Isoproterenol infusion into anesthetized dogs with cardiac pacing corrects the atrial and ventricular effective refractory periods caused by dofetilide. General treatment measures, override pacing, and magnesium therapy appear to be effective in the management of dofetilide-induced torsade de pointes.

**Drug Interactions** CYP3A3/4 enzyme substrate (minor).

Inhibitors of CYP3A3/4 (erythromycin, clarithromycin, azole antifungal agents, protease inhibitors, serotonin reuptake inhibitors, amiodarone, cannabinoids, diltiazem, grapefruit juice, nefazodone, norfloxacin, quinine, zafirlukast) should be used cautiously as they may increase dofetilide levels

Cimetidine, a cation transport system inhibitor, inhibits dofetilide's elimination and can cause a 58% increase in dofetilide's plasma levels; concomitant use is contraindicated

Diuretics and other drugs (aminoglycosides) which deplete potassium or magnesium may increase dofetilide toxicity (torsade de pointes)

Drugs which have been reported **not** to affect dofetilide include digoxin, amlodipine, phenytoin, glyburide, ranitidine, omeprazole, hormone replacement therapy (conjugated estrogens/medroxyprogesterone), antacid (aluminum/magnesium hydroxide), and theophylline

Drugs which prolong Q-T interval (including bepridil, cisapride, erythromycin, tricyclic antidepressants, phenothiazines, sparfloxacin, gatifloxacin, moxifloxacin): Use is contraindicated

Ketoconazole increases dofetilide's $C_{max}$ (53% males, 97% females) and the AUC (41% males, 69% females) when used concurrently; concomitant use is contraindicated

Renal cationic transport inhibitors (including triamterene, metformin, amiloride, prochlorperazine, megestrol) may increase dofetilide levels; coadminister with caution

Trimethoprim (alone or in combination with sulfamethoxazole) increases dofetilide's $C_{max}$ (103%) and AUC (93%); concomitant use is contraindicated

Verapamil causes an increase in dofetilide's peak plasma levels by 42%. In the supraventricular arrhythmia and a higher incidence of torsade de pointes was seen in patients on verapamil; concomitant use is contraindicated

**Usual Dosage** Adults: Oral:

**Note:** QTc must be determined prior to first dose (see Contraindications and Warnings/Precautions)

Initial: 500 mcg orally twice daily. Initial dosage must be adjusted in patients with estimated $Cl_{cr}$ <60 mL/minute. Dofetilide may be initiated at lower doses than recommended based on physician discretion.

Modification of dosage in response to initial dose:

QTc interval should be measured 2-3 hours after the initial dose. If the QTc >15% of baseline, or if the QTc is >500 msec (550 msec in patients with ventricular conduction abnormalities) dofetilide should be adjusted. If the starting dose is 500 mcg twice daily, then adjust to 250 mcg twice daily. If the starting dose was 250 mcg twice daily, then adjust to 125 mcg twice daily. If the starting dose was 125 mcg twice daily then adjust to 125 mcg every day.

Continued monitoring for doses 2-5:

QTc interval must be determined 2-3 hours after each subsequent dose of dofetilide for in-hospital doses 2-5. If the measured QTc is >500 msec (550 msec in patients with ventricular conduction abnormalities) dofetilide should be stopped.

**Dosage adjustment in renal impairment:**
- $Cl_{cr}$ >60 mL/minute: Administer 500 mcg twice daily
- $Cl_{cr}$ 40-60 mL/minute: Administer 250 mcg twice daily
- $Cl_{cr}$ 20-39 mL/minute: Administer 125 mcg twice daily
- $Cl_{cr}$ <20 mL/minute: Contraindicated in this group

**Elderly:** No specific dosage adjustments are recommended based on age; however, careful assessment of renal function is particularly important in this population

**Dosage adjustment in hepatic impairment:** No dosage adjustments required in Child-Pugh Class A and B; patients with severe hepatic impairment were not studied

**Patient Information** Take with or without food; take exactly the way it was prescribed; do not stop this medicine without talking with your physician; never take an extra dose; if you miss a dose just take your normal amount at the next scheduled time. If you take more medicine than you should call your physician now. If you cannot reach your physician, go to the nearest emergency room (take your medicine with you). Tell your physician about any new medicines before taking them; not all medicines mix well with this one. Call your physician now if you faint, become dizzy, have fast heartbeats, severe diarrhea, unusual sweating, vomiting, no appetite, or more thirst than normal. You may feel tired, weak, or have numbness, tingling, muscle cramps, constipation, vomiting, or rapid heartbeats if you have a low potassium level.

**Nursing Implications** Patient must be carefully instructed concerning how to take this medicine, what to do if a dose is missed, and the recognition of serious adverse events. Patients should be cautioned not to stop taking this medication without talking with their physician. Measure QTc as outlined in dosing information and discuss results with physician, monitor EKG for any tachyarrhythmias, and monitor for changes in renal function and signs/symptoms of electrolyte imbalance.

**Dosage Forms** Capsule: 125 mcg, 250 mcg, 500 mcg

- **DOK® [OTC]** *see* Docusate *on page 179*
- **Dolacet®** *see* Hydrocodone and Acetaminophen *on page 272*

## Dolasetron (dol A se tron)

**U.S. Brand Names** Anzemet®

**Pharmacologic Category** Selective 5-$HT_3$ Receptor Antagonist

**Use** Prevention of nausea and vomiting associated with emetogenic cancer chemotherapy, including initial and repeat courses; prevention of postoperative nausea and vomiting and treatment of postoperative nausea and vomiting (injectable form only)

**Effects on Mental Status** May cause drowsiness or dizziness

**Effects on Psychiatric Treatment** None reported

**Pregnancy Risk Factor** B

**Contraindications** Patients known to have hypersensitivity to the drug

**Warnings/Precautions** Dolasetron should be administered with caution in patients who have or may develop prolongation of cardiac conduction intervals, particularly $QT_c$ intervals. These include patients with hypokalemia or hypomagnesemia, patients taking diuretics with potential for inducing electrolyte abnormalities, patients with congenital Q-T syndrome, patients taking antiarrhythmic drugs or other drugs which lead to Q-T prolongation, and cumulative high-dose anthracycline therapy.

**Adverse Reactions** Dolasetron can cause electrocardiographic interval changes, which are related in frequency and magnitude to blood levels of the metabolite, hydrodolasetron

>2%:
- Cardiovascular: Hypertension
- Central nervous system: Headache, fatigue, dizziness, fever, chills and shivering
- Gastrointestinal: Diarrhea, abdominal pain
- Genitourinary: Urinary retention
- Hepatic: Transient increases in liver enzymes

**Overdosage/Toxicology**

Signs and symptoms: In animal toxicity studies, doses 6.3-12.6 times the recommended human dose based upon surface area were lethal and symptoms of acute poisoning included tremors, depression, and convulsions

Treatment: There is no known specific antidote for dolasetron and patients with suspected overdose should be managed with supportive therapy

**Drug Interactions** CYP2D6 and 3A3/4 enzyme substrate

Blood levels of the active metabolite are increased when dolasetron is coadministered with cimetidine, decreased with rifampin. Clearance of hydrodolasetron decreases when dolasetron is given with atenolol.

**Usual Dosage**

Children <2 years: Not recommended for use

Nausea and vomiting associated with chemotherapy (including initial and repeat courses):
- Children 2-16 years:
  - Oral: 1.8 mg/kg within 1 hour before chemotherapy; maximum: 100 mg/dose
  - I.V.: 1.8 mg/kg ~30 minutes before chemotherapy; maximum: 100 mg/dose
- Adults:
  - Oral: 100 mg within 1 hour before chemotherapy
  - I.V.: 1.8 mg/kg ~30 minutes before chemotherapy or may give 100 mg

Prevention of postoperative nausea and vomiting:
- Children 2-16 years:
  - Oral: 1.2 mg within 2 hours before surgery; maximum: 100 mg/dose
  - I.V.: 0.35 mg/kg (maximum: 12.5 mg) ~15 minutes before stopping anesthesia
- Adults:
  - Oral: 100 mg within 2 hours before surgery
  - I.V.: 12.5 mg ~15 minutes before stopping anesthesia

Treatment of postoperative nausea and vomiting: I.V. only:
- Children 2-16 years: 0.35 mg/kg as soon as needed
- Adults: 12.5 mg as soon as needed

**Dosing adjustment for elderly, renal/hepatic impairment:** No dosage adjustment is recommended

**Patient Information** This drug is given to reduce the incidence of nausea and vomiting. You may experience headache, drowsiness, or dizziness; request assistance when getting up or changing position and do not perform activities requiring alertness. Report immediately unusual pain, chills, or fever; severe headache or diarrhea; chest pain, palpitations, or tightness; swelling of throat or feeling of tightness in throat; or difficulty urinating.

**Nursing Implications** Dolasetron injection may be diluted in apple or apple-grape juice and taken orally

**Dosage Forms**

Injection, as mesylate: 20 mg/mL (0.625 mL, 5 mL)

Tablet, as mesylate: 50 mg, 100 mg

- **Dolene®** *see* Propoxyphene *on page 474*
- **Dolobid®** *see* Diflunisal *on page 168*
- **Dolophine®** *see* Methadone *on page 349*
- **Dolorac™ [OTC]** *see* Capsaicin *on page 89*
- **Domeboro® Topical [OTC]** *see* Aluminum Sulfate and Calcium Acetate *on page 28*

## Donepezil (don EH pa zil)

**Related Information**

Special Populations - Elderly *on page 662*

**U.S. Brand Names** Aricept®

**Synonyms** E2020

**Pharmacologic Category** Acetylcholinesterase Inhibitor; Cholinergic Agonist

**Use** Treatment of mild to moderate dementia of the Alzheimer's type

**Pregnancy Risk Factor** C

**Contraindications** Hypersensitivity to donepezil or piperidine derivatives

**Warnings/Precautions** Use with caution in patients with sick sinus syndrome or other supraventricular cardiac conduction abnormalities, in patients with seizures, COPD, or asthma; avoid use in nursing mothers. Use with caution in patients at risk of ulcer disease (ie, previous history of NSAID use), or in patients with bladder outlet obstruction. May cause diarrhea, nausea, and/or vomiting, which may be dose-related.

**Adverse Reactions**

>10%:
- Central nervous system: Headache
- Gastrointestinal: Nausea, diarrhea

1% to 10%:
- Cardiovascular: Syncope, chest pain, hypertension, atrial fibrillation, hypotension, hot flashes
- Central nervous system: Abnormal dreams, depression, dizziness, fatigue, insomnia, somnolence
- Dermatologic: Bruising
- Gastrointestinal: Anorexia, vomiting, weight loss, fecal incontinence, GI bleeding, bloating, epigastric pain
- Genitourinary: Frequent urination
- Neuromuscular & skeletal: Muscle cramps, arthritis, body pain

<1%: Abdominal pain, agitation, cholecystitis, confusion, convulsions, hallucinations, heart block, hemolytic anemia, hyponatremia, pancreatitis, rash

**Overdosage/Toxicology**

Signs and symptoms (seen in animals): Include reduced spontaneous movement, prone position, staggering gait, lacrimation, clonic convulsions, depressed respiration, salivation, miosis, tremors, fasciculations, and lower body surface temperature

Treatment: Includes general supportive measures. Tertiary anticholinergics, such as atropine, may be used as an antidote for overdosage. I.V. atropine sulfate titrated to effect is recommended; initial dose of 1 to 2 mg I.V. with subsequent doses based upon clinical response. Atypical increases in blood pressure and heart rate have been reported with other cholinomimetics when coadministered with quaternary anticholinergics such as glycopyrrolate.

**Drug Interactions** CYP2D6 and 3A3/4 enzyme substrate

Anticholinergic agents: Effects of donepezil may be inhibited by anticholinergic agents (benztropine)

Cholinergic agents: A synergistic effect may be seen with concurrent administration of succinylcholine or cholinergic agonists (bethanechol); excessive cholinergic stimulation and toxicity may occur; use caution

CYP2D6 inhibitors: Serum level and/or toxicity of donepezil may be increased; inhibitors include amiodarone, cimetidine, delavirdine, fluoxetine, paroxetine, propafenone, quinidine, and ritonavir; monitor for increased effect/toxicity

CYP3A3/4 inhibitors: Serum level and/or toxicity of donepezil may be increased; inhibitors include amiodarone, cimetidine, clarithromycin, erythromycin, delavirdine, diltiazem, dirithromycin, disulfiram, fluoxetine, fluvoxamine, grapefruit juice, indinavir, itraconazole, ketoconazole, metronidazole, nefazodone, nevirapine, propoxyfene, quinupristin-dalfopristin, ritonavir, saquinavir, verapamil, zafirlukast, zileuton; ketoconazole and quinidine inhibit donepezil's metabolism in vitro; monitor for altered clinical response

Enzyme inducers: Inducers of cytochrome P-450 enzymes may increase the rate of elimination of donepezil; monitor for altered clinical response; includes phenytoin, carbamazepine, dexamethasone, rifampin, and phenobarbital

**Mechanism of Action** Alzheimer's disease is characterized by cholinergic deficiency in the cortex and basal forebrain, which contributes to cognitive deficits. Donepezil reversibly and noncompetitively inhibits centrally-active acetylcholinesterase, the enzyme responsible for hydrolysis of acetylcholine. This appears to result in increased concentrations of acetylcholine available for synaptic transmission in the central nervous system.

**Pharmacodynamics/kinetics**

Absorption: Well absorbed

Protein binding: 96% mainly to albumin (75%) and $alpha_1$ acid glycoprotein (21%)

Metabolism: By CYP450 isoenzymes 2D6 and 3A4 and undergoes glucuronidation

Bioavailability: 100%

(Continued)

## Donepezil *(Continued)*

Half-life: 70 hours
Steady-state: 15 days
Time to peak plasma concentration: 3-4 hours
Elimination: Unchanged in urine and extensively metabolized to four major metabolites, two of which are active

**Usual Dosage** Adults: Initial: 5 mg/day at bedtime; may increase to 10 mg/day at bedtime after 4-6 weeks

**Monitoring Parameters** Behavior, mood, bowel function

**Patient Information** May be taken with or without food; donepezil is not a cure for Alzheimer's disease, but may slow the progression of symptoms

**Additional Information** Donepezil does not significantly elevate liver enzymes

**Dosage Forms** Tablet: 5 mg, 10 mg

♦ **Donnamar®** *see* Hyoscyamine *on page 279*

♦ **Donnapectolin-PG®** *see* Hyoscyamine, Atropine, Scopolamine, Kaolin, Pectin, and Opium *on page 280*

♦ **Donnatal®** *see* Hyoscyamine, Atropine, Scopolamine, and Phenobarbital *on page 279*

## Dopamine (DOE pa meen)

**U.S. Brand Names** Intropin® Injection

**Pharmacologic Category** Adrenergic Agonist Agent

**Use** Adjunct in the treatment of shock which persists after adequate fluid volume replacement

**Effects on Mental Status** None reported

**Effects on Psychiatric Treatment** Dopamine's effects may be enhanced by MAO inhibitors

**Usual Dosage** I.V. infusion (administration requires the use of an infusion pump):

Neonates: 1-20 mcg/kg/minute continuous infusion, titrate to desired response

Children: 1-20 mcg/kg/minute, maximum: 50 mcg/kg/minute continuous infusion, titrate to desired response

Adults: 1-5 mcg/kg/minute up to 50 mcg/kg/minute, titrate to desired response; infusion may be increased by 1-4 mcg/kg/minute at 10- to 30-minute intervals until optimal response is obtained

If dosages >20-30 mcg/kg/minute are needed, a more direct-acting pressor may be more beneficial (ie, epinephrine, norepinephrine)

**The hemodynamic effects of dopamine are dose-dependent:**

Low-dose: 1-3 mcg/kg/minute, increased renal blood flow and urine output

Intermediate-dose: 3-10 mcg/kg/minute, increased renal blood flow, heart rate, cardiac contractility, and cardiac output

High-dose: >10 mcg/kg/minute, alpha-adrenergic effects begin to predominate, vasoconstriction, increased blood pressure

**Dosage Forms**

Infusion, as hydrochloride, in $D_5W$: 0.8 mg/mL (250 mL, 500 mL); 1.6 mg/mL (250 mL, 500 mL); 3.2 mg/mL (250 mL, 500 mL)

Injection, as hydrochloride: 40 mg/mL (5 mL, 10 mL, 20 mL); 80 mg/mL (5 mL, 20 mL); 160 mg/mL (5 mL)

♦ **Dopar®** *see* Levodopa *on page 312*

♦ **Dopram® Injection** *see* Doxapram *on page 182*

♦ **Doral®** *see* Quazepam *on page 482*

♦ **Dormarex® 2 Oral [OTC]** *see* Diphenhydramine *on page 174*

♦ **Dormin® Oral [OTC]** *see* Diphenhydramine *on page 174*

## Dornase Alfa (DOOR nase AL fa)

**U.S. Brand Names** Pulmozyme®

**Pharmacologic Category** Enzyme

**Use** Management of cystic fibrosis patients to reduce the frequency of respiratory infections that require parenteral antibiotics, and to improve pulmonary function; has also demonstrated value in the treatment of chronic bronchitis

**Effects on Mental Status** None reported

**Effects on Psychiatric Treatment** None reported

**Usual Dosage** Children >5 years and Adults: Inhalation: 2.5 mg once daily through selected nebulizers in conjunction with a Pulmo-Aide® or a Pari-Proneb® compressor

**Dosage Forms** Solution, inhalation: 1 mg/mL (2.5 mL)

♦ **Dornomyl®** *see* Doxylamine *on page 186*

♦ **Doryx® Oral** *see* Doxycycline *on page 186*

## Dorzolamide (dor ZOLE a mide)

**Related Information**

Glaucoma Drug Therapy *on page 712*

**U.S. Brand Names** Trusopt®

**Pharmacologic Category** Carbonic Anhydrase Inhibitor; Ophthalmic Agent, Antiglaucoma

**Use** Lowers intraocular pressure to treat glaucoma in patients with ocular hypertension or open-angle glaucoma

**Effects on Mental Status** May cause drowsiness

**Effects on Psychiatric Treatment** None reported

**Usual Dosage** Adults: Glaucoma: Instill 1 drop in the affected eye(s) 3 times/day

**Dosage Forms** Solution, ophthalmic, as hydrochloride: 2%

## Dorzolamide and Timolol (dor ZOLE a mide & TYE moe lole)

**U.S. Brand Names** Cosopt™

**Pharmacologic Category** Beta Blocker; Carbonic Anhydrase Inhibitor

**Use** Lowers intraocular pressure to treat glaucoma in patients with ocular hypertension or open-angle glaucoma

**Effects on Mental Status** May cause drowsiness, dizziness, or fatigue; may rarely cause anxiety, depression, or hallucinations

**Effects on Psychiatric Treatment** Barbiturates and carbamazepine may decrease the effects of beta-blockers

**Usual Dosage** Adults: ophthalmic: One drop in eye(s) twice daily

**Dosage Forms** Solution, ophthalmic: Dorzolamide 2% and timolol 0.5% (5 mL, 10 mL)

♦ **DOS® Softgel® [OTC]** *see* Docusate *on page 179*

♦ **Dostinex®** *see* Cabergoline *on page 82*

♦ **Dovonex®** *see* Calcipotriene *on page 83*

## Doxacurium (doks a KYOO ri um)

**U.S. Brand Names** Nuromax® Injection

**Pharmacologic Category** Neuromuscular Blocker Agent, Nondepolarizing

**Use** Adjunct to general anesthesia; provides skeletal muscle relaxation during surgery. Doxacurium is a long-acting nondepolarizing neuromuscular blocker with virtually no cardiovascular side effects. The characteristics of this agent make it especially useful in procedures requiring careful maintenance of hemodynamic stability for prolonged periods.

**Effects on Mental Status** None reported

**Effects on Psychiatric Treatment** May decrease neuromuscular blockade, whereas lithium may increase it

**Usual Dosage** I.V. (in obese patients, use ideal body weight to calculate dose):

Children >2 years: Initial: 0.03-0.05 mg/kg followed by maintenance doses of 0.005-0.01 mg/kg after 30-45 minutes

Adults: Surgery: 0.05 mg/kg with thiopental/narcotic or 0.025 mg/kg with succinylcholine; maintenance doses of 0.005-0.01 mg/kg after 60-100 minutes

**Dosing adjustment in renal or hepatic impairment:** Reduce initial dose and titrate carefully as duration may be prolonged

**Dosage Forms** Injection, as chloride: 1 mg/mL (5 mL)

## Doxapram (DOKS a pram)

**U.S. Brand Names** Dopram® Injection

**Pharmacologic Category** Respiratory Stimulant; Stimulant

**Use** Respiratory and CNS stimulant; stimulates respiration in patients with drug-induced CNS depression or postanesthesia respiratory depression; in hospitalized patients with COPD associated with acute hypercapnia

**Effects on Mental Status** May cause CNS stimulation, restlessness, irritability, or hallucinations

**Effects on Psychiatric Treatment** May cause hypertensive crisis if used with MAOIs

**Pregnancy Risk Factor** B

**Contraindications** Hypersensitivity to doxapram or any component; epilepsy, cerebral edema, head injury, severe pulmonary disease, pheochromocytoma, cardiovascular disease, hypertension, hyperthyroidism

**Warnings/Precautions** May cause severe CNS toxicity, seizures. Should be used with caution in newborns as the U.S. product contains benzyl alcohol (0.9%). Doxapram is neither a nonspecific CNS depressant antagonist nor an opiate antagonist.

**Adverse Reactions** 1% to 10%:

Cardiovascular: Ectopic beats, hypotension, vasoconstriction, tachycardia, anginal pain, palpitations
Central nervous system: Headache
Gastrointestinal: Nausea, vomiting
Respiratory: Dyspnea

**Overdosage/Toxicology**
Signs and symptoms: Excessive increases in blood pressure, tachycardia, arrhythmias, muscle spasticity, dyspnea
Treatment: Supportive care is the preferred treatment; seizures are unlikely and can be treated with benzodiazepines; **doxapram is not dialyzable.**

**Drug Interactions** Increased toxicity (elevated blood pressure): Sympathomimetics, MAO inhibitors

Halothane, cyclopropane, and enflurane may sensitize the myocardium to catecholamine and epinephrine which is released at the initiation of doxapram, hence, separate discontinuation of anesthetics and start of doxapram by at least 10 minutes

**Usual Dosage** Not for use in newborns since doxapram contains a significant amount of benzyl alcohol (0.9%)

Neonatal apnea (apnea of prematurity): I.V.:
Initial: 1-1.5 mg/kg/hour
Maintenance: 0.5-2.5 mg/kg/hour, titrated to the lowest rate at which apnea is controlled
Adults: Respiratory depression following anesthesia: I.V.:
Initial: 0.5-1 mg/kg; may repeat at 5-minute intervals; maximum total dose: 2 mg/kg
I.V. infusion: Initial: 5 mg/minute until adequate response or adverse effects seen; decrease to 1-3 mg/minute; usual total dose: 0.5-4 mg/kg; maximum: 300 mg
Hemodialysis: Not dialyzable

**Patient Information** This drug is generally used in an emergency. Teaching should be appropriate to patient education. Someone will be observing response at all times.

**Dosage Forms** Injection, as hydrochloride: 20 mg/mL (20 mL)

## Doxazosin (doks AYE zoe sin)

**Related Information**
Pharmacotherapy of Urinary Incontinence *on page 758*

**U.S. Brand Names** Cardura®

**Pharmacologic Category** Alpha$_1$ Blockers

**Use** Treatment of hypertension alone or in conjunction with diuretics, cardiac glycosides, ACE inhibitors, or calcium antagonists (particularly appropriate for those with hypertension and other cardiovascular risk factors such as hypercholesterolemia and diabetes mellitus); treatment of urinary outflow obstruction and/or obstructive and irritative symptoms associated with benign prostatic hyperplasia (particularly useful in patients with troublesome symptoms who are unable or unwilling to undergo invasive procedures, but who require rapid symptomatic relief)

**Effects on Mental Status** Dizziness is common; may cause anxiety, nervousness, or sedation; rarely may cause depression

**Effects on Psychiatric Treatment** Psychotropics may potentiate the hypotensive effects of doxazosin

**Pregnancy Risk Factor** C

**Contraindications** Hypersensitivity to quinazolines (doxazosin, prazosin, terazosin) or any component

**Warnings/Precautions** Can cause significant orthostatic hypotension and syncope, especially with first dose. Prostate cancer should be ruled out before starting for BPH. May need dosage adjustment in severe hepatic dysfunction. Anticipate a similar effect if therapy is interrupted for a few days, if dosage is rapidly increased, or if another antihypertensive drug is introduced.

**Adverse Reactions**
>10%: Central nervous system: Dizziness
1% to 10%:
Cardiovascular: Palpitations, arrhythmia
Central nervous system: Vertigo, nervousness, somnolence, anxiety
Endocrine & metabolic: Decreased libido
Gastrointestinal: Nausea, vomiting, xerostomia, diarrhea, constipation
Neuromuscular & skeletal: Shoulder, neck, back pain
Ocular: Abnormal vision
Respiratory: Rhinitis
<1%: Abdominal discomfort, conjunctivitis, depression, dyspnea, epistaxis, flatulence, hypotension, incontinence, polyuria, sinusitis, tachycardia, tinnitus

**Overdosage/Toxicology**
Signs and symptoms: Severe hypotension, drowsiness, tachycardia
Treatment: Hypotension usually responds to I.V. fluids, Trendelenburg positioning, or parenteral vasoconstrictor; treatment is primarily supportive and symptomatic.

**Drug Interactions**
ACE inhibitors: Hypotensive effect may be increased
Beta-blockers: Hypotensive effect may be increased
Calcium channel blockers: Hypotensive effect may be increased
NSAIDs may reduce antihypertensive efficacy

**Usual Dosage** Oral:
Adults: 1 mg once daily in morning or evening; may be increased to 2 mg once daily. Thereafter titrate upwards, if needed, over several weeks, balancing therapeutic benefit with doxazosin-induced postural hypotension
Hypertension: Maximum dose: 16 mg/day
BPH: Maximum dose: 8 mg/day.
Elderly: Initial: 0.5 mg once daily

**Patient Information** Take as directed, at bedtime. Do not skip dose or discontinue without consulting prescriber. Follow recommended diet and exercise program. Do not use OTC medications which may affect blood pressure (eg, cough or cold remedies, diet pills, stay-awake medications) without consulting prescriber. This medication may cause drowsiness, dizziness, or impaired judgment (use caution when driving or engaging in tasks that require alertness until response to drug is known); postural hypotension (use caution when rising from sitting or lying position or when climbing stairs); or dry mouth or nausea (frequent mouth care or sucking lozenges may help). Report increased nervousness or depression; sudden weight gain (weigh yourself in the same clothes at the same time of day once a week); unusual or persistent swelling of ankles, feet, or extremities; palpitations or rapid heartbeat; muscle weakness, fatigue, or pain; or other persistent side effects.

**Nursing Implications** Syncope may occur usually within 90 minutes of the initial dose

**Dosage Forms** Tablet: 1 mg, 2 mg, 4 mg, 8 mg

## Doxepin (DOKS e pin)

**Related Information**
Antidepressant Agents Comparison Chart *on page 704*
Clinical Issues in the Use of Antidepressants *on page 627*
Discontinuation of Psychotropic Drugs - Withdrawal Symptoms and Recommendations *on page 798*
Federal OBRA Regulations Recommended Maximum Doses *on page 756*
Patient Information - Antidepressants (TCAs) *on page 640*
Substance-Related Disorders *on page 609*
Teratogenic Risks of Psychotropic Medications *on page 812*

**Generic Available** Yes

**U.S. Brand Names** Adapin® Oral; Sinequan® Oral; Zonalon® Topical Cream

**Canadian Brand Names** Apo®-Doxepin; Novo-Doxepin; Triadapin®

**Synonyms** Doxepin Hydrochloride

**Pharmacologic Category** Antidepressant, Tricyclic (Tertiary Amine); Topical Skin Product

**Use** Depression and/or anxiety
**Unlabeled use:** Analgesic for certain chronic and neuropathic pain
Topical: Short-term (<8 days) management of moderate pruritus in adults with atopic dermatitis or lichen simplex chronicus

**Pregnancy Risk Factor** C

**Contraindications** Hypersensitivity to this drug and similar chemical class; narrow angle glaucoma; urinary retention; use of monoamine oxidase inhibitors within 14 days; use in a patient during the acute recovery phase of MI

**Warnings/Precautions** Often causes sedation, which may result in impaired performance of tasks requiring alertness (ie, operating machinery or driving). Sedative effects may be additive with other CNS depressants and/or ethanol. The degree of sedation is very high relative to other antidepressants. May worsen psychosis in some patients or precipitate a shift to mania or hypomania in patients with bipolar disease. May increase the risks associated with electroconvulsive therapy. This agent should be discontinued, when possible, prior to elective surgery. Therapy should not be abruptly discontinued in patients receiving high doses for prolonged periods.

May cause orthostatic hypotension (risk is moderate relative to other antidepressants) - use with caution in patients at risk of hypotension or in patients where transient hypotensive episodes would be poorly tolerated (cardiovascular disease or cerebrovascular disease). The degree of anticholinergic blockade produced by this agent is high relative to other cyclic antidepressants - use caution in patients with benign prostatic hypertrophy, xerostomia, visual problems, constipation, or history of bowel obstruction.

Use caution in patients with depression, particularly if suicidal risk may be present. Use with caution in patients with a history of cardiovascular disease (including previous MI, stroke, tachycardia, or conduction abnormalities). The risk conduction abnormalities with this agent is moderate relative to other antidepressants. Use caution in patients with a previous seizure disorder or condition predisposing to seizures such as brain damage, alcoholism, or concurrent therapy with other drugs which lower the seizure threshold. Use with caution in hyperthyroid patients or those receiving thyroid supplementation. Use with caution in patients with hepatic or renal dysfunction and in elderly patients. Use in children <12 years of age has not been established.

**Adverse Reactions**
Cardiovascular: Hypotension, hypertension, tachycardia
Central nervous system: Drowsiness, dizziness, headache, disorientation, ataxia, confusion, seizure
Dermatologic: Alopecia, photosensitivity, rash, pruritus
(Continued)

## Doxepin *(Continued)*

Endocrine & metabolic: Breast enlargement, galactorrhea, SIADH, increase or decrease in blood sugar, increased or decreased libido
Gastrointestinal: Xerostomia, constipation, vomiting, indigestion, anorexia, aphthous stomatitis, nausea, unpleasant taste, weight gain, diarrhea, trouble with gums, decreased lower esophageal sphincter tone may cause GE reflux
Genitourinary: Urinary retention, testicular edema
Hematologic: Agranulocytosis, leukopenia, eosinophilia, thrombocytopenia, purpura
Neuromuscular & skeletal: Weakness, tremors, numbness, paresthesia, extrapyramidal symptoms, tardive dyskinesia
Ocular: Blurred vision
Otic: Tinnitus
Miscellaneous: Diaphoresis (excessive), allergic reactions

**Overdosage/Toxicology**
Signs and symptoms: Confusion, hallucinations, seizures, urinary retention, hypothermia, hypotension, tachycardia, cyanosis
Treatment:
Following initiation of essential overdose management, toxic symptoms should be treated
Ventricular arrhythmias often respond to systemic alkalinization with or without phenytoin 15-20 mg/kg (adults) (sodium bicarbonate 0.5-2 mEq/kg I.V.). Arrhythmias unresponsive to this therapy may respond to lidocaine 1 mg/kg I.V. followed by a titrated infusion. Physostigmine (1-2 mg I.V. slowly for adults or 0.5 mg I.V. slowly for children) may be indicated in reversing cardiac arrhythmias that are life-threatening,
Seizures usually respond to diazepam I.V. boluses (5-10 mg for adults up to 30 mg or 0.25-0.4 mg/kg/dose for children up to 10 mg/dose). If seizures are unresponsive or recur, phenytoin or phenobarbital may be required.

**Drug Interactions** CYP2D6 enzyme substrate
Altretamine: Concurrent use may cause orthostatic hypertension
Amphetamines: TCAs may enhance the effect of amphetamines; monitor for adverse CV effects
Anticholinergics: Combined use with TCAs may produce additive anticholinergic effects
Antihypertensives: TCAs may inhibit the antihypertensive response to bethanidine, clonidine, debrisoquin, guanadrel, guanethidine, guanabenz, guanfacine; monitor BP; consider alternate antihypertensive agent
Beta-agonists: When combined with TCAs may predispose patients to cardiac arrhythmias
Bupropion: May increase the levels of tricyclic antidepressants; based on limited information; monitor response
Carbamazepine: Tricyclic antidepressants may increase carbamazepine levels; monitor
Cholestyramine and colestipol: May bind TCAs and reduce their absorption; monitor for altered response
Clonidine: Abrupt discontinuation of clonidine may cause hypertensive crisis, amitriptyline may enhance the response
CNS depressants: Sedative effects may be additive with TCAs; monitor for increased effect; includes benzodiazepines, barbiturates, antipsychotics, ethanol and other sedative medications
CYP2D6 inhibitors: Serum levels and/or toxicity of some tricyclic antidepressants may be increased; inhibitors include amiodarone, cimetidine, delavirdine, fluoxetine, paroxetine, propafenone, quinidine, and ritonavir; monitor for increased effect/toxicity
Enzyme inducers: May increase the metabolism of TCAs resulting in decreased effect; includes carbamazepine, phenobarbital, phenytoin, and rifampin; monitor for decreased response
Epinephrine (and other direct alpha-agonists): The pressor response to I.V. epinephrine, norepinephrine, and phenylephrine may be enhanced in patients receiving TCAs; this combination is best avoided
Fenfluramine: May increase tricyclic antidepressant levels/effects
Hypoglycemic agents (including insulin): TCAs may enhance the hypoglycemic effects of tolazamide, chlorpropamide, or insulin; monitor for changes in blood glucose levels; reported with chlorpropamide, tolazamide, and insulin
Levodopa: Tricyclic antidepressants may decrease the absorption (bioavailability) of levodopa; rare hypertensive episodes have also been attributed to this combination
Linezolid: Hyperpyrexia, hypertension, tachycardia, confusion, seizures, and **deaths have been reported** with agents which inhibit MAO (serotonin syndrome); this combination should be avoided
Lithium: Concurrent use with a TCA may increase the risk for neurotoxicity
MAO inhibitors: Hyperpyrexia, hypertension, tachycardia, confusion, seizures, and **deaths have been reported** (serotonin syndrome); this combination should be avoided
Methylphenidate: Metabolism of TCAs may be decreased
Phenothiazines: Serum concentrations of some TCAs may be increased; in addition, TCAs may increase concentration of phenothiazines; monitor for altered clinical response
QTc prolonging agents: Concurrent use of tricyclic agents with other drugs which may prolong QTc interval may increase the risk of potentially fatal arrhythmias; includes type Ia and type III antiarrhythmics agents, selected quinolones (sparfloxacin, gatifloxacin, moxifloxacin, grepafloxacin), cisapride, and other agents
Sucralfate: Absorption of tricyclic antidepressants may be reduced with coadministration
Sympathomimetics, indirect-acting: Tricyclic antidepressants may result in a decreased sensitivity to indirect-acting sympathomimetics; includes dopamine and ephedrine; also see interaction with epinephrine (and direct-acting sympathomimetics)
Valproic acid: May increase serum concentrations/adverse effects of some tricyclic antidepressants
Warfarin (and other oral anticoagulants): TCAs may increase the anticoagulant effect in patients stabilized on warfarin; monitor INR

**Stability** Protect from light

**Mechanism of Action** Increases the synaptic concentration of serotonin and norepinephrine in the central nervous system by inhibition of their reuptake by the presynaptic neuronal membrane

**Pharmacodynamics/kinetics**
Peak effect (antidepressant): Usually more than 2 weeks; anxiolytic effects may occur sooner
Distribution: Crosses the placenta; appears in breast milk
Protein binding: 80% to 85%
Metabolism: Hepatic; metabolites include desmethyldoxepin (active)
Half-life: Adults: 6-8 hours
Elimination: Renal

**Usual Dosage**
Oral (entire daily dose may be given at bedtime):
Adolescents: Initial: 25-50 mg/day in single or divided doses; gradually increase to 100 mg/day
Adults: Initial: 30-150 mg/day at bedtime or in 2-3 divided doses; may gradually increase up to 300 mg/day; single dose should not exceed 150 mg; select patients may respond to 25-50 mg/day
**Dosing adjustment in hepatic impairment:** Use a lower dose and adjust gradually
Topical: Adults: Apply a thin film 4 times/day with at least 3- to 4-hour interval between applications

**Dietary Considerations** Alcohol: Additive CNS effect, avoid use

**Monitoring Parameters** Monitor blood pressure and pulse rate prior to and during initial therapy; monitor mental status, weight; EKG in older adults

**Reference Range** Therapeutic: 30-150 ng/mL; Toxic: >500 ng/mL; utility of serum level monitoring is controversial

**Test Interactions** ↑ glucose

**Patient Information** Avoid unnecessary exposure to sunlight; avoid alcohol ingestion; do not discontinue medication abruptly; may cause urine to turn blue-green; may cause drowsiness; can use sugarless gum or hard candy for dry mouth; full effect may not occur for 4-6 weeks

**Nursing Implications** May increase appetite; may cause drowsiness, raise bed rails, institute safety precautions

**Dosage Forms**
Capsule, as hydrochloride: 10 mg, 25 mg, 50 mg, 75 mg, 100 mg, 150 mg
Concentrate, oral, as hydrochloride: 10 mg/mL (120 mL)
Cream: 5% (30 g)

♦ **Doxepin Hydrochloride** *see* Doxepin *on page 183*

## Doxercalciferol (dox er kal si fe FEER ole)

**U.S. Brand Names** Hectorol®

**Pharmacologic Category** Vitamin D Analog

**Use** Reduction of elevated intact parathyroid hormone (iPTH) in the management of secondary hyperparathyroidism in patients on chronic hemodialysis

**Effects on Mental Status** Dizziness and malaise are common; may cause confusion or sleep disorders

**Effects on Psychiatric Treatment** Nausea and vomiting are common; use caution with SSRIs

**Pregnancy Risk Factor** B

**Contraindications** History of hypercalcemia or evidence of vitamin D toxicity; hyperphosphatemia should be corrected before initiating therapy

**Warnings/Precautions** Other forms of vitamin D should be discontinued when doxercalciferol is started. Overdose from vitamin D is dangerous and needs to be avoided. Careful dosage titration and monitoring can minimize risk. Hyperphosphatemia exacerbates secondary hyperparathyroidism, diminishing the effect of doxercalciferol. Hyperphosphatemia needs to be corrected for best results. Use with caution in patients with hepatic impairment. Safety and efficacy have not been established in pediatrics.

**Adverse Reactions** Some of the signs and symptoms of hypercalcemia include anorexia, nausea, vomiting, constipation, polyuria, weakness, fatigue, confusion, stupor, and coma.
>10%:
Central nervous system: Headache (28%), malaise (28%), dizziness (11.5%)
Cardiovascular: Edema (34.4%)
Gastrointestinal: Nausea/vomiting (34%)
Respiratory: Dyspnea (11.5%)

1% to 10%:
Central nervous system: Sleep disorder (3.3%)
Cardiovascular: Bradycardia (6.6%)
Neuromuscular & skeletal: Arthralgia (4.9%)
Gastrointestinal: Anorexia (4.9%), constipation (3.3%), dyspepsia (4.9%)
Dermatologic: Pruritus (8.2%)
Miscellaneous: Abscess (3.3%)

**Overdosage/Toxicology** Doxercalciferol, in excess, can cause hypercalcemia, hypercalciuria, hyperphosphatemia and oversuppression of PTH secretion. Some of the signs and symptoms of hypercalcemia include anorexia, nausea, vomiting, constipation, polyuria, weakness, fatigue, confusion, stupor, and coma. Following withdrawal of the drug and calcium supplements, hypercalcemia treatment consists of a low calcium diet and monitoring. Adjustments of calcium in the dialysis bath can also be made if necessary. When calcium levels normalize, then doxercalciferol can be restarted. Reduce each dose by at least 2.5 mcg. Monitor serum calcium levels closely.

**Drug Interactions**
Decreased effect: Cholestyramine, mineral oil (both reduce absorption)
Increased toxicity: Concurrent use of other vitamin D supplements, magnesium containing antacids and supplements (hypermagnesemia)

**Usual Dosage**
Adults: Oral:
If the iPTH >400 pg/mL, then the initial dose is 10 mcg 3 times/week at dialysis. The dose is adjusted at 8-week intervals based upon the iPTH levels.
If the iPTH level is decreased by 50% and >300 pg/mL, then the dose can be increased to 12.5 mcg 3 times/week for 8 more weeks. This titration process can continue at 8-week intervals up to a maximum dose of 20 mcg 3 times/week. Each increase should be by 2.5 mcg/dose.
If the iPTH is between 150-300 pg/mL, maintain the current dose.
If the iPTH is <100 pg/mL, then suspend the drug for 1 week. Resume doxercalciferol at a reduced dose. Decrease each dose (not weekly dose) by at least 2.5 mcg.
**Dosage adjustment in renal impairment:** No adjustment required
**Dosage adjustment in hepatic impairment:** Use caution in these patients; no guidelines for dosage adjustment

**Patient Information** Be clear on dose and directions for taking. Stop other vitamin D products. Do not miss doses. Avoid magnesium-containing antacids and supplements. Report headache, dizziness, weakness, sleepiness, severe nausea, vomiting, and difficulty thinking or concentrating to your health care provider. Do not take over-the-counter medicines or supplements without first consulting your health care provider. Follow diet and calcium supplements as directed by your health care provider.

**Dosage Forms** Capsule: 2.5 mcg

♦ **Doxil®** *see* Doxorubicin (Liposomal) *on page 185*

## Doxorubicin (doks oh ROO bi sin)

**U.S. Brand Names** Adriamycin PFS™; Adriamycin RDF®; Rubex®

**Pharmacologic Category** Antineoplastic Agent, Antibiotic

**Use** Treatment of leukemias, lymphomas, multiple myeloma, osseous and nonosseous sarcomas, mesotheliomas, germ cell tumors of the ovary or testis, and carcinomas of the head and neck, thyroid, lung, Wilms' tumor, breast, stomach, pancreas, liver, ovary, bladder, prostate, and uterus, neuroblastoma

**Effects on Mental Status** None reported

**Effects on Psychiatric Treatment** Myelosuppression is common; use caution with clozapine and carbamazepine

**Usual Dosage** Refer to individual protocols
I.V. (patient's ideal weight should be used to calculate body surface area):
Children: 35-75 mg/m$^2$ as a single dose, repeat every 21 days; **or** 20-30 mg/m$^2$ once weekly; **or** 60-90 mg/m$^2$ given as a continuous infusion over 96 hours every 3-4 weeks
Adults: 60-75 mg/m$^2$ as a single dose, repeat every 21 days **or** other dosage regimens like 20-30 mg/m$^2$/day for 2-3 days, repeat in 4 weeks **or** 20 mg/m$^2$ once weekly
The lower dose regimen should be given to patients with decreased bone marrow reserve, prior therapy or marrow infiltration with malignant cells
Currently, the maximum cumulative dose is 550 mg/m$^2$ or 450 mg/m$^2$ in patients who have received RT to the mediastinal areas; a baseline MUGA should be performed prior to initiating treatment. If the LVEF is <30% to 40%, therapy should not be instituted; LVEF should be monitored during therapy.
Doxorubicin has also been administered intraperitoneal (phase I in refractory ovarian cancer patients) and intra-arterially.
**Dosing adjustment in renal impairment:** Adjustments not required in mild to moderate renal failure
$Cl_{cr}$ <10 mL/minute: Reduce dose to 75% of normal dose in severe renal failure
Hemodialysis: Supplemental dose is not necessary
**Dosing adjustment in hepatic impairment:**
Bilirubin 1.2-3 mg/dL: Administer 50% of dose
Bilirubin 3.1-5 mg/dL: Administer 25% of dose
Bilirubin >5 mg/dL: Avoid use

**Dosage Forms**
Injection, as hydrochloride:
Aqueous, with NS: 2 mg/mL (5 mL, 10 mL, 25 mL)
Preservative free: 2 mg/mL (5 mL, 10 mL, 25 mL, 100 mL)
Powder for injection, as hydrochloride, lyophilized: 10 mg, 20 mg, 50 mg, 100 mg
Powder for injection, as hydrochloride, lyophilized, rapid dissolution formula: 10 mg, 20 mg, 50 mg, 150 mg

## Doxorubicin (Liposomal)
(doks oh ROO bi sin lip pah SOW mal)

**U.S. Brand Names** Doxil®

**Pharmacologic Category** Antineoplastic Agent, Anthracycline; Antineoplastic Agent, Antibiotic

**Use** Treatment of AIDS-related Kaposi's sarcoma in patients with disease that has progressed on prior combination chemotherapy or in patients who are intolerant to such therapy; treatment of metastatic carcinoma of the ovary in patients with disease that is refractory to both paclitaxel and platinum-based regimens
**Unlabeled use:** Breast cancer and solid tumors

**Effects on Mental Status** None reported

**Effects on Psychiatric Treatment** Myelosuppression is common; use caution with clozapine and carbamazepine

**Usual Dosage** Refer to individual protocols
I.V. (patient's ideal weight should be used to calculate body surface area): 20 mg/m$^2$ over 30 minutes, once every 3 weeks, for as long as patients respond satisfactorily and tolerate treatment.
AIDS-KS patients: I.V.: 20 mg/m$^2$/dose over 30 minutes once every 3 weeks for as long as patients respond satisfactorily and tolerate treatment
Breast cancer: I.V.: 20-80 mg/m$^2$/dose has been studied in a limited number of phase I/II trials
Ovarian cancer: I.V.: 50 mg/m$^2$/dose repeated every 4 weeks (minimum of 4 courses is recommended)
Solid tumors: I.V.: 50-60 mg/m$^2$/dose repeated every 3-4 weeks has been studied in a limited number of phase I/II trials

**Recommended dose modification guidelines:**
Palmar-Plantar erythrodysesthesia:
Toxicity Grade 1
Mild erythema, swelling, or desquamation not interfering with daily activities
Redose unless patient has experienced previous Grade 3 or 4 toxicity. If so, delay up to 2 weeks and decrease dose by 25%; return to original dosing interval.
Toxicity Grade 2
Erythema, desquamation, or swelling interfering with, but not precluding, normal physical activities; small blisters or ulcerations <2 cm in diameter
Delay dosing up to 2 weeks or until resolved to Grade 0-1. If after 2 weeks there is no resolution, liposomal doxorubicin should be discontinued.
Toxicity Grade 3
Blistering, ulceration, or swelling interfering with walking or normal daily activities; cannot wear regular clothing
Delay dosing up to 2 weeks or until resolved to Grade 0-1. Decrease dose by 25% and return to original dosing interval; if after 2 weeks there is no resolution, liposomal doxorubicin should be discontinued.
Toxicity Grade 4
Diffuse or local process causing infectious complications, or a bedridden state or hospitalization
Delay dosing up to 2 weeks or until resolved to Grade 0-1. Decrease dose by 25% and return to original dosing interval. If after 2 weeks there is no resolution, liposomal doxorubicin should be discontinued.
Stomatitis:
Toxicity Grade 1
Painless ulcers, erythema, or mild soreness
Redose unless patient has experienced previous Grade 3 or 4 toxicity. If so, delay up to 2 weeks and decrease by 25%. Return to original dosing interval.
Toxicity Grade 2
Painful erythema, edema, or ulcers, but can eat
Delay dosing up to 2 weeks or until resolved to Grade 0-1. If after 2 weeks there is no resolution, liposomal doxorubicin should be discontinued.
Toxicity Grade 3
Painful erythema, edema, or ulcers, but cannot eat
Delay dosing up to 2 weeks or until resolved to Grade 0-1. Decrease dose by 25% and return to original dosing interval. If after 2 weeks there is no resolution, liposomal doxorubicin should be discontinued.
Toxicity Grade 4
Requires parenteral or enteral support
(Continued)

## Doxorubicin (Liposomal) *(Continued)*

Delay dosing up to 2 weeks or until resolved to Grade 0-1. Decrease dose by 25% and return to original dosing interval. If after 2 weeks there is no resolution, liposomal doxorubicin should be discontinued.

**Dosing adjustment in hepatic impairment:**

Bilirubin 1.2-3 mg/dL or AST 60-180 units/L: Administer 50% of dose

Bilirubin >3 mg/dL: Administer 25% of dose

**Dosing adjustment in hematologic toxicity:**

Toxicity Grade 1

ANC 1500-1900; platelets 75,000-150,000: Resume treatment with no dose reduction

Toxicity Grade 2

ANC 1000-<1500; platelets 50,000-<75,000: Wait until ANC ≥1500 and platelets ≥75,000; redose with no dose reduction

Toxicity Grade 3

ANC 500-999; platelets 25,000-<50,000: Wait until ANC ≥1500 and platelets ≥75,000; redose with no dose reduction

Toxicity Grade 4

ANC <500; platelets <25,000: Wait until ANC ≥1500 and platelets ≥75,000; redose at 25% dose reduction or continue full dose with cytokine support

**Dosage Forms** Injection, as hydrochloride: 2 mg/mL (10 mL)

♦ **Doxychel® Injection** *see* Doxycycline *on page 186*

♦ **Doxychel® Oral** *see* Doxycycline *on page 186*

## Doxycycline (doks i SYE kleen)

**U.S. Brand Names** Bio-Tab® Oral; Doryx® Oral; Doxychel® Injection; Doxychel® Oral; Doxy® Oral; Monodox® Oral; Periostat®; Vibramycin® Injection; Vibramycin® Oral; Vibra-Tabs®

**Canadian Brand Names** Apo®-Doxy; Apo®-Doxy Tabs; Doxycin; Doxytec; Novo-Doxylin; Nu-Doxycycline

**Synonyms** Doxycycline Hyclate; Doxycycline Monohydrate

**Pharmacologic Category** Antibiotic, Tetracycline Derivative

**Use** Principally in the treatment of infections caused by susceptible *Rickettsia*, *Chlamydia*, and *Mycoplasma* along with uncommon susceptible gram-negative and gram-positive organisms; alternative to mefloquine for malaria prophylaxis; treatment for syphilis in penicillin-allergic patients; often active against vancomycin-resistant enterococci; used for community-acquired pneumonia and other common infections due to susceptible organisms; sclerosing agent for pleural effusions

**Effects on Mental Status** Tetracyclines have been reported to cause memory disturbance, mood stabilizing and antidepressant effects

**Effects on Psychiatric Treatment** May cause neutropenia; use caution with clozapine and carbamazepine; barbiturates and carbamazepine increase the clearance of doxycycline

**Pregnancy Risk Factor** D

**Contraindications** Hypersensitivity to doxycycline, tetracycline or any component; children <8 years of age; severe hepatic dysfunction

**Warnings/Precautions** Use of tetracyclines during tooth development may cause permanent discoloration of the teeth and enamel hypoplasia; prolonged use may result in superinfection; photosensitivity reaction may occur with this drug; avoid prolonged exposure to sunlight or tanning equipment. Do not administer to children ≤8 years of age.

**Adverse Reactions**

>10%: Miscellaneous: Discoloration of teeth in children

1% to 10%: Gastrointestinal: Esophagitis

<1%: Bulging fontanels in infants, diarrhea, eosinophilia, hepatotoxicity, increased intracranial pressure, nausea, neutropenia, phlebitis, photosensitivity, rash

**Overdosage/Toxicology**

Signs and symptoms: Nausea, anorexia, diarrhea

Treatment: Following GI decontamination, supportive care only; fluid support may be required for hypotension

**Drug Interactions** CYP3A3/4 enzyme substrate

Decreased effect with antacids containing aluminum, calcium, or magnesium

Iron and bismuth subsalicylate may decrease doxycycline bioavailability

Barbiturates, phenytoin, and carbamazepine decrease doxycycline's half-life

Increased effect of warfarin

**Usual Dosage** Oral, I.V.:

Children ≥8 years (<45 kg): 2-5 mg/kg/day in 1-2 divided doses, not to exceed 200 mg/day

Children >8 years (>45 kg) and Adults: 100-200 mg/day in 1-2 divided doses

Acute gonococcal infection: 200 mg immediately, then 100 mg at bedtime on the first day followed by 100 mg twice daily for 3 days **OR** 300 mg immediately followed by 300 mg in 1 hour

Primary and secondary syphilis: 300 mg/day in divided doses for ≥10 days

Uncomplicated chlamydial infections: 100 mg twice daily for ≥7 days

Endometritis, salpingitis, parametritis, or peritonitis: 100 mg I.V. twice daily with cefoxitin 2 g every 6 hours for 4 days and for ≥48 hours after patient improves; then continue with oral therapy 100 mg twice daily to complete a 10- to 14-day course of therapy

Sclerosing agent for pleural effusion injection: 500 mg as a single dose in 30-50 mL of NS or SWI

**Dosing adjustment in renal impairment:** $Cl_{cr}$ <10 mL/minute: 100 mg every 24 hours

Dialysis: Not dialyzable; 0% to 5% by hemo- and peritoneal methods or by continuous arteriovenous or venovenous hemofiltration (CAVH/CAVHD); no supplemental dosage necessary

**Patient Information** Take as directed, for the entire prescription, even if you are feeling better. Avoid alcohol and maintain adequate hydration (2-3 L/day of fluids unless instructed to restrict fluid intake). You may be very sensitive to sunlight; use sunblock, wear protective clothing and eyewear, or avoid exposure to direct sunlight. You may experience lightheadedness, dizziness, or drowsiness (use caution when driving or engaging in tasks that require alertness until response to drug is known); nausea or vomiting (small frequent meals, frequent mouth care, sucking lozenges, or chewing gum may help); or diarrhea (buttermilk, boiled milk, or yogurt may help). If diabetic, drug may cause false tests with Clinitest® urine glucose monitoring; use of glucose oxidase methods (Clinistix®) or serum glucose monitoring is preferable. Report skin rash or itching, easy bruising or bleeding, yellowing of skin or eyes, pale stool or dark urine, unhealed sores of mouth, itching or vaginal discharge, fever or chills, or unusual cough.

**Nursing Implications** Avoid extravasation

**Dosage Forms**

Capsule, as hyclate:

Doxychel®, Vibramycin®: 50 mg

Doxy®, Doxychel®, Vibramycin®: 100 mg

Periostat®: 20 mg

Capsule, as monohydrate (Monodox®): 50 mg, 100 mg

Capsule, coated pellets, as hyclate (Doryx®): 100 mg

Gel, for subgingival application: Atridox™: 50 mg in each 500 mg of blended formulation; 2-syringe system contains doxycycline syringe (50 mg) and delivery system syringe (450 mg) along with a blunt cannula

Powder for injection, as hyclate (Doxy®, Doxychel®, Vibramycin® IV): 100 mg, 200 mg

Powder for oral suspension, as monohydrate (raspberry flavor) (Vibramycin®): 25 mg/5 mL (60 mL)

Syrup, as calcium (raspberry-apple flavor) (Vibramycin®): 50 mg/5 mL (30 mL, 473 mL)

Tablet, as hyclate

Doxychel®: 50 mg

Bio-Tab®, Doxychel®, Vibra-Tabs®: 100 mg

♦ **Doxycycline Hyclate** *see* Doxycycline *on page 186*

♦ **Doxycycline Monohydrate** *see* Doxycycline *on page 186*

## Doxylamine (dox IL a meen)

**U.S. Brand Names** Alsadorm®; Dornomyl®; Doxysom®; Gittalun®; Hoggar® N; Mereprine®; Restaid®; Restavit®; Sedaplus®; Somnil®; Unisom®; Unisom® Nighttime Sleepaid

**Pharmacologic Category** Antihistamine

**Use** Sleep aid; antihistamine for hypersensitivity reactions and antiemetic

**Effects on Mental Status** Sedation is common; may cause paradoxical stimulation in children

**Effects on Psychiatric Treatment** Concurrent use with psychotropics may produce additive sedation and dry mouth

**Contraindications** Hypersensitivity to doxylamine or any component

**Adverse Reactions**

Cardiovascular: Tachycardia

Central nervous system: Sedation, paradoxical stimulation in children, hyperthermia

Gastrointestinal: Dry mucous membranes, constipation, nausea, vomiting

Genitourinary: Urinary retention

Neuromuscular & skeletal: Tremors

Ocular: Blurred vision, mydriasis

**Drug Interactions** CNS depressants, MAO inhibitors, tricyclic antidepressants, and phenothiazines can potentiate CNS depression

**Usual Dosage** Oral: Children >12 years and Adults: 25 mg at bedtime

**Dosage Forms** Tablet, as succinate: 25 mg

♦ **Doxy® Oral** *see* Doxycycline *on page 186*

♦ **Doxysom®** *see* Doxylamine *on page 186*

♦ **DPA** *see* Valproic Acid and Derivatives *on page 578*

♦ **D-Penicillamine** *see* Penicillamine *on page 424*

♦ **DPH** *see* Phenytoin *on page 441*

♦ **Dramamine® II [OTC]** *see* Meclizine *on page 335*

♦ **Dramamine® Oral [OTC]** *see* Dimenhydrinate *on page 173*

♦ **Drisdol® Oral** *see* Ergocalciferol *on page 198*

- **Dristan® Cold Caplets [OTC]** *see* Acetaminophen and Pseudoephedrine *on page 15*
- **Dristan® Long Lasting Nasal Solution [OTC]** *see* Oxymetazoline *on page 415*
- **Dristan® Sinus Caplets [OTC]** *see* Pseudoephedrine and Ibuprofen *on page 479*
- **Drithocreme®** *see* Anthralin *on page 45*
- **Drithocreme® HP 1%** *see* Anthralin *on page 45*
- **Dritho-Scalp®** *see* Anthralin *on page 45*
- **Drixomed®** *see* Dexbrompheniramine and Pseudoephedrine *on page 158*
- **Drixoral® [OTC]** *see* Dexbrompheniramine and Pseudoephedrine *on page 158*
- **Drixoral® Cough & Congestion Liquid Caps [OTC]** *see* Pseudoephedrine and Dextromethorphan *on page 479*
- **Drixoral® Cough Liquid Caps [OTC]** *see* Dextromethorphan *on page 160*
- **Drixoral® Cough & Sore Throat Liquid Caps [OTC]** *see* Acetaminophen and Dextromethorphan *on page 15*
- **Drixoral® Non-Drowsy [OTC]** *see* Pseudoephedrine *on page 478*
- **Drixoral® Syrup [OTC]** *see* Brompheniramine and Pseudoephedrine *on page 74*

## Dronabinol (droe NAB i nol)

**U.S. Brand Names** Marinol®

**Synonyms** Tetrahydrocannabinol; THC

**Pharmacologic Category** Antiemetic

**Use** When conventional antiemetics fail to relieve the nausea and vomiting associated with cancer chemotherapy, AIDS-related anorexia

**Effects on Mental Status** Drowsiness, anxiety, confusion, and mood changes are common; may cause depression or hallucinations

**Effects on Psychiatric Treatment** Concurrent use with barbiturates and benzodiazepines produce additive sedation

**Restrictions** C-II

**Pregnancy Risk Factor** C

**Contraindications** Use only for cancer chemotherapy-induced nausea; should not be used in patients with a history of schizophrenia or in patients with known hypersensitivity to dronabinol or any component

**Warnings/Precautions** Use with caution in patients with heart disease, hepatic disease, or seizure disorders; reduce dosage in patients with severe hepatic impairment

**Adverse Reactions**

>10%: Central nervous system: Drowsiness, dizziness, detachment, anxiety, difficulty concentrating, mood change

1% to 10%:

Cardiovascular: Orthostatic hypotension, tachycardia

Central nervous system: Ataxia, depression, headache, vertigo, hallucinations, memory lapse

Gastrointestinal: Xerostomia

Neuromuscular & skeletal: Paresthesia, weakness

<1%: Diaphoresis diarrhea, myalgia, nightmares, speech difficulties, syncope, tinnitus

**Overdosage/Toxicology** Signs and symptoms: Tachycardia, hypertension, and hypotension

**Drug Interactions** CYP2C18 and 3A3/4 enzyme substrate

Increased toxicity (drowsiness) with alcohol, barbiturates, benzodiazepines

**Usual Dosage** Oral:

Children: NCI protocol recommends 5 mg/m$^2$ starting 6-8 hours before chemotherapy and every 4-6 hours after to be continued for 12 hours after chemotherapy is discontinued

Adults: 5 mg/m$^2$ 1-3 hours before chemotherapy, then administer 5 mg/m$^2$/dose every 2-4 hours after chemotherapy for a total of 4-6 doses/day; dose may be increased up to a maximum of 15 mg/m$^2$/dose if needed (dosage may be increased by 2.5 mg/m$^2$ increments)

Appetite stimulant (AIDS-related): Initial: 2.5 mg twice daily (before lunch and dinner); titrate up to a maximum of 20 mg/day

**Dietary Considerations** Alcohol: Additive CNS effect, avoid use

**Patient Information** Take exactly as directed; do not increase dose or take more often than prescribed. Do not use alcohol or other depressant medications without consulting prescriber. You may experience psychotic reaction, impaired coordination or judgment, faintness, dizziness, or drowsiness (do not drive or engage in activities that require alertness and coordination until response to drug is known); clumsiness, unsteadiness, or muscular weakness (change position slowly and use caution when climbing stairs). Report excessive or persistent CNS changes (euphoria, anxiety, depression, memory lapse, bizarre though patterns, excitability, inability to control thoughts or behavior, fainting), respiratory difficulties, rapid heartbeat, or other adverse reactions.

**Nursing Implications** Raise bed rails, institute safety measures, assist with ambulation

**Dosage Forms** Capsule: 2.5 mg, 5 mg, 10 mg

## Droperidol (droe PER i dole)

**Related Information**

Discontinuation of Psychotropic Drugs - Withdrawal Symptoms and Recommendations *on page 798*

Patient Information - Antipsychotics (General) *on page 646*

**Generic Available** Yes

**U.S. Brand Names** Inapsine®

**Pharmacologic Category** Antiemetic

**Use** Tranquilizer and antiemetic in surgical and diagnostic procedures; preoperative medication; induction and adjunct in the maintenance of general and regional anesthesia; neuroleptanalgesia, in which droperidol is given concurrently with a narcotic analgesic (fentanyl) to aid in producing tranquility and decreasing anxiety and pain

**Unlabeled uses:** Agitation in psychiatric emergencies; antiemetic for cancer chemotherapy

**Pregnancy Risk Factor** C

**Contraindications** Hypersensitivity to droperidol or any component

**Warnings/Precautions** Safety in children <6 months of age has not been established; use with caution in patients with seizures, bone marrow suppression, or severe liver disease

Significant hypotension may occur, especially when the drug is administered parenterally; injection contains benzyl alcohol; injection also contains sulfites which may cause allergic reaction

Tardive dyskinesia (TD): TD is a chronic, potentially irreversible abnormal movement disorder associated with long-term use of antipsychotic medication. Movements may be choreiform, tonic, or athetotic and most commonly involve the face and mouth. Those at greater risk for developing TD are on prolonged antipsychotic therapy, older than 50 years of age, and with diabetes or primary affective disorder. TD prevalence estimates for neuroleptic-treated patients range from 10% to 15% in young patients, 12% to 25% in chronic patients, and 25% to 45% of state hospital patients.

Extrapyramidal syndromes: Extrapyramidal reactions are more common in elderly.

Acute dystonias are uncomfortable, involuntary muscle spasms of the face, neck, trunk, or extremities associated with antipsychotic treatment. Dystonias occur in 10% to 15% of patients on conventional antipsychotic medications, usually in the first several weeks of treatment.

Akathisia is a subjective feeling of restlessness seen in 10% to 40% of patients on typical antipsychotic medications. Patients may appear agitated, with frequent pacing and inability to keep their legs still.

Antipsychotic medication-associated parkinsonism is characterized by rigidity, bradykinesia, masked facies, drooling, and tremor. While not strictly an emergency the disabling symptoms occur subacutely within the first month of therapy on 10% to 15% of patients on typical antipsychotics.

Increased confusion, memory loss, psychotic behavior, and agitation frequently occur as a consequence of anticholinergic effects

Orthostatic hypotension is due to alpha-receptor blockade, the elderly are at greater risk for orthostatic hypotension

Antipsychotic associated sedation in nonpsychotic patients is extremely unpleasant due to feelings of depersonalization, derealization, and dysphoria

Life-threatening arrhythmias have occurred at therapeutic doses of antipsychotics

**Adverse Reactions**

Cardiovascular: Mild to moderate hypotension, tachycardia, hypertension, dizziness, chills, postoperative hallucinations

Central nervous system: Postoperative drowsiness, extrapyramidal reactions, shivering

Respiratory: Respiratory depression, apnea, muscular rigidity, laryngospasm, bronchospasm

**Overdosage/Toxicology**

Signs and symptoms: Hypotension, tachycardia, hallucinations, extrapyramidal symptoms

Treatment: Following initiation of essential overdose management, toxic symptom treatment and supportive treatment should be initiated. Hypotension usually responds to I.V. fluids or Trendelenburg positioning. If unresponsive to these measures, the use of a parenteral inotrope may be required (eg, norepinephrine 0.1-0.2 mcg/kg/minute titrated to response). Seizures commonly respond to diazepam (I.V. 5-10 mg bolus in adults every 15 minutes if needed up to a total of 30 mg; I.V. 0.25-0.4 mg/kg/dose up to a total of 10 mg in children) or to phenytoin or phenobarbital. Also critical cardiac arrhythmias often respond to I.V. phenytoin (15 mg/kg up to 1 g), while other antiarrhythmics can be used. Neuroleptics often cause extrapyramidal symptoms (eg, dystonic reactions) requiring management with diphenhydramine 1-2 mg/kg (adults) up to a maximum of 50 mg I.M. or I.V. slow push followed by a maintenance

(Continued)

## Droperidol *(Continued)*

dose for 48-72 hours. When these reactions are unresponsive to diphenhydramine, benztropine mesylate I.V. 1-2 mg (adults) may be effective. These agents are generally effective within 2-5 minutes.

**Drug Interactions**

CNS depressants: Sedative effects may be additive with other CNS depressants; monitor for increased effect; includes benzodiazepines, barbiturates, antipsychotics, ethanol, and other sedative medications

Cyclobenzaprine: Droperidol and cyclobenzaprine may have an additive effect on prolonging the Q-T interval; based on limited documentation; monitor

Inhalation anesthetics: Droperidol in combination with certain forms of induction anesthesia may produce peripheral vasodilitation and hypotension

Propofol: An increased incidence of postoperative nausea and vomiting have been reported following coadministration

**Stability**

Droperidol ampuls/vials should be stored at room temperature and protected from light

Stability of parenteral admixture at room temperature (25°C): 7 days

Standard diluent: 2.5 mg/50 mL $D_5W$

**Incompatible** with barbiturates

**Mechanism of Action** Butyrophenone derivative that produces tranquilization, sedation, and an antiemetic effect; other effects include alpha-adrenergic blockade, peripheral vascular dilation, and reduction of the pressor effect of epinephrine resulting in hypotension and decreased peripheral vascular resistance; may also reduce pulmonary artery pressure

**Pharmacodynamics/kinetics**

Following parenteral administration:

Peak effect: Within 30 minutes

Duration: 2-4 hours, may extend to 12 hours

Metabolism: In the liver

Half-life: Adults: 2.3 hours

Elimination: In urine (75%) and feces (22%)

**Usual Dosage** Titrate carefully to desired effect

Children 2-12 years:

Premedication: I.M.: 0.1-0.15 mg/kg; smaller doses may be sufficient for control of nausea or vomiting

Adjunct to general anesthesia: I.V. induction: 0.088-0.165 mg/kg

Nausea and vomiting: I.M., I.V.: 0.05-0.06 mg/kg/dose every 4-6 hours as needed

Adults:

Premedication: I.M.: 2.5-10 mg 30 minutes to 1 hour preoperatively

Adjunct to general anesthesia: I.V. induction: 0.22-0.275 mg/kg; maintenance: 1.25-2.5 mg/dose

Alone in diagnostic procedures: I.M.: Initial: 2.5-10 mg 30 minutes to 1 hour before; then 1.25-2.5 mg if needed

Nausea and vomiting: I.M., I.V.: 2.5-5 mg/dose every 3-4 hours as needed

Rapid tranquilization of agitated patient (administered every 30-60 minutes): I.M.: 2.5-5 mg; average total dose for tranquilization: 5-20 mg

**Monitoring Parameters** Blood pressure, heart rate, respiratory rate; observe for dystonias, extrapyramidal side effects, and temperature changes

**Patient Information** Avoid alcoholic beverages

**Dosage Forms** Injection: 2.5 mg/mL (1 mL, 2 mL, 5 mL, 10 mL)

## Droperidol and Fentanyl (droe PER i dole & FEN ta nil)

**U.S. Brand Names** Innovar®

**Synonyms** Fentanyl and Droperidol

**Pharmacologic Category** Analgesic, Narcotic

**Use** Produce and maintain analgesia and sedation during diagnostic or surgical procedures (neuroleptanalgesia and neuroleptanesthesia); adjunct to general anesthesia

**Effects on Mental Status** Drowsiness is common; may cause depression or extrapyramidal symptoms; rarely may produce delirium or hallucinations

**Effects on Psychiatric Treatment** Contraindicated within 14 days of MAOIs; concurrent use with psychotropics may produce additive sedation

**Pregnancy Risk Factor** C

**Contraindications** Hypersensitivity to droperidol or fentanyl; patients who have taken MAO inhibitors within 14 days

**Warnings/Precautions** Rapid I.V. injection can cause muscle rigidity, particularly involving those muscles of respiration; use with caution in patients with impaired hepatic and renal function, and pre-existing cardiac bradyarrhythmias; may cause muscle rigidity, laryngospasm, bronchospasm, apnea

**Adverse Reactions**

>10%:

Cardiovascular: Bradycardia, mild to moderate hypotension, tachycardia

Central nervous system: Drowsiness, nausea, vomiting, postoperative drowsiness

Respiratory: Respiratory depression

1% to 10%:

Cardiovascular: Cardiac arrhythmia, orthostatic hypotension, hypertension

Central nervous system: Confusion, CNS depression, extrapyramidal reactions

Gastrointestinal: Biliary spasm

Ocular: Blurred vision

Respiratory: Respiratory depression

**Overdosage/Toxicology** Treatment: Naloxone, resuscitative equipment, and oxygen should be available

**Drug Interactions** CNS depressant drugs may cause additive effects; may cause hypertensive crisis if given with MAO inhibitors

**Usual Dosage**

Children:

Premedication: I.M.: 0.03 mL/kg 30-60 minutes prior to surgery

Adjunct to general anesthesia: I.V.: Total dose: 0.05 mL/kg as slow infusion (1 mL/1-2 minutes) until sleep occurs

Adults:

Premedication: I.M.: 0.5-2 mL 30-60 minutes prior to surgery

Adjunct to general anesthesia: I.V.: 0.09-0.11 mL/kg as slow infusion (1 mL/1-2 minutes) until sleep occurs

**Patient Information** See individual agents

**Dosage Forms** Injection: Droperidol 2.5 mg and fentanyl 50 mcg per mL (2 mL, 5 mL)


♦ **Droxia™** *see* Hydroxyurea *on page 277*

♦ **Dr Scholl's Athlete's Foot [OTC]** *see* Tolnaftate *on page 555*

♦ **Dr Scholl's® Cracked Heel Relief Cream [OTC]** *see* Lidocaine *on page 317*

♦ **Dr Scholl's Maximum Strength Tritin [OTC]** *see* Tolnaftate *on page 555*

♦ **Dry Eyes® Solution [OTC]** *see* Artificial Tears *on page 48*

♦ **Dry Eye® Therapy Solution [OTC]** *see* Artificial Tears *on page 48*

♦ **Dryox® Gel [OTC]** *see* Benzoyl Peroxide *on page 62*

♦ **Dryox® Wash [OTC]** *see* Benzoyl Peroxide *on page 62*

♦ **Drysol™** *see* Aluminum Chloride Hexahydrate *on page 28*

♦ **DSCG** *see* Cromolyn Sodium *on page 142*

♦ **D-S-S® [OTC]** *see* Docusate *on page 179*

♦ **DTIC-Dome®** *see* Dacarbazine *on page 149*

♦ **DTO** *see* Opium Tincture *on page 406*

♦ **Duadacin® Capsule [OTC]** *see* Chlorpheniramine, Phenylpropanolamine, and Acetaminophen *on page 116*

♦ **Dulcolax® [OTC]** *see* Bisacodyl *on page 69*

♦ **Dull-C® [OTC]** *see* Ascorbic Acid *on page 48*

♦ **DuoCet™** *see* Hydrocodone and Acetaminophen *on page 272*

♦ **Duo-Cyp® Injection** *see* Estradiol and Testosterone *on page 205*

♦ **Duo-Trach®** *see* Lidocaine *on page 317*

♦ **Duotrate®** *see* Pentaerythritol Tetranitrate *on page 426*

♦ **DuP 753** *see* Losartan *on page 326*

♦ **Duphalac®** *see* Lactulose *on page 306*

♦ **Duracebrol®** *see* Nicergoline *on page 392*

♦ **Duraclon®** *see* Clonidine *on page 133*

♦ **Dura-Estrin® Injection** *see* Estradiol *on page 203*

♦ **Duragen® Injection** *see* Estradiol *on page 203*

♦ **Duragesic® Transdermal** *see* Fentanyl *on page 221*

♦ **Dura-Gest®** *see* Guaifenesin, Phenylpropanolamine, and Phenylephrine *on page 258*

♦ **Duralone® Injection** *see* Methylprednisolone *on page 359*

♦ **Duramist® Plus [OTC]** *see* Oxymetazoline *on page 415*

♦ **Duramorph® Injection** *see* Morphine Sulfate *on page 374*

♦ **Duraphyl™** *see* Theophylline Salts *on page 539*

♦ **Duratest® Injection** *see* Testosterone *on page 536*

♦ **Duratestrin® Injection** *see* Estradiol and Testosterone *on page 205*

♦ **Durathate® Injection** *see* Testosterone *on page 536*

♦ **Duration® Nasal Solution [OTC]** *see* Oxymetazoline *on page 415*

♦ **Duratuss-G®** *see* Guaifenesin *on page 256*

♦ **Dura-Vent®** *see* Guaifenesin and Phenylpropanolamine *on page 257*

♦ **Dura-Vent/DA®** *see* Chlorpheniramine, Phenylephrine, and Methscopolamine *on page 115*

- **Duricef®** *see* Cefadroxil *on page 97*
- **Durrax®** *see* Hydroxyzine *on page 278*
- **Duvoid®** *see* Bethanechol *on page 67*
- **DV® Vaginal Cream** *see* Dienestrol *on page 167*
- **Dwelle® Ophthalmic Solution [OTC]** *see* Artificial Tears *on page 48*
- **Dyazide®** *see* Hydrochlorothiazide and Triamterene *on page 271*
- **Dycill®** *see* Dicloxacillin *on page 165*
- **Dymelor®** *see* Acetohexamide *on page 17*
- **Dymenate® Injection** *see* Dimenhydrinate *on page 173*
- **Dynabac®** *see* Dirithromycin *on page 177*
- **Dynacin® Oral** *see* Minocycline *on page 367*
- **DynaCirc®** *see* Isradipine *on page 298*
- **Dynafed® IB [OTC]** *see* Ibuprofen *on page 280*
- **Dynafed®, Maximum Strength [OTC]** *see* Acetaminophen and Pseudoephedrine *on page 15*
- **Dyna-Hex® Topical [OTC]** *see* Chlorhexidine Gluconate *on page 111*
- **Dynapen®** *see* Dicloxacillin *on page 165*

## Dyphylline (DYE fi lin)

**U.S. Brand Names** Dilor®; Lufyllin®
**Pharmacologic Category** Theophylline Derivative
**Use** Bronchodilator in reversible airway obstruction due to asthma or COPD
**Effects on Mental Status** May cause nervousness, restlessness, or insomnia
**Effects on Psychiatric Treatment** May decrease serum lithium levels; monitor; barbiturates and carbamazepine may decrease dyphylline levels; may antagonize effects of benzodiazepines
**Usual Dosage**
Children: I.M.: 4.4-6.6 mg/kg/day in divided doses
Adults:
Oral: Up to 15 mg/kg 4 times/day, individualize dosage
I.M.: 250-500 mg, do not exceed total dosage of 15 mg/kg every 6 hours
**Dosing adjustment in renal impairment:**
$Cl_{cr}$ 50-80 mL/minute: Administer 75% of normal dose
$Cl_{cr}$ 10-50 mL/minute: Administer 50% of normal dose
$Cl_{cr}$ <10 mL/minute: Administer 25% of normal dose
**Dosage Forms**
Elixir:
Lufyllin®: 100 mg/15 mL with alcohol 20% (473 mL, 3780 mL)
Dilor®: 160 mg/15 mL with alcohol 18% (473 mL)
Injection (Dilor®, Lufyllin®): 250 mg/mL (2 mL)
Tablet: 200 mg, 400 mg
Dilor®, Lufyllin®: 200 mg, 400 mg

- **Dyrenium®** *see* Triamterene *on page 564*
- **7E3** *see* Abciximab *on page 12*
- **E2020** *see* Donepezil *on page 181*
- **Easprin®** *see* Aspirin *on page 49*
- **Eating Disorders** *see page 619*

## Echinacea

**Related Information**
Natural/Herbal Products *on page 746*
Natural Products, Herbals, and Dietary Supplements *on page 742*
Perspectives on the Safety of Herbal Medicines *on page 736*
**Synonyms** Black Susans; Comb Flower; *Echinacea angustifolia*; Indian Head; Purple Coneflower; Scury Root, American Coneflower; Snakeroot
**Pharmacologic Category** Herb
**Use** Prophylaxis and treatment of cold and flu; also used as an immunostimulant in herbal medicine; used to treat minor upper respiratory tract infections, urinary tract infections, wound/skin infections, arthritis, vaginal yeast infections
**Contraindications** Autoimmune diseases, such as collagen vascular disease (Lupus, RA), multiple sclerosis; allergy to sunflowers, daisies, ragweed; tuberculosis, HIV, AIDS, pregnancy, breast-feeding; parenteral administration only contraindicated per Commission E; oral use of Echinacea not contraindicated during pregnancy by Commission E
**Warnings/Precautions** May alter immunosuppression; persons allergic to sunflowers may display cross-allergy potential
**Adverse Reactions** May become immunosuppressive with continuous use over 6-8 weeks
Gastrointestinal: Tingling sensation of tongue
Miscellaneous: Allergic reactions (rarely)
Per Commission E: None known for oral and external use
**Overdosage/Toxicology** Treatment: Supportive therapy; can treat allergic manifestations with an antihistamine
**Drug Interactions** Theoretically may alter response to immunosuppressive therapy
**Usual Dosage** Continuous use should not exceed 8 weeks
Per Commission E: Expressed juice (of fresh herb): 6-9 mL/day
Capsule/tablet or tea form: 500 mg to 2 g 3 times/day
Liquid extract: 0.25-1 mL 3 times/day
Tincture: 1-2 mL 3 times/day
May be applied topically
**Additional Information** Persons allergic to sunflowers may display cross-allergy potential with this herb; a perennial daisy-like flowering plant 2-5 feet high usually found in the midwest and southeastern United States

- ***Echinacea angustifolia*** *see* Echinacea *on page 189*

## Echothiophate Iodide (ek oh THYE oh fate EYE oh dide)

**Related Information**
Glaucoma Drug Therapy *on page 712*
**U.S. Brand Names** Phospholine Iodide® Ophthalmic
**Pharmacologic Category** Ophthalmic Agent, Antiglaucoma; Ophthalmic Agent, Miotic
**Use** Reverse toxic CNS effects caused by anticholinergic drugs; used as miotic in treatment of open-angle glaucoma; may be useful in specific case of narrow-angle glaucoma; accommodative esotropia
**Effects on Mental Status** None reported
**Effects on Psychiatric Treatment** None reported
**Usual Dosage** Adults:
Ophthalmic: Glaucoma: Instill 1 drop twice daily into eyes with 1 dose just prior to bedtime; some patients have been treated with 1 dose daily or every other day
Accommodative esotropia:
Diagnosis: Instill 1 drop of 0.125% once daily into both eyes at bedtime for 2-3 weeks
Treatment: Use lowest concentration and frequency which gives satisfactory response, with a maximum dose of 0.125% once daily, although more intensive therapy may be used for short periods of time
**Dosage Forms** Powder for reconstitution, ophthalmic: 1.5 mg [0.03%] (5 mL); 3 mg [0.06%] (5 mL); 6.25 mg [0.125%] (5 mL); 12.5 mg [0.25%] (5 mL)

- **EC-Naprosyn®** *see* Naproxen *on page 384*
- **E-Complex-600® [OTC]** *see* Vitamin E *on page 586*

## Econazole (e KONE a zole)

**U.S. Brand Names** Spectazole™ Topical
**Canadian Brand Names** Ecostatin®
**Pharmacologic Category** Antifungal Agent, Topical
**Use** Topical treatment of tinea pedis (athlete's foot), tinea cruris (jock itch), tinea corporis (ringworm), tinea versicolor, and cutaneous candidiasis
**Effects on Mental Status** None reported
**Effects on Psychiatric Treatment** None reported
**Usual Dosage** Children and Adults: Topical:
Tinea pedis, tinea cruris, tinea corporis, tinea versicolor: Apply sufficient amount to cover affected areas once daily
Cutaneous candidiasis: Apply sufficient quantity twice daily (morning and evening)
Duration of treatment: Candidal infections and tinea cruris, versicolor, and corporis should be treated for 2 weeks and tinea pedis for 1 month; occasionally, longer treatment periods may be required
**Dosage Forms** Cream, as nitrate: 1% (15 g, 30 g, 85 g)

- **Econopred® Ophthalmic** *see* Prednisolone *on page 459*
- **Econopred® Plus Ophthalmic** *see* Prednisolone *on page 459*
- **Ecotrin® [OTC]** *see* Aspirin *on page 49*
- **Ecotrin® Low Adult Strength [OTC]** *see* Aspirin *on page 49*
- **Ed A-Hist® Liquid** *see* Chlorpheniramine and Phenylephrine *on page 114*
- **Edecrin®** *see* Ethacrynic Acid *on page 209*
- **Edex™** *see* Alprostadil *on page 27*

## Edrophonium (ed roe FOE nee um)

**U.S. Brand Names** Enlon® Injection; Reversol® Injection; Tensilon® Injection
**Pharmacologic Category** Antidote; Cholinergic Agonist; Diagnostic Agent, Myasthenia Gravis
**Use** Diagnosis of myasthenia gravis; differentiation of cholinergic crises from myasthenia crises; reversal of nondepolarizing neuromuscular blockers; treatment of paroxysmal atrial tachycardia
(Continued)

## Edrophonium *(Continued)*

**Effects on Mental Status** May cause drowsiness

**Effects on Psychiatric Treatment** None reported

**Usual Dosage** Usually administered I.V., however, if not possible, I.M. or S.C. may be used:

Infants:

I.M.: 0.5-1 mg

I.V.: Initial: 0.1 mg, followed by 0.4 mg if no response; total dose = 0.5 mg

Children:

Diagnosis: Initial: 0.04 mg/kg over 1 minute followed by 0.16 mg/kg if no response, to a maximum total dose of 5 mg for children <34 kg, or 10 mg for children >34 kg

I.M.:

<34 kg: 1 mg

>34 kg: 5 mg

Titration of oral anticholinesterase therapy: 0.04 mg/kg once given 1 hour after oral intake of the drug being used in treatment; if strength improves, an increase in neostigmine or pyridostigmine dose is indicated

Adults:

Diagnosis:

I.V.: 2 mg test dose administered over 15-30 seconds; 8 mg given 45 seconds later if no response is seen; test dose may be repeated after 30 minutes

I.M.: Initial: 10 mg; if no cholinergic reaction occurs, administer 2 mg 30 minutes later to rule out false-negative reaction

Titration of oral anticholinesterase therapy: 1-2 mg given 1 hour after oral dose of anticholinesterase; if strength improves, an increase in neostigmine or pyridostigmine dose is indicated

Reversal of nondepolarizing neuromuscular blocking agents (neostigmine with atropine usually preferred): I.V.: 10 mg over 30-45 seconds; may repeat every 5-10 minutes up to 40 mg

Termination of paroxysmal atrial tachycardia: I.V. rapid injection: 5-10 mg

Differentiation of cholinergic from myasthenic crisis: I.V.: 1 mg; may repeat after 1 minute. **Note:** Intubation and controlled ventilation may be required if patient has cholinergic crisis

**Dosing adjustment in renal impairment:** Dose may need to be reduced in patients with chronic renal failure

**Dosage Forms** Injection, as chloride: 10 mg/mL (1 mL, 10 mL, 15 mL)

♦ **ED-SPAZ®** *see* Hyoscyamine *on page 279*

♦ **Edstinyl®** *see* Ethinyl Estradiol *on page 210*

♦ **E.E.S.® Oral** *see* Erythromycin *on page 200*

## Efavirenz (e FAV e renz)

**U.S. Brand Names** Sustiva™

**Pharmacologic Category** Antiretroviral Agent, Reverse Transcriptase Inhibitor (Non-Nucleoside)

**Use** Treatment of HIV-1 infections in combination with at least two other antiretroviral agents. Also has some activity against hepatitis B virus and herpes viruses.

**Effects on Mental Status** May cause difficulty in concentration, insomnia, abnormal dreams, sedation, depression, nervousness, and fatigue. May rarely cause hallucinations, psychosis, anxiety, euphoria, emotional lability, agitation.

**Effects on Psychiatric Treatment** Should not be administered with other drugs known to be metabolized by the CYP3A4 system (midazolam, triazolam, ergot alkaloids) as combination may lead to life-threatening adverse effects

**Pregnancy Risk Factor** C

**Contraindications** Clinically significant hypersensitivity to any component of the formulation

**Warnings/Precautions** Do not use as single-agent therapy; avoid pregnancy; women of childbearing potential should undergo pregnancy testing prior to initiation of therapy; do not administer with other agents metabolized by cytochrome P-450 isoenzyme 3A4 including astemizole, cisapride, midazolam, triazolam or ergot alkaloids (potential for life-threatening adverse effects); history of mental illness/drug abuse (predisposition to psychological reactions); may cause depression and/or other psychiatric symptoms including impaired concentration, dizziness or drowsiness (avoid potentially hazardous tasks such as driving or operating machinery if these effects are noted); discontinue if severe rash (involving blistering, desquamation, mucosal involvement or fever) develops. Caution in patients with known or suspected hepatitis B or C infection (monitoring of liver function is recommended); hepatic impairment. Persistent elevations of serum transaminases >5 times the upper limit of normal should prompt evaluation - benefit of continued therapy should be weighed against possible risk of hepatotoxicity. Children are more susceptible to development of rash - prophylactic antihistamines may be used.

**Adverse Reactions**

2% to 10%:

Central nervous system: Dizziness (2% to 10%), inability to concentrate (0% to 9%), insomnia (0% to 7%), headache (5% to 6%) abnormal dreams (0% to 4%), somnolence (0% to 3%), depression (0% to 2%), anorexia (0% to 5%), nervousness (0% to 2%), fatigue (2% to 7%), hypoesthesia (1% to 2%)

Dermatologic: Rash (5% to 20%), pruritus (0% to 2%)

Gastrointestinal: Nausea (0% to 12%), vomiting (0% to 7%), diarrhea (2% to 12%), dyspepsia (0% to 4%), elevated transaminases (2% to 3%), abdominal pain (0% to 3%)

Miscellaneous: Increased sweating (0% to 2%)

<2%: Abnormal vision, agitation, alcohol intolerance, allergic reaction, alopecia, amnesia, anxiety, apathy, arthralgia, asthenia, asthma, ataxia, confusion, depersonalization, depression, diplopia, dry mouth, eczema, edema (peripheral), emotional lability, euphoria, fever, flatulence, flushing, folliculitis, hallucinations, hematuria, hepatitis, hot flashes, impaired coordination, increased cholesterol and triglycerides, malaise, migraine, myalgia, neuralgia, pain, palpitations, pancreatitis, paresthesia, parosmia, peripheral neuropathy, psychosis, renal calculus, seizures, skin exfoliation, speech disorder, syncope, tachycardia, taste disturbance, thrombophlebitis, tinnitus, tremor, urticaria, vertigo

Pediatric patients: Central nervous system reactions (9%), cough (25%), diarrhea (39%), fever (26%), nausea/vomiting (16%), rash (40%)

**Overdosage/Toxicology**

Increased central nervous system symptoms and involuntary muscle contractions have been reported in accidental overdose

Treatment is supportive, activated charcoal may enhance elimination; dialysis is unlikely to remove drug

**Drug Interactions**

Increased effect: CYP3A4, 2C9, 2C19 inhibitor; CYP3A4 inducer; coadministration with medications metabolized by these enzymes may lead to increased concentration-related effects. Astemizole, cisapride, midazolam, triazolam and ergot alkaloids may result in life-threatening toxicities. The AUC of nelfinavir is increased (20%); AUC of both ritonavir and efavirenz are increased by 20% during concurrent therapy. The AUC of ethinyl estradiol is increased 37% by efavirenz (clinical significance unknown). May increase effect of warfarin.

Decreased effect: Other inducers of this enzyme (including phenobarbital, rifampin and rifabutin) may decrease serum concentrations of efavirenz. Concentrations of indinavir may be reduced; dosage increase to 1000 mg 3 times/day is recommended. Concentrations of saquinavir may be decreased (use as sole protease inhibitor is not recommended). Plasma concentrations of clarithromycin are decreased (clinical significance unknown). May decrease effect of warfarin.

**Usual Dosage** Oral: Dosing at bedtime is recommended to limit central nervous system effects; should not be used as single-agent therapy

Children: Dosage is based on body weight

10 kg to <15 kg: 200 mg once daily

15 kg to <20 kg: 250 mg once daily

20 kg to <25 kg: 300 mg once daily

25 kg to <32.5 kg: 350 mg once daily

32.5 kg to <40 kg: 400 mg once daily

≥40 kg: 600 mg once daily

Adults: 600 mg once daily

**Dosing adjustment in renal impairment:** None recommended

**Dosing comments in hepatic impairment:** Limited clinical experience, use with caution

**Dietary Considerations** May be taken with or without food. Avoid high-fat meals when taking this medication. High-fat meals increase the absorption of efavirenz.

**Patient Information** Efavirenz is not a cure for HIV, nor will it reduce transmission of HIV. Take as directed (usually at bedtime to reduce CNS effects), with or without food. Do not alter dose or discontinue without consulting prescriber. Avoid high fat meals when taking this medication. Maintain adequate hydration (2-3 L/day of fluids unless instructed to restrict fluid intake). Avoid excessive alcohol (severe reaction), prescription, and OTC sedatives unless consulting prescriber. You may experience dry mouth, taste disturbances, nausea, or vomiting (small frequent meals or sucking hard candy may help - consult prescriber if nausea or vomiting persists); diarrhea (buttermilk, boiled milk, or yogurt may help); or dizziness, anxiety, tremor, impaired coordination (use caution when driving or engaging in tasks requiring alertness until response to drug is known); Report CNS changes (acute headache, abnormal dreams, sleepiness or fatigue, seizures, hallucinations, amnesia, emotional lability, confusion); sense of fullness or ringing in ears; vision changes or double vision; muscle pain, weakness, tremors, numbness, spasticity, or change in gait; skin rash or irritation; chest pain or palpitations; or other unusual effects related to this medication.

**Dosage Forms** Capsule: 50 mg, 100 mg, 200 mg

♦ **Effer-K™** *see* Potassium Bicarbonate and Potassium Citrate, Effervescent *on page 453*

♦ **Effer-Syllium® [OTC]** *see* Psyllium *on page 479*

♦ **Effexor®** *see* Venlafaxine *on page 582*

- **Effexor® XR** *see* Venlafaxine *on page 582*
- **Efidac/24® [OTC]** *see* Pseudoephedrine *on page 478*

## Eflornithine (ee FLOR ni theen)

**U.S. Brand Names** Ornidyl® Injection; Vaniqa™ Cream

**Pharmacologic Category** Antiprotozoal; Topical Skin Product

**Use**

Injection: Treatment of meningoencephalitic stage of *Trypanosoma brucei gambiense* infection (sleeping sickness)

Cream, females ≥12 years: Reduce unwanted hair from face and adjacent areas under the chin

**Effects on Mental Status** Dizziness is common

**Effects on Psychiatric Treatment** Leukopenia is common; use caution with clozapine and carbamazepine

**Usual Dosage**

Children ≥12 years and Adults: Females: Topical: Apply thin layer of cream to affected areas of face and adjacent chin twice daily, at least 8 hours apart

Adults: I.V. infusion: 100 mg/kg/dose given every 6 hours (over at least 45 minutes) for 14 days

**Dosing adjustment in renal impairment:** Injection: Dose should be adjusted although no specific guidelines are available

**Dosage Forms**

Cream, as hydrochloride: 13.9% (30 g)

Injection, as hydrochloride: 200 mg/mL (100 mL)

- **Efodine® [OTC]** *see* Povidone-Iodine *on page 456*
- **Efudex® Topical** *see* Fluorouracil *on page 231*
- **EHDP** *see* Etidronate Disodium *on page 215*
- **Elavil®** *see* Amitriptyline *on page 33*
- **Eldecort®** *see* Hydrocortisone *on page 273*
- **Eldepryl®** *see* Selegiline *on page 508*
- **Eldercaps® [OTC]** *see* Vitamins, Multiple *on page 587*
- **Eldopaque® [OTC]** *see* Hydroquinone *on page 276*
- **Eldopaque Forte®** *see* Hydroquinone *on page 276*
- **Eldoquin® [OTC]** *see* Hydroquinone *on page 276*
- **Eldoquin® Forte®** *see* Hydroquinone *on page 276*
- **Electrolyte Lavage Solution** *see* Polyethylene Glycol-Electrolyte Solution *on page 451*
- **Elevan®** *see* Deanol *on page 152*
- **Elimite™ Cream** *see* Permethrin *on page 432*
- **Elixophyllin®** *see* Theophylline Salts *on page 539*
- **Elixophyllin® SR** *see* Theophylline Salts *on page 539*
- **Ellence™** *see* Epirubicin *on page 196*
- **Elmiron®** *see* Pentosan Polysulfate Sodium *on page 429*
- **Elocon®** *see* Mometasone *on page 373*
- **Elspar®** *see* Asparaginase *on page 48*
- **Eltroxin®** *see* Levothyroxine *on page 316*
- **Emcyt®** *see* Estramustine *on page 205*
- **Emgel™ Topical** *see* Erythromycin, Ophthalmic/Topical *on page 202*
- **Eminase®** *see* Anistreplase *on page 45*
- **Emko® [OTC]** *see* Nonoxynol 9 *on page 398*
- **Empirin® [OTC]** *see* Aspirin *on page 49*
- **Empirin® With Codeine** *see* Aspirin and Codeine *on page 50*
- **Emulsified Dizac® Injection** *see* Diazepam *on page 161*
- **Emulsified Valium®** *see* Diazepam *on page 161*
- **E-Mycin® Oral** *see* Erythromycin *on page 200*
- **ENA 713** *see* Rivastigmine *on page 498*

## Enalapril (e NAL a pril)

**Related Information**

Angiotensin-Related Agents Comparison Chart *on page 700*

**U.S. Brand Names** Vasotec®; Vasotec® I.V.

**Canadian Brand Names** Apo®-Enalapril

**Synonyms** Enalaprilat; Enalapril Maleate

**Pharmacologic Category** Angiotensin-Converting Enzyme (ACE) Inhibitors

**Use** Management of mild to severe hypertension; treatment of congestive heart failure, left ventricular dysfunction after myocardial infarction

**Unlabeled use:** Hypertensive crisis, diabetic nephropathy, rheumatoid arthritis, diagnosis of anatomic renal artery stenosis, hypertension secondary to scleroderma renal crisis, diagnosis of aldosteronism, idiopathic edema, Bartter's syndrome, postmyocardial infarction for prevention of ventricular failure, severe congestive heart failure in infants, neonatal hypertension, acute pulmonary edema

**Effects on Mental Status** May cause drowsiness and dizziness; rarely may cause insomnia, confusion, depression

**Effects on Psychiatric Treatment** May rarely cause agranulocytosis; use caution with clozapine and carbamazepine; may decrease lithium clearance resulting in an increase in serum lithium levels and potential lithium toxicity; monitor serum lithium levels

**Pregnancy Risk Factor** C (1st trimester); D (2nd and 3rd trimester)

**Contraindications** Hypersensitivity to enalapril or enalaprilat; angioedema related to previous treatment with an ACE inhibitor; patients with idiopathic or hereditary angioedema; bilateral renal artery stenosis; primary hyperaldosteronism; pregnancy (2nd and 3rd trimesters)

**Warnings/Precautions** Anaphylactic reactions can occur. Angioedema can occur at any time during treatment (especially following first dose). Careful blood pressure monitoring with first dose (hypotension can occur especially in volume depleted patients). Dosage adjustment needed in renal impairment. Use with caution in hypovolemia; collagen vascular diseases; valvular stenosis (particularly aortic stenosis); hyperkalemia; or before, during, or immediately after anesthesia. Avoid rapid dosage escalation which may lead to renal insufficiency. Hypersensitivity reactions may be seen during hemodialysis with high-flux dialysis membranes (eg, AN69). Hyperkalemia may rarely occur. Neutropenia/agranulocytosis with myeloid hyperplasia can rarely occur. If patient has renal impairment then a baseline WBC with differential and serum creatinine should be evaluated and monitored closely during the first 3 months of therapy. Use with caution in unilateral renal artery stenosis and pre-existing renal insufficiency.

**Adverse Reactions**

1% to 10%:

Cardiovascular: Chest pain (2%), syncope (2%), hypotension (6.7%)

Central nervous system: Headache (2% to 5%), dizziness (4% to 8%), fatigue (2% to 3%)

Dermatologic: Rash (1.5%)

Gastrointestinal: Abnormal taste, abdominal pain, vomiting, nausea, diarrhea, anorexia, constipation

Neuromuscular & skeletal: Weakness

Respiratory (1% to 2%): Bronchitis, cough, dyspnea

<1%: Agranulocytosis, alopecia, anemia, angina pectoris, angioedema, asthma, ataxia, blurred vision, bronchospasm, cardiac arrest, confusion, conjunctivitis, CVA, depression, diaphoresis, drowsiness, dyspepsia, erythema multiforme, glossitis, gynecomastia, hemolysis with G-6-PD, hepatitis, hyperkalemia, hypoglycemia, ileus, impotence, insomnia, jaundice, myocardial infarction, nervousness, neutropenia, oliguria, orthostatic hypotension, palpitations, pancreatitis, paresthesia, pemphigus, pruritus, pulmonary edema, renal dysfunction, Stevens-Johnson syndrome, stomatitis, tinnitus, URI, urinary tract infection, urticaria, vertigo, xerostomia

**Overdosage/Toxicology**

Signs and symptoms: Mild hypotension has been the only toxic effect seen with acute overdose. Bradycardia may also occur; hyperkalemia occurs even with therapeutic doses, especially in patients with renal insufficiency and those taking NSAIDs.

Treatment: Following initiation of essential overdose management, toxic symptom treatment and supportive treatment should be initiated. Hypotension usually responds to I.V. fluids or Trendelenburg positioning.

**Drug Interactions** CYP3A3/4 enzyme substrate

Alpha$_1$ blockers: Hypotensive effect increased

Aspirin: The effects of ACE inhibitors may be blunted by aspirin administration, particularly at higher dosages

Diuretics: Hypovolemia due to diuretics may precipitate acute hypotensive events or acute renal failure

Insulin: Risk of hypoglycemia may be increased

Lithium: Risk of lithium toxicity may be increased; monitor lithium levels, especially in the first 4 weeks of therapy

Mercaptopurine: Risk of neutropenia may be increased

NSAIDs may decrease ACE inhibitor efficacy and/or increase risk of renal adverse effects

Potassium-sparing diuretics (amiloride, spironolactone, triamterene): Increased risk of hyperkalemia

Potassium supplements may increase the risk of hyperkalemia

Trimethoprim (high dose) may increase the risk of hyperkalemia

**Usual Dosage** Use lower listed initial dose in patients with hyponatremia, hypovolemia, severe congestive heart failure, decreased renal function, or in those receiving diuretics.

Infants and Children:

Investigational initial oral doses of **enalapril:** 0.1 mg/kg/day increasing as needed over 2 weeks to 0.5 mg/kg/day have been used to treat severe congestive heart failure in infants.

(Continued)

## Enalapril *(Continued)*

Investigational I.V. doses of **enalaprilat**: 5-10 mcg/kg/dose administered every 8-24 hours have been used for the treatment of neonatal hypertension. Monitor patients carefully; select patients may require higher doses.

Adults:

Oral: **Enalapril**

Hypertension: 2.5-5 mg/day then increase as required, usual therapeutic dose for hypertension: 10-40 mg/day in 1-2 divided doses. **Note:** Initiate with 2.5 mg if patient is taking a diuretic which cannot be discontinued. May add a diuretic if blood pressure cannot be controlled with enalapril alone.

Heart failure: As adjunct with diuretics and digitalis, initiate with 2.5 mg once or twice daily (usual range: 5-20 mg/day in 2 divided doses; maximum: 40 mg)

Asymptomatic left ventricular dysfunction: 2.5 mg twice daily, titrated as tolerated to 20 mg/day

I.V.: **Enalaprilat**

Hypertension: 1.25 mg/dose, given over 5 minutes every 6 hours; doses as high as 5 mg/dose every 6 hours have been tolerated for up to 36 hours. **Note:** If patients are concomitantly receiving diuretic therapy, begin with 0.625 mg I.V. over 5 minutes; if the effect is not adequate after 1 hour, repeat the dose and administer 1.25 mg at 6-hour intervals thereafter; if adequate, administer 0.625 mg I.V. every 6 hours.

Heart failure: Avoid I.V. administration in patients with unstable heart failure or those suffering acute myocardial infarction.

Conversion from I.V. to oral therapy if not concurrently on diuretics: 5 mg once daily; subsequent titration as needed; if concurrently receiving diuretics and responding to 0.625 mg I.V. every 6 hours, initiate with 2.5 mg/day.

**Dosing adjustment in renal impairment:**

Oral: Enalapril:

$Cl_{cr}$ 30-80 mL/minute: Administer 5 mg/day titrated upwards to maximum of 40 mg.

$Cl_{cr}$ <30 mL/minute: Administer 2.5 mg day; titrated upward until blood pressure is controlled.

For heart failure patients with sodium <130 mEq/L or serum creatinine >1.6 mg/dL, initiate dosage with 2.5 mg/day, increasing to twice daily as needed. Increase further in increments of 2.5 mg/dose at >4-day intervals to a maximum daily dose of 40 mg.

I.V.: Enalaprilat:

$Cl_{cr}$ >30 mL/minute: Initiate with 1.25 mg every 6 hours and increase dose based on response.

$Cl_{cr}$ <30 mL/minute: Initiate with 0.625 mg every 6 hours and increase dose based on response.

Hemodialysis: Moderately dialyzable (20% to 50%); administer dose postdialysis (eg, 0.625 mg I.V. every 6 hours) or administer 20% to 25% supplemental dose following dialysis; Clearance: 62 mL/minute.

Peritoneal dialysis: Supplemental dose is not necessary, although some removal of drug occurs.

**Dosing adjustment in hepatic impairment:** Hydrolysis of enalapril to enalaprilat may be delayed and/or impaired in patients with severe hepatic impairment, but the pharmacodynamic effects of the drug do not appear to be significantly altered; no dosage adjustment.

**Patient Information** Take exactly as directed; do not discontinue without consulting prescriber. Take first dose at bedtime. Take all doses on an empty stomach (30 minutes before or 2 hours after meals). This drug does not eliminate need for diet or exercise regimen as recommended by prescriber. Do not use potassium supplements or salt substitutes containing potassium without consulting prescriber. May cause dizziness, fainting, lightheadedness (use caution when driving or engaging in tasks that require alertness until response to drug is known); postural hypotension (use caution when rising from lying or sitting position or climbing stairs); nausea, vomiting, abdominal pain, dry mouth, or transient loss of appetite (small frequent meals, frequent mouth care, sucking lozenges, or chewing gum may help) - report if these persist. Report chest pain or palpitations; mouth sores; fever or chills; swelling of extremities, face, mouth, or tongue; skin rash; numbness, tingling, or pain in muscles; difficulty in breathing or unusual cough; or other persistent adverse reactions.

**Nursing Implications** May cause depression in some patients; discontinue if angioedema of the face, extremities, lips, tongue, or glottis occurs; watch for hypotensive effects within 1-3 hours of first dose or new higher dose

**Dosage Forms**

Injection, as enalaprilat: 1.25 mg/mL (1 mL, 2 mL)

Tablet, as maleate: 2.5 mg, 5 mg, 10 mg, 20 mg

## Enalapril and Diltiazem (e NAL a pril & dil TYE a zem)

**U.S. Brand Names** Teczem®

**Pharmacologic Category** Antihypertensive Agent, Combination

**Use** Treatment of hypertension, however, not indicated for initial treatment of hypertension; replacement therapy in patients receiving separate dosage forms (for patient convenience); when monotherapy with one component fails to achieve desired antihypertensive effect, or when dose-limiting adverse effects limit upward titration of monotherapy

**Effects on Mental Status** May cause drowsiness and dizziness, nervousness, or insomnia; rarely may cause confusion, depression

**Effects on Psychiatric Treatment** May rarely cause agranulocytosis; use caution with clozapine and carbamazepine; may decrease lithium clearance resulting in an increase in serum lithium levels and potential lithium toxicity; monitor serum lithium levels; carbamazepine levels may be increased; monitor levels

**Usual Dosage** Adults: Oral: One tablet daily, if further blood pressure control is required, increase dosage to two tablets daily

**Dosage Forms** Tablet, extended release: Enalapril maleate 5 mg and diltiazem maleate 180 mg

## Enalapril and Felodipine (e NAL a pril & fe LOE di peen)

**U.S. Brand Names** Lexxel™

**Pharmacologic Category** Antihypertensive Agent, Combination

**Use** Treatment of hypertension, however, not indicated for initial treatment of hypertension; replacement therapy in patients receiving separate dosage forms (for patient convenience); when monotherapy with one component fails to achieve desired antihypertensive effect, or when dose-limiting adverse effects limit upward titration of monotherapy

**Effects on Mental Status** May cause drowsiness and dizziness; rarely may cause nervousness, insomnia, confusion, or depression

**Effects on Psychiatric Treatment** May rarely cause agranulocytosis; use caution with clozapine and carbamazepine; may decrease lithium clearance resulting in an increase in serum lithium levels and potential lithium toxicity; monitor serum lithium levels; carbamazepine may decrease felodipine effect

**Usual Dosage** Adults: Oral: 1 tablet daily

**Dosage Forms** Tablet, extended release: Enalapril maleate 5 mg and felodipine 5 mg

## Enalapril and Hydrochlorothiazide
(e NAL a pril & hye droe klor oh THYE a zide)

**U.S. Brand Names** Vaseretic® 10-25

**Canadian Brand Names** Vaseretic®

**Pharmacologic Category** Antihypertensive Agent, Combination

**Use** Treatment of hypertension

**Effects on Mental Status** May cause drowsiness and dizziness; rarely may cause insomnia, confusion, and depression

**Effects on Psychiatric Treatment** May rarely cause agranulocytosis; use caution with clozapine and carbamazepine; may decrease lithium clearance resulting in an increase in serum lithium levels and potential lithium toxicity; monitor serum lithium levels

**Usual Dosage** Oral: Dose is individualized

**Dosage Forms** Tablet:

Enalapril maleate 5 mg and hydrochlorothiazide 12.5 mg

Enalapril maleate 10 mg and hydrochlorothiazide 25 mg

♦ **Enalaprilat** *see* Enalapril *on page 191*

♦ **Enalapril Maleate** *see* Enalapril *on page 191*

♦ **Enbrel®** *see* Etanercept *on page 209*

## Encainide (en KAY nide)

**U.S. Brand Names** Enkaid®

**Pharmacologic Category** Antiarrhythmic Agent, Class I-C

**Use** Ventricular arrhythmias; supraventricular arrhythmias

**Effects on Mental Status** Dizziness is common

**Effects on Psychiatric Treatment** Use beta-blockers with caution; may produce additive negative inotropic effect; caution with TCAs

**Contraindications** Hypersensitivity to encainide or any component; second or third degree A-V block; premature ventricular complexes; nonsustained ventricular arrhythmias; cardiogenic shock

**Warnings/Precautions** Can cause new or worsened arrhythmias; such proarrhythmic effects range from an increase in frequency of PVCs to the development of more severe ventricular tachycardia (ie, tachycardia that is more sustained or more resistant to conversion to sinus rhythm), with potentially fatal consequences; use with caution in patients with a history of congestive heart failure or myocardial dysfunction; use is recommended only in patients with life-threatening arrhythmias

**Adverse Reactions**

>10%:

Central nervous system: Dizziness

Ocular: Blurred vision

1% to 10%:

Cardiovascular: Chest pain congestive heart failure, ventricular tachycardia

Central nervous system: Headache

Gastrointestinal: Vomiting

Neuromuscular & skeletal: Weakness
Otic: Tinnitus

**Overdosage/Toxicology**

Signs and symptoms: Second or third degree A-V block, sinus arrest, hypotension, convulsions, widening of QRS complex

Treatment: Cardiac dysrhythmias and hypotension often respond to bolus I.V. injections of hypertonic sodium bicarbonate 1-2 mEq/kg, while conventional type I-A antiarrhythmics tend to worsen conduction defects, especially ventricular arrhythmias. In those patients displaying seizures along with conduction defects, phenytoin may be most effective in reducing these symptoms.

**Drug Interactions** CYP2D6 enzyme substrate; beta-blockers (possible negative inotropic effects)

**Usual Dosage** Adults: Oral: 25 mg every 8 hours; may increase to 35 mg every 8 hours after 3-5 days if needed; increase to 50 mg every 8 hours in another 3-5 days if response is not achieved

**Patient Information** Take as directed; do not change dose except from advice of your physician; report any chest pain and irregular heartbeats

**Dosage Forms** Capsule, as hydrochloride: 25 mg, 35 mg, 50 mg


- ♦ **Encare® [OTC]** *see* Nonoxynol 9 *on page 398*
- ♦ **Endal®** *see* Guaifenesin and Phenylephrine *on page 257*
- ♦ **End Lice® Liquid [OTC]** *see* Pyrethrins *on page 480*
- ♦ **Endocet®** *see* Oxycodone and Acetaminophen *on page 414*
- ♦ **Endolor®** *see* Butalbital Compound and Acetaminophen *on page 80*
- ♦ **Enduron®** *see* Methyclothiazide *on page 356*
- ♦ **Ener-B®** *see* Cyanocobalamin *on page 143*
- ♦ **Engerix-B®** *see* Hepatitis B Vaccine *on page 266*
- ♦ **English Hawthorn** *see* Hawthorn *on page 264*
- ♦ **Enisyl® [OTC]** *see* L-Lysine *on page 322*
- ♦ **Enkaid®** *see* Encainide *on page 192*
- ♦ **Enlon® Injection** *see* Edrophonium *on page 189*
- ♦ **Enomine®** *see* Guaifenesin, Phenylpropanolamine, and Phenylephrine *on page 258*
- ♦ **Enovil®** *see* Amitriptyline *on page 33*


## Enoxacin (en OKS a sin)

**U.S. Brand Names** Penetrex™

**Pharmacologic Category** Antibiotic, Quinolone

**Use** Treatment of complicated and uncomplicated urinary tract infections caused by susceptible gram-negative and gram-positive bacteria and uncomplicated urethral or cervical gonorrhea due to *N. gonorrhoeae*

**Effects on Mental Status** May cause dizziness; rarely may cause confusion, insomnia, or drowsiness; quinolones reported to cause restlessness, hallucinations, euphoria, depression, panic, and paranoia

**Effects on Psychiatric Treatment** Rarely causes leukopenia; use caution with clozapine and carbamazepine

**Pregnancy Risk Factor** C

**Contraindications** Hypersensitivity to enoxacin, any component, or other quinolones

**Warnings/Precautions** Use with caution in patients with a history of convulsions or epilepsy, renal dysfunction, psychosis, elevated intracranial pressure, prepubertal children, and pregnancy; nalidixic acid and ciprofloxacin (related compounds) have been associated with erosions of the cartilage in weight-bearing joints and other signs of arthropathy in immature animals and children; similar precautions are advised for enoxacin although no data is available; has rarely caused ruptured tendons (discontinue immediately with signs of inflammation or tendon pain)

**Adverse Reactions**

1% to 10%:

Central nervous system: Dizziness (<3%), headache (<2%), vertigo (3%)

Gastrointestinal: Nausea (2.9%), vomiting (6% to 9%), abdominal pain (1% to 2%), diarrhea (1% to 2%)

<1%: Acute renal failure, anemia, anorexia, arthralgia, chills, confusion, constipation, depression, drowsiness, dyspepsia, edema, eosinophilia, exfoliative dermatitis, fatigue, fever, flatulence, GI bleeding, hypo/hyperkalemia, increased liver enzymes, increased serum creatinine/BUN, insomnia, leukocytosis, leukopenia, palpitations, paresthesias, photosensitivity, proteinuria, pruritus, rash, restlessness, ruptured tendons, seizures, syncope, tremor, vaginitis, visual disturbances, xerostomia

**Overdosage/Toxicology**

Signs and symptoms: Acute renal failure, seizures

Treatment: GI decontamination and supportive care; diazepam for seizures; not removed by peritoneal or hemodialysis

**Drug Interactions** CYP1A2 enzyme inhibitor

Decreased effect of enoxacin with antacids (magnesium, aluminum), iron and zinc salts, sucralfate, bismuth salts, antineoplastics

Increased toxicity/levels of warfarin, cyclosporine, digoxin, caffeine, and theophylline with enoxacin

Increased levels of enoxacin with cimetidine, probenecid

**Usual Dosage** Adults: Oral:

Complicated urinary tract infection: 400 mg twice daily for 14 days

Cystitis: 200 mg twice daily for 7 days

Uncomplicated gonorrhea: 400 mg as single dose

**Dosing adjustment in renal impairment:** $Cl_{cr}$ <50 mL/minute: Administer 50% of dose

**Patient Information** Take as prescribed and for as long as directed. Take on an empty stomach (1 hour prior to or after meals). Do not use antacids within 2 hours of medication. Maintain adequate hydration (2-3 L/day of fluids unless instructed to restrict fluid intake). You may experience stomach discomfort (eat small, frequent meals) and dizziness or blurred vision (use caution when driving). May cause photosensitivity (use sunscreen, wear protective clothing and eyewear, and avoid direct sunlight). Report skin rash; visual changes; severe gastric upset; weakness; pain, inflammation, or rupture of tendon; or signs or symptoms of opportunistic infection (eg, white spots or sores in mouth or perineal area, itching or vaginal discharge, unhealed sores, fever).

**Dosage Forms** Tablet: 200 mg, 400 mg

## Enoxaparin (e noks ah PAIR in)

**U.S. Brand Names** Lovenox® Injection

**Pharmacologic Category** Low Molecular Weight Heparin

**Use** Prevention of deep vein thrombosis following hip or knee replacement surgery or abdominal surgery in patients at risk for thromboembolic complications; inpatient treatment of acute deep vein thrombosis with and without pulmonary embolism when administered in conjunction with warfarin sodium; outpatient treatment of acute deep vein thrombosis without pulmonary embolism when administered in conjunction with warfarin sodium; prevention of ischemic complications of unstable angina and non-Q wave myocardial infarction (when administered with aspirin)

**Effects on Mental Status** May cause confusion

**Effects on Psychiatric Treatment** None reported

**Usual Dosage** S.C.:

Prophylaxis of DVT following abdominal, hip replacement or knee replacement surgery:

Children: Safety and effectiveness have not been established.

Adults:

DVT prophylaxis in hip replacement:

30 mg twice daily: First dose within 12-24 hours after surgery and every 12 hours until risk of deep vein thrombosis has diminished or the patient is adequately anticoagulated on warfarin. Average duration of therapy: 7-10 days.

40 mg once daily: First dose within 9-15 hours before surgery and daily until risk of deep vein thrombosis has diminished or the patient is adequately anticoagulated on warfarin. Average duration of therapy: 7-10 days unless warfarin is not given concurrently, then 40 mg S.C. once daily should be continued for 3 more weeks (4 weeks total).

DVT prophylaxis in knee replacement:

30 mg twice daily: First dose within 12-24 hours after surgery and every 12 hours until risk of deep vein thrombosis has diminished. Average duration of therapy: 7-10 days; maximum course: 14 days.

Patients who weigh <100 lb or are >65 years of age: Some clinicians recommend 0.5 mg/kg/dose every 12 hours to reduce the risk of bleeding.

DVT prophylaxis in high-risk patients undergoing abdominal surgery: 40 mg once daily, with initial dose given 2 hours prior to surgery; usual duration: 7-10 days and up to 12 days has been tolerated in clinical trials.

Treatment of acute proximal DVT: Start warfarin within 72 hours and continue enoxaparin until INR is between 2.0 and 3.0 (usually 7 days).

Inpatient treatment of DVT with or without pulmonary embolism: Adults: S.C. 1 mg/kg/dose every 12 hours or 1.5 mg/kg once daily.

Outpatient treatment of DVT without pulmonary embolism: Adults: S.C.: 1 mg/kg/dose every 12 hours.

Prevention of ischemic complications with unstable angina or non-Q-wave myocardial infarction: S.C.: 1 mg/kg twice daily in conjunction with oral aspirin therapy (100-325 mg once daily); treatment should be continued for a minimum of 2 days and continued until clinical stabilization (usually 2-8 days).

**Dosing adjustment in renal impairment:** Total clearance is lower and elimination is delayed in patients with renal failure; adjustment may be necessary in elderly and patients with severe renal impairment.

Hemodialysis: Supplemental dose is not necessary.

Peritoneal dialysis: Significant drug removal is unlikely based on physiochemical characteristics.

**Dosage Forms** Injection, as sodium, preservative free:

Prefilled syringes: 30 mg/0.3 mL, 40 mg/0.4 mL

Graduated prefilled syringe: 60 mg/0.6 mL, 80 mg/0.8 mL, 100 mg/1.0 mL

Ampul: 30 mg/0.3 mL

## Entacapone (en TA ka pone)

**U.S. Brand Names** Comtan®

**Pharmacologic Category** Anti-Parkinson's Agent (COMT Inhibitor)

**Use** Adjunct to levodopa/carbidopa therapy in patients with idiopathic Parkinson's disease who experience "wearing-off" symptoms at the end of a dosing interval

**Pregnancy Risk Factor** C

**Pregnancy/Breast-Feeding Implications** Not recommended

**Contraindications** Hypersensitivity to the drug or any of its components

**Warnings/Precautions** Patient should not be treated concomitantly with entacapone and a nonselective MAO inhibitor. Orthostatic hypotension may be increased in patients on dopaminergic therapy in Parkinson's disease.

**Adverse Reactions**

>10%:

Gastrointestinal: Nausea (14%)

Neuromuscular & skeletal: Dyskinesia (25%), placebo (15%)

1% to 10%:

Central nervous system: Dizziness (8%), fatigue (6%), hallucinations (4%), anxiety (2%), somnolence (2%), agitation (1%)

Cardiovascular: Orthostatic hypotension (4.3%), syncope (1.2%)

Dermatologic: Purpura (2%)

Gastrointestinal: Diarrhea (10%), abdominal pain (8%), constipation (6%), vomiting (4%), dry mouth (3%), dyspepsia (2%), flatulence (2%), gastritis (1%), taste perversion (1%)

Genitourinary: Brown-orange urine discoloration (10%)

Neuromuscular & skeletal: Hyperkinesia (10%), hypokinesia (9%), back pain (4%), weakness (2%)

Miscellaneous: Increased sweating (2%), bacterial infection (1%)

Respiratory: Dyspnea (3%)

<1%: Hyperpyrexia and confusion (resembling neuroleptic malignant syndrome), pulmonary fibrosis, rhabdomyolysis, retroperitoneal fibrosis

**Note:** Approximately 14% of the 603 patients given entacapone in the double-blind, placebo-controlled trials discontinued treatment due to adverse events compared to 9% of the 400 patients who received placebo.

**Overdosage/Toxicology** There have been no reported cases of intentional or accidental overdose with this drug. COMT inhibition by entacapone treatment is dose-dependent.

**Drug Interactions** CYP1A2, 2A6, 2C9, 2C19, 2D6, 2E1, and 3A enzyme inhibitor, but only at high concentrations; not believed to be important clinically. These effects are seen only at concentrations higher than those achieved at recommended dosing.

Bromocriptine: Fibrotic complications (retroperitoneal or pulmonary fibrosis) have been associated with combinations of entacapone and bromocriptine

Catecholamines (and other drugs metabolized by COMT): Significant increases in cardiac effects or arrhythmias with drugs metabolized by COMT (eg, alpha-methyldopa, apomorphine, bitolterol, dobutamine, dopamine, epinephrine, isoproterenol, isoetharine, methyldopa, norepinephrine)

CNS depressants: Effects on mental status may be additive with other CNS depressants; includes barbiturates, benzodiazepines, TCAs, antipsychotics, ethanol, narcotic analgesics, and other sedative-hypnotics

Iron: Entacapone chelates iron and absorption may be limited; an iron supplement should not be administered at the same time as this agent

Levodopa: Therapeutic effects may be enhanced by entacapone

Linezolid: Due to MAO inhibition (see below); this combination should be avoided

MAO inhibitors: Concurrent use of nonselective MAO inhibitors with entacapone is contraindicated

Pergolide: Fibrotic complications (retroperitoneal or pulmonary fibrosis) have been associated with combinations of entacapone and pergolide

Selegiline: At low doses of selegiline, a selective MAO type B inhibitor, there does not appear to be an interaction with entacapone

**Note:** Caution with drugs that interfere with glucuronidation, intestinal, biliary excretion, intestinal beta-glucuronidase (eg, probenecid, cholestyramine, erythromycin, chloramphenicol, rifampicin, ampicillin)

**Mechanism of Action** Entacapone is a reversible and selective inhibitor of catechol-O-methyltransferase (COMT). When entacapone is taken with levodopa, the pharmacokinetics are altered, resulting in more sustained levodopa serum levels compared to levodopa taken alone. The resulting levels of levodopa provide for increased concentrations available for absorption across the blood-brain barrier, thereby providing for increased CNS levels of dopamine, the active metabolite of levodopa.

**Pharmacodynamics/kinetics**

Onset of action: Rapid

Peak effect: 1 hour

Absorption: Rapid

Distribution: $V_d$: 20 L after an I.V. dose at steady-state

Protein binding: 98% mainly to albumin

Metabolism: Isomerization to the cis-isomer, followed by direct glucuronidation of the parent and cis-isomer

Bioavailability: 35%

Half-life: 0.4-0.7 hours based on B-phase; 2.4 hours based on Y-phase

Time to peak serum concentration: 1 hour

Elimination: 10% in urine, 90% in feces

**Usual Dosage**

Adults: Oral: 200 mg dose, up to a maximum of 8 times/day; maximum daily dose: 1600 mg/day. Always administer with levodopa/carbidopa. To optimize therapy, the levodopa/carbidopa dosage must be reduced, usually by 25%. This reduction is usually necessary when the patient is taking more than 800 mg of levodopa daily.

**Dosage adjustment in hepatic impairment:** Treat with caution and monitor carefully; AUC and $C_{max}$ can be possibly doubled

**Dietary Considerations** Can take with or without food

**Administration** Always administer in association with levodopa/carbidopa; can be combined with both the immediate and sustained release formulations of levodopa/carbidopa. Can be taken with or without food. Should not be abruptly withdrawn from patient's therapy due to significant worsening of symptoms.

**Monitoring Parameters** Signs and symptoms of Parkinson's disease; liver function tests, blood pressure, patient's mental status

**Patient Information** Take only as prescribed; can be taken with or without food. Possible nausea, hallucinations, and change in color of urine (not clinically relevant) may occur. Do not drive a car or operate other complex machinery until there is sufficient experience with entacapone. Do not withdraw medication unless advised by healthcare professional.

**Dosage Forms** Tablet: 200 mg


- **Entertainer's Secret® Spray [OTC]** *see* Saliva Substitute *on page 502*
- **Entex®** *see* Guaifenesin, Phenylpropanolamine, and Phenylephrine *on page 258*
- **Entex® LA** *see* Guaifenesin and Phenylpropanolamine *on page 257*
- **Entex® PSE** *see* Guaifenesin and Pseudoephedrine *on page 257*
- **Entuss-D® Liquid** *see* Hydrocodone and Pseudoephedrine *on page 273*
- **Enulose®** *see* Lactulose *on page 306*
- **Enzone®** *see* Pramoxine and Hydrocortisone *on page 457*


## Ephedra

**Related Information**

Herbals That May Alter Metabolism and GI Absorption of Drugs *on page 745*

Natural Products, Herbals, and Dietary Supplements *on page 742*

Perspectives on the Safety of Herbal Medicines *on page 736*

**Synonyms** *Ephedra sinica*; Ma-Huang; Mormon Tea; Poptillo; Sea Grape; Squaw Tea

**Pharmacologic Category** Herb

**Use** Herbal medicinal uses include treatment for asthma, bronchitis, edema, arthritis, headache, fever, urticaria; also used for weight reduction and for euphoria

**Restrictions** Limit daily consumption to 120 mg total ephedra alkaloids in 4 equal doses

**Pregnancy Risk Factor** Contraindicated

**Contraindications** Per Commission E: Anxiety, restlessness, hypertension, glaucoma, impaired cerebral circulation, prostate adenoma with residual urine accumulation, pheochromocytoma, thyrotoxicosis

**Warnings/Precautions** AHPA warning as of March 1994 for ephedra product labels: "Seek advice from 2 healthcare professionals prior to use if you are pregnant or nursing, or if you have high blood pressure, heart or thyroid disease, diabetes, difficulty in urination due to prostate enlargement, or if taking two MAO inhibitors or any other prescription drug. Reduce or discontinue use if nervousness, tremor, sleeplessness, loss of appetite, or nausea occur. Not intended for use by persons <18 years of age. Keep out of reach of children."

**Adverse Reactions**

>10%: Central nervous system: Nervousness, restlessness, insomnia

<10%:

Cardiovascular: Hypertension, cardiomyopathy, vasculitis, cardiomegaly, palpitations, vasoconstriction

Central nervous system: CNS-stimulating effects, anxiety, fear, psychosis, tension, agitation, excitation, irritability, auditory and visual hallucinations, sympathetic storm

Gastrointestinal: Nausea, anorexia

Neuromuscular & skeletal: Tremors, weakness

**Overdosage/Toxicology**

Signs and symptoms: Dysrhythmias, CNS depression, depression, insomnia, dry skin, respiratory depression, vomiting, respiratory alkalosis, seizures, mydriasis

Decontamination: Lavage (within 1 hour)/activated charcoal with cathartic

Treatment: Supportive therapy; there is no specific antidote for ephedrine intoxication and the bulk of the treatment is supportive. Hyperactivity and agitation usually respond to reduced sensory input, however with extreme agitation haloperidol (2-5 mg I.M. for adults) may be required. Hyperthermia is best treated with external cooling measures, or when severe or unresponsive, muscle paralysis with pancuronium may be needed. Hypertension is usually transient and generally does not require treatment unless severe. For diastolic blood pressures >110 mm Hg, a nitroprusside infusion should be initiated. Seizures usually respond to diazepam or lorazepam I.V. and/or phenytoin maintenance regimens.

**Drug Interactions**

Antihypertensives (including calcium channel blockers and beta-blockers): Effects may be decreased by ephedra; contraindicated
Cardiac glycosides (digoxin): May precipitate arrhythmias; contraindicated
CNS stimulants: Effects/toxicity may be potentiated by ephedra
Guanethidine: Enhancement of sympathomimetic effect by ephedra
Halothane: May precipitate arrhythmias; contraindicated
Linezolid: Effect/toxicity may be enhanced and the sympathomimetic effect of ephedrine is potentiated; avoid concurrent administration
MAO inhibitors: Effect/toxicity may be enhanced and the sympathomimetic effect of ephedrine is potentiated; avoid concurrent administration

**Usual Dosage**

*E. sinica* extracts (with 10% alkaloid content): 125-250 mg 3 times/day
As a tea: Steeping 1 heaping teaspoon in 240 mL of boiling water for 10 minutes (equivalent to 15-30 mg of ephedrine)
Per Commission E: Single dose: Herb preparation corresponds to 15-30 mg total alkaloid (calculation as ephedrine)

**Patient Information** Considered unsafe by the FDA

**Additional Information** Erect evergreen shrubs growing up to 6 feet in height with rounded flowers blooming in early spring; while the fruits are nearly alkaloid free, the green stems and twigs contain the highest amount of ephedrine and pseudoephedrine; Mormon tea (*Ephedra nevadensis*) contains large amount of tannin, no ephedrine (but possibly t-norpseudoephedrine, a CNS stimulant) and can produce a mild diuresis along with constipation; in fact North and Central American ephedra species lack sympathomimetic alkaloids

♦ ***Ephedra sinica*** *see* Ephedra *on page 194*

## Ephedrine (e FED rin)

**Related Information**

Clozapine-Induced Side Effects *on page 780*

**U.S. Brand Names** Kondon's Nasal® [OTC]; Pretz-D® [OTC]

**Pharmacologic Category** Alpha/Beta Agonist

**Use** Treatment of bronchial asthma, nasal congestion, acute bronchospasm, idiopathic orthostatic hypotension

**Effects on Mental Status** Nervousness, anxiety, agitation, restlessness, and insomnia are common

**Effects on Psychiatric Treatment** Use with MAOIs may produce hypertensive crisis; avoid combination

**Pregnancy Risk Factor** C

**Contraindications** Hypersensitivity to ephedrine or any component, cardiac arrhythmias, angle-closure glaucoma, patients on other sympathomimetic agents

**Warnings/Precautions** Blood volume depletion should be corrected before ephedrine therapy is instituted; use caution in patients with unstable vasomotor symptoms, diabetes, hyperthyroidism, prostatic hypertrophy, or a history of seizures; also use caution in the elderly and those patients with cardiovascular disorders such as coronary artery disease, arrhythmias, and hypertension. Ephedrine may cause hypertension resulting in intracranial hemorrhage. Long-term use may cause anxiety and symptoms of paranoid schizophrenia. Avoid as a bronchodilator; generally not used as a bronchodilator since new $beta_2$ agents are less toxic. Use with caution in the elderly, since it crosses the blood-brain barrier and may cause confusion.

**Adverse Reactions**

>10%: Central nervous system: CNS stimulating effects, nervousness, anxiety, apprehension, fear, tension, agitation, excitation, restlessness, irritability, insomnia, hyperactivity

1% to 10%:
- Cardiovascular: Hypertension, tachycardia, palpitations, elevation or depression of blood pressure, unusual pallor
- Central nervous system: Dizziness, headache
- Gastrointestinal: Xerostomia, nausea, anorexia, GI upset, vomiting
- Genitourinary: Painful urination
- Neuromuscular & skeletal: Trembling, tremor (more common in the elderly), weakness
- Miscellaneous: Diaphoresis (increased)

<1%: Arrhythmias, chest pain, dyspnea

**Overdosage/Toxicology**

Signs and symptoms: Dysrhythmias, CNS excitation, respiratory depression, vomiting, convulsions

Treatment: There is no specific antidote for ephedrine intoxication and the bulk of the treatment is supportive. Hyperactivity and agitation usually respond to reduced sensory input; however, with extreme agitation, haloperidol (2-5 mg I.M. for adults) may be required. Hyperthermia is best treated with external cooling measures; or when severe or unresponsive, muscle paralysis with pancuronium may be needed. Hypertension is usually transient and generally does not require treatment unless severe. For diastolic blood pressures >110 mm Hg, a nitroprusside infusion should be initiated. Seizures usually respond to diazepam I.V. and/or phenytoin maintenance regimens.

**Drug Interactions**

Decreased effect: Alpha- and beta-adrenergic blocking agents decrease ephedrine vasopressor effects
Increased toxicity: Additive cardiostimulation with other sympathomimetic agents; theophylline → cardiostimulation; MAO inhibitors or atropine may increase blood pressure; cardiac glycosides or general anesthetics may increase cardiac stimulation

**Usual Dosage**

Children:
- Oral, S.C.: 3 mg/kg/day or 25-100 mg/m²/day in 4-6 divided doses every 4-6 hours
- I.M., slow I.V. push: 0.2-0.3 mg/kg/dose every 4-6 hours

Adults:
- Oral: 25-50 mg every 3-4 hours as needed
- I.M., S.C.: 25-50 mg, parenteral adult dose should not exceed 150 mg in 24 hours
- I.V.: 5-25 mg/dose slow I.V. push repeated after 5-10 minutes as needed, then every 3-4 hours not to exceed 150 mg/24 hours

**Patient Information** Use this medication exactly as directed; do not take more than recommended dosage. Avoid other stimulant prescriptive or OTC medications to avoid serious overdose reactions. Store this medication away from light. You may experience dizziness, blurred vision, restlessness (use caution when driving or engaging in tasks requiring alertness until response to drug is known); or difficulty urinating (empty bladder immediately before taking this medication). Report excessive nervousness or excitation, inability to sleep, facial flushing, pounding heartbeat, muscle tremors or weakness, chest pain or palpitations, bronchial irritation or coughing, or increased sweating.

**Nursing Implications** Do not administer unless solution is clear

**Dosage Forms**

Capsule, as sulfate: 25 mg, 50 mg
Injection, as sulfate: 25 mg/mL (1 mL); 50 mg/mL (1 mL, 10 mL)
Jelly, as sulfate (Kondon's Nasal®): 1% (20 g)
Spray, as sulfate (Pretz-D®): 0.25% (15 mL)

♦ **Epifrin®** *see* Epinephrine *on page 195*

♦ **Epilepsy Treatment** *see page 783*

♦ **E-Pilo-x® Ophthalmic** *see* Pilocarpine and Epinephrine *on page 445*

## Epinephrine (ep i NEF rin)

**Related Information**

Glaucoma Drug Therapy *on page 712*

**U.S. Brand Names** Adrenalin®; AsthmaHaler®; Bronitin®; Bronkaid® Mist [OTC]; Epifrin®; EpiPen® Auto-Injector; EpiPen® Jr Auto-Injector; Glaucon®; Primatene® Mist [OTC]; Sus-Phrine®

**Synonyms** Adrenaline; Epinephrine Bitartrate; Epinephrine Hydrochloride; Racemic Epinephrine

**Pharmacologic Category** Alpha/Beta Agonist; Antidote; Ophthalmic Agent, Antiglaucoma

**Use** Treatment of bronchospasms, anaphylactic reactions, cardiac arrest, management of open-angle (chronic simple) glaucoma

**Effects on Mental Status** Nervousness and restlessness are common; may cause insomnia

**Effects on Psychiatric Treatment** None reported; however, use cautiously with psychotropics that block alpha receptors (phenothiazines); may produce paradoxical hypotension

**Pregnancy Risk Factor** C

**Contraindications** Hypersensitivity to epinephrine or any component; cardiac arrhythmias, angle-closure glaucoma

**Warnings/Precautions** Use with caution in elderly patients, patients with diabetes mellitus, cardiovascular diseases (angina, tachycardia, myocardial infarction), thyroid disease, or cerebral arteriosclerosis, Parkinson's; some products contain sulfites as preservatives. Rapid I.V. infusion may cause death from cerebrovascular hemorrhage or cardiac arrhythmias. Oral inhalation of epinephrine is **not** the preferred route of administration.

**Adverse Reactions**

>10%:
- Cardiovascular: Tachycardia (parenteral), pounding heartbeat
- Central nervous system: Nervousness, restlessness

1% to 10%:
- Cardiovascular: Flushing, hypertension
- Central nervous system: Headache, dizziness, lightheadedness, insomnia
- Gastrointestinal: Nausea, vomiting
- Neuromuscular & skeletal: Weakness, trembling
- Miscellaneous: Diaphoresis (increased)

<1%: Acute urinary retention in patients with bladder outflow obstruction, anxiety, cardiac arrhythmias, chest pain, decreased renal and splanchnic blood flow, dry throat, increased myocardial oxygen consumption, pallor,

(Continued)

## Epinephrine *(Continued)*

precipitation of or exacerbation of narrow-angle glaucoma, sudden death, tachycardia, wheezing, xerostomia

**Overdosage/Toxicology**

Signs and symptoms: Hypertension which may result in subarachnoid hemorrhage and hemiplegia; symptoms of overdose include arrhythmias, unusually large pupils, pulmonary edema, renal failure, metabolic acidosis

Treatment: There is no specific antidote for epinephrine intoxication and the bulk of the treatment is supportive. Hyperactivity and agitation usually respond to reduced sensory input; however, with extreme agitation, haloperidol (2-5 mg I.M. for adults) may be required. Hyperthermia is best treated with external cooling measures; or when severe or unresponsive, muscle paralysis with pancuronium may be needed. Hypertension is usually transient and generally does not require treatment unless severe. For diastolic blood pressures >110 mm Hg, a nitroprusside infusion should be initiated. Seizures usually respond to diazepam I.V. and/or phenytoin maintenance regimens.

**Drug Interactions** Increased toxicity: Increased cardiac irritability if administered concurrently with halogenated inhalational anesthetics, beta-blocking agents, alpha-blocking agents

**Usual Dosage**

Neonates: Cardiac arrest: I.V.: Intratracheal: 0.01-0.03 mg/kg (0.1-0.3 mL/kg of **1:10,000** solution) every 3-5 minutes as needed; dilute intratracheal doses to 1-2 mL with normal saline

Infants and Children:

Bronchodilator: S.C.: 10 mcg/kg (0.01 mL/kg of **1:1000**) (single doses not to exceed 0.5 mg) **or** suspension (1:200): 0.005 mL/kg/dose (0.025 mg/kg/dose) to a maximum of 0.15 mL (0.75 mg for single dose) every 8-12 hours

Bradycardia:

I.V.: 0.01 mg/kg (0.1 mL/kg of **1:10,000** solution) every 3-5 minutes as needed (maximum: 1 mg/10 mL)

Intratracheal: 0.1 mg/kg (0.1 mL/kg of **1:1000** solution every 3-5 minutes); doses as high as 0.2 mg/kg may be effective

Asystole or pulseless arrest:

I.V. or intraosseous: **First dose**: 0.01 mg/kg (0.1 mL/kg of a **1:10,000** solution); **subsequent doses**: 0.1 mg/kg (0.1 mL/kg of a **1:1000** solution); doses as high as 0.2 mg/kg may be effective; repeat every 3-5 minutes

Intratracheal: 0.1 mg/kg (0.1 mL/kg of a **1:1000** solution); doses as high as 0.2 mg/kg may be effective

Hypersensitivity reaction: S.C.: 0.01 mg/kg every 15 minutes for 2 doses then every 4 hours as needed (single doses not to exceed 0.5 mg)

Refractory hypotension (refractory to dopamine/dobutamine): Continuous I.V. infusions of 0.1-1 mcg/kg/minute; titrate dosage to desired effect

Nebulization: 0.25-0.5 mL of 2.25% **racemic epinephrine** solution diluted in 3 mL normal saline, or L-epinephrine at an equivalent dose; racemic epinephrine 10 mg = 5 mg L-epinephrine; use lower end of dosing range for younger infants

Intranasal: Children ≥6 years and Adults: Apply locally as drops or spray or with sterile swab

Adults:

Asystole:

I.V.: 1 mg every 3-5 minutes; if this approach fails, alternative regimens include:

Intermediate: 2-5 mg every 3-5 minutes

Escalating: 1 mg, 3 mg, 5 mg at 3-minute intervals

High: 0.1 mg/kg every 3-5 minutes

Intratracheal: 1 mg (although optimal dose is unknown, doses of 2-2.5 times the I.V. dose may be needed)

Bronchodilator: I.M., S.C. (**1:1000**): 0.1-0.5 mg every 10-15 minutes to 4 hours

Hypersensitivity reaction: I.M., S.C.: 0.2-0.5 mg every 20 minutes to 4 hours (single dose maximum: 1 mg)

Refractory hypotension (refractory to dopamine/dobutamine): Continuous I.V. infusion 1 mcg/minute (range: 1-10 mcg/minute); titrate dosage to desired effect; severe cardiac dysfunction may require doses >10 mcg/minute (up to 0.1 mcg/kg/minute)

Nebulization: Instill 8-15 drops into nebulizer reservoirs; administer 1-3 inhalations 4-6 times/day

Ophthalmic: Instill 1-2 drops in eye(s) once or twice daily; when treating open-angle glaucoma, the concentration and dosage must be adjusted to the response of the patient

**Patient Information** Use this medication exactly as directed; do not take more than recommended dosage. Avoid other stimulant prescriptive or OTC medications to avoid serious overdose reactions. You may experience dizziness, blurred vision, restlessness (use caution when driving or engaging in tasks requiring alertness until response to drug is known); or difficulty urinating (empty bladder immediately before taking this medication). Report excessive nervousness or excitation, inability to sleep, facial flushing, pounding heartbeat, muscle tremors or weakness, chest pain or palpitations, bronchial irritation or coughing, or increased sweating.

Ophthalmic: Wash hands before instilling. Sit or lie down to instill. Open eye, look at ceiling, and instill prescribed amount of medication. Close eye and roll eye in all directions, and apply gentle pressure to inner corner of eye. Do not let tip of applicator touch eye or contaminate tip of applicator. Temporary stinging or burning may occur. Report persistent pain, burning, vision disturbances, swelling, itching, or worsening of condition.

Aerosol: Use aerosol or nebulizer as per instructions. Clear as much mucus as possible before use. Rinse mouth following each use. If more than one inhalation is necessary, wait 1 minute between inhalations. May cause restlessness or nervousness; use caution when driving or engaging in hazardous activities until response to medication is known. Report persistent nervousness, restlessness, sleeplessness, palpitations, tachycardia, chest pain, muscle tremors, dizziness, flushing, or if breathing difficulty persists.

Nasal: Instill 1 spray into each nostril 3-4 times a day. Report if symptoms worsen or nasal passages become irritated.

**Nursing Implications** Patients should be cautioned to avoid the use of over-the-counter epinephrine inhalation products; $beta_2$-adrenergic agents for inhalation are preferred

**Management of extravasation:** Use phentolamine as antidote; mix 5 mg with 9 mL of NS; inject a small amount of this dilution into extravasated area; blanching should reverse immediately. Monitor site; if blanching should recur, additional injections of phentolamine may be needed.

**Dosage Forms**

Aerosol, oral:

Bitartrate (AsthmaHaler®, Bronitin®, Medihaler-Epi®, Primatene® Suspension): 0.3 mg/spray [epinephrine base 0.16 mg/spray] (10 mL, 15 mL, 22.5 mL)

Bronkaid®: 0.5% (10 mL, 15 mL, 22.5 mL)

Primatene®: 0.2 mg/spray (15 mL, 22.5 mL)

Auto-injector:

EpiPen®: Delivers 0.3 mg I.M. of epinephrine 1:1000 (2 mL)

EpiPen® Jr.: Delivers 0.15 mg I.M. of epinephrine 1:2000 (2 mL)

Solution:

Inhalation:

Adrenalin®: 1% [10 mg/mL, 1:100] (7.5 mL)

AsthmaNefrin®, microNefrin®, Nephron®, S-2®: Racepinephrine 2% [epinephrine base 1.125%] (7.5 mL, 15 mL, 30 mL)

Vaponefrin®: Racepinephrine 2% [epinephrine base 1%] (15 mL, 30 mL)

Injection:

Adrenalin®: 0.01 mg/mL [1:100,000] (5 mL); 0.1 mg/mL [1:10,000] (3 mL, 10 mL); 1 mg/mL [1:1000] (1 mL, 2 mL, 30 mL)

Suspension (Sus-Phrine®): 5 mg/mL [1:200] (0.3 mL, 5 mL)

Nasal (Adrenalin®): 0.1% [1 mg/mL, 1:1000] (30 mL)

Ophthalmic, as borate (Epinal®): 0.5% (7.5 mL); 1% (7.5 mL)

Ophthalmic, as hydrochloride (Epifrin®, Glaucon®): 0.1% (1 mL, 30 mL); 0.5% (15 mL); 1% (1 mL, 10 mL, 15 mL); 2% (10 mL, 15 mL)

Topical (Adrenalin®): 0.1% [1 mg/mL, 1:1000] (10 mL, 30 mL)


- **Epinephrine Bitartrate** *see* Epinephrine *on page 195*
- **Epinephrine Hydrochloride** *see* Epinephrine *on page 195*
- **EpiPen® Auto-Injector** *see* Epinephrine *on page 195*
- **EpiPen® Jr Auto-Injector** *see* Epinephrine *on page 195*


## Epirubicin (ep i ROO bi sin)

**U.S. Brand Names** Ellence™

**Pharmacologic Category** Antineoplastic Agent, Anthracycline; Antineoplastic Agent, Antibiotic

**Use** As a component of adjuvant therapy following primary resection of primary breast cancer in patients with evidence of axillary node tumor involvement

**Effects on Mental Status** Lethargy is common

**Effects on Psychiatric Treatment** Leukopenia is common; use caution with clozapine and carbamazepine

**Usual Dosage**

Adults: I.V.:

Recommended starting dose: 100-120 mg/m$^2$. Epirubicin is given in repeated 3- to 4-week cycles with the total dose given on day 1 of each cycle or divided equally and given on days 1 and 8 of each cycle. Patients receiving the 120 mg/m$^2$ regimen should also receive prophylactic antibiotics with TMP-SMX or a fluoroquinolone.

As a component of adjuvant therapy in patients with axillary-node positive breast cancer:

CEF-120: 60 mg/m$^2$ on days 1 and 8 of cycle (in combination with cyclophosphamide and 5-fluorouracil); cycle is repeated every 28 days for 6 cycles

FEC-100: 100 mg/m$^2$ on day 1 of cycle (in combination with 5-fluorouracil and cyclophosphamide); cycle is repeated every 21 days for 6 cycles

Dosage adjustment in bone marrow dysfunction:
Patients with heavy pretreatment, pre-existing bone marrow depression, or the presence of neoplastic bone marrow infiltration: Consider lower starting doses of 75-90 mg/m$^2$
Dosage modifications after the first treatment cycle: Nadir platelet counts <50,000/mm$^3$, ANC <250/mm$^3$, neutropenic fever, or grades 3/4 nonhematologic toxicity: Reduce day 1 dose in subsequent cycles to 75% of the current cycle. Day 1 chemotherapy in subsequent courses of treatment should be delayed until platelet counts are ≥100,000/mm$^3$, ANC ≥1500/mm$^3$, and nonhematologic toxicities have recovered to ≤grade 1.
In addition, for patients receiving divided dose (day 1 and day 8) regimen:
Day 8 platelet counts 75,000-100,000/mm$^3$ and ANC 1000-1499/mm$^3$: Day 8 dose should be 75% of the day 1 dose
Day 8 platelet counts <75,000/mm$^3$, ANC <1000/mm$^3$, or grade 3 or 4 nonhematologic toxicity: Omit day 8 dose

**Dosage adjustment in renal impairment:** Severe renal impairment (serum creatinine >5 mg/dL): Lower doses should be considered

**Dosage adjustment in hepatic impairment:**
Bilirubin 1.2-3 mg/dL or AST 2-4 times the upper limit of normal: 50% of recommended starting dose
Bilirubin >3 mg/dL or AST >4 times the upper limit of normal: 25% of recommended starting dose

Elderly: Plasma clearance of epirubicin in elderly female patients was noted to be reduced by 35%. Although no initial dosage reduction is specifically recommended, particular care should be exercised in monitoring toxicity and adjusting subsequent dosage in elderly patients (particularly females >70 years of age).

**Dosage Forms** Injection: 2 mg/mL (50 mg/25 mL; 200 mg/100 mL)

- **Epitol®** *see* Carbamazepine *on page 90*
- **Epivir®** *see* Lamivudine *on page 306*
- **Epivir®-HBV™** *see* Lamivudine *on page 306*
- **EPO** *see* Epoetin Alfa *on page 197*

## Epoetin Alfa (e POE e tin AL fa)

**U.S. Brand Names** Epogen®; Procrit®
**Synonyms** EPO; Erythropoietin; *r*HuEPO-α
**Pharmacologic Category** Colony Stimulating Factor
**Use**
Treatment of anemia associated with chronic renal failure, including patients on dialysis (end-stage renal disease) and patients not on dialysis
Treatment of anemia related to zidovudine therapy in HIV-infected patients; in patients when the endogenous erythropoietin level is ≤500 mU/mL and the dose of zidovudine is ≤4200 mg/week
Treatment of anemia in cancer patients on chemotherapy; in patients with nonmyeloid malignancies where anemia is caused by the effect of the concomitantly administered chemotherapy; to decrease the need for transfusions in patients who will be receiving chemotherapy for a minimum of 2 months
Reduction of allogeneic block transfusion in surgery patients scheduled to undergo elective, noncardiac, nonvascular surgery
**Effects on Mental Status** Sedation is common; may cause dizziness
**Effects on Psychiatric Treatment** None reported
**Pregnancy Risk Factor** C
**Contraindications** Known hypersensitivity to albumin (human) or mammalian cell-derived products; uncontrolled hypertension
**Warnings/Precautions** Use with caution in patients with porphyria, hypertension, or a history of seizures; prior to and during therapy, iron stores must be evaluated. It is recommended that the epoetin dose be decreased if the hematocrit increase exceeds 4 points in any 2-week period.

**Pretherapy parameters:**
Serum ferritin >100 ng/dL
Transferrin saturation (serum iron/iron binding capacity x 100) of 20% to 30%
Iron supplementation (usual oral dosing of 325 mg 2-3 times/day) should be given during therapy to provide for increased requirements during expansion of the red cell mass secondary to marrow stimulation by EPO unless iron stores are already in excess
For patients with endogenous serum EPO levels which are inappropriately low for hemoglobin level, documentation of the serum EPO level will help indicate which patients may benefit from EPO therapy. Serum EPO levels can be ordered routinely from Clinical Chemistry (red top serum separator tube).

Listed are factors limiting response to epoetin alfa, and their mechanism:
- Iron deficiency: Limits hemoglobin synthesis
- Blood loss/hemolysis: Counteracts epoetin alfa-stimulated erythropoiesis
- Infection/inflammation: Inhibits iron transfer from storage to bone marrow; suppresses erythropoiesis through activated macrophages
- Aluminum overload: Inhibits iron incorporation into heme protein
- Bone marrow replacement; hyperparathyroidism; metastatic, neoplastic: Limits bone marrow volume
- Folic acid/vitamin $B_{12}$ deficiency: Limits hemoglobin synthesis
- Patient compliance: Self-administered epoetin alfa or iron therapy

Increased mortality has occurred when aggressive dosing is used in CHF or anginal patients undergoing hemodialysis. An Amgen-funded study determined that when patients were targeted for a hematocrit of 42% versus a less aggressive 30%, mortality was higher (35% versus 29%).
**Adverse Reactions**
>10%:
Cardiovascular: Hypertension
Central nervous system: Fatigue, headache, fever
1% to 10%:
Cardiovascular: Edema, chest pain
Gastrointestinal: Nausea, vomiting, diarrhea
Hematologic: Clotted access
Neuromuscular & skeletal: Arthralgias, weakness
<1%: CVA/TIA, hypersensitivity reactions, myocardial infarction, rash
**Overdosage/Toxicology**
Signs and symptoms: Include erythrocytosis
Treatment: Adequate airway and other supportive measures and agents for treating anaphylaxis should be present when I.V. drug is given
**Usual Dosage**
Chronic renal failure patients: I.V., S.C.:
Initial dose: 50-100 units/kg 3 times/week
Reduce dose by 25 units/kg when
1) hematocrit approaches 36% **or**
2) when hematocrit increases >4 points in any 2-week period
Increase dose if hematocrit does not increase by 5-6 points after 8 weeks of therapy and hematocrit is below suggested target range
Suggested target hematocrit range: 30% to 36%
Maintenance dose: Individualize to target range
Dialysis patients: Median dose: 75 units/kg 3 times/week
Nondialysis patients: Doses of 75-150 units/kg
Zidovudine-treated, HIV-infected patients: Patients with erythropoietin levels >500 mU/mL are **unlikely** to respond
Initial dose: I.V., S.C.: 100 units/kg 3 times/week for 8 weeks
Increase dose by 50-100 units/kg 3 times/week if response is not satisfactory in terms of reducing transfusion requirements or increasing hematocrit after 8 weeks of therapy
Evaluate response every 4-8 weeks thereafter and adjust the dose accordingly by 50-100 units/kg increments 3 times/week
If patients have not responded satisfactorily to a 300 unit/kg dose 3 times/week, it is unlikely that they will respond to higher doses
Stop dose if hematocrit exceeds 40% and resume treatment at a 25% dose reduction when hematocrit drops to 36%
Cancer patients on chemotherapy: Treatment of patients with erythropoietin levels >200 mU/mL is **not recommended**
Initial dose: S.C.: 150 units/kg 3 times/week
Dose adjustment: If response is not satisfactory in terms of reducing transfusion requirement or increasing hematocrit after 8 weeks of therapy, the dose may be increased up to 300 units/kg 3 times/week. If patients do not respond, it is unlikely that they will respond to higher doses.
If hematocrit exceeds 40%, hold the dose until it falls to 36% and reduce the dose by 25% when treatment is resumed
Surgery patients: Prior to initiating treatment, obtain a hemoglobin to establish that is is >10 mg/dL or ≤13 mg/dL
Initial dose: S.C.: 300 units/kg/day for 10 days before surgery, on the day of surgery, and for 4 days after surgery
Alternative dose: S.C.: 600 units/kg in once weekly doses (21, 14, and 7 days before surgery) plus a fourth dose on the day of surgery
**Patient Information** You will require frequent blood tests to determine appropriate dosage. Do not take other medications, vitamin or iron supplements, or make significant changes in your diet without consulting prescriber. Report signs or symptoms of edema (eg, swollen extremities, difficulty breathing, rapid weight gain), onset of severe headache, acute back pain, chest pain, or muscular tremors or seizure activity.
**Dosage Forms**
1 mL single-dose vials: Preservative-free solution
2000 units/mL
3000 units/mL
4000 units/mL
10,000 units/mL
2 mL multidose vials: Preserved solution: 10,000 units/mL

- **Epogen®** *see* Epoetin Alfa *on page 197*

## Epoprostenol (e poe PROST en ole)

**U.S. Brand Names** Flolan® Injection
(Continued)

## Epoprostenol *(Continued)*

**Pharmacologic Category** Plasma Volume Expander, Colloid; Prostaglandin

**Use** Long-term intravenous treatment of primary pulmonary hypertension associated with the scleroderma spectrum of disease in NYHA Class III and IV patients who are not responsive to conventional therapy

**Unlabeled use:** Other potential uses include pulmonary hypertension associated with ARDS, SLE, or CHF; neonatal pulmonary hypertension; cardiopulmonary bypass surgery; hemodialysis; atherosclerosis; peripheral vascular disorders; and neonatal purpura fulminans

**Effects on Mental Status** Anxiety, nervousness are common; may cause confusion, insomnia, or depression

**Effects on Psychiatric Treatment** Hypotensive effects may be exacerbated by low potency antipsychotics (chlorpromazine) and TCAs

**Usual Dosage** I.V.: The drug is administered by continuous intravenous infusion via a central venous catheter using an ambulatory infusion pump; during dose ranging it may be administered peripherally

**Acute dose ranging:** The initial infusion rate should be 2 ng/kg/minute by continuous I.V. and increased in increments of 2 ng/kg/minute every 15 minutes or longer until dose-limiting effects are elicited (such as chest pain, anxiety, dizziness, changes in heart rate, dyspnea, nausea, vomiting, headache, hypotension and/or flushing)

**Continuous chronic infusion:** Initial: 4 ng/kg/minute **less** than the maximum-tolerated infusion rate determined during acute dose ranging

If maximum-tolerated infusion rate is <5 ng/kg/minute, the chronic infusion rate should be ½ the maximum-tolerated acute infusion rate

**Dosage adjustments:** Dose adjustments in the chronic infusion rate should be based on persistence, recurrence, or worsening of patient symptoms of pulmonary hypertension

If symptoms persist or recur after improving, the infusion rate should be increased by 1-2 ng/kg/minute increments, every 15 minutes or greater; following establishment of a new chronic infusion rate, the patient should be observed and vital signs monitored.

**Preparation of infusion:** To make 100 mL of solution with the following concentrations:

3000 ng/mL:
Dissolve one 0.5 mg vial with 5 mL supplied diluent, withdraw 3 mL, and add to sufficient diluent to make a total of 100 mL.

5000 ng/mL:
Dissolve one 0.5 mg vial with 5 mL supplied diluent, withdraw entire vial contents, and add a sufficient volume of diluent to make a total of 100 mL.

10,000 ng/mL:
Dissolve two 0.5 mg vials each with 5 mL supplied diluent, withdraw entire vial contents, and add a sufficient volume of diluent to make a total of 100 mL.

15,000 ng/mL:
Dissolve one 1.5 mg vial with 5 mL supplied diluent, withdraw entire vial contents, and add a sufficient volume of diluent to make a total of 100 mL.

**Dosage Forms** Injection, as sodium: 0.5 mg/vial and 1.5 mg/vial, each supplied with 50 mL of sterile diluent

## Eprosartan (ep roe SAR tan)

**Related Information**

Angiotensin-Related Agents Comparison Chart *on page 700*

**U.S. Brand Names** Teveten®

**Pharmacologic Category** Angiotensin II Antagonists

**Use** Treatment of hypertension; may be used alone or in combination with other antihypertensives

**Effects on Mental Status** May cause fatigue or depression

**Effects on Psychiatric Treatment** Risk of lithium toxicity may be increased by eprosartan; monitor lithium levels

**Contraindications** Hypersensitivity to eprosartan or any component; sensitivity to other A-II receptor antagonists; bilateral renal artery stenosis; primary hyperaldosteronism; pregnancy (2nd and 3rd trimester)

**Warnings/Precautions** Avoid use or use a smaller dose in patients who are volume depleted; correct depletion first. Deterioration in renal function can occur with initiation. Use with caution in unilateral renal artery stenosis and pre-existing renal insufficiency; significant aortic/mitral stenosis. Safety and efficacy not established in pediatric patients.

**Adverse Reactions**

1% to 10%:

Central nervous system: Fatigue (2%), depression (1%)

Endocrine & metabolic: Hypertriglyceridemia (1%)

Gastrointestinal: Abdominal pain (2%)

Genitourinary: Urinary tract infection (1%)

Respiratory: Upper respiratory tract infection (8%), rhinitis (4%), pharyngitis (4%), cough (4%)

Miscellaneous: Viral infection (2%), injury (2%)

<1% (Limited to important or life-threatening symptoms): Alcohol intolerance, weakness, substernal chest pain, facial edema, peripheral edema, fatigue, fever, hot flushes, influenza-like symptoms, malaise, rigors, pain, angina pectoris, bradycardia, abnormal EKG, extrasystoles, atrial fibrillation, hypotension, tachycardia, palpitations, anorexia, constipation, dry mouth, esophagitis, flatulence, gastritis, gastroenteritis, gingivitis, nausea, periodontitis, toothache, vomiting, anemia, purpura, increased transaminases, increased creatine phosphokinase, diabetes mellitus, glycosuria, gout, hypercholesterolemia, hyperglycemia, hyperkalemia, hypokalemia, hyponatremia, arthritis, aggravated arthritis, arthrosis, skeletal pain, tendonitis, back pain, anxiety, ataxia, insomnia, migraine, neuritis, nervousness, paresthesia, somnolence, tremor, vertigo, herpes simplex, otitis externa, otitis media, asthma, epistaxis, eczema, furunculosis, pruritus, rash, maculopapular rash, increased sweating, conjunctivitis, abnormal vision, xerophthalmia, tinnitus, albuminuria, cystitis, hematuria, micturition frequency, polyuria, renal calculus, urinary incontinence, leg cramps, peripheral ischemia, increases in BUN or creatinine, leukopenia, neutropenia, thrombocytopenia

**Drug Interactions**

Lithium: Risk of toxicity may be increased by eprosartan; monitor lithium levels

Potassium-sparing diuretics (amiloride, potassium, spironolactone, triamterene): Increased risk of hyperkalemia

Potassium supplements may increase the risk of hyperkalemia

Trimethoprim (high dose) may increase the risk of hyperkalemia

**Usual Dosage** Adults: Oral: Dosage must be individualized; can administer once or twice daily with total daily doses of 400-800 mg. Usual starting dose is 600 mg once daily as monotherapy in patients who are euvolemic. Limited clinical experience with doses >800 mg.

**Dosage adjustment in renal impairment:** No starting dosage adjustment is necessary; however, carefully monitor the patient

**Dosage adjustment in hepatic impairment:** No starting dosage adjustment is necessary; however, carefully monitor the patient

Elderly: No starting dosage adjustment is necessary; however, carefully monitor the patient

**Dosage Forms** Tablet: 400 mg (scored), 600 mg

♦ **Epsom Salts** *see* Magnesium Sulfate *on page 331*

## Eptifibatide (ep TIF i ba tide)

**U.S. Brand Names** Integrilin®

**Pharmacologic Category** Antiplatelet Agent

**Use** Treatment of patients with acute coronary syndrome (UA/NQMI), including patients who are to be managed medically and those undergoing percutaneous coronary intervention (PCI including PTCA)

**Effects on Mental Status** None reported

**Effects on Psychiatric Treatment** Contraindicated in patients with a recent stroke (within 30 days)

**Usual Dosage** Adults: I.V.:

Acute coronary syndrome: Bolus of 180 mcg/kg over 1-2 minutes, begun as soon as possible following diagnosis, followed by a continuous infusion of 2 mcg/kg/minute (maximum: 15 mg/hour) until hospital discharge or initiation of CABG surgery, up to 72 hours. If a patient is to undergo a percutaneous coronary intervention (PCI) while receiving eptifibatide, consideration can be given to decreasing the infusion rate to 0.5 mcg/kg/minute at the time of the procedure. Infusion should be continued for an additional 20-24 hours after the procedure, allowing for up to 96 hours of therapy.

Percutaneous coronary intervention (PCI) in patients not presenting with an acute coronary syndrome: Bolus of 135 mcg/kg administered immediately before the initiation of PCI followed by a continuous infusion of 0.5 mcg/kg/minute for 20-24 hours.

**Dosing adjustment in renal impairment:** Adults: $S_{cr}$ >2 mg/dL and <4 mg/dL: Use 135 mcg/kg bolus and 0.5 mcg/kg/minute infusion.

**Dosage Forms** Injection: 0.75 mg/mL (100 mL); 2 mg/mL (10 mL)

♦ **Equagesic®** *see* Aspirin and Meprobamate *on page 51*

♦ **Equalactin® Chewable Tablet [OTC]** *see* Calcium Polycarbophil *on page 86*

♦ **Equanil®** *see* Meprobamate *on page 342*

♦ **Equilet® [OTC]** *see* Calcium Carbonate *on page 84*

♦ **Ercaf®** *see* Ergotamine *on page 200*

♦ **Ergamisol®** *see* Levamisole *on page 310*

♦ **Ergobel®** *see* Nicergoline *on page 392*

## Ergocalciferol (er goe kal SIF e role)

**U.S. Brand Names** Calciferol™ Injection; Calciferol™ Oral; Drisdol® Oral

**Canadian Brand Names** Ostoforte®; Radiostol®

**Synonyms** Activated Ergosterol; Viosterol; Vitamin $D_2$

**Pharmacologic Category** Vitamin D Analog

**Use** Treatment of refractory rickets, hypophosphatemia, hypoparathyroidism

**Effects on Mental Status** May cause irritability or drowsiness; may rarely cause psychosis

**Effects on Psychiatric Treatment** None reported

**Pregnancy Risk Factor** A (C if dose exceeds RDA recommendation)

**Contraindications** Hypercalcemia, hypersensitivity to ergocalciferol or any component; malabsorption syndrome; evidence of vitamin D toxicity

**Warnings/Precautions** Administer with extreme caution in patients with impaired renal function, heart disease, renal stones, or arteriosclerosis; must administer concomitant calcium supplementation; maintain adequate fluid intake; avoid hypercalcemia; renal function impairment with secondary hyperparathyroidism

**Adverse Reactions** Generally well tolerated

Percentage unknown: Anorexia, bone pain, cardiac arrhythmias, conjunctivitis, constipation, decreased libido (late), headache, hypercholesterolemia, hypertension (late), hyperthermia (late), increased BUN (late), increased LFTs (late), irritability, metallic taste, mild acidosis (late), myalgia, nausea, pancreatitis, photophobia (late), polydipsia (late), polyuria (late), pruritus, psychosis (rare), somnolence, vascular/nephrocalcinosis (rare) vomiting, weakness, weight loss (rare), xerostomia

**Overdosage/Toxicology**

Signs and symptoms of chronic overdose: Hypercalcemia, weakness, fatigue, lethargy, anorexia

Treatment: Following withdrawal of the drug and oral decontamination, treatment consists of bedrest, liberal intake of fluids, reduced calcium intake, and cathartic administration. Severe hypercalcemia requires I.V. hydration and forced diuresis with I.V. furosemide. Urine output should be monitored and maintained at >3 mL/kg/hour. I.V. saline can quickly and significantly increase excretion of calcium into urine. Calcitonin, mithramycin, and biphosphonates have all been used successfully to treat the more resistant cases of vitamin D-induced hypercalcemia.

**Drug Interactions**

Decreased effect: Cholestyramine, colestipol, mineral oil may decrease oral absorption

Increased effect: Thiazide diuretics may increase vitamin D effects

Increased toxicity: Cardiac glycosides may increase toxicity

**Usual Dosage** Oral dosing is preferred; I.M. therapy required with GI, liver, or biliary disease associated with malabsorption

Dietary supplementation (each mcg = 40 USP units):
- Premature infants: 10-20 mcg/day (400-800 units), up to 750 mcg/day (30,000 units)
- Infants and healthy Children: 10 mcg/day (400 units)
- Adults: 10 mcg/day (400 units)

Renal failure:
- Children: 100-1000 mcg/day (4000-40,000 units)
- Adults: 500 mcg/day (20,000 units)

Hypoparathyroidism:
- Children: 1.25-5 mg/day (50,000-200,000 units) and calcium supplements
- Adults: 625 mcg to 5 mg/day (25,000-200,000 units) and calcium supplements

Vitamin D-dependent rickets:
- Children: 75-125 mcg/day (3000-5000 units); maximum: 1500 mcg/day
- Adults: 250 mcg to 1.5 mg/day (10,000-60,000 units)

Nutritional rickets and osteomalacia:
- Children and Adults (with normal absorption): 25-125 mcg/day (1000-5000 units)
- Children with malabsorption: 250-625 mcg/day (10,000-25,000 units)
- Adults with malabsorption: 250-7500 mcg (10,000-300,000 units)

Vitamin D-resistant rickets:
- Children: Initial: 1000-2000 mcg/day (40,000-80,000 units) with phosphate supplements; daily dosage is increased at 3- to 4-month intervals in 250-500 mcg (10,000-20,000 units) increments
- Adults: 250-1500 mcg/day (10,000-60,000 units) with phosphate supplements

Familial hypophosphatemia: 10,000-80,000 units daily plus 1-2 g/day elemental phosphorus

Osteoporosis prophylaxis: Adults:
- 51-70 years of age: 400 units/day
- >70 years of age: 600 units/day
- Maximum daily dose: 2000 units/day

**Patient Information** Take exact dose prescribed; do not take more than recommended. Your prescriber may recommend a special diet; do not increase calcium intake without consulting prescriber. Avoid magnesium supplements or magnesium-containing antacids. You may experience nausea, vomiting, or metallic taste (frequent small meals, frequent mouth care, or sucking hard candy may help); hypotension (use caution when rising from sitting or lying position or when climbing stairs or bending over). Report chest pain or palpitations; acute headache, dizziness, or feeling of weakness; unresolved nausea or vomiting; persistent metallic taste; unrelieved muscle or bone pain; or CNS irritability.

**Nursing Implications** Monitor serum calcium, phosphorus, and BUN every 2 weeks

**Dosage Forms**

Capsule (Drisdol®): 50,000 units [1.25 mg]

Injection (Calciferol™): 500,000 units/mL [12.5 mg/mL] (1 mL)

Liquid (Calciferol™, Drisdol®): 8000 units/mL [200 mcg/mL] (60 mL)

Tablet (Calciferol™): 50,000 units [1.25 mg]

## Ergoloid Mesylates (ER goe loid MES i lates)

**U.S. Brand Names** Germinal®; Hydergine®; Hydergine® LC

**Synonyms** Dihydroergotoxine; Dihydrogenated Ergot Alkaloids

**Pharmacologic Category** Ergot Derivative

**Use** Treatment of cerebrovascular insufficiency in primary progressive dementia, Alzheimer's dementia, and senile onset

**Effects on Mental Status** None reported

**Effects on Psychiatric Treatment** Contraindicated in individuals with psychosis

**Pregnancy Risk Factor** C

**Contraindications** Acute or chronic psychosis, hypersensitivity to ergot or any component

**Warnings/Precautions** Exclude possibility that signs and symptoms of illness are from a potentially reversible and treatable condition

**Adverse Reactions** 1% to 10%:

Gastrointestinal: Transient nausea

Miscellaneous: Sublingual irritation

**Overdosage/Toxicology**

Signs and symptoms: Sinus bradycardia, blurred vision, headache, stomach cramps

Treatment: Chronic overdose usually manifests as signs and symptoms of extremity or organ ischemia; nitroprusside has been shown to reverse the vasoconstriction associated with ergot toxicity

**Drug Interactions** Increased toxicity with dopamine

**Usual Dosage** Adults: Oral: 1 mg 3 times/day up to 4.5-12 mg/day; up to 6 months of therapy may be necessary

**Patient Information** Do not chew or crush sublingual tablets, allow to dissolve under tongue

**Dosage Forms**

Capsule, liquid (Hydergine® LC): 1 mg

Liquid (Hydergine®): 1 mg/mL (100 mL)

Tablet: Oral: 0.5 mg
- Gerimal®, Hydergine®: 1 mg
- Sublingual: Gerimal®, Hydergine®: 0.5 mg, 1 mg

♦ **Ergomar®** *see* Ergotamine *on page 200*

♦ **Ergometrine Maleate** *see* Ergonovine *on page 199*

## Ergonovine (er goe NOE veen)

**U.S. Brand Names** Ergotrate® Maleate

**Synonyms** Ergometrine Maleate

**Pharmacologic Category** Ergot Derivative

**Use** Prevention and treatment of postpartum and postabortion hemorrhage caused by uterine atony or subinvolution

**Unlabeled use:** Migraine headaches, diagnostically to identify Prinzmetal's angina

**Effects on Mental Status** May cause dizziness

**Effects on Psychiatric Treatment** None reported

**Pregnancy Risk Factor** X

**Contraindications** Induction of labor, threatened spontaneous abortion, hypersensitivity to ergonovine or any component

**Warnings/Precautions** Use with caution in patients with sepsis, heart disease, hypertension, or with hepatic or renal impairment; restore uterine responsiveness in calcium-deficient patients who do not respond to ergonovine by I.V. calcium administration; avoid prolonged use; discontinue if ergotism develops

**Adverse Reactions**

1% to 10%: Gastrointestinal: Nausea, vomiting

<1%: Bradycardia, cerebrovascular accidents, diaphoresis, dizziness, dyspnea, ergotism, headache, hypertension (sometimes extreme - treat with I.V. chlorpromazine), myocardial infarction, palpitations, seizures, shock, thrombophlebitis, tinnitus, transient chest pain

**Overdosage/Toxicology**

Signs and symptoms: Gangrene (chronic), seizures (acute), chest pain, numbness in extremities, weak pulse, confusion, excitement, delirium, hallucinations

Treatment: Supportive following GI decontamination (for oral overdose). I.V. or intra-arterial nitroprusside for arterial venospasm; nitroglycerin for coronary vasospasm.

**Drug Interactions** No data reported

**Usual Dosage** Adults: I.M., I.V. (I.V. should be reserved for emergency use only): 0.2 mg, repeat dose in 2-4 hours as needed

**Patient Information** For angina diagnosis cardiologist will instruct patient about what to expect. For postpartum hemorrhage (an emergency situation) patient needs to know why the drug is being given and what side effects she might experience (eg, mild nausea and vomiting, dizziness, headache, ringing ears) and instructed to report difficulty breathing, acute (Continued)

## Ergonovine *(Continued)*

headache, or numbness and cold feeling in extremities, or severe abdominal cramping.

**Nursing Implications** I.V. use should be limited to patients with severe uterine bleeding or other life-threatening emergency situations

**Dosage Forms** Injection, as maleate: 0.2 mg/mL (1 mL)

## Ergotamine (er GOT a meen)

**U.S. Brand Names** Cafatine®; Cafatine-PB®; Cafergot®; Cafetrate®; Ercaf®; Ergomar®; Migranal®; Wigraine®

**Canadian Brand Names** Ergomar®; Gynergen®

**Synonyms** Ergotamine Tartrate; Ergotamine Tartrate and Caffeine

**Pharmacologic Category** Ergot Derivative

**Use** Abort or prevent vascular headaches, such as migraine or cluster

**Effects on Mental Status** Drowsiness and dizziness are common

**Effects on Psychiatric Treatment** Use caution with propranolol; vasoconstriction has been reported

**Pregnancy Risk Factor** X

**Contraindications** Hypersensitivity to ergotamine, caffeine, or any component; peripheral vascular disease, hepatic or renal disease, hypertension, peptic ulcer disease, sepsis; avoid during pregnancy; concurrent use with ritonavir, nelfinavir, and amprenavir

**Warnings/Precautions** Avoid prolonged administration or excessive dosage because of the danger of ergotism and gangrene; patients who take ergotamine for extended periods of time may become dependent on it. May be harmful due to reduction in cerebral blood flow; may precipitate angina, myocardial infarction, or aggravate intermittent claudication; therefore, not considered a drug of choice in the elderly.

**Adverse Reactions**

>10%:

Cardiovascular: Tachycardia, bradycardia, arterial spasm, claudication and vasoconstriction; rebound headache may occur with sudden withdrawal of the drug in patients on prolonged therapy; localized edema, peripheral vascular effects (numbness and tingling of fingers and toes)

Central nervous system: Drowsiness, dizziness

Gastrointestinal: Nausea, vomiting, diarrhea, xerostomia

1% to 10%:

Cardiovascular: Transient tachycardia or bradycardia, precordial distress and pain

Neuromuscular & skeletal: Weakness in the legs, abdominal or muscle pain, muscle pains in the extremities, paresthesia

**Overdosage/Toxicology**

Signs and symptoms: Vasospastic effects, nausea, vomiting, lassitude, impaired mental function, hypotension, hypertension, unconsciousness, seizures, shock, and death

Treatment: General supportive therapy, gastric lavage, or induction of emesis, activated charcoal, saline cathartic; keep extremities warm. Activated charcoal is effective at binding certain chemicals, and this is especially true for ergot alkaloids; treatment is symptomatic with heparin, vasodilators (nitroprusside); vasodilators should be used with caution to avoid exaggerating any pre-existing hypotension.

**Drug Interactions** Increased toxicity:

Propranolol: One case of severe vasoconstriction with pain and cyanosis has been reported

Erythromycin, troleandomycin, and other macrolide antibiotics: Monitor for signs of ergot toxicity

Ritonavir, amprenavir, and nelfinavir increase blood levels of ergot alkaloids; avoid concurrent use

**Usual Dosage**

Oral:

Cafergot®: 2 tablets at onset of attack; then 1 tablet every 30 minutes as needed; maximum: 6 tablets per attack; do not exceed 10 tablets/week.

Ergostat®: 1 tablet under tongue at first sign, then 1 tablet every 30 minutes, 3 tablets/24 hours, 5 tablets/week

Rectal (Cafergot® suppositories, Wigraine® suppositories, Cafatine® suppositories): 1 at first sign of an attack; follow with second dose after 1 hour, if needed; maximum: 2 per attack; do not exceed 5/week.

Nasal inhalation (Migranal®):One spray (0.5 mg) in each nostril, repeat with an additional spray in each nostril after 15 minute (total dose: 4 sprays or 2.0 mg)

**Patient Information** Take this drug as directed; do not increase dose or use more often than prescribed. If relief is not obtained, contact your prescriber. Avoid caffeine-containing products (eg, tea, coffee, colas, cocoa); caffeine increases GI absorption of ergotamines. May cause drowsiness (avoid activities requiring alertness until effects of medication are known). You may experience mild nausea/vomiting (you may have an antiemetic prescribed), mild weakness or numbness of extremities (avoid injury). Inspect your extremities for coldness, numbness, or injury. Report immediately extreme numbness, pain, tingling or weakness in extremities (toes, fingers), severe unresolved nausea or vomiting, difficulty breathing or irregular heartbeat.

Nasal inhaler: Follow directions for use on package insert. Prime inhaler before use. Wait 15 minutes between inhalations. Use no more than 4 inhalations (2 mg) for a single administration, and no more than 3 mg in a 24-hour period.

**Nursing Implications** Do not crush sublingual drug product

**Dosage Forms**

Suppository, rectal (Cafatine®, Cafergot®, Cafetrate®, Wigraine®): Ergotamine tartrate 2 mg and caffeine 100 mg (12s)

Tablet (Ercaf®, Wigraine®): Ergotamine tartrate 1 mg and caffeine 100 mg

Tablet, sublingual (Ergomar®): Ergotamine tartrate 2 mg


- **Ergotamine Tartrate** *see* Ergotamine *on page 200*
- **Ergotamine Tartrate and Caffeine** *see* Ergotamine *on page 200*
- **Ergotrate® Maleate** *see* Ergonovine *on page 199*
- **E•R•O Ear [OTC]** *see* Carbamide Peroxide *on page 92*
- **Eryc® Oral** *see* Erythromycin *on page 200*
- **Eryderm® Topical** *see* Erythromycin, Ophthalmic/Topical *on page 202*
- **Erygel® Topical** *see* Erythromycin, Ophthalmic/Topical *on page 202*
- **Erymax® Topical** *see* Erythromycin, Ophthalmic/Topical *on page 202*
- **EryPed® Oral** *see* Erythromycin *on page 200*
- **Ery-Tab® Oral** *see* Erythromycin *on page 200*


## Erythrityl Tetranitrate (e RI thri til te tra NYE trate)

**U.S. Brand Names** Cardilate®

**Pharmacologic Category** Vasodilator

**Use** Prophylaxis and long-term treatment of frequent or recurrent anginal pain and reduced exercise tolerance associated with angina pectoris

**Unlabeled use:** Reduce cardiac workload in CHF or following an MI; adjunct in treatment of Raynaud's disease

**Effects on Mental Status** May cause restlessness or dizziness

**Effects on Psychiatric Treatment** Hypotensive effects may be exacerbated by low potency antipsychotic (chlorpromazine) and TCAs

**Contraindications** Hypersensitivity to erythrityl tetranitrate or any component; severe anemia; angle-closure glaucoma; postural hypotension; cerebral hemorrhage; head trauma

**Warnings/Precautions** Use with caution in patients with hypertrophic cardiomyopathy, in patients with glaucoma, or volume depletion; tolerance may develop

**Adverse Reactions**

>10%: Central nervous system: Headache

1% to 10%: Cardiovascular: Tachycardia, hypotension, flushing

**Overdosage/Toxicology**

Signs and symptoms: Hypotension, tachycardia, flushing, diaphoresis, dizziness, syncope, nausea, confusion, increased intracranial pressure, methemoglobinemia, cyanosis, metabolic acidosis, seizures

Treatment: Following decontamination, keep patients recumbent, treat hypotension with fluids and pressors, treat methemoglobinemia with methylene-blue 1-2 mg/kg; epinephrine is ineffective in reversing hypotension.

**Drug Interactions** Sildenafil: Significant reduction of systolic and diastolic blood pressure with concurrent use. Do not give sildenafil within 24 hours of a nitrate preparation.

**Usual Dosage** Adults: Oral: 5 mg under the tongue or in the buccal pouch 3 times/day or 10 mg before meals or food, chewed 3 times/day, increasing in 2-3 days if needed. Dosages of up to 100 mg/day are tolerated. Some patients may need bedtime doses if they experience nocturnal symptoms.

**Patient Information** Do not change brands without consulting physician or pharmacist; notify physician if persistent headache, dizziness, or flushing occurs; seek medical help if chest pain is unresolved after 15 minutes; do not chew or swallow sublingual tablet

**Dosage Forms** Tablet, oral or sublingual: 10 mg


- **Erythrocin® Oral** *see* Erythromycin *on page 200*


## Erythromycin (er ith roe MYE sin)

**U.S. Brand Names** E.E.S.® Oral; E-Mycin® Oral; Eryc® Oral; EryPed® Oral; Ery-Tab® Oral; Erythrocin® Oral; Ilosone® Oral; PCE® Oral

**Canadian Brand Names** Apo®-Erythro E-C; Diomycin; Erybid™; Erythro-Base®; Novo-Rythro Encap; PMS-Erythromycin

**Synonyms** Erythromycin Base; Erythromycin Estolate; Erythromycin Ethylsuccinate; Erythromycin Gluceptate; Erythromycin Lactobionate; Erythromycin Stearate

**Pharmacologic Category** Antibiotic, Macrolide

**Use** Treatment of susceptible bacterial infections including *S. pyogenes*, some *S. pneumoniae*, some *S. aureus*, *M. pneumoniae*, *Legionella pneumophila*, diphtheria, pertussis, chancroid, *Chlamydia*, erythrasma, *N. gonorrhoeae*, *E. histolytica*, syphilis and nongonococcal urethritis, and

*Campylobacter* gastroenteritis; used in conjunction with neomycin for decontaminating the bowel; treatment of gastroparesis

**Effects on Mental Status** Macrolides have been reported to cause nightmares, confusion, anxiety, and mood lability

**Effects on Psychiatric Treatment** Contraindicated with pimozide; may increase concentration of bromocriptine, carbamazepine, and triazolam

**Pregnancy Risk Factor** B

**Contraindications** Hepatic impairment, known hypersensitivity to erythromycin or its components; pre-existing liver disease (erythromycin estolate); concomitant use with pimozide, terfenadine, astemizole, or cisapride

**Warnings/Precautions** Hepatic impairment with or without jaundice has occurred, it may be accompanied by malaise, nausea, vomiting, abdominal colic, and fever; discontinue use if these occur; avoid using erythromycin lactobionate in neonates since formulations may contain benzyl alcohol which is associated with toxicity in neonates; observe for superinfections

**Adverse Reactions**

>10%: Gastrointestinal: Abdominal pain, cramping, nausea, vomiting

1% to 10%:

- Gastrointestinal: Oral candidiasis
- Hepatic: Cholestatic jaundice
- Local: Phlebitis at the injection site
- Miscellaneous: Hypersensitivity reactions

<1%: Allergic reactions, cholestatic jaundice (most common with estolate), diarrhea, eosinophilia, fever, hypertrophic pyloric stenosis, rash, pseudomembranous colitis, thrombophlebitis, ventricular arrhythmias

**Overdosage/Toxicology**

Signs and symptoms: Nausea, vomiting, and diarrhea

Treatment: General and supportive care only

**Drug Interactions** CYP3A3/4 enzyme substrate; CYP1A2 and 3A3/4 enzyme inhibitor

Concurrent use of erythromycin and lovastatin and simvastatin may result in significantly increased levels and rhabdomyolysis

Death has been reported by potentiation of pimozide's cardiotoxicity when given concurrently with erythromycin; use is contraindicated

Erythromycin decreases clearance of carbamazepine, cyclosporine, triazolam, alfentanil, bromocriptine, digoxin (~10% of patients), disopyramide, ergot alkaloids, methylprednisolone; may decrease clearance of protease inhibitors

Erythromycin decreases metabolism of terfenadine, cisapride, and astemizole resulting in an increase in Q-T interval and potential heart failure

Erythromycin inhibits felodipine (and other dihydropyridine calcium antagonist) metabolism in the liver resulting in a twofold increase in levels and consequent toxicity

Erythromycin may decrease theophylline clearance and increase theophylline's half-life by up to 60% (patients on high-dose theophylline and erythromycin or who have received erythromycin for >5 days may be at higher risk)

Erythromycin may potentiate anticoagulant effect of warfarin and decrease metabolism of vinblastine

Protease inhibitors, like amprenavir and ritonavir, may increase erythromycin's serum concentration

Valproic acid: Erythromycin may increase serum concentrations of valproic acid; monitor

**Usual Dosage**

Infants and Children (Note: 400 mg ethylsuccinate = 250 mg base, stearate, or estolate salts):

- Oral: 30-50 mg/kg/day divided every 6-8 hours; may double doses in severe infections
- Preop bowel preparation: 20 mg/kg erythromycin base at 1, 2, and 11 PM on the day before surgery combined with mechanical cleansing of the large intestine and oral neomycin
- I.V.: Lactobionate: 20-40 mg/kg/day divided every 6 hours

Adults:

- Oral:
  - Base: 250-500 mg every 6-12 hours
  - Ethylsuccinate: 400-800 mg every 6-12 hours
- Preop bowel preparation: Oral: 1 g erythromycin base at 1, 2, and 11 PM on the day before surgery combined with mechanical cleansing of the large intestine and oral neomycin
- I.V.: Lactobionate: 15-20 mg/kg/day divided every 6 hours or 500 mg to 1 g every 6 hours, or given as a continuous infusion over 24 hours (maximum: 4 g/24 hours)

Children and Adults: Ophthalmic: Instill ½" (1.25 cm) 2-8 times/day depending on the severity of the infection

Dialysis: Slightly dialyzable (5% to 20%); no supplemental dosage necessary in hemo or peritoneal dialysis or in continuous arteriovenous or venovenous hemofiltration (CAVH/CAVHD)

Erythromycin has been used as a prokinetic agent to improve gastric emptying time and intestinal motility. In adults, 200 mg was infused I.V. initially followed by 250 mg orally 3 times/day 30 minutes before meals. In children, erythromycin 3 mg/kg I.V. has been infused over 60 minutes initially followed by 20 mg/kg/day orally in 3-4 divided doses before meals or before meals and at bedtime

**Dietary Considerations** Food: Increased drug absorption with meals. Drug may cause GI upset; may take with food.

**Patient Information** Take as directed, around-the-clock, with a full glass of water (not juice or milk), preferably on an empty stomach (1 hour before or 2 hours after meals). Take complete prescription even if you are feeling better. You may experience nausea, vomiting, or mouth sores (small frequent meals, frequent mouth care may help). Report skin rash or itching; easy bruising or bleeding; unhealed sores of mouth; itching or vaginal discharge; watery or bloody diarrhea; unresolved vomiting; yellowing of skin or eyes; easy fatigue; pale stool or dark urine; skin rash or itching; white plaques, sores, or fuzziness in mouth; or any change in hearing.

Ophthalmic: Wash hands before applying. Pull down lower eyelid gently, instill thin ribbon of ointment into lower lid, close eye, roll eyeball in all directions. Blurred vision and stinging is temporary. Report persistent pain, burning, vision disturbances, swelling, itching, or worsening of condition.

**Nursing Implications** Some formulations may contain benzyl alcohol as a preservative; use with extreme care in neonates; do not crush enteric coated drug product; GI upset, including diarrhea, is common; I.V. infusion may be very irritating to the vein; if phlebitis/pain occurs with used dilution, consider diluting further (eg, 1:5) and administer over ≥20-60 minutes, if fluid status of the patient will tolerate, or consider administering in larger available vein

**Dosage Forms**

Erythromycin base:

- Capsule, delayed release: 250 mg
- Capsule, delayed release, enteric coated pellets (Eryc®): 250 mg
- Ointment, ophthalmic: 0.55 mg (3.5 g)
- Tablet, delayed release: 333 mg
- Tablet, enteric coated (E-Mycin®, Ery-Tab®, E-Base®): 250 mg, 333 mg, 500 mg
- Tablet, film coated: 250 mg, 500 mg
- Tablet, polymer coated particles (PCE®): 333 mg, 500 mg

Erythromycin estolate:

- Capsule (Ilosone® Pulvules®): 250 mg
- Suspension, oral (Ilosone®): 125 mg/5 mL (480 mL); 250 mg/5 mL (480 mL)
- Tablet (Ilosone®): 500 mg

Erythromycin ethylsuccinate:

- Granules for oral suspension (EryPed®): 400 mg/5 mL (60 mL, 100 mL, 200 mL)
- Powder for oral suspension (E.E.S.®): 200 mg/5 mL (100 mL, 200 mL)
- Suspension, oral (E.E.S.®, EryPed®): 200 mg/5 mL (5 mL, 100 mL, 200 mL, 480 mL); 400 mg/5 mL (5 mL, 60 mL, 100 mL, 200 mL, 480 mL)
- Suspension, oral [drops] (EryPed®): 100 mg/2.5 mL (50 mL)
- Tablet (E.E.S.®): 400 mg
- Tablet, chewable (EryPed®): 200 mg

Erythromycin gluceptate: Injection: 1000 mg (30 mL)

Erythromycin lactobionate: Powder for injection: 500 mg, 1000 mg

Erythromycin stearate: Tablet, film coated (Eramycin®, Erythrocin®): 250 mg, 500 mg

## Erythromycin and Benzoyl Peroxide

(er ith roe MYE sin & BEN zoe il per OKS ide)

**U.S. Brand Names** Benzamycin®

**Pharmacologic Category** Topical Skin Product; Topical Skin Product, Acne

**Use** Topical control of acne vulgaris

**Effects on Mental Status** None reported

**Effects on Psychiatric Treatment** None reported

**Usual Dosage** Apply twice daily, morning and evening

**Dosage Forms** Gel: Erythromycin 30 mg and benzoyl peroxide 50 mg per g

## Erythromycin and Sulfisoxazole

(er ith roe MYE sin & sul fi SOKS a zole)

**U.S. Brand Names** Eryzole®; Pediazole®

**Pharmacologic Category** Antibiotic, Oxazolidinone; Antibiotic, Macrolide; Antibiotic, Sulfonamide Derivative

**Use** Treatment of susceptible bacterial infections of the upper and lower respiratory tract, otitis media in children caused by susceptible strains of *Haemophilus influenzae*, and many other infections in patients allergic to penicillin

**Effects on Mental Status** Macrolides have been reported to cause nightmares, confusion, anxiety, and mood lability; dizziness is common with sulfisoxazole; sulfonamides reported to cause restlessness, irritability, depression, euphoria, disorientation, panic, hallucinations, and delusions

**Effects on Psychiatric Treatment** Erythromycin is contraindicated with pimozide; may increase concentration of bromocriptine, carbamazepine, and triazolam; photosensitivity is common with sulfisoxazole; use caution with concurrent psychotropics; may cause leukopenia; caution with clozapine and carbamazepine

**Usual Dosage** Oral (dosage recommendation is based on the product's erythromycin content):

(Continued)

## Erythromycin and Sulfisoxazole *(Continued)*

Children ≥2 months: 50 mg/kg/day erythromycin and 150 mg/kg/day sulfisoxazole in divided doses every 6 hours; not to exceed 2 g erythromycin/day or 6 g sulfisoxazole/day for 10 days

Adults >45 kg: 400 mg erythromycin and 1200 mg sulfisoxazole every 6 hours

**Dosing adjustment in renal impairment** (sulfisoxazole must be adjusted in renal impairment):

$Cl_{cr}$ 10-50 mL/minute: Administer every 8-12 hours

$Cl_{cr}$ <10 mL/minute: Administer every 12-24 hours

**Dosage Forms** Suspension, oral: Erythromycin ethylsuccinate 200 mg and sulfisoxazole acetyl 600 mg per 5 mL (100 mL, 150 mL, 200 mL, 250 mL)

♦ **Erythromycin Base** *see* Erythromycin *on page 200*

♦ **Erythromycin Estolate** *see* Erythromycin *on page 200*

♦ **Erythromycin Ethylsuccinate** *see* Erythromycin *on page 200*

♦ **Erythromycin Gluceptate** *see* Erythromycin *on page 200*

♦ **Erythromycin Lactobionate** *see* Erythromycin *on page 200*

## Erythromycin, Ophthalmic/Topical

(er ith roe MYE sin TOP i kal)

**U.S. Brand Names** Akne-Mycin® Topical; A/T/S® Topical; Del-Mycin® Topical; Emgel™ Topical; Eryderm® Topical; Erygel® Topical; Erymax® Topical; E-Solve-2® Topical; ETS-2%® Topical; Ilotycin® Ophthalmic; Staticin® Topical; T-Stat® Topical

**Pharmacologic Category** Antibiotic, Ophthalmic; Antibiotic, Topical; Topical Skin Product; Topical Skin Product, Acne

**Use** Topical treatment of acne vulgaris

**Effects on Mental Status** None reported

**Effects on Psychiatric Treatment** None reported

**Usual Dosage**

Neonates:

Ophthalmic: Prophylaxis of neonatal gonococcal or chlamydial conjunctivitis: 0.5-1 cm ribbon of ointment should be instilled into each conjunctival sac

Children and Adults:

Ophthalmic: Instill one or more times daily depending on the severity of the infection

Topical: Apply 2% solution over the affected area twice daily after the skin has been thoroughly washed and patted dry

**Dosage Forms**

Gel: 2% (30 g, 60 g)

Gel (A/T/S®, Emgel™, Erygel®): 2% (27 g, 30 g, 60 g)

Ointment:

Ophthalmic: 0.5% [5 mg/g] (3.5 g)

Ilotycin®: 0.5% [5 mg/g] (3.5 g)

Topical (Akne-Mycin®): 2% (25 g)

Solution, topical:

Staticin®: 1.5% (60 mL)

Akne-Mycin®, A/T/S®, Del-Mycin®, EryDerm®, ETS-2%®, Romycin®, Theramycin Z®, T-Stat®: 2% (60 mL, 66 mL, 120 mL)

Pad (T-Stat®): 2% (60s)

Pledgets: 2% (60s)

Swab: 2% (60s)

♦ **Erythromycin Stearate** *see* Erythromycin *on page 200*

♦ **Erythropoietin** *see* Epoetin Alfa *on page 197*

♦ **Eryzole®** *see* Erythromycin and Sulfisoxazole *on page 201*

♦ **Esclim® Transdermal** *see* Estradiol *on page 203*

♦ **Eserine Salicylate** *see* Physostigmine *on page 444*

♦ **Esgic®** *see* Butalbital Compound and Acetaminophen *on page 80*

♦ **Esgic-Plus®** *see* Butalbital Compound and Acetaminophen *on page 80*

♦ **Esidrix®** *see* Hydrochlorothiazide *on page 271*

♦ **Eskalith®** *see* Lithium *on page 321*

♦ **Eskalith CR®** *see* Lithium *on page 321*

## Esmolol (ES moe lol)

**Related Information**

Beta-Blockers Comparison Chart *on page 709*

**U.S. Brand Names** Brevibloc® Injection

**Pharmacologic Category** Antiarrhythmic Agent, Class II; Beta Blocker, $Beta_1$ Selective

**Use** Treatment of supraventricular tachycardia, atrial fibrillation/flutter (primarily to control ventricular rate), and hypertension (especially perioperatively)

**Effects on Mental Status** May cause drowsiness, confusion, fatigue, or depression

**Effects on Psychiatric Treatment** Barbiturates may decease effects of esmolol

**Usual Dosage I.V. administration requires an infusion pump** (must be adjusted to individual response and tolerance):

Children: An extremely limited amount of information regarding esmolol use in pediatric patients is currently available.

Some centers have utilized doses of 100-500 mcg/kg given over 1 minute for control of supraventricular tachycardias.

Loading doses of 500 mcg/kg/minute over 1 minute with maximal doses of 50-250 mcg/kg/minute (mean = 173) have been used in addition to nitroprusside to treat postoperative hypertension after coarctation of aorta repair.

Adults: Loading dose: 500 mcg/kg over 1 minute; follow with a 50 mcg/kg/minute infusion for 4 minutes; if response is inadequate, rebolus with another 500 mcg/kg loading dose over 1 minute, and increase the maintenance infusion to 100 mcg/kg/minute. Repeat this process until a therapeutic effect has been achieved or to a maximum recommended maintenance dose of 200 mcg/kg/minute. Usual dosage range: 50-200 mcg/kg/minute with average dose of 100 mcg/kg/minute.

Esmolol: Hemodynamic effects of beta-blockade return to baseline within 20-30 minutes after discontinuing esmolol infusions.

Guidelines for withdrawal of therapy:

Transfer to alternative antiarrhythmic drug (propranolol, digoxin, verapamil).

Infusion should be reduced by 50% 30 minutes following the first dose of the alternative agent.

Following the second dose of the alternative drug, patient's response should be monitored and if control is adequate for the first hours, esmolol may be discontinued.

Dialysis: Not removed by hemo- or peritoneal dialysis; supplemental dose is not necessary.

**Dosage Forms** Injection, as hydrochloride: 10 mg/mL (10 mL); 250 mg/mL (10 mL)

♦ **E-Solve-2® Topical** *see* Erythromycin, Ophthalmic/Topical *on page 202*

♦ **Esoterica® Facial [OTC]** *see* Hydroquinone *on page 276*

♦ **Esoterica® Regular [OTC]** *see* Hydroquinone *on page 276*

♦ **Esoterica® Sensitive Skin Formula [OTC]** *see* Hydroquinone *on page 276*

♦ **Esoterica® Sunscreen [OTC]** *see* Hydroquinone *on page 276*

## Estazolam (es TA zoe lam)

**Related Information**

Anxiolytic/Hypnotic Use in Long-Term Care Facilities *on page 754*

Benzodiazepines Comparison Chart *on page 708*

Clinical Issues in the Use of Anxiolytics and Sedative/Hypnotics *on page 634*

Patient Information - Anxiolytics & Sedative Hypnotics (Benzodiazepines) *on page 653*

**Generic Available** Yes

**U.S. Brand Names** ProSom™

**Pharmacologic Category** Benzodiazepine

**Use** Short-term management of insomnia

**Restrictions** C-IV

**Pregnancy Risk Factor** X

**Contraindications** Hypersensitivity to this drug or any component of its formulation (cross-sensitivity with other benzodiazepines may exist); pregnancy

**Warnings/Precautions** Use with caution in elderly or debilitated patients, patients with hepatic disease (including alcoholics), or renal impairment. Use with caution in patients with respiratory disease or impaired gag reflex. Avoid use in patients with sleep apnea. As a hypnotic, should be used only after evaluation of potential causes of sleep disturbance. Failure of sleep disturbance to resolve after 7-10 days may indicate psychiatric or medical illness. A worsening of insomnia or the emergence of new abnormalities of thought or behavior may represent unrecognized psychiatric or medical illness and requires immediate and careful evaluation.

Causes CNS depression (dose-related) resulting in sedation, dizziness, confusion, or ataxia which may impair physical and mental capabilities. Patients must be cautioned about performing tasks which require mental alertness (ie, operating machinery or driving). Use with caution in patients receiving other CNS depressants or psychoactive agents. Effects with other sedative drugs or ethanol may be potentiated. Benzodiazepines have been associated with falls and traumatic injury and should be used with extreme caution in patients who are at risk of these events (especially the elderly).

Benzodiazepines have been associated with anterograde amnesia. Paradoxical reactions, including hyperactive or aggressive behavior, have been reported with benzodiazepines, particularly in adolescent/pediatric or psychiatric patients. Does not have analgesic, antidepressant, or antipsychotic properties.

Use caution in patients with depression, particularly if suicidal risk may be present. Use with caution in patients with a history of drug dependence. Benzodiazepines have been associated with dependence and acute withdrawal symptoms on discontinuation or reduction in dose. Acute withdrawal, including seizures, may be precipitated in patients after administration of flumazenil to patients receiving long-term benzodiazepine therapy.

**Adverse Reactions**

>10%:

Central nervous system: Somnolence

Neuromuscular & skeletal: Weakness

1% to 10%:

Cardiovascular: Flushing, palpitations

Central nervous system: Anxiety, confusion, dizziness, hypokinesia, abnormal coordination, hangover, agitation, amnesia, apathy, emotional lability, euphoria, hostility, seizure, sleep disorder, stupor, twitch

Dermatologic: Dermatitis, pruritus, rash, urticaria

Gastrointestinal: Xerostomia, constipation, decreased appetite, flatulence, gastritis, increased appetite, perverse taste

Genitourinary: Frequent urination, menstrual cramps, urinary hesitancy, urinary frequency, vaginal discharge/itching

Neuromuscular & skeletal: Paresthesia

Otic: Photophobia, eye pain, eye swelling

Respiratory: Cough, dyspnea, asthma, rhinitis, sinusitis

Miscellaneous: Diaphoresis

<1%: Allergic reactions, chills, drug dependence, fever, muscle spasm, myalgia, neck pain

**Overdosage/Toxicology**

Signs and symptoms: Respiratory depression, hypoactive reflexes, unsteady gait, hypotension

Treatment: Supportive; rarely is mechanical ventilation required

Flumazenil has been shown to selectively block the binding of benzodiazepines to CNS receptors, resulting in a reversal of benzodiazepine-induced CNS depression

**Drug Interactions** CYP3A3/4 enzyme substrate

CNS depressants: Sedative effects and/or respiratory depression may be additive with CNS depressants; includes ethanol, barbiturates, narcotic analgesics, and other sedative agents; monitor for increased effect

Enzyme inducers: Metabolism of some benzodiazepines may be increased, decreasing their therapeutic effect; consider using an alternative sedative/hypnotic agent; potential inducers include phenobarbital, phenytoin, carbamazepine, rifampin, and rifabutin

CYP3A3/4 inhibitors: Serum level and/or toxicity of some benzodiazepines may be increased; inhibitors include amiodarone, cimetidine, clarithromycin, erythromycin, delavirdine, diltiazem, dirithromycin, disulfiram, fluoxetine, fluvoxamine, grapefruit juice, indinavir, itraconazole, ketoconazole, nefazodone, nevirapine, propoxyfene, quinupristin-dalfopristin, ritonavir, saquinavir, verapamil, zafirlukast, zileuton; monitor for altered benzodiazepine response

Oral contraceptives: May decrease the clearance of some benzodiazepines (those which undergo oxidative metabolism); monitor for increased benzodiazepine effect

Theophylline: May partially antagonize some of the effects of benzodiazepines; monitor for decreased response; may require higher doses for sedation

**Mechanism of Action** Binds to stereospecific benzodiazepine receptors on the postsynaptic GABA neuron at several sites within the central nervous system, including the limbic system, reticular formation. Enhancement of the inhibitory effect of GABA on neuronal excitability results by increased neuronal membrane permeability to chloride ions. This shift in chloride ions results in hyperpolarization (a less excitable state) and stabilization.

**Pharmacodynamics/kinetics**

Studies have shown that the elderly are more sensitive to the effects of benzodiazepines as compared to younger adults

Metabolism: Rapid and extensive in the liver to inactive metabolites

Half-life: 10-24 hours (no significant changes in the elderly)

Peak serum levels: 0.5-1.6 hours

Elimination: <5% excreted unchanged in urine

**Usual Dosage** Adults: Oral: 1 mg at bedtime, some patients may require 2 mg; start at doses of 0.5 mg in debilitated or small elderly patients

**Dosing adjustment in hepatic impairment:** May be necessary

**Dietary Considerations** Alcohol: Additive CNS effect, avoid use

**Monitoring Parameters** Respiratory and cardiovascular status

**Patient Information** May cause daytime drowsiness, avoid alcohol and drugs with CNS depressant effects; avoid activities needing good psychomotor coordination until CNS effects are known; drug may cause physical or psychological dependence; avoid abrupt discontinuation after prolonged use

**Nursing Implications** Provide safety measures (ie, side rails, night light, and call button); remove smoking materials from area; supervise ambulation; avoid abrupt discontinuance in patients with prolonged therapy or seizure disorders

**Dosage Forms** Tablet: 1 mg, 2 mg

- **Esterified Estrogen and Methyltestosterone** *see* Estrogens and Methyltestosterone *on page 206*
- **Estivin® II Ophthalmic [OTC]** *see* Naphazoline *on page 383*
- **Estrace® Oral** *see* Estradiol *on page 203*
- **Estraderm® Transdermal** *see* Estradiol *on page 203*
- **Estra-D® Injection** *see* Estradiol *on page 203*

## Estradiol (es tra DYE ole)

**U.S. Brand Names** Alora™ Transdermal; Climara® Transdermal; Delestrogen® Injection; depGynogen® Injection; Depo®-Estradiol Injection; Depogen® Injection; Dioval® Injection; Dura-Estrin® Injection; Duragen® Injection; Esclim® Transdermal; Estrace® Oral; Estraderm® Transdermal; Estra-D® Injection; Estra-L® Injection; Estro-Cyp® Injection; Gynogen L.A.® Injection; Innofem®; Vagifem®; Vivelle® Transdermal

**Synonyms** Estradiol Cypionate; Estradiol Hemihydrate; Estradiol Transdermal; Estradiol Valerate

**Pharmacologic Category** Estrogen Derivative

**Use** Treatment of atrophic vaginitis, atrophic dystrophy of vulva, menopausal symptoms, female hypogonadism, ovariectomy, primary ovarian failure, inoperable breast cancer, inoperable prostatic cancer, mild to severe vasomotor symptoms associated with menopause, prevention of postmenopausal osteoporosis

**Effects on Mental Status** May cause anxiety or depression

**Effects on Psychiatric Treatment** None reported

**Pregnancy Risk Factor** X

**Contraindications** Hypersensitivity to estradiol or any component; known or suspected pregnancy; porphyria; abnormal genital bleeding of unknown etiology; known or suspected carcinoma of the breast (except in patients treated for metastatic disease); estrogen-dependent tumors; history of thrombophlebitis, thrombosis, or thromboembolic disorders associated with estrogen use

**Warnings/Precautions** Use with caution in patients with renal or hepatic insufficiency. Estrogens may cause premature closure of epiphyses in young individuals, in patients with a history of thromboembolism, stroke, myocardial infarction (especially >40 years of age who smoke), liver tumor, or hypertension.

Gallbladder disease may be increased by estrogens. In addition, estrogens may increase blood pressure or alter glucose regulation. Use with caution in patients with diseases which may be exacerbated by fluid retention, including asthma, epilepsy, migraine, CHF, and renal dysfunction. Estrogens have been associated with severe hypercalcemia in patients with bone metastases, and may cause severe elevations of triglycerides in patients with familial dyslipidemias. Use with caution in women with a history of pregnancy-associated jaundice or metabolic bone disease. May increase the risk of benign hepatic adenoma, which may cause significant consequences in the event of rupture.

Use vaginal tablets with caution in patients with severely atrophic vaginal mucosa or following gynecological surgery due to possible trauma from the applicator.

Estrogens have been reported to increase the risk of endometrial carcinoma; do not use estrogens during pregnancy. Before prescribing estrogen therapy to postmenopausal women, the risks and benefits must be weighed for each patient. Women should be informed of these risks and benefits, as well as possible side effects and the return of menstrual bleeding (when cycled with a progestin), and be involved in the decision to prescribe. Oral therapy may be more convenient for vaginal atrophy and stress incontinence.

**Adverse Reactions**

>10%:

Cardiovascular: Peripheral edema

Endocrine & metabolic: Enlargement of breasts (female and male), breast tenderness

Gastrointestinal: Nausea, anorexia, bloating

1% to 10%:

Central nervous system: Headache

Endocrine & metabolic: Increased libido (female), decreased libido (male)

Gastrointestinal: Vomiting, diarrhea

<1%: Amenorrhea, anxiety, breast tumors, change in menstrual flow, chloasma, cholestatic jaundice, decreased glucose tolerance, depression, dizziness, edema, folate deficiency, GI distress, hypercalcemia, increase in blood pressure, increased susceptibility to *Candida* infection, increased triglycerides and LDL, intolerance to contact lenses, melasma, myocardial infarction, pain at injection site, rash, stroke, thromboembolic disorders,

**Vaginal:** Trauma from applicator insertion may occur in women with severely atrophic vaginal mucosa

**Overdosage/Toxicology**

Signs and symptoms: Fluid retention, jaundice, thrombophlebitis, nausea, vomiting

(Continued)

## Estradiol *(Continued)*

Treatment: Toxicity is unlikely following single exposures of excessive doses, any treatment following emesis and charcoal administration should be supportive and symptomatic

**Drug Interactions** CYP1A2 and 3A3/4 enzyme substrate

Decreased effect: Rifampin decreases estrogen serum concentrations

Increased toxicity: Hydrocortisone increases corticosteroid toxic potential; increased potential for thromboembolic events with anticoagulants

**Usual Dosage** All dosage needs to be adjusted based upon the patient's response

Male:

Prostate cancer: Valerate: I.M.: ≥30 mg or more every 1-2 weeks

Prostate cancer (androgen-dependent, inoperable, progressing): Oral: 10 mg 3 times/day for at least 3 months

Female:

Oral:

Breast cancer (inoperable, progressing): 10 mg 3 times/day for at least 3 months

Osteoporosis prevention: 0.5 mg/day in a cyclic regimen (3 weeks on and 1 week off)

Hypogonadism, moderate to severe vasomotor symptoms: 1-2 mg/day in a cyclic regimen for 3 weeks on drug, then 1 week off

Treatment of moderate to severe vasomotor symptoms associated with menopause: 1-2 mg/day, adjusted as necessary to limit symptoms; administration should be cyclic (3 weeks on, 1 week off). Patients should be re-evaluated at 3- to 6-month intervals to determine if treatment is still necessary.

I.M.

Moderate to severe vasomotor symptoms associated with menopause: Cypionate: 1-5 mg every 3-4 weeks; Valerate: 10-20 mg every 4 weeks

Postpartum breast engorgement: Valerate: 10-25 mg at end of first stage of labor

Transdermal twice-weekly patch (Alora™, Esclim®, Estraderm®, Vivelle®):

Moderate to severe vasomotor symptoms associated with menopause, vulvar/vaginal atrophy, hypogonadism: Apply 0.05 mg patch initially (titrate dosage to response) applied twice weekly in a cyclic regimen, for 3 weeks on and 1 week off drug in patients with an intact uterus and continuously in patients without a uterus. Re-evaluate postmenopausal therapy at 3- to 6-month intervals to determine if treatment is still necessary.

Transdermal once-weekly patch (Climara®, Fempatch®):

Moderate to severe vasomotor symptoms associated with menopause: Apply 0.025-0.05 mg/day patch once weekly. Adjust dose as necessary to control symptoms. Patients should be re-evaluated at 3- to 6-month intervals to determine if treatment is still necessary.

Prevention of osteoporosis in postmenopausal women (approved indication for Climara®): Apply patch once weekly; minimum effective dose 0.025 mg/day; adjust response to therapy by biochemical markers and bone mineral density

Vaginal cream:

Atrophic vaginitis, kraurosis vulvae: Vaginal: Insert 2-4 g/day for 2 weeks then gradually reduce to ½ the initial dose for 2 weeks followed by a maintenance dose of 1 g 1-3 times/week

Vaginal ring (Estring®):

Postmenopausal vaginal atrophy, urogenital symptoms: Following insertion, Estring® should remain in place for 90 days

Vaginal tablets (Vagifem®):

Atrophic vaginitis: Initial: Insert 1 tablet once daily for 2 weeks; Maintenance: Insert 1 tablet twice weekly; attempts to discontinue or taper medication should be made at 3- to 6-month intervals

**Dosing adjustment in hepatic impairment:**

Mild to moderate liver impairment: Dosage reduction of estrogens is recommended

Severe liver impairment: **Not recommended**

**Patient Information** Use this drug in cycles or term as prescribed. Periodic gynecologic exam and breast exams are important. You may experience nausea or vomiting (small frequent meals may help); dizziness or mental depression (use caution when driving); photosensitivity (use sunscreen, wear protective clothing and eyewear, and avoid direct sunlight); rash; loss of scalp hair; enlargement/tenderness of breasts; increased/decreased libido. Report sudden acute pain in legs or calves, chest, or abdomen; shortness of breath; severe headache or vomiting; weakness or numbness of arms or legs; unusual vaginal bleeding; yellowing of skin or eyes; change in color of urine or stool; or easy bruising or bleeding.

Transdermal patch: Apply to clean dry skin. Do not apply transdermal patch to breasts. Apply to trunk of body (preferably abdomen). Rotate application sites. Aerosol topical corticosteroids may reduce allergic skin reaction; report persistent skin reaction.

Intravaginal cream: Insert high in vagina. Wash hands and applicator before and after use.

**Nursing Implications** Aerosol topical corticosteroids applied under the patch may reduce allergic reactions; do not apply transdermal system to breasts, but place on trunk of body (preferably abdomen); rotate application sites

**Dosage Forms**

Cream, vaginal (Estrace®): 0.1 mg/g (42.5 g)

Injection, as cypionate (depGynogen®, Depo®-Estradiol, Depogen®, Dura-Estrin®, Estra-D®, Estro-Cyp®, Estroject-L.A.®): 5 mg/mL (5 mL, 10 mL)

Injection, as valerate:

Valergen®: 10 mg/mL (5 mL, 10 mL); 20 mg/mL (1 mL, 5 mL, 10 mL); 40 mg/mL (5 mL, 10 mL)

Dioval®, Duragen®, Estra-L®, Gynogen L.A.®: 20 mg/mL (10 mL); 40 mg/mL (10 mL)

Tablet, micronized:

Estrace®: 1 mg, 2 mg

Gynodiol®: 0.5 mg, 1 mg, 1.5 mg, 2 mg

Transdermal system:

Alora™:

0.05 mg/24 hours [18 cm$^2$], total estradiol 1.5 mg

0.075 mg/24 hours [27 cm$^2$], total estradiol 2.3 mg

0.1 mg/24 hours [36 cm$^2$], total estradiol 3 mg

Climara®:

0.025 mg/24 hours [6.5 cm$^2$]

0.05 mg/24 hours [12.5 cm$^2$], total estradiol 3.9 mg

0.075 mg/24 hours [18.75 cm$^2$], total estradiol 5.85 mg

0.1 mg/24 hours [25 cm$^2$], total estradiol 7.8 mg

Esclim®:

0.025 mg/day

0.0375 mg/day

0.05 mg/day

0.075 mg/day

0.1 mg/day

Estraderm®:

0.05 mg/24 hours [10 cm$^2$], total estradiol 4 mg

0.1 mg/24 hours [20 cm$^2$], total estradiol 8 mg

Vivelle®:

0.0375 mg/day

0.05 mg/day

0.075 mg/day

0.1 mg/day

Vaginal ring (Estring®): 2 mg gradually released over 90 days

## Estradiol and Ethynodiol Diacetate

(ETH in il es tra DYE ole & e thye noe DYE ole dye AS e tate)

**U.S. Brand Names** Demulen®; Zovia®

**Pharmacologic Category** Contraceptive

**Use** Prevention of pregnancy; treatment of hypermenorrhea, endometriosis, female hypogonadism

**Effects on Mental Status** May cause anxiety or depression

**Effects on Psychiatric Treatment** None reported

**Usual Dosage** Oral: Adults: Female: Contraception:

Schedule 1 (Sunday starter): Dose begins on first Sunday after onset of menstruation; if the menstrual period starts on Sunday, take first tablet that very same day. **With a Sunday start, an additional method of contraception should be used until after the first 7 days of consecutive administration.**

For 21-tablet package: Dosage is 1 tablet daily for 21 consecutive days, followed by 7 days off of the medication; a new course begins on the 8th day after the last tablet is taken.

For 28-tablet package: Dosage is 1 tablet daily without interruption.

Schedule 2 (Day 1 starter): Dose starts on first day of menstrual cycle taking 1 tablet daily.

For 21-tablet package: Dosage is 1 tablet daily for 21 consecutive days, followed by 7 days off of the medication; a new course begins on the 8th day after the last tablet is taken.

For 28-tablet package: Dosage is 1 tablet daily without interruption.

If all doses have been taken on schedule and one menstrual period is missed, continue dosing cycle. If two consecutive menstrual periods are missed, pregnancy test is required before new dosing cycle is started.

**Missed doses monophasic formulations** (refer to package insert for complete information):

One dose missed: Take as soon as remembered or take 2 tablets next day

Two consecutive doses missed in the first 2 weeks: Take 2 tablets as soon as remembered or 2 tablets next 2 days. **An additional method of contraception should be used for 7 days after missed dose,**

Two consecutive doses missed in week 3 or three consecutive doses missed at any time: Schedule 1 (Sunday starter): Continue dose of 1 tablet daily until Sunday, then discard the rest of the pack, and a new pack should be started that same day. Schedule 2 (Day 1 starter): Current package should be discarded, and a new pack should be started that same day. **An additional method of contraception should be used for 7 days after missed doses.**

**Dosage Forms** Tablet:

1/35: Ethinyl estradiol 0.035 mg and ethynodiol diacetate 1 mg (21s, 28s)

1/50: Ethinyl estradiol 0.05 mg and ethynodiol diacetate 1 mg (21s, 28s)

## Estradiol and Norethindrone

(es tra DYE ole & nor eth IN drone)

**U.S. Brand Names** Activella™; CombiPatch™

**Pharmacologic Category** Estrogen Derivative

**Use** For use in women with an intact uterus

Tablet: Treatment of moderate to severe vasomotor symptoms associated with menopause; treatment of vulvar and vaginal atrophy; prophylaxis for postmenopausal osteoporosis

Transdermal patch: Treatment of moderate to severe vasomotor symptoms associated with menopause; treatment of vulvar and vaginal atrophy; treatment of hypoestrogenism due to hypogonadism, castration, or primary ovarian failure

**Effects on Mental Status** May cause anxiety or depression

**Effects on Psychiatric Treatment** None reported

**Usual Dosage** Adults:

Oral: 1 tablet daily

Transdermal patch:

Continuous combined regimen: Apply one patch twice weekly

Continuous sequential regimen: Apply estradiol-only patch for first 14 days of cycle, followed by one Combi-Patch® applied twice weekly for the remaining 14 days of a 28-day cycle

**Dosage Forms**

Tablet (Activella™): Estradiol 1 mg and norethindrone acetate 0.5 mg (28s)

Transdermal system (CombiPatch™):

9 sq cm: Estradiol 0.05 mg and norethindrone acetate 0.14 mg per day

16 sq cm: Estradiol 0.05 mg and norethindrone acetate 0.25 mg per day

## Estradiol and Testosterone

(es tra DYE ole & tes TOS ter one)

**U.S. Brand Names** Andro/Fem® Injection; Deladumone® Injection; depAndrogyn® Injection; Depo-Testadiol® Injection; Depotestogen® Injection; Duo-Cyp® Injection; Duratestrin® Injection; Valertest No.1® Injection

**Canadian Brand Names** Climacteron®

**Pharmacologic Category** Estrogen Derivative

**Use** Vasomotor symptoms associated with menopause; postpartum breast engorgement

**Effects on Mental Status** May cause anxiety or depression

**Effects on Psychiatric Treatment** None reported

**Dosage Forms** Injection:

Andro/Fem®, depAndrogyn®, Depo-Testadiol®, Depotestogen®, Duo-Cyp®, Duratestrin®: Estradiol cypionate 2 mg and testosterone cypionate 50 mg per mL in cottonseed oil (1 mL, 10 mL)

Androgyn L.A.®, Deladumone®, Estra-Testrin®, Valertest No.1®: Estradiol valerate 4 mg and testosterone enanthate 90 mg per mL in sesame oil (5 mL, 10 mL)

♦ **Estradiol Cypionate** *see* Estradiol *on page 203*

♦ **Estradiol Hemihydrate** *see* Estradiol *on page 203*

♦ **Estradiol Transdermal** *see* Estradiol *on page 203*

♦ **Estradiol Valerate** *see* Estradiol *on page 203*

♦ **Estra-L® Injection** *see* Estradiol *on page 203*

## Estramustine (es tra MUS teen)

**U.S. Brand Names** Emcyt®

**Synonyms** Estramustine Phosphate Sodium

**Pharmacologic Category** Antineoplastic Agent, Alkylating Agent

**Use** Palliative treatment of prostatic carcinoma (progressive or metastatic)

**Effects on Mental Status** May cause sedation or insomnia; rarely may cause depression

**Effects on Psychiatric Treatment** None reported

**Pregnancy Risk Factor** C

**Contraindications** Active thrombophlebitis or thromboembolic disorders, hypersensitivity to estramustine or any component, estradiol or nitrogen mustard

**Warnings/Precautions** The U.S. Food and Drug Administration (FDA) currently recommends that procedures for proper handling and disposal of antineoplastic agents be considered. Glucose tolerance may be decreased; elevated blood pressure may occur; exacerbation of peripheral edema or congestive heart disease may occur; use with caution in patients with impaired liver function, renal insufficiency, or metabolic bone diseases.

**Adverse Reactions**

>10%:

Cardiovascular: Edema

Gastrointestinal: Diarrhea, nausea, mild increases in AST (SGOT) or LDH

Endocrine & metabolic: Decreased libido, breast tenderness, breast enlargement

Respiratory: Dyspnea

1% to 10%:

Cardiovascular: Myocardial infarction

Central nervous system: Insomnia, lethargy

Gastrointestinal: Anorexia, flatulence

Hematologic: Leukopenia

Local: Thrombophlebitis

Neuromuscular & skeletal: Leg cramps

Respiratory: Pulmonary embolism

<1%: Cardiac arrest, depression, hot flashes, hypercalcemia, night sweats pigment changes, tinnitus

**Overdosage/Toxicology**

Signs and symptoms: Nausea, vomiting, myelosuppression

Treatment: There are no known antidotes, treatment is primarily symptomatic and supportive

**Drug Interactions** Decreased effect: Milk products and calcium-rich foods/drugs may impair the oral absorption of estramustine phosphate sodium

**Usual Dosage** Adults: Oral: 14 mg/kg/day (range: 10-16 mg/kg/day) in 3-4 divided doses for 30-90 days; some patients have been maintained for >3 years on therapy

**Patient Information** It may take several weeks to manifest effects of this medication. Store capsules in refrigerator. Do not take with milk or milk products. Preferable to take on empty stomach (1 hour before or 2 hours after meals). Small frequent meals, frequent mouth care may reduce incidence of nausea or vomiting. You may experience flatulence, diarrhea, decreased libido (reversible), breast tenderness or enlargement. Report sudden acute pain or cramping in legs or calves, chest pain, shortness of breath, weakness or numbness of arms or legs, difficulty breathing, or edema (increased weight, swelling of legs or feet).

**Dosage Forms** Capsule, as phosphate sodium: 140 mg

♦ **Estramustine Phosphate Sodium** *see* Estramustine *on page 205*

♦ **Estratab®** *see* Estrogens, Esterified *on page 207*

♦ **Estratest®** *see* Estrogens and Methyltestosterone *on page 206*

♦ **Estratest® H.S.** *see* Estrogens and Methyltestosterone *on page 206*

♦ **Estro-Cyp® Injection** *see* Estradiol *on page 203*

♦ **Estrogenic Substances, Conjugated** *see* Estrogens, Conjugated *on page 206*

## Estrogens and Medroxyprogesterone

(ES troe jenz & me DROKS ee proe JES te rone)

**U.S. Brand Names** Premphase™; Prempro™

**Pharmacologic Category** Estrogen Derivative

**Use** Women with an intact uterus for the treatment of moderate to severe vasomotor symptoms associated with the menopause; treatment of atrophic vaginitis; primary ovarian failure; osteoporosis prophylactic

**Effects on Mental Status** May cause insomnia, anxiety, or depression

**Effects on Psychiatric Treatment** Barbiturates and carbamazepine may decrease the effects of estrogens; estrogens may affect metabolism of benzodiazepines; monitor for clinical effect

**Pregnancy Risk Factor** X

**Contraindications** Pregnancy; thrombophlebitis; hypersensitivity to estrogens or medroxyprogesterone or any component; cerebral apoplexy; undiagnosed vaginal bleeding; thrombophlebitis; liver disease; carcinoma of the breast; estrogen dependent tumor

**Warnings/Precautions** Use with caution in patients with asthma, epilepsy, migraine, diabetes, cardiac or renal dysfunction. Estrogens may cause premature closure of the epiphyses in young individuals. Estrogens have been reported to increase the risk of endometrial carcinoma. Pretreatment exams should include Pap smear, physical exam of breasts and pelvic areas. May increase serum cholesterol and LDL, decrease HDL and triglycerides. Use of any progestin during the first 4 months of pregnancy is not recommended. May lead to severe hypercalcemia in patients with breast cancer and bone metastases. Occasional blood pressure increases during estrogen replacement therapy have been attributed to idiosyncratic reactions to estrogens.

**Adverse Reactions**

>10%:

Cardiovascular: Edema, peripheral edema

Endocrine & metabolic: Breakthrough bleeding, spotting, changes in menstrual flow, amenorrhea, enlargement of breasts, breast tenderness

Gastrointestinal: Anorexia, nausea, bloating

Local: Pain at injection site

Neuromuscular & skeletal: Weakness

1% to 10%:

Cardiovascular: Edema, central thrombosis

Central nervous system: Mental depression, fever, insomnia, headache

Dermatologic: Melasma, chloasma, allergic rash with or without pruritus

Endocrine & metabolic: Increased breast tenderness, increased libido

Gastrointestinal: Weight gain or loss, vomiting, diarrhea

Genitourinary: Changes in cervical erosion and secretions

Hepatic: Cholestatic jaundice

(Continued)

## Estrogens and Medroxyprogesterone *(Continued)*

Local: Thrombophlebitis
Respiratory: Embolism

**Overdosage/Toxicology**
Signs and symptoms: Fluid retention, jaundice, thrombophlebitis
Treatment: Toxicity is unlikely following single exposures of excessive doses, any treatment following emesis and charcoal administration should be supportive and symptomatic

**Drug Interactions**
Decreased effect: Rifampin, barbiturates, phenytoin, carbamazepine decrease estrogen serum concentrations; estrogens may decrease effect of sulfonylureas; aminoglutethimide may decrease effect by increasing hepatic metabolism
Estrogens may increase metabolism of some benzodiazepines (lorazepam, oxazepam, temazepam), but decrease metabolism of others
Increased toxicity: Hydrocortisone increases corticosteroid toxic potential; increases potential for thromboembolic events with anticoagulants

**Usual Dosage** Oral:
Premphase™: 1 maroon tablet/day for 28 days and 1 light purple tablet to be taken with the maroon tablet on days 15-28; for patients with moderate to severe vasomotor symptoms and vulvar and vaginal atrophy associated with menopause, re-evaluate patients at 3- and 6-month intervals to determine if treatment is still necessary; for prevention of osteoporosis, monitor patients for signs of endometrial cancer; rule out malignancy if unexplained vaginal bleeding occurs
Prempro™: Dosage as above with the exception that the white 2.5 mg Cycrin® tablet (medroxyprogesterone acetate) is taken on a daily basis with the maroon Premarin® tablet (conjugated estrogen) and not just on days 15-28

**Patient Information** Take this as prescribed; maintain schedule. If also taking supplemental calcium as part of osteoporosis prevention, consult prescriber for recommended amounts. Periodic gynecologic exam and breast exams are important. You may experience nausea or vomiting (small frequent meals may help); dizziness or mental depression (use caution when driving); rash, loss of scalp hair, enlargement/tenderness of breasts, or increased/decreased libido. Report significant swelling of extremities; sudden acute pain in legs or calves, chest or abdomen; shortness of breath; severe headache or vomiting; sudden blindness; weakness or numbness of arm or leg; unusual vaginal bleeding; yellowing of skin or eyes; or unusual bruising or bleeding.

**Dosage Forms**
Premphase™: Two separate tablets in therapy pack: Conjugated estrogens 0.625 mg [Premarin®] (28s) taken orally for 28 days and medroxyprogesterone acetate [Cycrin®] 5 mg (14s) which are taken orally with a Premarin® tablet on days 15 through 28
Prempro™: Conjugated estrogens 0.625 mg and medroxyprogesterone acetate 2.5 mg (14s)

## Estrogens and Methyltestosterone
(ES troe jenz & meth il tes TOS te rone)

**U.S. Brand Names** Estratest®; Estratest® H.S.; Premarin® With Methyltestosterone

**Synonyms** Conjugated Estrogen and Methyltestosterone; Esterified Estrogen and Methyltestosterone

**Pharmacologic Category** Estrogen Derivative

**Use** Atrophic vaginitis; hypogonadism; primary ovarian failure; vasomotor symptoms of menopause; prostatic carcinoma; osteoporosis prophylactic

**Effects on Mental Status** May cause depression

**Effects on Psychiatric Treatment** Barbiturates and carbamazepine may decrease the effects of estrogens; estrogens may affect metabolism of benzodiazepines; monitor for clinical effect

**Pregnancy Risk Factor** X

**Contraindications**
Conjugated estrogens: Known or suspected cancer of the breast, except in appropriately selected patients being treated for metastatic disease; known or suspected estrogen-dependent neoplasia; known or suspected pregnancy; undiagnosed abnormal genital bleeding; active thrombophlebitis or thromboembolic disorders; past history of thrombophlebitis, thrombosis, or thromboembolic disorders associated with previous estrogen use (except when used in the treatment of breast or prostatic malignancy); acute liver disease; chronic impaired liver function; neuro-ophthalmologic vascular disease
Testosterone: Contraindicated in patients hypersensitive to this agent, in males with breast carcinoma, during pregnancy (or in women who may become pregnant) and lactation, in the presence of extensive cardiac, hepatic, or renal disease, and with known or suspected carcinoma of the prostate gland in males

**Warnings/Precautions** Estrogens have been reported to increase the risk of endometrial carcinoma; do not use estrogens during pregnancy

**Adverse Reactions** 1% to 10%:
Cardiovascular: Increase in blood pressure, edema, thromboembolic disorder
Central nervous system: Depression, headache
Dermatologic: Chloasma, melasma
Endocrine & metabolic: Breast tenderness, change in menstrual flow, hypercalcemia
Gastrointestinal: Nausea, vomiting
Hepatic: Cholestatic jaundice

**Overdosage/Toxicology** Signs and symptoms: Fluid retention, jaundice, thrombophlebitis

**Usual Dosage** Adults: Female: Oral: Lowest dose that will control symptoms should be chosen, normally given 3 weeks on and 1 week off

**Patient Information** Women should inform their physicians if signs or symptoms of any of the following occur: thromboembolic or thrombotic disorders including sudden severe headache or vomiting, disturbance of vision or speech, loss of vision, numbness or weakness in an extremity, sharp or crushing chest pain, calf pain, shortness of breath, severe abdominal pain or mass, mental depression or unusual bleeding; women should discontinue taking the medication if they suspect they are pregnant or become pregnant.

**Dosage Forms** Tablet:
Estratest®, Menogen®: Esterified estrogen 1.25 mg and methyltestosterone 2.5 mg
Estratest® H.S., Menogen H.S.®: Esterified estrogen 0.625 mg and methyltestosterone 1.25 mg
Premarin® With Methyltestosterone: Conjugated estrogen 0.625 mg and methyltestosterone 5 mg; conjugated estrogen 1.25 mg and methyltestosterone 10 mg

## Estrogens, Conjugated (ES troe jenz, KON joo gate ed)

**Related Information**
Pharmacotherapy of Urinary Incontinence *on page 758*

**U.S. Brand Names** Premarin®

**Canadian Brand Names** C.E.S.™; Congest

**Synonyms** C.E.S.; Estrogenic Substances, Conjugated

**Pharmacologic Category** Estrogen Derivative

**Use** Atrophic vaginitis; hypogonadism; primary ovarian failure; vasomotor symptoms of menopause; prostatic carcinoma; osteoporosis prophylactic
**Unlabeled use:** Behavioral symptoms of dementia

**Effects on Mental Status** May rarely cause anxiety or depression

**Effects on Psychiatric Treatment** None reported

**Pregnancy Risk Factor** X

**Contraindications** Undiagnosed vaginal bleeding; hypersensitivity to estrogens or any component; thrombophlebitis, liver disease, known or suspected pregnancy, carcinoma of the breast, estrogen dependent tumor

**Warnings/Precautions** Use with caution in patients with asthma, epilepsy, migraine, diabetes, cardiac or renal dysfunction; estrogens may cause premature closure of the epiphyses in young individuals; safety and efficacy in children have not been established; estrogens have been reported to increase the risk of endometrial carcinoma; do not use estrogens during pregnancy

**Adverse Reactions**
>10%:
Cardiovascular: Peripheral edema
Endocrine & metabolic: Breast tenderness, hypercalcemia, enlargement of breasts
Gastrointestinal: Nausea, anorexia, bloating
1% to 10%:
Central nervous system: Headache
Endocrine & metabolic: Increased libido
Gastrointestinal: Vomiting, diarrhea
Local: Pain at injection site
<1%: Alterations in frequency and flow of menses, amenorrhea, anxiety, breast tumors, chloasma, cholestatic jaundice, decreased glucose tolerance, depression, dizziness, edema, GI distress, hypertension, increase in blood pressure, increased susceptibility to *Candida* infection, increased triglycerides and LDL, intolerance to contact lenses, melasma, myocardial infarction, rash, stroke, thromboembolic disorder

**Overdosage/Toxicology**
Signs and symptoms: Fluid retention, jaundice, thrombophlebitis
Treatment: Toxicity is unlikely following single exposures of excessive doses, any treatment following emesis and charcoal administration should be supportive and symptomatic

**Drug Interactions** CYP1A2 enzyme inducer
Decreased effect: Rifampin decreases estrogen serum concentrations
Increased toxicity:
Hydrocortisone increases corticosteroid toxic potential
Increased potential for thromboembolic events with anticoagulants

**Usual Dosage** Adolescents and Adults:
Male: Prostate cancer: Oral: 1.25-2.5 mg 3 times/day
Female:
Osteoporosis in postmenopausal women: Oral: 0.625 mg/day, cyclically (3 weeks on, 1 week off)
Dysfunctional uterine bleeding:
Stable hematocrit: Oral: 1.25 mg twice daily for 21 days; if bleeding persists after 48 hours, increase to 2.5 mg twice daily; if bleeding persists after 48 more hours, increase to 2.5 mg 4 times/day; some

recommend starting at 2.5 mg 4 times/day. (**Note:** Medroxyprogesterone acetate 10 mg/day is also given on days 17-21.)

Unstable hematocrit: Oral: I.V.: 5 mg 2-4 times/day; if bleeding is profuse, 20-40 mg every 4 hours up to 24 hours may be used. **Note:** A progestational-weighted contraception pill should also be given (eg, Ovral® 2 tablets stat and 1 tablet 4 times/day or medroxyprogesterone acetate 5-10 mg 4 times/day)

Alternatively: I.V.: 25 mg every 6-12 hours until bleeding stops

Hypogonadism: Oral: 2.5-7.5 mg/day for 20 days, off 10 days and repeat until menses occur. If bleeding does not occur by the end of this period, repeat dosage schedule. If bleeding occurs before the end of the 10-day period, begin a 20-day estrogen-progestin cyclic regimen with 2.5-7.5 mg estrogen daily in divided doses for 1-20 days. During the last 5 days of estrogen therapy, give an oral progestin. If bleeding occurs before this regimen is concluded, discontinue therapy and resume on day 5 of bleeding.

Moderate to severe vasomotor symptoms: Oral: 0.625 mg/day either cyclically or daily; alternatively, may give 1.25 mg/day cyclically

Postpartum breast engorgement: Oral: 3.75 mg every 4 hours for 5 doses, then 1.25 mg every 4 hours for 5 days

Atrophic vaginitis, kraurosis vulvae:

Oral: 0.3-1.25 mg or more daily depending on tissue response of the patient; administer cyclically (3 weeks of daily estrogen and 1 week off)

Vaginal: 2-4 g instilled/day 3 weeks on and 1 week off

Female castration and primary ovarian failure: Oral: 1.25 mg/day cyclically (3 weeks on, 1 week off). Adjust according to severity of symptoms and patient response. For maintenance, adjust to the lowest effective dose.

Male/Female: Uremic bleeding: I.V.: 0.6 mg/kg/dose daily for 5 days

**Dosing adjustment in hepatic impairment:**

Mild to moderate liver impairment: Dosage reduction of estrogens is recommended

Severe liver impairment: **Not recommended**

**Patient Information** Follow prescribed schedule and dose. Periodic gynecologic exam and breast exams are important with long-term use. Consult prescriber for specific dietary recommendations. You may experience nausea or vomiting (small frequent meals may help); dizziness or mental depression (use caution when driving); photosensitivity (use sunscreen, wear protective clothing and eyewear, and avoid direct sunlight); rash, loss of scalp hair (reversible); enlargement/tenderness of breasts (both male and female); increased (female)/decreased (male) libido; or headache (use of mild analgesic may help). Report swelling of extremities or unusual weight gain; chest pain or palpitations; sudden acute pain, warmth, or weakness in legs or calves; shortness of breath; severe headache or vomiting; or unusual vaginal bleeding, amenorrhea, or alterations in frequency and flow of menses.

Intravaginal cream: Insert high in vagina; wash hands and applicator before and after application.

**Nursing Implications** May also be administered intramuscularly; administer at bedtime to minimize occurrence of adverse effects; when administered I.V., drug should be administered slowly to avoid the occurrence of a flushing reaction

**Dosage Forms**

Cream, vaginal: 0.625 mg/g (42.5 g)

Injection: 25 mg (5 mL)

Tablet: 0.3 mg, 0.625 mg, 0.9 mg, 1.25 mg, 2.5 mg

## Estrogens, Conjugated (Synthetic)

(ES troe jenz, KON joo gate ed, sin THET ik)

**U.S. Brand Names** Cenestin™

**Pharmacologic Category** Estrogen Derivative

**Use** Treatment of moderate to severe vasomotor symptoms of menopause

**Effects on Mental Status** Insomnia, nervousness, depression, and dizziness are common

**Effects on Psychiatric Treatment** None reported

**Pregnancy Risk Factor** X

**Contraindications** Undiagnosed vaginal bleeding; hypersensitivity to estrogens or any component; thrombophlebitis, liver disease, known or suspected pregnancy, carcinoma of the breast, estrogen dependent tumor, thromboembolic disorders

**Warnings/Precautions** Use with caution in patients with a history of hypercalcemia, cardiac disease, and gallbladder disease. The addition of progestins may attenuate estrogen's effects on raising HDL and lowering LDL cholesterol. May increase blood pressure and serum triglycerides (in patients with familial dyslipidemias). Use caution in patients with hepatic disease or renal dysfunction; may increase risk of venous thromboembolism. Estrogens have been reported to increase the risk of endometrial carcinoma and may increase the risk of breast cancer. Safety and efficacy in children have not been established. Do not use estrogens during pregnancy.

**Adverse Reactions**

>10%:

Cardiovascular: Palpitation (21%), peripheral edema (10%)

Endocrine & metabolic: Breast pain (29%), menorrhagia (14%)

Central nervous system; Headache (68%), insomnia (42%), nervousness (28%), depression (28%), pain (11%), dizziness (11%)

Gastrointestinal: Abdominal pain (28%), flatulence (29%), nausea (18%), dyspepsia (10%)

Neuromuscular & skeletal: Myalgia (28%), arthralgia (25%), back pain (14%), paresthesia (33%)

Miscellaneous: Weakness (33%), infection (14%)

1% to 10%:

Gastrointestinal: Vomiting (7%), constipation (6%), diarrhea (6%)

Central nervous system: Hypertonia (6%), fever (1%)

Musculoskeletal: Leg cramps (10%)

Respiratory: Pharyngitis (8%), rhinitis (8%), cough (6%)

Additional adverse reactions associated with estrogen therapy include: Alopecia, alterations in frequency and flow of menses, aggravation of porphyria, amenorrhea, anxiety, breast enlargement, breast tenderness, breast tumors, changes in cervical secretions, changes in corneal curvature, changes in libido, cholestatic jaundice, chorea chloasma, decreased glucose tolerance, erythema multiforme, erythema nodosum, GI distress, hirsutism, hypercalcemia, hypertension, increase in blood pressure, increased susceptibility to *Candida* infection, increased triglycerides and LDL, intolerance to contact lenses, melasma, myocardial infarction, pancreatitis, rash, stroke, thromboembolic disorder, weight gain, weight loss

**Overdosage/Toxicology**

Symptoms of overdose include fluid retention, jaundice, thrombophlebitis

Toxicity is unlikely following single exposures of excessive doses, any treatment following emesis and charcoal administration should be supportive and symptomatic

**Drug Interactions** Specific drug interactions have not been conducted for the synthetic preparation; however,the following interactions have been noted for conjugated estrogens

Decreased effect: Rifampin decreases estrogen serum concentrations (other enzyme inducers may share this effect)

Increased toxicity:

Hydrocortisone increases corticosteroid toxic potential

Increased potential for thromboembolic events with anticoagulants

**Usual Dosage** Adolescents and Adults: Moderate to severe vasomotor symptoms: Oral: 0.625 mg/day; may be titrated up to 1.25 mg/day. Attempts to discontinue medication should be made at 3- to 6-month intervals.

**Patient Information** Follow prescribed schedule and dose. Periodic gynecologic exam and breast exams are important with long-term use. Consult prescriber for specific dietary recommendations. You may experience nausea or vomiting (small frequent meals may help); dizziness or mental depression (use caution when driving); photosensitivity (use sunscreen, wear protective clothing and eyewear, and avoid direct sunlight); rash, loss of scalp hair (reversible); enlargement/tenderness of breasts (both male and female); increased (female)/decreased (male) libido; or headache (use of mild analgesic may help). Report swelling of extremities or unusual weight gain; chest pain or palpitations; sudden acute pain, warmth, or weakness in legs or calves; shortness of breath; severe headache or vomiting; or unusual vaginal bleeding, amenorrhea, or alterations in frequency and flow of menses.

**Additional Information** Not biologically equivalent to conjugated estrogens from equine source. Contains 9 unique estrogenic compounds (equine source contains at least 10 active estrogenic compounds)

**Dosage Forms** Tablet: 0.625 mg, 1.25 mg

## Estrogens, Esterified (ES troe jenz, es TER i fied)

**U.S. Brand Names** Estratab®; Menest®

**Canadian Brand Names** Neo-Estrone®

**Pharmacologic Category** Estrogen Derivative

**Use** Atrophic vaginitis; hypogonadism; primary ovarian failure; vasomotor symptoms of menopause; prostatic carcinoma; osteoporosis prophylactic

**Effects on Mental Status** May rarely cause anxiety or depression

**Effects on Psychiatric Treatment** None reported

**Pregnancy Risk Factor** X

**Contraindications** Known or suspected cancer of the breast, except in appropriately selected patients being treated for metastatic disease; known or suspected estrogen-dependent neoplasia; known or suspected pregnancy; undiagnosed abnormal genital bleeding; active thrombophlebitis or thromboembolic disorders; past history of thrombophlebitis, thrombosis, or thromboembolic disorders associated with previous estrogen use except when used in the treatment of breast or prostatic malignancy

**Warnings/Precautions** Use with caution in patients with asthma, epilepsy, migraine, diabetes, cardiac or renal dysfunction; estrogens may cause premature closure of the epiphyses in young individuals; safety and efficacy in children have not been established; estrogens have been reported to increase the risk of endometrial carcinoma, do not use estrogens during pregnancy

**Adverse Reactions**

>10%:

Cardiovascular: Peripheral edema

(Continued)

## Estrogens, Esterified *(Continued)*

Endocrine & metabolic: Enlargement of breasts, breast tenderness
Gastrointestinal: Nausea, anorexia, bloating

1% to 10%:

Central nervous system: Headache
Endocrine & metabolic: Increased libido
Gastrointestinal: Vomiting, diarrhea

<1%: Alterations in frequency and flow of menses, amenorrhea, anxiety, breast tumors, chloasma, cholestatic jaundice, decreased glucose tolerance, depression, dizziness, edema, GI distress, hypertension, increased susceptibility to *Candida* infection, increased triglycerides and LDL, intolerance to contact lenses, melasma, myocardial infarction, rash, stroke, thromboembolism

**Overdosage/Toxicology**

Signs and symptoms of overdose include fluid retention, jaundice, thrombophlebitis

Treatment: Toxicity is unlikely following single exposures of excessive doses, any treatment following emesis and charcoal administration should be supportive and symptomatic

**Drug Interactions**

Decreased effect: Rifampin decreases estrogen serum concentrations

Increased toxicity:

Hydrocortisone increases corticosteroid toxic potential

Anticoagulants: Increases potential for thromboembolic events with anticoagulants

Carbamazepine, tricyclic antidepressants, and corticosteroids; increased thromboembolic potential with oral anticoagulants

**Usual Dosage** Adults: Oral:

Male: Prostate cancer (inoperable, progressing): 1.25-2.5 mg 3 times/day

Female:

Hypogonadism: 2.5-7.5 mg of estrogen daily for 20 days followed by a 10-day rest period. Administer cyclically (3 weeks on and 1 week off). If bleeding does not occur by the end of the 10-day period, begin an estrogen-progestin cyclic regimen of 2.5-7.5 mg/day in divided doses for 20 days. During the last days of estrogen therapy, give an oral progestin. If bleeding occurs before this regimen is concluded, discontinue therapy and resume on the fifth day of bleeding.

Moderate to severe vasomotor symptoms: 1.25 mg/day administered cyclically (3 weeks on and 1 week off). If patient has not menstruated within the last 2 months or more, cyclic administration is started arbitrary. If the patient is menstruating, cyclical administration is started on day 5 of the bleeding. For short-term use only and should be discontinued as soon as possible. Re-evaluate at 3- to 6-month intervals for tapering or discontinuation of therapy.

Atopic vaginitis and kraurosis vulvae: 0.3 to ≥1.25 mg/day, depending on the tissue response of the individual patient. Administer cyclically. For short-term use only and should be discontinued as soon as possible. Re-evaluate at 3- to 6-month intervals for tapering or discontinuation of therapy.

Breast cancer (inoperable, progressing): 10 mg 3 times/day for at least 3 months

Osteoporosis, in postmenopausal women: Initial: 0.3 mg/day and increase to a maximum daily dose of 1.25 mg/day; initiate therapy as soon as possible after menopause; cyclical therapy is recommended

Female castration and primary ovarian failure: 1.25 mg/day, cyclically. Adjust dosage up- or downward according to the severity of symptoms and patient response. For maintenance, adjust dosage to lowest level that will provide effective control.

**Dosing adjustment in hepatic impairment:**

Mild to moderate liver impairment: Dosage reduction of estrogens is recommended

Severe liver impairment: **Not recommended**

**Patient Information** Use this drug in cycles or term as prescribed. Take each day at the same time with food. Periodic gynecologic exam and breast exams are important. You may experience nausea or vomiting (small frequent meals may help); dizziness or mental depression (use caution when driving); rash; loss of scalp hair; enlargement/tenderness of breasts; or increased/decreased libido. Report significant swelling of extremities, sudden acute pain in legs or calves, chest, or abdomen; shortness of breath; severe headache or vomiting; weakness or numbness of arms or legs; or unusual vaginal bleeding.

**Dosage Forms** Tablet: 0.3 mg, 0.625 mg, 1.25 mg, 2.5 mg

## Estrone (ES trone)

**U.S. Brand Names** Aquest®; Kestrone®

**Canadian Brand Names** Femogen®; Neo-Estrone®; Oestrilin®

**Pharmacologic Category** Estrogen Derivative

**Use** Hypogonadism; primary ovarian failure; vasomotor symptoms of menopause; prostatic carcinoma; inoperable breast cancer, kraurosis vulvae, abnormal uterine bleeding due to hormone imbalance

**Effects on Mental Status** May rarely cause anxiety or depression

**Effects on Psychiatric Treatment** None reported

**Usual Dosage** Adults: I.M.:

Male: Prostatic carcinoma: 2-4 mg 2-3 times/week

Female:

Senile vaginitis and kraurosis vulvae: 0.1-0.5 mg 2-3 times/week; cyclical (3 weeks on and 1 week off)

Breast cancer (inoperable, progressing): 5 mg 3 or more times/week

Primary ovarian failure, hypogonadism: 0.1-1 mg/week, up to 2 mg/week in single or divided doses; cyclical (3 weeks on and 1 week off)

Abnormal uterine bleeding: Brief courses of intensive therapy: 2-5 mg/day for several days

**Dosing adjustment in hepatic impairment:**

Mild to moderate liver impairment: Dosage reduction of estrogens is recommended

Severe liver impairment: **Not recommended**

**Dosage Forms** Injection: 2 mg/mL (10 mL, 30 mL); 5 mg/mL (10 mL)

## Estropipate (ES troe pih pate)

**U.S. Brand Names** Ogen® Oral; Ogen® Vaginal; Ortho-Est® Oral

**Canadian Brand Names** Estrouis®

**Synonyms** Piperazine Estrone Sulfate

**Pharmacologic Category** Estrogen Derivative

**Use** Atrophic vaginitis; hypogonadism; primary ovarian failure; vasomotor symptoms of menopause; osteoporosis prophylactic

**Effects on Mental Status** May rarely cause anxiety or depression

**Effects on Psychiatric Treatment** None reported

**Pregnancy Risk Factor** X

**Contraindications** Thrombophlebitis, undiagnosed vaginal bleeding, hypersensitivity to estrogens or any component; pregnancy

**Warnings/Precautions** Use with caution in patients with asthma, epilepsy, migraine, diabetes, cardiac or renal dysfunction; estrogens may cause premature closure of the epiphyses in young individuals; safety and efficacy in children have not been established; estrogens have been reported to increase the risk of endometrial carcinoma, do not use estrogens during pregnancy

**Adverse Reactions**

>10%:

Cardiovascular: Peripheral edema
Endocrine & metabolic: Enlargement of breasts, breast tenderness
Gastrointestinal: Nausea, anorexia, bloating

1% to 10%:

Central nervous system: Headache
Endocrine & metabolic: Increased libido
Gastrointestinal: Vomiting, diarrhea

<1%: Alterations in frequency and flow of menses, amenorrhea, anxiety, breast tumors, chloasma, cholestatic jaundice, decreased glucose tolerance, depression, dizziness, edema, GI distress, hypertension, increased susceptibility to *Candida* infection, increased triglycerides and LDL, intolerance to contact lenses, melasma, myocardial infarction, rash, stroke, thromboembolism

**Overdosage/Toxicology**

Signs and symptoms: Fluid retention, jaundice, thrombophlebitis

Treatment: Toxicity is unlikely following single exposures of excessive doses, any treatment following emesis and charcoal administration should be supportive and symptomatic

**Drug Interactions**

Decreased effect: Rifampin decreases estrogen serum concentrations

Increased toxicity:

Hydrocortisone increases corticosteroid toxic potential

Anticoagulants: Increases potential for thromboembolic events with anticoagulants

Carbamazepine, tricyclic antidepressants, and corticosteroids; increased thromboembolic potential with oral anticoagulants

**Usual Dosage** Adults: Female:

Moderate to severe vasomotor symptoms: Oral: Usual dosage range: 0.75-6 mg estropipate daily. Use the lowest dose and regimen that will control symptoms, and discontinue as soon as possible. Attempt to discontinue or taper medication at 3- to 6-month intervals. If a patient with vasomotor symptoms has not menstruated within the last ≥2 months, start the cyclic administration arbitrarily. If the patient has menstruated, start cyclic administration on day 5 of bleeding.

Hypogonadism or primary ovarian failure: Oral: 1.5-9 mg/day for the first 3 weeks, followed by a rest period of 8-10 days. Repeat if bleeding does not occur by the end of the rest period. The duration of therapy necessary to product the withdrawal bleeding will vary according to the responsiveness of the endometrium. If satisfactory withdrawal bleeding does not occur, give an oral progestin in addition to estrogen during the third week of the cycle.

Osteoporosis prevention: Oral: 0.625 mg/day for 25 days of a 31-day cycle

Atrophic vaginitis or kraurosis vulvae: Vaginal: Instill 2-4 g/day 3 weeks on and 1 week off

**Dosing adjustment in hepatic impairment:**

Mild to moderate liver impairment: Dosage reduction of estrogens is recommended

Severe liver impairment: **Not recommended**

**Patient Information** It is important to maintain schedule of drug days and drug-free days. Periodic gynecologic exam and breast exams are important. You may experience nausea or vomiting (small frequent meals may help); dizziness or mental depression (use caution when driving); rash; loss of scalp hair; enlargement/tenderness of breasts; or increased/decreased libido. Report significant swelling of extremities, sudden acute pain in legs or calves, chest or abdomen; shortness of breath; severe headache or vomiting; weakness or numbness of arms or legs; or unusual vaginal bleeding.

Intravaginal cream: Insert high in vagina, wash hands and applicator before and after application.

**Dosage Forms**

Cream, vaginal: 0.15% [estropipate 1.5 mg/g] (42.5 g tube)

Tablet: 0.625 mg [estropipate 0.75 mg]; 1.25 mg [estropipate 1.5 mg]; 2.5 mg [estropipate 3 mg]; 5 mg [estropipate 6 mg]

♦ **Estrostep® 21** *see* Ethinyl Estradiol and Norethindrone *on page 212*

♦ **Estrostep® Fe** *see* Ethinyl Estradiol and Norethindrone *on page 212*

## Etanercept (et a NER cept)

**U.S. Brand Names** Enbrel®

**Pharmacologic Category** Antirheumatic, Disease Modifying

**Use** Reduction in signs and symptoms of moderately to severely active rheumatoid arthritis in patients who have had an inadequate response to one or more disease-modifying antirheumatic drugs (DMARDs).

**Effects on Mental Status** Dizziness is common; may cause depression

**Effects on Psychiatric Treatment** None reported

**Usual Dosage** S.C.:

Children: 0.4 mg/kg (maximum: 25 mg dose)

Adults: 25 mg given twice weekly; if the physician determines that it is appropriate, patients may self-inject after proper training in injection technique

Elderly: Although greater sensitivity of some elderly patients cannot be ruled out, no overall differences in safety or effectiveness were observed

**Dosage Forms** Powder for injection: 25 mg

♦ **Ethacrynate Sodium** *see* Ethacrynic Acid *on page 209*

## Ethacrynic Acid (eth a KRIN ik AS id)

**U.S. Brand Names** Edecrin®

**Synonyms** Ethacrynate Sodium

**Pharmacologic Category** Diuretic, Loop

**Use** Management of edema associated with congestive heart failure; hepatic cirrhosis or renal disease; short-term management of ascites due to malignancy, idiopathic edema, and lymphedema

**Effects on Mental Status** May cause dizziness; may rarely cause drowsiness, nervousness, or confusion

**Effects on Psychiatric Treatment** Rare reports of agranulocytosis; use caution with clozapine and carbamazepine; may increase serum lithium levels, however, more likely with thiazide diuretic

**Pregnancy Risk Factor** B

**Contraindications** Hypersensitivity to ethacrynic acid or any component; anuria; history of severe watery diarrhea caused by this product; infants

**Warnings/Precautions** Adjust dose to avoid dehydration. In cirrhosis, avoid electrolyte and acid/base imbalances that might lead to hepatic encephalopathy. Ototoxicity is associated with rapid I.V. administration, renal impairment, excessive doses, and concurrent use of other ototoxins. Has been associated with a higher incidence of ototoxicity than other loop diuretics. Hypersensitivity reactions can rarely occur. Monitor fluid status and renal function in an attempt to prevent oliguria, azotemia, and reversible increases in BUN and creatinine. Close medical supervision of aggressive diuresis required. Watch for and correct electrolyte disturbances. Coadministration of antihypertensives may increase the risk of hypotension. Increased risk of gastric hemorrhage associated with corticosteroid therapy.

**Adverse Reactions**

>10%: Gastrointestinal: Diarrhea

1% to 10%:

- Cardiovascular: Orthostatic hypotension
- Central nervous system: Headache
- Endocrine & metabolic: Hyponatremia, hypochloremic alkalosis, hypokalemia
- Gastrointestinal: Loss of appetite, nausea, vomiting
- Ocular: Blurred vision

<1%: Abnormal LFTs, agranulocytosis, chills, confusion, dysphagia, fatigue, fever, GI bleeding, gout, hematuria, hepatic dysfunction, hyperuricemia, irritation, jaundice, leukopenia, malaise, nervousness, ototoxicity (irreversible), pancreatitis, rash, renal injury, stomach cramps, thrombocytopenia

**Overdosage/Toxicology**

Signs and symptoms: Electrolyte depletion, volume depletion, dehydration, circulatory collapse

Treatment: Following GI decontamination, treatment is supportive; hypotension responds to fluids and Trendelenburg position

**Drug Interactions**

ACE inhibitors: Hypotensive effects and/or renal effects are potentiated by hypovolemia

Antidiabetic agents: Glucose tolerance may be decreased

Antihypertensive agents: Hypotensive effects may be enhanced

Cephaloridine or cephalexin: Nephrotoxicity may occur

Cholestyramine or colestipol may reduce bioavailability of ethacrynic acid

Clofibrate: Protein binding may be altered in hypoalbuminemic patients receiving ethacrynic acid, potentially increasing toxicity

Digoxin: Ethacrynic acid-induced hypokalemia may predispose to digoxin toxicity; monitor potassium

Indomethacin (and other NSAIDs) may reduce natriuretic and hypotensive effects of diuretics

Lithium: Renal clearance may be reduced; isolated reports of lithium toxicity have occurred; monitor lithium levels

NSAIDs: Risk of renal impairment may increase when used in conjunction with diuretics

Ototoxic drugs (aminoglycosides, cis platinum): Concomitant use of ethacrynic acid may increase risk of ototoxicity, especially in patients with renal dysfunction

Peripheral adrenergic-blocking drugs or ganglionic blockers: Effects may be increased

Salicylates (high-dose) with diuretics may predispose patients to salicylate toxicity due to reduced renal excretion or alter renal function

Sparfloxacin, gatifloxicin, and moxifloxacin: Risk of cardiotoxicity may be increased; avoid use

Thiazides: Synergistic diuretic effects occur

**Usual Dosage** I.V. formulation should be diluted in $D_5W$ or NS (1 mg/mL) and infused over several minutes.

Children: Oral: 1 mg/kg/dose once daily; increase at intervals of 2-3 days as needed, to a maximum of 3 mg/kg/day.

Adults:

Oral: 50-200 mg/day in 1-2 divided doses; may increase in increments of 25-50 mg at intervals of several days; doses up to 200 mg twice daily may be required with severe, refractory edema.

I.V.: 0.5-1 mg/kg/dose (maximum: 100 mg/dose); repeat doses not routinely recommended; however, if indicated, repeat doses every 8-12 hours.

**Dosing adjustment/comments in renal impairment:** $Cl_{cr}$ <10 mL/minute: Avoid use.

Dialysis: Not removed by hemo- or peritoneal dialysis; supplemental dose is not necessary.

**Patient Information** Take prescribed dose with food early in day. Include orange juice or bananas (or other potassium-rich foods) in your diet, but do not take potassium supplements without consulting prescriber. You may experience postural hypotension (use caution when rising from lying or sitting position, when climbing stairs, or when driving); lightheadedness, dizziness, or drowsiness (use caution driving or when engaging in hazardous activities); diarrhea (buttermilk, boiled milk, or yogurt may help); or decreased accommodation to heat (avoid excessive exercise in hot weather). Diabetics should monitor serum glucose closely (this medication may interfere with antidiabetic medications). Report changes in hearing or ringing in ears, persistent headache, unusual confusion or nervousness, abdominal pain or blood stool (black stool), palpitations, chest pain, rapid heartbeat, joint or muscle soreness or weakness, flu-like symptoms, skin rash or itching, or blurred vision. Report swelling of ankles or feet, weight changes of more than 3 lb/day, increased fatigue, or muscle cramping or trembling.

**Dosage Forms**

Powder for injection, as ethacrynate sodium: 50 mg (50 mL)

Tablet: 25 mg, 50 mg

## Ethambutol (e THAM byoo tole)

**U.S. Brand Names** Myambutol®

**Canadian Brand Names** Etibi®

**Pharmacologic Category** Antitubercular Agent

**Use** Treatment of tuberculosis and other mycobacterial diseases in conjunction with other antituberculosis agents

**Effects on Mental Status** May cause confusion and disorientation

**Effects on Psychiatric Treatment** None reported

**Pregnancy Risk Factor** B

**Contraindications** Hypersensitivity to ethambutol or any component; optic neuritis

**Warnings/Precautions** Use only in children whose visual acuity can accurately be determined and monitored (not recommended for use in children <13 years of age unless the benefit outweighs the risk); dosage modification required in patients with renal insufficiency

**Adverse Reactions**

1% to 10%:

- Central nervous system: Headache, confusion, disorientation
- Endocrine & metabolic: Acute gout or hyperuricemia
- Gastrointestinal: Abdominal pain, anorexia, nausea, vomiting

(Continued)

## Ethambutol *(Continued)*

<1%: Abnormal LFTs, anaphylaxis, fever, malaise, mental confusion, optic neuritis, peripheral neuritis, pruritus, rash

**Overdosage/Toxicology**

Signs and symptoms: Decrease in visual acuity, anorexia, joint pain, numbness of the extremities

Treatment: Following GI decontamination, treatment is supportive

**Drug Interactions** Decreased absorption with aluminum salts

**Usual Dosage** Oral:

Ethambutol is generally not recommended in children whose visual acuity cannot be monitored. However, ethambutol should be considered for all children with organisms resistant to other drugs, when susceptibility to ethambutol has been demonstrated, or susceptibility is likely.

**Note:** A four-drug regimen (isoniazid, rifampin, pyrazinamide, and either streptomycin or ethambutol) is preferred for the initial, empiric treatment of TB. When the drug susceptibility results are available, the regimen should be altered as appropriate.

Children and Adults:

Daily therapy: 15-25 mg/kg/day (maximum: 2.5 g/day)

Directly observed therapy (DOT): Twice weekly: 50 mg/kg (maximum: 2.5 g)

DOT: 3 times/week: 25-30 mg/kg (maximum: 2.5 g)

**Dosing interval in renal impairment:**

$Cl_{cr}$ 10-50 mL/minute: Administer every 24-36 hours

$Cl_{cr}$ <10 mL/minute: Administer every 48 hours

Hemodialysis: Slightly dialyzable (5% to 20%); Administer dose postdialysis

Peritoneal dialysis: Dose for $Cl_{cr}$ <10 mL/minute

Continuous arteriovenous or venovenous hemofiltration: Administer every 24-36 hours

**Patient Information** Take as scheduled, with meals. Avoid missing doses and do not discontinue without consulting prescriber. You may experience GI distress (frequent small meals and good oral care may help), dizziness, disorientation, drowsiness (avoid driving or engaging in tasks that require alertness until response to drug is known). You will need to have frequent ophthalmic exams and periodic medical check-ups to evaluate drug effects. Report changes in vision, numbness or tingling of extremities, or persistent loss of appetite.

**Dosage Forms** Tablet, as hydrochloride: 100 mg, 400 mg

♦ **ETH and C** *see* Terpin Hydrate and Codeine *on page 536*

## Ethaverine (eth AV er een)

**Pharmacologic Category** Vasodilator

**Use** Peripheral and cerebral vascular insufficiency associated with arterial spasm

**Effects on Mental Status** May cause drowsiness, dizziness, or depression

**Effects on Psychiatric Treatment** None reported

**Warnings/Precautions** Administer with caution to patients with glaucoma

**Adverse Reactions** <1%: Constipation, depression, diaphoresis, dizziness, drowsiness, flushing of the face, headache, hepatic hypersensitivity, hypotension, lethargy, nausea, pruritus, sedation, tachycardia, vertigo, xerostomia

**Usual Dosage** Adults: Oral: 100 mg 3 times/day

**Patient Information** May cause dizziness or drowsiness; use caution when driving or performing other tasks requiring alertness

**Dosage Forms**

Capsule, as hydrochloride: 100 mg

Tablet, as hydrochloride: 100 mg

## Ethchlorvynol (eth klor VI nole)

**Related Information**

Anxiolytic/Hypnotic Use in Long-Term Care Facilities *on page 754*

Clinical Issues in the Use of Anxiolytics and Sedative/Hypnotics *on page 634*

Federal OBRA Regulations Recommended Maximum Doses *on page 756*

**Generic Available** No

**U.S. Brand Names** Placidyl®

**Pharmacologic Category** Hypnotic, Miscellaneous

**Use** Short-term management of insomnia

**Restrictions** C-IV

**Pregnancy Risk Factor** C

**Contraindications** Porphyria; hypersensitivity to ethchlorvynol or any component

**Warnings/Precautions** Administer with caution to depressed or suicidal patients or to patients with a history of drug abuse; intoxication symptoms may appear with prolonged daily doses of as little as 1 g; withdrawal symptoms may be seen upon abrupt discontinuation; use with caution in the elderly and in patients with hepatic or renal dysfunction; use with caution in patients who have a history of paradoxical restlessness to barbiturates or alcohol; some products may contain tartrazine

**Adverse Reactions**

Cardiovascular: Hypotension, syncope

Central nervous system: Dizziness, facial numbness, mild hangover, excitement, ataxia, hysteria, prolonged hypnosis, mild stimulation, giddiness

Dermatologic: Rash, urticaria

Gastrointestinal: Indigestion, nausea, stomach pain, unpleasant aftertaste, vomiting

Hematologic: Thrombocytopenia

Hepatic: Cholestatic jaundice

Neuromuscular & skeletal: Weakness (severe)

Ocular: Blurred vision

**Overdosage/Toxicology**

Signs and symptoms: Prolonged deep coma, respiratory depression, hypothermia, bradycardia, hypotension, nystagmus

Treatment: Supportive in nature; hemoperfusion may be helpful in enhancing elimination

**Drug Interactions**

CNS depressants: Sedative effects may be additive with other CNS depressants; monitor for increased effect; includes benzodiazepines, barbiturates, antipsychotics, ethanol, and other sedative medications

Warfarin: May inhibit the hypoprothrombinemic response to warfarin via an unknown mechanism; monitor for altered anticoagulant effect or consider using a benzodiazepine

**Stability** Capsules should not be crushed and should not be refrigerated

**Mechanism of Action** Unknown; causes nonspecific depression of the reticular activating system

**Pharmacodynamics/kinetics**

Onset of action: 15-60 minutes

Duration: 5 hours

Absorption: Rapid from GI tract

Metabolism: In the liver

Half-life: 10-20 hours

Time to peak serum concentration: 2 hours

**Usual Dosage** Adults: Oral: 500-1000 mg at bedtime

**Dosing adjustment in renal impairment:** $Cl_{cr}$ <50 mL/minute: Avoid use

**Dietary Considerations** Alcohol: Additive CNS effect, avoid use

**Monitoring Parameters** Cardiac and respiratory function and abuse potential

**Reference Range** Therapeutic: 2-9 μg/mL; Toxic: >20 μg/mL

**Patient Information** May cause drowsiness, can impair judgment and coordination; avoid alcohol and other CNS depressants; ataxia can be reduced if taken with food, do not crush or refrigerate capsules

**Nursing Implications** Raise bed rails; institute safety measures; assist with ambulation

**Dosage Forms** Capsule: 200 mg, 500 mg, 750 mg

## Ethinyl Estradiol (ETH in il es tra DYE ole)

**U.S. Brand Names** Edstinyl®

**Pharmacologic Category** Estrogen Derivative

**Use** Hypogonadism; primary ovarian failure; vasomotor symptoms of menopause; prostatic carcinoma; breast cancer

**Effects on Mental Status** May rarely cause anxiety or depression

**Effects on Psychiatric Treatment** None reported

**Pregnancy Risk Factor** X

**Contraindications** Thrombophlebitis, undiagnosed vaginal bleeding, hypersensitivity to ethinyl estradiol or any component, pregnancy, estrogen-dependent neoplasia

**Warnings/Precautions** Use with caution in patients with asthma, seizure disorders, migraine, cardiac, renal or hepatic impairment, cerebrovascular disorders or history of breast cancer, past or present thromboembolic disease, smokers >35 years of age

**Adverse Reactions**

>10%:

Cardiovascular: Peripheral edema

Endocrine & metabolic: Enlargement of breasts, breast tenderness, bloating

Gastrointestinal: Nausea, anorexia

1% to 10%:

Central nervous system: Headache

Endocrine & metabolic: Increased libido

Gastrointestinal: Vomiting, diarrhea

<1%: Alterations in frequency and flow of menses, amenorrhea, anxiety, breast tumors, chloasma, cholestatic jaundice, decreased glucose tolerance, depression, dizziness, edema, GI distress, hypertension, increased susceptibility to *Candida* infection, increased triglycerides and LDL, intolerance to contact lenses, melasma, myocardial infarction, rash, stroke, thromboembolism

**Overdosage/Toxicology**

Signs and symptoms of overdose include fluid retention, jaundice, thrombophlebitis, nausea

Treatment: Toxicity is unlikely following single exposures of excessive doses, any treatment following emesis and charcoal administration should be supportive and symptomatic

**Drug Interactions** CYP3A3/4 and 3A5-7 enzyme substrate; CYP1A2 enzyme inhibitor

Increased toxicity: Carbamazepine, tricyclic antidepressants, and corticosteroids

Increased thromboembolic potential with oral anticoagulants

Decreased efficacy: Nelfinavir decreases ethinyl estradiol concentrations

**Usual Dosage** Adults: Oral:

Male: Prostatic cancer (inoperable, progressing): 0.15-2 mg/day for palliation

Female:

Hypogonadism: 0.05 mg 1-3 times/day during the first 2 weeks of a theoretical menstrual cycle. Follow with a progesterone during the last half of the arbitrary cycle. Continue for 3-6 months. The patient should not be treated for the following 2 months.

Vasomotor symptoms: Usual dosage range: 0.02-0.05 mg/day; give cyclically for short-term use only and use the lowest dose that will control symptoms. Discontinue as soon as possible and administer cyclically (3 weeks on and 1 week off). Attempt to discontinue or taper medication at 3- to 6-month intervals.

Breast cancer (inoperable, progressing): 1 mg 3 times/day for palliation

**Dosing adjustment in hepatic impairment:**

Mild to moderate liver impairment: Dosage reduction of estrogens is recommended

Severe liver impairment: **Not recommended**

**Patient Information** Take according to recommended schedule. It is important to maintain schedule of drug days and drug-free days. Periodic gynecologic exam and breast exams for females are important. You may experience nausea or vomiting (small frequent meals may help); dizziness or mental depression (use caution when driving); rash; loss of scalp hair; enlargement/tenderness of breasts; or increased/decreased libido. Report significant swelling in extremities, sudden acute pain in legs or calves, chest, or abdomen; shortness of breath; severe headache or vomiting; weakness or numbness of arms or legs; or unusual vaginal bleeding.

**Nursing Implications** Administer at bedtime to minimize occurrence of adverse effects

**Dosage Forms** Tablet: 0.02 mg, 0.05 mg, 0.5 mg

## Ethinyl Estradiol and Desogestrel

(ETH in il es tra DYE ole & des oh JES trel)

**U.S. Brand Names** Apri®; Desogen®; Mircette™; Ortho-Cept®

**Pharmacologic Category** Contraceptive

**Use** Prevention of pregnancy

**Effects on Mental Status** may cause depression, migraine, dizziness, anxiety, headache, and stroke

**Effects on Psychiatric Treatment** Barbiturates decrease the effects of oral contraceptives; may increase the toxicity of the benzodiazepines and TCAs

**Usual Dosage** Oral: Adults: Female: Contraception:

Schedule 1 (Sunday starter): Dose begins on first Sunday after onset of menstruation; if the menstrual period starts on Sunday, take first tablet that very same day. **With a Sunday start, an additional method of contraception should be used until after the first 7 days of consecutive administration.**

For 21-tablet package: Dosage is 1 tablet daily for 21 consecutive days, followed by 7 days off of the medication; a new course begins on the 8th day after the last tablet is taken.

For 28-tablet package: Dosage is 1 tablet daily without interruption.

Schedule 2 (Day 1 starter): Dose starts on first day of menstrual cycle taking 1 tablet daily.

For 21-tablet package: Dosage is 1 tablet daily for 21 consecutive days, followed by 7 days off of the medication; a new course begins on the 8th day after the last tablet is taken.

For 28-tablet package: Dosage is 1 tablet daily without interruption.

If all doses have been taken on schedule and one menstrual period is missed, continue dosing cycle. If two consecutive menstrual periods are missed, pregnancy test is required before new dosing cycle is started.

**Missed doses monophasic formulations** (refer to package insert for complete information):

One dose missed: Take as soon as remembered or take 2 tablets next day

Two consecutive doses missed in the first 2 weeks: Take 2 tablets as soon as remembered or 2 tablets next 2 days. **An additional method of contraception should be used for 7 days after missed dose.**

Two consecutive doses missed in week 3 or three consecutive doses missed at any time: Schedule 1 (Sunday starter): Continue to take 1 tablet daily until Sunday, then discard the rest of the pack, and a new pack is started that same day. Schedule 2 (Day 1 starter): Current pack should be discarded, and a new pack started that same day. **An additional method of contraception should be used for 7 days after missed dose.**

**Dosage Forms** Tablet:

Ethinyl estradiol 0.03 mg and desogestrel 0.15 mg (21s, 28s)

Miracette™: White tablets: Ethinyl estradiol 0.02 mg and desogestrel 0.15 mg; Yellow tablets: Ethinyl estradiol 0.01 mg (28s)

Apri®: Day 1-21: Ethinyl estradiol 0.03 mg and desogestrel 0.15 mg; day 22-28: placebo

## Ethinyl Estradiol and Fluoxymesterone

(eth i nil es tra DYE ole & floo oks i MES te rone)

**Pharmacologic Category** Androgen; Estrogen Derivative

**Use** Moderate to severe vasomotor symptoms of menopause, postpartum breast engorgement

**Effects on Mental Status** May cause depression, migraine, dizziness, anxiety, headache, and stroke

**Effects on Psychiatric Treatment** Barbiturates decrease the effects of oral contraceptives; may increase the toxicity of the benzodiazepines and TCAs

**Usual Dosage** Oral: 1-2 tablets at bedtime given cyclically, 3 weeks on and 1 week off

**Dosage Forms** Tablet: Ethinyl estradiol 0.02 mg and fluoxymesterone 1 mg

## Ethinyl Estradiol and Levonorgestrel

(ETH in il es tra DYE ole & LEE voe nor jes trel)

**U.S. Brand Names** Alesse™; Levlen®; Levlite®; Levora®; Nordette®; PREVEN™; Tri-Levlen®; Triphasil®

**Pharmacologic Category** Contraceptive

**Use** Prevention of pregnancy; treatment of hypermenorrhea, endometriosis, female hypogonadism

**Effects on Mental Status** May cause depression, migraine, dizziness, anxiety, headache, and stroke

**Effects on Psychiatric Treatment** Barbiturates decrease the effects of oral contraceptives; may increase the toxicity of the benzodiazepines and TCAs

**Usual Dosage** Oral: Adults: Female: Contraception:

Schedule 1 (Sunday starter): Dose begins on first Sunday after onset of menstruation; if the menstrual period starts on Sunday, take first tablet that very same day. **With a Sunday start, an additional method of contraception should be used until after the first 7 days of consecutive administration.**

For 21-tablet package: Dosage is 1 tablet daily for 21 consecutive days, followed by 7 days off of the medication; a new course begins on the 8th day after the last tablet is taken.

For 28-tablet package: Dosage is 1 tablet daily without interruption.

Schedule 2 (Day 1 starter): Dose starts on first day of menstrual cycle taking 1 tablet daily.

For 21-tablet package: Dosage is 1 tablet daily for 21 consecutive days, followed by 7 days off of the medication; a new course begins on the 8th day after the last tablet is taken.

For 28-tablet package: Dosage is 1 tablet daily without interruption.

If all doses have been taken on schedule and one menstrual period is missed, continue dosing cycle. If two consecutive menstrual periods are missed, pregnancy test is required before new dosing cycle is started.

**Missed doses monophasic formulations** (refer to package insert for complete information):

One dose missed: Take as soon as remembered or take 2 tablets next day

Two consecutive doses missed in the first 2 weeks: Take 2 tablets as soon as remembered or 2 tablets next 2 days. **An additional method of contraception should be used for 7 days after missed dose.**

Two consecutive doses missed in week 3 or three consecutive doses missed at any time: **An additional method of contraception must be used for 7 days after a missed dose:**

Schedule 1 (Sunday starter): Continue dose of 1 tablet daily until Sunday, then discard the rest of the pack, and a new pack should be started that same day.

Schedule 2 (Day 1 starter): Current pack should be discarded, and a new pack should be started that same day.

**Missed doses biphasic/triphasic formulations** (refer to package insert for complete information):

One dose missed: Take as soon as remembered or take 2 tablets next day.

Two consecutive doses missed in week 1 or week 2 of the pack: Take 2 tablets as soon as remembered and 2 tablets the next day. Resume taking 1 tablet daily until the pack is empty. **An additional method of contraception should be used for 7 days after a missed dose.**

Two consecutive doses missed in week 3 of the pack; **An additional method of contraception must be used for 7 days after a missed dose.**

Schedule 1 (Sunday Starter): Take 1 tablet every day until Sunday. Discard the remaining pack and start a new pack of pills on the same day.

(Continued)

## Ethinyl Estradiol and Levonorgestrel *(Continued)*

Schedule 2 (Day 1 starter): Discard the remaining pack and start a new pack the same day.

Three or more consecutive doses missed; **An additional method of contraception must be used for 7 days after a missed dose.**

Schedule 1 (Sunday Starter): Take 1 tablet every day until Sunday; on Sunday, discard the pack and start a new pack.

Schedule 2 (Day 1 Starter): Discard the remaining pack and begin new pack of tablets starting on the same day.

**Dosage Forms** Tablet:

Alesse™: Ethinyl estradiol 0.02 mg and levonorgestrel 0.1 mg (21s, 28s)

Levlen®, Levora®, Nordette®: Ethinyl estradiol 0.03 mg and levonorgestrel 0.15 mg (21s, 28s)

Tri-Levlen®, Triphasil®: Phase 1 (6 brown tablets): Ethinyl estradiol 0.03 mg and levonorgestrel 0.05 mg; Phase 2 (5 white tablets): Ethinyl estradiol 0.04 mg and levonorgestrel 0.075 mg; Phase 3 (10 yellow tablets): Ethinyl estradiol 0.03 mg and levonorgestrel 0.125 mg (21s, 28s)

PREVEN™: Ethinyl estradiol 0.05 mg and levonorgestrel 0.25 mg (4 pills per kit along with a pregnancy test)

## Ethinyl Estradiol and Norethindrone

(ETH in il es tra DYE ole & nor eth IN drone)

**U.S. Brand Names** Brevicon®; Estrostep® 21; Estrostep® Fe; Femhrt™; Genora® 0.5/35; Genora® 1/35; Jenest-28™; Loestrin®; Modicon™; N.E.E.® 1/35; Nelova™ 0.5/35E; Nelova™ 10/11; Norethin™ 1/35E; Norinyl® 1+35; Ortho-Novum® 1/35; Ortho-Novum® 7/7/7; Ortho-Novum® 10/11; Ovcon® 35; Ovcon® 50; Tri-Norinyl®

**Pharmacologic Category** Contraceptive

**Use** Prevention of pregnancy; treatment of hypermenorrhea, endometriosis, female hypogonadism, moderate to severe vasomotor symptoms associated with menopause; prevention of osteoporosis

**Effects on Mental Status** May cause depression, migraine, dizziness, anxiety, headache, and stroke

**Effects on Psychiatric Treatment** Barbiturates decrease the effects of oral contraceptives; may increase the toxicity of the benzodiazepines and TCAs

**Usual Dosage** Oral: Adults: Female: Contraception:

Schedule 1 (Sunday starter): Dose begins on first Sunday after onset of menstruation; if the menstrual period starts on Sunday, take first tablet that very same day. **With a Sunday start, an additional method of contraception should be used until after the first 7 days of consecutive administration.**

For 21-tablet package: Dosage is 1 tablet daily for 21 consecutive days, followed by 7 days off of the medication; a new course begins on the 8th day after the last tablet is taken.

For 28-tablet package: Dosage is 1 tablet daily without interruption.

Schedule 2 (Day 1 starter): Dose starts on first day of menstrual cycle taking 1 tablet daily.

For 21-tablet package: Dosage is 1 tablet daily for 21 consecutive days, followed by 7 days off of the medication; a new course begins on the 8th day after the last tablet is taken.

For 28-tablet package: Dosage is 1 tablet daily without interruption.

If all doses have been taken on schedule and one menstrual period is missed, continue dosing cycle. If two consecutive menstrual periods are missed, pregnancy test is required before new dosing cycle is started.

**Missed doses monophasic formulations** (refer to package insert for complete information):

One dose missed: Take as soon as remembered or take 2 tablets next day

Two consecutive doses missed in the first 2 weeks: Take 2 tablets as soon as remembered or 2 tablets next 2 days. **An additional method of contraception should be used for 7 days after missed dose.**

Two consecutive doses missed in week 3 or three consecutive doses missed at any time: **An additional method of contraception must be used for 7 days after a missed dose:**

Schedule 1 (Sunday starter): Continue dose of 1 tablet daily until Sunday, then discard the rest of the pack, and a new pack should be started that same day.

Schedule 2 (Day 1 starter): Current pack should be discarded, and a new pack should be started that same day.

**Missed doses biphasic/triphasic formulations** (refer to package insert for complete information):

One dose missed: Take as soon as remembered or take 2 tablets next day.

Two consecutive doses missed in week 1 or week 2 of the pack: Take 2 tablets as soon as remembered and 2 tablets the next day. Resume taking 1 tablet daily until the pack is empty. **An additional method of contraception should be used for 7 days after a missed dose.**

Two consecutive doses missed in week 3 of the pack; **An additional method of contraception must be used for 7 days after a missed dose.**

Schedule 1 (Sunday Starter): Take 1 tablet every day until Sunday. Discard the remaining pack and start a new pack of pills on the same day.

Schedule 2 (Day 1 starter): Discard the remaining pack and start a new pack the same day.

Three or more consecutive doses missed; **An additional method of contraception must be used for 7 days after a missed dose.**

Schedule 1 (Sunday Starter): Take 1 tablet every day until Sunday; on Sunday, discard the pack and start a new pack.

Schedule 2 (Day 1 Starter): Discard the remaining pack and begin new pack of tablets starting on the same day.

**Dosage Forms** Tablet:

Brevicon®, Genora® 0.5/35, Modicon™, Nelova™ 0.5/35E: Ethinyl estradiol 0.035 mg and norethindrone 0.5 mg (21s, 28s)

Estrostep®:

Triangular tablet (white): Ethinyl estradiol 0.02 mg and norethindrone acetate 1 mg

Square tablet (white): Ethinyl estradiol 0.03 mg and norethindrone acetate 1 mg

Round tablet (white): Ethinyl estradiol 0.035 mg and norethindrone acetate 1 mg

Estrostep® Fe:

Triangular tablet (white): Ethinyl estradiol 0.02 mg and norethindrone acetate 1 mg

Square tablet (white): Ethinyl estradiol 0.03 mg and norethindrone acetate 1 mg

Round tablet (white): Ethinyl estradiol 0.035 mg and norethindrone acetate 1 mg

Brown tablet: Ferrous fumarate 75 mg

Loestrin® 1.5/30: Ethinyl estradiol 0.03 mg and norethindrone acetate 1.5 mg (21s)

Loestrin® Fe 1.5/30: Ethinyl estradiol 0.03 mg and norethindrone acetate 1.5 mg with ferrous fumarate 75 mg in 7 inert tablets (28s)

Loestrin® 1/20: Ethinyl estradiol 0.02 mg and norethindrone acetate 1 mg (21s)

Loestrin® Fe 1/20: Ethinyl estradiol 0.02 mg and norethindrone acetate 1 mg with ferrous fumarate 75 mg in 7 inert tablets (28s)

Genora® 1/35, N.E.E.® 1/35, Nelova® 1/35E, Norethin™ 1/35E, Norinyl® 1+35, Ortho-Novum® 1/35: Ethinyl estradiol 0.035 mg and norethindrone 1 mg (21s, 28s)

Jenest-28™: Phase 1 (7 white tablets): Ethinyl estradiol 0.035 mg and norethindrone 0.5 mg; Phase 2 (14 peach tablets): Ethinyl estradiol 0.035 mg and norethindrone 1 mg and 7 green inert tablets (28s)

Ortho-Novum® 7/7/7: Phase 1 (7 white tablets): Ethinyl estradiol 0.035 mg and norethindrone 0.5 mg; Phase 2 (7 light peach tablets): Ethinyl estradiol 0.035 mg and norethindrone 0.75 mg; Phase 3 (7 peach tablets): Ethinyl estradiol 0.035 mg and norethindrone 1 mg (21s, 28s)

Ortho-Novum® 10/11: Phase 1 (10 white tablets): Ethinyl estradiol 0.035 mg and norethindrone 0.5 mg; Phase 2 (11 dark yellow tablets): Ethinyl estradiol 0.035 mg and norethindrone 1 mg (21s, 28s)

Ovcon® 35: Ethinyl estradiol 0.035 mg and norethindrone 0.4 mg (21s, 28s)

Ovcon® 50: Ethinyl estradiol 0.050 mg and norethindrone 1 mg (21s, 28s)

Tri-Norinyl®: Phase 1 (7 blue tablets): Ethinyl estradiol 0.035 mg and norethindrone 0.5 mg; Phase 2 (9 green tablets): Ethinyl estradiol 0.035 mg and norethindrone 1 mg; Phase 3 (5 blue tablets): Ethinyl estradiol 0.035 mg and norethindrone 0.5 mg (21s, 28s)

## Ethinyl Estradiol and Norgestimate

(ETH in il es tra DYE ole & nor JES ti mate)

**U.S. Brand Names** Ortho-Cyclen®; Ortho-Prefest®; Ortho Tri-Cyclen®

**Canadian Brand Names** Cyclen®; Tri-Cyclen®

**Pharmacologic Category** Contraceptive

**Use** Prevention of pregnancy

**Effects on Mental Status** May cause depression, migraine, dizziness, anxiety, headache, and stroke

**Effects on Psychiatric Treatment** Barbiturates decrease the effects of oral contraceptives; may increase the toxicity of the benzodiazepines and TCAs

**Usual Dosage** Oral: Adults: Female: Contraception:

Schedule 1 (Sunday starter): Dose begins on first Sunday after onset of menstruation; if the menstrual period starts on Sunday, take first tablet that very same day. **With a Sunday start, an additional method of contraception should be used until after the first 7 days of consecutive administration.**

For 21-tablet package: Dosage is 1 tablet daily for 21 consecutive days, followed by 7 days off of the medication; a new course begins on the 8th day after the last tablet is taken.

For 28-tablet package: Dosage is 1 tablet daily without interruption.

Schedule 2 (Day 1 starter): Dose starts on first day of menstrual cycle taking 1 tablet daily.

For 21-tablet package: Dosage is 1 tablet daily for 21 consecutive days, followed by 7 days off of the medication; a new course begins on the 8th day after the last tablet is taken.

For 28-tablet package: Dosage is 1 tablet daily without interruption.

If all doses have been taken on schedule and one menstrual period is missed, continue dosing cycle. If two consecutive menstrual periods are missed, pregnancy test is required before new dosing cycle is started.

**Missed doses monophasic formulations** (refer to package insert for complete information):

One dose missed: Take as soon as remembered or take 2 tablets next day

Two consecutive doses missed in the first 2 weeks: Take 2 tablets as soon as remembered or 2 tablets next 2 days. **An additional method of contraception should be used for 7 days after missed dose.**

Two consecutive doses missed in week 3 or three consecutive doses missed at any time: **An additional method of contraception must be used for 7 days after a missed dose:**

Schedule 1 (Sunday starter): Continue dose of 1 tablet daily until Sunday, then discard the rest of the pack, and a new pack should be started that same day.

Schedule 2 (Day 1 starter): Current pack should be discarded, and a new pack should be started that same day.

**Missed doses biphasic/triphasic formulations** (refer to package insert for complete information):

One dose missed: Take as soon as remembered or take 2 tablets next day.

Two consecutive doses missed in week 1 or week 2 of the pack: Take 2 tablets as soon as remembered and 2 tablets the next day. Resume taking 1 tablet daily until the pack is empty. **An additional method of contraception should be used for 7 days after a missed dose.**

Two consecutive doses missed in week 3 of the pack; **An additional method of contraception must be used for 7 days after a missed dose.**

Schedule 1 (Sunday Starter): Take 1 tablet every day until Sunday. Discard the remaining pack and start a new pack of pills on the same day.

Schedule 2 (Day 1 starter): Discard the remaining pack and start a new pack the same day.

Three or more consecutive doses missed; **An additional method of contraception must be used for 7 days after a missed dose.**

Schedule 1 (Sunday Starter): Take 1 tablet every day until Sunday; on Sunday, discard the pack and start a new pack.

Schedule 2 (Day 1 Starter): Discard the remaining pack and begin new pack of tablets starting on the same day.

**Dosage Forms** Tablet:

Ortho-Cyclen®: Ethinyl estradiol 0.035 mg and norgestimate 0.25 mg (21s, 28s)

Ortho Tri-Cyclen®: Phase 1 (7 white tablets): Ethinyl estradiol 0.035 mg and norgestimate 0.18 mg; Phase 2 (5 light blue tablets): Ethinyl estradiol 0.035 mg and norgestimate 0.215 mg; Phase 3 (10 blue tablets): Ethinyl estradiol 0.035 mg and norgestimate 0.25 mg (21s, 28s)

Ortho-Prefest®: 1 mg estradiol (#15) and 1 mg estradiol with 0.09 mg norgestimate (#15)

## Ethinyl Estradiol and Norgestrel

(ETH in il es tra DYE ole & nor JES trel)

**U.S. Brand Names** Lo/Ovral®; Ovral®

**Pharmacologic Category** Contraceptive

**Use** Prevention of pregnancy; oral: postcoital contraceptive or "morning after" pill; treatment of hypermenorrhea, endometriosis, female hypogonadism

**Effects on Mental Status** May cause depression, migraine, dizziness, anxiety, headache, and stroke

**Effects on Psychiatric Treatment** Barbiturates decrease the effects of oral contraceptives; may increase the toxicity of the benzodiazepines and TCAs

**Usual Dosage** Oral: Adults: Female: Contraception: Some products recommend starting with one schedule over the other (refer to product information for more details):

Schedule 1 (Sunday starter): Dose begins on first Sunday after onset of menstruation; if the menstrual period starts on Sunday, take first tablet that very same day. **With a Sunday start, an additional method of contraception should be used until after the first 7 days of consecutive administration.**

For 21-tablet package: Dosage is 1 tablet daily for 21 consecutive days, followed by 7 days off of the medication; a new course begins on the 8th day after the last tablet is taken.

For 28-tablet package: Dosage is 1 tablet daily without interruption.

Schedule 2 (Day 1 starter): Dose starts on first day of menstrual cycle taking 1 tablet daily.

For 21-tablet package: Dosage is 1 tablet daily for 21 consecutive days, followed by 7 days off of the medication; a new course begins on the 8th day after the last tablet is taken.

For 28-tablet package: Dosage is 1 tablet daily without interruption.

If all doses have been taken on schedule and one menstrual period is missed, continue dosing cycle. If two consecutive menstrual periods are missed, pregnancy test is required before new dosing cycle is started.

**Missed doses monophasic formulations** (refer to package insert for complete information):

One dose missed: Take as soon as remembered or take 2 tablets next day

Two consecutive doses missed in the first 2 weeks: Take 2 tablets as soon as remembered or 2 tablets next 2 days. **An additional method of contraception should be used for 7 days after missed dose.**

Two consecutive doses missed in week 3 or three consecutive doses missed at any time: Schedule 1 (Sunday starter): Continue to take 1 tablet daily until Sunday, then discard the rest of the pack, and a new pack is started that same day. Schedule 2 (Day 1 starter): Current pack should be discarded, and a new pack started that same day. **An additional method of contraception should be used for 7 days after missed dose.**

Postcoital contraception or "morning after" pill: Oral (50 mcg ethinyl estradiol and 0.5 mg norgestrel): 2 tablets at initial visit and 2 tablets 12 hours later

**Dosage Forms** Tablet:

Lo/Ovral®: Ethinyl estradiol 0.03 mg and norgestrel 0.3 mg (21s and 28s)

Ovral®: Ethinyl estradiol 0.05 mg and norgestrel 0.5 mg (21s and 28s)

Low-Ogestrel®: Bioequivalent to Lo/Ovral®

## Ethionamide (e thye on AM ide)

**U.S. Brand Names** Trecator®-SC

**Pharmacologic Category** Antitubercular Agent

**Use** Treatment of tuberculosis and other mycobacterial diseases, in conjunction with other antituberculosis agents, when first-line agents have failed or resistance has been demonstrated

**Effects on Mental Status** May cause drowsiness or dizziness; case reports of depression and psychosis

**Effects on Psychiatric Treatment** None reported

**Pregnancy Risk Factor** C

**Contraindications** Contraindicated in patients with severe hepatic impairment or in patients who are sensitive to the drug

**Warnings/Precautions** Use with caution in patients receiving cycloserine or isoniazid, in diabetics

**Adverse Reactions**

>10%: Gastrointestinal: Anorexia, nausea, vomiting

1% to 10%:

Cardiovascular: Postural hypotension

Central nervous system: Psychiatric disturbances, drowsiness

Gastrointestinal: Metallic taste, diarrhea

Hepatic: Hepatitis (5%), jaundice

Neuromuscular & skeletal: Weakness

<1%: Abdominal pain, alopecia, blurred vision, dizziness, gynecomastia, headache, hypoglycemia, hypothyroidism or goiter, olfactory disturbances, optic neuritis, peripheral neuritis, rash, seizures, stomatitis, thrombocytopenia

**Overdosage/Toxicology**

Signs and symptoms: Peripheral neuropathy, anorexia, joint pain

Treatment: Following GI decontamination, treatment is supportive; pyridoxine may be given to prevent peripheral neuropathy

**Drug Interactions** Cycloserine and isoniazid; increased hepatotoxicity with rifampin

**Usual Dosage** Oral:

Children: 15-20 mg/kg/day in 2 divided doses, not to exceed 1 g/day

Adults: 500-1000 mg/day in 1-3 divided doses

**Dosing adjustment in renal impairment:** $Cl_{cr}$ <50 mL/minute: Administer 50% of dose

**Patient Information** Take this medication as prescribed; avoid missing doses and do not discontinue without contacting prescriber. You will need to schedule regular medical checkups which will include blood tests. You may experience GI upset (small frequent meals may help), metallic taste and increased salivation (lozenges, frequent mouth care), dizziness, blurred vision (use caution when driving or engaging in tasks that require alertness until response to drug is known), postural hypotension (change position slowly), impotence and/or menstrual difficulties (these will go away when drug is discontinued). Report acute unresolved GI upset, changes in vision, numbness or pain in extremities, or unusual bleeding or bruising.

**Dosage Forms** Tablet, sugar coated: 250 mg

♦ **Ethmozine®** *see* Moricizine *on page 374*

## Ethosuximide (eth oh SUKS i mide)

**Related Information**

Anticonvulsants by Seizures Type *on page 703*

Epilepsy Treatment *on page 783*

Serum Drug Concentrations Commonly Monitored: Guidelines *on page 759*

**U.S. Brand Names** Zarontin®

**Synonyms** 2-ethyl-2-methylsuccinmide

**Pharmacologic Category** Anticonvulsant, Succinimide

**Use** Management of absence (petit mal) seizures

**Effects on Mental Status** May cause sedation, euphoria, insomnia, or hallucinations; may rarely cause depression

(Continued)

## Ethosuximide *(Continued)*

**Effects on Psychiatric Treatment** Barbiturates and carbamazepine may decrease the clinical effects of ethosuximide

**Contraindications** Hypersensitivity to ethosuximide

**Warnings/Precautions** Use with caution in patients with hepatic or renal disease; abrupt withdrawal of the drug may precipitate absence status; ethosuximide may increase tonic-clonic seizures in patients with mixed seizure disorders; ethosuximide must be used in combination with other anticonvulsants in patients with both absence and tonic-clonic seizures

**Adverse Reactions**

Central nervous system: Ataxia, drowsiness, sedation, dizziness, lethargy, euphoria, headache, irritability, hyperactivity, fatigue, night terrors, disturbance in sleep, inability to concentrate, aggressiveness, mental depression, paranoid psychosis

Dermatologic: Stevens-Johnson syndrome, SLE, rash, hirsutism

Endocrine & metabolic: Increased libido

Gastrointestinal: Weight loss, gastric upset, cramps, epigastric pain, diarrhea, nausea, vomiting, anorexia, abdominal pain

Genitourinary: Vaginal bleeding, microscopic hematuria

Hematologic: Leukopenia, agranulocytosis, pancytopenia, eosinophilia

Ocular: Myopia

Miscellaneous: Hiccups

**Overdosage/Toxicology**

Signs and symptoms: Acute overdosage can cause CNS depression, ataxia, stupor, coma, hypotension; chronic overdose can cause skin rash, confusion, ataxia, proteinuria, hepatic dysfunction, hematuria

Treatment: Supportive; hemoperfusion and hemodialysis may be useful

**Drug Interactions** CYP3A3/4 enzyme substrate; CYP3A3/4 enzyme inducer

CNS depressants: Sedative effects and/or respiratory depression may be additive with CNS depressants; includes ethanol, benzodiazepines, barbiturates, narcotic analgesics, and other sedative agents; monitor for increased effect

Enzyme inducers: Metabolism of ethosuximide may be increased, decreasing its therapeutic effect; consider using an alternative sedative/hypnotic agent; potential inducers include phenobarbital, phenytoin, carbamazepine, rifampin, and rifabutin

CYP3A3/4 inhibitors: Serum level and/or toxicity of ethosuximide may be increased; inhibitors include amiodarone, cimetidine, clarithromycin, erythromycin, delavirdine, diltiazem, dirithromycin, disulfiram, fluoxetine, fluvoxamine, grapefruit juice, indinavir, itraconazole, ketoconazole, nefazodone, nevirapine, propoxyfene, quinupristin-dalfopristin, ritonavir, saquinavir, verapamil, zafirlukast, zileuton; monitor for altered benzodiazepine response

Isoniazid: May inhibit hepatic metabolism of ethosuximide with a resultant increase in ethosuximide serum concentrations

Phenytoin: Ethosuximide may elevate phenytoin levels; phenytoin may decrease ethosuximide levels (see enzyme inducers)

Valproate acid: Has been reported to both increase and decrease ethosuximide levels

**Mechanism of Action** Increases the seizure threshold and suppresses paroxysmal spike-and-wave pattern in absence seizures; depresses nerve transmission in the motor cortex

**Pharmacodynamics/kinetics**

Time to peak serum concentration:

Capsule: Within 2-4 hours

Syrup: <2-4 hours

Distribution: Adults: $V_d$: 0.62-0.72 L/kg

Metabolism: ~80% metabolized in the liver to three inactive metabolites

Half-life:

Children: 30 hours

Adults: 50-60 hours

Elimination: Slowly excreted in urine as metabolites (50%) and as unchanged drug (10% to 20%); small amounts excreted in feces

**Usual Dosage** Oral:

Children 3-6 years: Initial: 250 mg/day (or 15 mg/kg/day) in 2 divided doses; increase every 4-7 days; usual maintenance dose: 15-40 mg/kg/day in 2 divided doses

Children >6 years and Adults: Initial: 250 mg twice daily; increase by 250 mg as needed every 4-7 days up to 1.5 g/day in 2 divided doses; usual maintenance dose: 20-40 mg/kg/day in 2 divided doses

**Monitoring Parameters** Seizure frequency, trough serum concentrations; CBC, platelets, liver enzymes, urinalysis

**Reference Range** Therapeutic: 40-100 µg/mL (SI: 280-710 µmol/L); Toxic: >150 µg/mL (SI: >1062 µmol/L)

**Test Interactions** ↑ alkaline phosphatase (S); positive Coombs' [direct]; ↓ calcium (S)

**Patient Information** Take with food; do not discontinue abruptly; may cause drowsiness and impair judgment

**Nursing Implications** Observe patient for excess sedation

**Dosage Forms**

Capsule: 250 mg

Syrup (raspberry flavor): 250 mg/5 mL (473 mL)

## Ethotoin (ETH oh toyn)

**U.S. Brand Names** Peganone®

**Synonyms** Ethylphenylhydantoin

**Pharmacologic Category** Anticonvulsant, Hydantoin

**Use** Generalized tonic-clonic or complex-partial seizures

**Effects on Mental Status** Drowsiness and dizziness are common; may cause insomnia or confusion

**Effects on Psychiatric Treatment** None reported

**Pregnancy Risk Factor** D

**Contraindications** Hepatic abnormalities; hematologic disorders; hypersensitivity to ethotoin

**Adverse Reactions**

>10%:

Central nervous system: Psychiatric changes, slurred speech, trembling, dizziness, drowsiness

Gastrointestinal: Constipation, nausea, vomiting

1% to 10%:

Central nervous system: Drowsiness, headache, insomnia

Dermatologic: Skin rash

Gastrointestinal: Anorexia, weight loss

Hematologic: Leukopenia

Hepatic: Hepatitis

Renal: Increase in serum creatinine

**Drug Interactions** May increase the metabolism of theophylline

**Usual Dosage** Oral:

Children: 30-60 mg/kg/day or 250 mg twice daily, may be increased up to 2-3 g/day

Adults: 250 mg 4 times/day after meals, may be increased up to 3 g/day in divided doses 4 times/day

**Patient Information** Take exactly as directed (do not increase dose or frequency or discontinue without consulting prescriber). While using this medication, do not use alcohol and other prescription or OTC medications (especially pain medications, sedatives, antihistamines, or hypnotics) without consulting prescriber. Maintain adequate hydration (2-3 L/day). You may experience drowsiness, dizziness, or blurred vision (use caution when driving or engaging in hazardous tasks); nausea, vomiting, loss of appetite, or dry mouth (small frequent meals, good mouth care, chewing gum, or sucking on lozenges may help); constipation (increased exercise, fluids, or dietary fruit and fiber may help). Diabetics need to monitor serum glucose closely (may alter antidiabetic medication requirements). If used for seizures, wear identification of epileptic status and medication. Report CNS changes, mentation changes, or changes in cognition; difficulty breathing or shortness of breath; muscle cramping, weakness, tremors, changes in gait; persistent GI symptoms (cramping, constipation, vomiting, anorexia); changes in urinary pattern, chest pain or palpitations, unusual bruising or bleeding (mouth, urine, stool); worsening of seizure activity, or loss of seizure control.

**Dosage Forms** Tablet: 250 mg, 500 mg

♦ **Ethoxynaphthamido Penicillin Sodium** *see* Nafcillin *on page 380*

♦ **2-ethyl-2-methylsuccinmide** *see* Ethosuximide *on page 213*

♦ **Ethylenediamine** *see* Theophylline Salts *on page 539*

## Ethylnorepinephrine (eth il nor ep i NEF rin)

**U.S. Brand Names** Bronkephrine® Injection

**Pharmacologic Category** Alpha/Beta Agonist

**Use** Bronchial asthma and reversible bronchospasm

**Effects on Mental Status** Nervousness is common; may cause insomnia, drowsiness, confusion, anxiety, or psychosis

**Effects on Psychiatric Treatment** None reported

**Pregnancy Risk Factor** C

**Contraindications** Cardiac arrhythmias; hypersensitivity to ethylnorepinephrine or any component

**Adverse Reactions**

>10%:

Cardiovascular: Tachycardia, pounding heart beat

Central nervous system: Nervousness, trembling

Gastrointestinal: Nausea

Neuromuscular & skeletal: Tremor

1% to 10%:

Cardiovascular: Hypertension or hypotension

Central nervous system: Dizziness, lightheadedness, headache, insomnia, drowsiness

Dermatologic: Flushing of face

Gastrointestinal: Xerostomia, heartburn, vomiting, abnormal taste

Genitourinary: Dysuria

Neuromuscular & skeletal: Muscle cramping, weakness

Respiratory: Coughing

Miscellaneous: Increased diaphoresis

**Usual Dosage** I.M., S.C.:

Children: Usually 0.1-0.5 mL, varies according to weight

Adults: 0.5-1 mL

**Dosage Forms** Injection, as hydrochloride: 2 mg/mL (1 mL)

♦ **Ethylphenylhydantoin** *see* Ethotoin *on page 214*

♦ **Ethyol®** *see* Amifostine *on page 30*

## Etidronate Disodium (e ti DROE nate dye SOW dee um)

**U.S. Brand Names** Didronel®

**Synonyms** EHDP; Sodium Etidronate

**Pharmacologic Category** Bisphosphonate Derivative

**Use** Symptomatic treatment of Paget's disease and heterotopic ossification due to spinal cord injury or after total hip replacement, hypercalcemia associated with malignancy

**Effects on Mental Status** None reported

**Effects on Psychiatric Treatment** None reported

**Pregnancy Risk Factor** B (oral)/C (parenteral)

**Contraindications** Patients with serum creatinine >5 mg/dL; hypersensitivity to biphosphonates

**Warnings/Precautions** Use with caution in patients with restricted calcium and vitamin D intake; dosage modification required in renal impairment; I.V. form may be nephrotoxic and should be used with caution, if at all, in patients with impaired renal function (serum creatinine: 2.5-4.9 mg/dL)

**Adverse Reactions**

1% to 10%:

Central nervous system: Fever, convulsions

Endocrine & metabolic: Hypophosphatemia, hypomagnesemia, fluid overload

Neuromuscular & skeletal: Bone pain

Respiratory: Dyspnea

<1%: Abnormal taste, angioedema, hypersensitivity reactions, increased risk of fractures, nephrotoxicity, occult blood in stools, pain, rash

**Overdosage/Toxicology**

Signs and symptoms: Diarrhea, nausea, vomiting, paresthesias, tetany, coma

Treatment: Antidote is calcium

**Drug Interactions** Foscarnet and plicamycin may have additive hypocalcemic effect

**Usual Dosage** Adults: Oral formulation should be taken on an empty stomach 2 hours before any meal.

Paget's disease: Oral

Initial: 5-10 mg/kg/day (not to exceed 6 months) or 11-20 mg/kg/day (not to exceed 3 months). Doses >10 mg/kg/day are **not** recommended.

Retreatment: Initiate only after etidronate-free period ≥90 days. Monitor patients every 3-6 months. Retreatment regimens are the same as for initial treatment.

Heterotopic ossification: Oral:

Caused by spinal cord injury: 20 mg/kg/day for 2 weeks, then 10 mg/kg/day for 10 weeks; total treatment period: 12 weeks

Complicating total hip replacement: 20 mg/kg/day for 1 month preoperatively then 20 mg/kg/day for 3 months postoperatively; total treatment period is 4 months

Hypercalcemia associated with malignancy:

I.V. (dilute dose in at least 250 mL NS): 7.5 mg/kg/day for 3 days; there should be at least 7 days between courses of treatment

Oral: Start 20 mg/kg/day on the last day of infusion and continue for 30-90 days

**Dosing adjustment in renal impairment:**

$S_{cr}$ 2.5-5 mg/dL: Use with caution

$S_{cr}$ >5 mg/dL: **Not recommended**

**Patient Information** Maintain adequate intake of calcium and vitamin D; take medicine on an empty stomach 2 hours before meals

**Nursing Implications** Ensure adequate hydration

**Dosage Forms**

Injection: 50 mg/mL (6 mL)

Tablet: 200 mg, 400 mg

## Etodolac (ee toe DOE lak)

**Related Information**

Nonsteroidal Anti-inflammatory Agents Comparison Chart *on page 722*

**U.S. Brand Names** Lodine®; Lodine® XL

**Synonyms** Etodolic Acid

**Pharmacologic Category** Nonsteroidal Anti-Inflammatory Agent (NSAID)

**Use** Acute and long-term use in the management of signs and symptoms of osteoarthritis and management of pain

**Unlabeled use:** Rheumatoid arthritis

**Effects on Mental Status** Dizziness is common; may cause nervousness; rarely produces confusion, depression, insomnia, or hallucinations

**Effects on Psychiatric Treatment** May rarely cause agranulocytosis; use caution with clozapine and carbamazepine; may decrease the clearance of lithium resulting in elevated serum levels and potential toxicity; monitor serum lithium levels

**Pregnancy Risk Factor** C (D if used in third trimester)

**Contraindications** Hypersensitivity to etodolac, aspirin, or other NSAIDs

**Warnings/Precautions** Use with caution in patients with congestive heart failure, hypertension, decreased renal or hepatic function, history of GI disease, or those receiving anticoagulants

**Adverse Reactions**

>10%:

Central nervous system: Dizziness

Dermatologic: Rash

Gastrointestinal: Abdominal cramps, heartburn, indigestion, nausea

1% to 10%:

Central nervous system: Headache, nervousness

Dermatologic: Itching

Endocrine & metabolic: Fluid retention

Gastrointestinal: Vomiting

Otic: Tinnitus

<1%: Acute renal failure, agranulocytosis, allergic rhinitis, anemia, angioedema, arrhythmia, aseptic meningitis, bone marrow suppression, blurred vision, confusion, congestive heart failure, conjunctivitis, cystitis, decreased hearing, drowsiness, dry eyes, epistaxis, erythema multiforme, gastritis, GI ulceration, hallucinations, hemolytic anemia, hepatitis, hot flashes, hypertension, insomnia, leukopenia, mental depression, peripheral neuropathy, polydipsia, polyuria, shortness of breath, Stevens-Johnson syndrome, tachycardia, thrombocytopenia, toxic amblyopia, toxic epidermal necrolysis, urticaria

**Overdosage/Toxicology**

Signs and symptoms: Acute renal failure, vomiting, drowsiness, leukocytes

Treatment: Management of a nonsteroidal anti-inflammatory drug (NSAID) intoxication is primarily supportive and symptomatic. Fluid therapy is commonly effective in managing the hypotension that may occur following an acute NSAID overdose, except when this is due to an acute blood loss.

**Drug Interactions**

ACE inhibitors: Effects may be reduced by NSAIDs; use lowest possible dose for shortest duration possible; monitor

Cholestyramine and colestipol: Absorption may be reduced by concurrent administration

Corticosteroids: May increase the risk of GI ulceration; use caution

Cyclosporine: Nephrotoxicity may be increased with concurrent NSAID use; monitor

Hydralazine: Antihypertensive effect may be decreased; avoid concurrent use

Lithium: Serum levels can be increased; avoid concurrent use if possible or monitor lithium levels and adjust dose. When NSAID is stopped, lithium may need adjustment again.

Loop diuretics: Therapeutic effects may be reduced by NSAIDs; avoid

Methotrexate: Toxicity may be increased by concurrent NSAID use; risk is limited in low-dose methotrexate regimens (such as for rheumatoid arthritis); prolonged leucovorin rescue may be required at antineoplastic doses; monitor

Thiazide diuretics: Antihypertensive effects are decreased; avoid concurrent use

Warfarin: INRs may be increased by some NSAIDs. This may depend, in part, on dose and duration; monitor INR closely. Use the lowest dose of NSAIDs possible and for the briefest duration.

**Usual Dosage** Single dose of 76-100 mg is comparable to the analgesic effect of aspirin 650 mg; in patients ≥65 years, no substantial differences in the pharmacokinetics or side-effects profile were seen compared with the general population

Adults: Oral:

Acute pain: 200-400 mg every 6-8 hours, as needed, not to exceed total daily doses of 1200 mg; for patients weighing <60 kg, total daily dose should not exceed 20 mg/kg/day

Osteoarthritis: Initial: 800-1200 mg/day given in divided doses: 400 mg 2 or 3 times/day; 300 mg 2, 3 or 4 times/day; 200 mg 3 or 4 times/day; total daily dose should not exceed 1200 mg; for patients weighing <60 kg, total daily dose should not exceed 20 mg/kg/day

**Patient Information** Take this medication exactly as directed; do not increase dose without consulting prescriber. Do not crush tablets or break capsules. Take with food or milk to reduce GI distress. Maintain adequate fluid intake (2-3 L/day of fluids unless instructed to restrict fluid intake). Do not use alcohol, aspirin, or aspirin-containing medication, and all other anti-inflammatory medications without consulting prescriber. You may experience anorexia, nausea, vomiting, or heartburn (frequent small meals, frequent mouth care, sucking lozenges, or chewing gum may help); drowsiness, dizziness, nervousness, or headache (use caution when driving or engaging in tasks requiring alertness until response to drug is known); fluid retention (weigh yourself weekly and report unusual (3-5 lb/week) weight gain). GI bleeding, ulceration, or perforation can occur with or without pain; discontinue medication and contact prescriber if persistent

(Continued)

## Etodolac *(Continued)*

abdominal pain or cramping, or blood in stool occurs. Report breathlessness, difficulty breathing, or unusual cough; chest pain, rapid heartbeat, palpitations; unusual bruising/bleeding; blood in urine, stool, mouth, or vomitus; swollen extremities; skin rash or itching; acute fatigue; or changes in hearing or ringing in ears.

**Dosage Forms**

Capsule (Lodine®): 200 mg, 300 mg
Tablet (Lodine®): 400 mg, 500 mg
Tablet, extended release (Lodine® XL): 400 mg, 500 mg, 600 mg

♦ **Etodolic Acid** *see* Etodolac *on page 215*

## Etomidate (e TOM i date)

**U.S. Brand Names** Amidate® Injection
**Pharmacologic Category** General Anesthetic
**Use** Induction of general anesthesia
**Effects on Mental Status** None reported
**Effects on Psychiatric Treatment** None reported
**Usual Dosage** Children >10 years and Adults: I.V.: 0.2-0.6 mg/kg over a period of 30-60 seconds for induction of anesthesia
**Dosage Forms** Injection: 2 mg/mL (10 mL, 20 mL)

♦ **Etopophos®** *see* Etoposide Phosphate *on page 216*

♦ **Etopophos® Injection** *see* Etoposide *on page 216*

## Etoposide (e toe POE side)

**U.S. Brand Names** Etopophos® Injection; Toposar® Injection; VePesid® Injection; VePesid® Oral
**Pharmacologic Category** Antineoplastic Agent, Natural Source (Plant) Derivative
**Use** Treatment of lymphomas, ANLL, lung, testicular, bladder, and prostate carcinoma, hepatoma, rhabdomyosarcoma, uterine carcinoma, neuroblastoma, mycosis fungoides, Kaposi's sarcoma, histiocytosis, gestational trophoblastic disease, Ewing's sarcoma, Wilms' tumor, and brain tumors
**Effects on Mental Status** May cause sedation
**Effects on Psychiatric Treatment** May cause myelosuppression; use caution with clozapine and carbamazepine
**Usual Dosage** Refer to individual protocols:

Oral: Twice the I.V. dose rounded to the nearest 50 mg given once daily if total dose ≤400 mg or in divided doses if >400 mg
Children: I.V.: 60-120 mg/m²/day for 3-5 days every 3-6 weeks
AML:
Remission induction: 150 mg/m²/day for 2-3 days for 2-3 cycles
Intensification or consolidation: 250 mg/m²/day for 3 days, courses 2-5
Brain tumor: 150 mg/m²/day on days 2 and 3 of treatment course
Neuroblastoma: 100 mg/m²/day over 1 hour on days 1-5 of cycle; repeat cycle every 4 weeks
BMT conditioning regimen used in patients with rhabdomyosarcoma or neuroblastoma: I.V. continuous infusion: 160 mg/m²/day for 4 days
Conditioning regimen for allogenic BMT: 60 mg/kg/dose as a single dose
Adults:
Small cell lung cancer:
Oral: Twice the I.V. dose rounded to the nearest 50 mg given once daily if tolerated
I.V.: 35 mg/m²/day for 4 days or 50 mg/m²/day for 5 days every 3-4 weeks total dose ≤400 mg/day or in divided doses if >400 mg/day
IVPB: 60-100 mg/m²/day for 3 days (with cisplatin)
CIV: 500 mg/m² over 24 hours every 3 weeks
Testicular cancer:
IVPB: 50-100 mg/m²/day for 5 days repeated every 3-4 weeks
I.V.: 100 mg/m² every other day for 3 doses repeated every 3-4 weeks
BMT/relapsed leukemia: I.V.: 2.4-3.5 g/m² or 25-70 mg/kg administered over 4-36 hours

**Dosing adjustment in renal impairment:**

$Cl_{cr}$ 10-50 mL/minute: Administer 75% of normal dose
$Cl_{cr}$ <10 mL minute: Administer 50% of normal dose
Hemodialysis: Supplemental dose is not necessary
Peritoneal dialysis: Supplemental dose is not necessary
CAPD effects: Unknown
CAVH effects: Unknown

**Dosing adjustment in hepatic impairment:**

Bilirubin 1.5-3 mg/dL or AST 60-180 units: Reduce dose by 50%
Bilirubin 3-5 mg/dL or AST >180 units: Reduce by 75%
Bilirubin >5 mg/dL: Do not administer

**Dosage Forms**

Capsule: 50 mg
Injection: 20 mg/mL (5 mL, 10 mL, 25 mL)

## Etoposide Phosphate (e toe POE side FOS fate)

**U.S. Brand Names** Etopophos®
**Pharmacologic Category** Antineoplastic Agent, Irritant; Antineoplastic Agent, Podophyllotoxin Derivative; Vesicant
**Use** Treatment of refractory testicular tumors and small cell lung cancer
**Effects on Mental Status** May cause sedation
**Effects on Psychiatric Treatment** May cause myelosuppression; use caution with clozapine and carbamazepine
**Usual Dosage** Refer to individual protocols. Adults:

Small cell lung cancer: I.V. (in combination with other approved chemotherapeutic drugs): **Equivalent doses of etoposide phosphate to an etoposide dosage** range of 35 mg/m²/day for 4 days to 50 mg/m²/day for 5 days. Courses are repeated at 3- to 4-week intervals after adequate recovery from any toxicity.
Testicular cancer: I.V. (in combination with other approved chemotherapeutic agents): **Equivalent dose of etoposide phosphate to etoposide dosage** range of 50-100 mg/m²/day on days 1-5 to 100 mg/m²/day on days 1, 3, and 5. Courses are repeated at 3- to 4-week intervals after adequate recovery from any toxicity.

**Dosage adjustment in renal impairment:**

$Cl_{cr}$ 15-50 mL/minute: Administer 75% of normal dose
$Cl_{cr}$ <15 mL minute: Data are not available and further dose reduction should be considered in these patients.
Hemodialysis: Supplemental dose is not necessary
Peritoneal dialysis: Supplemental dose is not necessary
CAPD effects: Unknown
CAVH effects: Unknown

**Dosage adjustment in hepatic impairment:**

Bilirubin 1.5-3 mg/dL or AST 60-180 units: Reduce dose by 50%
Bilirubin 3-5 mg/dL or AST >180 units: Reduce by 75%
Bilirubin >5 mg/dL: Do not administer

**Dosage Forms** Powder for injection, lyophilized: 119.3 mg (100 mg base)

♦ **Etrafon®** *see* Amitriptyline and Perphenazine *on page 34*

## Etretinate (e TRET i nate)

**U.S. Brand Names** Tegison®
**Pharmacologic Category** Antipsoriatic Agent
**Use** Treatment of severe recalcitrant psoriasis in patients intolerant of or unresponsive to standard therapies
**Effects on Mental Status** Sedation is common; may cause dizziness; may rarely cause confusion or depression
**Effects on Psychiatric Treatment** Concurrent use with psychotropics may produce additive sedation or dry mouth
**Pregnancy Risk Factor** X
**Contraindications** Pregnancy, known hypersensitivity to etretinate; because of the high likelihood of long lasting teratogenic effects, do not prescribe etretinate for women who are or who are likely to become pregnant while or after using the drug
**Warnings/Precautions** Not to be used in severe obesity or women of childbearing potential unless woman is capable of complying with effective contraceptive measures; therapy is normally begun on the second or third day of next normal menstrual period; effective contraception must be used for at least 1 month before beginning therapy, during therapy, and for 1 month after discontinuation of therapy; pregnancy test must be performed prior to starting therapy

**Adverse Reactions**

>10%:
Central nervous system: Fatigue, headache, fever
Dermatologic: Chapped lips, alopecia
Endocrine & metabolic: Hypercholesterolemia, hypertriglyceridemia
Gastrointestinal: Nausea, appetite change, xerostomia, sore tongue
Neuromuscular & skeletal: Hyperostosis, bone pain, arthralgia
Ocular: Eye irritation
Respiratory: Epistaxis
1% to 10%:
Cardiovascular: Edema
Central nervous system: Dizziness, lethargy
Hepatic: Hepatitis
Neuromuscular & skeletal: Myalgia
Ocular: Blurred vision
Otic: Otitis externa
Respiratory: Dyspnea
<1%: Amnesia, confusion, constipation, depression, diarrhea, dysuria, ear infection, flatulence, gingival bleeding, gout, hyperkinesia, hypertonia, kidney stones, mouth ulcers, phlebitis, photophobia, polyuria, pseudotumor cerebri, rhinorrhea, syncope, urticaria, weight loss

**Drug Interactions**

Increased effect: Milk increases absorption of etretinate
Increased toxicity: Additive toxicity with vitamin A

**Usual Dosage** Adults: Oral: Individualized; Initial: 0.75-1 mg/kg/day in divided doses, increase by 0.25 mg/kg/day at weekly intervals up to 1.5 mg/kg/day; maintenance dose established after 8-10 weeks of therapy 0.5-0.75 mg/kg/day
**Patient Information** Take with food. Do not take additional vitamin A supplements. You may experience dizziness, blurred vision, or fatigue; use

caution when driving or engaging in tasks that require alertness until response to drug is known. Report persistent severe nausea, abdominal pain, visual disturbances, yellowing of skin or eyes, unusual bruising or bleeding, muscle pain or cramping, or unusual nosebleeds.

**Dosage Forms** Capsule: 10 mg, 25 mg


- ♦ **ETS-2%® Topical** *see* Erythromycin, Ophthalmic/Topical *on page 202*
- ♦ **Eudal-SR®** *see* Guaifenesin and Pseudoephedrine *on page 257*
- ♦ **Eulexin®** *see* Flutamide *on page 236*
- ♦ **Evac-Q-Mag® [OTC]** *see* Magnesium Citrate *on page 330*
- ♦ **Evalose®** *see* Lactulose *on page 306*
- ♦ **Everone® Injection** *see* Testosterone *on page 536*
- ♦ **Evista®** *see* Raloxifene *on page 487*
- ♦ **E-Vitamin® [OTC]** *see* Vitamin E *on page 586*
- ♦ **Exact® Cream [OTC]** *see* Benzoyl Peroxide *on page 62*
- ♦ **Excedrin®, Extra Strength [OTC]** *see* Acetaminophen, Aspirin, and Caffeine *on page 15*
- ♦ **Excedrin® P.M. [OTC]** *see* Acetaminophen and Diphenhydramine *on page 15*
- ♦ **Exelderm® Topical** *see* Sulconazole *on page 522*
- ♦ **Exelon®** *see* Rivastigmine *on page 498*


## Exemestane (ex e MES tane)

**U.S. Brand Names** Aromasin®

**Pharmacologic Category** Antineoplastic Agent, Miscellaneous

**Use** Treatment of advanced breast cancer in postmenopausal women whose disease has progressed following tamoxifen therapy

**Effects on Mental Status** Drowsiness, depression, insomnia, and anxiety are common; may cause confusion

**Effects on Psychiatric Treatment** None reported

**Pregnancy Risk Factor** D

**Contraindications** Known hypersensitivity to exemestane or any component; pregnancy, or lactation

**Warnings/Precautions** Not indicated for premenopausal women; not to be given with estrogen-containing agents. Use with caution in hepatic impairment or renal insufficiency.

**Adverse Reactions**

>10% :

Central nervous system: Fatigue (22%), pain (13%), depression (13%), insomnia (11%), anxiety (10%)

Endocrine & metabolic: Hot flashes (13%)

Gastrointestinal: Nausea (18%)

1% to 10%:

Central nervous system: Dizziness (8%), headache (8%), fever (5%), hypoesthesia, confusion

Cardiovascular: Edema (7%), hypertension (5%), chest pain

Dermatologic: Rash, itching, alopecia

Gastrointestinal: Vomiting (7%), abdominal pain (6%), anorexia (6%), constipation (5%), diarrhea (4%), increased appetite (3%), dyspepsia

Genitourinary: urinary tract infection

Neuromuscular & skeletal: Weakness, paresthesia, pathological fracture, arthralgia

Miscellaneous: Influenza-like symptoms (6%), sweating (6%), lymphedema, infection

Respiratory: Dyspnea (10%), cough (6%), bronchitis, sinusitis, pharyngitis, rhinitis

<1%: Increase in transaminases and GGT

A dose-dependent decrease in sex-hormone binding globulin has been observed with daily doses of 25 mg or more. Serum luteinizing hormone and follicle-stimulating hormone levels have increased with this medicine.

**Overdosage/Toxicology** Daily doses as high as 800 mg have been used in healthy volunteers and 600 mg for 12 weeks in postmenopausal women with advanced breast cancer. If an overdose should occur, general supportive care would be indicated. Mice given 3200 mg/kg as a single dose died. This would be equivalent to 640 times the recommended human dose on a mg/m$^2$ basis. Rats and dogs died at higher single doses equivalent to 2000-4000 times the recommended human dose on a mg/m$^2$ basis.

**Drug Interactions** CYP3A4 substrate; however, ketoconazole, a CYP3A4 inhibitor, did not change the pharmacokinetics of exemestane. No other potential drug interactions have been evaluated.

**Usual Dosage** Adults; Oral: 25 mg once daily after a meal; treatment should continue until tumor progression is evident

**Dosing adjustment in renal/hepatic impairment:** Safety of chronic doses has not been studied

**Dietary Considerations** Plasma levels increased by 40% when exemestane was taken with a fatty meal

**Patient Information** Take after a meal; use caution if you have uncontrolled high blood pressure. Do not use in pregnancy or lactation. Avoid driving or doing other tasks or hobbies that require alertness until you know how this medicine affects you. Take at a similar time every day.

**Nursing Implications** Educate patient about getting blood pressure checked while on medicine, especially if there is a history of poor control. Encourage patient not to drive until she sees how the medicine affects her; it can cause fatigue and dizziness. Medication should be taken at a similar time every day and after a meal to decrease nausea and increase absorption.

**Dosage Forms** Tablet: 25 mg


- ♦ **Exhirud®** *see* Hirudin *on page 268*
- ♦ **Exidine® Scrub [OTC]** *see* Chlorhexidine Gluconate *on page 111*
- ♦ **Exna®** *see* Benzthiazide *on page 63*
- ♦ **Extendryl® SR** *see* Chlorpheniramine, Phenylephrine, and Methscopolamine *on page 115*
- ♦ **Extra Action Cough Syrup [OTC]** *see* Guaifenesin and Dextromethorphan *on page 257*
- ♦ **Extra Strength Adprin-B® [OTC]** *see* Aspirin *on page 49*
- ♦ **Extra Strength Bayer® Enteric 500 Aspirin [OTC]** *see* Aspirin *on page 49*
- ♦ **Extra Strength Bayer® Plus [OTC]** *see* Aspirin *on page 49*
- ♦ **Extra Strength Doan's® [OTC]** *see* Magnesium Salicylate *on page 331*
- ♦ **Extra Strength Dynafed® E.X. [OTC]** *see* Acetaminophen *on page 14*
- ♦ **Eye Balm** *see* Golden Seal *on page 254*
- ♦ **Eye-Lube-A® Solution [OTC]** *see* Artificial Tears *on page 48*
- ♦ **Eye Root** *see* Golden Seal *on page 254*
- ♦ **Eyesine® Ophthalmic [OTC]** *see* Tetrahydrozoline *on page 538*
- ♦ **Ezide®** *see* Hydrochlorothiazide *on page 271*


## Factor IX Complex (Human)

(FAK ter nyne KOM pleks HYU man)

**U.S. Brand Names** AlphaNine® SD; BeneFix™; Hemonyne®; Konȳne® 80; Profilnine® SD; Proplex® T

**Pharmacologic Category** Antihemophilic Agent; Blood Product Derivative

**Use**

Control bleeding in patients with factor IX deficiency (hemophilia B or Christmas disease) *NOTE: Factor IX concentrate containing ONLY factor IX is also available and preferable for this indication.*

Prevention/control of bleeding in hemophilia A patients with inhibitors to factor VIII

Prevention/control of bleeding in patients with factor VII deficiency

Emergency correction of the coagulopathy of warfarin excess in critical situations.

**Effects on Mental Status** May rarely cause sedation

**Effects on Psychiatric Treatment** None reported

**Usual Dosage** Children and Adults: Dosage is expressed in units of factor IX activity and must be individualized. I.V. only:

**Formula for units required to raise blood level %:**

Total blood volume (mL blood/kg) = 70 mL/kg (adults), 80 mL/kg (children)

Plasma volume = total blood volume (mL) x [1 - Hct (in decimals)]

For example, for a 70 kg adult with a Hct = 40%: Plasma volume = [70 kg x 70 mL/kg] x [1 - 0.4] = 2940 mL

To calculate number of units needed to increase level to desired range (highly individualized and dependent on patient's condition): Number of units = desired level increase [desired level - actual level] x plasma volume (in mL)

For example, for a 100% level in the above patient who has an actual level of 20%: Number of units needed = [1 (for a 100% level) - 0.2] x 2940 mL = 2352 units

As a general rule, the level of factor IX required for treatment of different conditions is listed below:

Minor spontaneous hemorrhage, prophylaxis:

Desired levels of factor IX for hemostasis: 15% to 25%

Initial loading dose to achieve desired level: <20-30 units/kg

Frequency of dosing: Once; repeated in 24 hours if necessary

Duration of treatment: Once; repeated if necessary

Major trauma or surgery:

Desired levels of factor IX for hemostasis: 25% to 50%

Initial loading dose to achieve desired level: <75 units/kg

Frequency of dosing: Every 18-30 hours, depending on half-life and measured factor IX levels

Duration of treatment: Up to 10 days, depending upon nature of insult

(Continued)

## Factor IX Complex (Human) *(Continued)*

**Factor VIII inhibitor patients:** 75 units/kg/dose; may be given every 6-12 hours

**Anticoagulant overdosage:** I.V.: 15 units/kg

**Dosage Forms** Injection:

AlphaNine® SD: Single dose vial

BeneFix™: 250 units, 500 units, 1000 units

Konÿne® 80: 20 mL, 40 mL

Hemonyne®: 20 mL, 40 mL

Profilnine® SD: Single dose vial

Proplex® T: 30 mL vial

## Factor IX, Purified (Human)

(FAK ter nyne, PURE eh fide HYU man)

**U.S. Brand Names** Mononine®

**Pharmacologic Category** Antihemophilic Agent; Blood Product Derivative

**Use**

Control bleeding in patients with factor IX deficiency (hemophilia B or Christmas disease)

Mononine® contains **nondetectable levels of factors II, VII, and X** (<0.0025 units per factor IX unit using standard coagulation assays) and is, therefore, **NOT INDICATED** for replacement therapy of any of these clotting factors

Mononine® is also **NOT INDICATED** in the treatment or reversal of coumarin-induced anticoagulation or in a hemorrhagic state caused by hepatitis-induced lack of production of liver dependent coagulation factors.

**Effects on Mental Status** May rarely cause sedation

**Effects on Psychiatric Treatment** None reported

**Usual Dosage** Children and Adults: Dosage is expressed in units of factor IX activity and must be individualized. I.V. only:

**Formula for units required to raise blood level %:**

Number of Factor IX Units Required = body weight (in kg) x desired Factor IX level increase (% normal) x 1 unit/kg

For example, for a 100% level a patient who has an actual level of 20%: Number of factor IX units needed = 70 kg x 80% x 1 Unit/kg = 5,600 Units

As a general rule, the level of factor IX required for treatment of different conditions is listed below:

Minor spontaneous hemorrhage, prophylaxis:

Desired levels of factor IX for hemostasis: 15% to 25%

Initial loading dose to achieve desired level: <20-30 units/kg

Frequency of dosing: Once; repeated in 24 hours if necessary

Duration of treatment: Once; repeated if necessary

Major trauma or surgery:

Desired levels of factor IX for hemostasis: 25% to 50%

Initial loading dose to achieve desired level: <75 units/kg

Frequency of dosing: Every 18-30 hours, depending on half-life and measured factor IX levels

Duration of treatment: Up to 10 days, depending upon nature of insult

**Dosage Forms** Factor IX units listed per vial and per lot to lot variation of factor IX

Injection: 250 units, 500 units, 1000 units

## Factor VIIa, Recombinant

(FAK ter SE ven aye, ree KOM be nant)

**U.S. Brand Names** Novo-Seven®

**Pharmacologic Category** Antihemophilic Agent; Blood Product Derivative

**Use** Treatment of bleeding episodes in patients with hemophilia A or B when inhibitors to Factor VIII or Factor IX are present

**Effects on Mental Status** None reported

**Effects on Psychiatric Treatment** None reported

**Usual Dosage** Children and Adults: I.V. administration only: 90 mcg/kg every 2 hours until hemostasis is achieved or until the treatment is judged ineffective. The dose and interval may be adjusted based upon the severity of bleeding and the degree of hemostasis achieved. The duration of therapy following hemostasis has not been fully established; for patients experiencing severe bleeds, dosing should be continued at 3- to 6-hour intervals after hemostasis has been achieved and the duration of dosing should be minimized.

In clinical trials, dosages have ranged from 35-120 mcg/kg and a decision on the final therapeutic dosages was reached within 8 hours in the majority of patients

**Dosage Forms** Powder for injection: 1.2 mg, 2.4 mg, 4.8 mg

♦ **Factrel®** *see* Gonadorelin *on page 254*

## Famciclovir (fam SYE kloe veer)

**U.S. Brand Names** Famvir™

**Pharmacologic Category** Antiviral Agent

**Use** Management of acute herpes zoster (shingles) and recurrent episodes of genital herpes; treatment of recurrent herpes simplex in immunocompetent patients

**Effects on Mental Status** May cause sedation

**Effects on Psychiatric Treatment** None reported

**Pregnancy Risk Factor** B

**Contraindications** Hypersensitivity to famciclovir

**Warnings/Precautions** Has not been studied in immunocompromised patients or patients with ophthalmic or disseminated zoster; dosage adjustment is required in patients with renal insufficiency ($Cl_{cr}$ <60 mL/minute) and in patients with noncompensated hepatic disease; safety and efficacy have not been established in children <18 years of age; animal studies indicated increases in incidence of carcinomas, mutagenic changes, and decreases in fertility with extremely large doses

**Adverse Reactions**

1% to 10%:

Central nervous system: Fatigue (4% to 6%), fever (1% to 3%), dizziness (3% to 5%), somnolence (1% to 2%), headache

Dermatologic: Pruritus (1% to 4%)

Gastrointestinal: Diarrhea (4% to 8%), vomiting (1% to 5%), constipation (1% to 5%), anorexia (1% to 3%), abdominal pain (1% to 4%), nausea

Neuromuscular & skeletal: Paresthesia (1% to 3%)

Respiratory: Sinusitis/pharyngitis (2%)

<1%: Arthralgia, rigors, upper respiratory infection

**Overdosage/Toxicology** Treatment: Supportive and symptomatic care is recommended; hemodialysis may enhance elimination

**Drug Interactions** Increased effect/toxicity:

Cimetidine: Penciclovir AUC may increase due to impaired metabolism

Digoxin: $C_{max}$ of digoxin increases by ~19%

Probenecid: Penciclovir serum levels significantly increase

Theophylline: Penciclovir AUC/$C_{max}$ may increase and renal clearance decrease, although not clinically significant

**Usual Dosage** Adults: Oral:

Acute herpes zoster: 500 mg every 8 hours for 7 days

Recurrent herpes simplex in immunocompetent patients: 125 mg twice daily for 5 days

Genital herpes:

Recurrent episodes: 125 mg twice daily for 5 days

Prophylaxis: 250 mg twice daily

**Dosing interval in renal impairment:**

$Cl_{cr}$ 40-59 mL/minute: Administer 500 mg every 12 hours

$Cl_{cr}$ 20-39 mL/minute: Administer 500 mg every 24 hours

$Cl_{cr}$ <20 mL/minute: Unknown

**Patient Information** Take for prescribed length of time, even if condition improves. Do not discontinue without consulting prescriber. This is not a cure for genital herpes. You may experience mild GI disturbances (eg, nausea, vomiting, constipation, or diarrhea), fatigue, headaches, or muscle aches and pains. If these are severe, contact prescriber.

**Dosage Forms** Tablet: 125 mg, 250 mg, 500 mg

## Famotidine (fa MOE ti deen)

**U.S. Brand Names** Pepcid®; Pepcid® AC Acid Controller [OTC]; Pepcid RPD™

**Canadian Brand Names** Apo®-Famotidine; Novo-Famotidine; Nu-Famotidine

**Pharmacologic Category** Histamine $H_2$ Antagonist

**Use**

Pepcid®: Therapy and treatment of duodenal ulcer, gastric ulcer, control gastric pH in critically ill patients, symptomatic relief in gastritis, gastroesophageal reflux, active benign ulcer, and pathological hypersecretory conditions

Pepcid® AC Acid Controller: Relieves heartburn, acid indigestion and sour stomach

**Effects on Mental Status** May cause dizziness or drowsiness; may rarely cause insomnia

**Effects on Psychiatric Treatment** May cause agranulocytosis; use caution with clozapine and carbamazepine

**Pregnancy Risk Factor** B

**Contraindications** Hypersensitivity to famotidine or other $H_2$-antagonists

**Warnings/Precautions** Modify dose in patients with renal impairment

**Adverse Reactions**

1% to 10%:

Central nervous system: Dizziness, headache

Gastrointestinal: Constipation, diarrhea

<1%: Abdominal discomfort, acne, agranulocytosis, allergic reaction, anorexia, belching, bradycardia, bronchospasm, drowsiness, dry skin, fatigue, fever, flatulence, hypertension, increased AST/ALT, increased BUN/creatinine, insomnia, neutropenia, palpitations, paresthesia,

proteinuria, pruritus, seizures, tachycardia, thrombocytopenia, urticaria, weakness

**Overdosage/Toxicology**

Signs and symptoms: Hypotension, tachycardia, vomiting, drowsiness

Treatment: Primarily symptomatic and supportive

**Drug Interactions** Decreased effect of ketoconazole, itraconazole

**Usual Dosage**

Children: Oral, I.V.: Doses of 1-2 mg/kg/day have been used; maximum dose: 40 mg

Adults:

Oral:

Duodenal ulcer, gastric ulcer: 40 mg/day at bedtime for 4-8 weeks

Hypersecretory conditions: Initial: 20 mg every 6 hours, may increase up to 160 mg every 6 hours

GERD: 20 mg twice daily for 6 weeks

I.V.: 20 mg every 12 hours

**Dosing adjustment in renal impairment:**

$Cl_{cr}$ <10 mL/minute: Administer every 24 hours or 50% of dose

**Patient Information** Take as directed, for full dose as prescribed, even if feeling better. Avoid alcohol and smoking (smoking decreases effectiveness of medication). You may experience some drowsiness or dizziness; use caution when driving or engaging in tasks that require alertness until response to drug is known. Increased exercise, increased dietary fluids, fruits, or fiber may reduce constipation; yogurt or buttermilk may help relieve diarrhea. Report acute headache, unresolved constipation or diarrhea, palpitations, black tarry stools, abdominal pain, rash, worsening of condition being treated, or recurrence of symptoms after therapy is completed.

**Dosage Forms**

Infusion, premixed in NS: 20 mg (50 mL)

Injection: 10 mg/mL (2 mL, 4 mL)

Powder for oral suspension (cherry-banana-mint flavor): 40 mg/5 mL (50 mL)

Tablet, film coated: 20 mg, 40 mg

Tablet, disintegrating: 20 mg, 40 mg

Pepcid® AC Acid Controller: 10 mg

- **Famvir™** *see* Famciclovir *on page 218*
- **Fansidar®** *see* Sulfadoxine and Pyrimethamine *on page 524*
- **Fareston®** *see* Toremifene *on page 557*
- **Fastin®** *see* Phentermine *on page 438*
- **5-FC** *see* Flucytosine *on page 228*
- **Featherfew** *see* Feverfew *on page 224*
- **Featherfoil** *see* Feverfew *on page 224*
- **Fedahist® Expectorant [OTC]** *see* Guaifenesin and Pseudoephedrine *on page 257*
- **Fedahist® Expectorant Pediatric [OTC]** *see* Guaifenesin and Pseudoephedrine *on page 257*
- **Fedahist® Tablet [OTC]** *see* Chlorpheniramine and Pseudoephedrine *on page 114*
- **Federal OBRA Regulations Recommended Maximum Doses** *see page 756*
- **Feen-A-Mint® [OTC]** *see* Bisacodyl *on page 69*
- **Feiba VH Immuno®** *see* Anti-inhibitor Coagulant Complex *on page 46*

## Felbamate (FEL ba mate)

**U.S. Brand Names** Felbatol®

**Pharmacologic Category** Anticonvulsant, Miscellaneous

**Use** Not as a first-line antiepileptic treatment; only in those patients who respond inadequately to alternative treatments and whose epilepsy is so severe that a substantial risk of aplastic anemia and/or liver failure is deemed acceptable in light of the benefits conferred by its use. Patient must be fully advised of risk and has signed written informed consent. Felbamate can be used as either monotherapy or adjunctive therapy in the treatment of partial seizures, with and without generalization, in adults with epilepsy, and as an adjunctive therapy in the treatment of partial and generalized seizures associated with Lennox-Gastaut syndrome in children.

**Effects on Mental Status** Anxiety and dizziness are common; may cause drowsiness, insomnia, or depression

**Effects on Psychiatric Treatment** Carbamazepine may decrease effects of felbamate; may increase effects of valproic acid

**Contraindications** Hypersensitivity to felbamate or its ingredients; use with caution in those patients who have demonstrated hypersensitivity reactions to other carbamates

**Warnings/Precautions** Use with caution in patients allergic to other carbamates (eg, meprobamate); antiepileptic drugs should not be suddenly discontinued because of the possibility of increasing seizure frequency; **reported 10 cases of aplastic anemia in the U.S. after 2½ to 6 months of therapy**; Carter Wallace and the FDA recommended the use of this agent be suspended unless withdrawal of the product would place a patient at greater risk as compared to the frequently fatal form of anemia

**Adverse Reactions**

>10%:

Central nervous system: Somnolence, headache, fatigue, dizziness

Gastrointestinal: Nausea, anorexia, vomiting, constipation

1% to 10%:

Cardiovascular: Chest pain, palpitations, tachycardia

Central nervous system: Depression or behavior changes, nervousness, anxiety, ataxia, stupor, malaise, agitation, psychological disturbances, aggressive reaction

Dermatologic: Skin rash, acne, pruritus

Gastrointestinal: Xerostomia, diarrhea, abdominal pain, weight gain, taste perversion

Neuromuscular & skeletal: Tremor, abnormal gait, paresthesia, myalgia

Ocular: Diplopia, abnormal vision

Respiratory: Sinusitis, pharyngitis

Miscellaneous: ALT increase

<1%: Euphoria, hallucinations, leukocytosis, leukopenia, lymphadenopathy, migraine, suicide attempts, thrombocytopenia, urticaria

**Overdosage/Toxicology**

Signs and symptoms: No serious adverse reactions have been reported

Treatment: Symptomatic

**Drug Interactions** CYP2C19 enzyme inhibitor

Carbamazepine: Felbamate may decrease carbamazepine levels and increase levels of the active metabolite of carbamazepine (10,11-epoxide) resulting in carbamazepine toxicity; monitor for signs of carbamazepine toxicity (dizziness, ataxia, nystagmus, drowsiness)

Enzyme inducers: May decrease serum felbamate concentrations; includes carbamazepine, phenytoin, and rifampin

Gabapentin: May increase serum concentrations of felbamate; monitor for increased effect

Oral contraceptives: Serum levels have been noted to decrease modestly in some patients receiving felbamate; clinical significance in terms of contraceptive failure has not been established

Phenytoin: Felbamate may increase serum concentrations, consider decreasing phenytoin dosage by 25%

Phenobarbital: Felbamate may increase serum concentrations, consider decreasing phenobarbital dosage by 25%

Valproic acid: Felbamate may increase serum concentrations; a decrease in valproic acid dosage may be necessary; monitor for valproic acid toxicity (confusion, irritability, restlessness)

**Stability** Store medication in tightly closed container at room temperature away from excessive heat

**Mechanism of Action** Mechanism of action is unknown but has properties in common with other marketed anticonvulsants; has weak inhibitory effects on GABA-receptor binding, benzodiazepine receptor binding, and is devoid of activity at the MK-801 receptor binding site of the NMDA receptor-ionophore complex.

**Pharmacodynamics/kinetics**

Absorption: Oral: Rapidly and almost completely absorbed after oral administration, food has no effect upon the tablet's absorption

Peak serum concentrations: Within 3 hours

$V_d$: 0.7-1 L/kg

Protein binding: 22% to 25%

Half-life: 20-23 hours average

Elimination: Cleared renally 40% to 50% as unchanged drug and 40% as inactive metabolites in the urine

**Usual Dosage**

Monotherapy: Children >14 years and Adults:

Initial: 1200 mg/day in divided doses 3 or 4 times/day; titrate previously untreated patients under close clinical supervision, increasing the dosage in 600 mg increments every 2 weeks to 2400 mg/day based on clinical response and thereafter to 3600 mg/day in clinically indicated

Conversion to monotherapy: Initiate at 1200 mg/day in divided doses 3 or 4 times/day, reduce the dosage of the concomitant anticonvulsant(s) by 20% to 33% at the initiation of felbamate therapy; at week 2, increase the felbamate dosage to 2400 mg/day while reducing the dosage of the other anticonvulsant(s) up to an additional 33% of their original dosage; at week 3, increase the felbamate dosage up to 3600 mg/day and continue to reduce the dosage of the other anticonvulsant(s) as clinically indicated

Adjunctive therapy: Children with Lennox-Gastaut and ages 2-14 years:

Week 1:

Felbamate: 15 mg/kg/day divided 3-4 times/day

Concomitant anticonvulsant(s): Reduce original dosage by 20% to 30%

Week 2:

Felbamate: 30 mg/kg/day divided 3-4 times/day

Concomitant anticonvulsant(s): Reduce original dosage up to an additional 33%

Week 3:

Felbamate: 45 mg//kg/day divided 3-4 times/day

Concomitant anticonvulsant(s): Reduce dosage as clinically indicated

(Continued)

## Felbamate *(Continued)*

Adjunctive therapy: Children >14 years and Adults:
- Week 1:
  - Felbamate: 1200 mg/day initial dose
  - Concomitant anticonvulsant(s): Reduce original dosage by 20% to 33%
- Week 2:
  - Felbamate: 2400 mg/day (Therapeutic range)
  - Concomitant anticonvulsant(s): Reduce original dosage by up to an additional 33%
- Week 3:
  - Felbamate: 3600 mg/day (Therapeutic range)
  - Concomitant anticonvulsant(s): Reduce original dosage as clinically indicated

**Monitoring Parameters** Monitor serum levels of concomitant anticonvulsant therapy

**Reference Range** Not necessary to routinely monitor serum drug levels, since dose should be titrated to clinical response

**Test Interactions** Blood urea nitrogen is slightly lower (1.25 mg/dL); may cause slightly elevated serum cholesterol level (about 7 mg/dL) in patients receiving about 2.6 g/day

**Patient Information** Shake oral suspension well before using

**Dosage Forms**
Suspension, oral: 600 mg/5 mL (240 mL, 960 mL)
Tablet: 400 mg, 600 mg

♦ **Felbatol®** *see* Felbamate *on page 219*

♦ **Feldene®** *see* Piroxicam *on page 449*

## Felodipine (fe LOE di peen)

**Related Information**
Calcium Channel Blocking Agents Comparison Chart *on page 710*

**U.S. Brand Names** Plendil®

**Canadian Brand Names** Renedil®

**Pharmacologic Category** Calcium Channel Blocker

**Use** Treatment of hypertension, congestive heart failure

**Effects on Mental Status** May cause dizziness; rarely may cause nervousness, insomnia, or depression

**Effects on Psychiatric Treatment** Carbamazepine may decrease felodipine effect

**Pregnancy Risk Factor** C

**Contraindications** Hypersensitivity to felodipine, any component, or other calcium channel blocker

**Warnings/Precautions** Watch for hypotension and syncope (can rarely occur). Reflex tachycardia may occur. Use caution in patients with heart failure particularly with concurrent beta-blocker use. Elderly patients and patients with hepatic impairment should start off with a lower dose. Peripheral edema is the most common side effect (occurs within 2-3 weeks of starting therapy). Safety and efficacy in children have not been established. Dosage titration should occur after 14 days on a given dose.

**Adverse Reactions**
- >10%:
  - Cardiovascular: Peripheral edema (22%)
  - Central nervous system: Headache (18%)
- 1% to 10%:
  - Cardiovascular: Chest pain, palpitations (2%), flushing (6%)
  - Central nervous system: Dizziness/lightheadedness (6%)
  - Dermatologic: Rash (1% to 2%)
  - Gastrointestinal: Constipation/diarrhea (1% to 2%), nausea (2%), abdominal pain (1% to 2%)
  - Neuromuscular & skeletal: Weakness (5%), paresthesia (2.5%)
  - Respiratory: Cough (3%), upper respiratory infection (5.5%)
- <1%: Anemia, angina, arrhythmia, A-V block, blurred vision, epistaxis, flatulence, gingival hyperplasia, hypotension, insomnia, marked elevations in LFTs, mental depression, micturition disorder, myocardial infarction, nervousness, pruritus, rhinitis, sexual disorder, shortness of breath, somnolence, syncope, tachycardia, vomiting, xerostomia

**Overdosage/Toxicology**
Signs and symptoms:
The primary cardiac symptoms of calcium blocker overdose includes hypotension and bradycardia. The hypotension is caused by peripheral vasodilation, myocardial depression, and bradycardia. Bradycardia results from sinus bradycardia, second- or third-degree atrioventricular block, or sinus arrest with junctional rhythm. Intraventricular conduction is usually not affected so QRS duration is normal (verapamil does prolong the P-R interval and bepridil prolongs the Q-T and may cause ventricular arrhythmias, including torsade de pointes).
The noncardiac symptoms include confusion, stupor, nausea, vomiting, metabolic acidosis and hyperglycemia. Following initial gastric decontamination, if possible, repeated calcium administration may promptly reverse the depressed cardiac contractility (but not sinus node depression or peripheral vasodilation); glucagon, epinephrine, and inamrinone may treat refractory hypotension; glucagon and epinephrine also increase the heart rate (outside the U.S., 4-aminopyridine may be available as an antidote); dialysis and hemoperfusion are not effective in enhancing elimination although repeat-dose activated charcoal may serve as an adjunct with sustained-release preparations.

**Drug Interactions** CYP3A3/4 enzyme substrate
- Azole antifungals (ketoconazole, itraconazole) may inhibit calcium channel blocker's metabolism; avoid this combination. Try an antifungal like terbinafine (if appropriate) or monitor closely for altered effect of the calcium channel blocker.
- Beta-blockers may have increased pharmacokinetic or pharmacodynamic interactions with felodipine
- Calcium may reduce the calcium channel blocker's effects, particularly hypotension
- Carbamazepine significantly reduces felodipine's bioavailability; avoid this combination
- Cimetidine may inhibit felodipine metabolism (AUC increased 50%); use caution
- Cyclosporine increases felodipine's serum concentration; avoid the combination or reduce dose of felodipine and monitor blood pressure
- Ethanol increases felodipine's absorption; watch for a greater hypotensive effect
- Erythromycin decreases felodipine's metabolism; monitor blood pressure
- Grapefruit juice increases the bioavailability of felodipine; monitor for altered felodipine effects
- Nafcillin decreases plasma concentration of felodipine; avoid this combination
- Rifampin increases the metabolism of the calcium channel blocker; adjust the dose of the calcium channel blocker to maintain efficacy

**Usual Dosage**
Adults: Oral: 2.5-10 mg once daily; usual initial dose: 5 mg; increase by 5 mg at 2-week intervals, as needed; maximum: 10 mg
Elderly: Begin with 2.5 mg/day
**Dosing adjustment/comments in hepatic impairment:** Begin with 2.5 mg/day; do not use doses >10 mg/day

**Dietary Considerations** Should be taken without food; the bioavailability of felodipine is influenced by the presence of food and has been shown to increase more than twofold when taken with concentrated grapefruit juice

**Patient Information** Take without food. Take as prescribed; do not stop abruptly without consulting prescriber immediately. Swallow whole; do not crush or chew. You may experience headache (if unrelieved, consult prescriber), nausea or vomiting (frequent small meals may help), constipation (increased dietary bulk and fluids may help), depression (should resolve when drug is discontinued). May cause dizziness or drowsiness; use caution when driving or engaging in tasks that require alertness until response to drug is known. Report any chest pain or swelling of hands or feet, respiratory distress, sudden weight gain, or unresolved constipation.

**Dosage Forms** Tablet, extended release: 2.5 mg, 5 mg, 10 mg

♦ **Femara™** *see* Letrozole *on page 309*

♦ **Femcet®** *see* Butalbital Compound and Acetaminophen *on page 80*

♦ **Femguard®** *see* Sulfabenzamide, Sulfacetamide, and Sulfathiazole *on page 522*

♦ **Femhrt™** *see* Ethinyl Estradiol and Norethindrone *on page 212*

♦ **Femiron® [OTC]** *see* Ferrous Fumarate *on page 223*

♦ **Femizole-7® [OTC]** *see* Clotrimazole *on page 135*

♦ **Femizol-M® [OTC]** *see* Miconazole *on page 364*

♦ **Femstat®** *see* Butoconazole *on page 81*

♦ **Fenesin™** *see* Guaifenesin *on page 256*

♦ **Fenesin™ DM** *see* Guaifenesin and Dextromethorphan *on page 257*

## Fenofibrate (fen oh FYE brate)

**U.S. Brand Names** TriCor™

**Canadian Brand Names** Apo®-Fenofibrate

**Synonyms** Procetofene; Proctofene

**Pharmacologic Category** Antilipemic Agent (Fibric Acid)

**Use** Adjunct to dietary therapy for the treatment of adults with very high elevations of serum triglyceride levels (types IV and V hyperlipidemia) who are at risk of pancreatitis and who do not respond adequately to a determined dietary effort; its efficacy can be enhanced by combination with other hypolipidemic agents that have a different mechanism of action; safety and efficacy may be greater than that of clofibrate; adjunct to dietary therapy for the reduction of low density lipoprotein cholesterol (LDL-C), total cholesterol (total-C), triglycerides, and apolipoprotein B (apo B) in adult patients with primary hypercholesterolemia or mixed dyslipidemia (Fredrickson types IIa and IIb)

**Effects on Mental Status** May rarely cause drowsiness or insomnia

**Effects on Psychiatric Treatment** None reported

**Pregnancy Risk Factor** C

**Contraindications** Hypersensitivity to fenofibrate or any component; hepatic or severe renal dysfunction including primary biliary cirrhosis and unexplained persistent liver function abnormalities; pre-existing gallbladder disease

**Warnings/Precautions** Hepatic transaminases can significantly elevate (dose-related). Regular monitoring of liver function tests is required. May cause cholelithiasis. Adjustments in warfarin therapy may be required with concurrent use. Use caution when combining fenofibrate with HMG-CoA reductase inhibitors (may lead to myopathy, rhabdomyolysis). The effect of CAD morbidity and mortality has not been established. Therapy should be withdrawn if an adequate response is not obtained after 2 months of therapy at the maximal daily dose (201 mg). Rare hypersensitivity reactions may occur. Dose adjustment is required for renal impairment and elderly patients. Safety and efficacy in children have not been established.

**Adverse Reactions**

>10%: Gastrointestinal: Nausea, gastric discomfort

1% to 10%:

Dermatologic: Skin reactions

Gastrointestinal: Constipation, diarrhea

<1%: Arthralgia, dizziness, fatigue, headache, insomnia, myalgia, transient increases in LFTs

**Overdosage/Toxicology**

Signs and symptoms: Nausea, vomiting, diarrhea, GI distress

Treatment: Following GI decontamination, treatment is supportive

**Drug Interactions**

Chlorpropamide: May increase risk of hypoglycemia.

Furosemide: Blood levels of furosemide and fibric acid derivatives (ie, clofibrate and fenofibrate) may be increased during concurrent dosing (particularly in hypoalbuminemia). Limited documentation; monitor for increased effect/toxicity.

HMG-CoA reductase inhibitors (atorvastatin, cerivastatin, fluvastatin, lovastatin, pravastatin, simvastatin) may increase the risk of myopathy and rhabdomyolysis. The manufacturer warns against concomitant use. However, combination therapy with statins has been used in some patients with resistant hyperlipidemias (with great caution).

Rifampin: Decreased fenofibrate blood levels

Warfarin: Increased hypoprothrombinemic response; monitor INRs closely when fenofibrate is initiated or discontinued

**Usual Dosage** Oral:

Adults:

Hypertriglyceridemia: Initial: 67 mg/day with meals, up to 200 mg/day

Hypercholesterolemia or mixed hyperlipidemia: Initial: 200 mg/day with meals

Elderly: Initial: 67 mg/day

**Dosage adjustment in renal impairment:** Decrease dose or increase dosing interval for patients with renal failure: Initial: 67 mg/day

**Patient Information** Take with food. Do not change dosage without consulting prescriber. Maintain diet and exercise program as prescribed. You may experience mild GI disturbances (eg, gas, diarrhea, constipation, nausea); inform prescriber if these are severe. Report skin rash or irritation, insomnia, unusual muscle pain or tremors, or persistent dizziness.

**Dosage Forms** Capsule: 67 mg

## Fenoldopam (fe NOL doe pam)

**U.S. Brand Names** Corlopam®

**Pharmacologic Category** Dopamine Agonist

**Use** Treatment of severe hypertension particularly I.V. and in patients with renal compromise; potential use for congestive heart failure

**Effects on Mental Status** May cause dizziness

**Effects on Psychiatric Treatment** Causes hypotension; caution with low potency antipsychotics and TCAs

**Usual Dosage** I.V.: Severe hypertension: Initial: 0.1 mcg/kg/minute; may be increased in increments of 0.05-0.2 mcg/kg/minute until target blood pressure is achieved; average rate: 0.25-0.5 mcg/kg/minute; usual length of treatment is 1-6 hours with tapering of 12% every 15-30 minutes

**Dosing adjustment in renal impairment:** None required

**Dosing adjustment in hepatic impairment:** None published

**Dosage Forms** Injection: 10 mg/mL (5 mL)

## Fenoprofen (fen oh PROE fen)

**Related Information**

Nonsteroidal Anti-inflammatory Agents Comparison Chart *on page 722*

**U.S. Brand Names** Nalfon®

**Pharmacologic Category** Nonsteroidal Anti-Inflammatory Agent (NSAID)

**Use** Symptomatic treatment of acute and chronic rheumatoid arthritis and osteoarthritis; relief of mild to moderate pain

**Effects on Mental Status** Dizziness is common; may cause nervousness; rarely may cause insomnia, confusion, depression, or hallucinations

**Effects on Psychiatric Treatment** May rarely cause may agranulocytosis; use caution with clozapine and carbamazepine; may decrease the clearance of lithium resulting in elevated serum levels and potential toxicity; monitor serum lithium levels; use acetaminophen, if possible, for pain

**Pregnancy Risk Factor** B (D if used in the 3rd trimester or near delivery)

**Contraindications** Known hypersensitivity to fenoprofen or other NSAIDs

**Warnings/Precautions** Use with caution in patients with congestive heart failure, dehydration, hypertension, decreased renal or hepatic function, history of GI disease, or those receiving anticoagulants

**Adverse Reactions**

>10%:

Central nervous system: Dizziness

Dermatologic: Rash

Gastrointestinal: Abdominal cramps, heartburn, indigestion, nausea

1% to 10%:

Central nervous system: Headache, nervousness

Dermatologic: Itching

Endocrine & metabolic: Fluid retention

Gastrointestinal: Vomiting

Otic: Tinnitus

<1%: Acute renal failure, agranulocytosis, allergic rhinitis, anemia, angioedema, arrhythmias, aseptic meningitis, bone marrow suppression, blurred vision, confusion, congestive heart failure, conjunctivitis, cystitis, decreased hearing, drowsiness, dry eyes, epistaxis, erythema multiforme, gastritis, GI ulceration, hallucinations, hemolytic anemia, hepatitis, hot flashes, hypertension, insomnia, leukopenia, mental depression, peripheral neuropathy, polydipsia, polyuria, shortness of breath, Stevens-Johnson syndrome, tachycardia, thrombocytopenia, toxic amblyopia, toxic epidermal necrolysis, urticaria

**Overdosage/Toxicology**

Signs and symptoms: Acute renal failure, vomiting, drowsiness, leukocytosis

Treatment: Management of a nonsteroidal anti-inflammatory drug (NSAID) intoxication is primarily supportive and symptomatic. Fluid therapy is commonly effective in managing the hypotension that may occur following an acute NSAID overdose, except when this is due to an acute blood loss.

**Drug Interactions**

ACE inhibitors: Effects may be reduced by NSAIDs; use lowest possible dose for shortest duration possible; monitor

Cholestyramine and colestipol: Absorption may be reduced by concurrent administration

Corticosteroids: May increase the risk of GI ulceration; use caution

Cyclosporine: Nephrotoxicity may be increased with concurrent NSAID use; monitor

Hydralazine: Antihypertensive effect may be decreased; avoid concurrent use

Lithium: Serum levels can be increased; avoid concurrent use if possible or monitor lithium levels and adjust dose. When NSAID is stopped, lithium may need adjustment again.

Loop diuretics: Therapeutic effects may be reduced by NSAIDs; avoid

Methotrexate: Toxicity may be increased by concurrent NSAID use; risk is limited in low-dose methotrexate regimens (such as for rheumatoid arthritis); prolonged leucovorin rescue may be required at antineoplastic doses; monitor

Thiazide diuretics: Antihypertensive effects are decreased; avoid concurrent use

Warfarin: INRs may be increased by some NSAIDs. This may depend, in part, on dose and duration; monitor INR closely. Use the lowest dose of NSAIDs possible and for the briefest duration.

**Usual Dosage** Adults: Oral:

Rheumatoid arthritis: 300-600 mg 3-4 times/day up to 3.2 g/day

Mild to moderate pain: 200 mg every 4-6 hours as needed

**Patient Information** Take this medication exactly as directed; do not increase dose without consulting prescriber. Do not crush tablets or break capsules. Take with food or milk to reduce GI distress. Maintain adequate fluid intake (2-3 L/day of fluids unless instructed to restrict fluid intake). Do not use alcohol, aspirin, or aspirin-containing medication, and all other anti-inflammatory medications without consulting prescriber. You may experience drowsiness, dizziness, nervousness, or headache (use caution when driving or engaging in tasks requiring alertness until response to drug is known); anorexia, nausea, vomiting, or heartburn (frequent small meals, frequent mouth care, sucking lozenges, or chewing gum may help); fluid retention (weigh yourself weekly and report unusual (3-5 lb/week) weight gain). GI bleeding, ulceration, or perforation can occur with or without pain; discontinue medication and contact prescriber if persistent abdominal pain or cramping, or blood in stool occurs. Report breathlessness, difficulty breathing, or unusual cough; chest pain, rapid heartbeat, palpitations; unusual bruising/bleeding; blood in urine, stool, mouth, or vomitus; swollen extremities; skin rash or itching; acute fatigue; or changes in hearing or ringing in ears.

**Dosage Forms**

Capsule, as calcium: 200 mg, 300 mg

Tablet, as calcium: 600 mg

## Fentanyl (FEN ta nil)

**Related Information**

Narcotic Agonists Comparison Chart *on page 720*

(Continued)

## Fentanyl *(Continued)*

**U.S. Brand Names** Actiq® Oral Transmucosal; Duragesic® Transdermal; Fentanyl Oralet®; Sublimaze® Injection

**Pharmacologic Category** Analgesic, Narcotic; General Anesthetic

**Use** Sedation, relief of pain, preoperative medication, adjunct to general or regional anesthesia, management of chronic pain (transdermal product)

**Effects on Mental Status** Drowsiness, sedation, and depression are common; may rarely cause paradoxical CNS excitement or delirium

**Effects on Psychiatric Treatment** Concurrent use with low potency antipsychotics and TCAs may produce additive hypotension

**Restrictions** C-II

**Pregnancy Risk Factor** B (D if used for prolonged periods or in high doses at term)

**Contraindications** Hypersensitivity to fentanyl or any component; increased intracranial pressure; severe respiratory depression; severe liver or renal insufficiency

Transmucosal is contraindicated in unmonitored settings where a risk of unrecognized hypoventilation exists or in treating acute or chronic pain

**Warnings/Precautions** Fentanyl shares the toxic potentials of opiate agonists, and precautions of opiate agonist therapy should be observed; use with caution in patients with bradycardia; rapid I.V. infusion may result in skeletal muscle and chest wall rigidity → impaired ventilation → respiratory distress → apnea, bronchoconstriction, laryngospasm; inject slowly over 3-5 minutes; nondepolarizing skeletal muscle relaxant may be required. Tolerance of drug dependence may result from extended use.

Transmucosal fentanyl: Fentanyl Oralet® is not indicated for use in unmonitored settings where there is a risk of unrecognized hypoventilation or in treating acute or chronic pain. Patients should be monitored by direct visual observation and by some means of measuring respiratory function such as pulse oximetry until they are recovered. Facilities for the administration of fluids, opioid antagonists, oxygen and resuscitation equipment (including facilities for endotracheal intubation) should be readily available.

Topical patches: Serum fentanyl concentrations may increase approximately one-third for patients with a body temperature of 40°C secondary to a temperature-dependent increase in fentanyl release from the system and increased skin permeability. Patients who experience adverse reactions should be monitored for at least 12 hours after removal of the patch.

The elderly may be particularly susceptible to the CNS depressant and constipating effects of narcotics

**Adverse Reactions**

>10%:
- Cardiovascular: Hypotension, bradycardia
- Central nervous system: CNS depression, drowsiness, sedation
- Gastrointestinal: Nausea, vomiting, constipation
- Respiratory: Respiratory depression

1% to 10%:
- Cardiovascular: Cardiac arrhythmias, orthostatic hypotension
- Central nervous system: Confusion
- Gastrointestinal: Biliary tract spasm
- Ocular: Miosis

<1%: ADH release, bronchospasm, circulatory depression, CNS excitation or delirium, cold/clammy skin, convulsions, dysesthesia, erythema, itching, laryngospasm, paradoxical dizziness, physical and psychological dependence with prolonged use, pruritus, rash, urinary tract spasm, urticaria

**Overdosage/Toxicology**

Signs and symptoms: CNS depression, respiratory depression, miosis

Treatment: Includes support of the patient's airway, establishment of an I.V. line, and administration of naloxone 2 mg I.V. (0.01 mg/kg for children) with repeat administration as necessary up to a total of 10 mg

**Drug Interactions** CYP3A3/4 enzyme substrate

Increased toxicity: CNS depressants, phenothiazines, tricyclic antidepressants may potentiate fentanyl's adverse effects

**Usual Dosage** Doses should be titrated to appropriate effects; wide range of doses, dependent upon desired degree of analgesia/anesthesia

Children 1-12 years:

Sedation for minor procedures/analgesia:

I.M., I.V.: 1-2 mcg/kg/dose; may repeat at 30- to 60-minute intervals. **Note:** Children 18-36 months of age may require 2-3 mcg/kg/dose

Transmucosal (dosage strength is based on patient weight): 5 mcg/kg if child is not fearful; fearful children and some younger children may require doses of 5-15 mcg/kg (which also carries an increased risk of hypoventilation); drug effect begins within 10 minutes, with sedation beginning shortly thereafter

Continuous sedation/analgesia: Initial I.V. bolus: 1-2 mcg/kg then 1 mcg/kg/hour; titrate upward; usual: 1-3 mcg/kg/hour

Pain control: Transdermal: Not recommended

Children >12 years and Adults:

Sedation for minor procedures/analgesia:

I.M., I.V.: 0.5-1 mcg/kg/dose; higher doses are used for major procedures

Transmucosal: 5 mcg/kg, suck on lozenge vigorously approximately 20-40 minutes before the start of procedure, drug effect begins within 10 minutes, with sedation beginning shortly thereafter.

Dosage recommendations for transmucosal fentanyl (Oralet®) based on patient age/weight:
- Children <2 years of age OR <10 kg: CONTRAINDICATED
- 10 kg: 5-10 mcg/kg/dose (100 mcg): 10-15 mcg/kg/dose (100 mcg)
- 15 kg: 5-10 mcg/kg/dose (100 mcg): 10-15 mcg/kg/dose (200 mcg)
- 20 kg: 5-10 mcg/kg/dose (100 or 200 mcg): 10-15 mcg/kg/dose (200 or 300 mcg)
- 25 kg: 5-10 mcg/kg/dose (200 mcg): 10-15 mcg/kg/dose (300 mcg)
- 30 kg: 5-10 mcg/kg/dose (300 mcg): 10-15 mcg/kg/dose (300 or 400 mcg)
- 35 kg: 5-10 mcg/kg/dose (300 mcg): 10-15 mcg/kg/dose (400 mcg)
- ≥40 kg; 5-10 mcg/dose (400 mcg): 10-15 mcg/dose (400 mcg)
- Adult dose: 400 mcg

Preoperative sedation, adjunct to regional anesthesia, postoperative pain: I.M., I.V.: 50-100 mcg/dose

Adjunct to general anesthesia: I.M., I.V.: 2-50 mcg/kg

General anesthesia without additional anesthetic agents: I.V. 50-100 mcg/kg with $O_2$ and skeletal muscle relaxant

Pain control: Transdermal: Initial: 25 mcg/hour system; if currently receiving opiates, convert to fentanyl equivalent and administer equianalgesic dosage titrated to minimize the adverse effects and provide analgesia. To convert patients from oral or parenteral opioids to Duragesic®, the previous 24-hour analgesic requirement should be calculated. This analgesic requirement should be converted to the equianalgesic oral morphine dose.

**Equianalgesic doses of opioid agonists*:**
- Codeine: 130 mg I.M.; 200 mg oral
- Hydromorphone: 1.5 mg I.M.; 7.5 mg oral
- Levorphanol: 2 mg I.M.; 4 mg oral
- Meperidine: 75 mg I.M.
- Methadone: 10 mg I.M.; 20 mg oral
- Morphine: 10 mg I.M.; 60 mg oral
- Oxycodone: 15 mg I.M.; 30 mg oral
- Oxymorphone: 1 mg I.M.; 10 mg rectal

*From *N Engl J Med*, 1985, 313:84-95.

**Corresponding doses of oral/intramuscular morphine and Duragesic®*:**
- 45-134 mg morphine oral/24 hours = 8-22 mg morphine I.M./24 hours = 25 mcg/hour Duragesic®
- 135-224 mg morphine oral/24 hours = 28-37 mg morphine I.M./24 hours = 50 mcg/hour Duragesic®
- 225-314 mg morphine oral/24 hours = 38-52 mg morphine I.M./24 hours = 75 mcg/hour Duragesic®
- 315-404 mg morphine oral/24 hours = 53-67 mg morphine I.M./24 hours = 100 mcg/hour Duragesic®
- 405-494 mg morphine oral/24 hours = 68-82 mg morphine I.M./24 hours = 125 mcg/hour Duragesic®
- 495-584 mg morphine oral/24 hours = 83-97 mg morphine I.M./24 hours = 150 mcg/hour Duragesic®
- 585-674 mg morphine oral/24 hours = 98-112 mg morphine I.M./24 hours = 175 mcg/hour Duragesic®
- 675-764 mg morphine oral/24 hours = 113-127 mg morphine I.M./24 hours = 200 mcg/hour Duragesic®
- 765-854 mg morphine oral/24 hours = 128-142 mg morphine I.M./24 hours = 225 mcg/hour Duragesic®
- 855-944 mg morphine oral/24 hours = 143-157 mg morphine I.M./24 hours = 250 mcg/hour Duragesic®
- 945-1034 mg morphine oral/24 hours = 158-172 mg morphine I.M./24 hours = 275 mcg/hour Duragesic®
- 1035-1124 mg morphine oral/24 hours = 173-187 mg morphine I.M./24 hours = 300 mcg/hour Duragesic®

*Product information, Duragesic® - Janssen Pharmaceuticals, January, 1991.

The dosage should not be titrated more frequently than every 3 days after the initial dose or every 6 days thereafter. The majority of patients are controlled on every 72-hour administration, however, a small number of patients require every 48-hour administration.

Elderly >65 years: Transmucosal: Dose should be reduced to 2.5-5 mcg/kg; elderly have been found to be twice as sensitive as younger patients to the effects of fentanyl

**Dosing adjustment in renal impairment:**
- $Cl_{cr}$ 10-50 mL/minute: Administer at 75% of normal dose
- $Cl_{cr}$ <10 mL/minute: Administer at 50% of normal dose

**Dietary Considerations**

Alcohol: Additive CNS effects, avoid or limit alcohol; watch for sedation

Food: Glucose may cause hyperglycemia; monitor blood glucose concentrations

**Patient Information** While using this medication, do not use alcohol and other prescription or OTC medications (especially sedatives, tranquilizers, antihistamines, or pain medications) without consulting prescriber. Maintain adequate hydration (2-3 L/day of fluids unless instructed to restrict fluid intake). May cause hypotension, dizziness, drowsiness, impaired coordination, or blurred vision (use caution when driving, climbing stairs, or changing position - rising from sitting or lying to standing, or when engaging in tasks requiring alertness until response to drug is known); nausea or vomiting (frequent mouth care, small frequent meals, chewing gum, or sucking lozenges may help); constipation (increased exercise, fluids, or dietary fruit and fiber may help - if constipation remains an unresolved problem, consult prescriber about use of stool softeners). Report acute dizziness, chest pain, slow or rapid heartbeat, acute headache; confusion or changes in mentation; changes in voiding frequency or amount, swelling of extremities, or unusual weight gain; shortness of breath or difficulty breathing; or changes in vision.

**Administration:** Transdermal: Apply to clean, dry skin, immediately after removing from package. Firmly press in place and hold for 20 seconds.

**Nursing Implications**

May cause rebound respiratory depression postoperatively

Patients with increased temperature may have increased fentanyl absorption transdermally, observe for adverse effects, dosage adjustment may be needed

Pharmacologic and adverse effects can be seen after discontinuation of transdermal system, observe patients for at least 12 hours after transdermal product removed; keep transdermal product (both used and unused) out of the reach of children

Do **not** use soap, alcohol, or other solvents to remove transdermal gel if it accidentally touches skin as they may increase transdermal absorption, use copious amounts of water For patients who have received transmucosal product within 6-12 hours, it is recommended that if other narcotics are required, they should be used at starting doses 1/4 to 1/3 those usually recommended.

**Dosage Forms**

Injection, preservative free, as citrate: 0.05 mg/mL (2 mL, 5 mL, 10 mL, 20 mL, 30 mL, 50 mL)

Lozenge, oral transmucosal, as citrate (raspberry flavored) mounted on a plastic radiopaque handle:

Actiq®: 200 mcg, 400 mcg, 600 mcg, 800 mcg, 1200 mcg, 1600 mcg

Fentanyl Oralet®: 100 mcg, 200 mcg, 300 mcg, 400 mcg

Transdermal system: 25 mcg/hour [10 $cm^2$]; 50 mcg/hour [20 $cm^2$]; 75 mcg/hour [30 $cm^2$]; 100 mcg/hour [40 $cm^2$] (all available in 5s)


- **Fentanyl and Droperidol** *see* Droperidol and Fentanyl *on page 188*
- **Fentanyl Oralet®** *see* Fentanyl *on page 221*
- **Feosol® [OTC]** *see* Ferrous Sulfate *on page 223*
- **Feostat® [OTC]** *see* Ferrous Fumarate *on page 223*
- **Ferancee® [OTC]** *see* Ferrous Sulfate and Ascorbic Acid *on page 224*
- **Feratab® [OTC]** *see* Ferrous Sulfate *on page 223*
- **Fergon® [OTC]** *see* Ferrous Gluconate *on page 223*
- **Fer-In-Sol® [OTC]** *see* Ferrous Sulfate *on page 223*
- **Fer-Iron® [OTC]** *see* Ferrous Sulfate *on page 223*
- **Fero-Grad 500® [OTC]** *see* Ferrous Sulfate and Ascorbic Acid *on page 224*
- **Fero-Gradumet® [OTC]** *see* Ferrous Sulfate *on page 223*
- **Ferospace® [OTC]** *see* Ferrous Sulfate *on page 223*
- **Ferralet® [OTC]** *see* Ferrous Gluconate *on page 223*
- **Ferralyn® Lanacaps® [OTC]** *see* Ferrous Sulfate *on page 223*
- **Ferra-TD® [OTC]** *see* Ferrous Sulfate *on page 223*


## Ferric Gluconate (FER ik GLOO koe nate)

**U.S. Brand Names** Ferrlecit®

**Pharmacologic Category** Iron Salt

**Use** Repletion of total body iron content in patients with iron deficiency anemia who are undergoing hemodialysis in conjunction with erythropoietin therapy

**Effects on Mental Status** May cause drowsiness, dizziness, insomnia, agitation

**Effects on Psychiatric Treatment** May cause hypotension; caution with low potency antipsychotics

**Usual Dosage** Adults:

Test dose (recommended): 2 mL diluted in 50 mL 0.9% sodium chloride over 60 minutes

Repletion of iron in hemodialysis patients: I.V.: 125 mg (10 mL) in 100 mL 0.9% sodium chloride over 1 hour during hemodialysis. Most patients will require a cumulative dose of 1 g elemental iron over approximately 8 sequential dialysis treatments to achieve a favorable response.

**Dosage Forms** Injection: 12.5 mg/mL (5 mL ampuls)


- **Ferrlecit®** *see* Ferric Gluconate *on page 223*
- **Ferro-Sequels® [OTC]** *see* Ferrous Fumarate *on page 223*


## Ferrous Fumarate (FER us FYOO ma rate)

**U.S. Brand Names** Femiron® [OTC]; Feostat® [OTC]; Ferro-Sequels® [OTC]; Fumasorb® [OTC]; Fumerin® [OTC]; Hemocyte® [OTC]; Ircon® [OTC]; Nephro-Fer™ [OTC]; Span-FF® [OTC]

**Pharmacologic Category** Iron Salt

**Use** Prevention and treatment of iron deficiency anemias

**Effects on Mental Status** None reported

**Effects on Psychiatric Treatment** Constipation is common; concurrent use with psychotropic agents may increase the risk

**Usual Dosage** Oral **(dose expressed in terms of elemental iron):**

Children:

Severe iron deficiency anemia: 4-6 mg Fe/kg/day in 3 divided doses

Mild to moderate iron deficiency anemia: 3 mg Fe/kg/day in 1-2 divided doses

Prophylaxis: 1-2 mg Fe/kg/day

Adults:

Iron deficiency: 60-100 mg twice daily up to 60 mg 2 times/day

Prophylaxis: 60-100 mg/day

To avoid GI upset, start with a single daily dose and increase by 1 tablet/day each week or as tolerated until desired daily dose is achieved

Elderly: 200 mg 3-4 times/day

**Dosage Forms** Amount of elemental iron is listed in brackets

Capsule, controlled release (Span-FF®): 325 mg [106 mg]

Drops (Feostat®): 45 mg/0.6 mL [15 mg/0.6 mL] (60 mL)

Suspension, oral (Feostat®): 100 mg/5 mL [33 mg/5 mL] (240 mL)

Tablet:

325 mg [106 mg]

Chewable (chocolate flavor) (Feostat®): 100 mg [33 mg]

Femiron®: 63 mg [20 mg]

Fumerin®: 195 mg [64 mg]

Fumasorb®, Ircon®: 200 mg [66 mg]

Hemocyte®: 324 mg [106 mg]

Nephro-Fer™: 350 mg [115 mg]

Timed release (Ferro-Sequels®): Ferrous fumarate 150 mg [50 mg] and docusate sodium 100 mg

## Ferrous Gluconate (FER us GLOO koe nate)

**U.S. Brand Names** Fergon® [OTC]; Ferralet® [OTC]; Simron® [OTC]

**Pharmacologic Category** Iron Salt

**Use** Prevention and treatment of iron deficiency anemias

**Effects on Mental Status** None reported

**Effects on Psychiatric Treatment** Constipation is common; concurrent use with psychotropic agents may increase the risk

**Usual Dosage** Oral **(dose expressed in terms of elemental iron):**

Children:

Severe iron deficiency anemia: 4-6 mg Fe/kg/day in 3 divided doses

Mild to moderate iron deficiency anemia: 3 mg Fe/kg/day in 1-2 divided doses

Prophylaxis: 1-2 mg Fe/kg/day

Adults:

Iron deficiency: 60 mg twice daily up to 60 mg 4 times/day

Prophylaxis: 60 mg/day

**Dosage Forms** Amount of elemental iron is listed in brackets

Capsule, soft gelatin (Simron®): 86 mg [10 mg]

Elixir (Fergon®): 300 mg/5 mL [34 mg/5 mL] with alcohol 7% (480 mL)

Tablet: 300 mg [34 mg]; 325 mg [38 mg]

Fergon®, Ferralet®: 320 mg [37 mg]

Sustained release (Ferralet® Slow Release): 320 mg [37 mg]

## Ferrous Sulfate (FER us SUL fate)

**U.S. Brand Names** Feosol® [OTC]; Feratab® [OTC]; Fer-In-Sol® [OTC]; Fer-Iron® [OTC]; Fero-Gradumet® [OTC]; Ferospace® [OTC]; Ferralyn® Lanacaps® [OTC]; Ferra-TD® [OTC]; Mol-Iron® [OTC]; Slow FE® [OTC]

**Canadian Brand Names** Apo®-Ferrous Sulfate; Ferodan®; PMS-Ferrous Sulfate

**Synonyms** $FeSO_4$

**Pharmacologic Category** Iron Salt

**Use** Prevention and treatment of iron deficiency anemias

**Effects on Mental Status** None reported

**Effects on Psychiatric Treatment** None reported

**Pregnancy Risk Factor** A

**Contraindications** Hemochromatosis, hemolytic anemia; known hypersensitivity to iron salts

**Warnings/Precautions** Administration of iron for >6 months should be avoided except in patients with continued bleeding, menorrhagia, or repeated pregnancies; avoid in patients with peptic ulcer, enteritis, or ulcerative colitis. Anemia in the elderly is often caused by "anemia of chronic disease" or associated with inflammation rather than blood loss. Iron stores are usually normal or increased, with a serum ferritin >50 ng/mL and a decreased total iron binding capacity. Hence, the "anemia of

(Continued)

## Ferrous Sulfate *(Continued)*

chronic disease" is not secondary to iron deficiency but the inability of the reticuloendothelial system to reclaim available iron stores.

**Adverse Reactions**

>10%: Gastrointestinal: GI irritation, epigastric pain, nausea, dark stool, vomiting, stomach cramping, constipation

1% to 10%:

Gastrointestinal: Heartburn, diarrhea

Genitourinary: Discoloration of urine

Miscellaneous: Liquid preparations may temporarily stain the teeth

<1%: Contact irritation

**Overdosage/Toxicology**

Signs and symptoms: Acute GI irritation; erosion of GI mucosa, hepatic and renal impairment, coma, hematemesis, lethargy, acidosis

Treatment: Following treatment for fluid losses, metabolic acidosis, and shock, a severe iron overdose may be treated with deferoxamine. Deferoxamine may be administered I.V. (80 mg/kg over 24 hours) or I.M. (40-90 mg/kg every 8 hours). Usual toxic dose of elemental iron: ≥35 mg/kg.

**Drug Interactions**

Decreased effect: Absorption of oral preparation of iron and tetracyclines are decreased when both of these drugs are given together; concurrent administration of antacids may decrease iron absorption; iron may decrease absorption of penicillamine when given at the same time; response to iron therapy may be delayed in patients receiving chloramphenicol; milk may decrease absorption of iron

Increased effect: Concurrent administration ≥200 mg vitamin C per 30 mg elemental Fe increases absorption of oral iron

**Usual Dosage** Oral:

Children **(dose expressed in terms of elemental iron):**

Severe iron deficiency anemia: 4-6 mg Fe/kg/day in 3 divided doses

Mild to moderate iron deficiency anemia: 3 mg Fe/kg/day in 1-2 divided doses

Prophylaxis: 1-2 mg Fe/kg/day up to a maximum of 15 mg/day

Adults **(dose expressed in terms of ferrous sulfate):**

Iron deficiency: 300 mg twice daily up to 300 mg 4 times/day or 250 mg (extended release) 1-2 times/day

Prophylaxis: 300 mg/day

**Patient Information** May color stool black, take between meals for maximum absorption; may take with food if GI upset occurs, do not take with milk or antacids; keep out of reach of children

**Dosage Forms** Amount of elemental iron is listed in brackets

Capsule:

Exsiccated, timed release (Feosol®): 159 mg [50 mg]

Exsiccated, timed release (Ferralyn® Lanacaps®, Ferra-TD®): 250 mg [50 mg]

Ferospace®: 250 mg [50 mg]

Drops, oral:

Fer-In-Sol®: 75 mg/0.6 mL [15 mg/0.6 mL] (50 mL)

Fer-Iron®: 125 mg/mL [25 mg/mL] (50 mL)

Elixir (Feosol®): 220 mg/5 mL [44 mg/5 mL] with alcohol 5% (473 mL, 4000 mL)

Syrup (Fer-In-Sol®): 90 mg/5 mL [18 mg/5 mL] with alcohol 5% (480 mL)

Tablet: 324 mg [65 mg]

Exsiccated (Feosol®) 200 mg [65 mg]

Exsiccated, timed release (Slow FE®): 160 mg [50 mg]

Feratab®: 300 mg [60 mg]

Mol-Iron®: 195 mg [39 mg]

Timed release (Fero-Gradumet®): 525 mg [105 mg]

## Ferrous Sulfate and Ascorbic Acid

(FER us SUL fate & a SKOR bik AS id)

**U.S. Brand Names** Ferancee® [OTC]; Fero-Grad 500® [OTC]

**Pharmacologic Category** Iron Salt; Vitamin

**Use** Treatment of iron deficiency in nonpregnant adults; treatment and prevention of iron deficiency in pregnant adults

**Effects on Mental Status** None reported

**Effects on Psychiatric Treatment** Constipation is common; concurrent use with psychotropic agents may increase the risk

**Usual Dosage** Adults: Oral: 1 tablet daily

**Dosage Forms** Amount of elemental iron is listed in brackets

Caplet, sustained release (Ferromar®): Ferrous fumarate 201.5 mg [65 mg] and ascorbic acid 200 mg

Tablet (Fero-Grad 500®): Ferrous sulfate 525 mg [105 mg] and ascorbic acid 500 mg

Chewable (Ferancee®): Ferrous fumarate 205 mg [67 mg] and ascorbic acid 150 mg

## Ferrous Sulfate, Ascorbic Acid, and Vitamin B-Complex

(FER us SUL fate, a SKOR bik AS id, & VYE ta min bee KOM pleks)

**U.S. Brand Names** Iberet®-Liquid [OTC]

**Pharmacologic Category** Iron Salt; Vitamin

**Use** Conditions of iron deficiency with an increased needed for B-complex vitamins and vitamin C

**Effects on Mental Status** None reported

**Effects on Psychiatric Treatment** Constipation is common; concurrent use with psychotropic agents may increase the risk

**Usual Dosage** Oral:

Children 1-3 years: 5 mL twice daily after meals

Children >4 years and Adults: 10 mL 3 times/day after meals

**Dosage Forms** Liquid:

Ferrous sulfate: 78.75 mg

Ascorbic acid: 375 mg

$B_1$: 4.5 mg

$B_2$: 4.5 mg

$B_3$: 22.5 mg

$B_5$: 7.5 mg

$B_6$: 3.75 mg

$B_{12}$: 18.75 mg all per 15 mL

## Ferrous Sulfate, Ascorbic Acid, Vitamin B-Complex, and Folic Acid

(FER us SUL fate, a SKOR bik AS id, VYE ta min bee KOM pleks, & FOE lik AS id)

**U.S. Brand Names** Iberet-Folic-500®

**Pharmacologic Category** Vitamin

**Use** Treatment of iron deficiency and prevention of concomitant folic acid deficiency where there is an associated deficient intake or increased need for B-complex vitamins

**Effects on Mental Status** None reported

**Effects on Psychiatric Treatment** Constipation is common; concurrent use with psychotropic agents may increase the risk

**Usual Dosage** Adults: Oral: 1 tablet daily

**Dosage Forms** Tablet, controlled release:

Ferrous sulfate: 105 mg

Ascorbic acid: 500 mg

$B_1$: 6 mg

$B_2$: 6 mg

$B_3$: 30 mg

$B_5$: 10 mg

$B_6$: 5 mg

$B_{12}$: 25 mcg

Folic acid: 800 mcg


- **Fertinex® Injection** *see* Follitropins *on page 239*
- **$FeSO_4$** *see* Ferrous Sulfate *on page 223*
- **Feverall™ [OTC]** *see* Acetaminophen *on page 14*
- **Feverall™ Sprinkle Caps [OTC]** *see* Acetaminophen *on page 14*


## Feverfew

**Related Information**

Natural/Herbal Products *on page 746*

Natural Products, Herbals, and Dietary Supplements *on page 742*

**Synonyms** Altamisa; Bachelor's Buttons; Featherfew; Featherfoil; Nosebleed; *Tanacetum parthenium*; Wild Quinine

**Pharmacologic Category** Herb

**Use** Prophylaxis and treatment of migraine headaches; menstrual complaints and fever

**Contraindications** Pregnancy, breast-feeding; children <2 years of age; allergies to feverfew and other members of the Asteraceae, daisy, ragweed, chamomile

**Warnings/Precautions** Use with caution in patients taking medications with serotonergic properties

**Adverse Reactions**

>10%: Gastrointestinal: Mouth ulcerations

<10%:

Dermatologic: Contact dermatitis

Gastrointestinal: Swelling of tongue, lips, abdominal pain, nausea, vomiting, loss of taste

Post-feverfew syndrome: Nervousness, insomnia, stiff joints, headache

**Overdosage/Toxicology**

Signs and symptoms: Nausea, vomiting, loss of taste, abdominal pain

Decontamination:

Oral: Do **not** induce emesis; dilute with milk or water

Dermal: Wash skin with soap and water

Treatment: Supportive therapy; treat contact dermatitis with diphenhydramine and/or steroids

**Drug Interactions** Use with caution in patients taking aspirin or anticoagulants due to increased potential for bleeding

**Usual Dosage** 125 mg of a preparation standardized to 0.2% parthenolide (250 mcg) once or twice daily

**Additional Information** Perennial bush which grows up to 3 feet tall with daisy-like yellow or white flowers; leaves are bitter tasting; contraindications in pregnancy and children <2 years of age

## Fexofenadine (feks oh FEN a deen)

**U.S. Brand Names** Allegra®

**Pharmacologic Category** Antihistamine

**Use** Nonsedating antihistamine indicated for the relief of seasonal allergic rhinitis and chronic idiopathic urticaria

**Effects on Mental Status** May cause drowsiness or dizziness

**Effects on Psychiatric Treatment** None reported

**Pregnancy Risk Factor** C

**Contraindications** Individuals demonstrating hypersensitivity to fexofenadine or any components of its formulation

**Warnings/Precautions** Safety and effectiveness in pediatric patients <12 years of age has not been established. Fexofenadine is classified in FDA pregnancy category C and no data is yet available evaluating its use in breast-feeding women.

**Adverse Reactions** 1% to 10%:

Central nervous system: Drowsiness (1.3%), fatigue (1.3%)

Endocrine & metabolic: Dysmenorrhea (1.5%)

Gastrointestinal: Nausea (1.5%), dyspepsia (1.3%)

Miscellaneous: Viral infection (2.5%)

**Drug Interactions** CYP3A3/4 enzyme substrate

Fexofenadine levels have increased with erythromycin (82% higher) and with ketoconazole (135% higher); this has not been associated with any increased incidence of side effects

In two separate studies, fexofenadine 120 mg twice daily (high doses) was coadministered with standard doses of erythromycin or ketoconazole to healthy volunteers and although fexofenadine peak plasma concentrations increased, no differences in adverse events or $QT_c$ intervals were observed. **It remains unknown if a similar interaction occurs with other azole antifungal agents (eg, itraconazole) or other macrolide antibiotics (eg, clarithromycin).**

**Usual Dosage** Oral:

Children 6-11 years: 30 mg twice daily (once daily in children with impaired renal function)

Children ≥12 years and Adults:

Seasonal allergic rhinitis: 60 mg twice daily **or** 180 mg once daily

Chronic idiopathic urticaria: 60 mg twice daily

**Dosing adjustment in renal impairment:** Recommended initial doses of 60 mg once daily

**Patient Information** Take as directed; do not exceed recommended dose. Store at room temperature in a dry place. Avoid use of other depressants, alcohol, or sleep-inducing medications unless approved by prescriber. You may experience mild drowsiness or dizziness (use caution when driving or engaging in tasks requiring alertness until response to drug is known); or nausea (frequent small meals, frequent mouth care, chewing gum, or sucking hard candy may help). Report persistent sedation or drowsiness, menstrual irregularities, or lack of improvement or worsening or condition.

**Dosage Forms** Capsule, as hydrochloride: 60 mg

## Fexofenadine and Pseudoephedrine
(feks oh FEN a deen & soo doe e FED rin)

**U.S. Brand Names** Allegra-D™

**Pharmacologic Category** Antihistamine/Decongestant Combination

**Use** Relief of symptoms associated with seasonal allergic rhinitis in adults and children 12 years of age and older. Symptoms treated effectively include sneezing, rhinorrhea, itchy nose/palate/ and/or throat, itchy/watery/ red eyes, and nasal congestion.

**Effects on Mental Status** May cause drowsiness or dizziness, nervousness, and insomnia; may rarely cause hallucinations

**Effects on Psychiatric Treatment** Contraindicated with MAOIs

**Usual Dosage** Oral: Adults: One tablet twice daily for adults and children 12 years of age and older. It is recommended that the administration with food should be avoided. A dose of one tablet once daily is recommended as the starting dose in patients with decreased renal function.

**Dosage Forms** Tablet, extended release: Fexofenadine hydrochloride 60 mg and pseudoephedrine hydrochloride 120 mg

- **Fiberall® Chewable Tablet [OTC]** *see* Calcium Polycarbophil *on page 86*
- **Fiberall® Powder [OTC]** *see* Psyllium *on page 479*
- **Fiberall® Wafer [OTC]** *see* Psyllium *on page 479*
- **FiberCon® Tablet [OTC]** *see* Calcium Polycarbophil *on page 86*
- **Fiber-Lax® Tablet [OTC]** *see* Calcium Polycarbophil *on page 86*

## Filgrastim (fil GRA stim)

**Related Information**

Clinical Issues in the Use of Antipsychotics *on page 630*

Clozapine-Induced Side Effects *on page 780*

**U.S. Brand Names** Neupogen®

**Synonyms** G-CSF; Granulocyte Colony Stimulating Factor

**Pharmacologic Category** Colony Stimulating Factor

**Use**

Patients with nonmyeloid malignancies receiving myelosuppressive anticancer drugs associated with a significant incidence of neutropenia (FDA-approved indication)

Cancer patients receiving bone marrow transplant (BMT) (FDA-approved indication)

Patients undergoing peripheral blood progenitor cell (PBPC) collection

Patients with severe chronic neutropenia (SCN) (FDA-approved indication)

Chronic administration in symptomatic patients with congenital neutropenia, cyclic neutropenia, or idiopathic neutropenic; filgrastim should not be started until the diagnosis of SCN is confirmed, as it may interfere with diagnostic efforts

Safety and efficacy of G-CSF given simultaneously with cytotoxic chemotherapy have not been established; concurrent treatment may increase myelosuppression; G-CSF should be avoided in patients receiving concomitant chemotherapy and radiation therapy

**Effects on Mental Status** None reported

**Effects on Psychiatric Treatment** May be used to treat clozapine-induced agranulocytosis; lithium may potentiate the release of neutrophils; use with caution

**Pregnancy Risk Factor** C

**Contraindications** Patients with known hypersensitivity to *E. coli*-derived proteins or G-CSF

**Warnings/Precautions** Complete blood count and platelet count should be obtained prior to chemotherapy. Do not use G-CSF in the period 12-24 hours before to 24 hours after administration of cytotoxic chemotherapy because of the potential sensitivity of rapidly dividing myeloid cells to cytotoxic chemotherapy. Precaution should be exercised in the usage of G-CSF in any malignancy with myeloid characteristics. G-CSF can potentially act as a growth factor for any tumor type, particularly myeloid malignancies. Tumors of nonhematopoietic origin may have surface receptors for G-CSF.

Allergic-type reactions have occurred in patients receiving G-CSF with first or later doses. Reactions tended to occur more frequently with intravenous administration and within 30 minutes of infusion. Most cases resolved rapidly with antihistamines, steroids, bronchodilators, and/or epinephrine. Symptoms recurred in >50% of patients on rechallenge.

**Adverse Reactions** Effects are generally mild and dose related

>10%:

Central nervous system: Neutropenic fever, fever

Dermatologic: Alopecia

Gastrointestinal: Nausea, vomiting, diarrhea, mucositis,

Splenomegaly: This occurs more commonly in patients with cyclic neutropenia/congenital agranulocytosis who received S.C. injections for a prolonged (>14 days) period of time; ~33% of these patients experience subclinical splenomegaly (detected by MRI or CT scan); ~3% of these patients experience clinical splenomegaly

Neuromuscular & skeletal: Medullary bone pain (24% incidence): This occurs most commonly in lower back pain, posterior iliac crest, and sternum and is controlled with non-narcotic analgesics

1% to 10%:

Cardiovascular: Chest pain, fluid retention

Central nervous system: Headache

Dermatologic: Skin rash

Gastrointestinal: Anorexia, stomatitis, constipation

Hematologic: Leukocytosis

Local: Pain at injection site

Neuromuscular & skeletal: Weakness

Respiratory: Dyspnea, cough, sore throat

<1%: Anaphylactic reaction, pericarditis, thrombophlebitis, transient supraventricular arrhythmia

**Overdosage/Toxicology**

Signs and symptoms: No clinical adverse effects seen with high dose producing ANC >10,000/mm$^3$; leukocytosis which was not associated with any clinical adverse effects

Treatment: After discontinuing the drug, there is a 50% decrease in circulating levels of neutrophils within 1-2 days, return to pretreatment levels within 1-7 days

**Drug Interactions** Drugs which may potentiate the release of neutrophils (eg, lithium) should be used with caution

**Usual Dosage** Children and Adults:

**Dosage should be based on actual body weight** (even in morbidly obese patients)

Existing clinical data suggest that starting G-CSF between 24 and 72 hours subsequent to chemotherapy may provide optimal neutrophil

(Continued)

## Filgrastim *(Continued)*

recover; continue therapy until the occurrence of an absolute neutrophil count of 10,000 µL after the neutrophil nadir

**The available data suggest that rounding the dose to the nearest vial size may enhance patient convenience and reduce costs without clinical detriment**

Neonates: 5-10 mcg/kg/day once daily for 3-5 days has been administered to neutropenic neonates with sepsis; there was a rapid and significant increase in peripheral neutrophil counts and the neutrophil storage pool

Children and Adults:

**Myelosuppressive chemotherapy** S.C. or I.V. infusion: 5 mcg/kg/day

Doses may be increased in increments of 5 mcg/kg for each chemotherapy cycle, according to the duration and severity of the absolute neutrophil count (ANC) nadir

Bone marrow transplant patients: 5-10 mcg/kg/day as an I.V. infusion of 4 or 24 hours or as continuous 24-hour S.C. infusion; administer first dose at least 24 hours after cytotoxic chemotherapy and at least 24 hours after bone marrow infusion; if ANC decreases <1000/mm$^3$ during the 5 mcg/kg/day dose, increase filgrastim to 10 mcg/kg/day and follow the recommended steps based on neutrophil response:

When ANC >1000/mm$^3$ for 3 consecutive days: Reduce Filgrastim dose to 5 mcg/kg/day

If ANC remains >1000/mm$^3$ for 3 more consecutive days: Discontinue filgrastim

If ANC decreases to <1000/mm$^3$ : Resume at 5 mcg/kg/day

If ANC decreases <1000/mm$^3$ during the 5 mcg/kg/day dose, increase filgrastim to 10 mcg/kg/day and follow the above steps

**Peripheral blood progenitor cell (PBPC) collection:** 10 mcg/kg/day either S.C. or a bolus or continuous I.V. infusion. It is recommended that G-CSF be given for at least 4 days before the first leukapheresis procedure and continued until the last leukapheresis; although the optimal duration of administration and leukapheresis schedule have not been established, administration of G-CSF for 6-7 days with leukaphereses on days 5,6 and 7 was found to be safe and effective; neutrophil counts should be monitored after 4 days of G-CSF, and G-CSF dose-modification should be considered for those patients who develop a white blood cell count >100,000/mm$^3$

**Severe chronic neutropenia:** S.C.:

Congenital neutropenia: 6 mcg/kg/dose twice daily

Idiopathic/cyclic neutropenia: 5 mcg/kg single dose daily

Chronic daily administration is required to maintain clinical benefit; adjust dose based on the patients' clinical course as well as ANC; in phase III studies, the target ANC was 1500-10,000/mm$^3$. Reduce the dose if the ANC is persistently >10,000/mm$^3$

Premature discontinuation of G-CSF therapy prior to the time of recovery from the expected neutrophil is generally not recommended; a transient increase in neutrophil counts is typically seen 1-2 days after initiation of therapy

Hemodialysis: Supplemental dose is not necessary

Peritoneal dialysis: Supplemental dose is not necessary

**Patient Information** Follow directions for proper storage and administration of S.C. medication. Never reuse syringes or needles. You may experience bone pain (request analgesic); nausea or vomiting (small frequent meals may help); hair loss (reversible); or sore mouth (frequent mouth care with soft toothbrush or cotton swab may help). Report unusual fever or chills; unhealed sores; severe bone pain; pain, redness, or swelling at injection site; unusual swelling of extremities or difficulty breathing; or chest pain and palpitations.

**Nursing Implications** Do not mix with sodium chloride solutions

**Dosage Forms** Injection, preservative free: 300 mcg/mL (1 mL, 1.6 mL)

## Finasteride (fi NAS teer ide)

**U.S. Brand Names** Proscar®

**Pharmacologic Category** Antiandrogen

**Use** Early data indicate that finasteride is useful in the treatment of symptomatic benign prostatic hyperplasia (BPH); male pattern baldness

**Unlabeled use:** Adjuvant monotherapy after radical prostatectomy in the treatment of prostatic cancer

**Effects on Mental Status** None reported

**Effects on Psychiatric Treatment** None reported

**Pregnancy Risk Factor** X

**Contraindications** History of hypersensitivity to drug, pregnancy, lactation, children

**Warnings/Precautions** A minimum of 6 months of treatment may be necessary to determine whether an individual will respond to finasteride. Use with caution in those patients with liver function abnormalities. Carefully monitor patients with a large residual urinary volume or severely diminished urinary flow for obstructive uropathy. These patients may not be candidates for finasteride therapy.

**Adverse Reactions** 1% to 10%:

Endocrine & metabolic: Decreased libido

Genitourinary: <4% incidence of impotence, decreased volume of ejaculate

**Drug Interactions** CYP3A3/4 enzyme substrate

**Usual Dosage** Adults: Male:

Benign prostatic hyperplasia: Oral: 5 mg/day as a single dose; clinical responses occur within 12 weeks to 6 months of initiation of therapy; long-term administration is recommended for maximal response

Male pattern baldness: Oral: 1 mg daily

**Dosing adjustment in renal impairment:** No dosage adjustment is necessary

**Dosing adjustment in hepatic impairment:** Use with caution in patients with liver function abnormalities because finasteride is metabolized extensively in the liver

**Dietary Considerations** Food: Administration with food may delay the rate and reduce the extent of oral absorption

**Patient Information** Results of therapy may take several months. Take as directed, with fluids, 30 minutes before or 2 hours after meals. You may experience decreased libido or impotence during therapy. Report any increase in urinary volume or voiding patterns occurs.

**Dosage Forms** Tablet, film coated: 1 mg, 5 mg


- **Fiorgen PF®** *see* Butalbital Compound and Aspirin *on page 80*
- **Fioricet®** *see* Butalbital Compound and Acetaminophen *on page 80*
- **Fiorinal®** *see* Butalbital Compound and Aspirin *on page 80*
- **Fiorinal® With Codeine** *see* Butalbital Compound and Codeine *on page 81*
- **Fisalamine** *see* Mesalamine *on page 344*
- **Fisifax®** *see* Nicergoline *on page 392*
- **FK506** *see* Tacrolimus *on page 529*
- **Flagyl®** *see* Metronidazole *on page 362*
- **Flagyl ER®** *see* Metronidazole *on page 362*
- **Flarex®** *see* Fluorometholone *on page 231*
- **Flatulex® [OTC]** *see* Simethicone *on page 512*
- **Flavorcee® [OTC]** *see* Ascorbic Acid *on page 48*


## Flavoxate (fla VOKS ate)

**U.S. Brand Names** Urispas®

**Pharmacologic Category** Antispasmodic Agent, Urinary

**Use** Antispasmodic to provide symptomatic relief of dysuria, nocturia, suprapubic pain, urgency, and incontinence due to detrusor instability and hyper-reflexia in elderly with cystitis, urethritis, urethrocystitis, urethrotrigonitis, and prostatitis

**Effects on Mental Status** Drowsiness is common; may cause nervousness

**Effects on Psychiatric Treatment** None reported

**Pregnancy Risk Factor** B

**Contraindications** Pyloric or duodenal obstruction, GI hemorrhage, GI obstruction; ileus; achalasia; obstructive uropathies of lower urinary tract (BPH)

**Warnings/Precautions** May cause drowsiness, vertigo, and ocular disturbances; administer cautiously in patients with suspected glaucoma

**Adverse Reactions**

>10%:

Central nervous system: Drowsiness

Gastrointestinal: Xerostomia, dry throat

1% to 10%:

Cardiovascular: Tachycardia, palpitations,

Central nervous system: Nervousness, fatigue, vertigo, headache, hyperpyrexia

Gastrointestinal: Constipation, nausea, vomiting

<1%: Confusion (especially in the elderly), increased intraocular pressure, leukopenia, rash

**Overdosage/Toxicology**

Signs and symptoms: Clumsiness, dizziness, drowsiness, flushing, hallucinations, irritability

Treatment: Supportive care only

**Drug Interactions** No data reported

**Usual Dosage** Children >12 years and Adults: Oral: 100-200 mg 3-4 times/day; reduce the dose when symptoms improve

**Patient Information** Take exactly as directed, with water, preferably on an empty stomach (1 hour before or 2 hours after meals). Do not use alcohol or OTC medications without consulting prescriber. You may experience mild drowsiness, nervousness, or dizziness (use caution when driving or engaging in tasks requiring alertness until response to drug is known); nausea, vomiting, dry mouth (small frequent meals, frequent oral care, chewing gum, or sucking hard candy may help); decreased ability to perspire (avoid extremes of heat); constipation (increased exercise or dietary fluid and fiber may help). Report vision changes (blurred vision); rapid heartbeat; or unresolved nausea, vomiting, or constipation.

**Dosage Forms** Tablet, film coated, as hydrochloride: 100 mg


- **Flaxedil®** *see* Gallamine Triethiodide *on page 245*

## Flecainide (fle KAY nide)

**U.S. Brand Names** Tambocor™
**Pharmacologic Category** Antiarrhythmic Agent, Class I-C
**Use** Prevention and suppression of documented life-threatening ventricular arrhythmias (eg, sustained ventricular tachycardia); controlling symptomatic, disabling supraventricular tachycardias in patients without structural heart disease in whom other agents fail
**Effects on Mental Status** Dizziness is common; may cause sedation; may rarely cause nervousness
**Effects on Psychiatric Treatment** Use beta-blockers with caution; may produce additive negative inotropic effect; use caution with TCAs; may affect cardiac conduction; CYP2D6 substrate; use caution with the SSRIs
**Pregnancy Risk Factor** C
**Contraindications** Hypersensitivity to flecainide or any component; pre-existing second- or third-degree AV block or with right bundle branch block when associated with a left hemiblock (bifascicular block) (except in patients with a functioning artificial pacemaker); cardiogenic shock; coronary artery disease (based on CAST study results); concurrent use of ritonavir or amprenavir
**Warnings/Precautions** Not recommend for patients with chronic atrial fibrillation. A worsening or new arrhythmia may occur (proarrhythmic effect). Use caution in heart failure (may precipitate or exacerbate CHF). Dose-related increases in PR, QRS, and Q-T intervals occur. Use with caution in sick sinus syndrome or with permanent pacemakers or temporary pacing wires (can increase endocardial pacing thresholds). Pre-existing hypokalemia or hyperkalemia should be corrected before initiation (can alter drug's effect). Cautious use in significant hepatic impairment.
**Adverse Reactions**
>10%:
Central nervous system: Dizziness (19%)
Ocular: Visual disturbances (16%)
Respiratory: Dyspnea (~10%)
1% to 10%:
Cardiovascular: Palpitations (6%), chest pain (5%), edema (3.5%), tachycardia (1% to 3%)
Central nervous system: Headache (4%), fatigue (8%), fever (1% to 3%), malaise (1% to 3%)
Dermatologic: Rash (1% to 3%)
Gastrointestinal: Nausea (9%), constipation, abdominal pain (3%), anorexia (1% to 3%)
Neuromuscular & skeletal: Tremor (5%), weakness (5%)
Ocular: Diplopia (1% to 3%)
<1%: Alopecia, angina, ataxia, A-V block, blood dyscrasias, bradycardia, congestive heart failure, eye pain, flatulence, flushing, heart block, hyper/hypotension, hypoesthesia, increased P-R, nervousness, paresthesia, photophobia, possible hepatic dysfunction, QRS duration, somnolence, tinnitus, vertigo, worsening ventricular arrhythmias, xerostomia
**Overdosage/Toxicology**
Signs and symptoms: Has a narrow therapeutic index and severe toxicity may occur slightly above the therapeutic range, especially if combined with other antiarrhythmic drugs. (Acute single ingestion of twice the daily therapeutic dose is life-threatening.) Symptoms of overdose include increases in P-R, QRS, Q-T intervals and amplitude of the T wave, A-V block, bradycardia, hypotension, ventricular arrhythmias (monomorphic or polymorphic ventricular tachycardia), and asystole; other symptoms include dizziness, blurred vision, headache, and GI upset.
Treatment: Supportive, using conventional treatment (fluids, positioning, anticonvulsants, antiarrhythmics). **Note:** Type Ia antiarrhythmic agents should not be used to treat cardiotoxicity caused by type Ic drugs; sodium bicarbonate may reverse QRS prolongation, bradycardia and hypotension; ventricular pacing may be needed; hemodialysis only of possible benefit for tocainide or flecainide overdose in patients with renal failure.
**Drug Interactions** CYP2D6 enzyme substrate
Cimetidine may decrease flecainide's metabolism; monitor cardiac status or use an alternative $H_2$-antagonist
Quinidine may decrease flecainide's metabolism; monitor cardiac status
Digoxin's serum concentration may increase slightly
Amiodarone increases in flecainide plasma levels; consider reducing flecainide dose by 25% to 33% with concurrent use
Amprenavir and ritonavir may increase cardiotoxicity of flecainide (decrease metabolism)
Propranolol (and possibly other beta-blockers) increases flecainide blood levels, and propranolol blood levels are increased with concurrent use; monitor for excessive negative inotropic effects
Urinary alkalinizers (antacids, sodium bicarbonate, acetazolamide) may increase flecainide blood levels
**Usual Dosage** Oral:
Children:
Initial: 3 mg/kg/day or 50-100 mg/m²/day in 3 divided doses
Usual: 3-6 mg/kg/day or 100-150 mg/m²/day in 3 divided doses; up to 11 mg/kg/day or 200 mg/m²/day for uncontrolled patients with subtherapeutic levels
Adults:
Life-threatening ventricular arrhythmias:
Initial: 100 mg every 12 hours
Increase by 50-100 mg/day (given in 2 doses/day) every 4 days; maximum: 400 mg/day.
Use of higher initial doses and more rapid dosage adjustments have resulted in an increased incidence of proarrhythmic events and congestive heart failure, particularly during the first few days. Do not use a loading dose. Use very cautiously in patients with history of congestive heart failure or myocardial infarction.
Prevention of paroxysmal supraventricular arrhythmias in patients with disabling symptoms but no structural heart disease:
Initial: 50 mg every 12 hours
Increase by 50 mg twice daily at 4-day intervals; maximum: 300 mg/day.
**Dosing adjustment in severe renal impairment:** $Cl_{cr}$ <35 mL/minute: Decrease initial dose to 50 mg every 12 hours; increase doses at intervals >4 days monitoring EKG levels closely.
Dialysis: Not dialyzable (0% to 5%) via hemo- or peritoneal dialysis; no supplemental dose necessary.
**Dosing adjustment/comments in hepatic impairment:** Monitoring of plasma levels is recommended because of significantly increased half-life.
When transferring from another antiarrhythmic agent, allow for 2-4 half-lives of the agent to pass before initiating flecainide therapy.
**Patient Information** Take exactly as directed, around-the-clock. Do not discontinue without consulting prescriber. You will require frequent monitoring while taking this medication. You may experience lightheadedness, nervousness, dizziness, visual disturbances (use caution when driving or engaging in tasks requiring alertness until response to drug is known); or nausea, vomiting, or loss of appetite (small frequent meals may help). Report palpitations, chest pain, excessively slow or rapid heartbeat; acute nervousness, headache, or fatigue; unusual weight gain; unusual cough; difficulty breathing; swelling of hands or ankles; or muscle tremor, numbness, or weakness.
**Dosage Forms** Tablet, as acetate: 50 mg, 100 mg, 150 mg


♦ **Fleet® Laxative [OTC]** *see* Bisacodyl *on page 69*
♦ **Fleet® Pain Relief [OTC]** *see* Pramoxine *on page 457*
♦ **Flexaphen®** *see* Chlorzoxazone *on page 120*
♦ **Flexeril®** *see* Cyclobenzaprine *on page 144*
♦ **Flolan® Injection** *see* Epoprostenol *on page 197*
♦ **Flomax®** *see* Tamsulosin *on page 531*
♦ **Flonase®** *see* Fluticasone *on page 237*
♦ **Florical® [OTC]** *see* Calcium Carbonate *on page 84*
♦ **Florinef® Acetate** *see* Fludrocortisone *on page 229*
♦ **Florone®** *see* Diflorasone *on page 168*
♦ **Florone E®** *see* Diflorasone *on page 168*
♦ **Floropryl® Ophthalmic** *see* Isoflurophate *on page 294*
♦ **Flovent®** *see* Fluticasone *on page 237*
♦ **Floxin®** *see* Ofloxacin *on page 403*


## Floxuridine (floks YOOR i deen)

**U.S. Brand Names** FUDR®
**Canadian Brand Names** Fludara®
**Pharmacologic Category** Antineoplastic Agent, Antimetabolite
**Use** Treatment of gastrointestinal adenocarcinoma metastatic to the liver
**Effects on Mental Status** May cause drowsiness
**Effects on Psychiatric Treatment** May rarely cause agranulocytosis; use caution with clozapine and carbamazepine
**Usual Dosage** Adults (refer to individual protocols):
Intra-arterial: Primarily by an implantable pump: 0.1-0.6 mg/kg/day continuous intra-arterial administration for 14 days then heparinized saline is given for 14 days; toxicity requires dose reduction
I.V.: 0.5-1 mg/kg/day for 6-15 days
**Dosage Forms**
Injection, preservative free: 100 mg/mL (5 mL)
Powder for injection: 500 mg (5 mL, 10 mL)


♦ **Flubenisolone** *see* Betamethasone *on page 65*


## Fluconazole (floo KOE na zole)

**U.S. Brand Names** Diflucan®
**Pharmacologic Category** Antifungal Agent, Oral; Antifungal Agent, Parenteral
**Use Indications for use in adult patients:** Oral or vaginal candidiasis unresponsive to nystatin or clotrimazole; nonlife-threatening *Candida*
(Continued)

## Fluconazole *(Continued)*

infections (eg, cystitis, esophagitis); treatment of hepatosplenic candidiasis and other *Candida* infections in persons unable to tolerate amphotericin B; treatment of cryptococcal infections; secondary prophylaxis for cryptococcal meningitis in persons with AIDS; antifungal prophylaxis in allogeneic bone marrow transplant recipients

Oral fluconazole should be used in persons able to tolerate oral medications; parenteral fluconazole should be reserved for patients who are both unable to take oral medications and are unable to tolerate amphotericin B (eg, due to hypersensitivity or renal insufficiency)

**Effects on Mental Status** May cause dizziness

**Effects on Psychiatric Treatment** None reported; CYP3A4 inhibitor; use caution with triazolam and alprazolam

**Pregnancy Risk Factor** C

**Contraindications** Known hypersensitivity to fluconazole or other azoles; concomitant administration with terfenadine

**Warnings/Precautions** Should be used with caution in patients with renal and hepatic dysfunction or previous hepatotoxicity from other azole derivatives. Patients who develop abnormal liver function tests during fluconazole therapy should be monitored closely and discontinued if symptoms consistent with liver disease develop. **Should be used with caution in patients receiving cisapride or astemizole.**

**Adverse Reactions**

1% to 10%:

Central nervous system: Headache

Dermatologic: Rash

Gastrointestinal: Nausea, vomiting, abdominal pain, diarrhea

<1%: Dizziness, hypokalemia, increased AST/ALT or alkaline phosphatase, pallor

**Overdosage/Toxicology**

Signs and symptoms: Decreased lacrimation, salivation, respiration and motility, urinary incontinence, cyanosis

Treatment: Includes supportive measures, a 3-hour hemodialysis will remove 50%

**Drug Interactions** CYP2C9 enzyme inducer; CYP2C9, 2C18, and 2C19 enzyme inhibitor and CYP3A3/4 enzyme inhibitor (weak)

Decreased effect: Rifampin and cimetidine decrease concentrations of fluconazole; fluconazole may decrease the effect of oral contraceptives

Increased effect/toxicity:

Coadministration with terfenadine or cisapride is contraindicated; use with caution with astemizole due to increased risk of significant cardiotoxicity

Hydrochlorothiazide may decrease fluconazole clearance

Fluconazole may also inhibit warfarin, phenytoin, cyclosporine, and theophylline, zidovudine, sulfonylureas, rifabutin, and warfarin clearance

Nephrotoxicity of tacrolimus may be increased

**Usual Dosage** The daily dose of fluconazole is the same for oral and I.V. administration

Neonates: First 2 weeks of life, especially premature neonates: Same dose as older children every 72 hours

Children: Once-daily dosing by indication:

Oropharyngeal candidiasis:

Day 1: 6 mg/kg; then 3 mg/kg for at least 14 days

Esophageal candidiasis:

Day 1: 6 mg/kg; then 3-12 mg/kg for a minimum of 21 days and for at least 2 weeks following resolution of symptoms

Systemic candidiasis:

6-12 mg/kg/day for at least 28 days

Cryptococcal meningitis:

Day 1: 12 mg/kg; then 6-12 mg/kg for at least 10-12 weeks after CSF culture becomes negative

Cryptococcal meningitis, relapse:

Day 1: 6 mg/kg; then 6 mg/kg for at least 10-12 weeks after CSF culture becomes negative

Adults: Oral, I.V.: Once-daily dosing by indication:

Oropharyngeal candidiasis:

Day 1: 200 mg; then 100 mg/day for at least 14 days

Esophageal candidiasis:

Day 1: 200 mg; then 100 mg/day for a minimum of 21 days and for at least 14 days following resolution of symptoms

Prevention of candidiasis in bone marrow transplant:

Day 1: 400 mg; then 400 mg/day for a minimum of 3 days before neutropenia, 7 days after neutrophils >1000 cells/mm$^3$

Candidiasis UTIs, peritonitis:

50-200 mg/day

Systemic candidiasis:

Day 1: 400 mg; then 200 mg/day for at least 28 days

Cryptococcal meningitis, acute:

Day 1: 400 mg; then 200 mg/day for at least 10-12 weeks after CSF culture becomes negative

Cryptococcal meningitis, relapse:

Day 1: 200 mg; then 200 mg/day for at least 10-12 weeks after CSF culture becomes negative

Vaginal candidiasis:

Day 1: 150 mg single dose

**Dosing adjustment/interval in renal impairment:**

No adjustment for vaginal candidiasis single-dose therapy

For multiple dosing, administer usual load then adjust daily doses

$Cl_{cr}$ 11-50 mL/minute: Administer 50% of recommended dose or administer every 48 hours

Hemodialysis: One dose after each dialysis

Continuous arteriovenous or venovenous hemodiafiltration (CAVH) effects: Dose as for $Cl_{cr}$ 10-50 mL/minute

**Patient Information** Take as directed, around-the-clock. Take full course of medication as ordered. Follow good hygiene measures to prevent reinfection. Frequent blood tests may be required. Maintain adequate hydration (2-3 L/day of fluids unless instructed to restrict fluid intake). You may experience headache, dizziness, drowsiness (use caution when driving or engaging in tasks that require alertness until response to drug is known); nausea, vomiting, or diarrhea (small frequent meals, frequent mouth care, sucking lozenges, or chewing gum may help). Report skin rash, redness, or irritation; persistent GI upset; urinary pattern changes; excessively dry eyes or mouth; changes in color of stool or urine.

**Dosage Forms**

Injection: 2 mg/mL (100 mL, 200 mL)

Powder for oral suspension: 10 mg/mL (35 mL); 40 mg/mL (35 mL)

Tablet: 50 mg, 100 mg, 150 mg, 200 mg

---

## Flucytosine (floo SYE toe seen)

**U.S. Brand Names** Ancobon®

**Canadian Brand Names** Ancotil®

**Synonyms** 5-FC; 5-Flurocytosine

**Pharmacologic Category** Antifungal Agent, Oral

**Use** Adjunctive treatment of susceptible fungal infections (usually *Candida* or *Cryptococcus*); synergy with amphotericin B for certain fungal infections (*Cryptococcus* spp., *Candida* spp.)

**Effects on Mental Status** May rarely cause drowsiness, confusion, or hallucinations

**Effects on Psychiatric Treatment** May cause bone marrow suppression; use caution with clozapine and carbamazepine

**Pregnancy Risk Factor** C

**Contraindications** Hypersensitivity to flucytosine or any component

**Warnings/Precautions** Use with extreme caution in patients with renal impairment, bone marrow suppression, or in patients with AIDS; dosage modification required in patients with impaired renal function

**Adverse Reactions**

1% to 10%:

Dermatologic: Rash

Gastrointestinal: Abdominal pain, diarrhea, loss of appetite, nausea, vomiting

Hematologic: Anemia, leukopenia, thrombocytopenia

Hepatic: Hepatitis, jaundice

<1%: Anaphylaxis, ataxia, bone marrow suppression, cardiac arrest, confusion, dizziness, drowsiness, elevated liver enzymes, hallucinations, headache, hearing loss, hypoglycemia, hypokalemia, paresthesia, parkinsonism, photosensitivity, psychosis, respiratory arrest, temporary growth failure

**Overdosage/Toxicology**

Signs and symptoms: Nausea, vomiting, diarrhea, bone marrow suppression

Treatment: Supportive

**Drug Interactions** Increased effect/toxicity with concurrent amphotericin administration; cytosine may inactivate flucytosine activity

**Usual Dosage** Children and Adults: Oral: 50-150 mg/kg/day in divided doses every 6 hours

**Dosing interval in renal impairment:** Use lower initial dose:

$Cl_{cr}$ >50 mL/minute: Administer every 12 hours

$Cl_{cr}$ 10-50 mL/minute: Administer every 16 hours

$Cl_{cr}$ <10 mL/minute: Administer every 24 hours

Hemodialysis: Dialyzable (50% to 100%); administer dose posthemodialysis

Peritoneal dialysis: Adults: Administer 0.5-1 g every 24 hours

Continuous arteriovenous or venovenous hemodiafiltration (CAVH) effects: Dose as for $Cl_{cr}$ 10-50 mL/minute

**Patient Information** Take capsules one at a time over a few minutes with food to reduce GI upset. Take full course of medication as ordered. Do not discontinue without consulting prescriber. Practice good hygiene measures to prevent reinfection. Frequent blood tests may be required. You may experience nausea and vomiting (small, frequent meals may help). Report rash, respiratory difficulty, CNS changes (eg, confusion, hallucinations, ataxia, acute headache), yellowing of skin or eyes, and changes in color of stool or urine, unresolved diarrhea or anorexia, or unusual bleeding or fatigue and weakness.

**Dosage Forms** Capsule: 250 mg, 500 mg

♦ **Fludara®** *see* Fludarabine *on page 229*

## Fludarabine (floo DARE a been)

**U.S. Brand Names** Fludara®

**Pharmacologic Category** Antineoplastic Agent, Antimetabolite

**Use** Treatment of chronic lymphocytic leukemia (B-cell) in patients who have not responded to other alkylating agent regimen

**Effects on Mental Status** Sedation is common

**Effects on Psychiatric Treatment** Myelosuppression is common; use caution with clozapine and carbamazepine; concurrent use with low potency antipsychotics and TCAs may produce additive sedation

**Usual Dosage** I.V.:

Children:

Acute leukemia: 10 mg/m$^2$ bolus over 15 minutes followed by continuous infusion of 30.5 mg/m$^2$/day over 5 days **or**

10.5 mg/m$^2$ bolus over 15 minutes followed by 30.5 mg/m$^2$/day over 48 hours followed by cytarabine has been used in clinical trials

Solid tumors: 9 mg/m$^2$ bolus followed by 27 mg/m$^2$/day continuous infusion over 5 days

Adults:

Chronic lymphocytic leukemia: 25 mg/m$^2$/day over a 30-minute period for 5 days; 5-day courses are repeated every 28 days days

Non-Hodgkin's lymphoma: Loading dose: 20 mg/m$^2$ followed by 30 mg/m$^2$/day for 48 hours

**Dosing in renal impairment:** $Cl_{cr}$ <50 mL/minute: Monitor closely for toxicity; dose reduction is indicated in patients with renal failure. However, no specific guidelines are available

**Dosage Forms** Powder for injection, as phosphate, lyophilized: 50 mg (6 mL)

## Fludrocortisone (floo droe KOR ti sone)

**Related Information**

Corticosteroids Comparison Chart *on page 711*

**U.S. Brand Names** Florinef® Acetate

**Synonyms** Fluohydrisone Acetate; Fluohydrocortisone Acetate; 9α-Fluorohydrocortisone Acetate

**Pharmacologic Category** Corticosteroid, Oral

**Use** Partial replacement therapy for primary and secondary adrenocortical insufficiency in Addison's disease; treatment of salt-losing adrenogenital syndrome

**Effects on Mental Status** May cause dizziness

**Effects on Psychiatric Treatment** Barbiturates and carbamazepine may decrease corticosteroid effects; useful in the management of psychotropic-induced hypotension

**Pregnancy Risk Factor** C

**Contraindications** Known hypersensitivity to fludrocortisone; systemic fungal infections

**Warnings/Precautions** Taper dose gradually when therapy is discontinued; use with caution with Addison's disease, sodium retention and potassium loss

**Adverse Reactions** 1% to 10%:

Cardiovascular: Hypertension, edema, congestive heart failure

Central nervous system: Convulsions, headache, dizziness

Dermatologic: Acne, rash, bruising

Endocrine & metabolic: Hypokalemic alkalosis, suppression of growth, hyperglycemia, HPA suppression

Gastrointestinal: Peptic ulcer

Neuromuscular & skeletal: Muscle weakness

Ocular: Cataracts

Miscellaneous: Diaphoresis

**Overdosage/Toxicology** Signs and symptoms: Hypertension, edema, hypokalemia, excessive weight gain. When consumed in excessive quantities, systemic hypercorticism and adrenal suppression may occur

Treatment: In those cases where systemic hypercorticism and adrenal suppression occur, discontinuation and withdrawal of the corticosteroid should be done judiciously

**Drug Interactions** Decreased effect:

Anticholinesterases effects are antagonized

Decreased corticosteroid effects by rifampin, barbiturates, and hydantoins

Decreased salicylate levels

**Usual Dosage** Oral:

Infants and Children: 0.05-0.1 mg/day

Adults: 0.1-0.2 mg/day with ranges of 0.1 mg 3 times/week to 0.2 mg/day

Addison's disease: Initial: 0.1 mg/day; if transient hypertension develops, reduce the dose to 0.05 mg/day. Preferred administration with cortisone (10-37.5 mg/day) or hydrocortisone (10-30 mg/day).

Salt-losing adrenogenital syndrome: 0.1-0.2 mg/day

**Patient Information** Take exactly as directed. Do not take more than prescribed dose and do not discontinue abruptly; consult prescriber. Take with or after meals. Take once-a-day dose with food in the morning. Limit intake of caffeine or stimulants. Maintain adequate nutrition; consult prescriber for possibility of special dietary recommendations. If diabetic, monitor serum glucose closely and notify prescriber of changes; this medication can alter hypoglycemic requirements. Notify prescriber if you are experiencing higher than normal levels of stress; medication may need adjustment. Periodic ophthalmic examinations will be necessary with long-term use. You will be susceptible to infection; avoid crowds or infected persons or persons with contagious diseases. You may experience insomnia or nervousness; use caution when driving or engaging in tasks requiring alertness until response to drug is known. Report weakness, change in menstrual pattern, vision changes, signs of hyperglycemia, signs of infection (eg, fever, chills, mouth sores, perianal itching, vaginal discharge), other persistent side effects, or worsening of condition.

**Dosage Forms** Tablet: 0.1 mg

◆ **Fluindostatin** *see* Fluvastatin *on page 237*

◆ **Flumadine®** *see* Rimantadine *on page 495*

## Flumazenil (FLO may ze nil)

**Related Information**

Clinical Issues in the Use of Anxiolytics and Sedative/Hypnotics *on page 634*

Special Populations - Elderly *on page 662*

Substance-Related Disorders *on page 609*

**Generic Available** No

**U.S. Brand Names** Romazicon™ Injection

**Canadian Brand Names** Anexate®

**Pharmacologic Category** Antidote

**Use** For complete or partial reverse of the sedative effects of benzodiazepine in cases where

1. general anesthesia has been induced and/or maintained with benzodiazepines
2. sedation has been produced with benzodiazepine for diagnostic and therapeutic procedures
3. management of benzodiazepine overdose

**Pregnancy Risk Factor** C

**Contraindications** Hypersensitivity to flumazenil or benzodiazepines; patients given benzodiazepines for control of potentially life-threatening conditions (eg, control of intracranial pressure or status epilepticus); patients who are showing signs of serious cyclic-antidepressant overdosage

**Warnings/Precautions**

Risk of seizures = high-risk patients:

Patients on benzodiazepines for long-term sedation

Tricyclic antidepressant overdose patients

Concurrent major sedative-hypnotic drug withdrawal

Recent therapy with repeated doses of parenteral benzodiazepines

Myoclonic jerking or seizure activity prior to flumazenil administration

**Hypoventilation: Does not reverse respiratory depression/hypoventilation or cardiac depression**

Resedation: Occurs more frequently in patients where a large single dose or cumulative dose of a benzodiazepine is administered along with a neuromuscular blocking agent and multiple anesthetic agents

**Flumazenil should be used with caution in the intensive care unit because of increased risk of unrecognized benzodiazepine dependence in such settings.**

**Adverse Reactions**

>10%: Gastrointestinal: Vomiting, nausea

1% to 10%:

Cardiovascular: Palpitations

Central nervous system: Headache, anxiety, nervousness, insomnia, abnormal crying, euphoria, depression, agitation, dizziness, emotional lability, ataxia, depersonalization, increased tears, dysphoria, paranoia

Endocrine & metabolic: Hot flashes

Gastrointestinal: Xerostomia

Local: Pain at injection site

Neuromuscular & skeletal: Tremor, weakness, paresthesia

Ocular: Abnormal vision, blurred vision

Respiratory: Dyspnea, hyperventilation

Miscellaneous: Diaphoresis

<1%: Abnormal hearing, arrhythmia, bradycardia, chest pain, confusion, generalized convulsions, hiccups, hypertension, shivering, somnolence, speech disorder, tachycardia, withdrawal syndrome

**Overdosage/Toxicology** Treatment: Management of suspected benzodiazepine overdose: 0.2 mg (2 mL) administered I.V. over 30 seconds; if desired level of consciousness is not obtained after 30 seconds, give 0.3 mg (3 mL) over another 30 seconds; further doses of 0.5 mg (5 mL) can be administered over 30 seconds at 1-minute intervals up to a cumulative dose of 3 mg (30 mL); on rare occasions, patients with partial response at 3 mg may require additional titration up to a total dose of 5 mg; if patient has not responded 5 minutes after cumulative dose of 5 mg, the major cause of sedation is likely not due to benzodiazepines.

**Drug Interactions Note:** Use with caution in overdosage involving mixed drug overdose; toxic effects may emerge (especially with cyclic antidepressants) with the reversal of the benzodiazepine effect by flumazenil

Benzodiazepines: Flumazenil may precipitate acute withdrawal reaction, including seizures, in patients who are habituated

(Continued)

## Flumazenil *(Continued)*

**Stability** For I.V. use only; **compatible** with $D_5W$, lactated Ringer's, or normal saline; once drawn up in the syringe or mixed with solution use within 24 hours; discard any unused solution after 24 hours

**Mechanism of Action** Competitively inhibits the activity at the benzodiazepine recognition site on the GABA/benzodiazepine receptor complex. Flumazenil does not antagonize the CNS effect of drugs affecting GABA-ergic neurons by means other than the benzodiazepine receptor (ethanol, barbiturates, general anesthetics) and does not reverse the effects of opioids

**Pharmacodynamics/kinetics**

Onset of action: 1-3 minutes; 80% response within 3 minutes

Peak effect: 6-10 minutes

Duration: Resedation occurs usually within 1 hour; duration is related to dose given and benzodiazepine plasma concentrations; reversal effects of flumazenil may wear off before effects of benzodiazepine

Distribution: 0.63-1.06 L/kg

Initial $V_d$: 0.5 L/kg

$V_{dss}$ 0.77-1.6 L/kg

Protein binding: 40% to 50%

Half-life, adults:

Alpha: 7-15 minutes

Terminal: 41-79 minutes

Elimination: Clearance dependent upon hepatic blood flow; hepatically eliminated, 0.2% unchanged in urine

**Usual Dosage** See table.

**Flumazenil**

| **Pediatric Dosage** Further studies are needed | |
|---|---|
| Pediatric dosage for **reversal of conscious sedation:** Intravenously through a freely running intravenous infusion into a large vein to minimize pain at the injection site | |
| Initial dose | 0.01 mg/kg over 15 seconds (maximum dose of 0.2 mg) |
| Repeat doses | 0.005-0.01 mg/kg (maximum dose of 0.2 mg) repeated at 1-minute intervals |
| Maximum total cumulative dose | 1 mg |
| Pediatric dosage for **management of benzodiazepine overdose:** Intravenously through a freely running intravenous infusion into a large vein to minimize pain at the injection site | |
| Initial dose | 0.01 mg/kg (maximum dose: 0.2 mg) |
| Repeat doses | 0.01 mg/kg (maximum dose of 0.2 mg) repeated at 1-minute intervals |
| Maximum total cumulative dose | 1 mg |
| In place of repeat bolus doses, follow-up continuous infusions of 0.005-0.01 mg/kg/h have been used; further studies are needed. | |
| **Adult Dosage** | |
| Adult dosage for **reversal of conscious sedation:** Intravenously through a freely running intravenous infusion into a large vein to minimize pain at the injection site | |
| Initial dose | 0.2 mg intravenously over 15 seconds |
| Repeat doses | If desired level of consciousness is not obtained, 0.2 mg may be repeated at 1-minute intervals. |
| Maximum total cumulative dose | 1 mg (usual dose 0.6-1 mg) **In the event of resedation:** Repeat doses may be given at 20-minute intervals with maximum of 1 mg/dose and 3 mg/h. |
| Adult dosage for **suspected benzodiazepine overdose:** Intravenously through a freely running intravenous infusion into a large vein to minimize pain at the injection site | |
| Initial dose | 0.2 mg intravenously over 30 seconds |
| Repeat doses | 0.5 mg over 30 seconds repeated at 1-minute intervals |
| Maximum total cumulative dose | 3 mg (usual dose 1-3 mg) Patients with a partial response at 3 mg may require additional titration up to a total dose of 5 mg. If a patient has not responded 5 minutes after cumulative dose of 5 mg, the major cause of sedation is not likely due to benzodiazepines. **In the event of resedation:** May repeat doses at 20-minute intervals with maximum of 1 mg/dose and 3 mg/h. |

Resedation: Repeated doses may be given at 20-minute intervals as needed; repeat treatment doses of 1 mg (at a rate of 0.5 mg/minute) should be given at any time and no more than 3 mg should be given in any hour. After intoxication with high doses of benzodiazepines, the duration of a single dose of flumazenil is not expected to exceed 1 hour; if desired, the period of wakefulness may be prolonged with repeated low intravenous doses of flumazenil, or by an infusion of 0.1-0.4 mg/hour. Most patients with benzodiazepine overdose will respond to a cumulative dose of 1-3 mg and doses >3 mg do not reliably produce additional effects. Rarely, patients with a partial response at 3 mg may require additional titration up to a total dose of 5 mg. **If a patient has not responded 5 minutes after receiving a cumulative dose of 5 mg, the major cause of sedation is not likely to be due to benzodiazepines.**

**Dosing in renal impairment:** Not significantly affected by renal failure ($Cl_{cr}$ <10 mL/minute) or hemodialysis beginning 1 hour after drug administration

**Dosing in hepatic impairment:** Initial dose of flumazenil used for initial reversal of benzodiazepine effects is not changed; however, subsequent doses in liver disease patients should be reduced in size or frequency

**Administration** For I.V. use only; give via freely running I.V. infusion into larger vein to decrease chance of pain, phlebitis

**Monitoring Parameters** Monitor patients for return of sedation or respiratory depression

**Patient Information** Flumazenil does not consistently reverse amnesia; do not engage in activities requiring alertness for 18-24 hours after discharge; resedation may occur in patients on long-acting benzodiazepines (such as diazepam)

**Nursing Implications** Compatible with $D_5W$, LR, NS

**Additional Information** Does **not** antagonize the CNS effects of other GABA agonists (such as ethanol, barbiturates, or general anesthetics), nor does it reverse narcotics

**Dosage Forms** Injection: 0.1 mg/mL (5 mL, 10 mL)

## Flunisolide (floo NIS oh lide)

**Related Information**

Asthma Guidelines *on page 773*

**U.S. Brand Names** AeroBid®-M Oral Aerosol Inhaler; AeroBid® Oral Aerosol Inhaler; Nasalide® Nasal Aerosol; Nasarel® Nasal Spray

**Canadian Brand Names** Bronalide®; Rhinalar®; Rhinaris®-F; Syn-Flunisolide

**Pharmacologic Category** Corticosteroid, Oral Inhaler; Corticosteroid, Nasal

**Use** Steroid-dependent asthma; nasal solution is used for seasonal or perennial rhinitis

**Effects on Mental Status** Dizziness and nervousness are common; may cause insomnia

**Effects on Psychiatric Treatment** None reported

**Pregnancy Risk Factor** C

**Contraindications** Known hypersensitivity to flunisolide, acute status asthmaticus; viral, tuberculosis, fungal or bacterial respiratory infections, or infections of nasal mucosa

**Warnings/Precautions** Use with caution in patients with hypothyroidism, cirrhosis, hypertension, congestive heart failure, ulcerative colitis, thromboembolic disorders; do not stop medication abruptly if on prolonged therapy; fatalities have occurred due to adrenal insufficiency in asthmatic patients during and after transfer from systemic corticosteroids to aerosol steroids; several months may be required for recovery of this syndrome; during this period, aerosol steroids do **not** provide the systemic steroid needed to treat patients having trauma, surgery or infections. When consumed in excessive quantities, systemic hypercorticism and adrenal suppression may occur; withdrawal and discontinuation of the corticosteroid should be done carefully. Controlled clinical studies have shown that inhaled and intranasal corticosteroids may cause a reduction in growth velocity in pediatric patients. Growth velocity provides a means of comparing the rate of growth among children of the same age.

In studies involving inhaled corticosteroids, the average reduction in growth velocity was approximately 1 cm (about 1/3 of an inch) per year. It appears that the reduction is related to dose and how long the child takes the drug.

FDA's Pulmonary and Allergy Drugs and Metabolic and Endocrine Drugs advisory committees discussed this issue at a July 1998 meeting. They recommended that the agency develop class-wide labeling to inform healthcare providers so they would understand this potential side effect and monitor growth routinely in pediatric patients who are treated with inhaled corticosteroids, intranasal corticosteroids or both.

Long-term effects of this reduction in growth velocity on final adult height are unknown. Likewise, it also has not yet been determined whether patients' growth will "catch up" if treatment in discontinued. Drug manufacturers will continue to monitor these drugs to learn more about long-term effects. Children are prescribed inhaled corticosteroids to treat asthma. Intranasal corticosteroids are generally used to prevent and treat allergy-related nasal symptoms.

Patients are advised not to stop using their inhaled or intranasal corticosteroids without first speaking to their healthcare providers about the benefits of these drugs compared to their risks.

**Adverse Reactions**

>10%:

Cardiovascular: Pounding heartbeat

Central nervous system: Dizziness, headache, nervousness
Dermatologic: Itching, rash
Endocrine & metabolic: Adrenal suppression, menstrual problems
Gastrointestinal: GI irritation, anorexia, sore throat, bitter taste
Local: Nasal burning, *Candida* infections of the nose or pharynx, atrophic rhinitis
Respiratory: Sneezing, coughing, upper respiratory tract infection, bronchitis, nasal congestion, nasal dryness
Miscellaneous: Increased susceptibility to infections

1% to 10%:
Central nervous system: Insomnia, psychic changes
Dermatologic: Acne, urticaria
Gastrointestinal: Increase in appetite, xerostomia, dry throat, loss of taste perception
Ocular: Cataracts
Respiratory: Epistaxis
Miscellaneous: Diaphoresis, loss of smell

<1%: Abdominal fullness, bronchospasm, shortness of breath

**Overdosage/Toxicology**
Signs and symptoms: When consumed in excessive quantities, systemic hypercorticism and adrenal suppression may occur
Treatment: In those cases when systemic hypercorticism and adrenal suppression occur, discontinuation and withdrawal of the corticosteroid should be done judiciously

**Drug Interactions** Expected interactions similar to other corticosteroids

**Usual Dosage**
Children >6 years:
Oral inhalation: 2 inhalations twice daily (morning and evening) up to 4 inhalations/day
Nasal: 1 spray each nostril twice daily (morning and evening), not to exceed 4 sprays/day each nostril

Adults:
Oral inhalation: 2 inhalations twice daily (morning and evening) up to 8 inhalations/day maximum
Nasal: 2 sprays each nostril twice daily (morning and evening); maximum dose: 8 sprays/day in each nostril

**Patient Information** Use as directed; do not use nasal preparations for oral inhalation. Do not increase dosage or discontinue abruptly without consulting prescriber. Review use of inhaler or spray with prescriber or follow package insert for directions. Keep oral inhaler clean and unobstructed. Always rinse mouth and throat after use of inhaler to prevent opportunistic infection. If you are also using an inhaled bronchodilator, wait 10 minutes before using this steroid aerosol. You may experience dizziness, anxiety, or blurred vision (rise slowly from sitting or lying position and use caution when driving or engaging in tasks requiring alertness until response to drug is known); or taste disturbance or aftertaste (frequent mouth care and mouth rinses may help). Report pounding heartbeat or chest pain; acute nervousness or inability to sleep; severe sneezing or nosebleed; difficulty breathing, sore throat, hoarseness, or bronchitis; respiratory difficulty or bronchospasms; disturbed menstrual pattern; vision changes; loss of taste or smell perception; or worsening of condition or lack of improvement.

**Administration:** Inhaler: Sit when using. Take deep breaths for 3-5 minutes, and clear nasal passages before administration (use decongestant as needed). Hold breath for 5-10 seconds after use, and wait 1-3 minutes between inhalations. Follow package insert instructions for use. Do not exceed maximum dosage. If also using inhaled bronchodilator, use before flunisolide. Rinse mouth and throat after use to reduce aftertaste and prevent candidiasis.

**Nursing Implications** Shake well before giving; do not use Nasalide® orally; throw out product after it has been opened for 3 months

**Dosage Forms**
Inhalant:
Nasal (Nasalide®, Nasarel™): 25 mcg/actuation [200 sprays] (25 mL)
Oral:
AeroBid®: 250 mcg/actuation [100 metered doses] (7 g)
AeroBid-M® (menthol flavor): 250 mcg/actuation [100 metered doses] (7 g)
Solution, spray: 0.025% [200 actuations] (25 mL)

## Fluocinolone (floo oh SIN oh lone)

**Related Information**
Corticosteroids Comparison Chart *on page 711*

**U.S. Brand Names** Derma-Smoothe/FS®; Fluonid®; Flurosyn®; FS Shampoo®; Synalar®; Synalar-HP®; Synemol®

**Canadian Brand Names** Lidemol®

**Pharmacologic Category** Corticosteroid, Topical

**Use** Relief of susceptible inflammatory dermatosis [low, medium, high potency topical corticosteroid]

**Effects on Mental Status** None reported

**Effects on Psychiatric Treatment** None reported

**Usual Dosage** Children and Adults: Topical: Apply a thin layer to affected area 2-4 times/day. Therapy should be discontinued when control is achieved; if no improvement is seen, reassessment of diagnosis may be necessary.

**Dosage Forms**
Cream, as acetonide: 0.01% (15 g, 60 g); 0.025% (15 g, 60 g)
Flurosyn®, Synalar®: 0.01% (15 g, 30 g, 60 g, 425 g)
Flurosyn®, Synalar®, Synemol®: 0.025% (15 g, 60 g, 425 g)
Synalar-HP®: 0.2% (12 g)
Ointment, topical, as acetonide: 0.025% (15 g, 60 g)
Flurosyn®, Synalar®: 0.025% (15 g, 30 g, 60 g, 425 g)
Oil, as acetonide (Derma-Smoothe/FS®): 0.01% (120 mL)
Shampoo, as acetonide (FS Shampoo®): 0.01% (180 mL)
Solution, topical, as acetonide: 0.01% (20 mL, 60 mL)
Fluonid®, Synalar®: 0.01% (20 mL, 60 mL)

## Fluocinonide (floo oh SIN oh nide)

**Related Information**
Corticosteroids Comparison Chart *on page 711*

**U.S. Brand Names** Lidex®; Lidex-E®

**Canadian Brand Names** Lyderm; Lydonide; Tiamol®; Topactin®; Topsyn®

**Pharmacologic Category** Corticosteroid, Topical

**Use** Anti-inflammatory, antipruritic, relief of inflammatory and pruritic manifestations [high potency topical corticosteroid]

**Effects on Mental Status** None reported

**Effects on Psychiatric Treatment** None reported

**Usual Dosage** Children and Adults: Topical: Apply thin layer to affected area 2-4 times/day depending on the severity of the condition. Therapy should be discontinued when control is achieved; if no improvement is seen, reassessment of diagnosis may be necessary.

**Dosage Forms**
Cream: 0.05% (15 g, 30 g, 60 g, 120 g)
Anhydrous, emollient (Lidex®): 0.05% (15 g, 30 g, 60 g, 120 g)
Aqueous, emollient (Lidex-E®): 0.05% (15 g, 30 g, 60 g, 120 g)
Gel, topical: 0.05% (15 g, 60 g)
Lidex®: 0.05% (15 g, 30 g, 60 g, 120 g)
Ointment, topical: 0.05% (15 g, 30 g, 60 g)
Lidex®: 0.05% (15 g, 30 g, 60 g, 120 g)
Solution, topical: 0.05% (20 mL, 60 mL)
Lidex®: 0.05% (20 mL, 60 mL)

♦ **Fluogen®** *see* Influenza Virus Vaccine *on page 287*

♦ **Fluohydrisone Acetate** *see* Fludrocortisone *on page 229*

♦ **Fluohydrocortisone Acetate** *see* Fludrocortisone *on page 229*

♦ **Fluonid®** *see* Fluocinolone *on page 231*

♦ **9α-Fluorohydrocortisone Acetate** *see* Fludrocortisone *on page 229*

## Fluorometholone (flure oh METH oh lone)

**U.S. Brand Names** Flarex®; Fluor-Op®; FML®; FML® Forte

**Pharmacologic Category** Corticosteroid, Ophthalmic; Corticosteroid, Topical

**Use** Inflammatory conditions of the eye, including keratitis, iritis, cyclitis, and conjunctivitis

**Effects on Mental Status** None reported

**Effects on Psychiatric Treatment** None reported

**Usual Dosage** Children >2 years and Adults: Ophthalmic:
Ointment: May be applied every 4 hours in severe cases; 1-3 times/day in mild to moderate cases
Solution: Instill 1-2 drops into conjunctival sac every hour during day, every 2 hours at night until favorable response is obtained, then use 1 drop every 4 hours; for mild to moderate inflammation, instill 1-2 drops into conjunctival sac 2-4 times/day

**Dosage Forms** Ophthalmic:
Ointment (FML®): 0.1% (3.5 g)
Suspension:
Flarex®, Fluor-Op®, FML®: 0.1% (2.5 mL, 5 mL, 10 mL)
FML® Forte: 0.25% (2 mL, 5 mL, 10 mL, 15 mL)

♦ **Fluor-Op®** *see* Fluorometholone *on page 231*

♦ **Fluoroplex® Topical** *see* Fluorouracil *on page 231*

## Fluorouracil (flure oh YOOR a sil)

**U.S. Brand Names** Adrucil® Injection; Efudex® Topical; Fluoroplex® Topical

**Pharmacologic Category** Antineoplastic Agent, Antimetabolite

**Use** Treatment of carcinoma of stomach, colon, rectum, breast, and pancreas; also used topically for management of multiple actinic keratoses and superficial basal cell carcinomas

**Effects on Mental Status** May cause drowsiness

**Effects on Psychiatric Treatment** Myelosuppression is common; use caution with clozapine and carbamazepine

(Continued)

## Fluorouracil *(Continued)*

**Usual Dosage** Refer to individual protocols

All dosages are based on the patient's actual weight. However, the estimated lean body mass (dry weight) is used if the patient is obese or if there has been a spurious weight gain due to edema, ascites or other forms of abnormal fluid retention.

Children and Adults:

I.V.: Initial: 400-500 mg/m²/day (12 mg/kg/day; maximum: 800 mg/day) for 4-5 days either as a single daily I.V. push or 4-day CIV

I.V.: Maintenance dose regimens:

200-250 mg/m² (6 mg/kg) every other day for 4 days repeated in 4 weeks

500-600 mg/m² (15 mg/kg) weekly as a CIV or I.V. push

I.V.: Concomitant with leucovorin:

370 mg/m²/day x 5 days

500-1000 mg/m² every 2 weeks

600 mg/m² weekly for 6 weeks

Although the manufacturer recommends no daily dose >800 mg, higher doses of up to 2 g/day are routinely administered by CIV; higher daily doses have been successfully used

Hemodialysis: Administer dose posthemodialysis

**Dosing adjustment/comments in hepatic impairment:** Bilirubin >5 mg/dL: Omit use

Topical:

Actinic or solar keratosis: Apply twice daily for 2-6 weeks

Superficial basal cell carcinomas: Apply 5% twice daily for at least 3-6 weeks and up to 10-12 weeks

**Dosage Forms**

Cream, topical:

Efudex®: 5% (25 g)

Fluoroplex®: 1% (30 g)

Injection (Adrucil®): 50 mg/mL (10 mL, 20 mL, 50 mL, 100 mL)

Solution, topical:

Efudex®: 2% (10 mL); 5% (10 mL)

Fluoroplex®: 1% (30 mL)

## Fluoxetine (floo OKS e teen)

**Related Information**

Antidepressant Agents Comparison Chart *on page 704*
Anxiety Disorders *on page 606*
Clinical Issues in the Use of Antidepressants *on page 627*
Discontinuation of Psychotropic Drugs - Withdrawal Symptoms and Recommendations *on page 798*
Mood Disorders *on page 600*
Patient Information - Antidepressants (SSRIs) *on page 639*
Pharmacokinetics of Selective Serotonin-Reuptake Inhibitors (SSRIs) *on page 723*
Special Populations - Pregnant and Breast-Feeding Patients *on page 668*
Teratogenic Risks of Psychotropic Medications *on page 812*

**Generic Available** Yes

**U.S. Brand Names** Prozac®; Sarafem™

**Synonyms** Fluoxetine Hydrochloride

**Pharmacologic Category** Antidepressant, Selective Serotonin Reuptake Inhibitor

**Use** Treatment of major depression; treatment of binge-eating and vomiting in patients with moderate-to-severe bulimia nervosa; obsessive-compulsive disorder; premenstrual dysphoric disorder (PMDD)

**Pregnancy Risk Factor** C

**Pregnancy/Breast-Feeding Implications** Breast-feeding is not recommended

**Contraindications** Hypersensitivity to this agent. Use of MAO inhibitors within prior 14 days; a MAO inhibitor should not be initiated until 5 weeks after the discontinuation of fluoxetine.

**Warnings/Precautions** Potential for severe reaction when used with MAO inhibitors - serotonin syndrome (hyperthermia, muscular rigidity, mental status changes/agitation, autonomic instability) may occur. Fluoxetine use has been associated with occurrences of significant rash and allergic events, including vasculitis, anaphylactoid reactions, and pulmonary inflammatory disease. May precipitate a shift to mania or hypomania in patients with bipolar disease. May cause insomnia, anxiety, nervousness or anorexia. Use with caution in patients where weight loss is undesirable. May impair cognitive or motor performance - caution operating hazardous machinery or driving. Use caution in patients with depression, particularly if suicidal risk may be present. Use caution in patients with a previous seizure disorder or condition predisposing to seizures such as brain damage, alcoholism, or concurrent therapy with other drugs which lower the seizure threshold. Use with caution in patients with hepatic or renal dysfunction and in elderly patients. May cause hyponatremia/SIADH. May increase the risks associated with electroconvulsive treatment. Use with caution in patients at risk of bleeding or receiving concurrent anticoagulant therapy - may cause impairment in platelet function. May alter glycemic control in patients with diabetes. Due to the long half-life of fluoxetine and its metabolites, the effects and interactions noted may persist for prolonged periods following discontinuation. May cause or exacerbate sexual dysfunction.

**Adverse Reactions** Predominant adverse effects are CNS and GI

>10%:

Central nervous system: Headache, nervousness, insomnia, anxiety, somnolence

Gastrointestinal: Nausea, diarrhea, xerostomia, anorexia

Neuromuscular & skeletal: Weakness

1% to 10%:

Cardiovascular: Vasodilation, palpitation, hypertension

Central nervous system: Amnesia, confusion, emotional lability, sleep disorder, dizziness, agitation, yawning

Dermatologic: Rash, pruritus

Endocrine & metabolic: SIADH, hypoglycemia, hyponatremia (elderly or volume-depleted patients)

Gastrointestinal: Dyspepsia, increased appetite, constipation, vomiting, flatulence, weight loss, weight gain

Genitourinary: Sexual dysfunction, urinary frequency

Neuromuscular & skeletal: Tremor

Ocular: Abnormal vision

Respiratory: Pharyngitis

Miscellaneous: Diaphoresis, fever, flu syndrome

<1%: Albuminuria, allergies, amenorrhea, anaphylactoid reactions, anemia, angina, aphthous stomatitis, arrhythmia, arthritis, asthma, bone pain, bursitis, CHF, cholelithiasis, colitis, dehydration, dysphagia, ecchymosis, edema, epistaxis, euphoria, extrapyramidal reactions (rare), gastritis, glossitis, gout, hallucinations, hiccups, hostility, hypercholesteremia, hyperventilation, hypokalemia, hypotension, hypothyroidism, leg cramps, myocardial infarction, suicidal ideation, syncope, tachycardia, visual disturbances

**Overdosage/Toxicology**

Signs and symptoms: Nausea, vomiting, agitation, hypomania, seizures

Treatment: Following initiation of essential overdose management, toxic symptoms should be treated. Seizures usually respond to diazepam I.V. boluses (5-10 mg for adults up to 30 mg or 0.25-0.4 mg/kg/dose for children up to 10 mg/dose). If seizures are unresponsive or recur, phenytoin or phenobarbital may be required.

**Drug Interactions** CYP2D6 enzyme substrate (minor), CYP3A3/4 enzyme substrate; CYP2C9 enzyme inducer; CYP1A2, 2C9, 2C19, 2D6, and 3A3/4 enzyme inhibitor

Amphetamines: SSRIs may increase the sensitivity to amphetamines, and amphetamines may increase the risk of serotonin syndrome

Benzodiazepines: Fluoxetine may inhibit the metabolism of alprazolam and diazepam resulting in elevated serum levels; monitor for increased sedation and psychomotor impairment

Beta-blockers: Fluoxetine may inhibit the metabolism of metoprolol and propranolol resulting in cardiac toxicity; monitor for bradycardia, hypotension, and heart failure if combination is used; not established for all beta-blockers (unlikely with atenolol or nadolol due to renal elimination)

Buspirone: Fluoxetine inhibits the reuptake of serotonin; combined use with a serotonin agonist (buspirone) may cause serotonin syndrome

Carbamazepine: Fluoxetine may inhibit the metabolism of carbamazepine resulting in increased carbamazepine levels and toxicity; monitor for altered carbamazepine response

Carvedilol: Serum concentrations may be increased; monitor carefully for increased carvedilol effect (hypotension and bradycardia)

Clozapine: Fluoxetine may increase serum levels of clozapine; levels may increase by 76%; monitor for increased effect/toxicity

Cyclosporine: Fluoxetine may increase serum levels of cyclosporine (and possibly tacrolimus); monitor

Cyproheptadine: May inhibit the effects of serotonin reuptake inhibitors (fluoxetine); monitor for altered antidepressant response; cyproheptadine acts as a serotonin agonist

Dextromethorphan: Fluoxetine inhibits the metabolism of dextromethorphan; visual hallucinations occurred in a patient receiving this combination; monitor for serotonin syndrome

Digoxin: Fluoxetine may increase serum levels of digoxin; monitor

Haloperidol: Fluoxetine may inhibit the metabolism of haloperidol and cause extrapyramidal symptoms (EPS); monitor patients for EPS if combination is utilized

HMG CoA reductase inhibitors: Fluoxetine may inhibit the metabolism of lovastatin and simvastatin resulting in myositis and rhabdomyolysis; these combinations are best avoided

Lithium: Patients receiving fluoxetine and lithium have developed neurotoxicity; if combination is used; monitor for neurotoxicity

Loop diuretics: Fluoxetine may cause hyponatremia; additive hyponatremic effects may be seen with combined use of a loop diuretic (bumetanide, furosemide, torsemide); monitor for hyponatremia

MAOIs: Fluoxetine should not be used with nonselective MAOIs (isocarboxazid, phenelzine); fatal reactions have been reported; wait 5 weeks after stopping fluoxetine before starting an MAOI and 2 weeks after stopping an MAOI before starting fluoxetine

Meperidine: Combined use with fluoxetine theoretically may increase the risk of serotonin syndrome

Nefazodone: May increase the risk of serotonin syndrome with SSRIs; monitor

Phenytoin: Fluoxetine inhibits the metabolism of phenytoin and may result in phenytoin toxicity; monitor for phenytoin toxicity (ataxia, confusion, dizziness, nystagmus, involuntary muscle movement)
Propafenone: Serum concentrations and/or toxicity may be increased by fluoxetine; avoid concurrent administration
Selegiline: Fluoxetine has been reported to cause mania or hypertension when combined with selegiline; this combination is best avoided. Concurrent use with SSRIs has also been reported to cause serotonin syndrome. As a MAO-B inhibitor, the risk of serotonin syndrome may be less than with nonselective MAO inhibitors.
Serotonin agonists: Theoretically may increase the risk of serotonin syndrome; includes sumatriptan, naratriptan, rizatriptan, and zolmitriptan
Sibutramine: May increase the risk of serotonin syndrome with SSRIs; avoid coadministration
SSRIs: Fluoxetine inhibits the reuptake of serotonin; combined use with other drugs which inhibit the reuptake may cause serotonin syndrome
Sympathomimetics: May increase the risk of serotonin syndrome with SSRIs
Tramadol: Fluoxetine combined with tramadol (serotonergic effects) may cause serotonin syndrome; monitor
Trazodone: Fluoxetine may inhibit the metabolism of trazodone resulting in increased toxicity; monitor
Tricyclic antidepressants: Fluoxetine inhibits the metabolism of tricyclic antidepressants (amitriptyline, desipramine, imipramine, nortriptyline) resulting is elevated serum levels; if combination is warranted, a low dose of TCA (10-25 mg/day) should be utilized
Tryptophan: Fluoxetine inhibits the reuptake of serotonin; combination with tryptophan, a serotonin precursor, may cause agitation and restlessness; this combination is best avoided
Valproic acid: Fluoxetine may increase serum levels of valproic acid; monitor
Venlafaxine: Sertraline may increase the risk of serotonin syndrome
Warfarin: Fluoxetine may alter the hypoprothombinemic response to warfarin; monitor

**Mechanism of Action** Inhibits CNS neuron serotonin reuptake; minimal or no effect on reuptake of norepinephrine or dopamine; does not significantly bind to alpha-adrenergic, histamine or cholinergic receptors

**Pharmacodynamics/kinetics**
Peak antidepressant effect: After >4 weeks
Absorption: Oral: Well absorbed
Metabolism: To norfluoxetine (active)
Half-life: Adults: 2-3 days for parent drug, 4-16 days for metabolite (norfluoxetine); due to long half-life, resolution of adverse reactions after discontinuation may be slow
Time to peak serum concentration: Within 6-8 hours
Elimination: In urine as fluoxetine (2.5% to 5%) and norfluoxetine (10%)

**Usual Dosage** Oral:
Children <18 years: Dose and safety not established; preliminary experience in children 6-14 years using initial doses of 20 mg/day have been reported
Adults: 20 mg/day in the morning; may increase after several weeks by 20 mg/day increments; maximum: 80 mg/day; doses >20 mg should be divided into morning and noon doses
Usual dosage range:
20-40 mg/day for depression
40-80 mg for OCD
60-80 mg/day for bulimia nervosa
**Note:** Lower doses of 5 mg/day have been used for initial treatment
Elderly: Some patients may require an initial dose of 10 mg/day with dosage increases of 10 and 20 mg every several weeks as tolerated; should not be taken at night unless patient experiences sedation
**Dosing adjustment in renal impairment:**
Single dose studies: Pharmacokinetics of fluoxetine and norfluoxetine were similar among subjects with all levels of impaired renal function, including anephric patients on chronic hemodialysis
Chronic administration: Additional accumulation of fluoxetine or norfluoxetine may occur in patients with severely impaired renal function
Hemodialysis: Not removed by hemodialysis
**Dosing adjustment in hepatic impairment:** Elimination half-life of fluoxetine is prolonged in patients with hepatic impairment; a lower or less frequent dose of fluoxetine should be used in these patients
Cirrhosis patients: Administer a lower dose or less frequent dosing interval
Compensated cirrhosis without ascites: Administer 50% of normal dose

**Dietary Considerations** Alcohol: Avoid use

**Monitoring Parameters** Signs and symptoms of depression, anxiety, sleep

**Reference Range**
Therapeutic: Fluoxetine: 100-800 ng/mL (SI: 289-2314 nmol/L); Norfluoxetine: 100-600 ng/mL (SI: 289-1735 nmol/L)
Toxic: Fluoxetine and norfluoxetine >2000 ng/mL

**Test Interactions** ↑ albumin in urine

**Patient Information** Take exactly as directed (do not increase dose or frequency); may take 2-3 weeks to achieve desired results; may cause physical and/or psychological dependence. Take once-a-day dose in the morning to reduce incidence of insomnia. Avoid excessive alcohol, caffeine, and other prescription or OTC medications not approved by prescriber. Maintain adequate hydration (2-3 L/day of fluids unless instructed to restrict fluid intake). You may experience drowsiness, lightheadedness, impaired coordination, dizziness, or blurred vision (use caution when driving or engaging in tasks requiring alertness until response to drug is known); constipation (increased exercise, fluids, or dietary fruit and fiber may help); anorexia (maintain regular dietary intake to avoid excessive weight loss); or postural hypotension (use caution when climbing stairs or changing position from lying or sitting to standing). If diabetic, monitor serum glucose closely (may cause hypoglycemia). Report persistent CNS effects (nervousness, restlessness, insomnia, anxiety, excitation, headache, sedation); rash or skin irritation; muscle cramping, tremors, or change in gait; respiratory depression or difficulty breathing; or worsening of condition.

**Nursing Implications** Offer patient sugarless hard candy for dry mouth

**Additional Information** EKG may reveal S-T segment depression; not shown to be teratogenic in rodents; 15-60 mg/day, buspirone and cyproheptadine, may be useful in treatment of sexual dysfunction during treatment with a selective serotonin reuptake inhibitor.

**Dosage Forms**
Capsule, as hydrochloride: 10 mg, 20 mg, 40 mg
Liquid, as hydrochloride (mint flavor): 20 mg/5 mL (120 mL)
Tablet, as hydrochloride: 10 mg, 20 mg

♦ **Fluoxetine Hydrochloride** *see* Fluoxetine *on page 232*

## Fluoxymesterone (floo oks i MES te rone)

**U.S. Brand Names** Halotestin®

**Pharmacologic Category** Androgen

**Use** Replacement of endogenous testicular hormone; in females, used as palliative treatment of breast cancer; stimulation of erythropoiesis, angioneurotic edema, postpartum breast engorgement

**Effects on Mental Status** None reported

**Effects on Psychiatric Treatment** May cause leukopenia; use caution with clozapine and carbamazepine

**Restrictions** C-III

**Pregnancy Risk Factor** X

**Contraindications** Serious cardiac disease, liver or kidney disease, hypersensitivity to fluoxymesterone or any component; pregnancy

**Warnings/Precautions** May accelerate bone maturation without producing compensatory gain in linear growth in children; in prepubertal children perform radiographic examination of the hand and wrist every 6 months to determine the rate of bone maturation and to assess the effect of treatment on the epiphyseal centers

**Adverse Reactions**
>10%:
Males: Priapism
Females: Menstrual problems (amenorrhea), virilism, breast soreness
Cardiovascular: Edema
Dermatologic: Acne
1% to 10%:
Males: Prostatic carcinoma, hirsutism (increase in pubic hair growth), impotence, testicular atrophy
Cardiovascular: Edema
Gastrointestinal: GI irritation, nausea, vomiting
Genitourinary: Prostatic hypertrophy
Hepatic: Hepatic dysfunction
<1%:
Males: Gynecomastia
Females: Amenorrhea
Cholestatic hepatitis, hepatic necrosis, hypercalcemia, hypersensitivity reactions, leukopenia, polycythemia

**Overdosage/Toxicology** Signs and symptoms: Abnormal liver function tests, water retention

**Drug Interactions**
Decreased effect:
Fluphenazine effectiveness with anticholinergics
Barbiturate levels and decreased fluphenazine effectiveness when given together
Increased toxicity:
Anticoagulants: Fluoxymesterone may suppress clotting factors II, V, VII, and X; therefore, bleeding may occur in patients on anticoagulant therapy
Cyclosporine: May elevate cyclosporine serum levels
Insulin: May enhance hypoglycemic effect of insulin therapy
May decrease blood glucose concentrations and insulin requirements in patients with diabetes
With ethanol, effects of both drugs may increase
EPSEs and other CNS effects may increase when coadministered with lithium
May potentiate the effects of narcotics including respiratory depression

**Usual Dosage** Adults: Oral:
Male:
Hypogonadism: 5-20 mg/day
(Continued)

## Fluoxymesterone *(Continued)*

Delayed puberty: 2.5-20 mg/day for 4-6 months

Female:

Inoperable breast carcinoma: 10-40 mg/day in divided doses for 1-3 months

Breast engorgement: 2.5 mg after delivery, 5-10 mg/day in divided doses for 4-5 days

**Patient Information** Take as directed; do not discontinue without consulting prescriber. Diabetics should monitor serum glucose closely and notify prescriber of changes; this medication can alter hypoglycemic requirements. You may experience acne, growth of body hair, loss of libido, impotence, or menstrual irregularity (usually reversible); nausea or vomiting (small frequent meals, frequent mouth care, sucking lozenges, or chewing gum may help). Report changes in menstrual pattern; deepening of voice or unusual growth of body hair; fluid retention (swelling of ankles, feet, or hands, difficulty breathing, or sudden weight gain); change in color of urine or stool; yellowing of eyes or skin; unusual bruising or bleeding; or other adverse reactions.

**Dosage Forms** Tablet: 2 mg, 5 mg, 10 mg

## Fluphenazine (floo FEN a zeen)

**Related Information**

Antipsychotic Agents Comparison Chart *on page 706*

Antipsychotic Medication Guidelines *on page 751*

Clinical Issues in the Use of Antipsychotics *on page 630*

Discontinuation of Psychotropic Drugs - Withdrawal Symptoms and Recommendations *on page 798*

Federal OBRA Regulations Recommended Maximum Doses *on page 756*

Liquid Compatibility With Antipsychotics and Mood Stabilizers *on page 718*

Patient Information - Antipsychotics (General) *on page 646*

Schizophrenia *on page 604*

Substance-Related Disorders *on page 609*

**Generic Available** Yes

**U.S. Brand Names** Permitil® Oral; Prolixin Decanoate® Injection; Prolixin Enanthate® Injection; Prolixin® Injection; Prolixin® Oral

**Canadian Brand Names** Apo®-Fluphenazine; Modecate®; Modecate® Enanthate; Moditen® Hydrochloride; PMS-Fluphenazine

**Synonyms** Fluphenazine Decanoate; Fluphenazine Enanthate; Fluphenazine Hydrochloride

**Pharmacologic Category** Antipsychotic Agent, Phenothazine, Piperazine

**Use** Management of manifestations of psychotic disorders and schizophrenia; depot formulation may offer improved outcome in individuals with psychosis who are noncompetent with oral antipsychotics

**Pregnancy Risk Factor** C

**Contraindications** Hypersensitivity to fluphenazine or any component (cross reactivity between phenothiazines may occur); severe CNS depression, coma, subcortical brain damage, blood dyscrasias, hepatic disease

**Warnings/Precautions** May be sedating, use with caution in disorders where CNS depression is a feature. Use with caution in Parkinson's disease. Caution in patients with hemodynamic instability; bone marrow suppression; predisposition to seizures; severe cardiac, renal, or respiratory disease. Esophageal dysmotility and aspiration have been associated with antipsychotic use - use with caution in patients at risk of pneumonia (ie, Alzheimer's disease). Caution in breast cancer or other prolactin-dependent tumors (may elevate prolactin levels). May alter temperature regulation or mask toxicity of other drugs due to antiemetic effects. May alter cardiac conduction; life-threatening arrhythmias have occurred with therapeutic doses of phenothiazines. Hypotension may occur, particularly with I.M. administration. May cause orthostatic hypotension - use with caution in patients at risk of this effect or those who would tolerate transient hypotensive episodes (cerebrovascular disease, cardiovascular disease, or other medications which may predispose). Adverse effects of depot injections may be prolonged.

Phenothiazines may cause anticholinergic effects (confusion, agitation, constipation, dry mouth, blurred vision, urinary retention). Therefore, they should be used with caution in patients with decreased gastrointestinal motility, urinary retention, BPH, xerostomia, or visual problems. Conditions which also may be exacerbated by cholinergic blockade include narrow-angle glaucoma (screening is recommended) and worsening of myasthenia gravis. Relative to other antipsychotics, fluphenazine has a low potency of cholinergic blockade.

May cause extrapyramidal reactions, including pseudoparkinsonism, acute dystonic reactions, akathisia and tardive dyskinesia (risk of these reactions is high relative to other antipsychotics). May be associated with neuroleptic malignant syndrome (NMS) or pigmentary retinopathy.

**Adverse Reactions**

Cardiovascular: Hypotension, tachycardia, fluctuations in blood pressure, hypertension, arrhythmias, edema

Central nervous system: Parkinsonian symptoms, akathisia, dystonias, tardive dyskinesia, dizziness, hyper-reflexia, headache, cerebral edema, drowsiness, lethargy, restlessness, excitement, bizarre dreams, EEG changes, depression, seizures, NMS, altered central temperature regulation

Dermatologic: Increased sensitivity to sun, rash, skin pigmentation, itching, erythema, urticaria, seborrhea, eczema, dermatitis

Endocrine & metabolic: Changes in menstrual cycle, breast pain, amenorrhea, galactorrhea, gynecomastia, changes in libido, elevated prolactin, SIADH

Gastrointestinal: Weight gain, loss of appetite, salivation, xerostomia, constipation, paralytic ileus, laryngeal edema

Genitourinary: Ejaculatory disturbances, impotence, polyuria, bladder paralysis, enuresis

Hematologic: Agranulocytosis, leukopenia, thrombocytopenia, nonthrombocytopenic purpura, eosinophilia, pancytopenia

Hepatic: Cholestatic jaundice, hepatotoxicity

Neuromuscular & skeletal: Trembling of fingers, SLE, facial hemispasm

Ocular: Pigmentary retinopathy, cornea and lens changes, blurred vision, glaucoma

Respiratory: Nasal congestion, asthma

**Overdosage/Toxicology**

Signs and symptoms: Deep sleep, hypotension or hypertension, dystonia, seizures, extrapyramidal symptoms, respiratory failure

Treatment: Following initiation of essential overdose management, toxic symptom treatment and supportive treatment should be initiated. Hypotension usually responds to I.V. fluids or Trendelenburg positioning. If unresponsive to these measures, the use of a parenteral inotrope may be required. Seizures commonly respond to diazepam (I.V. 5-10 mg bolus in adults every 15 minutes if needed up to a total of 30 mg; I.V. 0.25-0.4 mg/kg/dose up to a total of 10 mg in children) or to phenytoin or phenobarbital. Cardiac arrhythmias often respond to I.V. lidocaine while other antiarrhythmics can be used. Neuroleptics often cause extrapyramidal symptoms (eg, dystonic reactions) requiring management; benztropine mesylate I.V. 1-2 mg (adults) may be effective. These agents are generally effective within 2-5 minutes.

**Drug Interactions** CYP2D6 enzyme substrate; CYP2D6 enzyme inhibitor

Aluminum salts: May decrease the absorption of phenothiazines; monitor

Amphetamines: Efficacy may be diminished by antipsychotics; in addition, amphetamines may increase psychotic symptoms. Avoid concurrent use

Anticholinergics: May inhibit the therapeutic response to phenothiazines and excess anticholinergic effects may occur; includes benztropine, trihexyphenidyl, biperiden, and drugs with significant anticholinergic activity (TCAs, antihistamines, disopyramide)

Antihypertensives: Concurrent use of phenothiazines with an antihypertensive may produce additive hypotensive effects (particularly orthostasis)

Bromocriptine: Phenothiazines inhibit the ability of bromocriptine to lower serum prolactin concentrations

CNS depressants: Sedative effects may be additive with phenothiazines; monitor for increased effect; includes barbiturates, benzodiazepines, narcotic analgesics, ethanol, and other sedative agents

CYP2D6 inhibitors: Metabolism of phenothiazines may be decreased; increasing clinical effect or toxicity; inhibitors include amiodarone, cimetidine, delavirdine, fluoxetine, paroxetine, propafenone, quinidine, and ritonavir; monitor for increased effect/toxicity

Enzyme inducers: May enhance the hepatic metabolism of phenothiazines; larger doses may be required; includes rifampin, rifabutin, barbiturates, phenytoin, and cigarette smoking

Epinephrine: Chlorpromazine (and possibly other low potency antipsychotics) may diminish the pressor effects of epinephrine

Guanethidine and guanadrel: Antihypertensive effects may be inhibited by phenothiazines

Levodopa: Phenothiazines may inhibit the antiparkinsonian effect of levodopa; avoid this combination

Lithium: Phenothiazines may produce neurotoxicity with lithium; this is a rare effect

Phenytoin: May reduce serum levels of phenothiazines; phenothiazines may increase phenytoin serum levels

Propranolol: Serum concentrations of phenothiazines may be increased; propranolol also increases phenothiazine concentrations

Polypeptide antibiotics: Rare cases of respiratory paralysis have been reported with concurrent use of phenothiazines

QTc prolonging agents: Effects on QTc interval may be additive with phenothiazines, increasing the risk of malignant arrhythmias; includes type Ia antiarrhythmics, TCAs, and some quinolone antibiotics (sparfloxacin, moxifloxacin and gatifloxacin)

Sulfadoxine-pyrimethamine: May increase phenothiazine concentrations

Tricyclic antidepressants: Concurrent use may produce increased toxicity or altered therapeutic response

Trazodone: Phenothiazines and trazodone may produce additive hypotensive effects

Valproic acid: Serum levels may be increased by phenothiazines

**Stability** Avoid freezing; protect all dosage forms from light; clear or slightly yellow solutions may be used; should be dispensed in amber or opaque vials/bottles. Solutions may be diluted or mixed with fruit juices or other liquids but must be administered immediately after mixing; do not prepare bulk dilutions or store bulk dilutions.

**Mechanism of Action** Blocks postsynaptic mesolimbic dopaminergic $D_1$ and $D_2$ receptors in the brain; depresses the release of hypothalamic and hypophyseal hormones; believed to depress the reticular activating system thus affecting basal metabolism, body temperature, wakefulness, vasomotor tone, and emesis

**Pharmacodynamics/kinetics**

Following I.M. or S.C. administration (derivative dependent):

Decanoate (lasts the longest and requires more time for onset):

Onset of action: 24-72 hours

Peak neuroleptic effect: Within 48-96 hours

Hydrochloride salt (acts quickly and persists briefly):

Onset of activity: Within 1 hour

Duration: 6-8 hours

Distribution: Crosses the placenta; appears in breast milk

Metabolism: In the liver

Half-life: Derivative dependent:

Enanthate: 84-96 hours

Hydrochloride: 33 hours

Decanoate: 163-232 hours

**Usual Dosage** Adults:

Oral: 0.5-10 mg/day in divided doses at 6- to 8-hour intervals; some patients may require up to 40 mg/day

I.M.: 2.5-10 mg/day in divided doses at 6- to 8-hour intervals (parenteral dose is $^1/_3$ to $^1/_2$ the oral dose for the hydrochloride salts)

I.M. (decanoate): 12.5 mg every 2 weeks

Conversion from hydrochloride to decanoate I.M. 0.5 mL (12.5 mg) decanoate every 3 weeks is approximately equivalent to 10 mg hydrochloride/day

I.M. (enanthate): 12.5-25 mg every 2 weeks

Hemodialysis: Not dialyzable (0% to 5%)

**Dietary Considerations** Alcohol: Additive CNS effect, avoid use

**Administration** I.M. dose is 4-10 times the activity of oral dose; decanoate should be administered by Z track method

**Monitoring Parameters** EKG monitoring for 48 hours

**Reference Range** Therapeutic: 5-20 ng/mL (SI: 10-40 nmol/L)

**Test Interactions** ↑ cholesterol (S), glucose; ↓ uric acid (S)

**Patient Information** Avoid alcoholic beverages, may cause drowsiness, do not discontinue without consulting physician

**Nursing Implications** Avoid contact of oral solution or injection with skin (contact dermatitis); watch for hypotension when administering I.M. or I.V.; oral liquid to be diluted in the following **only**: water, saline, 7-UP®, homogenized milk, carbonated orange beverages, pineapple, apricot, prune, orange, V8® juice, tomato, and grapefruit juices

**Additional Information** Less sedative and hypotensive effects than chlorpromazine

**Dosage Forms**

Concentrate, as hydrochloride:

Permitil®: 5 mg/mL with alcohol 1% (118 mL)

Prolixin®: 5 mg/mL with alcohol 14% (120 mL)

Elixir, as hydrochloride (Prolixin®): 2.5 mg/5 mL with alcohol 14% (60 mL, 473 mL)

Injection, as decanoate (Prolixin Decanoate®): 25 mg/mL (1 mL, 5 mL)

Injection, as enanthate (Prolixin Enanthate®): 25 mg/mL (5 mL)

Injection, as hydrochloride (Prolixin®): 2.5 mg/mL (10 mL)

Tablet, as hydrochloride

Permitil®: 2.5 mg, 5 mg, 10 mg

Prolixin®: 1 mg, 2.5 mg, 5 mg, 10 mg

♦ **Fluphenazine Decanoate** *see* Fluphenazine *on page 234*

♦ **Fluphenazine Enanthate** *see* Fluphenazine *on page 234*

♦ **Fluphenazine Hydrochloride** *see* Fluphenazine *on page 234*

## Flurazepam (flure AZ e pam)

**Related Information**

Anxiolytic/Hypnotic Use in Long-Term Care Facilities *on page 754*

Benzodiazepines Comparison Chart *on page 708*

Federal OBRA Regulations Recommended Maximum Doses *on page 756*

Patient Information - Anxiolytics & Sedative Hypnotics (Benzodiazepines) *on page 653*

**Generic Available** Yes

**U.S. Brand Names** Dalmane®

**Canadian Brand Names** Apo®-Flurazepam; Novo-Flupam; PMS-Flupam; Somnol®; Som Pam®

**Synonyms** Flurazepam Hydrochloride

**Pharmacologic Category** Benzodiazepine

**Use** Short-term treatment of insomnia

**Restrictions** C-IV

**Pregnancy Risk Factor** X

**Contraindications** Hypersensitivity to this drug or any component of its formulation (cross-sensitivity with other benzodiazepines may exist); narrow-angle glaucoma; pregnancy

**Warnings/Precautions** Use with caution in elderly or debilitated patients, patients with hepatic disease (including alcoholics), or renal impairment. Active metabolites with extended half-lives may lead to delayed accumulation and adverse effects. Use with caution in patients with respiratory disease, or impaired gag reflex. Avoid use in patients with sleep apnea.

Causes CNS depression (dose-related) resulting in sedation, dizziness, confusion, or ataxia which may impair physical and mental capabilities. Patients must be cautioned about performing tasks which require mental alertness (ie, operating machinery or driving). Use with caution in patients receiving other CNS depressants or psychoactive agents. Effects with other sedative drugs or ethanol may be potentiated. Benzodiazepines have been associated with falls and traumatic injury and should be used with extreme caution in patients who are at risk of these events (especially the elderly).

Use caution in patients with depression, particularly if suicidal risk may be present. Use with caution in patients with a history of drug dependence. Benzodiazepines have been associated with dependence and acute withdrawal symptoms on discontinuation or reduction in dose. Acute withdrawal, including seizures, may be precipitated in patients after administration of flumazenil to patients receiving long-term benzodiazepine therapy.

As a hypnotic, should be used only after evaluation of potential causes of sleep disturbance. Failure of sleep disturbance to resolve after 7-10 days may indicate psychiatric or medical illness. A worsening of insomnia or the emergence of new abnormalities of thought or behavior may represent unrecognized psychiatric or medical illness and requires immediate and careful evaluation.

Benzodiazepines have been associated with anterograde amnesia. Paradoxical reactions, including hyperactive or aggressive behavior have been reported with benzodiazepines, particularly in adolescent/pediatric or psychiatric patients. Does not have analgesic, antidepressant, or antipsychotic properties.

**Adverse Reactions**

Cardiovascular: Palpitations, chest pain

Central nervous system: Drowsiness, ataxia, lightheadedness, memory impairment, depression, headache, hangover, confusion, nervousness, dizziness, falling, apprehension, irritability, euphoria, slurred speech, restlessness, hallucinations, paradoxical reactions, talkativeness

Dermatologic: Rash, pruritus

Gastrointestinal: Xerostomia, constipation, excessive salivation, heartburn, upset stomach, nausea, vomiting, diarrhea, increased or decreased appetite, bitter taste, weight gain or loss, increased salivation

Hematologic: Euphoria, granulocytopenia

Hepatic: Elevated AST/ALT, total bilirubin, alkaline phosphatase, cholestatic jaundice

Neuromuscular & skeletal: Dysarthria, body/joint pain, reflex slowing, weakness

Ocular: Blurred vision, burning eyes, difficulty focusing

Otic: Tinnitus

Respiratory: Apnea, shortness of breath

Miscellaneous: Diaphoresis, drug dependence

**Overdosage/Toxicology**

Signs and symptoms: Respiratory depression, hypoactive reflexes, unsteady gait, hypotension

Treatment: Supportive; rarely is mechanical ventilation required. Flumazenil has been shown to selectively block the binding of benzodiazepines to CNS receptors, resulting in a reversal of benzodiazepine-induced CNS depression.

**Drug Interactions** CYP3A3/4 enzyme substrate

CNS depressants: Sedative effects and/or respiratory depression may be additive with CNS depressants; includes ethanol, barbiturates, narcotic analgesics, and other sedative agents; monitor for increased effect

Enzyme inducers: Metabolism of some benzodiazepines may be increased, decreasing their therapeutic effect; consider using an alternative sedative/hypnotic agent; potential inducers include phenobarbital, phenytoin, carbamazepine, rifampin, and rifabutin

CYP3A3/4 inhibitors: Serum level and/or toxicity of some benzodiazepines may be increased; inhibitors include amiodarone, cimetidine, clarithromycin, erythromycin, delavirdine, diltiazem, dirithromycin, disulfiram, fluoxetine, fluvoxamine, grapefruit juice, indinavir, itraconazole, ketoconazole, nefazodone, nevirapine, propoxyfene, quinupristin-dalfopristin, ritonavir, saquinavir, verapamil, zafirlukast, zileuton; monitor for altered benzodiazepine response

Oral contraceptives: May decrease the clearance of some benzodiazepines (those which undergo oxidative metabolism); monitor for increased benzodiazepine effect

Theophylline: May partially antagonize some of the effects of benzodiazepines; monitor for decreased response; may require higher doses for sedation

**Stability** Store in light-resistant containers

**Mechanism of Action** Binds to stereospecific benzodiazepine receptors on the postsynaptic GABA neuron at several sites within the central nervous system, including the limbic system, reticular formation. Enhancement of the inhibitory effect of GABA on neuronal excitability results by increased neuronal membrane permeability to chloride ions. This shift in (Continued)

## Flurazepam *(Continued)*

chloride ions results in hyperpolarization (a less excitable state) and stabilization.

**Pharmacodynamics/kinetics**
Onset of hypnotic effect: 15-20 minutes
Peak: 3-6 hours
Duration of action: 7-8 hours
Metabolism: In the liver to N-desalkylflurazepam (active)
Half-life: Adults: 40-114 hours

**Usual Dosage** Oral:
Children:
<15 years: Dose not established
>15 years: 15 mg at bedtime
Adults: 15-30 mg at bedtime

**Dietary Considerations** Alcohol: Additive CNS effect, avoid use

**Monitoring Parameters** Respiratory and cardiovascular status

**Reference Range** Therapeutic: 0-4 ng/mL (SI: 0-9 nmol/L); Metabolite N-desalkylflurazepam: 20-110 ng/mL (SI: 43-240 nmol/L); Toxic: >0.12 µg/mL

**Test Interactions** ↑ liver enzymes

**Patient Information** Avoid alcohol and other CNS depressants; avoid activities needing good psychomotor coordination until CNS effects are known; drug may cause physical or psychological dependence; avoid abrupt discontinuation after prolonged use

**Nursing Implications** Provide safety measures (ie, side rails, night light, and call button); remove smoking materials from area; supervise ambulation; avoid abrupt discontinuance in patients with prolonged therapy or seizure disorders

**Additional Information** Abrupt discontinuation after sustained use (generally >10 days) may cause withdrawal symptoms

**Dosage Forms** Capsule, as hydrochloride: 15 mg, 30 mg

♦ **Flurazepam Hydrochloride** *see* Flurazepam *on page 235*

## Flurbiprofen (flure BI proe fen)

**Related Information**
Nonsteroidal Anti-inflammatory Agents Comparison Chart *on page 722*

**U.S. Brand Names** Ansaid® Oral; Ocufen® Ophthalmic

**Canadian Brand Names** Apo®-Flurbiprofen; Froben®; Froben-SR®; Novo-Flurprofen; Nu-Flurprofen

**Pharmacologic Category** Nonsteroidal Anti-Inflammatory Agent (NSAID)

**Use** Inhibition of intraoperative miosis; acute or long-term treatment of signs and symptoms of rheumatoid arthritis and osteoarthritis; prevention and management of postoperative ocular inflammation and postoperative cystoid macular edema remains to be determined

**Effects on Mental Status** Dizziness is common; may cause nervousness; may rarely cause drowsiness, confusion, depression, or hallucinations

**Effects on Psychiatric Treatment** May rarely cause agranulocytosis; use caution with clozapine and carbamazepine; may decrease the clearance of lithium resulting in elevated serum levels and potential toxicity; monitor serum lithium levels

**Pregnancy Risk Factor** C (D if used in third trimester)

**Contraindications** Dendritic keratitis, hypersensitivity to flurbiprofen or any component

**Warnings/Precautions** Should be used with caution in patients with a history of herpes simplex, keratitis, and patients who might be affected by inhibition of platelet aggregation; dehydration; slowing of corneal wound healing patients in whom asthma, rhinitis, or urticaria is precipitated by aspirin or other NSAIDs.

**Adverse Reactions**
Ophthalmic:
>10%: Ocular: Slowing of corneal wound healing, mild ocular stinging, itching and burning eyes, ocular irritation
1% to 10%: Ocular: Eye redness
Oral:
>10%:
Central nervous system: Dizziness
Dermatologic: Rash
Gastrointestinal: Abdominal cramps, heartburn, indigestion, nausea
1% to 10%:
Central nervous system: Headache, nervousness
Dermatologic: Itching
Endocrine & metabolic: Fluid retention
Gastrointestinal: Vomiting
Otic: Tinnitus
<1%: Acute renal failure, agranulocytosis, allergic rhinitis, anemia, angioedema, arrhythmias, aseptic meningitis, blurred vision, bone marrow suppression, confusion, congestive heart failure, conjunctivitis, cystitis, decreased hearing, drowsiness, dry eyes, epistaxis, erythema multiforme, gastritis, GI ulceration, hallucinations, hemolytic anemia, hepatitis, hot flashes, hypertension, insomnia, leukopenia, mental depression, peripheral neuropathy, polydipsia, polyuria, shortness of breath, Stevens-Johnson syndrome, tachycardia, thrombocytopenia, toxic amblyopia, toxic epidermal necrolysis, urticaria

**Overdosage/Toxicology**
Signs and symptoms: Apnea, metabolic acidosis, coma, and nystagmus; leukocytosis, renal failure
Treatment: Management of a nonsteroidal anti-inflammatory drug (NSAID) intoxication is primarily supportive and symptomatic. Fluid therapy is commonly effective in managing the hypotension that may occur following an acute NSAIDs overdose, except when this is due to an acute blood loss. Seizures tend to be very short-lived and often do not require drug treatment; although, recurrent seizures should be treated with I.V. diazepam. Since many of the NSAID undergo enterohepatic cycling, multiple doses of charcoal may be needed to reduce the potential for delayed toxicities.

**Drug Interactions** CYP2C9 enzyme substrate; CYP2C9 enzyme inhibitor
Decreased effect: When used concurrently with flurbiprofen, reports acetylcholine chloride and carbachol being ineffective; ACE inhibitor effects may be decreased by concurrent therapy with NSAIDs

**Usual Dosage**
Oral: Rheumatoid arthritis and osteoarthritis: 200-300 mg/day in 2-, 3-, or 4 divided doses
Ophthalmic: Instill 1 drop every 30 minutes, 2 hours prior to surgery (total of 4 drops to each affected eye)

**Patient Information**
Oral: Take this medication exactly as directed; do not increase dose without consulting prescriber. Do not crush tablets or break capsules. Take with food or milk to reduce GI distress. Maintain adequate fluid intake (2-3 L/day of fluids unless instructed to restrict fluid intake). Do not use alcohol, aspirin, or aspirin-containing medication, and all other anti-inflammatory medications without consulting prescriber. You may experience drowsiness, dizziness, nervousness, or headache (use caution when driving or engaging in tasks requiring alertness until response to drug is known); anorexia, nausea, vomiting, or heartburn (frequent small meals, frequent mouth care, sucking lozenges, or chewing gum may help); fluid retention (weigh yourself weekly and report unusual (3-5 lb/week) weight gain). GI bleeding, ulceration, or perforation can occur with or without pain; discontinue medication and contact prescriber if persistent abdominal pain or cramping, or blood in stool occurs. Report breathlessness, difficulty breathing, or unusual cough; chest pain, rapid heartbeat, palpitations; unusual bruising/bleeding; blood in urine, stool, mouth, or vomitus; swollen extremities; skin rash or itching; acute fatigue; changes in hearing or ringing in ears.
Ophthalmic: Wash hands before instilling. Sit or lie down to instill. Open eye, look at ceiling, and instill prescribed amount of medication. Close eye and roll eye in all directions, and apply gentle pressure to inner corner of eye. Do not let tip of applicator touch eye or contaminate tip of applicator. Use protective dark eyewear until healed; avoid direct sunlight. Temporary stinging or burning may occur. Report persistent pain, burning, redness, vision disturbances, swelling, itching, or worsening of condition.

**Nursing Implications** Care should be taken to avoid contamination of the solution container tip

**Dosage Forms**
Solution, ophthalmic, as sodium (Ocufen®): 0.03% (2.5 mL, 5 mL, 10 mL)
Tablet, as sodium (Ansaid®): 50 mg, 100 mg

♦ **5-Flurocytosine** *see* Flucytosine *on page 228*

♦ **Flurosyn®** *see* Fluocinolone *on page 231*

## Flutamide (FLOO ta mide)

**U.S. Brand Names** Eulexin®

**Canadian Brand Names** Novo-Flutamide

**Pharmacologic Category** Antiandrogen

**Use** In combination therapy with LHRH agonist analogues in treatment of metastatic prostatic carcinoma. A study has shown that the addition of flutamide to leuprolide therapy in patients with advanced prostatic cancer increased median actuarial survival time to 34.9 months versus 27.9 months with leuprolide alone. To achieve benefit to combination therapy, both drugs need to be started simultaneously.

**Effects on Mental Status** May rarely cause nervousness or confusion

**Effects on Psychiatric Treatment** None reported

**Pregnancy Risk Factor** D

**Contraindications** Known hypersensitivity to flutamide

**Warnings/Precautions** The U.S. Food and Drug Administration (FDA) currently recommends that procedures for proper handling and disposal of antineoplastic agents be considered. Animal data (based on using doses higher than recommended for humans) produced testicular interstitial cell adenoma. Do not discontinue therapy without physician's advice. May cause hepatic failure, which can be fatal. Serum transaminases should be monitored at baseline and monthly for the first four months of therapy, and periodically thereafter. These should also be repeated at the first sign and symptom of liver dysfunction. Use of flutamide is not recommended in patients with baseline elevation of transaminase levels (> twice the upper limit of normal). Flutamide should be discontinued immediately at any time if the patient develops jaundice or elevation in serum transaminase levels (>2 times upper limit of normal).

**Adverse Reactions**

>10%:

Gastrointestinal: Nausea, vomiting, diarrhea

Genitourinary: Impotence

Endocrine & metabolic: Loss of libido, hot flashes

1% to 10%:

Endocrine & metabolic: Gynecomastia

Gastrointestinal: Anorexia

Neuromuscular & skeletal: Numbness in extremities

<1%: Confusion, edema, drowsiness, hepatitis, hypertension, nervousness

**Overdosage/Toxicology**

Signs and symptoms: Hypoactivity, ataxia, anorexia, vomiting, slow respiration, lacrimation

Treatment: Management is supportive, dialysis not of benefit; induce vomiting

**Drug Interactions** CYP3A3/4 enzyme substrate

**Usual Dosage** Adults: Oral: 2 capsules every 8 hours for a total daily dose of 750 mg

**Patient Information** Take as directed; do not discontinue without consulting prescriber. You may experience decreased libido, impotence, swelling of breasts, or decreased appetite (small frequent meals may help). Report chest pain or palpitation; acute abdominal pain; pain, tingling, or numbness of extremities; swelling of extremities or unusual weight gain; difficulty breathing; or other persistent adverse effects.

**Dosage Forms** Capsule: 125 mg

♦ **Flutex®** *see* Triamcinolone *on page 563*

## Fluticasone (floo TIK a sone)

**Related Information**

Asthma Guidelines *on page 773*

Corticosteroids Comparison Chart *on page 711*

**U.S. Brand Names** Cutivate™; Flonase®; Flovent®

**Pharmacologic Category** Corticosteroid, Oral Inhaler; Corticosteroid, Nasal

**Use**

Inhalation: Maintenance treatment of asthma as prophylactic therapy. It is also indicated for patients requiring oral corticosteroid therapy for asthma to assist in total discontinuation or reduction of total oral dose. NOT indicated for the relief of acute bronchospasm.

Intranasal: Management of seasonal and perennial allergic rhinitis in patients ≥12 years of age

Topical: Relief of inflammation and pruritus associated with corticosteroid-responsive dermatoses [medium potency topical corticosteroid]

**Effects on Mental Status** None reported

**Effects on Psychiatric Treatment** None reported

**Usual Dosage**

Flovent® Rotadisk can now be used in children ≥4 years; Flovent® is still indicated for use ≥12 years of age

Topical product (Cutivate™) approved for use in pediatric patients ≥3 months of age

Children ≥4 years and Adolescents:

Intranasal: Initial: 1 spray (50 mcg/spray) per nostril once daily. Patients not adequately responding or patients with more severe symptoms may use 2 sprays (100 mcg) per nostril. Depending on response, dosage may be reduced to 50 mcg in each nostril daily. Total daily dosage should not exceed 2 sprays in each nostril (200 mcg)/day.

Adults:

Inhalation, Oral:

**Recommended Oral Inhalation Doses**

| Previous Therapy | Recommended Starting Dose | Recommended Highest Dose |
|---|---|---|
| Bronchodilator alone | 88 mcg twice daily | 440 mcg twice daily |
| Inhaled corticosteroids | 88–220 mcg twice daily | 440 mcg twice daily |
| Oral corticosteroids | 880 mcg twice daily | 880 mcg twice daily |

Intranasal: Initial: 2 sprays (50 mcg/spray) per nostril once daily; after the first few days, dosage may be reduced to 1 spray per nostril once daily for maintenance therapy; maximum total daily dose should not exceed 4 sprays (200 mcg)/day

Adults and Children ≥3 months of age: Topical: Apply sparingly in a thin film twice daily. Therapy should be discontinued when control is achieved. If no improvement is seen, reassessment of diagnosis may be necessary.

**Dosage Forms**

Spray, aerosol, oral inhalation (Flovent®): 44 mcg/actuation (7.9 g = 60 actuations or 13 g = 120 actuations), 110 mcg/actuation (13 g = 120 actuations); 220 mcg/actuation (13 g = 120 actuations)

Spray, intranasal (Flonase®): 50 mcg/actuation (16 g = 120 actuations)

Topical (Cutivate™):

Cream: 0.05% (15 g, 30 g, 60 g)

Ointment: 0.005% (15 g, 60 g )

## Fluvastatin (FLOO va sta tin)

**Related Information**

Lipid-Lowering Agents Comparison Chart *on page 717*

**U.S. Brand Names** Lescol®

**Synonyms** Fluindostatin

**Pharmacologic Category** Antilipemic Agent (HMG-CoA Reductase Inhibitor)

**Use** Adjunct to dietary therapy to decrease elevated serum total and LDL cholesterol concentrations in primary hypercholesterolemia

**Effects on Mental Status** May cause dizziness, insomnia, or drowsiness

**Effects on Psychiatric Treatment** None reported

**Pregnancy Risk Factor** X

**Contraindications** Hypersensitivity to fluvastatin or any component; active liver disease; unexplained persistent elevations of serum transaminases; pregnancy

**Warnings/Precautions** Liver function must be monitored by periodic laboratory assessment. Rhabdomyolysis with acute renal failure has occurred with other HMG-CoA reductase inhibitors. Risk is increased with concurrent use of clarithromycin, danazol, diltiazem, fluvoxamine, indinavir, nefazodone, nelfinavir, ritonavir, verapamil, troleandomycin, cyclosporine, fibric acid derivatives, erythromycin, niacin, or azole antifungals. The risk of combining any of these drugs with fluvastatin is minimal. Temporarily discontinue in any patient experiencing an acute or serious condition predisposing to renal failure secondary to rhabdomyolysis. Use caution in patients with previous liver disease or heavy alcohol use. Treatment in patients <18 years of age is not recommended.

**Adverse Reactions**

>10%: Respiratory: Upper respiratory infection (16%)

1% to 10%:

Central nervous system: Headache (9%), dizziness (2%), insomnia (2% to 3%), fatigue (2% to 3%)

Dermatologic: Rash (2% to 3%)

Gastrointestinal: Dyspepsia (8%), diarrhea (5%), nausea/vomiting (3%), constipation (2% to 3%), flatulence (2% to 3%), abdominal pain (5%)

Neuromuscular & skeletal: Back pain/myalgia (5% to 6%), arthropathy (2% to 4%)

Miscellaneous: Cold/flu symptoms (2% to 5%)

**Overdosage/Toxicology** Signs and symptoms: No symptomatology has been reported in cases of significant overdosage, however, supportive measure should be instituted, as required; dialyzability is not known

**Drug Interactions** CYP2C9 enzyme substrate; CYP2C9, 2C18, and 2C19 enzyme inhibitor

Cimetidine increases fluvastatin blood levels

Cholestyramine reduces fluvastatin absorption; separate administration times by at least 4 hours

Cholestyramine and colestipol (bile acid sequestrants): Cholesterol-lowering effects are additive

Clofibrate and fenofibrate may increase the risk of myopathy and rhabdomyolysis

Gemfibrozil: Increased risk of myopathy and rhabdomyolysis

Omeprazole increases fluvastatin blood levels

Ranitidine increases fluvastatin blood levels

Rifampin decreases fluvastatin blood levels

Ritonavir increases fluvastatin blood levels

Warfarin: Hypoprothrombinemic response is increased; monitor INR closely when fluvastatin is initiated or discontinued

**Usual Dosage** Adults: Oral:

Initial dose: 20-40 mg at bedtime

Usual dose: 20-80 mg at bedtime

**Note:** Splitting the 80 mg dose into a twice daily regimen may provide a modest improvement in LDL response. Maximum response occurs within 4-6 weeks. Decrease dose and monitor effects carefully in patients with hepatic insufficiency.

**Patient Information** Take at bedtime since highest rate of cholesterol synthesis occurs between midnight and 5 AM. Follow diet and exercise regimen as prescribed. Have periodic ophthalmic exam to check for cataract development. Avoid prolonged exposure to the sun and other ultraviolet light. Report unexplained muscle pain or weakness, especially if accompanied by fever or malaise.

**Dosage Forms** Capsule: 20 mg, 40 mg

## Fluvoxamine (floo VOKS ah meen)

**Related Information**

Antidepressant Agents Comparison Chart *on page 704*

Clinical Issues in the Use of Antidepressants *on page 627*

Discontinuation of Psychotropic Drugs - Withdrawal Symptoms and Recommendations *on page 798*

Patient Information - Antidepressants (SSRIs) *on page 639*

(Continued)

## Fluvoxamine *(Continued)*

Pharmacokinetics of Selective Serotonin-Reuptake Inhibitors (SSRIs) *on page 723*
Teratogenic Risks of Psychotropic Medications *on page 812*

**Generic Available** No

**U.S. Brand Names** Luvox®

**Canadian Brand Names** Apo®-Fluvoxamine

**Pharmacologic Category** Antidepressant, Selective Serotonin Reuptake Inhibitor

**Use** Treatment of obsessive-compulsive disorder (OCD)

**Unlabeled use:** Treatment of major depression; panic disorder

**Pregnancy Risk Factor** C

**Contraindications** Hypersensitivity to fluvoxamine; concurrent use with terfenadine, astemizole, pimozide, or cisapride; use of MAO inhibitors within 14 days

**Warnings/Precautions** Potential for severe reaction when used with MAO inhibitors - serotonin syndrome (hyperthermia, muscular rigidity, mental status changes/agitation, autonomic instability) may occur. May precipitate a shift to mania or hypomania in patients with bipolar disease. Has a low potential to impair cognitive or motor performance - caution operating hazardous machinery or driving. Use caution in patients with depression, particularly if suicidal risk may be present. Use caution in patients with a previous seizure disorder or condition predisposing to seizures such as brain damage, alcoholism, or concurrent therapy with other drugs which lower the seizure threshold. Use with caution in patients with hepatic or dysfunction and in elderly patients. May cause hyponatremia/SIADH. Use with caution in patients with renal insufficiency or other concurrent illness (cardiovascular disease). Use with caution in patients at risk of bleeding or receiving concurrent anticoagulant therapy, although not consistently noted, fluvoxamine may cause impairment in platelet function. May cause or exacerbate sexual dysfunction.

**Adverse Reactions**

>10%:

Central nervous system: Headache (22%), somnolence (22%), insomnia (21%), nervousness (12%), dizziness (11%)
Gastrointestinal: Nausea (40%), diarrhea (11%), xerostomia (14%)
Neuromuscular & skeletal: Weakness (14%)

1% to 10%:

Cardiovascular: Palpitations
Central nervous system: Somnolence, mania, hypomania, vertigo, abnormal thinking, agitation, anxiety, malaise, amnesia, yawning, hypertonia, CNS stimulation, depression
Endocrine & metabolic: Decreased libido
Gastrointestinal: Abdominal pain, vomiting, dyspepsia, constipation, abnormal taste, anorexia, flatulence
Genitourinary: Delayed ejaculation, impotence, anorgasmia, urinary frequency, urinary retention
Neuromuscular & skeletal: Tremors
Ocular: Blurred vision
Respiratory: Dyspnea
Miscellaneous: Diaphoresis

<1%: Acne, alopecia, anemia, angina, ataxia, bradycardia, delayed menstruation, dermatitis, dry skin, dysuria, elevated liver transaminases, extrapyramidal reactions, hyponatremia, lactation, leukocytosis, nocturia, seizures, SIADH, thrombocytopenia, urticaria

**Overdosage/Toxicology**

Signs and symptoms: Drowsiness, vomiting, diarrhea, dizziness, coma, tachycardia, bradycardia, hypotension, EKG abnormalities, liver function abnormalities, convulsions

Treatment: Primarily symptomatic and supportive; administration of activated charcoal may be as effective as emesis or lavage and should be considered; no specific antidotes for fluvoxamine; dialysis is not believed to be beneficial

**Drug Interactions** CYP1A2 enzyme substrate; CYP1A2, 2C9, 2C19, 2D6, and 3A3/4 enzyme inhibitor

Amphetamines: SSRIs may increase the sensitivity to amphetamines, and amphetamines may increase the risk of serotonin syndrome
Astemizole: Concurrent use is contraindicated
Benzodiazepines: Fluvoxamine may inhibit the metabolism of alprazolam, diazepam, and triazolam resulting in elevated serum levels; monitor for increased sedation and psychomotor impairment
Beta-blockers: Fluvoxamine may inhibit the metabolism of metoprolol and propranolol resulting in cardiac toxicity; monitor for bradycardia, hypotension, and heart failure if combination is used; not established for all beta-blockers (unlikely with atenolol or nadolol due to renal elimination)
Buspirone: Fluvoxamine inhibits the reuptake of serotonin; combined use with a serotonin agonist (buspirone) may cause serotonin syndrome; fluvoxamine may also increase serum concentrations of buspirone
Carbamazepine: Fluvoxamine may inhibit the metabolism of carbamazepine resulting in increased carbamazepine levels and toxicity; monitor for altered carbamazepine response
Carvedilol: Serum concentrations may be increased; monitor carefully for increased carvedilol effect (hypotension and bradycardia)
Cisapride: Concurrent use is contraindicated
Clozapine: Fluvoxamine inhibits the metabolism of clozapine; adjust clozapine dosage downward or use an alternative SSRI
Cyproheptadine: May inhibit the effects of serotonin reuptake inhibitors (fluvoxamine); monitor for altered antidepressant response; cyproheptadine acts as a serotonin agonist
Dextromethorphan: Fluvoxamine inhibits the metabolism of dextromethorphan; visual hallucinations occurred in a patient receiving this combination; monitor for serotonin syndrome
Haloperidol: Fluvoxamine may inhibit the metabolism of haloperidol and cause extrapyramidal symptoms (EPS); monitor patients for EPS if combination is utilized
HMG CoA reductase inhibitors: Fluvoxamine may inhibit the metabolism of lovastatin and simvastatin resulting in myositis and rhabdomyolysis; these combinations are best avoided
Lithium: Patients receiving SSRIs and lithium have developed neurotoxicity; if combination is used, monitor for neurotoxicity
Loop diuretics: Fluvoxamine may cause hyponatremia; additive hyponatremic effects may be seen with combined use of a loop diuretic (bumetanide, furosemide, torsemide); monitor for hyponatremia
MAOIs: Fluvoxamine should not be used with nonselective MAOIs (isocarboxazid, phenelzine); fatal reactions have been reported. Wait 5 weeks after stopping fluoxetine before starting an MAOI and 2 weeks after stopping an MAOI before starting fluoxetine.
Meperidine: Combined use with fluvoxamine theoretically may increase the risk of serotonin syndrome
Methadone: Fluvoxamine may increase serum concentrations of methadone; monitor for increased effect
Nefazodone: May increase the risk of serotonin syndrome with SSRIs
Pimozide: Concurrent use is contraindicated
Phenytoin: Fluvoxamine inhibits the metabolism of phenytoin and may result in phenytoin toxicity; monitor for phenytoin toxicity (ataxia, confusion, dizziness, nystagmus, involuntary muscle movement)
Propafenone: Serum concentrations and/or toxicity may be increased by fluoxetine; avoid concurrent administration
Quinidine: Serum concentrations may be increased with fluvoxamine; avoid concurrent use
Selegiline: SSRIs have been reported to cause mania or hypertension when combined with selegiline; this combination is best avoided. In addition, use with some SSRIs has been reported to cause serotonin syndrome. As a MAO-B inhibitor, the risk of serotonin syndrome may be less than with nonselective MAO inhibitors.
Serotonin agonists: Theoretically may increase the risk of serotonin syndrome; includes sumatriptan, naratriptan, rizatriptan, and zolmitriptan
Serotonin reuptake inhibitors: Combined use with other drugs which inhibit the reuptake may cause serotonin syndrome; monitor patient for altered response with nefazodone; avoid sibutramine combination
Sibutramine: May increase the risk of serotonin syndrome with SSRIs
Sympathomimetics: May increase the risk of serotonin syndrome with SSRIs
Tacrine: Fluvoxamine inhibits the metabolism of tacrine; use alternative SSRI
Tacrolimus: Fluvoxamine may inhibit the metabolism of tacrolimus; monitor for adverse effects; consider an alternative SSRI
Theophylline: Fluvoxamine inhibits the metabolism of theophylline; monitor for theophylline toxicity or use alternative SSRI
Tramadol: Fluvoxamine combined with tramadol (serotonergic effects) may cause serotonin syndrome; monitor
Trazodone: Fluvoxamine may inhibit the metabolism of trazodone resulting in increased toxicity; monitor
Tricyclic antidepressants Fluvoxamine inhibits the metabolism of tricyclic antidepressants (amitriptyline, desipramine, imipramine, nortriptyline) resulting is elevated serum levels; if combination is warranted, a low dose of TCA (10-25 mg/day) should be utilized
Tryptophan: Fluvoxamine inhibits the reuptake of serotonin; combination with tryptophan, a serotonin precursor, may cause agitation and restlessness; this combination is best avoided
Venlafaxine: Sertraline may increase the risk of serotonin syndrome
Warfarin: Fluvoxamine may alter the hypoprothombinemic response to warfarin; monitor

**Stability** Protect from high humidity and store at controlled room temperature 15°C to 30°C (59°F to 86°F); dispense in tight containers

**Mechanism of Action** Inhibits CNS neuron serotonin uptake; minimal or no effect on reuptake of norepinephrine or dopamine; does not significantly bind to alpha-adrenergic, histamine or cholinergic receptors

**Pharmacodynamics/kinetics**

Distribution: $V_d$: ~25 L/kg
Protein binding: ~80% (mostly albumin)
Metabolism: In liver
Bioavailability: 53%; not significantly affected by food
Half-life: 16 hours
Time to peak plasma concentration: 3 hours
Elimination: Excreted in urine

**Usual Dosage** Oral:

Adults: Initial: 50 mg at bedtime; adjust in 50 mg increments at 4- to 7-day intervals; usual dose range: 100-300 mg/day; divide total daily dose into 2 doses; administer larger portion at bedtime

Elderly or hepatic impairment: Reduce dose, titrate slowly

**Dietary Considerations**

Alcohol: Additive CNS effect, avoid use

Melatonin: The bioavailability of melatonin has been reported to be increased by fluvoxamine

**Monitoring Parameters** Signs and symptoms of depression, anxiety, weight gain or loss, nutritional intake, sleep

**Patient Information** Avoid alcoholic beverages; its favorable side effect profile makes it a useful alternative to the traditional agents; use sugarless hard candy for dry mouth; avoid alcoholic beverages, may cause drowsiness; improvement may take several weeks; rise slowly to prevent dizziness. As with all psychoactive drugs, fluvoxamine may impair judgment, thinking, or motor skills, so use caution when operating hazardous machinery, including automobiles, especially early on into therapy. Inform your physician of any concurrent medications you may be taking.

**Additional Information** Modify the initial dose and the subsequent dose titration in the elderly and hepatically impaired patients

**Dosage Forms** Tablet: 25 mg, 50 mg, 100 mg


- **Fluzone®** *see* Influenza Virus Vaccine *on page 287*
- **FML®** *see* Fluorometholone *on page 231*
- **FML® Forte** *see* Fluorometholone *on page 231*
- **FML-S® Ophthalmic Suspension** *see* Sulfacetamide Sodium and Fluorometholone *on page 523*
- **Foille® [OTC]** *see* Benzocaine *on page 61*
- **Foille® Medicated First Aid [OTC]** *see* Benzocaine *on page 61*
- **Folacin** *see* Folic Acid *on page 239*
- **Folate** *see* Folic Acid *on page 239*
- **Folex® PFS** *see* Methotrexate *on page 353*


## Folic Acid (FOE lik AS id)

**U.S. Brand Names** Folvite®

**Canadian Brand Names** Apo®-Folic; Flodine®; Novo-Folacid

**Synonyms** Folacin; Folate; Pteroylglutamic Acid

**Pharmacologic Category** Vitamin, Water Soluble

**Use** Treatment of megaloblastic and macrocytic anemias due to folate deficiency; dietary supplement to prevent neural tube defects

**Effects on Mental Status** May cause drowsiness

**Effects on Psychiatric Treatment** None reported

**Pregnancy Risk Factor** A (C if dose exceeds RDA recommendation)

**Contraindications** Pernicious, aplastic, or normocytic anemias

**Warnings/Precautions** Doses >0.1 mg/day may obscure pernicious anemia with continuing irreversible nerve damage progression. Resistance to treatment may occur with depressed hematopoiesis, alcoholism, deficiencies of other vitamins. Injection contains benzyl alcohol (1.5%) as preservative (use care in administration to neonates).

**Adverse Reactions** <1%: Allergic reaction, bronchospasm, general malaise, pruritus, rash, slight flushing

**Drug Interactions**

Decreased effect: In folate-deficient patients, folic acid therapy may increase phenytoin metabolism

Phenytoin, primidone, para-aminosalicylic acid, and sulfasalazine may decrease serum folate concentrations and cause deficiency

Oral contraceptives may also impair folate metabolism producing depletion, but the effect is unlikely to cause anemia or megaloblastic changes

Concurrent administration of chloramphenicol and folic acid may result in antagonism of the hematopoietic response to folic acid; dihydrofolate reductase inhibitors (eg, methotrexate, trimethoprim) may interfere with folic acid utilization

**Usual Dosage**

Infants: 0.1 mg/day

Children <4 years: Up to 0.3 mg/day

Children >4 years and Adults: 0.4 mg/day

Pregnant and lactating women: 0.8 mg/day

RDA:

Adult male: 0.15-0.2 mg/day

Adult female: 0.15-0.18 mg/day

**Patient Information** Take as prescribed. Toxicity can occur from elevated doses. Do not self medicate. Increase intake of foods high in folic acid (eg, dried beans, nuts, bran, vegetables, fruits) as recommended by prescriber. Excessive use of alcohol increases requirement for folic acid. May turn urine more intensely yellow. Report skin rash.

**Dosage Forms**

Injection, as sodium folate: 5 mg/mL (10 mL); 10 mg/mL (10 mL)

Folvite®: 5 mg/mL (10 mL)

Tablet: 0.1 mg, 0.4 mg, 0.8 mg, 1 mg

Folvite®: 1 mg


- **Folinic Acid** *see* Leucovorin *on page 309*
- **Follistim®** *see* Follitropins *on page 239*


## Follitropins (foe li TRO pins)

**U.S. Brand Names** Fertinex® Injection; Follistim®; Gonal-F®; Metrodin® Injection

**Pharmacologic Category** Gonadotropin; Ovulation Stimulator

**Use**

**Urofollitropin (Fertinex™):**

Polycystic ovary syndrome: Administered sequentially with hCG for the stimulation of follicular recruitment and development and the induction of ovulation in patients with polycystic ovary syndrome and infertility, who have failed to respond or conceive following adequate clomiphene citrate therapy

Follicle stimulation: Stimulation of the development of multiple follicles in ovulatory patients undergoing assisted reproductive technologies such as *in vitro* fertilization

**Follitropin alpha (Gonal-F™) / follitropin beta (Follistim™):**

Ovulation induction: Induction of ovulation and pregnancy in anovulatory infertile patients in whom the cause of infertility is functional and not caused by primary ovarian failure

Follicle stimulation: Stimulation of the development of multiple follicles in ovulatory patients undergoing assisted reproductive technologies such as *in vitro* fertilization

Spermatogenesis induction: Induction of spermatogenesis in men with primary and secondary hypogonadotropic hypogonadism in whom the cause of infertility is not due to primary testicular failure

**Effects on Mental Status** None reported

**Effects on Psychiatric Treatment** None reported

**Usual Dosage**

**Urofollitropin (Fertinex™):** Adults: S.C.:

Polycystic ovary syndrome: Initial recommended dose of the first cycle: 75 international units/day; consider dose adjustment after 5-7 days; additional dose adjustments may be considered based on individual patient response. The dose should not be increased more than twice in any cycle or by more than 75 international units per adjustment. To complete follicular development and affect ovulation in the absence of an endogenous LH surge, give 5000 to 10,000 units hCG, 1 day after the last dose of urofollitropin. Withhold hCG if serum estradiol is >2000 pg/mL.

Individualize the initial dose administered in subsequent cycles for each patient based on her response in the preceding cycle. Doses of >300 international units of FSH/day are not routinely recommended. As in the initial cycle, 5000 to 10,000 units of hCG must be given 1 day after the last dose of urofollitropin to complete follicular development and induce ovulation.

Give the lowest dose consistent with the expectation of good results. Over the course of treatment, doses may range between 75 to 300 international units/day depending on individual patient response. Administer urofollitropin until adequate follicular development as indicated by serum estradiol and vaginal ultrasonography. A response is generally evident after 5-7 days.

Encourage the couple to have intercourse daily, beginning on the day prior to the administration of hCG until ovulation becomes apparent from the indices employed for determination of progestational activity. Take care to ensure insemination.

Follicle stimulation: For Assisted Reproductive Technologies, initiate therapy with urofollitropin in the early follicular phase (cycle day 2 or 3) at a dose of 150 international units/day, until sufficient follicular development is attained. In most cases, therapy should not exceed 10 days.

**Follitropin alpha (Gonal-F®):** Adults: S.C.:

Ovulation induction: Initial recommended dose of the first cycle: 75 international units/day. Consider dose adjustment after 5-7 days; additional dose adjustments of up to 37.5 international units may be considered after 14 days. Further dose increases of the same magnitude can be made, if necessary, every 7 days. To complete follicular development and affect ovulation in the absence of an endogenous LH surge, give 5000 to 10,000 units hCG, 1 day after the last dose of follitropin alpha. Withhold hCG if serum estradiol is >2000 pg/mL.

Individualize the initial dose administered in subsequent cycles for each patient based on her response in the preceding cycle. Doses of >300 international units of FSH/day are not routinely recommended. As in the initial cycle, 5000 to 10,000 units of hCG must be given 1 day after the last dose of urofollitropin to complete follicular development and induce ovulation.

Give the lowest dose consistent with the expectation of good results. Over the course of treatment, doses may range between 75 to 300 international units/day depending on individual patient response. Administer urofollitropin until adequate follicular development as indicated by serum estradiol and vaginal ultrasonography. A response is generally evident after 5-7 days.

Encourage the couple to have intercourse daily, beginning on the day prior to the administration of hCG until ovulation becomes apparent from the indices employed for determination of progestational activity. Take care to ensure insemination.

Follicle stimulation: Initiate therapy with follitropin alpha in the early follicular phase (cycle day 2 or 3) at a dose of 150 international units/day,

(Continued)

## Follitropins *(Continued)*

until sufficient follicular development is attained. In most cases, therapy should not exceed 10 days.

In patients undergoing Assisted Reproductive Technologies, whose endogenous gonadotropin levels are suppressed, initiate follitropin alpha at a dose of 225 international units/day. Continue treatment until adequate follicular development is indicated as determined by ultrasound in combination with measurement of serum estradiol levels. Consider adjustments to dose after 5 days based on the patient's response; adjust subsequent dosage every 3-5 days by ≤75-150 international units additionally at each adjustment. Doses >450 international units/day are not recommended. Once adequate follicular development is evident, administer hCG (5000-10,000 units) to induce final follicular maturation in preparation for oocyte.

**Follitropin beta (Follistim™):** Adults: S.C. or I.M.:

Ovulation induction: Stepwise approach: Initiate therapy with 75 international units/day for up to 14 days. Increase by 37.5 international units at weekly intervals until follicular growth or serum estradiol levels indicate an adequate response. The maximum, individualized, daily dose that has been safely used for ovulation induction in patients during clinical trials is 300 international units. Treat the patient until ultrasonic visualizations or serum estradiol determinations indicate preovulatory conditions greater than or equal to normal values followed by 5000 to 10,000 units hCG.

During treatment and during a 2-week post-treatment period, examine patients at least every other day for signs of excessive ovarian stimulation. Discontinue follitropin beta administration if the ovaries become abnormally enlarged or abdominal pain occurs.

Encourage the couple to have intercourse daily, beginning on the day prior to the administration of hCG until ovulation becomes apparent from the indices employed for determination of progestational activity. Take care to ensure insemination.

Follicle stimulation: A starting dose of 150-225 international units of follitropin beta is recommended for at least the first 4 days of treatment. The dose may be adjusted for the individual patient based upon their ovarian response. Daily maintenance doses ranging from 75-300 international units for 6-12 days are usually sufficient, although longer treatment may be necessary. However, maintenance doses of up to 375-600 international units may be necessary according to individual response. The maximum daily dose used in clinical studies is 600 international units. When a sufficient number of follicles of adequate size are present, the final maturation of the follicles is induced by administering hCG at a dose of 5000-10,000 international units. Oocyte retrieval is performed 34-36 hours later. Withhold hCG in cases where the ovaries are abnormally enlarged on the last day of follitropin beta therapy.

**Dosage Forms**

Urofollitropin (Fertinex®): Powder for injection: 75 international units (1, 10, 100 mL ampuls with diluent), 150 international units (1 mL ampuls with diluent)

Follitropin alpha:

Gonal-F®: Powder for injection: 75 international units (1, 10, 100 mL ampuls with diluent), 150 international units (1 mL ampuls with diluent)

Gonal-F®: Injection: 37.5 FSH units

Follitropin beta (Follistim®): Powder for injection:: 75 international units (1, 5 mL vials with diluent)

♦ **Folvite®** *see* Folic Acid *on page 239*

## Fomepizole (foe ME pi zole)

**U.S. Brand Names** Antizol®

**Pharmacologic Category** Antidote

**Use** Ethylene glycol and methanol toxicity; may be useful in propylene glycol; unclear whether it is useful in disulfiram-ethanol reactions

**Effects on Mental Status** Dizziness is common; may cause drowsiness

**Effects on Psychiatric Treatment** None reported

**Usual Dosage** A loading dose of 15 mg/kg should be administered, followed by doses of 10 mg/kg every 12 hours for 4 doses, then 15 mg/kg every 12 hours thereafter until ethylene glycol levels have been reduced <20 mg/dL

Dialysis should be considered in addition to fomepizole in the case of renal failure, significant or worsening metabolic acidosis, or a measured ethylene glycol level of >50 mg/dL. Patients should be dialyzed to correct metabolic abnormalities and to lower the ethylene glycol level <50 mg/dL

Fomepizole is dialyzable and the frequency of dosing should be increased to every 4 hours during hemodialysis

**Dosage with hemodialysis:** See table.

| Dose at the Beginning of Hemodialysis | |
|---|---|
| **If <6 h since last fomepizole dose** | **If ≥6 h since last fomepizole dose** |
| Do not administer dose | Administer next scheduled dose |
| **Dosing During Hemodialysis** | |
| Dose every 4 h | |
| **Dosing at the Time Hemodialysis is Complete** | |
| **Time Between Last Dose and the End of Hemodialsysis** | |
| **<1 h** | Do not administer dose at the end of hemodialysis |
| **1-3 h** | Administer 1/2 of next scheduled dose |
| **>3 h** | Administer next scheduled dose |
| **Maintenance Dose When Off Hemodialysis** | |
| Give next scheduled dose 12 h from last dose administered | |

**Dosage Forms** Injection: 1 g/mL (1.5 mL)

♦ **Forane®** *see* Isoflurane *on page 294*

♦ **Formula Q®** *see* Quinine *on page 486*

♦ **5-Formyl Tetrahydrofolate** *see* Leucovorin *on page 309*

♦ **Fortaz®** *see* Ceftazidime *on page 101*

♦ **Fortovase®** *see* Saquinavir *on page 504*

♦ **Fosamax®** *see* Alendronate *on page 23*

## Foscarnet (fos KAR net)

**U.S. Brand Names** Foscavir® Injection

**Pharmacologic Category** Antiviral Agent

**Use**

Herpesvirus infections suspected to be caused by acyclovir - (HSV, VZV) or ganciclovir - (CMV) resistant strains (this occurs almost exclusively in immunocompromised persons, eg, with advanced AIDS), who have received prolonged treatment for a herpesvirus infection

CMV retinitis in persons with AIDS

Other CMV infections in persons unable to tolerate ganciclovir; may be given in combination with ganciclovir in patients who relapse after monotherapy with either drug

**Effects on Mental Status** Dizziness, anxiety, confusion, and depression are common; may rarely produce abnormal crying

**Effects on Psychiatric Treatment** Leukopenia is common; use caution with clozapine and carbamazepine

**Usual Dosage** Adolescents and Adults: I.V.:

CMV retinitis:

Induction treatment: 60 mg/kg/dose every 8 hours **or** 100 mg/kg every 12 hours for 14-21 days

Maintenance therapy: 90-120 mg/kg/day as a single infusion

Acyclovir-resistant HSV induction treatment: 40 mg/kg/dose every 8-12 hours for 14-21 days

**Dosage adjustment in renal impairment:**

Induction and maintenance dosing schedules based on creatinine clearance (mL/minute/kg):

**Induction Dosing:**

$Cl_{cr}$ <0.4: Not recommended

$Cl_{cr}$ ≥0.4-0.5:

HSV: 20 mg/kg every 24 hours (equivalent to 40 mg/kg q12h)
HSV: 35 mg/kg every 24 hours (equivalent to 40 mg/kg q8h)
CMV: 50 mg/kg every 24 hours (equivalent to 60 mg/kg q8h)
CMV: 50 mg/kg every 24 hours (equivalent to 90 mg/kg q12h)

$Cl_{cr}$ >0.5-0.6:

HSV: 25 mg/kg every 24 hours (equivalent to 40 mg/kg q12h)
HSV: 40 mg/kg every 24 hours (equivalent to 40 mg/kg q8h)
CMV: 60 mg/kg every 24 hours (equivalent to 60 mg/kg q8h)
CMV: 60 mg/kg every 24 hours (equivalent to 90 mg/kg q12h)

$Cl_{cr}$ >0.6-0.8:

HSV: 35 mg/kg every 24 hours (equivalent to 40 mg/kg q12h)
HSV: 25 mg/kg every 12 hours (equivalent to 40 mg/kg q8h)
CMV: 40 mg/kg every 12 hours (equivalent to 60 mg/kg q8h)
CMV: 80 mg/kg every 24 hours (equivalent to 90 mg/kg q12h)

$Cl_{cr}$ >0.8-1.0:

HSV: 20 mg/kg every 12 hours (equivalent to 40 mg/kg q12h)
HSV: 35 mg/kg every 12 hours (equivalent to 40 mg/kg q8h)
CMV: 50 mg/kg every 12 hours (equivalent to 60 mg/kg q8h)
CMV: 50 mg/kg every 12 hours (equivalent to 90 mg/kg q12h)

$Cl_{cr}$ >1.0-1.4:

HSV: 30 mg/kg every 12 hours (equivalent to 40 mg/kg q12h)
HSV: 30 mg/kg every 8 hours (equivalent to 40 mg/kg q8h)
CMV: 45 mg/kg every 8 hours (equivalent to 60 mg/kg q8h)
CMV: 70 mg/kg every 12 hours (equivalent to 90 mg/kg q12h)

$Cl_{cr}$ >1.4:

HSV: 40 mg/kg every 12 hours (equivalent to 40 mg/kg q12h)
HSV: 40 mg/kg every 8 hours (equivalent to 40 mg/kg q8h)
CMV: 60 mg/kg every 8 hours (equivalent to 60 mg q8h)
CMV: 90 mg/kg every 12 hours (equivalent to 90 mg/kg q12h)

**Maintenance dosing for CMV**

$Cl_{cr}$ <0.4: Not recommended

$Cl_{cr}$ ≥0.4-0.5:
50 mg/kg every 48 hours (equivalent to 90 mg/kg q24h);
65 mg/kg every 48 hours (equivalent to 120 mg/kg q24h)
$Cl_{cr}$ >0.5-0.6:
60 mg/kg every 48 hours (equivalent to 90 mg/kg q24h);
80 mg/kg every 48 hours (equivalent to 120 mg/kg q24h)
$Cl_{cr}$ >0.6-0.8:
80 mg/kg every 48 hours (equivalent to 90 mg/kg q24h);
105 mg/kg every 48 hours (equivalent to 120 mg/kg q24h)
$Cl_{cr}$ >0.8-1.0:
50 mg/kg every 24 hours (equivalent to 90 mg/kg q24h);
65 mg/kg every 24 hours (equivalent to 120 mg/kg q24h)
$Cl_{cr}$ >1.0-1.4:
70 mg/kg every 24 hours (equivalent to 90 mg/kg q24h);
90 mg/kg every 24 hours (equivalent to 120 mg/kg q24h)
$Cl_{cr}$ >1.4:
90 mg/kg every 24 hours (equivalent to 90 mg/kg q24h);
120 mg/kg every 24 hours (equivalent to 120 mg/kg q24h)

**Hemodialysis:**
Foscarnet is highly removed by hemodialysis (30% in 4 hours HD)
Doses of 50 mg/kg/dose posthemodialysis have been found to produce similar serum concentrations as doses of 90 mg/kg twice daily in patients with normal renal function
Doses of 60-90 mg/kg/dose loading dose (posthemodialysis) followed by 45 mg/kg/dose posthemodialysis (3 times/week) with the monitoring of weekly plasma concentrations to maintain peak plasma concentrations in the range of 400-800 μMolar has been recommended by some clinicians

Continuous arteriovenous or venovenous hemodiafiltration (CAVH) effects: Dose as for $Cl_{cr}$ 10-50 mL/minute

**Dosage Forms** Injection: 24 mg/mL (250 mL, 500 mL)

♦ **Foscavir® Injection** *see* Foscarnet *on page 240*

## Fosfomycin (fos foe MYE sin)

**U.S. Brand Names** Monurol™

**Synonyms** Fosfomycin Tromethamine

**Pharmacologic Category** Antibiotic, Miscellaneous

**Use** A single oral dose in the treatment of uncomplicated urinary tract infections in women due to susceptible strains of *E. coli* and *Enterococcus*; multiple doses have been investigated for complicated urinary tract infections in men; may have an advantage over other agents since it maintains high concentration in the urine for up to 48 hours

**Effects on Mental Status** May cause drowsiness

**Effects on Psychiatric Treatment** None reported

**Pregnancy Risk Factor** B

**Warnings/Precautions** Do not use more than the single dose to treat a single episode of acute cystitis. Repeated daily doses may increase the incidence of adverse events while producing no improved benefit.

**Adverse Reactions**
>1%:
Central nervous system: Headache
Dermatologic: Rash
Gastrointestinal: Diarrhea (2% to 8%), nausea, vomiting, epigastric discomfort, anorexia
<1%: Dizziness, drowsiness, fatigue, pruritus

**Drug Interactions**
Decreased effect: Antacids or calcium salts may cause precipitate formation and decrease fosfomycin absorption
Metoclopramide: Increased gastrointestinal motility may lower fosfomycin tromethamine serum concentrations and urinary excretion. This drug interaction possibly could be extrapolated to other medications which increase gastrointestinal motility.

**Usual Dosage** Adults: Urinary tract infections: Oral:
Female: Single dose of 3 g in 4 oz of water
Male: 3 g once daily for 2-3 days for complicated urinary tract infections
**Dosing adjustment in renal impairment:** Decrease dose; 80% removed by dialysis, repeat dose after dialysis
**Dosing adjustment in hepatic impairment:** No dosage decrease needed

**Patient Information** May be taken with or without food; avoid use of antacids or calcium salts within 4 hours before or 2 hours after taking fosfomycin; contact your physician if signs of allergy develop; if symptoms do not improve after 2-3 days, contact your healthcare provider

**Dosage Forms** Powder, as tromethamine: 3 g, to be mixed in 4 oz of water

♦ **Fosfomycin Tromethamine** *see* Fosfomycin *on page 241*

## Fosinopril (foe SIN oh pril)

**Related Information**
Angiotensin-Related Agents Comparison Chart *on page 700*

**U.S. Brand Names** Monopril®

**Pharmacologic Category** Angiotensin-Converting Enzyme (ACE) Inhibitors

**Use** Treatment of hypertension, either alone or in combination with other antihypertensive agents; treatment of congestive heart failure, left ventricular dysfunction after myocardial infarction

**Effects on Mental Status** May cause drowsiness or dizziness; may rarely cause insomnia

**Effects on Psychiatric Treatment** May rarely cause agranulocytosis; use caution with clozapine and carbamazepine; may decrease lithium clearance resulting in an increase in serum lithium levels and potential lithium toxicity; monitor serum lithium levels

**Pregnancy Risk Factor** C (1st trimester); D (2nd and 3rd trimester)

**Contraindications** Hypersensitivity to fosinopril or any component; angioedema related to previous treatment with an ACE inhibitor; patients with idiopathic or hereditary angioedema; bilateral renal artery stenosis; primary hyperaldosteronism; pregnancy (2nd and 3rd trimesters)

**Warnings/Precautions** Anaphylactic reactions can occur. Angioedema can occur at any time during treatment (especially following first dose). Careful blood pressure monitoring (hypotension can occur especially in volume depleted patients). Dosage adjustment needed in severe renal impairment ($Cl_{cr}$ <10 mL/minute). Use with caution in hypovolemia; collagen vascular diseases; valvular stenosis (particularly aortic stenosis); hyperkalemia; or before, during, or immediately after anesthesia. Avoid rapid dosage escalation which may lead to renal insufficiency. Hypersensitivity reactions may be seen during hemodialysis with high-flux dialysis membranes (eg, AN69). Hyperkalemia may rarely occur. Neutropenia/agranulocytosis with myeloid hyperplasia can rarely occur. If patient has renal impairment, then a baseline WBC with differential and serum creatinine should be evaluated and monitored closely during initial therapy. Use with caution in unilateral renal artery stenosis and pre-existing renal insufficiency. Safety and efficacy in pediatric patients have not been established.

**Adverse Reactions**
1% to 10%:
Cardiovascular: Orthostatic hypotension (especially after initial dose)
Central nervous system: Headache (3%), dizziness (1% to 2%), fatigue (1% to 2%)
Gastrointestinal: Diarrhea/nausea/vomiting (1% to 2%)
Respiratory: Cough (2%)
<1%: Abdominal distention, abnormal taste, agranulocytosis, anemia, angioedema, claudication, cold/flu symptoms, deterioration in renal function, drowsiness, dyspepsia, dysphagia, edema, hyperkalemia, hypertensive crisis, hypoglycemia, hypotension, impotence, insomnia, memory disturbance, muscle cramps, neutropenia, rash, syncope, tremor, vertigo

**Overdosage/Toxicology**
Signs and symptoms: Mild hypotension has been the only toxic effect seen with acute overdose; bradycardia may also occur. Hyperkalemia occurs even with therapeutic doses, especially in patients with renal insufficiency and those taking NSAIDs.
Treatment: Following initiation of essential overdose management, toxic symptom treatment and supportive treatment should be initiated. Hypotension usually responds to I.V. fluids or Trendelenburg positioning.

**Drug Interactions**
Alpha$_1$ blockers: Hypotensive effect increased
Aspirin: The effects of ACE inhibitors may be blunted by aspirin administration, particularly at higher dosages
Diuretics: Hypovolemia due to diuretics may precipitate acute hypotensive events or acute renal failure
Insulin: Risk of hypoglycemia may be increased
Lithium: Risk of lithium toxicity may be increased; monitor lithium levels, especially the first 4 weeks of therapy
Mercaptopurine: Risk of neutropenia may be increased
NSAIDs may decrease ACE inhibitor efficacy and/or increase risk of renal effects
Potassium-sparing diuretics (amiloride, spironolactone, triamterene): Increased risk of hyperkalemia
Potassium supplements may increase the risk of hyperkalemia
Trimethoprim (high dose) may increase the risk of hyperkalemia

**Usual Dosage** Adults: Oral:
Hypertension: Initial: 10 mg/day; most patients are maintained on 20-40 mg/day. May need to divide the dose into two if trough effect is inadequate; discontinue the diuretic, if possible 2-3 days before initiation of therapy; resume diuretic therapy carefully, if needed.
Heart failure: Initial: 10 mg/day (5 mg if renal dysfunction present) and increase, as needed, to a maximum of 40 mg once daily over several weeks; usual dose: 20-40 mg/day. If hypotension, orthostasis, or azotemia occur during titration, consider decreasing concomitant diuretic dose, if any.
**Dosing adjustment/comments in renal impairment:** None needed since hepatobiliary elimination compensates adequately diminished renal elimination.
Hemodialysis: Moderately dialyzable (20% to 50%)

**Patient Information** Take exactly as directed; do not discontinue without consulting prescriber. Take first dose at bedtime. This drug does not eliminate need for diet or exercise as recommended by prescriber. Do not use potassium supplements or salt substitutes containing potassium without consulting prescriber. May cause dizziness, fainting, lightheadedness (use caution when driving or engaging in tasks that require alertness until
(Continued)

## Fosinopril *(Continued)*

response to drug is known); postural hypotension (use caution when rising from lying or sitting position or climbing stairs); nausea, dry cough, diarrhea, or transient loss of appetite (small frequent meals, frequent mouth care, sucking lozenges, or chewing gum may help) - report if these persist; sexual dysfunction (will usually resolve). Report chest pain or palpitations; difficulty breathing or unusual cough; acute headache; or other persistent adverse reactions.

**Nursing Implications** May cause depression in some patients; discontinue if angioedema of the face, extremities, lips, tongue, or glottis occurs; watch for hypotensive effects within 1-3 hours of first dose or new higher dose

**Dosage Forms** Tablet: 10 mg, 20 mg

## Fosphenytoin (FOS fen i toyn)

**Related Information**

Phenytoin *on page 441*

**U.S. Brand Names** Cerebyx®

**Pharmacologic Category** Anticonvulsant, Hydantoin

**Use** Indicated for short-term parenteral administration when other means of phenytoin administration are unavailable, inappropriate or deemed less advantageous; the safety and effectiveness of fosphenytoin in this use has not been systematically evaluated for more than 5 days; may be used for the control of generalized convulsive status epilepticus and prevention and treatment of seizures occurring during neurosurgery

**Effects on Mental Status** May cause dizziness, drowsiness, or visual hallucinations

**Effects on Psychiatric Treatment** May cause neutropenia; use caution with clozapine and carbamazepine

**Pregnancy Risk Factor** D

**Contraindications** Hypersensitivity to phenytoin or fosphenytoin; occurrence of any rash while on treatment; the drug should not be resumed if rash is exfoliative, purpuric, or bullous; not recommended for use in children <4 years of age

**Warnings/Precautions** Use with caution in patients with severe cardiovascular, hepatic, renal disease or diabetes mellitus; avoid abrupt discontinuation; dosing should be slowly reduced to avoid precipitation of seizures; increased toxicity with nephrotic syndrome patient; may increase frequency of petit mal seizures; use with caution in patients with porphyria, fever, or hypothyroidism

**Adverse Reactions**

Percentage unknown: Pain on injection, sensory paresthesia (long-term treatment), nephrotic syndrome

>10%:

Central nervous system: Dizziness (31%), somnolence (21%), ataxia (11%)

Dermatologic: Pruritus (48.9%)

Ocular: Nystagmus (44%)

1% to 10%:

Cardiovascular: Hypotension (7.7%), vasodilation (>1%), tachycardia (2.2%)

Central nervous system: Stupor (7.7%), incoordination (4.4%), paresthesia (4.4%), choreoathetosis (4.4%), tremor (3.3%), agitation (3.3%)

Gastrointestinal: Nausea (>5%), vomiting (2%)

Ocular: Blurred vision (2%), diplopia (3.3%)

<1%: Acne, anemia (megaloblastic), diabetes insipidus, erythema multiforme, exfoliative dermatitis, lymphadenopathy, neutropenia, rash, thrombocytopenia

**Overdosage/Toxicology**

Signs and symptoms: Unsteady gait, tremors, hyperglycemia, chorea (extrapyramidal), gingival hyperplasia, gynecomastia, myoglobinuria, nephrotic syndrome, slurred speech, mydriasis, myoclonus, confusion, encephalopathy, hyperthermia, drowsiness, nausea, hypothermia, fever, hypotension, respiratory depression, leukopenia; neutropenia; agranulocytosis; granulocytopenia; hyper-reflexia, coma, systemic lupus erythematosus (SLE), ophthalmoplegia

Treatment: Supportive for hypotension; treat with I.V. fluids and place patient in Trendelenburg position; seizures may be controlled with lorazepam or diazepam 5-10 mg (0.25-0.4 mg/kg in children); intravenous albumin (25 g every 6 hours has been used to increase bound fraction of drug). Multiple dosing of activated charcoal may be effective; peritoneal dialysis, diuresis, hemodialysis, hemoperfusion, and plasmapheresis is of little value

**Drug Interactions** Refer to Phenytoin monograph

**Usual Dosage** **The dose, concentration in solutions, and infusion rates for fosphenytoin are expressed as phenytoin sodium equivalents; fosphenytoin should always be prescribed and dispensed in phenytoin sodium equivalents**

Status epilepticus: I.V.: Adults: Loading dose: Phenytoin equivalent: 15-20 mg/kg I.V. administered at 100-150 mg/minute

Nonemergent loading and maintenance dosing: I.V. or I.M.: Adults:

Loading dose: Phenytoin equivalent: 10-20 mg/kg I.V. or I.M. (maximum I.V. rate: 150 mg/minute)

Initial daily maintenance dose: Phenytoin equivalent: 4-6 mg/kg/day I.V. or I.M.

I.M. or I.V. substitution for oral phenytoin therapy: May be substituted for oral phenytoin sodium at the same total daily dose, however, Dilantin® capsules are ~90% bioavailable by the oral route; phenytoin, supplied as fosphenytoin, is 100% bioavailable by both the I.M. and I.V. routes; for this reason, plasma phenytoin concentrations may increase when I.M. or I.V. fosphenytoin is substituted for oral phenytoin sodium therapy; in clinical trials I.M. fosphenytoin was administered as a single daily dose utilizing either 1 or 2 injection sites; some patients may require more frequent dosing

**Dosing adjustments in renal/hepatic impairment**: Phenytoin clearance may be substantially reduced in cirrhosis and plasma level monitoring with dose adjustment advisable; free phenytoin levels should be monitored closely in patients with renal or hepatic disease or in those with hypoalbuminemia; furthermore, fosphenytoin clearance to phenytoin may be increased without a similar increase in phenytoin in these patients leading to increase frequency and severity of adverse events

**Patient Information** Patients may not be in a position to evaluate their response. If conscious or alert, advise patient to report signs or symptoms of palpitations, racing or falling heartbeat, difficulty breathing, acute faintness, or CNS disturbances (eg, somnolence, ataxia), and visual disturbances.

**Nursing Implications** I.V. injections should be followed by normal saline flushes through the same needle or I.V. catheter to avoid local irritation of the vein; must be diluted to concentrations <6 mg/mL, in normal saline, for I.V. infusion

**Dosage Forms** Injection, as sodium: 150 mg [equivalent to phenytoin sodium 100 mg] in 2 mL vials; 750 mg [equivalent to phenytoin sodium 500 mg] in 10 mL vials


♦ **Fostex® 10% BPO Gel [OTC]** *see* Benzoyl Peroxide *on page 62*

♦ **Fostex® 10% Wash [OTC]** *see* Benzoyl Peroxide *on page 62*

♦ **Fostex® Bar [OTC]** *see* Benzoyl Peroxide *on page 62*

♦ **Fragmin®** *see* Dalteparin *on page 150*

♦ **Frusemide** *see* Furosemide *on page 243*

♦ **FS Shampoo®** *see* Fluocinolone *on page 231*

♦ **FUDR®** *see* Floxuridine *on page 227*

♦ **Fulvicin® P/G** *see* Griseofulvin *on page 255*

♦ **Fulvicin-U/F®** *see* Griseofulvin *on page 255*

♦ **Fumasorb® [OTC]** *see* Ferrous Fumarate *on page 223*

♦ **Fumerin® [OTC]** *see* Ferrous Fumarate *on page 223*

♦ **Fungizone®** *see* Amphotericin B (Conventional) *on page 41*

♦ **Fungoid® Creme** *see* Miconazole *on page 364*

♦ **Fungoid® Tincture** *see* Miconazole *on page 364*

♦ **Furacin® Topical** *see* Nitrofurazone *on page 396*

♦ **Furadantin®** *see* Nitrofurantoin *on page 396*


## Furazolidone (fyoor a ZOE li done)

**U.S. Brand Names** Furoxone®

**Pharmacologic Category** Antiprotozoal

**Use** Treatment of bacterial or protozoal diarrhea and enteritis caused by susceptible organisms *Giardia lamblia* and *Vibrio cholerae*

**Effects on Mental Status** May cause drowsiness or dizziness

**Effects on Psychiatric Treatment** May rarely cause agranulocytosis; use caution with clozapine and carbamazepine; furazolidone inhibits MAO; caution with alcohol, anorexiants, antidepressants, meperidine, sympathomimetics, dopamine agonists, and tyramine-containing foods

**Pregnancy Risk Factor** C

**Contraindications** Known hypersensitivity to furazolidone; concurrent use of alcohol; patients <1 month of age because of the possibility of producing hemolytic anemia

**Warnings/Precautions** Use caution in patients with G-6-PD deficiency when administering large doses for prolonged periods; furazolidone inhibits monoamine oxidase

**Adverse Reactions**

>10%: Genitourinary: Discoloration of urine (dark yellow to brown)

1% to 10%:

Central nervous system: Headache

Gastrointestinal: Abdominal pain, diarrhea, nausea, vomiting

<1%: Agranulocytosis, arthralgia, disulfiram-like reaction after alcohol ingestion, dizziness, drowsiness, fever, hemolysis in patients with G-6-PD deficiency, hypoglycemia, leukopenia, malaise, orthostatic hypotension, rash

**Overdosage/Toxicology**

Signs and symptoms: Nausea, vomiting, serotonin crisis

Treatment: Supportive care only; serotonin crisis may require dantrolene/bromocriptine

**Drug Interactions**

Increases toxicity of sympathomimetic amines, tricyclic antidepressants, MAO inhibitors, meperidine, anorexiants, dextromethorphan, fluoxetine, paroxetine, sertraline, trazodone

Increased effect/toxicity of levodopa

Disulfiram-like reaction with alcohol

**Usual Dosage** Oral:

Children >1 month: 5-8 mg/kg/day in 4 divided doses for 7 days, not to exceed 400 mg/day or 8.8 mg/kg/day

Adults: 100 mg 4 times/day for 7 days

**Dietary Considerations**

Alcohol: Avoid use

Food: Marked elevation of blood pressure, hypertensive crisis, or hemorrhagic stroke may occur with foods high in amine content

**Patient Information** Take as directed. Avoid alcohol and tyramine-containing foods during and for 4 days following therapy. Do not take any other prescription or OTC medications without consulting prescriber. Your urine may turn dark brown or yellow (normal). If diabetic, use something other than Clinitest® for urine glucose testing. Report acute GI pain, unresolved diarrhea, unresolved nausea or vomiting, fever, dizziness, or unusual joint pain. Consult prescriber if condition is not resolved at the end of therapy.

**Dosage Forms**

Liquid: 50 mg/15 mL (60 mL, 473 mL)

Tablet: 100 mg

♦ **Furazosin** *see* Prazosin *on page 459*

## Furosemide (fyoor OH se mide)

**U.S. Brand Names** Lasix®

**Canadian Brand Names** Apo®-Furosemide; Furoside®; Novo-Semide; Uritol®

**Synonyms** Frusemide

**Pharmacologic Category** Diuretic, Loop

**Use** Management of edema associated with congestive heart failure and hepatic or renal disease; alone or in combination with antihypertensives in treatment of hypertension

**Effects on Mental Status** Dizziness is common

**Effects on Psychiatric Treatment** Orthostatic hypotension is common; use caution with low potency antipsychotics and TCAs; may rarely cause agranulocytosis; caution with clozapine and carbamazepine; may decrease renal clearance of lithium resulting in elevated serum levels and risk for toxicity; more common with thiazide diuretics; monitor lithium levels

**Pregnancy Risk Factor** C

**Contraindications** Hypersensitivity to furosemide, any component, or sulfonylureas; anuria; patients with hepatic coma or in states of severe electrolyte depletion until the condition improves or is corrected

**Warnings/Precautions** Adjust dose to avoid dehydration. In cirrhosis, avoid electrolyte and acid/base imbalances that might lead to hepatic encephalopathy. Ototoxicity is associated with rapid I.V. administration, renal impairment, excessive doses, and concurrent use of other ototoxins. Hypersensitivity reactions can rarely occur. Monitor fluid status and renal function in an attempt to prevent oliguria, azotemia, and reversible increases in BUN and creatinine. Close medical supervision of aggressive diuresis required. Monitor closely for electrolyte imbalances particularly hypokalemia. Watch for and correct electrolyte disturbances. Coadministration of antihypertensives may increase the risk of hypotension. Avoid use of medications in which the toxicity is enhanced by hypokalemia (including quinolones with Q-T prolongation). Use caution in patients with known hypersensitivity to sulfonamides or thiazides (due to possible cross-sensitivity); avoid in patients with history of severe reactions.

**Adverse Reactions**

>10%:

Cardiovascular: Orthostatic hypotension

Central nervous system: Dizziness

1% to 10%:

Central nervous system: Headache

Dermatologic: Photosensitivity

Endocrine & metabolic: Electrolyte imbalance (hypokalemia, hyponatremia, hypochloremia, hypercalciuria, hyperuricemia), alkalosis, dehydration

Gastrointestinal: Diarrhea, loss of appetite, stomach cramps or pain

Ocular: Blurred vision

<1%: Agranulocytosis, anemia, gout, hepatic dysfunction, interstitial nephritis, leukopenia, nausea, nephrocalcinosis, ototoxicity, pancreatitis, prerenal azotemia, rash, redness at injection site, thrombocytopenia, xanthopsia

**Overdosage/Toxicology**

Signs and symptoms of overdose include electrolyte imbalance, volume depletion, hypotension, dehydration, hypokalemia and hypochloremic alkalosis

Treatment: Following GI decontamination, treatment is supportive; hypotension responds to fluids and Trendelenburg position

**Drug Interactions**

ACE inhibitors: Hypotensive effects and/or renal effects are potentiated by hypovolemia

Antidiabetic agents: Glucose tolerance may be decreased

Antihypertensive agents: Hypotensive effects may be enhanced

Cephaloridine or cephalexin: Nephrotoxicity may occur

Cholestyramine or colestipol may reduce bioavailability of furosemide

Digoxin: Furosemide-induced hypokalemia may predispose to digoxin toxicity; monitor potassium

Fibric acid derivatives: Protein binding may be altered in hypoalbuminemic patients receiving furosemide, potentially increasing toxicity

Indomethacin (and other NSAIDs) may reduce natriuretic and hypotensive effects of furosemide

Lithium: Renal clearance may be reduced; isolated reports of lithium toxicity have occurred; monitor lithium levels

Metformin may decrease furosemide concentrations

Metformin blood levels may be increased by furosemide

NSAIDs: Risk of renal impairment may increase when used in conjunction with furosemide

Ototoxic drugs (aminoglycosides, cis-platinum): Concomitant use of furosemide may increase risk of ototoxicity, especially in patients with renal dysfunction

Peripheral adrenergic-blocking drugs or ganglionic blockers: Effects may be increased

Phenobarbital or phenytoin may reduce diuretic response to furosemide

Salicylates (high-dose) with furosemide may predispose patients to salicylate toxicity due to reduced renal excretion or alter renal function

Sparfloxacin, gatifloxacin, and moxifloxacin: Risk of hypokalemia and cardiotoxicity may be increased; avoid use

Succinylcholine: Action may be potentiated by furosemide

Sucralfate may limit absorption of furosemide, effects may be significantly decreased; separate oral administration by 2 hours

Thiazides: Synergistic diuretic effects occur

Tubocurarine: The skeletal muscle-relaxing effect may be attenuated by furosemide

**Usual Dosage**

Infants and Children:

Oral: 1-2 mg/kg/dose increased in increments of 1 mg/kg/dose with each succeeding dose until a satisfactory effect is achieved to a maximum of 6 mg/kg/dose no more frequently than 6 hours.

I.M., I.V.: 1 mg/kg/dose, increasing by each succeeding dose at 1 mg/kg/dose at intervals of 6-12 hours until a satisfactory response up to 6 mg/kg/dose.

Adults:

Oral: 20-80 mg/dose initially increased in increments of 20-40 mg/dose at intervals of 6-8 hours; usual maintenance dose interval is twice daily or every day; may be titrated up to 600 mg/day with severe edematous states.

I.M., I.V.: 20-40 mg/dose, may be repeated in 1-2 hours as needed and increased by 20 mg/dose until the desired effect has been obtained. Usual dosing interval: 6-12 hours; for acute pulmonary edema, the usual dose is 40 mg I.V. over 1-2 minutes. If not adequate, may increase dose to 80 mg.

Continuous I.V. infusion: Initial I.V. bolus dose of 0.1 mg/kg followed by continuous I.V. infusion doses of 0.1 mg/kg/hour doubled every 2 hours to a maximum of 0.4 mg/kg/hour if urine output is <1 mL/kg/hour have been found to be effective and result in a lower daily requirement of furosemide than with intermittent dosing. Other studies have used a rate of ≤4 mg/minute as a continuous I.V. infusion.

Elderly: Oral, I.M., I.V.: Initial: 20 mg/day; increase slowly to desired response.

Refractory heart failure: Oral, I.V.: Doses up to 8 g/day have been used.

**Dosing adjustment/comments in renal impairment:** Acute renal failure: High doses (up to 1-3 g/day - oral/I.V.) have been used to initiate desired response; avoid use in oliguric states.

Dialysis: Not removed by hemo- or peritoneal dialysis; supplemental dose is not necessary.

**Dosing adjustment/comments in hepatic disease:** Diminished natriuretic effect with increased sensitivity to hypokalemia and volume depletion in cirrhosis; monitor effects, particularly with high doses.

**Patient Information** Take as directed, with food or milk early in the day (daily), or if twice daily, take last dose in late afternoon in order to avoid sleep disturbance and achieve maximum therapeutic effect. Keep medication in original container, away from light; do not use discolored medication. Include bananas or orange juice (or other potassium-rich foods) in daily diet; do not take potassium supplements without advice of prescriber. Weigh yourself each day, at the same time, in the same clothes when beginning therapy, and weekly on long-term therapy; report unusual or unanticipated weight gain or loss. You may experience dizziness, blurred vision, or drowsiness; use caution when driving or engaging in tasks that require alertness until response to drug is known. Use caution when rising or changing position. You may experience sensitivity to sunlight; use sunblock or wear protective clothing and sunglasses. Report signs of

(Continued)

## Furosemide *(Continued)*

edema (eg, weight gains, swollen ankles, feet or hands), trembling, numbness or fatigue, any cramping or muscle weakness, palpitations, or unresolved nausea or vomiting.

**Dosage Forms**

Injection: 10 mg/mL (2 mL, 4 mL, 5 mL, 6 mL, 8 mL, 10 mL, 12 mL)
Solution, oral: 10 mg/mL (60 mL, 120 mL); 40 mg/5 mL (5 mL, 10 mL, 500 mL)
Tablet: 20 mg, 40 mg, 80 mg

♦ **Furoxone®** *see* Furazolidone *on page 242*

♦ **G-1®** *see* Butalbital Compound and Acetaminophen *on page 80*

## Gabapentin (GA ba pen tin)

**Related Information**

Anticonvulsants by Seizures Type *on page 703*
Mood Disorders *on page 600*
Mood Stabilizers *on page 719*
Serum Drug Concentrations Commonly Monitored: Guidelines *on page 759*

**Generic Available** No

**U.S. Brand Names** Neurontin®

**Pharmacologic Category** Anticonvulsant, Miscellaneous

**Use** Adjunct for treatment of partial seizures with and without secondarily generalized seizures in adults with epilepsy

**Unlabeled uses:** Bipolar disorder, chronic pain, social phobia

**Pregnancy Risk Factor** C

**Pregnancy/Breast-Feeding Implications**

Clinical effects on the fetus: No data on crossing the placenta; 4 reports of normal pregnancy outcomes; 1 report of infant with respiratory distress, pyloric stenosis, inguinal hernia following 1st trimester exposure to gabapentin plus carbamazepine; epilepsy itself, number of medications, genetic factors, or a combination of these probably influence the teratogenicity of anticonvulsant therapy

Breast-feeding/lactation: No data available

**Contraindications** Hypersensitivity to gabapentin or its ingredients

**Warnings/Precautions** Avoid abrupt withdrawal, may precipitate seizures; may be associated with a slight incidence (0.6%) of status epilepticus and sudden deaths (0.0038 deaths/patient year); use cautiously in patients with severe renal dysfunction; rat studies demonstrated an association with pancreatic adenocarcinoma in male rats; clinical implication unknown. May cause CNS depression, which may impair physical or mental abilities. Patients must be cautioned about performing tasks which require mental alertness (ie, operating machinery or driving). Effects with other sedative drugs or ethanol may be potentiated.

**Adverse Reactions**

>10%: Central nervous system: Somnolence, dizziness, ataxia, fatigue

1% to 10%:

- Cardiovascular: Peripheral edema
- Central nervous system: Nervousness, amnesia, depression, abnormal coordination, dysarthria, abnormal thinking, twitching
- Dermatologic: Pruritus
- Gastrointestinal: Dyspepsia, xerostomia, dry throat, constipation, appetite stimulation (weight gain)
- Genitourinary: Impotence
- Hematologic: Leukopenia
- Neuromuscular & skeletal: Back pain, myalgia, tremor
- Ocular: Diplopia, blurred vision, nystagmus
- Respiratory: Rhinitis, pharyngitis, coughing

**Overdosage/Toxicology**

Signs and symptoms: Acute overdosage up to 49 g has been reported; symptoms of acute overdose include double vision, slurred speech, drowsiness, lethargy, and diarrhea

Treatment: All patients recovered with supportive care

**Drug Interactions**

**Note:** Gabapentin does not generally modify plasma concentrations of standard anticonvulsant medications (ie, valproic acid, carbamazepine, phenytoin, or phenobarbital); see note on phenytoin

Antacids: Antacids reduce the bioavailability of gabapentin by 20%

Cimetidine: Cimetidine may increase gabapentin serum concentrations; clearance of gabapentin is decreased by 14%

Felbamate: Serum concentrations may be increased by gabapentin; monitor for increased felbamate effect/toxicity

Norethindrone: Gabapentin may increase $C_{max}$ of norethindrone by 13%

Phenytoin: Phenytoin serum concentrations may be increased by gabapentin; limited documentation; monitor

**Mechanism of Action** Exact mechanism of action is not known, but does have properties in common with other anticonvulsants; although structurally related to GABA, it does not interact with GABA receptors

**Pharmacodynamics/kinetics**

Absorption: Oral: 50% to 60%
Distribution: $V_d$: 0.6-0.8 L/kg
Protein binding: 0%
Half-life: 5-6 hours
Elimination: Renal, 56% to 80%

**Usual Dosage** If gabapentin is discontinued or if another anticonvulsant is added to therapy, it should be done slowly over a minimum of 1 week

Children >12 years and Adults: Oral:

- Initial: 300 mg 3 times/day, if necessary the dose may be increased using 300 or 400 mg capsules 3 times/day up to 1800 mg/day
- Total daily dosage range: 900-1800 mg/day administered in 3 divided doses at 8-hour intervals
- Pain: 300-1800 mg/day given in 3 divided doses has been the most common dosage range
- Bipolar disorder: 300-3000 mg/day given in 3 divided doses

**Dosing adjustment in renal impairment:**

- $Cl_{cr}$ >60 mL/minute: Administer 1200 mg/day
- $Cl_{cr}$ 30-60 mL/minute: Administer 600 mg/day
- $Cl_{cr}$ 15-30 mL/minute: Administer 300 mg/day
- $Cl_{cr}$ <15 mL/minute: Administer 150 mg/day

Hemodialysis: 200-300 mg after each 4-hour dialysis following a loading dose of 300-400 mg

**Dietary Considerations**

Food: Does not change rate or extent of absorption; take without regard to meals

Serum lipids: May see increases in total cholesterol, HDL cholesterol, and triglycerides. Hyperlipidemia and hypercholesterolemia have been reported with gabapentin.

**Administration** Administer first dose on first day at bedtime to avoid somnolence and dizziness

**Monitoring Parameters** Monitor serum levels of concomitant anticonvulsant therapy; routine monitoring of gabapentin levels is not mandatory

**Reference Range** Minimum effective serum concentration may be 2 µg/mL; **routine monitoring of drug levels is not required**

**Patient Information** Take only as prescribed; may cause dizziness, somnolence, and other symptoms and signs of CNS depression; do not operate machinery or drive a car until you have experience with the drug; may be administered without regard to meals

**Nursing Implications** Dosage must be adjusted for renal function and elderly often have reduced renal function

**Additional Information** If gabapentin is discontinued or if another anticonvulsant is added to therapy it should be done slowly over a minimum of 1 week. Gabapentin, like lithium, is renally eliminated.

**Dosage Forms**

Capsule: 100 mg, 300 mg, 400 mg
Solution, oral: 250 mg/5 mL
Tablet: 600 mg, 800 mg

♦ **Gabitril®** *see* Tiagabine *on page 547*

## Galantamine (ga LAN ta meen)

**U.S. Brand Names** Reminyl®

**Synonyms** Galantamine Hydrobromide

**Pharmacologic Category** Acetylcholinesterase Inhibitor (Central)

**Use Unlabeled use:** Dementia of the Alzheimer's type

**Contraindications** Bradycardia, asthma, epilepsy, hyperkinesia, ileus hypersensitivity to galantamine

**Warnings/Precautions** Use with caution in peptic ulcer disease, Parkinson's disease, pregnancy, heart disease, and hypotension

**Adverse Reactions** Placebo adjusted vs 24 mg

>10%: Gastrointestinal: Nausea, vomiting

1% to 10%:

- Central nervous system: Dizziness, anorexia
- Cardiovascular: Bradycardia
- Endocrine & metabolic: Weight loss
- Gastrointestinal: Diarrhea, abdominal pain
- Neuromuscular & skeletal: Tremor

**Mechanism of Action** Selective, reversible, and competitive inhibitor of acetylcholinesterase and allosterically modulates nicotinic acetylcholine receptors

**Pharmacodynamics/kinetics**

Duration: 3 hours; maximum inhibition of erythrocyte acetylcholinesterase approximately 40% at 1 hour post 10 mg oral dose; levels return to baseline at 30 hours

Distribution: 1.8-2.6 L/kg; levels in the brain are 2-3 times higher than in plasma

Protein binding: 18%

Metabolism: Linear, CYP2D6 and 3A4; metabolized to epigalanthaminone and galanthaminone both of which have acetylcholinesterase inhibitory activity 130 times less than galantamine

Bioavailability: 80% to 100%
Half-life: 6-8 hours
Time to peak: 45-120 minutes
Elimination: Renal (25%)

**Usual Dosage** Adults: Oral: 8 mg in 2 divided doses; titrate up to 16 mg/day in 2 divided doses over a 4-week period; maximum dose: 24 mg/day

**Monitoring Parameters** Mental status

**Additional Information NOTE:** This is a preliminary monograph; consult full prescribing information when it becomes available

♦ **Galantamine Hydrobromide** *see* Galantamine *on page 244*

## Gallamine Triethiodide (GAL a meen trye eth EYE oh dide)

**U.S. Brand Names** Flaxedil®

**Pharmacologic Category** Skeletal Muscle Relaxant

**Use** Produce skeletal muscle relaxation during surgery after general anesthesia has been induced

**Effects on Mental Status** None reported

**Effects on Psychiatric Treatment** None reported

**Usual Dosage** I.V.: 1 mg/kg then repeat dose of 0.5-1 mg/kg in 30-40 minutes for prolonged procedures

**Dosage Forms** Injection: 20 mg/mL (10 mL)

## Gallium Nitrate (GAL ee um NYE trate)

**U.S. Brand Names** Ganite™

**Pharmacologic Category** Antidote

**Use** Treatment of clearly symptomatic cancer-related hypercalcemia that has not responded to adequate hydration

**Effects on Mental Status** None reported

**Effects on Psychiatric Treatment** None reported

**Usual Dosage** Adults:

I.V. infusion (over 24 hours): 200 mg/m$^2$ for 5 consecutive days in 1 L of NS or $D_5W$

Mild hypercalcemia/few symptoms: 100 mg/m$^2$/day for 5 days in 1 L of NS or $D_5W$

**Dosing adjustment/comments in renal impairment:** $Cl_{cr}$ <30 mL/minute: Avoid use

**Dosage Forms** Injection: 25 mg/mL (20 mL)

♦ **Gamimune® N** *see* Immune Globulin, Intravenous *on page 284*

♦ **Gamma Benzene Hexachloride** *see* Lindane *on page 318*

♦ **Gammagard®** *see* Immune Globulin, Intravenous *on page 284*

♦ **Gammagard® S/D** *see* Immune Globulin, Intravenous *on page 284*

♦ **Gammar®-P I.V.** *see* Immune Globulin, Intravenous *on page 284*

## Ganciclovir (gan SYE kloe veer)

**U.S. Brand Names** Cytovene®; Vitrasert®

**Synonyms** DHPG Sodium; GCV Sodium; Nordeoxyguanosine

**Pharmacologic Category** Antiviral Agent

**Use**

Parenteral: Treatment of CMV retinitis in immunocompromised individuals, including patients with acquired immunodeficiency syndrome; prophylaxis of CMV infection in transplant patients; may be given in combination with foscarnet in patients who relapse after monotherapy with either drug

Oral: Alternative to the I.V. formulation for maintenance treatment of CMV retinitis in immunocompromised patients, including patients with AIDS, in whom retinitis is stable following appropriate induction therapy and for whom the risk of more rapid progression is balanced by the benefit associated with avoiding daily I.V. infusions.

Implant: Treatment of CMV retinitis

**Effects on Mental Status** May cause confusion; may rarely cause nervousness, psychosis, hallucinations, or disorientation

**Effects on Psychiatric Treatment** Leukopenia is common; use caution with clozapine and carbamazepine

**Pregnancy Risk Factor** C

**Contraindications** Absolute neutrophil count <500/mm$^3$; platelet count <25,000/mm$^3$; known hypersensitivity to ganciclovir or acyclovir

**Warnings/Precautions** Dosage adjustment or interruption of ganciclovir therapy may be necessary in patients with neutropenia and/or thrombocytopenia and patients with impaired renal function. Use with extreme caution in children since long-term safety has not been determined and due to ganciclovir's potential for long-term carcinogenic and adverse reproductive effects; ganciclovir may adversely affect spermatogenesis and fertility; due to its mutagenic potential, contraceptive precautions for female and male patients need to be followed during and for at least 90 days after therapy with the drug; take care to administer only into veins with good blood flow.

**Adverse Reactions**

>10%:

Central nervous system: Fever (38% to 48%)

Dermatologic: Rash (15% - oral, 10% - I.V.)

Gastrointestinal: Abdominal pain (17% to 19%), diarrhea (40%), nausea (25%), anorexia (15%), vomiting (13%)

Hematologic: Anemia (20% to 25%), leukopenia (30% to 40%)

1% to 10%:

Central nervous system: Confusion, neuropathy (8% to 9%), headache (4%)

Dermatologic: Pruritus (5%)

Hematologic: Thrombocytopenia (6%), neutropenia with ANC <500/mm$^3$ (5% - oral, 14% - I.V.)

Neuromuscular & skeletal: Paresthesia (6% to 10%), weakness (6%)

Miscellaneous: Sepsis (4% - oral, 15% - I.V.)

<1%: Alopecia, arrhythmia, ataxia, azotemia, coma, creatinine increased 2.5%, dizziness, dyspnea, edema, eosinophilia, hemorrhage, hypertension, hyphema, hypotension, increased LFTs, increased serum creatinine, inflammation or pain at injection site, malaise, nervousness, psychosis, retinal detachment, seizures, tremor, urticaria, uveitis (intravitreal implant), visual loss

**Overdosage/Toxicology**

Signs and symptoms: Neutropenia, vomiting, hypersalivation, bloody diarrhea, cytopenia, testicular atrophy

Treatment: Supportive; hemodialysis removes 50% of drug; hydration may be of some benefit

**Drug Interactions**

Decreased effect: Didanosine: A decrease in steady-state ganciclovir AUC may occur

Increased toxicity:

Immunosuppressive agents may increase cytotoxicity of ganciclovir

Imipenem/cilastatin may increase seizure potential

Zidovudine: Oral ganciclovir increased the AUC of zidovudine, although zidovudine decreases steady state levels of ganciclovir. Since both drugs have the potential to cause neutropenia and anemia, some patients may not tolerate concomitant therapy with these drugs at full dosage.

Probenecid: The renal clearance of ganciclovir is decreased in the presence of probenecid

Didanosine levels are increased with concurrent ganciclovir

Other nephrotoxic drugs (eg, amphotericin and cyclosporine) may have additive nephrotoxicity with ganciclovir

**Usual Dosage**

CMV retinitis: Slow I.V. infusion (dosing is based on total body weight):

Children >3 months and Adults:

Induction therapy: 5 mg/kg/dose every 12 hours for 14-21 days followed by maintenance therapy

Maintenance therapy: 5 mg/kg/day as a single daily dose for 7 days/week or 6 mg/kg/day for 5 days/week

CMV retinitis: Oral: 1000 mg 3 times/day with food **or** 500 mg 6 times/day with food

Prevention of CMV disease in patients with advanced HIV infection and normal renal function: Oral: 1000 mg 3 times/day with food

Prevention of CMV disease in transplant patients: Same initial and maintenance dose as CMV retinitis except duration of initial course is 7-14 days, duration of maintenance therapy is dependent on clinical condition and degree of immunosuppression

Intravitreal implant: One implant for 5- to 8-month period; following depletion of ganciclovir, as evidenced by progression of retinitis, implant may be removed and replaced

**Dosing adjustment in renal impairment:**

I.V. (Induction):

$Cl_{cr}$ 50-69 mL/minute: Administer 2.5 mg/kg/dose every 12 hours

$Cl_{cr}$ 25-49 mL/minute: Administer 2.5 mg/kg/dose every 24 hours

$Cl_{cr}$ 10-24 mL/minute: Administer 1.25 mg/kg/dose every 24 hours

$Cl_{cr}$ <10 mL/minute: Administer 1.25 mg/kg/dose 3 times/week following hemodialysis

I.V. (Maintenance):

$Cl_{cr}$ 50-69 mL/minute: Administer 2.5 mg/kg/dose every 24 hours

$Cl_{cr}$ 25-49 mL/minute: Administer 1.25 mg/kg/dose every 24 hours

$Cl_{cr}$ 10-24 mL/minute: Administer 0.625 mg/kg/dose every 24 hours

$Cl_{cr}$ <10 mL/minute: Administer 0.625 mg/kg/dose 3 times/week following hemodialysis

Oral:

$Cl_{cr}$ 50-69 mL/minute: Administer 1500 mg/day or 500 mg 3 times/day

$Cl_{cr}$ 25-49 mL/minute: Administer 1000 mg/day or 500 mg twice daily

$Cl_{cr}$ 10-24 mL/minute: Administer 500 mg/day

$Cl_{cr}$ <10 mL/minute: Administer 500 mg 3 times/week following hemodialysis

Hemodialysis effects: Dialyzable (50%) following hemodialysis; administer dose postdialysis. During peritoneal dialysis, dose as for $Cl_{cr}$ <10 mL/minute. During continuous arteriovenous or venovenous hemofiltration (CAVH/CAVHD), administer 2.5 mg/kg/dose every 24 hours.

**Patient Information** Ganciclovir is not a cure for CMV retinitis. For oral administration, take as directed and maintain adequate hydration (2-3 L/day of fluids unless instructed to restrict fluid intake). You will need frequent blood tests and regular ophthalmic exams while taking this drug. You may experience increased susceptibility to infection; avoid crowds or exposure to infectious persons. You may experience photosensitivity; use sunscreen, wear protective clothing and eyewear, and avoid direct sunlight. Report fever, chills, unusual bleeding or bruising, infection, or unhealed sores or white plaques in mouth.

(Continued)

## Ganciclovir *(Continued)*

**Nursing Implications** Must be prepared in vertical flow hood; use chemotherapy precautions during administration; discard appropriately

**Dosage Forms**

Capsule: 250 mg

Implant, intravitreal: 4.5 mg released gradually over 5-8 months

Powder for injection, lyophilized: 500 mg (10 mL)

## Ganirelix (ga ni REL ix)

**U.S. Brand Names** Antagon®

**Pharmacologic Category** Antigonadotropic Agent

**Use** Inhibits premature luteinizing hormone (LH) surges in women undergoing controlled ovarian hyperstimulation in fertility clinics

**Effects on Mental Status** None reported

**Effects on Psychiatric Treatment** None reported

**Usual Dosage** Adults: S.C.: 250 mcg/day during the early to midfollicular phase after initiating follicle-stimulating hormone; treatment should be continued daily until the day of chorionic gonadotropin administration

**Dosage Forms** Prefilled glass syringe: 250 mcg/0.5 mL with 27-gauge x 1/2 inch needle

♦ **Ganite™** *see* Gallium Nitrate *on page 245*

♦ **Gantanol®** *see* Sulfamethoxazole *on page 524*

♦ **Gantrisin®** *see* Sulfisoxazole *on page 526*

♦ **Garamycin® Injection** *see* Gentamicin *on page 248*

♦ **Garamycin® Ophthalmic** *see* Gentamicin *on page 248*

♦ **Garamycin® Topical** *see* Gentamicin *on page 248*

## Garlic

**Related Information**

Natural/Herbal Products *on page 746*

Natural Products, Herbals, and Dietary Supplements *on page 742*

**Synonyms** *Allium savitum*; Comphor of the Poor; Nectar of the Gods; Poor Mans Treacle; Rustic Treacle; Stinking Rose

**Pharmacologic Category** Herb

**Use** Herbal medicine used for lowering LDL cholesterol and triglycerides, and raising HDL cholesterol; protection against atherosclerosis, hypertension, antiseptic agent; may lower blood glucose and decrease thrombosis; potential anti-inflammatory and antitumor effects

**Warnings/Precautions** Cholesterol lowering and hypotensive effects may require months. Use with caution in patients receiving treatment for hyperglycemia or hypertension.

**Adverse Reactions**

Dermatologic: Skin blistering, eczema, systemic contact dermatitis, immunologic contact urticaria

Gastrointestinal: G.I. upset and changes in intestinal flora (in rare cases) per Commission E

Ocular: Lacrimation

Respiratory: Asthma (upon inhalation of garlic dust)

Miscellaneous: Allergic reactions (in rare cases); change in odor of skin and breath per Commission E

**Overdosage/Toxicology**

Signs and symptoms: Dizziness, lightheadedness, burning sensation of mouth, hematoma, nausea, sweating, leukocytosis; at doses >50 g daily - anorexia, diarrhea, emesis, and menorrhagia may develop

Decontamination:

Oral: Ipecac within 30 minutes or lavage within 1 hour acute ingestions >25 mL of garlic extract; dilute with milk or water; activated charcoal may prevent absorption

Ocular: Irrigate with saline

**Drug Interactions** Iodine uptake may be reduced with garlic ingestion; can exacerbate bleeding in patients taking aspirin or anticoagulant agents; may increase risk of hypoglycemia, may increase response to antihypertensives

**Usual Dosage** Adult dose: 4-12 mg allicin/day

Average daily dose for cardiovascular benefits: 0.25-1 g/kg or 1-4 cloves daily in an 80 kg individual in divided doses

Toxic dose: >5 cloves or >25 mL of extract can cause gastrointestinal symptoms

**Additional Information** 1% as active as penicillin as an antibiotic; number one over-the-counter medication in Germany; enteric-coated products may demonstrate best results

♦ **Gas-Ban DS® [OTC]** *see* Aluminum Hydroxide, Magnesium Hydroxide, and Simethicone *on page 28*

♦ **Gas Relief®** *see* Simethicone *on page 512*

♦ **Gastrocrom® Oral** *see* Cromolyn Sodium *on page 142*

♦ **Gastrosed™** *see* Hyoscyamine *on page 279*

♦ **Gas-X® [OTC]** *see* Simethicone *on page 512*

## Gatifloxacin (ga ti FLOKS a sin)

**U.S. Brand Names** Tequin™

**Pharmacologic Category** Antibiotic, Quinolone

**Use** Treatment of the following infections when caused by susceptible bacteria: Acute bacterial exacerbation of chronic bronchitis due to *S. pneumoniae, H. influenzae, H. parainfluenzae, M. catarrhalis*, or *S. aureus*; acute sinusitis due to *S. pneumoniae, H. influenzae*; community acquired pneumonia due to *S. pneumoniae, H. influenzae, H. parainfluenzae, M. catarrhalis, S. aureus, M. pneumoniae, C. pneumoniae*, or *L. pneumophilia*; uncomplicated urinary tract infections (cystitis) due to *E. coli, K. pneumoniae*, or *P. mirabilis*; complicated urinary tract infections due to *E. coli, K. pneumoniae*, or *P. mirabilis*; pyelonephritis due to *E. coli*; uncomplicated urethral and cervical gonorrhea; acute, uncomplicated rectal infections in women due to *N. gonorrhoeae*

**Effects on Mental Status** Gatifloxacin may cause dizziness, insomnia; may rarely produce abnormal thinking, agitation, anorexia, anxiety, asthenia, ataxia, confusion, depersonalization, depression, euphoria, hallucination, hostility, nervousness, panic attacks, paranoia, psychosis, somnolence, or stress

**Effects on Psychiatric Treatment** May have potential to prolong Q-T interval; should avoid in patients with uncorrected hypokalemia, or concurrent administration of other medications known to prolong the Q-T interval (antipsychotics, and tricyclic antidepressants)

**Pregnancy Risk Factor** C

**Contraindications** Hypersensitivity to gatifloxacin, other quinolone antibiotics, or any component

**Warnings/Precautions** Use with caution in patients with significant bradycardia or acute myocardial ischemia. May have potential to prolong Q-T interval; should avoid in patients with uncorrected hypokalemia, or concurrent administration of other medications known to prolong the Q-T interval (including class Ia and class III antiarrhythmics, cisapride, erythromycin, antipsychotics, and tricyclic antidepressants). Safety and effectiveness in pediatric patients (<18 years of age) have not been established. Experience in immature animals has resulted in permanent arthropathy. Use with caution in individuals at risk of seizures (CNS disorders or concurrent therapy with medications which may lower seizure threshold). Discontinue in patients who experience significant CNS adverse effects (dizziness, hallucinations, suicidal ideation or actions). Use caution in renal dysfunction (dosage adjustment required) and in severe hepatic insufficiency (no data available). Use caution in patients with diabetes - glucose regulation may be altered.

Severe hypersensitivity reactions, including anaphylaxis, have occurred with quinolone therapy. If an allergic reaction occurs (itching, urticaria, dyspnea, facial edema, loss of consciousness, tingling, cardiovascular collapse) discontinue drug immediately. Prolonged use may result in superinfection; pseudomembranous colitis may occur and should be considered in all patients who present with diarrhea. Tendon inflammation and/or rupture has been reported with other quinolone antibiotics. This has not been reported for gatifloxacin. Discontinue at first sign of tendon inflammation or pain.

**Adverse Reactions**

3% to 10%:

Central nervous system: Headache (3%), dizziness (3%)

Gastrointestinal: Nausea (8%), diarrhea (4%)

Genitourinary: Vaginitis (6%)

Local: Injection site reactions (5%)

0.1% to 3%: Allergic reaction, chills, fever, back pain, chest pain, palpitation, abdominal pain, constipation, dyspepsia, glossitis, oral candidiasis, stomatitis, mouth ulceration, vomiting, peripheral edema, abnormal dreams, insomnia, paresthesia, tremor, vasodilation, vertigo, dyspnea, pharyngitis, rash, sweating, abnormal vision, taste perversion, tinnitus, dysuria, hematuria, elevated serum transaminases, elevated alkaline phosphatase, increased serum bilirubin, increased serum amylase, tendonitis/tendon rupture

<0.1% (Limited to important or life-threatening symptoms): Abnormal thinking, agitation, alcohol intolerance, anorexia, anxiety, arthralgia, arthritis, asthenia, ataxia, bone pain, bradycardia, breast pain, bronchospasm, cheilitis, colitis, confusion, cyanosis, depersonalization, depression, diabetes mellitus, dry skin, dysphagia, ear pain, ecchymosis, edema, epistaxis, euphoria, eye pain, facial edema, flatulence, gastritis, gastrointestinal hemorrhage, gingivitis, halitosis, hallucination, hematemesis, hostility, hyperesthesia, hyperglycemia, hypertension, hypertonia, hyperventilation, hypoglycemia, leg cramps, lymphadenopathy, maculopapular rash, metrorrhagia, migraine, myalgia, myasthenia, neck pain, nervousness, panic attacks, paranoia, parosmia, pruritus, pseudomembranous colitis, psychosis, ptosis, rectal hemorrhage, seizures, somnolence, stress, tachycardia, taste disturbance, thirst, tongue edema, vesiculobullous rash

**Overdosage/Toxicology** Potential symptoms of overdose may include CNS excitation, seizures, Q-T prolongation, and arrhythmias (including torsade de pointes). Patients should be monitored by continuous EKG in the event of an overdose. Management is supportive and symptomatic. Not removed by dialysis.

**Drug Interactions**

Antineoplastic agents may decrease the absorption of quinolones

Calcium carbonate was not found to alter the absorption of gatifloxacin.

Cimetidine, and other $H_2$-antagonists may inhibit renal elimination of quinolones

Digoxin levels may be increased in some patients by gatifloxacin; monitor for increased effect/concentrations

Foscarnet has been associated with an increased risk of seizures with some quinolones

Gatifloxacin may prolong Q-T interval; avoid use with drugs which prolong Q-T interval (including class Ia and class III antiarrhythmics, erythromycin, cisapride, antipsychotics, and cyclic antidepressants).

$H_2$-antagonists and proton pump inhibitors may decrease absorption of some quinolones

Loop diuretics: Serum levels of some quinolones are increased by loop diuretic administration; may diminish renal excretion

Metal cations (magnesium, aluminum, iron, and zinc) bind quinolones in the gastrointestinal tract and inhibit absorption (by up to 98%). Antacids, electrolyte supplements, sucralfate, quinapril, and some didanosine formulations should be avoided. Gatifloxacin should be administered 4 hours before or 8 hours after these agents.

NSAIDs: The CNS stimulating effect of some quinolones may be enhanced, resulting in neuroexcitation and/or seizures; this effect has not been observed with gatifloxacin

Probenecid: Blocks renal secretion of gatifloxacin, increasing AUC and half-life

Warfarin: The hypoprothrombinemic effect of warfarin is enhanced by some quinolone antibiotics. No significant effect has been demonstrated for gatifloxacin; however, monitoring of the INR during concurrent therapy is recommended by the manufacturer.

**Usual Dosage** Adults: Oral, I.V.:

Acute bacterial exacerbation of chronic bronchitis; 400 mg every 24 hours for 7-10 days

Acute sinusitis: 400 mg every 24 hours for 10 days

Community acquired pneumonia: 400 mg every 24 hours for 7-14 days

Uncomplicated urinary tract infections (cystitis): 200-400 mg every 24 hours for 3 days

Complicated urinary tract infections: 400 mg every 24 hours for 7-10 days

Acute pyelonephritis: 400 mg every 24 hours for 7-10 days

Uncomplicated urethral gonorrhea in men, cervical or rectal gonorrhea in women: 400 mg single dose

**Dosage adjustment in renal impairment:** Creatinine clearance <40 mL/minute (or patients on hemodialysis/CAPD) should receive an initial dose of 400 mg, followed by a subsequent dose of 200 mg every 24 hours. Patients receiving single-dose or 3-day therapy for appropriate indications do not require dosage adjustment.

**Dosage adjustment in hepatic impairment:** No dosage adjustment is required in mild-moderate hepatic disease. No data are available in severe hepatic impairment (Child-Pugh Class C).

Elderly: No dosage adjustment is required based on age, however, assessment of renal function is particularly important in this population.

**Patient Information** May be taken with or without food. Drink plenty of fluids. Avoid exposure to direct sunlight during therapy and for several days following. Do not take antacids within 4 hours before or 2 hours after dosing. Contact your physician immediately if signs of allergy occur or if signs of tendon inflammation or pain occur. Do not discontinue therapy until your course has been completed. Take a missed dose as soon as possible, unless it is almost time for your next dose. Report immediately any pain, inflammation, or rupture of tendon.

**Dosage Forms**

Infusion: 2 mg/mL (100 mL, 200 mL)

Injection: 10 mg/mL (20 mL, 40 mL)

Tablet: 200 mg, 400 mg

- **Gaviscon®-2 Tablet [OTC]** *see* Aluminum Hydroxide and Magnesium Trisilicate *on page 28*
- **Gaviscon® Liquid [OTC]** *see* Aluminum Hydroxide and Magnesium Carbonate *on page 28*
- **Gaviscon® Tablet [OTC]** *see* Aluminum Hydroxide and Magnesium Trisilicate *on page 28*
- **G-CSF** *see* Filgrastim *on page 225*
- **GCV Sodium** *see* Ganciclovir *on page 245*
- **Gee Gee® [OTC]** *see* Guaifenesin *on page 256*
- **Gelpirin® [OTC]** *see* Acetaminophen, Aspirin, and Caffeine *on page 15*
- **Gelucast®** *see* Zinc Gelatin *on page 593*

## Gemcitabine (jem SIT a been)

**U.S. Brand Names** Gemzar®

**Pharmacologic Category** Antineoplastic Agent, Antimetabolite

**Use** Adenocarcinoma of the pancreas; first-line therapy for patients with locally advanced (nonresectable stage II of stage III) or metastatic (stage IV) adenocarcinoma of the pancreas (indicated for patients previously treated with 5-FU); combination with cisplatin for the first-line treatment of patients with inoperable, locally advanced (stage IIIA or IIIB) or metastatic (stage IV) nonsmall cell lung cancer

**Effects on Mental Status** None reported

**Effects on Psychiatric Treatment** Leukopenia is common; use caution with clozapine and carbamazepine

**Usual Dosage** Adults: I.V. (refer to individual protocols): 1000 mg/m$^2$ once weekly for up to 7 weeks (or until toxicity necessitates reducing or holding a dose), followed by a week of rest from treatment; subsequent cycles should consist of infusions once weekly for 3 consecutive weeks out of every 4 weeks

**Dosing reductions based on hematologic function:** Patients who complete an entire 7-week initial cycle of gemcitabine therapy or a subsequent 3-week cycle at a dose of 1000 mg/m$^2$ may have the dose for subsequent cycles increased by 25% (1250 mg/m$^2$), provided that the absolute granulocyte count and platelet nadirs exceed 1500 x 10$^6$/L and 100,000 x 10$^6$/L, respectively, and if nonhematologic toxicity has not been more than World Health Organization Grade 1

For patients who tolerate the subsequent course, at a dose of 1250 mg/m$^2$, the dose for the next cycle can be increased to 1500 mg/m$^2$, provided again that the AGC and platelet nadirs exceed 1500 x 10$^6$/L and 100,000 x 10$^6$/L, respectively, and again, if nonhematologic toxicity has not been greater than WHO Grade 1

**Dosing adjustment in renal/hepatic impairment:** Use with caution; gemcitabine has not been studied in patients with significant renal or hepatic dysfunction

**Dosage Forms** Powder for injection, as hydrochloride, lyophilized: 20 mg/mL (10 mL, 50 mL)

## Gemfibrozil (jem FI broe zil)

**Related Information**

Lipid-Lowering Agents Comparison Chart *on page 717*

**U.S. Brand Names** Lopid®

**Canadian Brand Names** Apo®-Gemfibrozil; Nu-Gemfibrozil

**Synonyms** CI-719

**Pharmacologic Category** Antilipemic Agent (Fibric Acid)

**Use** Treatment of hypertriglyceridemia in types IV and V hyperlipidemia for patients who are at greater risk for pancreatitis and who have not responded to dietary intervention

**Effects on Mental Status** May cause sedation; may rarely cause depression

**Effects on Psychiatric Treatment** None reported

**Pregnancy Risk Factor** C

**Contraindications** Hypersensitivity to gemfibrozil or any component; significant hepatic or renal dysfunction; primary biliary cirrhosis; pre-existing gallbladder disease

**Warnings/Precautions** Possible increased risk of malignancy and cholelithiasis. No evidence of cardiovascular mortality benefit. Anemia and leukopenia have been reported. Elevations in serum transaminases can be seen. Discontinue if lipid response not seen. Be careful in patient selection; this is not a first- or second-line choice. Other agents may be more suitable. Adjustments in warfarin therapy may be required with concurrent use. Use caution when combining gemfibrozil with HMG-CoA reductase inhibitors (may lead to myopathy, rhabdomyolysis). Renal function deterioration has been seen when used in patients with a serum creatinine >2.0 mg/dL. Safety and efficacy in pediatric patients have not been established.

**Adverse Reactions**

>10%:

Gastrointestinal: Dyspepsia (20%), abdominal pain (10%)

Hepatic: Cholelithiasis

1% to 10%:

Central nervous system: Fatigue (4%), vertigo (1.5%), headache (1.2%)

Dermatologic: Eczema/rash (1% to 2%)

Gastrointestinal: Diarrhea (7%), nausea/vomiting (2.5%), constipation (1.4%), acute appendicitis (1.2%)

<1%: Atrial fibrillation, blurred vision, dizziness, drowsiness, flatulence, hyperesthesia, mental depression, paresthesia, somnolence

**Overdosage/Toxicology**

Signs and symptoms: Abdominal pain, diarrhea, nausea, vomiting

Treatment: Following GI decontamination, treatment is supportive

**Drug Interactions** CYP3A3/4 enzyme substrate

Bexarotene's serum concentration is significantly increased; avoid concurrent use

Chlorpropamide: May increase risk of hypoglycemia

Cyclosporine's blood levels may be reduced; monitor cyclosporine levels and renal function

Furosemide: Increased blood levels of both in hypoalbuminemia

Glyburide (and possibly other sulfonylureas): The hypoglycemic effects may be increased

HMG-CoA reductase inhibitors (atorvastatin, cerivastatin, fluvastatin, lovastatin, pravastatin, simvastatin) may increase the risk of myopathy and

(Continued)

## Gemfibrozil *(Continued)*

rhabdomyolysis. The manufacturer warns against the concurrent use of lovastatin. However, combination therapy with statins has been used in some patients with resistant hyperlipidemias (with great caution).

Rifampin: Decreased gemfibrozil blood levels

Warfarin: Hypoprothrombinemic response increased; monitor INRs closely when gemfibrozil is initiated or discontinued

**Usual Dosage** Adults: Oral: 1200 mg/day in 2 divided doses, 30 minutes before breakfast and dinner

Hemodialysis: Not removed by hemodialysis; supplemental dose is not necessary

**Patient Information** You must return to provider for assessment of drug effectiveness. Should be taken 30 minutes before meals. Take with milk or meals if GI upset occurs. You may experience loss of appetite and flatulence (frequent small meals may help), muscle aches (mild, temporary pain relievers may be required), dizziness, faintness, or blurred vision (use caution when driving or engaging in tasks that require alertness until response to drug is known). Report severe stomach pain, nausea, vomiting, chills, sore throat, headache, and any vision changes.

**Dosage Forms**

Capsule: 300 mg

Tablet, film coated: 600 mg

## Gemtuzumab Ozogamicin (gem TUZ yu mab oh zog a MY sin)

**U.S. Brand Names** Mylotarg™

**Pharmacologic Category** Antineoplastic Agent, Natural Source (Plant) Derivative

**Use** Treatment of acute myeloid leukemia (CD33 positive) in first relapse in patients who are ≥60 years of age and who are not considered candidates for cytotoxic chemotherapy.

**Effects on Mental Status** Dizziness, insomnia, and depression are common

**Effects on Psychiatric Treatment** Hypotension is common; caution with low potency antipsychotics and TCAs; nausea and vomiting are common, use caution with the SSRIs. Neutropenia is common, use caution with carbamazepine and clozapine.

**Usual Dosage** I.V.: Adults ≥60 years: 9 mg/m$^2$, infused over 2 hours. The patient should receive diphenhydramine 50 mg and acetaminophen 650-1000 mg orally 1 hour prior to administration of each dose. Acetaminophen dosage should be repeated as needed every 4 hours for two additional doses. A full treatment course is a total of two doses administered with 14 days between doses. Full hematologic recovery is not necessary for administration of the second dose. There has been only limited experience with repeat courses of gemtuzumab ozogamicin.

**Dosage adjustment in renal impairment:** No recommendation (not studied)

**Dosage adjustment in hepatic impairment:** No recommendation (not studied)

**Dosage Forms** Powder for injection: 5 mg


- **Gemzar®** *see* Gemcitabine *on page 247*
- **Genabid®** *see* Papaverine *on page 419*
- **Genac® Tablet [OTC]** *see* Triprolidine and Pseudoephedrine *on page 572*
- **Genagesic®** *see* Guaifenesin and Phenylpropanolamine *on page 257*
- **Genahist® Oral** *see* Diphenhydramine *on page 174*
- **Genamin® Cold Syrup [OTC]** *see* Chlorpheniramine and Phenylpropanolamine *on page 114*
- **Genamin® Expectorant [OTC]** *see* Guaifenesin and Phenylpropanolamine *on page 257*
- **Genapap® [OTC]** *see* Acetaminophen *on page 14*
- **Genaspor® [OTC]** *see* Tolnaftate *on page 555*
- **Genatap® Elixir [OTC]** *see* Brompheniramine and Phenylpropanolamine *on page 74*
- **Genatuss® [OTC]** *see* Guaifenesin *on page 256*
- **Genatuss DM® [OTC]** *see* Guaifenesin and Dextromethorphan *on page 257*
- **Gencalc® 600 [OTC]** *see* Calcium Carbonate *on page 84*
- **Geneye® Ophthalmic [OTC]** *see* Tetrahydrozoline *on page 538*
- **Gen-K®** *see* Potassium Chloride *on page 453*
- **Genoptic® Ophthalmic** *see* Gentamicin *on page 248*
- **Genoptic® S.O.P. Ophthalmic** *see* Gentamicin *on page 248*
- **Genora® 0.5/35** *see* Ethinyl Estradiol and Norethindrone *on page 212*
- **Genora® 1/35** *see* Ethinyl Estradiol and Norethindrone *on page 212*
- **Genora® 1/50** *see* Mestranol and Norethindrone *on page 346*
- **Genotropin® Injection** *see* Human Growth Hormone *on page 269*
- **Genpril® [OTC]** *see* Ibuprofen *on page 280*
- **Gentacidin® Ophthalmic** *see* Gentamicin *on page 248*
- **Gentak® Ophthalmic** *see* Gentamicin *on page 248*


## Gentamicin (jen ta MYE sin)

**Related Information**

Serum Drug Concentrations Commonly Monitored: Guidelines *on page 759*

**U.S. Brand Names** Garamycin® Injection; Garamycin® Ophthalmic; Garamycin® Topical; Genoptic® Ophthalmic; Genoptic® S.O.P. Ophthalmic; Gentacidin® Ophthalmic; Gentak® Ophthalmic; G-myticin® Topical; Jenamicin® Injection

**Pharmacologic Category** Antibiotic, Aminoglycoside; Antibiotic, Ophthalmic; Antibiotic, Topical

**Use** Treatment of susceptible bacterial infections, normally gram-negative organisms including *Pseudomonas*, *Proteus*, *Serratia*, and gram-positive *Staphylococcus*; treatment of bone infections, respiratory tract infections, skin and soft tissue infections, as well as abdominal and urinary tract infections, endocarditis, and septicemia; used topically to treat superficial infections of the skin or ophthalmic infections caused by susceptible bacteria; prevention of bacterial endocarditis prior to dental or surgical procedures

**Effects on Mental Status** Dizziness is common; may cause drowsiness

**Effects on Psychiatric Treatment** May rarely cause agranulocytosis; use caution with clozapine and carbamazepine

**Usual Dosage** Individualization is critical because of the low therapeutic index

**Use of ideal body weight (IBW) for determining the mg/kg/dose appears to be more accurate than dosing on the basis of total body weight (TBW).**

In morbid obesity, dosage requirement may best be estimated using a dosing weight of IBW + 0.4 (TBW - IBW)

Initial and periodic peak and trough plasma drug levels should be determined, particularly in critically ill patients with serious infections or in disease states known to significantly alter aminoglycoside pharmacokinetics (eg, cystic fibrosis, burns, or major surgery)

Newborns: Intrathecal: 1 mg every day

Infants >3 months: Intrathecal: 1-2 mg/day

Infants and Children <5 years: I.M., I.V.: 2.5 mg/kg/dose every 8 hours*

Cystic fibrosis: 2.5 mg/kg/dose every 6 hours

Children >5 years: I.M., I.V.: 1.5-2.5 mg/kg/dose every 8 hours*

Prevention of bacterial endocarditis: Dental, oral, upper respiratory procedures, GI/GU procedures: 2 mg/kg with ampicillin (50 mg/kg) 30 minutes prior to procedure

*Some patients may require larger or more frequent doses (eg, every 6 hours) if serum levels document the need (ie, cystic fibrosis or febrile granulocytopenic patients)

Adults: I.M., I.V.:

Severe life-threatening infections: 2-2.5 mg/kg/dose

Urinary tract infections: 1.5 mg/kg/dose

Synergy (for gram-positive infections): 1 mg/kg/dose

Prevention of bacterial endocarditis:

Dental, oral, or upper respiratory procedures: 1.5 mg/kg not to exceed 80 mg with ampicillin (1-2 g) 30 minutes prior to procedure

GI/GU surgery: 1.5 mg/kg not to exceed 80 mg with ampicillin 2 g 30 minutes prior to procedure

Children and Adults:

Intrathecal: 4-8 mg/day

Ophthalmic:

Ointment: Instill 1/2" (1.25 cm) 2-3 times/day to every 3-4 hours

Solution: Instill 1-2 drops every 2-4 hours, up to 2 drops every hour for severe infections

Topical: Apply 3-4 times/day to affected area

Some clinicians suggest a daily dose of 4-7 mg/kg for all patients with normal renal function. This dose is at least as efficacious with similar, if not less, toxicity than conventional dosing.

**Dosing interval in renal impairment:**

$Cl_{cr}$ ≥60 mL/minute: Administer every 8 hours

$Cl_{cr}$ 40-60 mL/minute: Administer every 12 hours

$Cl_{cr}$ 20-40 mL/minute: Administer every 24 hours

$Cl_{cr}$ <20 mL/minute: Loading dose, then monitor levels

Hemodialysis: Dialyzable; removal by hemodialysis: 30% removal of aminoglycosides occurs during 4 hours of HD; administer dose after dialysis and follow levels

Removal by continuous ambulatory peritoneal dialysis (CAPD):

Administration via CAPD fluid:

Gram-negative infection: 4-8 mg/L (4-8 mcg/mL) of CAPD fluid

Gram-positive infection (ie, synergy): 3-4 mg/L (3-4 mcg/mL) of CAPD fluid

Administration via I.V., I.M. route during CAPD: Dose as for $Cl_{cr}$ <10 mL/minute and follow levels

Removal via continuous arteriovenous or venovenous hemofiltration (CAVH/CAVHD): Dose as for $Cl_{cr}$ 10-40 mL/minute and follow levels

**Dosing adjustment/comments in hepatic disease:** Monitor plasma concentrations

**Dosage Forms**

Cream, topical, as sulfate (Garamycin®, G-myticin®): 0.1% (15 g)

Infusion, in $D_5W$, as sulfate: 60 mg, 80 mg, 100 mg

Infusion, in NS, as sulfate: 40 mg, 60 mg, 80 mg, 90 mg, 100 mg, 120 mg

Injection, as sulfate: 40 mg/mL (1 mL, 1.5 mL, 2 mL)

Pediatric, as sulfate: 10 mg/mL (2 mL)

Intrathecal, preservative free, as sulfate (Garamycin®): 2 mg/mL (2 mL)

Ointment, as sulfate:

Ophthalmic: 0.3% [3 mg/g] (3.5 g)

Garamycin®, Genoptic® S.O.P., Gentacidin®, Gentak®: 0.3% [3 mg/g] (3.5 g)

Topical, as sulfate (Garamycin®, G-myticin®): 0.1% (15 g)

Solution, ophthalmic, as sulfate: 0.3% (5 mL, 15 mL)

Garamycin®, Genoptic®, Gentacidin®, Gentak®: 0.3% (1 mL, 5 mL, 15 mL)

- **Gen-XENE®** *see* Clorazepate *on page 134*
- **Geocillin®** *see* Carbenicillin *on page 92*
- **Gericin®** *see* Nitrendipine *on page 396*

## Germander

**Synonyms** *Teucrium chamaedrys*

**Pharmacologic Category** Herb

**Use** In folk medicine to treat obesity; digestive aid; gout; gall bladder conditions

**Adverse Reactions** Hepatic: Jaundice, liver function tests (elevated), hepatic necrosis (centrilobular)

**Overdosage/Toxicology**

Decontamination: Ipecac within 30 minutes or lavage (within 1 hour)/activated charcoal with cathartic

Treatment: Supportive therapy; although there are no human or animal data, due to the fact that glutathione depletion can result in increased hepatotoxicity in mice, there exists a rational to use N-acetylcysteine

**Usual Dosage** Daily dose: 600 mg to 1.62 g

**Patient Information** Considered unsafe

**Additional Information** Not reviewed by Commission E; not generally sold in the United States, mainly in Europe; plant is found in Eastern Europe and Mediterranean; dexamethasone or clotrimazole may increase hepatotoxicity; hepatotoxicity usually presents 3-18 hours after ingestion; blossoms are used in folk medicine in Europe, not in U.S.

**Dosage Forms**

Capsules: 200-275 mg (no longer marketed)

Herbal teas: ~1 g/bag of germander (no longer marketed)

- **Germinal®** *see* Ergoloid Mesylates *on page 199*
- **Gevrabon® [OTC]** *see* Vitamin B Complex *on page 586*
- **GG** *see* Guaifenesin *on page 256*
- **GG-Cen® [OTC]** *see* Guaifenesin *on page 256*
- **GI87084B** *see* Remifentanil *on page 490*

## Ginger

**Related Information**

Perspectives on the Safety of Herbal Medicines *on page 736*

**Synonyms** *Zingiber officinale*

**Pharmacologic Category** Herb

**Use** In herbal medicine as a digestive aid; for treatment of nausea (antiemetic) and motion sickness; also used as a menstruation promoter in Chinese herbal medicine; headaches, colds and flu; ginger oil is used as a flavoring agent in beverages and mouthwashes; may be useful in some forms of arthritis

**Contraindications** Gallstones per Commission E

**Warnings/Precautions** Use with caution in diabetics, patients on cardiac glycosides, and patients receiving anticoagulants

**Overdosage/Toxicology**

Signs and symptoms: May cause central nervous system depression in large doses

Decontamination: Lavage (within 1 hour)/activated charcoal with cathartic

**Drug Interactions** May alter response to cardiotonic, hypoglycemia, anticoagulant, antiplatelet agents

**Usual Dosage**

For preventing motion sickness or digestive aid: 1-4 g/day (250 mg of ginger root powder 4 times/day)

Per Commission E: 2-4 g/day or equivalent preparations

**Additional Information** Density of ginger oil is ~0.9; ginger is a perennial plant with green-purple flowers similar to orchids which grows in India, the Orient, and Jamaica; 8 oz of ginger ale contains ~1 g of ginger; ginger tea (1 cup) contains ~250 mg of ginger

## Ginkgo Biloba

**Related Information**

Natural/Herbal Products *on page 746*

Natural Products, Herbals, and Dietary Supplements *on page 742*

**Synonyms** CF100

**Pharmacologic Category** Herb

**Use** Dilates blood vessels; plant/leaf extract has been used in Europe for intermittent claudication, arterial insufficiency, and cerebral vascular disease (dementia); tinnitus, visual disorders, traumatic brain injury, vertigo of vascular origin

Per Commission E: Demential syndromes including memory deficits, etc (tinnitus, headache); depressive emotional conditions, primary degenerative dementia, vascular dementia, or both

**Unlabeled use:** Asthma, impotence (male)

**Contraindications** Pregnancy, patients with clotting disorders; hypersensitivity to ginkgo biloba preparations per Commission E

**Warnings/Precautions** Use with caution following recent surgery or trauma; effects may require 1-2 months

**Adverse Reactions**

Cardiovascular: Palpitations, bilateral subdural hematomas

Central nervous system: Headache (very seldom per Commission E), dizziness, seizures (in children), restlessness

Dermatologic: Urticaria, cheilitis

Gastrointestinal: Nausea, diarrhea, vomiting, stomatitis, proctitis; very seldom stomach or intestinal upsets (per Commission E)

Ocular: Hyphema

Miscellaneous: Allergic skin reactions (very seldom per Commission E)

**Overdosage/Toxicology**

Decontamination:

Dermal: Washing skin within 10 minutes may prevent dermal allergic contact dermatitis; remove all clothing

Oral: Lavage (within 1 hour)/activated charcoal (laxative not needed)

Treatment: Supportive therapy; although human data are lacking, since the central nervous system effects may be due to 4-*o*-methylpyridoxine (an antipyridoxine compound), pyridoxine may be useful after ingestion of ginkgo seeds or kernels in children; topical corticosteroids can be used for skin reactions

**Drug Interactions**

Acetylcholinesterase inhibitors: Effect and/or toxicity may be increased with concurrent administration

Antiplatelet agents: Effects on platelet aggregation may be potentiated by ginkgo

MAO inhibitors: Effect/toxicity may be enhanced by ginkgo

Linezolid: Effect/toxicity may be enhanced by ginkgo

Warfarin: Anticoagulant effects may be potentiated by antiplatelet activity of ginkgo

**Usual Dosage** Beneficial effects for cerebral ischemia in the elderly occur after one month of use

Usual dosage: ~40 mg 3 times/day with meals; 60-80 mg twice daily to 3 times/day depending on indication; maximum dose: 360 mg/day

Cerebral ischemia: 120 mg/day in 2-3 divided doses (24% flavonoid-glycoside extract, 6% terpene glycosides)

**Additional Information** Seeds and pulp are poisonous; beneficial effects for cerebral ischemia in the elderly occur after one month of use. Grown on plantations, leaves are extracted with organic solvent (acetone) to a potency of 24% flavonoids and 6% terpenoids. Can increase alpha waves and decrease slow potentials in EEG. An Oriental deciduous tree with plum-like fruits (in autumn) and flowers in spring. May reach a height of 125' (20' girth) and is found in the U.S., Europe, China, and Japan. Cross-reactivity for contact dermatitis due to the fruit pulp exists with poison ivy and poison oak; the dermatological symptoms may last for 10 days, inner bark is used as a whitish brown cloth dye. Leaf extract has been used in herbal medicine to treat dementia, chronic tinnitus, vertigo, cochlear deafness, and impotence.

## Ginseng

**Related Information**

Natural/Herbal Products *on page 746*

Natural Products, Herbals, and Dietary Supplements *on page 742*

**Synonyms** *P. quinquefolium L.*; *P. trifolius L.*

**Pharmacologic Category** Herb

**Use** A popular ingredient in herbal teas; has been advocated for its antistress and adaptogenic effects although these effects have not been scientifically confirmed, there's much "suggestive" scientific literature

**Contraindications** Estrogen-receptor positive breast cancer

**Warnings/Precautions** Nervousness may occur during first few days; use with caution in hypertensives, diabetes; avoid long-term use

**Adverse Reactions**

Cardiovascular: Tachycardia, hypertension, sinus tachycardia

(Continued)

## Ginseng *(Continued)*

Central nervous system: Nervousness, agitation, mania, headache, sciatic nerve inflammation

Dermatologic: Stevens Johnson syndrome

Endocrine & metabolic: Hypoglycemia, vaginal bleeding, breast nodules

**Overdosage/Toxicology**

Signs and symptoms: Ginseng abuse syndrome (noted in patients ingesting 3-15 g/day for up to 2 years) is characterized by morning diarrhea, insomnia, euphoria, edema, nervousness, and skin eruptions

Decontamination: Usually decontamination is not required for ingestions <3 g; lavage (within 1 hour)/activated charcoal can be utilized

**Drug Interactions**

**Note:** Drug interaction potential may vary by species (Panax vs Siberian ginseng)

Antihypertensives: Effect on blood pressure may be antagonized or potentiated (orthostasis); monitor BP

Antiplatelet agents: Effects on platelet aggregation may be potentiated by ginseng

Barbiturates: Effects may be potentiated by Siberian ginseng

CNS stimulants: Effects may be potentiated by ginseng

Digoxin: Serum levels may be increased by Siberian ginseng

Estrogens: Effects may be potentiated by Siberian ginseng

Hypoglycemics (including insulin): Effects may be potentiated by Siberian ginseng (not Panax)

Sympathomimetics: Effects may be potentiated by ginseng

Warfarin: Anticoagulant effects may be potentiated by antiplatelet activity of ginseng

**Usual Dosage** Avoid long-term use

Herbal tea: Usually about 1.75 g; 0.5-2 g/day

Dried root: 0.6-3 g/day of dried root or equivalent preparations

Ethanolic extract: 0.5-6 mL 1-3 times/day

Root: 1-2 g/day

Extract: (7% ginsenosides) 100-300 mg 3 times/day

**Additional Information** There are three forms of ginseng (American, Asian, and Siberian); each has slightly different properties. In the U.S., the root crop of ginseng is obtained from *Panax quinquefolius* L (American ginseng) or *Panax trifolius* L (Dwarf ginseng). The plants are found in woody areas and are about 3 feet tall with yellow-green flowers and red/yellow fruits (from June to July). Additional information can be obtained from:

Ginseng Board of Wisconsin
16-H Menard Plaza
Wausau, Wisconsin 54401
(715) 845-7300

Capsules: 100-200 mg ginseng claimed per capsule (0.4-23.2 mg of ginsenoside noted per capsule). Most brands contain <8% concentration of ginsenoside/capsule.

♦ **Gittalun®** *see* Doxylamine *on page 186*

## Glatiramer (gla TIR a mer)

**U.S. Brand Names** Copaxone®

**Synonyms** Copolymer-1

**Pharmacologic Category** Biological, Miscellaneous

**Use** Relapsing-remitting type multiple sclerosis; studies indicate that it reduces the frequency of attacks and the severity of disability; appears to be most effective for patients with minimal disability

**Effects on Mental Status** May cause anxiety or depression

**Effects on Psychiatric Treatment** None reported

**Pregnancy Risk Factor** B

**Contraindications** Previous hypersensitivity to any component of the copolymer formulation

**Adverse Reactions**

>10%:

Cardiovascular: Chest pain (26%)

Local: Pain

1% to 10%:

Cardiovascular: Chest tightness, flushing, tachycardia, vasodilitation

Central nervous system: Anxiety, depression, dizziness

Dermatologic: Erythema (4%), urticaria

Hematologic: Transient eosinophilia

Local: Injection site reactions (6.5%)

Neuromuscular & skeletal: Tremor

Respiratory: Dyspnea

Miscellaneous: Diaphoresis, unintended pregnancy

**Overdosage/Toxicology** Signs and symptoms: Well tolerated; no serious toxicities can be anticipated

**Usual Dosage** Adults: S.C.: 20 mg daily

**Patient Information** It is essential to provide the patient with proper handling and reconstitution instruction, since they will most likely have to self-administer the drug for an extended period

**Dosage Forms** Injection: Single-use vials containing 20 mg of glatiramer and 40 mg mannitol; packaged in 2 mL vials along with 1 mL vial of diluent (sterile water for injection)

♦ **Glaucoma Drug Therapy** *see page 712*

♦ **Glaucon®** *see* Epinephrine *on page 195*

♦ **GlaucTabs®** *see* Methazolamide *on page 351*

♦ **Glibenclamide** *see* Glyburide *on page 252*

## Glimepiride (GLYE me pye ride)

**Related Information**

Diabetes Mellitus Treatment *on page 782*

Hypoglycemic Drugs and Thiazolidinedione Information *on page 714*

**U.S. Brand Names** Amaryl®

**Pharmacologic Category** Antidiabetic Agent (Sulfonylurea)

**Use**

Management of noninsulin-dependent diabetes mellitus (type 2) as an adjunct to diet and exercise to lower blood glucose

Use in combination with insulin to lower blood glucose in patients whose hyperglycemia cannot be controlled by diet and exercise in conjunction with an oral hypoglycemic agent

**Effects on Mental Status** None reported

**Effects on Psychiatric Treatment** May rarely cause agranulocytosis; use caution with clozapine and carbamazepine; phenothiazines and TCAs may antagonize glimepiride hypoglycemic effects; MAOIs and TCAs may enhance hypoglycemic effects

**Pregnancy Risk Factor** C

**Contraindications** Hypersensitivity to glimepiride or any component, other sulfonamides; diabetic ketoacidosis (with or without coma)

**Warnings/Precautions** All sulfonylurea drugs are capable of producing severe hypoglycemia. Hypoglycemia is more likely to occur when caloric intake is deficient, after severe or prolonged exercise, when alcohol is ingested, or when more than one glucose-lowering drug is used.

Product labeling states oral hypoglycemic drugs may be associated with an increased cardiovascular mortality as compared to treatment with diet alone or diet plus insulin. Data to support this association are limited, and several studies, including a large prospective trial (UKPDS) have not supported an association.

**Adverse Reactions**

1% to 10%: Central nervous system: Headache

<1%: Agranulocytosis, anorexia, aplastic anemia, blood dyscrasias, bone marrow suppression, cholestatic jaundice, constipation, diarrhea, diuretic effect, edema, epigastric fullness, heartburn, hemolytic anemia, hypoglycemia, hyponatremia, nausea, photosensitivity, rash, thrombocytopenia, urticaria, vomiting

**Overdosage/Toxicology**

Signs and symptoms: Low blood sugar, tingling of lips and tongue, nausea, yawning, confusion, agitation, tachycardia, sweating, convulsions, stupor, and coma

Treatment: Intoxications with sulfonylureas can cause hypoglycemia and are best managed with glucose administration (oral for milder hypoglycemia or by injection in more severe forms). Patients should be monitored for a minimum of 24-48 hours after ingestion.

**Drug Interactions** CYP2C9 enzyme substrate

Decreased effects: Cholestyramine, hydantoins, rifampin, thiazide diuretics, urinary alkalines, charcoal

Increased effects: $H_2$-antagonists, anticoagulants, androgens, beta-blockers, fluconazole, salicylates, gemfibrozil, sulfonamides, tricyclic antidepressants, probenecid, MAO inhibitors, methyldopa, NSAIDs, salicylates, sulfonamides, chloramphenicol, coumarins, probenecid, MAO inhibitors, digitalis glycosides, urinary acidifiers

Increased toxicity: Cimetidine may increase hypoglycemic effects; certain drugs tend to produce hyperglycemia and may lead to loss of control. These drugs include the thiazides and other diuretics, corticosteroids, phenothiazines, thyroid products, estrogens, oral contraceptives, phenytoin, nicotinic acid, sympathomimetics, and isoniazid.

**Usual Dosage** Oral (allow several days between dose titrations):

Adults: Initial: 1-2 mg once daily, administered with breakfast or the first main meal; usual maintenance dose: 1-4 mg once daily; after a dose of 2 mg once daily, increase in increments of 2 mg at 1- to 2-week intervals based upon the patient's blood glucose response to a maximum of 8 mg once daily

Elderly: Initial: 1 mg/day

Combination with insulin therapy (fasting glucose level for instituting combination therapy is in the range of >150 mg/dL in plasma or serum depending on the patient): 8 mg once daily with the first main meal

After starting with low-dose insulin, upward adjustments of insulin can be done approximately weekly as guided by frequent measurements of fasting blood glucose. Once stable, combination-therapy patients should monitor their capillary blood glucose on an ongoing basis, preferably daily.

**Dosing adjustment/comments in renal impairment:** $Cl_{cr}$ <22 mL/minute: Initial starting dose should be 1 mg and dosage increments should be based on fasting blood glucose levels

**Dosing adjustment in hepatic impairment:** No data available

**Patient Information** This medication is used to control diabetes; it is not a cure. Other components of treatment plan are important: follow prescribed diet, medication, and exercise regimen. Take exactly as directed; 30 minutes before meal(s) at the same time each day. Do not change dose or discontinue without consulting prescriber. Avoid alcohol while taking this medication; could cause severe reaction. Inform prescriber of all other prescription or OTC medications you are taking; do not introduce new medication without consulting prescriber. Do not take other medication within 2 hours of this medication unless so advised by prescriber. If you experience hypoglycemic reaction, contact prescriber immediately. Maintain regular dietary intake and exercise routine and always carry quick source of sugar with you. You may experience side effects during first weeks of therapy (headache, nausea); consult prescriber if these persist. Report severe or persistent side effects, extended vomiting or flu-like symptoms, skin rash, easy bruising or bleeding, or change in color of urine or stool.

**Nursing Implications** Patients who are NPO may need to have their dose held to avoid hypoglycemia

**Dosage Forms** Tablet: 1 mg, 2 mg, 4 mg

## Glipizide (GLIP i zide)

**Related Information**

Hypoglycemic Drugs and Thiazolidinedione Information *on page 714*

**U.S. Brand Names** Glucotrol®; Glucotrol® XL

**Synonyms** Glydiazinamide

**Pharmacologic Category** Antidiabetic Agent (Sulfonylurea)

**Use** Management of noninsulin-dependent diabetes mellitus (type 2)

**Effects on Mental Status** None reported

**Effects on Psychiatric Treatment** May rarely cause agranulocytosis; use caution with clozapine and carbamazepine; phenothiazines and TCAs may antagonize glipizide hypoglycemic effects; MAOIs and TCAs may enhance hypoglycemic effects

**Pregnancy Risk Factor** C

**Contraindications** Hypersensitivity to glipizide or any component, other sulfonamides, type 1 diabetes mellitus

**Warnings/Precautions** Use with caution in patients with severe hepatic disease; a useful agent since few drug to drug interactions and not dependent upon renal elimination of active drug

Product labeling states oral hypoglycemic drugs may be associated with an increased cardiovascular mortality as compared to treatment with diet alone or diet plus insulin. Data to support this association are limited, and several studies, including a large prospective trial (UKPDS) have not supported an association.

**Adverse Reactions**

>10%:

Central nervous system: Headache

Gastrointestinal: Anorexia, nausea, vomiting, diarrhea, epigastric fullness, constipation, heartburn

1% to 10%: Dermatologic: Rash, urticaria, photosensitivity

<1%: Agranulocytosis, aplastic anemia, blood dyscrasias, bone marrow suppression, cholestatic jaundice, diuretic effect edema, hemolytic anemia, hypoglycemia, hyponatremia, thrombocytopenia

**Overdosage/Toxicology**

Signs and symptoms: Low blood sugar, tingling of lips and tongue, nausea, yawning, confusion, agitation, tachycardia, sweating, convulsions, stupor, and coma

Treatment: Intoxications with sulfonylureas can cause hypoglycemia and are best managed with glucose administration (oral for milder hypoglycemia or by injection in more severe forms)

**Drug Interactions**

Decreased effects: Beta-blockers, cholestyramine, hydantoins, rifampin, thiazide diuretics, urinary alkalines, charcoal

Increased effects: $H_2$-antagonists, anticoagulants, androgens, fluconazole, salicylates, gemfibrozil, sulfonamides, tricyclic antidepressants, probenecid, MAO inhibitors, methyldopa, digitalis glycosides, urinary acidifiers

Increased toxicity: Cimetidine may increase hypoglycemic effects

**Usual Dosage** Oral (allow several days between dose titrations): Give ~30 minutes before a meal to obtain the greatest reduction in postprandial hyperglycemia

Adults: Initial: 5 mg/day; adjust dosage at 2.5-5 mg daily increments as determined by blood glucose response at intervals of several days. Maximum recommended once-daily dose: 15 mg; maximum recommended total daily dose: 40 mg.

Elderly: Initial: 2.5 mg/day; increase by 2.5-5 mg/day at 1- to 2-week intervals

**Dosing adjustment/comments in renal impairment:** $Cl_{cr}$ <10 mL/minute: Some investigators recommend not using

**Dosing adjustment in hepatic impairment:** Initial dosage should be 2.5 mg/day

**Dietary Considerations**

Alcohol: A disulfiram-like reaction characterized by flushing, headache, nausea, vomiting, sweating, or tachycardia; avoid use

Food: Food delays absorption by 40%; take glipizide before meals

Glucose: Decreases blood glucose concentration. Hypoglycemia may occur. Educate patients how to detect and treat hypoglycemia. Monitor for signs and symptoms of hypoglycemia. Administer glucose if necessary. Evaluate patient's diet and exercise regimen. May need to decrease or discontinue dose of sulfonylurea.

Sodium: Reports of hyponatremia and SIADH. Those at increased risk include patients on medications or who have medical conditions that predispose them to hyponatremia. Monitor sodium serum concentration and fluid status. May need to restrict water intake.

**Patient Information** This medication is used to control diabetes; it is not a cure. Other components of treatment plan are important: follow prescribed diet, medication, and exercise regimen. Take exactly as directed; 30 minutes before meal(s) at the same time each day. Do not chew or crush extended release tablets. Do not change dose or discontinue without consulting prescriber. Avoid alcohol while taking this medication; could cause severe reaction. Inform prescriber of all other prescription or OTC medications you are taking; do not introduce new medication without consulting prescriber. Do not take other medication within 2 hours of this medication unless so advised by prescriber. If you experience hypoglycemic reaction, contact prescriber immediately. Maintain regular dietary intake and exercise routine and always carry quick source of sugar with you. You may be more sensitive to sunlight (use sunscreen, wear protective clothing and eyewear, and avoid direct sunlight). You may experience side effects during first weeks of therapy (headache, nausea); consult prescriber if these persist. Report severe or persistent side effects, extended vomiting, diarrhea, or constipation; flu-like symptoms; skin rash; easy bruising or bleeding; or change in color of urine or stool.

**Nursing Implications** Patients who are NPO may need to have their dose held to avoid hypoglycemia

**Dosage Forms**

Tablet: 5 mg, 10 mg

Tablet, extended release: 5 mg, 10 mg

♦ **Glucagen®** *see* Glucagon *on page 251*

## Glucagon (GLOO ka gon)

**U.S. Brand Names** Glucagen®

**Pharmacologic Category** Antidote; Diagnostic Agent, Gastrointestinal

**Use** Management of hypoglycemia; diagnostic aid in the radiologic examination of GI tract when a hypnotic state is needed; used with some success as a cardiac stimulant in management of severe cases of beta-adrenergic blocking agent overdosage

**Effects on Mental Status** None reported

**Effects on Psychiatric Treatment** None reported

**Pregnancy Risk Factor** B

**Contraindications** Hypersensitivity to glucagon or any component

**Warnings/Precautions** Use with caution in patients with a history of insulinoma and/or pheochromocytoma

**Adverse Reactions** 1% to 10%:

Cardiovascular: Hypotension

Dermatologic: Urticaria

Gastrointestinal: Nausea, vomiting

Respiratory: Respiratory distress

**Overdosage/Toxicology** Signs and symptoms: Hypokalemia, nausea, vomiting

**Drug Interactions** Increased toxicity: Oral anticoagulant - hypoprothrombinemic effects may be increased possibly with bleeding

**Usual Dosage**

Hypoglycemia or insulin shock therapy: I.M., I.V., S.C.:

Children: 0.025-0.1 mg/kg/dose, not to exceed 1 mg/dose, repeated in 20 minutes as needed

Adults: 0.5-1 mg, may repeat in 20 minutes as needed

**If patient fails to respond to glucagon, I.V. dextrose must be given**

Diagnostic aid: Adults: I.M., I.V.: 0.25-2 mg 10 minutes prior to procedure

**Patient Information** Identify appropriate support person to administer glucagon if necessary. Follow prescribers instructions for administering glucagon. Review diet, insulin administration, and testing procedures with prescriber or diabetic educator.

**Dosage Forms** Powder for injection, lyophilized: 1 mg [1 unit]; 10 mg [10 units]

♦ **Glucocerebrosidase** *see* Alglucerase *on page 23*

♦ **Glucophage®** *see* Metformin *on page 348*

## Glucosamine

**Pharmacologic Category** Nutritional Supplement

**Use** Osteoarthritis, rheumatoid arthritis, tendonitis, gout, bursitis

**Adverse Reactions** Gastrointestinal: Very few effects (eg, flatulence, nausea)

(Continued)

## Glucosamine *(Continued)*

**Drug Interactions** None known

**Usual Dosage** 500 mg of the sulfate form 3 times/day

**Additional Information** Both a sulfate and a hydrochloride salt are available. Glucosamine appears more highly absorbed when administered in the sulfate form, and sulfate is also an important mineral in cartilage.

## Glucose, Instant (GLOO kose, IN stant)

**U.S. Brand Names** B-D Glucose® [OTC]; Glutose® [OTC]; Insta-Glucose® [OTC]

**Pharmacologic Category** Antihypoglycemic Agent

**Use** Management of hypoglycemia

**Effects on Mental Status** None reported

**Effects on Psychiatric Treatment** None reported

**Usual Dosage** Adults: Oral: 10-20 g

**Dosage Forms**

Gel, oral (Glutose®, Insta-Glucose®): Dextrose 40% (25 g, 30.8 g, 80 g)
Tablet, chewable (B-D Glucose®): 5 g

♦ **Glucotrol®** *see* Glipizide *on page 251*

♦ **Glucotrol® XL** *see* Glipizide *on page 251*

♦ **Glucovance™** *see* Glyburide and Metformin *on page 253*

## Glutethimide (gloo TETH i mide)

**Related Information**

Anxiolytic/Hypnotic Use in Long-Term Care Facilities *on page 754*
Clinical Issues in the Use of Anxiolytics and Sedative/Hypnotics *on page 634*
Federal OBRA Regulations Recommended Maximum Doses *on page 756*

**Pharmacologic Category** Hypnotic, Miscellaneous

**Use** Short-term treatment of insomnia

**Effects on Mental Status** Sedation is common; may cause confusion; may rarely produce paradoxical reaction

**Effects on Psychiatric Treatment** Concurrent use with other psychotropics may produce additive sedation

**Restrictions** C-II

**Contraindications** Hypersensitivity to glutethimide; porphyria

**Adverse Reactions**

>10%: Central nervous system: Daytime drowsiness
1% to 10%:
- Central nervous system: Confusion, headache
- Dermatologic: Skin rash
- Gastrointestinal: Nausea, vomiting
- Ocular: Blurred vision

**Drug Interactions** Decreased effect of anticoagulants

**Usual Dosage** Oral:

Adults: 250-500 mg at bedtime, dose may be repeated but not less than 4 hours before intended awakening; maximum: 1 g/day
Elderly/debilitated patients: Total daily dose should not exceed 500 mg

**Dosage Forms** Tablet: 250 mg

♦ **Glutose® [OTC]** *see* Glucose, Instant *on page 252*

♦ **Glyate® [OTC]** *see* Guaifenesin *on page 256*

♦ **Glybenclamide** *see* Glyburide *on page 252*

♦ **Glybenzcyclamide** *see* Glyburide *on page 252*

## Glyburide (GLYE byoor ide)

**Related Information**

Diabetes Mellitus Treatment *on page 782*
Hypoglycemic Drugs and Thiazolidinedione Information *on page 714*

**U.S. Brand Names** Diaβeta®; Glynase™ PresTab™; Micronase®

**Canadian Brand Names** Albert® Glyburide; Apo®-Glyburide; Euglucon®; Gen-Glybe; Novo-Glyburide; Nu-Glyburide

**Synonyms** Glibenclamide; Glybenclamide; Glybenzcyclamide

**Pharmacologic Category** Antidiabetic Agent (Sulfonylurea)

**Use** Management of noninsulin-dependent diabetes mellitus (type 2)

**Effects on Mental Status** Dizziness is common

**Effects on Psychiatric Treatment** May rarely cause agranulocytosis; use caution with clozapine and carbamazepine; phenothiazines and TCAs may antagonize glimepiride hypoglycemic effects; MAOIs and TCAs may enhance hypoglycemic effects

**Pregnancy Risk Factor** C

**Contraindications** Hypersensitivity to glyburide or any component, or other sulfonamides; type 1 diabetes mellitus, diabetic ketoacidosis with or without coma

**Warnings/Precautions** Elderly: Rapid and prolonged hypoglycemia (>12 hours) despite hypertonic glucose injections have been reported; age and hepatic and renal impairment are independent risk factors for hypoglycemia; dosage titration should be made at weekly intervals. Use with caution in patients with renal and hepatic impairment, malnourished or debilitated conditions, or adrenal or pituitary insufficiency.

Product labeling states oral hypoglycemic drugs may be associated with an increased cardiovascular mortality as compared to treatment with diet alone or diet plus insulin. Data to support this association are limited, and several studies, including a large prospective trial (UKPDS) have not supported an association.

**Adverse Reactions**

>10%:
- Central nervous system: Headache, dizziness
- Gastrointestinal: Nausea, epigastric fullness, heartburn, constipation, diarrhea, anorexia
- Ocular: Blurred vision

1% to 10%: Dermatologic: Pruritus, rash, urticaria, photosensitivity reaction

<1%: Agranulocytosis, aplastic anemia, arthralgia, bone marrow suppression, cholestatic jaundice, diuretic effect, hemolytic anemia, hypoglycemia, leukopenia, nocturia, paresthesia, thrombocytopenia

**Overdosage/Toxicology**

Signs and symptoms: Severe hypoglycemia, seizures, cerebral damage, tingling of lips and tongue, nausea, yawning, confusion, agitation, tachycardia, sweating, convulsions, stupor, and coma

Treatment: Intoxications with sulfonylureas can cause hypoglycemia and are best managed with glucose administration (oral for milder hypoglycemia or by injection in more severe forms)

**Drug Interactions** CYP3A3/4 enzyme substrate

Decreased effect: Thiazides may decrease effectiveness of glyburide

Increased effect: Possible interaction between glyburide and fluoroquinolone antibiotics has been reported resulting in a potentiation of hypoglycemic action of glyburide

Increased toxicity:
- Since this agent is highly protein bound, the toxic potential is increased when given concomitantly with other highly protein bound drugs (ie, phenylbutazone, oral anticoagulants, hydantoins, salicylates, NSAIDs, beta-blockers, sulfonamides) - increase hypoglycemic effect
- Alcohol increases disulfiram reactions
- Phenylbutazone can increase hypoglycemic effects
- Certain drugs tend to produce hyperglycemia and may lead to loss of control (ie, thiazides and other diuretics, corticosteroids, phenothiazines, thyroid products, estrogens, oral contraceptives, phenytoin, nicotinic acid, sympathomimetics, calcium channel blocking drugs, and isoniazid)

Possible interactions between glyburide and coumarin derivatives have been reported that may either potentiate or weaken the effects of coumarin derivatives

**Usual Dosage** Oral:

Adults:
- Initial: 2.5-5 mg/day, administered with breakfast or the first main meal of the day. In patients who are more sensitive to hypoglycemic drugs, start at 1.25 mg/day.
- Increase in increments of no more than 2.5 mg/day at weekly intervals based on the patient's blood glucose response
- Maintenance: 1.25-20 mg/day given as single or divided doses; maximum: 20 mg/day
- Elderly: Initial: 1.25-2.5 mg/day, increase by 1.25-2.5 mg/day every 1-3 weeks

Micronized tablets (Glynase PresTab™): Adults:
- Initial: 1.5-3 mg/day, administered with breakfast or the first main meal of the day in patients who are more sensitive to hypoglycemic drugs, start at 0.75 mg/day. Increase in increments of no more than 1.5 mg/day in weekly intervals based on the patient's blood glucose response.
- Maintenance: 0.75-12 mg/day given as a single dose or in divided doses. Some patients (especially those receiving >6 mg/day) may have a more satisfactory response with twice-daily dosing.

**Dosing adjustment/comments in renal impairment:** $Cl_{cr}$ <50 mL/minute: **Not recommended**

**Dosing adjustment in hepatic impairment:** Use conservative initial and maintenance doses and avoid use in severe disease

**Dietary Considerations**

Alcohol: A disulfiram-like reaction characterized by flushing, headache, nausea, vomiting, sweating, or tachycardia; avoid use

Food: Food does not affect absorption; glyburide may be taken with food
- Glucose: Decreases blood glucose concentration. Hypoglycemia may occur. Educate patients how to detect and treat hypoglycemia. Monitor for signs and symptoms of hypoglycemia. Administer glucose if necessary. Evaluate patient's diet and exercise regimen. May need to decrease or discontinue dose of sulfonylurea.
- Sodium: Reports of hyponatremia and SIADH. Those at increased risk include patients on medications or who have medical conditions that predispose them to hyponatremia. Monitor sodium serum concentration and fluid status. May need to restrict water intake.

**Patient Information** This medication is used to control diabetes; it is not a cure. Other components of treatment plan are important: follow prescribed diet, medication, and exercise regimen. Take exactly as directed; 30 minutes before meal(s) at the same time each day. Do not change dose or discontinue without consulting prescriber. Avoid alcohol while taking this medication; could cause severe reaction. Inform prescriber of all other prescription or OTC medications you are taking; do not introduce new medication without consulting prescriber. Do not take other medication within 2 hours of this medication unless so advised by prescriber. If you experience hypoglycemic reaction, contact prescriber immediately. Maintain regular dietary intake and exercise routine and always carry quick source of sugar with you. You may be more sensitive to sunlight (use sunscreen, wear protective clothing and eyewear, and avoid direct sunlight). You may experience side effects during first weeks of therapy (headache, nausea); consult prescriber if these persist. Report severe or persistent side effects, extended vomiting or flu-like symptoms, skin rash, easy bruising or bleeding, or change in color of urine or stool.

**Nursing Implications** Patients who are anorexic or NPO, may need to have their dose held to avoid hypoglycemia

**Dosage Forms**
Tablet (Diaβeta®, Micronase®): 1.25 mg, 2.5 mg, 5 mg
Tablet, micronized (Glynase™ PresTab™): 1.5 mg, 3 mg, 6 mg

## Glyburide and Metformin (GLYE byoor ide & met FOR min)

**U.S. Brand Names** Glucovance™

**Pharmacologic Category** Antidiabetic Agent, Oral; Antidiabetic Agent (Sulfonylurea)

**Use** Initial therapy for management of type 2 (noninsulin-dependent) diabetes mellitus when hyperglycemia cannot be managed with diet and exercise alone. Second-line therapy for management of type 2 (noninsulin-dependent) diabetes mellitus when hyperglycemia cannot be managed with a sulfonylurea or metformin along with diet and exercise.

**Effects on Mental Status** Dizziness is common; may cause sedation

**Effects on Psychiatric Treatment** May rarely cause agranulocytosis; use caution with clozapine and carbamazepine; phenothiazines and TCAs may antagonize glyburide's hypoglycemic effects; MAOIs and TCAs may enhance hypoglycemic effects; concurrent use with psychotropics may produce additive sedation

**Usual Dosage** Adults: Oral: Dose should be individualized based on effectiveness and tolerance; titrate to minimum effective dose needed to achieve blood glucose control; **do not exceed maximum recommended doses**

Initial therapy: Glucovance™ 1.25 mg/250 mg once daily with a meal; patients with Hb $A_{1c}$ >9% or fasting plasma glucose (FPG) >200 mg/dL may start with Glucovance™ 1.25 mg/250 mg twice daily with meals

Dosage increases may be made every 2 weeks, in increments of Glucovance™ 1.25 mg/250 mg, until a dose of glyburide 10 mg/metformin 2000 mg per day has been reached

**Due to increased risk of hypoglycemia, do not start with Glucovance™ 5 mg/500 mg.**

Second-line therapy: Patients previously treated with a sulfonylurea or metformin alone: Starting dose: Glucovance™ 2.5 mg/500 mg or Glucovance™ 5 mg/500 mg twice daily with the morning and evening meals; doses may be increased in increments no larger than glyburide 5 mg/metformin 500 mg, up to a maximum dose of glyburide 20 mg/metformin 2000 mg.

When switching patients previously on a sulfonylurea and metformin together, do not exceed the daily dose of glyburide (or glyburide equivalent) or metformin.

**Dosage adjustment in renal impairment:** Risk of lactic acidosis increases with degree of renal impairment; contraindicated in renal disease or renal dysfunction

**Dosage adjustment in hepatic impairment:** Use conservative initial and maintenance doses and avoid use in severe hepatic disease

Elderly: Conservative doses are recommended in the elderly due to potentially decreased renal function; **do not titrate to maximum dose**; should not be used in patients ≥80 years of age unless renal function is verified as normal

**Dosage Forms** Tablet, film-coated:
Glucovance™ 1.25 mg/250 mg: Glyburide 1.25 mg and metformin hydrochloride 250 mg
Glucovance™ 2.5 mg/500 mg: Glyburide 2.5 mg and metformin hydrochloride 500 mg
Glucovance™ 5 mg/500 mg: Glyburide 5 mg and metformin hydrochloride 500 mg


♦ **Glycerol Guaiacolate** *see* Guaifenesin *on page 256*

♦ **Glycerol-T®** *see* Theophylline and Guaifenesin *on page 539*

♦ **Glyceryl Trinitrate** *see* Nitroglycerin *on page 397*

♦ **Glycofed®** *see* Guaifenesin and Pseudoephedrine *on page 257*


## Glycopyrrolate (glye koe PYE roe late)

**U.S. Brand Names** Robinul®; Robinul® Forte

**Synonyms** Glycopyrronium Bromide

**Pharmacologic Category** Anticholinergic Agent

**Use** Adjunct in treatment of peptic ulcer disease; inhibit salivation and excessive secretions of the respiratory tract preoperatively; reversal of neuromuscular blockade; control of upper airway secretions

**Effects on Mental Status** May rarely cause drowsiness, confusion, amnesia

**Effects on Psychiatric Treatment** Concurrent use with other psychotropics may produce additive sedation and dry mouth

**Pregnancy Risk Factor** B

**Contraindications** Narrow-angle glaucoma, acute hemorrhage, tachycardia, hypersensitivity to glycopyrrolate or any component; ulcerative colitis, obstructive uropathy, paralytic ileus, obstructive disease of GI tract

**Warnings/Precautions** Not recommended in children <12 years of age for the management of peptic ulcer; infants, patients with Down syndrome, and children with spastic paralysis or brain damage may be hypersensitive to antimuscarine effects. Use caution in elderly, patients with autonomic neuropathy, hepatic or renal disease, ulcerative colitis may predispose megacolon, hyperthyroidism, CAD, CHF, arrhythmias, tachycardia, BPH, hiatal hernia, with reflux.

**Adverse Reactions**
>10%:
Dermatologic: Dry skin
Gastrointestinal: Constipation, dry throat, xerostomia
Local: Irritation at injection site
Respiratory: Dry nose
Miscellaneous: Diaphoresis (decreased)
1% to 10%:
Dermatologic: Increased sensitivity to light
Endocrine & metabolic: Decreased flow of breast milk
Gastrointestinal: Dysphagia
<1%: Ataxia, bloated feeling, blurred vision, confusion, drowsiness, dysuria, fatigue, headache, increased intraocular pain, loss of memory, nausea, orthostatic hypotension, palpitations, rash, tachycardia, ventricular fibrillation, vomiting, weakness

**Overdosage/Toxicology**
Signs and symptoms: Blurred vision, urinary retention, tachycardia, absent bowel sounds
Treatment: Anticholinergic toxicity is caused by strong binding of the drug to cholinergic receptors. For anticholinergic overdose with severe life-threatening symptoms, physostigmine 1-2 mg (0.5 or 0.02 mg/kg for children) S.C. or I.V., slowly may be given to reverse these effects.

**Drug Interactions**
Decreased effect of levodopa
Increased toxicity with amantadine, cyclopropane

**Usual Dosage**
Children:
Control of secretions:
Oral: 40-100 mcg/kg/dose 3-4 times/day
I.M., I.V.: 4-10 mcg/kg/dose every 3-4 hours; maximum: 0.2 mg/dose or 0.8 mg/24 hours
Intraoperative: I.V.: 4 mcg/kg not to exceed 0.1 mg; repeat at 2- to 3-minute intervals as needed
Preoperative: I.M.:
<2 years: 4.4-8.8 mcg/kg 30-60 minutes before procedure
>2 years: 4.4 mcg/kg 30-60 minutes before procedure
Children and Adults: Reverse neuromuscular blockade: I.V.: 0.2 mg for each 1 mg of neostigmine or 5 mg of pyridostigmine administered
Adults:
Intraoperative: I.V.: 0.1 mg repeated as needed at 2- to 3-minute intervals
Preoperative: I.M.: 4.4 mcg/kg 30-60 minutes before procedure
Peptic ulcer:
Oral: 1-2 mg 2-3 times/day
I.M., I.V.: 0.1-0.2 mg 3-4 times/day

**Patient Information** Take as directed before meals; do not increase dose and do not discontinue without consulting prescriber. Void before taking medication. You may experience dizziness or blurred vision (use caution when driving or engaging in tasks that require alertness until response to drug is known); dry mouth (sucking on lozenges may help); photosensitivity (wear dark glasses in bright sunlight); or impotence (temporary). Report excessive and persistent anticholinergic effects (blurred vision, headache, flushing, tachycardia, nervousness, constipation, dizziness, insomnia, mental confusion or excitement, dry mouth, altered taste perception, dysphagia, palpitations, bradycardia, urinary hesitancy or retention, impotence, decreased sweating).

**Dosage Forms**
Injection, as bromide: 0.2 mg/mL (1 mL, 2 mL, 5 mL, 20 mL)
Robinul®: 0.2 mg/mL (1 mL, 2 mL, 5 mL, 20 mL)
Tablet, as bromide:
Robinul®: 1 mg
Robinul® Forte: 2 mg


♦ **Glycopyrronium Bromide** *see* Glycopyrrolate *on page 253*

♦ **Glycotuss® [OTC]** *see* Guaifenesin *on page 256*

- **Glycotuss-dM® [OTC]** *see* Guaifenesin and Dextromethorphan *on page 257*
- ***Glycyrrhiza glabra*** *see* Licorice *on page 317*
- **Glydiazinamide** *see* Glipizide *on page 251*
- **Glynase™ PresTab™** *see* Glyburide *on page 252*
- **Gly-Oxide® Oral [OTC]** *see* Carbamide Peroxide *on page 92*
- **Glyset™** *see* Miglitol *on page 367*
- **Glytuss® [OTC]** *see* Guaifenesin *on page 256*
- **GM-CSF** *see* Sargramostim *on page 504*
- **G-myticin® Topical** *see* Gentamicin *on page 248*
- **Goatweed** *see* St Johns Wort *on page 519*


## Golden Seal

**Related Information**

Herbals That May Alter Metabolism and GI Absorption of Drugs *on page 745*

Natural/Herbal Products *on page 746*

**Synonyms** Eye Balm; Eye Root; *Hydrastis canadensis*; Indian Eye: Orange Root; Jaundice Root; Tumeric Root; Yellow Indian Paint; Yellow Root

**Pharmacologic Category** Herb

**Use** Gastrointestinal and peripheral vascular activity; also used in sterile eye washes, as a mouthwash, laxative, hemorrhoids, and to stop postpartum hemorrhage. Efficacy not established in clinical studies; has been used to treat mucosal inflammation/gastritis

**Contraindications** Pregnancy, breast-feeding

**Warnings/Precautions** Should not be used in patients with hypertension, glaucoma, diabetes, history of stroke, or heart disease

**Adverse Reactions** Generally high doses:

Central nervous system: Stimulation/agitation

Gastrointestinal: Nausea, vomiting, diarrhea, mouth and throat irritation

Neuromuscular & skeletal: Extremity numbness

Respiratory: Respiratory failure

**Overdosage/Toxicology**

Signs and symptoms: Hypotension, respiratory depression, seizures, nausea, vomiting, diarrhea, uterine contractions, brown discoloration of urine, mydriasis, paresthesia

Decontamination: activated charcoal with cathartic

Treatment: Supportive therapy; benzodiazepines can be utilized for seizure control

**Drug Interactions** May interfere with vitamin B absorption

**Usual Dosage**

Root: 0.5-1 g 3 times/day

Solid form: Usual dosage: 5-10 grains

**Additional Information** Perennial with green-white flowers and dark red berries (from April to May) that is found from Vermont to Arkansas

## Gold Sodium Thiomalate (gold SOW dee um thye oh MAL ate)

**U.S. Brand Names** Aurolate®

**Pharmacologic Category** Gold Compound

**Use** Treatment of progressive rheumatoid arthritis

**Effects on Mental Status** None reported

**Effects on Psychiatric Treatment** May rarely cause agranulocytosis; use caution with clozapine and carbamazepine

**Usual Dosage** I.M.:

Children: Initial: Test dose of 10 mg is recommended, followed by 1 mg/kg/week for 20 weeks; maintenance: 1 mg/kg/dose at 2- to 4-week intervals thereafter for as long as therapy is clinically beneficial and toxicity does not develop. Administration for 2-4 months is usually required before clinical improvement is observed.

Adults: 10 mg first week; 25 mg second week; then 25-50 mg/week until 1 g cumulative dose has been given; if improvement occurs without adverse reactions, administer 25-50 mg every 2-3 weeks for 2-20 weeks, then every 3-4 weeks indefinitely

**Dosing adjustment in renal impairment:**

$Cl_{cr}$ 50-80 mL/minute: Administer 50% of normal dose

$Cl_{cr}$ <50 mL/minute: Avoid use

**Dosage Forms** Injection: 25 mg/mL (1 mL); 50 mg/mL (1 mL, 2 mL, 10 mL)


- **GoLYTELY®** *see* Polyethylene Glycol-Electrolyte Solution *on page 451*


## Gonadorelin (goe nad oh REL in)

**U.S. Brand Names** Factrel®; Lutrepulse®

**Pharmacologic Category** Diagnostic Agent, Gonadotrophic Hormone; Gonadotropin

**Use** Evaluation of the functional capacity and response of gonadotrophic hormones; evaluate abnormal gonadotropin regulation as in precocious puberty and delayed puberty. Lutrepulse®: Induction of ovulation in females with hypothalamic amenorrhea.

**Effects on Mental Status** None reported

**Effects on Psychiatric Treatment** Antipsychotics may decrease the effects of gonadorelin

**Usual Dosage**

Diagnostic test: Children >12 years and Adults (female): I.V., S.C. hydrochloride salt: 100 mcg administered in women during early phase of menstrual cycle (day 1-7)

Primary hypothalamic amenorrhea: Female adults: Acetate: I.V.: 5 mcg every 90 minutes via Lutrepulse® pump kit at treatment intervals of 21 days (pump will pulsate every 90 minutes for 7 days)

**Dosage Forms**

Injection, as acetate (Lutrepulse®): 0.8 mg, 3.2 mg

Injection, as hydrochloride (Factrel®): 100 mcg, 500 mcg


- **Gonak™ [OTC]** *see* Hydroxypropyl Methylcellulose *on page 277*
- **Gonal-F®** *see* Follitropins *on page 239*
- **Gonic®** *see* Chorionic Gonadotropin *on page 122*
- **Goniosol® [OTC]** *see* Hydroxypropyl Methylcellulose *on page 277*
- **Goody's® Headache Powders** *see* Acetaminophen, Aspirin, and Caffeine *on page 15*
- **Gormel® Creme [OTC]** *see* Urea *on page 576*


## Goserelin (GOE se rel in)

**U.S. Brand Names** Zoladex® Implant

**Pharmacologic Category** Antineoplastic Agent, Miscellaneous; Gonadotropin Releasing Hormone Analog; Luteinizing Hormone-Releasing Hormone Analog

**Use**

Prostate carcinoma: Palliative treatment of advanced carcinoma of the prostate. An alternative treatment of prostatic cancer when orchiectomy or estrogen administration are either not indicated or unacceptable to the patient. Combination with flutamide for the management of locally confined stage T2b-T4 (stage B2-C) carcinoma of the prostate.

3.6 mg implant **only**:

Endometriosis: Management of endometriosis, including pain relief and reduction of endometriotic lesions for the duration of therapy

Advanced breast cancer: Palliative treatment of advanced breast cancer in pre- and perimenopausal women. Estrogen and progesterone receptor values may help to predict whether goserelin therapy is likely to be beneficial.

**Note:** The 10.8 mg implant is not indicated in women as the data are insufficient to support reliable suppression of serum estradiol

**Effects on Mental Status** May cause sedation or insomnia

**Effects on Psychiatric Treatment** Sexual dysfunction is common; concurrent use with SSRIs may produce additive dysfunction

**Usual Dosage**

Adults: S.C.:

Monthly implant: 3.6 mg injected into upper abdomen every 28 days; do not try to aspirate with the goserelin syringe; if the needle is in a large vessel, blood will immediately appear in syringe chamber. While a delay of a few days is permissible, attempt to adhere to the 28-day schedule.

3-month implant: 10.8 mg injected into the upper abdominal wall every 12 weeks; do not try to aspirate with the goserelin syringe; if the needle is in a large vessel, blood will immediately appear in syringe chamber. While a delay of a few days is permissible, attempt to adhere to the 12-week schedule.

Prostate carcinoma: Intended for long-term administration

Endometriosis: Recommended duration: 6 months; retreatment is not recommended since safety data is not available. If symptoms recur after a course of therapy, and further treatment is contemplated, consider monitoring bone mineral density. Currently, there are no clinical data on the effect of treatment of benign gynecological conditions with goserelin for periods >6 months.

**Dosing adjustment in renal/hepatic impairment:** No adjustment is necessary

**Dosage Forms** Injection, implant: 3.6 mg single dose disposable syringe with 16-gauge hypodermic needle; 10.8 mg single dose disposable syringe with 14-gauge hypodermic needle


- **GP 47680** *see* Oxcarbazepine *on page 411*
- ***G. palidiflora*** *see* Licorice *on page 317*
- **GR1222311X** *see* Ranitidine Bismuth Citrate *on page 488*


## Granisetron (gra NI se tron)

**U.S. Brand Names** Kytril™

**Synonyms** BRL 43694

**Pharmacologic Category** Selective 5-$HT_3$ Receptor Antagonist

**Use** Prophylaxis and treatment of chemotherapy-related emesis; may be prescribed for patients who are refractory to or have severe adverse reactions to standard antiemetic therapy. Granisetron may be prescribed for young patients (ie, <45 years of age who are more likely to develop extrapyramidal reactions to high-dose metoclopramide) who are to receive highly emetogenic chemotherapeutic agents as listed:

Agents with high emetogenic potential (>90%) (dose/m$^2$):
- Amifostine
- Azacitidine
- Carmustine ≥200 mg/m$^2$
- Cisplatin ≥50 mg/m$^2$
- Cyclophosphamide ≥1 g/m$^2$
- Cytarabine ≥1500 mg/m$^2$
- Dacarbazine ≥500 mg/m$^2$
- Dactinomycin
- Doxorubicin ≥60 mg/m$^2$
- Lomustine ≥60 mg/m$^2$
- Mechlorethamine
- Melphalan ≥100 mg/m$^2$
- Streptozocin
- Thiotepa ≥100 mg/m$^2$

**or** two agents classified as having high or moderately high emetogenic potential as listed:

Agents with moderately high emetogenic potential (60% to 90%) (dose/m$^2$):
- Carboplatin 200-400 mg/m$^2$
- Carmustine <200 mg/m$^2$
- Cisplatin <50 mg/m$^2$
- Cyclophosphamide 600-999 mg/m$^2$
- Dacarbazine <500 mg/m$^2$
- Doxorubicin 21-59 mg/m$^2$
- Hexamethyl melamine
- Ifosfamide ≥5000 mg/m$^2$
- Lomustine <60 mg/m$^2$
- Methotrexate ≥250 mg/m$^2$
- Pentostatin
- Procarbazine

Granisetron should not be prescribed for chemotherapeutic agents with a low emetogenic potential (eg, bleomycin, busulfan, cyclophosphamide <1000 mg, etoposide, 5-fluorouracil, vinblastine, vincristine)

**Effects on Mental Status** May cause anxiety or insomnia

**Effects on Psychiatric Treatment** None reported

**Pregnancy Risk Factor** B

**Contraindications** Previous hypersensitivity to granisetron

**Warnings/Precautions** Use with caution in patients with liver disease or in pregnant patients

**Adverse Reactions**

>10%: Central nervous system: Headache

1% to 10%:
- Cardiovascular: Hyper/hypotension
- Central nervous system: Dizziness, insomnia, anxiety
- Gastrointestinal: Constipation, abdominal pain, diarrhea
- Neuromuscular & skeletal: Weakness

<1%: Agitation, arrhythmias, hot flashes, liver enzyme elevations, somnolence

**Drug Interactions** CYP3A3/4 enzyme substrate

**Usual Dosage**

I.V.: Children and Adults: 10 mcg/kg for 1-3 doses. Doses should be administered as a single IVPB over 5 minutes to 1 hour or by undiluted IV push over 30 seconds, given just prior to chemotherapy (15-60 minutes before); as intervention therapy for breakthrough nausea and vomiting, during the first 24 hours following chemotherapy, 2 or 3 repeat infusions (same dose) have been administered, separated by at least 10 minutes

Oral: Adults: 1 mg twice daily; the first 1 mg dose should be given up to 1 hour before chemotherapy, and the second tablet, 12 hours after the first; alternatively may give a single dose of 2 mg, up to 1 hour before chemotherapy

**Note: Granisetron should only be given on the day(s) of chemotherapy**

**Dosing interval in renal impairment:** Creatinine clearance values have no relationship to granisetron clearance

**Dosing interval in hepatic impairment:** Kinetic studies in patients with hepatic impairment showed that total clearance was approximately halved, however, standard doses were very well tolerated

**Patient Information** This drug will be administered on days when you receive chemotherapy to reduce nausea and vomiting. If outpatient chemotherapy, you may be given oral medication to take after return home; take as directed. You may experience drowsiness; use caution when driving. For persistent acute headache request analgesic from prescriber. Frequent mouth care, chewing gum, or sucking on lozenges may relieve persistent nausea. Report unrelieved headache, fever, diarrhea, or constipation.

**Nursing Implications** Doses should be given at least 15 minutes prior to initiation of chemotherapy

**Dosage Forms**

Injection: 1 mg/mL

Tablet: 1 mg (2s), (20s)

♦ **Granulocyte Colony Stimulating Factor** *see* Filgrastim *on page 225*

♦ **Granulocyte-Macrophage Colony Stimulating Factor** *see* Sargramostim *on page 504*

♦ **Green Ginger** *see* Wormwood *on page 588*

## Grepafloxacin (*Voluntarily Withdrawn From Market*) (grep a FLOX a sin)

**U.S. Brand Names** Raxar®

**Pharmacologic Category** Antibiotic, Quinolone

**Use** Treatment of acute bacterial exacerbations of chronic bronchitis caused by *Haemophilus influenzae*, *Streptococcus pneumoniae*, or *Moraxella catarrhalis*; community-acquired pneumonia caused by *Mycoplasma pneumoniae* or the organisms previously mentioned; uncomplicated gonorrhea caused by *Neisseria gonorrhoeae*, and nongonococcal cervicitis and urethritis caused by *Chlamydia trachomatis*

*In vitro* studies suggest similar or lesser activity against *Enterobacteriaceae* and *P. aeruginosa* but greater activity against gram-positive cocci, especially *S. pneumoniae*, and some anaerobes and *Chlamydia* spp.

**Effects on Mental Status** May cause drowsiness or dizziness; quinolones reported to cause restlessness, hallucinations, euphoria, depression, panic, and paranoia

**Effects on Psychiatric Treatment** None reported

**Pregnancy Risk Factor** C

**Contraindications** Previous hypersensitivity to grepafloxacin and other quinolone derivatives; in patients with hepatic failure; given concomitantly with class I and III antiarrhythmics or bepridil due to the potential risk of cardiac arrhythmias (including torsade de pointes); patients with $QT_c$ prolongation and use with drugs which prolong $QT_c$ interval

**Warnings/Precautions** Use caution in patients with cerebral arteriosclerosis or epilepsy, and in patients with GI disorders or hepatic or renal dysfunction; there is no data to support safety and efficacy in children <18 years of age

**Adverse Reactions** Percentage unknown: Abdominal pain, diarrhea, dizziness, emesis due to medicinal taste, fatigue, headache, hepatotoxicity (ie, elevated serum transaminases), hypersensitivity, nausea, syncope

**Drug Interactions** CYP1A2 enzyme substrate

Antacids decrease grepafloxacin levels by 60%; grepafloxacin decreases theophylline clearance by 50%; may inhibit the metabolism of other drugs metabolized by cytochrome P-450 enzymes; may have additive effect of QTc prolongation when administered with other agent that may prolong QTc interval

**Usual Dosage** Oral:
- Bronchitis: 400-600 mg/day for 10 days
- Community-acquired pneumonia: 600 mg/day for 10 days
- Nongonococcal urethritis or cervicitis: 400 mg/day for 7 days
- Uncomplicated gonorrhea: 400 mg as a single dose

**Patient Information** Take per recommended schedule; complete full course of therapy and do not skip doses. Take on an empty stomach (1 hour before or 2 hours after meals, dairy products, antacids, or other medications). Maintain adequate hydration (2-3 L/day of fluids unless instructed to restrict fluid intake). Diabetics should monitor glucose levels closely; this medication may alter effect of oral hypoglycemic agents. You may experience dizziness, lightheadedness, anxiety, insomnia, or confusion (use caution when driving or engaging in tasks that require alertness until response to drug is known); photosensitivity (use sunscreen, wear protective clothing and eyewear, and avoid direct sunlight). Report immediately any CNS disturbances (hallucinations, agitation, confusion, seizures), chest pain, or palpitations. Report persistent GI disturbances; muscle or tendon pain, swelling, or redness; signs of opportunistic infection (sore throat, chills, fever, burning, itching on urination, vaginal discharge, white plaques in mouth); or worsening of condition.

**Dosage Forms** Tablet, as hydrochloride: 200 mg, 400 mg, 600 mg

♦ **Grifulvin® V** *see* Griseofulvin *on page 255*

♦ **Grisactin® Ultra** *see* Griseofulvin *on page 255*

## Griseofulvin (gri see oh FUL vin)

**U.S. Brand Names** Fulvicin® P/G; Fulvicin-U/F®; Grifulvin® V; Grisactin® Ultra; Gris-PEG®

**Canadian Brand Names** Grisovin®-FP

**Synonyms** Griseofulvin Microsize; Griseofulvin Ultramicrosize

**Pharmacologic Category** Antifungal Agent, Oral

**Use** Treatment of susceptible tinea infections of the skin, hair, and nails

**Effects on Mental Status** May cause dizziness, confusion, or insomnia

**Effects on Psychiatric Treatment** May rarely cause leukopenia; use caution with clozapine and carbamazepine; barbiturates may decrease levels of griseofulvin

(Continued)

## Griseofulvin *(Continued)*

**Pregnancy Risk Factor** C

**Contraindications** Hypersensitivity to griseofulvin or any component; severe liver disease, porphyria (interferes with porphyrin metabolism)

**Warnings/Precautions** Safe use in children <2 years of age has not been established; during long-term therapy, periodic assessment of hepatic, renal, and hematopoietic functions should be performed; may cause fetal harm when administered to pregnant women; avoid exposure to intense sunlight to prevent photosensitivity reactions; hypersensitivity cross reaction between penicillins and griseofulvin is possible

**Adverse Reactions**

>10%: Dermatologic: Rash, urticaria

1% to 10%:

Central nervous system: Headache, fatigue, dizziness, insomnia, mental confusion

Dermatologic: Photosensitivity

Gastrointestinal: Nausea, vomiting, epigastric distress, diarrhea

Miscellaneous: Oral thrush

<1%: Angioneurotic edema, GI bleeding, hepatotoxicity, leukopenia, menstrual toxicity, nephrosis, proteinuria

**Overdosage/Toxicology**

Signs and symptoms: Lethargy, vertigo, blurred vision, nausea, vomiting, diarrhea

Treatment: Following GI decontamination, treatment is supportive

**Drug Interactions**

Decreased effect:

Barbiturates may decrease levels of griseofulvin

Decreased warfarin, cyclosporine, and salicylate activity with griseofulvin

Griseofulvin decreases oral contraceptive effectiveness

Increased toxicity: With alcohol → tachycardia and flushing

**Usual Dosage** Oral:

Children:

Microsize: 10-20 mg/kg/day in single or 2 divided doses

Ultramicrosize: >2 years: 5-10 mg/kg/day in single or 2 divided doses

Adults:

Microsize: 500-1000 mg/day in single or divided doses

Ultramicrosize: 330-375 mg/day in single or divided doses; doses up to 750 mg/day have been used for infections more difficult to eradicate such as tinea unguium

Duration of therapy depends on the site of infection:

Tinea corporis: 2-4 weeks

Tinea capitis: 4-6 weeks or longer

Tinea pedis: 4-8 weeks

Tinea unguium: 3-6 months or longer

**Patient Information** Take as directed; around-the-clock with food. Take full course of medication; do not discontinue without notifying prescriber. Avoid alcohol while taking this drug (disulfiram reactions). Practice good hygiene measures to prevent reinfection. Frequent blood tests may be required with prolonged therapy. You may experience nausea and vomiting (small, frequent meals may help); confusion, dizziness, drowsiness (use caution when driving or engaging in tasks that require alertness until response to drug is known); nausea, vomiting, or diarrhea (small frequent meals, frequent mouth care, sucking lozenges, or chewing gum may help); increased sensitivity to sun (use sunscreen, wear protective clothing and eyewear, and avoid excessive exposure to direct sunlight). Report skin rash, respiratory difficulty, CNS changes (confusion, dizziness, acute headache), changes in color of stool or urine, white plaques in mouth, or worsening of condition.

**Dosage Forms**

Microsize:

Capsule: 125 mg, 250 mg

Suspension, oral (Grifulvin® V): 125 mg/5 mL with alcohol 0.2% (120 mL)

Tablet:

Fulvicin-U/F®, Grifulvin® V: 250 mg

Fulvicin-U/F®, Grifulvin® V, Grisactin-500®: 500 mg

Ultramicrosize:

Tablet:

Fulvicin® P/G: 165 mg, 330 mg

Fulvicin® P/G, Grisactin® Ultra, Gris-PEG®: 125 mg, 250 mg

Grisactin® Ultra: 330 mg

♦ **Griseofulvin Microsize** *see* Griseofulvin *on page 255*

♦ **Griseofulvin Ultramicrosize** *see* Griseofulvin *on page 255*

♦ **Gris-PEG®** *see* Griseofulvin *on page 255*

♦ **Guaifed® [OTC]** *see* Guaifenesin and Pseudoephedrine *on page 257*

♦ **Guaifed-PD®** *see* Guaifenesin and Pseudoephedrine *on page 257*

## Guaifenesin (gwye FEN e sin)

**U.S. Brand Names** Anti-Tuss® Expectorant [OTC]; Breonesin® [OTC]; Diabetic Tussin® EX [OTC]; Duratuss-G®; Fenesin™; Gee Gee® [OTC]; Genatuss® [OTC]; GG-Cen® [OTC]; Glyate® [OTC]; Glycotuss® [OTC]; Glytuss® [OTC]; Guaifenex® LA; GuiaCough® Expectorant [OTC]; Guiatuss® [OTC]; Halotussin® [OTC]; Humibid® L.A.; Humibid® Sprinkle; Hytuss® [OTC]; Hytuss-2X® [OTC]; Liquibid®; Medi-Tuss® [OTC]; Monafed®; Muco-Fen-LA®; Mytussin® [OTC]; Naldecon® Senior EX [OTC]; Organidin® NR; Pneumomist®; Respa-GF®; Robitussin® [OTC]; Scot-Tussin® [OTC]; Siltussin® [OTC]; Sinumist®-SR Capsulets®; Touro Ex®; Tusibron® [OTC]; Uni-tussin® [OTC]

**Canadian Brand Names** Balminil® Expectorant; Calmylin Expectorant

**Synonyms** GG; Glycerol Guaiacolate

**Pharmacologic Category** Expectorant

**Use** Temporary control of cough due to minor throat and bronchial irritation

**Effects on Mental Status** May cause drowsiness

**Effects on Psychiatric Treatment** None reported

**Pregnancy Risk Factor** C

**Contraindications** Hypersensitivity to guaifenesin or any component

**Warnings/Precautions** Not for persistent cough such as occurs with smoking, asthma, or emphysema or cough accompanied by excessive secretions

**Adverse Reactions** 1% to 10%:

Central nervous system: Drowsiness, headache

Dermatologic: Rash

Gastrointestinal: Nausea, vomiting, stomach pain

**Overdosage/Toxicology**

Signs and symptoms: Vomiting, lethargy, coma, respiratory depression

Treatment: Supportive

**Drug Interactions** Disulfiram, MAO inhibitors, metronidazole, procarbazine

**Usual Dosage** Oral:

Children:

<2 years: 12 mg/kg/day in 6 divided doses

2-5 years: 50-100 mg every 4 hours, not to exceed 600 mg/day

6-11 years: 100-200 mg every 4 hours, not to exceed 1.2 g/day

Children >12 years and Adults: 200-400 mg every 4 hours to a maximum of 2.4 g/day

**Patient Information** Take only as prescribed; do not exceed prescribed dose or frequency. Do not chew or crush timed release capsule. Maintain adequate hydration (2-3 L/day of fluids unless instructed to restrict fluid intake). You may experience some drowsiness (use caution when driving or engaging in tasks requiring alertness until response to drug is known). Report excessive drowsiness, difficulty breathing, or lack of improvement or worsening or condition.

**Dosage Forms**

Caplet, sustained release (Touro Ex®): 600 mg

Capsule (Breonesin®, GG-Cen®, Hytuss-2X®): 200 mg

Capsule, sustained release (Humibid® Sprinkle): 300 mg

Liquid:

Diabetic Tussin EX®, Organidin® NR, Tusibron®: 100 mg/5 mL (118 mL)

Naldecon® Senior EX: 200 mg/5 mL (118 mL, 480 mL)

Syrup (Anti-Tuss® Expectorant, Genatuss®, Glyate®, GuiaCough® Expectorant, Guiatuss®, Halotussin®, Malotuss®, Medi-Tuss®, Mytussin®, Robitussin®, Scot-Tussin®, Siltussin®, Tusibron®, Uni-Tussin®): 100 mg/5 mL with alcohol 3.5% (30 mL, 120 mL, 240 mL, 473 mL, 946 mL)

Tablet:

Duratuss-G®: 1200 mg

Gee Gee®, Glytuss®, Organidin® NR: 200 mg

Glycotuss®, Hytuss®: 100 mg

Sustained release:

Fenesin™, Guaifenex LA®, Humibid® L.A., Liquibid®, Monafed®, Muco-Fen-LA®, Pneumomist®, Respa-GF®, Sinumist®-SR Capsulets®: 600 mg

## Guaifenesin and Codeine (gwye FEN e sin & KOE deen)

**U.S. Brand Names** Brontex® Liquid; Brontex® Tablet; Cheracol®; Guaituss AC®; Guiatussin® With Codeine; Mytussin® AC; Robafen® AC; Robitussin® A-C; Tussi-Organidin® NR

**Pharmacologic Category** Antitussive; Cough Preparation; Expectorant

**Use** Temporary control of cough due to minor throat and bronchial irritation

**Effects on Mental Status** Drowsiness is common; may cause confusion, headache, dizziness, lightheadedness, false feeling of well being, restlessness, paradoxical CNS stimulation, or malaise; may rarely cause hallucinations, mental depression, nightmares, or insomnia

**Effects on Psychiatric Treatment** Constipation and drowsiness are common, this effect may be additive when used concurrently with psychotropics

**Restrictions** C-V

**Usual Dosage** Oral:

Children:

2-6 years: 1-1.5 mg/kg codeine/day divided into 4 doses administered every 4-6 hours (maximum: 30 mg/24 hours)

6-12 years: 5 mL every 4 hours, not to exceed 30 mL/24 hours

Children >12 years and Adults: 5-10 mL every 4-8 hours not to exceed 60 mL/24 hours

**Dosage Forms**

Liquid (Brontex®): Guaifenesin 75 mg and codeine phosphate 2.5 mg per 5 mL

Syrup (Cheracol®, Guaituss AC®, Guiatussin® with Codeine, Mytussin® AC, Robafen® AC, Robitussin® A-C, Tussi-Organidin® NR): Guaifenesin 100 mg and codeine phosphate 10 mg per 5 mL (60 mL, 120 mL, 480 mL)

Tablet (Brontex®): Guaifenesin 300 mg and codeine phosphate 10 mg

## Guaifenesin and Dextromethorphan

(gwye FEN e sin & deks troe meth OR fan)

**U.S. Brand Names** Benylin® Expectorant [OTC]; Cheracol® D [OTC]; Clear Tussin® 30; Contac® Cough Formula Liquid [OTC]; Diabetic Tussin DM® [OTC]; Extra Action Cough Syrup [OTC]; Fenesin™ DM; Genatuss DM® [OTC]; Glycotuss-dM® [OTC]; Guaifenex® DM; GuiaCough® [OTC]; Guiatuss-DM® [OTC]; Halotussin® DM [OTC]; Humibid® DM [OTC]; Iobid DM®; Kolephrin® GG/DM [OTC]; Monafed® DM; Muco-Fen-DM®; Mytussin® DM [OTC]; Naldecon® Senior DX [OTC]; Phanatuss® Cough Syrup [OTC]; Phenadex® Senior [OTC]; Respa®-DM; Rhinosyn-DMX® [OTC]; Robafen DM® [OTC]; Robitussin®-DM [OTC]; Safe Tussin® 30 [OTC]; Scot-Tussin® Senior Clear [OTC]; Siltussin DM® [OTC]; Synacol® CF [OTC]; Syracol-CF® [OTC]; Tolu-Sed® DM [OTC]; Tusibron-DM® [OTC]; Tuss-DM® [OTC]; Tussi-Organidin® DM NR; Uni-tussin® DM [OTC]; Vicks® 44E [OTC]; Vicks® Pediatric Formula 44E [OTC]

**Pharmacologic Category** Antitussive; Cough Preparation; Expectorant

**Use** Temporary control of cough due to minor throat and bronchial irritation

**Effects on Mental Status** May cause drowsiness

**Effects on Psychiatric Treatment** Concurrent use with psychotropics may produce additive sedation

**Usual Dosage** Oral:

Children: Dextromethorphan: 1-2 mg/kg/24 hours divided 3-4 times/day

Children >12 years and Adults: 5 mL every 4 hours or 10 mL every 6-8 hours not to exceed 40 mL/24 hours

**Dosage Forms**

Syrup:

Benylin® Expectorant: Guaifenesin 100 mg and dextromethorphan hydrobromide 5 mg per 5 mL (118 mL, 236 mL)

Cheracol® D, Clear Tussin® 30, Genatuss® DM, Mytussin® DM, Robitussin®-DM, Siltussin DM®, Tolu-Sed® DM, Tussi-Organidin® DM NR: Guaifenesin 100 mg and dextromethorphan hydrobromide 10 mg per 5 mL (5 mL, 10 mL, 120 mL, 240 mL, 360 mL, 480 mL, 3780 mL)

Contac® Cough Formula Liquid: Guaifenesin 67 mg and dextromethorphan hydrobromide 10 mg per 5 mL (120 mL)

Extra Action Cough Syrup, GuiaCough®, Guiatuss DM®, Halotussin® DM, Rhinosyn-DMX®, Tusibron-DM®, Uni Tussin® DM: Guaifenesin 100 mg and dextromethorphan hydrobromide 15 mg per 5 mL (120 mL, 240 mL, 480 mL)

Kolephrin® GG/DM: Guaifenesin 150 mg and dextromethorphan hydrobromide 10 mg per 5 mL (120 mL)

Naldecon® Senior DX: Guaifenesin 200 mg and dextromethorphan hydrobromide 15 mg per 5 mL (118 mL, 480 mL)

Phanatuss®: Guaifenesin 85 mg and dextromethorphan hydrobromide 10 mg per 5 mL

Vicks® 44E: Guaifenesin 66.7 mg and dextromethorphan hydrobromide 6.7 mg per 5 mL

Tablet:

Extended release

Guaifenex DM®, Iobid DM®, Fenesin™ DM, Humibid® DM, Monafed® DM, Respa®-DM: Guaifenesin 600 mg and dextromethorphan hydrobromide 30 mg

Glycotuss-dM®: Guaifenesin 100 mg and dextromethorphan hydrobromide 10 mg

Queltuss®: Guaifenesin 100 mg and dextromethorphan hydrobromide 15 mg

Syracol-CF®: Guaifenesin 200 mg and dextromethorphan hydrobromide 15 mg

Tuss-DM®: Guaifenesin 200 mg and dextromethorphan hydrobromide 10 mg

## Guaifenesin and Phenylephrine

(gwye FEN e sin & fen il EF rin)

**U.S. Brand Names** Deconsal® Sprinkle®; Endal®; Sinupan®

**Pharmacologic Category** Decongestant; Expectorant

**Use** Symptomatic relief of those respiratory conditions where tenacious mucous plugs and congestion complicate the problem such as sinusitis, pharyngitis, bronchitis, asthma, and as an adjunctive therapy in serous otitis media

**Effects on Mental Status** Guaifenesin may cause drowsiness; phenylephrine may cause anxiety or restlessness

**Effects on Psychiatric Treatment** Concurrent use with psychotropics may produce additive sedation or lessen the effects of anxiolytics depending on whether the effects of guaifenesin or phenylephrine predominate; concurrent use with MAOIs may result in hypertensive crisis; avoid combination

**Usual Dosage** Oral: Adults: 1 or 2 every 12 hours

**Dosage Forms**

Capsule, sustained release:

Deconsal® Sprinkle®: Guaifenesin 300 mg and phenylephrine hydrochloride 10 mg

Sinupan®: Guaifenesin 200 mg and phenylephrine hydrochloride 40 mg

Tablet, timed release (Endal®): Guaifenesin 300 mg and phenylephrine hydrochloride 20 mg

## Guaifenesin and Phenylpropanolamine

(gwye FEN e sin & fen il proe pa NOLE a meen)

**U.S. Brand Names** Ami-Tex LA®; Coldlac-LA®; Conex® [OTC]; Contuss® XT; Dura-Vent®; Entex® LA; Genagesic®; Genamin® Expectorant [OTC]; Guaifenex® PPA 75; Guaipax®; Myminic® Expectorant [OTC]; Naldecon-EX® Children's Syrup [OTC]; Nolex® LA; Partuss® LA; Phenylfenesin® L.A.; Profen II®; Profen LA®; Rymed-TR®; Silaminic® Expectorant [OTC]; Sildicon-E® [OTC]; Snaplets-EX® [OTC]; Triaminic® Expectorant [OTC]; Tri-Clear® Expectorant [OTC]; Triphenyl® Expectorant [OTC]; ULR-LA®; Vicks® DayQuil® Sinus Pressure & Congestion Relief [OTC]

**Pharmacologic Category** Decongestant; Expectorant

**Use** Symptomatic relief of those respiratory conditions where tenacious mucous plugs and congestion complicate the problem such as sinusitis, pharyngitis, bronchitis, asthma, and as an adjunctive therapy in serous otitis media

**Effects on Mental Status** Guaifenesin may cause drowsiness; phenylpropanolamine may cause anxiety or restlessness

**Effects on Psychiatric Treatment** Concurrent use with psychotropics may produce additive sedation or lessen the effects of anxiolytics depending on whether the effects of guaifenesin or phenylpropanolamine predominate; concurrent use with MAOIs may result in hypertensive crisis; avoid combination

**Usual Dosage** Oral:

Children:

2-6 years: 2.5 mL every 4 hours

6-12 years: ½ tablet every 12 hours or 5 mL every 4 hours

Children >12 years and Adults: 1 tablet every 12 hours or 10 mL every 4 hours

**Dosage Forms**

Caplet:

Vicks® DayQuil® Sinus Pressure & Congestion Relief: Guaifenesin 200 mg and phenylpropanolamine hydrochloride 25 mg

Gentab-LA®, Rymed-TR®: Guaifenesin 400 mg and phenylpropanolamine hydrochloride 75 mg

Drops:

Fedahist® Expectorant Pediatric: Guaifenesin 40 mg and phenylpropanolamine hydrochloride 7.5 mg per mL (30 mL)

Sildicon-E®: Guaifenesin 30 mg and phenylpropanolamine hydrochloride 6.25 mg per mL (30 mL)

Granules (Snaplets-EX®): Guaifenesin 50 mg and phenylpropanolamine hydrochloride 6.25 mg (pack)

Liquid:

Conex®, Genamin® Expectorant, Myminic® Expectorant, Silaminic® Expectorant, Theramine® Expectorant, Triaminic® Expectorant, Tri-Clear® Expectorant, Triphenyl® Expectorant: Guaifenesin 100 mg and phenylpropanolamine hydrochloride 12.5 mg per 5 mL (120 mL, 240 mL, 480 mL, 3780 mL)

Naldecon-EX® Children's Syrup: Guaifenesin 100 mg and phenylpropanolamine hydrochloride 6.25 mg per 5 mL (120 mL)

Tablet, extended release:

Ami-Tex LA®, Contuss® XT, Entex® LA, Guaipax®, Nolex® LA, Partuss® LA, Phenylfenesin® L.A., ULR-LA®: Guaifenesin 400 mg and phenylpropanolamine hydrochloride 75 mg

Dura-Vent®, Profen-LA®: Guaifenesin 600 mg and phenylpropanolamine hydrochloride 75 mg

Coldloc-LA®, Guaifenex® PPA 75, Profen II®: Guaifenesin 600 mg and phenylpropanolamine hydrochloride 37.5 mg

## Guaifenesin and Pseudoephedrine

(gwye FEN e sin & soo doe e FED rin)

**U.S. Brand Names** Congess® Jr; Congess® Sr; Congestac®; Deconsal® II; Defen®-LA; Entex® PSE; Eudal-SR®; Fedahist® Expectorant [OTC]; Fedahist® Expectorant Pediatric [OTC]; Glycofed®; Guaifed® [OTC]; Guaifed-PD®; Guaifenex® PSE; GuaiMax-D®; Guaitab®; Guaivent®; Guai-Vent/PSE®; Guiatuss PE® [OTC]; Halotussin® PE [OTC]; Histalet® X; Maxifed®; Maxifed-G®; Nasabid™; Respa-1st®; Respaire®-60 SR; Respaire®-120 SR; Robitussin-PE® [OTC]; Robitussin® Severe Congestion Liqui-Gels® [OTC]; Ru-Tuss® DE; Rymed®; Sinufed® Timecelles®; Touro LA®; Tuss-LA®; V-Dec-M®; Versacaps®; Zephrex®; Zephrex LA®

**Pharmacologic Category** Decongestant; Expectorant

**Use** Enhance the output of respiratory tract fluid and reduce mucosal congestion and edema in the nasal passage

**Effects on Mental Status** Guaifenesin may cause drowsiness; pseudoephedrine may cause anxiety or restlessness

(Continued)

## Guaifenesin and Pseudoephedrine *(Continued)*

**Effects on Psychiatric Treatment** Concurrent use with psychotropics may produce additive sedation or lessen the effects of anxiolytics depending on whether the effects of guaifenesin or pseudoephedrine predominate; concurrent use with MAOIs may result in hypertensive crisis; avoid combination

**Usual Dosage** Oral:

Children:

2-6 years: 2.5 mL every 4 hours not to exceed 15 mL/24 hours

6-12 years: 5 mL every 4 hours not to exceed 30 mL/24 hours

Children >12 years and Adults: 10 mL every 4 hours not to exceed 60 mL/24 hours

**Dosage Forms**

Capsule:

Guai-Vent™: Guaifenesin 250 mg and pseudoephedrine hydrochloride 120 mg

Robitussin® Severe Congestion Liqui-Gels®: Guaifenesin 200 mg and pseudoephedrine hydrochloride 30 mg

Rymed®: Guaifenesin 250 mg and pseudoephedrine hydrochloride 30 mg

Capsule, extended release:

Congess® Jr: Guaifenesin 125 mg and pseudoephedrine hydrochloride 60 mg

Nasabid®: Guaifenesin 250 mg and pseudoephedrine hydrochloride 90 mg

Congess® SR, Guaifed®, Respaire®-120 SR: Guaifenesin 250 mg and pseudoephedrine hydrochloride 120 mg

Guaifed-PD®, Sinufed® Timecelles®, Versacaps®: Guaifenesin 300 mg and pseudoephedrine hydrochloride 60 mg

Respaire®-60 SR: Guaifenesin 200 mg and pseudoephedrine hydrochloride 60 mg

Tuss-LA® Capsule: Guaifenesin 500 mg and pseudoephedrine hydrochloride 120 mg

Drops, oral (Fedahist® Expectorant Pediatric): Guaifenesin 40 mg and pseudoephedrine hydrochloride 7.5 mg per mL (30 mL)

Syrup:

Fedahist® Expectorant, Guaifed®: Guaifenesin 200 mg and pseudoephedrine hydrochloride 30 mg per 5 mL (120 mL, 240 mL)

Guiatuss® PE, Halotussin® PE, Robitussin-PE®, Rymed®: Guaifenesin 100 mg and pseudoephedrine hydrochloride 30 mg per 5 mL (120 mL, 240 mL, 480 mL)

Histalet® X: Guaifenesin 200 mg and pseudoephedrine hydrochloride 45 mg per 5 mL (473 mL)

Tablet:

Congestac®, Guiatab®, Zephrex®: Guaifenesin 400 mg and pseudoephedrine hydrochloride 60 mg

Glycofed®: Guaifenesin 100 mg and pseudoephedrine hydrochloride 30 mg

Tablet, extended release:

Deconsal® II, Defen-L.A.®, Respa-1st®: Guaifenesin 600 mg and pseudoephedrine hydrochloride 60 mg

Entex® PSE, Guaifenex PSE®, GuaiMax-D®, Guai-Vent/PSE™, Ru-Tuss® DE, Sudex®, Zephrex LA®: Guaifenesin 600 mg and pseudoephedrine hydrochloride 120 mg

Eudal-SR®, Histalet® X, Touro LA®: Guaifenesin 400 mg and pseudoephedrine hydrochloride 120 mg

Maxifed®: Guaifenesin 550 mg and pseudoephedrine hydrochloride 80 mg

Maxifed-G®: Guaifenesin 550 mg and pseudoephedrine hydrochloride 60 mg

Tuss-LA® Tablet, V-Dec-M®: Guaifenesin 5 mg and pseudoephedrine hydrochloride 120 mg

## Guaifenesin, Phenylpropanolamine, and Dextromethorphan

(gwye FEN e sin, fen il proe pa NOLE a meen, & deks troe meth OR fan)

**U.S. Brand Names** Anatuss® [OTC]; Guiatuss CF® [OTC]; Naldecon® DX Adult Liquid [OTC]; Profen II DM®; Robafen® CF [OTC]; Robitussin-CF® [OTC]; Siltussin-CF® [OTC]; TRIKOF-D®

**Pharmacologic Category** Cough Preparation; Decongestant; Expectorant

**Use** Temporarily relieves nasal congestion and controls cough due to minor throat and bronchial irritation; helps loosen phlegm and thin bronchial secretions to make coughs more productive

**Effects on Mental Status** Guaifenesin and dextromethorphan may cause drowsiness or dizziness; phenylpropanolamine may cause anxiety or restlessness

**Effects on Psychiatric Treatment** Concurrent use with psychotropics may produce additive sedation or lessen the effects of anxiolytics depending on whether the effects of guaifenesin/dextromethorphan or phenylpropanolamine predominate; concurrent use with MAOIs may result in hypertensive crisis; avoid combination

**Usual Dosage** Oral:

Children:

2-6 years: 2.5 mL every 4 hours not to exceed 15 mL/24 hours

6-12 years: 5 mL every 4 hours not to exceed 30 mL/24 hours

Children >12 years and Adults: 10 mL every 4 hours not to exceed 60 mL/24 hours

**Dosage Forms**

Syrup:

Anatuss®: Guaifenesin 100 mg, phenylpropanolamine hydrochloride 25 mg, and dextromethorphan hydrobromide 15 mg per 5 mL (120 mL, 473 mL)

Guiatuss® CF, Robafen® CF, Robitussin-CF®: Guaifenesin 100 mg, phenylpropanolamine hydrochloride 12.5 mg, and dextromethorphan hydrobromide 10 mg per 5 mL (120 mL, 240 mL, 360 mL, 480 mL)

Naldecon® DX Adult: Guaifenesin 200 mg, phenylpropanolamine hydrochloride 12.5 mg, and dextromethorphan hydrobromide 10 mg per 5 mL (120 mL, 473 mL)

Siltussin-CF®: Guaifenesin 100 mg, phenylpropanolamine hydrochloride 12.5 mg, and dextromethorphan hydrobromide 10 mg per 5 mL

Tablet (Anatuss®): Guaifenesin 100 mg, phenylpropanolamine hydrochloride 25 mg, and dextromethorphan hydrobromide 15 mg

Tablet, timed-release (TRIKOF-D®): Guaifenesin 600 mg, phenylpropanolamine hydrochloride 37.5 mg, and dextromethorphan hydrobromide 30 mg

## Guaifenesin, Phenylpropanolamine, and Phenylephrine

(gwye FEN e sin, fen il proe pa NOLE a meen, & fen il EF rin)

**U.S. Brand Names** Coldloc®; Contuss®; Dura-Gest®; Enomine®; Entex®; Guaifenex®; Guiatex®

**Pharmacologic Category** Decongestant; Expectorant

**Use** Temporary relief of nasal congestion, running nose, sneezing, itching of nose and throat, and itchy, watery eyes due to common cold, hay fever, or other upper respiratory allergies

**Effects on Mental Status** Guaifenesin may cause drowsiness or dizziness; phenylpropanolamine/phenylephrine may cause anxiety or restlessness

**Effects on Psychiatric Treatment** Concurrent use with psychotropics may produce additive sedation or lessen the effects of anxiolytics depending on whether the effects of guaifenesin or phenylpropanolamine/phenylephrine predominate; concurrent use with MAOIs may result in hypertensive crisis; avoid combination

**Usual Dosage** Children >12 years and Adults: 1 capsule/tablet or 10 mL 4 times/day (every 6 hours) with food or fluid

**Dosage Forms**

Capsule (Contuss®, Dura-Gest®, Enomine®, Entex®, Guiatex®, ULR®): Guaifenesin 200 mg, phenylpropanolamine hydrochloride 45 mg, and phenylephrine hydrochloride 5 mg

Liquid (Coldloc®, Contuss®, Entex®, Guaifenex®): Guaifenesin 100 mg, phenylpropanolamine hydrochloride 20 mg, and phenylephrine hydrochloride 5 mg per 5 mL (118 mL, 480 mL)

Tablet (Respinol-G®): Guaifenesin 200 mg, phenylpropanolamine hydrochloride 45 mg, and phenylephrine hydrochloride 5 mg

## Guaifenesin, Pseudoephedrine, and Codeine

(gwye FEN e sin, soo doe e FED rin, & KOE deen)

**U.S. Brand Names** Codafed® Expectorant; Cycofed® Pediatric; Decohistine® Expectorant; Deproist® Expectorant With Codeine; Dihistine® Expectorant; Guiatuss DAC®; Guiatussin® DAC; Halotussin® DAC; Isoclor® Expectorant; Mytussin® DAC; Nucofed®; Nucofed® Pediatric Expectorant; Nucotuss®; Phenhist® Expectorant; Robitussin®-DAC; Ryna-CX®; Tussar® SF Syrup

**Pharmacologic Category** Antitussive/Decongestant/Expectorant

**Use** Temporarily relieves nasal congestion and controls cough due to minor throat and bronchial irritation; helps loosen phlegm and thin bronchial secretions to make coughs more productive

**Effects on Mental Status** Guaifenesin may cause drowsiness or dizziness; pseudoephedrine may cause anxiety or restlessness; codeine may cause drowsiness; may cause euphoria, confusion, insomnia, hallucinations, or depression

**Effects on Psychiatric Treatment** Concurrent use with psychotropics may produce additive sedation or lessen the effects of anxiolytics depending on whether the effects of guaifenesin/codeine or pseudoephedrine predominate; concurrent use with MAOIs may result in hypertensive crisis; avoid combination

**Restrictions** C-III; C-V

**Usual Dosage** Oral:

Children 6-12 years: 5 mL every 4 hours, not to exceed 40 mL/24 hours

Children >12 years and Adults: 10 mL every 4 hours, not to exceed 40 mL/24 hours

**Dosage Forms**

Liquid:

C-III: Nucofed®, Nucotuss®: Guaifenesin 200 mg, pseudoephedrine hydrochloride 60 mg, and codeine phosphate 20 mg per 5 mL (480 mL)

C-V: Codafed® Expectorant, Decohistine® Expectorant, Deproist® Expectorant with Codeine, Dihistine® Expectorant, Guiatuss DAC®, Guiatussin® DAC, Halotussin® DAC, Isoclor® Expectorant, Mytussin® DAC, Nucofed® Pediatric Expectorant, Phenhist® Expectorant, Robitussin®-DAC, Ryna-CX®, Tussar® SF: Guaifenesin 100 mg, pseudoephedrine hydrochloride 30 mg, and codeine phosphate 10 mg per 5 mL (120 mL, 480 mL, 4000 mL)

## Guaifenesin, Pseudoephedrine, and Dextromethorphan

(gwye FEN e sin, soo doe e FED rin, & deks troe meth OR fan)

**U.S. Brand Names** Anatuss® DM [OTC]; Dimacol® Caplets [OTC]; Maxifed® DM; Rhinosyn-X® Liquid [OTC]; Ru-Tuss® Expectorant [OTC]; Sudafed® Cold & Cough Liquid Caps [OTC]

**Pharmacologic Category** Antitussive/Decongestant/Expectorant

**Use** Temporarily relieves nasal congestion and controls cough due to minor throat and bronchial irritation; helps loosen phlegm and thin bronchial secretions to make coughs more productive

**Effects on Mental Status** Guaifenesin may cause drowsiness or dizziness; pseudoephedrine may cause anxiety or restlessness; dextromethorphan may cause drowsiness

**Effects on Psychiatric Treatment** Concurrent use with psychotropics may produce additive sedation or lessen the effects of anxiolytics depending on whether the effects of guaifenesin/dextromethorphan or pseudoephedrine predominate; concurrent use with MAOIs may result in hypertensive crisis; avoid combination

**Usual Dosage** Adults: Oral: 2 capsules (caplets) or 10 mL every 4 hours

**Dosage Forms**

Caplets (Dimacol®): Guaifenesin 100 mg, pseudoephedrine hydrochloride 30 mg, and dextromethorphan hydrobromide 10 mg

Capsule (Sudafed® Cold & Cough Liquid Caps): Guaifenesin 100 mg, pseudoephedrine hydrochloride 30 mg, and dextromethorphan hydrobromide 10 mg

Liquid (Anatuss® DM, Novahistine® DMX Liquid, Rhinosyn-X® Liquid, Ru-Tuss® Expectorant): Guaifenesin 100 mg, pseudoephedrine hydrochloride 30 mg, and dextromethorphan hydrobromide 10 mg per 5 mL

Tablet, sustained relief (Maxifed® DM): Guaifenesin 550 mg, pseudoephedrine hydrochloride 60 mg, and dextromethorphan hydrobromide 30 mg


- ♦ **Guaifenex®** *see* Guaifenesin, Phenylpropanolamine, and Phenylephrine *on page 258*
- ♦ **Guaifenex® DM** *see* Guaifenesin and Dextromethorphan *on page 257*
- ♦ **Guaifenex® LA** *see* Guaifenesin *on page 256*
- ♦ **Guaifenex® PPA 75** *see* Guaifenesin and Phenylpropanolamine *on page 257*
- ♦ **Guaifenex® PSE** *see* Guaifenesin and Pseudoephedrine *on page 257*
- ♦ **GuaiMax-D®** *see* Guaifenesin and Pseudoephedrine *on page 257*
- ♦ **Guaipax®** *see* Guaifenesin and Phenylpropanolamine *on page 257*
- ♦ **Guaitab®** *see* Guaifenesin and Pseudoephedrine *on page 257*
- ♦ **Guaituss AC®** *see* Guaifenesin and Codeine *on page 256*
- ♦ **Guaivent®** *see* Guaifenesin and Pseudoephedrine *on page 257*
- ♦ **Guai-Vent/PSE®** *see* Guaifenesin and Pseudoephedrine *on page 257*


## Guanabenz (GWAHN a benz)

**U.S. Brand Names** Wytensin®

**Pharmacologic Category** $Alpha_2$ Agonist

**Use** Management of hypertension

**Effects on Mental Status** Drowsiness and dizziness are common; may cause anxiety or depression

**Effects on Psychiatric Treatment** Has been used to treat ADHD; concurrent use with psychotropics may produce additive sedation and dry mouth; TCAs may decrease the hypotensive effect of guanabenz

**Pregnancy Risk Factor** C

**Contraindications** Hypersensitivity to guanabenz or any component

**Warnings/Precautions** Use with caution in severe hepatic or renal failure. Avoid in pregnancy and breast-feeding. Safety and efficacy for use in children <12 years of age have not been demonstrated. Use with caution in patients with severe coronary insufficiency, recent MI or cerebrovascular disease. Abrupt discontinuation can result in rebound hypertension. Avoid use in CNS disease, elderly or with other CNS depressants (can cause sedation and drowsiness alone). May cause significant orthostasis.

**Adverse Reactions**

>10%:

Central nervous system: Drowsiness or sedation, dizziness
Gastrointestinal: Xerostomia
Neuromuscular & skeletal: Weakness

1% to 10%:

Cardiovascular: Chest pain, edema
Central nervous system: Headache
Endocrine & metabolic: Decreased sexual ability
Gastrointestinal: Nausea

**Overdosage/Toxicology**

Signs and symptoms: CNS depression, hypothermia, apnea, lethargy, diarrhea, hypotension, bradycardia

Treatment: Primarily supportive and symptomatic. Hypotension usually responds to I.V. fluids, Trendelenburg positioning, or vasoconstrictors. CNS depression and/or apnea may respond to naloxone I.V. 0.4-2 mg, with repeats as needed.

**Drug Interactions**

TCAs decrease the hypotensive effect of guanabenz

Hypoglycemic symptoms may be reduced. Educate patient about decreased signs and symptoms of hypoglycemia or avoid use in patients with frequent episodes of hypoglycemia.

Nitroprusside and guanabenz have additive hypotensive effects

Noncardioselective beta-blockers (nadolol, propranolol, timolol) may exacerbate rebound hypertension when guanabenz is withdrawn. The beta-blocker should be withdrawn first. The gradual withdrawal of guanabenz or a cardioselective beta-blocker could be substituted.

**Usual Dosage** Adults: Oral: Initial: 4 mg twice daily; increase in increments of 4-8 mg/day every 1-2 weeks to a maximum of 32 mg twice daily.

**Dosing adjustment in hepatic impairment:** Probably necessary

**Patient Information** May impair alertness, judgment, coordination; do not abruptly discontinue; do not discontinue without notifying physician

**Dosage Forms** Tablet, as acetate: 4 mg, 8 mg

## Guanadrel (GWAHN a drel)

**U.S. Brand Names** Hylorel®

**Pharmacologic Category** False Neurotransmitter

**Use** Considered a second line agent in the treatment of hypertension, usually with a diuretic

**Effects on Mental Status** Sedation is common; may cause confusion; may rarely cause depression

**Effects on Psychiatric Treatment** Contraindicated with MAOIs; TCAs and phenothiazines may decrease the hypotensive effects of guanadrel

**Pregnancy Risk Factor** B

**Contraindications** Hypersensitivity to guanadrel or any component; known or suspected pheochromocytoma; concurrent use or within 1 week of any monoamine oxidase inhibitor; exacerbation of CHF

**Warnings/Precautions** Orthostatic hypotension is common. Avoid using other drugs that cause orthostatic hypotension (alpha-blocking agents or reserpine). Discontinue 48-72 hours before elective surgery (reduces potential for vascular collapse). If emergency surgery required, notify anesthesiologist of the drug regimen. Avoid using tricyclic antidepressants and indirect-acting sympathomimetics (can reverse the blood pressure lowering effects). Use cautiously in asthma (may aggravate condition), CHF (sodium and water retention), and PUD (may aggravate condition). Safety and efficacy have not been established in pediatric patients. Dosage adjustment required with renal dysfunction.

**Adverse Reactions**

>10%:

Cardiovascular: Palpitations, chest pain, peripheral edema
Central nervous system: Fatigue, headache, faintness, drowsiness, confusion
Gastrointestinal: Increased bowel movements, gas pain, constipation, anorexia, weight gain/loss
Genitourinary: Nocturia, urinary frequency, ejaculation disturbances
Neuromuscular & skeletal: Paresthesia, aching limbs, leg cramps, backache, arthralgia
Ocular: Visual disturbances
Respiratory: Shortness of breath, coughing

1% to 10%:

Cardiovascular: Orthostatic hypotension
Central nervous system: Psychological problems, depression, sleep disorders
Gastrointestinal: Increased bowel movements, glossitis, nausea, vomiting, xerostomia
Genitourinary: Impotence
Renal: Hematuria

**Overdosage/Toxicology**

Signs and symptoms: Hypotension, blurred vision, dizziness, syncope

Treatment: Primarily supportive and symptomatic; hypotension usually responds to I.V. fluids, Trendelenburg positioning or vasoconstrictors

**Drug Interactions**

Increased toxicity of direct-acting amines (epinephrine, norepinephrine) by guanadrel; the hypotensive effect of guanadrel may be potentiated

(Continued)

## Guanadrel *(Continued)*

Increased effect of beta-blockers, vasodilators

Amphetamines, related sympathomimetics, and methylphenidate decrease the antihypertensive response to guanadrel; consider an alternative antihypertensive with different mechanism of action. Reassess the need for amphetamine, related sympathomimetic, or methylphenidate; consider alternatives.

Ephedrine may inhibit the antihypertensive response to guanadrel; consider an alternative antihypertensive with different mechanism of action; reassess the need for ephedrine

MAO inhibitors may cause severe hypertension; give at least 1 week apart

Norepinephrine/phenylephrine have exaggerated pressor response; monitor blood pressure closely

Phenothiazines may inhibit the antihypertensive response to guanadrel; consider an alternative antihypertensive with different mechanism of action

TCAs decrease hypotensive effect of guanadrel

**Usual Dosage** Oral:

Adults: Initial: 10 mg/day (5 mg twice daily); adjust dosage weekly or monthly until blood pressure is controlled, usual dosage: 20-75 mg/day, given twice daily. For larger dosage, 3-4 times/day dosing may be needed.

Elderly: Initial: 5 mg once daily

**Dosing interval in renal impairment:**

$Cl_{cr}$ 10-50 mL/minute: Administer every 12-24 hours.

$Cl_{cr}$ <10 mL/minute: Administer every 24-48 hours.

**Patient Information** May cause orthostatic hypotension, sit or lie down at the first sign of dizziness or weakness; rise slowly from sitting or lying, especially for prolonged periods; take no new prescription or OTC medication without contacting your physician or pharmacist

**Dosage Forms** Tablet, as sulfate: 10 mg, 25 mg

## Guanethidine (gwahn ETH i deen)

**U.S. Brand Names** Ismelin®

**Canadian Brand Names** Apo®-Guanethidine

**Pharmacologic Category** False Neurotransmitter

**Use** Treatment of moderate to severe hypertension

**Effects on Mental Status** Sedation is common; may cause confusion; may rarely cause depression

**Effects on Psychiatric Treatment** Contraindicated with MAOIs; TCAs and antipsychotics may decrease the hypotensive effects of guanethidine

**Pregnancy Risk Factor** C

**Contraindications** Hypersensitivity to guanethidine or any component; known or suspected pheochromocytoma; concurrent use or within 1 week of any monoamine oxidase inhibitor; exacerbation of CHF (unrelated to HTN)

**Warnings/Precautions** Orthostatic hypotension is common. Avoid using other drugs that cause orthostatic hypotension (alpha-blocking agents or reserpine). Discontinue 2 weeks before elective surgery (reduces potential for vascular collapse). If emergency surgery required, notify anesthesiologist of the drug regimen. Fever reduces dosage requirements. Avoid using tricyclic antidepressants and indirect-acting sympathomimetics (can reverse the blood pressure lowering effects). Use cautiously in asthma (may aggravate condition), CHF (sodium and water retention), renal dysfunction (can worsen renal function), recent MI, cerebrovascular disease with encephalopathy, and PUD (may aggravate condition). Safety and efficacy have not been established in pediatric patients. Dosage adjustment required with severe renal dysfunction.

**Adverse Reactions**

>10%:

Cardiovascular: Palpitations, chest pain, peripheral edema

Central nervous system: Fatigue, headache, faintness, drowsiness, confusion

Gastrointestinal: Increased bowel movements, gas pain, constipation, anorexia, weight gain/loss

Genitourinary: Nocturia, urinary frequency, impotence, ejaculation disturbances

Neuromuscular & skeletal: Paresthesia, aching limbs, leg cramps, backache, arthralgia

Ocular: Visual disturbances

Respiratory: Shortness of breath, coughing

1% to 10%:

Cardiovascular: Orthostatic hypotension

Central nervous system: Psychological problems, depression, sleep disorders

Gastrointestinal: Increased bowel movements, glossitis, nausea, vomiting, xerostomia

Renal: Hematuria

**Overdosage/Toxicology**

Signs and symptoms: Hypotension, blurred vision, dizziness, syncope

Treatment: Hypotension usually responds to I.V. fluids, Trendelenburg positioning or vasoconstrictors; treatment is primarily supportive and symptomatic

**Drug Interactions**

TCAs decrease hypotensive effect of guanethidine

Phenothiazines may inhibit the antihypertensive response to guanethidine consider an alternative antihypertensive with different mechanism of action.

Amphetamines, related sympathomimetics, and methylphenidate decrease the antihypertensive response to guanethidine; consider an alternative antihypertensive with different mechanism of action. Reassess the need for amphetamine, related sympathomimetic, or methylphenidate; consider alternatives.

Ephedrine may inhibit the antihypertensive response to guanethidine; consider an alternative antihypertensive with different mechanism of action. Reassess the need for ephedrine.

Norepinephrine/phenylephrine have exaggerated pressor response; monitor blood pressure closely

Oral contraceptives may decrease hypotensive effect; avoid concurrent use

Minoxidil may cause severe orthostatic hypotension; avoid concurrent use

Enflurane may cause hypotension; avoid concurrent use

**Usual Dosage** Oral:

Children: Initial: 0.2 mg/kg/day; increase by 0.2 mg/kg/day at 7- to 10-day intervals to a maximum of 3 mg/kg/day.

Adults:

Ambulatory patients: Initial: 10 mg/day; increase at 5- to 7-day intervals to an average of 25-50 mg/day.

Hospitalized patients: Initial: 25-50 mg/day; increase by 25-50 mg/day or every other day to desired therapeutic response.

Elderly: Initial: 5 mg once daily

**Dosing interval in renal impairment:** $Cl_{cr}$ <10 mL/minute: Administer every 24-36 hours.

**Patient Information** Take as directed. Do not skip dose or discontinue without consulting prescriber. Store medication container away from light. Follow recommended diet and exercise program. Do not use OTC medications which may affect blood pressure (eg, cough or cold remedies, diet pills, stay-awake medications) without consulting prescriber. This medication may cause drowsiness, dizziness, or impaired judgment (use caution when driving or engaging in tasks that require alertness until response to drug is known); decreased libido or sexual function (will resolve when drug is discontinued); postural hypotension (use caution when rising from sitting or lying position or when climbing stairs - this may be worse in early morning, during hot weather, following exercise, or with alcohol use); or dry mouth or nausea (frequent mouth care or sucking lozenges may help). Report difficulty, pain, or burning on urination; increased nervousness or depression; sudden weight gain (weigh yourself in the same clothes at the same time of day once a week); unusual or persistent swelling of ankles, feet, or extremities; wet cough or respiratory difficulty; chest pain or palpitations; muscle weakness, fatigue, or pain; or other persistent side effects.

**Dosage Forms** Tablet, as monosulfate: 10 mg, 25 mg

## Guanfacine (GWAHN fa seen)

**U.S. Brand Names** Tenex®

**Pharmacologic Category** $Alpha_2$ Agonist

**Use** Management of hypertension

**Effects on Mental Status** Drowsiness is common; may cause insomnia or dizziness, may rarely cause confusion or depression

**Effects on Psychiatric Treatment** Has been used to treat ADHD; concurrent use with psychotropics may produce additive sedation and dry mouth; TCAs may decrease the hypotensive effect of guanfacine

**Pregnancy Risk Factor** B

**Contraindications** Hypersensitivity to guanfacine or any component

**Warnings/Precautions** Use caution with severe coronary insufficiency, recent MI, cerebrovascular disease, or chronic renal or hepatic disease. Abrupt discontinuation can result in nervousness, anxiety and rarely, rebound hypertension (occurs 2-4 days after withdrawal). Avoid use in CNS disease, elderly, or with other CNS depressants (can cause sedation and drowsiness alone). Safety and efficacy in children <12 years of age have not been demonstrated. May cause orthostasis.

**Adverse Reactions**

>10%:

Central nervous system: Somnolence, dizziness

Gastrointestinal: Xerostomia, constipation

1% to 10%:

Central nervous system: Fatigue, headache, insomnia

Endocrine & metabolic: Decreased sexual ability

Gastrointestinal: Nausea, vomiting

Ocular: Conjunctivitis

**Overdosage/Toxicology**

Signs and symptoms: CNS depression, hypothermia, apnea, lethargy, diarrhea, hypotension, bradycardia

Treatment: Primarily supportive and symptomatic. Hypotension usually responds to I.V. fluids, Trendelenburg positioning or vasoconstrictors. Naloxone may be utilized in treating CNS depression and/or apnea.

**Drug Interactions**
Hypoglycemic symptoms may be decreased. Educate patient about decreased signs and symptoms of hypoglycemia or avoid use in patients with frequent episodes of hypoglycemia.
Nitroprusside and guanfacine have additive hypotensive effects
Noncardioselective beta-blockers (nadolol, propranolol, timolol) may exacerbate rebound hypertension when guanfacine is withdrawn. The beta-blocker should be withdrawn first. The gradual withdrawal of guanfacine or a cardioselective beta-blocker could be substituted.
TCAs decrease the hypotensive effect of guanfacine

**Usual Dosage** Adults: Oral: 1 mg usually at bedtime, may increase if needed at 3- to 4-week intervals; 1 mg/day is most common dose

**Patient Information** May impair alertness, judgment, coordination; do not abruptly discontinue; do not discontinue without notifying physician

**Dosage Forms** Tablet, as hydrochloride: 1 mg, 2 mg

- **GuiaCough® [OTC]** *see* Guaifenesin and Dextromethorphan *on page 257*
- **GuiaCough® Expectorant [OTC]** *see* Guaifenesin *on page 256*
- **Guiatex®** *see* Guaifenesin, Phenylpropanolamine, and Phenylephrine *on page 258*
- **Guiatuss® [OTC]** *see* Guaifenesin *on page 256*
- **Guiatuss CF® [OTC]** *see* Guaifenesin, Phenylpropanolamine, and Dextromethorphan *on page 258*
- **Guiatuss DAC®** *see* Guaifenesin, Pseudoephedrine, and Codeine *on page 258*
- **Guiatuss-DM® [OTC]** *see* Guaifenesin and Dextromethorphan *on page 257*
- **Guiatussin® DAC** *see* Guaifenesin, Pseudoephedrine, and Codeine *on page 258*
- **Guiatussin® With Codeine** *see* Guaifenesin and Codeine *on page 256*
- **Guiatuss PE® [OTC]** *see* Guaifenesin and Pseudoephedrine *on page 257*
- ***G. uralensis*** *see* Licorice *on page 317*
- **G-well®** *see* Lindane *on page 318*
- **Gynecort® [OTC]** *see* Hydrocortisone *on page 273*
- **Gyne-Lotrimin® [OTC]** *see* Clotrimazole *on page 135*
- **Gyne-Sulf®** *see* Sulfabenzamide, Sulfacetamide, and Sulfathiazole *on page 522*
- **Gynogen L.A.® Injection** *see* Estradiol *on page 203*
- **Gynol II® [OTC]** *see* Nonoxynol 9 *on page 398*
- **Habitrol™ Patch** *see* Nicotine *on page 392*

## *Haemophilus* b Conjugate and Hepatitis b Vaccine

(he MOF i lus bee KON joo gate & hep a TYE tis bee vak SEEN)

**U.S. Brand Names** Comvax®

**Pharmacologic Category** Vaccine

**Use**
Immunization against invasive disease caused by *H. influenzae* type b and against infection caused by all known subtypes of hepatitis B virus in infants 8 weeks to 15 months of age born of $HB_sAg$-negative mothers
Infants born of $HB_sAg$-positive mothers or mothers of unknown $HB_sAg$ status should receive hepatitis B immune globulin and hepatitis B vaccine (Recombinant) at birth and should complete the hepatitis B vaccination series given according to a particular schedule

**Effects on Mental Status** May cause irritability or lethargy

**Effects on Psychiatric Treatment** May lessen or potentiate the effects of anxiolytics or mood stabilizers

**Usual Dosage** Infants (>8 weeks of age): I.M.: 0.5 mL at 2, 4, and 12-15 months of age (total of 3 doses)

If the recommended schedule cannot be followed, the interval between the first two doses should be at least 2 months and the interval between the second and third dose should be as close as possible to 8-11 months.
*Modified Schedule:* Children who receive one dose of hepatitis B vaccine at or shortly after birth may receive Comvax™ on a schedule of 2,4, and 12-15 months of age

**Dosage Forms** Injection: 7.5 mcg *Haemophilus* b PRP and 5 mcg $HB_sAg$/0.5 mL

## *Haemophilus* b Conjugate Vaccine

(hem OF fi lus bee KON joo gate vak SEEN)

**U.S. Brand Names** HibTITER®; OmniHIB™; PedvaxHIB™; ProHIBiT®

**Pharmacologic Category** Vaccine

**Use** Routine immunization of children 2 months to 5 years of age against invasive disease caused by *H. influenzae*

Unimmunized children ≥5 years of age with a chronic illness known to be associated with increased risk of *Haemophilus influenzae* type b disease, specifically, persons with anatomic or functional asplenia or sickle cell anemia or those who have undergone splenectomy, should receive Hib vaccine.

*Haemophilus* b conjugate vaccines are not indicated for prevention of bronchitis or other infections due to *H. influenzae* in adults; adults with specific dysfunction or certain complement deficiencies who are at especially high risk of *H. influenzae* type b infection (HIV-infected adults); patients with Hodgkin's disease (vaccinated at least 2 weeks before the initiation of chemotherapy or 3 months after the end of chemotherapy)

**Effects on Mental Status** May cause irritability or lethargy

**Effects on Psychiatric Treatment** May lessen or potentiate the effects of anxiolytics or mood stabilizers

**Usual Dosage** Children: I.M.: 0.5 mL as a single dose should be administered according to one of the following "brand-specific" schedules; do not inject I.V.

**Vaccination schedule for *Haemophilus* b conjugate vaccines, by product/age:**
It is not currently recommended that the various *Haemophilus* b conjugate vaccines be interchanged (ie, the same brand should be used throughout the entire vaccination series). If the health care provider does not know which vaccine was previously used, it is prudent that an infant, 2-6 months of age, be given a primary series of three doses.

**HibTITER®:**
Age at 1st dose: 2-6 months:
Primary series: 3 doses, 2 months apart; booster: 15 months (at least 2 months after previous dose)
Age at 1st dose: 7-11 months:
Primary series: 2 doses, 2 months apart; booster: 15 months (at least 2 months after previous dose)
Age at 1st dose: 12-14 months:
Primary series: 1 dose; booster: 15 months (at least 2 months after previous dose)
Age at 1st dose: 15-60 months:
Primary series: 1 dose; no booster

**PedvaxHIB™:**
Age at 1st dose: 2-6 months:
Primary series: 2 doses, 2 months apart; booster: 12 months (at least 2 months after previous dose)
Age at 1st dose: 7-11 months:
Primary series: 2 doses, 2 months apart; booster: 15 months (at least 2 months after previous dose)
Age at 1st dose: 12-14 months:
Primary series: 1 dose; booster: 15 months (at least 2 months after previous dose)
Age at 1st dose: 15-60 months:
Primary series: 1 dose; no booster

**ProHIBiT®:**
Age at 1st dose: 15-60 months:
Primary series: 1 dose; no booster

**Dosage Forms** Injection:
ActHIB®, HibTITER®, OmniHIB™: Capsular oligosaccharide 10 mcg and diphtheria $CRM_{197}$ protein ~25 mcg per 0.5 mL (0.5 mL, 2.5 mL, 5 mL)
PedvaxHIB™: Purified capsular polysaccharide 15 mcg and *Neisseria meningitidis* OMPC 250 mcg per dose (0.5 mL)
ProHIBiT®: Purified capsular polysaccharide 25 mcg and conjugated diphtheria toxoid protein 18 mcg per dose (0.5 mL, 2.5 mL, 5 mL)
TriHIBit® vaccine [Tripedia® vaccine used to reconstitute ActHIB®]: 0.5 mL

## Halazepam (hal AZ e pam)

**Related Information**
Anxiolytic/Hypnotic Use in Long-Term Care Facilities *on page 754*
Benzodiazepines Comparison Chart *on page 708*
Federal OBRA Regulations Recommended Maximum Doses *on page 756*
Patient Information - Anxiolytics & Sedative Hypnotics (Benzodiazepines) *on page 653*

**Generic Available** No

**U.S. Brand Names** Paxipam®

**Pharmacologic Category** Benzodiazepine

**Use** Management of anxiety disorders
**Unlabeled use:** Hostility; schizophrenia; alcohol withdrawal

**Restrictions** C-IV

**Pregnancy Risk Factor** D

**Contraindications** Hypersensitivity to this drug or any component of its formulation (cross-sensitivity with other benzodiazepines may exist); narrow-angle glaucoma; pregnancy

**Warnings/Precautions** Use with caution in elderly or debilitated patients, patients with hepatic disease (including alcoholics), or renal impairment. Active metabolites with extended half-lives may lead to delayed accumulation and adverse effects. Use with caution in patients with respiratory disease, or impaired gag reflex. Avoid use in patients with sleep apnea.
(Continued)

## Halazepam *(Continued)*

Causes CNS depression (dose-related) resulting in sedation, dizziness, confusion, or ataxia which may impair physical and mental capabilities. Patients must be cautioned about performing tasks which require mental alertness (ie, operating machinery or driving). Use with caution in patients receiving other CNS depressants or psychoactive agents. Effects with other sedative drugs or ethanol may be potentiated. Benzodiazepines have been associated with falls and traumatic injury and should be used with extreme caution in patients who are at risk of these events (especially the elderly).

Use caution in patients with depression, particularly if suicidal risk may be present. Use with caution in patients with a history of drug dependence. Benzodiazepines have been associated with dependence and acute withdrawal symptoms on discontinuation or reduction in dose. Acute withdrawal, including seizures, may be precipitated after administration of flumazenil to patients receiving long-term benzodiazepine therapy.

Benzodiazepines have been associated with anterograde amnesia. Paradoxical reactions, including hyperactive or aggressive behavior, have been reported with benzodiazepines, particularly in adolescent/pediatric or psychiatric patients. Does not have analgesic, antidepressant, or antipsychotic properties.

**Adverse Reactions**

>10%: Central nervous system: Drowsiness

1% to 10%:

Cardiovascular: Tachycardia, hypotension, bradycardia

Central nervous system: Confusion, headache, apathy, euphoria, disorientation

Dermatologic: Dermatitis, rash

Gastrointestinal: Increased salivation, xerostomia, nausea, sense of seasickness, constipation

Ocular: Blurred vision

<1%: Blood dyscrasias, drug dependence menstrual irregularities, reflex slowing

**Overdosage/Toxicology** Treatment: Supportive; rarely is mechanical ventilation required; flumazenil has been shown to selectively block the binding of benzodiazepines to CNS receptors, resulting in a reversal of benzodiazepine-induced sedation; however, its use may not alter the course of overdose

**Drug Interactions** CYP3A3/4 enzyme substrate

CNS depressants: Sedative effects and/or respiratory depression may be additive with CNS depressants; includes ethanol, barbiturates, narcotic analgesics, and other sedative agents; monitor for increased effect

Enzyme inducers: Metabolism of some benzodiazepines may be increased, decreasing their therapeutic effect; consider using an alternative sedative/hypnotic agent; potential inducers include phenobarbital, phenytoin, carbamazepine, rifampin, and rifabutin

CYP3A3/4 inhibitors: Serum level and/or toxicity of some benzodiazepines may be increased; inhibitors include amiodarone, cimetidine, clarithromycin, erythromycin, delavirdine, diltiazem, dirithromycin, disulfiram, fluoxetine, fluvoxamine, grapefruit juice, indinavir, itraconazole, ketoconazole, nefazodone, nevirapine, propoxyfene, quinupristin-dalfopristin, ritonavir, saquinavir, verapamil, zafirlukast, zileuton; monitor for altered benzodiazepine response

Oral contraceptives: May decrease the clearance of some benzodiazepines (those which undergo oxidative metabolism); monitor for increased benzodiazepine effect

Theophylline: May partially antagonize some of the effects of benzodiazepines; monitor for decreased response; may require higher doses for sedation

**Mechanism of Action** Binds to stereospecific benzodiazepine receptors on the postsynaptic GABA neuron at several sites within the central nervous system, including the limbic system, reticular formation. Enhancement of the inhibitory effect of GABA on neuronal excitability results by increased neuronal membrane permeability to chloride ions. This shift in chloride ions results in hyperpolarization (a less excitable state) and stabilization.

**Pharmacodynamics/kinetics**

Half-life:

Parent: 14 hours

Active metabolite (desmethyldiazepam): 50-100 hours

Peak level: 1-3 hours

Elimination: <1% excreted unchanged in urine

**Usual Dosage** Oral:

Adults: 20-40 mg 3-4 times/day; optimal dosage usually ranges from 80-160 mg/day. If side effects occur with the starting dose, lower the dose.

Elderly ≥70 years or debilitated patients: 20 mg 1-2 times/day and adjust dose accordingly

**Monitoring Parameters** Respiratory, cardiovascular and mental status, symptoms of anxiety

**Patient Information** Avoid alcohol and other CNS depressants; may cause drowsiness; avoid activities needing good psychomotor coordination until CNS effects are known; may cause physical or psychological dependence; avoid abrupt discontinuation after prolonged use

**Additional Information** Halazepam offers no significant advantage over other benzodiazepines

**Dosage Forms** Tablet: 20 mg, 40 mg

## Halcinonide (hal SIN oh nide)

**Related Information**

Corticosteroids Comparison Chart *on page 711*

**U.S. Brand Names** Halog®; Halog®-E

**Pharmacologic Category** Corticosteroid, Topical

**Use** Inflammation of corticosteroid-responsive dermatoses [high potency topical corticosteroid]

**Effects on Mental Status** None reported

**Effects on Psychiatric Treatment** None reported

**Usual Dosage** Children and Adults: Topical: Apply sparingly 1-3 times/day, occlusive dressing may be used for severe or resistant dermatoses; a thin film of cream or ointment is effective; do not overuse. Therapy should be discontinued when control is achieved; if no improvement is seen, reassessment of diagnosis may be necessary.

**Dosage Forms**

Cream (Halog®): 0.025% (15 g, 60 g, 240 g); 0.1% (15 g, 30 g, 60 g, 240 g)

Cream, emollient base (Halog®-E) : 0.1% (15 g, 30 g, 60 g)

Ointment, topical (Halog®): 0.1% (15 g, 30 g, 60 g, 240 g)

Solution (Halog®): 0.1% (20 mL, 60 mL)


- **Halcion®** *see* Triazolam *on page 565*
- **Haldol®** *see* Haloperidol *on page 263*
- **Haldol® Decanoate** *see* Haloperidol *on page 263*
- **Halenol® Children's [OTC]** *see* Acetaminophen *on page 14*
- **Haley's M-O® [OTC]** *see* Magnesium Hydroxide and Mineral Oil Emulsion *on page 330*
- **Halfan®** *see* Halofantrine *on page 262*
- **Halfprin® 81® [OTC]** *see* Aspirin *on page 49*
- **Hallucinogenic Drugs** *see page 713*


## Halobetasol (hal oh BAY ta sol)

**Related Information**

Corticosteroids Comparison Chart *on page 711*

**U.S. Brand Names** Ultravate™ Topical

**Pharmacologic Category** Corticosteroid, Topical

**Use** Relief of inflammatory and pruritic manifestations of corticosteroid-response dermatoses [very high potency topical corticosteroid]

**Effects on Mental Status** None reported

**Effects on Psychiatric Treatment** None noted

**Usual Dosage** Children and Adults: Topical: Apply sparingly to skin twice daily, rub in gently and completely; treatment should not exceed 2 consecutive weeks and total dosage should not exceed 50 g/week. Therapy should be discontinued when control is achieved; if no improvement is seen, reassessment of diagnosis may be necessary.

**Dosage Forms**

Cream, as propionate: 0.05% (15 g, 45 g)

Ointment, topical, as propionate: 0.05% (15 g, 45 g)

## Halofantrine (ha loe FAN trin)

**U.S. Brand Names** Halfan®

**Pharmacologic Category** Antimalarial Agent

**Use** Treatment of mild to moderate acute malaria caused by susceptible strains of *Plasmodium falciparum* and *Plasmodium vivax*

**Effects on Mental Status** May cause drowsiness

**Effects on Psychiatric Treatment** None reported

**Pregnancy Risk Factor** C

**Contraindications** Family history of congenital QTc prolongation; hypersensitivity to halofantrine

**Warnings/Precautions** Monitor closely for decreased hematocrit and hemoglobin, patients with chronic liver disease

**Adverse Reactions**

>10%: Dermatologic: Pruritus

1% to 10%:

Cardiovascular: Edema

Central nervous system: Malaise, headache

Gastrointestinal: Nausea, vomiting

Hematologic: Leukocytosis

Hepatic: Elevated LFTs

Local: Tenderness

Neuromuscular & skeletal: Myalgia

Respiratory: Cough

Miscellaneous: Lymphadenopathy

<1%: Anaphylactic shock, asthma, hypoglycemia, hypotension, sterile abscesses, tachycardia, urticaria

**Drug Interactions** CYP2D6 and 3A3/4 enzyme substrate

Increased toxicity (QTc interval prolongation) with other agents that cause QTc interval prolongation, especially mefloquine

**Usual Dosage** Oral:

Children <40 kg: 8 mg/kg every 6 hours for 3 doses; repeat in 1 week

Adults: 500 mg every 6 hours for 3 doses; repeat in 1 week

**Patient Information** Take on an empty stomach; avoid high fat meals; notify physician of persistent nausea, vomiting, abdominal pain, light stools, dark urine

**Nursing Implications** Monitor closely for jaundice, other signs of hepatotoxicity

**Dosage Forms** Tablet, as hydrochloride: 250 mg

♦ **Halog®** *see* Halcinonide *on page 262*

♦ **Halog®-E** *see* Halcinonide *on page 262*

## Haloperidol (ha loe PER i dole)

**Related Information**

Antipsychotic Agents Comparison Chart *on page 706*
Antipsychotic Medication Guidelines *on page 751*
Clinical Issues in the Use of Antipsychotics *on page 630*
Discontinuation of Psychotropic Drugs - Withdrawal Symptoms and Recommendations *on page 798*
Federal OBRA Regulations Recommended Maximum Doses *on page 756*
Liquid Compatibility With Antipsychotics and Mood Stabilizers *on page 718*
Mood Disorders *on page 600*
Patient Information - Antipsychotics (General) *on page 646*
Schizophrenia *on page 604*
Special Populations - Elderly *on page 662*
Special Populations - Mentally Retarded Patients *on page 665*
Special Populations - Pregnant and Breast-Feeding Patients *on page 668*
Substance-Related Disorders *on page 609*

**Generic Available** Yes

**U.S. Brand Names** Haldol®; Haldol® Decanoate

**Canadian Brand Names** Haldol® LA; Peridol

**Synonyms** Haloperidol Decanoate; Haloperidol Lactate

**Pharmacologic Category** Antipsychotic Agent, Butyrophenone

**Use** Treatment of psychoses; control of tics and vocal utterances of Tourette's disorder in children and adults; severe behavioral problems in children

**Unlabeled use:** May be used for the emergency sedation of severely agitated or delirious patients

**Pregnancy Risk Factor** C

**Contraindications** Hypersensitivity to haloperidol or any component; Parkinson's disease; severe CNS depression, bone marrow suppression, severe cardiac or hepatic disease; coma

**Warnings/Precautions** Hypotension may occur, particularly with parenteral administration. Decanoate form should never be administered I.V. Avoid in thyrotoxicosis. May be sedating, use with caution in disorders where CNS depression is a feature. Caution in patients with hemodynamic instability, predisposition to seizures, subcortical brain damage, renal or respiratory disease. Esophageal dysmotility and aspiration have been associated with antipsychotic use - use with caution in patients at risk of pneumonia (ie, Alzheimer's disease). Caution in breast cancer or other prolactin-dependent tumors (may elevate prolactin levels). May alter temperature regulation or mask toxicity of other drugs due to antiemetic effects. May alter cardiac conduction - life-threatening arrhythmias have occurred with therapeutic doses of antipsychotics. Adverse effects of decanoate may be prolonged. May cause orthostatic hypotension - use with caution in patients at risk of this effect or those who would tolerate transient hypotensive episodes (cerebrovascular disease, cardiovascular disease, or other medications which may predispose). Some tablets contain tartrazine.

May cause anticholinergic effects (confusion, agitation, constipation, dry mouth, blurred vision, urinary retention). Therefore, they should be used with caution in patients with decreased gastrointestinal motility, urinary retention, BPH, xerostomia, or visual problems. Conditions which also may be exacerbated by cholinergic blockade include narrow-angle glaucoma (screening is recommended) and worsening of myasthenia gravis. Relative to other neuroleptics, haloperidol has a low potency of cholinergic blockade.

May cause extrapyramidal reactions, including pseudoparkinsonism, acute dystonic reactions, akathisia, and tardive dyskinesia (risk of these reactions is high relative to other neuroleptics). May be associated with neuroleptic malignant syndrome (NMS) or pigmentary retinopathy.

**Adverse Reactions**

Cardiovascular: Hypotension, hypertension, tachycardia, arrhythmias, abnormal T waves with prolonged ventricular repolarization

Central nervous system: Restlessness, anxiety, extrapyramidal reactions, dystonic reactions, pseudoparkinsonian signs and symptoms, tardive dyskinesia, neuroleptic malignant syndrome (NMS), altered central temperature regulation, akathisia, tardive dystonia, insomnia, euphoria, agitation, drowsiness, depression, lethargy, headache, confusion, vertigo, seizures

Dermatologic: Hyperpigmentation, pruritus, rash, contact dermatitis, alopecia, photosensitivity (rare)

Endocrine & metabolic: Amenorrhea, galactorrhea, gynecomastia, sexual dysfunction, lactation, breast engorgement, mastalgia, menstrual irregularities, hyperglycemia, hypoglycemia, hyponatremia

Gastrointestinal: Nausea, vomiting, anorexia, constipation, diarrhea, hypersalivation, dyspepsia, xerostomia

Genitourinary: Urinary retention, priapism

Hematologic: Cholestatic jaundice, obstructive jaundice

Ocular: Blurred vision

Respiratory: Laryngospasm, bronchospasm

Miscellaneous: Heat stroke, diaphoresis

**Overdosage/Toxicology**

Signs and symptoms: deep sleep, dystonia, agitation, dysrhythmias, extrapyramidal symptoms

Treatment: Following initiation of essential overdose management, toxic symptom treatment and supportive treatment should be initiated. Also critical cardiac arrhythmias often respond to I.V. lidocaine, while other antiarrhythmics can be used. Neuroleptics often cause extrapyramidal symptoms (eg, dystonic reactions) requiring management with benztropine mesylate I.V. 1-2 mg (adult) may be effective. These agents are generally effective within 2-5 minutes.

**Drug Interactions** CYP1A2 (minor), CYP2D6 (minor); and CYP3A3/4 enzyme substrate; CYP2D6 and CYP3A3/4 enzyme inhibitor

Anticholinergics: May inhibit the therapeutic response to haloperidol and excess anticholinergic effects may occur; tardive dyskinesias have also been reported; includes benztropine and trihexyphenidyl

Antihypertensives: Concurrent use of haloperidol with an antihypertensive may produce additive hypotensive effects (particularly orthostasis)

Bromocriptine: Antipsychotics inhibit the ability of bromocriptine to lower serum prolactin concentrations

Chloroquine: Serum concentrations of haloperidol may be increased by chloroquine

CNS depressants: Sedative effects may be additive; monitor for increased effect; includes barbiturates, benzodiazepines, narcotic analgesics, ethanol and other sedative agents

CYP3A3/4 inhibitors: Serum level and/or toxicity of haloperidol may be increased; inhibitors include amiodarone, cimetidine, clarithromycin, erythromycin, delavirdine, diltiazem, dirithromycin, disulfiram, fluoxetine, fluvoxamine, grapefruit juice, indinavir, itraconazole, ketoconazole, metronidazole, nefazodone, nevirapine, propoxyfene, ritonavir, saquinavir, verapamil, zafirlukast, zileuton; monitor for increased response

Enzyme inducers: May enhance the hepatic metabolism of haloperidol, decreasing its effects; larger doses of haloperidol may be required; includes barbiturates, carbamazepine, phenytoin, rifampin, and rifabutin

Indomethacin: Haloperidol in combination with indomethacin may result in drowsiness, tiredness, and confusion; monitor for adverse effects

Inhalation anesthetics: Haloperidol in combination with certain forms of induction anesthesia may produce peripheral vasodilitation and hypotension

Levodopa: Haloperidol may inhibit the antiparkinsonian effect of levodopa; avoid this combination

Lithium: Haloperidol may produce neurotoxicity with lithium; this is a rare effect

Methyldopa: Effect of haloperidol may be altered; enhanced effects, as well as reduced efficacy have been reported

Nefazodone: Haloperidol and nefazodone may produce additive CNS toxicity, including sedation

Propranolol: Serum concentrations of haloperidol may be increased

Quinidine: May increase haloperidol concentrations; monitor for EPS and/or QTc prolongation

SSRIs: Fluoxetine, fluvoxamine, and paroxetine may inhibit the metabolism of haloperidol resulting in EPS; monitor for EPS

Sulfadoxine-pyrimethamine: May increase fluphenazine concentrations

Tricyclic antidepressants: Concurrent use may produce increased toxicity or altered therapeutic response

Trazodone: Haloperidol and trazodone may produce additive hypotensive effects

**Stability**

Protect oral dosage forms from light

Haloperidol lactate injection should be stored at controlled room temperature and protected from light, freezing and temperatures >40°C; exposure to light may cause discoloration and the development of a grayish-red precipitate over several weeks

Haloperidol lactate may be administered IVPB or I.V. infusion in $D_5W$ solutions; NS solutions should not be used due to reports of decreased stability and incompatibility

Standardized dose: 0.5-100 mg/50-100 mL $D_5W$

Stability of standardized solutions is 38 days at room temperature (24°C)

**Mechanism of Action** Blocks postsynaptic mesolimbic dopaminergic $D_1$ and $D_2$ receptors in the brain; depresses the release of hypothalamic and hypophyseal hormones; believed to depress the reticular activating system

(Continued)

## Haloperidol *(Continued)*

thus affecting basal metabolism, body temperature, wakefulness, vasomotor tone, and emesis

**Pharmacodynamics/kinetics**

Onset of sedation: I.V.: Within 1 hour
Duration of action: ~3 weeks for decanoate form
Distribution: Crosses the placenta; appears in breast milk
Protein binding: 90%
Metabolism: In the liver to inactive compounds
Bioavailability: Oral: 60%
Half-life: 20 hours
Time to peak serum concentration: 20 minutes
Elimination: 33% to 40% excreted in urine within 5 days; an additional 15% excreted in feces

**Usual Dosage**

Children: 3-12 years (15-40 kg): Oral:
Initial: 0.05 mg/kg/day or 0.25-0.5 mg/day given in 2-3 divided doses; increase by 0.25-0.5 mg every 5-7 days; maximum: 0.15 mg/kg/day
Usual maintenance:
Agitation or hyperkinesia: 0.01-0.03 mg/kg/day once daily
Nonpsychotic disorders: 0.05-0.075 mg/kg/day in 2-3 divided doses
Psychotic disorders: 0.05-0.15 mg/kg/day in 2-3 divided doses
Children 6-12 years: I.M. (as lactate): 1-3 mg/dose every 4-8 hours to a maximum of 0.15 mg/kg/day; change over to oral therapy as soon as able
Adults:
Oral: 0.5-5 mg 2-3 times/day; usual maximum: 30 mg/day
I.M. (as lactate): 2-5 mg every 4-8 hours as needed
I.M. (as decanoate): Initial: 10-20 times the daily oral dose administered at 4-week intervals
Maintenance dose: 10-15 times initial oral dose; used to stabilize psychiatric symptoms
Sedation in the Intensive Care Unit:
I.M./IVP/IVPB: May repeat bolus doses after 30 minutes until calm achieved then administer 50% of the maximum dose every 6 hours
Mild agitation: 0.5-2 mg
Moderate agitation: 2.5-5 mg
Severe agitation: 10-20 mg
Oral: Agitation: 5-10 mg
Continuous intravenous infusion (100 mg/100 mL $D_5W$): Rates of 1-40 mg/hour have been used
Rapid tranquilization of agitated patient (administer every 30-60 minutes):
Oral: 5-10 mg
I.M.: 5 mg
Average total dose for tranquilization: 10-20 mg
Elderly (nonpsychotic patients, dementia behavior):
Initial: Oral: 0.25-0.5 mg 1-2 times/day; increase dose at 4- to 7-day intervals by 0.25-0.5 mg/day; increase dosing intervals (twice daily, 3 times/day, etc) as necessary to control response or side effects
Hemodialysis/peritoneal dialysis: Supplemental dose is not necessary

**Dietary Considerations** Alcohol: Additive CNS effect, avoid use

**Administration** The decanoate injectable formulation should be administered I.M. only via Z track method, **do not administer decanoate I.V.** Dilute the oral concentrate with water or juice before administration

**Monitoring Parameters** Monitor orthostatic blood pressures after initiation of therapy or a dose increase; observe for tremor and abnormal movement or posturing (extrapyramidal symptoms)

**Reference Range** Therapeutic: 5-15 ng/mL (SI: 10-30 nmol/L) (psychotic disorders - less for Tourette's and mania); Toxic: >42 ng/mL (SI: >84 nmol/L). Rarely monitored in most clinical settings.

**Test Interactions** ↓ cholesterol (S)

**Patient Information** May cause drowsiness, restlessness, avoid alcohol and other CNS depressants, rise slowly from recumbent position; use of supportive stockings may help prevent orthostatic hypotension; do not alter dosage or discontinue without consulting physician; oral concentrate must be diluted in 2-4 oz of liquid (water, fruit juice, carbonated drinks, milk, or pudding)

**Nursing Implications** Avoid skin contact with oral suspension or solution; may cause contact dermatitis

**Additional Information** May be used for the emergency sedation of severely agitated or delirious patients

**Dosage Forms**

Concentrate, oral, as lactate: 2 mg/mL (5 mL, 10 mL, 15 mL, 120 mL, 240 mL)
Injection, as decanoate: 50 mg/mL (1 mL, 5 mL); 100 mg/mL (1 mL, 5 mL)
Injection, as lactate: 5 mg/mL (1 mL, 2 mL, 2.5 mL, 10 mL)
Tablet: 0.5 mg, 1 mg, 2 mg, 5 mg, 10 mg, 20 mg


- **Haloperidol Decanoate** *see* Haloperidol *on page 263*
- **Haloperidol Lactate** *see* Haloperidol *on page 263*


## Haloprogin (ha loe PROE jin)

**U.S. Brand Names** Halotex®

**Pharmacologic Category** Antifungal Agent, Topical

**Use** Topical treatment of tinea pedis (athlete's foot), tinea cruris (jock itch), tinea corporis (ringworm), tinea manuum caused by *Trichophyton rubrum, Trichophyton tonsurans, Trichophyton mentagrophytes, Microsporum canis*, or *Epidermophyton floccosum*; topical treatment of *Malassezia furfur*

**Effects on Mental Status** None reported

**Effects on Psychiatric Treatment** None reported

**Usual Dosage** Topical: Children and Adults: Apply liberally twice daily for 2-3 weeks; intertriginous areas may require up to 4 weeks of treatment

**Dosage Forms**

Cream: 1% (15 g, 30 g)
Solution, topical: 1% with alcohol 75% (10 mL, 30 mL)


- **Halotestin®** *see* Fluoxymesterone *on page 233*
- **Halotex®** *see* Haloprogin *on page 264*
- **Halotussin® [OTC]** *see* Guaifenesin *on page 256*
- **Halotussin® DAC** *see* Guaifenesin, Pseudoephedrine, and Codeine *on page 258*
- **Halotussin® DM [OTC]** *see* Guaifenesin and Dextromethorphan *on page 257*
- **Halotussin® PE [OTC]** *see* Guaifenesin and Pseudoephedrine *on page 257*
- **Haltran® [OTC]** *see* Ibuprofen *on page 280*
- **Havrix®** *see* Hepatitis A Vaccine *on page 266*
- **Haw** *see* Hawthorn *on page 264*


## Hawthorn

**Related Information**

Natural/Herbal Products *on page 746*
Natural Products, Herbals, and Dietary Supplements *on page 742*

**Synonyms** *Crataegus laevigata*; *Crataegus monogyna*; *Crataegus oxyacantha*; *Crataegus pinnatifida*; English Hawthorn; Haw; Maybush; Whitehorn

**Pharmacologic Category** Herb

**Use** In herbal medicine to treat cardiovascular abnormalities (arrhythmia, angina), increased cardiac output, increased contractility of heart muscle; also used as a sedative

**Contraindications** Pregnancy and breast-feeding

**Adverse Reactions**

Cardiovascular: Hypotension, bradycardia, hypertension
Central nervous system: Depression, fatigue, sedation
Dermatologic: Rash
Gastrointestinal: Nausea

**Overdosage/Toxicology**

Signs and symptoms: Hypotension, CNS depression, syncope
Decontamination: Lavage (within 1 hour)/activated charcoal with cathartic
Treatment: Supportive therapy; treat hypotension with I.V. crystalloid infusion and placement in Trendelenburg position; vasopressor agents can be used in refractory cases

**Drug Interactions** Antihypertensives (effect enhanced), digoxin; effects with Viagra® unknown

**Usual Dosage** Daily dose of total flavonoids: ~10 mg
Per Commission E: 160-900 mg native water-ethanol extract (ethanol 45% v/v or methanol 70% v/v, drug-extract ratio: 4-7:1, with defined flavonoid or procyanidin content), corresponding to 30-168.7 mg procyanidins, calculated as epicatechin, or 3.5-19.8 mg flavonoids, calculated as hyperoside in accordance with DAB 10 [German pharmacopoeia #10] in 2 or 3 individual doses; duration of administration: 6 weeks minimum

**Additional Information** A small deciduous tree which can grow up to 25 feet; its white, strongly aromatic flowers bloom in mid to late spring; tincture has a bitter taste


- **Hayfebrol® Liquid [OTC]** *see* Chlorpheniramine and Pseudoephedrine *on page 114*
- **H-BIG®** *see* Hepatitis B Immune Globulin *on page 266*
- **25-HCC** *see* Calcifediol *on page 83*
- **HCFA Guidelines for Unnecessary Drugs in Long-Term Care Facilities** *see page 757*
- **hCG** *see* Chorionic Gonadotropin *on page 122*
- **HCTZ** *see* Hydrochlorothiazide *on page 271*
- **Heartline® [OTC]** *see* Aspirin *on page 49*
- **Hectorol®** *see* Doxercalciferol *on page 184*
- ***Helicobacter pylori* Treatment** *see page 784*
- **Helidac™** *see* Bismuth Subsalicylate, Metronidazole, and Tetracycline *on page 69*
- **Helixate®** *see* Antihemophilic Factor (Recombinant) *on page 46*

♦ **Hemabate™** *see* Carboprost Tromethamine *on page 93*

## Hemin (HEE min)

**U.S. Brand Names** Panhematin®

**Pharmacologic Category** Blood Modifiers

**Use** Treatment of recurrent attacks of acute intermittent porphyria (AIP) only after an appropriate period of alternate therapy has been tried

**Effects on Mental Status** None reported

**Effects on Psychiatric Treatment** Avoid concurrent use with barbiturates

**Usual Dosage** I.V.: 1-4 mg/kg/day administered over 10-15 minutes for 3-14 days; may be repeated no earlier than every 12 hours; not to exceed 6 mg/kg in any 24-hour period

**Dosage Forms** Powder for injection, preservative free: 313 mg/vial [hematin 7 mg/mL] (43 mL)

♦ **Hemocyte® [OTC]** *see* Ferrous Fumarate *on page 223*

♦ **Hemofil® M** *see* Antihemophilic Factor (Human) *on page 45*

♦ **Hemonyne®** *see* Factor IX Complex (Human) *on page 217*

♦ **Hemril-HC® Uniserts®** *see* Hydrocortisone *on page 273*

## Heparin (HEP a rin)

**U.S. Brand Names** Hepflush-10®; Hep-Lock®

**Synonyms** Heparin Calcium; Heparin Lock Flush; Heparin Sodium

**Pharmacologic Category** Anticoagulant

**Use** Prophylaxis and treatment of thromboembolic disorders

**Effects on Mental Status** None reported

**Effects on Psychiatric Treatment** None reported

**Pregnancy Risk Factor** C

**Contraindications** Hypersensitivity to heparin or any component; severe thrombocytopenia; uncontrolled active bleeding except when due to DIC; suspected intracranial hemorrhage; not for I.M. use; not for use when appropriate monitoring parameters cannot be obtained

**Warnings/Precautions** Use cautiously in patients with a documented hypersensitivity reaction and only in life-threatening situations. Hemorrhage is the most common complication. Monitor for signs and symptoms of bleeding. Certain patients are at increased risk of bleeding. Risk factors include bacterial endocarditis; congenital or acquired bleeding disorders; active ulcerative or angiodysplastic GI diseases; severe uncontrolled hypertension; hemorrhagic stroke; or use shortly after brain, spinal, or ophthalmology surgery; patient treated concomitantly with platelet inhibitors; conditions associated with increased bleeding tendencies (hemophilia, vascular purpura); recent GI bleeding; thrombocytopenia or platelet defects; severe liver disease; hypertensive or diabetic retinopathy; or in patients undergoing invasive procedures. A higher incidence of bleeding has been reported in patients >60 years of age, particularly women. They are also more sensitive to the dose.

Patients who develop thrombocytopenia on heparin may be at risk of developing a new thrombus ("White-clot syndrome"). Hypersensitivity reactions can occur. Osteoporosis can occur following long-term use (>6 months). Monitor for hyperkalemia. Discontinue therapy and consider alternatives if platelets are <100,000/mm$^3$. Patients >60 years of age may require lower doses of heparin.

Some preparations contain benzyl alcohol as a preservative. In neonates, large amounts of benzyl alcohol (>100 mg/kg/day) have been associated with fatal toxicity (gasping syndrome). The use of preservative-free heparin is, therefore, recommended in neonates. Some preparations contain sulfite which may cause allergic reactions.

Heparin does not possess fibrinolytic activity and, therefore, cannot lyse established thrombi; discontinue heparin if hemorrhage occurs; severe hemorrhage or overdosage may require protamine

**Adverse Reactions**

>10%:
- Dermatologic: Unexplained bruising
- Gastrointestinal: Constipation, vomiting of blood
- Hematologic: Hemorrhage, blood in urine, bleeding from gums

1% to 10%:
- Cardiovascular: Chest pain
- Genitourinary: Frequent or persistent erection
- Neuromuscular & skeletal: Peripheral neuropathy
- Miscellaneous: Allergic reactions

<1%: Chills, elevated liver enzymes, fever, headache, irritation, nausea, ulceration, urticaria, vomiting; thrombocytopenia (heparin-associated thrombocytopenia occurs in <1% of patients, immune thrombocytopenia occurs with progressive fall in platelet counts and, in some cases, thromboembolic complications; daily platelet counts for 5-7 days at initiation of therapy may help detect the onset of this complication); cutaneous necrosis have been rarely reported with deep S.C. injections, osteoporosis (chronic therapy effect)

**Overdosage/Toxicology**

Signs and symptoms: The primary symptom of overdose is bleeding

Treatment: Antidote is protamine; dose 1 mg per 1 mg (100 units) of heparin. Discontinue all heparin if evidence of progressive immune thrombocytopenia occurs.

**Drug Interactions**

Cephalosporins which contain the MTT side chain may increase the risk of hemorrhage

Drugs which affect platelet function (eg, aspirin, NSAIDs, dipyridamole, ticlopidine, clopidogrel) may potentiate the risk of hemorrhage

Nitroglycerin (I.V.) may decrease heparin's anticoagulant effect. This interaction has not been validated in some studies, and may only occur at high nitroglycerin dosages.

Penicillins (parenteral) may prolong bleeding time via inhibition of platelet aggregation, potentially increasing the risk of hemorrhage

Thrombolytic agents increase the risk of hemorrhage

Warfarin: Risk of bleeding may be increased during concurrent therapy. Heparin is commonly continued during the initiation of warfarin therapy to assure anticoagulation and to protect against possible transient hypercoagulability

Other drugs reported to increase heparin's anticoagulant effect include antihistamines, tetracycline, quinine, nicotine, and cardiac glycosides (digoxin)

**Usual Dosage**

Line flushing: When using daily flushes of heparin to maintain patency of single and double lumen central catheters, 10 units/mL is commonly used for younger infants (eg, <10 kg) while 100 units/mL is used for older infants, children, and adults. Capped PVC catheters and peripheral heparin locks require flushing more frequently (eg, every 6-8 hours). Volume of heparin flush is usually similar to volume of catheter (or slightly greater). Additional flushes should be given when stagnant blood is observed in catheter, after catheter is used for drug or blood administration, and after blood withdrawal from catheter.

Addition of heparin (0.5-1 unit/mL) to peripheral and central TPN has been shown to increase duration of line patency. The final concentration of heparin used for TPN solutions may need to be decreased to 0.5 units/mL in small infants receiving larger amounts of volume in order to avoid approaching therapeutic amounts. Arterial lines are heparinized with a final concentration of 1 unit/mL.

Children:
- Intermittent I.V.: Initial: 50-100 units/kg, then 50-100 units/kg every 4 hours
- I.V. infusion: Initial: 50 units/kg, then 15-25 units/kg/hour; increase dose by 2-4 units/kg/hour every 6-8 hours as required

Adults:
- Prophylaxis (low-dose heparin): S.C.: 5000 units every 8-12 hours
- Intermittent I.V.: Initial: 10,000 units, then 50-70 units/kg (5000-10,000 units) every 4-6 hours
- I.V. infusion: 50 units/kg to start, then 15-25 units/kg/hour as continuous infusion; increase dose by 5 units/kg/hour every 4 hours as required according to PTT results, usual range: 10-30 units/hour
  - Weight-based protocol: 80 units/kg I.V. push followed by continuous infusion of 18 units/kg/hour. Using a Standard Heparin Solution (25,000 units/500mL $D_5W$), the following infusion rates can be used to achieve the listed doses.
  - For a dose of:
    - 400 units/hour: Infuse at 8 mL/hour
    - 500 units/hour: Infuse at 10 mL/hour
    - 600 units/hour: Infuse at 12 mL/hour
    - 700 units/hour: Infuse at 14 mL/hour
    - 800 units/hour: Infuse at 16 mL/hour
    - 900 units/hour: Infuse at 18 mL/hour
    - 1000 units/hour: Infuse at 20 mL/hour
    - 1100 units/hour: Infuse at 22 mL/hour
    - 1200 units/hour: Infuse at 24 mL/hour
    - 1300 units/hour: Infuse at 26 mL/hour
    - 1400 units/hour: Infuse at 28 mL/hour
    - 1500 units/hour: Infuse at 30 mL/hour
    - 1600 units/hour: Infuse at 32 mL/hour
    - 1700 units/hour: Infuse at 34 mL/hour
    - 1800 units/hour: Infuse at 36 mL/hour
    - 1900 units/hour: Infuse at 38 mL/hour
    - 2000 units/hour: Infuse at 40 mL/hour

**Dosing adjustments in the elderly:** May be more sensitive to a given dose.

**Patient Information** This drug can only be administered by injection. You may have a tendency to bleed easily while taking this drug; brush teeth with soft brush, floss with waxed floss, use electric razor, avoid scissors or sharp knives, and potentially harmful activities. May discolor urine or stool. Report CNS changes (fever, confusion), unusual fever, persistent nausea or GI upset, unusual bleeding or bruising (bleeding gums, nosebleed, blood in urine, dark stool), pain in joints or back, swelling or pain at injection site.

(Continued)

## Heparin *(Continued)*

**Dosage Forms**

Heparin sodium:

Lock flush injection:

Beef lung source: 10 units/mL (1 mL, 2 mL, 2.5 mL, 3 mL, 5 mL, 10 mL, 30 mL); 100 units/mL (1 mL, 2 mL, 2.5 mL, 3 mL, 5 mL, 10 mL, 30 mL)

Porcine intestinal mucosa source: 10 units/mL (1 mL, 2 mL, 10 mL, 30 mL); 100 units/mL (1 mL, 2 mL, 10 mL, 30 mL)

Porcine intestinal mucosa source, preservative free: 10 units/mL (1 mL, 10 mL); 100 units/mL (1 mL)

Multiple-dose vial injection:

Beef lung source, with preservative: 1000 units/mL (5 mL, 10 mL, 30 mL); 5000 units/mL (10 mL); 10,000 units/mL (4 mL, 5 mL, 10 mL); 20,000 units/mL (2 mL, 5 mL, 10 mL); 40,000 units/mL (5 mL)

Porcine intestinal mucosa source, with preservative: 1000 units/mL (10 mL, 30 mL); 5000 units/mL (10 mL); 10,000 units/mL (4 mL); 20,000 units/mL (2 mL, 5 mL)

Single-dose vial injection:

Beef lung source: 1000 units/mL (1 mL); 5000 units/mL (1 mL); 10,000 units/mL (1 mL); 20,000 units/mL (1 mL); 40,000 units/mL (1 mL)

Porcine intestinal mucosa: 1000 units/mL (1 mL); 5000 units/mL (1 mL); 10,000 units/mL (1 mL); 20,000 units/mL (1 mL); 40,000 units/ mL (1 mL)

Unit dose injection:

Porcine intestinal mucosa source, with preservative: 1000 units/dose (1 mL, 2 mL); 2500 units/dose (1 mL); 5000 units/dose (0.5 mL, 1 mL); 7500 units/dose (1 mL); 10,000 units/dose (1 mL); 15,000 units/ dose (1 mL); 20,000 units/dose (1 mL)

Heparin sodium infusion, porcine intestinal mucosa source:

$D_5W$: 40 units/mL (500 mL); 50 units/mL (250 mL, 500 mL); 100 units/mL (100 mL, 250 mL)

NaCl 0.45%: 2 units/mL (500 mL, 1000 mL); 50 units/mL (250 mL); 100 units/mL (250 mL)

NaCl 0.9%: 2 units/mL (500 mL, 1000 mL); 5 units/mL (1000 mL); 50 units/mL (250 mL, 500 mL, 1000 mL)

Heparin calcium:

Unit dose injection, porcine intestinal mucosa, preservative free (Calciparine®): 5000 units/dose (0.2 mL); 12,500 units/dose (0.5 mL); 20,000 units/dose (0.8 mL)

♦ **Heparin Calcium** *see* Heparin *on page 265*

♦ **Heparin Lock Flush** *see* Heparin *on page 265*

♦ **Heparin Sodium** *see* Heparin *on page 265*

## Hepatitis A Vaccine (hep a TYE tis aye vak SEEN)

**U.S. Brand Names** Havrix®

**Pharmacologic Category** Vaccine

**Use** For populations desiring protection against hepatitis A or for populations at high risk of exposure to hepatitis A virus (travelers to developing countries, household and sexual contacts of persons infected with hepatitis A), child day care employees, patients with chronic liver disease, illicit drug users, male homosexuals, institutional workers (eg, institutions for the mentally and physically handicapped persons, prisons, etc), and health-care workers who may be exposed to hepatitis A virus (eg, laboratory employees); protection lasts for approximately 15 years

**Effects on Mental Status** None reported

**Effects on Psychiatric Treatment** None reported

**Usual Dosage** I.M.:

Havrix®:

Children 2-18 years: 720 ELISA units (administered as 2 injections of 360 ELISA units [0.5 mL]) 15-30 days prior to travel with a booster 6-12 months following primary immunization; the deltoid muscle should be used for I.M. injection

Adults: 1440 ELISA units(1 mL) 15-30 days prior to travel with a booster 6-12 months following primary immunization; injection should be in the deltoid

VAQTA®:

Children 2-17 years: 25 units (0.5 mL) with 25 units (0.5 mL) booster to be given 6-18 months after primary immunization

Adults: 50 units (1 mL) with 50 units (1 mL) booster to be given 6 months after primary immunization

**Dosage Forms**

Injection: 360 ELISA units/0.5 mL (0.5 mL); 1440 ELISA units/mL (1 mL)

Injection, pediatric: 720 ELISA units/0.5 mL (0.5 mL)

Injection (VAQTA®): 50 units/mL (1 mL)

## Hepatitis B Immune Globulin
(hep a TYE tis bee i MYUN GLOB yoo lin)

**U.S. Brand Names** H-BIG®; HyperHep®

**Pharmacologic Category** Immune Globulin

**Use** Provide prophylactic passive immunity to hepatitis B infection to those individuals exposed; newborns of mothers known to be hepatitis B surface antigen positive; hepatitis B immune globulin is not indicated for treatment of active hepatitis B infections and is ineffective in the treatment of chronic active hepatitis B infection

**Effects on Mental Status** May cause dizziness or drowsiness

**Effects on Psychiatric Treatment** Sedative effects may be additive with concurrent psychotropic use

**Usual Dosage** I.M.:

Newborns: Hepatitis B: 0.5 mL as soon after birth as possible (within 12 hours); may repeat at 3 months in order for a higher rate of prevention of the carrier state to be achieved; at this time an active vaccination program with the vaccine may begin

Adults: Postexposure prophylaxis: 0.06 mL/kg as soon as possible after exposure (ie, within 24 hours of needlestick, ocular, or mucosal exposure or within 14 days of sexual exposure); usual dose: 3-5 mL; repeat at 28-30 days after exposure

**Note:** HBIG may be administered at the same time (but at a different site) or up to 1 month preceding hepatitis B vaccination without impairing the active immune response

**Dosage Forms** Injection:

H-BIG®: 4 mL, 5 mL

HyperHep®: 0.5 mL, 1 mL, 5 mL

## Hepatitis B Vaccine (hep a TYE tis bee vak SEEN)

**U.S. Brand Names** Engerix-B®; Recombivax HB®

**Pharmacologic Category** Vaccine

**Use** Immunization against infection caused by all known subtypes of hepatitis B virus, in individuals considered at high risk of potential exposure to hepatitis B virus or $HB_sAg$-positive materials; see list below.

**Pre-exposure Prophylaxis for Hepatitis B**

Health care workers*

- Special patient groups (eg, adolescents, infants born to $HB_sAg$-positive mothers, military personnel, etc): Hemodialysis patients**, recipients of certain blood products***
- Lifestyle factors: Homosexual and bisexual men, intravenous drug abusers, heterosexually active persons with multiple sexual partners or recently acquired sexually transmitted diseases
- Environmental factors: Household and sexual contacts of HBV carriers, prison inmates, clients and staff of institutions for the mentally handicapped, residents, immigrants and refugees from areas with endemic HBV infection, international travelers at increased risk of acquiring HBV infection

*The risk of hepatitis B virus (HBV) infection for health care workers varies both between hospitals and within hospitals. Hepatitis B vaccination is recommended for all health care workers with blood exposure.

**Hemodialysis patients often respond poorly to hepatitis B vaccination; higher vaccine doses or increased number of doses are required. A special formulation of one vaccine is now available for such persons (Recombivax HB®, 40 mcg/mL). The anti-$HB_s$ (antibody to hepatitis B surface antigen) response of such persons should be tested after they are vaccinated, and those who have not responded should be revaccinated with 1-3 additional doses.

Patients with chronic renal disease should be vaccinated as early as possible, ideally before they require hemodialysis. In addition, their anti-$HB_s$ levels should be monitored at 6-12 month intervals to assess the need for revaccination.

***Patients with hemophilia should be immunized subcutaneously, not intramuscularly.

**Effects on Mental Status** Malaise and fatigue are common; may rarely cause lightheadedness, somnolence, insomnia, irritability, agitation, anorexia

**Effects on Psychiatric Treatment** Sedative effects may be additive with concurrent psychotropic use

**Usual Dosage** Routine immunization regimen of three I.M. hepatitis B vaccine doses, by product/age:

**Recombivax HB®**

Birth* to 10 years: Initial dose 0.25 mL**; repeat in 1 month and 6 months

11-19 years: Initial dose 0.5 mL; repeat in 1 month and 6 months

≥20 years: Initial dose 1 mL; repeat in 1 month and 6 months

**Energix-B®**

Birth* to 10 years: Initial dose 0.5 mL; repeat in 1 month and 6 months

11-19 years: Initial dose 1 mL; repeat in 1 month and 6 months

≥20 years: Initial dose 1 mL; repeat in 1 month and 6 months

Dialysis or immunocompromised patients: Initial dose 2 mL***; repeat in 1 month and 6 months

*Infants born of $HB_sAg$, **negative** mothers

**0.5 mL of the 5 mcg/0.5 mL (adolescent/high-risk infant) product or 0.5 mL of the 25 mcg/0.5 mL pediatric formulation

***Two 1 mL doses given at different sites.

**Postexposure prophylaxis recommended dosage for infants born to $HB_sAg$-positive mothers, by product/age:**

**Engerix-B®** (pediatric product dose 10 mcg/0.5 mL):
Give 0.5 mL within 7 days. Alternately, the first dose may be given at birth at the same time as HBIG, but give in the opposite anterolateral thigh. This may better ensure vaccine absorption.
Repeat 0.5 mL at 1 month and 6 months.

**Recombivax HB®** (high-risk infant product dose 5 mcg/0.5 mL):
Give 0.25 mL within 7 days, or 0.5 mL of the pediatric product (0.25 mcg/0.5 mL). Alternately, the first dose may be given at birth at the same time as HBIG, but give in the opposite anterolateral thigh. This may better ensure vaccine absorption.
Repeat 0.25 mL at 1 month and 6 months, or with 0.5 mL if using the pediatric product (0.25 mcg/0.5 mL)

**Hepatitis B immune globulin:**
Give 0.5 mL at birth

**Note:** An alternate regimen is administration of the vaccine at birth, within 7 days of birth, and 1, 2, and 12 months later.

Dialysis regimen: Use Recombivax HB® formulation (40 mcg/mL); initial: 40 mcg/mL, then at 1 and 6 months; revaccination: if anti-$HB_s$ <10 mIU/mL ≥1-2 months after 3rd dose

**Dosage Forms** Injection:
Recombinant DNA (Engerix-B®)
Pediatric formulation: Hepatitis B surface antigen 10 mcg/0.5 mL (0.5 mL)
Adult formulation: Hepatitis B surface antigen 20 mcg/mL (1 mL)
Recombinant DNA (Recombivax HB®):
Pediatric formulation: Hepatitis B surface antigen 2.5 mg/0.5 mL (0.5 mL/3 mL)
Adolescent/high-risk infant formulation: Hepatitis B surface antigen 5 mcg/0.5 mL (0.5 mL)
Adult formulation: Hepatitis B surface antigen 10 mcg/mL (1 mL, 3 mL)
Dialysis formulation, recombinant DNA: Hepatitis B surface antigen 40 mcg/mL (1 mL)


♦ **Hepflush-10®** *see* Heparin *on page 265*

♦ **Hep-Lock®** *see* Heparin *on page 265*

♦ **Heptalac®** *see* Lactulose *on page 306*

♦ **Herbals That May Alter Metabolism and GI Absorption of Drugs** *see page 745*

♦ **Herb-of-Grace** *see* Rue *on page 501*

♦ **Herceptin®** *see* Trastuzumab *on page 560*


## Heroin (HAIR oh in)

**Related Information**
Hallucinogenic Drugs *on page 713*

**Synonyms** Acetomorphine; Diacetylmorphine; Diamorphine Hydrochloride

**Pharmacologic Category** Analgesic, Narcotic

**Use** Most commonly a drug of abuse in the United States; used as an analgesic agent or cough suppressant in Britain

**Effects on Mental Status** May cause sedation, euphoria, depression, paranoia, hallucinations

**Effects on Psychiatric Treatment** May counteract psychotropic intended effect

**Contraindications** Hypersensitivity to morphine or diamorphine; acute respiratory depression

**Warnings/Precautions** May provoke hypertension and tachycardia in patients with pheochromocytoma; use with caution in renal/liver insufficiency, diarrhea associated with antibiotics; pulmonary disease, gallbladder disease, hypothyroidism, inflammatory bowel disease, prostatic hypertrophy, increased intracranial pressure

**Adverse Reactions**
Cardiovascular: Hypotension, congestive heart failure
Central nervous system: Lethargy, coma, euphoria, hallucinations, CNS depression, depression, paranoia
Dermatologic: Pemphigus
Gastrointestinal: Constipation, xerostomia, nausea, vomiting, Ogilvie's syndrome, esophageal sphincter tone (decreased)
Genitourinary: Urinary retention
Hematologic: Thrombocytopenia, progressive spongiform leukoencephalopathy, leukoencephalopathy
Neuromuscular & skeletal: Myoclonus, rhabdomyolysis
Ocular: Miosis, photophobia
Renal: Renal failure, proteinuria
Respiratory: Apnea, respiratory depression, bronchospasm (upon nasal insufflation), pulmonary edema, aspiration

**Drug Interactions** Subcutaneous absorption may be delayed when coadministered with cocaine

**Usual Dosage**
Analgesia (in Europe):
Oral: 5-10 mg
I.M., S.C.: 5 mg (usually I.V. dose)
As a drug of abuse: Nasal insufflation, I.V., S.C.: Up to 200 mg; usual dose: ~2 mg


♦ **Hetrazan®** *see* Diethylcarbamazine *on page 167*

♦ **Hexachlorocyclohexane** *see* Lindane *on page 318*

♦ **Hexadrol®** *see* Dexamethasone *on page 157*

♦ **Hexadrol® Phosphate** *see* Dexamethasone *on page 157*

♦ **Hexalen®** *see* Altretamine *on page 27*

♦ **Hexamethylenetetramine** *see* Methenamine *on page 351*


## Hexobarbital (hex oh BAR bi tal)

**Related Information**
Patient Information - Anxiolytics & Sedative Hypnotics (Barbiturates) *on page 654*

**U.S. Brand Names** Pre-Sed®

**Pharmacologic Category** Barbiturate

**Use** Preoperative medication; short-term sedation for diagnostic and minor surgical procedures; potentiating agent for analgesic; postoperative medication; patients suffering from mental and emotional stress that cannot fall asleep

**Restrictions** C-III

**Pregnancy Risk Factor** D

**Contraindications** Hypersensitivity to barbiturates or any component of the formulation; marked hepatic impairment; dyspnea or airway obstruction; porphyria

**Warnings/Precautions** Potential for drug dependency exists, abrupt cessation may precipitate withdrawal, including status epilepticus in epileptic patients. Do not administer to patients in acute pain. Use caution in elderly, debilitated, renally impaired, hepatic dysfunction or pediatric patients. May cause paradoxical responses, including agitation and hyperactivity, particularly in acute pain and pediatric patients. Use with caution in patients with depression or suicidal tendencies, or in patients with a history of drug abuse. Tolerance, psychological and physical dependence may occur with prolonged use. May cause CNS depression, which may impair physical or mental abilities. Patients must cautioned about performing tasks which require mental alertness (operating machinery or driving). Effects with other sedative drugs or ethanol may be potentiated. May cause respiratory depression or hypotension; use with caution in hemodynamically unstable patients or patients with respiratory disease.

**Drug Interactions** CYP2C9 and 2C19 enzyme substrate
**Note:** Barbiturates are enzyme inducers; patients should be monitored when these drugs are started or stopped for a decreased or increased therapeutic effect respectively
Acetaminophen: Barbiturates may enhance the hepatotoxic potential of acetaminophen overdoses
Antiarrhythmics: Barbiturates may increase the metabolism of antiarrhythmics, decreasing their clinical effect; includes disopyramide, propafenone, and quinidine
Anticonvulsants: Barbiturates may increase the metabolism of anticonvulsants; includes ethosuximide, felbamate (possibly), lamotrigine, phenytoin, tiagabine, topiramate, and zonisamide; does not appear to affect gabapentin or levetiracetam
Antineoplastics: Limited evidence suggests that enzyme-inducing anticonvulsant therapy may reduce the effectiveness of some chemotherapy regimens (specifically in ALL); teniposide and methotrexate may be cleared more rapidly in these patients
Antipsychotics: Barbiturates may enhance the metabolism (decrease the efficacy) of antipsychotics; monitor for altered response; dose adjustment may be needed
Beta-blockers: Metabolism of beta-blockers may be increased and clinical effect decreased; atenolol and nadolol are unlikely to interact given their renal elimination
Calcium channel blockers: Barbiturates may enhance the metabolism of calcium channel blockers, decreasing their clinical effect
Chloramphenicol: Barbiturates may increase the metabolism of chloramphenicol and chloramphenicol may inhibit barbiturate metabolism; monitor for altered response
Cimetidine: Barbiturates may enhance the metabolism of cimetidine, decreasing its clinical effect
CNS depressants: Sedative effects and/or respiratory depression with barbiturates may be additive with other CNS depressants; monitor for increased effect; includes ethanol, sedatives, antidepressants, narcotic analgesics, and benzodiazepines
Corticosteroids: Barbiturates may enhance the metabolism of corticosteroids, decreasing their clinical effect
Cyclosporine: Levels may be decreased by barbiturates; monitor
(Continued)

## Hexobarbital *(Continued)*

Immunosuppressants: Barbiturates may enhance the metabolism of immunosuppressants, decreasing its clinical effect; includes both cyclosporine and tacrolimus
Doxycycline: Barbiturates may enhance the metabolism of doxycycline, decreasing its clinical effect; higher dosages may be required
Estrogens: Barbiturates may increase the metabolism of estrogens and reduce their efficacy
Felbamate may inhibit the metabolism of barbiturates and barbiturates may increase the metabolism of felbamate
Griseofulvin: Barbiturates may impair the absorption of griseofulvin, and griseofulvin metabolism may be increased by barbiturates, decreasing clinical effect
Guanfacine: Effect may be decreased by barbiturates
Loop diuretics: Metabolism may be increased and clinical effects decreased; established for furosemide, effect with other loop diuretics not established
MAOIs: Metabolism of barbiturates may be inhibited, increasing clinical effect or toxicity of the barbiturates
Methadone: Barbiturates may enhance the metabolism of methadone resulting in methadone withdrawal
Methoxyflurane: Barbiturates may enhance the nephrotoxic effects of methoxyflurane
Oral contraceptives: Barbiturates may enhance the metabolism of oral contraceptives, decreasing their clinical effect; an alternative method of contraception should be considered
Theophylline: Barbiturates may increase metabolism of theophylline derivatives and decrease their clinical effect
Tricyclic antidepressants: Barbiturates may increase metabolism of tricyclic antidepressants and decrease their clinical effect; sedative effects may be additive
Valproic acid: Metabolism of barbiturates may be inhibited by valproic acid; monitor for excessive sedation; a dose reduction may be needed
Warfarin: Barbiturates inhibit the hypoprothrombinemic effects of oral anticoagulants via increased metabolism; this combination should generally be avoided

**Mechanism of Action** Interferes with transmission of impulses from the thalamus to the cortex of the brain resulting in an imbalance in central inhibitory and facilitatory mechanisms

**Pharmacodynamics/kinetics** Duration of action: ~1 hour

**Usual Dosage** Oral:
Children 6 to 12 years: One-fourth (1/4) to one-half (1/2) tablet ~15 minutes before procedure
Children >12 years: One-half (1/2) to one tablet ~15 minutes before procedure
Adults: 1-2 tablets ~15 minutes before procedure

**Additional Information** This tranquilizer has a rapid 10-minute onset time and ultra-short duration of one hour. Developed exclusively for the dental industry to help reduce chair time. A comfortable patient will return and talk about the ease of his appointment.

**Dosage Forms** Tablet, scored: 260 mg


♦ **Hibiclens® Topical [OTC]** *see* Chlorhexidine Gluconate *on page 111*

♦ **Hibistat® Topical [OTC]** *see* Chlorhexidine Gluconate *on page 111*

♦ **HibTITER®** *see Haemophilus* b Conjugate Vaccine *on page 261*

♦ **Hi-Cor® 1.0** *see* Hydrocortisone *on page 273*

♦ **Hi-Cor® 2.5** *see* Hydrocortisone *on page 273*

♦ **Hiprex®** *see* Methenamine *on page 351*

♦ **Hirucreme®** *see* Hirudin *on page 268*


## Hirudin (he RUE din)

**U.S. Brand Names** Exhirud®; Hirucreme®
**Pharmacologic Category** False Neurotransmitter
**Effects on Mental Status** None reported
**Effects on Psychiatric Treatment** None reported
**Adverse Reactions** Hematologic: Bleeding, hemorrhage, disseminated intravascular coagulation (DIC)
**Usual Dosage** I.V.:
Bolus: 0.1-0.4 mg/kg
Infusion: 0.06-0.15 mg/kg/hour


♦ **Histalet Forte® Tablet** *see* Chlorpheniramine, Pyrilamine, Phenylephrine, and Phenylpropanolamine *on page 116*

♦ **Histalet® Syrup [OTC]** *see* Chlorpheniramine and Pseudoephedrine *on page 114*

♦ **Histalet® X** *see* Guaifenesin and Pseudoephedrine *on page 257*

♦ **Histatab® Plus Tablet [OTC]** *see* Chlorpheniramine and Phenylephrine *on page 114*

♦ **Hista-Vadrin® Tablet** *see* Chlorpheniramine, Phenylephrine, and Phenylpropanolamine *on page 115*

♦ **Histerone® Injection** *see* Testosterone *on page 536*

♦ **Histolyn-CYL® Injection** *see* Histoplasmin *on page 268*


## Histoplasmin (his toe PLAZ min)

**U.S. Brand Names** Histolyn-CYL® Injection
**Pharmacologic Category** Diagnostic Agent
**Use** Diagnosing histoplasmosis; to assess cell-mediated immunity
**Effects on Mental Status** None reported
**Effects on Psychiatric Treatment** None reported
**Usual Dosage** Adults: Intradermally: 0.1 mL of 1:100 dilution into volar surface of forearm; induration of ≥5 mm in diameter indicates a positive reaction
**Dosage Forms** Injection: 1:100 (0.1 mL, 1.3 mL)


♦ **Histor-D® Syrup** *see* Chlorpheniramine and Phenylephrine *on page 114*

♦ **Histor-D® Timecelles®** *see* Chlorpheniramine, Phenylephrine, and Methscopolamine *on page 115*


## Histrelin (his TREL in)

**U.S. Brand Names** Supprelin™ Injection
**Pharmacologic Category** Gonadotropin Releasing Hormone Analog; Luteinizing Hormone-Releasing Hormone Analog
**Use** Treatment of central idiopathic precocious puberty; treatment of estrogen-associated gynecological disorders such as acute intermittent porphyria, endometriosis, leiomyomata uteri, and premenstrual syndrome
**Effects on Mental Status** May cause mood swings
**Effects on Psychiatric Treatment** None reported
**Usual Dosage**
Central idiopathic precocious puberty: S.C.: Usual dose is 10 mcg/kg/day given as a single daily dose at the same time each day
Acute intermittent porphyria in women: S.C.: 5 mcg/day
Endometriosis: S.C.: 100 mcg/day
Leiomyomata uteri: S.C.: 20-50 mcg/day or 4 mcg/kg/day
**Dosage Forms** Injection: 7-day kits of single use: 120 mcg/0.6 mL; 300 mcg/0.6 mL; 600 mcg/0.6 mL


♦ **Histussin D® Liquid** *see* Hydrocodone and Pseudoephedrine *on page 273*

♦ **Hivid®** *see* Zalcitabine *on page 590*

♦ **HMS Liquifilm®** *see* Medrysone *on page 336*

♦ **Hoggar® N** *see* Doxylamine *on page 186*

♦ **Hold® DM [OTC]** *see* Dextromethorphan *on page 160*


## Homatropine (hoe MA troe peen)

**U.S. Brand Names** AK-Homatropine® Ophthalmic; Isopto® Homatropine Ophthalmic
**Pharmacologic Category** Anticholinergic Agent, Ophthalmic; Ophthalmic Agent, Mydriatic
**Use** Producing cycloplegia and mydriasis for refraction; treatment of acute inflammatory conditions of the uveal tract
**Effects on Mental Status** May cause drowsiness
**Effects on Psychiatric Treatment** None reported
**Usual Dosage**
Children:
Mydriasis and cycloplegia for refraction: Instill 1 drop of 2% solution immediately before the procedure; repeat at 10-minute intervals as needed
Uveitis: Instill 1 drop of 2% solution 2-3 times/day
Adults:
Mydriasis and cycloplegia for refraction: Instill 1-2 drops of 2% solution or 1 drop of 5% solution before the procedure; repeat at 5- to 10-minute intervals as needed; maximum of 3 doses for refraction
Uveitis: Instill 1-2 drops of 2% or 5% 2-3 times/day up to every 3-4 hours as needed
**Dosage Forms** Solution, ophthalmic, as hydrobromide:
2% (1 mL, 5 mL); 5% (1 mL, 2 mL, 5 mL)
AK-Homatropine®: 5% (15 mL)
Isopto® Homatropine 2% (5 mL, 15 mL); 5% (5 mL, 15 mL)

## Hops

**Related Information**
Herbals That May Alter Metabolism and GI Absorption of Drugs *on page 745*
**Synonyms** *Humulus lupulus*
**Pharmacologic Category** Herb
**Use** In herbal medicine as a sleep aid (sometimes combined with valerian root)

Per Commission E: Mood disturbances such as restlessness and anxiety, sleep disturbances

**Adverse Reactions** None known relating to herb (as per Commission E); Dermatologic: Contact dermatitis (upon exposure to extracts)

**Overdosage/Toxicology** Decontamination:

Oral: **Do not** induce emesis; lavage (within 1 hour)/activated charcoal with cathartic

Dermal: Wash with soap and water

**Drug Interactions** CNS depressants: Sedative effects may be additive with CNS depressants; includes ethanol, barbiturates, narcotic analgesics, and other sedative agents; monitor for increased effect

**Usual Dosage** Per Commission E: Single dose: 0.5 g

**Additional Information** A perennial, climbing vine with heights up to 25 feet found in Germany and Pacific Northwest; loses most of its activity (85%) after 9 months of storage; not to be confused with Wild Hops (*Bryonia*)

♦ **H.P. Acthar® Gel** *see* Corticotropin *on page 140*

♦ **Humalog®** *see* Insulin Preparations *on page 287*

♦ **Humalog® Mix 50/50™** *see* Insulin Preparations *on page 287*

♦ **Humalog® Mix 75/25™** *see* Insulin Preparations *on page 287*

## Human Growth Hormone (HYU man grothe HOR mone)

**U.S. Brand Names** Genotropin® Injection; Humatrope® Injection; Norditropin® Injection; Nutropin® AQ Injection; Nutropin® Injection; Protropin® Injection; Saizen® Injection; Serostim® Injection

**Pharmacologic Category** Growth Hormone

**Use**

Children:

Long-term treatment of growth failure from lack of adequate endogenous growth hormone secretion; long-term treatment of short stature associated with Turner's syndrome; treatment of pediatric patients with Prader-Willi syndrome

Nutropin®: Treatment of growth failure associated with chronic renal insufficiency up until the time of renal transplantation

Adults: Indicated for the replacement of endogenous growth hormone in patients with adult growth hormone deficiency who meet both of the following criteria:

Biochemical diagnosis of adult growth hormone deficiency by means of a subnormal response to a standard growth hormone stimulation test (peak growth hormone ≤5 µg/L)

**and**

Adult-onset: Patients who have adult growth hormone deficiency wither alone or with multiple hormone deficiencies (hypopituitarism) as a result of pituitary disease, hypothalamic disease, surgery, radiation therapy, or trauma,

**or**

Childhood-onset: Patients who were growth hormone deficient during childhood, confirmed as an adult before replacement therapy is initiated

**Effects on Mental Status** None reported

**Effects on Psychiatric Treatment** None reported

**Usual Dosage**

Children (individualize dose):

Somatrem (Protropin®): I.M., S.C.: Up to 0.1 mg (0.26 units)/kg/dose 3 times/week

Somatropin (Genotropin®): S.C.: Weekly dosage of 0.16-0.24 mg/kg divided into 6-7 doses

Somatropin (Humatrope®): I.M., S.C.: Up to 0.06 mg (0.16 units)/kg/dose 3 times/week

Somatropin (Nutropin®): S.C.:

Growth hormone inadequacy: Weekly dosage of 0.3 mg/kg (0.78 units/kg) divided into daily doses; pubertal patients: ≤0.7 mg/kg/week divided daily

Chronic renal insufficiency: Weekly dosage of 0.35 mg/kg (0.91 units/kg) divided into daily injections

Therapy should be discontinued when patient has reached satisfactory adult height, when epiphyses have fused, or when the patient ceases to respond

Growth of 5 cm/year or more is expected, if growth rate does not exceed 2.5 cm in a 6-month period, double the dose for the next 6 months, if there is still no satisfactory response, discontinue therapy

Somatropin (Nutropin® Depot™): S.C.:

Once-monthly injection: 1.5 mg/kg body weight administered on the same day of each month; patients >15 kg will require more than one injection per dose

Twice-monthly injection: 0.75 mg/kg body weight administered twice each month on the same days of each month (eg, days 1 and 15 of each month); patients >30 kg will require more than one injection per dose

Turner's syndrome: S.C.: Weekly dosage of up to 0.375 mg/kg divided into equal doses 3-7 times per week

Adults: Growth hormone deficiency: S.C.: ≤0.006 mg/kg/day; dose may be increased according to individual requirements, up to a maximum of 0.025 mg/kg/day in patients <35 years of age, or up to a maximum of 0.0125 mg/kg/day in patients ≥35 years of age. To minimize adverse events in older or overweight patients, reduced dosages may be necessary. During therapy, dosage should be decreased if required by the occurrence of side effects or excessive IGF-I levels.

**Dosage Forms** Powder for injection (lyophilized):

Somatropin:

Genotropin®: 1.5 mg ~4.5 units (5 mL); 5.8 mg ~17.4 units (5 mL)

Humatrope®: 5 mg ~15 units

Norditropin®: 4 mg ~12 units; 8 mg ~24 units

Nutropin®: 5 mg ~15 units (10 mL); 10 mg ~30 units (10 mL)

Nutropin® AQ: 10 mg ~30 units (2 mL)

Saizen® (rDNA origin): 5 mg ~15 units

Serostim®: 5 mg ~15 units (5 mL); 6 mg ~18 units (5 mL)

Somatrem, Protropin®: 5 mg ~15 units (10 mL); 10 mg ~30 units (10 mL)

♦ **Humate-P®** *see* Antihemophilic Factor (Human) *on page 45*

♦ **Humatin®** *see* Paromomycin *on page 421*

♦ **Humatrope® Injection** *see* Human Growth Hormone *on page 269*

♦ **Humegon™** *see* Menotropins *on page 340*

♦ **Humex®** *see* Carbinoxamine *on page 92*

♦ **Humibid® DM [OTC]** *see* Guaifenesin and Dextromethorphan *on page 257*

♦ **Humibid® L.A.** *see* Guaifenesin *on page 256*

♦ **Humibid® Sprinkle** *see* Guaifenesin *on page 256*

♦ **Humorsol® Ophthalmic** *see* Demecarium *on page 153*

♦ **Humulin® 50/50** *see* Insulin Preparations *on page 287*

♦ **Humulin® 70/30** *see* Insulin Preparations *on page 287*

♦ **Humulin® L** *see* Insulin Preparations *on page 287*

♦ **Humulin® N** *see* Insulin Preparations *on page 287*

♦ ***Humulus lupulus*** *see* Hops *on page 268*

♦ **Hurricaine®** *see* Benzocaine *on page 61*

## Hyaluronidase (hye al yoor ON i dase)

**U.S. Brand Names** Wydase® Injection

**Pharmacologic Category** Antidote

**Use** Increases the dispersion and absorption of other drugs; increases rate of absorption of parenteral fluids given by hypodermoclysis; enhances diffusion of locally irritating or toxic drugs in the management of I.V. extravasation

**Effects on Mental Status** May cause dizziness

**Effects on Psychiatric Treatment** None reported

**Usual Dosage**

Infants and Children:

Management of I.V. extravasation: Reconstitute the 150 unit vial of lyophilized powder with 1 mL normal saline; take 0.1 mL of this solution and dilute with 0.9 mL normal saline to yield 15 units/mL; using a 25- or 26-gauge needle, five 0.2 mL injections are made subcutaneously or intradermally into the extravasation site at the leading edge, changing the needle after each injection

Hypodermoclysis:

S.C.: 1 mL (150 units) is added to 1000 mL of infusion fluid and 0.5 mL (75 units) in injected into each clysis site at the initiation of the infusion

I.V.: 15 units is added to each 100 mL of I.V. fluid to be administered

Children <3 years: Limit volume of single clysis to 200 mL

Premature Infants: Do not exceed 25 mL/kg/day and not >2 mL/minute

Adults: Absorption and dispersion of drugs: 150 units are added to the vehicle containing the drug

**Dosage Forms**

Injection, stabilized solution: 150 units/mL (1 mL, 10 mL)

Powder for injection, lyophilized: 150 units, 1500 units

♦ **Hyate®:C** *see* Antihemophilic Factor (Porcine) *on page 45*

♦ **Hybalamin®** *see* Hydroxocobalamin *on page 276*

♦ **Hybolin™ Decanoate Injection** *see* Nandrolone *on page 383*

♦ **Hybolin™ Improved Injection** *see* Nandrolone *on page 383*

♦ **Hycamtin™** *see* Topotecan *on page 556*

♦ **HycoClear Tuss®** *see* Hydrocodone and Guaifenesin *on page 272*

♦ **Hycodan®** *see* Hydrocodone and Homatropine *on page 273*

♦ **Hycomine®** *see* Hydrocodone and Phenylpropanolamine *on page 273*

♦ **Hycomine® Compound** *see* Hydrocodone, Chlorpheniramine, Phenylephrine, Acetaminophen and Caffeine *on page 273*

♦ **Hycomine® Pediatric** *see* Hydrocodone and Phenylpropanolamine *on page 273*

♦ **Hycort®** *see* Hydrocortisone *on page 273*

♦ **Hycotuss® Expectorant Liquid** *see* Hydrocodone and Guaifenesin *on page 272*

♦ **Hydergine®** *see* Ergoloid Mesylates *on page 199*

♦ **Hydergine® LC** *see* Ergoloid Mesylates *on page 199*

## Hydralazine (hye DRAL a zeen)

**U.S. Brand Names** Apresoline®

**Canadian Brand Names** Apo®-Hydralazine; Novo-Hylazin; Nu-Hydral

**Pharmacologic Category** Vasodilator

**Use** Management of moderate to severe hypertension, congestive heart failure, hypertension secondary to pre-eclampsia/eclampsia; treatment of primary pulmonary hypertension

**Effects on Mental Status** May cause drowsiness

**Effects on Psychiatric Treatment** Concurrent use with MAOIs may result in significant decrease in blood pressure; use cautiously

**Pregnancy Risk Factor** C

**Contraindications** Hypersensitivity to hydralazine or any component; mitral valve rheumatic heart disease

**Warnings/Precautions** May cause a drug-induced lupus-like syndrome (more likely on larger doses, longer duration). Adjust dose in severe renal dysfunction. Use with caution in CAD (increase in tachycardia may increase myocardial oxygen demand). Use with caution in pulmonary hypertension (may cause hypotension). Tartrazine may be in some products (do not use in sensitive individuals). Patients may be poorly compliant because of frequent dosing.

Monitor blood pressure closely following I.V. administration. Response may be delayed and unpredictable in some patients. Titrate cautiously to response. Hydralazine-induced fluid and sodium retention may require addition or increased dosage of a diuretics.

**Adverse Reactions**

>10%:
- Cardiovascular: Palpitations, flushing, tachycardia, angina pectoris
- Central nervous system: Headache
- Gastrointestinal: Nausea, vomiting, diarrhea, anorexia

1% to 10%:
- Cardiovascular: Hypotension, redness or flushing of face
- Gastrointestinal: Constipation
- Ocular: Lacrimation
- Respiratory: Dyspnea, nasal congestion

<1%: Arthralgias, dizziness, edema, fever, malaise, peripheral neuritis, positive ANA, positive LE cells, rash, weakness

**Note:** Because of blunted beta-receptor response, the elderly are less likely to experience reflex tachycardia; this puts them at greater risk for orthostatic hypotension

**Overdosage/Toxicology**

Signs and symptoms: Hypotension, tachycardia, shock

Treatment: Hypotension usually responds to I.V. fluid, Trendelenburg positioning or vasoconstrictors; treatment is primarily supportive and symptomatic

**Drug Interactions**

Beta-blockers (metoprolol, propranolol) serum concentrations and pharmacologic effects may be increased; monitor cardiovascular status

NSAIDs may decrease the hemodynamic effects of hydralazine; avoid use if possible or closely monitor cardiovascular status

Propranolol increases hydralazine's serum concentrations; acebutolol, atenolol, and nadolol (low hepatic clearance or no first-pass metabolism) are unlikely to be affected

**Usual Dosage**

Children:

Oral: Initial: 0.75-1 mg/kg/day in 2-4 divided doses; increase over 3-4 weeks to maximum of 7.5 mg/kg/day in 2-4 divided doses; maximum daily dose: 200 mg/day

I.M., I.V.: 0.1-0.2 mg/kg/dose (not to exceed 20 mg) every 4-6 hours as needed, up to 1.7-3.5 mg/kg/day in 4-6 divided doses

Adults:

Oral: Hypertension:

Initial dose: 10 mg 4 times/day for first 2-4 days; increase to 25 mg 4 times/day for the balance of the first week

Increase by 10-25 mg/dose gradually to 50 mg 4 times/day; 300 mg/day may be required for some patients

Oral: Congestive heart failure:

Initial dose: 10-25 mg 3 times/day

Target dose: 75 mg 3 times/day

Maximum dose: 100 mg 3 times/day

I.M., I.V.:

Hypertension: Initial: 10-20 mg/dose every 4-6 hours as needed, may increase to 40 mg/dose; change to oral therapy as soon as possible.

Pre-eclampsia/eclampsia: 5 mg/dose then 5-10 mg every 20-30 minutes as needed.

Elderly: Oral: Initial: 10 mg 2-3 times/day; increase by 10-25 mg/day every 2-5 days.

**Dosing interval in renal impairment:**

$Cl_{cr}$ 10-50 mL/minute: Administer every 8 hours.

$Cl_{cr}$ <10 mL/minute: Administer every 8-16 hours in fast acetylators and every 12-24 hours in slow acetylators.

Hemodialysis: Supplemental dose is not necessary.

Peritoneal dialysis: Supplemental dose is not necessary.

**Dietary Considerations** Food enhances bioavailability of hydralazine

**Patient Information** Take as directed, with meals. Do not use alcohol or OTC medication without consulting prescriber. Weigh daily at the same time, in the same clothes. Report weight gain >5 lb/week, swelling of feet or ankles. May cause dizziness or weakness; change position slowly when rising from sitting or lying position and avoid driving or activities requiring alertness until response to drug is known. You may experience nausea (small frequent meals may help), impotence (reversible), or constipation (fluids, exercise, dietary fiber may help). This medication does not replace other antihypertensive interventions; follow instructions for diet and lifestyle changes. Report flu-like symptoms, difficulty breathing, skin rash, blackened stool, or numbness and tingling of extremities.

**Nursing Implications** Aid with ambulation, rising may cause orthostasis

**Dosage Forms**

Injection, as hydrochloride: 20 mg/mL (1 mL)

Tablet, as hydrochloride: 10 mg, 25 mg, 50 mg, 100 mg

## Hydralazine and Hydrochlorothiazide
(hye DRAL a zeen & hye droe klor oh THYE a zide)

**U.S. Brand Names** Apresazide®

**Pharmacologic Category** Antihypertensive Agent, Combination

**Use** Management of moderate to severe hypertension and treatment of congestive heart failure

**Effects on Mental Status** May cause drowsiness or depression

**Effects on Psychiatric Treatment** Concurrent use with MAOIs may result in significant decrease in blood pressure, use cautiously; may decrease lithium clearance resulting in an increase in serum lithium levels and potential lithium toxicity; monitor serum lithium levels

**Usual Dosage** Adults: Oral: 1 capsule twice daily

**Dosage Forms** Capsule:

25/25: Hydralazine hydrochloride 25 mg and hydrochlorothiazide 25 mg

50/50: Hydralazine hydrochloride 50 mg and hydrochlorothiazide 50 mg

100/50: Hydralazine hydrochloride 100 mg and hydrochlorothiazide 50 mg

## Hydralazine, Hydrochlorothiazide, and Reserpine
(hye DRAL a zeen, hye droe klor oh THYE a zide, & re SER peen)

**U.S. Brand Names** Hydrap-ES®; Marpres®; Ser-Ap-Es®

**Pharmacologic Category** Antihypertensive Agent, Combination

**Use** Hypertensive disorders

**Effects on Mental Status** May cause drowsiness, depression, dizziness, headache, nightmares, nervousness, fatigue, dull sensorium, paradoxical anxiety

**Effects on Psychiatric Treatment** Concurrent use with MAOIs may result in significant decrease in blood pressure or alternatively hypertensive crisis; avoid use; may decrease lithium clearance resulting in an increase in serum lithium levels and potential lithium toxicity; monitor serum lithium levels. Use caution in patients with depression, as reserpine may worsen it or lessen the effect of the antidepressant.

**Usual Dosage** Adults: Oral: 1-2 tablets 3 times/day

**Dosage Forms** Tablet: Hydralazine 25 mg, hydrochlorothiazide 15 mg, and reserpine 0.1 mg

♦ **Hydramyn® Syrup [OTC]** *see* Diphenhydramine *on page 174*

♦ **Hydrap-ES®** *see* Hydralazine, Hydrochlorothiazide, and Reserpine *on page 270*

♦ ***Hydrastis canadensis*** *see* Golden Seal *on page 254*

♦ **Hydrated Chloral** *see* Chloral Hydrate *on page 107*

♦ **Hydrate® Injection** *see* Dimenhydrinate *on page 173*

♦ **Hydrea®** *see* Hydroxyurea *on page 277*

♦ **Hydrocet®** *see* Hydrocodone and Acetaminophen *on page 272*

## Hydrochloric Acid (hye droe KLOR ik AS id)

**Pharmacologic Category** Gastrointestinal Agent, Miscellaneous

**Use** Although hydrochloric acid is neither approved nor disapproved by the Food and Drug Administration for management of metabolic alkalosis, it has proven to be highly effective in the medical literature. Indications for hydrochloric acid include severe metabolic alkalosis (pH >7.55) or symptoms of alkalotic toxicity unresponsive to fluid and electrolyte administration and inability to tolerate a large sodium and fluid load. This would include patients with decompensated heart failure, acute renal failure with oliguria or compromised liver function

**Effects on Mental Status** None reported

**Effects on Psychiatric Treatment** None reported

**Usual Dosage** The dose of hydrochloric acid (HCl) to be administered has been based upon several methods, including bicarbonate excess, chloride deficit, and base excess. Calculation of the amount of HCl needed to correct alkalosis has varied significantly. HCl is usually infused as a 0.1 N solution administered via a central venous catheter.

**Dosage Forms**

Liquid: 500 mL, 2500 mL

Liquid, diluted: 500 mL, 2500 mL

## Hydrochlorothiazide (hye droe klor oh THYE a zide)

**U.S. Brand Names** Esidrix®; Ezide®; HydroDIURIL®; Hydro-Par®; Microzide™; Oretic®

**Canadian Brand Names** Apo®-Hydro; Diuchlor®; Neo-Codema®; Novo-Hydrazide; Urozide®

**Synonyms** HCTZ

**Pharmacologic Category** Diuretic, Thiazide

**Use** Management of mild to moderate hypertension; treatment of edema in congestive heart failure and nephrotic syndrome

**Effects on Mental Status** None reported

**Effects on Psychiatric Treatment** Used to treat lithium-induced diabetes insipidus; monitor for hypokalemia; may decrease lithium clearance resulting in an increase in serum lithium levels and potential lithium toxicity; monitor serum lithium levels

**Pregnancy Risk Factor** B (per manufacturer); D (based on expert analysis)

**Contraindications** Hypersensitivity to hydrochlorothiazide or any component, thiazides, or sulfonamide-derived drugs; anuria; renal decompensation; pregnancy

**Warnings/Precautions** Avoid in severe renal disease (ineffective). Electrolyte disturbances (hypokalemia, hypochloremic alkalosis, hyponatremia) can occur. Use with caution in severe hepatic dysfunction; hepatic encephalopathy can be caused by electrolyte disturbances. Gout can be precipitate in certain patients with a history of gout, a familial predisposition to gout, or chronic renal failure. Cautious use in diabetics; may see a change in glucose control. Hypersensitivity reactions can occur. Can cause SLE exacerbation or activation. Use with caution in patients with moderate or high cholesterol concentrations. Photosensitization may occur. Correct hypokalemia before initiating therapy.

**Adverse Reactions**

1% to 10%: Endocrine & metabolic: Hypokalemia

<1%: Fluid and electrolyte imbalances, hyperglycemia, hypotension, photosensitivity, prerenal azotemia, rarely blood dyscrasias

**Overdosage/Toxicology**

Signs and symptoms: Hypermotility, diuresis, lethargy, confusion, muscle weakness

Treatment: Following GI decontamination, therapy is supportive with I.V. fluids, electrolytes, and I.V. pressors if needed

**Drug Interactions**

Angiotensin-converting enzyme inhibitors: Increased hypotension if aggressively diuresed with a thiazide diuretic

Beta-blockers increase hyperglycemic effects in Type 2 diabetes mellitus

Cyclosporine and thiazides can increase the risk of gout or renal toxicity; avoid concurrent use

Digoxin toxicity can be exacerbated if a thiazide induces hypokalemia or hypomagnesemia

Lithium toxicity can occur by reducing renal excretion of lithium; monitor lithium concentration and adjust as needed

Neuromuscular blocking agents can prolong blockade; monitor serum potassium and neuromuscular status

NSAIDs can decrease the efficacy of thiazides reducing the diuretic and antihypertensive effects

**Usual Dosage** Oral (effect of drug may be decreased when used every day):

Children (In pediatric patients, chlorothiazide may be preferred over hydrochlorothiazide as there are more dosage formulations (eg, suspension) available):

<6 months: 2-3 mg/kg/day in 2 divided doses

>6 months: 2 mg/kg/day in 2 divided doses

Adults: 25-100 mg/day in 1-2 doses

Maximum: 200 mg/day

Elderly: 12.5-25 mg once daily

Minimal increase in response and more electrolyte disturbances are seen with doses >50 mg/day.

**Dosing adjustment/comments in renal impairment:** $Cl_{cr}$ 25-50 mL/minute: Not effective

**Patient Information** This medication does not replace other antihypertensive recommendations (diet and lifestyle changes). Take as directed, with meals, early in the day to avoid nocturia. Avoid alcohol or OTC medication unless approved by prescriber. Include bananas and/or orange juice in daily diet; do not take potassium supplements unless recommended by prescriber. May cause dizziness or postural hypotension (use caution when rising from sitting or lying position, when driving, climbing stairs, or engaging in tasks that require alertness until response to drug is known); nausea or vomiting (small frequent meals, frequent mouth care, sucking lozenges, or chewing gum may help); impotence (reversible); constipation (increased exercise or dietary fruit, fiber, or fluids will help); photosensitivity (use sunscreen, wear protective clothing and eyewear, and avoid direct sunlight). If diabetic, monitor serum glucose closely; this medication may increase serum glucose levels. Report persistent flu-like symptoms, chest pain, palpitations, muscle cramping, difficulty breathing, skin rash or itching, unusual bruising or easy bleeding, or excessive fatigue.

**Nursing Implications** Take blood pressure with patient lying down and standing

**Dosage Forms**

Capsule: 12.5 mg

Solution, oral (mint flavor): 50 mg/5 mL (50 mL)

Tablet: 25 mg, 50 mg, 100 mg

## Hydrochlorothiazide and Reserpine

(hye droe klor oh THYE a zide & re SER peen)

**U.S. Brand Names** Hydropres®; Hydro-Serp®; Hydroserpine®

**Pharmacologic Category** Antihypertensive Agent, Combination

**Use** Management of mild to moderate hypertension; treatment of edema in congestive heart failure and nephrotic syndrome

**Effects on Mental Status** May cause drowsiness, depression, dizziness, headache, nightmares, nervousness, fatigue, dull sensorium, paradoxical anxiety

**Effects on Psychiatric Treatment** Concurrent use with MAOIs may result in hypertensive crisis, avoid use; may decrease lithium clearance resulting in an increase in serum lithium levels and potential lithium toxicity, monitor serum lithium levels. Use caution in patients with depression, as reserpine may worsen it or lessen the effect of the antidepressant.

**Usual Dosage** Adults: Oral: 1-2 tablets once or twice daily

**Dosage Forms** Tablet:

25: Hydrochlorothiazide 25 mg and reserpine 0.125 mg

50: Hydrochlorothiazide 50 mg and reserpine 0.125 mg

## Hydrochlorothiazide and Spironolactone

(hye droe klor oh THYE a zide & speer on oh LAK tone)

**U.S. Brand Names** Aldactazide®

**Canadian Brand Names** Apo®-Spirozide; Novo-Spirozine

**Pharmacologic Category** Antihypertensive Agent, Combination

**Use** Management of mild to moderate hypertension; treatment of edema in congestive heart failure and nephrotic syndrome, and cirrhosis of the liver accompanied by edema and/or ascites

**Effects on Mental Status** May cause lethargy or anorexia

**Effects on Psychiatric Treatment** May decrease lithium clearance resulting in an increase in serum lithium levels and potential lithium toxicity; monitor serum lithium levels

**Usual Dosage** Oral:

Children: 1.66-3.3 mg/kg/day (of spironolactone) in 2-4 divided doses

Adults: 1-8 tablets in 1-2 divided doses

**Dosage Forms** Tablet:

25/25: Hydrochlorothiazide 25 mg and spironolactone 25 mg

50/50: Hydrochlorothiazide 50 mg and spironolactone 50 mg

## Hydrochlorothiazide and Triamterene

(hye droe klor oh THYE a zide & trye AM ter een)

**U.S. Brand Names** Dyazide®; Maxzide®

**Canadian Brand Names** Apo®-Triazide; Novo-Triamzide; Nu-Triazide

**Pharmacologic Category** Antihypertensive Agent, Combination; Diuretic, Potassium Sparing; Diuretic, Thiazide

**Use** Management of mild to moderate hypertension; treatment of edema in congestive heart failure and nephrotic syndrome

**Effects on Mental Status** May cause lethargy or anorexia

**Effects on Psychiatric Treatment** May decrease lithium clearance resulting in an increase in serum lithium levels and potential lithium toxicity; monitor serum lithium levels

**Usual Dosage** Adults: Oral:

Triamterene/hydrochlorothiazide 37.5 mg/25 mg: 1-2 tablets/capsules once daily

Triamterene/hydrochlorothiazide 75 mg/50 mg: ½-1 tablet daily

**Dosage Forms**

Capsule (Dyazide®): Hydrochlorothiazide 25 mg and triamterene 37.5 mg

Tablet:

Maxzide®-25: Hydrochlorothiazide 25 mg and triamterene 37.5 mg

Maxzide®: Hydrochlorothiazide 50 mg and triamterene 75 mg

♦ **Hydrocil® [OTC]** *see* Psyllium *on page 479*

♦ **Hydro-Cobex®** *see* Hydroxocobalamin *on page 276*

## Hydrocodone and Acetaminophen

(hye droe KOE done & a seet a MIN oh fen)

**U.S. Brand Names** Anexsia®; Anodynos-DHC®; Bancap HC®; Co-Gesic®; Dolacet®; DuoCet™; Hydrocet®; Hydrogesic®; Hy-Phen®; Lorcet®; Lorcet®-HD; Lorcet® Plus; Lortab®; Margesic® H; Medipain 5®; Norco™; Stagesic®; T-Gesic®; Vicodin®; Vicodin® ES; Vicodin® HP; Zydone®

**Canadian Brand Names** Vapocet®

**Synonyms** Acetaminophen and Hydrocodone

**Pharmacologic Category** Analgesic, Narcotic

**Use** Relief of moderate to severe pain; antitussive (hydrocodone)

**Effects on Mental Status** Sedation is common; may cause confusion; may rarely cause hallucinations

**Effects on Psychiatric Treatment** May result in loss of pain control when used in combination with SSRIs (especially paroxetine and fluoxetine); concurrent use with psychotropics may produce additive sedation

**Restrictions** C-III

**Pregnancy Risk Factor** C

**Contraindications** CNS depression, hypersensitivity to hydrocodone, acetaminophen or any component; severe respiratory depression

**Warnings/Precautions** Use with caution in patients with hypersensitivity reactions to other phenanthrene derivative opioid agonists (morphine, hydrocodone, hydromorphone, levorphanol, oxycodone, oxymorphone); tablets contain metabisulfite which may cause allergic reactions; tolerance or drug dependence may result from extended use

**Adverse Reactions**

>10%:
- Cardiovascular: Hypotension
- Central nervous system: Lightheadedness, dizziness, sedation, drowsiness, fatigue
- Neuromuscular & skeletal: Weakness

1% to 10%:
- Cardiovascular: Bradycardia
- Central nervous system: Confusion
- Gastrointestinal: Nausea, vomiting
- Genitourinary: Decreased urination
- Respiratory: Shortness of breath, dyspnea

<1%: Anorexia, biliary tract spasm, diplopia, hallucinations, histamine release, hypertension, miosis, physical and psychological dependence with prolonged use, urinary tract spasm, xerostomia

**Overdosage/Toxicology**

Signs and symptoms of overdose include hepatic necrosis, blood dyscrasias, respiratory depression

Treatment: Acetylcysteine 140 mg/kg orally (loading) followed by 70 mg/kg every 4 hours for 17 doses. Therapy should be initiated based upon laboratory analysis suggesting high probability of hepatotoxic potential. Naloxone (2 mg I.V.) can also be used to reverse the toxic effects of the opiate. Activated charcoal is effective at binding certain chemicals, and this is especially true for acetaminophen.

**Drug Interactions**

Decreased effect with phenothiazines

Increased effect with dextroamphetamine

Increased toxicity with CNS depressants, TCAs; effect of warfarin may be enhanced

**Usual Dosage** Oral (doses should be titrated to appropriate analgesic effect):

Children:
- Antitussive (hydrocodone): 0.6 mg/kg/day in 3-4 divided doses
  - A single dose should not exceed 10 mg in children >12 years, 5 mg in children 2-12 years, and 1.25 mg in children <2 years of age
- Analgesic (acetaminophen): Refer to Acetaminophen monograph

Adults: Analgesic: 1-2 tablets or capsules every 4-6 hours or 5-10 mL solution every 4-6 hours as needed for pain

**Patient Information** If self-administered, use exactly as directed (do not increase dose or frequency); may cause physical and/or psychological dependence. Take with food or milk. While using this medication, do not use alcohol and other prescription or OTC medications (especially sedatives, tranquilizers, antihistamines, or pain medications) without consulting prescriber. Maintain adequate hydration (2-3 L/day of fluids unless instructed to restrict fluid intake). May cause dizziness, lightheadedness, confusion, or drowsiness (use caution when driving, climbing stairs, or changing position - rising from sitting or lying to standing, or when engaging in tasks requiring alertness until response to drug is known); nausea or vomiting (frequent mouth care, frequent sips of fluids, chewing gum, or sucking lozenges may help). Report chest pain or palpitations; persistent dizziness, shortness of breath, or difficulty breathing; unusual bleeding or bruising; or unusual fatigue and weakness.

**Nursing Implications** Observe patient for excessive sedation, respiratory depression

**Dosage Forms**

Capsule:
- Bancap HC®, Dolacet®, Hydrocet®, Hydrogesic®, Lorcet®-HD, Margesic® H, Medipain 5®, Norcet®, Stagesic®, T-Gesic®, Zydone®: Hydrocodone bitartrate 5 mg and acetaminophen 500 mg

Elixir (tropical fruit punch flavor) (Lortab®): Hydrocodone bitartrate 2.5 mg and acetaminophen 167 mg per 5 mL with alcohol 7% (480 mL)

Solution, oral (tropical fruit punch flavor) (Lortab®): Hydrocodone bitartrate 2.5 mg and acetaminophen 167 mg per 5 mL with alcohol 7% (480 mL)

Tablet: Hydrocodone bitartrate 5 mg and acetaminophen 400 mg; hydrocodone bitartrate 7.5 mg and acetaminophen 400 mg; hydrocodone bitartrate 10 mg and acetaminophen 400 mg; hydrocodone bitartrate 5 mg and acetaminophen 500 mg; hydrocodone bitartrate 7.5 mg and acetaminophen 750 mg; hydrocodone bitartrate 7.5 mg and acetaminophen 500 mg; hydrocodone bitartrate 7.5 mg and acetaminophen 650 mg; hydrocodone bitartrate 10 mg and acetaminophen 650 mg
- Lortab® 2.5/500: Hydrocodone bitartrate 2.5 mg and acetaminophen 500 mg
- Anexsia® 5/500, Anodynos-DHC®, Co-Gesic®, DuoCet™, DHC®; Hy-Phen®, Lorcet®, Lortab®® 5/500, Vicodin®: Hydrocodone bitartrate 5 mg and acetaminophen 500 mg
- Lortab® 7.5/500: Hydrocodone bitartrate 7.5 mg and acetaminophen 500 mg
- Anexsia® 7.5/650, Lorcet® Plus: Hydrocodone bitartrate 7.5 mg and acetaminophen 650 mg
- Vicodin® ES: Hydrocodone bitartrate 7.5 mg and acetaminophen 750 mg
- Norco™: Hydrocodone bitartrate 10 mg and acetaminophen 325 mg
- Lortab® 10/500: Hydrocodone bitartrate 10 mg and acetaminophen 500 mg
- Lorcet® 10/650: Hydrocodone bitartrate 10 mg and acetaminophen 650 mg
- Vicodin® HP: Hydrocodone bitartrate 10 mg and acetaminophen 660 mg
- Zydone®: Hydrocodone bitartrate 5 mg and acetaminophen 400 mg; hydrocodone bitartrate 7.5 mg and acetaminophen 400 mg; Hydrocodone bitartrate 10 mg and acetaminophen 400 mg

## Hydrocodone and Aspirin (hye droe KOE done & AS pir in)

**U.S. Brand Names** Alor® 5/500; Azdone®; Damason-P®; Lortab® ASA; Panasal® 5/500

**Pharmacologic Category** Analgesic, Narcotic

**Use** Relief of moderate to moderately severe pain

**Effects on Mental Status** Sedation is common; may cause confusion or dizziness; may rarely cause hallucinations

**Effects on Psychiatric Treatment** May result in loss of pain control when used in combination with SSRIs (especially paroxetine and fluoxetine); concurrent use with psychotropics may produce additive sedation

**Restrictions** C-III

**Usual Dosage** Adults: Oral: 1-2 tablets every 4-6 hours as needed for pain

**Dosage Forms** Tablet: Hydrocodone bitartrate 5 mg and aspirin 500 mg

## Hydrocodone and Chlorpheniramine

(hye droe KOE done & klor fen IR a meen)

**U.S. Brand Names** Tussionex®

**Pharmacologic Category** Antihistamine/Antitussive

**Use** Symptomatic relief of cough and allergy

**Effects on Mental Status** Sedation is common; may cause confusion, dizziness, excitability, nervousness, fatigue, or depression; may rarely cause hallucinations

**Effects on Psychiatric Treatment** May result in loss of pain control when used in combination with SSRIs (especially paroxetine and fluoxetine); concurrent use with psychotropics may produce additive sedation or dry mouth

**Restrictions** C-III

**Usual Dosage** Oral:

Children 6-12 years: 2.5 mL every 12 hours; do not exceed 5 mL/24 hours

Adults: 5 mL every 12 hours; do not exceed 10 mL/24 hours

**Dosage Forms** Syrup, alcohol free: Hydrocodone polistirex 10 mg and chlorpheniramine polistirex 8 mg per 5 mL (480 mL, 900 mL)

## Hydrocodone and Guaifenesin

(hye droe KOE done & gwye FEN e sin)

**U.S. Brand Names** Codiclear® DH; HycoClear Tuss®; Hycotuss® Expectorant Liquid; Kwelcof®

**Pharmacologic Category** Antitussive/Expectorant

**Use** Symptomatic relief of nonproductive coughs associated with upper and lower respiratory tract congestion

**Effects on Mental Status** May cause drowsiness, sedation, mental clouding, mental impairment, anxiety, fear, dysphoria, dizziness, psychotic dependence, mood changes

**Effects on Psychiatric Treatment** Concurrent use with psychotropics may produce additive sedation

**Restrictions** C-III

**Usual Dosage** Oral:

Children:
- <2 years: 0.3 mg/kg/day (hydrocodone) in 4 divided doses
- 2-12 years: 2.5 mL every 4 hours, after meals and at bedtime

>12 years: 5 mL every 4 hours, after meals and at bedtime
Adults: 5 mL every 4 hours, after meals and at bedtime, not to exceed 30 mL in a 24-hour period

**Dosage Forms** Liquid: Hydrocodone bitartrate 5 mg and guaifenesin 100 mg per 5 mL (120 mL, 480 mL)

## Hydrocodone and Homatropine

(hye droe KOE done & hoe MA troe peen)

**U.S. Brand Names** Hycodan®; Hydromet®; Oncet®; Tussigon®

**Pharmacologic Category** Antitussive

**Use** Symptomatic relief of cough

**Effects on Mental Status** Lightheadedness, dizziness, sedation, drowsiness, and fatigue are common; may cause confusion; may rarely cause hallucinations

**Effects on Psychiatric Treatment** Concurrent use with psychotropics may produce additive sedation

**Restrictions** C-III

**Usual Dosage** Oral (based on hydrocodone component):

Children: 0.6 mg/kg/day in 3-4 divided doses; do not administer more frequently than every 4 hours

A single dose should not exceed 1.25 mg in children <2 years of age, 5 mg in children 2-12 years, and 10 mg in children >12 years

Adults: 5-10 mg every 4-6 hours, a single dose should not exceed 15 mg; do not administer more frequently than every 4 hours

**Dosage Forms**

Syrup (Hycodan®, Hydromet®): Hydrocodone bitartrate 5 mg and homatropine methylbromide 1.5 mg per 5 mL (120 mL, 480 mL, 4000 mL)

Tablet (Hycodan®, Oncet®, Tussigon®): Hydrocodone bitartrate 5 mg and homatropine methylbromide 1.5 mg

## Hydrocodone and Ibuprofen

(hye droe KOE done & eye byoo PROE fen)

**U.S. Brand Names** Vicoprofen®

**Pharmacologic Category** Analgesic, Narcotic

**Use** Short-term (generally <10 days) management of moderate to severe acute pain; is not indicated for treatment of such conditions as osteoarthritis or rheumatoid arthritis

**Effects on Mental Status** Sedation, drowsiness, and fatigue are common; may cause nervousness or confusion; may rarely cause hallucinations, depression, or insomnia

**Effects on Psychiatric Treatment** Hypotension is common and may be potentiated by low potency antipsychotics and other psychotropics. May rarely cause agranulocytosis, caution with clozapine and carbamazepine. Sedation may be additive with psychotropics. Ibuprofen may inhibit the clearance of lithium resulting in elevated serum lithium levels; may need to adjust dosage downward.

**Restrictions** C-III

**Usual Dosage** Adults: Oral: 1-2 tablets every 4-6 hours as needed for pain; maximum: 5 tablets/day

**Dosage Forms** Tablet: Hydrocodone bitartrate 7.5 mg and ibuprofen 200 mg

## Hydrocodone and Phenylpropanolamine

(hye droe KOE done & fen il proe pa NOLE a meen)

**U.S. Brand Names** Codamine®; Codamine® Pediatric; Hycomine®; Hycomine® Pediatric; Hydrocodone PA® Syrup

**Pharmacologic Category** Antitussive/Decongestant

**Use** Symptomatic relief of cough and nasal congestion

**Effects on Mental Status** May cause sedation, drowsiness, mental clouding, lethargy, impairment mental performance, anxiety, fear, dysphoria, dizziness, psychic dependence, mood changes

**Effects on Psychiatric Treatment** Contraindicated with MAOIs

**Restrictions** C-III

**Usual Dosage** Oral:

Children 6-12 years: 2.5 mL every 4 hours, up to 6 doses/24 hours
Adults: 5 mL every 4 hours, up to 6 doses/24 hours

**Dosage Forms** Syrup:

Codamine®, Hycomine®: Hydrocodone bitartrate 5 mg and phenylpropanolamine hydrochloride 25 mg per 5 mL (480 mL)

Codamine® Pediatric, Hycomine® Pediatric: Hydrocodone bitartrate 2.5 mg and phenylpropanolamine hydrochloride 12.5 mg per 5 mL (480 mL)

## Hydrocodone and Pseudoephedrine

(hye droe KOE done & soo doe e FED rin)

**U.S. Brand Names** Detussin® Liquid; Entuss-D® LIquid; Histussin D® Liquid; Tyrodone® Liquid

**Pharmacologic Category** Cough and Cold Combination

**Use** Symptomatic relief of cough due to colds, etc

**Effects on Mental Status** May cause sedation, drowsiness, mental clouding, lethargy, impairment of mental performance, anxiety, fear, dysphoria, dizziness, psychic dependence, mood changes

**Effects on Psychiatric Treatment** Contraindicated with MAOIs

**Usual Dosage** Oral: Adults: 5 mL four times/day

**Dosage Forms** Liquid:

Entuss-D®: Hydrocodone bitartrate 5 mg and pseudoephedrine hydrochloride 30 mg per 5 mL

Detussin®, Histussin D®, Tyrodone®: Hydrocodone bitartrate 5 mg and pseudoephedrine hydrochloride 60 mg per 5 mL

## Hydrocodone, Chlorpheniramine, Phenylephrine, Acetaminophen and Caffeine

(hye droe KOE done, klor fen IR a meen, fen il EF rin, a seet a MIN oh fen, & KAF een)

**U.S. Brand Names** Hycomine® Compound

**Pharmacologic Category** Antitussive

**Use** Symptomatic relief of cough and symptoms of upper respiratory infection

**Effects on Mental Status** Sedation is common; may cause confusion, dizziness, excitability, nervousness, fatigue, anxiety, restlessness, or depression; may rarely cause hallucinations

**Effects on Psychiatric Treatment** May result in loss of pain control when used in combination with SSRIs (especially paroxetine and fluoxetine); concurrent use with psychotropics may produce additive sedation or dry mouth. Concurrent use with MAOIs may result in hypertensive crisis; avoid combination; barbiturates and carbamazepine may increase the hepatotoxic potential of acetaminophen.

**Usual Dosage** Adults: Oral: 1 tablet every 4 hours, up to 4 times/day

**Dosage Forms** Tablet: Hydrocodone bitartrate 5 mg, chlorpheniramine maleate 2 mg, phenylephrine hydrochloride 10 mg, acetaminophen 250 mg, and caffeine 30 mg

♦ **Hydrocodone PA® Syrup** *see* Hydrocodone and Phenylpropanolamine *on page 273*

## Hydrocodone, Phenylephrine, Pyrilamine, Phenindamine, Chlorpheniramine, and Ammonium Chloride

(hye droe KOE done, fen il EF rin, peer IL a meen, fen IN da meen, klor fen IR a meen, & a MOE nee um KLOR ide)

**U.S. Brand Names** P-V-Tussin®

**Pharmacologic Category** Antihistamine/Decongestant/Antitussive

**Use** Symptomatic relief of cough and nasal congestion

**Effects on Mental Status** May cause sedation, drowsiness, mental clouding, lethargy, impairment of mental performance, anxiety, fear, dysphoria, dizziness, psychic dependence, mood changes

**Effects on Psychiatric Treatment** Contraindicated with MAOIs

**Usual Dosage** Adults: Oral: 10 mL every 4-6 hours, up to 40 mL/day

**Dosage Forms** Syrup: Hydrocodone bitartrate 2.5 mg, phenylephrine hydrochloride 5 mg, pyrilamine maleate 6 mg, phenindamine tartrate 5 mg, chlorpheniramine maleate 2 mg, and ammonium chloride 50 mg per 5 mL with alcohol 5% (480 mL, 3780 mL)

## Hydrocodone, Pseudoephedrine, and Guaifenesin

(hye droe KOE done, soo doe e FED rin & gwye FEN e sin)

**U.S. Brand Names** Cophene XP®; Detussin® Expectorant; SRC® Expectorant; Tussafin® Expectorant

**Pharmacologic Category** Antitussive/Decongestant/Expectorant

**Use** Symptomatic relief of irritating, nonproductive cough associated with respiratory conditions such as bronchitis, bronchial asthma, tracheobronchitis, and the common cold

**Effects on Mental Status** May cause drowsiness, fear, anxiety, tenseness, restlessness, insomnia, hallucinations, CNS depression

**Effects on Psychiatric Treatment** Contraindicated with MAOIs

**Restrictions** C-III

**Usual Dosage** Adults: Oral: 5 mL every 4-6 hours

**Dosage Forms**

Liquid: Hydrocodone bitartrate 2.5 mg, pseudoephedrine hydrochloride 15 mg, and guaifenesin 100 mg per 5 mL (25 mL, 473 mL)

Liquid: Hydrocodone bitartrate 5 mg, pseudoephedrine hydrochloride 60 mg, and guaifenesin 200 mg per 5 mL with alcohol 12.5% (480 mL)

♦ **Hydrocort®** *see* Hydrocortisone *on page 273*

## Hydrocortisone (hye droe KOR ti sone)

**Related Information**

Corticosteroids Comparison Chart *on page 711*

(Continued)

## Hydrocortisone *(Continued)*

**U.S. Brand Names** Aeroseb-HC®; A-hydroCort®; Ala-Cort®; Ala-Scalp®; Anucort-HC® Suppository; Anuprep HC® Suppository; Anusol® HC 1 [OTC]; Anusol® HC 2.5% [OTC]; Anusol-HC® Suppository; Caldecort®; Caldecort® Anti-Itch Spray; Clocort® Maximum Strength; CortaGel® [OTC]; Cortaid® Maximum Strength [OTC]; Cortaid® With Aloe [OTC]; Cort-Dome®; Cortef®; Cortef® Feminine Itch; Cortenema®; Cortifoam®; Cortizone®-5 [OTC]; Cortizone®-10 [OTC]; Delcort®; Dermacort®; Dermarest Dricort®; DermiCort®; Dermolate® [OTC]; Dermtex® HC With Aloe; Eldecort®; Gynecort® [OTC]; Hemril-HC® Uniserts®; Hi-Cor® 1.0; Hi-Cor® 2.5; Hycort®; Hydrocort®; Hydrocortone® Acetate; Hydrocortone® Phosphate; HydroTex® [OTC]; Hytone®; LactiCare-HC®; Lanacort® [OTC]; Locoid®; Nutracort®; Orabase® HCA; Pandel®; Penecort®; Procort® [OTC]; Proctocort™; Scalpicin®; Solu-Cortef®; S-T Cort®; Synacort®; Tegrin®-HC [OTC]; Westcort®

**Pharmacologic Category** Corticosteroid, Oral; Corticosteroid, Parenteral; Corticosteroid, Rectal

**Use** Management of adrenocortical insufficiency; relief of inflammation of corticosteroid-responsive dermatoses (low and medium potency topical corticosteroid); adjunctive treatment of ulcerative colitis

**Effects on Mental Status** Insomnia and nervousness are common; rare reports of delirium, euphoria, hallucinations, and mood swings

**Effects on Psychiatric Treatment** Barbiturates may increase the metabolism of hydrocortisone; lithium has been used to treat mood swings associated with hydrocortisone

**Pregnancy Risk Factor** C

**Contraindications** Serious infections, except septic shock or tuberculous meningitis; known hypersensitivity to hydrocortisone; viral, fungal, or tubercular skin lesions

**Warnings/Precautions**

Use with caution in patients with hyperthyroidism, cirrhosis, nonspecific ulcerative colitis, hypertension, osteoporosis, thromboembolic tendencies, CHF, convulsive disorders, myasthenia gravis, thrombophlebitis, peptic ulcer, diabetes

Acute adrenal insufficiency may occur with abrupt withdrawal after long-term therapy or with stress; young pediatric patients may be more susceptible to adrenal axis suppression from topical therapy

Because of the risk of adverse effects, systemic corticosteroids should be used cautiously in the elderly, in the smallest possible dose, and for the shortest possible time

**Adverse Reactions**

>10%:
- Central nervous system: Insomnia, nervousness
- Gastrointestinal: Increased appetite, indigestion

1% to 10%:
- Dermatologic: Hirsutism
- Endocrine & metabolic: Diabetes mellitus
- Neuromuscular & skeletal: Arthralgia
- Ocular: Cataracts
- Respiratory: Epistaxis

<1%: Abdominal distention, acne, amenorrhea, bone growth suppression, bruising, Cushing's syndrome, delirium, dermatitis, edema, euphoria, hallucinations, headache, hyperglycemia, hyperpigmentation, hypersensitivity reactions, hypertension, hypokalemia, immunosuppression, mood swings, muscle wasting, pancreatitis, peptic ulcer, seizures, skin atrophy, sodium and water retention, ulcerative esophagitis

**Overdosage/Toxicology**

Signs and symptoms: Cushingoid appearance (systemic), muscle weakness (systemic), osteoporosis (systemic) all with long-term use only. When consumed in excessive quantities for prolonged periods, systemic hypercorticism and adrenal suppression may occur.

Treatment: In those cases where hypercorticism and adrenal suppression occur, discontinuation and withdrawal of the corticosteroid should be done judiciously.

**Drug Interactions** CYP2D6 and 3A3/4 enzyme substrate

Decreased effect:
- Insulin decreases hypoglycemic effect
- Phenytoin, phenobarbital, ephedrine, and rifampin increase metabolism of hydrocortisone and decrease steroid blood level

Increased toxicity:
- Oral anticoagulants change prothrombin time; potassium-depleting diuretics increase risk of hypokalemia
- Cardiac glucosides increase risk of arrhythmias or digitalis toxicity secondary to hypokalemia

**Usual Dosage** Dose should be based on severity of disease and patient response

Acute adrenal insufficiency: I.M., I.V.:
- Infants and young Children: Succinate: 1-2 mg/kg/dose bolus, then 25-150 mg/day in divided doses every 6-8 hours
- Older Children: Succinate: 1-2 mg/kg bolus then 150-250 mg/day in divided doses every 6-8 hours
- Adults: Succinate: 100 mg I.V. bolus, then 300 mg/day in divided doses every 8 hours or as a continuous infusion for 48 hours; once patient is stable change to oral, 50 mg every 8 hours for 6 doses, then taper to 30-50 mg/day in divided doses

Chronic adrenal corticoid insufficiency: Adults: Oral: 20-30 mg/day

Anti-inflammatory or immunosuppressive:
- Infants and Children:
  - Oral: 2.5-10 mg/kg/day **or** 75-300 mg/m²/day every 6-8 hours
  - I.M., I.V.: Succinate: 1-5 mg/kg/day **or** 30-150 mg/m²/day divided every 12-24 hours
- Adolescents and Adults: Oral, I.M., I.V.: Succinate: 15-240 mg every 12 hours

Congenital adrenal hyperplasia: Oral: Initial: 30-36 mg/m²/day with 1/3 of dose every morning and 2/3 every evening or 1/4 every morning and mid-day and 1/2 every evening; maintenance: 20-25 mg/m²/day in divided doses

Physiologic replacement: Children:
- Oral: 0.5-0.75 mg/kg/day **or** 20-25 mg/m²/day every 8 hours
- I.M.: Succinate: 0.25-0.35 mg/kg/day **or** 12-15 mg/m²/day once daily

Shock: I.M., I.V.: Succinate:
- Children: Initial: 50 mg/kg, then repeated in 4 hours and/or every 24 hours as needed
- Adolescents and Adults: 500 mg to 2 g every 2-6 hours

Status asthmaticus: Children and Adults: I.V.: Succinate: 1-2 mg/kg/dose every 6 hours for 24 hours, then maintenance of 0.5-1 mg/kg every 6 hours

Rheumatic diseases:
- Adults: Intralesional, intra-articular, soft tissue injection: Acetate:
  - Large joints: 25 mg (up to 37.5 mg)
  - Small joints: 10-25 mg
- Tendon sheaths: 5-12.5 mg
- Soft tissue infiltration: 25-50 mg (up to 75 mg)
- Bursae: 25-37.5 mg
- Ganglia: 12.5-25 mg

Dermatosis: Children >2 years and Adults: Topical: Apply to affected area 3-4 times/day (Buteprate: Apply once or twice daily). Therapy should be discontinued when control is achieved; if no improvement is seen, reassessment of diagnosis may be necessary.

Ulcerative colitis: Adults: Rectal: 10-100 mg 1-2 times/day for 2-3 weeks

**Patient Information**

Systemic: Take as directed; do not increase doses and do not stop abruptly without consulting prescribed. Dosage of systemic hydrocortisone is usually tapered off gradually. Take oral dose with food to reduce GI upset. Hydrocortisone may cause immunosuppression and mask symptoms of infection; avoid exposure to contagion and notify prescriber of any signs of infection (eg, fever, chills, sore throat, injury) and notify dentist or surgeon (if necessary) that you are taking this medication. You may experience increased appetite, indigestion, or increased nervousness. Report any sudden weight gain (>5 lb/week), swelling of extremities or difficulty breathing, abdominal pain, severe vomiting, black or tarry stools, fatigue, anorexia, weakness, or unusual mood swings.

Topical: Before applying, wash area gently and thoroughly. Apply gel, cream, or ointment in thin film to cleansed area and rub in gently until medication vanishes. Avoid exposing affected area to sunlight; you will be more sensitive and severe sunburn may occur. Consult prescriber if breast-feeding.

Rectal: Insert suppository gently as high as possible with gloved finger while lying down. Avoid injury with long or sharp fingernails. Remain in resting position for 10 minutes after insertion.

**Dosage Forms**

**Hydrocortisone acetate:**
- Aerosol, rectal: 10% (20 g)
- Cream, topical: 0.5% (15 g, 22.5 g, 30 g); 1% (15 g, 30 g, 120 g)
- Ointment, topical: 0.5% (15 g, 30 g); 1% (15 g, 21 g, 30 g)
- Injection, suspension: 25 mg/mL (5 mL, 10 mL); 50 mg/mL (5 mL, 10 mL)
- Suppositories, rectal: 10 mg, 25 mg

**Hydrocortisone base:**
- Aerosol, topical: 0.5% (45 g, 58 g); 1% (45 mL)
- Cream, rectal: 1% (30 g); 2.5% (30 g)
- Cream, topical: 0.5% (15 g, 30 g, 60 g, 120 g, 454 g); 1% (15 g, 20 g, 30 g, 60 g, 90 g, 120 g, 240 g, 454 g); 2.5% (15 g, 20 g, 30 g, 60 g, 120 g, 240 g, 454 g)
- Gel, topical: 0.5% (15 g, 30 g); 1% (15 g, 30 g)
- Lotion, topical: 0.25% (120 mL); 0.5% (30 mL, 60 mL, 120 mL); 1% (60 mL, 118 mL, 120 mL); 2% (30 mL) ; 2.5% (60 mL, 120 mL)
- Ointment, rectal: 1% (30 g)
- Ointment, topical: 0.5% (30 g) ; 1% (15 g, 20 g, 28 g, 30 g, 60 g, 120 g, 240 g, 454 g); 2.5% (20 g, 30 g)
- Paste: 0.5% (5 g)
- Solution, topical: 1% (45 mL, 75 mL, 120 mL)
- Suspension, rectal: 100 mg/60 mL (7s)
- Tablet, oral: 5 mg, 10 mg, 20 mg

**Hydrocortisone buteprate:** Cream: 1% (15 g, 45 g)

**Hydrocortisone butyrate:**
- Cream: 0.1% (15 g, 45 g)
- Ointment, topical: 0.1% (15 g, 45 g)
- Solution, topical: 0.1% (20 mL, 50 mL)

**Hydrocortisone cypionate:**
- Suspension, oral: 10 mg/5 mL (120 mL)

**Hydrocortisone sodium phosphate:**
Injection, I.M./I.V./S.C.: 50 mg/mL (2 mL, 10 mL)
**Hydrocortisone sodium succinate:**
Injection, IM/I.V.: 100 mg, 250 mg, 500 mg, 1000 mg
**Hydrocortisone valerate:**
Cream, topical: 0.2% (15 g, 45 g, 60 g)
Ointment, topical: 0.2% (15 g, 45 g, 60 g, 120 g)

- **Hydrocortone® Acetate** *see* Hydrocortisone *on page 273*
- **Hydrocortone® Phosphate** *see* Hydrocortisone *on page 273*
- **Hydro-Crysti-12®** *see* Hydroxocobalamin *on page 276*
- **HydroDIURIL®** *see* Hydrochlorothiazide *on page 271*

## Hydroflumethiazide (hye droe floo meth EYE a zide)

**U.S. Brand Names** Diucardin®; Saluron®

**Pharmacologic Category** Diuretic, Thiazide

**Use** Management of mild to moderate hypertension; treatment of edema in congestive heart failure and nephrotic syndrome

**Effects on Mental Status** May cause drowsiness

**Effects on Psychiatric Treatment** May rarely cause agranulocytosis; use caution with clozapine and carbamazepine; may decrease lithium clearance resulting in an increase in serum lithium levels and potential lithium toxicity; monitor serum lithium levels

**Pregnancy Risk Factor** C

**Contraindications** Hypersensitivity to hydroflumethiazide or any component, thiazides, or sulfonamide-derived drugs; anuria; renal decompensation

**Warnings/Precautions** Avoid in severe renal disease (ineffective). Electrolyte disturbances (hypokalemia, hypochloremic alkalosis, hyponatremia) can occur. Use with caution in severe hepatic dysfunction; hepatic encephalopathy can be caused by electrolyte disturbances. Gout can be precipitate in certain patients with a history of gout, a familial predisposition to gout, or chronic renal failure. Cautious use in diabetics; may see a change in glucose control. Hypersensitivity reactions can occur. Can cause SLE exacerbation or activation. Use with caution in patients with moderate or high cholesterol concentrations. Photosensitization may occur. Correct hypokalemia before initiating therapy.

**Adverse Reactions**
1% to 10%: Endocrine & metabolic: Hypokalemia
<1%: Agranulocytosis, anorexia, aplastic anemia, drowsiness, fluid and electrolyte imbalances (hypocalcemia, hypomagnesemia, hyponatremia), hemolytic anemia, hepatitis, hyperglycemia, hypotension, leukopenia, paresthesia, photosensitivity, polyuria, prerenal azotemia, rarely blood dyscrasias, rash, thrombocytopenia, uremia

**Overdosage/Toxicology**
Signs and symptoms: Hypermotility, diuresis, lethargy
Treatment: Following GI decontamination, therapy is supportive with I.V. fluids, electrolytes, and I.V. pressors if needed

**Drug Interactions**
Angiotensin-converting enzyme inhibitors: Increased hypotension if aggressively diuresed with a thiazide diuretic
Beta-blockers increase hyperglycemic effects in Type 2 diabetes mellitus
Cyclosporine and thiazides can increase the risk of gout or renal toxicity; avoid concurrent use
Digoxin toxicity can be exacerbated if a thiazide induces hypokalemia or hypomagnesemia
Lithium toxicity can occur by reducing renal excretion of lithium; monitor lithium concentration and adjust as needed
Neuromuscular blocking agents can prolong blockade; monitor serum potassium and neuromuscular status
NSAIDs can decrease the efficacy of thiazides reducing the diuretic and antihypertensive effects

**Usual Dosage** Oral:
Children (not approved): 1 mg/kg/24 hours
Adults:
Edema:
Initial: 50 mg 1-2 times/day
Maintenance: 25-200 mg/day (use divided doses when >100 mg/day)
Hypertension:
Initial: 50 mg twice daily
Maintenance: 50-100 mg/day; maximum: 200 mg/day

**Patient Information** May be taken with food or milk; take early in day to avoid nocturia; take the last dose of multiple doses no later than 6 PM unless instructed otherwise. A few people who take this medication become more sensitive to sunlight and may experience skin rash, redness, itching or severe sunburn, especially if sun block SPF ≥15 is not used on exposed skin areas.

**Nursing Implications** Take blood pressure with patient lying down and standing

**Dosage Forms** Tablet: 50 mg

## Hydroflumethiazide and Reserpine
(hye droe floo meth EYE a zide & re SER peen)

**U.S. Brand Names** Salutensin®

**Pharmacologic Category** Antihypertensive Agent, Combination

**Use** Management of hypertension

**Effects on Mental Status** May cause dizziness, headache, nightmares, nervousness, drowsiness, fatigue, mental depression, parkinsonism, dull sensorium, syncope, paradoxical anxiety

**Effects on Psychiatric Treatment** May rarely cause agranulocytosis; use caution with clozapine and carbamazepine; may decrease lithium clearance resulting in an increase in serum lithium levels and potential lithium toxicity, monitor serum lithium levels; contraindicated in those with depression or undergoing ECT; avoid concurrent use with MAOIs

**Usual Dosage** As determined by individual titration, usually 1 tablet once or twice daily

**Dosage Forms**
Tablet (Salutensin®): Hydroflumethiazide 50 mg and reserpine 0.125 mg
Tablet (Hydro-Fluserpine®, Salutensin-Demi®): Hydroflumethiazide 25 mg and reserpine 0.125 mg

- **Hydrogesic®** *see* Hydrocodone and Acetaminophen *on page 272*
- **Hydromet®** *see* Hydrocodone and Homatropine *on page 273*

## Hydromorphone (hye droe MOR fone)

**Related Information**
Narcotic Agonists Comparison Chart *on page 720*

**U.S. Brand Names** Dilaudid®; Dilaudid-5®; Dilaudid-HP®; HydroStat IR®

**Canadian Brand Names** Hydromorph Contin®; PMS-Hydromorphone

**Synonyms** Dihydromorphinone

**Pharmacologic Category** Analgesic, Narcotic

**Use** Management of moderate to severe pain; antitussive at lower doses

**Effects on Mental Status** Drowsiness and dizziness are common; may cause nervousness or restlessness; may rarely cause hallucinations or depression

**Effects on Psychiatric Treatment** Concurrent use with psychotropics may produce additive sedation

**Restrictions** C-II

**Pregnancy Risk Factor** B (D if used for prolonged periods or in high doses at term)

**Contraindications** Hypersensitivity to hydromorphone or any component or other phenanthrene derivative

**Warnings/Precautions** Tablet and cough syrup contain tartrazine which may cause allergic reactions; hydromorphone shares toxic potential of opiate agonists, and precaution of opiate agonist therapy should be observed; extreme caution should be taken to avoid confusing the highly concentrated injection with the less concentrated injectable product, injection contains benzyl alcohol; use with caution in patients with hypersensitivity to other phenanthrene opiates, in patients with respiratory disease, or severe liver or renal failure; tolerance or drug dependence may result from extended use

**Adverse Reactions**
Percentage unknown: Antidiuretic hormone release, biliary tract spasm, urinary tract spasm, miosis, histamine release, physical and psychological dependence, increased AST, ALT
>10%:
Cardiovascular: Palpitations, hypotension, peripheral vasodilation
Central nervous system: Dizziness, lightheadedness, drowsiness
Gastrointestinal: Anorexia
1% to 10%:
Cardiovascular: Tachycardia, bradycardia, flushing of face
Central nervous system: CNS depression, increased intracranial pressure, fatigue, headache, nervousness, restlessness
Gastrointestinal: Nausea, vomiting, constipation, stomach cramps, xerostomia
Genitourinary: Decreased urination, ureteral spasm
Hepatic: Increased LFTs
Neuromuscular & skeletal: Trembling, weakness
Respiratory: Respiratory depression, dyspnea, shortness of breath
<1%: Hallucinations, mental depression, paralytic ileus, pruritus, rash, urticaria

**Overdosage/Toxicology**
Signs and symptoms: CNS depression, respiratory depression, miosis, apnea, pulmonary edema, convulsions
Treatment: Maintain airway, establish I.V. line; naloxone 2 mg I.V. (0.01 mg/kg for children) with repeat administration as necessary up to a total of 10 mg

**Drug Interactions** Increased toxicity: CNS depressants, phenothiazines, tricyclic antidepressants may potentiate the adverse effects of hydromorphone

(Continued)

## Hydromorphone *(Continued)*

**Usual Dosage**

Doses should be titrated to appropriate analgesic effects; when changing routes of administration, note that oral doses are less than half as effective as parenteral doses (may be only one-fifth as effective)

Pain: Older Children and Adults:

Oral, I.M., I.V., S.C.: 1-4 mg/dose every 4-6 hours as needed; usual adult dose: 2 mg/dose

Rectal: 3 mg every 6-8 hours

Antitussive: Oral:

Children 6-12 years: 0.5 mg every 3-4 hours as needed

Children >12 years and Adults: 1 mg every 3-4 hours as needed

**Dosing adjustment in hepatic impairment:** Should be considered

**Dietary Considerations**

Alcohol: Additive CNS effects, avoid or limit alcohol; watch for sedation

Food: Glucose may cause hyperglycemia; monitor blood glucose concentrations

**Patient Information** If self-administered, use exactly as directed (do not increase dose or frequency); may cause physical and/or psychological dependence. While using this medication, do not use alcohol and other prescription or OTC medications (especially sedatives, tranquilizers, antihistamines, or pain medications) without consulting prescriber. Maintain adequate hydration (2-3 L/day of fluids unless instructed to restrict fluid intake). May cause dizziness, drowsiness, impaired coordination, or blurred vision (use caution when driving, climbing stairs, or changing position - rising from sitting or lying to standing, or when engaging in tasks requiring alertness until response to drug is known); loss of appetite, nausea, or vomiting (frequent mouth care, small frequent meals, chewing gum, or sucking lozenges may help); constipation (increased exercise, fluids, or dietary fruit and fiber may help - if constipation remains an unresolved problem, consult prescriber about use of stool softeners). Report chest pain, slow or rapid heartbeat, acute dizziness, or persistent headache; swelling of extremities or unusual weight gain; changes in urinary elimination; acute headache; back or flank pain or spasms; or other adverse reactions.

**Nursing Implications** Observe patient for oversedation, respiratory depression, implement safety measures

**Dosage Forms**

Injection, as hydrochloride:

Dilaudid®: 1 mg/mL (1 mL); 2 mg/mL (1 mL, 20 mL); 3 mg/mL (1 mL); 4 mg/mL (1 mL)

Dilaudid-HP®: 10 mg/mL (1 mL, 2 mL, 5 mL)

Liquid, as hydrochloride: 5 mg/5 mL (480 mL)

Powder for injection, as hydrochloride: (Dilaudid-HP®): 250 mg

Suppository, rectal, as hydrochloride: 3 mg (6s)

Tablet, as hydrochloride: 1 mg, 2 mg, 3 mg, 4 mg, 8 mg

♦ **Hydromox®** *see* Quinethazone *on page 485*

♦ **Hydro-Par®** *see* Hydrochlorothiazide *on page 271*

♦ **Hydrophed®** *see* Theophylline, Ephedrine, and Hydroxyzine *on page 539*

♦ **Hydropres®** *see* Hydrochlorothiazide and Reserpine *on page 271*

## Hydroquinone (HYE droe kwin one)

**U.S. Brand Names** Ambi® Skin Tone [OTC]; Eldopaque® [OTC]; Eldopaque Forte®; Eldoquin® [OTC]; Eldoquin® Forte®; Esoterica® Facial [OTC]; Esoterica® Regular [OTC]; Esoterica® Sensitive Skin Formula [OTC]; Esoterica® Sunscreen [OTC]; Melanex®; Porcelana® [OTC]; Porcelana® Sunscreen [OTC]; Solaquin® [OTC]; Solaquin Forte®

**Canadian Brand Names** Neostrata™ HQ; Ultraquin™

**Pharmacologic Category** Depigmenting Agent

**Use** Gradual bleaching of hyperpigmented skin conditions

**Effects on Mental Status** None reported

**Effects on Psychiatric Treatment** None reported

**Usual Dosage** Children >12 years and Adults: Topical: Apply thin layer and rub in twice daily

**Dosage Forms**

Cream, topical:

Esoterica® Sensitive Skin Formula: 1.5% (85 g)

Eldopaque®, Eldoquin®, Esoterica® Facial, Esoterica® Regular, Porcelana®: 2% (14.2 g, 28.4 g, 60 g, 85 g, 120 g)

Eldopaque Forte®, Eldoquin® Forte®, Melquin HP®: 4% (14.2 g, 28.4 g)

Cream, topical, with sunscreen:

Esoterica® Sunscreen, Porcelana®, Solaquin®: 2% (28.4 g, 120 g)

Melpaque HP®, Nuquin HP®, Solaquin Forte®: 4% (14.2 g, 28.4 g)

Gel, topical, with sunscreen (Solaquin Forte®): 4% (14.2 g, 28.4 g)

Solution, topical (Melanex®): 3% (30 mL)

♦ **Hydro-Serp®** *see* Hydrochlorothiazide and Reserpine *on page 271*

♦ **Hydroserpine®** *see* Hydrochlorothiazide and Reserpine *on page 271*

♦ **HydroStat IR®** *see* Hydromorphone *on page 275*

♦ **HydroTex® [OTC]** *see* Hydrocortisone *on page 273*

## Hydroxocobalamin (hye droks oh koe BAL a min)

**U.S. Brand Names** Alphamin®; Codroxomin®; Hybalamin®; Hydro-Cobex®; Hydro-Crysti-12®; LA-12®

**Canadian Brand Names** Acti-$B_{12}$®

**Pharmacologic Category** Vitamin, Water Soluble

**Use** Treatment of pernicious anemia, vitamin $B_{12}$ deficiency, increased $B_{12}$ requirements due to pregnancy, thyrotoxicosis, hemorrhage, malignancy, liver or kidney disease

**Effects on Mental Status** None reported

**Effects on Psychiatric Treatment** None reported

**Usual Dosage** Vitamin $B_{12}$ deficiency: I.M.:

Children: 1-5 mg given in single doses of 100 mcg over 2 or more weeks, followed by 30-50 mcg/month

Adults: 30 mcg/day for 5-10 days, followed by 100-200 mcg/month

**Dosage Forms** Injection: 1000 mcg/mL (10 mL, 30 mL)

## Hydroxyamphetamine (hye droks ee am FET a meen)

**U.S. Brand Names** Paredrine®

**Pharmacologic Category** Adrenergic Agonist Agent

**Use** Produce mydriasis in diagnostic eye examination

**Effects on Mental Status** None reported

**Effects on Psychiatric Treatment** None reported

**Usual Dosage** Instill 1-2 drops into conjunctival sac

**Dosage Forms** Solution, as hydrobromide: 1%

## Hydroxyamphetamine and Tropicamide

(hye droks ee am FET a meen & troe PIK a mide)

**U.S. Brand Names** Paremyd® Ophthalmic

**Pharmacologic Category** Adrenergic Agonist Agent

**Use** Mydriasis with cycloplegia

**Effects on Mental Status** None reported

**Effects on Psychiatric Treatment** None reported

**Usual Dosage** Ophthalmic: Adults: Instill 1-2 drops into conjunctival sac(s)

**Dosage Forms** Solution, ophthalmic: Hydroxyamphetamine hydrobromide 1% and tropicamide 0.25% (5 mL, 15 mL)

♦ **Hydroxycarbamide** *see* Hydroxyurea *on page 277*

## Hydroxychloroquine (hye droks ee KLOR oh kwin)

**U.S. Brand Names** Plaquenil®

**Pharmacologic Category** Aminoquinoline (Antimalarial)

**Use** Suppresses and treats acute attacks of malaria; treatment of systemic lupus erythematosus and rheumatoid arthritis

**Effects on Mental Status** May cause dizziness or nervousness

**Effects on Psychiatric Treatment** May rarely cause agranulocytosis; use caution with clozapine and carbamazepine

**Pregnancy Risk Factor** C

**Contraindications** Retinal or visual field changes attributable to 4-aminoquinolines; hypersensitivity to hydroxychloroquine, 4-aminoquinoline derivatives, or any component

**Warnings/Precautions** Use with caution in patients with hepatic disease, G-6-PD deficiency, psoriasis, and porphyria; long-term use in children is not recommended; perform baseline and periodic (6 months) ophthalmologic examinations; test periodically for muscle weakness

**Adverse Reactions**

>10%:

Central nervous system: Headache

Dermatologic: Itching

Gastrointestinal: Diarrhea, loss of appetite, nausea, stomach cramps, vomiting

Ocular: Ciliary muscle dysfunction

1% to 10%:

Central nervous system: Dizziness, lightheadedness, nervousness, restlessness

Dermatologic: Bleaching of hair, rash, discoloration of skin (black-blue)

Ocular: Ocular toxicity, keratopathy, retinopathy

<1%: Agranulocytosis, aplastic anemia, emotional changes, neuromyopathy, neutropenia, ototoxicity, seizures, thrombocytopenia

**Overdosage/Toxicology**

Signs and symptoms: Headache, drowsiness, visual changes, cardiovascular collapse, and seizures followed by respiratory and cardiac arrest

Treatment: Symptomatic; urinary alkalinization will enhance renal elimination

**Drug Interactions**

Chloroquine and other 4-aminoquinolones may be decreased due to GI binding with kaolin or magnesium trisilicate

Increased effect: Cimetidine increases levels of chloroquine and probably other 4-aminoquinolones

**Usual Dosage** Note: Hydroxychloroquine sulfate 200 mg is equivalent to 155 mg hydroxychloroquine base and 250 mg chloroquine phosphate.

Oral:

Children:

Chemoprophylaxis of malaria: 5 mg/kg (base) once weekly; should not exceed the recommended adult dose; begin 2 weeks before exposure; continue for 4-6 weeks after leaving endemic area; if suppressive therapy is not begun prior to the exposure, double the initial dose and give in 2 doses, 6 hours apart

Acute attack: 10 mg/kg (base) initial dose; followed by 5 mg/kg at 6, 24, and 48 hours

JRA or SLE: 3-5 mg/kg/day divided 1-2 times/day; avoid exceeding 7 mg/kg/day

Adults:

Chemoprophylaxis of malaria: 310 mg base weekly on same day each week; begin 2 weeks before exposure; continue for 4-6 weeks after leaving endemic area; if suppressive therapy is not begun prior to the exposure, double the initial dose and give in 2 doses, 6 hours apart

Acute attack: 620 mg first dose day 1; 310 mg in 6 hours day 1; 310 mg in 1 dose day 2; and 310 mg in 1 dose on day 3

Rheumatoid arthritis: 310-465 mg/day to start taken with food or milk; increase dose until optimum response level is reached; usually after 4-12 weeks dose should be reduced by 1/2 and a maintenance dose of 155-310 mg/day given

Lupus erythematosus: 310 mg every day or twice daily for several weeks depending on response; 155-310 mg/day for prolonged maintenance therapy

**Patient Information** It is important to complete full course of therapy which may take up to 6 months for full effect. May be taken with meals to decrease GI upset and bitter aftertaste. Avoid alcohol. You should have regular ophthalmic exams (every 4-6 months) if using this medication over extended periods. You may experience skin discoloration (blue/black), hair bleaching, or skin rash. If you have psoriasis, you may experience exacerbation. You may experience dizziness, headache, nervousness, or light-headedness (use caution when driving or engaging in tasks requiring alertness until response to drug is known); nausea, vomiting, or loss of appetite (small frequent meals, frequent mouth care, sucking lozenges, or chewing gum may help); or increased sensitivity to sunlight (wear dark glasses and protective clothing, use sunblock, and avoid direct exposure to sunlight). Report vision changes, rash or itching, persistent diarrhea or GI disturbances, change in hearing acuity or ringing in the ears, chest pain or palpitation, CNS changes, unusual fatigue, easy bruising or bleeding, or any other persistent adverse reactions.

**Nursing Implications** Periodic blood counts and eye examinations are recommended when patient is on chronic therapy

**Dosage Forms** Tablet, as sulfate: 200 mg [base 155 mg]

♦ **25-Hydroxycholecalciferol** *see* Calcifediol *on page 83*

## Hydroxyprogesterone (hye droks ee proe JES te rone)

**U.S. Brand Names** Hylutin® Injection; Hyprogest® 250 Injection

**Pharmacologic Category** Progestin

**Use** Treatment of amenorrhea, abnormal uterine bleeding, endometriosis, uterine carcinoma

**Effects on Mental Status** May cause insomnia or depression

**Effects on Psychiatric Treatment** None reported

**Usual Dosage** Adults: Female: I.M.: *Long-acting progestin*

Amenorrhea: 375 mg; if no bleeding, begin cyclic treatment with estradiol valerate

Production of secretory endometrium and desquamation: (Medical D and C): 125-250 mg administered on day 10 of cycle; repeat every 7 days until suppression is no longer desired.

Uterine carcinoma: 1 g one or more times/day (1-7 g/week) for up to 12 weeks

**Dosage Forms** Injection:

125 mg/mL (10 mL)

Hylutin®, Hyprogest®: 250 mg/mL (5 mL)

## Hydroxypropyl Cellulose

(hye droks ee PROE pil SEL yoo lose)

**U.S. Brand Names** Lacrisert®

**Pharmacologic Category** Ophthalmic Agent, Miscellaneous

**Use** Dry eyes

**Effects on Mental Status** None reported

**Effects on Psychiatric Treatment** None reported

**Usual Dosage** Adults: Ophthalmic: Apply once daily into the inferior cul-de-sac beneath the base of tarsus, not in apposition to the cornea nor beneath the eyelid at the level of the tarsal plate

**Dosage Forms** Insert, ophthalmic: 5 mg

## Hydroxypropyl Methylcellulose

(hye droks ee PROE pil meth il SEL yoo lose)

**U.S. Brand Names** Gonak™ [OTC]; Goniosol® [OTC]

**Pharmacologic Category** Ophthalmic Agent, Miscellaneous

**Use** Ophthalmic surgical aid in cataract extraction and intraocular implantation; gonioscopic examinations

**Effects on Mental Status** None reported

**Effects on Psychiatric Treatment** None reported

**Usual Dosage** Introduced into anterior chamber of eye with 20-gauge or larger cannula

**Dosage Forms** Solution: 2.5% (15 mL)

## Hydroxyurea (hye droks ee yoor EE a)

**U.S. Brand Names** Droxia™; Hydrea®

**Synonyms** Hydroxycarbamide

**Pharmacologic Category** Antineoplastic Agent, Antimetabolite

**Use** CML in chronic phase; radiosensitizing agent in the treatment of primary brain tumors, head and neck tumors, uterine cervix and nonsmall cell lung cancer, psoriasis, sickle cell anemia and other hemoglobinopathies; treatment of hematologic conditions such as essential thrombocythemia, polycythemia vera, hypereosinophilia, and hyperleukocytosis due to acute leukemia. Has shown activity against renal cell cancer, melanoma, ovarian cancer, head and neck cancer, and prostate cancer. Management of sickle cell anemia - to reduce the frequency of painful crises and to reduce the need for blood transfusions in adult patients with sickle cell anemia with recurrent moderate to severe painful crises (generally at least 3 during the preceding 12 months). Has been used in combination with didanosine and other antiretrovirals in the treatment of HIV.

**Effects on Mental Status** Drowsiness is common; may rarely cause disorientation and hallucinations

**Effects on Psychiatric Treatment** Myelosuppression is common; use caution with clozapine and carbamazepine

**Pregnancy Risk Factor** D

**Contraindications** Severe anemia, severe bone marrow suppression; WBC <2500/mm$^3$ or platelet count <100,000/mm$^3$; hypersensitivity to hydroxyurea

**Warnings/Precautions** The U.S. Food and Drug Administration (FDA) currently recommends that procedures for proper handling and disposal of antineoplastic agents be considered. Use with caution in patients with renal impairment, in patients who have received prior irradiation therapy, and in the elderly.

**Adverse Reactions**

>10%:

Central nervous system: Drowsiness

Gastrointestinal: Mild to moderate nausea and vomiting may occur, as well as diarrhea, constipation, mucositis, ulceration of the GI tract, anorexia, and stomatitis

Hematologic: Myelosuppression: Dose-limiting toxicity, causes a rapid drop in leukocyte count (seen in 4-5 days in nonhematologic malignancy and more rapidly in leukemia); thrombocytopenia and anemia occur less often; reversal of WBC count occurs rapidly, but the platelet count may take 7-10 days to recover

WBC: Moderate

Platelets: Moderate

Onset (days): 7

Nadir (days): 10

Recovery (days): 21

1% to 10%:

Dermatologic: Dermatologic changes (hyperpigmentation, erythema of the hands and face, maculopapular rash, or dry skin), alopecia

Hepatic: Abnormal LFTs and hepatitis

Renal: Increased creatinine and BUN due to impairment of renal tubular function

Miscellaneous: Carcinogenic potential

<1%: Disorientation, dizziness, dyspnea, dysuria, elevated hepatic enzymes, facial erythema, fever, hallucination, headache, hyperuricemia, neurotoxicity, rarely acute diffuse pulmonary infiltrates, seizures

**Overdosage/Toxicology**

Signs and symptoms: Myelosuppression, facial swelling, hallucinations, disorientation

Treatment: Supportive

**Drug Interactions**

Increased effect: Zidovudine, zalcitabine, didanosine: Synergy

Increased toxicity:

Fluorouracil: The potential for neurotoxicity may increase with concomitant administration

Cytarabine: Modulation of its metabolism and cytotoxicity → reduction of cytarabine dose is recommended

**Usual Dosage** Oral (refer to individual protocols): All dosage should be based on ideal or actual body weight, whichever is less:

(Continued)

## Hydroxyurea *(Continued)*

Children:

No FDA-approved dosage regimens have been established; dosages of 1500-3000 mg/m$^2$ as a single dose in combination with other agents every 4-6 weeks have been used in the treatment of pediatric astrocytoma, medulloblastoma, and primitive neuroectodermal tumors

CML: Initial: 10-20 mg/kg/day once daily; adjust dose according to hematologic response

Adults: Dose should always be titrated to patient response and WBC counts; usual oral doses range from 10-30 mg/kg/day or 500-3000 mg/day; if WBC count falls to <2500 cells/mm$^3$, or the platelet count to <100,000/mm$^3$, therapy should be stopped for at least 3 days and resumed when values rise toward normal

Solid tumors:

Intermittent therapy: 80 mg/kg as a single dose every third day

Continuous therapy: 20-30 mg/kg/day given as a single dose/day

Concomitant therapy with irradiation: 80 mg/kg as a single dose every third day starting at least 7 days before initiation of irradiation

Resistant chronic myelocytic leukemia: 20-30 mg/kg/day divided daily

HIV: 1000-1500 mg daily in a single dose or divided doses

Sickle cell anemia (moderate/severe disease): Initial: 15 mg/kg/day, increased by 5 mg/kg every 12 weeks if blood counts are in an acceptable range until the maximum tolerated dose of 35 mg/kg/day is achieved or the dose that does not produce toxic effects

*Acceptable range:*

Neutrophils ≥2500 cells/mm$^3$

Platelets ≥95,000/mm$^3$

Hemoglobin >5.3 g/dL, and

Reticulocytes ≥95,000/mm$^3$ if the hemoglobin concentration is <9 g/dL

*Toxic range:*

Neutrophils <2000 cells/mm$^3$

Platelets <80,000/mm$^3$

Hemoglobin <4.5 g/dL

Reticulocytes <80,000/mm$^3$ if the hemoglobin concentration is <9 g/dL

Monitor for toxicity every 2 weeks; if toxicity occurs, stop treatment until the bone marrow recovers; restart at 2.5 mg/kg/day less than the dose at which toxicity occurs; if no toxicity occurs over the next 12 weeks, then the subsequent dose should be increased by 2.5 mg/kg/day; reduced dosage of hydroxyurea alternating with erythropoietin may decrease myelotoxicity and increase levels of fetal hemoglobin in patients who have not been helped by hydroxyurea alone

**Dosing adjustment in renal impairment:**

$Cl_{cr}$ 10-50 mL/minute: Administer 50% of normal dose

$Cl_{cr}$ <10 mL/minute: Administer 20% of normal dose

Hemodialysis: Supplemental dose is not necessary. Hydroxyurea is a low molecular weight compound with high aqueous solubility that may be freely dialyzable, however, clinical studies confirming this hypothesis have not been performed; peak serum concentrations are reached within 2 hours after oral administration and by 24 hours, the concentration in the serum is zero

CAPD effects: Unknown

CAVH effects: Unknown

**Patient Information** Take capsules exactly on schedule directed by prescriber (dosage and timing will be specific to purpose of therapy). Contents of capsule may be emptied into a glass of water and taken immediately. You will require frequent monitoring and blood tests while taking this medication to assess effectiveness and monitor adverse reactions. You will be susceptible to infection; avoid crowds, infected persons, and persons with contagious diseases. You may experience nausea, vomiting, or loss of appetite (small frequent meals, frequent mouth care, sucking lozenges, or chewing gum may help); constipation (increased exercise, fluid, or dietary fiber may help); diarrhea (buttermilk, boiled milk, or yogurt may help); mouth sores (frequent mouth care will help). Report persistent vomiting, diarrhea, constipation, stomach pain, or mouth sores; skin rash, redness, irritation, or sores; painful or difficult urination; increased confusion, depression, hallucinations, lethargy, or seizures; persistent fever or chills, unusual fatigue, white plaques in mouth, vaginal discharge, or unhealed sores; unusual lassitude, weakness, or muscle tremors; easy bruising/bleeding; or blood in vomitus, stool, or urine. People not taking hydroxyurea should not be exposed to it; if powder from capsule is spilled, wipe up with damp, disposable towel immediately, and discard the towel in a closed container, such as a plastic bag. Wash hands thoroughly.

**Dosage Forms**

Capsule (Droxia™): 200 mg, 300 mg, 400 mg

Capsule: 500 mg

♦ **25-Hydroxyvitamin D$_3$** *see* Calcifediol *on page 83*

## Hydroxyzine (hye DROKS i zeen)

**Related Information**

Anxiolytic/Hypnotic Use in Long-Term Care Facilities *on page 754*

Clinical Issues in the Use of Anxiolytics and Sedative/Hypnotics *on page 634*

Federal OBRA Regulations Recommended Maximum Doses *on page 756*

Nonbenzodiazepine Anxiolytics and Hypnotics *on page 721*

**Generic Available** Yes

**U.S. Brand Names** Anxanil®; Atarax®; Atozine®; Durrax®; Hy-Pam®; Hyzine-50®; Neucalm®; Quiess®; Rezine®; Vamate®; Vistacon-50®; Vistaquel®; Vistaril®; Vistazine®

**Canadian Brand Names** Apo®-Hydroxyzine; Multipax®; Novo-Hydroxyzin; PMS-Hydroxyzine

**Synonyms** Hydroxyzine Hydrochloride; Hydroxyzine Pamoate

**Pharmacologic Category** Antiemetic; Antihistamine

**Use** Treatment of anxiety; as a preoperative sedative; as an antipruritic

**Unlabeled uses:** Antiemetic; alcohol withdrawal symptoms

**Pregnancy Risk Factor** C

**Contraindications** Hypersensitivity to hydroxyzine or any component

**Warnings/Precautions** Causes sedation, caution must be used in performing tasks which require alertness (ie, operating machinery or driving). Sedative effects of CNS depressants or ethanol are potentiated. S.C., intra-arterial, and I.V. administration are not recommended since thrombosis and digital gangrene can occur; extravasation can result in sterile abscess and marked tissue induration; should be used with caution in patients with narrow-angle glaucoma, prostatic hypertrophy, and bladder neck obstruction; should also be used with caution in patients with asthma or COPD.

Anticholinergic effects are not well tolerated in the elderly. Hydroxyzine may be useful as a short-term antipruritic, but it is not recommended for use as a sedative or anxiolytic in the elderly.

**Adverse Reactions**

Central nervous system: Drowsiness, headache, fatigue, nervousness, dizziness

Respiratory: Thickening of bronchial secretions

Gastrointestinal: Xerostomia

Neuromuscular & skeletal: Tremor, paresthesia, seizure

Ocular: Blurred vision

**Overdosage/Toxicology**

Signs and symptoms: Seizures, sedation, hypotension; there is no specific treatment for an antihistamine overdose, however, most of its clinical toxicity is due to anticholinergic effects; anticholinesterase inhibitors may be useful by reducing acetylcholinesterase

Treatment: For anticholinergic overdose with severe life-threatening symptoms, physostigmine 1-2 mg (0.5 or 0.02 mg/kg for children) I.V., slowly may be given to reverse these effects.

**Drug Interactions**

Amantadine, rimantadine: Central and/or peripheral anticholinergic syndrome can occur when administered with amantadine or rimantadine

Anticholinergic agents: Central and/or peripheral anticholinergic syndrome can occur when administered with narcotic analgesics, phenothiazines and other antipsychotics (especially with high anticholinergic activity), tricyclic antidepressants, quinidine and some other antiarrhythmics, and antihistamines

Antipsychotics: Hydroxyzine may antagonize the therapeutic effects of antipsychotics

CNS depressants: Sedative effects of hydroxyzine may be additive with CNS depressants; includes ethanol, benzodiazepines, barbiturates, narcotic analgesics, and other sedative agents; monitor for increased effect

**Stability** Protect from light; store at 15°C to 30°C and protected from freezing; I.V. is **incompatible** when mixed with aminophylline, amobarbital, chloramphenicol, dimenhydrinate, heparin, penicillin G, pentobarbital, phenobarbital, phenytoin, ranitidine, sulfisoxazole, vitamin B complex with C

**Mechanism of Action** Competes with histamine for $H_1$-receptor sites on effector cells in the gastrointestinal tract, blood vessels, and respiratory tract. Possesses skeletal muscle relaxing, bronchodilator, antihistamine, antiemetic, and analgesic properties.

**Pharmacodynamics/kinetics**

Onset of effect: Within 15-30 minutes

Duration: 4-6 hours

Absorption: Oral: Rapid

Metabolism: Exact fate is unknown

Half-life: 3-7 hours

Time to peak serum concentration: Within 2 hours

**Usual Dosage**

Children:

Oral: 0.6 mg/kg/dose every 6 hours

I.M.: 0.5-1 mg/kg/dose every 4-6 hours as needed

Adults:

Antiemetic: I.M.: 25-100 mg/dose every 4-6 hours as needed

Anxiety: Oral: 25-100 mg 4 times/day; maximum dose: 600 mg/day
Preoperative sedation:
Oral: 50-100 mg
I.M.: 25-100 mg
Management of pruritus: Oral: 25 mg 3-4 times/day

**Dosing interval in hepatic impairment:** Change dosing interval to every 24 hours in patients with primary biliary cirrhosis

**Dietary Considerations** Alcohol: Additive CNS effect, avoid use

**Administration** For I.M. administration in children, injections should be made into the midlateral muscles of the thigh; S.C., intra-arterial, and I.V. administration **not** recommended since thrombosis and digital gangrene can occur

**Monitoring Parameters** Relief of symptoms, mental status, blood pressure

**Reference Range** Plasma hydroxyzine level of 5.6-41.8 µg/dL (13.2-102.0 nmol/L) therapeutic for pruritus in children; peak plasma level is 73 µg/L after 0.7 mg/kg dose in adults

**Patient Information** Will cause drowsiness, avoid alcohol and other CNS depressants, avoid driving and other hazardous tasks until the CNS effects are known

**Nursing Implications** Extravasation can result in sterile abscess and marked tissue induration; provide safety measures (ie, side rails, night light, and call button); remove smoking materials from area; supervise ambulation

**Additional Information**
Hydroxyzine hydrochloride: Anxanil®, Atarax®, Hydroxacen®, Quiess®, Vistaril® injection, Vistazine®
Hydroxyzine pamoate: Hy-Pam®, Vistaril® capsule and suspension

**Dosage Forms**
Hydroxyzine hydrochloride:
Injection: 25 mg/mL (1 mL, 2 mL, 10 mL); 50 mg/mL (1 mL, 2 mL, 10 mL)
Syrup: 10 mg/5 mL (120 mL, 480 mL, 4000 mL)
Tablet: 10 mg, 25 mg, 50 mg, 100 mg
Hydroxyzine pamoate:
Capsule: 25 mg, 50 mg, 100 mg
Suspension, oral: 25 mg/5 mL (120 mL, 480 mL)


♦ **Hydroxyzine Hydrochloride** *see* Hydroxyzine *on page 278*

♦ **Hydroxyzine Pamoate** *see* Hydroxyzine *on page 278*

♦ **Hygroton®** *see* Chlorthalidone *on page 119*

♦ **Hylorel®** *see* Guanadrel *on page 259*

♦ **Hylutin® Injection** *see* Hydroxyprogesterone *on page 277*

♦ **Hyoscine** *see* Scopolamine *on page 506*


## Hyoscyamine (hye oh SYE a meen)

**U.S. Brand Names** Anaspaz®; A-Spas® S/L; Cystospaz®; Cystospaz-M®; Donnamar®; ED-SPAZ®; Gastrosed™; Levbid®; Levsin®; Levsinex®; Levsin/SL®

**Synonyms** *l*-Hyoscyamine Sulfate

**Pharmacologic Category** Anticholinergic Agent

**Use** Treatment of GI tract disorders caused by spasm, adjunctive therapy for peptic ulcers

**Effects on Mental Status** May cause drowsiness; may rarely cause restlessness, amnesia, or delirium

**Effects on Psychiatric Treatment** Concurrent use with psychotropics may produce additive sedation and dry mouth

**Pregnancy Risk Factor** C

**Contraindications** Narrow-angle glaucoma, obstructive uropathy, obstructive GI tract disease, myasthenia gravis, known hypersensitivity to belladonna alkaloids

**Warnings/Precautions** Use with caution in children with spastic paralysis; use with caution in elderly patients. Low doses cause a paradoxical decrease in heart rates. Some commercial products contain sodium metabisulfite, which can cause allergic-type reactions. May accumulate with multiple inhalational administration, particularly in the elderly. Heat prostration may occur in hot weather. Use with caution in patients with autonomic neuropathy, prostatic hypertrophy, hyperthyroidism, congestive heart failure, cardiac arrhythmias, chronic lung disease, biliary tract disease.

**Adverse Reactions**
>10%:
Dermatologic: Dry skin
Gastrointestinal: Dry throat, xerostomia
Local: Irritation at injection site
Respiratory: Dry nose
Miscellaneous: Diaphoresis (decreased)
1% to 10%:
Dermatologic: Photosensitivity
Gastrointestinal: Constipation, dysphagia
Ocular: Blurred vision, mydriasis
<1%: Ataxia, delirium, dysuria, fatigue, headache, increased intraocular pressure, lightheadedness, memory loss, orthostatic hypotension, palpitations, rash, restlessness, tremor

**Overdosage/Toxicology**
Signs and symptoms: Dilated, unreactive pupils; blurred vision; hot, dry flushed skin; dryness of mucous membranes; difficulty in swallowing, foul breath, diminished or absent bowel sounds, urinary retention, tachycardia, hyperthermia, hypertension, increased respiratory rate
Treatment: Anticholinergic toxicity is caused by strong binding of the drug to cholinergic receptors. Anticholinesterase inhibitors reduce acetylcholinesterase, the enzyme that breaks down acetylcholine and thereby allows acetylcholine to accumulate and compete for receptor binding with the offending anticholinergic. For anticholinergic overdose with severe life-threatening symptoms, physostigmine 1-2 mg (0.5 or 0.02 mg/kg for children) S.C. or I.V., slowly may be given to reverse these effects.

**Drug Interactions**
Decreased effect with antacids
Increased toxicity with amantadine, antimuscarinics, haloperidol, phenothiazines, TCAs, MAO inhibitors

**Usual Dosage**
Children: Oral, S.L.: Dose as listed, based on age (y) and weight (kg); repeat dose every 4 hours as needed
Children <2 years:
2.3 kg: 12.5 mcg; maximum 75mcg/24 hours
3.4 kg: 16.7 mcg; maximum 100 mcg/24 hours
5 kg: 20.8 mcg; maximum 125 mcg/24 hours
7 kg: 25 mcg; maximum 150 mcg/24 hours
10 kg: 31.3-33.3 mcg; maximum 200 mcg/24 hours
15 kg: 45.8 mcg; maximum 275 mcg/24 hour
Children 2-10 years:
10 kg: 31.3-33.3 mcg; do not exceed 0.75 mg/24 hours
20 kg: 62.5 mcg; do not exceed 0.75 mg/24 hours
40 kg: 93.8 mcg; do not exceed 0.75 mg/24 hours
50 kg: 125 mcg; do not exceed 0.75 mg/24 hours
Adults:
Oral or S.L.: 0.125-0.25 mg 3-4 times/day before meals or food and at bedtime
Oral: 0.375-0.75 mg (timed release) every 12 hours
I.M., I.V., S.C.: 0.25-0.5 mg every 6 hours

**Patient Information** Take as directed before meals; do not increase dose and do not discontinue without consulting prescriber. Void before taking medication. You may experience dizziness or blurred vision (use caution when driving or engaging in tasks that require alertness until response to drug is known); dry mouth (sucking on lozenges may help); photosensitivity (wear dark glasses in bright sunlight); or impotence (temporary). Report chest pain or palpitations, or excessive and persistent anticholinergic effects (blurred vision, headache, flushing, tachycardia, nervousness, constipation, dizziness, insomnia, mental confusion or excitement, hyperthermia, dry mouth, altered taste perception, dysphagia, palpitations, bradycardia, urinary hesitancy or retention, impotence, decreased sweating).

**Nursing Implications** Observe for tachycardia if patient has cardiac problems.

**Dosage Forms**
Capsule, as sulfate, timed release (Cystospaz-M®, Levsinex®): 0.375 mg
Elixir, as sulfate (Levsin®): 0.125 mg/5 mL with alcohol 20% (480 mL)
Injection, as sulfate (Levsin®): 0.5 mg/mL (1 mL, 10 mL)
Solution, oral (Gastrosed™, Levsin®): 0.125 mg/mL (15 mL)
Tablet, as sulfate:
Anaspaz®, Gastrosed™, Levsin®, Neoquess®: 0.125 mg
Cystospaz®: 0.15 mg
Extended release (Levbid®): 0.375 mg

## Hyoscyamine, Atropine, Scopolamine, and Phenobarbital

(hye oh SYE a meen, A troe peen, skoe POL a meen & fee noe BAR bi tal)

**U.S. Brand Names** Barbidonna®; Bellatal®; Donnatal®; Hyosophen®; Spasmolin®

**Pharmacologic Category** Anticholinergic Agent; Antispasmodic Agent, Gastrointestinal

**Use** Adjunct in treatment of peptic ulcer disease, irritable bowel, spastic colitis, spastic bladder, and renal colic

**Effects on Mental Status** May rarely cause confusion, drowsiness, headache, loss of memory, fatigue, ataxia

**Effects on Psychiatric Treatment** Anticholinergic effects are common and may be increased with concurrent psychotropic use

**Usual Dosage** Oral:
Children 2-12 years: Kinesed® dose: ½ to 1 tablet 3-4 times/day
Children: Donnatal® elixir: 0.1 mL/kg/dose every 4 hours; maximum dose: 5 mL **OR** see below for alternative dose (mL) based on weight (kg):
4.5 kg: 0.5 mL every 4 hours OR 0.75 mL every 6 hours
10 kg: 1 mL every 4 hours OR 1.5 mL every 6 hours
14 kg: 1.5 mL every 4 hours OR 2 mL every 6 hours
(Continued)

## Hyoscyamine, Atropine, Scopolamine, and Phenobarbital *(Continued)*

23 kg: 2.5 mL every 4 hours OR 3.8 mL every 6 hours
34 kg: 3.8 mL every 4 hours OR 5 mL every 6 hours
≥45 kg: 5 mL every 4 hours OR 7.5 mL every 6 hours

Adults: 1-2 capsules or tablets 3-4 times/day; or 1 Donnatal® Extentab® in sustained release form every 12 hours; or 5-10 mL elixir 3-4 times/day or every 8 hours

**Dosage Forms**

Capsule (Donnatal®, Spasmolin®): Hyoscyamine sulfate 0.1037 mg, atropine sulfate 0.0194 mg, scopolamine hydrobromide 0.0065 mg, and phenobarbital 16.2 mg

Elixir (Donnatal®, Hyosophen®, Spasmophen®): Hyoscyamine sulfate 0.1037 mg, atropine sulfate 0.0194 mg, scopolamine hydrobromide 0.0065 mg, and phenobarbital 16.2 mg per 5 mL (120 mL, 480 mL, 4000 mL)

Tablet:

Barbidonna®: Hyoscyamine hydrobromide 0.1286 mg, atropine sulfate 0.025 mg, scopolamine hydrobromide 0.0074 mg, and phenobarbital 16 mg

Barbidonna® No. 2: Hyoscyamine hydrobromide 0.1286 mg, atropine sulfate 0.025 mg, scopolamine hydrobromide 0.0074 mg, and phenobarbital 32 mg

Donnatal®, Hyosophen®: Hyoscyamine sulfate 0.1037 mg, atropine sulfate 0.0194 mg, scopolamine hydrobromide 0.0065 mg, and phenobarbital 16.2 mg

Long-acting (Donnatal®): Hyoscyamine sulfate 0.3111 mg, atropine sulfate 0.0582 mg, scopolamine hydrobromide 0.0195 mg, and phenobarbital 48.6 mg

Spasmophen®: Hyoscyamine sulfate 0.1037 mg, atropine sulfate 0.0194 mg, scopolamine hydrobromide 0.0065 mg, and phenobarbital 15 mg

## Hyoscyamine, Atropine, Scopolamine, Kaolin, and Pectin

(hye oh SYE a meen, A troe peen, skoe POL a meen, KAY oh lin & PEK tin)

**Pharmacologic Category** Anticholinergic Agent; Antidiarrheal

**Use** Antidiarrheal; also used in gastritis, enteritis, colitis, and acute gastrointestinal upsets, and nausea which may accompany any of these conditions

**Effects on Mental Status** None reported

**Effects on Psychiatric Treatment** Anticholinergic effects are common and may be increased with concurrent psychotropic use

**Usual Dosage** Oral:

Children:
10-20 lb: 2.5 mL
20-30 lb: 5 mL
>30 lb: 5-10 mL

Adults:
Diarrhea: 30 mL at once and 15-30 mL with each loose stool
Other conditions: 15 mL every 3 hours as needed

**Dosage Forms** Suspension, oral: Hyoscyamine sulfate 0.1037 mg, atropine sulfate 0.0194 mg, scopolamine hydrobromide 0.0065 mg, kaolin 6 g, and pectin 142.8 mg per 30 mL

## Hyoscyamine, Atropine, Scopolamine, Kaolin, Pectin, and Opium

(hye oh SYE a meen, A troe peen, skoe POL a meen, KAY oh lin, PEK tin, & OH pee um)

**U.S. Brand Names** Donnapectolin-PG®; Kapectolin PG®

**Pharmacologic Category** Anticholinergic Agent; Antidiarrheal

**Use** Treatment of diarrhea

**Effects on Mental Status** May rarely cause confusion, drowsiness, headache, loss of memory, fatigue, ataxia

**Effects on Psychiatric Treatment** Anticholinergic effects are common and may be increased with concurrent psychotropic use

**Restrictions** C-V

**Usual Dosage**

Children 6-12 years: Initial: 10 mL, then, 5-10 mL every 3 hours thereafter

Alternate children's dosing recommendations based on body weight:
10 lb: 2.5 mL
20 lb: 5 mL
≥ 30 lb: 5-10 mL

Do not administer more than 4 doses in any 24-hour period

Children >12 years and Adults: Initial: 30 mL (1 fluid oz) followed by 15 mL every 3 hours

**Dosage Forms** Suspension, oral: Hyoscyamine sulfate 0.1037 mg, atropine sulfate 0.0194 mg, scopolamine hydrobromide 0.0065 mg, kaolin 6 g, pectin 142.8 mg, and powdered opium 24 mg per 30 mL with alcohol 5%


- **Hyosophen®** *see* Hyoscyamine, Atropine, Scopolamine, and Phenobarbital *on page 279*
- **Hy-Pam®** *see* Hydroxyzine *on page 278*
- ***Hypercium perforatum*** *see* St Johns Wort *on page 519*
- **HyperHep®** *see* Hepatitis B Immune Globulin *on page 266*
- **Hyperlipidemia Treatment** *see page 785*
- **Hyperstat® I.V.** *see* Diazoxide *on page 163*
- **Hypertension Treatment** *see page 788*
- **Hy-Phen®** *see* Hydrocodone and Acetaminophen *on page 272*
- **Hypoglycemic Drugs and Thiazolidinedione Information** *see page 714*
- **HypoTears PF Solution [OTC]** *see* Artificial Tears *on page 48*
- **HypoTears Solution [OTC]** *see* Artificial Tears *on page 48*
- **Hyprogest® 250 Injection** *see* Hydroxyprogesterone *on page 277*
- **Hyrexin-50® Injection** *see* Diphenhydramine *on page 174*
- **Hytakerol®** *see* Dihydrotachysterol *on page 171*
- **Hytinic® [OTC]** *see* Polysaccharide-Iron Complex *on page 452*
- **Hytone®** *see* Hydrocortisone *on page 273*
- **Hytrin®** *see* Terazosin *on page 534*
- **Hytuss® [OTC]** *see* Guaifenesin *on page 256*
- **Hytuss-2X® [OTC]** *see* Guaifenesin *on page 256*
- **Hyzaar®** *see* Losartan and Hydrochlorothiazide *on page 327*
- **Hyzine-50®** *see* Hydroxyzine *on page 278*
- **Iberet-Folic-500®** *see* Ferrous Sulfate, Ascorbic Acid, Vitamin B-Complex, and Folic Acid *on page 224*
- **Iberet®-Liquid [OTC]** *see* Ferrous Sulfate, Ascorbic Acid, and Vitamin B-Complex *on page 224*
- **Ibidomide Hydrochloride** *see* Labetalol *on page 304*
- **IBU®** *see* Ibuprofen *on page 280*
- **Ibuprin® [OTC]** *see* Ibuprofen *on page 280*


## Ibuprofen (eye byoo PROE fen)

**Related Information**

Nonsteroidal Anti-inflammatory Agents Comparison Chart *on page 722*

**U.S. Brand Names** Advil® [OTC]; Advil® Migraine Liqui-Gels [OTC]; Bayer® Select® Pain Relief Formula [OTC]; Children's Advil® Oral Suspension [OTC]; Children's Motrin® Oral Suspension [OTC]; Dynafed® IB [OTC]; Genpril® [OTC]; Haltran® [OTC]; IBU®; Ibuprin® [OTC]; Ibuprohm® [OTC]; Junior Strength Motrin® [OTC]; Menadol® [OTC]; Midol® IB [OTC]; Motrin®; Motrin® IB [OTC]; Motrin® Migraine Pain [OTC]; Nuprin® [OTC]; Saleto-200® [OTC]; Saleto-400®; Saleto-600®; Saleto-800®

**Canadian Brand Names** Actiprofen®; Apo®-Ibuprofen; Novo-Profen®; Nu-Ibuprofen

**Synonyms** *p*-Isobutylhydratropic Acid

**Pharmacologic Category** Nonsteroidal Anti-Inflammatory Agent (NSAID)

**Use** Inflammatory diseases and rheumatoid disorders including juvenile rheumatoid arthritis, mild to moderate pain, fever, dysmenorrhea, gout, ankylosing spondylitis, acute migraine headache

**Effects on Mental Status** Drowsiness and dizziness are common; may cause nervousness; may rarely cause insomnia, confusion, hallucinations, or depression

**Effects on Psychiatric Treatment** May rarely cause agranulocytosis; use caution with clozapine and carbamazepine; may decrease lithium clearance resulting in an increase in serum lithium levels and potential lithium toxicity; monitor serum lithium levels

**Pregnancy Risk Factor** B (D if used in the 3rd trimester)

**Contraindications** Hypersensitivity to ibuprofen, any component, aspirin, or other nonsteroidal anti-inflammatory drugs (NSAIDs)

**Warnings/Precautions** Do not exceed 3200 mg/day; use with caution in patients with congestive heart failure, dehydration, hypertension, decreased renal or hepatic function, history of GI disease (bleeding or ulcers), or those receiving anticoagulants; safety and efficacy in children <6 months of age have not yet been established; elderly are a high-risk population for adverse effects from nonsteroidal anti-inflammatory agents. As much as 60% of elderly can develop peptic ulceration and/or hemorrhage asymptomatically.

Use lowest effective dose for shortest period possible. Use of NSAIDs can compromise existing renal function especially when $Cl_{cr}$ is <30 mL/minute. CNS adverse effects such as confusion, agitation, and hallucination are generally seen in overdose or high dose situations; but elderly may demonstrate these adverse effects at lower doses than younger adults.

**Adverse Reactions**

>10%:

Central nervous system: Dizziness, fatigue

Dermatologic: Rash, urticaria
Gastrointestinal: Abdominal cramps, heartburn, indigestion, nausea
1% to 10%:
Central nervous system: Headache, nervousness
Dermatologic: Itching
Endocrine & metabolic: Fluid retention
Gastrointestinal: Dyspepsia, vomiting, abdominal pain, peptic ulcer, GI bleed, GI perforation
Otic: Tinnitus
<1%: Acute renal failure, agranulocytosis, allergic rhinitis, anemia, arrhythmias, aseptic meningitis, blurred vision, bone marrow suppression, confusion, congestive heart failure, conjunctivitis, cystitis, decreased hearing, drowsiness, dry eyes, edema, epistaxis, erythema multiforme, gastritis, GI ulceration, hallucinations, hemolytic anemia, hepatitis, hot flashes, hypertension, inhibition of platelet aggregation, insomnia, leukopenia, mental depression, neutropenia, peripheral neuropathy, polydipsia, polyuria, shortness of breath, Stevens-Johnson syndrome, tachycardia, thrombocytopenia, toxic amblyopia, toxic epidermal necrolysis, vision changes

**Overdosage/Toxicology**
Signs and symptoms: Apnea, metabolic acidosis, coma, and nystagmus; leukocytosis, renal failure
Treatment: Management of a nonsteroidal anti-inflammatory drug (NSAID) intoxication is primarily supportive and symptomatic. Fluid therapy is commonly effective in managing the hypotension that may occur following an acute NSAID overdose, except when this is due to an acute blood loss. Seizures tend to be very short-lived and often do not require drug treatment; although, recurrent seizures should be treated with I.V. diazepam. Since many of the NSAIDs undergo enterohepatic cycling, multiple doses of charcoal may be needed to reduce the potential for delayed toxicities.

**Drug Interactions** CYP2C8 and 2C9 enzyme substrate
ACE inhibitors: Effects may be reduced by NSAIDs; use lowest possible dose for shortest duration possible; monitor
Aspirin: May decrease ibuprofen serum concentrations
Cholestyramine and colestipol: Absorption may be reduced by concurrent administration
Corticosteroids: May increase the risk of GI ulceration; use caution
Cyclosporine: Nephrotoxicity may be increased with concurrent NSAID use; monitor
CYP2C9 inhibitors: May increase in diclofenac concentrations; inhibitors include amiodarone, cimetidine, fluvoxamine, metronidazole, omeprazole, sulfonamides, valproic acid, and zafirlukast
Hydralazine: Antihypertensive effect may be decreased; avoid concurrent use
Lithium: Serum levels can be increased; avoid concurrent use if possible or monitor lithium levels and adjust dose. When NSAID is stopped, lithium may need adjustment again.
Loop diuretics: Therapeutic effects may be reduced by NSAIDs; avoid
Methotrexate: Toxicity may be increased by concurrent NSAID use; risk is limited in low-dose methotrexate regimens (such as for rheumatoid arthritis); prolonged leucovorin rescue may be required at antineoplastic doses; monitor
Thiazide diuretics: Antihypertensive effects are decreased; avoid concurrent use
Warfarin: INRs may be increased by some NSAIDs. This may depend, in part, on dose and duration; monitor INR closely. Use the lowest dose of NSAIDs possible and for the briefest duration.

**Usual Dosage** Oral:
Children:
Antipyretic: 6 months to 12 years: Temperature <102.5°F (39°C): 5 mg/kg/dose; temperature >102.5°F: 10 mg/kg/dose given every 6-8 hours; maximum daily dose: 40 mg/kg/day
Juvenile rheumatoid arthritis: 30-70 mg/kg/24 hours divided every 6-8 hours
<20 kg: Maximum: 400 mg/day
20-30 kg: Maximum: 600 mg/day
30-40 kg: Maximum: 800 mg/day
>40 kg: Adult dosage
Start at lower end of dosing range and titrate upward; maximum: 2.4 g/day
Analgesic: 4-10 mg/kg/dose every 6-8 hours
Adults:
Inflammatory disease: 400-800 mg/dose 3-4 times/day; maximum dose: 3.2 g/day
Analgesia/pain/fever/dysmenorrhea: 200-400 mg/dose every 4-6 hours; maximum daily dose: 1.2 g (unless directed by physician)
**Dosing adjustment/comments in severe hepatic impairment:** Avoid use

**Dietary Considerations** Food: May decrease the rate but not the extent of oral absorption; drug may cause GI upset, bleeding, ulceration, perforation; take with food or milk to minimize GI upset

**Patient Information** If self-administered, use exactly as directed (do not increase dose or frequency); adverse reactions can occur with overuse. Do not take longer than 3 days for fever, or 10 days for pain without consulting medical advisor. Take with food or milk. While using this medication, do not use alcohol, excessive amounts of vitamin C, or salicylate containing foods (curry powder, prunes, raisins, tea, or licorice), other prescription or OTC medications containing aspirin or salicylate, or other NSAIDs without consulting prescriber. Maintain adequate hydration (2-3 L/day of fluids unless instructed to restrict fluid intake). May discolor urine (red/pink). You may experience nausea, vomiting, gastric discomfort (frequent mouth care, small frequent meals, chewing gum, sucking lozenges may help). GI bleeding, ulceration, or perforation can occur with or without pain. Stop taking medication and report ringing in ears; persistent cramping or pain in stomach; unresolved nausea or vomiting; difficulty breathing or shortness of breath; unusual bruising or bleeding (mouth, urine, stool); skin rash; unusual swelling of extremities; chest pain; or palpitations.

**Nursing Implications** Do not crush tablet

**Dosage Forms**
Caplet: 100 mg
Drops, oral (berry flavor): 40 mg/mL (15 mL)
Suspension, oral: 100 mg/5 mL [OTC] (60 mL, 120 mL, 480 mL)
Suspension, oral, drops: 40 mg/mL [OTC]
Tablet: 100 mg [OTC], 200 mg [OTC], 300 mg, 400 mg, 600 mg, 800 mg
Tablet, chewable: 50 mg, 100 mg

♦ **Ibuprohm® [OTC]** *see* Ibuprofen *on page 280*

## Ibutilide (i BYOO ti lide)

**U.S. Brand Names** Corvert®
**Pharmacologic Category** Antiarrhythmic Agent, Class III
**Use** Acute termination of atrial fibrillation or flutter of recent onset; the effectiveness of ibutilide has not been determined in patients with arrhythmias >90 days in duration
**Effects on Mental Status** None reported
**Effects on Psychiatric Treatment** Concurrent use with phenothiazine and antidepressants may produce prolongation of the Q-T interval; use combination with caution; consider a nonphenothiazine antipsychotic
**Usual Dosage** I.V.: Initial:
<60 kg: 0.01 mg/kg over 10 minutes
≥60 kg: 1 mg over 10 minutes
If the arrhythmia does not terminate within 10 minutes after the end of the initial infusion, a second infusion of equal strength may be infused over a 10-minute period
**Dosage Forms** Injection, as fumarate: 0.1 mg/mL (10 mL)

♦ **ICI 204, 219** *see* Zafirlukast *on page 589*

♦ **Idamycin®** *see* Idarubicin *on page 281*

## Idarubicin (eye da ROO bi sin)

**U.S. Brand Names** Idamycin®
**Pharmacologic Category** Antineoplastic Agent, Antibiotic
**Use** In combination treatment of acute myeloid leukemia (AML), this includes classifications M1 through M7 of the French-American-British (FAB) classification system; also used for the treatment of acute lymphocytic leukemia (ALL) in children
**Effects on Mental Status** None reported
**Effects on Psychiatric Treatment** Leukopenia is common; use caution with clozapine and carbamazepine
**Usual Dosage** I.V.:
Children:
Leukemia: 10-12 mg/m² once daily for 3 days and repeat every 3 weeks
Solid tumors: 5 mg/m² once daily for 3 days and repeat every 3 weeks
Adults: 12 mg/m²/day for 3 days by slow (10-15 minutes) intravenous injection in combination with Ara-C
The Ara-C may be given as 100 mg/m²/day by continuous infusion for 7 days or as Ara-C 25 mg/m² bolus followed by Ara-C 200 mg/m²/day for 5 days continuous infusion
**Dosing adjustment in renal impairment:** Dose reduction is recommended
Serum creatinine ≥2 mg/dL: Reduce dose by 25%
Hemodialysis: Significant drug removal is unlikely based on physiochemical characteristics
Peritoneal dialysis: Significant drug removal is unlikely based on physiochemical characteristics
**Dosing adjustment/comments in hepatic impairment:**
Bilirubin 1.5-5.0 mg/dL or AST 60-180 units/L: Reduce dose 50%
Bilirubin >5 mg/dL or AST >180 units/L: Do not administer
**Dosage Forms** Powder for injection, lyophilized, as hydrochloride: 5 mg, 10 mg

♦ **Ifex®** *see* Ifosfamide *on page 281*

## Ifosfamide (eye FOSS fa mide)

**U.S. Brand Names** Ifex®
(Continued)

## Ifosfamide *(Continued)*

**Pharmacologic Category** Antineoplastic Agent, Alkylating Agent

**Use** In combination with certain other antineoplastics in treatment of lung cancer, Hodgkin's and non-Hodgkin's lymphoma, breast cancer, acute and chronic lymphocytic leukemia, ovarian cancer, testicular cancer, and sarcomas, pancreatic and gastric carcinoma, osteosarcoma

**Effects on Mental Status** Sedation, confusion, and hallucinations are common

**Effects on Psychiatric Treatment** May cause myelosuppression; use caution with clozapine and carbamazepine; barbiturates and chloral hydrate may increase the metabolism of ifosfamide

**Usual Dosage** I.V. (refer to individual protocols):

Children: 1200-1800 mg/m²/day for 3-5 days every 21-28 days

Adults:

Doses may be given as 50 mg/kg/day **or** 700-2000 mg/m²/day for 5 days

Alternatives include 2400 mg/m²/day for 3 days **or** 5000 mg/m² as a single dose

Doses of 700-900 mg/m²/day for 5 days may be given IVP; courses may be repeated every 3-4 weeks

To prevent bladder toxicity, ifosfamide should be given with extensive hydration consisting of at least 2 L of oral or I.V. fluid per day. A protector, such as mesna, should also be used to prevent hemorrhagic cystitis. The dose-limiting toxicity is hemorrhagic cystitis and ifosfamide should be used in conjunction with a uroprotective agent.

**Dosing adjustment in renal impairment:**

$S_{cr}$ >3.0 mg/dL: Withhold drug

$S_{cr}$ 2.1-3.0 mg/dL: Reduce dose by 25% to 50%

**Dosing adjustment in hepatic impairment:** Although no specific guidelines are available, it is possible that higher doses are indicated in hepatic disease. One author [Falkson G, et al, "An Extended Phase II Trial of Ifosfamide Plus Mesna in Malignant Mesothelioma," *Invest New Drugs*: 1992;10:337-343.] recommended the following dosage adjustments:

AST >300 or bilirubin >3.0 mg/dL: Decrease ifosfamide dose by 75%

**Dosage Forms** Powder for injection: 1 g, 3 g


- ***Ilex paraguariensis*** *see* Maté *on page 333*
- **Ilopan-Choline® Oral** *see* Dexpanthenol *on page 158*
- **Ilopan® Injection** *see* Dexpanthenol *on page 158*
- **Ilosone® Oral** *see* Erythromycin *on page 200*
- **Ilotycin® Ophthalmic** *see* Erythromycin, Ophthalmic/Topical *on page 202*
- **Ilozyme®** *see* Pancrelipase *on page 418*
- **Imdur™** *see* Isosorbide Mononitrate *on page 297*


## Imiglucerase (imi GLOO ser ase)

**U.S. Brand Names** Cerezyme®

**Pharmacologic Category** Enzyme

**Use** Long-term enzyme replacement therapy for patients with Type 1 Gaucher's disease

**Effects on Mental Status** May cause dizziness

**Effects on Psychiatric Treatment** None reported

**Usual Dosage** I.V.: 2.5 units/kg 3 times a week up to as much as 60 units/kg administered as frequently as once a week or as infrequently as every 4 weeks; 60 units/kg administered every 2 weeks is the most common dose

**Dosage Forms** Powder for injection, preservative free (lyophilized): 212 units [equivalent to a withdrawal dose of 200 units]

## Imipenem and Cilastatin (i mi PEN em & sye la STAT in)

**U.S. Brand Names** Primaxin®

**Pharmacologic Category** Antibiotic, Carbapenem

**Use** Treatment of respiratory tract, urinary tract, intra-abdominal, gynecologic, bone and joint, skin structure, and polymicrobic infections as well as bacterial septicemia and endocarditis. Antibacterial activity includes resistant gram-negative bacilli (*Pseudomonas aeruginosa* and *Enterobacter* sp), gram-positive bacteria (methicillin-sensitive *Staphylococcus aureus* and *Streptococcus* sp) and anaerobes.

**Effects on Mental Status** Reports of encephalopathy

**Effects on Psychiatric Treatment** May rarely cause neutropenia; use caution with clozapine and carbamazepine

**Usual Dosage** Dosing based on imipenem component:

Children: I.V.:

3 months to 3 years: 25 mg/kg every 6 hours; maximum: 2 g/day

≥3 years: 15 mg/kg/every 6 hours

Adults: I.V.:

Mild to moderate infection: 250-500 mg every 6-8 hours

Severe infections with only **moderately susceptible** organisms: 1 g every 6-8 hours

Mild to moderate infection **only**: I.M.: 500-750 mg every 12 hours (**Note:** 750 mg is recommended for intra-abdominal and more severe respiratory, dermatologic, or gynecologic infections; total daily I.M. dosages >1500 mg are not recommended; deep I.M. injection should be carefully made into a large muscle mass only)

**Dosing adjustment in renal impairment:** Dosing based on creatinine clearance (mL/min/1.73 m²). Dose (mg) and frequency listed below:

$Cl_{cr}$ 30-70: 500 mg every 8 hours

$Cl_{cr}$ 20-30: 500 mg every 12 hours

$Cl_{cr}$ 5-20: 250 mg every 12 hours

Hemodialysis: Imipenem (**not cilastatin**) is moderately dialyzable (20% to 50%); administer dose postdialysis

Peritoneal dialysis: Dose as for $Cl_{cr}$ <10 mL/minute

Continuous arteriovenous or venovenous hemofiltration (CAVH/CAVHD): Dose as for $Cl_{cr}$ 20-30 mL/minute; monitor for seizure activity; imipenem is well removed by CAVH but cilastatin is not; removes 20 mg of imipenem per liter of filtrate per day

**Dosage Forms** Powder for injection:

I.M.:

Imipenem 500 mg and cilastatin 500 mg

Imipenem 750 mg and cilastatin 750 mg

I.V.:

Imipenem 250 mg and cilastatin 250 mg

Imipenem 500 mg and cilastatin 500 mg

## Imipramine (im IP ra meen)

**Related Information**


Antidepressant Agents Comparison Chart *on page 704*

Anxiety Disorders *on page 606*

Clinical Issues in the Use of Antidepressants *on page 627*

Discontinuation of Psychotropic Drugs - Withdrawal Symptoms and Recommendations *on page 798*

Federal OBRA Regulations Recommended Maximum Doses *on page 756*

Patient Information - Antidepressants (TCAs) *on page 640*

Pharmacotherapy of Urinary Incontinence *on page 758*

Serum Drug Concentrations Commonly Monitored: Guidelines *on page 759*

Substance-Related Disorders *on page 609*

Teratogenic Risks of Psychotropic Medications *on page 812*


**Generic Available** Yes: Tablet

**U.S. Brand Names** Janimine®; Tofranil®; Tofranil-PM®

**Canadian Brand Names** Apo®-Imipramine; Novo-Pramine; PMS-Imipramine

**Synonyms** Imipramine Hydrochloride; Imipramine Pamoate

**Pharmacologic Category** Antidepressant, Tricyclic (Tertiary Amine)

**Use** Treatment of various forms of depression

**Unlabeled use:** Enuresis in children; analgesic for certain chronic and neuropathic pain; panic disorder

**Pregnancy Risk Factor** D

**Contraindications** Hypersensitivity to imipramine (cross-reactivity with other dibenzodiazepines may occur); use of monoamine oxidase inhibitors within 14 days; use in a patient during the acute recovery phase of MI

**Warnings/Precautions** May cause sedation, resulting in impaired performance of tasks requiring alertness (ie, operating machinery or driving). Sedative effects may be additive with other CNS depressants and/or ethanol. The degree of sedation is high relative to other antidepressants. May worsen psychosis in some patients or precipitate a shift to mania or hypomania in patients with bipolar disease. May increase the risks associated with electroconvulsive therapy. This agent should be discontinued, when possible, prior to elective surgery. Therapy should not be abruptly discontinued in patients receiving high doses for prolonged periods.

May cause orthostatic hypotension (risk is very high relative to other antidepressants) - use with caution in patients at risk of hypotension or in patients where transient hypotensive episodes would be poorly tolerated (cardiovascular disease or cerebrovascular disease). The degree of anticholinergic blockade produced by this agent is high relative to other cyclic antidepressants - use caution in patients with urinary retention, benign prostatic hypertrophy, narrow-angle glaucoma, xerostomia, visual problems, constipation, or history of bowel obstruction.

Use caution in patients with depression, particularly if suicidal risk may be present. Use with caution in patients with a history of cardiovascular disease (including previous MI, stroke, tachycardia, or conduction abnormalities). The risk of conduction abnormalities with this agent is high relative to other antidepressants. EKG monitoring is recommended if high dosages are used. Use caution in patients with a previous seizure disorder or condition predisposing to seizures such as brain damage, alcoholism, or concurrent therapy with other drugs which lower the seizure threshold. Use with caution in hyperthyroid patients or those receiving thyroid supplementation. Use with caution in patients with hepatic or renal dysfunction and in elderly patients. Has been associated with photosensitization.

**Adverse Reactions**

Cardiovascular: Orthostatic hypotension, arrhythmias, tachycardia, hypertension, palpitations, myocardial infarction, heart block, EKG changes, CHF, stroke

Central nervous system: Dizziness, drowsiness, headache, agitation, insomnia, nightmares, hypomania, psychosis, fatigue, confusion, hallucinations, disorientation, delusions, anxiety, restlessness, seizures

Endocrine & metabolic: Gynecomastia, breast enlargement, galactorrhea, increase or decrease in libido, increase or decrease in blood sugar, SIADH

Gastrointestinal: Nausea, unpleasant taste, weight gain, xerostomia, constipation, ileus, stomatitis, abdominal cramps, vomiting, anorexia, epigastric disorders, diarrhea, black tongue, weight loss

Genitourinary: Urinary retention, impotence

Neuromuscular & skeletal: Weakness, numbness, tingling, paresthesias, incoordination, ataxia, tremor, peripheral neuropathy, extrapyramidal symptoms

Ocular: Blurred vision, disturbances of accommodation, mydriasis

Otic: Tinnitus

Miscellaneous: Diaphoresis

<1%: Agranulocytosis, alopecia, cholestatic jaundice, eosinophilia, increased liver enzymes, itching, petechiae, photosensitivity, purpura, rash, thrombocytopenia, urticaria

**Overdosage/Toxicology**

Signs and symptoms: Confusion, hallucinations, constipation, cyanosis, tachycardia, urinary retention, ventricular tachycardia, seizures

Treatment: Following initiation of essential overdose management, toxic symptoms should be treated. Ventricular arrhythmias often respond to concurrent systemic alkalinization (sodium bicarbonate 0.5-2 mEq/kg I.V.). Arrhythmias unresponsive to this therapy may respond to lidocaine 1 mg/kg I.V. followed by a titrated infusion. Physostigmine (1-2 mg I.V. slowly for adults or 0.5 mg I.V. slowly for children) may be indicated in reversing cardiac arrhythmias that are life-threatening. Seizures usually respond to diazepam I.V. boluses (5-10 mg for adults up to 30 mg or 0.25-0.4 mg/kg/dose for children up to 10 mg/dose). If seizures are unresponsive or recur, phenytoin or phenobarbital may be required.

**Drug Interactions** CYP1A2, 2C9, 2C19, 2D6, and 3A3/4 enzyme substrate

Altretamine: Concurrent use may cause orthostatic hypertension

Amphetamines: TCAs may enhance the effect of amphetamines; monitor for adverse CV effects

Anticholinergics: Combined use with TCAs may produce additive anticholinergic effects

Antihypertensives: TCAs may inhibit the antihypertensive response to bethanidine, clonidine, debrisoquin, guanadrel, guanethidine, guanabenz, guanfacine; monitor BP; consider alternate antihypertensive agent

Beta-agonists: When combined with TCAs may predispose patients to cardiac arrhythmias

Bupropion: May increase the levels of tricyclic antidepressants; based on limited information; monitor response

Carbamazepine: Tricyclic antidepressants may increase carbamazepine levels; monitor

Cholestyramine and colestipol: May bind TCAs and reduce their absorption; monitor for altered response

Clonidine: Abrupt discontinuation of clonidine may cause hypertensive crisis, amitriptyline may enhance the response

CNS depressants: Amitriptyline may be additive with or may potentiate sedation; sedative effects may be additive with TCAs; monitor for increased effect; includes benzodiazepines, barbiturates, antipsychotics, ethanol and other sedative medications

CYP2C8/9 inhibitors: Serum levels and/or toxicity of some tricyclic antidepressants may be increased; inhibitors include amiodarone, cimetidine, fluvoxamine, some NSAIDs, metronidazole, ritonavir, sulfonamides, troglitazone, valproic acid, and zafirlukast; monitor for increased effect/ toxicity

CYP2D6 inhibitors: Serum levels and/or toxicity of some tricyclic antidepressants may be increased; inhibitors include amiodarone, cimetidine, delavirdine, fluoxetine, paroxetine, propafenone, quinidine, and ritonavir; monitor for increased effect/toxicity

CYP3A3/4 inhibitors: Serum level and/or toxicity of some tricyclic antidepressants may be increased; inhibitors include amiodarone, cimetidine, clarithromycin, erythromycin, delavirdine, diltiazem, dirithromycin, disulfiram, fluoxetine, fluvoxamine, grapefruit juice, indinavir, itraconazole, ketoconazole, nefazodone, nevirapine, propoxyfene, quinupristin-dalfopristin, ritonavir, saquinavir, verapamil, zafirlukast, zileuton; monitor for altered effects; a decrease in TCA dosage may be required

Enzyme inducers: May increase the metabolism of TCAs resulting in decreased effect; includes carbamazepine, phenobarbital, phenytoin, and rifampin; monitor for decreased response

Epinephrine (and other direct alpha-agonists): The pressor response to I.V. epinephrine, norepinephrine, and phenylephrine may be enhanced in patients receiving TCAs; this combination is best avoided

Fenfluramine: May increase tricyclic antidepressant levels/effects

Hypoglycemic agents (including insulin): TCAs may enhance the hypoglycemic effects of tolazamide, chlorpropamide, or insulin; monitor for changes in blood glucose levels; reported with chlorpropamide, tolazamide, and insulin

Levodopa: Tricyclic antidepressants may decrease the absorption (bioavailability) of levodopa; rare hypertensive episodes have also been attributed to this combination

Linezolid: Hyperpyrexia, hypertension, tachycardia, confusion, seizures, and **deaths have been reported** with agents which inhibit MAO (serotonin syndrome); this combination should be avoided

Lithium: Concurrent use with a TCA may increase the risk for neurotoxicity

MAO inhibitors: Hyperpyrexia, hypertension, tachycardia, confusion, seizures, and **deaths have been reported** (serotonin syndrome); this combination should be avoided

Methylphenidate: Metabolism of TCAs may be decreased

Phenothiazines: Serum concentrations of some TCAs may be increased; in addition, TCAs may increase concentration of phenothiazines; monitor for altered clinical response

QTc prolonging agents: Concurrent use of tricyclic agents with other drugs which may prolong QTc interval may increase the risk of potentially fatal arrhythmias; includes type Ia and type III antiarrhythmics agents, selected quinolones (sparfloxacin, gatifloxacin, moxifloxacin, grepafloxacin), cisapride, and other agents

Sucralfate: Absorption of tricyclic antidepressants may be reduced with coadministration

Sympathomimetics, indirect-acting: Tricyclic antidepressants may result in a decreased sensitivity to indirect-acting sympathomimetics; includes dopamine and ephedrine; also see interaction with epinephrine (and direct-acting sympathomimetics)

Valproic acid: May increase serum concentrations/adverse effects of some tricyclic antidepressants

Warfarin (and other oral anticoagulants): TCAs may increase the anticoagulant effect in patients stabilized on warfarin; monitor INR

**Stability** Solutions stable at a pH of 4-5; turns yellowish or reddish on exposure to light. Slight discoloration does not affect potency; marked discoloration is associated with loss of potency. Capsules stable for 3 years following date of manufacture.

**Mechanism of Action** Traditionally believed to increase the synaptic concentration of serotonin and/or norepinephrine in the central nervous system by inhibition of their reuptake by the presynaptic neuronal membrane. However, additional receptor effects have been found including desensitization of adenyl cyclase, down regulation of beta-adrenergic receptors, and down regulation of serotonin receptors.

**Pharmacodynamics/kinetics**

Peak antidepressant effect: Usually ≥2 weeks

Absorption: Oral: Well absorbed

Distribution: Crosses the placenta

Metabolism: In the liver by microsomal enzymes to desipramine (active) and other metabolites; significant first-pass metabolism

Half-life: 6-18 hours

Elimination: Almost all compounds following metabolism are excreted in urine

**Usual Dosage**

Children: Oral:

Depression: 1.5 mg/kg/day with dosage increments of 1 mg/kg every 3-4 days to a maximum dose of 5 mg/kg/day in 1-4 divided doses; monitor carefully especially with doses ≥3.5 mg/kg/day

Enuresis: ≥6 years: Initial: 10-25 mg at bedtime, if inadequate response still seen after 1 week of therapy, increase by 25 mg/day; dose should not exceed 2.5 mg/kg/day or 50 mg at bedtime if 6-12 years of age or 75 mg at bedtime if ≥12 years of age

Adjunct in the treatment of cancer pain: Initial: 0.2-0.4 mg/kg at bedtime; dose may be increased by 50% every 2-3 days up to 1-3 mg/kg/dose at bedtime

Adolescents: Oral: Initial: 25-50 mg/day; increase gradually; maximum: 100 mg/day in single or divided doses

Adults:

Oral: Initial: 25 mg 3-4 times/day, increase dose gradually, total dose may be given at bedtime; maximum: 300 mg/day

I.M.: Initial: Up to 100 mg/day in divided doses; change to oral as soon as possible

Elderly: Initial: 10-25 mg at bedtime; increase by 10-25 mg every 3 days for inpatients and weekly for outpatients if tolerated; average daily dose to achieve a therapeutic concentration: 100 mg/day; range: 50-150 mg/day

**Dietary Considerations** Alcohol: Additive CNS effect, avoid use

**Monitoring Parameters** Monitor blood pressure and pulse rate prior to and during initial therapy; EKG in older adults, CBC; evaluate mental status

**Reference Range** Therapeutic: Imipramine and desipramine: 150-250 ng/mL (SI: 530-890 nmol/L); desipramine: 150-300 ng/mL (SI: 560-1125 nmol/L); Toxic: >500 ng/mL (SI: 446-893 nmol/L); utility of serum level monitoring controversial

**Test Interactions** ↑ glucose

**Patient Information** May require 4-6 weeks to achieve desired effect; avoid alcohol ingestion; do not discontinue medication abruptly; may cause urine to turn blue-green; may cause drowsiness, avoid alcohol and other CNS depressants; dry mouth may be helped by sips of water, sugarless gum, or hard candy; rise slowly to avoid dizziness

(Continued)

## Imipramine *(Continued)*

**Nursing Implications** Raise bed rails, institute safety measures

**Dosage Forms**

Capsule, as pamoate (Tofranil-PM®): 75 mg, 100 mg, 125 mg, 150 mg

Injection, as hydrochloride (Tofranil®): 12.5 mg/mL (2 mL)

Tablet, as hydrochloride (Janimine®, Tofranil®): 10 mg, 25 mg, 50 mg

♦ **Imipramine Hydrochloride** *see* Imipramine *on page 282*

♦ **Imipramine Pamoate** *see* Imipramine *on page 282*

## Imiquimod (i mi KWI mod)

**U.S. Brand Names** Aldara™

**Pharmacologic Category** Skin and Mucous Membrane Agent; Topical Skin Product

**Use** Treatment of external genital and perianal warts/condyloma acuminata in adults

**Effects on Mental Status** None reported

**Effects on Psychiatric Treatment** None reported

**Usual Dosage** Adults: Topical: Apply 3 times/week prior to normal sleeping hours and leave on the skin for 6-10 hours. Following treatment period, remove cream by washing the treated area with mild soap and water. Examples of 3 times/week application schedules are: Monday, Wednesday, Friday; or Tuesday, Thursday, Saturday. Continue imiquimod treatment until there is total clearance of the genital/perianal warts for ≤16 weeks. A rest period of several days may be taken if required by the patient's discomfort or severity of the local skin reaction. Treatment may resume once the reaction subsides.

Nonocclusive dressings such as cotton gauze or cotton underwear may be used in the management of skin reactions. Handwashing before and after cream application is recommended. Imiquimod is packaged in single-use packets that contain sufficient cream to cover a wart area of up to 20 $cm^2$; avoid use of excessive amounts of cream. Instruct patients to apply imiquimod to external or perianal warts. Apply a thin layer to the wart area and rub in until the cream is no longer visible. Do not occlude the application site.

**Dosage Forms** Cream, topical: 5% (250 mg single dose packets in boxes of 12)

♦ **Imitrex®** *see* Sumatriptan *on page 528*

## Immune Globulin, Intramuscular

(i MYUN GLOB yoo lin, IN tra MUS kyoo ler)

**Pharmacologic Category** Immune Globulin

**Use** Household and sexual contacts of persons with hepatitis A, measles, varicella, and possibly rubella; travelers to high-risk areas outside tourist routes; staff, attendees, and parents of diapered attendees in day-care center outbreaks

For travelers, IG is not an alternative to careful selection of foods and water; immune globulin can interfere with the antibody response to parenterally administered live virus vaccines. Frequent travelers should be tested for hepatitis A antibody, immune hemolytic anemia, and neutropenia (with ITP, I.V. route is usually used).

**Effects on Mental Status** None reported

**Effects on Psychiatric Treatment** None reported

**Usual Dosage** I.M.:

Hepatitis A:

Pre-exposure prophylaxis upon travel into endemic areas (hepatitis A vaccine preferred):

0.02 mL/kg for anticipated risk 1-3 months

0.06 mL/kg for anticipated risk >3 months

Repeat approximate dose every 4-6 months if exposure continues

Postexposure prophylaxis: 0.02 mL/kg given within 2 weeks of exposure

Measles:

Prophylaxis: 0.25 mL/kg/dose (maximum dose: 15 mL) given within 6 days of exposure followed by live attenuated measles vaccine in 3 months or at 15 months of age (whichever is later)

For patients with leukemia, lymphoma, immunodeficiency disorders, generalized malignancy, or receiving immunosuppressive therapy: 0.5 mL/kg (maximum dose: 15 mL)

Poliomyelitis: Prophylaxis: 0.3 mL/kg/dose as a single dose

Rubella: Prophylaxis: 0.55 mL/kg/dose within 72 hours of exposure

Varicella:: Prophylaxis: 0.6-1.2 mL/kg (varicella zoster immune globulin preferred) within 72 hours of exposure

IgG deficiency: 1.3 mL/kg, then 0.66 mL/kg in 3-4 weeks

Hepatitis B: Prophylaxis: 0.06 mL/kg/dose (HBIG preferred)

**Dosage Forms** Injection: I.M.: 165±15 mg (of protein)/mL (2 mL, 10 mL)

## Immune Globulin, Intravenous

(i MYUN GLOB yoo lin, IN tra VEE nus)

**U.S. Brand Names** Gamimune® N; Gammagard®; Gammagard® S/D; Gammar®-P I.V.; Polygam® S/D; Sandoglobulin®; Venoglobulin®-I; Venoglobulin®-S

**Pharmacologic Category** Immune Globulin

**Use** Treatment of immunodeficiency sufficiency (hypogammaglobulinemia, agammaglobulinemia, IgG subclass deficiencies, severe combined immunodeficiency syndromes (SCIDS), Wiskott-Aldrich syndrome), idiopathic thrombocytopenic purpura; used in conjunction with appropriate anti-infective therapy *to prevent or modify acute bacterial or viral infections* in patients with iatrogenically-induced or disease-associated immunodepression; *chronic lymphocytic leukemia (CLL) - chronic prophylaxis autoimmune neutropenia, bone marrow transplantation patients, autoimmune hemolytic anemia or neutropenia, refractory dermatomyositis/polymyositis, autoimmune diseases* (myasthenia gravis, SLE, bullous pemphigoid, severe rheumatoid arthritis), Guillain-Barré syndrome; pediatric HIV infection to decrease frequency of serious bacterial infections

**Effects on Mental Status** None reported

**Effects on Psychiatric Treatment** None reported

**Usual Dosage** Children and Adults: I.V.:

**Dosages should be based on ideal body weight** and not actual body weight in morbidly obese patients; approved doses and regimens may vary between brands; check manufacturer guidelines

Primary immunodeficiency disorders: 200-400 mg/kg every 4 weeks or as per monitored serum IgG concentrations

Chronic lymphocytic leukemia (CLL): 400 mg/kg/dose every 3 weeks

Idiopathic thrombocytopenic purpura (ITP): Maintenance dose:

400 mg/kg/day for 2-5 consecutive days; or 1000 mg/kg every other day for 3 doses, if needed or

1000 mg/kg/day for 2 consecutive days; or up to 2000 mg/kg/day over 2-7 consecutive days

Chronic ITP: 400-2000 mg/kg/dose as needed to maintain appropriate platelet counts

Kawasaki disease:

400 mg/kg/day for 4 days within 10 days of onset of fever

800 mg/kg/day for 1-2 days within 10 days of onset of fever

2 g/kg for one dose only

Acquired immunodeficiency syndrome (patients must be symptomatic):

200-250 mg/kg/dose every 2 weeks

400-500 mg/kg/dose every month or every 4 weeks

Pediatric HIV: 400 mg/kg every 28 days

Autoimmune hemolytic anemia and neutropenia: 1000 mg/kg/dose for 2-3 days

Autoimmune diseases: 400 mg/kg/day for 4 days

Bone marrow transplant: 500 mg/kg beginning on days 7 and 2 pretransplant, then 500 mg/kg/week for 90 days post-transplant

Adjuvant to severe cytomegalovirus infections: 500 mg/kg/dose every other day for 7 doses

Severe systemic viral and bacterial infections: Children: 500-1000 mg/kg/week

Prevention of gastroenteritis: Infants and Children: Oral: 50 mg/kg/day divided every 6 hours

Guillain-Barré syndrome:

400 mg/kg/day for 4 days

1000 mg/kg/day for 2 days

2000 mg/kg/day for one day

Refractory dermatomyositis: 2 g/kg/dose every month x 3-4 doses

Refractory polymyositis: 1 g/kg/day x 2 days every month x 4 doses

Chronic inflammatory demyelinating polyneuropathy:

400 mg/kg/day for 5 doses once each month

800 mg/kg/day for 3 doses once each month

1000 mg/kg/day for 2 days once each month

**Dosing adjustment/comments in renal impairment:** $Cl_{cr}$ <10 mL/minute: Avoid use

**Dosage Forms**

Injection: Gamimune® N: 5% [50 mg/mL] (10 mL, 50 mL, 100 mL, 250 mL); 10% [100 mg/mL] (10 mL, 50 mL, 100 mL, 200 mL)

Powder for injection, lyophilized:

Gammar®-P I.V. (5% IgG and 3% albumin): 1 g, 2.5 g, 5 g, 10 g

Polygam®: 0.5 g, 2.5 g, 5 g, 10 g

Sandoglobulin®: 1 g, 3 g, 6 g, 12 g

Venoglobulin®-I: 0.5 g, 2.5 g, 5 g, 10 g

Detergent treated:

Gammagard® S/D: 2.5 g, 5 g, 10 g

Polygam® S/D: 2.5 g, 5 g, 10 g

Venoglobulin®-S: 5% [50 mg/mL] (50 mL, 100 mL, 200 mL); 10% [100 mg/mL] (50 mL, 100 mL, 200 mL)

♦ **Imodium®** *see* Loperamide *on page 324*

♦ **Imodium® A-D [OTC]** *see* Loperamide *on page 324*

♦ **Impulse Control Disorders** *see page 622*

♦ **Imuran®** *see* Azathioprine *on page 55*

## Inamrinone (eye NAM ri none)

**U.S. Brand Names** Inocor®

**Pharmacologic Category** Phosphodiesterase Enzyme Inhibitor

**Use** Infrequently used as a last resort, short-term therapy in patients with intractable heart failure

**Effects on Mental Status** None reported

**Effects on Psychiatric Treatment** May cause hypotension which may be exacerbated by psychotropics

**Usual Dosage** Dosage is based on clinical response (**Note:** Dose should not exceed 10 mg/kg/24 hours).

Infants, Children, and Adults: 0.75 mg/kg I.V. bolus over 2-3 minutes followed by maintenance infusion of 5-10 mcg/kg/minute; I.V. bolus may need to be repeated in 30 minutes.

**Dosing adjustment in renal failure:** $Cl_{cr}$ <10 mL/minute: Administer 50% to 75% of dose.

**Dosage Forms** Injection, as lactate: 5 mg/mL (20 mL)

♦ **I-Naphline® Ophthalmic** *see* Naphazoline *on page 000*

♦ **Inapsine®** *see* Droperidol *on page 187*

## Indapamide (in DAP a mide)

**U.S. Brand Names** Lozol®

**Canadian Brand Names** Apo®-Indapadmide; Lozide®

**Pharmacologic Category** Diuretic, Thiazide

**Use** Management of mild to moderate hypertension; treatment of edema in congestive heart failure and nephrotic syndrome

**Effects on Mental Status** May rarely cause mood changes

**Effects on Psychiatric Treatment** May decrease lithium clearance resulting in an increase in serum lithium levels and potential lithium toxicity; monitor serum lithium levels

**Pregnancy Risk Factor** B (per manufacturer); D (based on expert analysis)

**Contraindications** Hypersensitivity to indapamide or any component, thiazides, or sulfonamide-derived drugs; anuria; renal decompensation; pregnancy (based on expert analysis)

**Warnings/Precautions** Use with caution in severe renal disease. Electrolyte disturbances (hypokalemia, hypochloremic alkalosis, hyponatremia) can occur. Use with caution in severe hepatic dysfunction; hepatic encephalopathy can be caused by electrolyte disturbances. Gout can be precipitate in certain patients with a history of gout, a familial predisposition to gout, or chronic renal failure. Cautious use in diabetics; may see a change in glucose control. I.V. use is generally not recommended (but is available). Hypersensitivity reactions can occur. Can cause SLE exacerbation or activation. Use with caution in patients with moderate or high cholesterol concentrations. Photosensitization may occur. Correct hypokalemia before initiating therapy.

**Adverse Reactions**

1% to 10%: Endocrine & metabolic: Hypokalemia

<1%: Arrhythmia, fluid and electrolyte imbalances (hypocalcemia, hypomagnesemia, hyponatremia), hyperglycemia, hypotension, increased thirst, mood changes, numbness or paresthesia in hands, feet or lips, muscle cramps or pain, photosensitivity, prerenal azotemia, rarely blood dyscrasias, shortness of breath, unusual weakness, weak pulse, xerostomia

**Overdosage/Toxicology**

Signs and symptoms: Lethargy, diuresis, hypermotility, confusion, muscle weakness

Treatment: Following GI decontamination, therapy is supportive with I.V. fluids, electrolytes, and I.V. pressors if needed

**Drug Interactions**

Angiotensin-converting enzyme inhibitors: Increased hypotension if aggressively diuresed with a thiazide diuretic

Beta-blockers increase hyperglycemic effects in Type 2 diabetes mellitus

Cyclosporine and thiazides can increase the risk of gout or renal toxicity; avoid concurrent use

Digoxin toxicity can be exacerbated if a thiazide induces hypokalemia or hypomagnesemia

Lithium toxicity can occur by reducing renal excretion of lithium; monitor lithium concentration and adjust as needed

Neuromuscular blocking agents can prolong blockade; monitor serum potassium and neuromuscular status

NSAIDs can decrease the efficacy of thiazides reducing the diuretic and antihypertensive effects

**Usual Dosage** Adults: Oral:

Edema: 2.5-5 mg/day. **Note:** There is little therapeutic benefit to increasing the dose >5 mg/day; there is, however, an increased risk of electrolyte disturbances

Hypertension: 1.25 mg in the morning, may increase to 5 mg/day by increments of 1.25-2.5 mg; consider adding another antihypertensive and decreasing the dose if response is not adequate

**Patient Information** Take as directed, early in the day (last dose late afternoon). Do not exceed recommended dosage. Noninsulin-dependent diabetics should monitor serum glucose closely (medication may decrease effect of oral hypoglycemics). Monitor weight on a regular basis. Report sudden or excessive weight gain, swelling of ankles or hands, or difficulty breathing. You may experience dizziness, weakness, or drowsiness; use caution when changing position (rising from sitting or lying position) and when driving or engaging in tasks that require alertness until response to drug is known. Use may experience sensitivity to sunlight (use sunblock, wear protective clothing or sunglasses), impotence (reversible), dry mouth or thirst (frequent mouth care, chewing gum or sucking on lozenges may help). Report unusual bleeding, palpitations, numbness or tingling or cramping.

**Nursing Implications** Take blood pressure with patient lying down and standing; may increase serum glucose in diabetic patients

**Dosage Forms** Tablet: 1.25 mg, 2.5 mg

♦ **Inderal®** *see* Propranolol *on page 475*

♦ **Inderal® LA** *see* Propranolol *on page 475*

♦ **Inderide®** *see* Propranolol and Hydrochlorothiazide *on page 476*

♦ **Indian Eye: Orange Root** *see* Golden Seal *on page 254*

♦ **Indian Head** *see* Echinacea *on page 189*

## Indinavir (in DIN a veer)

**Related Information**

Protease Inhibitors *on page 724*

**U.S. Brand Names** Crixivan®

**Pharmacologic Category** Antiretroviral Agent, Protease Inhibitor

**Use** Treatment of HIV infection; should always be used as part of a multidrug regimen (at least three antiretroviral agents)

**Effects on Mental Status** May cause insomnia; may rarely cause dizziness or drowsiness

**Effects on Psychiatric Treatment** Contraindicated with midazolam and triazolam; use caution with other benzodiazepines; may produce additive sedation and respiratory depression

**Pregnancy Risk Factor** C

**Contraindications** Hypersensitivity to the drug or its components

**Warnings/Precautions** Because indinavir may cause nephrolithiasis/urolithiasis the drug should be discontinued if signs and symptoms occur. Indinavir should not be administered concurrently with terfenadine, astemizole, cisapride, lovastatin, simvastatin, triazolam, and midazolam because of competition for metabolism of these drugs through the CYP3A4 system, and potential serious or life-threatening events. Patients with hepatic insufficiency due to cirrhosis should have dose reduction. Warn patients about fat redistribution that can occur.

**Adverse Reactions** Protease inhibitors cause dyslipidemia which includes elevated cholesterol and triglycerides and a redistribution of body fat centrally to cause "protease paunch", buffalo hump, facial atrophy, and breast enlargement. These agents also cause hyperglycemia.

1% to 10%:

Central nervous system: Headache (5.6%), insomnia (3.1%)

Gastrointestinal: Mild elevation of indirect bilirubin (10%), abdominal pain (8.7%), nausea (11.7%), diarrhea/vomiting (4% to 5%), taste perversion (2.6%)

Neuromuscular & skeletal: Weakness (3.6%), flank pain (2.6%)

Renal: Kidney stones (2% to 3%)

<1%: Anorexia, decreased hemoglobin, dizziness, malaise, somnolence, xerostomia

**Drug Interactions** CYP3A3/4 enzyme substrate; CYP3A3/4 enzyme inhibitor

Decreased effect: Concurrent use of rifampin and rifabutin may decrease the effectiveness of indinavir (dosage increase of indinavir is recommended), dosage decreases of rifampin/rifabutin are recommended; the efficacy of protease inhibitors may be decreased when given with nevirapine or efavirenz.

Increased toxicity: Gastric pH is lowered and absorption may be decreased when didanosine and indinavir are taken <1 hour apart; a reduction of dose is often required when coadministered with ketoconazole; astemizole and cisapride should be avoided with indinavir due to life-threatening cardiotoxicity; benzodiazepines with indinavir may result in prolonged sedation and respiratory depression; ketoconazole, itraconazole, nelfinavir, ritonavir, and delavirdine increased indinavir levels. Indinavir inhibits the metabolism of HMG-CoA reductase inhibitors (atorvastatin, cerivastatin, lovastatin, simvastatin) which increases the risk of myopathy. Indinavir increases the AUC of amprenavir.

**Drug-Herb interactions:** St John's wort (hypericum) appears to induce CYP3A enzymes and has lead to 57% reductions in indinavir AUCs and 81% reductions in trough serum concentrations, which may lead to treatment failures

**Usual Dosage** Adults: Oral: 800 mg every 8 hours

(Continued)

## Indinavir *(Continued)*

**Dosage adjustment in hepatic impairment:** 600 mg every 8 hours with mild/medium impairment due to cirrhosis or with ketoconazole coadministration

**Dietary Considerations** Meals high in calories, fat, and protein result in a significant decrease in drug levels; grapefruit juice may decrease indinavir's AUC

**Patient Information** Take as directed, around-the-clock, with a large glass of water, preferably 1 hour before or 2 hours after meals. Maintain adequate hydration (2-3 L/day of fluids unless instructed to restrict fluid intake). If indinavir and didanosine are prescribed together, take at least 1 hour apart on an empty stomach.

**Nursing Implications** Administer around-the-clock to avoid significant fluctuation in serum levels; administer with plenty of water

**Dosage Forms** Capsule: 200 mg, 333 mg, 400 mg


♦ **Indochron E-R®** *see* Indomethacin *on page 286*

♦ **Indocin®** *see* Indomethacin *on page 286*

♦ **Indocin® I.V.** *see* Indomethacin *on page 286*

♦ **Indocin® SR** *see* Indomethacin *on page 286*

♦ **Indometacin** *see* Indomethacin *on page 286*


## Indomethacin (in doe METH a sin)

**Related Information**

Nonsteroidal Anti-inflammatory Agents Comparison Chart *on page 722*

**U.S. Brand Names** Indochron E-R®; Indocin®; Indocin® I.V.; Indocin® SR

**Canadian Brand Names** Apo®-Indomethacin; Indocid®; Indocid® SR; Novo-Methacin; Nu-Indo; Pro-Indo®

**Synonyms** Indometacin; Indomethacin Sodium Trihydrate

**Pharmacologic Category** Nonsteroidal Anti-Inflammatory Agent (NSAID)

**Use** Management of inflammatory diseases and rheumatoid disorders; moderate pain; acute gouty arthritis; I.V. form used as alternative to surgery for closure of patent ductus arteriosus in neonates

**Effects on Mental Status** Dizziness is common; may cause nervousness; may rarely cause sedation, confusion, depression, and hallucinations

**Effects on Psychiatric Treatment** May cause bone marrow suppression; use caution with clozapine and carbamazepine; may decrease lithium clearance resulting in an increase in serum lithium levels and potential lithium toxicity; monitor serum lithium levels

**Pregnancy Risk Factor** B (D if used longer than 48 hours or after 34-week gestation)

**Contraindications** Hypersensitivity to indomethacin, any component, aspirin, or other nonsteroidal anti-inflammatory drugs (NSAIDs); active GI bleeding, ulcer disease; premature neonates with necrotizing enterocolitis, impaired renal function, active bleeding, thrombocytopenia

**Warnings/Precautions** Use with caution in patients with cardiac dysfunction, dehydration, hypertension, renal or hepatic impairment, epilepsy, history of GI bleeding, patients receiving anticoagulants, and for treatment of JRA in children (fatal hepatitis has been reported); may have adverse effects on fetus; may affect platelet and renal function in neonates; elderly are a high-risk population for adverse effects from nonsteroidal anti-inflammatory agents. As much as 60% of elderly can develop peptic ulceration and/or hemorrhage asymptomatically.

Use lowest effective dose for shortest period possible. Use of NSAIDs can compromise existing renal function especially when $Cl_{cr}$ is <30 mL/minute.

CNS adverse effects such as confusion, agitation, and hallucination are generally seen in overdose or high-dose situations; but elderly may demonstrate these adverse effects at lower doses than younger adults.

**Adverse Reactions**

>10%:
- Central nervous system: Dizziness
- Dermatologic: Rash
- Gastrointestinal: Nausea, epigastric pain, abdominal pain, anorexia, GI bleeding, ulcers, perforation, abdominal cramps, heartburn, indigestion

1% to 10%:
- Central nervous system: Headache, nervousness
- Dermatologic: Itching
- Endocrine & metabolic: Fluid retention
- Gastrointestinal: Vomiting
- Otic: Tinnitus

<1%: Agranulocytosis, allergic rhinitis, anemia, angioedema, arrhythmias, aseptic meningitis, blurred vision, bone marrow suppression, confusion, congestive heart failure, conjunctivitis, corneal opacities, cystitis, decreased hearing, depression, dilutional hyponatremia (I.V.), drowsiness, dry eyes, epistaxis, erythema multiforme, fatigue, gastritis, GI ulceration, hallucinations, hemolytic anemia, hepatitis, hot flashes, hyperkalemia, hypersensitivity reactions, hypertension, hypoglycemia (I.V.), inhibition of platelet aggregation, leukopenia, oliguria, peripheral neuropathy, polydipsia, polyuria, renal failure, shortness of breath, somnolence, Stevens-Johnson syndrome, tachycardia, thrombocytopenia, toxic amblyopia, toxic epidermal necrolysis, urticaria

**Drug Interactions** CYP2C9 enzyme substrate

ACE inhibitors: Effects may be reduced by NSAIDs; use lowest possible dose for shortest duration possible; monitor

Cholestyramine and colestipol: Absorption may be reduced by concurrent administration

Corticosteroids: May increase the risk of GI ulceration; use caution

Cyclosporine: Nephrotoxicity may be increased with concurrent NSAID use; monitor

CYP2C9 inhibitors: May increase in diclofenac concentrations; inhibitors include amiodarone, cimetidine, fluvoxamine, metronidazole, omeprazole, sulfonamides, valproic acid, and zafirlukast

Hydralazine: Antihypertensive effect may be decreased; avoid concurrent use

Lithium: Serum levels can be increased; avoid concurrent use if possible or monitor lithium levels and adjust dose. When NSAID is stopped, lithium may need adjustment again.

Loop diuretics: Therapeutic effects may be reduced by NSAIDs; avoid

Methotrexate: Toxicity may be increased by concurrent NSAID use; risk is limited in low-dose methotrexate regimens (such as for rheumatoid arthritis); prolonged leucovorin rescue may be required at antineoplastic doses; monitor

Thiazide diuretics: Antihypertensive effects are decreased; avoid concurrent use

Warfarin: INRs may be increased by some NSAIDs. This may depend, in part, on dose and duration; monitor INR closely. Use the lowest dose of NSAIDs possible and for the briefest duration.

**Usual Dosage**

Patent ductus arteriosus: Neonates: I.V.: Initial: 0.2 mg/kg; followed with: 2 doses of 0.1 mg/kg at 12- to 24-hour intervals if age <48 hours at time of first dose; 0.2 mg/kg 2 times if 2-7 days old at time of first dose; or 0.25 mg/kg 2 times if over 7 days at time of first dose; discontinue if significant adverse effects occur. Dose should be withheld if patient has anuria or oliguria.

Analgesia:
- Children: Oral: Initial: 1-2 mg/kg/day in 2-4 divided doses; maximum: 4 mg/kg/day; not to exceed 150-200 mg/day
- Adults: Oral, rectal: 25-50 mg/dose 2-3 times/day; maximum dose: 200 mg/day; extended release capsule should be given on a 1-2 times/day schedule

**Dietary Considerations**

Food: May decrease the rate but not the extent of oral absorption. Drug may cause GI upset, bleeding, ulceration, perforation; take with food or milk to minimize GI upset.

Potassium: Hyperkalemia has been reported. The elderly and those with renal insufficiency are at greatest risk. Monitor potassium serum concentration in those at greatest risk. Avoid salt substitutes.

Sodium: Hyponatremia from sodium retention. Suspect secondary to suppression of renal prostaglandin. Monitor serum concentration and fluid status. May need to restrict fluid.

**Patient Information**

Oral: Take this medication exactly as directed; do not increase dose without consulting prescriber. Do not crush, break, or chew capsules. Take with food or milk to reduce GI distress. Maintain adequate fluid intake (2-3 L/day of fluids unless instructed to restrict fluid intake).

Rectal: Suppositories do not need to be refrigerated. Wash hands before inserting unwrapped suppository high up in rectum. Wearing glove is recommended. (Use caution to avoid damage with long fingernails.)

Do not use alcohol, aspirin, or aspirin-containing medication, and all other anti-inflammatory medications without consulting prescriber. You may experience drowsiness, dizziness, nervousness, or headache (use caution when driving or engaging in tasks requiring alertness until response to drug is known); anorexia, nausea, vomiting, or heartburn (frequent small meals, frequent oral care, sucking lozenges, or chewing gum may help); fluid retention (weigh yourself weekly and report unusual (3-5 lb/week) weight gain). May discolor stool (green). GI bleeding, ulceration, or perforation can occur with or without pain; discontinue medication and contact prescriber if persistent abdominal pain or cramping, or blood in stool occurs. Report breathlessness, difficulty breathing, or unusual cough; chest pain, rapid heartbeat, palpitations; unusual bruising/bleeding; blood in urine, stool, gums, or vomitus; swollen extremities; skin rash, irritation, or itching; acute fatigue; or changes in hearing or ringing in ears.

**Nursing Implications** Extended release capsules must be swallowed intact

**Dosage Forms**

Capsule: 25 mg, 50 mg
- Indocin®: 25 mg, 50 mg

Capsule, sustained release (Indocin® SR): 75 mg

Powder for injection, as sodium trihydrate (Indocin® I.V.): 1 mg

Suppository, rectal (Indocin®): 50 mg

Suspension, oral (Indocin®): 25 mg/5 mL (5 mL, 10 mL, 237 mL, 500 mL)


♦ **Indomethacin Sodium Trihydrate** *see* Indomethacin *on page 286*

♦ **Infants Feverall™ [OTC]** *see* Acetaminophen *on page 14*

- **Infants' Silapap® [OTC]** *see* Acetaminophen *on page 14*
- **Infasurf®** *see* Calfactant *on page 86*
- **InFeD™ Injection** *see* Iron Dextran Complex *on page 293*
- **Infergen®** *see* Interferon Alfacon-1 *on page 289*
- **Inflamase® Forte Ophthalmic** *see* Prednisolone *on page 459*
- **Inflamase® Mild Ophthalmic** *see* Prednisolone *on page 459*

## Infliximab (in FLIKS e mab)

**U.S. Brand Names** Remicade™

**Pharmacologic Category** Monoclonal Antibody

**Use** Treatment of moderately to severely active Crohn's disease for the reduction of the signs and symptoms in patients who have an inadequate response to conventional therapy or for the treatment of patients with fistulizing Crohn's disease for the reduction in the number of draining enterocutaneous fistula(s)

**Effects on Mental Status** Fatigue is common; may cause dizziness

**Effects on Psychiatric Treatment** None reported

**Usual Dosage**

Moderately to severely active Crohn's disease: Adults: I.V.: 5 mg/kg as a single infusion over a minimum of 2 hours

Fistulizing Crohn's disease: 5 mg/kg as an infusion over a minimum of 2 hours, dose repeated at 2 and 6 weeks after the initial infusion

**Dosing adjustment in renal impairment:** No specific adjustment recommended

**Dosing adjustment in hepatic impairment:** No specific adjustment recommended

**Dosage Forms** Powder for injection: 100 mg

## Influenza Virus Vaccine (in floo EN za VYE rus vak SEEN)

**U.S. Brand Names** Fluogen®; Fluzone®

**Canadian Brand Names** Fluviral S/F®

**Synonyms** Influenza Virus Vaccine (inactivated whole-virus); Influenza Virus Vaccine (split-virus) Influenza Virus Vaccine (purified surface antigen)

**Pharmacologic Category** Vaccine

**Use** Provide active immunity to influenza virus strains contained in the vaccine; for high-risk persons, previous year vaccines should not be used to prevent present year influenza

Groups at Increased Risk for Influenza Related Complications:

- Persons ≥65 years of age
- Residents of nursing homes and other chronic-care facilities that house persons of any age with chronic medical conditions
- Adults and children with chronic disorders of the pulmonary or cardiovascular systems, including children with asthma
- Adults and children who have required regular medical follow-up or hospitalization during the preceding year because of chronic metabolic diseases (including diabetes mellitus), renal dysfunction, hemoglobinopathies, or immunosuppression (including immunosuppression caused by medications)

Children and teenagers (6 months to 18 years of age) who are receiving long-term aspirin therapy and therefore, may be at risk for developing Reye's syndrome after influenza

**Effects on Mental Status** None reported

**Effects on Psychiatric Treatment** None reported

**Pregnancy Risk Factor** C

**Contraindications** Persons with allergy history to eggs or egg products, chicken, chicken feathers or chicken dander, hypersensitivity to thimerosal, influenza virus vaccine or any component, presence of acute respiratory disease or other active infections or illnesses, delay immunization in a patient with an active neurological disorder

**Warnings/Precautions** Although there is no evidence of maternal or fetal risk when vaccine is given in pregnancy, waiting until the 2nd or 3rd trimester to vaccinate the pregnant woman with a high-risk condition may be reasonable. Antigenic response may not be as great as expected in patients requiring immunosuppressive drug; hypersensitivity reactions may occur; because of potential for febrile reactions, risks and benefits must carefully be considered in patients with history of febrile convulsions; influenza vaccines from previous seasons must not be used; patients with sulfite sensitivity may be affected by this product.

**Adverse Reactions All serious adverse reactions must be reported to the U.S. Department of Health and Human Services (DHHS) Vaccine Adverse Event Reporting System (VAERS) 1-800-822-7967.**

1% to 10%:

Central nervous system: Fever, malaise

Local: Tenderness, redness, or induration at the site of injection (<33%)

<1%: Allergic reactions, anaphylactoid reactions (most likely to residual egg protein), angioedema, asthma, Guillain-Barré syndrome, fever, myalgia, urticaria

**Drug Interactions**

Decreased effect with immunosuppressive agents; some manufacturers and clinicians recommend that the flu vaccine not be administered with the DTP for the potential for increased febrile reactions (specifically whole-cell pertussis), and that one should wait at least 3 days. ACIP recommends that children at high risk for influenza may get the vaccine concomitantly with DTP.

Increased effect/toxicity of theophylline and warfarin possible

**Usual Dosage** I.M.:

Children:

6-35 months: 1-2 doses of 0.25 mL with ≥4 weeks between doses and the last dose administered before December

3-8 years: 1-2 doses of 0.5 mL (in anterolateral aspect of thigh) with ≥4 weeks between doses and the last dose administered before December

Children ≥9 years and Adults: 0.5 mL each year of appropriate vaccine for the year, one dose is all that is necessary; administer in late fall to allow maximum titers to develop by peak epidemic periods usually occurring in early December

**Note:** The split virus or purified surface antigen is recommended for children ≤12 years of age; if the child has received at least one dose of the 1978-79 or later vaccine, one dose is sufficient

**Patient Information** Be aware of possible adverse effects

**Dosage Forms** Injection:

Purified surface antigen (Flu-Imune®): 5 mL

Split-virus (Fluogen®, Fluzone®): 0.5 mL, 5 mL

Whole-virus (Fluzone®): 5 mL

- **Influenza Virus Vaccine (inactivated whole-virus)** *see* Influenza Virus Vaccine *on page 287*
- **Influenza Virus Vaccine (split-virus) Influenza Virus Vaccine (purified surface antigen)** *see* Influenza Virus Vaccine *on page 287*
- **Infumorph™ Injection** *see* Morphine Sulfate *on page 374*
- **INH** *see* Isoniazid *on page 294*
- **Innofem®** *see* Estradiol *on page 203*
- **Innohep®** *see* Tinzaparin *on page 550*
- **Innovar®** *see* Droperidol and Fentanyl *on page 188*
- **Inocor®** *see* Inamrinone *on page 285*
- **Insta-Char® [OTC]** *see* Charcoal *on page 106*
- **Insta-Glucose® [OTC]** *see* Glucose, Instant *on page 252*

## Insulin Preparations (IN su lin prep a RAY shuns)

**U.S. Brand Names** Humalog®; Humalog® Mix 50/50™; Humalog® Mix 75/25™; Humulin® 50/50; Humulin® 70/30; Humulin® L; Humulin® N; Lantus®; Lente® Iletin® I; Lente® Iletin® II; Lente® Insulin; Lente® L; Novolin® 70/30; Novolin® L; Novolin® N; Novolin® R; NovoLog™; NPH Iletin® I; NPH-N; Pork NPH Iletin® II; Pork Regular Iletin® II; Regular (Concentrated) Iletin® II U-500; Regular Iletin® I; Regular Insulin; Regular Purified Pork Insulin; Velosulin® BR Human (Buffered); Velosulin® Human

**Pharmacologic Category** Antidiabetic Agent (Insulin); Antidote

**Use** Treatment of insulin-dependent diabetes mellitus, also noninsulin-dependent diabetes mellitus unresponsive to treatment with diet and/or oral hypoglycemics; to assure proper utilization of glucose and reduce glucosuria in nondiabetic patients receiving parenteral nutrition whose glucosuria cannot be adequately controlled with infusion rate adjustments or those who require assistance in achieving optimal caloric intakes; hyperkalemia (regular insulin only; use with glucose to shift potassium into cells to lower serum potassium levels)

**Effects on Mental Status** May cause drowsiness or confusion

**Effects on Psychiatric Treatment** MAOIs may enhance the hypoglycemic effects of insulin; TCAs may antagonize the effects of insulin

**Pregnancy Risk Factor** B; C (insulin glargine - Lantus® per manufacturer)

**Warnings/Precautions** Hypoglycemia is the most common adverse effect of insulin. The timing of hypoglycemia differs among various insulin formulations. Any change of insulin should be made cautiously; changing manufacturers, type and/or method of manufacture, may result in the need for a change of dosage; human insulin differs from animal-source insulin; regular insulin is the only insulin to be used I.V.; hypoglycemia may result from increased work or exercise without eating; use of long-acting insulin preparations (insulin glargine, Ultralente®, insulin U) may delay recovery from hypoglycemia

In type 1 diabetes, insulin lispro (Humalog®) should be used in combination with a long-acting insulin. However, in type 2 diabetes it may be used without a long-acting insulin when used in combination with a sulfonylurea.

Use with caution in renal or hepatic impairment

Insulin aspart (NovoLog™): Safety and efficacy of use in children has not been established

**Adverse Reactions** 1% to 10%:

Cardiovascular: Palpitation, tachycardia, pallor

(Continued)

## Insulin Preparations *(Continued)*

Central nervous system: Fatigue, mental confusion, loss of consciousness, headache, hypothermia
Dermatologic: Urticaria, redness
Endocrine & metabolic: Hypoglycemia
Gastrointestinal: Hunger, nausea, numbness of mouth
Local: Itching, edema, stinging, or warmth at injection site, atrophy or hypertrophy of S.C. fat tissue
Neuromuscular & skeletal: Muscle weakness, paresthesia, tremors
Ocular: Transient presbyopia or blurred vision, blurred vision
Miscellaneous: Diaphoresis, anaphylaxis

**Overdosage/Toxicology**
Signs and symptoms: Tachycardia, anxiety, hunger, tremors, pallor, headache, motor dysfunction, speech disturbances, sweating, palpitations, coma, death
Treatment: Antidote is glucose and glucagon, if necessary

**Drug Interactions**
Drugs which **DECREASE** hypoglycemic effect of insulin:
Contraceptives (oral), corticosteroids, dextrothyroxine, diltiazem, dobutamine, epinephrine, niacin, smoking, thiazide diuretics, thyroid hormone

Drugs which **INCREASE** hypoglycemic effect of insulin:
Alcohol, alpha-blockers, anabolic steroids, beta-blockers*, clofibrate, fenfluramine, guanethidine, MAO inhibitors, pentamidine, phenylbutazone, salicylates, sulfinpyrazone, tetracyclines
*Nonselective beta-blockers may delay recovery from hypoglycemic episodes and mask signs/symptoms of hypoglycemia. Cardioselective agents may be alternatives.

**Usual Dosage** Dose requires continuous medical supervision; may administer I.V. (regular), I.M., S.C.

Diabetes mellitus: The number and size of daily doses, time of administration, and diet and exercise require continuous medical supervision. In addition, specific formulations may require distinct administration procedures.
Lispro should be given within 15 minutes before or immediately after a meal
Human regular insulin should be given within 30-60 minutes before a meal.
Intermediate-acting insulins may be administered 1-2 times/day.
Long-acting insulins may be administered once daily.
Insulin glargine (Lantus®) should be administered subcutaneously once daily at bedtime. Maintenance doses should be administered subcutaneously and sites should be rotated to prevent lipodystrophy.
Children and Adults: 0.5-1 unit/kg/day in divided doses
Adolescents (growth spurts): 0.8-1.2 units/kg/day in divided doses
Adjust dose to maintain premeal and bedtime blood glucose of 80-140 mg/dL (children <5 years: 100-200 mg/dL)
Insulin glargine (Lantus®):
Type 2 diabetes (patient not already on insulin): 10 units once daily, adjusted according to patient response (range in clinical study 2-100 units/day)
Patients already receiving insulin: In clinical studies, when changing to insulin glargine from once-daily NPH or Ultralente® insulin, the initial dose was not changed; when changing from twice-daily NPH to once daily insulin glargine, the total daily dose was reduced by 20% and adjusted according to patient response

Hyperkalemia: Administer calcium gluconate and $NaHCO_3$ first then 50% dextrose at 0.5-1 mL/kg and insulin 1 unit for every 4-5 g dextrose given
Diabetic ketoacidosis: Children and Adults: Regular insulin: I.V. loading dose: 0.1 unit/kg, then maintenance continuous infusion: 0.1 unit/kg/hour (range: 0.05-0.2 units/kg/hour depending upon the rate of decrease of serum glucose - too rapid decrease of serum glucose may lead to cerebral edema).
Optimum rate of decrease (serum glucose): 80-100 mg/dL/hour
**Note:** Newly diagnosed patients with IDDM presenting in DKA and patients with blood sugars <800 mg/dL may be relatively "sensitive" to insulin and should receive loading and initial maintenance doses approximately $^1/_2$ of those indicated above.

**Dosing adjustment in renal impairment (regular):** Insulin requirements are reduced due to changes in insulin clearance or metabolism
$Cl_{cr}$ 10-50 mL/minute: Administer at 75% of normal dose
$Cl_{cr}$ <10 mL/minute: Administer at 25% to 50% of normal dose and monitor glucose closely
Hemodialysis: Because of a large molecular weight (6000 daltons), insulin is not significantly removed by either peritoneal or hemodialysis
Supplemental dose is not necessary
Peritoneal dialysis: Supplemental dose is not necessary
Continuous arteriovenous or venovenous hemofiltration effects: Supplemental dose is not necessary

**Dietary Considerations**
Alcohol: Increase in hypoglycemic effect of insulin; monitor blood glucose concentration; avoid or limit use
Food:
Potassium: Shifts potassium from extracellular to intracellular space. Decreases potassium serum concentration; monitor potassium serum concentration.
Sodium: SIADH; water retention and dilutional hyponatremia may occur. Patients at greatest risk are those with CHF or hepatic cirrhosis. Monitor sodium serum concentration and fluid status.

**Patient Information** This medication is used to control diabetes; it is not a cure. Other components of treatment plan are important: follow prescribed diet, medication, and exercise regimen. Take exactly as directed. Do not change dose or discontinue unless so advised by prescriber. Inform prescriber of all other prescription or OTC medications you are taking; do not introduce new medication without consulting prescriber. If you experience hypoglycemic reaction, contact prescriber immediately. Maintain regular dietary intake and exercise routine and always carry quick source of sugar with you. Report adverse side effects, including chest pain or palpitations; persistent fatigue, confusion, headache; skin rash or redness; numbness of mouth, lips, or tongue; muscle weakness or tremors; changes in vision; difficulty breathing; or nausea, vomiting, or flu-like symptoms. With insulin aspart (NovoLog™), you must start eating within 5-10 minutes after injection.

**Nursing Implications** Patients using human insulin may be less likely to recognize hypoglycemia than if they use pork insulin, patients on pork insulin that have low blood sugar exhibit hunger and sweating; regular insulin is the only form for I.V. use. Patients who are unable to accurately draw up their dose will need assistance such as prefilled syringes.

**Dosage Forms** All insulins are 100 units/mL (10 mL) except where indicated:
RAPID-ACTING:
**Insulin lispro rDNA origin:** Humalog® *[Lilly]* (1.5 mL, 10 mL)
**Insulin aspart injection:** NovoLog™ *[Novo Nordisk]* (3 mL, 10 mL)
**Insulin injection** (Regular Insulin)
Beef and pork: Regular Iletin® I *[Lilly]*
Human:
rDNA: Humulin® R *[Lilly]*, Novolin® R *[Novo Nordisk]*
Semisynthetic: Velosulin® Human *[Novo Nordisk]*
rDNA Human, Buffered: Velosulin® BR
Pork: Regular Insulin *[Novo Nordisk]*
Purified pork:
Pork Regular Iletin® II *[Lilly]*, Regular Purified Pork Insulin *[Novo Nordisk]*
Regular (Concentrated) Iletin® II U-500 (*Lilly*): 500 units/mL

INTERMEDIATE-ACTING:
**Insulin zinc suspension** (Lente)
Beef and pork: Lente® Iletin® I *[Lilly]*
Human, rDNA: Humulin® L *[Lilly]*, Novolin® L *[Novo Nordisk]*
Purified pork: Lente® Iletin® II *[Lilly]*, Lente® L *[Novo Nordisk]*

**Isophane insulin suspension** (NPH)
Beef and pork: NPH Iletin® I *[Lilly]*
Human, rDNA: Humulin® N *[Lilly]*, Novolin® N *[Novo Nordisk]*
Purified pork: Pork NPH Iletin® II *[Lilly]*, NPH-N *[Novo Nordisk]*

LONG-ACTING:
**Insulin zinc suspension, extended** (Ultralente®)
Human, rDNA: Humulin® U [Lilly]
**Insulin glargine,** rDNA: Lantus® *[Avantis Pharmaceuticals Inc]*

COMBINATIONS:
**Isophane insulin suspension and insulin injection**
Isophane insulin suspension (50%) and insulin injection (50%) human (rDNA): Humulin® 50/50 *[Lilly]*
Isophane insulin suspension (70%) and insulin injection (30%) human (rDNA): Humulin® 70/30 *[Lilly]*, Novolin® 70/30 *[Novo Nordisk]*
**Insulin lispro protamine suspension and insulin lispro injection**
Insulin lispro protamine suspension (50%) and insulin lispro injection (50%) (rDNA): Humalog® Mix 50/50™ *[ Lilly]*
Insulin lispro protamine suspension (75%) and insulin lispro injection (25%) (rDNA): Humalog® Mix 75/25™ *[Lilly]*

♦ **Intal® Nebulizer Solution** *see* Cromolyn Sodium *on page 142*

♦ **Intal® Oral Inhaler** *see* Cromolyn Sodium *on page 142*

♦ **Integrilin®** *see* Eptifibatide *on page 198*

## Interferon Alfa-2a (in ter FEER on AL fa too aye)

**U.S. Brand Names** Roferon-A®

**Pharmacologic Category** Biological Response Modulator

**Use** Patients >18 years of age: Hairy cell leukemia, AIDS-related Kaposi's sarcoma, chronic myelogenous leukemia (CML), chronic hepatitis C, adjuvant treatment to surgery for primary or recurrent malignant melanoma; multiple unlabeled uses; indications and dosage regimens are specific for a particular brand of interferon

**Effects on Mental Status** Dizziness and drowsiness are common; may rarely cause delirium or depression

**Effects on Psychiatric Treatment** May cause leukopenia; use caution with clozapine and carbamazepine; concurrent use with psychotropics may produce additive sedation and dry mouth

**Usual Dosage** Refer to individual protocols

Infants and Children: Hemangiomas of infancy, pulmonary hemangiomatosis: S.C.: 1-3 million units/m²/day once daily

Adults >18 years: I.M., S.C.:

Hairy cell leukemia:

Induction: 3 million units/day for 16-24 weeks.

Maintenance: 3 million units 3 times/week (may be treated for up to 20 consecutive weeks)

AIDS-related Kaposi's sarcoma:

Induction: 36 million units/day for 10-12 weeks

Maintenance: 36 million units 3 times/week (may begin with dose escalation from 3-9-18 million units each day over 3 consecutive days followed by 36 million units/day for the remainder of the 10-12 weeks of induction)

If severe adverse reactions occur, modify dosage (50% reduction) or temporarily discontinue therapy until adverse reactions abate

**Dosage Forms**

Injection: 3 million units/mL (1 mL); 6 million units/mL (3 mL); 9 million units/mL (0.9 mL, 3 mL); 36 million units/mL (1 mL)

Powder for injection: 6 million units/mL when reconstituted

## Interferon Alfa-2b (in ter FEER on AL fa too bee)

**U.S. Brand Names** Intron® A

**Pharmacologic Category** Biological Response Modulator

**Use** Hairy-cell leukemia in patients >18 years, condylomata acuminata, AIDS-related Kaposi's sarcoma in patients >18 years, chronic non-A/non-B/C hepatitis in patients >18 years, chronic hepatitis B in patients >18 years (indications and dosage are specific for a particular brand of interferon)

**Effects on Mental Status** Dizziness and drowsiness are common; may rarely cause delirium or depression

**Effects on Psychiatric Treatment** May cause leukopenia; use caution with clozapine and carbamazepine; concurrent use with psychotropics may produce additive sedation and dry mouth

**Usual Dosage** Adults (refer to individual protocols):

Hairy cell leukemia: I.M., S.C.: 2 million units/m² 3 times/week for 2 to ≥6 months of therapy

AIDS-related Kaposi's sarcoma: I.M., S.C. (use 50 million international unit vial): 30 million units/m² 3 times/week

*Condylomata acuminata*: Intralesionally (use 10 million international unit vial): 1 million units/lesion 3 times/week for 4-8 weeks; not to exceed 5 million units per treatment (maximum: 5 lesions at one time)

Chronic hepatitis C (non-A/non-B): I.M., S.C.: 3 million units 3 times/week for approximately a 6-month course

Chronic hepatitis B: I.M., S.C.: 5 million international units/day or 10 million international units 3 times/week for 16 weeks; if severe adverse reactions occur, reduce dosage 50% or temporarily discontinue therapy until adverse reactions abate; when platelet/granulocyte count returns to normal, reinstitute therapy

Hemodialysis: Supplemental dose is not necessary

Peritoneal dialysis: Supplemental dose is not necessary

**Dosage Forms**

Injection, albumin free: 3 million units (0.5 mL); 5 million units (0.5 mL); 10 million units (1 mL); 25 million units

Powder for injection, lyophilized: 18 million units, 50 million units

## Interferon Alfa-2b and Ribavirin Combination Pack
(in ter FEER on AL fa too bee & rye ba VYE rin com bi NAY shun pak)

**U.S. Brand Names** Rebetron™

**Pharmacologic Category** Antiviral Agent; Biological Response Modulator

**Use** The combination therapy of oral ribavirin with interferon alfa-2b, recombinant (Intron® A) injection is indicated for the treatment of chronic hepatitis C in patients with compensated liver disease who have relapsed after alpha interferon therapy.

**Effects on Mental Status** None reported

**Effects on Psychiatric Treatment** None reported

**Usual Dosage** The recommended dosage of combination therapy is 3 million int. units of Intron® A injected subcutaneously 3 times/week and 1000-1200 mg of Rebetol® capsules administered orally in a divided daily (morning and evening) dose for 24 weeks; patients weighing 75 kg (165 pounds) or less should receive 1000 mg of Rebetol® daily (2 x 200 mg capsules in the morning and 3 x 200 mg capsules in the evening); while patients weighing more than 75 kg should receive 1200 mg of Rebetol® daily (3 x 200 mg capsules in the morning and 3 x 200 mg capsules in the evening)

**Dosage Forms** Combination package:

For patients ≤75 kg:

Each Rebetron™ combination package consists of:

A box containing 6 vials of Intron® A (3 million int. units in 0.5 mL per vial) and 6 syringes and alcohol swabs; two boxes containing 35 Rebetol® 200 mg capsules each for a total of 70 capsules (5 capsules per blister card)

One 18 million int. units multidose vial of Intron® A injection (22.8 million int. units per 3.8 mL; 3 million int. units/0.5 mL) and 6 syringes and alcohol swabs; two boxes containing 35 Rebetol® 200 mg capsules each for a total of 70 capsules (5 capsules per blister card)

One 18 million int. units Intron® A injection multidose pen (22.5 million int. units per 1.5 mL; 3 million int. units/0.2 mL) and 6 disposable needles and alcohol swabs; two boxes containing 35 Rebetol® 200 mg capsules each for a total of 70 capsules (5 capsules per blister card)

For patients >75 kg:

A box containing 6 vials of Intron® A injection (3 million int. units in 0.5 mL per vial) and 6 syringes and alcohol swabs; two boxes containing 42 Rebetol® 200 mg capsules each for a total of 84 capsules (6 capsules per blister card)

One 18 million int. units multidose vial of Intron® A injection (22.5 million int. units per 3.8 mL; 3 million int. units/0.5 mL) and 6 syringes and alcohol swabs; two boxes containing 42 Rebetol® 200 mg capsules each for a total of 84 capsules (6 capsules per blister card)

One 18 million int. units Intron® A injection multidose pen (22.5 million int. units per 1.5 mL; 3 million int. units/0.2 mL) and 6 disposable needles and alcohol swabs; two boxes containing 42 Rebetol® 200 mg capsules each for a total of 84 capsules (6 capsules per blister card)

For Rebetol® dose reduction:

A box containing 6 vials of Intron® A injection (3 million int. units in 0.5 mL per vial) and 6 syringes and alcohol swabs; one box containing 42 Rebetol® 200 mg capsules (6 capsules per blister card)

One 18 million int. units multidose vial of Intron® A injection (22.8 million int. units per 3.8 mL; 3 million int. units/0.5 mL) and 6 syringes and alcohol swabs; one box containing 42 Rebetol® 200 mg capsules (6 capsules per blister card)

One 18 million int. units Introl® A injection multidose pen (22.5 million int. units per 1.5 mL; 3 million int. units/0.2 mL) and 6 disposable needles and alcohol swabs; one box containing 42 Rebetol® 200 mg capsules (6 capsules per blister card)

## Interferon Alfacon-1 (in ter FEER on AL fa con one)

**U.S. Brand Names** Infergen®

**Pharmacologic Category** Interferon

**Use** Treatment of chronic hepatitis C virus (HCV) infection in patients ≥18 years of age with compensated liver disease and anti-HCV serum antibodies or HCV RNA.

**Usual Dosage** Adults ≥18 years: S.C.:

Chronic HCV infection: 9 mcg 3 times/week for 24 weeks; allow 48 hours between doses

Patients who have previously tolerated interferon therapy but did not respond or relapsed: 15 mcg 3 times/week for 6 months

Dose reduction for toxicity: Dose should be held in patients who experience a severe adverse reaction, and treatment should be stopped or decreased if the reaction does not become tolerable.

Doses were reduced from 9 mcg to 7.5 mcg in the pivotal study.

For patients receiving 15 mcg/dose, doses were reduced in 3 mcg increments. Efficacy is decreased with doses <7.5 mcg

**Dosage adjustment in renal impairment:** No information available.

**Dosage adjustment in hepatic impairment:** Avoid use in decompensated hepatic disease.

Elderly: No information available.

**Dosage Forms** Injection, preservative free:

Prefilled syringe, single dose: 30 mcg/mL (0.3 mL, 0.5 mL)

Vial, single dose: 30 mcg/mL (0.3 mL, 0.5 mL)

## Interferon Alfa-n3 (in ter FEER on AL fa en-three)

**U.S. Brand Names** Alferon® N

**Pharmacologic Category** Biological Response Modulator

**Use** Patients ≥18 years of age: Condylomata acuminata, intralesional treatment of refractory or recurring genital or venereal warts; useful in patients who do not respond or are not candidates for usual treatments; indications and dosage regimens are specific for a particular brand of interferon

**Effects on Mental Status** Dizziness and drowsiness are common; may rarely cause delirium or depression

**Effects on Psychiatric Treatment** May cause leukopenia; use caution with clozapine and carbamazepine; concurrent use with psychotropics may produce additive sedation and dry mouth

**Usual Dosage** Adults: Inject 250,000 units (0.05 mL) in each wart twice weekly for a maximum of 8 weeks; therapy should not be repeated for at least 3 months after the initial 8-week course of therapy

**Dosage Forms** Injection: 5 million units (1 mL)

## Interferon Beta-1a (in ter FEER on BAY ta won aye)

**U.S. Brand Names** Avonex™

**Pharmacologic Category** Biological Response Modulator

(Continued)

## Interferon Beta-1a *(Continued)*

**Use** Treatment of relapsing forms of multiple sclerosis (MS); to slow the accumulation of physical disability and decrease the frequency of clinical exacerbations

**Effects on Mental Status** May cause sedation, depression, suicidal ideation, anxiety, agitation, or confusion

**Effects on Psychiatric Treatment** May cause leukopenia; use caution with clozapine and carbamazepine; concurrent use with psychotropics may produce additive sedation

**Pregnancy Risk Factor** C

**Contraindications** History of hypersensitivity to natural or recombinant interferon beta, human albumin, or any other component of the formulation

**Warnings/Precautions** Interferon beta-1a should be used with caution in patients with a history of depression, seizures, or cardiac disease; because its use has not been evaluated during lactation, its use in breast-feeding mothers may not be safe and should be warned against

**Adverse Reactions** 1% to 10%:

Cardiovascular: CHF (rare), tachycardia, syncope

Central nervous system: Headache, lethargy, depression, emotional lability, anxiety, suicidal ideations, somnolence, agitation, confusion

Dermatologic: Alopecia (rare)

Endocrine & metabolic: Hypocalcemia

Gastrointestinal: Nausea, anorexia, vomiting, diarrhea, chronic weight loss

Hematologic: Leukopenia, thrombocytopenia, anemia (frequent, dose-related, but not usually severe)

Hepatic: Elevated liver enzymes (mild, transient)

Local: Pain/redness at injection site (80%)

Neuromuscular & skeletal: Weakness

Ocular: Retinal toxicity/visual changes

Renal: Elevated BUN and $S_{cr}$

Miscellaneous: Flu-like syndrome (fever, nausea, malaise, myalgia) occurs in most patients, but is usually controlled by acetaminophen or NSAIDs; dose related abortifacient activity was reported in Rhesus monkeys

**Overdosage/Toxicology**

Signs and symptoms: CNS depression, obtundation, flu-like symptoms, myelosuppression

Treatment: Supportive

**Drug Interactions** Decreases clearance of zidovudine thus increasing zidovudine toxicity

**Usual Dosage** Adults >18 years: I.M.: 30 mcg once weekly

**Patient Information** This is not a cure for MS; you will continue to receive regular treatment and follow-up for MS. Use as directed; do not change dosage or schedule of administration without consulting prescriber. Maintain adequate hydration (2-3 L/day of fluids unless instructed to restrict fluid intake). You may experience flu-like syndrome (acetaminophen may help); nausea, vomiting, or loss of appetite (frequent small meals, frequent mouth care, sucking lozenges, or chewing gum may help); drowsiness, dizziness, agitation, or abnormal thinking (use caution when driving or engaging in tasks requiring alertness until response to drug is known). Report unusual bruising or bleeding; persistent abdominal disturbances; unusual fatigue; muscle pain or tremors; chest pain or palpitations, swelling of extremities; visual disturbances; pain, swelling, or redness at injection site; or other unusual symptoms.

**Nursing Implications** Patient should be informed of possible side effects, especially depression, suicidal ideations, and the risk of abortion; flu-like symptoms such as chills, fever, malaise, diaphoresis, and myalgia are common

**Dosage Forms** Powder for injection, lyophilized: 33 mcg [6.6 million units]

## Interferon Beta-1b (in ter FEER on BAY ta won bee)

**U.S. Brand Names** Betaseron®

**Pharmacologic Category** Biological Response Modulator

**Use** Reduces the frequency of clinical exacerbations in ambulatory patients with relapsing-remitting multiple sclerosis (MS)

**Effects on Mental Status** May cause sedation, depression, suicidal ideation, anxiety, agitation, or confusion

**Effects on Psychiatric Treatment** May cause leukopenia; use caution with clozapine and carbamazepine; concurrent use with psychotropics may produce additive sedation

**Pregnancy Risk Factor** C

**Contraindications** Hypersensitivity to *E. coli* derived products, natural or recombinant interferon beta, albumin human or any other component of the formulation

**Warnings/Precautions** The safety and efficacy of interferon beta-1b in chronic progressive MS have not been evaluated; use in breast-feeding women is not recommended; flu-like symptoms complex (ie, myalgia, fever, chills, malaise, sweating) is reported in 53% of patients who receive interferon beta-1b

**Adverse Reactions** Due to the pivotal position of interferon in the immune system, toxicities can affect nearly every organ system: Injection site reactions, injection site necrosis, flu-like symptoms, menstrual disorders, depression (with suicidal ideations), somnolence, palpitations, peripheral vascular disorders, hypertension, blood dyscrasias, dyspnea, laryngitis, cystitis, gastrointestinal complaints, seizures, headache, and liver enzyme elevations

**Overdosage/Toxicology**

Signs and symptoms: CNS depression, obtundation, flu-like symptoms, myelosuppression

Treatment: Supportive

**Drug Interactions** Decreases clearance of zidovudine thus increasing zidovudine toxicity

**Usual Dosage** S.C.:

Children <18 years: Not recommended

Adults >18 years: 0.25 mg (8 million units) every other day

**Patient Information** This is not a cure for MS; you will continue to receive regular treatment and follow-up for MS. Use as directed; do not change dosage or schedule of administration without consulting prescriber. Maintain adequate hydration (2-3 L/day of fluids unless instructed to restrict fluid intake). You may experience flu-like syndrome (acetaminophen may help); nausea, vomiting, or loss of appetite (frequent small meals, frequent mouth care, sucking lozenges, or chewing gum may help); drowsiness, dizziness, agitation, or abnormal thinking (use caution when driving or engaging in tasks requiring alertness until response to drug is known). Report unusual bruising or bleeding; persistent abdominal disturbances; unusual fatigue; muscle pain or tremors; chest pain or palpitations, swelling of extremities; visual disturbances; pain, swelling, or redness at injection site; or other unusual symptoms.

**Nursing Implications** Patient should be informed of possible side effects, especially depression, suicidal ideations, and the risk of abortion; flu-like symptoms such as chills, fever, malaise, sweating, and myalgia are common

**Dosage Forms** Powder for injection, lyophilized: 0.3 mg [9.6 million units]

## Interferon Gamma-1b (in ter FEER on GAM ah won bee)

**U.S. Brand Names** Actimmune®

**Pharmacologic Category** Biological Response Modulator

**Use** Reduce frequency and severity of serious infections associated with chronic granulomatous disease; delay time to disease progression in patients with severe, malignant osteopetrosis

**Effects on Mental Status** Sedation is common; may rarely cause depression

**Effects on Psychiatric Treatment** May cause leukopenia; use caution with clozapine and carbamazepine; concurrent use with psychotropics may produce additive sedation

**Usual Dosage** If severe reactions occur, modify dose (50% reduction) or therapy should be discontinued until adverse reactions improve.

Chronic granulomatous disease: Children >1 year and Adults: S.C.:

BSA ≤0.5 $m^2$: 1.5 mcg/kg/dose 3 times/week

BSA >0.5 $m^2$: 50 mcg/$m^2$ (1 million int. units/$m^2$) 3 times/week

Severe, malignant osteopetrosis: Children >1 year: S.C.:

BSA ≤0.5 $m^2$: 1.5 mcg/kg/dose 3 times/week

BSA >0.5 $m^2$: 50 mcg/$m^2$ (1 million int. units/$m^2$) 3 times/week

**Dosage Forms** Injection: 100 mcg [3 million units]


- **Intron® A** *see* Interferon Alfa-2b *on page 289*
- **Intropin® Injection** *see* Dopamine *on page 182*
- **Inversine®** *see* Mecamylamine *on page 334*
- **Invirase®** *see* Saquinavir *on page 504*
- **Iobid DM®** *see* Guaifenesin and Dextromethorphan *on page 257*
- **Iodex® [OTC]** *see* Povidone-Iodine *on page 456*
- **Iodex-p® [OTC]** *see* Povidone-Iodine *on page 456*


## Iodinated Glycerol (EYE oh di nay ted GLI ser ole)

**Pharmacologic Category** Expectorant

**Use** Mucolytic expectorant in adjunctive treatment of bronchitis, bronchial asthma, pulmonary emphysema, cystic fibrosis, or chronic sinusitis

**Effects on Mental Status** None reported

**Effects on Psychiatric Treatment** May result in increased toxicity when used with disulfiram, MAO inhibitors, CNS depressants, and lithium

**Usual Dosage** Oral:

Children: Up to 30 mg 4 times/day

Adults: 60 mg 4 times/day

**Dosage Forms** Organically bound iodine in brackets

Elixir: 60 mg/5 mL [30 mg/5 mL] (120 mL, 480 mL)

Solution: 50 mg/mL [25 mg/mL] (30 mL)

Tablet: 30 mg [15 mg]

## Iodine (EYE oh dyne)

**Pharmacologic Category** Topical Skin Product

**Use** Used topically as an antiseptic in the management of minor, superficial skin wounds and has been used to disinfect the skin preoperatively

**Effects on Mental Status** None reported
**Effects on Psychiatric Treatment** None reported
**Usual Dosage** Apply topically as necessary to affected areas of skin
**Dosage Forms**
Solution: 2%
Tincture: 2%

## Iodoquinol (eye oh doe KWIN ole)

**U.S. Brand Names** Yodoxin®
**Canadian Brand Names** Diodoquin®
**Synonyms** Diiodohydroxyquin
**Pharmacologic Category** Amebicide
**Use** Treatment of acute and chronic intestinal amebiasis; asymptomatic cyst passers; *Blastocystis hominis* infections; ineffective for amebic hepatitis or hepatic abscess
**Effects on Mental Status** May cause agitation or amnesia
**Effects on Psychiatric Treatment** None reported
**Pregnancy Risk Factor** C
**Contraindications** Known hypersensitivity to iodine or iodoquinol; hepatic damage; pre-existing optic neuropathy
**Warnings/Precautions** Optic neuritis, optic atrophy, and peripheral neuropathy have occurred following prolonged use; avoid long-term therapy
**Adverse Reactions**
>10%: Gastrointestinal: Diarrhea, nausea, vomiting, stomach pain
1% to 10%:
Central nervous system: Fever, chills, agitation, retrograde amnesia, headache
Dermatologic: Rash, urticaria
Endocrine & metabolic: Thyroid gland enlargement
Neuromuscular & skeletal: Peripheral neuropathy, weakness
Ocular: Optic neuritis, optic atrophy, visual impairment
Miscellaneous: Itching of rectal area
**Overdosage/Toxicology**
Signs and symptoms:
Chronic overdose can result in vomiting, diarrhea, abdominal pain, metallic taste, paresthesias, paraplegia, and loss of vision; can lead to destruction of the long fibers of the spinal cord and optic nerve
Acute overdose: Delirium, stupor, coma, amnesia
Treatment: Following GI decontamination, treatment is symptomatic
**Drug Interactions** No data reported
**Usual Dosage** Oral:
Children: 30-40 mg/kg/day (maximum: 650 mg/dose) in 3 divided doses for 20 days; not to exceed 1.95 g/day
Adults: 650 mg 3 times/day after meals for 20 days; not to exceed 1.95 g/day
**Patient Information** Take as directed; complete full course of therapy. Maintain adequate hydration (2-3 L/day of fluids unless instructed to restrict fluid intake) and nutrition. If GI upset occurs, small frequent meals, frequent mouth care, sucking lozenges, or chewing gum may help. Report unresolved or severe nausea or vomiting, skin rash, fever, or fatigue.
**Nursing Implications** Tablets may be crushed and mixed with applesauce or chocolate syrup
**Dosage Forms**
Powder: 25 g
Tablet: 210 mg, 650 mg

## Iodoquinol and Hydrocortisone
(eye oh doe KWIN ole & hye droe KOR ti sone)

**U.S. Brand Names** Vytone® Topical
**Pharmacologic Category** Antifungal Agent, Topical; Corticosteroid, Topical
**Use** Treatment of eczema; infectious dermatitis; chronic eczematoid otitis externa; mycotic dermatoses
**Effects on Mental Status** None reported
**Effects on Psychiatric Treatment** None reported
**Usual Dosage** Apply 3-4 times/day. Therapy should be discontinued when control is achieved; if no improvement is seen, reassessment of diagnosis may be necessary.
**Dosage Forms** Cream: Iodoquinol 1% and hydrocortisone 1% (30 g)


- **Iofed®** *see* Brompheniramine and Pseudoephedrine *on page 74*
- **Iofed® PD** *see* Brompheniramine and Pseudoephedrine *on page 74*
- **Ionamin®** *see* Phentermine *on page 438*
- **Iopidine®** *see* Apraclonidine *on page 47*
- **I-Paracaine®** *see* Proparacaine *on page 473*


## Ipecac Syrup (IP e kak SIR up)

**Pharmacologic Category** Antidote
**Use** Treatment of acute oral drug overdosage and in certain poisonings
**Effects on Mental Status** May cause sedation
**Effects on Psychiatric Treatment** Combination with chlorpromazine has been associated with dystonic reactions
**Pregnancy Risk Factor** C
**Contraindications** Do not use in unconscious patients when time elapsed since exposure is >1 hour, patients with no gag reflex; following ingestion of strong bases or acids, volatile oils; when seizures are likely
**Warnings/Precautions** Do not confuse ipecac syrup with ipecac fluid extract, which is 14 times more potent; use with caution in patients with cardiovascular disease and bulimics; may not be effective in antiemetic overdose
**Adverse Reactions** 1% to 10%:
Cardiovascular: Cardiotoxicity
Central nervous system: Lethargy
Gastrointestinal: Protracted vomiting, diarrhea
Neuromuscular & skeletal: Myopathy
**Overdosage/Toxicology**
Signs and symptoms: Diarrhea, persistent vomiting, hypotension, atrial fibrillation
Treatment: Activated charcoal, gastric lavage
**Drug Interactions**
Decreased effect: Activated charcoal, milk, carbonated beverages
Increased toxicity: Phenothiazines (chlorpromazine has been associated with serious dystonic reactions)
**Usual Dosage** Oral:
Children:
6-12 months: 5-10 mL followed by 10-20 mL/kg of water; repeat dose one time if vomiting does not occur within 20 minutes
1-12 years: 15 mL followed by 10-20 mL/kg of water; repeat dose one time if vomiting does not occur within 20 minutes
If emesis does not occur within 30 minutes after second dose, ipecac must be removed from stomach by gastric lavage
Adults: 15-30 mL followed by 200-300 mL of water; repeat dose one time if vomiting does not occur within 20 minutes
**Patient Information** The Poison Control Center should be contacted before administration. Take only as directed; do not take more than recommended or more often than recommended. Follow with 8 oz of water. If vomiting does not occur within 30 minutes, contact the Poison Control Center or emergency services again. Do not administer if vomiting. If vomiting occurs after taking, do not eat or drink until vomiting subsides.
**Nursing Implications** Do **not** administer to unconscious patients; patients should be kept active and moving following administration of ipecac; if vomiting does not occur after second dose, gastric lavage may be considered to remove ingested substance
**Dosage Forms** Syrup: 70 mg/mL (15 mL, 30 mL, 473 mL, 4000 mL)


- **I-Pentolate®** *see* Cyclopentolate *on page 145*
- **I-Phrine® Ophthalmic Solution** *see* Phenylephrine *on page 439*


## Ipratropium (i pra TROE pee um)

**U.S. Brand Names** Atrovent®
**Pharmacologic Category** Anticholinergic Agent
**Use** Anticholinergic bronchodilator used in bronchospasm associated with COPD, bronchitis, and emphysema; symptomatic relief of rhinorrhea associated with the common cold and allergic and nonallergic rhinitis
**Effects on Mental Status** Nervousness, dizziness, and fatigue are common; may cause insomnia
**Effects on Psychiatric Treatment** Concurrent use with psychotropics may produce additive anticholinergic effects
**Pregnancy Risk Factor** B
**Contraindications** Hypersensitivity to atropine or its derivatives
**Warnings/Precautions** Not indicated for the initial treatment of acute episodes of bronchospasm; use with caution in patients with narrow-angle glaucoma, prostatic hypertrophy, or bladder neck obstruction; ipratropium has not been specifically studied in the elderly, but it is poorly absorbed from the airways and appears to be safe in this population.
**Adverse Reactions Note:** Ipratropium is poorly absorbed from the lung, so systemic effects are rare
>10%:
Central nervous system: Nervousness, dizziness, fatigue, headache
Gastrointestinal: Nausea, xerostomia, stomach upset
Respiratory: Cough
1% to 10%:
Cardiovascular: Palpitations, hypotension
Central nervous system: Insomnia
Genitourinary: Urinary retention
Neuromuscular & skeletal: Trembling
Ocular: Blurred vision
Respiratory: Nasal congestion
<1%: Rash, stomatitis, urticaria
(Continued)

## Ipratropium *(Continued)*

**Overdosage/Toxicology**

Signs and symptoms: Dry mouth, drying of respiratory secretions, cough, nausea, GI distress, blurred vision or impaired visual accommodation, headache, nervousness

Treatment: Acute overdosage with ipratropium by inhalation is unlikely since it is so poorly absorbed. However, if poisoning occurs, it can be treated like any other anticholinergic toxicity. An anticholinergic overdose with severe life-threatening symptoms may be treated with physostigmine 1-2 mg (0.5 or 0.02 mg/kg for children) S.C. or I.V., slowly.

**Drug Interactions**

Increased effect with albuterol

Increased toxicity with anticholinergics or drugs with anticholinergic properties, dronabinol

**Usual Dosage**

Nebulization:

Infants and Children ≤12 years: 125-250 mcg 3 times/day

Children >12 years and Adults: 500 mcg (one unit-dose vial) 3-4 times/day with doses 6-8 hours apart

Metered dose inhaler:

Children 3-12 years: 1-2 inhalations 3 times/day, up to 6 inhalations/24 hours

Children >12 years and Adults: 2 inhalations 4 times/day, up to 12 inhalations/24 hours

Nasal spray:

Symptomatic relief of rhinorrhea associated with the common cold (safety and efficacy of use beyond 4 days in patients with the common cold have not been established):

Children 5-11 years: 0.06%: 2 sprays in each nostril 3 times/day

Children ≥5 years and Adults: 0.06%: 2 sprays in each nostril 3-4 times/day

Symptomatic relief of rhinorrhea associated with allergic/nonallergic rhinitis: Children ≥6 years and Adults: 0.03%: 2 sprays in each nostril 2-3 times/day

**Patient Information** Use exactly as directed. Do not use more often than recommended. Store solution away from light. Maintain adequate hydration (2-3 L/day of fluids unless instructed to restrict fluid intake). You may experience sensitivity to heat (avoid extremes in temperature); nervousness, dizziness, or fatigue (use caution when driving or engaging in tasks requiring alertness until response to drug is known); dry mouth, unpleasant taste, stomach upset (frequent small meals, frequent mouth care, chewing gum, or sucking hard candy may help); or difficulty urinating (always void before treatment). Report unresolved GI upset, dizziness or fatigue, vision changes, palpitations, persistent inability to void, nervousness, or insomnia.

**Administration:** Inhaler: Follow instructions for use accompanying the product. Close eyes when administering ipratropium; blurred vision may result if sprayed into eyes. Effects are enhanced by holding breath 10 seconds after inhalation; wait at least 1 full minute between inhalations.

Nebulizer: Wash hands before and after treatment. Wash and dry nebulizer after each treatment. Twist open the top of one unit dose vial and squeeze the contents into the nebulizer reservoir. Connect the nebulizer reservoir to the mouthpiece or face mask. Connect the nebulizer reservoir to the mouthpiece or face mask. Connect nebulizer to compressor. Sit in a comfortable, upright position. Place mouthpiece in your mouth or put on the face mask and turn on the compressor. If a face mask is used, avoid leakage around the mask (temporary blurring of vision, worsening of narrow-angle glaucoma, or eye pain may occur if mist gets into eyes). Breathe calmly and deeply until no more mist is formed in the nebulizer (about 5 minutes). At this point, treatment is finished.

**Dosage Forms** Solution, as bromide:

Inhalation: 18 mcg/actuation (14 g)

Nasal spray: 0.03% (30 mL); 0.06% (15 mL)

Nebulizing: 0.02% (2.5 mL)

## Ipratropium and Albuterol

(i pra TROE pee um & al BYOO ter ole)

**U.S. Brand Names** Combivent®

**Pharmacologic Category** Bronchodilator

**Use** Treatment of chronic obstructive pulmonary disease (COPD) in those patients that are currently on a regular bronchodilator who continue to have bronchospasms and require a second bronchodilator

**Effects on Mental Status** Nervousness, dizziness, fatigue, headache are common; may cause insomnia or anxiety

**Effects on Psychiatric Treatment** May produce additive anticholinergic effects if used concurrently with psychotropics; effect of propranolol may be reduced; cardiovascular effects (tachycardia, palpitations) may be increased with MAOIs, TCAs, and amphetamines

**Usual Dosage** Adults: 2 inhalations 4 times/day, maximum of 12 inhalations/24 hours

**Dosage Forms** Aerosol: Ipratropium bromide 18 mcg and albuterol sulfate 103 mcg per actuation [200 doses] (14.7 g)

♦ **Iproveratril Hydrochloride** *see* Verapamil *on page 583*

## Irbesartan (ir be SAR tan)

**Related Information**

Angiotensin-Related Agents Comparison Chart *on page 700*

**U.S. Brand Names** Avapro®

**Pharmacologic Category** Angiotensin II Antagonists

**Use** Treatment of hypertension alone or in combination with other antihypertensives

**Effects on Mental Status** May cause anxiety, dizziness, nervousness

**Effects on Psychiatric Treatment** None reported

**Pregnancy Risk Factor** C (1st trimester); D (2nd and 3rd trimesters)

**Contraindications** Hypersensitivity to irbesartan or any component; hypersensitivity to other A-II receptor antagonists; primary hyperaldosteronism; bilateral renal artery stenosis; pregnancy (2nd and 3rd trimesters)

**Warnings/Precautions** Avoid use or use smaller doses in patients who are volume depleted; correct depletion first. Deterioration in renal function can occur with initiation. Use with caution in unilateral renal artery stenosis and pre-existing renal insufficiency; significant aortic/mitral stenosis. Safety and efficacy have not been established in pediatric patients.

**Adverse Reactions** 1% to 10%:

Cardiovascular: Edema, chest pain, tachycardia

Central nervous system: Dizziness, headache, fatigue, anxiety, nervousness

Dermatologic: Rash

Gastrointestinal: Diarrhea, dyspepsia/heartburn, nausea, vomiting, abdominal pain

Genitourinary: Urinary tract infection

Neuromuscular & skeletal: Pain, trauma

Respiratory: Upper respiratory infection, cough, sinus disorder, pharyngitis, rhinitis, influenza

**Overdosage/Toxicology**

Signs and symptoms: Most likely manifestation of an overdosage would be hypotension and tachycardia; bradycardia could occur from parasympathetic (vagal) stimulation

Treatment: If symptomatic hypotension should occur, institute supportive treatment

**Drug Interactions** CYP2C9 enzyme substrate

Inhibitors of CYP2C9 may increase blood levels

Lithium: Risk of toxicity may be increased by irbesartan; monitor lithium levels

Potassium-sparing diuretics (amiloride, potassium, spironolactone, triamterene): Increased risk of hyperkalemia

Potassium supplements may increase the risk of hyperkalemia

Trimethoprim (high dose) may increase the risk of hyperkalemia

**Usual Dosage** Adults: Oral: 150 mg once daily with or without food; patients may be titrated to 300 mg once daily

**Patient Information** Take exactly as directed; do not discontinue without consulting prescriber. Take first dose at bedtime. This drug does not eliminate need for diet or exercise regimen as recommended by prescriber. May cause dizziness, fainting, lightheadedness (use caution when driving or engaging in tasks that require alertness until response to drug is known); nausea, vomiting, or abdominal pain (small frequent meals, frequent mouth care, sucking lozenges, or chewing gum may help); diarrhea (buttermilk, boiled milk, yogurt may help). Report chest pain or palpitations, skin rash, fluid retention (swelling of extremities), difficulty in breathing or unusual cough, or other persistent adverse reactions.

**Dosage Forms** Tablet: 75 mg, 150 mg, 300 mg

## Irbesartan and Hydrochlorothiazide

(ir be SAR tan & hye droe klor oh THYE a zide)

**U.S. Brand Names** Avapro® HCT

**Pharmacologic Category** Antihypertensive Agent, Combination

**Use** Combination therapy for the management of hypertension

**Effects on Mental Status** May cause anxiety, dizziness, nervousness

**Effects on Psychiatric Treatment** May decrease lithium clearance resulting in an increase in serum lithium levels and potential lithium toxicity; monitor serum lithium levels

**Dosage Forms** Tablet: Irbesartan 75 mg and hydrochlorothiazide 12.5 mg; irbesartan 150 mg and hydrochlorothiazide 12.5 mg; irbesartan 300 mg and hydrochlorothiazide 12.5 mg

♦ **Ircon® [OTC]** *see* Ferrous Fumarate *on page 223*

## Irinotecan (eye rye no TEE kan)

**U.S. Brand Names** Camptosar®

**Pharmacologic Category** Antineoplastic Agent, Natural Source (Plant) Derivative

**Use** A component of first-line therapy in combination with 5-fluorouracil and leucovorin for the treatment of metastatic carcinoma of the colon or rectum; treatment of metastatic carcinoma of the colon or rectum which has recurred or progressed following fluorouracil-based therapy

**Unlabeled use:** Lung cancer (small cell and nonsmall cell), cervical cancer, gastric cancer, pancreatic cancer, leukemia, lymphoma

**Effects on Mental Status** Dizziness and insomnia are common

**Effects on Psychiatric Treatment** May cause myelosuppression; use caution with clozapine and carbamazepine; concurrent use with prochlorperazine has produced akathisia

**Usual Dosage** Refer to individual protocols; courses may be repeated indefinitely as long as the patient continues to experience clinical benefit: Adults: I.V.:

**Single-agent therapy:**

Weekly regimen: 125 mg/m² over 90 minutes on days 1, 8, 15, and 22, followed by a 2-week rest

Once-every-3-week regimen: 350 mg/m² over 90 minutes, once every 3 weeks

A reduction in the starting dose by one dose level may be considered for patients ≥65 years of age, prior pelvic/abdominal radiotherapy, performance status of 2, or increased bilirubin (dosing for patients with a bilirubin >2 mg/dL cannot be recommended based on lack of data per manufacturer)

Depending on the patient's ability to tolerate therapy, doses should be adjusted in increments of 25-50 mg/m². Irinotecan doses may range 50-150 mg/m².

**Combination therapy with 5-FU and leucovorin:** Six-week (42-day) cycle (next cycle beginning on day 45):

125 mg/m² over 90 minutes on days 1, 8, 15, and 22; to be given in combination with bolus leucovorin and 5-FU (leucovorin administered immediately following irinotecan; 5-FU immediately following leucovorin)

180 mg/m² over 90 minutes on days 1, 15, and 22; to be given in combination with infusional leucovorin and bolus/infusion 5-FU (leucovorin administered immediately following irinotecan; 5-FU immediately following leucovorin)

**Note: For all regimens:** It is recommended that new courses begin only after the granulocyte count recovers to ≥1500/mm³, the platelet count recovers to ≥100,000/mm³, and treatment-related diarrhea has fully resolved. Treatment should be delayed 1-2 weeks to allow for recovery from treatment-related toxicities. If the patient has not recovered after a 2-week delay, consideration should be given to discontinuing irinotecan.

**Dosing adjustment for toxicities:** A decrease in dose level corresponds to a decrease in irinotecan dosage by 25-50 mg/m²; specific dose levels corresponding to individual protocols should be consulted.

The following are examples of dosing adjustments cited by the manufacturer:

Standard dose: 125 mg/m²
- Dose level -1: 100 mg/m²
- Dose level -2: 75 mg/m²

Standard dose: 180 mg/m²
- Dose level -1: 150 mg/m²
- Dose level -2: 120 mg/m²

Standard dose: 350 mg/m²
- Dose level -1: 300 mg/m²
- Dose level -2: 250 mg/m²

**Dosing adjustment in renal impairment:** Effects have not been evaluated

**Dosing adjustment in hepatic impairment:**

AUC of irinotecan and SN-38 have been reported to be higher in patients with known hepatic tumor involvement. The manufacturer recommends that no change in dosage or administration be made for patients with liver metastases and normal hepatic function.

In patients with a combined history of prior pelvic/abdominal irradiation and modestly elevated total serum bilirubin levels (1.0-2.0 mg/dL) prior to treatment with irinotecan, there may be substantially increased likelihood of grade 3 or 4 neutropenia. Consideration may be given to starting irinotecan at a lower dose (eg, 100 mg/m²) in such patients. Definite recommendations regarding the most appropriate starting dose in patients who have pretreatment total serum bilirubin elevations >2.0 mg/dL are not available, but it is likely that lower starting doses will need to be considered in such patients.

**Dosage Forms** Injection: 20 mg/mL (5 mL)

## Iron Dextran Complex (EYE ern DEKS tran KOM pleks)

**U.S. Brand Names** Dexferrum® Injection; InFeD™ Injection

**Canadian Brand Names** Infufer®

**Pharmacologic Category** Iron Salt

**Use** Treatment of microcytic hypochromic anemia resulting from iron deficiency in whom oral administration is infeasible or ineffective

**Effects on Mental Status** May cause dizziness

**Effects on Psychiatric Treatment** None reported

**Pregnancy Risk Factor** C

**Contraindications** Hypersensitivity to iron dextran, all anemias that are not involved with iron deficiency, hemochromatosis, hemolytic anemia

**Warnings/Precautions** Use with caution in patients with history of asthma, hepatic impairment, rheumatoid arthritis; not recommended in children <4 months of age; deaths associated with parenteral administration following anaphylactic-type reactions have been reported; use only in patients where the iron deficient state is not amenable to oral iron therapy. A test dose of 0.5 mL I.V. or I.M. should be given to observe for adverse reactions. Anemia in the elderly is often caused by "anemia of chronic disease" or associated with inflammation rather than blood loss. Iron stores are usually normal or increased, with a serum ferritin >50 ng/mL and a decreased total iron binding capacity. I.V. administration of iron dextran is often preferred over I.M. in the elderly secondary to a decreased muscle mass and the need for daily injections.

**Adverse Reactions**

>10%:
- Cardiovascular: Flushing
- Central nervous system: Dizziness, fever, headache, pain
- Gastrointestinal: Nausea, vomiting, metallic taste
- Local: Staining of skin at the site of I.M. injection
- Miscellaneous: Diaphoresis

1% to 10%:
- Cardiovascular: Hypotension (1% to 2%)
- Dermatologic: Urticaria (1% to 2%), phlebitis (1% to 2%)
- Gastrointestinal: Diarrhea
- Genitourinary: Discoloration of urine

<1%: Arthralgia, cardiovascular collapse, chills, leukocytosis, lymphadenopathy, respiratory difficulty

**Note:** Diaphoresis, urticaria, arthralgia, fever, chills, dizziness, headache, and nausea may be delayed 24-48 hours after I.V. administration or 3-4 days after I.M. administration

Anaphylactoid reactions: Respiratory difficulties and cardiovascular collapse have been reported and occur most frequently within the first several minutes of administration

**Overdosage/Toxicology**

Signs and symptoms: Erosion of GI mucosa, pulmonary edema, hyperthermia, convulsions, tachycardia, hepatic and renal impairment, coma, hematemesis, lethargy, tachycardia, acidosis, serum Fe level >300 mcg/mL requires treatment of overdose due to severe toxicity

Treatment: Although rare, if a severe iron overdose (when the serum iron concentration exceeds the total iron-binding capacity) occurs, it may be treated with deferoxamine. Deferoxamine may be administered I.V. (80 mg/kg over 24 hours) or I.M. (40-90 mg/kg every 8 hours).

**Drug Interactions** Decreased effect with chloramphenicol

**Usual Dosage** I.M. (Z-track method should be used for I.M. injection), I.V.:

A 0.5 mL test dose (0.25 mL in infants) should be given prior to starting iron dextran therapy; total dose should be divided into a daily schedule for I.M., total dose may be given as a single continuous infusion

Iron deficiency anemia: Dose (mL) = 0.0476 x LBW (kg) x (normal hemoglobin - observed hemoglobin) + (1 mL/5 kg of LBW to maximum of 14 mL for iron stores)

Iron replacement therapy for blood loss: Replacement iron (mg) = blood loss (mL) x hematocrit

Maximum daily dose (can administer total dose at one time I.V.):
- Infants <5 kg: 25 mg iron (0.5 mL)
- Children:
  - 5-10 kg: 50 mg iron (1 mL)
  - 10-50 kg: 100 mg iron (2 mL)
- Adults >50 kg: 100 mg iron (2 mL)

**Patient Information** You will need frequent blood tests while on this therapy. If you have rheumatoid arthritis you may experience increased swelling or joint pain; consult prescriber for medication adjustment. If you experience dizziness or severe headache, use caution when driving or engaging in tasks that require alertness until response to drug is known. Small frequent meals, frequent mouth care, sucking lozenges, or chewing gum may relieve nausea and metallic taste. You may experience increased sweating. Report acute GI problems, fever, difficulty breathing, rapid heartbeat, yellowing of skin or eyes, or swelling of hands and feet.

**Dosage Forms** Injection: 50 mg/mL (2 mL, 10 mL)


- **ISD** *see* Isosorbide Dinitrate *on page 296*
- **ISDN** *see* Isosorbide Dinitrate *on page 296*
- **Ismelin®** *see* Guanethidine *on page 260*
- **ISMN** *see* Isosorbide Mononitrate *on page 297*
- **Ismo®** *see* Isosorbide Mononitrate *on page 297*
- **Ismotic®** *see* Isosorbide *on page 296*
- **Isobamate** *see* Carisoprodol *on page 94*
- **Isocaine® HCl** *see* Mepivacaine *on page 342*

## Isocarboxazid (eye soe kar BOKS a zid)

**Related Information**

Clinical Issues in the Use of Antidepressants *on page 627*
Patient Information - Antidepressants (MAOIs) *on page 644*

**Generic Available** No

**U.S. Brand Names** Marplan®

**Pharmacologic Category** Antidepressant, Monoamine Oxidase Inhibitor

**Use** Symptomatic treatment of atypical, nonendogenous or neurotic depression

**Pregnancy Risk Factor** C

**Contraindications** Uncontrolled hypertension; hypersensitivity to isocarboxazid; pheochromocytoma; congestive heart failure; severe renal or hepatic impairment

**Adverse Reactions**

>10%:
- Cardiovascular: Orthostatic hypotension
- Central nervous system: Drowsiness
- Endocrine & metabolic: Decreased sexual ability
- Neuromuscular & skeletal: Weakness, trembling
- Ocular: Blurred vision

1% to 10%:
- Cardiovascular: Tachycardia, peripheral edema
- Central nervous system: Nervousness, chills
- Dermatologic: Xerostomia
- Gastrointestinal: Diarrhea, anorexia, constipation

<1%:
- Central nervous system: Parkinsonian syndrome
- Hematologic: Leukopenia
- Hepatic: Hepatitis

**Drug Interactions**

Amphetamines: MAOIs in combination with amphetamines may result in severe hypertensive reaction; these combinations are best avoided

Anorexiants: Concurrent use of anorexiants may result in serotonin syndrome; these combinations are best avoided; includes dexfenfluramine, fenfluramine, or sibutramine

Barbiturates: MAOIs may inhibit the metabolism of barbiturates and prolong their effect

CNS stimulants: MAOIs in combination with stimulants (methylphenidate) may result in severe hypertensive reaction; these combinations are best avoided

Dextromethorphan: Concurrent use of MAOIs may result in serotonin syndrome; these combinations are best avoided

Disulfiram: MAOIs may produce delirium in patients receiving disulfiram; monitor

Guanadrel and guanethidine: MAOIs inhibit the antihypertensive response to guanadrel or guanethidine; use an alternative antihypertensive agent

Hypoglycemic agents: MAOIs may produce hypoglycemia in patients with diabetes; monitor

Levodopa: MAOIs in combination with levodopa may result in hypertensive reactions; monitor

Lithium: MAOIs in combination with lithium have resulted in malignant hyperpyrexia; this combination is best avoided

Meperidine: May cause serotonin syndrome when combined with an MAO inhibitor; avoid this combination

Nefazodone: Concurrent use of MAOIs may result in serotonin syndrome; these combinations are best avoided

Norepinephrine: MAOIs may increase the pressor response of norepinephrine (effect is generally small); monitor

Reserpine: MAOIs in combination with reserpine may result in hypertensive reactions; monitor

Serotonin agonists: Theoretically, may increase the risk of serotonin syndrome; includes sumatriptan, naratriptan, rizatriptan, and zolmitriptan

SSRIs: May cause serotonin syndrome when combined with an MAO inhibitor; avoid this combination

Succinylcholine: MAOIs may prolong the muscle relaxation produced by succinylcholine via decreased plasma pseudocholinesterase

Sympathomimetics (indirect-acting): MAOIs in combination with sympathomimetics such as dopamine, metaraminol, phenylephrine, and decongestants (pseudoephedrine) may result in severe hypertensive reaction; these combinations are best avoided

Tramadol: May increase the risk of seizures and serotonin syndrome in patients receiving an MAOI

Trazodone: Concurrent use of MAOIs may result in serotonin syndrome; these combinations are best avoided

Tricyclic antidepressants: May cause serotonin syndrome when combined with an MAO inhibitor; avoid this combination

Tyramine: Foods (eg, cheese) and beverages (eg, ethanol) containing tyramine, should be avoided in patients receiving an MAOI; hypertensive crisis may result

Venlafaxine: Concurrent use of MAOIs may result in serotonin syndrome; these combinations are best avoided

**Mechanism of Action** Thought to act by increasing endogenous concentrations of epinephrine, norepinephrine, dopamine, and serotonin through inhibition of the enzyme (monoamine oxidase) responsible for the breakdown of these neurotransmitters

**Usual Dosage** Adults: Oral: 10 mg 3 times/day; reduce to 10-20 mg/day in divided doses when condition improves

**Patient Information** Avoid tyramine-containing foods and drinks

**Dosage Forms** Tablet: 10 mg

♦ **Isoclor® Expectorant** *see* Guaifenesin, Pseudoephedrine, and Codeine *on page 258*

♦ **Isocom®** *see* Acetaminophen, Isometheptene, and Dichloralphenazone *on page 16*

## Isoetharine (eye soe ETH a reen)

**U.S. Brand Names** Arm-a-Med® Isoetharine; Beta-2®; Bronkometer®; Bronkosol®; Dey-Lute® Isoetharine

**Pharmacologic Category** Adrenergic Agonist Agent; Bronchodilator; Sympathomimetic

**Use** Bronchodilator in bronchial asthma and for reversible bronchospasm occurring with bronchitis and emphysema

**Effects on Mental Status** May cause dizziness, lightheadedness, headache, nervousness, or insomnia

**Effects on Psychiatric Treatment** Beta-blockers may decrease the effects of isoetharine

**Usual Dosage** Treatments are not usually repeated more than every 4 hours, except in severe cases

Nebulizer: Children: 0.01 mL/kg; minimum dose 0.1 mL; maximum dose: 0.5 mL diluted in 2-3 mL normal saline

Inhalation: Oral: Adults: 1-2 inhalations every 4 hours as needed

**Dosage Forms**

Aerosol, oral, as mesylate: 340 mcg/metered spray

Solution, inhalation, as hydrochloride: 0.062% (4 mL); 0.08% (3.5 mL); 0.1% (2.5 mL, 5 mL); 0.125% (4 mL); 0.167% (3 mL); 0.17% (3 mL); 0.2% (2.5 mL); 0.25% (2 mL, 3.5 mL); 0.5% (0.5 mL); 1% (0.5 mL, 0.25 mL, 10 mL, 14 mL, 30 mL)

## Isoflurane (eye soe FLURE ane)

**U.S. Brand Names** Forane®

**Pharmacologic Category** General Anesthetic

**Use** General induction and maintenance of anesthesia (inhalation)

**Effects on Mental Status** None reported

**Effects on Psychiatric Treatment** None reported

**Usual Dosage** 1.5% to 3%

**Dosage Forms** Solution: 100 mL, 125 mL, 250 mL

## Isoflurophate (eye soe FLURE oh fate)

**Related Information**

Glaucoma Drug Therapy *on page 712*

**U.S. Brand Names** Floropryl® Ophthalmic

**Pharmacologic Category** Acetylcholinesterase Inhibitor (Central); Ophthalmic Agent, Antiglaucoma; Ophthalmic Agent, Miotic

**Use** Treat primary open-angle glaucoma and conditions that obstruct aqueous outflow and to treat accommodative convergent strabismus

**Effects on Mental Status** None reported

**Effects on Psychiatric Treatment** None reported

**Usual Dosage** Adults: Ophthalmic:

Glaucoma: Instill 0.25" strip in eye every 8-72 hours

Strabismus: Instill 0.25" strip to each eye every night for 2 weeks then reduce to 0.25" every other night to once weekly for 2 months

**Dosage Forms** Ointment, ophthalmic: 0.025% in polyethylene mineral oil gel (3.5 g)

♦ **Isollyl® Improved** *see* Butalbital Compound and Aspirin *on page 80*

## Isoniazid (eye soe NYE a zid)

**U.S. Brand Names** Laniazid® Oral

**Canadian Brand Names** PMS-Isoniazid

**Synonyms** INH; Isonicotinic Acid Hydrazide

**Pharmacologic Category** Antitubercular Agent

**Use** Treatment of susceptible tuberculosis infections and prophylactically to those individuals exposed to tuberculosis

**Effects on Mental Status** May cause drowsiness or dizziness; may rarely cause depression or psychosis; reports of insomnia, restlessness, disorientation, hallucinations, delusions, obsessive-compulsive symptoms, and exacerbation of schizophrenia

**Effects on Psychiatric Treatment** Isoniazid may impair the metabolism of carbamazepine and oxidatively metabolized benzodiazepines; monitor for adverse effects

**Pregnancy Risk Factor** C

**Contraindications** Acute liver disease; hypersensitivity to isoniazid or any component; previous history of hepatic damage during isoniazid therapy

**Warnings/Precautions** Use with caution in patients with renal impairment and chronic liver disease. Severe and sometimes fatal hepatitis may occur or develop even after many months of treatment; patients must report any prodromal symptoms of hepatitis, such as fatigue, weakness, malaise, anorexia, nausea, or vomiting. Children with low milk and low meat intake should receive concomitant pyridoxine therapy. Periodic ophthalmic examinations are recommended even when usual symptoms do not occur; pyridoxine (10-50 mg/day) is recommended in individuals likely to develop peripheral neuropathies.

**Adverse Reactions**

>10%:

Gastrointestinal: Loss of appetite, nausea, vomiting, stomach pain

Hepatic: Mild increased LFTs (10% to 20%)

Neuromuscular & skeletal: Weakness, peripheral neuropathy (dose-related incidence, 10% to 20% incidence with 10 mg/kg/day)

1% to 10%:

Central nervous system: Dizziness, slurred speech, lethargy

Hepatic: Progressive liver damage (increases with age; 2.3% in patients >50 years of age)

Neuromuscular & skeletal: Hyper-reflexia

<1%: Arthralgia, blood dyscrasias, blurred vision, fever, loss of vision, mental depression, psychosis, rash, seizures

**Overdosage/Toxicology**

Signs and symptoms: Nausea, vomiting, slurred speech, dizziness, blurred vision, hallucinations, stupor, coma, intractable seizures, onset of metabolic acidosis is 30 minutes to 3 hours. Because of the severe morbidity and high mortality rates with isoniazid overdose, patients who are asymptomatic after an overdose, should be monitored for 4-6 hours.

Treatment: Pyridoxine has been shown to be effective in the treatment of intoxication, especially when seizures occur. Pyridoxine I.V. is administered on a milligram to milligram dose. If the amount of isoniazid ingested is unknown, 5 g of pyridoxine should be given over 3-5 minutes and may be followed by an additional 5 g in 30 minutes. Treatment is supportive; may require airway protection, ventilation; diazepam for seizures, sodium bicarbonate for acidosis; forced diuresis and hemodialysis can result in more rapid removal.

**Drug Interactions** CYP2E1 enzyme substrate; CYP2E1 enzyme inducer; and CYP1A2, 2C, 2C9, 2C18, 2C19, and 3A3/4 enzyme inhibitor

Decreased effect of ketoconazole with isoniazid

Decreased effect/levels of isoniazid with aluminum salts

Increased toxicity/levels of oral anticoagulants, carbamazepine, cycloserine, meperidine, hydantoins, hepatically metabolized benzodiazepines with isoniazid; reaction with disulfiram occurs; enflurane with isoniazid may result in renal failure especially in rapid acetylators

Increased hepatic toxicity with alcohol or with rifampin and isoniazid

**Usual Dosage** Recommendations often change due to resistant strains and newly developed information; consult *MMWR* for current CDC recommendations: **Oral** (injectable is available for patients who are unable to either take or absorb oral therapy):

**Note:** A four-drug regimen (isoniazid, rifampin, pyrazinamide, and either streptomycin or ethambutol) is preferred for the initial, empiric treatment of TB. When the drug susceptibility results are available, the regimen should be altered as appropriate.

Infants and Children:

Prophylaxis: 10 mg/kg/day in 1-2 divided doses (maximum: 300 mg/day) 6 months in patients who do not have HIV infection and 12 months in patients who have HIV infection

Treatment:

Daily therapy: 10-20 mg/kg/day in 1-2 divided doses (maximum: 300 mg/day)

Directly observed therapy (DOT): Twice weekly therapy: 20-40 mg/kg (maximum: 900 mg/day); 3 times/week therapy: 20-40 mg/kg (maximum: 900 mg)

Adults:

Prophylaxis: 300 mg/day for 6 months in patients who do not have HIV infection and 12 months in patients who have HIV infection

Treatment:

Daily therapy: 5 mg/kg/day given daily (usual dose: 300 mg/day); 10 mg/kg/day in 1-2 divided doses in patients with disseminated disease

Directly observed therapy (DOT): Twice weekly therapy: 15 mg/kg (maximum: 900 mg); 3 times/week therapy: 15 mg/kg (maximum: 900 mg)

**Note:** Concomitant administration of 6-50 mg/day pyridoxine is recommended in malnourished patients or those prone to neuropathy (eg, alcoholics, diabetics)

**Hemodialysis:** Dialyzable (50% to 100%)

Administer dose postdialysis

**Peritoneal dialysis effects:** Dose for $Cl_{cr}$ <10 mL/minute

**Continuous arteriovenous or venovenous hemofiltration (CAVH/CAVHD):** Dose for $Cl_{cr}$ <10 mL/minute

**Dosing adjustment in hepatic impairment:** Dose should be reduced in severe hepatic disease

**Patient Information** Best if taken on an empty stomach (1 hour before or 2 hours after meals). Avoid missing any dose and do not discontinue without notifying prescriber. Avoid alcohol and tyramine-containing foods (eg, fish, preserved meats or sausages, tuna, sauerkraut, aged cheeses, broad beans, liver pate, wine, protein supplements, etc). Increase dietary intake of folate, niacin, magnesium. If diabetic, use serum testing (isoniazid may affect Clinitest® results). You may experience GI distress (taking dose with meals may help). Use caution to prevent injury. You will need to have frequent ophthalmic exams and periodic medical check-ups to evaluate drug effects. Report tingling or numbness in hands or feet, loss of sensation, unusual weakness, fatigue, nausea or vomiting, dark colored urine, change in urinary pattern, yellowing skin or eyes, or change in color of stool.

**Dosage Forms**

Injection: 100 mg/mL (10 mL)

Syrup (orange flavor): 50 mg/5 mL (473 mL)

Tablet: 50 mg, 100 mg, 300 mg

♦ **Isonicotinic Acid Hydrazide** *see* Isoniazid *on page 294*

♦ **Isonipecaine Hydrochloride** *see* Meperidine *on page 341*

♦ **Isopap®** *see* Acetaminophen, Isometheptene, and Dichloralphenazone *on page 16*

♦ **Isoprenaline Hydrochloride** *see* Isoproterenol *on page 295*

## Isopropamide (eye soe PROE pa mide)

**U.S. Brand Names** Darbid®

**Pharmacologic Category** Anticholinergic Agent; Antispasmodic Agent, Gastrointestinal

**Use** Adjunctive therapy for peptic ulcer, irritable bowel syndrome

**Effects on Mental Status** May cause confusion, amnesia, drowsiness, or insomnia

**Effects on Psychiatric Treatment** Concurrent use with psychotropics may produce additive sedation and dry mouth

**Usual Dosage** Children >12 years and Adults: Oral: 5-10 mg every 12 hours; dose may be increased up to 10 mg twice daily or more

**Dosage Forms** Tablet, as iodide: 5 mg

## Isoproterenol (eye soe proe TER e nole)

**U.S. Brand Names** Arm-a-Med® Isoproterenol; Dey-Dose® Isoproterenol; Isuprel®; Medihaler-Iso®

**Synonyms** Isoprenaline Hydrochloride; Isoproterenol Hydrochloride; Isoproterenol Sulfate

**Pharmacologic Category** $Beta_1$/$Beta_2$ Agonist

**Use** Treatment of reversible airway obstruction as in asthma or COPD; used parenterally in ventricular arrhythmias due to A-V nodal block; hemodynamically compromised bradyarrhythmias or atropine-resistant bradyarrhythmias; temporary use in third degree A-V block until pacemaker insertion; low cardiac output; vasoconstrictive shock states

**Effects on Mental Status** Insomnia and restlessness are common

**Effects on Psychiatric Treatment** None reported

**Pregnancy Risk Factor** C

**Contraindications** Angina, pre-existing cardiac arrhythmias (ventricular); tachycardia or A-V block caused by cardiac glycoside intoxication; allergy to sulfites or isoproterenol or other sympathomimetic amines

**Warnings/Precautions** Elderly patients, diabetics, renal or cardiovascular disease, hyperthyroidism; excessive or prolonged use may result in decreased effectiveness

**Adverse Reactions**

>10%:

Central nervous system: Insomnia, restlessness

Gastrointestinal: Dry throat, xerostomia, discoloration of saliva (pinkish-red)

1% to 10%:

Cardiovascular: Flushing of the face or skin, ventricular arrhythmias, tachycardias, profound hypotension, hypertension

Central nervous system: Nervousness, anxiety, dizziness, headache, lightheadedness

Gastrointestinal: Vomiting, nausea

Neuromuscular & skeletal: Trembling, tremor, weakness

Miscellaneous: Diaphoresis

<1%: Arrhythmias, chest pain, paradoxical bronchospasm

**Overdosage/Toxicology**

Signs and symptoms: Tremors, nausea, vomiting, hypotension; beta-adrenergic stimulation can cause increased heart rate, decreased blood pressure, and CNS excitation

Treatment: Heart rate can be treated with beta-blockers, decreased blood pressure can be treated with pure alpha-adrenergic agents, diazepam 0.07 mg/kg can be used for excitation, seizures

**Drug Interactions** Increased toxicity: Sympathomimetic agents may cause headaches and elevate blood pressure; general anesthetics may cause arrhythmias

(Continued)

## Isoproterenol *(Continued)*

**Usual Dosage**

Children:

Bronchodilation: Inhalation: Metered dose inhaler: 1-2 metered doses up to 5 times/day

Bronchodilation (using 1:200 inhalation solution) 0.01 mL/kg/dose every 4 hours as needed (maximum: 0.05 mL/dose) diluted with NS to 2 mL

Sublingual: 5-10 mg every 3-4 hours, not to exceed 30 mg/day

Cardiac arrhythmias: I.V.: Start 0.1 mcg/kg/minute (usual effective dose 0.2-2 mcg/kg/minute)

Adults:

Bronchodilation: Inhalation: Metered dose inhaler: 1-2 metered doses 4-6 times/day

Bronchodilation: 1-2 inhalations of a 0.25% solution, no more than 2 inhalations at any one time (1-5 minutes between inhalations); no more than 6 inhalations in any hour during a 24-hour period; maintenance therapy: 1-2 inhalations 4-6 times/day. Alternatively: 0.5% solution via hand bulb nebulizer is 5-15 deep inhalations repeated once in 5-10 minutes if necessary; treatments may be repeated up to 5 times/day.

Sublingual: 10-20 mg every 3-4 hours; not to exceed 60 mg/day

Cardiac arrhythmias: I.V.: 5 mcg/minute initially, titrate to patient response (2-20 mcg/minute)

Shock: I.V.: 0.5-5 mcg/minute; adjust according to response

**Patient Information**

Sublingual: Do not chew or swallow tables, let them dissolve under the tongue.

Inhalant: Shake canister before use. Administer pressurized inhalation during the second half of inspiration. If more than one dose is necessary, wait at least 1 full minute between inhalations; second inhalation is best delivered after 5-10 minutes. Do not use more often than recommended. Store solution away from light or excess heat or cold.

You may experience nervousness, dizziness, or fatigue. Use caution when driving or engaging in tasks requiring alertness until response to drug is known. Frequent small meals may reduce the incidence of nausea or vomiting. Report chest pain, rapid heartbeat or palpitations, unresolved/persistent GI upset, dizziness, fatigue, trembling, increased anxiety, sleeplessness, or difficulty breathing.

**Nursing Implications** Elderly may find it useful to utilize a spacer device when using a metered dose inhaler

**Dosage Forms**

Inhalation:

Aerosol: 0.2% (1:500) (15 mL, 22.5 mL); 0.25% (1:400) (15 mL)

Solution for nebulization: 0.031% (4 mL); 0.062% (4 mL); 0.25% (0.5 mL, 30 mL); 0.5% (0.5 mL, 10 mL, 60 mL); 1% (10 mL)

Injection: 0.2 mg/mL (1:5000) (1 mL, 5 mL, 10 mL)

Tablet, sublingual: 10 mg, 15 mg


- **Isoproterenol Hydrochloride** *see* Isoproterenol *on page 295*
- **Isoproterenol Sulfate** *see* Isoproterenol *on page 295*
- **Isoptin®** *see* Verapamil *on page 583*
- **Isoptin® SR** *see* Verapamil *on page 583*
- **Isopto® Atropine Ophthalmic** *see* Atropine *on page 53*
- **Isopto® Carbachol Ophthalmic** *see* Carbachol *on page 90*
- **Isopto® Carpine Ophthalmic** *see* Pilocarpine *on page 445*
- **Isopto® Cetamide® Ophthalmic** *see* Sulfacetamide *on page 522*
- **Isopto® Cetapred® Ophthalmic** *see* Sulfacetamide Sodium and Prednisolone *on page 523*
- **Isopto® Homatropine Ophthalmic** *see* Homatropine *on page 268*
- **Isopto® Hyoscine Ophthalmic** *see* Scopolamine *on page 506*
- **Isopto® Plain Solution [OTC]** *see* Artificial Tears *on page 48*
- **Isopto® Tears Solution [OTC]** *see* Artificial Tears *on page 48*
- **Isordil®** *see* Isosorbide Dinitrate *on page 296*


## Isosorbide (eye soe SOR bide)

**U.S. Brand Names** Ismotic®

**Pharmacologic Category** Diuretic, Osmotic; Ophthalmic Agent, Antiglaucoma; Ophthalmic Agent, Osmotic

**Use** Short-term emergency treatment of acute angle-closure glaucoma and short-term reduction of intraocular pressure prior to and following intraocular surgery; may be used to interrupt an acute glaucoma attack; preferred agent when need to avoid nausea and vomiting

**Effects on Mental Status** May cause confusion or disorientation; may rarely cause drowsiness, dizziness, or irritability

**Effects on Psychiatric Treatment** None reported

**Pregnancy Risk Factor** B

**Contraindications** Severe renal disease, anuria, severe dehydration, acute pulmonary edema, severe cardiac decompensation, known hypersensitivity to isosorbide

**Warnings/Precautions** Use with caution in patients with impending pulmonary edema and in the elderly due to the elderly's predisposition to dehydration and the fact that they frequently have concomitant diseases which may be aggravated by the use of isosorbide; hypernatremia and dehydration may begin to occur after 72 hours of continuous administration. Maintain fluid/electrolyte balance with multiple doses; monitor urinary output; if urinary output declines, need to review clinical status.

**Adverse Reactions**

1% to 10%:

Central nervous system: Headache, confusion, disorientation

Gastrointestinal: Vomiting

<1%: Abdominal/gastric discomfort (infrequently), anorexia, dizziness, hiccups, hypernatremia, hyperosmolarity, irritability, lethargy, lightheadedness, nausea, rash, syncope, thirst, vertigo

**Overdosage/Toxicology**

Signs and symptoms: Dehydration, hypotension, hyponatremia

Treatment: General supportive care, fluid administration, electrolyte balance, discontinue agent

**Drug Interactions** No data reported

**Usual Dosage** Adults: Oral: Initial: 1.5 g/kg with a usual range of 1-3 g/kg 2-4 times/day as needed

**Patient Information** This is for short-term treatment, it is not for long-term use. Pour over cracked ice and sip. Take all of medication. You may experience frequent urination (maintain adequate hydration); gastric upset (small frequent meals may help); dizziness, drowsiness, or confusion (use caution when driving); or dry mouth (chewing gum, frequent oral care, sucking on lozenges may help). Report difficulty breathing, unrelieved headache, changes in CNS (eg, confusion or disorientation). Consult prescriber if breast-feeding.

**Nursing Implications** Palatability may be improved if poured over ice and sipped

**Dosage Forms** Solution: 45% [450 mg/mL] (220 mL)

## Isosorbide Dinitrate (eye soe SOR bide dye NYE trate)

**U.S. Brand Names** Dilatrate®-SR; Isordil®; Sorbitrate®

**Canadian Brand Names** Apo®-ISDN; Cedocard®-SR; Coradur®

**Synonyms** ISD; ISDN

**Pharmacologic Category** Vasodilator

**Use** Prevention and treatment of angina pectoris; for congestive heart failure; to relieve pain, dysphagia, and spasm in esophageal spasm with GE reflux

**Effects on Mental Status** May cause dizziness

**Effects on Psychiatric Treatment** None reported

**Pregnancy Risk Factor** C

**Contraindications** Hypersensitivity to isosorbide dinitrate or any component; hypersensitivity to organic nitrates; concurrent use with sildenafil; angle-closure glaucoma (intraocular pressure may be increased); head trauma or cerebral hemorrhage (increase intracranial pressure); severe anemia

**Warnings/Precautions** Severe hypotension can occur. Use with caution in volume depletion, hypotension, and right ventricular infarctions. Paradoxical bradycardia and increased angina pectoris can accompany hypotension. Postural hypotension can also occur. Tolerance does develop to nitrates and appropriate dosing is needed to minimize this. Safety and efficacy have not been established in pediatric patients. Nitrate may aggravate angina caused by hypertrophic cardiomyopathy. Avoid concurrent use with sildenafil.

**Adverse Reactions**

>10%:

Cardiovascular: Flushing, postural hypotension

Central nervous system: Headache, lightheadedness, dizziness

Neuromuscular & skeletal: Weakness

1% to 10%: Dermatologic: Drug rash, exfoliative dermatitis

<1%: Methemoglobinemia (overdose), nausea, vomiting

**Overdosage/Toxicology**

Signs and symptoms: Most common include hypotension, throbbing headache, tachycardia, and flushing. Methemoglobinemia may occur with massive doses; hypotension may aggravate symptoms of cardiac ischemia or cerebrovascular disease and may even cause seizures (rare).

Treatment: Consists of placing patient in recumbent position and administering fluids; alpha-adrenergic vasopressors may be required; treat methemoglobinemia with oxygen and methylene blue at a dose of 1-2 mg/kg I.V. slowly.

**Drug Interactions** Sildenafil: Significant reduction of systolic and diastolic blood pressure with concurrent use; do not give sildenafil within 24 hours of a nitrate preparation

**Usual Dosage** Adults (elderly should be given lowest recommended daily doses initially and titrate upward): Oral:

Angina: 5-40 mg 4 times/day or 40 mg every 8-12 hours in sustained-release dosage form

Congestive heart failure:
Initial dose: 10 mg 3 times/day
Target dose: 40 mg 3 times/day
Maximum dose: 80 mg 3 times/day
Sublingual: 2.5-10 mg every 4-6 hours
Chew: 5-10 mg every 2-3 hours

**Tolerance to nitrate effects develops with chronic exposure**

Dose escalation does not overcome this effect. Tolerance can only be overcome by short periods of nitrate absence from the body. Short periods (14 hours) or nitrate withdrawal help minimize tolerance.

Hemodialysis: During hemodialysis, administer dose postdialysis or administer supplemental 10-20 mg dose

Peritoneal dialysis: Supplemental dose is not necessary

**Patient Information** Take as directed, at the same time each day. Do not chew or swallow sublingual tablets; allow them to dissolve under your tongue. Do not change brands without consulting prescriber. Do not discontinue abruptly. Keep medication in original container, tightly closed. Avoid alcohol; combination may cause severe hypotension. Take medication while sitting down and use caution when changing position (rise from sitting or lying position slowly). May cause dizziness; use caution when driving or engaging in hazardous activities until response to drug is known. If chest pain is unresolved in 15 minutes, seek emergency medical help at once. Report acute headache, rapid heartbeat, unusual restlessness or dizziness, muscular weakness, or blurring vision.

**Nursing Implications** 8- to 12-hour nitrate-free interval is needed each day to prevent tolerance

**Dosage Forms**

Capsule, sustained release: 40 mg
Tablet:
Chewable: 5 mg, 10 mg
Oral: 5 mg, 10 mg, 20 mg, 30 mg, 40 mg
Sublingual: 2.5 mg, 5 mg, 10 mg
Sustained release: 40 mg

## Isosorbide Mononitrate (eye soe SOR bide mon oh NYE trate)

**U.S. Brand Names** Imdur™; Ismo®; Monoket®

**Synonyms** ISMN

**Pharmacologic Category** Vasodilator

**Use** Long-acting metabolite of the vasodilator isosorbide dinitrate used for the prophylactic treatment of angina pectoris

**Effects on Mental Status** May cause dizziness; may rarely cause drowsiness, agitation, anxiety, confusion, nervousness, or insomnia

**Effects on Psychiatric Treatment** None reported

**Pregnancy Risk Factor** C

**Contraindications** Hypersensitivity to isosorbide or any component; hypersensitivity to organic nitrates; concurrent use with sildenafil; angle-closure glaucoma (intraocular pressure may be increased); head trauma or cerebral hemorrhage (increase intracranial pressure); severe anemia

**Warnings/Precautions** Severe hypotension can occur. Use with caution in volume depletion, hypotension, and right ventricular infarctions. Paradoxical bradycardia and increased angina pectoris can accompany hypotension. Orthostatic hypotension can also occur. Alcohol can accentuate this. Tolerance does develop to nitrates and appropriate dosing is needed to minimize this (drug-free interval). Safety and efficacy have not been established in pediatric patients. Nitrates may aggravate angina caused by hypertrophic cardiomyopathy. Avoid concurrent use with sildenafil.

**Adverse Reactions**

>10%: Central nervous system: Headache

1% to 10%: Gastrointestinal: Dizziness, nausea, vomiting

<1%: Abdominal pain, agitation, angina pectoris, anxiety, arrhythmias, arthralgia, atrial fibrillation, blurred vision, bronchitis, cold sweat confusion, diarrhea, diplopia, dyscoordination, dyspepsia, dysuria, edema, hypoesthesia, hypotension, impotence, increased appetite, insomnia, malaise, methemoglobinemia (rarely with very high doses), neck stiffness, nervousness, nightmares, palpitations, pneumonia, polyuria, postural hypotension, premature ventricular contractions, pruritus, rash, rigors, supraventricular tachycardia, syncope, tenesmus, tooth disorder, upper respiratory tract infection, weakness

**Overdosage/Toxicology**

Signs and symptoms: Most common include hypotension, throbbing headache, tachycardia, and flushing. Methemoglobinemia may occur with massive doses; hypotension may aggravate symptoms of cardiac ischemia or cerebrovascular disease and may even cause seizures (rare).

Treatment: Consists of placing patient in recumbent position and administering fluids; alpha-adrenergic vasopressors may be required; treat methemoglobinemia with oxygen and methylene blue at a dose of 1-2 mg/kg I.V. slowly.

**Drug Interactions** Sildenafil: Significant reduction of systolic and diastolic blood pressure with concurrent use; do not give sildenafil within 24 hours of a nitrate preparation

**Usual Dosage** Geriatrics (start with lowest recommended dose) and Adults: Oral:

Regular tablet: 5-10 mg twice daily with the two doses given 7 hours apart (eg, 8 AM and 3 PM) to decrease tolerance development; then titrate to 10 mg twice daily in first 2-3 days.

Extended release tablet (Imdur™): Initial: 30-60 mg given in morning as a single dose; titrate upward as needed, giving at least 3 days between increases; maximum daily single dose: 240 mg

**Dosing adjustment in renal impairment:** Not necessary for elderly or patients with altered renal or hepatic function.

Tolerance to nitrate effects develops with chronic exposure. Dose escalation does not overcome this effect. Tolerance can only be overcome by short periods of nitrate absence from the body. Short periods (10-12 hours) of nitrate withdrawal help minimize tolerance. General recommendations are to take the last dose of short-acting agents no later than 7 PM; administer 2 times/day rather than 4 times/day. Administer sustained release tablet (Imdur™) once daily in the morning.

**Dietary Considerations** Alcohol: Has been found to exhibit additive effects of this variety

**Patient Information** Take as directed, at the same time each day. Do not chew or crush extended release capsules; swallow with 8 oz of water. Do not change brands without consulting prescriber. Do not discontinue abruptly. Keep medication in original container, tightly closed. Avoid alcohol; combination may cause severe hypotension. Take medication while sitting down and use caution when changing position (rise from sitting or lying position slowly). May cause dizziness; use caution when driving or engaging in hazardous activities until response to drug is known. If chest pain is unresolved in 15 minutes, seek emergency medical help at once. Report acute headache, rapid heartbeat, unusual restlessness or dizziness, muscular weakness, or blurring vision.

**Nursing Implications** Do not crush; 8- to 12-hour nitrate-free interval is needed each day to prevent tolerance

**Dosage Forms**

Tablet (Ismo®, Monoket®): 10 mg, 20 mg
Tablet, extended release (Imdur™): 30 mg, 60 mg, 120 mg

## Isotretinoin (eye soe TRET i noyn)

**U.S. Brand Names** Accutane®

**Canadian Brand Names** Isotrex®

**Synonyms** 13-*cis*-Retinoic Acid

**Pharmacologic Category** Retinoic Acid Derivative

**Use** Treatment of severe recalcitrant cystic and/or conglobate acne unresponsive to conventional therapy

**Unlabeled use:** Treatment of children with metastatic neuroblastoma or leukemia that does not respond to conventional therapy

**Effects on Mental Status** May cause sedation, depression, or psychosis; may rarely cause suicidal ideation

**Effects on Psychiatric Treatment** May increase the clearance of carbamazepine

**Pregnancy Risk Factor** X

**Contraindications** Sensitivity to parabens, vitamin A, or other retinoids; patients who are pregnant or intend to become pregnant during treatment

**Warnings/Precautions** Use with caution in patients with diabetes mellitus, hypertriglyceridemia; acute pancreatitis and fatal hemorrhagic pancreatitis (rare) have been reported; **not to be used in women of childbearing potential** unless woman is capable of complying with effective contraceptive measures; therapy is begun after two negative pregnancy tests; effective contraception must be used for at least 1 month before beginning therapy, during therapy, and for 1 month after discontinuation of therapy. Prescriptions should be written for no more than a 1-month supply, and pregnancy testing and counseling should be repeated monthly. Because of the high likelihood of teratogenic effects (~20%), do not prescribe isotretinoin for women who are or who are likely to become pregnant while using the drug. Isolated reports of depression, psychosis and rarely suicidal thoughts and actions have been reported during isotretinoin usage. Discontinuation of treatment alone may not be sufficient, further evaluation may be necessary. Cases of pseudotumor cerebri (benign intracranial hypertension) have been reported, some with concomitant use of tetracycline (avoid using together). Patients with papilledema, headache, nausea, vomiting, and visual disturbances should be referred to a neurologist and treatment with isotretinoin discontinued. Hearing impairment, which can continue after therapy is discontinued, may occur. Clinical hepatitis, elevated liver enzymes, inflammatory bowel disease, skeletal hyperostosis, premature epiphyseal closure, vision impairment, corneal opacities, and decreased night vision have also been reported with the use of isotretinoin.

**Adverse Reactions**

>10%:

Dermatologic: Redness, cheilitis, inflammation of lips, dry skin, pruritus, photosensitivity
Endocrine & metabolic: Increased serum concentration of triglycerides
Gastrointestinal: Xerostomia
Local: Burning
Neuromuscular & skeletal: Bone pain, arthralgia, myalgia
Ocular: Itching eyes
Respiratory: Epistaxis, dry nose

(Continued)

## Isotretinoin *(Continued)*

1% to 10%:

Cardiovascular: Facial edema, pallor

Central nervous system: Fatigue, headache, mental depression, hypothermia

Dermatologic: Skin peeling on hands or soles of feet, rash, cellulitis

Endocrine & metabolic: Fluid imbalance, acidosis

Gastrointestinal: Stomach upset

Hepatic: Ascites

Neuromuscular & skeletal: Flank pain

Ocular: Dry eyes, photophobia

Miscellaneous: Lymph disorders

<1%: Alopecia, anorexia, bleeding of gums, cataracts, conjunctivitis, corneal opacities, decrease in hemoglobin and hematocrit, hepatitis, hyperuricemia, increase in erythrocyte sedimentation rate, inflammatory bowel syndrome, mood change, nausea, optic neuritis, pruritus, pseudomotor cerebri, vomiting, xerostomia

**Overdosage/Toxicology** Signs and symptoms: Headache, vomiting, flushing, abdominal pain, ataxia; all signs and symptoms have been transient

**Drug Interactions**

Decreased effect: Increased clearance of carbamazepine

Increased toxicity: Avoid other vitamin A products; may interfere with medications used to treat hypertriglyceridemia

**Usual Dosage** Oral:

Children: Maintenance therapy for neuroblastoma: 100-250 mg/m$^2$/day in 2 divided doses has been used investigationally

Children and Adults: 0.5-2 mg/kg/day in 2 divided doses (dosages as low as 0.05 mg/kg/day have been reported to be beneficial) for 15-20 weeks or until the total cyst count decreases by 70%, whichever is sooner

**Dosing adjustment in hepatic impairment:** Dose reductions empirically are recommended in hepatitis disease

**Patient Information** Use exactly as directed; do not take more than recommended. Capsule can be chewed and swallowed, swallowed, or opened with a large needle and contents sprinkled on applesauce or ice cream. Do not take any other vitamin A products, limit vitamin A intake, and increase exercise during therapy. Exacerbations of acne may occur during first weeks of therapy. You may experience headache, loss of night vision, lethargy, or visual disturbances (use caution when driving or engaging in tasks requiring alertness until response to drug is known); photosensitivity (use sunscreen, wear protective clothing and eyewear, and avoid direct sunlight); dry mouth or nausea (small frequent meals, sucking hard candy, or chewing gum may may help); dryness, redness, or itching of skin, eye irritation, or increased sensitivity to contact lenses (wear regular glasses). Discontinue therapy and report acute vision changes, rectal bleeding, abdominal cramping, or unresolved diarrhea.

**Nursing Implications** Capsules can be swallowed, or chewed and swallowed. The capsule may be opened with a large needle and the contents placed on applesauce or ice cream for patients unable to swallow the capsule.

**Dosage Forms** Capsule: 10 mg, 20 mg, 40 mg

## Isoxsuprine (eye SOKS syoo preen)

**U.S. Brand Names** Vasodilan®

**Pharmacologic Category** Vasodilator

**Use** Treatment of peripheral vascular diseases, such as arteriosclerosis obliterans and Raynaud's disease

**Effects on Mental Status** None reported

**Effects on Psychiatric Treatment** None reported

**Pregnancy Risk Factor** C

**Contraindications** Presence of arterial bleeding; do not administer immediately postpartum

**Warnings/Precautions** May cause hypotension in elderly

**Adverse Reactions** 1% to 10%: Gastrointestinal: Nausea, vomiting

**Overdosage/Toxicology**

Signs and symptoms: Hypotension, flushing; vasodilation mediated second to alpha-adrenergic stimulation or direct smooth muscle effects

Treatment: Treat with I.V. fluids, alpha-adrenergic pressors may be required

**Drug Interactions** May enhance effects of other vasodilators/hypotensive agents; use with caution in elderly

**Usual Dosage** Adults: 10-20 mg 3-4 times/day; start with lower dose in elderly due to potential hypotension

**Patient Information** May cause skin rash; discontinue use if rash occurs; arise slowly from prolonged sitting or lying position

**Dosage Forms** Tablet, as hydrochloride: 10 mg, 20 mg

## Isradipine (iz RA di peen)

**Related Information**

Calcium Channel Blocking Agents Comparison Chart *on page 710*

**U.S. Brand Names** DynaCirc®

**Pharmacologic Category** Calcium Channel Blocker

**Use** Treatment of hypertension

**Effects on Mental Status** May cause dizziness or drowsiness

**Effects on Psychiatric Treatment** None reported

**Pregnancy Risk Factor** C

**Contraindications** Hypersensitivity to isradipine or any component; hypotension (<90 mm Hg systolic)

**Warnings/Precautions** Use cautiously in CHF, hypertrophic cardiomyopathy (IHSS), and in hepatic dysfunction. Safety and efficacy have not been established in pediatric patients. Adjust doses at 2- to 4-week intervals.

**Adverse Reactions**

>10%: Central nervous system: Headache (14%)

1% to 10%:

Cardiovascular: Edema (7%), palpitations (4%), flushing (2.6%), angina (2.4%), tachycardia (1.5%), hypotension

Central nervous system: Dizziness (7%), fatigue (4%)

Dermatologic: Rash (1.5%)

Gastrointestinal: Nausea (1.8%), abdominal discomfort (1.7%), vomiting/diarrhea (1%)

Neuromuscular & skeletal: Weakness (1% to 2%)

Respiratory: Dyspnea (1.8%)

<1%: Abnormal EKG, atrial and ventricular fibrillation, A-V block, cough, disturbed sleep, foot cramps, heart failure, leukopenia, myocardial infarction, nocturia, numbness, paresthesia, pruritus, TIAs, urticaria, visual disturbance, xerostomia

**Overdosage/Toxicology**

Signs and symptoms:

The primary cardiac symptoms of calcium blocker overdose includes hypotension and bradycardia. The hypotension is caused by peripheral vasodilation, myocardial depression, and bradycardia. Bradycardia results from sinus bradycardia, second- or third-degree atrioventricular block, or sinus arrest with junctional rhythm. Intraventricular conduction is usually not affected so QRS duration is normal (verapamil does prolong the P-R interval and bepridil prolongs the Q-T and may cause ventricular arrhythmias, including torsade de pointes).

The noncardiac symptoms include confusion, stupor, nausea, vomiting, metabolic acidosis and hyperglycemia. Following initial gastric decontamination, if possible, repeated calcium administration may promptly reverse the depressed cardiac contractility (but not sinus node depression or peripheral vasodilation); glucagon, epinephrine, and inamrinone may treat refractory hypotension; glucagon and epinephrine also increase the heart rate (outside the U.S., 4-aminopyridine may be available as an antidote); dialysis and hemoperfusion are not effective in enhancing elimination although repeat-dose activated charcoal may serve as an adjunct with sustained-release preparations.

**Drug Interactions** CYP3A3/4 enzyme substrate

Azole antifungals may inhibit the calcium channel blocker's metabolism; avoid this combination. Try an antifungal like terbinafine (if appropriate) or monitor closely for altered effect of the calcium channel blocker.

Beta-blockers may have increased pharmacokinetic or pharmacodynamic interactions with isradipine

Calcium may reduce the calcium channel blocker's effects, particularly hypotension

Rifampin increases the metabolism of the calcium channel blocker; adjust the dose of the calcium channel blocker to maintain efficacy

**Usual Dosage** Adults: 2.5 mg twice daily; antihypertensive response occurs in 2-3 hours; maximal response in 2-4 weeks; increase dose at 2- to 4-week intervals at 2.5-5 mg increments; usual dose range: 5-20 mg/day. **Note:** Most patients show no improvement with doses >10 mg/day except adverse reaction rate increases

**Patient Information** Take as prescribed; do not stop abruptly without consulting prescriber immediately. You may experience headache (if unrelieved, consult prescriber), nausea or vomiting (frequent small meals may help), constipation (increased dietary bulk and fluids may help), or depression (should resolve when drug is discontinued). May cause dizziness or drowsiness; use caution when driving or engaging in tasks that require alertness until response to drug is known. Report unrelieved headache, vomiting, constipation, palpitations, swelling of hands or feet, or sudden weight gain.

**Dosage Forms** Capsule: 2.5 mg, 5 mg

♦ **Isuprel®** *see* Isoproterenol *on page 295*

♦ **Itch-X® [OTC]** *see* Pramoxine *on page 457*

## Itraconazole (i tra KOE na zole)

**U.S. Brand Names** Sporanox®

**Pharmacologic Category** Antifungal Agent, Oral

**Use** Treatment of susceptible fungal infections in immunocompromised and immunocompetent patients including blastomycosis and histoplasmosis; indicated for aspergillosis, and onychomycosis of the toenail; treatment of onychomycosis of the fingernail without concomitant toenail infection via a pulse-type dosing regimen; has activity against *Aspergillus*, *Candida*, *Coccidioides*, *Cryptococcus*, *Sporothrix*, tinea unguium

Oral solution (not capsules) is marketed for oral and esophageal candidiasis

Useful in superficial mycoses including dermatophytoses (eg, tinea capitis), pityriasis versicolor, sebopsoriasis, vaginal and chronic mucocutaneous candidiases; systemic mycoses including candidiasis, meningeal and disseminated cryptococcal infections, paracoccidioidomycosis, coccidioidomycoses; miscellaneous mycoses such as sporotrichosis, chromomycosis, leishmaniasis, fungal keratitis, alternariosis, zygomycosis

Intravenous solution is indicated in the treatment of blastomycosis, histoplasmosis (nonmeningeal), and aspergillosis (in patients intolerant or refractory to amphotericin B therapy)

**Effects on Mental Status** May cause sedation

**Effects on Psychiatric Treatment** None reported

**Pregnancy Risk Factor** C

**Contraindications** Known hypersensitivity to other azoles; concurrent administration with astemizole, cisapride, lovastatin, midazolam, simvastatin, or triazolam

**Warnings/Precautions** Rare cases of serious cardiovascular adverse event, including death, ventricular tachycardia and torsade de pointes have been observed due to increased terfenadine and cisapride concentrations induced by itraconazole; patients who develop abnormal liver function tests during itraconazole therapy should be monitored and therapy discontinued if symptoms of liver disease develop

**Adverse Reactions** Listed incidences are for higher doses appropriate for systemic fungal infections

>10%: Gastrointestinal: Nausea (10.6%)

1% to 10%:

Cardiovascular: Edema (3.5%), hypertension (3.2%)

Central nervous system: Headache (4%), fatigue (2% to 3%), malaise (1.2%), fever (2.5%)

Dermatologic: Rash (8.6%)

Endocrine & metabolic: Decreased libido (1.2%), hypertriglyceridemia

Gastrointestinal: Abdominal pain (1.5%), vomiting (5%), diarrhea (3%)

Hepatic: Abnormal LFTs (2.7%), hepatitis

<1%: Adrenal suppression, albuminuria, anorexia, dizziness, gynecomastia, hypokalemia, impotence, pruritus, somnolence

**Overdosage/Toxicology**

Signs and symptoms: Overdoses are well tolerated

Treatment: Following decontamination, if possible, supportive measures only are required; dialysis is not effective

**Drug Interactions** CYP3A3/4 enzyme substrate; CYP3A3/4 enzyme inhibitor

Decreased effect:

Decreased serum levels with carbamazepine, didanosine, isoniazid, phenobarbital, phenytoin, rifabutin, and rifampin; may cause a decreased effect of oral contraceptives; alternative birth control is recommended

Decreased/undetectable serum levels with rifampin - **should not be administered concomitantly with rifampin**

Absorption requires gastric acidity; therefore, antacids, $H_2$-antagonists (cimetidine and ranitidine), proton pump inhibitors like omeprazole, and sucralfate significantly reduce bioavailability resulting in treatment failures and should not be administered concomitantly; amphotericin B or fluconazole should be used instead

Increased toxicity:

Itraconazole may increase protease inhibitors' serum concentrations.

May increase cyclosporine or tacrolimus levels (by 50%) when high doses are used

Itraconazole increases serum levels of lovastatin (possibly 20-fold) and other HMG-CoA inhibitors due to inhibition of CYP3A4

May increase phenytoin serum concentration

May inhibit warfarin's metabolism

May increase digoxin serum levels

May increase astemizole, busulfan, cisapride, terfenadine, and vinca alkaloid levels - **concomitant administration is not recommended** due to increased risk of cardiotoxicity

Itraconazole may increase astemizole levels resulting in prolonged Q-T intervals - concomitant administration is contraindicated

Itraconazole may increase levels of cisapride - concomitant administration is contraindicated due to increased risk of cardiotoxicity

May increase amlodipine, benzodiazepine, buspirone, corticosteroids, and oral hypoglycemic levels; use with caution in patients prescribed medications eliminated by CYP3A4 metabolism

**Usual Dosage** Oral: Capsule: Absorption is best if taken with food, therefore, it is best to administer itraconazole after meals; Solution: Should be taken on an empty stomach. Absorption of both products is significantly increased when taken with a cola beverage.

Children: Efficacy and safety have not been established; a small number of patients 3-16 years of age have been treated with 100 mg/day for systemic fungal infections with no serious adverse effects reported

Adults:

Oral:

Blastomycosis/histoplasmosis: 200 mg once daily, if no obvious improvement or there is evidence of progressive fungal disease, increase the dose in 100 mg increments to a maximum of 400 mg/day; doses >200 mg/day are given in 2 divided doses; length of therapy varies from 1 day to >6 months depending on the condition and mycological response

Aspergillosis: 200-400 mg/day

Onychomycosis: 200 mg once daily for 12 consecutive weeks

Life-threatening infections: Loading dose: 200 mg 3 times/day (600 mg/day) should be given for the first 3 days of therapy

Oropharyngeal and esophageal candidiasis: Oral solution: 100-200 mg once daily

I.V.: 200 mg twice daily for 4 doses, followed by 200 mg daily

**Dosing adjustment in renal impairment:** Not necessary; itraconazole injection is not recommended in patients with $Cl_{cr}$ <30 mL/minute

Hemodialysis: Not dialyzable

**Dosing adjustment in hepatic impairment:** May be necessary, but specific guidelines are not available

**Dietary Considerations** Food increases absorption of capsule and decreases absorption of the solution

**Patient Information** Take as directed, around-the-clock, with food. Take full course of medication; do not discontinue without notifying prescriber. Practice good hygiene measures to prevent reinfection. If diabetic, test serum glucose regularly (can cause hypoglycemia when given with sulfonylureas). Frequent blood tests may be required with prolonged therapy. You may experience dizziness or drowsiness (use caution when driving or engaging in tasks that require alertness until response to drug is known); nausea, vomiting, or diarrhea (small frequent meals, frequent mouth care, sucking lozenges, or chewing gum may help). Report skin rash or other persistent adverse reactions.

**Dosage Forms**

Capsule: 100 mg

Injection kit: 10 mg/mL - 25 mL ampul, one 50 mL (100 mL capacity) bag 0.9% sodium chloride, one filtered infusion set

Solution, oral: 100 mg/10 mL (150 mL)

♦ **I-Tropine® Ophthalmic** *see* Atropine *on page 53*

## Ivermectin (eye ver MEK tin)

**U.S. Brand Names** Stromectol®

**Pharmacologic Category** Antibiotic, Miscellaneous

**Use** Treatment of the following infections: Strongyloidiasis of the intestinal tract due the nematode parasite *Strongyloides stercoralis*. Onchocerciasis due to the nematode parasite *Onchocerca volvulus*. Ivermectin is only active against the immature form of *Onchocerca volvulus*, and the intestinal forms of *Strongyloides stercoralis*. Ivermectin has been used for other parasitic infections including *Ascaris lumbricoides*, bancroftian filariasis, *Brugia malayi*, scabies, *Enterobius vermicularis*, *Mansonella ozzardi*, *Trichuris trichiura*.

**Effects on Mental Status** May cause dizziness, drowsiness, or insomnia

**Effects on Psychiatric Treatment** May cause leukopenia; use caution with clozapine and carbamazepine

**Pregnancy Risk Factor** C

**Contraindications** Hypersensitivity to ivermectin or any component

**Warnings/Precautions** Data have shown that antihelmintic drugs like ivermectin may cause cutaneous and/or systemic reactions (Mazzoti reaction) of varying severity including ophthalmological reactions in patients with onchocerciasis. These reactions are probably due to allergic and inflammatory responses to the death of microfilariae. Patients with hyperreactive onchodermatitis may be more likely than others to experience severe adverse reactions, especially edema and aggravation of the onchodermatitis. Repeated treatment may be required in immunocompromised patients (eg, HIV); control of extraintestinal strongyloidiasis may necessitate suppressive (once monthly) therapy

**Adverse Reactions**

Percentage unknown: Abdominal pain, blurred vision, diarrhea, dizziness, eosinophilia, headache, hyperthermia, hypotension, increased ALT/AST, insomnia, leukopenia, limbitis, mild conjunctivitis, mild EKG changes, myalgia, nausea, peripheral and facial edema, pruritus, punctate opacity, rash, somnolence, transient tachycardia, tremor, urticaria, vertigo, vomiting, weakness

Mazzotti reaction (with onchocerciasis): Pruritus, edema, rash, fever, lymphadenopathy, ocular damage

**Overdosage/Toxicology**

Signs and symptoms: Accidental intoxication with, or significant exposure to unknown quantities of veterinary formulations of ivermectin in humans, either by ingestion, inhalation, injection, or exposure to body surfaces, has resulted in the following adverse effects: rash, edema, headache, dizziness, asthenia, nausea, vomiting, and diarrhea; other adverse effects that have been reported include seizure and ataxia

Treatment: Supportive; usual methods for decontamination are recommended

**Usual Dosage** Oral:

Children ≥5 years: 150 mcg/kg as a single dose; treatment for onchocerciasis may need to be repeated every 3-12 months until the adult worms die

(Continued)

## Ivermectin *(Continued)*

Adults:

Strongyloidiasis: 200 mcg/kg as a single dose; follow-up stool examinations

Onchocerciasis: 150 mcg/kg as a single dose; retreatment may be required every 3-12 months until the adult worms die

**Patient Information** If infected with strongyloidiasis, repeated stool examinations are required to document clearance of the organisms; repeated follow-up and retreatment is usually required in the treatment of onchocerciasis

**Nursing Implications** Ensure that patients take ivermectin with water

**Dosage Forms** Tablet: 6 mg


- **Janimine®** *see* Imipramine *on page 282*
- **Jaundice Root** *see* Golden Seal *on page 254*
- **Jenamicin® Injection** *see* Gentamicin *on page 248*
- **Jenest-28™** *see* Ethinyl Estradiol and Norethindrone *on page 212*
- **Jesuit's Tea** *see* Maté *on page 333*
- **Junior Strength Motrin® [OTC]** *see* Ibuprofen *on page 280*
- **Junior Strength Panadol® [OTC]** *see* Acetaminophen *on page 14*
- **Just Tears® Solution [OTC]** *see* Artificial Tears *on page 48*
- **K+ 10®** *see* Potassium Chloride *on page 453*
- **Kabikinase®** *see* Streptokinase *on page 520*
- **Kadian™ Capsule** *see* Morphine Sulfate *on page 374*
- **Kalcinate®** *see* Calcium Gluconate *on page 85*


## Kanamycin (kan a MYE sin)

**U.S. Brand Names** Kantrex®

**Pharmacologic Category** Antibiotic, Aminoglycoside

**Use**

Oral: Preoperative bowel preparation in the prophylaxis of infections and adjunctive treatment of hepatic coma (oral kanamycin is not indicated in the treatment of systemic infections); treatment of susceptible bacterial infection including gram-negative aerobes, gram-positive *Bacillus* as well as some mycobacteria

Parenteral: Rarely used in antibiotic irrigations during surgery

**Effects on Mental Status** May cause drowsiness or dizziness; case reports of delirium and psychosis with aminoglycosides

**Effects on Psychiatric Treatment** May cause agranulocytosis; use caution with clozapine and carbamazepine

**Pregnancy Risk Factor** D

**Contraindications** Hypersensitivity to kanamycin or any component or other aminoglycosides

**Warnings/Precautions** Use with caution in patients with pre-existing renal insufficiency, vestibular or cochlear impairment, myasthenia gravis, conditions which depress neuromuscular transmission

Parenteral aminoglycosides are associated with nephrotoxicity or ototoxicity; the ototoxicity may be proportional to the amount of drug given and the duration of treatment; tinnitus or vertigo are indications of vestibular injury and impending hearing loss; renal damage is usually reversible

**Adverse Reactions** Percentage unknown: Agranulocytosis, anorexia, burning, diarrhea (most common with oral form), drowsiness, dyspnea, edema, enterocolitis, erythema, granulocytopenia, headache, increased salivation, malabsorption syndrome with prolonged and high-dose therapy of hepatic coma, muscle cramps, nausea, nephrotoxicity, neurotoxicity, ototoxicity (auditory), ototoxicity (vestibular), photosensitivity, pseudomotor cerebri, rash, redness, skin itching, stinging, thrombocytopenia, tremors, vomiting, weakness, weight loss

**Overdosage/Toxicology**

Signs and symptoms: Ototoxicity, nephrotoxicity, and neuromuscular toxicity

Treatment: Treatment of choice following a single acute overdose appears to be the maintenance of good urine output of at least 3 mL/kg/hour. Dialysis is of questionable value in the enhancement of aminoglycoside elimination. If required, hemodialysis is preferred over peritoneal dialysis in patients with normal renal function. Careful hydration may be all that is required to promote diuresis and, therefore, the enhancement of the drug's elimination.

**Drug Interactions**

Increased toxicity:

Penicillins, cephalosporins, amphotericin B, diuretics may increase nephrotoxicity; polypeptide antibiotics may increase risk of respiratory paralysis and renal dysfunction

Neuromuscular blocking agents with oral kanamycin may increase neuromuscular blockade; a small increase in warfarin's effect may occur due to decreased absorption of vitamin K

Decreased toxicity: Methotrexate with kanamycin (oral) may be less well absorbed as may digoxin (minor) and vitamin A

**Usual Dosage**

Children: Infections: I.M., I.V.: 15 mg/kg/day in divided doses every 8-12 hours

Adults:

Infections: I.M., I.V.: 5-7.5 mg/kg/dose in divided doses every 8-12 hours (<15 mg/kg/day)

Preoperative intestinal antisepsis: Oral: 1 g every 4-6 hours for 36-72 hours

Hepatic coma: Oral: 8-12 g/day in divided doses

Intraperitoneal: After contamination in surgery: 500 mg diluted in 20 mL distilled water; other irrigations: 0.25% solutions

Aerosol: 250 mg 2-4 times/day (250 mg diluted with 3 mL of NS and nebulized)

**Dosing adjustment/interval in renal impairment:**

$Cl_{cr}$ 50-80 mL/minute: Administer 60% to 90% of dose or administer every 8-12 hours

$Cl_{cr}$ 10-50 mL/minute: Administer 30% to 70% of dose or administer every 12 hours

$Cl_{cr}$ <10 mL/minute: Administer 20% to 30% of dose or administer every 24-48 hours

Hemodialysis: Dialyzable (50% to 100%)

**Patient Information** It is important to maintain adequate hydration (2-3 L/day of fluids unless instructed to restrict fluid intake). Report change in hearing acuity, ringing or roaring in ears, alteration in balance, vertigo, feeling of fullness in head; pain, tingling, or numbness of any body part; change in urinary pattern or decrease in urine; signs of opportunistic infection (eg, white plaques in mouth, vaginal discharge, unhealed sores, sore throat, unusual fever, chills); pain, redness, or swelling at injection site; skin rash; or other adverse reactions.

**Dosage Forms**

Capsule, as sulfate: 500 mg

Injection, as sulfate:

Pediatric: 75 mg (2 mL)

Adults: 500 mg (2 mL); 1 g (3 mL)


- **Kantrex®** *see* Kanamycin *on page 300*
- **Kaochlor®** *see* Potassium Chloride *on page 453*
- **Kaochlor® SF** *see* Potassium Chloride *on page 453*
- **Kaodene® [OTC]** *see* Kaolin and Pectin *on page 300*


## Kaolin and Pectin (KAY oh lin & PEK tin)

**U.S. Brand Names** Kaodene® [OTC]; Kao-Spen® [OTC]; Kapectolin® [OTC]

**Canadian Brand Names** Donnagel®-MB

**Synonyms** Pectin and Kaolin

**Pharmacologic Category** Antidiarrheal

**Use** Treatment of uncomplicated diarrhea

**Effects on Mental Status** None reported

**Effects on Psychiatric Treatment** May decrease absorption of beta-blockers

**Pregnancy Risk Factor** C

**Contraindications** Hypersensitivity to kaolin or pectin

**Warnings/Precautions** Not to be used for self-medication for diarrhea for >48 hours, in presence of high fever in infants and children <3 years of age; do not use for diarrhea associated with pseudomembraneous enterocolitis or in diarrhea caused by toxigenic bacteria

**Adverse Reactions** 1% to 10%: Gastrointestinal: Constipation, fecal impaction

**Overdosage/Toxicology** Signs and symptoms: May cause bowel impaction and obstruction

**Drug Interactions** May decrease absorption of many drugs, including chloroquine, atenolol, metoprolol, propranolol, diflunisal, isoniazid, penicillamine, clindamycin, digoxin (give kaolin/pectin 2 hours before or 4 hours after medication)

**Usual Dosage** Oral:

Children:

<6 years: Do not use

6-12 years: 30-60 mL after each loose stool

Adults: 60-120 mL after each loose stool

**Patient Information** Shake well

**Dosage Forms** Suspension, oral: Kaolin 975 mg and pectin 22 mg per 5 mL

## Kaolin and Pectin With Opium

(KAY oh lin & PEK tin with OH pee um)

**U.S. Brand Names** Parepectolin®

**Canadian Brand Names** Donnagel®-PG Capsule; Donnagel®-PG Suspension

**Pharmacologic Category** Antidiarrheal

**Use** Symptomatic relief of diarrhea

**Effects on Mental Status** None reported

**Effects on Psychiatric Treatment** May decrease absorption of beta-blockers
**Restrictions** C-V
**Usual Dosage** Oral:
Children:
3-6 years: 7.5 mL with each loose bowel movement, not to exceed 30 mL in 12 hours
6-12 years: 5-10 mL with each loose bowel movement, not to exceed 40 mL in 12 hours
Children >12 years and Adults: 15-30 mL with each loose bowel movement, not to exceed 120 mL in 12 hours
**Dosage Forms** Suspension, oral: Kaolin 5.5 g, pectin 162 mg, and opium 15 mg per 30 mL [3.7 mL paregoric] (240 mL)

- ♦ **Kaon®** *see* Potassium Gluconate *on page 454*
- ♦ **Kaon-Cl®** *see* Potassium Chloride *on page 453*
- ♦ **Kaon-Cl-10®** *see* Potassium Chloride *on page 453*
- ♦ **Kaopectate® Advanced Formula [OTC]** *see* Attapulgite *on page 53*
- ♦ **Kaopectate® II [OTC]** *see* Loperamide *on page 324*
- ♦ **Kaopectate® Maximum Strength Caplets** *see* Attapulgite *on page 53*
- ♦ **Kao-Spen® [OTC]** *see* Kaolin and Pectin *on page 300*
- ♦ **Kapectolin® [OTC]** *see* Kaolin and Pectin *on page 300*
- ♦ **Kapectolin PG®** *see* Hyoscyamine, Atropine, Scopolamine, Kaolin, Pectin, and Opium *on page 280*
- ♦ **Kasof® [OTC]** *see* Docusate *on page 179*

## Kava

**Related Information**
Natural Products, Herbals, and Dietary Supplements *on page 742*
Perspectives on the Safety of Herbal Medicines *on page 736*
**Synonyms** Awa; Kew; *Piper methysticum*; Tonga
**Pharmacologic Category** Herb
**Use** Conditions of nervous anxiety, stress, and restlessness per Commission E; used for sleep inducement and to reduce anxiety
**Restrictions** Not more than 3 months without medical advice per Commission E
**Contraindications** Per Commission E: Pregnancy, breast-feeding, endogenous depression. "Extended continuous intake can cause a temporary yellow discoloration of skin, hair and nails. In this case, further application must be discontinued. In rare cases, allergic skin reactions occur. Also, accommodative disturbances (eg, enlargement of the pupils and disturbances of the oculomotor equilibrium) have been described."
**Adverse Reactions**
Central nervous system: Euphoria, depression, somnolence
Dermatologic: Skin discoloration (prolonged use)
Neuromuscular & skeletal: Muscle weakness
Ocular: Eye disturbances
**Overdosage/Toxicology**
Signs and symptoms: Ataxia, deafness, yellow skin discoloration, sedation, extrapyramidal effects
Decontamination: Lavage (within 1 hour)/activated charcoal with cathartic
Treatment: Supportive therapy; can treat extrapyramidal reactions with benztropine and/or diphenhydramine
**Drug Interactions**
Alprazolam (and potentially all benzodiazepines): A case report of coma following concurrent alprazolam and kava has been reported. Combinations should be avoided
CNS depressants: Sedative effects may be additive with CNS depressants; includes ethanol, barbiturates, narcotic analgesics, and other sedative agents; monitor for increased effect
Levodopa: Effects may be antagonized by kava
**Usual Dosage** Per Commission E: Herb and preparations equivalent to 60-120 mg kavalactones
**Additional Information** Social and ceremonial drink in South Pacific Islands; has medicinal use as a GU antiseptic, antipyretic, diuretic, local anesthetic, and muscle relaxant agent; shrubs can grow 8-20 feet tall with green stems and rounded fruit; characteristic yellow discoloration rash resembles pellagra, but does not respond to nicotinamide.

- ♦ **Kay Ciel®** *see* Potassium Chloride *on page 453*
- ♦ **K+ Care®** *see* Potassium Chloride *on page 453*
- ♦ **KCl** *see* Potassium Chloride *on page 453*
- ♦ **K-Dur® 10** *see* Potassium Chloride *on page 453*
- ♦ **K-Dur® 20** *see* Potassium Chloride *on page 453*
- ♦ **Keflex®** *see* Cephalexin *on page 103*
- ♦ **Keftab®** *see* Cephalexin *on page 103*
- ♦ **Kefurox® Injection** *see* Cefuroxime *on page 102*
- ♦ **Kefzol®** *see* Cefazolin *on page 97*
- ♦ **Kemadrin®** *see* Procyclidine *on page 467*
- ♦ **Kenacort®** *see* Triamcinolone *on page 563*
- ♦ **Kenaject-40®** *see* Triamcinolone *on page 563*
- ♦ **Kenalog®** *see* Triamcinolone *on page 563*
- ♦ **Kenalog-10®** *see* Triamcinolone *on page 563*
- ♦ **Kenalog-40®** *see* Triamcinolone *on page 563*
- ♦ **Kenalog® H** *see* Triamcinolone *on page 563*
- ♦ **Kenalog® in Orabase®** *see* Triamcinolone *on page 563*
- ♦ **Kenonel®** *see* Triamcinolone *on page 563*
- ♦ **Keoxifene Hydrochloride** *see* Raloxifene *on page 487*
- ♦ **Keppra®** *see* Levetiracetam *on page 311*
- ♦ **Keralyt® Gel** *see* Salicylic Acid and Propylene Glycol *on page 502*
- ♦ **Kerlone® Oral** *see* Betaxolol *on page 66*
- ♦ **Kestrone®** *see* Estrone *on page 208*
- ♦ **Ketalar® Injection** *see* Ketamine *on page 301*

## Ketamine (KEET a meen)

**U.S. Brand Names** Ketalar® Injection
**Pharmacologic Category** General Anesthetic
**Use** Induction of anesthesia; short surgical procedures; dressing changes
**Effects on Mental Status** Vivid dreams and hallucinations common
**Effects on Psychiatric Treatment** Contraindicated in patients with psychotic disorders; barbiturates and hydroxyzine may increase the effects of ketamine; avoid combination
**Restrictions** C-III
**Usual Dosage** Used in combination with anticholinergic agents to decrease hypersalivation
Children:
Oral: 6-10 mg/kg for 1 dose (mixed in 0.2-0.3 mL/kg of cola or other beverage) given 30 minutes before the procedure
I.M.: 3-7 mg/kg
I.V.: Range: 0.5-2 mg/kg, use smaller doses (0.5-1 mg/kg) for sedation for minor procedures; usual induction dosage: 1-2 mg/kg
Continuous I.V. infusion: Sedation: 5-20 mcg/kg/minute
Adults:
I.M.: 3-8 mg/kg
I.V.: Range: 1-4.5 mg/kg; usual induction dosage: 1-2 mg/kg
Children and Adults: Maintenance: Supplemental doses of $^1/_3$ to $^1/_2$ of initial dose
**Dosage Forms** Injection, as hydrochloride: 10 mg/mL (20 mL, 25 mL, 50 mL); 50 mg/mL (10 mL); 100 mg/mL (5 mL)

## Ketobemidone (kee toe BE meh done)

**U.S. Brand Names** Cliradon®; Ketogan®
**Synonyms** Cetobemidone
**Pharmacologic Category** Analgesic, Narcotic
**Use** Pain relief in the postoperative period and during acute myocardial infarction; premedication for anesthesia
**Effects on Mental Status** May cause sedation, confusion, or euphoria
**Effects on Psychiatric Treatment** Concurrent use with psychotropic may produce additive sedation
**Contraindications** Hypersensitivity to ketobemidone or acute respiratory depression
**Warnings/Precautions** Use with caution in patients with renal, pulmonary, or hepatic disease, increased intracranial pressure, prostatic hypertrophy, gastrointestinal surgery
**Adverse Reactions**
Central nervous system: Lethargy, headache, confusion, sedation, dizziness, euphoria
Gastrointestinal: Ileus, nausea, vomiting, xerostomia, obstipation, constipation
Genitourinary: Urinary retention
Neuromuscular & skeletal: Smooth muscle spasm
Ocular: Blurred vision
Respiratory: Cough, apnea
**Usual Dosage**
I.M.: 5-7.5 mg every 6 hours
I.V.:
Patient-controlled analgesia: 2-3 mg over one minute with each dose allowable per 15 minutes
Postoperative pain: 3 mg/hour decreasing to 0.75 mg/hour after shivering cessation
Oral: 5-15 mg every 3-6 hours
(Continued)

## Ketobemidone *(Continued)*

Rectal: 10 mg every 3-4 hours

**Dosage Forms**

Injection: 5 mg/mL
Suppository: 10 mg
Tablet: 5 mg

## Ketoconazole (kee toe KOE na zole)

**U.S. Brand Names** Nizoral®; Nizoral® A-D Shampoo [OTC]

**Pharmacologic Category** Antifungal Agent, Oral; Antifungal Agent, Topical

**Use** Treatment of susceptible fungal infections, including candidiasis, oral thrush, blastomycosis, histoplasmosis, paracoccidioidomycosis, coccidioidomycosis, chromomycosis, candiduria, chronic mucocutaneous candidiasis, as well as, certain recalcitrant cutaneous dermatophytoses; used topically for treatment of tinea corporis, tinea cruris, tinea versicolor, and cutaneous candidiasis, seborrheic dermatitis

**Effects on Mental Status** May cause drowsiness, dizziness, or depression

**Effects on Psychiatric Treatment** May cause leukopenia; use caution with clozapine and carbamazepine

**Pregnancy Risk Factor** C

**Contraindications** Hypersensitivity to ketoconazole or any component; CNS fungal infections (due to poor CNS penetration); coadministration with terfenadine, astemizole, or cisapride is contraindicated due to risk of potentially fatal cardiac arrhythmias

**Warnings/Precautions** Rare cases of serious cardiovascular adverse event, including death, ventricular tachycardia and torsade de pointes have been observed due to increased terfenadine concentrations induced by ketoconazole. Use with caution in patients with impaired hepatic function; has been associated with hepatotoxicity, including some fatalities; perform periodic liver function tests; high doses of ketoconazole may depress adrenocortical function.

**Adverse Reactions**

Oral:
1% to 10%:
Dermatologic: Pruritus (1.5%)
Gastrointestinal: Nausea/vomiting (3% to 10%), abdominal pain (1.2%)
<1%: Bulging fontanelles, chills, depression, diarrhea, dizziness, fever, gynecomastia, headache, hemolytic anemia, hepatotoxicity, impotence, leukopenia, photophobia, somnolence, thrombocytopenia
Cream: Severe irritation, pruritus, stinging (~5%)
Shampoo: Increases in normal hair loss, irritation (<1%), abnormal hair texture, scalp pustules, mild dryness of skin, itching, oiliness/dryness of hair

**Overdosage/Toxicology**

Signs and symptoms: Dizziness, headache, nausea, vomiting, diarrhea; overdoses are well tolerated
Treatment: Supportive measures and gastric decontamination

**Drug Interactions** CYP3A3/4 enzyme substrate; CYP1A2, 2C, 2C9, 2C18, 2C19, 3A3/4, and 3A5-7 enzyme inhibitor

Decreased effect:
Decreased ketoconazole serum levels with isoniazid and phenytoin; decreased/undetectable serum levels with rifampin - **should not be administered concomitantly with rifampin**; theophylline and oral hypoglycemic serum levels may be decreased
Absorption requires gastric acidity; therefore, antacids, $H_2$-antagonists (cimetidine and ranitidine), omeprazole, and sucralfate significantly reduce bioavailability resulting in treatment failures; should not be administered concomitantly

Increased toxicity:
May increase cyclosporine levels (by 50%) when high doses are used
Inhibits warfarin metabolism resulting in increased anticoagulant effect
Increases corticosteroid bioavailability and decreases steroid clearance
Increases amprenavir, phenytoin, digoxin, terfenadine, astemizole, indinavir and cisapride concentrations; **concomitant administration with astemizole or cisapride is contraindicated**; may significantly increase levels and toxicity of lovastatin and simvastatin due to CYP3A4 inhibition; a disulfiram-type reaction may occur with concomitant ethanol

**Usual Dosage**

Oral:
Children ≥2 years: 3.3-6.6 mg/kg/day as a single dose for 1-2 weeks for candidiasis, for at least 4 weeks in recalcitrant dermatophyte infections, and for up to 6 months for other systemic mycoses
Adults: 200-400 mg/day as a single daily dose for durations as stated above
Shampoo: Apply twice weekly for 4 weeks with at least 3 days between each shampoo
Topical: Rub gently into the affected area once daily to twice daily
**Dosing adjustment in hepatic impairment:** Dose reductions should be considered in patients with severe liver disease
Hemodialysis: Not dialyzable (0% to 5%)

**Patient Information**

Oral: May take with food; at least 2 hours before any antacids. Take full course of medication as directed; some infections may require long periods of therapy. Frequent blood tests may be required with long-term therapy. Practice good hygiene measures to reduce incidence of reinfection. If diabetic, test serum glucose regularly. You may experience nausea and vomiting (small frequent meals, frequent mouth care, sucking lozenges, or chewing gum may help); headache (mild analgesic may be necessary); or dizziness (use caution when driving). Report unresolved headache, rash or itching, yellowing of eyes or skin, changes in color of urine or stool, chest pain or palpitations, or sense of fullness or ringing in ears.

Topical: Wash and dry area before applying medication thinly. Do not cover with occlusive dressing. Report severe skin irritation or if condition does not improve.

Shampoo: Allow 3 days between shampoos. You may experience some hair loss, scalp irritation, itching, change in hair texture, or scalp pustules. Report severe side effects or if infestation persists.

**Nursing Implications** Administer 2 hours prior to antacids to prevent decreased absorption due to the high pH of gastric contents

**Dosage Forms**

Cream: 2% (15 g, 30 g, 60 g)
Shampoo: 1% (207 mL); 2% (120 mL)
Tablet: 200 mg

♦ **Ketogan®** *see* Ketobemidone *on page 301*

## Ketoprofen (kee toe PROE fen)

**Related Information**

Nonsteroidal Anti-inflammatory Agents Comparison Chart *on page 722*

**U.S. Brand Names** Actron® [OTC]; Orudis®; Orudis® KT [OTC]; Oruvail®

**Canadian Brand Names** Apo®-Keto; Apo®-Keto-E; Novo-Keto-EC; Nu-Ketoprofen; Nu-Ketoprofen-E; Orafen; PMS-Ketoprofen; Rhodis™; Rhodis-EC™

**Pharmacologic Category** Nonsteroidal Anti-Inflammatory Agent (NSAID)

**Use** Acute and long-term treatment of rheumatoid arthritis and osteoarthritis; primary dysmenorrhea; mild to moderate pain

**Effects on Mental Status** Dizziness is common; may cause nervousness; may rarely cause insomnia, confusion, depression, or hallucinations

**Effects on Psychiatric Treatment** May rarely cause agranulocytosis; use caution with clozapine and carbamazepine; may decrease lithium clearance resulting in an increase in serum lithium levels and potential lithium toxicity; monitor serum lithium levels

**Pregnancy Risk Factor** B (D if used in third trimester)

**Contraindications** Known hypersensitivity to ketoprofen or other NSAIDs/aspirin

**Warnings/Precautions** Use with caution in patients with congestive heart failure, dehydration, hypertension, decreased renal or hepatic function, history of GI disease (bleeding or ulcers), or those receiving anticoagulants; safety and efficacy in children <6 months of age have not yet been established

**Adverse Reactions**

>10%:
Central nervous system: Dizziness
Dermatologic: Rash
Gastrointestinal: Abdominal cramps, heartburn, indigestion, nausea
1% to 10%:
Central nervous system: Headache, nervousness
Dermatologic: Itching
Endocrine & metabolic: Fluid retention
Gastrointestinal: Vomiting
Otic: Tinnitus
<1%: Acute renal failure, agranulocytosis, allergic rhinitis, anemia, angioedema, arrhythmias, aseptic meningitis, blurred vision, bone marrow suppression, confusion, congestive heart failure, conjunctivitis, cystitis, decreased hearing, drowsiness, dry eyes, epistaxis, erythema multiforme, gastritis, GI ulceration, hallucinations, hemolytic anemia, hepatitis, hot flashes, hypertension, insomnia, leukopenia, mental depression, peripheral neuropathy, polydipsia, polyuria, shortness of breath, Stevens-Johnson syndrome, tachycardia, thrombocytopenia, toxic amblyopia, toxic epidermal necrolysis, urticaria

**Overdosage/Toxicology**

Signs and symptoms: Apnea, metabolic acidosis, coma, and nystagmus; leukocytosis, renal failure
Treatment: Management of a nonsteroidal anti-inflammatory drug (NSAID) intoxication is primarily supportive and symptomatic. Fluid therapy is commonly effective in managing the hypotension that may occur following an acute NSAID overdose, except when this is due to an acute blood loss. Seizures tend to be very short-lived and often do not require drug treatment. Although, recurrent seizures should be treated with I.V. diazepam. Since many of the NSAIDs undergo enterohepatic cycling,

multiple doses of charcoal may be needed to reduce the potential for delayed toxicities.

**Drug Interactions** CYP2C and 2C9 enzyme inhibitor

ACE inhibitors: Effects may be reduced by NSAIDs; use lowest possible dose for shortest duration possible; monitor

Cholestyramine and colestipol: Absorption may be reduced by concurrent administration

Corticosteroids: May increase the risk of GI ulceration; use caution

Cyclosporine: Nephrotoxicity may be increased with concurrent NSAID use; monitor

CYP2C9 inhibitors: May increase in diclofenac concentrations; inhibitors include amiodarone, cimetidine, fluvoxamine, metronidazole, omeprazole, sulfonamides, valproic acid, and zafirlukast

CYP2C9 substrates: Coadministration of drugs metabolized by CYP2C9 may result in increased serum concentrations of these agents

Hydralazine: Antihypertensive effect may be decreased; avoid concurrent use

Lithium: Serum levels can be increased; avoid concurrent use if possible or monitor lithium levels and adjust dose. When NSAID is stopped, lithium may need adjustment again.

Loop diuretics: Therapeutic effects may be reduced by NSAIDs; avoid

Methotrexate: Toxicity may be increased by concurrent NSAID use; risk is limited in low-dose methotrexate regimens (such as for rheumatoid arthritis); prolonged leucovorin rescue may be required at antineoplastic doses; monitor

Thiazide diuretics: Antihypertensive effects are decreased; avoid concurrent use

Warfarin: INRs may be increased by some NSAIDs. This may depend, in part, on dose and duration; monitor INR closely. Use the lowest dose of NSAIDs possible and for the briefest duration.

**Usual Dosage** Oral:

Children 3 months to 14 years: Fever: 0.5-1 mg/kg every 6-8 hours

Children >12 years and Adults:

- Rheumatoid arthritis or osteoarthritis: 50-75 mg 3-4 times/day up to a maximum of 300 mg/day
- Mild to moderate pain: 25-50 mg every 6-8 hours up to a maximum of 300 mg/day

**Patient Information** Take this medication exactly as directed; do not increase dose without consulting prescriber. Do not crush tablets or break capsules. Take with food or milk to reduce GI distress. Maintain adequate fluid intake (2-3 L/day of fluids unless instructed to restrict fluid intake). Do not use alcohol, aspirin, or aspirin-containing medication, and all other anti-inflammatory medications without consulting prescriber. You may experience drowsiness, dizziness, nervousness, or headache (use caution when driving or engaging in tasks requiring alertness until response to drug is known); anorexia, nausea, vomiting, or heartburn (frequent small meals, frequent mouth care, sucking lozenges, or chewing gum may help); fluid retention (weigh yourself weekly and report unusual (3-5 lb/week) weight gain). GI bleeding, ulceration, or perforation can occur with or without pain; discontinue medication and contact prescriber if persistent abdominal pain or cramping, or blood in stool occurs. Report breathlessness, difficulty breathing, or unusual cough; chest pain, rapid heartbeat, palpitations; unusual bruising/bleeding; blood in urine, stool, mouth, or vomitus; swollen extremities; skin rash or itching; acute fatigue; or changes in hearing or ringing in ears.

**Dosage Forms**

Capsule (Orudis®): 25 mg, 50 mg, 75 mg

Actron®, Orudis® KT [OTC]: 12.5 mg

Capsule, extended release (Oruvail®): 100 mg, 200 mg

## Ketorolac Tromethamine (KEE toe role ak troe METH a meen)

**Related Information**

Nonsteroidal Anti-inflammatory Agents Comparison Chart *on page 722*

**U.S. Brand Names** Acular® Ophthalmic; Toradol® Injection; Toradol® Oral

**Pharmacologic Category** Nonsteroidal Anti-Inflammatory Agent (NSAID)

**Use** Short-term (<5 days) management of pain; first parenteral NSAID for analgesia; 30 mg provides the analgesia comparable to 12 mg of morphine or 100 mg of meperidine

**Effects on Mental Status** May cause drowsiness or dizziness; may rarely produce depression

**Effects on Psychiatric Treatment** May decrease lithium clearance resulting in an increase in serum lithium levels and potential lithium toxicity; monitor serum lithium levels

**Pregnancy Risk Factor** B (D if used in the 3rd trimester)

**Contraindications** In patients who have developed nasal polyps, angioedema, or bronchospastic reactions to other NSAIDs, active peptic ulcer disease, recent GI bleeding or perforation, patients with advanced renal disease or risk of renal failure, labor and delivery, nursing mothers, patients with hypersensitivity to ketorolac, aspirin, or other NSAIDs, **prophylaxis before major surgery**, suspected or confirmed cerebrovascular bleeding, hemorrhagic diathesis, concurrent ASA or other NSAIDs, epidural or intrathecal administration, concomitant probenecid

**Warnings/Precautions** Use extra caution and reduce dosages in the elderly because it is cleared renally somewhat slower, and the elderly are also more sensitive to the renal effects of NSAIDs; use with caution in patients with congestive heart failure, hypertension, decreased renal or hepatic function, history of GI disease (bleeding or ulcers), or those receiving anticoagulants

**Adverse Reactions**

Percentage unknown: Renal impairment, wound bleeding (with I.M.), postoperative hematomas

1% to 10%:

- Cardiovascular: Edema
- Central nervous system: Drowsiness, dizziness, headache, pain
- Gastrointestinal: Nausea, dyspepsia, diarrhea, gastric ulcers, indigestion
- Local: Pain at injection site
- Miscellaneous: Diaphoresis (increased)

<1%: Aphthous stomatitis, change in vision, dyspnea, mental depression, oliguria, peptic ulceration, purpura, rectal bleeding

**Overdosage/Toxicology**

Signs and symptoms: Diarrhea, pallor, vomiting, labored breathing, apnea, metabolic acidosis, leukocytosis, renal failure

Treatment: Management of a nonsteroidal anti-inflammatory drug (NSAID) intoxication is primarily supportive and symptomatic. Fluid therapy is commonly effective in managing the hypotension that may occur following an acute NSAID overdose, except when this is due to an acute blood loss. Seizures tend to be very short-lived and often do not require drug treatment; although, recurrent seizures should be treated with I.V. diazepam. Since many of the NSAIDs undergo enterohepatic cycling, multiple doses of charcoal may be needed to reduce the potential for delayed toxicities. NSAIDs are highly bound to plasma proteins; therefore, hemodialysis and peritoneal dialysis are not useful.

**Drug Interactions**

ACE inhibitors: Effects may be reduced by NSAIDs; use lowest possible dose for shortest duration possible; monitor

Cholestyramine and colestipol: Absorption may be reduced by concurrent administration

Corticosteroids: May increase the risk of GI ulceration; use caution

Cyclosporine: Nephrotoxicity may be increased with concurrent NSAID use; monitor

Hydralazine: Antihypertensive effect may be decreased; avoid concurrent use

Lithium: Serum levels can be increased; avoid concurrent use if possible or monitor lithium levels and adjust dose. When NSAID is stopped, lithium may need adjustment again.

Loop diuretics: Therapeutic effects may be reduced by NSAIDs; avoid

Methotrexate: Toxicity may be increased by concurrent NSAID use; risk is limited in low-dose methotrexate regimens (such as for rheumatoid arthritis); prolonged leucovorin rescue may be required at antineoplastic doses; monitor

Thiazide diuretics: Antihypertensive effects are decreased; avoid concurrent use

Warfarin: INRs may be increased by some NSAIDs. This may depend, in part, on dose and duration; monitor INR closely. Use the lowest dose of NSAIDs possible and for the briefest duration.

**Usual Dosage Note:** The use of ketorolac in children <16 years of age is outside of product labeling

Children 2-16 years: Dosing guidelines are not established; **do not exceed adult doses**

- Single-dose treatment:
  - I.M., I.V.: 0.4-1 mg/kg as a single dose; **Note:** Limited information exists. Single I.V. doses of 0.5 mg/kg, 0.75 mg/kg, 0.9 mg/kg and 1 mg/kg have been studied in children 2-16 years of age for postoperative analgesia. One study (Maunuksela, 1992) used a titrating dose starting with 0.2 mg/kg up to a total of 0.5 mg/kg (median dose required: 0.4 mg/kg).
  - Oral: One study used 1 mg/kg as a single dose for analgesia in 30 children (mean ± SD age: 3 ± 2.5 years) undergoing bilateral myringotomy
- Multiple-dose treatment: I.M., I.V., Oral: No pediatric studies exist; one report (Buck, 1994) of the clinical experience with ketorolac in 112 children, 6 months to 19 years of age (mean: 9 years), described usual I.V. maintenance doses of 0.5 mg/kg every 6 hours (mean dose: 0.52 mg/kg; range: 0.17-1 mg/kg)

Adults (pain relief usually begins within 10 minutes with parenteral forms):

- Oral: 10 mg every 4-6 hours as needed for a maximum of 40 mg/day; on day of transition from I.M. to oral: maximum oral dose: 40 mg (or 120 mg combined oral and I.M.); maximum 5 days administration
- I.M.: Initial: 30-60 mg, then 15-30 mg every 6 hours as needed for up to 5 days maximum; maximum dose in the first 24 hours: 150 mg with 120 mg/24 hours for up to 5 days total
- I.V.: Initial: 30 mg, then 15-30 mg every 6 hours as needed for up to 5 days **maximum**; maximum daily dose: 120 mg for up to 5 days total
- Ophthalmic: Instill 1 drop in eye(s) 4 times/day for up to 7 days

Elderly >65 years: Renal insufficiency or weight <50 kg:

- I.M.: 30 mg, then 15 mg every 6 hours

(Continued)

## Ketorolac Tromethamine *(Continued)*

I.V.: 15 mg every 6 hours as needed for up to 5 days total; maximum daily dose: 60 mg

**Dietary Considerations**

Potassium: Hyperkalemia has been reported. The elderly and those with renal insufficiency are at greatest risk. Monitor potassium serum concentration in those at greatest risk. Avoid salt substitutes.

Sodium: Hyponatremia from sodium retention. Suspect secondary to suppression of renal prostaglandin. Monitor serum concentration and fluid status. May need to restrict fluid.

**Patient Information** If self-administered, use exactly as directed (do not increase dose or frequency); adverse reactions can occur with overuse. Do not take longer than 5 days without consulting medical advisor. Take with food or milk. While using this medication, do not use alcohol, other prescription or OTC medications including aspirin, aspirin-containing medications, or other NSAIDs without consulting prescriber. Maintain adequate hydration (2-3 L/day of fluids unless instructed to restrict fluid intake). You may experience nausea, vomiting, gastric discomfort (frequent mouth care, small frequent meals, chewing gum, or sucking lozenges may help). GI bleeding, ulceration, or perforation can occur with or without pain. Stop taking medication and report ringing in ears; persistent cramping or pain in stomach; unresolved nausea or vomiting; difficulty breathing or shortness of breath; unusual bruising or bleeding (mouth, urine, stool); skin rash; unusual swelling of extremities; chest pain; or palpitations.

Ophthalmic: Instill drops as often as recommended. Wash hands before instilling. Sit or lie down to instill. Open eye, look at ceiling, and instill prescribed amount of solution. Close eye and roll eye in all directions, and apply gentle pressure to inner corner of eye for 1-2 minutes after instillation. Do not let tip of applicator touch eye or contaminate tip of applicator. Temporary stinging or blurred vision may occur. Report persistent pain, burning, double vision, swelling, itching, worsening of condition. Inform prescriber if you are or intend to be pregnant. Do not breast-feed.

**Nursing Implications** Monitor for signs of pain relief, such as an increased appetite and activity

**Dosage Forms**

Injection: 15 mg/mL (1 mL); 30 mg/mL (1 mL, 2 mL)

Solution, ophthalmic: 0.5% (5 mL)

Tablet: 10 mg

## Ketotifen (kee toe TYE fen)

**U.S. Brand Names** Zaditor™

**Pharmacologic Category** Antihistamine, $H_1$ Blocker, Ophthalmic

**Use** Temporary prevention of eye itching due to allergic conjunctivitis

**Effects on Mental Status** None reported

**Effects on Psychiatric Treatment** May cause dry eyes which can be exacerbated by anticholinergic agents or psychotropics with significant anticholinergic activity

**Usual Dosage** Adults: Instill 1 drop in the affected eye (s) every 8-12 hours

**Dosage Forms** Solution, ophthalmic: 0.025% (5 mL)


- **Kevadon®** *see* Thalidomide *on page 538*
- **Kew** *see* Kava *on page 301*
- **Key-Pred® Injection** *see* Prednisolone *on page 459*
- **Key-Pred-SP® Injection** *see* Prednisolone *on page 459*
- **K-G®** *see* Potassium Gluconate *on page 454*
- **KI** *see* Potassium Iodide *on page 454*
- **K-Ide®** *see* Potassium Bicarbonate and Potassium Citrate, Effervescent *on page 453*
- **Kinevac®** *see* Sincalide *on page 513*
- **Klamath Weed** *see* St Johns Wort *on page 519*
- **K-Lease®** *see* Potassium Chloride *on page 453*
- **Klerist-D® Tablet [OTC]** *see* Chlorpheniramine and Pseudoephedrine *on page 114*
- **Klonopin™** *see* Clonazepam *on page 132*
- **K-Lor™** *see* Potassium Chloride *on page 453*
- **Klor-Con®** *see* Potassium Chloride *on page 453*
- **Klor-Con® 8** *see* Potassium Chloride *on page 453*
- **Klor-Con® 10** *see* Potassium Chloride *on page 453*
- **Klor-Con®/25** *see* Potassium Chloride *on page 453*
- **Klor-con®/EF** *see* Potassium Bicarbonate and Potassium Citrate, Effervescent *on page 453*
- **Klorvess®** *see* Potassium Chloride *on page 453*
- **Klotrix®** *see* Potassium Chloride *on page 453*
- **K-Lyte®** *see* Potassium Bicarbonate and Potassium Citrate, Effervescent *on page 453*
- **K-Lyte®/Cl** *see* Potassium Chloride *on page 453*
- **K-Norm®** *see* Potassium Chloride *on page 453*
- **Koāte®-HP** *see* Antihemophilic Factor (Human) *on page 45*
- **Koāte®-HS** *see* Antihemophilic Factor (Human) *on page 45*
- **Kogenate®** *see* Antihemophilic Factor (Recombinant) *on page 46*
- **Kolephrin® GG/DM [OTC]** *see* Guaifenesin and Dextromethorphan *on page 257*
- **Konakion® Injection** *see* Phytonadione *on page 444*
- **Kondon's Nasal® [OTC]** *see* Ephedrine *on page 195*
- **Konsyl® [OTC]** *see* Psyllium *on page 479*
- **Konsyl-D® [OTC]** *see* Psyllium *on page 479*
- **Konȳne® 80** *see* Factor IX Complex (Human) *on page 217*
- **Koromex® [OTC]** *see* Nonoxynol 9 *on page 398*
- **K-Phos® Neutral** *see* Potassium Phosphate and Sodium Phosphate *on page 456*
- **K-Tab®** *see* Potassium Chloride *on page 453*
- **Ku-Zyme® HP** *see* Pancrelipase *on page 418*
- **K-Vescent®** *see* Potassium Bicarbonate and Potassium Citrate, Effervescent *on page 453*
- **Kwelcof®** *see* Hydrocodone and Guaifenesin *on page 272*
- **Kytril™** *see* Granisetron *on page 254*
- ***L*-3-Hydroxytyrosine** *see* Levodopa *on page 312*
- **LA-12®** *see* Hydroxocobalamin *on page 276*


## Labetalol (la BET a lole)

**Related Information**

Beta-Blockers Comparison Chart *on page 709*

**U.S. Brand Names** Normodyne®; Trandate®

**Synonyms** Ibidomide Hydrochloride

**Pharmacologic Category** Alpha-/Beta- Blocker

**Use** Treatment of mild to severe hypertension; I.V. for hypertensive emergencies

**Effects on Mental Status** Dizziness is common; may cause sedation

**Effects on Psychiatric Treatment** Barbiturates may decrease effects of beta-blockers; low potency antipsychotic and TCAs may potentiate the hypotensive effects of beta-blockers

**Pregnancy Risk Factor** C (per manufacturer); D (in second or third trimester, based on expert analysis)

**Contraindications** Hypersensitivity to labetalol or any component; sinus bradycardia; heart block greater than first degree (except in patients with a functioning artificial pacemaker); cardiogenic shock; bronchial asthma; uncompensated cardiac failure; pregnancy (2nd and 3rd trimesters)

**Warnings/Precautions** Use only with extreme caution in compensated heart failure and monitor for a worsening of the condition. Avoid abrupt discontinuation in patients with a history of CAD; slowly wean while monitoring for signs and symptoms of ischemia. Use caution with concurrent use of beta-blockers and either verapamil or diltiazem; bradycardia or heart block can occur. Avoid concurrent I.V. use of both agents. Patients with bronchospastic disease should not receive beta-blockers. Labetalol may be used with caution in patients with nonallergic bronchospasm (chronic bronchitis, emphysema). Use cautiously in diabetics because it can mask prominent hypoglycemic symptoms. Can mask signs of thyrotoxicosis. Can cause fetal harm when administered in pregnancy. Use cautiously in the hepatically impaired. Use caution when using I.V. labetalol and halothane concurrently (significant myocardial depression).

**Adverse Reactions**

1% to 10%:

Cardiovascular: Orthostatic hypotension (dose-related, usual 1% to 5%), edema (1%)

Central nervous system: Dizziness (11%), fatigue (2% to 5%), vertigo (2%), headache (2%)

Endocrine & metabolic: Decreased sexual ability (1% to 2%)

Gastrointestinal: Nausea (1% to 4%), stomach discomfort (3%), abnormal taste (1%)

Neuromuscular & skeletal: Paresthesia (1% to 2%)

Respiratory: Dyspnea (2%), nasal congestion (1% to 3%)

<1%: Diarrhea, drowsiness, rash (1%), vision abnormality, vomiting

**Overdosage/Toxicology**

Signs and symptoms: Cardiac disturbances, CNS toxicity, bronchospasm, hypoglycemia and hyperkalemia. The most common cardiac symptoms include hypotension and bradycardia; atrioventricular block, intraventricular conduction disturbances, cardiogenic shock, and asystole may occur with severe overdose, especially with membrane-depressant drugs (eg, propranolol); CNS effects include convulsions, coma, and respiratory arrest is commonly seen with propranolol and other membrane-depressant and lipid-soluble drugs.

Treatment: Symptomatic treatment of seizures, hypotension, hyperkalemia and hypoglycemia; bradycardia and hypotension resistant to atropine, isoproterenol or pacing may respond to glucagon; wide QRS defects caused by the membrane-depressant poisoning may respond to hypertonic sodium bicarbonate; repeat-dose charcoal, hemoperfusion, or hemodialysis may be helpful in removal of only those beta-blockers with a small $V_d$, long half-life or low intrinsic clearance (acebutolol, atenolol, nadolol, sotalol)

**Drug Interactions** CYP2D6 substrate/inhibitor

Inhibitors of CYP2D6 including quinidine, paroxetine, and propafenone are likely to increase blood levels of labetalol

Alpha-blockers (prazosin, terazosin): Concurrent use of beta-blockers may increase risk of orthostasis

Cimetidine increases the bioavailability of labetalol

Halothane, isoflurane, enflurane (possibly other inhalational anesthetics): Excessive hypotension may occur

NSAIDs may reduce antihypertensive efficacy of labetalol

NSAIDs (ibuprofen, indomethacin, naproxen, piroxicam) may reduce the antihypertensive effects of beta-blockers

Salicylates may reduce the antihypertensive effects of beta-blockers

Sulfonylureas: Effects may be decreased by beta-blockers

Verapamil or diltiazem may have synergistic or additive pharmacological effects when taken concurrently with beta-blockers; avoid concurrent I.V. use

**Usual Dosage** Due to limited documentation of its use, labetalol should be initiated cautiously in pediatric patients with careful dosage adjustment and blood pressure monitoring.

Children:

Oral: Limited information regarding labetalol use in pediatric patients is currently available in literature. Some centers recommend initial oral doses of 4 mg/kg/day in 2 divided doses. Reported oral doses have started at 3 mg/kg/day and 20 mg/kg/day and have increased up to 40 mg/kg/day.

I.V., intermittent bolus doses of 0.3-1 mg/kg/dose have been reported.

For treatment of pediatric hypertensive emergencies, initial continuous infusions of 0.4-1 mg/kg/hour with a maximum of 3 mg/kg/hour have been used. Administration requires the use of an infusion pump.

Adults:

Oral: Initial: 100 mg twice daily, may increase as needed every 2-3 days by 100 mg until desired response is obtained; usual dose: 200-400 mg twice daily; may require up to 2.4 g/day.

I.V.: 20 mg (0.25 mg/kg for an 80 kg patient) IVP over 2 minutes; may administer 40-80 mg at 10-minute intervals, up to 300 mg total dose.

I.V. infusion: Initial: 2 mg/minute; titrate to response up to 300 mg total dose, if needed. Administration requires the use of an infusion pump.

I.V. infusion (500 mg/250 mL $D_5W$) rates:

1 mg/minute: 30 mL/hour
2 mg/minute: 60 mL/hour
3 mg/minute: 90 mL/hour
4 mg/minute: 120 mL/hour
5 mg/minute: 150 mL/hour
6 mg/minute: 180 mL/hour

Dialysis: Not removed by hemo- or peritoneal dialysis; supplemental dose is not necessary.

**Dosage adjustment in hepatic impairment:** Dosage reduction may be necessary.

**Patient Information** For I.V. use in emergency situations - patient information is included in general instruction. Oral: Take as directed, with meals. Do not skip dose or discontinue without consulting prescriber. Follow recommended diet and exercise program. Do not use alcohol or OTC medications which may affect blood pressure (eg, cough or cold remedies, diet pills, stay-awake medications) without consulting prescriber. If diabetic, monitor serum glucose closely and notify prescriber of changes; this medication can alter hypoglycemic requirements. You may experience drowsiness, dizziness, or impaired judgment (use caution when driving or engaging in tasks that require alertness until response to drug is known); postural hypotension (use caution when rising from sitting or lying position or when climbing stairs); dry mouth, nausea, or loss of appetite (frequent mouth care or sucking lozenges may help); or sexual dysfunction (reversible, may resolve with continued use). Report altered CNS status (eg, fatigue, depression, numbness or tingling of fingers, toes, or skin); palpitations or slowed heartbeat; difficulty breathing; edema or cold extremities; or other persistent side effects.

**Dosage Forms**

Injection, as hydrochloride: 5 mg/mL (20 mL, 40 mL, 60 mL)

Tablet, as hydrochloride: 100 mg, 200 mg, 300 mg

♦ **LaBID®** *see* Theophylline Salts *on page 539*

♦ **Laboratory Values** *see page 748*

♦ **Lac-Hydrin®** *see* Lactic Acid With Ammonium Hydroxide *on page 305*

♦ **Lacril® Ophthalmic Solution [OTC]** *see* Artificial Tears *on page 48*

♦ **Lacrisert®** *see* Hydroxypropyl Cellulose *on page 277*

♦ **LactAid® [OTC]** *see* Lactase *on page 305*

## Lactase (LAK tase)

**U.S. Brand Names** Dairy Ease® [OTC]; LactAid® [OTC]; Lactrase® [OTC]

**Canadian Brand Names** Dairyaid

**Pharmacologic Category** Nutritional Supplement

**Use** Help digest lactose in milk for patients with lactose intolerance

**Effects on Mental Status** None reported

**Effects on Psychiatric Treatment** None reported

**Usual Dosage** Oral:

Capsule: 1-2 capsules taken with milk or meal; pretreat milk with 1-2 capsules/quart of milk

Liquid: 5-15 drops/quart of milk

Tablet: 1-3 tablets with meals

**Dosage Forms**

Caplet: 3000 FCC lactase units

Capsule: 250 mg

Liquid: 1250 neutral lactase units/5 drops

Tablet, chewable: 3300 FCC lactase units

## Lactic Acid and Sodium-PCA
(LAK tik AS id & SOW dee um-pee see aye)

**U.S. Brand Names** LactiCare® [OTC]

**Pharmacologic Category** Topical Skin Product

**Use** Lubricate and moisturize the skin counteracting dryness and itching

**Effects on Mental Status** None reported

**Effects on Psychiatric Treatment** None reported

**Usual Dosage** Apply as needed

**Dosage Forms** Lotion, topical: Lactic acid 5% and sodium-PCA 2.5% (240 mL)

## Lactic Acid With Ammonium Hydroxide
(LAK tik AS id with a MOE nee um hye DROKS ide)

**U.S. Brand Names** Lac-Hydrin®

**Pharmacologic Category** Topical Skin Product

**Use** Treatment of moderate to severe xerosis and ichthyosis vulgaris

**Effects on Mental Status** None reported

**Effects on Psychiatric Treatment** None reported

**Usual Dosage** Shake well; apply to affected areas, use twice daily, rub in well

**Dosage Forms** Lotion: Lactic acid 12% with ammonium hydroxide (150 mL)

♦ **LactiCare® [OTC]** *see* Lactic Acid and Sodium-PCA *on page 305*

♦ **LactiCare-HC®** *see* Hydrocortisone *on page 273*

♦ **Lactinex® [OTC]** *see Lactobacillus acidophilus* and *Lactobacillus bulgaricus on page 305*

## *Lactobacillus acidophilus* and *Lactobacillus bulgaricus*
(lak toe ba SIL us as i DOF fil us & lak toe ba SIL us bul GAR i cus)

**U.S. Brand Names** Bacid® [OTC]; Lactinex® [OTC]; MoreDophilus® [OTC]; Pro-Bionate® [OTC]; Superdophilus® [OTC]

**Canadian Brand Names** Fermalac®

**Pharmacologic Category** Antidiarrheal

**Use** Treatment of uncomplicated diarrhea particularly that caused by antibiotic therapy; re-establish normal physiologic and bacterial flora of the intestinal tract

**Effects on Mental Status** None reported

**Effects on Psychiatric Treatment** None reported

**Contraindications** Allergy to milk or lactose

**Warnings/Precautions** Discontinue if high fever present; do not use in children <3 years of age

**Adverse Reactions** 1% to 10%: Gastrointestinal: Intestinal flatus

**Drug Interactions** No data reported

**Usual Dosage** Children >3 years and Adults: Oral:

Capsules: 2 capsules 2-4 times/day

Granules: 1 packet added to or taken with cereal, food, milk, fruit juice, or water, 3-4 times/day

Powder: 1 teaspoonful daily with liquid

Tablet, chewable: 4 tablets 3-4 times/day; may follow each dose with a small amount of milk, fruit juice, or water

**Patient Information** Granules may be added to or taken with cereal, food, milk, fruit juice, or water.

**Dosage Forms**

Capsule: 50s, 100s

(Continued)

## *Lactobacillus acidophilus* and *Lactobacillus bulgaricus* *(Continued)*

Granules: 1 g/packet (12 packets/box)
Powder: 12 oz
Tablet, chewable: 50s

- **Lactoflavin** *see* Riboflavin *on page 492*
- **Lactrase® [OTC]** *see* Lactase *on page 305*

## Lactulose (LAK tyoo lose)

**Related Information**
Laxatives, Classification and Properties *on page 716*

**U.S. Brand Names** Cephulac®; Cholac®; Chronulac®; Constilac®; Constulose®; Duphalac®; Enulose®; Evalose®; Heptalac®; Lactulose PSE®

**Pharmacologic Category** Ammonium Detoxicant; Laxative, Miscellaneous

**Use** Adjunct in the prevention and treatment of portal-systemic encephalopathy (PSE); treatment of chronic constipation

**Effects on Mental Status** None reported

**Effects on Psychiatric Treatment** None reported

**Pregnancy Risk Factor** B

**Contraindications** Patients with galactosemia and require a low galactose diet, hypersensitivity to any component

**Warnings/Precautions** Use with caution in patients with diabetes mellitus; monitor periodically for electrolyte imbalance when lactulose is used >6 months or in patients predisposed to electrolyte abnormalities (eg, elderly); patients receiving lactulose and an oral anti-infective agent should be monitored for possible inadequate response to lactulose

**Adverse Reactions**
>10%: Gastrointestinal: Flatulence, diarrhea (excessive dose)
1% to 10%: Gastrointestinal: Abdominal discomfort, nausea, vomiting

**Overdosage/Toxicology**
Signs and symptoms: Diarrhea, abdominal pain, hypochloremic alkalosis, dehydration, hypotension, hypokalemia
Treatment: Supportive care

**Drug Interactions** Decreased effect: Oral neomycin, laxatives, antacids

**Usual Dosage** Diarrhea may indicate overdosage and responds to dose reduction
Prevention of portal systemic encephalopathy (PSE): Oral:
Infants: 2.5-10 mL/day divided 3-4 times/day; adjust dosage to produce 2-3 stools/day
Older Children: Daily dose of 40-90 mL divided 3-4 times/day; if initial dose causes diarrhea, then reduce it immediately; adjust dosage to produce 2-3 stools/day
Constipation:
Children: 5 g/day (7.5 mL) after breakfast
Adults:
Acute PSE:
Oral: 20-30 g (30-45 mL) every 1-2 hours to induce rapid laxation; adjust dosage daily to produce 2-3 soft stools; doses of 30-45 mL may be given hourly to cause rapid laxation, then reduce to recommended dose; usual daily dose: 60-100 g (90-150 mL) daily
Rectal administration: 200 g (300 mL) diluted with 700 mL of $H_2O$ or NS; administer rectally via rectal balloon catheter and retain 30-60 minutes every 4-6 hours
Constipation: Oral: 15-30 mL/day increased to 60 mL/day if necessary

**Patient Information** Not for long-term use. Take as directed, alone, or diluted with water, juice or milk, or take with food. Laxative results may not occur for 24-48 hours; do not take more often than recommended or for a longer time than recommended. Do not use any other laxatives while taking lactulose. Increased fiber, fluids, and exercise may help reduce constipation. Do not use if experiencing abdominal pain, nausea, or vomiting. Diarrhea may indicate overdose. May cause flatulence, belching, or abdominal cramping. Report persistent or severe diarrhea or abdominal cramping.

**Nursing Implications** Dilute lactulose in water, usually 60-120 mL, prior to administering through a gastric or feeding tube

**Dosage Forms** Syrup: 10 g/15 mL (15 mL, 30 mL, 237 mL, 473 mL, 946 mL, 1890 mL)

- **Lactulose PSE®** *see* Lactulose *on page 306*
- **Lamictal®** *see* Lamotrigine *on page 306*
- **Lamictal® CD** *see* Lamotrigine *on page 306*
- **Lamisil® AT™ Topical** *see* Terbinafine *on page 535*
- **Lamisil® Dermgel** *see* Terbinafine *on page 535*
- **Lamisil® Topical** *see* Terbinafine *on page 535*

## Lamivudine (la MI vyoo deen)

**U.S. Brand Names** Epivir®; Epivir®-HBV™

**Synonyms** 3TC

**Pharmacologic Category** Antiretroviral Agent, Reverse Transcriptase Inhibitor (Non-Nucleoside)

**Use** Treatment of HIV infection when antiretroviral therapy is warranted; should always be used as part of a multidrug regimen (at least three antiretroviral agents); indicated for the treatment of chronic hepatitis B associated with evidence of hepatitis B viral replication and active liver inflammation

**Effects on Mental Status** Fatigue and insomnia are common; may cause dizziness or depression

**Effects on Psychiatric Treatment** May rarely cause neutropenia; use caution with clozapine and carbamazepine

**Pregnancy Risk Factor** C

**Contraindications** Hypersensitivity to lamivudine or any component

**Warnings/Precautions** A decreased dosage is recommended in patients with renal dysfunction since AUC, $C_{max}$, and half-life increased with diminishing renal function; use with extreme caution in children with history of pancreatitis or risk factors for development of pancreatitis. Do not use as monotherapy in treatment of HIV.

**Adverse Reactions**
>10%:
Central nervous system: Headache, insomnia, malaise, fatigue, pain
Gastrointestinal: Nausea, diarrhea, vomiting
Neuromuscular & skeletal: Peripheral neuropathy, paresthesia
Respiratory: Nasal signs and symptoms, cough
1% to 10%:
Central nervous system: Dizziness, depression, fever, chills
Dermatologic: Rashes
Gastrointestinal: Anorexia, abdominal pain, dyspepsia, increased amylase
Hematologic: Neutropenia, anemia
Hepatic: Elevated AST/ALT
Neuromuscular & skeletal: Myalgia, arthralgia
<1%: Hyperbilirubinemia, pancreatitis, thrombocytopenia

**Overdosage/Toxicology**
Signs and symptoms: Very limited information is available although there have been no clinical signs or symptoms noted and hematologic tests remained normal in overdose
Treatment: No antidote is available; unknown dialyzability

**Drug Interactions** Increased effect: Zidovudine concentrations increase (~39%) with coadministration with lamivudine; trimethoprim/sulfamethoxazole increases lamivudine's AUC and decreases its renal clearance by 44% and 29%, respectively; although the AUC was not significantly affected, absorption of lamivudine was slowed and $C_{max}$ was 40% lower when administered to patients in the fed versus the fasted state

**Usual Dosage** Oral: Use with at least two other antiretroviral agents when treating HIV
Children 3 months to 12 years: 4 mg/kg twice daily (maximum: 150 mg twice daily)
Adolescents 12-16 years and Adults: 150 mg twice daily
Prevention of HIV following needlesticks: 150 mg twice daily (with zidovudine and a protease inhibitor)
Adults <50 kg: 2 mg/kg twice daily
Treatment of hepatitis B: 100 mg/day
**Dosing interval in renal impairment in patients >16 years for HIV:**
$Cl_{cr}$ 30-49 mL/minute: Administer 150 mg once daily
$Cl_{cr}$ 15-29 mL/minute: Administer 150 mg first dose, then 100 mg once daily
$Cl_{cr}$ 5-14 mL/minute: Administer 150 mg first dose, then 50 mg once daily
$Cl_{cr}$ <5 mL/minute: Administer 50 mg first dose, then 25 mg once daily
**Dosing interval in renal impairment in patients with hepatitis B:**
$Cl_{cr}$ 30-49: Administer 100 mg first dose then 50 mg once daily
$Cl_{cr}$ 15-29: Administer 100 mg first dose then 25 mg once daily
$Cl_{cr}$ 5-14: Administer 35 mg first dose then 15 mg once daily
$Cl_{cr}$ <5: Administer 35 mg first dose then 10 mg once daily
Dialysis: No data available

**Patient Information** This is not a cure for AIDS or AIDS complex, nor will it reduce the risk of transmission to others. Long-term effects are unknown. You will need frequent blood tests to adjust dosage for maximum therapeutic effect. Take as directed for full course of therapy; do not discontinue (even if feeling better). You may experience loss of appetite; change in taste (sucking on lozenges, chewing gum, or small frequent meals may help); dizziness or numbness (use caution when driving or engaging in tasks that require alertness until response to drug is known); headache, fever, or muscle pain (an analgesic may be recommended). Report persistent lethargy, acute headache, severe nausea or vomiting, difficulty breathing, loss of sensation, or rash.

**Dosage Forms**
Solution, oral: 5 mg/mL (240 mL); 10 mg/mL (240 mL)
Tablet: 100 mg, 150 mg

## Lamotrigine (la MOE tri jeen)

**Related Information**
Anticonvulsants by Seizures Type *on page 703*

Mood Disorders *on page 600*
Mood Stabilizers *on page 719*

**Generic Available** No

**U.S. Brand Names** Lamictal®; Lamictal® CD

**Synonyms** BW-430C; LTG

**Pharmacologic Category** Anticonvulsant, Miscellaneous

**Use** Adjunctive therapy in the treatment of partial seizures in adults with epilepsy (safety and effectiveness in children <16 years of age have not been established); adjunctive therapy in the generalized seizures of Lennox-Gastaut syndrome in pediatric and adult patients; conversion to monotherapy in adults with partial seizures who are receiving treatment with a single enzyme-inducing antiepileptic drug

**Unlabeled use:** Bipolar disorder

**Effects on Mental Status** May cause sedation

**Effects on Psychiatric Treatment** Currently being studied in bipolar disorder; may be particularly useful for depressive phase of bipolar illness; valproic acid decreases clearance of lamotrigine; carbamazepine may decrease effects of lamotrigine

**Pregnancy Risk Factor** C

**Contraindications** Hypersensitivity to lamotrigine or any component

**Warnings/Precautions** Lactation, impaired renal, hepatic, or cardiac function; avoid abrupt cessation, taper over at least 2 weeks if possible. Severe and potentially life-threatening skin rashes have been reported; this appears to occur most frequently in pediatric patients. May cause CNS depression, which may impair physical or mental abilities. Patients must be cautioned about performing tasks which require mental alertness (ie, operating machinery or driving). Effects with other sedative drugs or ethanol may be potentiated.

**Adverse Reactions**

>10%:

Central nervous system: Headache, nausea, dizziness, ataxia, somnolence
Ocular: Diplopia, blurred vision
Respiratory: Rhinitis

1% to 10%:

Cardiovascular: Hot flashes, palpitations
Central nervous system: Depression, anxiety, irritability, confusion, speech disorder, difficulty concentrating, emotional lability, malaise, seizure, incoordination, insomnia
Dermatologic: Hypersensitivity rash, Stevens-Johnson syndrome, angioedema, pruritus, alopecia, acne
Gastrointestinal: Abdominal pain, vomiting, diarrhea, dyspepsia, constipation, psoriasis, xerostomia
Genitourinary: Vaginitis, amenorrhea
Neuromuscular & skeletal: Tremor, arthralgia, joint pain
Ocular: Nystagmus, diplopia
Renal: Hematuria
Respiratory: Cough

Miscellaneous: Flu syndrome, fever

**Overdosage/Toxicology**

Decontamination: Lavage/activated charcoal with cathartic
Enhancement of elimination: Multiple dosing of activated charcoal may be useful

**Drug Interactions**

Acetaminophen: May reduce serum concentrations of lamotrigine; mechanism not defined; of clinical concern only with chronic acetaminophen dosing (not single doses)
Carbamazepine: Lamotrigine may increase the epoxide metabolite of carbamazepine resulting in toxicity
Enzyme inducers: Carbamazepine, phenytoin, phenobarbital may decrease concentrations of lamotrigine
Sertraline: Toxicity has been reported following the addition of sertraline; limited documentation; monitor
Valproic acid: Inhibits the metabolism of lamotrigine; lamotrigine enhances the metabolism of valproic acid

**Mechanism of Action** A triazine derivative which inhibits release of glutamate (an excitatory amino acid) and inhibits voltage-sensitive sodium channels, which stabilizes neuronal membranes. Lamotrigine has weak inhibitory effect on the $5HT_3$ receptor; *in vitro* inhibits dihydrofolate reductase.

**Pharmacodynamics/kinetics**

Distribution: $V_d$: 1.1 L/kg
Protein binding: 55%
Metabolism: Hepatic and renal
Half-life: 24 hours; increases to 59 hours with concomitant valproic acid therapy; decreases with concomitant phenytoin or carbamazepine therapy to 15 hours
Peak levels: Within 1-4 hours
Elimination: In urine as the glucuronide conjugate

**Usual Dosage** Oral:

Adults: Initial dose: 50 mg/day for 2 weeks, then 100 mg in 2 doses for 2 weeks; thereafter, daily dose can be increased by 100 mg every 1-2 weeks to 300-500 mg/day given in 2 divided doses
With concomitant valproic acid therapy and other antiepileptic drugs: 25 mg every other day for 2 weeks; 25 mg/day for 2 weeks; thereafter, dose may be increased by 25-50 mg/day every 1-2 weeks to 150 mg/day given in 2 divided doses

**Dietary Considerations** Food: Has no effect on absorption, take without regard to meals; drug may cause GI upset

**Monitoring Parameters** Seizure, frequency and duration, serum levels of concurrent anticonvulsants, hypersensitivity reactions, especially rash

**Reference Range** Therapeutic range: 2-4 μg/mL

**Patient Information** Notify physician immediately if skin rash develops or seizure control worsens; may cause dizziness or sedation; avoid activities needing good psychomotor activities until CNS effects are known; avoid abrupt discontinuation

**Additional Information** Low water solubility

**Dosage Forms**

Tablet: 25 mg, 100 mg, 150 mg, 200 mg
Tablet, dispersible, chewable: 5 mg, 25 mg


- **Lamprene®** *see* Clofazimine *on page 130*
- **Lanacane® [OTC]** *see* Benzocaine *on page 61*
- **Lanacort® [OTC]** *see* Hydrocortisone *on page 273*
- **Lanaphilic® Topical [OTC]** *see* Urea *on page 576*
- **Laniazid® Oral** *see* Isoniazid *on page 294*


## Lanolin, Cetyl Alcohol, Glycerin, and Petrolatum

(LAN oh lin, SEE til AL koe hol, GLIS er in, & pe troe LAY tum)

**U.S. Brand Names** Lubriderm® [OTC]

**Pharmacologic Category** Topical Skin Product

**Use** Treatment of dry skin

**Effects on Mental Status** None reported

**Effects on Psychiatric Treatment** None reported

**Usual Dosage** Topical: Apply to skin as necessary

**Dosage Forms** Lotion: 480 mL


- **Lanorinal®** *see* Butalbital Compound and Aspirin *on page 80*
- **Lanoxicaps®** *see* Digoxin *on page 169*
- **Lanoxin®** *see* Digoxin *on page 169*


## Lansoprazole (lan SOE pra zole)

**U.S. Brand Names** Prevacid®

**Pharmacologic Category** Proton Pump Inhibitor

**Use** Short-term treatment (up to 4 weeks) for healing and symptom relief of active duodenal ulcers (should not be used for maintenance therapy of duodenal ulcers); as part of a multiple drug regimen for *H. pylori* eradication; short-term treatment of symptomatic GERD; up to 8 weeks of treatment for all grades of erosive esophagitis (8 additional weeks can be given for incompletely healed esophageal erosions or for recurrence); and long-term treatment of pathological hypersecretory conditions, including Zollinger-Ellison syndrome

**Effects on Mental Status** May cause drowsiness or dizziness

**Effects on Psychiatric Treatment** None reported

**Pregnancy Risk Factor** B

**Contraindications** Should not be taken by anyone with a known hypersensitivity to lansoprazole or any of the formulation's components

**Warnings/Precautions** Liver disease may require dosage reductions

**Adverse Reactions**

1% to 10%:

Central nervous system: Fatigue, dizziness, headache
Gastrointestinal: Abdominal pain, diarrhea, nausea, increased appetite, hypergastrinoma

<1%: Proteinuria, rash, tinnitus

**Overdosage/Toxicology**

Signs and symptoms: Hypothermia, sedation, convulsions, decreased respiratory rate demonstrated in animals only
Treatment: Supportive; not dialyzable

**Drug Interactions** CYP2C19 enzyme substrate, CYP3A3/4 enzyme substrate (minor)

Decreased effect: Ketoconazole, itraconazole, and other drugs dependent upon acid for absorption; theophylline clearance increased slightly; sucralfate delays and reduces lansoprazole absorption by 30%

**Usual Dosage**

Duodenal ulcer: 15 mg once daily for 4 weeks; maintenance therapy: 15 mg once daily
Gastric ulcer: 30 mg once daily for up to 8 weeks
GERD: 15 mg once daily for up to 8 weeks
Erosive esophagitis: 30 mg once daily for up to 8 weeks, continued treatment for an additional 8 weeks may be considered for recurrence or for patients that do not heal after the first 8 weeks of therapy. Maintenance therapy: 15 mg once daily.
Hypersecretory conditions: Initial: 60 mg once daily; adjust dose based upon patient response and to reduce acid secretion to <10 mEq/hour (5

(Continued)

## Lansoprazole *(Continued)*

mEq/hour in patients with prior gastric surgery); doses of 90 mg twice daily have been used; administer doses >120 mg/day in divided doses.

*Helicobacter pylori*-associated antral gastritis: 30 mg/day for 2 weeks (in combination with 1 g amoxicillin and 500 mg clarithromycin given twice daily for 14 days). Alternatively, in patients allergic to or intolerant of clarithromycin or in whom resistance to clarithromycin is known or suspected, lansoprazole 30 mg every 8 hours and amoxicillin 1 g every 8 hours may be given for 2 weeks

**Dosing adjustment in hepatic impairment:** Dose reduction is necessary for severe hepatic impairment

**Patient Information** Take as directed, before eating. Do not crush or chew granules. Patients who may have difficulty swallowing capsules may open the delayed-release capsules and sprinkle the contents on applesauce, pudding, cottage cheese, yogurt, or Ensure. Report unresolved fatigue, diarrhea, or constipation, and appetite changes.

**Dosage Forms** Capsule, delayed release: 15 mg, 30 mg

## Lansoprazole, Amoxicillin, and Clarithromycin

(lan SOE pra zole, a moks i SIL in, & kla RITH roe mye sin)

**U.S. Brand Names** Prevpac™

**Pharmacologic Category** Antibiotic, Oxazolidinone; Antibiotic, Penicillin; Gastrointestinal Agent, Miscellaneous

**Use** Eradication of *H. pylori* to reduce the risk of recurrent duodenal ulcer

**Effects on Mental Status** May cause drowsiness or dizziness; rarely large doses may produce confusion, hallucinations, and depression; penicillins have been reported to cause apprehension, illusions, agitation, insomnia, depersonalization, and encephalopathy; macrolides have been reported to cause nightmares, confusion, anxiety, and mood lability

**Effects on Psychiatric Treatment** Disulfiram may increase amoxicillin levels; macrolides are contraindicated with pimozide and increase carbamazepine and triazolam levels; monitor for signs of toxicity

**Dosage Forms** The package contains:

Amoxicillin: 500 mg capsules
Clarithromycin: 500 mg tablets
Lansoprazole: 30 mg capsules

♦ **Lantus®** *see* Insulin Preparations *on page 287*

♦ **Largon® Injection** *see* Propiomazine *on page 473*

♦ **Lariam®** *see* Mefloquine *on page 337*

♦ **Larodopa®** *see* Levodopa *on page 312*

♦ ***Larrea tridentata*** *see* Chaparral *on page 106*

♦ **Lasix®** *see* Furosemide *on page 243*

♦ **Lassar's Zinc Paste** *see* Zinc Oxide *on page 593*

## Latanoprost (la TAN oh prost)

**Related Information**

Glaucoma Drug Therapy *on page 712*

**U.S. Brand Names** Xalatan®

**Pharmacologic Category** Ophthalmic Agent, Antiglaucoma; Prostaglandin, Ophthalmic

**Use** Reduction of elevated intraocular pressure in patients with open-angle glaucoma and ocular hypertension who are intolerant of the other IOP lowering medications or insufficiently responsive (failed to achieve target IOP determined after multiple measurements over time) to another IOP lowering medication

**Effects on Mental Status** None reported

**Effects on Psychiatric Treatment** None reported

**Usual Dosage** Adults: Ophthalmic: 1 drop (1.5 mcg) in the affected eye(s) once daily in the evening; do not exceed the once daily dosage because it has been shown that more frequent administration may decrease the IOP lowering effect

**Dosage Forms** Solution, ophthalmic: 0.005% (2.5 mL)

♦ **Laxatives, Classification and Properties** *see page 716*

♦ **L-Carnitine** *see* Levocarnitine *on page 312*

♦ **L-Deprenyl** *see* Selegiline *on page 508*

♦ ***L*-Dopa** *see* Levodopa *on page 312*

♦ **Lederplex® [OTC]** *see* Vitamin B Complex *on page 586*

## Leflunomide (le FLU no mide)

**U.S. Brand Names** Arava™

**Pharmacologic Category** Antimetabolite

**Use** Treatment of active rheumatoid arthritis to reduce signs and symptoms and to retard structural damage as evidenced by x-ray erosions and joint space narrowing

**Effects on Mental Status** May cause dizziness, malaise, anxiety, depression, or insomnia

**Effects on Psychiatric Treatment** May rarely cause leukopenia, caution with clozapine and carbamazepine

**Usual Dosage**

Adults: Oral: Initial: 100 mg/day for 3 days, followed by 20 mg/day; dosage may be decreased to 10 mg/day in patients who have difficulty tolerating the 20 mg dose. Due to the long half-life of the active metabolite, plasma levels may require a prolonged period to decline after dosage reduction.

**Dosing adjustment in renal impairment:** No specific dosage adjustment is recommended. There is no clinical experience in the use of leflunomide in patients with renal impairment. The free fraction of MI is doubled in dialysis patients. Patients should be monitored closely for adverse effects requiring dosage adjustment.

**Dosing adjustment in hepatic impairment:** No specific dosage adjustment is recommended. Since the liver is involved in metabolic activation and subsequent metabolism/elimination of leflunomide, patients with hepatic impairment should be monitored closely for adverse effects requiring dosage adjustment.

Guidelines for dosage adjustment or discontinuation based on the severity and persistence of ALT elevation secondary to leflunomide have been developed. For ALT elevations >2 times the upper limit of normal, dosage reduction to 10 mg/day may allow continued administration. Cholestyramine 8 g 3 times/day for 1-3 days may be administered to decrease plasma levels. If elevations >2 times but ≤3 times the upper limit of normal persist, liver biopsy is recommended. If elevations >3 times the upper limit of normal persist despite cholestyramine administration and dosage reduction, leflunomide should be discontinued and drug elimination should be enhanced with additional cholestyramine as indicated.

Elderly: Although hepatic function may decline with age, no specific dosage adjustment is recommended. Patients should be monitored closely for adverse effects which may require dosage adjustment.

**Dosage Forms** Tablet: 10 mg, 20 mg, 100 mg

## Lemon Grass Oil

**Pharmacologic Category** Herb

**Use** Perfumes; flavoring agent; used also as a hypotensive and carminative in folk medicine

**Overdosage/Toxicology**

Signs and symptoms: Mucosal irritation, allergic contact dermatitis, skin irritation with citral concentrations >8%, CNS depression at high doses

Decontamination:

Oral: Dilute with milk or water

Dermal: Wash with cool water (warm water may increase severity of reactions)

Ocular: Irrigate copiously with saline

**Usual Dosage** Acceptable daily intake for food: 500 mcg of citral

**Additional Information** Not widely used in U.S. market as an herbal dietary supplement; plant is a perennial grass native to Ceylon and Southern India

♦ **Lente® Iletin® I** *see* Insulin Preparations *on page 287*

♦ **Lente® Iletin® II** *see* Insulin Preparations *on page 287*

♦ **Lente® Insulin** *see* Insulin Preparations *on page 287*

♦ **Lente® L** *see* Insulin Preparations *on page 287*

## Lepirudin (leh puh ROO din)

**U.S. Brand Names** Refludan™

**Pharmacologic Category** Anticoagulant

**Use** Indicated for anticoagulation in patient with heparin-induced thrombocytopenia (HIT) and associated thromboembolic disease in order to prevent further thromboembolic complications

**Unlabeled use:** Prevention or reduction of ischemic complications associated with unstable angina

**Effects on Mental Status** None reported

**Effects on Psychiatric Treatment** Contraindicated in patients with a recent stroke

**Usual Dosage** Adults: Maximum dose: Do not exceed 0.21 mg/kg/hour unless an evaluation of coagulation abnormalities limiting response has been completed. **Dosing is weight-based, however patients weighing >110 kg should not receive doses greater than the recommended dose for a patient weighing 110 kg (44 mg bolus and initial maximal infusion rate of 16.5 mg/hour).**

Heparin-induced thrombocytopenia: Bolus dose: 0.4 mg/kg IVP (over 15-20 seconds), followed by continuous infusion at 0.15 mg/kg/hour; bolus and infusion must be reduced in renal insufficiency

Concomitant use with thrombolytic therapy: Bolus dose: 0.2 mg/kg IVP (over 15-20 seconds), followed by continuous infusion at 0.1 mg/kg/hour

Dosing adjustments during infusions: Monitor first APTT 4 hours after the start of the infusion. Subsequent determinations of APTT should be obtained at least once daily during treatment. More frequent monitoring is recommended in renally impaired patients. Any APTT ratio measurement out of range (1.5-2.5) should be confirmed prior to adjusting dose, unless a clinical need for immediate reaction exists. If the APTT is below target range, increase infusion by 20%. If the APTT is in excess of the target range, decrease infusion rate by 50%. A repeat APTT should be obtained 4 hours after any dosing change.

Use in patients scheduled for switch to oral anticoagulants: Reduce lepirudin dose gradually to reach APTT ratio just above 1.5 before starting warfarin therapy; as soon as INR reaches 2.0, lepirudin therapy should be discontinued.

**Dosing adjustment in renal impairment**: All patients with a creatinine clearance of <60 mL/minute or a serum creatinine of >1.5 mg should receive a reduction in lepirudin dosage; there is only limited information on the therapeutic use of lepirudin in HIT patients with significant renal impairment; the following dosage recommendations are mainly based on single-dose studies in a small number of patients with renal impairment.

Initial: Bolus dose: 0.2 mg/kg IVP (over 15-20 seconds), followed by adjusted infusion based on renal function; refer to the following infusion rate adjustments based on creatinine clearance (mL/minute) and serum creatinine (mg/dL):

**Lepirudin infusion rates in patients with renal impairment:**

$Cl_{cr}$ 45-60; $S_{cr}$ 1.6-2.0:
Adjust rate to 50% of standard infusion rate: 0.075 mg/kg/hour

$Cl_{cr}$ 30-44; $S_{cr}$ 2.1-3.0:
Adjust rate to 30% of standard infusion rate: 0.045 mg/kg/hour

$Cl_{cr}$ 15-29; $S_{cr}$ 3.1-6.0:
Adjust rate to 15% of standard infusion rate: 0.0225 mg/kg/hour

$Cl_{cr}$ <15; $S_{cr}$ >6.0: Avoid or STOP infusion.

**Note: Acute renal failure or hemodialysis:** Infusion is to be avoided or stopped. Following the bolus dose, additional bolus doses of 0.1 mg/kg may be administered every other day (only if APTT falls below lower therapeutic limit).

**Dosage Forms** Injection: 50 mg vials

◆ **Lergefin®** *see* Carbinoxamine *on page 92*

◆ **Lescol®** *see* Fluvastatin *on page 237*

## Letrozole (LET roe zole)

**U.S. Brand Names** Femara™

**Pharmacologic Category** Antineoplastic Agent, Miscellaneous; Aromatase Inhibitor

**Use** Treatment of advanced breast cancer in postmenopausal women with disease progression following antiestrogen therapy

**Effects on Mental Status** May cause drowsiness or dizziness

**Effects on Psychiatric Treatment** None reported

**Pregnancy Risk Factor** D

**Contraindications** Hypersensitivity to letrozole or any of its excipients

**Warnings/Precautions** Letrozole was not mutagenic in *in vitro* tests but was observed to be a potential clastogen in *in vitro* assays. Repeated dosing caused sexual inactivity in females and atrophy in the reproductive tract in males and females at doses of 0.6 mg/kg, 0.1 mg/kg, and 0.03 mg/kg in mice, rats, and dogs, respectively (~1 mg/kg, 0.4 mg/kg, and 0.4 mg/kg the maximum recommended human doses, respectively).

Moderate decreases in lymphocyte counts, of uncertain clinical significance, were observed in some patients receiving letrozole 2.5 mg. This depression was transient in ~50% of those affected. Two patients on letrozole developed thrombocytopenia; relationship to the drug was unclear.

Increases in AST, ALT, and GGT ≥5 times the upper limit of normal (ULN) and of bilirubin ≥1.5 times the ULN were most often associated with metastatic disease in the liver.

**Adverse Reactions**

>10%: Gastrointestinal: Nausea

1% to 10%:
- Central nervous system: Headache, somnolence, dizziness
- Dermatologic: Hot flashes, rash, pruritus
- Gastrointestinal: Vomiting, constipation, diarrhea, abdominal pain, anorexia, dyspepsia
- Neuromuscular: Arthralgia
- Respiratory: Dyspnea, coughing

<1%: Thromboembolic events, vaginal bleeding

**Overdosage/Toxicology**

Signs and symptoms: No experience with letrozole overdose has been reported. In single-dose studies, the highest dose used was 30 mg, which was well tolerated. Lethality was observed in mice and rats following single oral doses that were ≥2000 mg/kg (~4000 to 8000 times the maximum daily doses recommended in humans); death was associated with reduced motor activity, ataxia, and dyspnea. Lethality was observed in cats following single I.V. doses that were ≥10 mg/kg (~50 times the maximum daily dose recommended in humans): death was preceded by depressed blood pressure and arrhythmias.

Treatment: Firm recommendations for treatment are not possible; emesis could be induced if the patient is alert. In general, supportive care and frequent monitoring of vital signs are appropriate.

**Drug Interactions** CYP3A3/4 and 2A6 enzyme substrate; CYP2A6 and 2C19 enzyme inhibitor

**Usual Dosage** Oral (refer to individual protocols):

Adults: 2.5 mg once daily without regard to meals; continue treatment until tumor progression is evident. Patients treated with letrozole do not require glucocorticoid or mineralocorticoid replacement therapy.

**Dosage adjustment in renal impairment:** No dosage adjustment is required in patients with renal impairment if $Cl_{cr}$ ≥10 mL/minute

**Dosage adjustment in hepatic impairment:** No dosage adjustment is recommended for patients with mild-to-moderate hepatic impairment. Patients with severe impairment of liver function have not been studied; dose patients with severe impairment of liver function with caution.

**Patient Information** Take as directed, without regard to food. You may experience nausea, vomiting, or loss of appetite (frequent mouth care, frequent small meals, chewing gum, or sucking lozenges may help); musculoskeletal pain or headache (mild analgesics may offer relief); sleepiness, fatigue, or dizziness (use caution when driving, climbing stairs, or engaging in tasks that require alertness until response to drug is known); constipation (increased exercise, or dietary fruit or fluids may help); diarrhea (boiled milk or yogurt may help); loss of hair (will grow back). Report chest pain, palpitations, or swollen extremities; vaginal bleeding or hot flashes; unusual coughing or difficulty breathing; severe nausea; muscle pain; or skin rash.

**Dosage Forms** Tablet: 2.5 mg

## Leucovorin (loo koe VOR in)

**U.S. Brand Names** Wellcovorin®

**Synonyms** Calcium Leucovorin; Citrovorum Factor; Folinic Acid; 5-Formyl Tetrahydrofolate

**Pharmacologic Category** Antidote; Vitamin, Water Soluble

**Use** Antidote for folic acid antagonists (methotrexate [>100 mg/m²], trimethoprim, pyrimethamine); treatment of megaloblastic anemias when folate is deficient as in infancy, sprue, pregnancy, and nutritional deficiency when oral folate therapy is not possible; in combination with fluorouracil in the treatment of malignancy

**Effects on Mental Status** None reported

**Effects on Psychiatric Treatment** None reported

**Pregnancy Risk Factor** C

**Contraindications** Pernicious anemia or vitamin $B_{12}$ deficient megaloblastic anemias; should **NOT** be administered Intrathecally/Intraventricularly

**Warnings/Precautions** Use with caution in patients with a history of hypersensitivity

**Adverse Reactions** <1%: Anaphylactoid reactions, erythema, pruritus, rash, thrombocytosis, urticaria, wheezing

**Drug Interactions** Increased toxicity of fluorouracil

**Usual Dosage** Children and Adults:

Treatment of folic acid antagonist overdosage (eg, pyrimethamine or trimethoprim): Oral: 2-15 mg/day for 3 days or until blood counts are normal or 5 mg every 3 days; doses of 6 mg/day are needed for patients with platelet counts <100,000/mm³

Folate-deficient megaloblastic anemia: I.M.: 1 mg/day

Megaloblastic anemia secondary to congenital deficiency of dihydrofolate reductase: I.M.: 3-6 mg/day

Rescue dose (rescue therapy should start within 24 hours of MTX therapy): I.V.: 10 mg/m² to start, then 10 mg/m² every 6 hours orally for 72 hours until serum MTX concentration is $<10^{-8}$ molar; if serum creatinine 24 hours after methotrexate is elevated 50% or more above the pre-MTX serum creatinine **or** the serum MTX concentration is $>5 \times 10^{-6}$ molar (see graph), increase dose to 100 mg/m²/dose (preservative-free) every 3 hours until serum methotrexate level is $<1 \times 10^{-8}$ molar

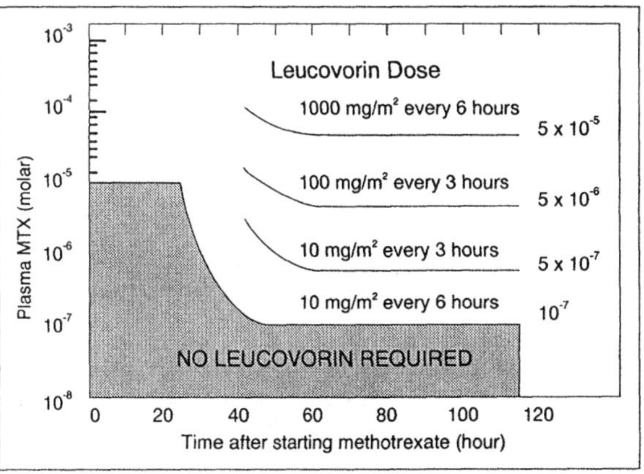

Investigational: Post I.T. methotrexate: Oral, I.V.: 12 mg/m² as a single dose; post high-dose methotrexate: 100-1000 mg/m²/dose until the serum methotrexate level is less than 1 x $10^{-7}$ molar

**The drug should be given parenterally instead of orally in patients with GI toxicity, nausea, vomiting, and when individual doses are >25 mg**

**Patient Information** Take as directed, at evenly spaced intervals around-the-clock. Maintain hydration (2-3 L of water/day while taking for rescue therapy). For folic acid deficiency, eat foods high in folic acid (eg, meat proteins, bran, dried beans, asparagus, green leafy vegetables). Report respiratory difficulty, lethargy, or rash or itching.

**Dosage Forms**

Injection, as calcium: 3 mg/mL (1 mL)
Powder for injection, as calcium: 25 mg, 50 mg, 100 mg, 350 mg
Powder for oral solution, as calcium: 1 mg/mL (60 mL)
Tablet, as calcium: 5 mg, 10 mg, 15 mg, 25 mg

♦ **Leukeran®** *see* Chlorambucil *on page 108*

♦ **Leukine™** *see* Sargramostim *on page 504*

## Leuprolide (loo PROE lide)

**U.S. Brand Names** Lupron®; Lupron Depot®; Lupron Depot-3® Month; Lupron Depot-4® Month; Lupron Depot-Ped®

**Pharmacologic Category** Antineoplastic Agent, Miscellaneous; Luteinizing Hormone-Releasing Hormone Analog

**Use** Palliative treatment of advanced prostate carcinoma (alternative when orchiectomy or estrogen administration are not indicated or are unacceptable to the patient); combination therapy with flutamide for treating metastatic prostatic carcinoma; endometriosis (3.75 mg depot only); central precocious puberty (may be used an agent to treat precocious puberty because of its effect in lowering levels of LH and FSH, testosterone, and estrogen).

**Unlabeled use:** Treatment of breast, ovarian, and endometrial cancer; leiomyoma uteri; infertility; prostatic hypertrophy

**Effects on Mental Status** Depression is common; may cause drowsiness, dizziness, or insomnia

**Effects on Psychiatric Treatment** None reported

**Usual Dosage** Requires parenteral administration

Children: Precocious puberty:
S.C.: 20-45 mcg/kg/day
I.M. (Depot®) formulation: 0.3 mg/kg/dose given every 28 days
≤25 kg: 7.5 mg
>25-37.5 kg: 11.25 mg
>37.5 kg: 15 mg

Adults:
Male: Advanced prostatic carcinoma:
Implant (Viadur®): One subcutaneous implant for 12 months; must be removed after 12 months of hormonal therapy; another implant may be inserted to continue therapy
S.C.: 1 mg/day **or**
I.M., Depot® (suspension): 7.5 mg/dose given monthly (every 28-33 days)
Female: Endometriosis: I.M., Depot® (suspension): 3.75 mg monthly for up to 6 months

**Dosage Forms**

Injection: 5 mg/mL (2.8 mL)
Powder for injection (depot):
Depot®: 3.75 mg, 7.5 mg
Depot-3® Month: 11.25 mg, 22.5 mg
Depot-4® Month: 30 mg
Depot-Ped™: 7.5 mg, 11.25 mg, 15 mg

♦ **Leustatin™** *see* Cladribine *on page 127*

## Levalbuterol (leve al BYOO ter ole)

**U.S. Brand Names** Xopenex™

**Synonyms** R-albuterol

**Pharmacologic Category** $Beta_2$ Agonist

**Use** Treatment or prevention of bronchospasm in adults and adolescents 12 years of age and older with reversible obstructive airway disease.

**Effects on Mental Status** May cause nervousness, anxiety, and dizziness; may rarely cause insomnia

**Effects on Psychiatric Treatment** Effects of anxiolytics may be ameliorated; cardiac effects may be potentiated with MAOIs and TCAs

**Pregnancy Risk Factor** C

**Contraindications** Patients with known hypersensitivity to levalbuterol or any of the formulation's components

**Warnings/Precautions** May provoke paradoxical bronchospasm (similar to other bronchodilators). Immediate hypersensitivity reactions have occurred, including angioedema, oropharyngeal edema, urticaria, rash, and anaphylaxis. Use with caution in patients with cardiovascular disease, including coronary artery disease, hypertension and a history of arrhythmias (may increase heart rate, blood pressure or other symptoms, including EKG changes). Do not use doses higher than recommended - fatalities have been associated with excessive use of other sympathomimetics. The need to use bronchodilators more frequently than usual should prompt an evaluation of the need for additional anti-inflammatory medication. Additional anti-inflammatory medication (such as corticosteroids) may be required to control asthma. Use with caution in diabetic patients and in patients with hypokalemia. Use with caution during labor and delivery. Safety and efficacy in patients <12 years of age not established.

**Adverse Reactions** Events reported include those ≥2% with incidence higher than placebo.

>10%:
Endocrine and metabolic: Increased serum glucose, decreased serum potassium
Respiratory: Viral infection (6.9% to 12.3%), rhinitis (2.7% to 11.1%)

>2% to <10%:
Central nervous system: Nervousness (2.8% to 9.6%), tremor (0 to 6.8%), anxiety (0 to 2.7%), dizziness (1.4% to 2.7%), migraine (0 to 2.7%), pain (1.4% to 2.8%)
Cardiovascular: Tachycardia (2.7% to 2.8%)
Respiratory: Cough (1.4% to 4.1%), nasal edema (1.4% to 2.8%), sinusitis (1.4% to 4.2%)
Gastrointestinal: Dyspepsia (1.4% to 2.7%)
Neuromuscular & skeletal: Leg cramps (0 to 2.7%)
Miscellaneous: Flu-like syndrome (1.4% to 4.2%), accidental injury (0 to 2.7%)

<2%: Abnormal EKG, anxiety, asthma exacerbation, chest pain, chills, diarrhea, dyspepsia, gastroenteritis, hypertension, hypesthesia (hand), hypotension, insomnia, itching eyes, lymphadenopathy, myalgia, nausea, oropharyngeal dryness, paresthesia, sweating, syncope, vomiting, wheezing

**Overdosage/Toxicology** Symptoms of overdose include tachycardia, tremor, hypertension, angina and seizures. Hypokalemia also may occur. Cardiac arrest and death may be associated with abuse of beta-agonist bronchodilators. Treatment includes immediate discontinuation and symptomatic and supportive therapies. Cautious use of beta-adrenergic blocking agents may be considered in severe cases.

**Drug Interactions**

Decreased effect: Beta-blockers (particularly nonselective agents) block the effect of levalbuterol. Digoxin levels may be decreased

Increased effect/toxicity: May add to effects of medications which deplete potassium (eg, loop or thiazide diuretics). Cardiac effects may be potentiated in patients receiving MAOIs, tricyclic antidepressants, sympathomimetics (eg, amphetamine, dobutamine), inhaled anesthetics (eg, enflurane)

**Usual Dosage**

Pediatric: Safety and efficacy in patients <12 years of age not established.

Children >12 years and Adults: Inhalation: 0.63 mg 3 times/day at intervals of 6-8 hours, via nebulization. Dosage may be increased to 1.25 mg 3 times/day with close monitoring for adverse effects. Most patients gain optimal benefit from regular use

Elderly: Only a small number of patients have been studied. Although greater sensitivity of some elderly patients cannot be ruled out, no overall differences in safety or effectiveness were observed. An initial dose of 0.63 mg should be used in all patients >65 years of age.

**Administration** Administered ONLY via nebulization. Safety and efficacy were established when administered with the following nebulizers: PARI LC Jet™, PARI LC Plus™, as well as the following compressors: PARI Master®, and Dura-Neb® 2000.

**Patient Information** If a previously effective regimen fails to provide expected relief, medical advice should be sought immediately.

**Dosage Forms** Solution, inhalation: 0.63 mg/3 mL, 1.25 mg/3 mL

## Levamisole (lee VAM i sole)

**U.S. Brand Names** Ergamisol®

**Pharmacologic Category** Immune Modulator

**Use** Adjuvant treatment with fluorouracil in Dukes stage C colon cancer

**Effects on Mental Status** May cause sedation, dizziness, depression, nervousness, or insomnia

**Effects on Psychiatric Treatment** May produce leukopenia; use caution with clozapine and carbamazepine

**Pregnancy Risk Factor** C

**Contraindications** Previous hypersensitivity to the drug

**Warnings/Precautions** Agranulocytosis can occur asymptomatically and flu-like symptoms can occur without hematologic adverse effects; frequent hematologic monitoring is necessary

**Adverse Reactions**

>10%: Gastrointestinal: Nausea, diarrhea

1% to 10%:
Cardiovascular: Edema
Central nervous system: Fatigue, fever, dizziness, headache, somnolence, depression, nervousness, insomnia
Dermatologic: Dermatitis, alopecia

Gastrointestinal: Stomatitis, vomiting, anorexia, abdominal pain, constipation, taste perversion
Hematologic: Leukopenia
Neuromuscular & skeletal: Rigors, arthralgia, myalgia, paresthesia
Miscellaneous: Infection
<1%: Abnormal tearing, altered sense of smell, anemia, anxiety, blurred vision, chest pain, conjunctivitis, dyspepsia, epistaxis, flatulence, granulocytopenia, pruritus, thrombocytopenia, urticaria

**Overdosage/Toxicology** Treatment: Following decontamination is symptomatic and supportive

**Drug Interactions**
Increased toxicity/serum levels of phenytoin
Disulfiram-like reaction with alcohol

**Usual Dosage** Adults: Oral: Initial: 50 mg every 8 hours for 3 days, then 50 mg every 8 hours for 3 days every 2 weeks (fluorouracil is always given concomitantly)

**Dosing adjustment in hepatic impairment:** May be necessary in patients with liver disease, but no specific guidelines are available

**Patient Information** Take as directed, at regular intervals around-the-clock. Avoid alcohol (may cause disulfiram-like effect). Avoid all aspirin containing medications. You may experience GI upset (small frequent meals may help); diarrhea (request medication); sensitivity to sun (use sunblock, wear protective clothing, and avoid direct sun); or dizziness, drowsiness, or impaired judgment (use caution when driving, climbing stairs, or engaging in tasks requiring alertness until response to drug is known). You will be more susceptible to infection; avoid crowds or infected persons. Report chills or fever, confusion, persistent or violent vomiting, persistent diarrhea, or respiratory difficulty.

**Dosage Forms** Tablet, as base: 50 mg

♦ **Levaquin™** *see* Levofloxacin *on page 314*

♦ **Levatol®** *see* Penbutolol *on page 423*

♦ **Levbid®** *see* Hyoscyamine *on page 279*

## Levetiracetam (lev e tir AS e tam)

**U.S. Brand Names** Keppra®

**Pharmacologic Category** Anticonvulsant, Miscellaneous

**Use** Indicated as adjunctive therapy in the treatment of partial onset seizures in adults with epilepsy

**Effects on Mental Status** Associated with somnolence and fatigue, psychosis, hallucinations, psychotic depression, and other behavioral symptoms (agitation, hostility, anxiety, apathy, emotional lability, depersonalization, and depression)

**Effects on Psychiatric Treatment** May cause leukopenia, use caution with clozapine and carbamazepine

**Pregnancy Risk Factor** C

**Contraindications** Should not be administered to patients who have previously exhibited hypersensitivity to levetiracetam or any of the inactive ingredients in the tablets

**Warnings/Precautions** Associated with the occurrence of central nervous system adverse events; somnolence and fatigue, which were treated by discontinuation, reduction, or hospitalization; coordination difficulty was treated by reduction, and only one patient was hospitalized. Behavioral abnormalities, such as psychosis, hallucinations, psychotic depression and other behavioral symptoms (agitation, hostility, anxiety, apathy, emotional lability, depersonalization, and depression) were treated by reduction of dose and in some cases hospitalization. Levetiracetam should be withdrawn gradually to minimize the potential of increased seizure frequency.

**Adverse Reactions**
>10%:
Central nervous system: Somnolence (14.8% vs 8.4% with placebo)
Neuromuscular & skeletal: Weakness (14.7% vs 9.1% with placebo)
<10%:
Central nervous system: Psychotic symptoms (0.7%), amnesia (2% vs 1% with placebo), ataxia (3% vs 1% with placebo), depression (4% vs 2% with placebo), dizziness (9% vs 4% with placebo), emotional lability (2%), nervousness (4% vs 2% with placebo), vertigo (3% vs 1% with placebo)
Hematologic: Decreased erythrocyte counts (3.2%), decreased leukocytes (2.4-3.2%)
Neuromuscular & skeletal: Ataxia and other coordination difficulties (3.4% vs 1.6% with placebo), pain (7% vs 6% with placebo)
Ophthalmic: Diplopia (2% vs 1% with placebo)

**Drug Interactions**
Anticonvulsants: No interaction was observed in pharmacokinetic trials with other anticonvulsants, including phenytoin, carbamazepine, valproic acid, phenobarbital, lamotrigine, gabapentin, and primidone
CNS depressants: Sedative effects may be additive with other CNS depressants; monitor for increased effect; includes ethanol, barbiturates, sedatives, antidepressants, narcotic analgesics, and benzodiazepines
Probenecid: The renal clearance of an inactive levetiracetam metabolite is reduced during coadministration

**Usual Dosage**
Adults: Initial: 500 mg twice daily; additional dosing increments may be given (1000 mg/day additional every 2 weeks) to a maximum recommended daily dose of 3000 mg
**Dosing adjustment in renal impairment:**
$Cl_{cr}$ >80 mL/min: 500-1500 mg every 12 hours
$Cl_{cr}$ 50-80 mL/min: 500-1000 mg every 12 hours
$Cl_{cr}$ 30-50 mL/min: 250-750 mg every 12 hours
$Cl_{cr}$ <30 mL/min: 250-500 mg every 12 hours
End-stage renal disease patients using dialysis: 500-2000 mg every 24 hours

**Patient Information** Notify your physician and/or pharmacist if you become pregnant during therapy with levetiracetam; be advised that levetiracetam may cause dizziness and somnolence and accordingly, you should not drive or operate machinery or engage in other hazardous activities until sufficient experience has been gained on levetiracetam to gauge whether it adversely affects your performance of these activities

**Dosage Forms** Tablet: 250 mg, 500 mg, 750 mg

♦ **Levlen®** *see* Ethinyl Estradiol and Levonorgestrel *on page 211*

♦ **Levlite®** *see* Ethinyl Estradiol and Levonorgestrel *on page 211*

## Levobetaxolol (lee voe be TAX oh lol)

**Related Information**
Glaucoma Drug Therapy *on page 712*

**U.S. Brand Names** Betaxon®

**Pharmacologic Category** Beta Blocker, $Beta_1$ Selective; Ophthalmic Agent, Antiglaucoma

**Use** Lowering of intraocular pressure in patients with chronic open-angle glaucoma or ocular hypertension

**Effects on Mental Status** may rarely cause anxiety, dizziness, or vertigo

**Effects on Psychiatric Treatment** Concurrent use with psychotropics may increase the risk for hypotension

**Usual Dosage** Adults: Ophthalmic: Instill 1 drop in affected eye(s) twice daily

**Dosage Forms** Solution, ophthalmic: 0.5% (5 mL, 10 mL, 15 mL)

## Levobunolol (lee voe BYOO noe lole)

**Related Information**
Glaucoma Drug Therapy *on page 712*

**U.S. Brand Names** AKBeta®; Betagan® Liquifilm®

**Pharmacologic Category** Beta Blocker, Nonselective; Ophthalmic Agent, Antiglaucoma

**Use** To lower intraocular pressure in chronic open-angle glaucoma or ocular hypertension

**Effects on Mental Status** May cause dizziness

**Effects on Psychiatric Treatment** May increase the effects of oral beta-blockers

**Usual Dosage** Adults: Instill 1 drop in the affected eye(s) 1-2 times/day

**Dosage Forms** Solution, ophthalmic, as hydrochloride: 0.25% (5 mL, 10 mL, 15 mL); 0.5% (2 mL, 5 mL, 10 mL, 15 mL)

## Levobupivacaine (LEE voe byoo PIV a kane)

**U.S. Brand Names** Chirocaine®

**Pharmacologic Category** Local Anesthetic, Injectable

**Use** Production of local or regional anesthesia for surgery and obstetrics, and for postoperative pain management

**Effects on Mental Status** May cause anxiety, dizziness or somnolence; may rarely cause confusion

**Effects on Psychiatric Treatment** Fluvoxamine and nefazodone may increase the levels of levobupivacaine; carbamazepine and barbiturates may lower levels

**Usual Dosage** Adults: **Note:** Rapid injection of a large volume of local anesthetic solution should be avoided. Fractional (incremental) doses are recommended.

**Guidelines (individual response varies):**

**Surgical anesthesia:**
**Epidural for surgery**: Concentration 0.5% to 0.75%; volume 10-20 mL; dose 50-150 mg; moderate to complete motor block
**Epidural - C-section**: Concentration 0.5%; volume 20-30 mL; dose 100-150 mg; moderate to complete motor block
**Peripheral nerve**: Concentration 0.25% to 0.5%; volume 0.4 mL/kg (30 mL); dose 1-2 mg/kg (75-150 mg); moderate to complete motor block
**Ophthalmic**: Concentration 0.75%; volume 5-15 mL; dose 37.5-112.5 mg; moderate to complete motor block
**Local infiltration**: Concentration 0.25%; volume 60 mL; dose 150 mg; motor block - not applicable

**Pain management:** Levobupivacaine can be used epidurally with fentanyl or clonidine; dilutions for epidural administration should be made with

(Continued)

## Levobupivacaine *(Continued)*

preservative free 0.9% saline according to standard hospital procedures for sterility

**Labor analgesia (epidural bolus):** Concentration 0.25%; volume 10-20 mL; dose 25-50 mg; minimal to moderate motor block

**Postoperative pain (epidural infusion):** Concentration 0.125% to 0.25%; volume 4-10 mL/hour; dose 5-25 mg/hour; minimal to moderate motor block; **Note:** 0.125% concentration is to be used only as adjunct therapy in combination with fentanyl or clonidine

**Maximum dosage:** Epidural doses up to 375 mg have been administered incrementally to patients during a surgical procedure

Intraoperative block and postoperative pain: 695 mg in 24 hours

Postoperative epidural infusion over 24 hours: 570 mg

Single-fractionated injection for brachial plexus block: 300 mg

**Dosage Forms** Injection: 2.5 mg/mL (10 mL, 30 mL); 5.0 mg/mL (10 mL, 30 mL); 7.5 mg/mL (10 mL, 30 mL)

## Levocabastine (LEE voe kab as teen)

**U.S. Brand Names** Livostin®

**Pharmacologic Category** Antihistamine; Antihistamine, $H_1$ Blocker, Ophthalmic

**Use** Treatment of allergic conjunctivitis

**Effects on Mental Status** May cause drowsiness

**Effects on Psychiatric Treatment** None reported

**Usual Dosage** Children >12 years and Adults: Instill 1 drop in affected eye(s) 4 times/day for up to 2 weeks

**Dosage Forms** Suspension, ophthalmic, as hydrochloride: 0.05% (2.5 mL, 5 mL, 10 mL)

## Levocarnitine (lee voe KAR ni teen)

**U.S. Brand Names** Carnitor® Injection; Carnitor® Oral; VitaCarn® Oral

**Synonyms** L-Carnitine

**Pharmacologic Category** Dietary Supplement

**Use**

Oral: Primary systemic carnitine deficiency; acute and chronic treatment of patients with an inborn error of metabolism which results in secondary carnitine deficiency

I.V. Acute and chronic treatment of patients with an inborn error of metabolism which results in secondary carnitine deficiency; prevention and treatment of carnitine deficiency in patients with end stage renal disease who are undergoing hemodialysis.

**Effects on Mental Status** None reported

**Effects on Psychiatric Treatment** None reported

**Warnings/Precautions** Caution in patients with seizure disorders or in those at risk of seizures (CNS mass or medications which may lower seizure threshold). Both new-onset seizure activity as well as an increased frequency of seizures has been observed.

**Adverse Reactions** 1% to 10%:

Gastrointestinal: Nausea, vomiting, abdominal cramps, diarrhea

Neuromuscular & skeletal: Myasthenia

Miscellaneous: Body odor

**Drug Interactions** Valproic acid, sodium benzoate

**Usual Dosage**

Oral:

Infants/Children: Initial: 50 mg/kg/day; titrate to 50-100 mg/kg/day in divided doses with a maximum dose of 3 g/day

Adults: 990 mg (oral tablets) 2-3 times/day or 1-3 g/day (oral solution)

I.V.:

Metabolic disorders: 50 mg/kg as a slow 2- to 3-minute I.V. bolus or by I.V. infusion

Severe metabolic crisis:

A loading dose of 50 mg/kg followed by an equivalent dose over the following 24 hours administered as every 3 hours or every 4 hours (never less than every 6 hours either by infusion or by intravenous injection)

All subsequent daily doses are recommended to be in the range of 50 mg/kg or as therapy may require

The highest dose administered has been 300 mg/kg

It is recommended that a plasma carnitine concentration be obtained prior to beginning parenteral therapy accompanied by weekly and monthly monitoring

ESRD patients on hemodialysis:

Predialysis levocarnitine concentrations below normal (40-50 μmol/L): 10-20 mg/kg dry body weight as a slow 2- to 3-minute bolus after each dialysis session

Dosage adjustments should be guided by predialysis trough levocarnitine concentrations and downward dose adjustments (to 5 mg/kg after dialysis) may be made as early as every 3rd or 4th week of therapy

**Patient Information** The oral solution should be consumed slowly and spaced evenly throughout the day to improve tolerance

**Dosage Forms**

Capsule: 250 mg

Injection: 1 g/5 mL (5 mL)

Liquid (cherry flavor): 100 mg/mL (10 mL)

Tablet: 330 mg

## Levodopa (lee voe DOE pa)

**Related Information**

Discontinuation of Psychotropic Drugs - Withdrawal Symptoms and Recommendations *on page 798*

**Generic Available** No

**U.S. Brand Names** Dopar®; Larodopa®

**Synonyms** *L*-3-Hydroxytyrosine; *L*-Dopa

**Pharmacologic Category** Anti-Parkinson's Agent (Dopamine Agonist)

**Use** Treatment of Parkinson's disease

**Unlabeled use:** Diagnostic agent for growth hormone deficiency

**Pregnancy Risk Factor** C

**Contraindications** Hypersensitivity to levodopa or any component; narrow-angle glaucoma; use of MAO inhibitors within prior 14 days (however, may be administered concomitantly with the manufacturer's recommended dose of an MAO inhibitor with selectivity for MAO type B); history of melanoma or any undiagnosed skin lesions

**Warnings/Precautions** Use with caution in patients with history of cardiovascular disease (including myocardial infarction and arrhythmias); pulmonary diseases such as asthma, psychosis, wide-angle glaucoma, peptic ulcer disease; as well as in renal, hepatic, or endocrine disease. Sudden discontinuation of levodopa may cause a worsening of Parkinson's disease. Elderly may be more sensitive to CNS effects of levodopa. May cause or exacerbate dyskinesias. May cause orthostatic hypotension; Parkinson's disease patients appear to have an impaired capacity to respond to a postural challenge. Use with caution in patients at risk of hypotension (such as those receiving antihypertensive drugs) or where transient hypotensive episodes would be poorly tolerated (cardiovascular disease or cerebrovascular disease). Observe patients closely for development of depression with concomitant suicidal tendencies. Safety and effectiveness in pediatric patients have not been established. Some products may contain tartrazine. Dopaminergic agents have been associated with a syndrome resembling neuroleptic malignant syndrome on withdrawal or significant dosage reduction after long-term use. Pyridoxine may reverse effects of levodopa. Toxic reactions have occurred with dextromethorphan.

**Adverse Reactions**

Cardiovascular: Orthostatic hypotension, arrhythmias, chest pain, hypertension, syncope, palpitations, phlebitis

Central nervous system: Dizziness, anxiety, confusion, nightmares, headache, hallucinations, on-off phenomenon, decreased mental acuity, memory impairment, disorientation, delusions, euphoria, agitation, somnolence, insomnia, gait abnormalities, nervousness, ataxia, EPS, falling

Gastrointestinal: Anorexia, nausea, vomiting, constipation, GI bleeding, duodenal ulcer, diarrhea, dyspepsia, taste alterations, sialorrhea, heartburn

Genitourinary: Discoloration of urine, urinary frequency

Hematologic: Hemolytic anemia, agranulocytosis, thrombocytopenia, leukopenia, decreased hemoglobin and hematocrit, abnormalities in AST and ALT, LDH, bilirubin, BUN, Coombs' test

Neuromuscular & skeletal: Choreiform and involuntary movements, paresthesia, bone pain, shoulder pain, muscle cramps, weakness

Ocular: Blepharospasm

Renal: Difficult urination

Respiratory: Dyspnea, cough

Miscellaneous: Hiccups, discoloration of sweat

**Overdosage/Toxicology**

Signs and symptoms: Palpitations, arrhythmias, spasms, hypertension or hypotension

Treatment: Use fluids judiciously to maintain pressures; may precipitate a variety of arrhythmias

**Drug Interactions**

Antacids: Levodopa absorption may be increased; monitor

Anticholinergics: May reduce the efficacy of levodopa, possibly due to reduced gastrointestinal absorption (also see tricyclic antidepressants); limited evidence of clinical significance; monitor

Antipsychotics: May inhibit the antiparkinsonian effects of levodopa via dopamine receptor blockade; use antipsychotics with low dopamine blockade (clozapine, olanzapine, quetiapine)

Benzodiazepines: May inhibit the antiparkinsonian effects of levodopa; monitor for reduced effect

Clonidine: May reduce the efficacy of levodopa; monitor

Furazolidine: May increase the effect/toxicity of levodopa; hypertensive episodes have been reported; monitor

Iron salts: Binds levodopa and reduces its bioavailability; separate doses of iron and levodopa

Linezolid: Due to MAO inhibition (see below), this agent is best avoided

MAO inhibitors: Concurrent use of levodopa with nonselective MAOIs may result in hypertensive reactions via an increased storage and release of dopamine, norepinephrine, or both; use with carbidopa to minimize reactions if combination is necessary; otherwise avoid combination

L-methionine: May inhibit levodopa's antiparkinsonian effects; monitor for reduced effect

Metoclopramide: May increase the absorption/effect of levodopa; hypertensive episodes have been reported. Levodopa antagonizes metoclopramide's effects on lower esophageal sphincter pressure; avoid use of metoclopramide for reflux, monitor response to levodopa carefully if used.

Methyldopa: May potentiate the effects of levodopa; levodopa may increase the hypotensive response to methyldopa; monitor

Papaverine: May decrease the efficacy of levodopa; includes other similar agents (ethaverine); monitor

Penicillamine: May increase serum concentrations of levodopa; monitor for increased effect

Phenytoin: May inhibit levodopa's antiparkinsonian effects; monitor for reduced effect

Pyridoxine: May inhibit levodopa's antiparkinsonian effects; monitor for reduced effect

Spiramycin: May inhibit levodopa's antiparkinsonian effects; monitor for reduced effect

Tacrine: May inhibit the effects of levodopa via enhanced cholinergic activity; monitor for reduced effect

Tricyclic antidepressants: May decrease the absorption (bioavailability) of levodopa; rare hypertensive episodes have also been attributed to this combination

**Mechanism of Action** Increases dopamine levels in the brain, then stimulates dopaminergic receptors in the basal ganglia to improve the balance between cholinergic and dopaminergic activity

**Pharmacodynamics/kinetics**

Time to peak serum concentration: Oral: 1-2 hours

Metabolism: Majority of drug is peripherally decarboxylated to dopamine; small amounts of levodopa reach the brain where it is also decarboxylated to active dopamine

Half-life: 1.2-2.3 hours

Elimination: Primarily in urine (80%) as dopamine, norepinephrine, and homovanillic acid

**Usual Dosage** Oral:

Children (administer as a single dose to evaluate growth hormone deficiency):

0.5 g/m$^2$ **or**

<30 lb: 125 mg

30-70 lb: 250 mg

>70 lb: 500 mg

Adults: 500-1000 mg/day in divided doses every 6-12 hours; increase by 100-750 mg/day every 3-7 days until response or total dose of 8000 mg is reached

A significant therapeutic response may not be obtained for 6 months

**Administration** Administer with meals to decrease GI upset

**Monitoring Parameters** Serum growth hormone concentration

**Reference Range** Peak serum level of 3.2 mg/L occurs after ingestion of 200 mg levodopa

**Test Interactions** False-positive reaction for urinary glucose with Clinitest®; false-negative reaction using Clinistix®; false-positive urine ketones with Acetest®, Ketostix®, Labstix®

**Patient Information** Avoid vitamins with $B_6$ (pyridoxine); can take with food to prevent GI upset; do not stop taking this drug even if you do not think it is working; dizziness, lightheadedness, fainting may occur when you get up from a sitting or lying position.

**Nursing Implications** Give with meals to decrease GI upset; sustained-release product should not be crushed

**Additional Information** Single dose is not usually associated with the above adverse reactions

**Dosage Forms**

Capsule: 100 mg, 250 mg, 500 mg

Tablet: 100 mg, 250 mg, 500 mg

## Levodopa and Carbidopa (lee voe DOE pa & kar bi DOE pa)

**Generic Available** Yes

**U.S. Brand Names** Sinemet®; Sinemet® CR

**Synonyms** Carbidopa and Levodopa

**Pharmacologic Category** Anti-Parkinson's Agent (Dopamine Agonist)

**Use** Idiopathic Parkinson's disease; postencephalitic parkinsonism; symptomatic parkinsonism

**Pregnancy Risk Factor** C

**Contraindications** Known hypersensitivity to levodopa, carbidopa, or any component; narrow-angle glaucoma; use of MAO inhibitors within prior 14 days (however may be administered concomitantly with the manufacturer's recommended dose of an MAO inhibitor with selectivity for MAO type B); history of melanoma or undiagnosed skin lesions

**Warnings/Precautions** Use with caution in patients with history of cardiovascular disease (including myocardial infarction and arrhythmias); pulmonary diseases such as asthma, psychosis, wide-angle glaucoma, peptic ulcer disease; as well as in renal, hepatic, or endocrine disease. Sudden discontinuation of levodopa may cause a worsening of Parkinson's disease. Elderly may be more sensitive to CNS effects of levodopa. May cause or exacerbate dyskinesias. May cause orthostatic hypotension; Parkinson's disease patients appear to have an impaired capacity to respond to a postural challenge; use with caution in patients at risk of hypotension (such as those receiving antihypertensive drugs) or where transient hypotensive episodes would be poorly tolerated (cardiovascular disease or cerebrovascular disease). Observe patients closely for development of depression with concomitant suicidal tendencies. Some products may contain tartrazine. Has been associated with a syndrome resembling neuroleptic malignant syndrome on withdrawal or significant dosage reduction after long-term use. Toxic reactions have occurred with dextromethorphan. Protein in the diet should be distributed throughout the day to avoid fluctuations in levodopa absorption.

**Adverse Reactions**

Cardiovascular: Orthostatic hypotension, arrhythmias, chest pain, hypertension, syncope, palpitations, phlebitis

Central nervous system: Dizziness, anxiety, confusion, nightmares, headache, hallucinations, on-off phenomenon, decreased mental acuity, memory impairment, disorientation, delusions, euphoria, agitation, somnolence, insomnia, gait abnormalities, nervousness, ataxia, EPS, falling

Gastrointestinal: Anorexia, nausea, vomiting, constipation, GI bleeding, duodenal ulcer, diarrhea, dyspepsia, taste alterations, sialorrhea, heartburn

Genitourinary: Discoloration of urine, urinary frequency

Hematologic: Hemolytic anemia, agranulocytosis, thrombocytopenia, leukopenia, decreased hemoglobin and hematocrit, abnormalities in AST and ALT, LDH, bilirubin, BUN, Coombs' test

Neuromuscular & skeletal: Choreiform and involuntary movements, paresthesia, bone pain, shoulder pain, muscle cramps, weakness

Ocular: Blepharospasm

Renal: Difficult urination

Respiratory: Dyspnea, cough

Miscellaneous: Hiccups, discoloration of sweat

**Overdosage/Toxicology**

Signs and symptoms: Palpitations, arrhythmias, spasms, hypotension; may cause hypertension or hypotension

Treatment: Use fluids judiciously to maintain pressures; may precipitate a variety of arrhythmias

**Drug Interactions**

Antacids: Levodopa absorption may be increased; monitor

Anticholinergics: May reduce the efficacy of levodopa, possibly due to reduced gastrointestinal absorption (also see tricyclic antidepressants); limited evidence of clinical significance; monitor

Antipsychotics: May inhibit the antiparkinsonian effects of levodopa via dopamine receptor blockade; use antipsychotics with low dopamine blockade (clozapine, olanzapine, quetiapine)

Benzodiazepines: May inhibit the antiparkinsonian effects of levodopa; monitor for reduced effect

Clonidine: May reduce the efficacy of levodopa; monitor

Furazolidine: May increase the effect/toxicity of levodopa; hypertensive episodes have been reported; monitor

Iron salts: Binds levodopa and reduces its bioavailability; separate doses of iron and levodopa

Linezolid: Due to MAO inhibition (see below), this agent is best avoided

MAO inhibitors: Concurrent use of levodopa with nonselective MAOIs may result in hypertensive reactions via an increased storage and release of dopamine, norepinephrine, or both; use with carbidopa to minimize reactions if combination is necessary, otherwise avoid combination.

L-methionine: May inhibit levodopa's antiparkinsonian effects; monitor for reduced effect

Metoclopramide: May increase the absorption/effect of levodopa; hypertensive episodes have been reported. Levodopa antagonizes metoclopramide's effects on lower esophageal sphincter pressure. Avoid use of metoclopramide for reflux, monitor response to levodopa carefully if used.

Methyldopa: May potentiate the effects of levodopa; levodopa may increase the hypotensive response to methyldopa; monitor

Papaverine: May decrease the efficacy of levodopa; includes other similar agents (ethaverine); monitor

Penicillamine: May increase serum concentrations of levodopa; monitor for increased effect

Phenytoin: May inhibit levodopa's antiparkinsonian effects; monitor for reduced effect

Pyridoxine: May inhibit levodopa's antiparkinsonian effects; monitor for reduced effect

Spiramycin: May inhibit levodopa's antiparkinsonian effects; monitor for reduced effect

Tacrine: May inhibit the effects of levodopa via enhanced cholinergic activity; monitor for reduced effect

Tricyclic antidepressants: May decrease the absorption (bioavailability) of levodopa; rare hypertensive episodes have also been attributed to this combination

(Continued)

## Levodopa and Carbidopa *(Continued)*

**Mechanism of Action** Parkinson's symptoms are due to a lack of striatal dopamine; levodopa circulates in the plasma to the blood-brain-barrier (BBB), where it crosses, to be converted by striatal enzymes to dopamine; carbidopa inhibits the peripheral plasma breakdown of levodopa by inhibiting its decarboxylation, and thereby increases available levodopa at the BBB

**Pharmacodynamics/kinetics**

**Carbidopa:**

Absorption: Oral: 40% to 70%
Protein binding: 36%
Half-life: 1-2 hours
Elimination: Excreted unchanged

**Levodopa:**

Absorption: May be decreased if given with a high protein meal
Half-life: 1.2-2.3 hours
Elimination: Primarily in urine (80%) as dopamine, norepinephrine, and homovanillic acid

**Usual Dosage** Oral:

Adults: Initial: 25/100 2-4 times/day, increase as necessary to a maximum of 200/2000 mg/day
Elderly: Initial: 25/100 twice daily, increase as necessary

**Conversion from Sinemet® to Sinemet® CR (50/200):** (Sinemet® [total daily dose of levodopa] / Sinemet® CR)

300-400 mg / 1 tablet twice daily
500-600 mg / 1½ tablets twice daily or one 3 times/day
700-800 mg / 4 tablets in 3 or more divided doses
900-1000 mg / 5 tablets in 3 or more divided doses

Intervals between doses of Sinemet® CR should be 4-8 hours while awake

**Administration** Administer with meals to decrease GI upset

**Monitoring Parameters** Blood pressure, standing and sitting/supine; symptoms of parkinsonism, dyskinesias, mental status

**Test Interactions** False-positive reaction for urinary glucose with Clinitest®; false-negative reaction using Clinistix®; false-positive urine ketones with Acetest®, Ketostix®, Labstix®

**Patient Information** Avoid vitamins with $B_6$ (pyridoxine); do not stop taking this drug even if you do not think it is working; take on an empty stomach if possible; if GI distress occurs, take with meals; sustained release product should not be crushed; rise carefully from lying or sitting position as dizziness, lightheadedness, or fainting may occur

**Nursing Implications** Space doses evenly over the waking hours; give with meals to decrease GI upset; sustained release product should not be crushed

**Additional Information** 50-100 mg/day of carbidopa is needed to block the peripheral conversion of levodopa to dopamine. "On-off" (a clinical syndrome characterized by sudden periods of drug activity/inactivity), can be managed by giving smaller, more frequent doses of Sinemet® or adding a dopamine agonist or selegiline; when adding a new agent, doses of Sinemet® can usually be decreased. Protein in the diet should be distributed throughout the day to avoid fluctuations in levodopa absorption. Levodopa is the drug of choice when rigidity is the predominant presenting symptom.

**Dosage Forms** Tablet:

10/100: Carbidopa 10 mg and levodopa 100 mg
25/100: Carbidopa 25 mg and levodopa 100 mg
25/250: Carbidopa 25 mg and levodopa 250 mg
Sustained release: Carbidopa 25 mg and levodopa 100 mg; carbidopa 50 mg and levodopa 200 mg

♦ **Levo-Dromoran®** *see* Levorphanol *on page 315*

## Levofloxacin (lee voe FLOKS a sin)

**U.S. Brand Names** Levaquin™

**Pharmacologic Category** Antibiotic, Quinolone

**Use** Acute maxillary sinusitis due to *S. pneumoniae*, *H. influenzae*, or *M. catarrhalis*; uncomplicated urinary tract infection due to *E. coli*, *K. pneumoniae*, or *S. saprophyticus*; also for acute bacterial exacerbation of chronic bronchitis and community-acquired pneumonia due to *S. aureus*, *S. pneumoniae* (including penicillin-resistant strains), *H. influenzae*, *H. parainfluenzae*, or *M. catarrhalis*, *C. pneumoniae*, *L. pneumophila*, or *M. pneumoniae*; may be used for uncomplicated skin and skin structure infection (due to *S. aureus* or *S. pyogenes*) and complicated urinary tract infection due to gram-negative *Enterobacter* sp, including acute pyelonephritis (caused by *E. coli*)

**Effects on Mental Status** May cause dizziness or insomnia; quinolones reported to cause restlessness, hallucinations, euphoria, depression, panic, and paranoia

**Effects on Psychiatric Treatment** May cause leukopenia; use caution with clozapine and carbamazepine; inhibits CYP1A2 isoenzyme; caution with clozapine and other psychotropics; monitor for adverse effects

**Pregnancy Risk Factor** C

**Contraindications** Hypersensitivity to levofloxacin, any component, or other quinolones; pregnancy, lactation

**Warnings/Precautions** Not recommended in children <18 years of age; other quinolones have caused transient arthropathy in children; CNS stimulation may occur (tremor, restlessness, confusion, and very rarely hallucinations or seizures); use with caution in patients with known or suspected CNS disorders or renal dysfunction; prolonged use may result in superinfection; if an allergic reaction (itching, urticaria, dyspnea, pharyngeal or facial edema, loss of consciousness, tingling, cardiovascular collapse) occurs, discontinue the drug immediately; use caution to avoid possible photosensitivity reactions during and for several days following fluoroquinolone therapy; pseudomembranous colitis may occur and should be considered in patients who present with diarrhea

Quinolones have been associated with tendonitis and tendon rupture (discontinue at first signs or symptoms of tendon pain)

Rare cases of torsade de pointes have been reported in patients receiving levofloxacin. Use caution in patients with bradycardia, hypokalemia, hypomagnesemia, or in those receiving concurrent therapy with Class Ia or Class III antiarrhythmics.

**Adverse Reactions**

>1%:

Central nervous system: Dizziness, headache, insomnia
Dermatologic: Rash
Gastrointestinal: Nausea, vomiting, increased transaminases
Hematologic: Leukopenia, thrombocytopenia
Neuromuscular & skeletal: Tremor, arthralgia

<1%: Quinolones have been associated with tendonitis and tendon rupture

**Overdosage/Toxicology**

Signs and symptoms: Acute renal failure, seizures
Treatment: Should include GI decontamination and supportive care; not removed by peritoneal or hemodialysis

**Drug Interactions** CYP1A2 enzyme inhibitor (minor) CYP1A2 enzyme inhibitor (minor)

Antineoplastic agents may decrease the absorption of quinolones
Cimetidine, and other $H_2$-antagonists may inhibit renal elimination of quinolones
Foscarnet has been associated with an increased risk of seizures with some quinolones
Loop diuretics: Serum levels of some quinolones are increased by loop diuretic administration; may diminish renal excretion
Metal cations (magnesium, aluminum, iron, and zinc) bind quinolones in the gastrointestinal tract and inhibit absorption (by up to 98%). Antacids, electrolyte supplements, sucralfate, quinapril, and some didanosine formulations should be avoided. Levofloxacin should be administered 4 hours before or 8 hours after these agents.
NSAIDs: The CNS stimulating effect of some quinolones may be enhanced, resulting in neuroexcitation and/or seizures
Probenecid: Blocks renal secretion of quinolones, increasing concentrations
Warfarin: The hypoprothrombinemic effect of warfarin is enhanced by some quinolone antibiotics. Levofloxacin does not alter warfarin kinetics, but may alter the gastrointestinal flora; monitor INR closely during therapy.

**Usual Dosage** Adults: Oral, I.V. (infuse I.V. solution over 60 minutes):

Acute bacterial exacerbation of chronic bronchitis: 500 mg every 24 hours for at least 7 days
Community acquired pneumonia: 500 mg every 24 hours for 7-14 days
Acute maxillary sinusitis: 500 mg every 24 hours for 10-14 days
Uncomplicated skin infections: 500 mg every 24 hours for 7-10 days
Uncomplicated urinary tract infections: 250 mg once daily for 3 days
Complicated urinary tract infections include acute pyelonephritis: 250 mg every 24 hours for 10 days

**Dosing adjustment in renal impairment:**

$Cl_{cr}$ 20-49 mL/minute: Administer 250 mg every 24 hours (initial: 500 mg)
$Cl_{cr}$ 10-19 mL/minute: Administer 250 mg every 48 hours (initial: 500 mg for most infections; 250 mg for renal infections)

Hemodialysis/CAPD: 250 mg every 48 hours (initial: 500 mg)

**Patient Information** Oral: Take per recommended schedule, preferably on an empty stomach (1 hour before or 2 hours after meals). Maintain adequate hydration (2-3 L/day of fluids unless instructed to restrict fluid intake). Take complete prescription; do not skip doses. Do not take with antacids; separate by 2 hours. You may experience dizziness, lightheadedness, or confusion; use caution when driving or engaging in tasks that require alertness until response to drug is known. Small frequent meals and frequent mouth care may reduce nausea or vomiting. You may experience photosensitivity; use sunscreen, wear protective clothing and eyewear, and avoid direct sunlight. Report palpitations or chest pain, persistent diarrhea, GI disturbances or abdominal pain, muscle tremor or pain, yellowing of eyes or skin, easy bruising or bleeding, unusual fatigue, fever, chills, signs of infection, or worsening of condition. Report immediately any rash; itching; unusual CNS changes; pain, inflammation, or rupture of tendon; or any facial swelling.

**Nursing Implications** Infuse I.V. solutions over 60 minutes

**Dosage Forms**

Infusion, in $D_5W$: 5 mg/mL (50 mL, 100 mL)
Injection: 25 mg/mL (20 mL)
Tablet: 250 mg, 500 mg

- **Levomepromazine** *see* Methotrimeprazine *on page 354*

## Levomethadyl Acetate Hydrochloride
(lee voe METH a dil AS e tate hye droe KLOR ide)

**Related Information**
Addiction Treatments *on page 772*
**Generic Available** No
**U.S. Brand Names** ORLAAM®
**Pharmacologic Category** Analgesic, Narcotic
**Use** Management of opiate dependence
**Restrictions** C-II; must be dispensed in a designated clinic setting only
**Pregnancy Risk Factor** C
**Warnings/Precautions** Not recommended for use outside of the treatment of opiate addiction; shall be dispensed only by treatment programs approved by FDA, DEA, and the designated state authority. Approved treatment programs shall dispense and use levomethadyl in oral form only and according to the treatment requirements stipulated in federal regulations. Failure to abide by these requirements may result in injunction precluding operation of the program, seizure of the drug supply, revocation of the program approval, and possible criminal prosecution.
**Adverse Reactions**
>10%:
Central nervous system: Malaise
Miscellaneous: Flu syndrome
1% to 10%:
Central nervous system: CNS depression, sedation, chills, abnormal dreams, anxiety, euphoria, headache, insomnia, nervousness, hypesthesia
Endocrine & metabolic: Hot flashes (males 2:1)
Gastrointestinal: Abdominal pain, constipation, diarrhea, xerostomia, nausea, vomiting
Genitourinary: Urinary tract spasm, difficult ejaculation, impotence, decreased sex drive
Neuromuscular & skeletal: Arthralgia, back pain, weakness
Ocular: Miosis, blurred vision
<1%: Myalgia, postural hypotension, tearing
**Drug Interactions**
CNS depressants: Sedative, tranquilizers, propoxyphene, antidepressants, benzodiazepines, alcohol used in combination with levomethadyl may result in serious overdose
Enzyme inducers: Carbamazepine, phenobarbital, rifampin, phenytoin may enhance the metabolism of levomethadyl leading to an increase in levomethadyl peak effect and shorten its duration of action
Enzyme inhibitors: Erythromycin, cimetidine, and ketoconazole may slow the onset, lower the activity, and/or increase the duration of action of levomethadyl
Meperidine: May be ineffective in patients taking levomethadyl
Opiate antagonists and partial antagonists: Levomethadyl used in combination with naloxone, naltrexone, pentazocine, nalbuphine, butorphanol, and buprenorphine may result in withdrawal symptoms
**Stability** Store at room temperature
**Mechanism of Action** A synthetic opioid agonist with actions similar to morphine; principal actions are analgesia and sedation. Its clinical effects in the treatment of opiate abuse occur through two mechanisms: 1) cross sensitivity for opiates of the morphine type, suppressing symptoms of withdrawal in opiate-dependent persons; 2) with chronic oral administration, can produce sufficient tolerance to block the subjective high of usual doses of parenterally administered opiates
**Pharmacodynamics/kinetics**
Protein binding: 80%
Metabolism: Hepatic to L-alpha-noracetylmethadol and L-alpha-dinoracetylmethadol (active metabolites)
Half-life: 35-60 hours
Time to peak serum concentration: 1.5-6 hours
Elimination: Renal products as methadol and normethadol
**Usual Dosage** Adults: Oral: 20-40 mg 3 times/week, with ranges of 10 mg to as high as 140 mg 3 times/week; always dilute before administration and mix with diluent prior to dispensing
**Monitoring Parameters** Patient adherence with regimen and avoidance of illicit substances; random drug testing is recommended
**Reference Range** A 60 mg dose can result in a peak serum level of 130 ng/mL; at 24 hours, it is 50 ng/mL
**Test Interactions** Can cause positive opiate urine screen
**Nursing Implications** Drug administration and dispensing is to take place in an authorized clinic setting only; can potentially cause Q-T prolongation on EKG (not dose related)
**Dosage Forms** Solution, oral: 10 mg/mL (474 mL)

## Levonorgestrel (LEE voe nor jes trel)

**U.S. Brand Names** Norplant® Implant; Plan B™
**Synonyms** D-Norgestrel
**Pharmacologic Category** Contraceptive
**Use** Prevention of pregnancy. The net cumulative 5-year pregnancy rate for levonorgestrel implant use has been reported to be from 1.5-3.9 pregnancies/100 users. Norplant® is a very efficient, yet reversible, method of contraception. The long duration of action may be particularly advantageous in women who desire an extended period of contraceptive protection without sacrificing the possibility of future fertility.
**Effects on Mental Status** May cause nervousness or dizziness
**Effects on Psychiatric Treatment** Carbamazepine may decrease the effects of levonorgestrel
**Pregnancy Risk Factor** X
**Contraindications** Women with undiagnosed abnormal uterine bleeding, hemorrhagic diathesis, known or suspected pregnancy, active hepatic disease, active thrombophlebitis, thromboembolic disorders, or known or suspected carcinoma of the breast
**Warnings/Precautions** Patients presenting with lower abdominal pain should be evaluated for follicular atresia and ectopic pregnancy
**Adverse Reactions**
>10%: Hormonal: Prolonged menstrual flow, spotting
1% to 10%:
Central nervous system: Headache, nervousness, dizziness
Dermatologic: Dermatitis, acne
Endocrine & metabolic: Amenorrhea, irregular menstrual cycles, scanty bleeding, breast discharge
Gastrointestinal: Nausea, change in appetite, weight gain
Genitourinary: Vaginitis, leukorrhea
Local: Pain or itching at implant site
Neuromuscular & skeletal: Myalgia
<1%: Infection at implant site
**Overdosage/Toxicology** Can result if >6 capsules are *in situ*
Signs and symptoms: Include uterine bleeding irregularities and fluid retention
Treatment: Includes removal of all implanted capsules
**Drug Interactions** Decreased effect: Carbamazepine/phenytoin
**Usual Dosage** Total administration doses (implanted): 216 mg in 6 capsules which should be implanted during the first 7 days of onset of menses subdermally in the upper arm; each Norplant® silastic capsule releases 80 mcg of drug/day for 6-18 months, following which a rate of release of 25-30 mcg/day is maintained for ≤5 years; capsules should be removed by end of 5th year
Emergency contraception: One 0.75 mg tablet as soon as possible within 72 hours of unprotected sex; a second 0.75 mg tablet should be taken 12 hours after the first dose
**Patient Information** Do not attempt to remove implants - see prescriber. You may experience photosensitivity (use sunscreen, wear protective clothing and eyewear, and avoid direct sunlight); dizziness or sleeplessness (use caution when driving or engaging in hazardous tasks until response to drug is known); skin rash, change in skin color, loss of hair, or unusual menses (breakthrough bleeding, irregularity, excessive bleeding - these should resolve after the first month). Report swelling, pain, or excessive feelings of warmth in calves, sudden acute headache, or visual disturbance, unusual nausea or vomiting, and any loss of feeling in arms or legs, unusual menses (if they persist past first month), and irritation at insertion site.
**Dosage Forms** Capsule, subdermal implantation: 36 mg (6s)

- **Levophed® Injection** *see* Norepinephrine *on page 398*
- **Levoprome®** *see* Methotrimeprazine *on page 354*
- **Levora®** *see* Ethinyl Estradiol and Levonorgestrel *on page 211*

## Levorphanol (lee VOR fa nole)

**Related Information**
Narcotic Agonists Comparison Chart *on page 720*
**U.S. Brand Names** Levo-Dromoran®
**Synonyms** Levorphan Tartrate
**Pharmacologic Category** Analgesic, Narcotic
**Use** Relief of moderate to severe pain; also used parenterally for preoperative sedation and an adjunct to nitrous oxide/oxygen anesthesia; 2 mg levorphanol produces analgesia comparable to that produced by 10 mg of morphine
**Effects on Mental Status** Drowsiness and dizziness are common; may cause nervousness, restlessness, or confusion; may rarely cause depression, hallucinations, or paradoxical CNS stimulation
**Effects on Psychiatric Treatment** Concurrent use with psychotropics may produce additive sedation
**Restrictions** C-II
**Pregnancy Risk Factor** B (D if used for prolonged periods or in high doses at term)
**Contraindications** Hypersensitivity to levorphanol or any component
**Warnings/Precautions** Use with caution in patients with hypersensitivity reactions to other phenanthrene derivative opioid agonists (morphine, hydrocodone, hydromorphone, levorphanol, oxycodone, oxymorphone); respiratory diseases including asthma, emphysema, COPD or severe liver or renal insufficiency; some preparations contain sulfites which may cause

(Continued)

## Levorphanol *(Continued)*

allergic reactions; tolerance or dependence may result from extended use; dextromethorphan has equivalent antitussive activity but has much lower toxicity in accidental overdose. Elderly may be particularly susceptible to the CNS depressant and constipating effects of narcotics.

**Adverse Reactions**

>10%:

Cardiovascular: Palpitations, hypotension, bradycardia, peripheral vasodilation

Central nervous system: CNS depression, fatigue, drowsiness, dizziness

Dermatologic: Pruritus

Gastrointestinal: Nausea, vomiting

Neuromuscular & skeletal: Weakness

1% to 10%:

Central nervous system: Nervousness, headache, restlessness, anorexia, malaise, confusion

Gastrointestinal: Stomach cramps, xerostomia, constipation

Endocrine & metabolic: Antidiuretic hormone release

Gastrointestinal: Biliary tract spasm

Genitourinary: Decreased urination, urinary tract spasm

Local: Pain at injection site

Ocular: Miosis

Respiratory: Respiratory depression

<1%: Hallucinations, histamine release, increased intracranial pressure, mental depression, paradoxical CNS stimulation, paralytic ileus, physical and psychological dependence rash, urticaria

**Overdosage/Toxicology**

Signs and symptoms: CNS depression, respiratory depression, miosis, apnea, pulmonary edema, convulsions

Treatment: Naloxone 2 mg I.V. (0.01 mg/kg for children) with repeat administration as necessary up to a total of 10 mg

**Drug Interactions** Increased toxicity: CNS depressants increase CNS depression

**Usual Dosage** Adults:

Oral: 2 mg every 6-24 hours as needed

S.C.: 2 mg, up to 3 mg if necessary, every 6-8 hours

**Dosing adjustment in hepatic disease:** Reduction is necessary in patients with liver disease

**Dietary Considerations**

Alcohol: Additive CNS effects, avoid or limit alcohol; watch for sedation

Food: Glucose may cause hyperglycemia; monitor blood glucose concentrations

**Patient Information** If self-administered, use exactly as directed (do not increase dose or frequency); may cause physical and/or psychological dependence. While using this medication, do not use alcohol and other prescription or OTC medications (especially sedatives, tranquilizers, antihistamines, or pain medications) without consulting prescriber. Maintain adequate hydration (2-3 L/day of fluids unless instructed to restrict fluid intake). May cause hypotension, dizziness, drowsiness, impaired coordination, or blurred vision (use caution when driving, climbing stairs, or changing position - rising from sitting or lying to standing, or when engaging in tasks requiring alertness until response to drug is known); loss of appetite, nausea, or vomiting (frequent mouth care, small frequent meals, chewing gum, or sucking lozenges may help); constipation (increased exercise, fluids, or dietary fruit and fiber may help - if constipation remains an unresolved problem, consult prescriber about use of stool softeners). Report chest pain, slow or rapid heartbeat, acute dizziness, or persistent headache; swelling of extremities or unusual weight gain; changes in urinary elimination; acute headache; back or flank pain or spasms; blurred vision; skin rash; or shortness of breath.

**Nursing Implications** Observe patient for excessive sedation, respiratory depression; implement safety measures, assist with ambulation

**Dosage Forms**

Injection, as tartrate: 2 mg/mL (1 mL, 10 mL)

Tablet, as tartrate: 2 mg

♦ **Levorphan Tartrate** *see* Levorphanol *on page 315*

♦ **Levo-T™** *see* Levothyroxine *on page 316*

♦ **Levothroid®** *see* Levothyroxine *on page 316*

## Levothyroxine (lee voe thye ROKS een)

**U.S. Brand Names** Eltroxin®; Levo-T™; Levothroid®; Levoxyl®; Synthroid®; Unithroid™

**Canadian Brand Names** Eltroxin®; PMS-Levothyroxine Sodium

**Synonyms** *L*-Thyroxine Sodium; $T_4$

**Pharmacologic Category** Thyroid Product

**Use** Replacement or supplemental therapy in hypothyroidism; some clinicians suggest levothyroxine is the drug of choice for replacement therapy

**Effects on Mental Status** May rarely cause nervousness or insomnia

**Effects on Psychiatric Treatment** Used to augment antidepressants; TCAs may increase toxic potential of both drugs

**Pregnancy Risk Factor** A

**Contraindications** Recent myocardial infarction or thyrotoxicosis, uncorrected adrenal insufficiency, hypersensitivity to levothyroxine sodium or any component

**Warnings/Precautions** Ineffective for weight reduction; high doses may produce serious or even life-threatening toxic effects particularly when used with some anorectic drugs. Use with caution and reduce dosage in patients with angina pectoris or other cardiovascular disease; levothyroxine tablets contain tartrazine dye which may cause allergic reactions in susceptible individuals; use cautiously in elderly since they may be more likely to have compromised cardiovascular functions. Patients with adrenal insufficiency, myxedema, diabetes mellitus and insipidus may have symptoms exaggerated or aggravated; thyroid replacement requires periodic assessment of thyroid status. Chronic hypothyroidism predisposes patients to coronary artery disease.

**Adverse Reactions** <1%: Abdominal cramps, alopecia, ataxia, cardiac arrhythmias, changes in menstrual cycle, chest pain, constipation, diaphoresis, diarrhea, fever, hand tremors, headache, increased appetite, insomnia, myalgia, nervousness, palpitations, shortness of breath, tachycardia, tremor, weight loss

**Overdosage/Toxicology**

Signs and symptoms: Chronic overdose may cause hyperthyroidism, weight loss, nervousness, sweating, tachycardia, insomnia, heat intolerance, menstrual irregularities, palpitations, psychosis, fever; acute overdose may cause fever, hypoglycemia, CHF, unrecognized adrenal insufficiency

Treatment: Chronic overdose is treated by withdrawal of the drug; massive overdose may require beta-blockers for increased sympathomimetic activity. Reduce dose or temporarily discontinue therapy; normal hypothalamic-pituitary-thyroid axis will return to normal in 6-8 weeks; serum $T_4$ levels do not correlate well with toxicity; in massive acute ingestion, reduce GI absorption, administer general supportive care; treat congestive heart failure with digitalis glycosides; excessive adrenergic activity (tachycardia) require propranolol 1-3 mg I.V. over 10 minutes or 80-160 mg orally/day; fever may be treated with acetaminophen.

**Drug Interactions**

Aluminum and magnesium containing antacids, calcium carbonate, simethicone, or sucralfate: May decrease T4 absorption; separate dose from levothyroxine by at least 4 hours

Antidiabetic agents (biguanides, meglitinides, sulfonylureas, thiazolidinediones, insulin): Changes in thyroid function may alter requirements of antidiabetic agent; monitor closely at initiation of therapy, or when dose is changed or discontinued

Cholestyramine and colestipol: Decrease T4 absorption; separate dose from levothyroxine by at least 4 hours

CYP enzyme inducers: May increase the metabolism of T3 and T4; inducers include barbiturates, carbamazepine, phenytoin, and rifampin/rifabutin

Digoxin: Digoxin levels may be reduced in hyperthyroidism; therapeutic effect may be reduced; impact of thyroid replacement should be monitored

Iron: Decrease T4 absorption; separate dose from levothyroxine by at least 4 hours

Kayexalate®: Decrease T4 absorption; separate dose from levothyroxine by at least 4 hours

Ketamine: May cause marked hypertension and tachycardia, monitor

Ritonavir: May alter response to levothyroxine (limited documentation/case report); monitor

Somatrem, Somatropin: Excessive thyroid replacement leads to accelerated epiphyseal closure; inadequate replacement interferes with growth response. Effect of thyroid replacement not specifically evaluated; use caution.

SSRI antidepressants: May need to increase dose of levothyroxine when SSRI is added to a previously stabilized patient

Sympathomimetics: Effects of sympathomimetic agent or levothyroxine may be increased; risk of coronary insufficiency is increased in patients with coronary artery disease when these agents are used together

Theophylline, caffeine: Decreased theophylline clearance in hypothyroid patients; monitor during thyroid replacement

Tricyclic and tetracyclic antidepressants: Therapeutic and toxic effects of levothyroxine and the antidepressant are increased.

Warfarin (and other oral anticoagulants): The hypoprothrombic response to warfarin may be altered by a change in thyroid function or replacement. Replacement may dramatically increase response to warfarin. However, initiation of warfarin in a patient stabilized on a dose of levothyroxine does not appear to require a significantly different approach.

**NOTE:** Several medications have effects on thyroid production or conversion. The impact in thyroid replacement has not been specifically evaluated, but patient response should be monitored. Methimazole decreases thyroid hormone secretion, while propylthiouracil decrease thyroid hormone secretion and decreases conversion of T4 to T3. Beta-adrenergic antagonists: Decrease conversion of T4 to T3 (dose related, propranolol ≥160 mg/day); patients may be clinically euthyroid. Iodide, iodine-containing radiographic contrast agents may decrease thyroid hormone secretion; may also increase thyroid hormone secretion, especially in patients with Graves' disease. Other agents reported to impact on thyroid production/conversion include include aminoglutethimide, amiodarone, chloral hydrate, diazepam, ethionamide, interferon-alfa, interleukin-2, lithium, lovastatin (case report), glucocorticoids (dose-related), 6-mercaptopurine, sulfonamides, thiazide diuretics, and tolbutamide. In addition, a number of medications have been noted to cause transient depression in TSH secretion (usually dose-related), which may complicate interpretation of monitoring tests for levothyroxine, including corticosteroids, octreotide, and dopamine. In addition, metoclopramide may increase TSH secretion.

**Usual Dosage**

Children: Congenital hypothyroidism:

Oral:

0-6 months: 8-10 mcg/kg/day **or** 25-50 mcg/day

6-12 months: 6-8 mcg/kg/day **or** 50-75 mcg/day

1-5 years: 5-6 mcg/kg/day **or** 75-100 mcg/day

6-12 years: 4-5 mcg/kg/day **or** 100-150 mcg/day

>12 years: 2-3 mcg/kg/day **or** ≥150 mcg/day

I.M., I.V.: 50% to 75% of the oral dose

Adults:

Oral: Initial: 0.05 mg/day, then increase by increments of 25 mcg/day at intervals of 2-3 weeks; average adult dose: 100-200 mcg/day; maximum dose: 200 mcg/day

I.M., I.V.: 50% of the oral dose

Myxedema coma or stupor: I.V.: 200-500 mcg one time, then 100-300 mcg the next day if necessary

Thyroid suppression therapy: Oral: 2-6 mcg/kg/day for 7-10 days

**Dietary Considerations** Should be administered on an empty stomach; limit intake of goitrogenic foods (asparagus, cabbage, peas, turnip greens, broccoli, spinach, Brussels sprouts, lettuce, soybeans). Soybean flour (infant formula), walnuts, and dietary fiber may decrease absorption of levothyroxine from GI tract.

**Patient Information** Thyroid replacement therapy is generally for life. Take as directed, in the morning before breakfast. Do not change brands and do not discontinue without consulting prescriber. Consult prescriber if drastically increasing or decreasing intake of goitrogenic food (eg, asparagus, cabbage, peas, turnip greens, broccoli, spinach, Brussels sprouts, lettuce, soybeans). Report chest pain, rapid heart rate, palpitations, heat intolerance, excessive sweating, increased nervousness, agitation, or lethargy.

**Nursing Implications** I.V. form must be prepared immediately prior to administration; should not be admixed with other solutions

**Dosage Forms**

Powder for injection, as sodium, lyophilized: 200 mcg/vial (6 mL, 10 mL); 500 mcg/vial (6 mL, 10 mL)

Tablet, as sodium: 25 mcg, 50 mcg, 75 mcg, 88 mcg, 100 mcg, 112 mcg, 125 mcg, 150 mcg, 175 mcg, 200 mcg, 300 mcg

♦ **Levoxyl®** *see* Levothyroxine *on page 316*

♦ **Levsin®** *see* Hyoscyamine *on page 279*

♦ **Levsinex®** *see* Hyoscyamine *on page 279*

♦ **Levsin/SL®** *see* Hyoscyamine *on page 279*

♦ **Levulan® Kerastick™** *see* Aminolevulinic Acid *on page 31*

♦ **Lexxel™** *see* Enalapril and Felodipine *on page 192*

♦ ***l*-Hyoscyamine Sulfate** *see* Hyoscyamine *on page 279*

♦ **Librax®** *see* Clidinium and Chlordiazepoxide *on page 128*

♦ **Libritabs®** *see* Chlordiazepoxide *on page 109*

♦ **Librium®** *see* Chlordiazepoxide *on page 109*

♦ **Lice-Enz® Shampoo [OTC]** *see* Pyrethrins *on page 480*

## Licorice

**Related Information**

Natural/Herbal Products *on page 746*

Natural Products, Herbals, and Dietary Supplements *on page 742*

Perspectives on the Safety of Herbal Medicines *on page 736*

**Synonyms** *Glycyrrhiza glabra*; *G. palidiflora*; *G. uralensis*; Sweet Root

**Pharmacologic Category** Herb

**Use** Foodstuff in chewing gum, chewing tobacco, cough preparations

Per Commission E: Catarrhs of the upper respiratory tract and gastric/duodenal ulcers

**Restrictions** Per Commission E: Not more than 4-6 weeks administration without medical advice; there is no objection of using licorice as a flavoring agent up to maximum daily dose: 100 mg glycyrrhizin

**Pregnancy Risk Factor** Contraindicated per Commission E

**Contraindications** Per Commission E: Cholestatic liver disorders, liver cirrhosis, hypertonia, hypokalemia, severe kidney insufficiency, pregnancy

**Adverse Reactions**

Cardiovascular: Hypertension

Central nervous system: Headache, seizures, tetany

Endocrine & metabolic: Amenorrhea, hyponatremia, hypokalemia, hypomagnesemia

Neuromuscular & skeletal: Myopathy, carpopedal spasms, rhabdomyolysis

Ocular: Bilateral ptosis

Renal: Myoglobinuria

Per Commission E: On prolonged use and with higher doses, mineral corticoid effects may occur in the form of sodium and water retention and potassium loss, accompanied by hypertension, edema, and hypokalemia, and in rare cases, myoglobinuria

**Overdosage/Toxicology** Treatment: Supportive therapy; fluid/electrolyte (especially potassium) replacement; spironolactone (1 g/day in divided doses) also may be useful in reversing electrolyte abnormalities; tetany can be treated with magnesium sulfate

**Drug Interactions**

Attenuated effect of strychnine, tetrodoxine, nicotine, cocaine, barbiturates, pilocarpine, urethane, epinephrine, and ephedrine through glucuronic-like conjugation action; traditional emmenagogue; increases progesterone and cortisol half-life; concomitant use of furosemide can exacerbate hypokalemia

Per Commission E: Potassium loss due to other drugs (eg, thiazide diuretics), can be increased; with potassium loss, sensitivity to digitalis glycosides increases

**Usual Dosage**

100 g (equivalent to 700 mg of glycyrrhizinic acid) of licorice found in 2-4 licorice twists; toxic effect can be seen if ingested daily (2-3 twists) for 2-4 weeks

Per Commission E: 5-15 g root/day, equivalent to 200-600 mg glycyrrhizin; succus liquiritiae (juice): 0.5-1 g for catarrhs of upper respiratory tract; 1.5-3 g for gastric/duodenal ulcers; equivalent preparations

**Patient Information** Considered unsafe

**Additional Information** Syndrome of pseudoprimary hyperaldosteronism is a complication of chronic licorice ingestion; serum potassium as low as 0.9 mmol/L has been noted

♦ **Lidex®** *see* Fluocinonide *on page 231*

♦ **Lidex-E®** *see* Fluocinonide *on page 231*

## Lidocaine (LYE doe kane)

**Related Information**

Serum Drug Concentrations Commonly Monitored: Guidelines *on page 759*

**U.S. Brand Names** Anestacon®; Dermaflex® Gel; Dilocaine®; Dr Scholl's® Cracked Heel Relief Cream [OTC]; Duo-Trach®; LidoPen® Auto-Injector; Nervocaine®; Octocaine®; Solarcaine® Aloe Extra Burn Relief [OTC]; Xylocaine®; Zilactin-L® [OTC]

**Canadian Brand Names** PMS-Lidocaine Viscous; Xylocard®

**Pharmacologic Category** Analgesic, Topical; Antiarrhythmic Agent, Class I-B; Local Anesthetic

**Use** Local anesthetic and acute treatment of ventricular arrhythmias from myocardial infarction, cardiac manipulation, digitalis intoxication; topical local anesthetic; drug of choice for ventricular ectopy, ventricular tachycardia, ventricular fibrillation; for pulseless VT or VF preferably administer **after** defibrillation and epinephrine; control of premature ventricular contractions, wide-complex PSVT

**Effects on Mental Status** May rarely cause agitation, anxiety, euphoria, or hallucinations

**Effects on Psychiatric Treatment** None reported

**Usual Dosage**

Topical: Apply to affected area as needed; maximum: 3 mg/kg/dose; do not repeat within 2 hours

Injectable local anesthetic: Varies with procedure, degree of anesthesia needed, vascularity of tissue, duration of anesthesia required, and physical condition of patient; maximum: 4.5 mg/kg/dose; do not repeat within 2 hours

I.M.: Adults: 300 mg (best in deltoid muscle; only 10% solution)

Children: Endotracheal, I.O., I.V.: Loading dose: 1 mg/kg; may repeat in 10-15 minutes x 2 doses; after loading dose, start I.V. continuous infusion 20-50 mcg/kg/minute (300 mcg/kg/minute per American Heart Association)

Use 20 mcg/kg/minute in patients with shock, hepatic disease, mild congestive heart failure (CHF)

Moderate to severe CHF may require 1/2 loading dose and lower infusion rates to avoid toxicity

Adults: Antiarrhythmic:

I.V.: 1-1.5 mg/kg bolus over 2-3 minutes; may repeat doses of 0.5-0.75 mg/kg in 5-10 minutes up to a total of 3 mg/kg; continuous infusion: 1-4 mg/minute

I.V. (2 g/250 mL $D_5W$) infusion rates (infusion pump should be used for I.V. infusion administration):

1 mg/minute: 7 mL/hour

2 mg/minute: 15 mL/hour

3 mg/minute: 21 mL/hour

4 mg/minute: 30 mL/hour

Ventricular fibrillation (after defibrillation and epinephrine): Initial dose: 1.5 mg/kg, may repeat boluses as above; follow with continuous infusion after return of perfusion

Prevention of ventricular fibrillation: I.V.: Initial bolus: 0.5 mg/kg; repeat every 5-10 minutes to a total dose of 2 mg/kg

(Continued)

## Lidocaine *(Continued)*

Refractory ventricular fibrillation: Repeat 1.5 mg/kg bolus may be given 3-5 minutes after initial dose

Endotracheal: 2-2.5 times the I.V. dose

**Decrease dose in patients with CHF, shock, or hepatic disease**

**Dosing adjustment/comments in hepatic disease:** Reduce dose in acute hepatitis and decompensated cirrhosis by 50%

Dialysis: Not dialyzable (0% to 5%) by hemo- or peritoneal dialysis; supplemental dose not necessary; supplemental dose is not necessary

**Dosage Forms**

Cream, as hydrochloride: 2% (56 g)

Injection, as hydrochloride: 0.5% [5 mg/mL] (50 mL); 1% [10 mg/mL] (2 mL, 5 mL, 10 mL, 20 mL, 30 mL, 50 mL); 1.5% [15 mg/mL] (20 mL); 2% [20 mg/mL] (2 mL, 5 mL, 10 mL, 20 mL, 30 mL, 50 mL); 4% [40 mg/mL] (5 mL); 10% [100 mg/mL] (10 mL); 20% [200 mg/mL] (10 mL, 20 mL)

Injection, as hydrochloride:

I.M. use: 10% [100 mg/mL] (3 mL, 5 mL)

Direct I.V.: 1% [10 mg/mL] (5 mL, 10 mL); 20 mg/mL (5 mL)

I.V. admixture, preservative free: 4% [40 mg/mL] (25 mL, 30 mL); 10% [100 mg/mL] (10 mL); 20% [200 mg/mL] (5 mL, 10 mL)

I.V. infusion, in $D_5W$: 0.2% [2 mg/mL] (500 mL); 0.4% [4 mg/mL] (250 mL, 500 mL, 1000 mL); 0.8% [8 mg/mL] (250 mL, 500 mL)

Gel, , as hydrochloride, topical: 2% (30 mL); 2.5% (15 mL)

Liquid, as hydrochloride, topical: 2.5% (7.5 mL)

Liquid, as hydrochloride, viscous: 2% (20 mL, 100 mL)

Ointment, as hydrochloride, topical: 2.5% [OTC], 5% (35 g)

Solution, as hydrochloride, topical: 2% (15 mL, 240 mL); 4% (50 mL)

♦ **LidoPen® Auto-Injector** *see* Lidocaine *on page 317*

♦ **Limbitrol®** *see* Amitriptyline and Chlordiazepoxide *on page 34*

♦ **Lincocin® Injection** *see* Lincomycin *on page 318*

♦ **Lincocin® Oral** *see* Lincomycin *on page 318*

## Lincomycin (lin koe MYE sin)

**U.S. Brand Names** Lincocin® Injection; Lincocin® Oral; Lincorex® Injection

**Pharmacologic Category** Antibiotic, Macrolide

**Use** Treatment of susceptible bacterial infections, mainly those caused by streptococci and staphylococci resistant to other agents

**Effects on Mental Status** May cause dizziness

**Effects on Psychiatric Treatment** May cause granulocytopenia; use caution with clozapine and carbamazepine

**Contraindications** Minor bacterial infections or viral infections; hypersensitivity to lincomycin or any component or clindamycin

**Warnings/Precautions** Can cause severe and possibly fatal colitis; characterized by severe persistent diarrhea, severe abdominal cramps and, possibly, the passage of blood and mucus; discontinue drug if significant diarrhea occurs; severe hepatic disease

**Adverse Reactions** 1% to 10%: Gastrointestinal: Nausea, vomiting, diarrhea

**Overdosage/Toxicology**

Signs and symptoms: Diarrhea, abdominal cramps

Treatment: Following oral decontamination, treatment is supportive

**Drug Interactions**

Decreased effect with erythromycin

Increased activity/toxicity of neuromuscular blocking agents

**Usual Dosage**

Children >1 month:

Oral: 30-60 mg/kg/day in divided doses every 8 hours

I.M.: 10 mg/kg every 8-12 hours

I.V.: 10-20 mg/kg/day in divided doses every 8-12 hours

Adults:

Oral: 500 mg every 6-8 hours

I.M.: 600 mg every 12-24 hours

I.V.: 600-1 g every 8-12 hours up to 8 g/day

**Dosing interval in renal impairment:**

$Cl_{cr}$ 10-50 mL/minute: Administer every 6-12 hours

$Cl_{cr}$ <10 mL/minute: Administer every 12 hours

**Dosing adjustment in hepatic impairment:** Reductions are indicated

**Patient Information** Report any severe diarrhea immediately and do not take antidiarrheal medication; take each oral dose with a full glass of water; finish all medication; do not skip doses; store capsules in a light-proof container

**Dosage Forms**

Capsule, as hydrochloride: 250 mg, 500 mg

Injection, as hydrochloride: 300 mg/mL (2 mL, 10 mL)

♦ **Lincorex® Injection** *see* Lincomycin *on page 318*

## Lindane (LIN dane)

**U.S. Brand Names** G-well®

**Canadian Brand Names** Hexit®; Kwellada™; PMS-Lindane

**Synonyms** Benzene Hexachloride; Gamma Benzene Hexachloride; Hexachlorocyclohexane

**Pharmacologic Category** Antiparasitic Agent, Topical; Pediculocide; Scabicidal Agent

**Use** Treatment of scabies (*Sarcoptes scabiei*), *Pediculus capitis* (head lice), and *Pediculus pubis* (crab lice); FDA recommends reserving lindane as a second-line agent or with inadequate response to other therapies

**Effects on Mental Status** May cause dizziness or restlessness

**Effects on Psychiatric Treatment** May cause aplastic anemia; use caution with clozapine and carbamazepine

**Pregnancy Risk Factor** B

**Contraindications** Hypersensitivity to lindane or any component; premature neonates; acutely inflamed skin or raw, weeping surfaces

**Warnings/Precautions Not considered a drug of first choice**; use with caution in infants and small children, and patients with a history of seizures; avoid contact with face, eyes, mucous membranes, and urethral meatus. Because of the potential for systemic absorption and CNS side effects, lindane should be used with caution; consider permethrin or crotamiton agent first.

**Adverse Reactions** <1%: Aplastic anemia, ataxia, burning and stinging, cardiac arrhythmia, contact dermatitis, dizziness, eczematous eruptions, headache, hematuria, hepatitis, nausea, pulmonary edema, restlessness, seizures, skin and adipose tissue may act as repositories, vomiting

**Overdosage/Toxicology**

Signs and symptoms: Vomiting, restlessness, ataxia, seizures, arrhythmias, pulmonary edema, hematuria, hepatitis. Absorbed through skin and mucous membranes and GI tract, has occasionally caused serious CNS, hepatic and renal toxicity when used excessively for prolonged periods, or when accidental ingestion has occurred

Treatment: If ingested, perform gastric lavage and general supportive measures; diazepam 0.01 mg/kg can be used to control seizures.

**Drug Interactions** Increased toxicity: Oil-based hair dressing may increase toxic potential

**Usual Dosage** Children and Adults: Topical:

Scabies: Apply a thin layer of lotion or cream and massage it on skin from the neck to the toes (head to toe in infants). For adults, bathe and remove the drug after 8-12 hours; for children, wash off 6-8 hours after application (for infants, wash off 6 hours after application); repeat treatment in 7 days if lice or nits are still present

Pediculosis, capitis and pubis: 15-30 mL of shampoo is applied and lathered for 4-5 minutes; rinse hair thoroughly and comb with a fine tooth comb to remove nits; repeat treatment in 7 days if lice or nits are still present

**Patient Information** For external use only. Do not apply to face and avoid getting in eyes. Do not apply immediately after hot soapy bath. Apply from neck to toes. Bathe to remove drug after 8-12 hours. Repeat in 7 days if lice or nits are still present. Clothing and bedding must be washed in hot water or dry cleaned to kill nits. Wash combs and brushes with lindane shampoo and thoroughly rinse. May need to treat all members of household and all sexual contacts concurrently. Report if condition persists or infection occurs.

**Dosage Forms**

Cream: 1% (60 g, 454 g)

Lotion: 1% (60 mL, 473 mL, 4000 mL)

Shampoo: 1% (60 mL, 473 mL, 4000 mL)

## Linezolid (li NE zoh lid)

**U.S. Brand Names** Zyvox™

**Pharmacologic Category** Antibiotic, Oxazolidinone

**Use** Treatment of vancomycin-resistant *Enterococcus faecium* (VRE) infections, nosocomial pneumonia caused by *Staphylococcus aureus* including MRSA or *Streptococcus pneumoniae* (penicillin-susceptible strains only), complicated and uncomplicated skin and skin structure infections, and community-acquired pneumonia caused by susceptible gram-positive organisms.

**Effects on Mental Status** May cause insomnia and dizziness

**Effects on Psychiatric Treatment** Has mild monoamine oxidase inhibitor properties and has the potential to have the same interactions as other MAOIs; thrombocytopenia has been reported and may be dependent on duration of therapy (generally >2 weeks of treatment), caution with valproic acid; avoid use with serotonergic agents such as TCAs, venlafaxine, trazodone, sibutramine, meperidine, dextromethorphan, and SSRIs; may cause leukopenia, use caution with clozapine and carbamazepine

**Pregnancy Risk Factor** C

**Contraindications** Allergy to linezolid or any other component

**Warnings/Precautions** Linezolid has mild monoamine oxidase inhibitor properties and has the potential to have the same interactions as other MAOIs; use with caution in uncontrolled hypertension, pheochromocytoma, carcinoid syndrome, or untreated hyperthyroidism; thrombocytopenia has been reported and may be dependent on duration of therapy (generally >2 weeks of treatment); avoid use with serotonergic agents such as TCAs, venlafaxine, trazodone, sibutramine, meperidine, dextromethorphan, and SSRIs; consider alternatives before initiating outpatient treatment (unnecessary use may lead the development of resistance to linezolid)

**Adverse Reactions**

1% to 10%:

Cardiovascular: Hypertension (1% to 3%)

Central nervous system: Headache (0.5% to 11%), insomnia (3%), dizziness (0.4% to 2%), fever (2%)

Dermatologic: Rash (2%)

Gastrointestinal: Nausea (3% to 10%), diarrhea (3% to 11%), vomiting (1% to 4%), constipation (2%), taste alteration (1% to 2%), tongue discoloration (0.2% to 1%), oral moniliasis (0.4% to 1%), pancreatitis

Genitourinary: Vaginal moniliasis (1% to 2%)

Hematologic: Thrombocytopenia (0.3% to 10%), anemia, leukopenia, neutropenia

Hepatic: Abnormal LFTs (0.4% to 1%)

Miscellaneous: Fungal infections (0.1% to 2%)

<1%: *C. difficile*-related complications, increase in creatinine, dyspepsia, localized abdominal pain, pruritus

**Overdosage/Toxicology** Treatment includes supportive care; hemodialysis may improve elimination (30% of a dose is removed during a 3-hour hemodialysis session)

**Drug Interactions** Linezolid is a reversible, nonselective inhibitor of MAO

Adrenergic agents (eg, phenylpropanolamine, pseudoephedrine, sympathomimetic agents, vasopressor or dopaminergic agents) may cause hypertension

Serotonergic agents (eg, TCAs, venlafaxine, trazodone, sibutramine, meperidine, dextromethorphan, and SSRIs) may cause a serotonin syndrome (eg, hyperpyrexia, cognitive dysfunction) when used concomitantly

**Usual Dosage** Adults:

Oral, I.V.:

VRE infections: 600 mg every 12 hours for 14-28 days

Nosocomial pneumonia, complicated skin and skin structure infections, community-acquired pneumonia including concurrent bacteremia: 600 mg every 12 hours for 10-14 days

Oral: Uncomplicated skin and skin structure infections: 400 mg every 12 hours for 10-14 days

**Dosage adjustment in renal impairment:** No specific adjustment recommended. The two primary metabolites may accumulate in patients with renal impairment but the clinical significance is unknown. Weigh the risk of accumulation of metabolites versus the benefit of therapy. Both linezolid and the two metabolites are eliminated by dialysis. Linezolid should be given after hemodialysis.

**Dosage adjustment in hepatic impairment:** No dosage adjustment required for mild to moderate hepatic insufficiency (Child-Pugh class A or B). Use in severe hepatic insufficiency has not been adequately evaluated.

Elderly: No dosage adjustment required

**Dietary Considerations** Take with or without food. Suspension contains 20 mg phenylalanine per teaspoonful.

**Patient Information** Take with or without food. Take with food if medicine causes stomach upset. Tell your healthcare provider if you have hypertension or are taking any cold remedy or decongestant. Limit quantities of tyramine-containing foods. Gently mix suspension. Store at room temperature.

**Nursing Implications** Administer intravenous infusion over 30-120 minutes. Do not mix or infuse with other medications. The yellow color of the injection may intensify over time without affecting potency.

**Dosage Forms**

Infusion: 200 mg (100 mL); 400 mg (200 mL); 600 mg (300 mL)

Suspension, oral (orange-flavored): 20 mg/mL (150 mL)

Tablet: 400 mg, 600 mg

♦ **Lioresal®** *see* Baclofen *on page 57*

## Liothyronine (lye oh THYE roe neen)

**Related Information**

Mood Disorders *on page 600*

**U.S. Brand Names** Cytomel® Oral; Triostat™ Injection

**Synonyms** Liothyronine Sodium; Sodium *L*-Triiodothyronine; $T_3$ Sodium

**Pharmacologic Category** Thyroid Product

**Use** Replacement or supplemental therapy in hypothyroidism, management of nontoxic goiter, chronic lymphocytic thyroiditis, as an adjunct in thyrotoxicosis and as a diagnostic aid; **levothyroxine is recommended for chronic therapy**; although previously thought to benefit cardiac patients with severely reduced fractions, liothyronine injection is no longer considered beneficial

**Effects on Mental Status** May cause nervousness or insomnia

**Effects on Psychiatric Treatment** Used to augment antidepressants

**Pregnancy Risk Factor** A

**Contraindications** Recent myocardial infarction or thyrotoxicosis, hypersensitivity to liothyronine sodium or any component, undocumented or uncorrected adrenal insufficiency

**Warnings/Precautions** Ineffective for weight reduction; high doses may produce serious or even life-threatening toxic effects particularly when used with some anorectic drugs. Use with extreme caution in patients with angina pectoris or other cardiovascular disease (including hypertension) or coronary artery disease; use with caution in elderly patients since they may be more likely to have compromised cardiovascular function. Patients with adrenal insufficiency, myxedema, diabetes mellitus and insipidus may have symptoms exaggerated or aggravated; thyroid replacement requires periodic assessment of thyroid status. Chronic hypothyroidism predisposes patients to coronary artery disease.

**Adverse Reactions** <1%: Abdominal cramps, alopecia, ataxia, cardiac arrhythmias, changes in menstrual cycle, chest pain, constipation, diaphoresis, diarrhea, fever, hand tremors, headache, increased appetite, insomnia, myalgia, nervousness, palpitations, shortness of breath, tachycardia, tremor, weight loss

**Overdosage/Toxicology**

Signs and symptoms: Chronic overdose may cause hyperthyroidism, weight loss, nervousness, sweating, tachycardia, insomnia, heat intolerance, menstrual irregularities, palpitations, psychosis, fever; acute overdose may cause fever, hypoglycemia, CHF, unrecognized adrenal insufficiency.

Treatment: Reduce dose or temporarily discontinue therapy; normal hypothalamic-pituitary-thyroid axis will return to normal in 6-8 weeks; serum $T_4$ levels do not correlate well with toxicity. In massive acute ingestion, reduce GI absorption, administer general supportive care; treat congestive heart failure with digitalis glycosides; excessive adrenergic activity (tachycardia) requires propranolol 1-3 mg I.V. over 10 minutes or 80-160 mg orally/day; fever may be treated with acetaminophen.

**Drug Interactions**

Decreased effect:

Cholestyramine resin may decrease absorption

Antidiabetic drug requirements are increased

Estrogens may increase thyroid requirements

Increased effect: Increased oral anticoagulant effects

**Usual Dosage**

Congenital hypothyroidism: Children: Oral: 5 mcg/day increase by 5 mcg every 3-4 days until the desired response is achieved. Usual maintenance dose: 20 mcg/day for infants, 50 mcg/day for children 1-3 years of age, and adult dose for children >3 years.

Hypothyroidism: Oral:

Adults: 25 mcg/day increase by increments of 12.5-25 mcg/day every 1-2 weeks to a maximum of 100 mcg/day; usual maintenance dose: 25-75 mcg/day

Elderly: Initial: 5 mcg/day, increase by 5 mcg/day every 1-2 weeks; usual maintenance dose: 25-75 mcg/day

$T_3$ suppression test: Oral: 75-100 mcg/day for 7 days; use lowest dose for elderly

Myxedema: Oral: Initial: 5 mcg/day; increase in increments of 5-10 mcg/day every 1-2 weeks. When 25 mcg/day is reached, dosage may be increased at intervals of 12.5-25 mcg/day every 1-2 weeks. Usual maintenance dose: 50-100 mcg/day.

Myxedema coma: I.V.: 25-50 mcg

Patients with known or suspected cardiovascular disease: 10-20 mcg

**Note:** Normally, at least 4 hours should be allowed between doses to adequately assess therapeutic response and no more than 12 hours should elapse between doses to avoid fluctuations in hormone levels. Oral therapy should be resumed as soon as the clinical situation has been stabilized and the patient is able to take oral medication. If levothyroxine rather than liothyronine sodium is used in initiating oral therapy, the physician should bear in mind that there is a delay of several days in the onset of levothyroxine activity and that I.V. therapy should be discontinued gradually.

**Patient Information** Take as directed; do not change brands of medication or discontinue without consulting prescriber. Do not change diet without consulting prescriber. Report chest pain, increased heartbeat, palpitations, excessive weight gain or loss, change in level of energy (increased or decreased), excessive sweating, or intolerance to heat.

**Dosage Forms**

Injection, as sodium: 10 mcg/mL (1 mL)

Tablet, as sodium: 5 mcg, 25 mcg, 50 mcg

♦ **Liothyronine Sodium** *see* Liothyronine *on page 319*

## Liotrix (LYE oh triks)

**U.S. Brand Names** Thyrolar®

**Synonyms** $T_3/T_4$ Liotrix

**Pharmacologic Category** Thyroid Product

**Use** Replacement or supplemental therapy in hypothyroidism (uniform mixture of $T_4$:$T_3$ in 4:1 ratio by weight); little advantage to this product exists and cost is not justified

**Effects on Mental Status** May cause nervousness or insomnia

**Effects on Psychiatric Treatment** None reported

**Pregnancy Risk Factor** A

(Continued)

## Liotrix *(Continued)*

**Contraindications** Hypersensitivity to liotrix or any component; recent myocardial infarction or thyrotoxicosis, uncomplicated by hypothyroidism; uncorrected adrenal insufficiency, hypersensitivity to active or extraneous constituents

**Warnings/Precautions** Ineffective for weight reduction; high doses may produce serious or even life-threatening toxic effects particularly when used with some anorectic drugs; use cautiously in patients with pre-existing cardiovascular disease (angina, CHD), elderly since they may be more likely to have compromised cardiovascular function

**Adverse Reactions** <1%: Abdominal cramps, alopecia, ataxia, cardiac arrhythmias, changes in menstrual cycle, chest pain, constipation, diaphoresis, diarrhea, excessive bone loss with overtreatment (excess thyroid replacement), fever, hand tremors, headache, heat intolerance, increased appetite, insomnia, myalgia, nervousness, palpitations, shortness of breath, tachycardia, tremor, vomiting, weight loss

**Overdosage/Toxicology**

Signs and symptoms: Chronic overdose may cause weight loss, nervousness, sweating, tachycardia, insomnia, heat intolerance, menstrual irregularities, palpitations, psychosis, fever; acute overdose may cause fever, hypoglycemia, CHF, unrecognized adrenal insufficiency

Treatment: Reduce dose or temporarily discontinue therapy; normal hypothalamic-pituitary-thyroid axis will return to normal in 6-8 weeks; serum $T_4$ levels do not correlate well with toxicity. In massive acute ingestion, reduce GI absorption, administer general supportive care; treat congestive heart failure with digitalis glycosides; excessive adrenergic activity (tachycardia) require propranolol 1-3 mg I.V. over 10 minutes or 80-160 mg orally/day; fever may be treated with acetaminophen.

**Drug Interactions**

Decreased effect:
- Thyroid hormones increase hypoglycemic drug requirements
- Phenytoin → clinical lymphothyroidism
- Cholestyramine may decrease drug absorption

Increased effect: Increased oral anticoagulant effect

Increased toxicity: Tricyclic antidepressants may increase potential of both drugs

**Usual Dosage** Oral:

Congenital hypothyroidism:
- Children (dose of $T_4$ or levothyroxine/day):
  - 0-6 months: 8-10 mcg/kg or 25-50 mcg/day
  - 6-12 months: 6-8 mcg/kg or 50-75 mcg/day
  - 1-5 years: 5-6 mcg/kg or 75-100 mcg/day
  - 6-12 years: 4-5 mcg/kg or 100-150 mcg/day
  - >12 years: 2-3 mcg/kg or >150 mcg/day

Hypothyroidism (dose of thyroid equivalent):
- Adults: 30 mg/day (15 mg/day if cardiovascular impairment), increasing by increments of 15 mg/day at 2- to 3-week intervals to a maximum of 180 mg/day (usual maintenance dose: 60-120 mg/day)
- Elderly: Initial: 15 mg, adjust dose at 2- to 4-week intervals by increments of 15 mg

**Patient Information** Do not change brands without physician's knowledge; report immediately to physician any chest pain, increased pulse, palpitations, heat intolerances, excessive sweating; do not discontinue without notifying your physician; replacement therapy will be for life; take as a single dose before breakfast

**Dosage Forms** Tablet: 15 mg, 30 mg, 60 mg, 120 mg, 180 mg [thyroid equivalent]


- ♦ **Lipancreatin** *see* Pancrelipase *on page 418*
- ♦ **Lipid-Lowering Agents Comparison Chart** *see page 717*
- ♦ **Lipitor®** *see* Atorvastatin *on page 52*
- ♦ **Lipovite® [OTC]** *see* Vitamin B Complex *on page 586*
- ♦ **Liquibid®** *see* Guaifenesin *on page 256*
- ♦ **Liqui-Char® [OTC]** *see* Charcoal *on page 106*
- ♦ **Liquid Antidote** *see* Charcoal *on page 106*
- ♦ **Liquid Compatibility With Antipsychotics and Mood Stabilizers** *see page 718*
- ♦ **Liquid Pred®** *see* Prednisone *on page 461*
- ♦ **Liquifilm® Forte Solution [OTC]** *see* Artificial Tears *on page 48*
- ♦ **Liquifilm® Tears Solution [OTC]** *see* Artificial Tears *on page 48*
- ♦ **Liquiprin® [OTC]** *see* Acetaminophen *on page 14*


## Lisinopril (lyse IN oh pril)

**Related Information**

Angiotensin-Related Agents Comparison Chart *on page 700*

**U.S. Brand Names** Prinivil®; Zestril®

**Canadian Brand Names** Apo®-Lisinopril

**Pharmacologic Category** Angiotensin-Converting Enzyme (ACE) Inhibitors

**Use** Treatment of hypertension, either alone or in combination with other antihypertensive agents; adjunctive therapy in treatment of CHF (afterload reduction); treatment of hemodynamically stable patients within 24 hours of acute myocardial infarction, to improve survival; treatment of acute myocardial infarction within 24 hours in hemodynamically stable patients to improve survival; treatment of left ventricular dysfunction after myocardial infarction

**Effects on Mental Status** May cause dizziness or fatigue; may rarely cause sedation, insomnia, or depression

**Effects on Psychiatric Treatment** May cause neutropenia; use caution with clozapine and carbamazepine; may decrease lithium clearance resulting in an increase in serum lithium levels and potential lithium toxicity; monitor serum lithium levels

**Pregnancy Risk Factor** C (1st trimester); D (2nd and 3rd trimester)

**Contraindications** Hypersensitivity to lisinopril or any component; angioedema related to previous treatment with an ACE inhibitor; bilateral renal artery stenosis; primary hyperaldosteronism; pregnancy (2nd and 3rd trimesters)

**Warnings/Precautions** Anaphylactic reactions can occur. Angioedema can occur at any time during treatment (especially following first dose). Careful blood pressure monitoring with first dose (hypotension can occur especially in volume depleted patients). Dosage adjustment needed in renal impairment. Use with caution in hypovolemia; collagen vascular diseases; valvular stenosis (particularly aortic stenosis); hyperkalemia; or before, during, or immediately after anesthesia. Avoid rapid dosage escalation, which may lead to renal insufficiency. Neutropenia/agranulocytosis with myeloid hyperplasia can rarely occur. If patient has renal impairment then a baseline WBC with differential and serum creatinine should be evaluated and monitored closely during the first 3 months of therapy. Hypersensitivity reactions may be seen during hemodialysis with high-flux dialysis membranes (eg, AN69). Deterioration in renal function can occur with initiation. Use with caution in unilateral renal artery stenosis and pre-existing renal insufficiency.

**Adverse Reactions**

1% to 10%:
- Cardiovascular: Hypotension (1% to 5%)
- Central nervous system: Dizziness (6%), headache (5%), fatigue (3%)
- Dermatologic: Rash (1.5%)
- Gastrointestinal: Diarrhea/vomiting/nausea (1% to 3%)
- Renal: Increased BUN/serum creatinine (transient)
- Respiratory: Upper respiratory symptoms, cough (3% to 5%)

<1%: Abdominal pain, angina pectoris, angioedema, anorexia, arthralgia, blurred vision, bone marrow suppression, bronchitis, chest discomfort (~1%), constipation, depression, diaphoresis fever, flatulence, flushing, gout, hepatitis, insomnia, malaise, myocardial infarction, neutropenia, orthostatic hypotension, palpitations, pancreatitis, peripheral edema, pharyngeal pain, pruritus, rhythm disturbances, shoulder pain, sinusitis, somnolence, syncope, tachycardia, urticaria, vasculitis, xerostomia

**Overdosage/Toxicology**

Signs and symptoms: Mild hypotension has been the only toxic effect seen with acute overdose. Bradycardia may also occur; hyperkalemia occurs even with therapeutic doses, especially in patients with renal insufficiency and those taking NSAIDs.

Treatment: Following initiation of essential overdose management, toxic symptom treatment and supportive treatment should be initiated. Hypotension usually responds to I.V. fluids or Trendelenburg positioning.

**Drug Interactions**
- Allopurinol: Case reports (rare) indicate a possible increased risk of hypersensitivity reactions when combined with lisinopril
- $Alpha_1$ blockers: Hypotensive effect increased
- Aspirin: The effects of ACE inhibitors may be blunted by aspirin administration, particularly at higher dosages
- Diuretics: Hypovolemia due to diuretics may precipitate acute hypotensive events or acute renal failure
- Insulin: Risk of hypoglycemia may be increased
- Lithium: Risk of lithium toxicity may be increased; monitor lithium levels, especially the first 4 weeks of therapy
- Mercaptopurine: Risk of neutropenia may be increased
- NSAIDs may decrease ACE inhibitor efficacy and/or increase adverse renal effects
- Potassium-sparing diuretics (amiloride, spironolactone, triamterene): Increased risk of hyperkalemia
- Potassium supplements may increase the risk of hyperkalemia
- Trimethoprim (high dose) may increase the risk of hyperkalemia

**Usual Dosage**

Hypertension:
- Adults: Initial: 10 mg/day; increase doses 5-10 mg/day at 1- to 2-week intervals; maximum daily dose: 40 mg
- Elderly: Initial: 2.5-5 mg/day; increase doses 2.5-5 mg/day at 1- to 2-week intervals; maximum daily dose: 40 mg
- Patients taking diuretics should have them discontinued 2-3 days prior to initiating lisinopril if possible. Restart diuretic after blood pressure is stable if needed. If diuretic cannot be discontinued prior to therapy, begin with 5 mg with close supervision until stable blood pressure. In patients with hyponatremia (<130 mEq/L), start dose at 2.5 mg/day,

Congestive heart failure: Adults: 5 mg initially with diuretics and digitalis; may be increase in no greater than 10 mg increments at intervals no less than 2 weeks to a maximum of 40 mg/day. Usual maintenance: 5-40 mg/day as a single dose

Acute myocardial infarction (within 24 hours in hemodynamically stable patients): Oral: 5 mg immediately, then 5 mg at 24 hours, 10 mg at 48 hours, and 10 mg every day thereafter for 6 weeks. Patients should continue to receive standard treatments such as thrombolytics, aspirin, and beta-blockers.

**Dosing adjustment in renal impairment:**

$Cl_{cr}$ 10-50 mL/minute: Administer 50% to 75% of normal dose.

$Cl_{cr}$ <10 mL/minute: Administer 25% to 50% of normal dose.

Hemodialysis: Dialyzable (50%)

**Patient Information** Take exactly as directed; do not discontinue without consulting prescriber. Take first dose at bedtime. This drug does not eliminate need for diet or exercise regimen as recommended by prescriber. Do not take potassium supplements or salt substitutes containing potassium without consulting prescriber. May cause dizziness, fainting, lightheadedness (use caution when driving or engaging in tasks that require alertness until response to drug is known); postural hypotension (use caution when rising from lying or sitting position or climbing stairs); nausea, vomiting, abdominal pain, dry mouth, or transient loss of appetite (small frequent meals, frequent mouth care, sucking lozenges, or chewing gum may help) - report if these persist. Report chest pain or palpitations; mouth sores; fever or chills; skin rash; numbness, tingling, or pain in muscles; difficulty in breathing or unusual cough; or other persistent adverse reactions.

**Nursing Implications** May cause depression in some patients; discontinue if angioedema of the face, extremities, lips, tongue, or glottis occurs; watch for hypotensive effects within 1-3 hours of first dose or new higher dose

**Dosage Forms** Tablet: 2.5 mg, 5 mg, 10 mg, 20 mg, 40 mg

## Lisinopril and Hydrochlorothiazide

(lyse IN oh pril & hye droe klor oh THYE a zide)

**U.S. Brand Names** Prinzide®; Zestoretic®

**Pharmacologic Category** Antihypertensive Agent, Combination

**Use** Treatment of hypertension

**Effects on Mental Status** May cause dizziness or fatigue; may rarely cause sedation, insomnia, or depression

**Effects on Psychiatric Treatment** May cause neutropenia; use caution with clozapine and carbamazepine; may decrease lithium clearance resulting in an increase in serum lithium levels and potential lithium toxicity; monitor serum lithium levels

**Usual Dosage** Adults: Oral: Dosage is individualized; see each component for appropriate dosing suggestions

**Dosage Forms** Tablet:

Lisinopril 10 mg and hydrochlorothiazide 12.5 mg

[12.5]-Lisinopril 20 mg and hydrochlorothiazide 12.5 mg

[25]-Lisinopril 20 mg and hydrochlorothiazide 25 mg

♦ **Lithane®** *see* Lithium *on page 321*

## Lithium (LITH ee um)

**Related Information**

Clinical Issues in the Use of Mood Stabilizers *on page 632*

Impulse Control Disorders *on page 622*

Liquid Compatibility With Antipsychotics and Mood Stabilizers *on page 718*

Mood Disorders *on page 600*

Mood Stabilizers *on page 719*

Patient Information - Mood Stabilizers (Lithium) *on page 649*

Personality Disorders *on page 625*

Serum Drug Concentrations Commonly Monitored: Guidelines *on page 759*

Special Populations - Children and Adolescents *on page 663*

Special Populations - Elderly *on page 662*

Special Populations - Pregnant and Breast-Feeding Patients *on page 668*

Teratogenic Risks of Psychotropic Medications *on page 812*

**Generic Available** Yes

**U.S. Brand Names** Eskalith®; Eskalith CR®; Lithane®; Lithobid®; Lithonate®; Lithotabs®

**Synonyms** Lithium Carbonate; Lithium Citrate

**Pharmacologic Category** Lithium

**Use** Management of bipolar disorders

**Unlabeled uses:** Potential augmenting agent for antidepressants; aggression; post-traumatic stress disorder

**Pregnancy Risk Factor** D

**Contraindications** Hypersensitivity to lithium or any component; severe cardiovascular or renal disease; severe debilitation, dehydration, or sodium depletion

**Warnings/Precautions** Lithium toxicity is closely related to serum levels and can occur at therapeutic doses; serum lithium determinations are required to monitor therapy. Use with caution in patients with cardiovascular or thyroid disease, or in patients receiving medications which alter sodium excretion (eg, diuretics, ACE inhibitors, NSAIDs). Some elderly patients may be extremely sensitive to the effects of lithium, see Usual Dosage and Reference Range. Chronic therapy results in diminished renal concentrating ability (nephrogenic DI). Changes in renal function should be monitored, and re-evaluation of treatment may be necessary.

Use with caution in patients receiving neuroleptic medications - a syndrome resembling NMS has been associated with concurrent therapy. Lithium may impair the patient's alertness, affecting the ability to operate machinery or driving a vehicle. Neuromuscular blocking agents should be administered with caution - the response may be prolonged.

Higher serum concentrations may be required and tolerated during an acute manic phase; however, the tolerance decreases when symptoms subside. Normal fluid and salt intake must be maintained during therapy.

**Adverse Reactions**

Cardiovascular: Cardiac arrhythmias, hypotension, sinus node dysfunction, flattened or inverted T waves (reversible), edema

Central nervous system: Dizziness, vertigo, slurred speech, blackout spells, seizures, sedation, restlessness, confusion, psychomotor retardation, stupor, coma, dystonia, fatigue, lethargy, headache, pseudotumor cerebri

Dermatologic: Dry or thinning of hair, folliculitis, alopecia, exacerbation of psoriasis, rash

Endocrine & metabolic: Euthyroid goiter and/or hypothyroidism, hyperthyroidism, hyperglycemia, diabetes insipidus

Gastrointestinal: Polydipsia, anorexia, nausea, vomiting, diarrhea, xerostomia, metallic taste, weight gain

Genitourinary: Incontinence, polyuria, glycosuria, oliguria, albuminuria

Hematologic: Leukocytosis

Neuromuscular & skeletal: Tremor, muscle hyperirritability, ataxia, choreoathetoid movements, hyperactive deep tendon reflexes

Ocular: Nystagmus, blurred vision

Miscellaneous: Discoloration of fingers and toes

**Overdosage/Toxicology**

Signs and symptoms: Sedation, confusion, tremors, joint pain, visual changes, seizures, coma

Treatment: There is no specific antidote for lithium poisoning. In the acute ingestion following initiation of essential overdose management, correction of fluid and electrolyte imbalances should be commenced.

Hemodialysis is the treatment of choice for severe intoxications

Charcoal is ineffective

**Drug Interactions**

ACE inhibitors: May increase the risk of lithium toxicity via sodium depletion; monitor

Angiotensin receptor antagonists (losartan): May reduce the renal clearance of lithium; monitor

Carbamazepine: Concurrent use of lithium with carbamazepine, diltiazem may increase the risk for neurotoxicity; monitor

Carbonic anhydrase inhibitors: May decrease lithium levels; includes acetazolamide; monitor

Calcium channel blockers (diltiazem and verapamil): May increase the risk for neurotoxicity; monitor; does not appear to involve dihydropyridine class

Chlorpromazine: May lower serum concentrations of both drugs; monitor

Haloperidol: May increase the risk for neurotoxicity; monitor

Iodine salts: May enhance the hypothyroid effects of lithium; monitor

Loop diuretics: May decrease the renal excretion of lithium, leading to toxicity; monitor

MAOIs: Should generally be avoided due to use reports of fatal malignant hyperpyrexia when combined with lithium

Methyldopa: May increase the risk for neurotoxicity; monitor

Metronidazole: May increase lithium toxicity (rare); monitor

Neuromuscular blocking agents: Lithium may potentiate the response to neuromuscular blockade, resulting in prolonged blockade and possible delayed recovery

NSAIDs: Renal lithium excretion may be decreased leading to increased serum lithium concentrations; sulindac and aspirin may be the exceptions; monitor

Phenothiazines: May increase the risk for neurotoxicity; monitor

Phenytoin: May enhance lithium toxicity; monitor

Selegiline: Risk of severe reactions when combined with MAO inhibitors may be decreased when administered with selective MAO type B inhibitor, particularly at selegiline doses <10 mg/day; however, theoretical risk is still present

SSRIs: May increase the risk for neurotoxicity; monitor; effect noted with fluoxetine, fluvoxamine

Sibutramine: Combined use of lithium with sibutramine may increase the risk of serotonin syndrome; this combination is best avoided

Sodium-containing products: Bicarbonate and/or high sodium intake may reduce serum lithium concentrations via enhanced excretion; monitor

Sympathomimetics: Lithium may blunt the pressor response to sympathomimetics (epinephrine, phenylephrine, norepinephrine)

Tetracyclines: May increase lithium levels; monitor

(Continued)

## Lithium *(Continued)*

Theophylline: May increase real clearance of lithium, resulting in a decrease in serum lithium concentrations; monitor
Thiazide diuretics: May increase serum lithium concentration via sodium depletion and decreased lithium clearance; a lithium dose reduction of 50% is commonly recommended
Tricyclic antidepressants: May increase the risk for neurotoxicity; monitor

**Mechanism of Action** Alters cation transport across cell membrane in nerve and muscle cells and influences reuptake of serotonin and/or norepinephrine; second messenger systems involving the phosphatidylinositol cycle are inhibited; postsynaptic D2 receptor supersensitivity is inhibited

**Pharmacodynamics/kinetics**
Distribution: $V_d$: Initial: 0.3-0.4 L/kg; $V_{dss}$: 0.7-1 L/kg; crosses the placenta; appears in breast milk at 35% to 50% the concentrations in serum
Half-life: 18-24 hours; can increase to more than 36 hours in elderly or patients with renal impairment
Time to peak serum concentration (nonsustained release product): Within 0.5-2 hours following oral absorption
Elimination: 90% to 98% of dose excreted in urine as unchanged drug; other excretory routes include feces (1%) and sweat (4% to 5%)

**Usual Dosage** Oral: Monitor serum concentrations and clinical response (efficacy and toxicity) to determine proper dose
Children 6-12 years: 15-60 mg/kg/day in 3-4 divided doses; dose not to exceed usual adult dosage
Adults: 900-2400 mg/day in 3-4 divided doses or 900-1800 mg/day in two divided doses of sustained release
Elderly: Initial dose: 300 mg twice daily; increase weekly in increments of 300 mg/day, monitoring levels; rarely need >900-1200 mg/day
**Dosing adjustment in renal impairment:**
$Cl_{cr}$ 10-50 mL/minute: Administer 50% to 75% of normal dose
$Cl_{cr}$ <10 mL/minute: Administer 25% to 50% of normal dose
Hemodialysis: Dialyzable (50% to 100%)

**Administration** Administer with meals to decrease GI upset

**Monitoring Parameters** Serum lithium every 4-5 days during initial therapy; draw lithium serum concentrations 12 hours postdose; renal, thyroid, and cardiovascular function; fluid status; serum electrolytes; CBC with differential, urinalysis; monitor for signs of toxicity; b-HCG pregnancy test for all females not known to be sterile

**Reference Range** Therapeutic: 0.6-1.2 mEq/L (SI: 0.6-1.2 mmol/L); for acute mania: 0.9-1.2 mEq/L (SI: 0.9-1.2 mmol/L); for protection against future episodes in most patients with bipolar disorder: 0.6-0.9 mEq/L. A higher rate of relapse is described in subjects who are maintained below 0.4 mEq/L (SI: 0.4 mmol/L); Toxic: >2 mEq/L (SI: >2 mmol/L).

**Test Interactions** ↑ calcium (S), glucose, magnesium, potassium (S); ↓ thyroxine (S)

**Patient Information** Avoid tasks requiring psychomotor coordination until the CNS effects are known, blood level monitoring is required to determine the proper dose; maintain a steady salt and fluid intake especially during the summer months; do not crush or chew slow or extended release dosage form, swallow whole

**Nursing Implications** Give with meals to decrease GI upset; avoid dehydration

**Additional Information**
Lithium citrate: Cibalith-S®
Lithium carbonate: Eskalith®, Lithane®, Lithobid®, Lithonate®, Lithotabs®

**Dosage Forms**
Capsule, as carbonate: 150 mg, 300 mg, 600 mg
Syrup, as citrate: 300 mg/5 mL (5 mL, 10 mL, 480 mL)
Tablet, as carbonate: 300 mg
Tablet:
Controlled release, as carbonate: 450 mg
Slow release, as carbonate: 300 mg


♦ **Lithium Carbonate** *see* Lithium *on page 321*

♦ **Lithium Citrate** *see* Lithium *on page 321*

♦ **Lithobid®** *see* Lithium *on page 321*

♦ **Lithonate®** *see* Lithium *on page 321*

♦ **Lithotabs®** *see* Lithium *on page 321*

♦ **Livostin®** *see* Levocabastine *on page 312*


## L-Lysine (el LYE seen)

**U.S. Brand Names** Enisyl® [OTC]; Lycolan® Elixir [OTC]
**Pharmacologic Category** Nutritional Supplement
**Use** Improves utilization of vegetable proteins
**Effects on Mental Status** None reported
**Effects on Psychiatric Treatment** None reported
**Usual Dosage** Adults: Oral: 334-1500 mg/day
**Dosage Forms** l-lysine hydrochloride:
Capsule: 500 mg
Elixir: 100 mg/15 mL with glycine 1800 mg/15 mL and alcohol 12%
Tablet: 312 mg, 334 mg, 500 mg, 1000 mg


♦ **8-*L*-Lysine Vasopressin** *see* Lypressin *on page 329*

♦ ***Lobela inflata*** *see* Lobelia *on page 322*


## Lobelia

**Synonyms** *Lobela inflata*
**Pharmacologic Category** Herb
**Use** Primary use is in homeopathic products; in herbal medicine used as an expectorant; relief of muscle spasms; also incorporated (in doses of 2-4 mg) in tablets/lozenges or chewing gum to aid in smoking cessation

**Overdosage/Toxicology**
Signs and symptoms: Hypothermia, hypertension, respiratory depression, coma, paralysis, seizures, euphoria, nausea, vomiting, abdominal pain, salivation, dermal irritation, tachycardia, diaphoresis
Decontamination:
Oral: **Do not** induce emesis; lavage (within 1 hour)/ingestions >8 mg of lobeline, 50 mg of dried herb or 1 mL of tincture of lobelia; activated charcoal with cathartic can then be used
Occular: Irrigate with saline copiously
Dermal: Wash with soap and water
Treatment: Supportive therapy; seizures can be treated with benzodiazepines; phenobarbital or phenytoin can be used for refractory seizures; hypotension can be treated with intravenous fluid bolus (10-20 mL/kg) and placement in Trendelenburg position; dopamine or norepinephrine can be used for refractory cases

**Usual Dosage**
Toxic dose:
Dried herb: 50 mg
Lobelia, tincture: 1 mL
Lobeline: 8 mg
Toxic daily dose: >20 mg
Therapeutic dose:
Lobeline hydrochloride:
S.C.: 10 mg (up to 20 mg/day)
I.V.: 3 mg (maximum daily dose: 20 mg)
Lobeline sulfate: 2-4 mg

**Patient Information** Considered unsafe; nicotine-like effect; use only for short-term and <50 mg

**Additional Information** Not reviewed by Commission E; found in eastern North America with small, pale blue flowers; acrid/bitter taste; can cause euphoria; an annual weed which grows by roadsides and in open woods; irritating odor; contains 6% piperidine alkaloids


♦ **LoCHOLEST®** *see* Cholestyramine Resin *on page 120*

♦ **LoCHOLEST® Light** *see* Cholestyramine Resin *on page 120*

♦ **Locoid®** *see* Hydrocortisone *on page 273*

♦ **Lodine®** *see* Etodolac *on page 215*

♦ **Lodine® XL** *see* Etodolac *on page 215*


## Lodoxamide Tromethamine

(loe DOKS a mide troe METH a meen)

**U.S. Brand Names** Alomide® Ophthalmic
**Pharmacologic Category** Mast Cell Stabilizer
**Use** Treatment of vernal keratoconjunctivitis, vernal conjunctivitis, and vernal keratitis
**Effects on Mental Status** May cause drowsiness or dizziness
**Effects on Psychiatric Treatment** None reported
**Pregnancy Risk Factor** B
**Contraindications** Hypersensitivity to any component of product
**Warnings/Precautions** Safety and efficacy in children <2 years of age have not been established; not for injection; not for use in patients wearing soft contact lenses during treatment

**Adverse Reactions**
>10%: Local: Transient burning, stinging, discomfort
1% to 10%:
Central nervous system: Headache
Ocular: Blurred vision, corneal erosion/ulcer, eye pain, corneal abrasion, blepharitis
<1%: Dizziness, dry nose, nausea, rash, sneezing, somnolence, stomach discomfort

**Overdosage/Toxicology**
Signs and symptoms: Feeling of warmth of flushing, headache, dizziness, fatigue, sweating, nausea, loose stools, and urinary frequency/urgency
Treatment: Consider emesis in the event of accidental ingestion

**Drug Interactions** No data reported
**Usual Dosage** Children >2 years and Adults: Instill 1-2 drops in eye(s) 4 times/day for up to 3 months
**Patient Information** Do not wear soft contact lenses during treatment
**Dosage Forms** Solution, ophthalmic: 0.1% (10 mL)


♦ **Loestrin®** *see* Ethinyl Estradiol and Norethindrone *on page 212*

- **Logen®** *see* Diphenoxylate and Atropine *on page 175*
- **Lomanate®** *see* Diphenoxylate and Atropine *on page 175*

## Lomefloxacin (loe me FLOKS a sin)

**U.S. Brand Names** Maxaquin®

**Pharmacologic Category** Antibiotic, Quinolone

**Use** Lower respiratory infections, acute bacterial exacerbation of chronic bronchitis, skin infections, sexually transmitted diseases, and urinary tract infections caused by *E. coli, K. pneumoniae, P. mirabilis, P. aeruginosa*; also has gram-positive activity including *S. pneumoniae* and some staphylococci

**Effects on Mental Status** Dizziness is common; may cause sedation; quinolones reported to cause restlessness, confusion, depression, paranoia, euphoria, panic, and hallucinations

**Effects on Psychiatric Treatment** Inhibits CYP1A2 isoenzyme; use caution with clozapine and other psychotropics; monitor for adverse effects

**Pregnancy Risk Factor** C

**Contraindications** Hypersensitivity to lomefloxacin or other members of the quinolone group such as nalidixic acid, oxolinic acid, cinoxacin, norfloxacin, and ciprofloxacin; avoid use in children <18 years of age due to association of other quinolones with transient arthropathies

**Warnings/Precautions** Use with caution in patients with epilepsy or other CNS diseases which could predispose them to seizures.

**Adverse Reactions**

1% to 10%:

Central nervous system: Headache, dizziness

Dermatologic: Photosensitivity

Gastrointestinal: Nausea

<1%: Abdominal pain, abnormal taste, allergic reaction, angina pectoris, anuria, arrhythmia, back pain, bradycardia, cardiac failure, chest pain, chills, coma, constipation, convulsions, cough, cyanosis, decreased heat tolerance, diaphoresis (increased), discoloration of tongue, dyspnea, dysuria, earache, edema, epistaxis, extrasystoles, facial edema, fatigue, flatulence, flu-like symptoms, flushing, gout, hematuria, hyperkinesia, hypertension, hypoglycemia, hypotension, increased fibrinolysis, leg cramps, malaise, myalgia, myocardial infarction, paresthesias, purpura, rash, syncope, tachycardia, thirst, thrombocytopenia, tremor, urinary disorders, vertigo, vomiting, weakness, xerostomia

**Overdosage/Toxicology**

Signs and symptoms: Acute renal failure, seizures

Treatment: GI decontamination and supportive care; diazepam for seizures; not removed by peritoneal or hemodialysis

**Drug Interactions**

Decreased effect: Decreased absorption with antacids containing aluminum, magnesium, and/or calcium (by up to 98% if given at the same time), sucralfate, didanosine, divalent and trivalent cations

Increased toxicity/serum levels: Quinolones cause increased levels of caffeine, warfarin, cyclosporine, and theophylline; cimetidine, probenecid increase quinolone levels

**Usual Dosage**

Lower respiratory and urinary tract infections (UTI): Adults: Oral: 400 mg once daily for 10-14 days

Urinary tract infection (UTI) due to susceptible organisms:

Uncomplicated cystitis caused by *Escherichia coli*: Adult female: Oral: 400 mg once daily for 3 successive days

Uncomplicated cystitis caused by *Klebsiella pneumoniae, Proteus mirabilis*, or *Staphylococcus saprophyticus*: Adult female: 400 mg once daily for 10 successive days

Complicated UTI caused by *Escherichia coli, Klebsiella penumoniae, Proteus mirabilis*, or *Pseudomonas aeruginosa*: Adults: Oral: 400 mg once daily for 14 successive days

Surgical prophylaxis: 400 mg 2-6 hours before surgery

Uncomplicated gonorrhea: 400 mg as a single dose

No dosage adjustment is needed for elderly patients with normal renal function

**Dosing adjustment in renal impairment:**

$Cl_{cr}$ 11-39 mL/minute: Loading dose: 400 mg; then 200 mg every day

Hemodialysis: Same as above

**Dietary Considerations** May be taken without regard to meals

**Patient Information** Take as directed, preferably on an empty stomach 1 hour before or 2 hours after meals. Complete entire prescription even if feeling better. Maintain adequate hydration (2-3 L/day of fluids unless instructed to restrict fluid intake). You may experience dizziness or drowsiness; use caution when driving or engaging in tasks that require alertness until response to drug is known. You may experience photosensitivity (use sunscreen, wear protective clothing and eyewear, and avoid direct sunlight). Can take in the evening to reduce risk of photosensitivity. Report any signs of opportunistic infection (eg, fever, chills, vaginal itching or foul-smelling vaginal discharge, oral thrush, easy bruising). Report immediately any signs of allergic reaction (eg, rash, itching or tingling of skin); join pain; difficulty breathing; CNS changes (excitability, seizures); pain, inflammation, or rupture of tendon; or abdominal cramping or pain.

**Dosage Forms** Tablet, as hydrochloride: 400 mg

- **Lomotil®** *see* Diphenoxylate and Atropine *on page 175*

## Lomustine (loe MUS teen)

**U.S. Brand Names** CeeNU®

**Synonyms** CCNU

**Pharmacologic Category** Antineoplastic Agent, Alkylating Agent

**Use** Treatment of brain tumors and Hodgkin's disease, non-Hodgkin's lymphoma, melanoma, renal carcinoma, lung cancer, colon cancer

**Effects on Mental Status** May rarely cause sedation or disorientation

**Effects on Psychiatric Treatment** Myelosuppression is common; avoid usage with clozapine and carbamazepine; concurrent use with phenobarbital may result in diminished efficacy of both drugs

**Pregnancy Risk Factor** D

**Contraindications** Hypersensitivity to lomustine or any component

**Warnings/Precautions** The U.S. Food and Drug Administration (FDA) currently recommends that procedures for proper handling and disposal for antineoplastic agents be considered. Bone marrow suppression, notably thrombocytopenia and leukopenia, may lead to bleeding and overwhelming infections in an already compromised patient; will last for at least 6 weeks after a dose, do not administer courses more frequently than every 6 weeks because the toxicity is cumulative. Use with caution in patients with depressed platelet, leukocyte or erythrocyte counts, liver function abnormalities.

**Adverse Reactions**

>10%:

Gastrointestinal: Nausea and vomiting occur 3-6 hours after oral administration; this is due to a centrally mediated mechanism, not a direct effect on the GI lining; if vomiting occurs, it is not necessary to replace the dose unless it occurs immediately after drug administration

Emetic potential:

<60 mg: Moderately high (60% to 90%)

≥60 mg: High (>90%)

Time course of nausea/vomiting: Onset: 2-6 hours; Duration: 4-6 hours

Hematologic: Myelosuppression: Anemia; effects occur 4-6 weeks after a dose and may persist for 1-2 weeks

WBC: Moderate

Platelets: Severe

Onset (days): 14

Nadir (weeks): 4-5

Recovery (weeks): 6

1% to 10%:

Central nervous system: Neurotoxicity

Dermatologic: Skin rash

Gastrointestinal: Stomatitis, diarrhea

Hematologic: Anemia

<1%: Alopecia, ataxia, disorientation, dysarthria, hepatotoxicity, lethargy, pulmonary fibrosis with cumulative doses >600 mg, renal failure

**Overdosage/Toxicology**

Signs and symptoms: Nausea, vomiting, leukopenia; there are no known antidotes

Treatment: Primarily symptomatic and supportive

**Drug Interactions** CYP2D6 enzyme inhibitor

Decreased effect with phenobarbital, resulting in decreased efficacy of both drugs

Increased toxicity with cimetidine, reported to cause bone marrow suppression or to potentiate the myelosuppressive effects of lomustine

**Usual Dosage** Oral (refer to individual protocols):

Children: 75-150 mg/m$^2$ as a single dose every 6 weeks; subsequent doses are readjusted after initial treatment according to platelet and leukocyte counts

Adults: 100-130 mg/m$^2$ as a single dose every 6 weeks; readjust after initial treatment according to platelet and leukocyte counts

With compromised marrow function: Initial dose: 100 mg/m$^2$ as a single dose every 6 weeks

Repeat courses should only be administered after adequate recovery: WBC >4000 and platelet counts >100,000

**Subsequent dosing adjustment based on nadir:**

Leukocytes 2000-2900/mm$^3$, platelets 25,000-74,999/mm$^3$: Administer 70% of prior dose

Leukocytes <2000/mm$^3$, platelets <25,000/mm$^3$: Administer 50% of prior dose

**Dosage adjustment in renal impairment:**

$Cl_{cr}$ 10-50 mL/minute: Administer 75% of normal dose

$Cl_{cr}$ <10 mL/minute: Administer 50% of normal dose

Hemodialysis: Supplemental dose is not necessary

Peritoneal dialysis: Significant drug removal is unlikely based on physiochemical characteristics

**Patient Information** Take with fluids on an empty stomach; do not eat or drink for 2 hours following administration. Do not use alcohol, aspirin, or aspirin-containing medications and OTC medications without consulting prescriber. Maintain adequate fluid balance (2-3 L/day of fluids unless instructed to restrict fluid intake). May cause hair loss (reversible); easy bleeding or bruising (use soft toothbrush or cotton swabs and frequent mouth care, use electric razor, avoid sharp knives or scissors); increased

(Continued)

## Lomustine *(Continued)*

susceptibility to infection (avoid crowds or exposure to infection - do not have any vaccinations unless approved by prescriber). Report unusual bleeding or bruising or persistent fever or sore throat; blood in urine, stool, or vomitus; delayed healing of any wounds; skin rash; yellowing of skin or eyes; changes in color of urine of stool.

**Dosage Forms**
Capsule: 10 mg, 40 mg, 100 mg
Dose Pack: 10 mg (2s); 100 mg (2s); 40 mg (2s)

♦ **Loniten®** *see* Minoxidil *on page 368*

♦ **Lonox®** *see* Diphenoxylate and Atropine *on page 175*

♦ **Lo/Ovral®** *see* Ethinyl Estradiol and Norgestrel *on page 213*

## Loperamide (loe PER a mide)

**U.S. Brand Names** Diar-aid® [OTC]; Imodium®; Imodium® A-D [OTC]; Kaopectate® II [OTC]; Pepto® Diarrhea Control [OTC]

**Canadian Brand Names** PMS-Loperamine

**Pharmacologic Category** Antidiarrheal

**Use** Treatment of acute diarrhea and chronic diarrhea associated with inflammatory bowel disease; chronic functional diarrhea (idiopathic), chronic diarrhea caused by bowel resection or organic lesions; to decrease the volume of ileostomy discharge

**Unlabeled use:** Treatment of traveler's diarrhea in combination with trimethoprim-sulfamethoxazole (co-trimoxazole) (3 days therapy)

**Effects on Mental Status** May cause drowsiness or dizziness

**Effects on Psychiatric Treatment** Concurrent use with psychotropics may produce additive sedation and dry mouth

**Pregnancy Risk Factor** B

**Contraindications** Patients who must avoid constipation, diarrhea resulting from some infections, or in patients with pseudomembranous colitis, hypersensitivity to specific drug or component, bloody diarrhea

**Warnings/Precautions** Large first-pass metabolism, use with caution in hepatic dysfunction; should not be used if diarrhea accompanied by high fever, blood in stool

**Adverse Reactions** Percentage unknown: Abdominal cramping, abdominal distention, constipation, dizziness, drowsiness, fatigue, nausea, rash, sedation, vomiting, xerostomia

**Overdosage/Toxicology**
Signs and symptoms: CNS and respiratory depression, gastrointestinal cramping, constipation, GI irritation, nausea, vomiting; overdosage is noted when daily doses approximate 60 mg of loperamide
Treatment: Gastric lavage followed by 100 g activated charcoal through a nasogastric tube. Monitor for signs of CNS depression; if they occur, administer naloxone 2 mg I.V. (0.01 mg/kg for children) with repeat administration as necessary up to a total of 10 mg.

**Drug Interactions** Increased toxicity: CNS depressants, phenothiazines, tricyclic antidepressants may potentiate the adverse effects

**Usual Dosage** Oral:
Children:
Acute diarrhea: Initial doses (in first 24 hours):
2-6 years: 1 mg 3 times/day
6-8 years: 2 mg twice daily
8-12 years: 2 mg 3 times/day
Maintenance: After initial dosing, 0.1 mg/kg doses after each loose stool, but not exceeding initial dosage
Chronic diarrhea: 0.08-0.24 mg/kg/day divided 2-3 times/day, maximum: 2 mg/dose
Adults: Initial: 4 mg (2 capsules), followed by 2 mg after each loose stool, up to 16 mg/day (8 capsules)

**Patient Information** Do not take more than 8 capsules or 80 mL in 24 hours. May cause drowsiness. If acute diarrhea lasts longer than 48 hours, consult prescriber. Do not take if diarrhea is bloody.

**Nursing Implications** Therapy for chronic diarrhea should not exceed 10 days

**Dosage Forms**
Caplet, as hydrochloride: 2 mg
Capsule, as hydrochloride: 2 mg
Liquid, oral, as hydrochloride: 1 mg/5 mL (60 mL, 90 mL, 120 mL)
Tablet, as hydrochloride: 2 mg

♦ **Lopid®** *see* Gemfibrozil *on page 247*

♦ **Lopressor®** *see* Metoprolol *on page 362*

♦ **Loprox®** *see* Ciclopirox *on page 122*

♦ **Lorabid™** *see* Loracarbef *on page 324*

## Loracarbef (lor a KAR bef)

**U.S. Brand Names** Lorabid™

**Pharmacologic Category** Antibiotic, Carbacephem

**Use** Infections caused by susceptible organisms involving the respiratory tract, acute otitis media, sinusitis, skin and skin structure, bone and joint, and urinary tract and gynecologic

**Effects on Mental Status** May cause nervousness; cephalosporins reported to cause illusions, delusion, depersonalization, and euphoria

**Effects on Psychiatric Treatment** May cause neutropenia; use caution with clozapine and carbamazepine

**Pregnancy Risk Factor** B

**Contraindications** Patients with a history of hypersensitivity to loracarbef or cephalosporins

**Warnings/Precautions** Modify dosage in patients with severe renal impairment; prolonged use may result in superinfection; use with caution in patients with a previous history of hypersensitivity to other beta-lactam antibiotics (eg, penicillins, cephalosporins)

**Adverse Reactions**
>1%: Gastrointestinal: Diarrhea
<1%: Arthralgia, candidiasis, cholestatic jaundice, eosinophilia, headache, hemolytic anemia, interstitial nephritis, nausea, nephrotoxicity with transient elevations of BUN/creatinine, nervousness, neutropenia, positive Coombs' test, pruritus, pseudomembranous colitis, rash, seizures (with high doses and renal dysfunction), serum sickness, slightly increased AST/ALT, Stevens-Johnson syndrome, thrombocytopenia, urticaria, vomiting

**Overdosage/Toxicology**
Signs and symptoms: Abdominal discomfort, diarrhea
Treatment: Supportive care only

**Drug Interactions**
Increased effect: Probenecid may decrease cephalosporin elimination
Increased toxicity: Furosemide, aminoglycosides may be a possible additive to nephrotoxicity

**Usual Dosage** Oral:
Children:
Acute otitis media: 15 mg/kg twice daily for 10 days
Pharyngitis and impetigo: 7.5-15 mg/kg twice daily for 10 days
Adults:
Uncomplicated urinary tract infections: 200 mg once daily for 7 days
Skin and soft tissue: 200-400 mg every 12-24 hours
Uncomplicated pyelonephritis: 400 mg every 12 hours for 14 days
Upper/lower respiratory tract infection: 200-400 mg every 12-24 hours for 7-14 days

**Dosing comments in renal impairment:**
$Cl_{cr}$ 10-49 mL/minute: 50% of usual dose at usual interval or usual dose given half as often
$Cl_{cr}$ <10 mL/minute: Administer usual dose every 3-5 days
Hemodialysis: Doses should be administered after dialysis sessions

**Patient Information** Take as directed, preferably on an empty stomach (30 minutes before or 2 hours after meals). Take entire prescription even if feeling better. Maintain adequate hydration (2-3 L/day of fluids unless instructed to restrict fluid intake). You may experience nausea, vomiting, or anorexia (small frequent meals, frequent mouth care, sucking lozenges, or chewing gum may help). Report immediately any signs of skin rash, joint or back pain, or difficulty breathing. Report unusual fever, chills, vaginal itching or foul-smelling vaginal discharge, or easy bruising or bleeding.

**Dosage Forms**
Capsule: 200 mg, 400 mg
Suspension, oral: 100 mg/5 mL (50 mL, 100 mL); 200 mg/5 mL (50 mL, 100 mL)

## Loratadine (lor AT a deen)

**U.S. Brand Names** Claritin® RediTabs®; Claritin® Syrup; Claritin® Tablets

**Synonyms** SCH-29851

**Pharmacologic Category** Antihistamine

**Use** Relief of nasal and non-nasal symptoms of seasonal allergic rhinitis

**Effects on Mental Status** Drowsiness is common; may cause anxiety or depression

**Effects on Psychiatric Treatment** None reported

**Pregnancy Risk Factor** B

**Contraindications** Hypersensitivity to loratadine or any of its components

**Warnings/Precautions** Patients with liver impairment or renal impairment ($Cl_{cr}$ <30 mL/minute) should start with a lower dose (10 mg every other day), since their ability to clear the drug will be reduced; use with caution in lactation. Safety and efficacy in children <6 years of age have not been established.

**Adverse Reactions**
>10%:
Central nervous system: Headache, somnolence, fatigue
Gastrointestinal: Xerostomia
1% to 10%:
Cardiovascular: Hypotension, hypertension, palpitations, tachycardia
Central nervous system: Anxiety, depression
Endocrine & metabolic: Breast pain
Neuromuscular & skeletal: Hyperkinesia, arthralgias
Respiratory: Nasal dryness, pharyngitis, dyspnea
Miscellaneous: Diaphoresis

**Overdosage/Toxicology**

Signs and symptoms: Somnolence, tachycardia, headache

Treatment: No specific antidote is available, treatment is first decontamination, then symptomatic and supportive; loratadine is not eliminated by dialysis

**Drug Interactions** CYP2D6 and 3A3/4 enzyme substrate

Increased plasma concentrations of loratadine and its active metabolite with ketoconazole; erythromycin increases the AUC of loratadine and its active metabolite; no change in $QT_c$ interval was seen

Increased toxicity: Procarbazine, other antihistamines, alcohol

**Usual Dosage** Children ≥6 years and Adults: Oral: 10 mg/day on an empty stomach

**Dosing interval in hepatic impairment:** 10 mg every other day to start

**Patient Information** Take as directed; do not exceed recommended dose. Avoid use of other depressants, alcohol, or sleep-inducing medications unless approved by prescriber. You may experience drowsiness or dizziness (use caution when driving or engaging in tasks requiring alertness until response to drug is known); or dry mouth or nausea (frequent small meals, frequent mouth care, chewing gum, or sucking hard candy may help). Report persistent dizziness, sedation, or seizures; chest pain, rapid heartbeat, or palpitations; swelling of face, mouth, lips, or tongue; difficulty breathing; changes in urinary pattern; yellowing of skin or eyes, dark urine, or pale stool; or lack of improvement or worsening or condition.

**Dosage Forms**

Syrup: 1 mg/mL (480 mL)

Tablet: 10 mg

Rapid-disintegrating tablets: 10 mg (RediTabs®)

## Loratadine and Pseudoephedrine

(lor AT a deen & soo doe e FED rin)

**Generic Available** No

**U.S. Brand Names** Claritin-D® 12-Hour; Claritin-D® 24-Hour

**Canadian Brand Names** Chlor-Tripolon® N.D.; Claritin® Extra

**Pharmacologic Category** Antihistamine/Decongestant Combination

**Use** Temporary relief of symptoms of seasonal allergic rhinitis and nasal congestion

**Effects on Mental Status** Dizziness, drowsiness, nervousness, and insomnia are common; may cause anxiety or depression; may rarely cause hallucinations

**Effects on Psychiatric Treatment** Contraindicated with MAOIs

**Usual Dosage** Children ≥12 years and Adults: Oral:

Claritin-D® 12-Hour: 1 tablet every 12 hours

Claritin-D® 24-Hour: 1 tablet daily

**Dosage adjustment in renal impairment:**

Claritin-D® 12-Hour: 1 tablet daily

Claritin-D® 24-Hour: 1 tablet every other day

**Dosage Forms** Tablet:

Extended release, 12-hour: Loratadine 5 mg and pseudoephedrine sulfate 120 mg

Extended release, 24-hour: Loratadine 10 mg and pseudoephedrine sulfate 240 mg

## Lorazepam (lor A ze pam)

**Related Information**

Agents for Treatment of Extrapyramidal Symptoms *on page 638*
Anxiolytic/Hypnotic Use in Long-Term Care Facilities *on page 754*
Benzodiazepines Comparison Chart *on page 708*
Clinical Issues in the Use of Anxiolytics and Sedative/Hypnotics *on page 634*
Federal OBRA Regulations Recommended Maximum Doses *on page 756*
Mood Disorders *on page 600*
Patient Information - Anxiolytics & Sedative Hypnotics (Benzodiazepines) *on page 653*
Personality Disorders *on page 625*
Schizophrenia *on page 604*
Secondary Mental Disorders *on page 616*
Substance-Related Disorders *on page 609*

**Generic Available** Yes

**U.S. Brand Names** Ativan®

**Canadian Brand Names** Apo®-Lorazepam; Novo-Lorazepam; Nu-Loraz; PMS-Lorazepam; Pro-Lorazepam®

**Pharmacologic Category** Benzodiazepine

**Use**

Oral: Management of anxiety disorders or short-term relief of the symptoms of anxiety or anxiety associated with depressive symptoms

I.V.: Status epilepticus, preanesthesia

**Unlabeled uses:** Alcohol detoxification; insomnia; psychogenic catatonia; partial complex seizures; antiemetic adjunct

**Restrictions** C-IV

**Pregnancy Risk Factor** D

**Pregnancy/Breast-Feeding Implications**

Clinical effects on the fetus: Crosses the placenta. Respiratory depression or hypotonia if administered near time of delivery.

Breast-feeding/lactation: Crosses into breast milk and no data on clinical effects on the infant. American Academy of Pediatrics states **may be of concern.**

**Contraindications** Hypersensitivity to this drug or any component of its formulation (cross-sensitivity with other benzodiazepines may exist); acute narrow-angle glaucoma; sleep apnea (parenteral); intra-arterial injection of parenteral formulation; severe respiratory insufficiency (except during mechanical ventilation); pregnancy

**Warnings/Precautions** Use with caution in elderly or debilitated patients, patients with hepatic disease (including alcoholics) or renal impairment. Use with caution in patients with respiratory disease or impaired gag reflex. Initial doses in elderly or debilitated patients should not exceed 2 mg. Prolonged lorazepam use may have a possible relationship to GI disease, including esophageal dilation.

The parenteral formulation of lorazepam contains polyethylene glycol and propylene glycol. Each agent has been associated with specific toxicities when administered in prolonged infusions at high dosages. Also contains benzyl alcohol - avoid rapid injection in neonates or prolonged infusions. Intra-arterial injection or extravasation should be avoided. Concurrent administration with scopolamine results in an increased risk of hallucinations, sedation, and irrational behavior.

Causes CNS depression (dose-related) resulting in sedation, dizziness, confusion, or ataxia which may impair physical and mental capabilities. Patients must be cautioned about performing tasks which require mental alertness (ie, operating machinery or driving). Use with caution in patients receiving other CNS depressants or psychoactive agents. Effects with other sedative drugs or ethanol may be potentiated. Benzodiazepines have been associated with falls and traumatic injury and should be used with extreme caution in patients who are at risk of these events (especially the elderly).

Lorazepam may cause anterograde amnesia. Paradoxical reactions, including hyperactive or aggressive behavior have been reported with benzodiazepines, particularly in adolescent/pediatric or psychiatric patients. Does not have analgesic, antidepressant, or antipsychotic properties.

Use caution in patients with depression, particularly if suicidal risk may be present. Use with caution in patients with a history of drug dependence. Benzodiazepines have been associated with dependence and acute withdrawal symptoms on discontinuation or reduction in dose. Acute withdrawal, including seizures, may be precipitated after administration of flumazenil to patients receiving long-term benzodiazepine therapy.

As a hypnotic agent, should be used only after evaluation of potential causes of sleep disturbance. Failure of sleep disturbance to resolve after 7-10 days may indicate psychiatric or medical illness. A worsening of insomnia or the emergence of new abnormalities of thought or behavior may represent unrecognized psychiatric or medical illness and requires immediate and careful evaluation.

**Adverse Reactions**

>10%:

Central nervous system: Sedation

Respiratory: Respiratory depression

1% to 10%:

Cardiovascular: Hypotension

Central nervous system: Confusion, dizziness, akathisia, unsteadiness, headache, depression, disorientation, amnesia

Dermatologic: Dermatitis, rash

Gastrointestinal: Weight gain or loss, nausea, changes in appetite

Neuromuscular & skeletal: Weakness

Respiratory: Nasal congestion, hyperventilation, apnea

<1%: Blood dyscrasias, increased salivation, menstrual irregularities, physical and psychological dependence with prolonged use, reflex slowing

**Overdosage/Toxicology**

Signs and symptoms: Confusion, coma, hypoactive reflexes, dyspnea, labored breathing

Treatment for benzodiazepine overdose is supportive. Rarely is mechanical ventilation required.

Flumazenil has been shown to selectively block the binding of benzodiazepines to CNS receptors, resulting in a reversal of benzodiazepine-induced CNS depression but not respiratory depression

**Drug Interactions** CYP3A3/4 enzyme substrate

CNS depressants: Sedative effects and/or respiratory depression may be additive with CNS depressants; includes ethanol, barbiturates, narcotic analgesics, and other sedative agents; monitor for increased effect

CYP3A3/4 inhibitors: Serum level and/or toxicity of some benzodiazepines may be increased; inhibitors include amiodarone, cimetidine, clarithromycin, erythromycin, delavirdine, diltiazem, dirithromycin, disulfiram, fluoxetine, fluvoxamine, grapefruit juice, indinavir, itraconazole, ketoconazole, metronidazole, nefazodone, nevirapine, propoxyfene, quinupristin-dalfopristin, ritonavir, saquinavir, verapamil, zafirlukast, zileuton; monitor for altered benzodiazepine response

(Continued)

## Lorazepam *(Continued)*

Enzyme inducers: Metabolism of some benzodiazepines may be increased, decreasing their therapeutic effect; consider using an alternative sedative/hypnotic agent; potential inducers include phenobarbital, phenytoin, carbamazepine, rifampin, and rifabutin

Levodopa: Lorazepam may decrease the antiparkinsonian efficacy of levodopa (limited documentation); monitor

Loxapine: There are rare reports of significant respiratory depression, stupor, and/or hypotension with concomitant use of loxapine and lorazepam; use caution if concomitant administration of loxapine and CNS drugs is required

Oral contraceptives: May decrease the clearance of some benzodiazepines (those which undergo oxidative metabolism); monitor for increased benzodiazepine effect

Scopolamine: May increase the incidence of sedation, hallucinations, and irrational behavior; reported only with parenteral lorazepam

Theophylline: May partially antagonize some of the effects of benzodiazepines; monitor for decreased response; may require higher doses for sedation

**Stability**

Intact vials should be refrigerated, protected from light; do not use discolored or precipitate containing solutions

May be stored at room temperature for up to 60 days

Stability of parenteral admixture at room temperature (25°C): 24 hours

Standard diluent: 1 mg/100 mL $D_5W$

I.V. is **incompatible** when administered in the same line with foscarnet, ondansetron, sargramostim

**Mechanism of Action** Binds to stereospecific benzodiazepine receptors on the postsynaptic GABA neuron at several sites within the central nervous system, including the limbic system, reticular formation. Enhancement of the inhibitory effect of GABA on neuronal excitability results by increased neuronal membrane permeability to chloride ions. This shift in chloride ions results in hyperpolarization (a less excitable state) and stabilization.

**Pharmacodynamics/kinetics**

Onset of hypnosis: I.M.: 20-30 minutes

Duration: 6-8 hours

Absorption: Oral, I.M.: Prompt following administration

Distribution: Crosses the placenta; appears in breast milk

$V_d$:

Neonates: 0.76 L/kg

Adults: 1.3 L/kg

Protein binding: 85%, free fraction may be significantly higher in elderly

Metabolism: In the liver to inactive compounds

Half-life:

Neonates: 40.2 hours

Older Children: 10.5 hours

Adults: 12.9 hours

Elderly: 15.9 hours

End-stage renal disease: 32-70 hours

Elimination: Urinary excretion and minimal fecal clearance

**Usual Dosage**

Antiemetic:

Children 2-15 years: I.V.: 0.05 mg/kg (up to 2 mg/dose) prior to chemotherapy

Adults: Oral, I.V.: 0.5-2 mg every 4-6 hours as needed

Anxiety and sedation:

Infants and Children: Oral, I.V.: Usual: 0.05 mg/kg/dose (range: 0.02-0.09 mg/kg) every 4-8 hours

Adults: Oral: 1-10 mg/day in 2-3 divided doses; usual dose: 2-6 mg/day in divided doses

Elderly: 0.5-4 mg/day

Insomnia: Adults: Oral: 2-4 mg at bedtime

Preoperative: Adults:

I.M.: 0.05 mg/kg administered 2 hours before surgery; maximum: 4 mg/dose

I.V.: 0.044 mg/kg 15-20 minutes before surgery; usual maximum: 2 mg/dose

Operative amnesia: Adults: I.V.: Up to 0.05 mg/kg; maximum: 4 mg/dose

Status epilepticus: I.V.:

Infants and Children: 0.1 mg/kg slow I.V. over 2-5 minutes, do not exceed 4 mg/single dose; may repeat second dose of 0.05 mg/kg slow I.V. in 10-15 minutes if needed

Adolescents: 0.07 mg/kg slow I.V. over 2-5 minutes; maximum: 4 mg/dose; may repeat in 10-15 minutes

Adults: 4 mg/dose given slowly over 2-5 minutes; may repeat in 10-15 minutes; usual maximum dose: 8 mg

Rapid tranquilization of agitated patient (administer every 30-60 minutes):

Oral: 1-2 mg

I.M.: 0.5-1 mg

Average total dose for tranquilization: 4-8 mg

**Dietary Considerations** Alcohol: Additive CNS depression has been reported with benzodiazepines; avoid or limit alcohol

**Administration**

Lorazepam may be administered by I.M. or I.V.

I.M.: Should be administered deep into the muscle mass

I.V.: Do not exceed 2 mg/minute or 0.05 mg/kg over 2-5 minutes

Dilute I.V. dose with equal volume of compatible diluent ($D_5W$, NS, SWI)

Injection must be made slowly with repeated aspiration to make sure the injection is not intra-arterial and that perivascular extravasation has not occurred

**Monitoring Parameters** Respiratory and cardiovascular status, blood pressure, heart rate, symptoms of anxiety

**Reference Range** Therapeutic: 50-240 ng/mL (SI: 156-746 nmol/L)

**Test Interactions** May increase the results of liver function tests

**Patient Information** Advise patient of potential for physical and psychological dependence with chronic use; do not use alcohol; advise patient of possible retrograde amnesia after I.V. or I.M. use; will cause drowsiness, impairment of judgment or coordination

**Nursing Implications** Keep injectable form in the refrigerator; **inadvertent intra-arterial injection may produce arteriospasm resulting in gangrene which may require amputation;** emergency resuscitative equipment should be available when administering by I.V.; prior to I.V. use, lorazepam injection must be diluted with an equal amount of compatible diluent; injection must be made slowly with repeated aspiration to make sure the injection is not intra-arterial and that perivascular extravasation has not occurred; provide safety measures (ie, side rails, night light, and call button); supervise ambulation

**Additional Information** Oral doses >0.09 mg/kg produced ↑ ataxia without ↑ sedative benefit vs lower doses; preferred anxiolytic when I.M. route needed

**Dosage Forms**

Injection: 2 mg/mL (1 mL, 10 mL); 4 mg/mL (1 mL, 10 mL)

Solution, oral concentrated, alcohol and dye free: 2 mg/mL (30 mL)

Tablet: 0.5 mg, 1 mg, 2 mg


♦ **Lorcet®** *see* Hydrocodone and Acetaminophen *on page 272*

♦ **Lorcet®-HD** *see* Hydrocodone and Acetaminophen *on page 272*

♦ **Lorcet® Plus** *see* Hydrocodone and Acetaminophen *on page 272*

♦ **Loroxide® [OTC]** *see* Benzoyl Peroxide *on page 62*

♦ **Lortab®** *see* Hydrocodone and Acetaminophen *on page 272*

♦ **Lortab® ASA** *see* Hydrocodone and Aspirin *on page 272*


## Losartan (loe SAR tan)

**Related Information**

Angiotensin-Related Agents Comparison Chart *on page 700*

**U.S. Brand Names** Cozaar®

**Synonyms** DuP 753; Losartan Potassium; MK594

**Pharmacologic Category** Angiotensin II Antagonists

**Use** Treatment of hypertension with or without concurrent use of thiazide diuretics

**Effects on Mental Status** May cause dizziness or insomnia; may rarely cause anxiety, confusion, depression, and sleep disorders

**Effects on Psychiatric Treatment** Barbiturates may decrease the effects of losartan

**Pregnancy Risk Factor** C (1st trimester); D (2nd and 3rd trimester)

**Contraindications** Hypersensitivity to losartan or any component; hypersensitivity to other A-II receptor antagonists; primary hyperaldosteronism; bilateral renal artery stenosis; pregnancy (2nd and 3rd trimesters)

**Warnings/Precautions** Avoid use or use a smaller dose in patients who are volume depleted; correct depletion first. Deterioration in renal function can occur with initiation. Use with caution in unilateral renal artery stenosis and pre-existing renal insufficiency; significant aortic/mitral stenosis.

**Adverse Reactions**

1% to 10%:

Cardiovascular: Hypotension without reflex tachycardia

Central nervous system: Dizziness, insomnia

Endocrine & metabolic: Hyperkalemia

Gastrointestinal: Diarrhea, dyspepsia

Hematologic: Slight decreases in hemoglobin and hematocrit

Neuromuscular & skeletal: Back/leg pain, myalgia

Renal: Hypouricemia (with large doses)

Respiratory: Cough (less than ACE inhibitors), nasal congestion, sinus disorders, sinusitis

<1%: Abnormal taste, alopecia, angina, anorexia, anxiety; arm, hip, shoulder, and knee pain; ataxia, blurred vision, bronchitis, bruising, burning and stinging eyes, confusion, conjunctivitis, constipation, CVA, decreased libido, decreased visual acuity, depression, dermatitis, diaphoresis, dream abnormality, dry skin, dyspnea, epistaxis, erythema, facial edema, fever, fibromyalgia, flatulence, flushing, gastritis, gout, headache, impotence, joint edema, migraine, mild increases in BUN/creatinine, muscle weakness, nocturia, orthostatic effects, palpitations, paresthesia, pharyngeal discomfort, photosensitivity, polyuria, pruritus, rash, respiratory congestion, rhinitis, second degree A-V block, sinus bradycardia, sleep disorders, slightly elevated LFTs and bilirubin, tachycardia, tinnitus, tremor, urinary tract infection, urticaria, vertigo, vomiting

**Overdosage/Toxicology**
Signs and symptoms may occur with very significant overdosages including hypotension and tachycardia
Treatment: Supportive

**Drug Interactions** CYP2C9 substrate and CYP3A3/4 substrate
Inhibitors of CYP2C9 or CYP3A3/4 may increase blood levels
Fluconazole (and possibly other azoles) decreases the plasma level of losartan's active metabolite; monitor for decreased efficacy
Lithium: Risk of toxicity may be increased by losartan; monitor lithium levels
Potassium-sparing diuretics (amiloride, potassium, spironolactone, triamterene): Increased risk of hyperkalemia
Potassium supplements may increase the risk of hyperkalemia
Rifampin may reduce antihypertensive efficacy of losartan
Trimethoprim (high dose) may increase the risk of hyperkalemia

**Usual Dosage**
Oral: The usual starting dose is 50 mg once daily. Can be administered once or twice daily with total daily doses ranging from 25 mg to 100 mg.
Usual initial doses in patients receiving diuretics or those with intravascular volume depletion: 25 mg
Patients not receiving diuretics: 50 mg
**Dosing adjustment in renal impairment**: None necessary
**Dosing adjustment in hepatic impairment or geriatric patients**: Reduce the initial dose to 25 mg; divide dosage intervals into two.
Not removed via hemodialysis

**Patient Information** Take exactly as directed; do not discontinue without consulting prescriber. Take first dose at bedtime. This drug does not eliminate need for diet or exercise regimen as recommended by prescriber. May cause dizziness, fainting, lightheadedness (use caution when driving or engaging in tasks that require alertness until response to drug is known); diarrhea (buttermilk, boiled milk, yogurt may help). Report chest pain or palpitations; unrelenting headache; swelling of extremities, face, or tongue; difficulty in breathing or unusual cough; flu-like symptoms; or other persistent adverse reactions

**Nursing Implications** Observe for symptomatic hypotension and tachycardia especially in patients with CHF; hyponatremia, high-dose diuretics, or severe volume depletion

**Dosage Forms** Tablet, film coated, as potassium: 25 mg, 50 mg

## Losartan and Hydrochlorothiazide
(loe SAR tan & hye droe klor oh THYE a zide)

**U.S. Brand Names** Hyzaar®
**Pharmacologic Category** Antihypertensive Agent, Combination
**Use** Treatment of hypertension
**Effects on Mental Status** May cause dizziness or insomnia; may rarely cause anxiety, confusion, depression, and sleep disorders
**Effects on Psychiatric Treatment** Barbiturates may decrease the effects of losartan; may decrease lithium clearance resulting in an increase in serum lithium levels and potential lithium toxicity; monitor serum lithium levels
**Usual Dosage** Adults: Oral: 1 tablet daily
**Dosage Forms** Tablet: Losartan potassium 50 mg and hydrochlorothiazide 12.5 mg; losartan potassium 100 mg and hydrochlorothiazide 25 mg

- **Losartan Potassium** *see* Losartan *on page 326*
- **Lotemax®** *see* Loteprednol *on page 327*
- **Lotensin®** *see* Benazepril *on page 60*
- **Lotensin® HCT** *see* Benazepril and Hydrochlorothiazide *on page 61*

## Loteprednol (loe te PRED nol)

**U.S. Brand Names** Alrex™; Lotemax®
**Pharmacologic Category** Corticosteroid, Ophthalmic
**Use**
0.2% suspension (Alrex™): Temporary relief of signs and symptoms of seasonal allergic conjunctivitis
0.5% suspension (Lotemax®): Inflammatory conditions (treatment of steroid-responsive inflammatory conditions of the palpebral and bulbar conjunctiva, cornea, and anterior segment of the globe such as allergic conjunctivitis, acne rosacea, superficial punctate keratitis, herpes zoster keratitis, iritis, cyclitis, selected infective conjunctivitis, when the inherent hazard of steroid use is accepted to obtain an advisable diminution in edema and inflammation) and treatment of postoperative inflammation following ocular surgery
**Effects on Mental Status** None reported
**Effects on Psychiatric Treatment** None reported
**Usual Dosage** Adults: Ophthalmic:
0.2% suspension (Alrex™): Instill 1 drop into affected eye(s) 4 times/day
0.5% suspension (Lotemax®):
Inflammatory conditions: Apply 1-2 drops into the conjunctival sac of the affected eye(s) 4 times/day. During the initial treatment within the first week, the dosing may be increased up to 1 drop every hour. Advise patients not to discontinue therapy prematurely. If signs and symptoms fail to improve after 2 days, re-evaluate the patient.
Postoperative inflammation: Apply 1-2 drops into the conjunctival sac of the operated eye(s) 4 times/day beginning 24 hours after surgery and continuing throughout the first 2 weeks of the postoperative period
**Dosage Forms** Suspension, ophthalmic, as etabonate:
0.2% (Alrex™): 5 mL, 10 mL
0.5% (Lotemax®): 2.5 mL, 5 mL, 10 mL, 15 mL

- **Lotrel®** *see* Amlodipine and Benazepril *on page 35*
- **Lotrimin®** *see* Clotrimazole *on page 135*
- **Lotrimin® AF Cream [OTC]** *see* Clotrimazole *on page 135*
- **Lotrimin® AF Lotion [OTC]** *see* Clotrimazole *on page 135*
- **Lotrimin® AF Powder [OTC]** *see* Miconazole *on page 364*
- **Lotrimin® AF Solution [OTC]** *see* Clotrimazole *on page 135*
- **Lotrimin® AF Spray Liquid [OTC]** *see* Miconazole *on page 364*
- **Lotrimin® AF Spray Powder [OTC]** *see* Miconazole *on page 364*
- **Lotrisone®** *see* Betamethasone and Clotrimazole *on page 66*
- **Lotronex®** *see* Alosetron *on page 25*

## Lovastatin (LOE va sta tin)

**Related Information**
Lipid-Lowering Agents Comparison Chart *on page 717*
**U.S. Brand Names** Mevacor®
**Canadian Brand Names** Apo®-Lovastatin
**Synonyms** Mevinolin; Monacolin K
**Pharmacologic Category** Antilipemic Agent (HMG-CoA Reductase Inhibitor)
**Use** Adjunct to dietary therapy to decrease elevated serum total and LDL cholesterol concentrations in primary hypercholesterolemia; primary prevention of coronary artery disease (patients without symptomatic disease with average to moderately elevated total and LDL cholesterol and below average HDL cholesterol)
**Effects on Mental Status** May cause dizziness
**Effects on Psychiatric Treatment** None reported
**Pregnancy Risk Factor** X
**Contraindications** Hypersensitivity to lovastatin or any component; active liver disease; unexplained persistent elevations of serum transaminases; pregnancy
**Warnings/Precautions** Liver function must be monitored by periodic laboratory assessment. Rhabdomyolysis with acute renal failure has occurred. Risk is increased with concurrent use of clarithromycin, danazol, diltiazem, fluvoxamine, indinavir, nefazodone, nelfinavir, ritonavir, verapamil, troleandomycin, cyclosporine, fibric acid derivatives, erythromycin, niacin, or azole antifungals. Weigh the risk versus benefit when combining any of these drugs with lovastatin. Temporarily discontinue in any patient experiencing an acute or serious condition predisposing to renal failure secondary to rhabdomyolysis. Use with caution in patients who consume large amounts of alcohol or have a history of liver disease.
**Adverse Reactions**
1% to 10%:
Central nervous system: Headache, dizziness
Dermatologic: Rash, pruritus
Gastrointestinal: Flatulence, abdominal pain, cramps, diarrhea, pancreatitis, constipation, nausea, dyspepsia, heartburn
Neuromuscular & skeletal: Myalgia, increased CPK
<1%: Abnormal taste, blurred vision, gynecomastia, lenticular opacities, myositis
**Overdosage/Toxicology**
Signs and symptoms: Very few adverse events
Treatment: Symptomatic
**Drug Interactions** CYP3A3/4 substrate
Inhibitors of CYP3A3/4 (clarithromycin, cyclosporine, danazol, diltiazem, fluvoxamine, erythromycin, fluconazole, itraconazole, ketoconazole, miconazole, nefazodone,amprenavir, indinavir, nelfinavir, ritonavir, saquinavir, troleandomycin, and verapamil) increase lovastatin blood levels; may increase the risk of lovastatin-induced myopathy and rhabdomyolysis.
Cholestyramine reduces absorption of several HMG-CoA reductase inhibitors. Separate administration times by at least 4 hours.
Cholestyramine and colestipol (bile acid sequestrants): Cholesterol-lowering effects are additive
Clofibrate and fenofibrate may increase the risk of myopathy and rhabdomyolysis
Gemfibrozil: Increased risk of myopathy and rhabdomyolysis
Grapefruit juice may inhibit metabolism of lovastatin via CYP3A3/4; avoid high dietary intakes of grapefruit juice
Isradipine may decrease lovastatin blood levels
Niacin may increase risk of myopathy and rhabdomyolysis
(Continued)

## Lovastatin *(Continued)*

Warfarin effect (hypoprothrombinemic response) may be increased; monitor INR closely when lovastatin is initiated or discontinued

**Usual Dosage** Adults: Oral: Initial: 20 mg with evening meal, then adjust at 4-week intervals; maximum dose: 80 mg/day; before initiation of therapy, patients should be placed on a standard cholesterol-lowering diet for 3-6 months and the diet should be continued during drug therapy

**Patient Information** Take with evening meal (highest rate of cholesterol synthesis occurs from midnight to morning). If sleep disturbances occur, take earlier in the day. Do not change dosage without consulting prescriber. Maintain diet and exercise program as identified by prescriber. Have periodic ophthalmic exams while taking lovastatin (check for cataracts). You may experience mild GI disturbances (eg, gas, diarrhea, constipation); inform prescriber if these are severe or if you experience severe muscle pain, weakness, or tenderness.

**Nursing Implications** Urge patient to adhere to cholesterol-lowering diet

**Dosage Forms** Tablet: 10 mg, 20 mg, 40 mg

♦ **Lovenox® Injection** *see* Enoxaparin *on page 193*

## Loxapine (LOKS a peen)

**Related Information**

Antipsychotic Medication Guidelines *on page 751*
Clinical Issues in the Use of Antipsychotics *on page 630*
Discontinuation of Psychotropic Drugs - Withdrawal Symptoms and Recommendations *on page 798*
Federal OBRA Regulations Recommended Maximum Doses *on page 756*
Liquid Compatibility With Antipsychotics and Mood Stabilizers *on page 718*
Patient Information - Antipsychotics (General) *on page 646*

**Generic Available** Yes

**U.S. Brand Names** Loxitane®; Loxitane® C; Loxitane® I.M.

**Canadian Brand Names** Loxapac®

**Synonyms** Loxapine Hydrochloride; Loxapine Succinate; Oxilapine Succinate

**Pharmacologic Category** Antipsychotic Agent, Dibenzoxazepine

**Use** Management of psychotic disorders

**Pregnancy Risk Factor** C

**Contraindications** Hypersensitivity to loxapine or any component; severe CNS depression and coma

**Warnings/Precautions** May cause hypotension, particularly with I.M. administration. Moderately sedating, use with caution in disorders where CNS depression is a feature. Use with caution in Parkinson's disease. Caution in patients with hemodynamic instability; bone marrow suppression; predisposition to seizures; subcortical brain damage; severe cardiac, hepatic, renal or respiratory disease. Esophageal dysmotility and aspiration have been associated with antipsychotic use - use with caution in patients at risk of pneumonia (ie, Alzheimer's disease). Caution in breast cancer or other prolactin-dependent tumors (may elevate prolactin levels). May alter temperature regulation or mask toxicity of other drugs due to antiemetic effects. May alter cardiac conduction; life-threatening arrhythmias have occurred with therapeutic doses of phenothiazines. May cause orthostatic hypotension - use with caution in patients at risk of this effect or those who would tolerate transient hypotensive episodes (cerebrovascular disease, cardiovascular disease, or other medications which may predispose). Safety and effectiveness of loxapine in pediatric patients have not been established.

Phenothiazines may cause anticholinergic effects (confusion, agitation, constipation, dry mouth, blurred vision, urinary retention); therefore, they should be used with caution in patients with decreased gastrointestinal motility, urinary retention, BPH, xerostomia, or visual problems. Conditions which also may be exacerbated by cholinergic blockade include narrow-angle glaucoma (screening is recommended) and worsening of myasthenia gravis. Relative to other antipsychotics, loxapine has a low potency of cholinergic blockade.

May cause extrapyramidal reactions, including pseudoparkinsonism, acute dystonic reactions, akathisia, and tardive dyskinesia (risk of these reactions is moderate-high relative to other neuroleptics). May be associated with neuroleptic malignant syndrome (NMS) or pigmentary retinopathy.

**Adverse Reactions**

Cardiovascular: Orthostatic hypotension, tachycardia, arrhythmias, abnormal T-waves with prolonged ventricular repolarization, hypertension, hypotension, lightheadedness, syncope

Central nervous system: Drowsiness, extrapyramidal reactions (dystonia, akathisia, pseudoparkinsonism, tardive dyskinesia, akinesia), dizziness, faintness, ataxia, insomnia, agitation, tension, seizures, slurred speech, confusion, headache, neuroleptic malignant syndrome (NMS), altered central temperature regulation

Dermatologic: Rash, pruritus, photosensitivity, dermatitis, alopecia, seborrhea

Endocrine & metabolic: Enlargement of breasts, galactorrhea, amenorrhea, gynecomastia, menstrual irregularity

Gastrointestinal: Xerostomia, constipation, nausea, vomiting, nasal congestion, weight gain or loss, adynamic ileus, polydipsia

Genitourinary: Urinary retention, sexual dysfunction

Hematologic: Agranulocytosis, leukopenia, thrombocytopenia

Neuromuscular & skeletal: Weakness

Ocular: Blurred vision

**Overdosage/Toxicology**

Signs and symptoms: Deep sleep, dystonia, agitation, dysrhythmias, extrapyramidal symptoms, hypotension, seizures

Treatment:

Following initiation of essential overdose management, toxic symptom treatment and supportive treatment should be initiated

Hypotension usually responds to I.V. fluids or Trendelenburg positioning. If unresponsive to these measures, the use of a parenteral inotrope may be required (eg, norepinephrine 0.1-0.2 mcg/kg/minute titrated to response).

Seizures commonly respond to diazepam (I.V. 5-10 mg bolus in adults every 15 minutes if needed up to a total of 30 mg; I.V. 0.25-0.4 mg/kg/dose up to a total of 10 mg in children) or to phenytoin or phenobarbital.

Critical cardiac arrhythmias often respond to I.V. phenytoin (15 mg/kg up to 1 gram), while other antiarrhythmics can be used

Neuroleptics often cause extrapyramidal symptoms (eg, dystonic reactions) requiring management with diphenhydramine 1-2 mg/kg (adults) up to a maximum of 50 mg I.M. or I.V. slow push followed by a maintenance dose for 48-72 hours. When these reactions are unresponsive to diphenhydramine, benztropine mesylate I.V. 1-2 mg (adults) may be effective. These agents are generally effective within 2-5 minutes.

**Drug Interactions**

Aluminum salts: May decrease the absorption of antipsychotics; monitor

Amphetamines: Efficacy may be diminished by antipsychotics; in addition, amphetamines may increase psychotic symptoms; avoid concurrent use

Anticholinergics: May inhibit the therapeutic response to antipsychotics and excess anticholinergic effects may occur; includes benztropine, trihexyphenidyl, biperiden, and drugs with significant anticholinergic activity (TCAs, antihistamines, disopyramide)

Antihypertensives: Concurrent use of antipsychotics with an antihypertensive may produce additive hypotensive effects (particularly orthostasis)

Bromocriptine: Antipsychotics inhibit the ability of bromocriptine to lower serum prolactin concentrations

CNS depressants: Sedative effects may be additive with antipsychotics; monitor for increased effect; includes barbiturates, benzodiazepines, narcotic analgesics, ethanol, and other sedative agents

Enzyme inducers: May enhance the hepatic metabolism of antipsychotics. Larger doses may be required; includes rifampin, rifabutin, barbiturates, phenytoin, and cigarette smoking

Epinephrine: Chlorpromazine (and possibly other low potency antipsychotics) may diminish the pressor effects of epinephrine

Guanethidine and guanadrel: Antihypertensive effects may be inhibited by antipsychotics

Levodopa: Antipsychotics may inhibit the antiparkinsonian effect of levodopa; avoid this combination

Lithium: Antipsychotics may produce neurotoxicity with lithium; this is a rare effect

Phenytoin: May reduce serum levels of antipsychotics; antipsychotics may increase phenytoin serum levels

Propranolol: Serum concentrations of antipsychotics may be increased; propranolol also increases antipsychotic concentrations

QTc prolonging agents: Effects on QTc interval may be additive with antipsychotics, increasing the risk of malignant arrhythmias. Includes type Ia antiarrhythmics, TCAs, and some quinolone antibiotics (sparfloxacin, moxifloxacin and gatifloxacin)

Sulfadoxine-pyrimethamine: May increase antipsychotic concentrations

Tricyclic antidepressants: Concurrent use may produce increased toxicity or altered therapeutic response

Trazodone: Antipsychotics and trazodone may produce additive hypotensive effects

Valproic acid: Serum levels may be increased by antipsychotics

**Stability** Protect from light; dispense in amber or opaque vials

**Mechanism of Action** Blocks postsynaptic mesolimbic D1 and D2 receptors in the brain, and also possesses serotonin 5HT2 blocking activity

**Pharmacodynamics/kinetics**

Onset of neuroleptic effect: Oral: Within 20-30 minutes

Peak effect: 1.5-3 hours

Duration: ~12 hours

Metabolism: Hepatic to glucuronide conjugates

Half-life, biphasic:

Initial: 5 hours

Terminal: 12-19 hours

Elimination: In urine, and to a smaller degree, feces

**Usual Dosage** Adults:

Oral: 10 mg twice daily, increase dose until psychotic symptoms are controlled; usual dose range: 20-100 mg/day in divided doses 2-4 times/day; dosages >250 mg/day are not recommended

Elderly: 20-60 mg/day

I.M.: 12.5-50 mg every 4-6 hours or longer as needed and change to oral therapy as soon as possible
Rapid tranquilization of agitated patient:
Oral: 25 mg
I.M.: 10-15 mg
Average total dose for tranquilization: 30-60 mg

**Dietary Considerations** Alcohol: Additive CNS effect, avoid use

**Administration** Injectable is for I.M. use only

**Monitoring Parameters** EKG, CBC, blood pressure, electrolytes, pH

**Reference Range** Not useful

**Test Interactions** False-positives for phenylketonuria, amylase, uroporphyrins, urobilinogen; ↑ liver function tests, cholesterol (S), prolactin, glucose; ↓ uric acid (S)

**Patient Information** May cause drowsiness; avoid alcoholic beverages; may impair judgment or coordination; may cause photosensitivity; avoid excessive sunlight; do not stop taking without consulting physician

**Additional Information**
Loxapine hydrochloride: Loxitane® C oral concentrate, Loxitane® IM
Loxapine succinate: Loxitane® capsule

**Dosage Forms**
Capsule, as succinate: 5 mg, 10 mg, 25 mg, 50 mg
Concentrate, oral, as hydrochloride: 25 mg/mL (120 mL dropper bottle)
Injection, as hydrochloride: 50 mg/mL (1 mL)


- **Loxapine Hydrochloride** *see* Loxapine *on page 328*
- **Loxapine Succinate** *see* Loxapine *on page 328*
- **Loxitane®** *see* Loxapine *on page 328*
- **Loxitane® C** *see* Loxapine *on page 328*
- **Loxitane® I.M.** *see* Loxapine *on page 328*
- **Lozol®** *see* Indapamide *on page 285*
- **L-PAM** *see* Melphalan *on page 339*
- **L-Sarcolysin** *see* Melphalan *on page 339*
- **LTG** *see* Lamotrigine *on page 306*
- ***L*-Thyroxine Sodium** *see* Levothyroxine *on page 316*
- **Lubriderm® [OTC]** *see* Lanolin, Cetyl Alcohol, Glycerin, and Petrolatum *on page 307*
- **LubriTears® Solution [OTC]** *see* Artificial Tears *on page 48*
- **Ludiomil®** *see* Maprotiline *on page 332*
- **Lufyllin®** *see* Dyphylline *on page 189*
- **Lugol's Solution** *see* Potassium Iodide *on page 454*
- **Luminal®** *see* Phenobarbital *on page 435*
- **Lupron®** *see* Leuprolide *on page 310*
- **Lupron Depot®** *see* Leuprolide *on page 310*
- **Lupron Depot-3® Month** *see* Leuprolide *on page 310*
- **Lupron Depot-4® Month** *see* Leuprolide *on page 310*
- **Lupron Depot-Ped®** *see* Leuprolide *on page 310*
- **Lutrepulse®** *see* Gonadorelin *on page 254*
- **Luvox®** *see* Fluvoxamine *on page 237*
- **LY170053** *see* Olanzapine *on page 403*
- **LY-237216** *see* Dirithromycin *on page 177*
- **Lycolan® Elixir [OTC]** *see* L-Lysine *on page 322*


## Lyme Disease Vaccine (LIME dee seas vak SEEN)

**U.S. Brand Names** LYMErix™

**Pharmacologic Category** Vaccine

**Use** Active immunization against Lyme disease in individuals between 15-70 years of age. Individuals most at risk are those who live, work, or travel to *B. burgdorferi*-infected, tick-infested, grassy/wooded areas.

**Effects on Mental Status** May cause fatigue or dizziness

**Effects on Psychiatric Treatment** None reported

**Usual Dosage** Adults: I.M.: Vaccination with 3 doses of 30 mcg (0.5 mL), administered at 0, 1, and 12 months, is recommended for optimal protection

**Dosage Forms** Injection:
Vial: 30 mcg/0.5 mL
Prefilled syringe (Tip-Lok™): 30 mcg/0.5 mL


- **LYMErix™** *see* Lyme Disease Vaccine *on page 329*


## Lymphocyte Immune Globulin
(LIM foe site i MYUN GLOB yoo lin)

**U.S. Brand Names** Atgam®

**Pharmacologic Category** Immunosuppressant Agent

**Use** Prevention and treatment of acute renal and other solid organ allograft rejection; treatment of moderate to severe aplastic anemia in patients not considered suitable candidates for bone marrow transplantation; prevention of graft-versus-host disease following bone marrow transplantation

**Effects on Mental Status** May cause malaise

**Effects on Psychiatric Treatment** Leukopenia is common use caution with clozapine and carbamazepine

**Usual Dosage** An intradermal skin test is recommended prior to administration of the initial dose of ATG; use 0.1 mL of a 1:1000 dilution of ATG in normal saline. A positive skin reaction consists of a wheal ≥10 mm in diameter. If a positive skin test occurs, the first infusion should be administered in a controlled environment with intensive life support immediately available. A systemic reaction precludes further administration of the drug. The absence of a reaction does **not** preclude the possibility of an immediate sensitivity reaction.

First dose: Premedicate with diphenhydramine 50 mg orally 30 minutes prior to and hydrocortisone 100 mg I.V. 15 minutes prior to infusion and acetaminophen 650 mg 2 hours after start of infusion
Children: I.V.:
Aplastic anemia protocol: 10-20 mg/kg/day for 8-14 days; then administer every other day for 7 more doses; addition doses may be given every other day for 21 total doses in 28 days
Renal allograft: 5-25 mg/kg/day
Adults: I.V.:
Aplastic anemia protocol: 10-20 mg/kg/day for 8-14 days, then administer every other day for 7 more doses
Renal allograft:
Rejection prophylaxis: 15 mg/kg/day for 14 days followed by 14 days of alternative day therapy at the same dose; the first dose should be administered within 24 hours before or after transplantation
Rejection treatment: 10-15 mg/kg/day for 14 days, then administer every other day for 10-14 days up to 21 doses in 28 days

**Dosage Forms** Injection: 50 mg of equine IgG/mL (5 mL)


- **Lyphocin®** *see* Vancomycin *on page 580*


## Lypressin (lye PRES in)

**U.S. Brand Names** Diapid® Nasal Spray

**Synonyms** 8-*L*-Lysine Vasopressin

**Pharmacologic Category** Antidiuretic Hormone Analog

**Use** Controls or prevents signs and complications of neurogenic diabetes insipidus

**Effects on Mental Status** May cause dizziness

**Effects on Psychiatric Treatment** Carbamazepine may produce prolongation of antidiuretic effects

**Pregnancy Risk Factor** C

**Contraindications** Known hypersensitivity to lypressin

**Warnings/Precautions** Use with caution in patients with coronary artery disease

**Adverse Reactions**
1% to 10%:
Cardiovascular: Chest tightness
Central nervous system: Dizziness, headache
Endocrine & metabolic: Water intoxication
Gastrointestinal: Abdominal cramping, increased bowel movements
Local: Irritation or burning
Respiratory: Coughing, dyspnea, rhinorrhea, nasal congestion
<1%: Inadvertent inhalation

**Overdosage/Toxicology** Signs and symptoms: Drowsiness, headache, confusion, weight gain, hypertension; systemic toxicity is unlikely to occur from the nasal spray

**Drug Interactions** Increased effect: Chlorpropamide, clofibrate, carbamazepine → prolongation of antidiuretic effects

**Usual Dosage** Children and Adults: Instill 1-2 sprays into one or both nostrils whenever frequency of urination increases or significant thirst develops; usual dosage is 1-2 sprays 4 times/day; range: 1 spray/day at bedtime to 10 sprays each nostril every 3-4 hours

**Patient Information** To control nocturia, an additional dose may be given at bedtime. Notify prescriber if drowsiness, fatigue, headache, shortness of breath, abdominal cramps, or severe nasal irritation occurs.

**Dosage Forms** Spray: 0.185 mg/mL (equivalent to 50 USP posterior pituitary units/mL) (8 mL)


- **Lysodren®** *see* Mitotane *on page 369*
- **Maalox® [OTC]** *see* Aluminum Hydroxide and Magnesium Hydroxide *on page 28*
- **Maalox® Anti-Gas [OTC]** *see* Simethicone *on page 512*

◆ **Maalox® Therapeutic Concentrate [OTC]** *see* Aluminum Hydroxide and Magnesium Hydroxide *on page 28*

◆ **Macrobid®** *see* Nitrofurantoin *on page 396*

◆ **Macrodantin®** *see* Nitrofurantoin *on page 396*

## Magaldrate (MAG al drate)

**U.S. Brand Names** Riopan® [OTC]
**Pharmacologic Category** Antacid
**Use** Symptomatic relief of hyperacidity associated with peptic ulcer, gastritis, peptic esophagitis and hiatal hernia
**Effects on Mental Status** None reported
**Effects on Psychiatric Treatment** None reported
**Usual Dosage** Adults: Oral: 540-1080 mg between meals and at bedtime
**Dosage Forms** Suspension, oral: 540 mg/5 mL (360 mL)

## Magaldrate and Simethicone
(MAG al drate & sye METH i kone)

**U.S. Brand Names** Riopan Plus® [OTC]
**Canadian Brand Names** Riopan® Plus Extra Strength
**Pharmacologic Category** Antacid; Antiflatulent
**Use** Relief of hyperacidity associated with peptic ulcer, gastritis, peptic esophagitis and hiatal hernia which are accompanied by symptoms of gas
**Effects on Mental Status** None reported
**Effects on Psychiatric Treatment** Constipation is common; concurrent use with psychotropics may produce additive effects
**Usual Dosage** Adults: Oral: 5-10 mL between meals and at bedtime
**Dosage Forms** Suspension, oral: Magaldrate 480 mg and simethicone 20 mg per 5 mL (360 mL)

◆ **Magalox Plus® [OTC]** *see* Aluminum Hydroxide, Magnesium Hydroxide, and Simethicone *on page 28*

◆ **Magan®** *see* Magnesium Salicylate *on page 331*

## Magnesium (mag NEE zhum)

**Related Information**
Laxatives, Classification and Properties *on page 716*
**U.S. Brand Names** Magonate® [OTC]
**Pharmacologic Category** Magnesium Salt
**Use** Dietary supplement for treatment of magnesium deficiencies
**Effects on Mental Status** None reported
**Effects on Psychiatric Treatment** None reported
**Contraindications** Patients with heart block; severe renal disease
**Warnings/Precautions** Use with caution in patients with impaired renal function; hypermagnesemia and toxicity may occur due to decreased renal clearance of absorbed magnesium
**Adverse Reactions** 1% to 10%: Gastrointestinal: Diarrhea (excessive dose)
**Overdosage/Toxicology**
Signs and symptoms: Hypermagnesemia rarely occurs after acute or chronic overexposure except in patients with renal insufficiency or massive overdose; moderate toxicity causes nausea, vomiting, weakness, and cutaneous flushing; larger doses cause cardiac conduction abnormalities, hypotension, severe muscle weakness, and lethargy; very high levels cause coma, respiratory arrest, and asystole.
Treatment: Includes replacing fluid and electrolyte losses caused by excessive catharsis; while there is no specific antidote and treatment is supportive, administration of I.V. calcium may temporarily alleviate respiratory depression; hemodialysis rapidly removes magnesium and is the only route of elimination in anuric patients (hemoperfusion and repeat-dose charcoal are not effective).
**Drug Interactions**
Increased effect of nondepolarizing neuromuscular blockers
Decreased absorption of aminoquinolones, digoxin, nitrofurantoin, penicillamine, and tetracyclines may occur with magnesium salts
**Usual Dosage** The recommended dietary allowance (RDA) of magnesium is 4.5 mg/kg which is a total daily allowance of 350-400 mg for adult men and 280-300 mg for adult women. During pregnancy the RDA is 300 mg and during lactation the RDA is 355 mg.

Dietary supplement: Oral:
Children: 3-6 mg/kg/day in divided doses 3-4 times/day; maximum: 400 mg/day
Adults: 54-483 mg/day in divided doses; refer to product labeling

**Dosing in renal impairment:** Patients in severe renal failure should not receive magnesium due to toxicity from accumulation. Patients with a $Cl_{cr}$ <25 mL/minute receiving magnesium should be monitored by serum magnesium levels.
**Dosage Forms**
Gluconate:
Liquid: 54 mg/5 mL as magnesium
Tablet: 500 mg (elemental magnesium 27 mg)
Oxide:
Capsule: 140 mg (84.5 mg magnesium)
Tablet: 400 mg (241.3 mg magnesium)
Chloride: Tablet, sustained release: 535 mg (64 mg magnesium)
Amino acids chelate: Tablet: 500 mg (100 mg magnesium)

## Magnesium Chloride (mag NEE zhum KLOR ide)

**U.S. Brand Names** Slow-Mag® [OTC]
**Pharmacologic Category** Magnesium Salt
**Use** Correct or prevent hypomagnesemia
**Effects on Mental Status** May cause somnolence
**Effects on Psychiatric Treatment** Concurrent use with psychotropics may produce additive sedation
**Usual Dosage**
Oral: Adults: Dietary supplement: 54-283 mg/day in divided doses
I.V. in TPN:
Children: 2-10 mEq/day
The usual recommended pediatric maintenance intake of magnesium ranges from 0.2-0.6 mEq/kg/day. The dose of magnesium may also be based on the caloric intake; on that basis, 3-10 mEq/day of magnesium are needed; maximum maintenance dose: 8-16 mEq/day
Adults: 8-24 mEq/day
**Dosage Forms**
Injection: 200 mg/mL [1.97 mEq/mL] (30 mL, 50 mL)
Tablet: Elemental magnesium 64 mg

## Magnesium Citrate (mag NEE zhum SIT rate)

**U.S. Brand Names** Evac-Q-Mag® [OTC]
**Pharmacologic Category** Laxative, Saline; Magnesium Salt
**Use** Evacuation of bowel prior to certain surgical and diagnostic procedures or overdose situations
**Effects on Mental Status** None reported
**Effects on Psychiatric Treatment** None reported
**Usual Dosage** Cathartic: Oral:
Children:
<6 years: 0.5 mL/kg up to a maximum of 200 mL repeated every 4-6 hours until stools are clear
6-12 years: 100-150 mL
Adults ≥12 years: ½ to 1 full bottle (120-300 mL)
**Dosage Forms** Solution, oral: 300 mL

## Magnesium Hydroxide (mag NEE zhum hye DROKS ide)

**Related Information**
Laxatives, Classification and Properties *on page 716*
**U.S. Brand Names** Phillips'® Milk of Magnesia [OTC]
**Pharmacologic Category** Antacid; Laxative, Saline; Magnesium Salt
**Use** Short-term treatment of occasional constipation and symptoms of hyperacidity, magnesium replacement therapy
**Effects on Mental Status** None reported
**Effects on Psychiatric Treatment** None reported
**Usual Dosage** Oral:
Average daily intakes of dietary magnesium have declined in recent years due to processing of food; the latest estimate of the average American dietary intake was 349 mg/day
Laxative:
<2 years: 0.5 mL/kg/dose
2-5 years: 5-15 mL/day or in divided doses
6-12 years: 15-30 mL/day or in divided doses
≥12 years: 30-60 mL/day or in divided doses
Antacid:
Children: 2.5-5 mL as needed up to 4 times/day
Adults: 5-15 mL up to 4 times/day as needed
**Dosing in renal impairment:** Patients in severe renal failure should not receive magnesium due to toxicity from accumulation. Patients with a $Cl_{cr}$ <25 mL/minute receiving magnesium should be monitored by serum magnesium levels.
**Dosage Forms**
Liquid: 390 mg/5 mL (10 mL, 15 mL, 20 mL, 30 mL, 100 mL, 120 mL, 180 mL, 360 mL, 720 mL)
Liquid, concentrate: 10 mL equivalent to 30 mL milk of magnesia USP
Suspension, oral: 2.5 g/30 mL (10 mL, 15 mL, 30 mL)
Tablet: 300 mg, 600 mg

## Magnesium Hydroxide and Mineral Oil Emulsion
(mag NEE zhum hye DROKS ide & MIN er al oyl e MUL shun)

**U.S. Brand Names** Haley's M-O® [OTC]
**Pharmacologic Category** Laxative

**Use** Short-term treatment of occasional constipation
**Effects on Mental Status** None reported
**Effects on Psychiatric Treatment** None reported
**Usual Dosage** Adults: Oral: 5-45 mL at bedtime
**Dosage Forms** Suspension, oral: Equivalent to magnesium hydroxide 24 mL/mineral oil emulsion 6 mL (30 mL unit dose)

## Magnesium Oxide (mag NEE zhum OKS ide)

**U.S. Brand Names** Maox®
**Pharmacologic Category** Antacid; Electrolyte Supplement, Oral; Laxative, Saline; Magnesium Salt
**Use** Short-term treatment of occasional constipation and symptoms of hyperacidity
**Effects on Mental Status** May rarely cause depression
**Effects on Psychiatric Treatment** None reported
**Usual Dosage** Adults: Oral:
Dietary supplement: 20-40 mEq (1-2 tablets) 2-3 times
Antacid: 140 mg 3-4 times/day **or** 400-840 mg/day
Laxative: 2-4 g at bedtime with full glass of water
**Dosing in renal impairment:** Patients in severe renal failure should not receive magnesium due to toxicity from accumulation. Patients with a $Cl_{cr}$ <25 mL/minute should be monitored by serum magnesium levels.
**Note:** Oral magnesium is not generally adequate for repletion in patients with serum magnesium concentrations <1.5 mEq/L
**Dosage Forms**
Capsule: 140 mg
Tablet: 400 mg, 425 mg

## Magnesium Salicylate (mag NEE zhum sa LIS i late)

**U.S. Brand Names** Doan's®, Original [OTC]; Extra Strength Doan's® [OTC]; Magan®; Mobidin®
**Pharmacologic Category** Salicylate
**Use** Mild to moderate pain, fever, various inflammatory conditions
**Effects on Mental Status** None reported
**Effects on Psychiatric Treatment** None reported
**Usual Dosage** Oral: Adults: 650 mg 4 times daily or 1090 mg 3 times daily; may increase to 3.6-4.8 mg/day in 3 or 4 divided doses
**Dosage Forms**
Caplet:
Doan's®, Original: 325 mg
Extra Strength Doan's®: 500 mg
Tablet:
Magan®: 545 mg
Mobidin®: 600 mg

## Magnesium Sulfate (mag NEE zhum SUL fate)

**Synonyms** Epsom Salts
**Pharmacologic Category** Antacid; Anticonvulsant, Miscellaneous; Electrolyte Supplement, Parenteral; Laxative, Saline; Magnesium Salt
**Use** Treatment and prevention of hypomagnesemia and in seizure prevention in severe pre-eclampsia or eclampsia, pediatric acute nephritis; also used as short-term treatment of constipation, postmyocardial infarction, and torsade de pointes
**Effects on Mental Status** May cause sedation or CNS depression
**Effects on Psychiatric Treatment** Concurrent use with psychotropics may produce additive CNS depression
**Pregnancy Risk Factor** B
**Contraindications** Heart block, serious renal impairment, myocardial damage, hepatitis, Addison's disease
**Warnings/Precautions** Use with caution in patients with impaired renal function (accumulation of magnesium which may lead to magnesium intoxication); use with caution in digitalized patients (may alter cardiac conduction leading to heart block); monitor serum magnesium level, respiratory rate, deep tendon reflex, renal function when $MgSO_4$ is administered parenterally
**Adverse Reactions** 1% to 10%:
Serum magnesium levels >3 mg/dL:
Central nervous system: Depressed CNS
Gastrointestinal: Diarrhea
Neuromuscular & skeletal: Blocked peripheral neuromuscular transmission leading to anticonvulsant effects
Serum magnesium levels >5 mg/dL:
Cardiovascular: Flushing
Central nervous system: Somnolence
Serum magnesium levels >12.5 mg/dL:
Cardiovascular: Complete heart block
Respiratory: Respiratory paralysis
**Overdosage/Toxicology**
Signs and symptoms of overdose: Usually present with serum level >4 mEq/L
Serum magnesium >4 mEq/L: Deep tendon reflexes may be depressed
Serum magnesium ≥10 mEq/L: Deep tendon reflexes may disappear, respiratory paralysis may occur, heart block may occur
Serum level >12 mEq/L may be fatal, serum level ≥10 mEq/L may cause complete heart block
Treatment: I.V. calcium (5-10 mEq) 1-2 g calcium gluconate will reverse respiratory depression or heart block; in extreme cases, peritoneal dialysis or hemodialysis may be required
**Drug Interactions**
Decreased effect: Nifedipine decreased blood pressure and neuromuscular blockade
Increased toxicity: Aminoglycosides increased neuromuscular blockade; CNS depressants increased CNS depression; neuromuscular antagonists, betamethasone (pulmonary edema), ritodrine increased cardiotoxicity
**Usual Dosage** The recommended dietary allowance (RDA) of magnesium is 4.5 mg/kg which is a total daily allowance of 350-400 mg for adult men and 280-300 mg for adult women. During pregnancy the RDA is 300 mg and during lactation the RDA is 355 mg. Average daily intakes of dietary magnesium have declined in recent years due to processing of food. The latest estimate of the average American dietary intake was 349 mg/day. Dose represented as $MgSO_4$ unless stated otherwise.
**Note:** Serum magnesium is poor reflection of repletional status as the majority of magnesium is intracellular; serum levels may be transiently normal for a few hours after a dose is given, therefore, aim for consistently high normal serum levels in patients with normal renal function for most efficient repletion
Hypomagnesemia:
Neonates: I.V.: 25-50 mg/kg/dose (0.2-0.4 mEq/kg/dose) every 8-12 hours for 2-3 doses
Children: I.M., I.V.: 25-50 mg/kg/dose (0.2-0.4 mEq/kg/dose) every 4-6 hours for 3-4 doses, maximum single dose: 2000 mg (16 mEq), may repeat if hypomagnesemia persists (higher dosage up to 100 mg/kg/dose $MgSO_4$ I.V. has been used); maintenance: I.V.: 30-60 mg/kg/day (0.25-0.5 mEq/kg/day)
Adults:
Oral: 3 g every 6 hours for 4 doses as needed
I.M., I.V.: 1 g every 6 hours for 4 doses; for severe hypomagnesemia: 8-12 g $MgSO_4$/day in divided doses has been used
Management of seizures and hypertension: Children: I.M., I.V.: 20-100 mg/kg/dose every 4-6 hours as needed; in severe cases doses as high as 200 mg/kg/dose have been used
Eclampsia, pre-eclampsia: Adults:
I.M.: 1-4 g every 4 hours
I.V.: Initial: 4 g, then switch to I.M. or 1-4 g/hour by continuous infusion
Maximum dose should not exceed 30-40 g/day; maximum rate of infusion: 1-2 g/hour
Maintenance electrolyte requirements:
Daily requirements: 0.2-0.5 mEq/kg/24 hours or 3-10 mEq/1000 kcal/24 hours
Maximum: 8-16 mEq/24 hours
Cathartic: Oral:
Children: 0.25 g/kg every 4-6 hours
Adults: 10-15 g in a glass of water
**Dosing adjustment/comments in renal impairment:** $Cl_{cr}$ <25 mL/minute: Do not administer or monitor serum magnesium levels carefully
**Patient Information** Take in divided doses; report diarrhea (>5 stools/day) or changes in mental function to physician, nurse, or pharmacist
**Dosage Forms**
Granules: ~40 mEq magnesium/5 g (240 g)
Injection: 100 mg/mL (20 mL); 125 mg/mL (8 mL); 250 mg/mL (150 mL); 500 mg/mL (2 mL, 5 mL, 10 mL, 30 mL, 50 mL)
Solution, oral: 50% [500 mg/mL] (30 mL)


- **Magonate® [OTC]** *see* Magnesium *on page 330*
- **Ma-Huang** *see* Ephedra *on page 194*
- **Malarone™** *see* Atovaquone and Proguanil *on page 52*
- **Mallamint® [OTC]** *see* Calcium Carbonate *on page 84*
- **Mallazine® Eye Drops [OTC]** *see* Tetrahydrozoline *on page 538*
- **Mallisol® [OTC]** *see* Povidone-Iodine *on page 456*
- **Mandol®** *see* Cefamandole *on page 97*


## Mannitol (MAN i tole)

**U.S. Brand Names** Osmitrol® Injection; Resectisol® Irrigation Solution
**Synonyms** *D*-Mannitol
**Pharmacologic Category** Diuretic, Osmotic
**Use** Reduction of increased intracranial pressure associated with cerebral edema; promotion of diuresis in the prevention and/or treatment of oliguria or anuria due to acute renal failure; reduction of increased intraocular pressure; promoting urinary excretion of toxic substances; genitourinary irrigant in transurethral prostatic resection or other transurethral surgical procedures
(Continued)

## Mannitol *(Continued)*

**Effects on Mental Status** May cause dizziness

**Effects on Psychiatric Treatment** Has been used to treat lithium toxicity/overdose but its overall effect in lowering serum lithium level is minimum; if toxicity is severe, hemodialysis is the treatment of choice

**Pregnancy Risk Factor** C

**Contraindications** Severe renal disease (anuria), dehydration, or active intracranial bleeding, severe pulmonary edema or congestion, hypersensitivity to any component

**Warnings/Precautions** Should not be administered until adequacy of renal function and urine flow is established; cardiovascular status should also be evaluated; do not administer electrolyte-free mannitol solutions with blood

**Adverse Reactions**

>10%:
- Central nervous system: Headache
- Gastrointestinal: Nausea, vomiting
- Genitourinary: Polyuria

1% to 10%:
- Central nervous system: Dizziness
- Dermatologic: Rash
- Ocular: Blurred vision

<1%: Allergic reactions chills, circulatory overload, congestive heart failure, convulsions, dehydration and hypovolemia secondary to rapid diuresis, dysuria, fluid and electrolyte imbalance, headache, pulmonary edema, tissue necrosis, water intoxication, xerostomia

**Overdosage/Toxicology**

Signs and symptoms: Polyuria, hypotension, cardiovascular collapse, pulmonary edema, hyponatremia, hypokalemia, oliguria, seizures

Treatment: Increased electrolyte excretion and fluid overload can occur; hemodialysis will clear mannitol and reduce osmolality

**Drug Interactions** Lithium toxicity (with diuretic-induced hyponatremia)

**Usual Dosage** I.V.:

Children:
- Test dose (to assess adequate renal function): 200 mg/kg over 3-5 minutes to produce a urine flow of at least 1 mL/kg for 1-3 hours
- Initial: 0.5-1 g/kg
- Maintenance: 0.25-0.5 g/kg given every 4-6 hours

Adults:
- Test dose (to assess adequate renal function): 12.5 g (200 mg/kg) over 3-5 minutes to produce a urine flow of at least 30-50 mL of urine per hour over the next 2-3 hours
- Initial: 0.5-1 g/kg
- Maintenance: 0.25-0.5 g/kg every 4-6 hours; usual adult dose: 20-200 g/24 hours
- Intracranial pressure: Cerebral edema: 1.5-2 g/kg/dose I.V. as a 15% to 20% solution over ≥30 minutes; maintain serum osmolality 310-320 mOsm/kg
- Preoperative for neurosurgery: 1.5-2 g/kg administered 1-1.5 hours prior to surgery
- Transurethral irrigation: Use urogenital solution as required for irrigation

**Patient Information** This medication can only be given by infusion. Report immediately any muscle weakness, numbness, tingling, acute headache, nausea, dizziness, blurred vision, eye pain, difficulty breathing, chest pain, or pain at infusion site.

**Nursing Implications** Avoid extravasation; crenation and agglutination of red blood cells may occur if administered with whole blood

**Dosage Forms**

Injection: 5% [50 mg/mL] (1000 mL); 10% [100 mg/mL] (500 mL, 1000 mL); 15% [150 mg/mL] (150 mL, 500 mL); 20% [200 mg/mL] (150 mL, 250 mL, 500 mL); 25% [250 mg/mL] (50 mL)

Solution, urogenital: 0.54% [5.4 mg/mL] (2000 mL)

♦ **Mantoux** *see* Tuberculin Purified Protein Derivative *on page 575*

♦ **Maolate®** *see* Chlorphenesin *on page 113*

♦ **Maox®** *see* Magnesium Oxide *on page 331*

♦ **Mapap® [OTC]** *see* Acetaminophen *on page 14*

## Maprotiline (ma PROE ti leen)

**Related Information**

Antidepressant Agents Comparison Chart *on page 704*
Clinical Issues in the Use of Antidepressants *on page 627*
Discontinuation of Psychotropic Drugs - Withdrawal Symptoms and Recommendations *on page 798*
Federal OBRA Regulations Recommended Maximum Doses *on page 756*
Patient Information - Antidepressants (TCAs) *on page 640*
Teratogenic Risks of Psychotropic Medications *on page 812*

**Generic Available** Yes

**U.S. Brand Names** Ludiomil®

**Synonyms** Maprotiline Hydrochloride

**Pharmacologic Category** Antidepressant, Tetracyclic

**Use** Treatment of depression and anxiety associated with depression

**Unlabeled use:** Bulimia; duodenal ulcers; enuresis; urinary symptoms of multiple sclerosis; pain; panic attacks; schizophrenia; tension headache; cocaine withdrawal

**Pregnancy Risk Factor** B

**Contraindications** Hypersensitivity to maprotiline; use of monoamine oxidase inhibitors within 14 days; use in a patient during the acute recovery phase of MI

**Warnings/Precautions** May cause sedation, resulting in impaired performance of tasks requiring alertness (ie, operating machinery or driving). Sedative effects may be additive with other CNS depressants and/or ethanol. The degree of sedation is high relative to other antidepressants. May worsen psychosis in some patients or precipitate a shift to mania or hypomania in patients with bipolar disease. May increase the risks associated with electroconvulsive therapy. This agent should be discontinued, when possible, prior to elective surgery. Therapy should not be abruptly discontinued in patients receiving high doses for prolonged periods.

May cause orthostatic hypotension (risk is moderate relative to other antidepressants) - use with caution in patients at risk of hypotension or in patients where transient hypotensive episodes would be poorly tolerated (cardiovascular disease or cerebrovascular disease). The degree of anticholinergic blockade produced by this agent is moderate relative to other cyclic antidepressants, however, caution should still be used in patients with urinary retention, benign prostatic hypertrophy, narrow-angle glaucoma, xerostomia, visual problems, constipation, or history of bowel obstruction.

Use caution in patients with depression, particularly if suicidal risk may be present. Use with caution in patients with a history of cardiovascular disease (including previous MI, stroke, tachycardia, or conduction abnormalities). The risk conduction abnormalities with this agent is moderate relative to other antidepressants. Use caution in patients with a previous seizure disorder or condition predisposing to seizures such as brain damage, alcoholism, or concurrent therapy with other drugs which lower the seizure threshold. Use with caution in hyperthyroid patients or those receiving thyroid supplementation. Use with caution in patients with hepatic or renal dysfunction and in elderly patients.

**Adverse Reactions**

>10%:
- Central nervous system: Drowsiness
- Gastrointestinal: Xerostomia

1% to 10%:
- Central nervous system: Insomnia, nervousness, anxiety, agitation, dizziness, fatigue, headache
- Gastrointestinal: Constipation, nausea
- Neuromuscular & skeletal: Tremor, weakness
- Ocular: Blurred vision

<1%: Abdominal cramps, accommodation disturbances, akathisia, arrhythmias, ataxia, bitter taste, breast enlargement, confusion, decreased libido, delusions, diaphoresis (excessive), diarrhea, disorientation, dysarthria, dysphagia, edema of testicles, epigastric distress, EPS, exacerbation of psychosis, hallucinations, heart block, hyperglycemia, hypertension, hypomania, hypotension, impotence, mania, motor hyperactivity, mydriasis, nightmares, numbness, palpitations, petechiae, photosensitivity, rash, restlessness, seizures, syncope, tachycardia, tingling, tinnitus, urinary retention, vomiting, weight gain or loss

**Overdosage/Toxicology**

Signs and symptoms: Agitation, confusion, hallucinations, urinary retention, hypothermia, hypotension, seizures, ventricular tachycardia

Treatment:
- Following initiation of essential overdose management, toxic symptoms should be treated
- Ventricular arrhythmias often respond to systemic alkalinization (sodium bicarbonate 0.5-2 mEq/kg I.V.). Arrhythmias unresponsive to this therapy may respond to lidocaine 1 mg/kg I.V. followed by a titrated infusion. Physostigmine (1-2 mg I.V. slowly for adults or 0.5 mg I.V. slowly for children) may be indicated in reversing cardiac arrhythmias that are life-threatening.
- Seizures usually respond to diazepam I.V. boluses (5-10 mg for adults up to 30 mg or 0.25-0.4 mg/kg/dose for children up to 10 mg/dose). If seizures are unresponsive or recur, phenytoin or phenobarbital may be required.

**Drug Interactions** CYP1A2 and 2D6 enzyme substrate

Altretamine: Concurrent use may cause orthostatic hypertension

Amphetamines: Cyclic antidepressants may enhance the effect of amphetamines; monitor for adverse CV effects

Anticholinergics: Combined use with cyclic antidepressants may produce additive anticholinergic effects

Antihypertensives: Cyclic antidepressants may inhibit the antihypertensive response to bethanidine, clonidine, debrisoquin, guanadrel, guanethidine, guanabenz, guanfacine; monitor BP; consider alternate antihypertensive agent

Beta-agonists: When combined with cyclic antidepressants may predispose patients to cardiac arrhythmias

Bupropion: May increase the levels of cyclic antidepressants; based on limited information; monitor response
Carbamazepine: Cyclic antidepressants may increase carbamazepine levels; monitor
Cholestyramine and colestipol: May bind cyclic antidepressants and reduce their absorption; monitor for altered response
Clonidine: Abrupt discontinuation of clonidine may cause hypertensive crisis, cyclic antidepressants may enhance the response
CNS depressants: Sedative effects may be additive with cyclic antidepressants; monitor for increased effect; includes benzodiazepines, barbiturates, antipsychotics, ethanol and other sedative medications
CYP1A2 inhibitors: Serum levels and/or toxicity of some cyclic antidepressants may be increased; inhibitors include cimetidine, ciprofloxacin, fluvoxamine, isoniazid, ritonavir, and zileutin
CYP2D6 inhibitors: Serum levels and/or toxicity of some cyclic antidepressants may be increased; inhibitors include amiodarone, cimetidine, delavirdine, fluoxetine, paroxetine, propafenone, quinidine, and ritonavir; monitor for increased effect/toxicity
Enzyme inducers: May increase the metabolism of cyclic antidepressants resulting in decreased effect; includes carbamazepine, phenobarbital, phenytoin, and rifampin; monitor for decreased response
Epinephrine (and other direct alpha-agonists): The pressor response to I.V. epinephrine, norepinephrine, and phenylephrine may be enhanced in patients receiving cyclic antidepressants; this combination is best avoided
Fenfluramine: May increase cyclic antidepressant levels/effects
Hypoglycemic agents (including insulin): Hypoglycemic effects may be enhanced, profound hypoglycemia has been reported; monitor for changes in blood glucose levels; reported with chlorpropamide, tolazamide, and insulin
Levodopa: Cyclic antidepressants may decrease the absorption (bioavailability) of levodopa; rare hypertensive episodes have also been attributed to this combination
Linezolid: Hyperpyrexia, hypertension, tachycardia, confusion, seizures, and **deaths have been reported** with agents which inhibit MAO (serotonin syndrome); this combination should be avoided
Lithium: Concurrent use with a cyclic antidepressant may increase the risk for neurotoxicity
MAO inhibitors: Hyperpyrexia, hypertension, tachycardia, confusion, seizures, and **deaths have been reported** (serotonin syndrome); this combination should be avoided
Methylphenidate: Metabolism of maprotiline may be decreased
Phenothiazines: Serum concentrations of some TCAs may be increased; in addition, TCAs may increase concentration of phenothiazines; monitor for altered clinical response
QTc prolonging agents: Concurrent use of cyclic agents with other drugs which may prolong QTc interval may increase the risk of potentially fatal arrhythmias; includes type Ia and type III antiarrhythmics agents, selected quinolones (sparfloxacin, gatifloxacin, moxifloxacin, grepafloxacin), cisapride, and other agents
Sucralfate: Absorption of cyclic antidepressants may be reduced with coadministration.
Sympathomimetics, indirect-acting: Cyclic antidepressants may result in a decreased sensitivity to indirect-acting sympathomimetics; includes dopamine and ephedrine; also see interaction with epinephrine (and direct-acting sympathomimetics)
Valproic acid: May increase serum concentrations/adverse effects of some cyclic antidepressants
Warfarin (and other oral anticoagulants): Cyclic antidepressants may increase the anticoagulant effect in patients stabilized on warfarin; monitor INR

**Mechanism of Action** Traditionally believed to increase the synaptic concentration of norepinephrine in the central nervous system by inhibition of their reuptake by the presynaptic neuronal membrane. However, additional receptor effects have been found including desensitization of adenyl cyclase, down regulation of beta-adrenergic receptors, and down regulation of serotonin receptors.

**Pharmacodynamics/kinetics**
Absorption: Slow
Protein binding: 88%
Metabolism: In the liver to active and inactive compounds
Half-life: 27-58 hours (mean, 43 hours)
Time to peak serum concentration: Within 12 hours
Elimination: In urine (70%) and feces (30%)

**Usual Dosage** Oral:
Children 6-14 years: 10 mg/day, increase to a maximum daily dose of 75 mg
Adults: 75 mg/day to start, increase by 25 mg every 2 weeks up to 150-225 mg/day; given in 3 divided doses or in a single daily dose
Elderly: Initial: 25 mg at bedtime, increase by 25 mg every 3 days for inpatients and weekly for outpatients if tolerated; usual maintenance dose: 50-75 mg/day, higher doses may be necessary in nonresponders

**Dietary Considerations** Alcohol: Additive CNS effect, avoid use

**Monitoring Parameters** Monitor blood pressure and pulse rate prior to and during initial therapy; evaluate mood and somatic complaints; monitor appetite and weight; EKG in older adults

**Reference Range** Therapeutic: 200-600 ng/mL (SI: 721-2163 nmol/L)

**Patient Information** Avoid alcohol ingestion; do not discontinue medication abruptly; may cause drowsiness; full effect may not occur for 4-6 weeks; dry mouth may be helped by sips of water, sugarless gum, or hard candy; rise slowly to avoid dizziness

**Nursing Implications** May increase appetite and possibly a craving for sweets; often requires 4-6 weeks for therapeutic effects to be seen; severe constipation and urinary retention are possible; urge patient to report symptoms of stomatitis, and xerostomia; observe seizure precautions

**Additional Information** Odorless, bitter tasting; seizures rarely seen 5-30 hours postdrug ingestion

**Dosage Forms** Tablet, as hydrochloride: 25 mg, 50 mg, 75 mg


- ♦ **Maprotiline Hydrochloride** *see* Maprotiline *on page 332*
- ♦ **Maranox® [OTC]** *see* Acetaminophen *on page 14*
- ♦ **Marax®** *see* Theophylline, Ephedrine, and Hydroxyzine *on page 539*
- ♦ **Marcaine®** *see* Bupivacaine *on page 76*
- ♦ **Marcillin®** *see* Ampicillin *on page 42*
- ♦ **Marezine® [OTC]** *see* Cyclizine *on page 144*
- ♦ **Margesic® H** *see* Hydrocodone and Acetaminophen *on page 272*


## Margosa Oil

**Pharmacologic Category** Herb

**Use** A folk remedy in India, Japan, and Southeast Asia; antihelminthic, insecticidal, or analgesic agent; an extract from the dried stem bark and tree leaves of *Azadirachta indica* (Neem tree)

**Adverse Reactions**
Cardiovascular: Reye's-like syndrome, cerebral edema
Central nervous system: Lethargy, seizures, coma
Endocrine & metabolic: Metabolic acidosis
Gastrointestinal: Vomiting (15 minutes to 4 hours)
Hematology: Leukocytosis
Hepatic: Steatosis of the liver
Neuromuscular & skeletal: Tremor
Respiratory: Tachypnea, dyspnea

**Overdosage/Toxicology**
Decontamination: Do **not** induce emesis; lavage within 1 hour (if spontaneous emesis has not already occurred), activated charcoal with cathartic
Treatment: Supportive therapy; benzodiazepines have been used to treat seizures; paraldehyde has also been used to terminate seizures; mannitol and/or dexamethasone should be used to treat cerebral edema

**Additional Information** Not generally available in U.S. market; not listed with Commission E; some Neem extracts are used as ingredients in imported (from India) toothpastes and in natural cosmetics, but **not** as a dietary supplement for oral consumption


- ♦ **Marinol®** *see* Dronabinol *on page 187*
- ♦ **Marplan®** *see* Isocarboxazid *on page 294*
- ♦ **Marpres®** *see* Hydralazine, Hydrochlorothiazide, and Reserpine *on page 270*
- ♦ **Marthritic®** *see* Salsalate *on page 503*
- ♦ **Massengill® Medicated Douche w/Cepticin [OTC]** *see* Povidone-Iodine *on page 456*


## Maté

**Synonyms** *Ilex paraguariensis*; Jesuit's Tea; Paraguay Tea; St Bartholomew's Tea

**Pharmacologic Category** Herb

**Use** Herbal medicine as a depurative, stimulant, diuretic, urinary tract infection, kidney and bladder stones, CHF
Per Commission E: Physical fatigue

**Adverse Reactions**
Cardiovascular: Tachycardia
Central nervous system: Fever, disorientation
Dermatologic: Flushed skin
Gastrointestinal: Xerostomia
Genitourinary: Urinary retention
Ocular: Mydriasis
Miscellaneous: Incidence of esophageal cancer and bladder cancer increased when used with tobacco (in chronic users)

**Overdosage/Toxicology**
Decontamination: Lavage (within 1 hour)/activated charcoal with cathartic
Treatment: Supportive therapy; physostigmine (0.5 mg in children, up to 4 mg in adult as a total dose) has been used to treat severe anticholinergic toxicity due to ingestion of Paraguay tea contaminated with anticholinergic agents. This modality should not be used for treating effects of caffeine exposure.

**Drug Interactions** CYP1A2, 2E1, and 3A3/4 enzyme substrate
(Continued)

## Maté *(Continued)*

**Note:** Contains significant amounts of caffeine; interactions noted are for caffeine content

Adenosine: Caffeine may antagonize the cardiovascular effects of adenosine

Beta-agonists: Therapeutic effect of beta-agonists (bronchodilation) and toxicity (tachycardia, tremor) may be additive; use caution

CYP1A2 inhibitors: Metabolism of caffeine may be decreased, increasing clinical effect or toxicity; inhibitors include cimetidine, ciprofloxacin, fluvoxamine, isoniazid, ritonavir, and zileutin

CNS stimulants: Effects on CNS stimulation are additive with caffeine; cardiovascular side effects may also be additive; includes phenylpropanolamine, amphetamines, methylphenidate and others

Disulfiram: May increase the effects of caffeine

Theophylline: Therapeutic effect of theophylline (respiratory stimulation, bronchodilation) and toxicity (tachycardia, tremor, possible seizures) may be additive; avoid combinations

**Usual Dosage**

One cup of maté (6 ounces) is equivalent to 25-50 mg of caffeine

Per Commission E: Daily dose: 3 g of drug (dried herb); equivalent preparations

**Additional Information** A climbing evergreen shrub which can grow to 20 feet; native to South American countries; greenish white flowers with small deep red berries; leaves contain as much as 2% caffeine along with theophylline (0.05%); apnea has occurred in an infant after breast-feeding from a mother ingesting maté; teas should be used with caution in patients with elevated blood pressure, diabetes or ulcer disease


- ***Matricaria chamomilla*** *see* Chamomile *on page 106*
- ***Matricarta recutita*** *see* Chamomile *on page 106*
- **Matulane®** *see* Procarbazine *on page 465*
- **Mavik®** *see* Trandolapril *on page 558*
- **Maxair™ Inhalation Aerosol** *see* Pirbuterol *on page 448*
- **Maxalt®** *see* Rizatriptan *on page 498*
- **Maxalt-MLT™** *see* Rizatriptan *on page 498*
- **Maxaquin®** *see* Lomefloxacin *on page 323*
- **Maxidex®** *see* Dexamethasone *on page 157*
- **Maxifed®** *see* Guaifenesin and Pseudoephedrine *on page 257*
- **Maxifed® DM** *see* Guaifenesin, Pseudoephedrine, and Dextromethorphan *on page 259*
- **Maxifed-G®** *see* Guaifenesin and Pseudoephedrine *on page 257*
- **Maxiflor®** *see* Diflorasone *on page 168*
- **Maximum Strength Anbesol® [OTC]** *see* Benzocaine *on page 61*
- **Maximum Strength Desenex® Antifungal Cream [OTC]** *see* Miconazole *on page 364*
- **Maximum Strength Dex-A-Diet® [OTC]** *see* Phenylpropanolamine *on page 440*
- **Maximum Strength Dexatrim® [OTC]** *see* Phenylpropanolamine *on page 440*
- **Maximum Strength Maalox® [OTC]** *see* Aluminum Hydroxide, Magnesium Hydroxide, and Simethicone *on page 28*
- **Maximum Strength Nytol® [OTC]** *see* Diphenhydramine *on page 174*
- **Maximum Strength Orajel® [OTC]** *see* Benzocaine *on page 61*
- **Maxipime®** *see* Cefepime *on page 98*
- **Maxitrol®** *see* Neomycin, Polymyxin B, and Dexamethasone *on page 389*
- **Maxivate®** *see* Betamethasone *on page 65*
- **Maxolon®** *see* Metoclopramide *on page 360*
- **Maxzide®** *see* Hydrochlorothiazide and Triamterene *on page 271*
- **Maybush** *see* Hawthorn *on page 264*
- **Mazanor®** *see* Mazindol *on page 334*


## Mazindol (MAY zin dole)

**U.S. Brand Names** Mazanor®; Sanorex®

**Pharmacologic Category** Anorexiant

**Use** Short-term adjunct in exogenous obesity

**Restrictions** C-IV

**Contraindications** Hypersensitivity to mazindol

**Adverse Reactions**

Cardiovascular: Palpitation, tachycardia, edema

Central nervous system: Insomnia, overstimulation, dizziness, dysphoria, drowsiness, depression, headache, restlessness

Dermatologic: Rash, clamminess

Endocrine & metabolic: Changes in libido

Gastrointestinal: Nausea, constipation, vomiting, xerostomia, unpleasant taste, diarrhea, abdominal cramps

Genitourinary: Dysuria, polyuria, impotence

Neuromuscular & skeletal: Tremor, weakness

Ocular: Blurred vision, corneal opacities

Miscellaneous: Diaphoresis (excessive)

**Drug Interactions**

Antipsychotics: Efficacy of CNS stimulants may be decreased by antipsychotics; in addition, amphetamines may induce an increase in psychotic symptoms in some patients

Furazolidine: Amphetamine-like compounds may induce hypertensive episodes in patients receiving furazolidone

Guanethidine: Amphetamine-like compounds inhibit the antihypertensive response to guanethidine; probably also may occur with guanadrel

MAOIs: Severe hypertensive episodes have occurred with amphetamines when used in patients receiving MAOIs; likely to occur with related compounds; concurrent use or use within 14 days is contraindicated

Norepinephrine: Amphetamine-like compounds may enhance the pressor response to norepinephrine

Sibutramine: Concurrent use of sibutramine and amphetamine-like compounds may cause severe hypertension and tachycardia; use is contraindicated (benzphetamine)

SSRIs: Amphetamine-like compounds may increase the potential for serotonin syndrome when used concurrently with selective serotonin reuptake inhibitors (including fluoxetine, fluvoxamine, paroxetine, and sertraline)

**Mechanism of Action** An isoindole with pharmacologic activity similar to amphetamine; produces CNS stimulation in humans and animals and appears to work primarily in the limbic system

**Pharmacodynamics/kinetics**

Half-life: 33-55 hours

Elimination: Renal

**Usual Dosage** Oral: Adults: Initial dose, 1 mg once daily and adjust to patient response; usual dose is 1 mg 3 times daily, 1 hour before meals, or 2 mg once daily, 1 hour before lunch; take with meals to avoid GI discomfort

**Dosage Forms** Tablet:

Mazanor®: 1 mg

Sanorex®: 1 mg, 2 mg


- **Mebaral®** *see* Mephobarbital *on page 342*


## Mebendazole (me BEN da zole)

**U.S. Brand Names** Vermox®

**Pharmacologic Category** Anthelmintic

**Use** Treatment of pinworms (*Enterobius vermicularis*), whipworms (*Trichuris trichiura*), roundworms (*Ascaris lumbricoides*), and hookworms (*Ancylostoma duodenale*)

**Effects on Mental Status** May cause dizziness

**Effects on Psychiatric Treatment** Carbamazepine may decrease the effects of mebendazole; may rarely cause neutropenia; use caution with clozapine and carbamazepine

**Usual Dosage** Children and Adults: Oral:

Pinworms: 100 mg as a single dose; may need to repeat after 2 weeks; treatment should include family members in close contact with patient

Whipworms, roundworms, hookworms: One tablet twice daily, morning and evening on 3 consecutive days; if patient is not cured within 3-4 weeks, a second course of treatment may be administered

Capillariasis: 200 mg twice daily for 20 days

**Dosing adjustment in hepatic impairment:** Dosage reduction may be necessary in patients with liver dysfunction

Hemodialysis: Not dialyzable (0% to 5%)

**Dosage Forms** Tablet, chewable: 100 mg

## Mecamylamine (mek a MIL a meen)

**Related Information**

Substance-Related Disorders *on page 609*

**U.S. Brand Names** Inversine®

**Pharmacologic Category** Ganglionic Blocking Agent

**Use** Treatment of moderately severe to severe hypertension and in uncomplicated malignant hypertension

**Unlabeled use:** Tourette's syndrome

**Effects on Mental Status** May cause drowsiness, confusion, or depression

**Effects on Psychiatric Treatment** None reported

**Pregnancy Risk Factor** C

**Contraindications** Coronary insufficiency, pyloric stenosis, glaucoma, uremia, recent myocardial infarction, unreliable, uncooperative patients

**Warnings/Precautions** Use with caution in patients receiving sulfonamides or antibiotics that cause neuromuscular blockade; use with caution in patients with impaired renal function, previous CNS abnormalities, prostatic hypertrophy, bladder obstruction, or urethral strictive; do not abruptly discontinue

**Adverse Reactions** Percentage unknown: Bloating, blurred vision, convulsions, confusion, decreased sexual ability, drowsiness, dysuria, enlarged pupils, frequent stools - followed by severe constipation, loss of appetite, mental depression, nausea, postural hypotension, shortness of breath, trembling; uncontrolled movements of hands, arms, legs, or face; vomiting, xerostomia

**Overdosage/Toxicology**

Signs and symptoms: Hypotension, nausea, vomiting, urinary retention, constipation. Signs and symptoms are a direct result of ganglionic blockade.

Treatment: Supportive; pressor amines may be used to correct hypotension; use caution as patients will be unusually sensitive to these agents.

**Drug Interactions** Increased effect with sulfonamides and antibiotics that cause neuromuscular blockade; action of mecamylamine may be increased by anesthesia, other antihypertensives, and alcohol

**Usual Dosage** Adults: Oral: 2.5 mg twice daily after meals for 2 days, increased by increments of 2.5 mg at intervals ≥2 days until desired blood pressure response is achieved; average daily dose: 25 mg (usually in 3 divided doses)

**Note:** Reduce dosage of other antihypertensives when combined with mecamylamine with exception of thiazide diuretics which may be maintained at usual dose while decreasing mecamylamine by 50%

**Dosing adjustment/comments in renal impairment:** Use with caution, if at all, although no specific guidelines are available

**Patient Information** Take after meals at the same time each day; notify physician immediately if frequent loose bowel movements occur; rise slowly from sitting or lying for prolonged periods; do not restrict salt intake

**Nursing Implications** Check frequently for orthostatic hypotension; aid with ambulation

**Dosage Forms** Tablet, as hydrochloride: 2.5 mg

## Mechlorethamine (me klor ETH a meen)

**U.S. Brand Names** Mustargen® Hydrochloride

**Pharmacologic Category** Antineoplastic Agent, Alkylating Agent

**Use** Combination therapy of Hodgkin's disease and malignant lymphomas; non-Hodgkin's lymphoma; palliative treatment of bronchogenic, breast and ovarian carcinoma; may be used by intracavitary injection for treatment of metastatic tumors; pleural and other malignant effusions; topical treatment of mycosis fungoides

**Effects on Mental Status** May cause dizziness

**Effects on Psychiatric Treatment** Leukopenia is common; avoid use with clozapine and carbamazepine

**Usual Dosage** Refer to individual protocols. Dosage should be based on ideal dry weight; the presence of edema or ascites must be considered so that dosage will be based on actual weight unaugmented by these conditions

Children and Adults: MOPP: I.V.: 6 mg/m$^2$ on days 1 and 8 of a 28-day cycle

Adults:

I.V.: 0.4 mg/kg **OR** 12-16 mg/m$^2$ for one dose **OR** divided into 0.1 mg/kg/day for 4 days, repeated at 4- to 6-week intervals

Intracavitary: 10-20 mg diluted in 10 mL of SWI or 0.9% sodium chloride

Intrapericardially: 0.2-0.4 mg/kg diluted in up to 100 mL of 0.9% sodium chloride

Hemodialysis: Not removed; supplemental dosing is not required

Peritoneal dialysis: Not removed; supplemental dosing is not required

Topical mechlorethamine has been used in the treatment of cutaneous lesions of mycosis fungoides. A skin test should be performed prior to treatment with the topical preparation to detect sensitivity and possible irritation (use fresh mechlorethamine 0.1 mg/mL and apply over a 3 x 5 cm area of normal skin).

**Dosage Forms** Powder for injection, as hydrochloride: 10 mg

♦ **Meclan® Topical** *see* Meclocycline *on page 335*

## Meclizine (MEK li zeen)

**U.S. Brand Names** Antivert®; Antrizine®; Bonine® [OTC]; Dizmiss® [OTC]; Dramamine® II [OTC]; Meni-D®; Ru-Vert-M®; Vergon® [OTC]

**Pharmacologic Category** Antihistamine

**Use** Prevention and treatment of symptoms of motion sickness; management of vertigo with diseases affecting the vestibular system

**Effects on Mental Status** Drowsiness is common; may cause dizziness or nervousness; may rarely cause sedation or depression

**Effects on Psychiatric Treatment** Concurrent use with psychotropic may produce additive sedation and dry mouth

**Pregnancy Risk Factor** B

**Contraindications** Hypersensitivity to meclizine or any component; pregnancy

**Warnings/Precautions** Use with caution in patients with angle-closure glaucoma, prostatic hypertrophy, pyloric or duodenal obstruction, or bladder neck obstruction; use with caution in hot weather, and during exercise; elderly may be at risk for anticholinergic side effects such as glaucoma, prostatic hypertrophy, constipation, gastrointestinal obstructive disease; if vertigo does not respond in 1-2 weeks, it is advised to discontinue use

**Adverse Reactions**

>10%:

Central nervous system: Slight to moderate drowsiness

Respiratory: Thickening of bronchial secretions

1% to 10%:

Central nervous system: Headache, fatigue, nervousness, dizziness

Gastrointestinal: Appetite increase, weight gain, nausea, diarrhea, abdominal pain, xerostomia

Neuromuscular & skeletal: Arthralgia

Respiratory: Pharyngitis

<1%: Angioedema, blurred vision, bronchospasm, depression, epistaxis, hepatitis, hypotension, myalgia, palpitations, paresthesia, photosensitivity, rash, sedation, tremor, urinary retention

**Overdosage/Toxicology**

Signs and symptoms: CNS depression, confusion, nervousness, hallucinations, dizziness, blurred vision, nausea, vomiting, hyperthermia

Treatment: There is no specific treatment for an antihistamine overdose, however, most of its clinical toxicity is due to anticholinergic effects. For anticholinergic overdose with severe life-threatening symptoms, physostigmine 1-2 mg (0.5 or 0.02 mg/kg for children) I.V., slowly may be given to reverse these effects.

**Drug Interactions** Increased toxicity: CNS depressants, neuroleptics, anticholinergics

**Usual Dosage** Children >12 years and Adults: Oral:

Motion sickness: 12.5-25 mg 1 hour before travel, repeat dose every 12-24 hours if needed; doses up to 50 mg may be needed

Vertigo: 25-100 mg/day in divided doses

**Dietary Considerations** Alcohol: Additive CNS effect, avoid use

**Patient Information** Take exactly as prescribed; do not increase dose. Avoid alcohol, other CNS depressants, sleeping aids without consulting prescriber. You may experience dizziness, drowsiness, or blurred vision (use caution when driving or engaging in tasks that require alertness until response to drug is known); dry mouth (frequent mouth care, sucking lozenges, or chewing gum may help); constipation (increased dietary fluid, fiber, and fruit and exercise may help); heat intolerance (avoid excessive exercise, hot environments, maintain adequate fluid intake). Report CNS change (hallucination, confusion, nervousness); sudden or unusual weight gain; unresolved nausea or diarrhea; chest pain or palpitations; muscle pain; or changes in urinary pattern.

**Dosage Forms**

Capsule, as hydrochloride: 15 mg, 25 mg, 30 mg

Tablet, as hydrochloride: 12.5 mg, 25 mg, 50 mg

Tablet, as hydrochloride:

Chewable: 25 mg

Film coated: 25 mg

## Meclocycline (me kloe SYE kleen)

**U.S. Brand Names** Meclan® Topical

**Pharmacologic Category** Antibiotic, Topical; Topical Skin Product, Acne

**Use** Topical treatment of inflammatory acne vulgaris

**Effects on Mental Status** None reported

**Effects on Psychiatric Treatment** None reported

**Usual Dosage** Children >11 years and Adults: Topical: Apply generously to affected areas twice daily

**Dosage Forms** Cream, topical, as sulfosalicylate: 1% (20 g, 45 g)

## Meclofenamate (me kloe fen AM ate)

**Related Information**

Nonsteroidal Anti-inflammatory Agents Comparison Chart *on page 722*

**U.S. Brand Names** Meclomen®

**Pharmacologic Category** Nonsteroidal Anti-Inflammatory Agent (NSAID)

**Use** Treatment of inflammatory disorders

**Effects on Mental Status** Dizziness is common; may cause drowsiness, confusion, hallucinations, or depression

**Effects on Psychiatric Treatment** May rarely cause agranulocytosis; use caution with clozapine or carbamazepine; may decrease lithium clearance resulting in an increase in serum lithium levels and potential lithium toxicity; monitor serum lithium levels

**Pregnancy Risk Factor** B (D if used in the 3rd trimester)

**Contraindications** Active GI bleeding, ulcer disease, hypersensitivity to aspirin, meclofenamate, or other NSAIDs

**Warnings/Precautions** May have adverse effects on fetus; use with caution with dehydration

(Continued)

## Meclofenamate *(Continued)*

**Adverse Reactions**

>10%:

Central nervous system: Dizziness

Dermatologic: Rash

Gastrointestinal: Abdominal cramps, heartburn, indigestion, nausea

1% to 10%:

Central nervous system: Headache, nervousness

Dermatologic: Itching

Endocrine & metabolic: Fluid retention

Gastrointestinal: Vomiting

Otic: Tinnitus

<1%: Acute renal failure, agranulocytosis, allergic rhinitis, anemia, angioedema, arrhythmias, aseptic meningitis, blurred vision, bone marrow suppression, confusion, congestive heart failure, conjunctivitis, cystitis, decreased hearing, drowsiness, dry eyes, epistaxis, erythema multiforme, gastritis, GI ulceration, hallucinations, hemolytic anemia, hepatitis, hot flashes, hypertension, insomnia, leukopenia, mental depression, peripheral neuropathy, polydipsia, polyuria, shortness of breath, Stevens-Johnson syndrome, tachycardia, thrombocytopenia, toxic amblyopia, toxic epidermal necrolysis, urticaria

**Overdosage/Toxicology**

Signs and symptoms: Drowsiness, lethargy, nausea, vomiting, seizures, paresthesia, headache, dizziness, GI bleeding, cerebral edema, cardiac arrest, tinnitus

Treatment: Management of a nonsteroidal anti-inflammatory drug (NSAID) intoxication is primarily supportive and symptomatic. Fluid therapy is commonly effective in managing the hypotension that may occur following an acute NSAID overdose, except when this is due to an acute blood loss. Seizures tend to be very short-lived and often do not require drug treatment. Although, recurrent seizures should be treated with I.V. diazepam. Since many of the NSAID undergo enterohepatic cycling, multiple doses of charcoal may be needed to reduce the potential for delayed toxicities.

**Drug Interactions**

ACE inhibitors: Effects may be reduced by NSAIDs; use lowest possible dose for shortest duration possible; monitor

Cholestyramine and colestipol: Absorption may be reduced by concurrent administration

Corticosteroids: May increase the risk of GI ulceration; use caution

Cyclosporine: Nephrotoxicity may be increased with concurrent NSAID use; monitor

Hydralazine: Antihypertensive effect may be decreased; avoid concurrent use

Lithium: Serum levels can be increased; avoid concurrent use if possible or monitor lithium levels and adjust dose. When NSAID is stopped, lithium may need adjustment again.

Loop diuretics: Therapeutic effects may be reduced by NSAIDs; avoid

Methotrexate: Toxicity may be increased by concurrent NSAID use; risk is limited in low-dose methotrexate regimens (such as for rheumatoid arthritis); prolonged leucovorin rescue may be required at antineoplastic doses; monitor

Thiazide diuretics: Antihypertensive effects are decreased; avoid concurrent use

Warfarin: INRs may be increased by some NSAIDs. This may depend, in part, on dose and duration; monitor INR closely; use the lowest dose of NSAIDs possible and for the briefest duration

**Usual Dosage** Children >14 years and Adults: Oral:

Mild to moderate pain: 50 mg every 4-6 hours, not to exceed 400 mg/day

Rheumatoid arthritis/osteoarthritis: 200-400 mg/day in 3-4 equal doses

**Patient Information** Take with food, milk, or with antacids

**Nursing Implications** Should be used for short-term only (<7 days); advise patient to report persistent GI discomfort, sore throat, fever, or malaise

**Dosage Forms** Capsule, as sodium: 50 mg, 100 mg


- **Meclomen®** *see* Meclofenamate *on page 335*
- **Medicinal Carbon** *see* Charcoal *on page 106*
- **Medicinal Charcoal** *see* Charcoal *on page 106*
- **Medigesic®** *see* Butalbital Compound and Acetaminophen *on page 80*
- **Medihaler-Iso®** *see* Isoproterenol *on page 295*
- **Medipain 5®** *see* Hydrocodone and Acetaminophen *on page 272*
- **Medi-Quick® Topical Ointment [OTC]** *see* Bacitracin, Neomycin, and Polymyxin B *on page 57*
- **Medi-Tuss® [OTC]** *see* Guaifenesin *on page 256*
- **Medralone® Injection** *see* Methylprednisolone *on page 359*
- **Medrol® Oral** *see* Methylprednisolone *on page 359*


## Medroxyprogesterone (me DROKS ee proe JES te rone)

**U.S. Brand Names** Amen® Oral; Curretab® Oral; Cycrin® Oral; Depo-Provera® Injection; Provera® Oral

**Canadian Brand Names** Novo-Medrone

**Synonyms** Acetoxymethylprogesterone; Methylacetoxyprogesterone

**Pharmacologic Category** Contraceptive; Progestin

**Use** Endometrial carcinoma or renal carcinoma as well as secondary amenorrhea or abnormal uterine bleeding due to hormonal imbalance; prevention of pregnancy

**Effects on Mental Status** May cause insomnia or depression

**Effects on Psychiatric Treatment** None reported

**Pregnancy Risk Factor** X

**Contraindications** Pregnancy, thrombophlebitis; hypersensitivity to medroxyprogesterone or any component; cerebral apoplexy, undiagnosed vaginal bleeding, liver dysfunction

**Warnings/Precautions** Use with caution in patients with depression, diabetes, epilepsy, asthma, migraines, renal or cardiac dysfunction; pretreatment exams should include PAP smear, physical exam of breasts and pelvic areas. May increase serum cholesterol, LDL, decrease HDL and triglycerides; use of any progestin during the first 4 months of pregnancy is not recommended; monitor patient closely for loss of vision, sudden onset of proptosis, diplopia, migraine, and signs and symptoms of thromboembolic disorders.

**Adverse Reactions**

>10%:

Cardiovascular: Edema

Endocrine & metabolic: Breakthrough bleeding, spotting, changes in menstrual flow, amenorrhea

Gastrointestinal: Anorexia

Local: Pain at injection site

Neuromuscular & skeletal: Weakness

1% to 10%:

Cardiovascular: Embolism, central thrombosis

Central nervous system: Mental depression, fever, insomnia

Dermatologic: Melasma or chloasma, allergic rash with or without pruritus

Endocrine & metabolic: Changes in cervical erosion and secretions, increased breast tenderness

Gastrointestinal: Weight gain or loss

Hepatic: Cholestatic jaundice

Local: Thrombophlebitis

**Overdosage/Toxicology**

Signs and symptoms; Toxicity is unlikely following single exposures of excessive doses

Treatment: Supportive treatment is adequate in most cases

**Drug Interactions** Decreased effect: Aminoglutethimide may decrease effects by increasing hepatic metabolism

**Usual Dosage**

Adolescents and Adults: Oral:

Amenorrhea: 5-10 mg/day for 5-10 days or 2.5 mg/day

Abnormal uterine bleeding: 5-10 mg for 5-10 days starting on day 16 or 21 of cycle

Accompanying cyclic estrogen therapy, postmenopausal: 2.5-10 mg the last 10-13 days of estrogen dosing each month

Adults: I.M.:

Endometrial or renal carcinoma: 400-1000 mg/week

Contraception: 150 mg every 3 months

**Dosing adjustment in hepatic impairment:** Dose needs to be lowered in patients with alcoholic cirrhosis

**Patient Information** Follow dosage schedule and do not take more than prescribed. You may experience sensitivity to sunlight (use sunblock, wear protective clothing and eyewear, and avoid extensive exposure to direct sunlight); dizziness, anxiety, depression (use caution when driving or engaging in tasks that require alertness until response to drug is known); changes in appetite (maintain adequate hydration and diet - 2-3 L/day of fluids unless instructed to restrict fluid intake); decreased libido or increased body hair (reversible when drug is discontinued); hot flashes (cool clothes and environment may help). May cause discoloration of stool (green). Report swelling of face, lips, or mouth; absence or altered menses; abdominal pain; vaginal itching, irritation, or discharge; heat, warmth, redness, or swelling of extremities; or sudden onset change in vision.

**Nursing Implications** Patients should receive a copy of the patient labeling for the drug

**Dosage Forms**

Injection, suspension: 100 mg/mL (5 mL); 150 mg/mL (1 mL); 400 mg/mL (1 mL, 2.5 mL, 10 mL)

Tablet: 2.5 mg, 5 mg, 10 mg

## Medrysone (ME dri sone)

**U.S. Brand Names** HMS Liquifilm®

**Pharmacologic Category** Corticosteroid, Ophthalmic

**Use** Treatment of allergic conjunctivitis, vernal conjunctivitis, episcleritis, ophthalmic epinephrine sensitivity reaction

**Effects on Mental Status** None reported

**Effects on Psychiatric Treatment** None reported

**Usual Dosage** Children and Adults: Ophthalmic: Instill 1 drop in conjunctival sac 2-4 times/day up to every 4 hours; may use every 1-2 hours during first 1-2 days

**Dosage Forms** Solution, ophthalmic: 1% (5 mL, 10 mL)

## Mefenamic Acid (me fe NAM ik AS id)

**Related Information**

Nonsteroidal Anti-inflammatory Agents Comparison Chart *on page 722*

**U.S. Brand Names** Ponstel®

**Canadian Brand Names** Apo®-Mefenamic; Ponstan®

**Pharmacologic Category** Nonsteroidal Anti-Inflammatory Agent (NSAID)

**Use** Short-term relief of mild to moderate pain including primary dysmenorrhea

**Effects on Mental Status** Dizziness is common; may cause nervousness, may rarely cause confusion, hallucination, or depression

**Effects on Psychiatric Treatment** May rarely cause agranulocytosis; use caution with clozapine or carbamazepine; may decrease lithium clearance resulting in an increase in serum lithium levels and potential lithium toxicity; monitor serum lithium levels

**Pregnancy Risk Factor** C

**Contraindications** Known hypersensitivity to mefenamic acid or other NSAIDs

**Warnings/Precautions** May have adverse effects on fetus

**Adverse Reactions**

>10%:

Central nervous system: Dizziness

Dermatologic: Rash

Gastrointestinal: Abdominal cramps, heartburn, indigestion, nausea

1% to 10%:

Central nervous system: Headache, nervousness

Dermatologic: Itching

Endocrine & metabolic: Fluid retention

Gastrointestinal: Vomiting

Otic: Tinnitus

<1%: Acute renal failure, agranulocytosis, allergic rhinitis, anemia, angioedema, arrhythmias, aseptic meningitis, blurred vision, bone marrow suppression, confusion, congestive heart failure, conjunctivitis, cystitis, decreased hearing, drowsiness, dry eyes, epistaxis, erythema multiforme, gastritis, GI ulceration, hallucinations, hemolytic anemia, hepatitis, hot flashes, hypertension, insomnia, leukopenia, mental depression, peripheral neuropathy, polydipsia, polyuria, shortness of breath, Stevens-Johnson syndrome, tachycardia, thrombocytopenia, toxic amblyopia, toxic epidermal necrolysis, urticaria

**Overdosage/Toxicology**

Signs and symptoms: CNS stimulation, agitation, seizures

Treatment: Management of a nonsteroidal anti-inflammatory drug (NSAID) intoxication is primarily supportive and symptomatic. Fluid therapy is commonly effective in managing the hypotension that may occur following an acute NSAIDs overdose, except when this is due to an acute blood loss. Seizures tend to be very short-lived and often do not require drug treatment. Although, recurrent seizures should be treated with I.V. diazepam. Since many of the NSAID undergo enterohepatic cycling, multiple doses of charcoal may be needed to reduce the potential for delayed toxicities.

**Drug Interactions** CYP2C9 enzyme substrate

ACE inhibitors: Effects may be reduced by NSAIDs; use lowest possible dose for shortest duration possible; monitor

Cholestyramine and colestipol: Absorption may be reduced by concurrent administration

Corticosteroids: May increase the risk of GI ulceration; use caution

Cyclosporine: Nephrotoxicity may be increased with concurrent NSAID use; monitor

CYP2C9 inhibitors: May increase serum concentrations; inhibitors include amiodarone, cimetidine, fluvoxamine, metronidazole, omeprazole, sulfonamides, valproic acid, and zafirlukast

Hydralazine: Antihypertensive effect may be decreased; avoid concurrent use

Lithium: Serum levels can be increased; avoid concurrent use if possible or monitor lithium levels and adjust dose. When NSAID is stopped, lithium may need adjustment again.

Loop diuretics: Therapeutic effects may be reduced by NSAIDs; avoid

Methotrexate: Toxicity may be increased by concurrent NSAID use; risk is limited in low-dose methotrexate regimens (such as for rheumatoid arthritis); prolonged leucovorin rescue may be required at antineoplastic doses; monitor

Thiazide diuretics: Antihypertensive effects are decreased; avoid concurrent use

Warfarin: INRs may be increased by some NSAIDs. This may depend, in part, on dose and duration; monitor INR closely. Use the lowest dose of NSAIDs possible and for the briefest duration.

**Usual Dosage** Children >14 years and Adults: Oral: 500 mg to start then 250 mg every 4 hours as needed; maximum therapy: 1 week

**Dosing adjustment/comments in renal impairment:** Not recommended for use

**Patient Information** Take with food, milk, or with antacids; extended release capsules must be swallowed intact

**Dosage Forms** Capsule: 250 mg

## Mefloquine (ME floe kwin)

**U.S. Brand Names** Lariam®

**Pharmacologic Category** Antimalarial Agent

**Use** Treatment of acute malarial infections and prevention of malaria

**Effects on Mental Status** May cause dizziness, insomnia, or difficulty concentrating; may rarely cause anxiety, confusion, hallucination, or depression

**Effects on Psychiatric Treatment** Concurrent use with valproic acid may valproate blood levels; monitor levels

**Pregnancy Risk Factor** C

**Contraindications** Hypersensitivity to any component

**Warnings/Precautions** Caution is warranted with lactation; discontinue if unexplained neuropsychiatric disturbances occur, caution in epilepsy patients or in patients with significant cardiac disease. If mefloquine is to be used for a prolonged period, periodic evaluations including liver function tests and ophthalmic examinations should be performed. (Retinal abnormalities have not been observed with mefloquine in humans; however, it has with long-term administration to rats.) In cases of life-threatening, serious, or overwhelming malaria infections due to *Plasmodium falciparum*, patients should be treated with intravenous antimalarial drug. Mefloquine may be given orally to complete the course. Caution should be exercised with regard to driving, piloting airplanes, and operating machines since dizziness, disturbed sense of balance; neuropsychiatric reactions have been reported with mefloquine.

**Adverse Reactions**

1% to 10%:

Central nervous system: Difficulty concentrating, headache, insomnia, lightheadedness, vertigo

Gastrointestinal: Vomiting (3%), diarrhea, stomach pain, nausea

Ocular: Visual disturbances

Otic: Tinnitus

<1%: Anxiety, bradycardia, confusion, dizziness, extrasystoles, hallucinations, mental depression, psychosis, seizures, syncope

**Overdosage/Toxicology**

Signs and symptoms: Vomiting, diarrhea; cardiotoxic

Treatment: Following GI contamination supportive care only

**Drug Interactions**

Decreased effect of valproic acid

Increased toxicity of beta-blockers; chloroquine, quinine, and quinidine (hold treatment until at least 12 hours after these later drugs)

**Usual Dosage** Oral:

Children: Malaria prophylaxis:

15-19 kg: 1/4 tablet

20-30 kg: 1/2 tablet

31-45 kg: 3/4 tablet

>45 kg: 1 tablet

Administer weekly starting 1 week before travel, continuing weekly during travel and for 4 weeks after leaving endemic area

Adults:

Treatment of mild to moderate malaria infection: 5 tablets (1250 mg) as a single dose with at least 8 oz of water

Malaria prophylaxis: 1 tablet (250 mg) weekly starting 1 week before travel, continuing weekly during travel and for 4 weeks after leaving endemic area

**Patient Information** Take on schedule as directed, with a full 8 oz glass of water. Ophthalmic exams will be necessary when used long-term. When taking for prophylaxis, begin 1 week before traveling to endemic areas, continue during travel period, and for 4 weeks following return. You may experience GI distress (frequent small meals may help). You may experience dizziness, changes in mentation, insomnia, headache, visual disturbances (use caution when driving or engaging in tasks that require alertness until response to drug is known).

**Dosage Forms** Tablet, as hydrochloride: 250 mg


- **Mefoxin®** *see* Cefoxitin *on page 99*
- **Mega B® [OTC]** *see* Vitamin B Complex *on page 586*
- **Megace®** *see* Megestrol *on page 338*
- **Megaton™ [OTC]** *see* Vitamin B Complex *on page 586*

## Megestrol (me JES trole)

**U.S. Brand Names** Megace®

**Pharmacologic Category** Antineoplastic Agent, Miscellaneous; Progestin

**Use** Palliative treatment of breast and endometrial carcinomas, appetite stimulation, and promotion of weight gain in cachexia

**Effects on Mental Status** May cause insomnia or depression

**Effects on Psychiatric Treatment** May rarely cause myelosuppression; use caution with clozapine and carbamazepine

**Pregnancy Risk Factor** X

**Contraindications** Hypersensitivity to megestrol or any component; pregnancy

**Warnings/Precautions** The U.S. Food and Drug Administration (FDA) currently recommends that procedures for proper handling and disposal of antineoplastic agents be considered. Use during the first few months of pregnancy is not recommended. Use with caution in patients with a history of thrombophlebitis. Elderly females may have vaginal bleeding or discharge and need to be forewarned of this side effect and inconvenience.

**Adverse Reactions**

>10%:
- Cardiovascular: Edema
- Endocrine & metabolic: Breakthrough bleeding and amenorrhea, spotting, changes in menstrual flow
- Neuromuscular & skeletal: Weakness

1% to 10%:
- Central nervous system: Insomnia, depression, fever, headache
- Dermatologic: Allergic rash with or without pruritus, melasma or chloasma, rash, and rarely alopecia
- Endocrine & metabolic: Changes in cervical erosion and secretions, increased breast tenderness, changes in vaginal bleeding pattern, edema, fluid retention, hyperglycemia
- Gastrointestinal: Weight gain (not attributed to edema or fluid retention), nausea, vomiting, stomach cramps
- Hepatic: Cholestatic jaundice, hepatotoxicity
- Hematologic: Myelosuppressive:
  - WBC: None
  - Platelets: None
- Local: Thrombophlebitis
- Neuromuscular & skeletal: Carpal tunnel syndrome
- Respiratory: Hyperpnea

**Overdosage/Toxicology** Toxicity is unlikely following simple exposures of excessive doses

**Drug Interactions** No data reported

**Usual Dosage** Adults: Oral (refer to individual protocols):

Female:
- Breast carcinoma: 40 mg 4 times/day
- Endometrial: 40-320 mg/day in divided doses; use for 2 months to determine efficacy; maximum doses used have been up to 800 mg/day
- Uterine bleeding: 40 mg 2-4 times/day

Male/Female: HIV-related cachexia: Initial dose: 800 mg/day; daily doses of 400 and 800 mg/day were found to be clinically effective

**Dosing adjustment in renal impairment:** No data available; however, the urinary excretion of megestrol acetate administered in doses of 4-90 mg ranged from 56% to 78% within 10 days

Hemodialysis: Megestrol acetate has not been tested for dialyzability; however, due to its low solubility, it is postulated that dialysis would not be an effective means of treating an overdose

**Patient Information** Follow dosage schedule and do not take more than prescribed. You may experience sensitivity to sunlight (use sunblock, wear protective clothing, and avoid extended exposure to direct sunlight); dizziness, anxiety, depression (use caution when driving or engaging in tasks that require alertness until response to drug is known); change in appetite (maintain adequate hydration and diet - 2-3 L/day of fluids unless instructed to restrict fluid intake); decreased libido or increased body hair (reversible when drug is discontinued); hot flashes (cool clothes and environment may help). Report swelling of face, lips, or mouth; absence or altered menses; abdominal pain; vaginal itching, irritation, or discharge; heat, warmth, redness, or swelling of extremities; or sudden onset change in vision.

**Dosage Forms**

Suspension, oral: 40 mg/mL with alcohol 0.06% (236.6 mL)

Tablet: 20 mg, 40 mg

## Melaleuca Oil

**Pharmacologic Category** Herb

**Use** Marketed as having fungicidal, bactericidal properties; also used as a topical dermal agent for burns

**Overdosage/Toxicology**

Signs and symptoms: CNS depression, ataxia, aspiration pneumonitis, lethargy

Decontamination: Activated charcoal with cathartic

**Usual Dosage** Minimal toxic dose: Infant: <10 mL

**Additional Information** Found in New South Wales (Australia) on the north coast in swampy lowlands, this paper-bark tree can grow up to 20 ft high; the tree may also be found in southern U.S. (Florida), Spain, or Portugal; nutmeg odor; has been used to treat acne vulgaris, athlete's foot, and vaginitis

Oral: Mildly toxic

Dermal: Very mild irritant; no dermal sensitization; no phototoxicity

♦ **Melanex®** *see* Hydroquinone *on page 276*

## Melatonin (mel ah TOE nin)

**Related Information**

Clinical Issues in the Use of Anxiolytics and Sedative/Hypnotics *on page 634*

Perspectives on the Safety of Herbal Medicines *on page 736*

**Synonyms** N-Acetyl-5-methoxytryptamine

**Pharmacologic Category** Hormone; Hypnotic, Miscellaneous

**Use** Sleep disorders (insomnia), circadian rhythm disturbances (ie, jet lag); only FDA approval (as an orphan drug) is for treatment of circadian rhythm sleep disorders in blind people with no light perception

**Adverse Reactions** Percentage unknown:
- Central nervous system: Drowsiness, dysphoria (especially in depressed patients), giddiness, headache
- Dermatologic: Pruritus
- Gastrointestinal: Nausea
- Miscellaneous: Increase in alkaline phosphatase

**Drug Interactions**
- CNS depressants: Sedative effects may be additive with other sedative agents; monitor for increased effect; includes benzodiazepines, barbiturates, antipsychotics, antihistamines, ethanol, and other sedative medications
- Fluvoxamine: The bioavailability of melatonin has been reported to be increased by fluvoxamine
- Nifedipine: Melatonin has been reported to decrease the antihypertensive efficacy of nifedipine

**Mechanism of Action** A hormone produced and secreted in the pineal gland causes an increase in hypothalamus aminobutyric acid and serotonin. Increased secretion occurs during dark hours; decreases neopterin release; counteracts apoptosis; increases thymus activity

**Pharmacodynamics/kinetics**

Absorption: Rapid

Peak plasma level: 1 hour

**Usual Dosage** Oral:
- Jet lag: 5 mg/day (at 6 PM) for 1 week starting 3 days before the flight
- Hypnotic effects: Oral: 0.1-0.3 mg (daytime); 1-10 mg (nighttime)
- Insomnia: 5-75 mg at night have been used

**Reference Range** Mean baseline melatonin serum levels 80 pg/mL (range: 0-200) between 2-4 AM. Elevated endogenous levels seen after 9 AM; after a 2.5 mg oral dose, plasma melatonin level may be as high as 8.50 pg/mL.

**Dosage Forms**

Tablet: 3 mg

Tablet, sublingual: 2.5 mg

♦ **Mellaril®** *see* Thioridazine *on page 544*

♦ **Mellaril-S®** *see* Thioridazine *on page 544*

## Meloxicam (mel OX ee cam)

**U.S. Brand Names** Mobic®

**Pharmacologic Category** Nonsteroidal Anti-Inflammatory Agent (NSAID)

**Use** Relief of signs and symptoms of osteoarthritis

**Effects on Mental Status** May cause dizziness; may rarely cause abnormal dreams, anxiety, confusion, depression, nervousness, and somnolence

**Effects on Psychiatric Treatment** Rare reports of agranulocytosis, use caution with clozapine and carbamazepine; lithium levels can be increased; avoid concurrent use if possible or monitor lithium levels and adjust dose. When NSAID is stopped, lithium will need adjustment again.

**Pregnancy Risk Factor** C (D in third trimester)

**Contraindications** Hypersensitivity to meloxicam or any component, aspirin, or other nonsteroidal anti-inflammatory drugs (NSAIDs)

**Warnings/Precautions** Gastrointestinal irritation, ulceration, bleeding, and perforation may occur with NSAIDs. Serious complications may occur without prior symptoms of gastrointestinal distress. Use with caution in patients with a history of GI disease (bleeding or ulcers), decreased renal function, hepatic disease, congestive heart failure, dehydration, hypertension, or asthma. Use with caution in elderly patients. Anaphylactoid reactions may occur, even with no prior exposure to meloxicam. Use in advanced renal disease is not recommended. May alter platelet function; use with caution in patients receiving anticoagulants or with hemostatic disorders. Safety and efficacy in pediatric patients have not been established.

**Adverse Reactions**

1% to 10%:

Cardiovascular: Edema (2% to 5%)

Central nervous system: Headache and dizziness occurred in 2% to 8% of patients, but occurred less frequently than placebo in controlled trials

Dermatologic: Rash (1% to 3%)

Gastrointestinal: Diarrhea (3% to 8%), dyspepsia (5%), nausea (4%), flatulence (3%), abdominal pain (2% to 3%)

Respiratory: Upper respiratory infection (2% to 3%), pharyngitis (1% to 3%)

Miscellaneous: Flu-like symptoms (4% to 5%), falls (3%)

<2%: Allergic reaction, anaphylactic reaction, shock, fatigue, hot flashes, malaise, syncope, weight changes, angina, cardiac failure, hypertension, hypotension, myocardial infarction, vasculitis, seizures, paresthesia, tremor, vertigo, colitis, xerostomia, duodenal ulcer, gastric ulcer, gastritis, gastroesophageal reflux, gastrointestinal hemorrhage, hematemesis, intestinal perforation, melena, pancreatitis, duodenal perforation, gastric perforation, ulcerative stomatitis, arrhythmia, palpitations, tachycardia, agranulocytosis, leukopenia, purpura, thrombocytopenia, increased ALT, increased AST, hyperbilirubinemia, increased GGT, hepatitis, jaundice, hepatic failure, dehydration, abnormal dreams, anxiety, confusion, depression, nervousness, somnolence, asthma, bronchospasm, dyspnea, alopecia, angioedema, bullous eruption, erythema multiforme, photosensitivity reaction, pruritus, Stevens-Johnson syndrome, toxic epidermal necrolysis, urticaria, abnormal vision, conjunctivitis, taste perversion, tinnitus, albuminuria, increased BUN, increased creatinine, hematuria, interstitial nephritis, renal failure

**Overdosage/Toxicology** Symptoms of overdose include lethargy, drowsiness, nausea, vomiting, and epigastric pain. Rarely, severe symptoms have been associated with NSAID overdose including apnea, metabolic acidosis, coma, nystagmus, seizures, leukocytosis, and renal failure. Management of nonsteroidal anti-inflammatory (NSAID) intoxication is supportive and symptomatic. Since meloxicam undergoes enterohepatic cycling, multiple doses of charcoal may be needed to reduce the potential for delayed toxicities. Cholestyramine has been shown to increase meloxicam clearance.

**Drug Interactions** CYP2C8 and 2C9 enzyme substrate; CYP2C9 enzyme inhibitor

ACE inhibitors: Effects may be reduced by NSAIDs; use lowest possible dose for shortest duration possible; monitor

Cholestyramine and colestipol: Absorption may be reduced by concurrent administration

Corticosteroids: May increase the risk of GI ulceration; use caution

Cyclosporine: Nephrotoxicity may be increased with concurrent NSAID use; monitor

CYP2C9 inhibitors: May increase concentrations; inhibitors include amiodarone, cimetidine, fluvoxamine, metronidazole, omeprazole, sulfonamides, valproic acid, and zafirlukast

CYP2C9 substrates: Coadministration of drugs metabolized by CYP2C9 may result in increased serum concentrations of these agents

Hydralazine: Antihypertensive effect may be decreased; avoid concurrent use

Lithium: Serum levels can be increased; avoid concurrent use if possible or monitor lithium levels and adjust dose. When NSAID is stopped, lithium may need adjustment again.

Loop diuretics: Therapeutic effects may be reduced by NSAIDs; avoid

Methotrexate: Toxicity may be increased by concurrent NSAID use; risk is limited in low-dose methotrexate regimens (such as for rheumatoid arthritis); prolonged leucovorin rescue may be required at antineoplastic doses; monitor

Thiazide diuretics: Antihypertensive effects are decreased; avoid concurrent use

Warfarin: INRs may be increased by some NSAIDs. This may depend, in part, on dose and duration; monitor INR closely. Use the lowest dose of NSAIDs possible and for the briefest duration.

**Usual Dosage** Adults: Oral: Initial: 7.5 mg once daily; some patients may receive additional benefit from an increased dose of 15 mg once daily

**Dosage adjustment in renal impairment:** No specific dosage adjustment is recommended for mild to moderate renal impairment; avoid use in significant renal impairment

**Dosage adjustment in hepatic impairment:** No specific adjustment is recommended in hepatic impairment; patients with severe hepatic impairment have not been adequately studied

Elderly: Increased concentrations may occur in elderly patients (particularly in females); however, no specific dosage adjustment is recommended

**Dietary Considerations** Should be taken with food or milk to minimize gastrointestinal irritation

**Patient Information** If self-administered, use exactly as directed (do not increase dose or frequency); adverse reactions can occur with overuse. Take with food or milk. While using this medication, do not use alcohol, excessive amounts of vitamin C, or salicylate-containing foods (curry powder, prunes, raisins, tea, or licorice), other prescription or OTC medications containing aspirin or salicylate, or other NSAIDs without consulting prescriber. Maintain adequate hydration (2-3 L/day of fluids unless instructed to restrict fluid intake). You may experience nausea, vomiting, gastric discomfort (frequent mouth care, small frequent meals, chewing gum, sucking lozenges may help). GI bleeding, ulceration, or perforation can occur with or without pain. Stop taking medication and report ringing in ears; persistent cramping or pain in stomach; unresolved nausea or vomiting; difficulty breathing or shortness of breath; unusual bruising or bleeding (mouth, urine, stool); skin rash; unusual swelling of extremities; chest pain; or palpitations.

**Dosage Forms** Tablet: 7.5 mg

## Melphalan (MEL fa lan)

**U.S. Brand Names** Alkeran®

**Synonyms** L-PAM; L-Sarcolysin; Phenylalanine Mustard

**Pharmacologic Category** Antineoplastic Agent, Alkylating Agent

**Use** Palliative treatment of multiple myeloma and nonresectable epithelial ovarian carcinoma; neuroblastoma, rhabdomyosarcoma, breast cancer

**Effects on Mental Status** None reported

**Effects on Psychiatric Treatment** Myelosuppression is common; avoid concurrent use with clozapine and carbamazepine

**Pregnancy Risk Factor** D

**Contraindications** Hypersensitivity to melphalan or any component; severe bone marrow suppression; patients whose disease was resistant to prior therapy

**Warnings/Precautions** The U.S. Food and Drug Administration (FDA) currently recommends that procedures for proper handling and disposal for antineoplastic agents be considered. Is potentially mutagenic, carcinogenic, and teratogenic; produces amenorrhea. Reduce dosage or discontinue therapy if leukocyte count <3000/mm$^3$ or platelet count <100,000/mm$^3$; use with caution in patients with bone marrow suppression, impaired renal function, or who have received prior chemotherapy or irradiation; will cause amenorrhea. Toxicity to immunosuppressives is increased in elderly. Start with lowest recommended adult doses. Signs of infection, such as fever and WBC rise, may not occur. Lethargy and confusion may be more prominent signs of infection.

**Adverse Reactions**

>10%:

Hematologic: Myelosuppressive: Leukopenia and thrombocytopenia are the most common effects of melphalan. Irreversible bone marrow failure has been reported.

WBC: Moderate

Platelets: Moderate

Onset (days): 7

Nadir (days): 8-10 and 27-32

Recovery (days): 42-50

Second malignancies: Reported are melphalan more frequently

1% to 10%:

Cardiovascular: Vasculitis

Dermatologic: Vesiculation of skin, alopecia, pruritus, rash

Endocrine & metabolic: SIADH, sterility and amenorrhea

Gastrointestinal: Nausea and vomiting are mild; stomatitis and diarrhea are infrequent

Genitourinary: Bladder irritation, hemorrhagic cystitis

Hematologic: Anemia, agranulocytosis, hemolytic anemia

Respiratory: Pulmonary fibrosis, interstitial pneumonitis

Miscellaneous: Hypersensitivity

**Overdosage/Toxicology** Signs and symptoms: Hypocalcemia, pulmonary fibrosis, nausea and vomiting, bone marrow suppression

**Drug Interactions**

Decreased effect: Cimetidine® and other $H_2$-antagonists: The reduction in gastric pH has been reported to decrease bioavailability of melphalan by 30%

Increased toxicity: Cyclosporine: Increased incidence of nephrotoxicity

**Usual Dosage**

Oral (refer to individual protocols); dose should always be adjusted to patient response and weekly blood counts:

Children: 4-20 mg/m$^2$/day for 1-21 days

Adults:

Multiple myeloma: 6 mg/day initially adjusted as indicated **or** 0.15 mg/kg/day for 7 days **or** 0.25 mg/kg/day for 4 days; repeat at 4- to 6-week intervals

Ovarian carcinoma: 0.2 mg/kg/day for 5 days, repeat every 4-5 weeks

Intravenous (refer to individual protocols):

Children:

Pediatric rhabdomyosarcoma: 10-35 mg/m$^2$/dose every 21-28 days

High-dose melphalan with bone marrow transplantation for neuroblastoma: 70-100 mg/m$^2$/day on day 7 and 6 before BMT **or** 140-220 mg/m$^2$ single dose before BMT **or** 50 mg/m$^2$/day for 4 days **or** 70 mg/m$^2$/day for 3 days

Adults:

Multiple myeloma: 16 mg/m$^2$ administered at 2-week intervals for 4 doses, then repeat monthly as per protocol for multiple myeloma

**Dosing adjustment in renal impairment:**

$Cl_{cr}$ 10-50 mL/minute: Administer at 75% of normal dose

(Continued)

## Melphalan *(Continued)*

$Cl_{cr}$ <10 mL/minute: Administer at 50% of normal dose

**or**

BUN >30 mg/dL: Reduce dose by 50%

Serum creatinine >1.5 mg/dL: Reduce dose by 50%

Hemodialysis: Unknown

CAPD effects: Unknown

CAVH effects: Unknown

**Patient Information** Infusion: Report promptly any pain, irritation, or redness at infusion site. Oral: Preferable to take on an empty stomach, 1 hour prior to or 2 hours after meals. Do not take alcohol, aspirin or aspirin-containing medications, and OTC medications without consulting prescriber. Inform prescriber of all prescription medication you are taking. Maintain adequate fluid balance (2-3 L/day of fluids unless instructed to restrict fluid intake). May cause hair loss (reversible); easy bleeding or bruising (use soft toothbrush or cotton swabs and frequent mouth care, use electric razor, avoid sharp knives or scissors); increased susceptibility to infection (avoid crowds or exposure to infection - do not have any vaccinations unless approved by prescriber). Report unusual bleeding or bruising or persistent fever or sore throat; blood in urine, stool, or vomitus; delayed healing of any wounds; skin rash; yellowing of skin or eyes; changes in color of urine or black stool; pain or burning on urination; respiratory difficulty; or other severe adverse reactions.

**Nursing Implications** Avoid skin contact with I.V. formulation

**Dosage Forms**

Powder for injection: 50 mg

Tablet: 2 mg

♦ **Memoq®** *see* Nicergoline *on page 392*

♦ **Menadol® [OTC]** *see* Ibuprofen *on page 280*

♦ **Menest®** *see* Estrogens, Esterified *on page 207*

♦ **Meni-D®** *see* Meclizine *on page 335*

## Meningococcal Polysaccharide Vaccine, Groups A, C, Y, and W-135

(me NIN joe kok al pol i SAK a ride vak SEEN, groops aye, see, why, & dubl yoo won thur tee fyve)

**U.S. Brand Names** Menomune®-A/C/Y/W-135

**Pharmacologic Category** Vaccine

**Use**

Immunization of persons 2 years of age and above in epidemic or endemic areas as might be determined in a population delineated by neighborhood, school, dormitory, or other reasonable boundary. The prevalent serogroup in such a situation should match a serogroup in the vaccine. Individuals at particular high-risk include persons with terminal component complement deficiencies and those with anatomic or functional asplenia.

Travelers visiting areas of a country that are recognized as having hyper-endemic or epidemic meningococcal disease

Vaccinations should be considered for household or institutional contacts of persons with meningococcal disease as an adjunct to appropriate antibiotic chemoprophylaxis as well as medical and laboratory personnel at risk of exposure to meningococcal disease

**Effects on Mental Status** May cause drowsiness

**Effects on Psychiatric Treatment** None reported

**Pregnancy Risk Factor** C

**Contraindications** Children <2 years of age

**Warnings/Precautions** Patients who undergo splenectomy secondary to trauma or nonlymphoid tumors respond well; however, those asplenic patients with lymphoid tumors who receive either chemotherapy or irradiation respond poorly; pregnancy, unless there is substantial risk of infection.

**Adverse Reactions All serious adverse reactions must be reported to the U.S. Department of Health and Human Services (DHHS) Vaccine Adverse Event Reporting System (VAERS) 1-800-822-7967.**

>10%:

Central nervous system: Pain (17.5% to 24%)

Dermatologic: Erythema (0.8% to 31.7%), induration (4.8% to 8.3%)

Local: Tenderness (24% to 29%)

1% to 10%: Central nervous system: Headache (1.2% to 4.1%), malaise (≤2.6%), fever (0.4% to 3.1%), chills (≤1.7%)

**Drug Interactions** Decreased effect with administration of immunoglobulin within 1 month

**Usual Dosage** One dose S.C. (0.5 mL); the need for booster is unknown

**Patient Information** Inform patients about common side effects; patients should report serious and unusual effects to physician

**Nursing Implications** Epinephrine 1:1000 should be available to control allergic reaction

**Dosage Forms** Injection: 10 dose, 50 dose

♦ **Menomune®-A/C/Y/W-135** *see* Meningococcal Polysaccharide Vaccine, Groups A, C, Y, and W-135 *on page 340*

## Menotropins (men oh TROE pins)

**U.S. Brand Names** Humegon™; Pergonal®; Repronex™

**Pharmacologic Category** Gonadotropin; Ovulation Stimulator

**Use** Sequentially with hCG to induce ovulation and pregnancy in the infertile woman with functional anovulation or in patients who have previously received pituitary suppression; used with hCG in men to stimulate spermatogenesis in those with primary hypogonadotropic hypogonadism

**Effects on Mental Status** None reported

**Effects on Psychiatric Treatment** None reported

**Pregnancy Risk Factor** X

**Contraindications** Primary ovarian failure, overt thyroid and adrenal dysfunction, abnormal bleeding, pregnancy, men with normal urinary gonadotropin concentrations, elevated gonadotropin levels indicating primary testicular failure

**Warnings/Precautions** Advise patient of frequency and potential hazards of multiple pregnancy; to minimize the hazard of abnormal ovarian enlargement, use the lowest possible dose

**Adverse Reactions**

Male:

>10%: Endocrine & metabolic: Gynecomastia

1% to 10%: Erythrocytosis (shortness of breath, dizziness, anorexia, syncope, epistaxis)

Female:

>10%:

Endocrine & metabolic: Ovarian enlargement

Gastrointestinal: Abdominal distention

Local: Pain/rash at injection site

1% to 10%: Ovarian hyperstimulation syndrome

<1%: Febrile reactions, pain, thromboembolism

**Overdosage/Toxicology** Signs and symptoms: Ovarian hyperstimulation

**Drug Interactions** Clomiphene may ↓ amount of HMG needed to induce ovulation (Gonadorelin, Factrel®) should not be used with drugs that stimulate ovulation

**Usual Dosage** Adults: I.M.:

Male: Following pretreatment with hCG, 1 ampul 3 times/week and hCG 2000 units twice weekly until sperm is detected in the ejaculate (4-6 months) then may be increased to 2 ampuls of menotropins (150 units FSH/150 units LH) 3 times/week

Female: 1 ampul/day (75 units of FSH and LH) for 9-12 days followed by 10,000 units hCG 1 day after the last dose; repeated at least twice at same level before increasing dosage to 2 ampuls (150 units FSH/150 units LH)

Repronex™: I.M., S.C.:

Infertile patients with oligo-anovulation: Initial: 150 int. units daily for the first 5 days of treatment. Adjustments should not be made more frequently than once every 2 days and should not exceed 75-150 int. units per adjustment. Maximum daily dose should not exceed 450 int. units and dosing beyond 12 days is not recommended. If patient's response to Repronex™ is appropriate, hCG 5000-10,000 units should be given one day following the last dose of Repronex™.

Assisted reproductive technologies: Initial (in patients who have received GnRH agonist or antagonist pituitary suppression): 225 int. units; adjustments in dose should not be made more frequently than once every 2 days and should not exceed more than 75-50 int. units per adjustment. The maximum daily doses of Repronex™ given should not exceed 450 int. units and dosing beyond 12 days is not recommended. Once adequate follicular development is evident, hCG (5000-10,000 units) should be administered to induce final follicular maturation in preparation for oocyte retrieval.

**Patient Information** Self injection: Follow prescriber's recommended schedule for injections. Multiple ovulations resulting in multiple pregnancies have been reported. Male infertility and/or breast enlargement may occur. Report pain at injection site; enlarged breasts (male); difficulty breathing; nosebleeds; acute abdominal discomfort; or fever, pain, redness, or swelling of calves.

**Dosage Forms** Injection:

Follicle stimulating hormone activity 75 units and luteinizing hormone activity 75 units per 2 mL ampul

Follicle stimulating hormone activity 150 units and luteinizing hormone activity 150 units per 2 mL ampul

♦ **Mentax®** *see* Butenafine *on page 81*

♦ ***Mentha pulegium*** *see* Pennyroyal Oil *on page 426*

## Mepenzolate (me PEN zoe late)

**U.S. Brand Names** Cantil®

**Pharmacologic Category** Anticholinergic Agent; Antispasmodic Agent, Gastrointestinal

**Use** Management of peptic ulcer disease; inhibit salivation and excessive secretions in respiratory tract preoperatively

**Effects on Mental Status** May rarely cause confusion, amnesia, drowsiness, nervousness, or insomnia

**Effects on Psychiatric Treatment** Concurrent use with psychotropics may produce additive drowsiness or anticholinergic side effects (dry mouth)

**Usual Dosage** Adults: Oral: 25-50 mg 4 times/day with meal and at bedtime

**Dosage Forms** Tablet, as bromide: 25 mg

♦ **Mepergan®** *see* Meperidine and Promethazine *on page 341*

## Meperidine (me PER i deen)

**Related Information**

Narcotic Agonists Comparison Chart *on page 720*

**U.S. Brand Names** Demerol®

**Synonyms** Isonipecaine Hydrochloride; Pethidine Hydrochloride

**Pharmacologic Category** Analgesic, Narcotic

**Use** Management of moderate to severe pain; adjunct to anesthesia and preoperative sedation

**Effects on Mental Status** Sedation is common; may cause nervousness or confusion; may rarely produce depression, hallucinations, or paradoxical CNS stimulation

**Effects on Psychiatric Treatment** Sedation is common; may cause nervousness or confusion; may rarely produce depression, hallucinations, or paradoxical CNS stimulation

**Restrictions** C-II

**Pregnancy Risk Factor** B (D if used for prolonged periods or in high doses at term)

**Contraindications** Hypersensitivity to meperidine or any component; patients receiving MAO inhibitors presently or in the past 14 days

**Warnings/Precautions** Use with caution in patients with pulmonary, hepatic, renal disorders, or increased intracranial pressure; use with caution in patients with renal failure or seizure disorders or those receiving high-dose meperidine; normeperidine (an active metabolite and CNS stimulant) may accumulate and precipitate twitches, tremors, or seizures; some preparations contain sulfites which may cause allergic reaction; not recommended as a drug of first choice for the treatment of chronic pain in the elderly due to the accumulation of normeperidine; for acute pain, its use should be limited to 1-2 doses; tolerance or drug dependence may result from extended use

**Adverse Reactions**

>10%:

- Cardiovascular: Hypotension
- Central nervous system: Fatigue, drowsiness, dizziness
- Gastrointestinal: Nausea, vomiting, constipation
- Neuromuscular & skeletal: Weakness
- Miscellaneous: Histamine release

1% to 10%:

- Central nervous system: Nervousness, headache, restlessness, malaise, confusion
- Gastrointestinal: Anorexia, stomach cramps, xerostomia, biliary spasm
- Genitourinary: Ureteral spasms, decreased urination
- Local: Pain at injection site
- Respiratory: Dyspnea, shortness of breath

<1%: Hallucinations, increased intracranial pressure, mental depression, paradoxical CNS stimulation, paralytic ileus, physical and psychological dependence, rash, urticaria

**Overdosage/Toxicology**

Signs and symptoms: CNS depression, respiratory depression, mydriasis, bradycardia, pulmonary edema, chronic tremors, CNS excitability, seizures

Treatment: Includes support of the patient's airway, establishment of an I.V. line, and administration of naloxone 2 mg I.V. (0.01 mg/kg for children) with repeat administration as necessary up to a total of 10 mg.

**Drug Interactions** CYP2D6 enzyme substrate

Decreased effect: Phenytoin may decrease the analgesic effects

Increased toxicity: May aggravate the adverse effects of isoniazid; MAO inhibitors, fluoxetine, and other serotonin uptake inhibitors greatly potentiate the effects of meperidine; acute opioid overdosage symptoms can be seen, including severe toxic reactions; CNS depressants, tricyclic antidepressants, phenothiazines may potentiate the effects of meperidine

**Usual Dosage** Doses should be titrated to appropriate analgesic effect; when changing route of administration, note that oral doses are about half as effective as parenteral dose

Children: Oral, I.M., I.V., S.C.: 1-1.5 mg/kg/dose every 3-4 hours as needed; 1-2 mg/kg as a single dose preoperative medication may be used; maximum 100 mg/dose

Adults: Oral, I.M., I.V.: S.C.: 50-150 mg/dose every 3-4 hours as needed

Elderly:

- Oral: 50 mg every 4 hours
- I.M.: 25 mg every 4 hours

**Dosing adjustment in renal impairment:**

- $Cl_{cr}$ 10-50 mL/minute: Administer at 75% of normal dose
- $Cl_{cr}$ <10 mL/minute: Administer at 50% of normal dose

**Dosing adjustment/comments in hepatic disease:** Increased narcotic effect in cirrhosis; reduction in dose more important for oral than I.V. route

**Dietary Considerations**

Alcohol: Additive CNS effects, avoid or limit alcohol; watch for sedation

Food: Glucose may cause hyperglycemia; monitor blood glucose concentrations

**Patient Information** If self-administered, use exactly as directed (do not increase dose or frequency); may cause physical and/or psychological dependence. While using this medication, do not use alcohol and other prescription or OTC medications (especially sedatives, tranquilizers, antihistamines, or pain medications) without consulting prescriber. Maintain adequate hydration (2-3 L/day of fluids unless instructed to restrict fluid intake). May cause hypotension, dizziness, drowsiness, impaired coordination, or blurred vision (use caution when driving, climbing stairs, or changing position - rising from sitting or lying to standing, or when engaging in tasks requiring alertness until response to drug is known); loss of appetite, nausea, or vomiting (frequent mouth care, small frequent meals, chewing gum, or sucking lozenges may help); constipation (increased exercise, fluids, or dietary fruit and fiber may help - if constipation remains an unresolved problem, consult prescriber about use of stool softeners). Report chest pain, slow or rapid heartbeat, acute dizziness or persistent headache; changes in mental status; swelling of extremities or unusual weight gain; changes in urinary elimination; acute headache; back or flank pain or muscle spasms; blurred vision; skin rash; or shortness of breath.

**Dosage Forms**

Injection, as hydrochloride:

- Multiple-dose vials: 50 mg/mL (30 mL); 100 mg/mL (20 mL)
- Single-dose: 10 mg/mL (5 mL, 10 mL, 30 mL); 25 mg/dose (0.5 mL, 1 mL); 50 mg/dose (1 mL); 75 mg/dose (1 mL, 1.5 mL); 100 mg/dose (1 mL)

Syrup, as hydrochloride: 50 mg/5 mL (500 mL)

Tablet, as hydrochloride: 50 mg, 100 mg

## Meperidine and Promethazine
(me PER i deen & proe METH a zeen)

**U.S. Brand Names** Mepergan®

**Pharmacologic Category** Analgesic, Narcotic

**Use** Management of moderate to severe pain

**Effects on Mental Status** Sedation is common; may cause nervousness or confusion; may rarely produce depression, hallucinations, or paradoxical CNS stimulation

**Effects on Psychiatric Treatment** CYP2D6 enzyme substrate; may aggravate the adverse effects of MAO inhibitors, fluoxetine, and other serotonin uptake inhibitors. CNS depressants, tricyclic antidepressants, and phenothiazines may potentiate the effects of meperidine. Phenothiazines inhibit the ability of bromocriptine to lower serum prolactin concentrations; benztropine (and other anticholinergics) may inhibit the therapeutic response to promethazine and excess anticholinergic effects may occur.

**Usual Dosage** Adults:

- Oral: One (1) capsule every 4-6 hours
- I.M.: Inject 1-2 mL every 3-4 hours

**Dosage Forms**

Capsule: Meperidine hydrochloride 50 mg and promethazine hydrochloride 25 mg

Injection: Meperidine hydrochloride 25 mg and promethazine hydrochloride 25 per mL (2 mL, 10 mL)

## Mephentermine (me FEN ter meen)

**U.S. Brand Names** Wyamine® Sulfate Injection

**Pharmacologic Category** Adrenergic Agonist Agent

**Use** Treatment of hypotension secondary to ganglionic blockade or spinal anesthesia; may be used as an emergency measure to maintain blood pressure until whole blood replacement becomes available

**Effects on Mental Status** None reported

**Effects on Psychiatric Treatment** None reported

**Usual Dosage**

Hypotension: I.M., I.V.:

- Children: 0.4 mg/kg
- Adults: 0.5 mg/kg

Hypotensive emergency: I.V. infusion: 20-60 mg

**Dosage Forms** Injection, as sulfate: 15 mg/mL (2 mL, 10 mL); 30 mg/mL (10 mL)

## Mephenytoin (me FEN i toyn)

**Related Information**

Phenytoin *on page 441*

**U.S. Brand Names** Mesantoin®

**Synonyms** Methoin; Methylphenylethylhydantoin; Phenantoin

(Continued)

## Mephenytoin *(Continued)*

**Pharmacologic Category** Anticonvulsant, Hydantoin

**Use** Treatment of tonic-clonic and partial seizures in patients who are uncontrolled with less toxic anticonvulsants; usually used in combination with other anticonvulsants

**Effects on Mental Status** Drowsiness and dizziness are common; may cause insomnia; may rarely cause confusion

**Effects on Psychiatric Treatment** May cause leukopenia; use caution with clozapine or carbamazepine; may induce hepatic enzymes; caution with concurrent psychotropics; monitor for altered response

**Contraindications** Hypersensitivity to mephenytoin, other hydantoins, or any component

**Warnings/Precautions** Fatal irreversible aplastic anemia has occurred; abrupt withdrawal may precipitate seizures; may increase frequency of petit mal seizures; use with caution in patients with liver disease or porphyria; usually listed in combination with other anticonvulsants

**Adverse Reactions**

>10%:

Central nervous system: Psychiatric changes, slurred speech, trembling, dizziness, drowsiness

Gastrointestinal: Constipation, nausea, vomiting

1% to 10%:

Central nervous system: Headache, insomnia

Dermatologic: Skin rash

Gastrointestinal: Anorexia, weight loss

Hematologic: Leukopenia

Hepatic: Hepatitis

Renal: Increase in serum creatinine

**Overdosage/Toxicology**

Signs and symptoms: Restlessness, dizziness, drowsiness, nausea, vomiting, nystagmus, ataxia, dysarthria, tremor, slurred speech, hypotension, respiratory depression, coma

Treatment: Supportive

**Drug Interactions** Refer to Phenytoin monograph

**Usual Dosage** Oral:

Children: 3-15 mg/kg/day in 3 divided doses; usual maintenance dose: 100-400 mg/day in 3 divided doses

Adults: Initial dose: 50-100 mg/day given daily; increase by 50-100 mg at weekly intervals; usual maintenance dose: 200-600 mg/day in 3 divided doses; maximum: 800 mg/day

**Patient Information** Take with food, avoid alcoholic beverages; may cause dizziness, drowsiness, and impair coordination or judgment

**Dosage Forms** Tablet: 100 mg

## Mephobarbital (me foe BAR bi tal)

**Related Information**

Patient Information - Anxiolytics & Sedative Hypnotics (Barbiturates) *on page 654*

**U.S. Brand Names** Mebaral®

**Synonyms** Methylphenobarbital

**Pharmacologic Category** Barbiturate

**Use** Sedative; treatment of grand mal and petit mal epilepsy

**Effects on Mental Status** Dizziness and drowsiness are common; may cause confusion, nervousness, depression, nightmares, or insomnia; may rarely cause hallucinations

**Effects on Psychiatric Treatment** May rarely cause agranulocytosis; use caution with clozapine and carbamazepine; may induce hepatic enzymes resulting in an increase or decrease effect of concurrent psychotropic; monitor to altered response

**Restrictions** C-IV

**Pregnancy Risk Factor** D

**Contraindications** Hypersensitivity to mephobarbital, other barbiturates, or any component; pre-existing CNS depression; respiratory depression; severe uncontrolled pain; history of porphyria

**Warnings/Precautions** Use with caution in patients with renal impairment, pulmonary insufficiency, or hepatic dysfunction; sometimes used in specific patients who have excessive sedation or hyperexcitability from phenobarbital; abrupt withdrawal may precipitate status epilepticus

**Adverse Reactions**

>10%: Central nervous system: Dizziness, lightheadedness, drowsiness, "hangover" effect

1% to 10%:

Central nervous system: Confusion, mental depression, unusual excitement, nervousness, faint feeling, headache, insomnia, nightmares

Gastrointestinal: Constipation, nausea, vomiting

**Overdosage/Toxicology**

Signs and symptoms: CNS depression, respiratory depression, hypothermia, tachycardia, hypotension

Treatment: Repeated oral doses of activated charcoal significantly reduce the half-life of barbiturates resulting from an enhancement of nonrenal elimination. The usual dose is 30-60 g every 4-6 hours for 3-4 days unless the patient has no bowel movement causing the charcoal to remain in the GI tract. Assure adequate hydration and renal function. Urinary alkalinization with I.V. sodium bicarbonate also helps to enhance elimination. Hemodialysis or hemoperfusion is of uncertain value. Patients in stage IV coma due to high serum barbiturate levels may require charcoal hemoperfusion.

**Drug Interactions** CYP2C, 2C8, and 2C19 enzyme substrate

Antineoplastics: Limited evidence suggests that enzyme-inducing anticonvulsant therapy may reduce the effectiveness of some chemotherapy regimens (specifically in ALL); teniposide and methotrexate may be cleared more rapidly in these patients

**Usual Dosage** Oral:

Epilepsy:

Children: 6-12 mg/kg/day in 2-4 divided doses

Adults: 200-600 mg/day in 2-4 divided doses

Sedation:

Children:

<5 years: 16-32 mg 3-4 times/day

>5 years: 32-64 mg 3-4 times/day

Adults: 32-100 mg 3-4 times/day

**Dosing adjustment in renal or hepatic impairment:** Use with caution and reduce dosages

**Patient Information** May cause drowsiness, may impair coordination and judgment; do not discontinue abruptly; notify physician of dark urine, pale stools, jaundice, abdominal pain, persistent nausea, and vomiting; do not skip doses

**Dosage Forms** Tablet: 32 mg, 50 mg, 100 mg

♦ **Mephyton® Oral** *see* Phytonadione *on page 444*

## Mepivacaine (me PIV a kane)

**U.S. Brand Names** Carbocaine®; Isocaine® HCl; Polocaine®

**Pharmacologic Category** Local Anesthetic

**Use** Local anesthesia by nerve block; infiltration in dental procedures; **not** for use in spinal anesthesia

**Effects on Mental Status** May rarely cause anxiety, restlessness, confusion, drowsiness

**Effects on Psychiatric Treatment** None reported

**Usual Dosage** Children and Adults: Injectable local anesthetic: Varies with procedure, degree of anesthesia needed, vascularity of tissue, duration of anesthesia required, and physical condition of patient

**Dosage Forms** Injection, as hydrochloride: 1% [10 mg/mL] (30 mL, 50 mL); 1.5% [15 mg/mL] (30 mL); 2% [20 mg/mL] (20 mL, 50 mL); 3% [30 mg/mL] (1.8 mL)

## Meprobamate (me proe BA mate)

**Related Information**

Anxiolytic/Hypnotic Use in Long-Term Care Facilities *on page 754*

Federal OBRA Regulations Recommended Maximum Doses *on page 756*

**Generic Available** Yes

**U.S. Brand Names** Equanil®; Miltown®; Neuramate®

**Canadian Brand Names** Apo®-Meprobamate; Meditran®; Novo-Mepro

**Pharmacologic Category** Antianxiety Agent, Miscellaneous

**Use** Management of anxiety disorders

**Unlabeled uses:** Demonstrated value for muscle contraction; headache; premenstrual tension; external sphincter spasticity; muscle rigidity; opisthotonos-associated with tetanus

**Restrictions** C-IV

**Pregnancy Risk Factor** D

**Contraindications** Acute intermittent porphyria; hypersensitivity to meprobamate, related compounds (including carisoprodol), or any component; pre-existing CNS depression; narrow-angle glaucoma; severe uncontrolled pain; pregnancy

**Warnings/Precautions** Physical and psychological dependence and abuse may occur; abrupt cessation may precipitate withdrawal. Use with caution in patients with depression or suicidal tendencies, or in patients with a history of drug abuse. May cause CNS depression, which may impair physical or mental abilities. Patients must be cautioned about performing tasks which require mental alertness (ie, operating machinery or driving). Effects with other sedative drugs or ethanol may be potentiated. Not recommended in children <6 years of age; allergic reaction may occur in patients with history of dermatological condition (usually by fourth dose). Use with caution in patients with renal or hepatic impairment, or with a history of seizures. Use caution in the elderly as it may cause confusion, cognitive impairment, or excessive sedation.

**Adverse Reactions**

Cardiovascular: Syncope, peripheral edema, palpitations, tachycardia, arrhythmia

Central nervous system: Drowsiness, ataxia, dizziness, paradoxical excitement, confusion, slurred speech, headache, euphoria, chills, vertigo, paresthesia, overstimulation

Dermatologic: Rashes, purpura, dermatitis, Stevens-Johnson syndrome, petechiae, ecchymosis

Gastrointestinal: Diarrhea, vomiting, nausea

Hematologic: Leukopenia, eosinophilia, agranulocytosis, aplastic anemia
Neuromuscular & skeletal: Weakness
Ocular: Blurred vision, impairment of accommodation
Renal: Renal failure
Respiratory: Wheezing, dyspnea, bronchospasm, angioneurotic edema

**Drug Interactions** CNS depressants: Sedative effects may be additive with other CNS depressants; monitor for increased effect; includes barbiturates, benzodiazepines, narcotic analgesics, ethanol, and other sedative agents

**Mechanism of Action** Affects the thalamus and limbic system; also appears to inhibit multineuronal spinal reflexes

**Pharmacodynamics/kinetics**
Onset of sedation: Oral: Within 1 hour
Distribution: Crosses the placenta; appears in breast milk
Metabolism: Promptly in the liver
Half-life: 10 hours
Elimination: In urine (8% to 20% as unchanged drug) and feces (10% as metabolites)

**Usual Dosage** Oral:
Children 6-12 years: 100-200 mg 2-3 times/day
Sustained release: 200 mg twice daily
Adults: 400 mg 3-4 times/day, up to 2400 mg/day
Sustained release: 400-800 mg twice daily
**Dosing interval in renal impairment:**
$Cl_{cr}$ 10-50 mL/minute: Administer every 9-12 hours
$Cl_{cr}$ <10 mL/minute: Administer every 12-18 hours
Hemodialysis: Moderately dialyzable (20% to 50%)
**Dosing adjustment in hepatic impairment:** Probably necessary in patients with liver disease

**Dietary Considerations** Alcohol: Additive CNS effect, avoid use

**Monitoring Parameters** Mental status

**Reference Range** Therapeutic: 6-12 µg/mL (SI: 28-55 µmol/L); Toxic: >60 µg/mL (SI: >275 µmol/L)

**Patient Information** May cause drowsiness; avoid alcoholic beverages

**Nursing Implications** Assist with ambulation

**Additional Information** Withdrawal should be gradual over 1-2 weeks; benzodiazepine and buspirone are better choices for treatment of anxiety disorders

**Dosage Forms**
Capsule, sustained release: 200 mg, 400 mg
Tablet: 200 mg, 400 mg, 600 mg

♦ **Mepron™** *see* Atovaquone *on page 52*

## Mequinol and Tretinoin (ME kwi nol & TRET i noyn)

**U.S. Brand Names** Solagé™ Topical Solution

**Pharmacologic Category** Retinoic Acid Derivative; Vitamin A Derivative; Vitamin, Topical

**Use** Treatment of solar lentigines; the efficacy of using Solagé™ daily for >24 weeks has not been established. The local cutaneous safety of Solagé™ in non-Caucasians has not been adequately established.

**Effects on Mental Status** None reported

**Effects on Psychiatric Treatment** Photosensitizing drugs such as psychotropics can further increase sun sensitivity; avoid concurrent use

**Usual Dosage** Adults: Topical: Apply twice daily to solar lentigines using the applicator tip while avoiding application to the surrounding skin. Separate application by at least 8 hours or as directed by physician.

**Dosage Forms** Liquid, topical: Mequinol 2% and tretinoin 0.01% (30 mL)

## Mercaptopurine (mer kap toe PYOOR een)

**U.S. Brand Names** Purinethol®

**Synonyms** 6-Mercaptopurine; 6-MP

**Pharmacologic Category** Antineoplastic Agent, Antimetabolite

**Use** Treatment of acute leukemias (ALL or AML) maintenance therapy

**Effects on Mental Status** None reported

**Effects on Psychiatric Treatment** May cause leukopenia; use caution with clozapine or carbamazepine

**Pregnancy Risk Factor** D

**Contraindications** Hypersensitivity to mercaptopurine or any component; patients whose disease showed prior resistance to mercaptopurine or thioguanine; severe liver disease, severe bone marrow suppression

**Warnings/Precautions** The U.S. Food and Drug Administration (FDA) currently recommends that procedures for proper handling and disposal of antineoplastic agents be considered. Mercaptopurine may cause birth defects; potentially carcinogenic; adjust dosage in patients with renal impairment or hepatic failure; use with caution in patients with prior bone marrow suppression; patients may be at risk for pancreatitis. Toxicity to immunosuppressives is increased in elderly. Start with lowest recommended adult doses. Signs of infection, such as fever and WBC rise, may not occur. Lethargy and confusion may be more prominent signs of infection.

**Adverse Reactions**
>10%: Hepatic: 6-MP can cause an intrahepatic cholestasis and focal centrilobular necrosis manifested as hyperbilirubinemia, increased alkaline phosphatase, and increased AST. This may be dose related, occurring more frequently at doses >2.5 mg/kg/day; jaundice is noted 1-2 months into therapy, but has ranged from 1 week to 8 years.
1% to 10%:
Dermatologic: Hyperpigmentation, rash
Endocrine & metabolic: Hyperuricemia
Gastrointestinal: Nausea, vomiting, diarrhea, stomatitis, anorexia, stomach pain, and mucositis may require parenteral nutrition and dose reduction; 6-TG is less GI toxic than 6-MP
Hematologic: Leukopenia, thrombocytopenia, anemia may occur at high doses
Myelosuppressive:
WBC: Moderate
Platelets: Moderate
Onset (days): 7-10
Nadir (days): 14
Recovery (days): 21
Renal: Renal toxicity
<1%: Drug fever, dry and scaling rash, eosinophilia, glossitis, tarry stools

**Overdosage/Toxicology** Signs and symptoms:
Immediate: Nausea, vomiting
Delayed: Bone marrow suppression, hepatic necrosis, gastroenteritis

**Drug Interactions**
Decreased effect: Warfarin: 6-MP inhibits the anticoagulation effect of warfarin by an unknown mechanism
Increased toxicity:
Allopurinol: Can cause increased levels of 6-MP by inhibition of xanthine oxidase; decrease dose of 6-MP by 75% when both drugs are used concomitantly; seen only with oral 6-MP usage, not with I.V.; may potentiate effect of bone marrow suppression (reduce 6-MP to 25% of dose)
Doxorubicin: Synergistic liver toxicity with 6-MP in >50% of patients, which resolved with discontinuation of the 6-MP
Hepatotoxic drugs: Any agent which could potentially alter the metabolic function of the liver could produce higher drug levels and greater toxicities from either 6-MP or 6-TG

**Usual Dosage** Oral (refer to individual protocols):
Children: Maintenance: 75 mg/m²/day given once daily
Adults:
Induction: 2.5-5 mg/kg/day (100-200 mg)
Maintenance: 1.5-2.5 mg/kg/day **OR** 80-100 mg/m²/day given once daily
Elderly: Due to renal decline with age, start with lower recommended doses for adults
**Dosing adjustment in renal or hepatic impairment:** Dose should be reduced to avoid accumulation, but specific guidelines are not available
Hemodialysis: Removed; supplemental dosing is usually required

**Patient Information** Take daily dose at the same time each day. Preferable to take an on empty stomach (1 hour before or 2 hours after meals). Maintain adequate hydration (2-3 L/day of fluids unless instructed to restrict fluid intake). You may experience nausea and vomiting, diarrhea, or loss of appetite (frequent small meals may help/request medication) or weakness or lethargy (use caution when driving or engaging in tasks that require alertness until response to drug is known). Use good oral care to reduce incidence of mouth sores. You may be more susceptible to infection (avoid crowds or exposure to infection). May cause headache (request medication). Report signs of opportunistic infection (eg, fever, chills, sore throat, burning urination, fatigue); bleeding (eg, tarry stools, easy bruising); unresolved mouth sores, nausea, or vomiting; swelling of extremities, difficulty breathing, or unusual weight gain.

**Dosage Forms** Tablet, scored: 50 mg

♦ **6-Mercaptopurine** *see* Mercaptopurine *on page 343*

♦ **Mercapturic Acid** *see* Acetylcysteine *on page 18*

## Mercuric Oxide (mer KYOOR ik OKS ide)

**Synonyms** Yellow Mercuric Oxide

**Pharmacologic Category** Antibiotic, Ophthalmic

**Use** Treatment of irritation and minor infections of the eyelids

**Effects on Mental Status** None reported

**Effects on Psychiatric Treatment** None reported

**Warnings/Precautions** Prolonged use may cause serious mercury poisoning

**Usual Dosage** Apply small amount to inner surface of lower eyelid once or twice daily

**Dosage Forms** Ointment, ophthalmic: 1%, 2% [OTC]

♦ **Mereprine®** *see* Doxylamine *on page 186*

♦ **Meridia®** *see* Sibutramine *on page 511*

## Meropenem (mer oh PEN em)

**U.S. Brand Names** Merrem® I.V.

**Pharmacologic Category** Antibiotic, Carbapenem

**Use** Intra-abdominal infections (complicated appendicitis and peritonitis) caused by viridans group streptococci, *E. coli*, *K. pneumoniae*, *P. aeruginosa*, *B. fragilis*, *B. thetaiotaomicron*, and *Peptostreptococcus* sp; also indicated for bacterial meningitis in pediatric patients >3 months of age caused by *S. pneumoniae*, *H. influenzae*, and *N. meningitidis*; meropenem has also been used to treat soft tissue infections, febrile neutropenia, and urinary tract infections

**Effects on Mental Status** May rarely cause agitation, confusion, insomnia, hallucinations, or depression

**Effects on Psychiatric Treatment** None reported

**Usual Dosage** I.V.:

Neonates:

Preterm: 20 mg/kg/dose every 12 hours (may be increased to 40 mg/kg/dose if treating a highly resistant organism such as *Pseudomonas aeruginosa*)

Full-term (<3 months of age): 20 mg/kg/dose every 8 hours (may be increased to 40 mg/kg/dose if treating a highly resistant organism such as *Pseudomonas aeruginosa*)

Children >3 months (<50 kg):

Intra-abdominal infections: 20 mg/kg every 8 hours (maximum dose: 1 g every 8 hours)

Meningitis: 40 mg/kg every 8 hours (maximum dose: 2 g every 8 hours)

Children >50 kg:

Intra-abdominal infections: 1 g every 8 hours

Meningitis: 2 g every 8 hours

Adults: 1 g every 8 hours

**Dosing adjustment in renal impairment:** Adults:

$Cl_{cr}$ 26-50 mL/minute: Administer 1 g every 12 hours

$Cl_{cr}$ 10-25 mL/minute: Administer 500 mg every 12 hours

$Cl_{cr}$ <10 mL/minute: Administer 500 mg every 24 hours

Dialysis: Meropenem and its metabolites are readily dialyzable

Continuous arteriovenous or venovenous hemodiafiltration (CAVH) effects: Dose as $Cl_{cr}$ 10-50 mL/minute

**Dosage Forms**

Infusion: 500 mg (100 mL); 1 g (100 mL)

Infusion, ADD-vantage®: 500 mg (15 mL); 1 g (15 mL)

Injection: 25 mg/mL (20 mL); 33.3 mg/mL (30 mL)

♦ **Merrem® I.V.** *see* Meropenem *on page 344*

## Mesalamine (me SAL a meen)

**U.S. Brand Names** Asacol® Oral; Pentasa® Oral; Rowasa® Rectal

**Synonyms** 5-Aminosalicylic Acid; 5-ASA; Fisalamine; Mesalazine

**Pharmacologic Category** 5-Aminosalicylic Acid Derivative

**Use**

Oral: Remission and treatment of mildly to moderately active ulcerative colitis

Rectal: Treatment of active mild to moderate distal ulcerative colitis, proctosigmoiditis, or proctitis

**Effects on Mental Status** Malaise is common

**Effects on Psychiatric Treatment** None reported

**Pregnancy Risk Factor** B

**Contraindications** Known hypersensitivity to mesalamine, sulfasalazine, sulfites, or salicylates

**Warnings/Precautions** Pericarditis should be considered in patients with chest pain; pancreatitis should be considered in any patient with new abdominal complaints. Elderly may have difficulty administering and retaining rectal suppositories. Given renal function decline with aging, monitor serum creatinine often during therapy. Use caution in patients with impaired hepatic function.

**Adverse Reactions**

>10%:

Central nervous system: Headache, malaise

Gastrointestinal: Abdominal pain, cramps, flatulence, gas

1% to 10%: Dermatologic: Alopecia, rash

<1%: Acute intolerance syndrome (bloody diarrhea, severe abdominal cramps, severe headache), anal irritation

**Overdosage/Toxicology**

Signs and symptoms: Decreased motor activity, diarrhea, vomiting, renal function impairment

Treatment: Supportive; emesis, gastric lavage, and follow with activated charcoal slurry

**Drug Interactions** Decreased effect: Decreased digoxin bioavailability

**Usual Dosage** Adults (usual course of therapy is 3-6 weeks):

Oral:

Capsule: 1 g 4 times/day

Tablet: 800 mg 3 times/day

Retention enema: 60 mL (4 g) at bedtime, retained overnight, approximately 8 hours

Rectal suppository: Insert 1 suppository in rectum twice daily

Some patients may require rectal and oral therapy concurrently

**Patient Information** Take as directed. Oral: Do not chew or break tablets. Enemas: Shake well before using, retain for 8 hours or as long as possible. Suppository: After removing foil wrapper, insert high in rectum without excessive handling (warmth will melt suppository). You may experience flatulence, headache, or hair loss (reversible). Report abdominal pain, unresolved diarrhea, severe headache, or chest pain.

**Nursing Implications** Provide patient with copy of mesalamine administration instructions

**Dosage Forms**

Capsule, controlled release (Pentasa®): 250 mg

Suppository, rectal (Rowasa®): 500 mg

Suspension, rectal (Rowasa®): 4 g/60 mL (7s)

Tablet, enteric coated (Asacol®): 400 mg

♦ **Mesalazine** *see* Mesalamine *on page 344*

♦ **Mesantoin®** *see* Mephenytoin *on page 341*

## Mesna (MES na)

**U.S. Brand Names** Mesnex™

**Pharmacologic Category** Antidote

**Use** Detoxifying agent used as a protectant against hemorrhagic cystitis induced by ifosfamide and cyclophosphamide

**Effects on Mental Status** May cause malaise

**Effects on Psychiatric Treatment** None reported

**Usual Dosage** Children and Adults (refer to individual protocols); oral dose is approximately equivalent to 2 times the I.V. dose

I.V.:

Ifosfamide: 20% W/W of ifosfamide dose 15 minutes before ifosfamide administration and 4 and 8 hours after each dose of ifosfamide; **total daily dose is 60% to 100% of ifosfamide**; for high dose ifosfamide: 20% W/W 15 minutes before ifosfamide administration, and every 3 hours for 3-6 doses, some regimens use up to 160% of the total ifosfamide dose

Cyclophosphamide: 20% W/W of cyclophosphamide dose 15 minutes prior to cyclophosphamide administration and 4 and 8 hours after each dose of cyclophosphamide; **total daily dose = 60% to 200% of cyclophosphamide dose**

Oral: 40% W/W of the ifosfamide or cyclophosphamide agent dose in 3 doses at 4-hour intervals **OR** 20 mg/kg/dose every 4 hours x 3 (oral mesna is not recommended for the first dose before ifosfamide or cyclophosphamide)

**Dosage Forms** Injection: 100 mg/mL (2 mL, 4 mL, 10 mL)

♦ **Mesnex™** *see* Mesna *on page 344*

## Mesoridazine (mez oh RID a zeen)

**Related Information**

Antipsychotic Agents Comparison Chart *on page 706*

Antipsychotic Medication Guidelines *on page 751*

Clinical Issues in the Use of Antipsychotics *on page 630*

Discontinuation of Psychotropic Drugs - Withdrawal Symptoms and Recommendations *on page 798*

Federal OBRA Regulations Recommended Maximum Doses *on page 756*

Liquid Compatibility With Antipsychotics and Mood Stabilizers *on page 718*

Patient Information - Antipsychotics (General) *on page 646*

**Generic Available** No

**U.S. Brand Names** Serentil®

**Synonyms** Mesoridazine Besylate

**Pharmacologic Category** Antipsychotic Agent, Phenothazine, Piperidine

**Use** Schizophrenia; behavioral problems in mental deficiency and chronic brain syndrome; alcoholism (acute and chronic); psychoneurotic manifestations (anxiety, tension)

**Pregnancy Risk Factor** C

**Contraindications** Hypersensitivity to mesoridazine or any component (cross reactivity between phenothiazines may occur); severe CNS depression and coma

**Warnings/Precautions** May cause hypotension, particularly with I.M. administration. Highly sedating, use with caution in disorders where CNS depression is a feature. Use with caution in Parkinson's disease. Caution in patients with hemodynamic instability; bone marrow suppression; predisposition to seizures; subcortical brain damage; severe cardiac, hepatic, renal, or respiratory disease. Esophageal dysmotility and aspiration have been associated with antipsychotic use - use with caution in patients at risk of pneumonia (ie, Alzheimer's disease). Caution in breast cancer or other prolactin-dependent tumors (may elevate prolactin levels). May alter temperature regulation or mask toxicity of other drugs due to antiemetic effects. May alter cardiac conduction; life-threatening arrhythmias have occurred with therapeutic doses of phenothiazines. May cause orthostatic hypotension - use with caution in patients at risk of this effect or those who would tolerate transient hypotensive episodes (cerebrovascular disease, cardiovascular disease, or other medications which may predispose).

Phenothiazines may cause anticholinergic effects (confusion, agitation, constipation, dry mouth, blurred vision, urinary retention). Therefore, they should be used with caution in patients with decreased gastrointestinal motility, urinary retention, BPH, xerostomia, or visual problems. Conditions which also may be exacerbated by cholinergic blockade include narrow-angle glaucoma (screening is recommended) and worsening of myasthenia gravis. Relative to other antipsychotics, mesoridazine has a high potency of cholinergic blockade.

May cause extrapyramidal reactions, including pseudoparkinsonism, acute dystonic reactions, akathisia, and tardive dyskinesia (risk of these reactions is low relative to other neuroleptics). May be associated with neuroleptic malignant syndrome (NMS) or pigmentary retinopathy (particularly at doses >1 g/day).

**Adverse Reactions**

Cardiovascular: Hypotension, orthostatic hypotension, tachycardia, Q-T prolongation, syncope, edema

Central nervous system: Pseudoparkinsonism, akathisia, dystonias, tardive dyskinesia, dizziness, drowsiness, restlessness, ataxia, slurred speech, neuroleptic malignant syndrome (NMS), impairment of temperature regulation, lowering of seizure threshold

Dermatologic: Increased sensitivity to sun, rash, itching, angioneurotic edema, dermatitis, discoloration of skin (blue-gray)

Endocrine & metabolic: Changes in menstrual cycle, changes in libido, gynecomastia, lactation, galactorrhea

Gastrointestinal: Constipation, xerostomia, weight gain, nausea, vomiting, stomach pain

Genitourinary: Difficulty in urination, ejaculatory disturbances, impotence, enuresis, incontinence, priapism, urinary retention

Hematologic: Agranulocytosis, leukopenia, eosinophilia, thrombocytopenia, anemia, aplastic anemia

Hepatic: Cholestatic jaundice, hepatotoxicity

Neuromuscular & skeletal: Weakness, tremor, rigidity

Ocular: Pigmentary retinopathy, photophobia, blurred vision, cornea and lens changes

Respiratory: Nasal congestion

Miscellaneous: Diaphoresis (decreased)

**Overdosage/Toxicology**

Signs and symptoms: Deep sleep, coma, extrapyramidal symptoms, abnormal involuntary muscle movements, hypotension

Treatment:

Following initiation of essential overdose management, toxic symptom treatment and supportive treatment should be initiated

Hypotension usually responds to I.V. fluids or Trendelenburg positioning. If unresponsive to these measures, the use of a parenteral inotrope may be required.

Seizures commonly respond to diazepam (I.V. 5-10 mg bolus in adults every 15 minutes if needed up to a total of 30 mg; I.V. 0.25-0.4 mg/kg/dose up to a total of 10 mg in children) or to phenytoin or phenobarbital.

Critical cardiac arrhythmias often respond to I.V. phenytoin (15 mg/kg up to 1 g), while other antiarrhythmics can be used.

Extrapyramidal symptoms (eg, dystonic reactions) can be managed with benztropine mesylate I.V. 1-2 mg (adults)

**Drug Interactions** CYP1A2, 2D6, and 3A3/4 enzyme substrate; CYP2D6 enzyme inhibitor

Aluminum salts: May decrease the absorption of phenothiazines; monitor

Amphetamines: Efficacy may be diminished by antipsychotics; in addition, amphetamines may increase psychotic symptoms; avoid concurrent use

Anticholinergics: May inhibit the therapeutic response to phenothiazines and excess anticholinergic effects may occur; includes benztropine, trihexyphenidyl, biperiden, and drugs with significant anticholinergic activity (TCAs, antihistamines, disopyramide)

Antihypertensives: Concurrent use of phenothiazines with an antihypertensive may produce additive hypotensive effects (particularly orthostasis)

Bromocriptine: Phenothiazines inhibit the ability of bromocriptine to lower serum prolactin concentrations

Chloroquine: Serum concentrations of chlorpromazine may be increased by chloroquine

CNS depressants: Sedative effects may be additive with phenothiazines; monitor for increased effect; includes barbiturates, benzodiazepines, narcotic analgesics, ethanol, and other sedative agents

CYP1A2 inhibitors: Metabolism of phenothiazines may be decreased; increasing clinical effect or toxicity. Inhibitors include cimetidine, ciprofloxacin, fluvoxamine, isoniazid, ritonavir, and zileutin

CYP2D6 inhibitors: Metabolism of phenothiazines may be decreased; increasing clinical effect or toxicity; inhibitors include amiodarone, cimetidine, delavirdine, fluoxetine, paroxetine, propafenone, quinidine, and ritonavir; monitor for increased effect/toxicity

CYP3A3/4 inhibitors: Metabolism of phenothiazines may be decreased; increasing clinical effect or toxicity; inhibitors include amiodarone, cimetidine, clarithromycin, erythromycin, delavirdine, diltiazem, dirithromycin, disulfiram, fluoxetine, fluvoxamine, grapefruit juice, indinavir, itraconazole, ketoconazole, nefazodone, nevirapine, propoxyfene, quinupristin-dalfopristin, ritonavir, saquinavir, verapamil, zafirlukast, zileuton

Enzyme inducers: May enhance the hepatic metabolism of phenothiazines; larger doses may be required. Includes rifampin, rifabutin, barbiturates, phenytoin, and cigarette smoking

Epinephrine: Chlorpromazine (and possibly other low potency antipsychotics) may diminish the pressor effects of epinephrine

Guanethidine and guanadrel: Antihypertensive effects may be inhibited by chlorpromazine

Levodopa: Chlorpromazine may inhibit the antiparkinsonian effect of levodopa; avoid this combination

Lithium: Chlorpromazine may produce neurotoxicity with lithium; this is a rare effect

Phenytoin: May reduce serum levels of phenothiazines; phenothiazines may increase phenytoin serum levels

Propranolol: Serum concentrations of phenothiazines may be increased; propranolol also increases phenothiazine concentrations

Polypeptide antibiotics: Rare cases of respiratory paralysis have been reported with concurrent use of phenothiazines

QTc prolonging agents: Effects on QTc interval may be additive with phenothiazines, increasing the risk of malignant arrhythmias; includes type Ia antiarrhythmics, TCAs, and some quinolone antibiotics (sparfloxacin, moxifloxacin and gatifloxacin)

Sulfadoxine-pyrimethamine: May increase phenothiazine concentrations

Tricyclic antidepressants: Concurrent use may produce increased toxicity or altered therapeutic response

Trazodone: Phenothiazines and trazodone may produce additive hypotensive effects

Valproic acid: Serum levels may be increased by phenothiazines

**Stability** Protect all dosage forms from light; clear or slightly yellow solutions may be used; should be dispensed in amber or opaque vials/bottles. Solutions may be diluted or mixed with fruit juices or other liquids but must be administered immediately after mixing; do not prepare bulk dilutions or store bulk dilutions.

**Mechanism of Action** Blockade of postsynaptic CNS dopamine$_2$ receptors in the mesolimbic and mesocortical areas

**Pharmacodynamics/kinetics**

Duration of action: 4-6 hours

Absorption: Very erratic with oral tablet; oral liquids much more dependable

Protein binding: 91% to 99%

Half-life: 24-48 hours

Time to peak serum concentration: 2-4 hours

Time to steady-state serum: 4-7 days

Elimination: In urine

**Usual Dosage** Concentrate may be diluted just prior to administration with distilled water, acidified tap water, orange or grape juice; do not prepare and store bulk dilutions

Adults:

Oral: 25-50 mg 3 times/day; maximum: 100-400 mg/day

I.M.: Initial: 25 mg, repeat in 30-60 minutes as needed; optimal dosage range: 25-200 mg/day

Hemodialysis: Not dialyzable (0% to 5%)

**Dietary Considerations** Alcohol: Additive CNS effect, avoid use

**Administration** Watch for hypotension when administering I.M. or I.V., dilute oral concentration before administering; do not mix oral solutions of mesoridazine and lithium, these oral liquids are incompatible when mixed

**Monitoring Parameters** Orthostatic blood pressures; tremors, gait changes, abnormal movement in trunk, neck, buccal area or extremities; monitor target behaviors for which the agent is given; monitor hepatic function (especially if fever with flu-like symptoms)

**Reference Range** Not useful

**Test Interactions** ↑ cholesterol (S), glucose; ↓ uric acid (S); false-positive pregnancy test

**Patient Information** May cause drowsiness or restlessness, avoid alcohol and other CNS depressants; do not alter dosage or discontinue without consulting physician; avoid excessive/intense sunlight, yearly ophthalmic examinations are necessary

**Nursing Implications** Watch for hypotension when administering I.M. or I.V., dilute oral concentration before administering

**Additional Information** Coadministration of two or more antipsychotics does not improve clinical response and may increase the potential for adverse effects

**Dosage Forms**

Injection, as besylate: 25 mg/mL (1 mL)

Liquid, oral, as besylate: 25 mg/mL (118 mL)

Tablet, as besylate: 10 mg, 25 mg, 50 mg, 100 mg

♦ **Mesoridazine Besylate** *see* Mesoridazine *on page 344*

♦ **Mestinon® Injection** *see* Pyridostigmine *on page 481*

♦ **Mestinon® Oral** *see* Pyridostigmine *on page 481*

## Mestranol and Norethindrone

(MES tra nole & nor eth IN drone)

**U.S. Brand Names** Genora® 1/50; Nelova® 1/50M; Norethin 1/50M; Norinyl® 1+50; Ortho-Novum® 1/50

**Synonyms** Norethindrone and Mestranol

**Pharmacologic Category** Contraceptive

**Use** Prevention of pregnancy; treatment of hypermenorrhea, endometriosis, female hypogonadism [monophasic oral contraceptive]

**Effects on Mental Status** May cause anxiety or depression

**Effects on Psychiatric Treatment** Hepatic metabolism of TCAs, benzodiazepines (oxidatively metabolized) and beta-blockers may be decreased by oral contraceptives; monitor increased/toxic effects; may increase the clearance of benzodiazepines (glucuronidation); barbiturates may increase the metabolism of oral contraceptives resulting in decreased effectiveness

**Pregnancy Risk Factor** X

**Contraindications** Known or suspected breast cancer, undiagnosed abnormal vaginal bleeding, carcinoma of the breast, estrogen-dependent tumor, pregnancy

**Warnings/Precautions** Use with caution in patients with a history of thromboembolism, stroke, myocardial infarction, liver tumor, hypertension, cardiac, renal or hepatic insufficiency; use of any progestin during the first 4 months of pregnancy is not recommended; risk of cardiovascular side effects increases in those women who smoke cigarettes and in women >35 years of age

**Adverse Reactions**

>10%:

Cardiovascular: Peripheral edema

Central nervous system: Headache

Endocrine: Enlargement of breasts, breast tenderness, increased libido

Gastrointestinal: Nausea, anorexia, bloating

1% to 10%: Gastrointestinal: Vomiting, diarrhea

<1%: Alterations in frequency and flow of menses, amenorrhea, anxiety, breast tumors, chloasma, cholestatic jaundice, decreased glucose tolerance, depression, dizziness, edema, GI distress, hypertension, increased susceptibility to *Candida* infection, increased triglycerides and LDL, intolerance to contact lenses, melasma, myocardial infarction, rash, stroke, thromboembolism

See tables.

**Achieving Proper Hormonal Balance in an Oral Contraceptive**

| Estrogen | | Progestin | |
|---|---|---|---|
| **Excess** | **Deficiency** | **Excess** | **Deficiency** |
| Nausea, bloating | Early or midcycle breakthrough bleeding | Increased appetite | Late breakthrough bleeding |
| Cervical mucorrhea, polyposis | Increased spotting | Weight gain | Amenorrhea |
| Melasma | Hypomenorrhea | Tiredness, fatigue | Hypermenorrhea |
| Migraine headache | | Hypomenorrhea | |
| Breast fullness or tenderness | | Acne, oily scalp* | |
| Edema | | Hair loss, hirsutism* | |
| Hypertension | | Depression | |
| | | Monilial vaginitis | |
| | | Breast regression | |

*Result of androgenic activity of progestins.

**Pharmacological Effects of Progestins Used in Oral Contraceptives**

| | Progestin | Estrogen | Antiestrogen | Androgen |
|---|---|---|---|---|
| Norgestrel/ levonorgestrel | +++ | 0 | ++ | +++ |
| Ethynodiol diacetate | ++ | +* | +* | + |
| Norethindrone acetate | + | + | +++ | + |
| Norethindrone | + | +* | +* | + |
| Norethynodrel | + | +++ | 0 | 0 |

*Has estrogenic effect at low doses; may have antiestrogenic effect at higher doses.

+++ = pronounced effect

++ = moderate effect

+ = slight effect

0 = no effect

**Overdosage/Toxicology**

Signs and symptoms: Toxicity is unlikely following single exposures of excessive doses

Treatment: Any treatment following emesis and charcoal administration should be supportive and symptomatic

**Drug Interactions**

Decreased effect:

Tetracyclines, penicillins, griseofulvin, rifampin, acetaminophen, barbiturates, hydantoins may increase contraceptive failures

Decreases acetaminophen, estrogen levels, and anticoagulants

Increased toxicity: Increases benzodiazepines, caffeine, metoprolol, theophyllines, and tricyclic antidepressants

**Usual Dosage** Oral: Adults: Female: Contraception:

Schedule 1 (Sunday starter): Dose begins on first Sunday after onset of menstruation; if the menstrual period starts on Sunday, take first tablet that very same day. **With a Sunday start, an additional method of contraception should be used until after the first 7 days of consecutive administration.**

For 21-tablet package: Dosage is 1 tablet daily for 21 consecutive days, followed by 7 days off of the medication; a new course begins on the 8th day after the last tablet is taken.

For 28-tablet package: Dosage is 1 tablet daily without interruption.

Schedule 2 (Day 1 starter): Dose starts on first day of menstrual cycle taking 1 tablet daily.

For 21-tablet package: Dosage is 1 tablet daily for 21 consecutive days, followed by 7 days off of the medication; a new course begins on the 8th day after the last tablet is taken.

For 28-tablet package: Dosage is 1 tablet daily without interruption.

If all doses have been taken on schedule and one menstrual period is missed, continue dosing cycle. If two consecutive menstrual periods are missed, pregnancy test is required before new dosing cycle is started.

**Missed doses monophasic formulations** (refer to package insert for complete information):

One dose missed: Take as soon as remembered or take 2 tablets next day

Two consecutive doses missed in the first 2 weeks: Take 2 tablets as soon as remembered or 2 tablets next 2 days. **An additional method of contraception should be used for 7 days after missed dose.**

Two consecutive doses missed in week 3 or three consecutive doses missed at any time: **An additional method of contraception must be used for 7 days after a missed dose:**

Schedule 1 (Sunday starter): Continue dose of 1 tablet daily until Sunday, then discard the rest of the pack, and a new pack should be started that same day.

Schedule 2 (Day 1 starter): Current pack should be discarded, and a new pack should be started that same day.

**Patient Information** Take exactly as directed; use additional method of birth control during first week of administration of first cycle; photosensitivity may occur

Women should inform their physicians if signs or symptoms of any of the following occur thromboembolic or thrombotic disorders including sudden severe headache or vomiting, disturbance of vision or speech, loss of vision, numbness or weakness in an extremity, sharp or crushing chest pain, calf pain, shortness of breath, severe abdominal pain or mass, mental depression or unusual bleeding

Missed doses: Refer to package insert for instructions. When any doses are missed, additional contraceptive methods should be used (see Usual Dosage and package insert).

Women should discontinue taking the medication if they suspect they are pregnant or if they become pregnant.

**Nursing Implications** Administer at bedtime to minimize occurrence of adverse effects

**Dosage Forms** Tablet: Mestranol 0.05 mg and norethindrone 1 mg (21s and 28s)

## Mestranol and Norethynodrel

(MES tra nole & nor e THYE noe drel)

**Synonyms** Norethynodrel and Mestranol

**Pharmacologic Category** Contraceptive

**Use** Treatment of hypermenorrhea, endometriosis, female hypogonadism

**Effects on Mental Status** May cause anxiety, dizziness, or depression

**Effects on Psychiatric Treatment** Hepatic metabolism of TCAs, benzodiazepines (oxidatively metabolized) and beta-blockers may be decreased by oral contraceptives; monitor increased/toxic effects; may increase the clearance of benzodiazepines (glucuronidation); barbiturates may increase the metabolism of oral contraceptives resulting in decreased effectiveness

**Contraindications** Known or suspected breast cancer; undiagnosed abnormal vaginal bleeding; carcinoma of the breast; estrogen-dependent tumors

**Warnings/Precautions** In patients with a history of thromboembolism, stroke, myocardial infarction, liver tumor, hypertension, cardiac, renal or hepatic insufficiency; use of any progestin during the first 4 months of pregnancy is not recommended; risk of cardiovascular side effects increases in those women who smoke cigarettes and in women >35 years of age

**Adverse Reactions**

>10%:

Cardiovascular: Peripheral edema

Endocrine & metabolic: Enlargement of breasts, breast tenderness

Gastrointestinal: Nausea, anorexia, bloating

1% to 10%:

Central nervous system: Headache

Endocrine & metabolic: Increased libido

Gastrointestinal: Vomiting, diarrhea

**Overdosage/Toxicology**

Signs and symptoms: Toxicity is unlikely following single exposures of excessive doses

Treatment: Any treatment following emesis and charcoal administration should be supportive and symptomatic

**Drug Interactions**

Decreased effect with barbiturates, hydantoins (phenytoin, rifampin, antibiotics), penicillins, tetracyclines, griseofulvin

Increased toxicity of acetaminophen, anticoagulants, benzodiazepines, caffeine, corticosteroids, metoprolol, theophylline, tricyclic antidepressants

**Usual Dosage** Adults: Female: Oral:

Endometriosis: 5-10 mg/day for 2 weeks beginning on day 5 of menstrual cycle; increase by 5-10 mg increments at 2-week intervals up to 20 mg/day for 6-9 months

Hypermenorrhea: 20-30 mg/day until bleeding is controlled, then reduce to 10 mg/day and continue through day 24 of cycle; administer 5-10 mg/day from day 5 through day 24 of next 2-3 cycles

**Patient Information** Patients should inform their physicians if signs or symptoms of any of the following occur: Thromboembolic or thrombotic disorders including sudden severe headache or vomiting, disturbance of vision or speech, loss of vision, numbness or weakness in an extremity, sharp or crushing chest pain, calf pain, shortness of breath, severe abdominal pain or mass, mental depression, or unusual bleeding.

**Dosage Forms** Tablet:

5 mg: Mestranol 0.075 mg and norethynodrel 5 mg

10 mg: Mestranol 0.150 mg and norethynodrel 9.85 mg


- **Metadate ER®** *see* Methylphenidate *on page 357*
- **Metahydrin®** *see* Trichlormethiazide *on page 565*
- **Metamucil® [OTC]** *see* Psyllium *on page 479*
- **Metamucil® Instant Mix [OTC]** *see* Psyllium *on page 479*
- **Metaprel®** *see* Metaproterenol *on page 347*


## Metaproterenol (met a proe TER e nol)

**U.S. Brand Names** Alupent®; Arm-a-Med® Metaproterenol; Dey-Dose® Metaproterenol; Metaprel®; Prometa®

**Synonyms** Orciprenaline Sulfate

**Pharmacologic Category** $Beta_2$ Agonist

**Use** Bronchodilator in reversible airway obstruction due to asthma or COPD; because of its delayed onset of action (1 hour) and prolonged effect (4 or more hours), this may not be the drug of choice for assessing response to a bronchodilator

**Effects on Mental Status** Nervousness is common; may cause dizziness, restlessness, or insomnia

**Effects on Psychiatric Treatment** Concurrent use with TCAs and MAOIs may result in additive toxicity

**Pregnancy Risk Factor** C

**Contraindications** Hypersensitivity to metaproterenol or any components, pre-existing cardiac arrhythmias associated with tachycardia

**Warnings/Precautions** Use with caution in patients with hypertension, CHF, hyperthyroidism, CAD, diabetes, or sensitivity to sympathomimetics; excessive prolonged use may result in decreased efficacy or increased toxicity and death; use caution in patients with pre-existing cardiac arrhythmias associated with tachycardia. Metaproterenol has more $beta_1$ activity than other sympathomimetics such as albuterol and, therefore, may no longer be the beta agonist of first choice. All patients should utilize a spacer device when using a metered dose inhaler. Oral use should be avoided due to the increased incidence of adverse effects.

**Adverse Reactions**

>10%:

Central nervous system: Nervousness

Neuromuscular & skeletal: Tremor

1% to 10%:

Cardiovascular: Tachycardia, palpitations, hypertension

Central nervous system: Headache, dizziness

Gastrointestinal: Nausea, vomiting, bad taste

Neuromuscular & skeletal: Trembling, muscle cramps, weakness

Respiratory: Coughing

Miscellaneous: Diaphoresis (increased)

<1%: Paradoxical bronchospasm

**Overdosage/Toxicology**

Signs and symptoms: Angina, arrhythmias, tremor, dry mouth, insomnia; beta-adrenergic stimulation can increase and cause increased heart rate, decreased blood pressure, decreased CNS excitation

Treatment: In cases of overdose, supportive therapy should be instituted, and prudent use of a cardioselective beta-adrenergic blocker (eg, atenolol or metoprolol) should be considered, keeping in mind the potential for induction of bronchoconstriction in an asthmatic individual. Dialysis has not been shown to be of value in the treatment of an overdose with this agent. Diazepam 0.07 mg/kg can be used for excitation seizures.

**Drug Interactions**

Decreased effect: Beta-blockers

Increased toxicity: Sympathomimetics, TCAs, MAO inhibitors

**Usual Dosage**

Oral:

Children:

<2 years: 0.4 mg/kg/dose given 3-4 times/day; in infants, the dose can be given every 8-12 hours

2-6 years: 1-2.6 mg/kg/day divided every 6 hours

6-9 years: 10 mg/dose 3-4 times/day

Children >9 years and Adults: 20 mg 3-4 times/day

Elderly: Initial: 10 mg 3-4 times/day, increasing as necessary up to 20 mg 3-4 times/day

Inhalation: Children >12 years and Adults: 2-3 inhalations every 3-4 hours, up to 12 inhalations in 24 hours

Nebulizer:

Infants and Children: 0.01-0.02 mL/kg of 5% solution; minimum dose: 0.1 mL; maximum dose: 0.3 mL diluted in 2-3 mL normal saline every 4-6 hours (may be given more frequently according to need)

Adolescents and Adults: 5-20 breaths of full strength 5% metaproterenol or 0.2 to 0.3 mL 5% metaproterenol in 2.5-3 mL normal saline until nebulized every 4-6 hours (can be given more frequently according to need)

**Patient Information** Use exactly as directed. Do not use more often than recommended. Maintain adequate hydration (2-3 L/day of fluids unless instructed to restrict fluid intake). You may experience nervousness, dizziness, or fatigue (use caution when driving or engaging in tasks requiring alertness until response to drug is known); dry mouth, unpleasant aftertaste, stomach upset (frequent small meals, frequent mouth care, chewing gum, or sucking hard candy may help); or increased perspiration. Report unresolved GI upset; dizziness or fatigue; vision changes; chest pain, rapid heartbeat, or palpitations; nervousness or insomnia; muscle cramping or tremor; or unusual cough.

**Administration:**

Self-administered inhalation: Store canister upside down; do not freeze. Shake canister before using. Sit when using medication. Close eyes when administering metaproterenol to avoid spray getting into eyes. Exhale slowly and completely through nose; inhale deeply through mouth while administering aerosol. Hold breath for 1-3 seconds after inhalation. Wait at least 1 full minute between inhalations. Wash mouthpiece between use. If more than one inhalation medication is used, use bronchodilator first and wait 5 minutes between medications.

Self-administered nebulizer: Wash hands before and after treatment. Wash and dry nebulizer after each treatment. Twist open the top of one unit dose vial and squeeze contents into nebulizer reservoir. Connect nebulizer reservoir to the mouthpiece or face-mask. Connect nebulizer to compressor. Sit in comfortable, upright position. Place mouthpiece in your mouth or put on face-mask and turn on compressor. If face-mask is used, avoid leakage around the mask to avoid mist getting into eyes which may cause vision problems. Breath calmly and deeply until no more mist is formed in nebulizer (about 5 minutes). At this point treatment is finished.

**Nursing Implications** Do not use solutions for nebulization if they are brown or contain a precipitate; before using, the inhaler must be shaken well

**Dosage Forms**

Aerosol, oral, as sulfate: 0.65 mg/dose (5 mL, 10 mL)

Solution for inhalation, as sulfate, preservative free: 0.4% [4 mg/mL] (2.5 mL); 0.6% [6 mg/mL] (2.5 mL); 5% [50 mg/mL] (10 mL, 30 mL)

Syrup, as sulfate: 10 mg/5 mL (480 mL)

Tablet, as sulfate: 10 mg, 20 mg

## Metaraminol (met a RAM i nole)

**U.S. Brand Names** Aramine®

**Pharmacologic Category** $Alpha_1$ Agonist

**Use** Acute hypotensive crisis in the treatment of shock

**Effects on Mental Status** None reported

**Effects on Psychiatric Treatment** Contraindicated with MAOIs; the pressor effect of direct-acting vasopressors may be potentiated by the TCAs

**Usual Dosage**

Children:

I.M.: 0.01 mg/kg as a single dose

I.V.: 0.01 mg/kg as a single dose or intravenous infusion of 5 mcg/kg/minute

Adults:

Prevention of hypotension: I.M., S.C.: 2-10 mg

Adjunctive treatment of hypotension: I.V.: 15-100 mg in 250-500 mL NS or 5% dextrose in water

Severe shock: I.V.: 0.5-5 mg direct I.V. injection followed by intravenous infusion of 15-100 mg in 250-500 mL NS or $D_5W$; may also be administered endotracheally

**Dosage Forms** Injection, as bitartrate: 10 mg/mL (10 mL)

## Metaxalone (me TAKS a lone)

**U.S. Brand Names** Skelaxin®

**Pharmacologic Category** Skeletal Muscle Relaxant

**Use** Relief of discomfort associated with acute, painful musculoskeletal conditions

**Effects on Mental Status** Drowsiness and dizziness are common; may cause paradoxical stimulation

**Effects on Psychiatric Treatment** May cause leukopenia; use caution with clozapine and carbamazepine; concurrent use with psychotropics may produce additive sedation

**Pregnancy Risk Factor** C

**Contraindications** Impaired hepatic or renal function, known hypersensitivity to metaxalone, history of drug-induced hemolytic anemias or other anemias

**Warnings/Precautions** Use with caution in patients with impaired hepatic function

**Adverse Reactions**

>10%:

Gastrointestinal: Nausea, vomiting, stomach cramps

Central nervous system: Paradoxical stimulation, headache, drowsiness, dizziness

<1%: Allergic dermatitis, anaphylaxis, hemolytic anemia, hepatotoxicity, leukopenia

**Overdosage/Toxicology** Signs and symptoms: No major toxicities have been reported

**Drug Interactions** Increased effect of alcohol, CNS depressants

**Usual Dosage** Children >12 years and Adults: Oral: 800 mg 3-4 times/day

**Patient Information** Avoid alcohol and other CNS depressants; may cause drowsiness, impairment of judgment, or coordination; notify physician of dark urine, pale stools, yellowing of eyes, severe nausea, vomiting, or abdominal pain

**Nursing Implications** Raise bed rails, institute safety measures, assist with ambulation

**Dosage Forms** Tablet: 400 mg

## Metformin (met FOR min)

**Related Information**

Diabetes Mellitus Treatment *on page 782*

Hypoglycemic Drugs and Thiazolidinedione Information *on page 714*

**U.S. Brand Names** Glucophage®

**Canadian Brand Names** Novo-Metformin

**Pharmacologic Category** Antidiabetic Agent (Biguanide)

**Use** Management of noninsulin-dependent diabetes mellitus (type 2) as monotherapy when hyperglycemia cannot be managed on diet alone. May be used concomitantly with a sulfonylurea when diet and metformin or sulfonylurea alone do not result in adequate glycemic control.

**Unlabeled use:** Data suggests that some patients with NIDDM with secondary failure to sulfonylurea therapy may obtain significant improvement in metabolic control when metformin in combination with insulin and a sulfonylurea is used in lieu of insulin alone

**Effects on Mental Status** None reported

**Effects on Psychiatric Treatment** May cause leukopenia; use caution with clozapine and carbamazepine; concurrent use with psychotropics may produce additive sedation

**Pregnancy Risk Factor** B

**Contraindications** Hypersensitivity to metformin or any component; renal disease or renal dysfunction (serum creatinine ≥1.5 mg/dL in males or ≥1.4 mg/dL in females or creatinine clearance <60 mL/minute) which may also result from conditions such as cardiovascular collapse, acute myocardial infarction, and septicemia; acute or chronic metabolic acidosis with or without coma (including diabetic ketoacidosis); should be temporarily withheld (at the time of or prior to the procedure and withheld for 48 hours subsequent to the procedure and reinstituted only after renal function has been re-evaluated and found to be normal) in patients undergoing radiologic studies involving the parenteral administration of iodinated contrast materials (potential for acute alteration in renal function)

**Warnings/Precautions** Administration of oral antidiabetic drugs has been reported to be associated with increased cardiovascular mortality as compared to treatment with diet alone or diet plus insulin. Metformin is substantially excreted by the kidney - the risk of accumulation and lactic acidosis increases with the degree of impairment of renal function. Patients with renal function below the limit of normal for their age should not receive metformin. In elderly patients, renal function should be monitored regularly. Use of concomitant medications that may affect renal function (ie, affect tubular secretion) may affect metformin disposition. Therapy should be suspended for any surgical procedures. Avoid use in patients with impaired liver function. Metformin should be discontinued at the time of or prior to the procedure in patients undergoing radiologic studies in which intravascular iodinated contrast materials are utilized, and withheld for 48 hours subsequent to the procedure, and reinstituted only after renal function has been re-evaluated and found to be normal.

**Adverse Reactions**

>10%: Gastrointestinal: Anorexia, nausea, vomiting, diarrhea, epigastric fullness, constipation, heartburn

1% to 10%:

Dermatologic: Rash, urticaria, photosensitivity

Miscellaneous: Decreased vitamin $B_{12}$ levels

<1%: Agranulocytosis, aplastic anemia, blood dyscrasias, bone marrow suppression, hemolytic anemia, thrombocytopenia

**Overdosage/Toxicology**

Signs and symptoms: Hypoglycemia has not been observed with ingestions of up to 85 g of metformin, although lactic acidosis has occurred in such circumstances

Treatment: Metformin is dialyzable with a clearance of up to 170 mL/minute; hemodialysis may be useful for removal of accumulated drug from patients in whom metformin overdosage is suspected

**Drug Interactions**

Decreased effect: Drugs which tend to produce hyperglycemia (eg, diuretics, corticosteroids, phenothiazines, thyroid products, estrogens, oral contraceptives, phenytoin, nicotinic acid, sympathomimetics, calcium channel blocking drugs, isoniazid) may lead to a loss of glycemic control

Increased effect: Furosemide increased the metformin plasma and blood $C_{max}$ without altering metformin renal clearance in a single dose study

Increased toxicity:

Cationic drugs (eg, amiloride, digoxin, morphine, procainamide, quinidine, quinine, ranitidine, triamterene, trimethoprim, and vancomycin) which are eliminated by renal tubular secretion could have the potential for interaction with metformin by competing for common renal tubular transport systems

Cimetidine increases (by 60%) peak metformin plasma and whole blood concentrations

**Usual Dosage** Oral (allow 1-2 weeks between dose titrations): Generally, clinically significant responses are not seen at doses <1500 mg daily; however, a lower recommended starting dose and gradual increased dosage is recommended to minimize gastrointestinal symptoms

Adults:

500 mg tablets: Initial: 500 mg twice daily (give with the morning and evening meals). Dosage increases should be made in increments of 1 tablet every week, given in divided doses, up to a maximum of 2500 mg/day. Doses of up to 2000 mg/day may be given twice daily. If a dose of 2500 mg/day is required, it may be better tolerated 3 times/day (with meals).

850 mg tablets: Initial: 850 mg once daily (give with the morning meal). Dosage increases should be made in increments of 1 tablet every **other** week, given in divided doses, up to a maximum of 2550 mg/day. Usual maintenance dose: 850 mg twice daily (with the morning and evening meals). Some patients may be given 850 mg 3 times/day (with meals).

Elderly: The initial and maintenance dosing should be conservative, due to the potential for decreased renal function. Generally, elderly patients should not be titrated to the maximum dose of metformin.

**Transfer from other antidiabetic agents:** No transition period is generally necessary except when transferring from chlorpropamide. When transferring from chlorpropamide, care should be exercised during the first 2 weeks because of the prolonged retention of chlorpropamide in the body, leading to overlapping drug effects and possible hypoglycemia.

**Concomitant metformin and oral sulfonylurea therapy:** If patients have not responded to 4 weeks of the maximum dose of metformin monotherapy, consideration to a gradual addition of an oral sulfonylurea while continuing metformin at the maximum dose, even if prior primary or secondary failure to a sulfonylurea has occurred.

**Dosing adjustment/comments in renal impairment:** The plasma and blood half-life of metformin is prolonged and the renal clearance is decreased in proportion to the decrease in creatinine clearance. Metformin is contraindicated in the presence of renal dysfunction defined as a serum creatinine >1.5 mg/dL in males or >1.4 mg/dL in females or an abnormal creatinine clearance.

**Dosing adjustment in hepatic impairment:** No studies have been conducted, however, metformin should be avoided because the presence of liver disease is a risk factor for the development of lactic acidosis during metformin therapy.

**Dietary Considerations**

Alcohol: Incidence of lactic acidosis may be increased; avoid or limit use

Food: Food decreases the extent and slightly delays the absorption. Drug may cause GI upset; take with food to decrease GI upset.

Glucose: Decreases blood glucose concentration. Hypoglycemia does not usually occur unless a patient is predisposed. Monitor blood glucose concentration. Exercise caution with administration in patients predisposed to hypoglycemia (eg, cases of reduced caloric intake, strenuous exercise without repletion of calories, alcohol ingestion or when metformin is combined with another oral antidiabetic agent).

Vitamin $B_{12}$: Decreases absorption of Vitamin $B_{12}$; monitor for signs and symptoms of vitamin $B_{12}$ deficiency

Folic acid: Decreases absorption of folic acid; monitor for signs and symptoms of folic acid deficiency

**Patient Information** This medication is used to control diabetes; it is not a cure. Other components of treatment plan are important: follow prescribed diet, medication, and exercise regimen. Take exactly as directed; with meal(s) at the same time each day. Do not change dose or discontinue without consulting prescriber. Avoid alcohol while taking this medication; could cause severe reaction. Inform prescriber of all other prescription or OTC medications you are taking; do not introduce new medication without consulting prescriber. Do not take other medication within 2 hours of this medication unless so advised by prescriber. Maintain regular dietary intake and exercise routine and always carry quick source of sugar with you. You may experience side effects during first weeks of therapy (headache, nausea); consult prescriber if these persist. Report severe or persistent side effects, extended vomiting or flu-like symptoms, skin rash, easy bruising or bleeding, or change in color of urine or stool.

**Nursing Implications** Patients who are NPO may need to have their dose held to avoid hypoglycemia

**Dosage Forms** Tablet, as hydrochloride: 500 mg, 625 mg, 750 mg, 850 mg, 1000 mg

## Methadone (METH a done)

**Related Information**

Addiction Treatments *on page 772*
Narcotic Agonists Comparison Chart *on page 720*
Substance-Related Disorders *on page 609*

**Generic Available** Yes

**U.S. Brand Names** Dolophine®

**Canadian Brand Names** Methadose®

**Synonyms** Methadone Hydrochloride

**Pharmacologic Category** Analgesic, Narcotic

**Use** Management of severe pain; detoxification and maintenance treatment of narcotic addiction

**Restrictions** C-II

**Pregnancy Risk Factor** B (D if used for prolonged periods or in high doses at term)

**Contraindications** Hypersensitivity to methadone or any component

**Warnings/Precautions** Because methadone's effects on respiration last much longer than its analgesic effects, the dose must be titrated slowly; because of its long half-life and risk of accumulation, it is not considered a drug of first choice in the elderly, who may be particularly susceptible to its CNS depressant and constipating effects. May cause respiratory depression - use caution in patients with respiratory disease or pre-existing respiratory depression. Potential for drug dependency exists, abrupt cessation may precipitate withdrawal. Use caution in elderly, debilitated, or pediatric patients. Use with caution in patients with depression or suicidal tendencies, or in patients with a history of drug abuse. Tolerance or psychological and physical dependence may occur with prolonged use. Use with caution in patients with hepatic, pulmonary, or renal function impairment. May cause CNS depression, which may impair physical or mental abilities. Patients must cautioned about performing tasks which require mental alertness (ie, operating machinery or driving). Effects with other sedative drugs or ethanol may be potentiated. Elderly may be more sensitive to CNS depressant and constipating effects. Use with caution in patients with head injury or increased ICP, biliary tract dysfunction or pancreatitis; history of ileus or bowel obstruction, glaucoma, hyperthyroidism, adrenal insufficiency, prostatic hypertrophy or urinary stricture, CNS depression, toxic psychosis, alcoholism, delirium tremens, or kyphoscoliosis. Tablets are to be used only for oral administration and must not be used for injection.

**Adverse Reactions**

Cardiovascular: Bradycardia, peripheral vasodilation, cardiac arrest, syncope, faintness

Central nervous system: Euphoria, dysphoria, headache, insomnia, agitation, disorientation, drowsiness, dizziness, lightheadedness, sedation

Dermatologic: Pruritus, urticaria, rash

Endocrine & metabolic: Decreased libido

Gastrointestinal: Nausea, vomiting, constipation, anorexia, stomach cramps, xerostomia, biliary tract spasm

Genitourinary: Urinary retention or hesitancy, antidiuretic effect, impotence

Neuromuscular & skeletal: Weakness

Ocular: Miosis, visual disturbances

Respiratory: Respiratory depression, respiratory arrest

Miscellaneous: Physical and psychological dependence

**Overdosage/Toxicology**

Signs and symptoms: Respiratory depression, CNS depression, miosis, hypothermia, circulatory collapse, convulsions

Treatment: Naloxone 2 mg I.V. (0.01 mg/kg for children) with repeat administration as necessary up to a total of 10 mg

**Drug Interactions** CYP1A2, 2D6, and 3A3/4 enzyme substrate; CYP2D6 inhibitor

CYP1A2 inhibitors: Serum level and/or toxicity of methadone may be increased, increasing clinical effect or toxicity; inhibitors include cimetidine, ciprofloxacin, fluvoxamine, isoniazid, ritonavir, and zileutin

CYP2D6 inhibitors: Serum level and/or toxicity of methadone may be increased, increasing clinical effect or toxicity; inhibitors include amiodarone, cimetidine, delavirdine, fluoxetine, paroxetine, propafenone, quinidine, and ritonavir; monitor for increased effect/toxicity

CYP3A3/4 inhibitors: Serum level and/or toxicity of methadone may be increased; inhibitors include amiodarone, cimetidine, clarithromycin, erythromycin, delavirdine, diltiazem, dirithromycin, disulfiram, fluoxetine, fluvoxamine, grapefruit juice, indinavir, itraconazole, ketoconazole, metronidazole, nefazodone, nevirapine, propoxyfene, quinupristin-dalfopristin, ritonavir, saquinavir, verapamil, zafirlukast, zileuton; monitor for altered response

Enzyme inducers: Barbiturates, carbamazepine, phenytoin, primidone, and rifampin may decrease serum methadone concentrations via enhanced hepatic metabolism; monitor for methadone withdrawal; larger doses of methadone may be required

Somatostatin: Therapeutic effect of methadone may be decreased; limited documentation; monitor

Zidovudine: serum concentrations may be increased by methadone; monitor

**Stability** Highly **incompatible** with all other I.V. agents when mixed together

**Mechanism of Action** Binds to opiate receptors in the CNS, causing inhibition of ascending pain pathways, altering the perception of and response to pain; produces generalized CNS depression

**Pharmacodynamics/kinetics**

Oral:
- Onset of analgesia: Within 0.5-1 hour
- Duration: 6-8 hours, increases to 22-48 hours with repeated doses

Parenteral:
- Onset of effect: Within 10-20 minutes
- Peak effect: Within 1-2 hours

Distribution: Crosses the placenta; appears in breast milk

Protein binding: 80% to 85%

Metabolism: In the liver (N-demethylation)

Half-life: 15-29 hours, may be prolonged with alkaline pH

Elimination: In urine (<10% as unchanged drug); increased renal excretion with urine pH <6

**Usual Dosage** Doses should be titrated to appropriate effects

Children: Analgesia:
- Oral, I.M., S.C.: 0.7 mg/kg/24 hours divided every 4-6 hours as needed or 0.1-0.2 mg/kg every 4-12 hours as needed; maximum: 10 mg/dose
- I.V.: 0.1 mg/kg every 4 hours initially for 2-3 doses, then every 6-12 hours as needed; maximum: 10 mg/dose

Adults:
- Analgesia: Oral, I.M., S.C.: 2.5-10 mg every 3-8 hours as needed, up to 5-20 mg every 6-8 hours
- Detoxification: Oral: 15-40 mg/day; should not exceed 21 days and may not be repeated earlier than 4 weeks after completion of preceding course
- Maintenance of opiate dependence: Oral: 20-120 mg/day

**Dosing adjustment in renal impairment:** $Cl_{cr}$ <10 mL/minute: Administer at 50% to 75% of normal dose

**Dosing adjustment/comments in hepatic disease:** Avoid in severe liver disease

**Important note:** Methadone accumulates with repeated doses and dosage may need to be adjusted downward after 3-5 days to prevent toxic effects. Some patients may benefit from every 8- to 12-hour dosing interval (pain control).

**Monitoring Parameters** Pain relief, respiratory and mental status, blood pressure

**Reference Range** Therapeutic: 100-400 ng/mL (SI: 0.32-1.29 μmol/L); Toxic: >2 μg/mL (SI: >6.46 μmol/L)

**Test Interactions** ↑ thyroxine (S), aminotransferase [ALT (SGPT)/AST (SGOT)] (S)

**Patient Information** May cause drowsiness, avoid alcohol and other CNS depressants

**Nursing Implications** Observe patient for excessive sedation, respiratory depression, implement safety measures, assist with ambulation

**Dosage Forms**

Injection, as hydrochloride: 10 mg/mL (1 mL, 10 mL, 20 mL)

Solution, as hydrochloride:
- Oral: 5 mg/5 mL (5 mL, 500 mL); 10 mg/5 mL (500 mL)
- Oral, concentrate: 10 mg/mL (30 mL)

Tablet, as hydrochloride: 5 mg, 10 mg

Tablet, dispersible, as hydrochloride: 40 mg

♦ **Methadone Hydrochloride** *see* Methadone *on page 349*

♦ **Methaminodiazepoxide Hydrochloride** *see* Chlordiazepoxide *on page 109*

## Methamphetamine (meth am FET a meen)

**Related Information**

Patient Information - Stimulants *on page 652*
Stimulant Agents Used for ADHD *on page 728*

(Continued)

## Methamphetamine *(Continued)*

Substance-Related Disorders *on page 609*

**U.S. Brand Names** Desoxyn®; Desoxyn Gradumet®

**Synonyms** Desoxyephedrine Hydrochloride; Methamphetamine Hydrochloride

**Pharmacologic Category** Stimulant

**Use** Treatment of ADHD; exogenous obesity (short-term adjunct)

**Unlabeled use:** Narcolepsy

**Restrictions** C-II

**Pregnancy Risk Factor** C

**Contraindications** Known hypersensitivity or idiosyncrasy to sympathomimetic amines; patients with advanced arteriosclerosis, symptomatic cardiovascular disease, moderate to severe hypertension (stage II or III), hyperthyroidism, glaucoma, agitated states; patients with a history of drug abuse; use during or within 14 days following MAO inhibitor therapy; stimulant medications are contraindicated for use in children with attention deficit/hyperactivity disorders and concomitant Tourette's syndrome or tics

**Warnings/Precautions** Use with caution in patients with bipolar disorder, diabetes mellitus, cardiovascular disease, seizure disorders, insomnia, porphyria, or mild hypertension (stage I). May exacerbate symptoms of behavior and thought disorder in psychotic patients. Potential for drug dependency exists - avoid abrupt discontinuation in patients who have received for prolonged periods. Use in weight reduction programs only when alternative therapy has been ineffective. Products may contain tartrazine - use with caution in potentially sensitive individuals. Stimulant use in children has been associated with growth suppression.

**Adverse Reactions**

Cardiovascular: Hypertension, tachycardia, palpitations

Central nervous system: Restlessness, headache, exacerbation of motor and phonic tics and Tourette's syndrome, dizziness, psychosis, dysphoria, overstimulation, euphoria, insomnia

Dermatologic: Rash, urticaria

Endocrine & metabolic: Change in libido

Gastrointestinal: Diarrhea, nausea, vomiting, stomach cramps, constipation, anorexia, weight loss, xerostomia, unpleasant taste

Genitourinary: Impotence

Neuromuscular & skeletal: Tremor

Miscellaneous: Suppression of growth in children, tolerance and withdrawal with prolonged use

**Overdosage/Toxicology**

Signs and symptoms: Seizures, hyperactivity, coma, hypertension

Treatment: There is no specific antidote for amphetamine intoxication and the bulk of the treatment is supportive. Hyperactivity and agitation usually respond to reduced sensory input, however with extreme agitation haloperidol (2-5 mg I.M. for adults) may be required. Hyperthermia is best treated with external cooling measures, or when severe or unresponsive, muscle paralysis with pancuronium may be needed. Hypertension is usually transient and generally does not require treatment unless severe. For diastolic blood pressures >110 mm Hg, a nitroprusside infusion should be initiated. Seizures usually respond to diazepam IVP and/or phenytoin maintenance regimens.

**Drug Interactions** CYP2D6 enzyme substrate

Acidifiers: Very large doses of potassium acid phosphate or ammonium chloride may increase the renal elimination of amphetamines due to urinary acidification

Alkalinizers: Large doses of sodium bicarbonate or other alkalinizers may increase renal tubular reabsorption (decreased elimination) and diminish the effect of amphetamine; includes potassium or sodium citrate and acetate

Antipsychotics: Efficacy of amphetamines may be decreased by antipsychotics; in addition, amphetamines may induce an increase in psychotic symptoms in some patients

CYP2D6 inhibitors: Serum levels and/or toxicity of methamphetamine may be increased; inhibitors include amiodarone, cimetidine, delavirdine, fluoxetine, paroxetine, propafenone, quinidine, and ritonavir; monitor for increased effect/toxicity

Enzyme inducers: Metabolism of amphetamine may be increased; decreasing clinical effect; inducers include barbiturates, carbamazepine, phenytoin, and rifampin

Furazolidine: Amphetamines may induce hypertensive episodes in patients receiving furazolidone

Guanethidine: Amphetamines inhibit the antihypertensive response to guanethidine; probably also may occur with guanadrel

MAOIs: Severe hypertensive episodes have occurred with amphetamine when used in patients receiving MAOIs; concurrent use or use within 14 days is contraindicated

Norepinephrine: Amphetamines enhance the pressor response to norepinephrine

Sibutramine: Concurrent use of sibutramine and amphetamines may cause severe hypertension and tachycardia; use is contraindicated (benzphetamine)

SSRIs: Amphetamines may increase the potential for serotonin syndrome when used concurrently with selective serotonin reuptake inhibitors (including fluoxetine, fluvoxamine, paroxetine, and sertraline)

Tricyclic antidepressants: Concurrent of amphetamines with TCAs may result in hypertension and CNS stimulation; avoid this combination

**Mechanism of Action** A sympathomimetic amine related to ephedrine and amphetamine with CNS stimulant activity; peripheral actions include elevation of systolic and diastolic blood pressure and weak bronchodilator and respiratory stimulant action

**Usual Dosage**

Attention deficit disorder: Children >6 years: 2.5-5 mg 1-2 times/day, may increase by 5 mg increments weekly until optimum response is achieved, usually 20-25 mg/day

Exogenous obesity: Children >12 years and Adults: 5 mg, 30 minutes before each meal; long-acting formulation: 10-15 mg in morning; treatment duration should not exceed a few weeks

**Monitoring Parameters** Heart rate, respiratory rate, blood pressure, and CNS activity

**Reference Range** Therapeutic: 20-30 ng/mL

**Test Interactions** False-positives by immunoassay can be seen with ranitidine, phenylpropanolamine, brompheniramine, chlorpromazine, fluspirilene, or pipothiazine coingestion

**Patient Information** Take during day to avoid insomnia; do not discontinue abruptly, may cause physical and psychological dependence with prolonged use; do not crush or chew extended release tablet

**Nursing Implications** Dose should not be given in evening or at bedtime; do not crush extended release tablet

**Additional Information** Illicit methamphetamine may contain lead; alkalinizing urine can result in longer methamphetamine half-life and elevated blood level; ephedrine is a precursor in the illicit manufacture of methamphetamine; ephedrine is extracted by dissolving ephedrine tablets in water or alcohol (50,000 tablets can result in 1 kg of ephedrine); conversion to methamphetamine occurs at a rate of 50% to 70% of the weight of ephedrine. 3,4-methylene dioxymethamphetamine (slang: XTC, Ecstasy, Adam) affects the serotinergic, dopaminergic, and noradrenergic pathways. As such, it can cause the serotonin syndrome associated with malignant hyperthermia and rhabdomyolysis.

**Dosage Forms**

Tablet, as hydrochloride: 5 mg

Tablet, extended release, as hydrochloride (Gradumet®): 5 mg, 10 mg, 15 mg

♦ **Methamphetamine Hydrochloride** *see* Methamphetamine *on page 349*

## Methantheline (meth AN tha leen)

**U.S. Brand Names** Banthine®

**Synonyms** Methanthelinium Bromide

**Pharmacologic Category** Anticholinergic Agent

**Use** Adjunctive treatment of peptic ulcer, irritable bowel syndrome, pancreatitis, ureteral and urinary bladder spasm; to reduce duodenal motility during diagnostic radiologic procedures and treatment of an uninhibited neurogenic bladder

**Effects on Mental Status** May cause confusion, amnesia, drowsiness, nervousness, or insomnia

**Effects on Psychiatric Treatment** Concurrent use with psychotropics may produce additive sedation or dry mouth

**Contraindications** Angle-closure glaucoma; hypersensitivity to methantheline

**Adverse Reactions**

>10%:

- Dermatologic: Dry skin
- Gastrointestinal: Constipation, xerostomia, dry throat
- Respiratory: Dry nose
- Miscellaneous: Decreased diaphoresis

1% to 10%: Gastrointestinal: Dysphagia

**Usual Dosage** Oral:

Neonates: 12.5 mg twice daily then 3 times/day

Children:

- <1 year: 12.5-25 mg 4 times/day
- >1 year: 12.5-50 mg 4 times/day

Adults: 50-100 mg every 6 hours

**Dosage Forms** Tablet, as bromide: 50 mg

♦ **Methanthelinium Bromide** *see* Methantheline *on page 350*

## Metharbital (meth AR bi tal)

**Synonyms** Metharbitone

**Pharmacologic Category** Anticonvulsant, Barbiturate

**Use** Control of grand mal, petit mal, myoclonic and mixed types of seizures

**Effects on Mental Status** Sedation is common; may cause cognitive impairment or paradoxical excitement

**Effects on Psychiatric Treatment** Concurrent use with psychotropics may produce additive sedation

**Contraindications** Suspected pregnancy; status asthmaticus; hypersensitivity to metharbital (barbiturates)

**Adverse Reactions** 1% to 10%:
- Cardiovascular: Hypotension, circulatory collapse
- Central nervous system: Drowsiness, paradoxical excitement, hyperkinetic activity, cognitive impairment, defects in general comprehension, short-term memory deficits, decreased attention span, ataxia
- Dermatologic: Skin eruptions, skin rash, exfoliative dermatitis
- Hematologic: Megaloblastic anemia
- Hepatic: Hepatitis
- Ocular: Vision color changes (yellow tinge), ptosis
- Respiratory: Apnea (especially with rapid I.V. use), respiratory depression
- Miscellaneous: Psychological and physical dependence

**Usual Dosage** Oral:
- Children: 5-15 mg/kg/day or 50 mg 1-3 times/day
- Adults: 100 mg 1-3 times/day, adjust dosage to obtain optimal effect

**Dosage Forms** Tablet: 100 mg

◆ **Metharbitone** *see* Metharbital *on page 350*

## Methazolamide (meth a ZOE la mide)

**Related Information**
Glaucoma Drug Therapy *on page 712*

**U.S. Brand Names** GlaucTabs®; Neptazane®

**Pharmacologic Category** Carbonic Anhydrase Inhibitor; Diuretic, Carbonic Anhydrase Inhibitor; Ophthalmic Agent, Antiglaucoma

**Use** Adjunctive treatment of open-angle or secondary glaucoma; short-term therapy of narrow-angle glaucoma when delay of surgery is desired

**Effects on Mental Status** Sedation is common; may cause dizziness or depression

**Effects on Psychiatric Treatment** May rarely cause bone marrow suppression; use caution with clozapine and carbamazepine; may increase lithium excretion but overall effect is minimal; if lithium toxicity is severe, hemodialysis is the treatment of choice

**Pregnancy Risk Factor** C

**Contraindications** Marked kidney or liver dysfunction, severe pulmonary obstruction, hypersensitivity to methazolamide or any component

**Warnings/Precautions** Sulfonamide-type reactions, melena, anorexia, nausea, vomiting, constipation, hematuria, glycosuria, urinary frequency, renal colic, renal calculi, crystalluria, polyuria, hepatic insufficiency, various CNS effects, transient myopia, bone marrow suppression, thrombocytopenia/purpura, hemolytic anemia, leukopenia, pancytopenia, agranulocytosis, urticaria, pruritus, rash, Stevens-Johnson syndrome, weight loss, fever, acidosis; use with caution in patients with respiratory acidosis and diabetes mellitus; impairment of mental alertness and/or physical coordination. Malaise and complaints of tiredness and myalgia are signs of excessive dosing and acidosis in the elderly.

**Adverse Reactions**

>10%:
- Central nervous system: Malaise
- Gastrointestinal: Metallic taste, anorexia
- Genitourinary: Polyuria
- Neuromuscular & skeletal: Weakness

1% to 10%:
- Central nervous system: Mental depression, drowsiness, dizziness
- Genitourinary: Crystalluria

<1%: Black tarry stools, bone marrow suppression, constipation, dysuria, fatigue, fever, GI irritation, headache, hyperchloremic metabolic acidosis, hyperglycemia, hypersensitivity, hypokalemia, loss of smell, myopia, paresthesia, rash, seizures, Stevens-Johnson syndrome, sulfonamide rash, tinnitus, trembling, unsteadiness, xerostomia

**Drug Interactions**

Increased toxicity:
- May induce hypokalemia which would sensitize a patient to digitalis toxicity
- May increase the potential for salicylate toxicity
- Hypokalemia may be compounded with concurrent diuretic use or steroids
- Primidone absorption may be delayed

Decreased effect: Increased lithium excretion and altered excretion of other drugs by alkalinization of the urine, such as amphetamines, quinidine, procainamide, methenamine, phenobarbital, salicylates

**Usual Dosage** Adults: Oral: 50-100 mg 2-3 times/day

**Patient Information** Take with food; swallow whole, do not chew or crush. You may experience gastrointestinal upset and loss of appetite; frequent small meals are advised to reduce these effects and the metallic taste that sometimes occurs with this medication. You may experience lightheadedness, depression, dizziness, or weakness for a few days; use caution when driving or engaging in tasks that require alertness until response to drug is known. Report excessive tiredness; loss of appetite; cramping, pain, or weakness in muscles; acute GI symptoms; changes in CNS (depression, drowsiness); difficulty or pain on urination; visual changes; or skin rash.

**Nursing Implications** May cause an alteration in taste, especially when drinking carbonated beverages

**Dosage Forms** Tablet: 25 mg, 50 mg

## Methdilazine (meth DIL a zeen)

**U.S. Brand Names** Tacaryl®

**Pharmacologic Category** Antihistamine

**Use** Symptomatic relief of pruritus associated with urticaria; neuroallergic, atopic, contact, poison ivy or eczematous dermatitis; pruritus ani or drug rash

**Effects on Mental Status** Sedation is common; may cause dizziness or nervousness; may rarely cause insomnia or depression

**Effects on Psychiatric Treatment** Concurrent use with psychotropics may produce additive sedation

**Contraindications** Acute asthmatic attack; dehydrated children; hypersensitivity to methdilazine

**Adverse Reactions**

>10%:
- Central nervous system: Slight to moderate drowsiness
- Respiratory: Thickening of bronchial secretions

1% to 10%:
- Central nervous system: Headache, fatigue, nervousness, dizziness
- Gastrointestinal: Appetite increase, weight increase, nausea, diarrhea, abdominal pain, xerostomia
- Neuromuscular & skeletal: Arthralgia
- Respiratory: Pharyngitis

**Overdosage/Toxicology**

Signs and symptoms: Hypotension, cardiac arrhythmias

Treatment: There is no specific treatment for an antihistamine overdose, however, most of its clinical toxicity is due to anticholinergic effects. Anticholinesterase inhibitors may be useful by reducing acetylcholinesterase. Anticholinesterase inhibitors include physostigmine, neostigmine, pyridostigmine and edrophonium. For anticholinergic overdose with severe life-threatening symptoms, physostigmine 1-2 mg (0.5 or 0.02 mg/kg for children) I.V., slowly may be given to reverse these effects. Hypotension second to alpha-adrenergic blockade should be treated with I.V. fluids and alpha-adrenergic pressors.

**Usual Dosage** Oral:
- Children >3 years: 4 mg 2-4 times/day
- Adults: 8 mg 2-4 times/day
- Not dialyzable (0% to 5%)

**Patient Information** May cause drowsiness; avoid alcohol and other CNS depressants; notify physician if muscle stiffness or restlessness occurs

**Dosage Forms**
- Syrup, as hydrochloride: 4 mg/5 mL (473 mL)
- Tablet, as hydrochloride: 8 mg
- Tablet, chewable: 3.6 mg [methdilazine hydrochloride 4 mg]

## Methenamine (meth EN a meen)

**U.S. Brand Names** Hiprex®; Urex®

**Canadian Brand Names** Dehydral™; Hip-Rex™; Urasal®

**Synonyms** Hexamethylenetetramine; Methenamine Hippurate; Methenamine Mandelate

**Pharmacologic Category** Antibiotic, Miscellaneous

**Use** Prophylaxis or suppression of recurrent urinary tract infections; urinary tract discomfort secondary to hypermotility

**Effects on Mental Status** None reported

**Effects on Psychiatric Treatment** None reported

**Pregnancy Risk Factor** C

**Contraindications** Severe dehydration, renal insufficiency, hepatic insufficiency in patients receiving hippurate salt, hypersensitivity to methenamine or any component; patients receiving sulfonamides

**Warnings/Precautions** Use with caution in patients with hepatic disease, gout, and the elderly; doses of 8 g/day for 3-4 weeks may cause bladder irritation, some products may contain tartrazine; methenamine should not be used to treat infections outside of the lower urinary tract. Use care to maintain an acid pH of the urine, especially when treating infections due to urea splitting organisms (eg, *Proteus* and strains of *Pseudomonas*); reversible increases in LFTs have occurred during therapy especially in patients with hepatic dysfunction.

**Adverse Reactions**

1% to 10%:
- Dermatologic: Rash (3.5%)
- Gastrointestinal: Nausea, dyspepsia (3.5%)
- Genitourinary: Dysuria (3.5%)

<1%: Bladder irritation, crystalluria (especially with large doses), increased AST/ALT (reversible, rare)

**Drug Interactions**

Decreased effect: Sodium bicarbonate and acetazolamide will decrease effect secondary to alkalinization of urine

Increased toxicity: Sulfonamides (may precipitate)

**Usual Dosage** Oral:

Children:
- <6 years: 0.25 g/30 lb 4 times/day

(Continued)

## Methenamine *(Continued)*

6-12 years:

Hippurate: 25-50 mg/kg/day divided every 12 hours or 0.5-1 g twice daily

Mandelate: 50-75 mg/kg/day divided every 6 hours or 0.5 g 4 times/day

Children >12 years and Adults:

Hippurate: 1 g twice daily

Mandelate: 1 g 4 times/day after meals and at bedtime

**Dosing adjustment/comments in renal impairment:** $Cl_{cr}$ <50 mL/minute: Avoid use

**Patient Information** Take per recommended schedule, at regular intervals around-the-clock. Complete full course of therapy; do not skip doses. Maintain adequate hydration (2-3 L/day of fluids unless instructed to restrict fluid intake). Avoid excessive citrus fruits, milk, or alkalizing medications. You may experience nausea or vomiting or GI upset (small frequent meals, frequent mouth care, sucking lozenges, or chewing gum may help). Report pain on urination or blood in urine, skin rash, other persistent adverse effects, or if condition does not improve.

**Nursing Implications** Urine should be acidic (pH <5.5) for maximum effect

**Dosage Forms**

Suspension, oral: 0.5 g/5 mL (480 mL)

Tablet, as hippurate (Hiprex®, Urex®): 1 g (Hiprex® contains tartrazine dye)

Tablet, as mandelate, enteric coated: 500 mg, 1 g

♦ **Methenamine Hippurate** *see* Methenamine *on page 351*

♦ **Methenamine Mandelate** *see* Methenamine *on page 351*

♦ **Methergine®** *see* Methylergonovine *on page 357*

## Methicillin (meth i SIL in)

**U.S. Brand Names** Staphcillin®

**Pharmacologic Category** Antibiotic, Penicillin

**Use** Treatment of susceptible bacterial infections such as osteomyelitis, septicemia, endocarditis, and CNS infections due to penicillinase-producing strains of *Staphylococcus*; other antistaphylococcal penicillins are usually preferred

**Effects on Mental Status** Penicillins reported to cause apprehension, illusions, hallucinations, depersonalization, agitation, insomnia, and encephalopathy

**Effects on Psychiatric Treatment** May cause leukopenia; use caution with clozapine and carbamazepine

**Usual Dosage** I.M., I.V.:

Infants:

>7 days and >2000 g: 100 mg/kg/day in divided doses every 6 hours (for meningitis: 200 mg/kg/day)

>7 days and <2000 g: 75 mg/kg/day in divided doses every 8 hours (for meningitis: 150 mg/kg/day)

<7 days and >2000 g: Same as above

<7 days and <2000 g: 50 mg/kg/day in divided doses every 12 hours (for meningitis: 100 mg/kg/day)

Children: 100-300 mg/kg/day in divided doses every 4-6 hours

Adults: 4-12 g/day in divided doses every 4-6 hours

**Dosing interval in renal impairment:**

$Cl_{cr}$ 10-50 mL/minute: Administer every 6-8 hours

$Cl_{cr}$ <10 mL/minute: Administer every 8-12 hours

Hemodialysis: Not dialyzable (0% to 5%)

**Dosage Forms** Powder for injection, as sodium: 1 g, 4 g, 6 g, 10 g

## Methimazole (meth IM a zole)

**U.S. Brand Names** Tapazole®

**Synonyms** Thiamazole

**Pharmacologic Category** Antithyroid Agent

**Use** Palliative treatment of hyperthyroidism, return the hyperthyroid patient to a normal metabolic state prior to thyroidectomy, and to control thyrotoxic crisis that may accompany thyroidectomy. The use of antithyroid thioamides is as effective in elderly as they are in younger adults; however, the expense, potential adverse effects, and inconvenience (compliance, monitoring) make them undesirable. The use of radioiodine due to ease of administration and less concern for long-term side effects and reproduction problems (some older males) makes it a more appropriate therapy.

**Effects on Mental Status** May cause dizziness or drowsiness

**Effects on Psychiatric Treatment** Leukopenia is common; use caution with clozapine and carbamazepine; concurrent use with lithium may increase the effects on the thyroid

**Pregnancy Risk Factor** D

**Contraindications** Hypersensitivity to methimazole or any component, nursing mothers (per manufacturer; however, expert analysis and the American Academy of Pediatrics state this drug may be used with caution in nursing mothers)

**Warnings/Precautions** Use with extreme caution in patients receiving other drugs known to cause myelosuppression particularly agranulocytosis, patients >40 years of age; avoid doses >40 mg/day (↑ myelosuppression); may cause acneiform eruptions or worsen the condition of the thyroid

**Adverse Reactions**

>10%:

Central nervous system: Fever

Hematologic: Leukopenia

1% to 10%:

Central nervous system: Dizziness

Gastrointestinal: Nausea, vomiting, stomach pain, abnormal taste

Hematologic: Agranulocytosis

Miscellaneous: SLE-like syndrome

<1%: Alopecia, aplastic anemia, arthralgia, cholestatic jaundice, constipation, drowsiness, edema, goiter, headache, nephrotic syndrome, paresthesia, pruritus, rash, swollen salivary glands, thrombocytopenia, urticaria, vertigo, weight gain

**Overdosage/Toxicology**

Signs and symptoms: Nausea, vomiting, epigastric distress, headache, fever, arthralgia, pruritus, edema, pancytopenia, and signs of hypothyroidism

Treatment: Management of overdose is supportive

**Drug Interactions** Increased toxicity: Iodinated glycerol, lithium, potassium iodide; anticoagulant activity increased

**Usual Dosage** Oral: Administer in 3 equally divided doses at approximately 8-hour intervals

Children: Initial: 0.4 mg/kg/day in 3 divided doses; maintenance: 0.2 mg/kg/day in 3 divided doses up to 30 mg/24 hours maximum

Alternatively: Initial: 0.5-0.7 mg/kg/day **or** 15-20 mg/m²/day in 3 divided doses

Maintenance: 1/3 to 2/3 of the initial dose beginning when the patient is euthyroid

Maximum: 30 mg/24 hours

Adults: Initial: 15 mg/day for mild hyperthyroidism; 30-40 mg/day in moderately severe hyperthyroidism; 60 mg/day in severe hyperthyroidism; maintenance: 5-15 mg/day

Adjust dosage as required to achieve and maintain serum $T_3$, $T_4$, and TSH levels in the normal range. An elevated $T_3$ may be the sole indicator of inadequate treatment. An elevated TSH indicates excessive antithyroid treatment.

**Dosing adjustment in renal impairment:** Adjustment is not necessary

**Patient Information** Take as directed, at the same time each day around-the-clock; do not miss doses or make up missed doses. This drug will need to be taken for an extended period of time to achieve appropriate results. You may experience nausea or vomiting (small frequent meals may help), dizziness or drowsiness (use caution when driving or engaging in tasks that require alertness until response to drug is known). Report rash, fever, unusual bleeding or bruising, unresolved headache, yellowing of eyes or skin, or changes in color of urine or feces, unresolved malaise.

**Dosage Forms** Tablet: 5 mg, 10 mg

## Methocarbamol (meth oh KAR ba mole)

**U.S. Brand Names** Robaxin®

**Pharmacologic Category** Skeletal Muscle Relaxant

**Use** Treatment of muscle spasm associated with acute painful musculoskeletal conditions, supportive therapy in tetanus

**Effects on Mental Status** Drowsiness and dizziness are common

**Effects on Psychiatric Treatment** May rarely cause leukopenia; use caution with clozapine and carbamazepine; concurrent use with psychotropics may produce additive sedation

**Pregnancy Risk Factor** C

**Contraindications** Renal impairment, hypersensitivity to methocarbamol or any component

**Warnings/Precautions** Rate of injection should not exceed 3 mL/minute; solution is hypertonic; avoid extravasation; use with caution in patients with a history of seizures

**Adverse Reactions**

>10%: Central nervous system: Drowsiness, dizziness, lightheadedness

1% to 10%:

Cardiovascular: Flushing of face, bradycardia

Dermatologic: Allergic dermatitis

Gastrointestinal: Nausea, vomiting

Ocular: Nystagmus

Respiratory: Nasal congestion

<1%: Allergic manifestations, blurred vision, convulsions, leukopenia, pain at injection site, renal impairment, syncope, thrombophlebitis

**Overdosage/Toxicology**

Signs and symptoms: Cardiac arrhythmias, nausea, vomiting, drowsiness, coma

Treatment: Treatment is supportive following attempts to enhance drug elimination. Hypotension should be treated with I.V. fluids and/or Trendelenburg positioning. Dialysis and hemoperfusion and osmotic diuresis have all been useful in reducing serum drug concentrations. The patient should be observed for possible relapses due to incomplete gastric emptying.

**Drug Interactions** Increased effect/toxicity with CNS depressants

**Usual Dosage**

Children: Recommended **only** for use in tetanus I.V.: 15 mg/kg/dose or 500 mg/m²/dose, may repeat every 6 hours if needed; maximum dose: 1.8 g/m²/day for 3 days only

Adults: Muscle spasm:

Oral: 1.5 g 4 times/day for 2-3 days, then decrease to 4-4.5 g/day in 3-6 divided doses

I.M., I.V.: 1 g every 8 hours if oral not possible

**Dosing adjustment/comments in renal impairment:** Do not administer parenteral formulation to patients with renal dysfunction

**Dietary Considerations** Alcohol: Additive CNS effect, avoid use

**Patient Information** Take exactly as directed. Do not increase dose or discontinue without consulting prescriber. Do not use alcohol, prescriptive or OTC antidepressants, sedatives, or pain medications without consulting prescriber. You may experience drowsiness, dizziness, lightheadedness (avoid driving or engaging in tasks requiring alertness until response to drug is known); or nausea or vomiting (small, frequent meals, frequent mouth care, or sucking hard candy may help). Report excessive drowsiness or mental agitation, chest pain, skin rash, swelling of mouth/face, difficulty speaking, or vision disturbances.

**Nursing Implications** Monitor closely for extravasation of I.V. injection

**Dosage Forms**

Injection: 100 mg/mL in polyethylene glycol 50% (10 mL)

Tablet: 500 mg, 750 mg

## Methohexital (meth oh HEKS i tal)

**Related Information**

Patient Information - Anxiolytics & Sedative Hypnotics (Barbiturates) *on page 654*

**U.S. Brand Names** Brevital® Sodium

**Canadian Brand Names** Brietal Sodium®

**Synonyms** Methohexital Sodium

**Pharmacologic Category** Barbiturate

**Use** Induction and maintenance of general anesthesia for short procedures

**Can be used in pediatric patients >1 month of age as follows:** For rectal or intramuscular induction of anesthesia prior to the use of other general anesthetic agents, as an adjunct to subpotent inhalational anesthetic agents for short surgical procedures, or for short surgical, diagnostic, or therapeutic procedures associated with minimal painful stimuli

**Effects on Mental Status** Drowsiness is common

**Effects on Psychiatric Treatment** Used as induction anesthesia for electroconvulsive therapy (ECT); concurrent use with psychotropics may produce additive CNS depression

**Restrictions** C-IV

**Pregnancy Risk Factor** C

**Contraindications** Porphyria, hypersensitivity to methohexital or any component

**Warnings/Precautions** Use with extreme caution in patients with liver impairment, asthma, cardiovascular instability

**Adverse Reactions**

>10%: Local: Pain on I.M. injection

1% to 10%: Gastrointestinal: Cramping, diarrhea, rectal bleeding

<1%: Apnea, coughing, headache, hemolytic anemia, hiccups, hypotension, involuntary muscle movement, laryngospasm, nausea, peripheral vascular collapse, radial nerve palsy, respiratory depression, rigidity, seizures, thrombophlebitis, tremor, twitching, vomiting

**Overdosage/Toxicology**

Signs and symptoms: Apnea, tachycardia, hypotension

Treatment: Primarily supportive with mechanical ventilation if needed

**Drug Interactions**

Antineoplastics: Limited evidence suggests that enzyme-inducing anticonvulsant therapy may reduce the effectiveness of some chemotherapy regimens (specifically in ALL); teniposide and methotrexate may be cleared more rapidly in these patients

CNS depressants worsen CNS depression

**Usual Dosage** Doses must be titrated to effect

Children 3-12 years:

I.M.: Preop: 5-10 mg/kg/dose

I.V.: Induction: 1-2 mg/kg/dose

Rectal: Preop/induction: 20-35 mg/kg/dose; usual 25 mg/kg/dose; administer as 10% aqueous solution

Adults: I.V.: Induction: 50-120 mg to start; 20-40 mg every 4-7 minutes

**Dosing adjustment/comments in hepatic impairment:** Lower dosage and monitor closely

**Patient Information** May cause drowsiness

**Nursing Implications** Avoid extravasation or intra-arterial administration

**Dosage Forms** Injection, as sodium: 500 mg, 2.5 g, 5 g

◆ **Methohexital Sodium** *see* Methohexital *on page 353*

◆ **Methoin** *see* Mephenytoin *on page 341*

## Methotrexate (meth oh TREKS ate)

**U.S. Brand Names** Folex® PFS; Rheumatrex®

**Synonyms** Amethopterin; MTX

**Pharmacologic Category** Antineoplastic Agent, Antimetabolite

**Use** Treatment of trophoblastic neoplasms; leukemias; psoriasis; rheumatoid arthritis; breast, head and neck, and lung carcinomas; osteosarcoma; sarcomas; carcinoma of gastric, esophagus, testes; lymphomas

**Effects on Mental Status** May cause drowsiness or dizziness

**Effects on Psychiatric Treatment** Leukopenia is common; avoid clozapine and carbamazepine

**Pregnancy Risk Factor** D

**Contraindications** Hypersensitivity to methotrexate or any component; severe renal or hepatic impairment; pre-existing profound bone marrow suppression in patients with psoriasis or rheumatoid arthritis, alcoholic liver disease, AIDS, pre-existing blood dyscrasias

**Warnings/Precautions** The U.S. Food and Drug Administration (FDA) currently recommends that procedures for proper handling and disposal of antineoplastic agents be considered

May cause photosensitivity type reaction. When given concomitantly with radiotherapy may increase the risk of soft tissue necrosis and osteonecrosis. Reduce dosage in patients with renal or hepatic impairment; drain ascites and pleural effusions prior to treatment; use with caution in patients with peptic ulcer disease, ulcerative colitis, pre-existing bone marrow suppression. Monitor closely for pulmonary disease; use with caution in the elderly.

Because of the possibility of severe toxic reactions, fully inform patient of the risks involved. Do not use in women of childbearing age unless benefit outweighs risks; may cause hepatotoxicity, fibrosis, and cirrhosis, along with marked bone marrow depression. Death from intestinal perforation may occur. Risk of hepatotoxicity may be increased when administered with other hepatotoxic drugs (eg, azathioprine, retinoids, sulfasalazine).

Patients should receive 1-2 L of I.V. fluid prior to initiation of high-dose methotrexate. Patients should receive sodium bicarbonate to alkalinize their urine during and after high-dose methotrexate (urine SG <1.010 and pH >7 should be maintained for at least 24 hours after infusion).

Toxicity to methotrexate or any immunosuppressive is increased in elderly; must monitor carefully. For rheumatoid arthritis and psoriasis, immunosuppressive therapy should only be used when disease is active and less toxic, traditional therapy is ineffective. Recommended doses should be reduced when initiating therapy in elderly due to possible decreased metabolism, reduced renal function, and presence of interacting diseases and drugs.

Methotrexate penetrates slowly into 3rd space fluids, such as pleural effusions or ascites, and exits slowly from these compartments (slower than from plasma).

**Adverse Reactions**

>10%:

Central nervous system (with I.T. administration only):

Arachnoiditis: Acute reaction manifested as severe headache, nuchal rigidity, vomiting, and fever; may be alleviated by reducing the dose

Subacute toxicity: 10% of patients treated with 12-15 mg/m² of I.T. MTX may develop this in the second or third week of therapy; consists of motor paralysis of extremities, cranial nerve palsy, seizures, or coma. This has also been seen in pediatric cases receiving very high-dose I.V. MTX (when enough MTX can get across into the CSF).

Demyelinating encephalopathy: Seen months or years after receiving MTX; usually in association with cranial irradiation or other systemic chemotherapy

Dermatologic: Reddening of skin

Endocrine & metabolic: Hyperuricemia, defective oogenesis or spermatogenesis

Gastrointestinal: Ulcerative stomatitis, glossitis, gingivitis, nausea, vomiting, diarrhea, anorexia, intestinal perforation, mucositis (dose-dependent; appears in 3-7 days after therapy, resolving within 2 weeks)

Emetic potential:

<100 mg: Moderately low (10% to 30%)

≥100 mg or <250 mg: Moderate (30% to 60%)

≥250 mg: Moderately high (60% to 90%)

Hematologic: Leukopenia, thrombocytopenia

Renal: Renal failure, azotemia, nephropathy

Respiratory: Pharyngitis

1% to 10%:

Cardiovascular: Vasculitis

Central nervous system: Dizziness, malaise, encephalopathy, seizures, fever, chills

Dermatitis: Alopecia, rash, photosensitivity, depigmentation or hyperpigmentation of skin

Endocrine & metabolic: Diabetes

Genitourinary: Cystitis

Hematologic: Hemorrhage

(Continued)

## Methotrexate *(Continued)*

Myelosuppressive: This is the primary dose-limiting factor (along with mucositis) of MTX; occurs about 5-7 days after MTX therapy, and should resolve within 2 weeks
WBC: Mild
Platelets: Moderate
Onset (days): 7
Nadir (days): 10
Recovery (days): 21
Hepatic: Cirrhosis and portal fibrosis have been associated with chronic MTX therapy; acute elevation of liver enzymes are common after high-dose MTX, and usually resolve within 10 days
Neuromuscular & skeletal: Arthralgia
Ocular: Blurred vision
Renal: Renal dysfunction: Manifested by an abrupt rise in serum creatinine and BUN and a fall in urine output; more common with high-dose MTX, and may be due to precipitation of the drug. The best treatment is prevention: Aggressively hydrate with 3 L/m²/day starting 12 hours before therapy and continue for 24-36 hours; alkalinize the urine by adding 50 mEq of bicarbonate to each liter of fluid; keep urine flow >100 mL/hour and urine pH >7.
Respiratory: Pneumonitis: Associated with fever, cough, and interstitial pulmonary infiltrates; treatment is to withhold MTX during the acute reaction
Miscellaneous: Anaphylaxis, decreased resistance to infection

**Overdosage/Toxicology**
Signs and symptoms: Nausea, vomiting, alopecia, melena, renal failure
Treatment: Antidote: Leucovorin; administer as soon as toxicity is seen; administer 10 mg/m² orally or parenterally; follow with 10 mg/m² orally every 6 hours for 72 hours. After 24 hours following methotrexate administration, if the serum creatinine is ≥50% premethotrexate serum creatinine, increase leucovorin dose to 100 mg/m² every 3 hours until serum MTX level is <5 x $10^{-8}$M. Hydration and alkalinization may be used to prevent precipitation of MTX or MTX metabolites in the renal tubules. Toxicity in low dose range is negligible, but may present mucositis and mild bone marrow suppression; severe bone marrow toxicity can result from overdose. Neither peritoneal nor hemodialysis have been shown to ↑ elimination. Leucovorin should be administered intravenously, never intrathecally, for over doses of intrathecal methotrexate.

**Drug Interactions**
Anticonvulsants: Enzyme-inducing therapy (including phenobarbital or phenytoin) may increase the rate of methotrexate clearance; some data suggest an association with reduced effectiveness in ALL
Decreased effect:
Corticosteroids: Reported to decrease uptake of MTX into leukemia cells. Administration of these drugs should be separated by 12 hours. Dexamethasone has been reported to not affect methotrexate influx into cells.
Decreases phenytoin, 5-FU
Increased toxicity:
Live virus vaccines → vaccinia infections
Vincristine: Inhibits MTX efflux from the cell, leading to increased and prolonged MTX levels in the cell; the dose of VCR needed to produce this effect is not achieved clinically
Organic acids: Salicylates, sulfonamides, probenecid, and high doses of penicillins compete with MTX for transport and reduce renal tubular secretion. Salicylates and sulfonamides may also displace MTX from plasma proteins, ↑ MTX levels.
Ara-C: Increases formation of the Ara-C nucleotide can occur when MTX precedes Ara-C, thus promoting the action of Ara-C
Cyclosporine: CSA and MTX interfere with each others renal elimination, which may result in increased toxicity
Nonsteroidal anti-inflammatory drugs (NSAIDs): Should not be used during moderate or high-dose methotrexate due to increased and prolonged methotrexate levels may increase toxicity
Hepatotoxic agents (azathioprine, retinoids, sulfasalazine) may increase the risk of hepatotoxic reactions

**Usual Dosage** Refer to individual protocols. May be administered orally, I.M., intra-arterially, intrathecally, or I.V.

Leucovorin may be administered concomitantly or within 24 hours of methotrexate - refer to Leucovorin Calcium for details
Children:
Dermatomyositis: Oral: 15-20 mg/m²/week as a single dose once weekly or 0.3-1 mg/kg/dose once weekly
Juvenile rheumatoid arthritis: Oral, I.M.: 5-15 mg/m²/week as a single dose **or** as 3 divided doses given 12 hours apart
Antineoplastic dosage range:
Oral, I.M.: 7.5-30 mg/m²/week **or** every 2 weeks
I.V.: 10-18,000 mg/m² bolus dosing **or** continuous infusion over 6-42 hours
Dosing schedules listed below:
**Conventional Dose:**
15-20 mg/m² oral twice weekly
30-50 mg/m² oral, I.V. weekly
15 mg/day for 5 days oral, I.M. every 2-3 weeks
**Intermediate Dose:**
50-150 mg/m² I.V. push every 2-3 weeks
240 mg/m²* I.V. infusion every 4-7 days
0.5-1 g/m²* I.V. infusion every 2-3 weeks
**High Dose:**
1-12 g/m²* I.V. infusion every 1-3 weeks
*Followed with leucovorin rescue - refer to leucovorin monograph for details.
Pediatric solid tumors (high-dose): I.V.:
<12 years: 12 g/m² (dosage range: 12-18 g)
≥12 years: 8 g/m² (maximum: 18 g)
Acute lymphocytic leukemia (intermediate-dose): I.V.: Loading: 100 mg/m² over 1 hour, followed by a 35-hour infusion of 900 mg/m²/day
Meningeal leukemia: I.T.: 10-15 mg/m² (maximum dose: 15 mg) **or**
≤3 months: 3 mg/dose
4-11 months: 6 mg/dose
1 year: 8 mg/dose
2 years: 10 mg/dose
≥3 years: 12 mg/dose
I.T. doses are prepared with preservative-free MTX only. Hydrocortisone may be added to the I.T. preparation; total volume should range from 3-6 mL. Doses should be repeated at 2- to 5-day intervals until CSF counts return to normal followed by a dose once weekly for 2 weeks then monthly thereafter.
Adults: I.V.: Range is wide from 30-40 mg/m²/week to 100-12,000 mg/m² with leucovorin rescue
Doses **not** requiring leucovorin rescue range from 30-40 mg/m² I.V. or I.M. repeated weekly, or oral regimens of 10 mg/m² twice weekly
**High-dose MTX is considered to be >100 mg/m²** and can be as high as 1500-7500 mg/m². These doses **require** leucovorin rescue. Patients receiving doses ≥1000 mg/m² should have their urine alkalinized with bicarbonate or Bicitra® prior to and following MTX therapy.
Trophoblastic neoplasms: Oral, I.M.: 15-30 mg/day for 5 days; repeat in 7 days for 3-5 courses
Head and neck cancer: Oral, I.M., I.V.: 25-50 mg/m² once weekly
Rheumatoid arthritis: Oral: 7.5 mg once weekly **OR** 2.5 mg every 12 hours for 3 doses/week; not to exceed 20 mg/week
Psoriasis: Oral: 2.5-5 mg/dose every 12 hours for 3 doses given weekly **or** Oral, I.M.: 10-25 mg/dose given once weekly
Ectopic pregnancy: I.M./I.V.: 50 mg/m² single-dose without leucovorin rescue
Elderly: Rheumatoid arthritis/psoriasis: Oral: Initial: 5 mg once weekly; if nausea occurs, split dose to 2.5 mg every 12 hours for the day of administration; dose may be increased to 7.5 mg/week based on response, not to exceed 20 mg/week
**Dosing adjustment in renal impairment:**
$Cl_{cr}$ 61-80 mL/minute: Reduce dose to 75% of usual dose
$Cl_{cr}$ 51-60 mL/minute: Reduce dose to 70% of usual dose
$Cl_{cr}$ 10-50 mL/minute: Reduce dose to 30% to 50% of usual dose
$Cl_{cr}$ <10 mL/minute: Avoid use
Hemodialysis: Not dialyzable (0% to 5%); supplemental dose is not necessary
Peritoneal dialysis: Supplemental dose is not necessary
**Dosage adjustment in hepatic impairment:**
Bilirubin 3.1-5 mg/dL OR AST >180 units: Administer 75% of usual dose
Bilirubin >5 mg/dL: Do not use

**Dietary Considerations** Alcohol: Avoid use

**Patient Information** Avoid alcohol to prevent serious side effects. Avoid intake of extra dietary folic acid, maintain adequate hydration (2-3 L/day of fluids unless instructed to restrict fluid intake) and adequate nutrition (frequent small meals may help). You may experience nausea and vomiting (small frequent meals may help or request antiemetic from prescriber); drowsiness, tingling, numbness, or blurred vision (avoid driving or engaging in tasks that require alertness until response to drug is known); mouth sores (frequent oral care is necessary); loss of hair; permanent sterility; skin rash; photosensitivity (use sunscreen, wear protective clothing and eyewear, and avoid direct sunlight). Report black or tarry stools, fever, chills, unusual bleeding or bruising, shortness of breath or difficulty breathing, yellowing of skin or eyes, dark or bloody urine, or acute joint pain or other side effects you may experience.

**Dosage Forms**
Injection, as sodium: 2.5 mg/mL (2 mL); 25 mg/mL (2 mL, 4 mL, 8 mL, 10 mL)
Injection, as sodium, preservative free: 25 mg (2 mL, 4 mL, 8 mL, 10 mL)
Powder, for injection: 20 mg, 25 mg, 50 mg, 100 mg, 250 mg, 1 g
Tablet, as sodium: 2.5 mg
Tablet, as sodium, dose pack: 2.5 mg (4 cards with 2, 3, 4, 5, or 6 tablets each)

## Methotrimeprazine (meth oh trye MEP ra zeen)

**U.S. Brand Names** Levoprome®
**Canadian Brand Names** Nozinan®
**Synonyms** Levomepromazine
**Pharmacologic Category** Analgesic, Non-narcotic

**Use** Relief of moderate to severe pain in nonambulatory patients; for analgesia and sedation when respiratory depression is to be avoided, as in obstetrics; preanesthetic for producing sedation, somnolence and relief of apprehension and anxiety

**Effects on Mental Status** Is a phenothiazine; dizziness and extrapyramidal symptoms are common; may rarely cause neuroleptic malignant syndrome

**Effects on Psychiatric Treatment** Contraindicated with MAOIs and patient with hypersensitivity to phenothiazines; may rarely cause agranulocytosis; use caution with clozapine and carbamazepine

**Pregnancy Risk Factor** C

**Contraindications** Severe cardiac, renal, or hepatic disease; history of convulsive disorders; concurrent use of MAO inhibitors; significant hypotension; children <12 years of age; hypersensitivity to methotrimeprazine or phenothiazines, sulfite sensitivity

**Warnings/Precautions** Use with caution in patients receiving antihypertensive agents and in the elderly; if used longer than 30 days monitor for hematologic adverse effects

**Adverse Reactions**

>10%:

Cardiovascular: Hypotension, orthostatic hypotension

Central nervous system: Pseudoparkinsonism, akathisia, dystonias, dizziness

Gastrointestinal: Constipation

Neuromuscular & skeletal: Tardive dyskinesia

Ocular: Pigmentary retinopathy

Respiratory: Nasal congestion

Miscellaneous: Decreased diaphoresis

1% to 10%:

Central nervous system: Dizziness

Dermatologic: Increased sensitivity to sun, skin rash

Endocrine & metabolic: Changes in menstrual cycle, ejaculatory disturbances, changes in libido, pain in breasts

Gastrointestinal: Weight gain, nausea, vomiting, stomach pain

Genitourinary: Dysuria

Neuromuscular & skeletal: Trembling of fingers

**Drug Interactions** Increased toxicity: Additive effects with other CNS-depressants

**Usual Dosage** Adults: I.M.:

Sedation analgesia: 10-20 mg every 4-6 hours as needed

Preoperative medication: 2-20 mg, 45 minutes to 3 hours before surgery

Postoperative analgesia: 2.5-7.5 mg every 4-6 hours is suggested as necessary since residual effects of anesthetic may be present

Pre- and postoperative hypotension: I.M.: 5-10 mg

**Dosing adjustment/comments in renal or hepatic impairment:** Administer cautiously although no specific guidelines are available

**Patient Information** May cause drowsiness, rise slowly after sitting or lying after administration

**Dosage Forms** Injection, as hydrochloride: 20 mg/mL (10 mL)

## Methoxamine (meth OKS a meen)

**U.S. Brand Names** Vasoxyl®

**Pharmacologic Category** Alpha$_1$ Agonist

**Use** Treatment of hypotension occurring during general anesthesia; to terminate episodes of supraventricular tachycardia; treatment of shock

**Effects on Mental Status** None reported

**Effects on Psychiatric Treatment** Psychotropics may alter pressor response; monitor blood pressure

**Usual Dosage** Adults:

Emergencies: I.V.: 3-5 mg

Supraventricular tachycardia: I.V.: 10 mg

During spinal anesthesia: I.M.: 10-20 mg

**Dosage Forms** Injection, as hydrochloride: 20 mg/mL (1 mL)

## Methoxsalen (meth OKS a len)

**U.S. Brand Names** Oxsoralen®; Oxsoralen-Ultra®

**Synonyms** Methoxypsoralen; 8-Methoxypsoralen; 8-MOP

**Pharmacologic Category** Psoralen

**Use**

Oral: Symptomatic control of severe, recalcitrant disabling psoriasis, not responsive to other therapy when to diagnosis has been supported by biopsy. Administer only in conjunction with a schedule of controlled doses of long wave ultraviolet (UV) radiation; also used with long wave ultraviolet (UV) radiation for repigmentation of idiopathic vitiligo.

Topical: Repigmenting agent in vitiligo, used in conjunction with controlled doses of UVA or sunlight

**Effects on Mental Status** May cause nervousness, dizziness, or depression

**Effects on Psychiatric Treatment** Concurrent use with psychotropics may produce additive photosensitivity

**Pregnancy Risk Factor** C

**Contraindications** Diseases associated with photosensitivity, cataract, invasive squamous cell cancer, known hypersensitivity to methoxsalen (psoralens), and children <12 years of age

**Warnings/Precautions** Family history of sunlight allergy or chronic infections; lotion should only be applied under direct supervision of a physician and should not be dispensed to the patient; for use only if inadequate response to other forms of therapy, serious burns may occur from UVA or sunlight even through glass if dose and or exposure schedule is not maintained; some products may contain tartrazine; use caution in patients with hepatic or cardiac disease

**Adverse Reactions**

>10%:

Dermatologic: Itching

Gastrointestinal: Nausea

1% to 10%:

Cardiovascular: Severe edema, hypotension

Central nervous system: Nervousness, vertigo, depression

Dermatologic: Painful blistering, burning, and peeling of skin; pruritus, freckling, hypopigmentation, rash, cheilitis, erythema

Neuromuscular & skeletal: Loss of muscle coordination

**Overdosage/Toxicology**

Signs and symptoms: Nausea, severe burns

Treatment: Follow accepted treatment of severe burns; keep room darkened until reaction subsides (8-24 hours or more)

**Drug Interactions** Increased toxicity: Concomitant therapy with other photosensitizing agents such as anthralin, coal tar, griseofulvin, phenothiazines, nalidixic acid, sulfanilamides, tetracyclines, thiazides

**Usual Dosage**

Psoriasis: Adults: Oral: 10-70 mg 1½-2 hours before exposure to ultraviolet light, 2-3 times at least 48 hours apart; dosage is based upon patient's body weight and skin type

Vitiligo: Children >12 years and Adults:

Oral: 20 mg 2-4 hours before exposure to UVA light or sunlight; limit exposure to 15-40 minutes based on skin basic color and exposure

Topical: Apply lotion 1-2 hours before exposure to UVA light, no more than once weekly

**Patient Information** This medication is used in conjunction with specific ultraviolet treatment. Follow prescriber's directions exactly for oral medication which can be taken with food or milk to reduce nausea. Consult prescriber for specific dietary instructions. Avoid use of any other skin treatments unless approved by prescriber. Control exposure to direct sunlight as per prescriber's instructions. If sunlight cannot be avoided, use sunblock (consult prescriber for specific SPF level), wear protective clothing and wraparound protective eyewear. Consult prescriber immediately if burning, blistering, or skin irritation occur.

**Dosage Forms**

Capsule: 10 mg

Lotion: 1% (30 mL)

Solution: 20 mcg/mL

♦ **Methoxypsoralen** *see* Methoxsalen *on page 355*

♦ **8-Methoxypsoralen** *see* Methoxsalen *on page 355*

## Methscopolamine (meth skoe POL a meen)

**U.S. Brand Names** Pamine®

**Pharmacologic Category** Anticholinergic Agent

**Use** Adjunctive therapy in the treatment of peptic ulcer

**Effects on Mental Status** May rarely cause drowsiness, confusion, amnesia, or nervousness

**Effects on Psychiatric Treatment** Concurrent use with psychotropics may produce additive sedation and dry mouth

**Contraindications** Anticholinergic drugs decrease both esophageal and gastric motility and relax the lower esophageal sphincter and are contraindicated in the presence of reflux esophagitis; glaucoma; obstructed uropathy; obstructed disease of the GI tract (pyloroduodenal stenosis); paralytic ileus; intestinal atony of elderly or debilitated individuals; unstable cardiovascular status in acute hemorrhage; severe ulcerative colitis; toxic megacolon; complicated ulcerative colitis; myasthenia gravis; hypersensitivity to methscopolamine or related drugs

**Adverse Reactions**

>10%:

Dermatologic: Dry skin

Gastrointestinal: Constipation, xerostomia, dry

Respiratory: Dry nose

Miscellaneous: Decreased diaphoresis

1% to 10%: Gastrointestinal: Dysphagia

**Drug Interactions** No data reported

**Usual Dosage** Adults: Oral: 2.5 mg 30 minutes before meals or food and 2.5-5 mg at bedtime

**Dosage Forms** Tablet, as bromide: 2.5 mg

## Methsuximide (meth SUKS i mide)

**U.S. Brand Names** Celontin®

**Pharmacologic Category** Anticonvulsant, Succinimide

**Use** Control of absence (petit mal) seizures that are refractory to other drugs

**Unlabeled use:** Partial complex (psychomotor) seizures

**Contraindications** Hypersensitivity to methsuximide

**Warnings/Precautions** Use with caution in patients with hepatic or renal disease; abrupt withdrawal of the drug may precipitate absence status; methsuximide may increase tonic-clonic seizures in patients with mixed seizure disorders; methsuximide must be used in combination with other anticonvulsants in patients with both absence and tonic-clonic seizures

**Adverse Reactions**

Cardiovascular: Hyperemia

Central nervous system: Ataxia, dizziness, drowsiness, headache, aggressiveness, mental depression, irritability, nervousness, insomnia, confusion, psychosis, suicidal behavior, auditory hallucinations

Dermatologic: Stevens-Johnson syndrome, rash, urticaria

Gastrointestinal: Anorexia, nausea, vomiting, weight loss, diarrhea, epigastric and abdominal pain, constipation

Genitourinary: Proteinuria

Hematologic: Leukopenia, pancytopenia, eosinophilia, monocytosis

Ocular: Blurred vision, photophobia, peripheral edema

**Overdosage/Toxicology**

Signs and symptoms: Acute overdosage can cause CNS depression, ataxia, stupor, coma, hypotension; chronic overdose can cause skin rash, confusion, ataxia, proteinuria, hepatic dysfunction, hematuria

Treatment: Supportive; hemoperfusion and hemodialysis may be useful

**Drug Interactions**

CNS depressants: Sedative effects and/or respiratory depression may be additive with CNS depressants; includes ethanol, benzodiazepines, barbiturates, narcotic analgesics, and other sedative agents; monitor for increased effect

Enzyme inducers: Metabolism of succimides may be increased, decreasing their therapeutic effect; consider using an alternative sedative/hypnotic agent; potential inducers include phenobarbital, phenytoin, carbamazepine, rifampin, and rifabutin

CYP3A3/4 inhibitors: Serum level and/or toxicity of succimides may be increased; inhibitors include amiodarone, cimetidine, clarithromycin, erythromycin, delavirdine, diltiazem, dirithromycin, disulfiram, fluoxetine, fluvoxamine, grapefruit juice, indinavir, itraconazole, ketoconazole, nefazodone, nevirapine, propoxyfene, quinupristin-dalfopristin, ritonavir, saquinavir, verapamil, zafirlukast, zileuton; monitor for altered benzodiazepine response

**Stability** Protect from high temperature

**Mechanism of Action** Increases the seizure threshold and suppresses paroxysmal spike-and-wave pattern in absence seizures; depresses nerve transmission in the motor cortex

**Pharmacodynamics/kinetics**

Metabolism: Rapidly demethylated in the liver to N-desmethylmethsuximide (active metabolite)

Half-life: 2-4 hours

Time to peak serum concentration: Oral: Within 1-3 hours

Elimination: <1% excreted in urine as unchanged drug

**Usual Dosage** Oral:

Children: Initial: 10-15 mg/kg/day in 3-4 divided doses; increase weekly up to maximum of 30 mg/kg/day

Adults: 300 mg/day for the first week; may increase by 300 mg/day at weekly intervals up to 1.2 g/day in 2-4 divided doses/day

**Monitoring Parameters** CBC, hepatic function tests, urinalysis

**Reference Range** Therapeutic: 10-40 μg/mL (SI: 53-212 μmol/L); Toxic: >40 μg/mL (SI: >212 μmol/L)

**Test Interactions** ↑ alkaline phosphatase (S); positive Coombs' [direct]; ↓ calcium (S)

**Patient Information** Take with food; do not discontinue abruptly; may cause drowsiness and impair judgment

**Nursing Implications** Observe patient for excess sedation

**Additional Information** May cause drowsiness; periodic blood test monitoring required

**Dosage Forms** Capsule: 150 mg, 300 mg

## Methyclothiazide (meth i kloe THYE a zide)

**U.S. Brand Names** Aquatensen®; Enduron®

**Pharmacologic Category** Diuretic, Thiazide

**Use** Management of mild to moderate hypertension; treatment of edema in congestive heart failure and nephrotic syndrome

**Effects on Mental Status** May cause drowsiness

**Effects on Psychiatric Treatment** May rarely cause agranulocytosis; use caution with clozapine and carbamazepine; may cause photosensitivity; use psychotropics with caution; may decrease lithium clearance resulting in an increase in serum lithium levels and potential lithium toxicity; monitor serum lithium levels

**Pregnancy Risk Factor** B

**Contraindications** Hypersensitivity to methyclothiazide or any component, thiazides, or sulfonamide-derived drugs; anuria; renal decompensation

**Warnings/Precautions** Avoid in severe renal disease (ineffective). Electrolyte disturbances (hypokalemia, hypochloremic alkalosis, hyponatremia) can occur. Use with caution in severe hepatic dysfunction; hepatic encephalopathy can be caused by electrolyte disturbances. Gout can be precipitate in certain patients with a history of gout, a familial predisposition to gout, or chronic renal failure. Cautious use in diabetics; may see a change in glucose control. Hypersensitivity reactions can occur. Can cause SLE exacerbation or activation. Use with caution in patients with moderate or high cholesterol concentrations. Photosensitization may occur. Correct hypokalemia before initiating therapy.

**Adverse Reactions**

1% to 10%: Endocrine & metabolic: Hypokalemia

<1%: Agranulocytosis, anorexia, aplastic anemia, drowsiness, fluid and electrolyte imbalances (hypocalcemia, hypomagnesemia, hyponatremia), hemolytic anemia, hepatitis, hyperglycemia, hypotension, leukopenia, nausea, paresthesia, photosensitivity, polyuria, prerenal azotemia, rarely blood dyscrasias, rash, thrombocytopenia, uremia vomiting

**Overdosage/Toxicology**

Signs and symptoms: Hypermotility, diuresis, lethargy

Treatment: GI decontamination and supportive care; fluids for hypovolemia

**Drug Interactions**

Angiotensin-converting enzyme inhibitors: Increased hypotension if aggressively diuresed with a thiazide diuretic

Beta-blockers increase hyperglycemic effects in Type 2 diabetes mellitus

Cyclosporine and thiazides can increase the risk of gout or renal toxicity; avoid concurrent use

Digoxin toxicity can be exacerbated if a thiazide induces hypokalemia or hypomagnesemia

Lithium toxicity can occur by reducing renal excretion of lithium; monitor lithium concentration and adjust as needed

Neuromuscular blocking agents can prolong blockade; monitor serum potassium and neuromuscular status

NSAIDs can decrease the efficacy of thiazides reducing the diuretic and antihypertensive effects

**Usual Dosage** Adults: Oral:

Edema: 2.5-10 mg/day

Hypertension: 2.5-5 mg/day; may add another antihypertensive if 5 mg is not adequate after a trial of 8-12 weeks of therapy

**Patient Information** Take exactly as directed - with meals. May take early in day to avoid nocturia. Include bananas or orange juice in daily diet but do not take dietary supplements without advice or consultation of prescriber. Do not use alcohol or OTC medication without consulting prescriber. Weigh weekly at the same time, in the same clothes. Report weight gain >5 lb/week. May cause dizziness or weakness; change position slowly when rising from sitting or lying position and avoid driving or tasks requiring alertness until response to drug is known. You may experience nausea or loss of appetite (small frequent meals may help), impotence (reversible), constipation (fluids, exercise, dietary fiber may help), photosensitivity (use sunscreen, wear protective clothing and eyewear, and avoid direct sunlight). This medication does not replace other antihypertensive interventions; follow instructions for diet and lifestyle changes. Report flu-like symptoms, headache, joint soreness or weakness, difficulty breathing, skin rash, or excessive fatigue, swelling of extremities, or difficulty breathing.

**Nursing Implications** Assess weight, I & O reports daily to determine fluid loss; take blood pressure with patient lying down and standing

**Dosage Forms** Tablet: 2.5 mg, 5 mg

♦ **Methylacetoxyprogesterone** *see* Medroxyprogesterone *on page 336*

## Methyldopa (meth il DOE pa)

**U.S. Brand Names** Aldomet®

**Canadian Brand Names** Apo®-Methyldopa; Dopamet®; Medimet®; Novo-Medopa®; Nu-Medopa

**Pharmacologic Category** False Neurotransmitter

**Use** Management of moderate to severe hypertension

**Effects on Mental Status** May cause drowsiness, dizziness, anxiety, nightmares, or depression

**Effects on Psychiatric Treatment** Contraindicated with MAOIs; may rarely cause leukopenia; use caution with clozapine and carbamazepine; associated with lithium toxicity; use alternative antihypertensive agent; methyldopa may interact with psychotropics; monitor blood pressure and clinical status

**Pregnancy Risk Factor** B (oral); C (I.V.)

**Contraindications** Hypersensitivity to methyldopa or any component; active hepatic disease; liver disorders previously associated with use of methyldopa; on monoamine oxidase inhibitors; bisulfite allergy if using oral suspension or injectable

**Warnings/Precautions** Monitor for hemolytic anemia, positive Coombs' test, and liver dysfunction. A diuretic may be needed for weight gain or edema management. Its CNS side effects prevent it from being used frequently. It is the drug of choice for treatment of hypertension in pregnancy. Do use oral suspension or injectable if bisulfite allergy.

**Adverse Reactions**

Percentage unknown: Anxiety, "black" tongue, bradycardia (sinus), chills, cholestasis or hepatitis and heptocellular injury, cirrhosis, colitis, decreased libido, depression, diarrhea, drowsiness, drug fever, dyspnea, fever, gynecomastia, headache, hyperprolactinemia, increased liver enzymes, jaundice, memory lapse, mental depression, nausea, nightmares, orthostatic hypotension, pancreatitis, paresthesias, peripheral edema, rash, sedation, sexual dysfunction, SLE-like syndrome, sodium retention, vertigo, vomiting, weakness, xerostomia

>10%: Hematologic: Positive Coombs' test (20% to 43%)

<1%: Thrombocytopenia, hemolytic anemia (0.1% to 0.2%), leukopenia, transient leukopenia or granulocytopenia

**Overdosage/Toxicology**

Signs and symptoms: Hypotension, sedation, bradycardia, dizziness, constipation or diarrhea, flatus, nausea, vomiting

Treatment: Hypotension usually responds to I.V. fluids, Trendelenburg positioning, or vasoconstrictors. Treatment is primarily supportive and symptomatic; can be removed by hemodialysis.

**Drug Interactions**

Barbiturates and TCAs may reduce response to methyldopa

Beta-blockers, MAO inhibitors, phenothiazines, and sympathomimetics: Hypertension, sometimes severe, may occur

Iron supplements can interact and cause a significant **increase** in blood pressure

Lithium: Methyldopa may increase lithium toxicity; monitor lithium levels

Tolbutamide, haloperidol, anesthetics, and levodopa effects/toxicity are increased with methyldopa

**Usual Dosage**

Children:

Oral: Initial: 10 mg/kg/day in 2-4 divided doses; increase every 2 days as needed to maximum dose of 65 mg/kg/day; do not exceed 3 g/day.

I.V.: 5-10 mg/kg/dose every 6-8 hours up to a total dose of 65 mg/kg/24 hours or 3 g/24 hours

Adults:

Oral: Initial: 250 mg 2-3 times/day; increase every 2 days as needed; usual dose 1-1.5 g/day in 2-4 divided doses; maximum dose: 3 g/day.

I.V.: 250-500 mg every 6-8 hours; maximum dose: 1 g every 6 hours

**Dosing interval in renal impairment:**

$Cl_{cr}$ >50 mL/minute: Administer every 8 hours.

$Cl_{cr}$ 10-50 mL/minute: Administer every 8-12 hours.

$Cl_{cr}$ <10 mL/minute: Administer every 12-24 hours.

Hemodialysis: Slightly dialyzable (5% to 20%)

**Patient Information** Take as directed. Do not skip dose or discontinue without consulting prescriber. Follow recommended diet and exercise program. Do not use OTC medications which may affect blood pressure (eg, cough or cold remedies, diet pills, stay-awake medications) without consulting prescriber. This medication may cause altered color of urine (normal); drowsiness, dizziness, or impaired judgment (use caution when driving or engaging in tasks that require alertness until response to drug is known); postural hypotension (use caution when rising from sitting or lying position or when climbing stairs); or dry mouth or nausea (frequent mouth care or sucking lozenges may help). Report altered CNS status (eg, nightmares, depression, anxiety, increased nervousness); sudden weight gain (weigh yourself in the same clothes at the same time of day once a week); unusual or persistent swelling of ankles, feet, or extremities; palpitations or rapid heartbeat; persistent weakness, fatigue, or unusual bleeding; or other persistent side effects.

**Nursing Implications** Transient sedation or depression may be common for first 72 hours of therapy; usually disappears over time; infuse over 30 minutes; assist with ambulation

**Dosage Forms**

Injection, as methyldopate hydrochloride: 50 mg/mL (5 mL, 10 mL)

Suspension, oral: 250 mg/5 mL (5 mL, 473 mL)

Tablet: 125 mg, 250 mg, 500 mg

## Methyldopa and Hydrochlorothiazide

(meth il DOE pa & hye droe klor oh THYE a zide)

**U.S. Brand Names** Aldoril®

**Canadian Brand Names** Aldoril®-15; Aldoril®-25; Apo®-Methazide; Novo-Doparil; PMS-Dopazide

**Pharmacologic Category** Antihypertensive Agent, Combination

**Use** Management of moderate to severe hypertension

**Effects on Mental Status** May cause drowsiness, dizziness, anxiety, nightmares, or depression

**Effects on Psychiatric Treatment** Contraindicated with MAOIs; may rarely cause leukopenia; use caution with clozapine and carbamazepine; associated with lithium toxicity; use alternative antihypertensive agent; methyldopa may interact with psychotropics; monitor blood pressure and clinical status; thiazides may decrease lithium clearance resulting in an increase in serum lithium levels and potential lithium toxicity; monitor serum lithium levels

**Usual Dosage** Oral: 1 tablet 2-3 times/day for first 48 hours, then decrease or increase at intervals of not less than 2 days until an adequate response is achieved

**Dosage Forms** Tablet:

15: Methyldopa 250 mg and hydrochlorothiazide 15 mg

25: Methyldopa 250 mg and hydrochlorothiazide 25 mg

D30: Methyldopa 500 mg and hydrochlorothiazide 30 mg

D50: Methyldopa 500 mg and hydrochlorothiazide 50 mg

♦ **Methylergometrine Maleate** *see* Methylergonovine *on page 357*

## Methylergonovine (meth il er goe NOE veen)

**U.S. Brand Names** Methergine®

**Synonyms** Methylergometrine Maleate

**Pharmacologic Category** Ergot Derivative

**Use** Prevention and treatment of postpartum and postabortion hemorrhage caused by uterine atony or subinvolution

**Effects on Mental Status** May rarely cause dizziness or hallucinations

**Effects on Psychiatric Treatment** None reported

**Pregnancy Risk Factor** C

**Contraindications** Induction of labor, threatened spontaneous abortion, hypertension, toxemia, hypersensitivity to methylergonovine or any component, pregnancy

**Warnings/Precautions** Use caution in patients with sepsis, obliterative vascular disease, hepatic, or renal involvement, hypertension; administer with extreme caution if using I.V.

**Adverse Reactions**

>10%: Cardiovascular: Hypertension

1% to 10%: Gastrointestinal: Nausea, vomiting

<1%: Diaphoresis, diarrhea, dizziness, dyspnea, foul taste, hallucinations, headache, hematuria, leg cramps, nasal congestion, palpitations, seizures, temporary chest pain, thrombophlebitis, tinnitus, water intoxication

**Overdosage/Toxicology**

Signs and symptoms: Vasospastic effects, nausea, vomiting, lassitude, impaired mental function, hypotension, hypertension, unconsciousness, seizures, shock, and death

Treatment: General supportive therapy, gastric lavage, or induction of emesis, activated charcoal, saline cathartic; keep extremities warm. Activated charcoal is effective at binding certain chemicals, and this is especially true for ergot alkaloids; treatment is symptomatic with heparin, vasodilators (nitroprusside); vasodilators should be used with caution to avoid exaggerating any pre-existing hypotension.

**Drug Interactions** Augmented effects may occur with concurrent use of methylergonovine and vasoconstrictors or ergot alkaloids

**Usual Dosage** Adults:

Oral: 0.2 mg 3-4 times/day for 2-7 days

I.M.: 0.2 mg after delivery of anterior shoulder, after delivery of placenta, or during puerperium; may be repeated as required at intervals of 2-4 hours

I.V.: Same dose as I.M., but should not be routinely administered I.V. because of possibility of inducing sudden hypertension and cerebrovascular accident

**Patient Information** This drug will generally not be needed for more than a week. You may experience nausea and vomiting (small frequent meals may help), dizziness, headache, or ringing in the ears (will reverse when drug is discontinued). Report any respiratory difficulty, acute headache, or numb cold extremities, or severe abdominal cramping.

**Nursing Implications** Ampuls containing discolored solution should not be used

**Dosage Forms**

Injection, as maleate: 0.2 mg/mL (1 mL)

Tablet, as maleate: 0.2 mg

♦ **Methylin™** *see* Methylphenidate *on page 357*

♦ **Methylin™ ER** *see* Methylphenidate *on page 357*

♦ **Methylmorphine** *see* Codeine *on page 137*

## Methylphenidate (meth il FEN i date)

**Related Information**

Clinical Issues in the Use of Stimulants *on page 637*
Clozapine-Induced Side Effects *on page 780*
Patient Information - Stimulants *on page 652*
Sleep Disorders *on page 620*
Special Populations - Children and Adolescents *on page 663*
Special Populations - Elderly *on page 662*
Stimulant Agents Used for ADHD *on page 728*

**Generic Available** Yes

**U.S. Brand Names** Concerta™; Metadate ER®; Methylin™; Methylin™ ER; Ritalin®; Ritalin-SR®

**Canadian Brand Names** PMS-Methylphenidate; Riphenidate

**Synonyms** Methylphenidate Hydrochloride

**Pharmacologic Category** Stimulant

(Continued)

## Methylphenidate *(Continued)*

**Use** Treatment of attention deficit disorder; symptomatic management of narcolepsy

**Unlabeled use:** Depression (especially elderly or medically ill)

**Restrictions** C-II

**Pregnancy Risk Factor** C

**Contraindications** Known hypersensitivity or idiosyncrasy to sympathomimetic amines; marked anxiety, tension, and agitation; patients with advanced arteriosclerosis, symptomatic cardiovascular disease, moderate to severe hypertension (stage II or III), hyperthyroidism, glaucoma; patients with a history of drug abuse; use during or within 14 days following MAO inhibitor therapy; stimulant medications are contraindicated for use in children with attention deficit/hyperactivity disorders and concomitant Tourette's syndrome or tics

**Warnings/Precautions** Safety and efficacy in children <6 years of age not established. Use with caution in patients with bipolar disorder, diabetes mellitus, cardiovascular disease, seizure disorders, insomnia, porphyria, or mild hypertension (stage I). May exacerbate symptoms of behavior and thought disorder in psychotic patients. Do not use to treat severe depression or fatigue states. Potential for drug dependency exists - avoid abrupt discontinuation in patients who have received for prolonged periods. Stimulant use has been associated with growth suppression. Concerta™ should not be used in patients with pre-existing severe gastrointestinal narrowing (small bowel disease, short gut syndrome, history of peritonitis, cystic fibrosis, chronic intestinal pseudo-obstruction, Meckel's diverticulum)

**Adverse Reactions**

Cardiovascular: Tachycardia, bradycardia, angina, hypertension, hypotension, palpitations, cardiac arrhythmias

Central nervous system: Nervousness, insomnia, headache, dyskinesia, toxic psychosis, Tourette's syndrome, NMS, dizziness, drowsiness

Dermatologic: Rash

Endocrine & metabolic: Growth retardation

Gastrointestinal: Nausea, vomiting, anorexia, nausea, abdominal pain, weight loss

Hematologic: Thrombocytopenia, anemia, leukopenia

Ocular: Blurred vision

Respiratory: Upper respiratory tract infection, increased cough, pharyngitis, sinusitis

Miscellaneous: Hypersensitivity reactions

**Overdosage/Toxicology**

Symptoms of overdose include vomiting, agitation, tremors, hyperpyrexia, muscle twitching, hallucinations, tachycardia, mydriasis, sweating, palpitations

There is no specific antidote for methylphenidate intoxication and the bulk of the treatment is supportive. Hyperactivity and agitation usually respond to reduced sensory input or benzodiazepines, however, with extreme agitation haloperidol (2-5 mg I.M. for adults) may be required. Hyperthermia is best treated with external cooling measures, or when severe or unresponsive, muscle paralysis with pancuronium may be needed. Hypertension is usually transient and generally does not require treatment unless severe. For diastolic blood pressures >110 mm Hg, a nitroprusside infusion should be initiated. Seizures usually respond to diazepam I.V. and/or phenytoin maintenance regimens.

**Drug Interactions**

Guanethidine: Methylphenidate inhibits the antihypertensive response to guanethidine; probably also may occur with guanadrel

Linezolid: Due to MAO inhibition (see below), concurrent use with methylphenidate should generally be avoided

MAO inhibitors: Severe hypertensive episodes have occurred with amphetamine when used in patients receiving nonselective MAOIs; methylphenidate may be less likely to interact, or reactions may be less severe; use with caution only when warranted

Phenytoin: Serum levels may be increased by methylphenidate (in some patients); monitor

Selegiline: When selegiline is used at low dosages (<10 mg/day), an interaction with methylphenidate is less likely than with nonselective MAO inhibitors (see above), but theoretically possible; monitor

Sibutramine: Potential for reactions noted with amphetamines (severe hypertension and tachycardia) appears to be low; use with caution

Tricyclic antidepressants: Methylphenidate may increase serum concentrations of some tricyclic agents; clinical reports of toxicity are limited; dosage reduction of tricyclic antidepressants may be required; monitor

Venlafaxine: NMS has been reported in a patient receiving methylphenidate and venlafaxine

Warfarin: Methylphenidate may decrease metabolism of coumarin anticoagulants; effect has not been confirmed in all studies; monitor INR

**Stability**

Tablets: Do not store above 30°C (86°F); protect from light

Sustained release tablets: Do not store above 30°C (86°F); protect from moisture

Osmotic controlled release tablets (Concerta™): Store at 27°C (77°F); protect from humidity

**Mechanism of Action** Mild CNS stimulant; blocks the reuptake mechanism of dopaminergic neurons; appears to stimulate the cerebral cortex and subcortical structures similar to amphetamines

**Pharmacodynamics/kinetics**

Immediate release tablet:
- Peak cerebral stimulation effect: Within 2 hours
- Duration: 3-6 hours

Sustained release tablet:
- Peak effect: Within 4-7 hours
- Duration: 8 hours

Osmotic release tablet (Concerta™):
- Peak effect: Initial: 1-2 hours; $C_{max}$: 6-8 hours

Absorption: Readily absorbed from GI tract

Metabolism: In liver via de-esterification to an active metabolite

Half-life: 2-4 hours

Elimination: 90% in urine as metabolites and unchanged drug

**Usual Dosage** Oral: (Discontinue periodically to re-evaluate or if no improvement occurs within 1 month)

Children ≥6 years: Attention deficit disorder: Initial: 0.3 mg/kg/dose or 2.5-5 mg/dose given before breakfast and lunch; increase by 0.1 mg/kg/dose or by 5-10 mg/day at weekly intervals; usual dose: 0.5-1 mg/kg/day; maximum dose: 2 mg/kg/day or 60 mg/day; extended release product: Take once daily

Concerta™:

Children not currently taking methylphenidate:
- Initial: 18 mg once daily in the morning
- Adjustment: May increase to 54 mg/day; dose may be adjusted at weekly intervals

Children currently taking methylphenidate: **Note:** Dosing based on current regimen and clinical judgment; suggested dosing listed below:
- Patients taking methylphenidate 5 mg 2-3 times/day or 20 mg/day sustained release formulation: Initial dose: 18 mg once every morning (maximum: 54 mg/day)
- Patients taking methylphenidate 10 mg 2-3 times/day or 40 mg/day sustained release formulation: Initial dose: 36 mg once every morning (maximum: 54 mg/day)
- Patients taking methylphenidate 15 mg 2-3 times/day or 60 mg/day sustained release formulation: Initial dose: 54 mg once every morning (maximum: 54 mg/day)

Adults:
- Narcolepsy: 10 mg 2-3 times/day, up to 60 mg/day
- Depression: Initial: 2.5 mg every morning before 9 AM; dosage may be increased by 2.5-5 mg every 2-3 days as tolerated to a maximum of 20 mg/day; may be divided (ie, 7 AM and 12 noon), but should not be given after noon; do not use sustained release product

**Monitoring Parameters** Blood pressure, heart rate, signs and symptoms of depression

**Reference Range** Therapeutic: 5-40 ng/mL

**Test Interactions** False-positives by immunoassay can be seen with ranitidine, phenylpropanolamine, brompheniramine, chlorpromazine, fluspirilene, or pipothiazine coingestion. May also show up as a postive test for amphetamine.

**Patient Information** Take exactly as directed; do not change dosage or discontinue without consulting prescriber. Response may take some time. Do not crush or chew sustained release dosage forms. Tablets and sustained release tablets should be taken 30-45 minutes before meals. Concerta™ may be taken with or without food, but must be taken with water, milk, or juice. Avoid alcohol, caffeine, or other stimulants. Maintain adequate fluid intake (2-3 L/day of fluids unless instructed to restrict fluid intake). You may experience decreased appetite or weight loss (small frequent meals may help maintain adequate nutrition); restlessness, impaired judgment, or dizziness, especially during early therapy (use caution when driving or engaging in tasks requiring alertness until response to drug is known); Report unresolved rapid heartbeat; excessive agitation, nervousness, insomnia, tremors, or dizziness; blackened stool; skin rash or irritation; or altered gait or movement. Concerta™ tablet shell may appear intact in stool; this is normal.

**Nursing Implications** Do not crush or allow patient to chew sustained release dosage forms; to effectively avoid insomnia, dosing should be completed by noon.

Concerta™ tablet shell may appear intact in stool; this is normal. Must be taken with water, milk, or juice.

**Additional Information** Concerta™ is an osmotic controlled release formulation (OROS®) of methylphenidate. The tablet has an immediate-release overcoat that provides an initial dose of methylphenidate within 1 hour. The overcoat covers a trilayer core. The trilayer core is composed of two layers containing the drug and excipients, and one layer of osmotic components. As water from the gastrointestinal tract enters the core, the osmotic components expand and methylphenidate is released.

Treatment with methylphenidate should include "drug holidays" or periodic discontinuation in order to assess the patient's requirements and to decrease tolerance and limit suppression of linear growth and weight; specific patients may require 3 doses/day for treatment of ADHD (ie, additional dose at 4 PM)

**Dosage Forms**
Tablet, as hydrochloride: 5 mg, 10 mg, 20 mg
Methylin™, Ritalin®: 5 mg, 10 mg, 20 mg
Tablet, as hydrochloride, sustained release: 20 mg
Methylin ER™: 10 mg, 20 mg
Methylin ER™, Ritalin-SR®: 20 mg
Tablet, as hydrochloride, sustained release (once-daily) (Concerta™): 18 mg, 36 mg

♦ **Methylphenidate Hydrochloride** *see* Methylphenidate *on page 357*

♦ **Methylphenobarbital** *see* Mephobarbital *on page 342*

♦ **Methylphenylethylhydantoin** *see* Mephenytoin *on page 341*

♦ **Methylphenyl Isoxazolyl Penicillin** *see* Oxacillin *on page 408*

♦ **Methylphytyl Napthoquinone** *see* Phytonadione *on page 444*

## Methylprednisolone (meth il pred NIS oh lone)

**Related Information**
Corticosteroids Comparison Chart *on page 711*

**U.S. Brand Names** Adlone® Injection; A-methaPred® Injection; depMedalone® Injection; Depoject® Injection; Depo-Medrol® Injection; Depopred® Injection; D-Med® Injection; Duralone® Injection; Medralone® Injection; Medrol® Oral; M-Prednisol® Injection; Solu-Medrol® Injection

**Synonyms** 6-α-Methylprednisolone; Methylprednisolone Acetate; Methylprednisolone Sodium Succinate

**Pharmacologic Category** Corticosteroid, Parenteral

**Use** Primarily as an anti-inflammatory or immunosuppressant agent in the treatment of a variety of diseases including those of hematologic, allergic, inflammatory, neoplastic, and autoimmune origin. Prevention and treatment of graft-versus-host disease following allogeneic bone marrow transplantation.

**Effects on Mental Status** Nervousness and insomnia are common; may rarely cause delirium, mood swings, euphoria, or hallucinations

**Effects on Psychiatric Treatment** Barbiturates may increase the clearance of methylprednisolone

**Pregnancy Risk Factor** C

**Contraindications** Serious infections, except septic shock or tuberculous meningitis; known hypersensitivity to methylprednisolone; viral, fungal, or tubercular skin lesions; administration of live virus vaccines. Methylprednisolone formulations containing benzyl alcohol preservative are contraindicated in infants.

**Warnings/Precautions** Use with caution in patients with hyperthyroidism, cirrhosis, nonspecific ulcerative colitis, hypertension, osteoporosis, thromboembolic tendencies, CHF, convulsive disorders, myasthenia gravis, thrombophlebitis, peptic ulcer, diabetes; because of the risk of adverse effects, systemic corticosteroids should be used cautiously in the elderly, in the smallest possible dose, and for the shortest possible time

Acute adrenal insufficiency may occur with abrupt withdrawal after long-term therapy or with stress; young pediatric patients may be more susceptible to adrenal axis suppression from topical therapy

**Adverse Reactions**
>10%:
Central nervous system: Insomnia, nervousness
Gastrointestinal: Increased appetite, indigestion
1% to 10%:
Dermatologic: Hirsutism
Endocrine & metabolic: Diabetes mellitus, adrenal suppression, hyperlipidemia
Hematologic: Transient leukocytosis
Neuromuscular & skeletal: Arthralgia
Ocular: Cataracts, glaucoma
Miscellaneous: Infections
<1%: Abdominal distention, acne, alkalosis, amenorrhea, arrhythmias, avascular necrosis, bruising, Cushing's syndrome, delirium, edema, euphoria, fractures, glucose intolerance, growth suppression, hallucinations, headache, hyperglycemia, hyperpigmentation, hypersensitivity reactions, hypertension, hypokalemia, intractable hiccups, mood swings, muscle weakness, nausea, osteoporosis, pancreatitis, peptic ulcer, pituitary-adrenal axis suppression, pseudotumor cerebri, psychoses, secondary malignancy, seizures, skin atrophy, sodium and water retention, ulcerative esophagitis, vertigo, vomiting

**Overdosage/Toxicology**
Signs and symptoms: Cushingoid appearance (systemic), muscle weakness (systemic), osteoporosis (systemic) all with long-term use only. When consumed in excessive quantities for prolonged periods, systemic hypercorticism and adrenal suppression may occur.
Treatment: In those cases where systemic hypercorticism and adrenal suppression occur, discontinuation and withdrawal of the corticosteroid should be done judiciously

**Drug Interactions** CYP3A enzyme inducer
Decreased effect:
Phenytoin, phenobarbital, rifampin increase clearance of methylprednisolone
Potassium depleting diuretics enhance potassium depletion
Increased toxicity:
Skin test antigens, immunizations decrease response and increase potential infections
Methylprednisolone may increase circulating glucose levels and may need adjustments of insulin or oral hypoglycemics

**Usual Dosage** Dosing should be based on the lesser of ideal body weight or actual body weight

**Only sodium succinate may be given I.V.;** methylprednisolone sodium succinate is highly soluble and has a rapid effect by I.M. and I.V. routes. Methylprednisolone acetate has a low solubility and has a sustained I.M. effect.

Children:
Anti-inflammatory or immunosuppressive: Oral, I.M., I.V. (sodium succinate): 0.5-1.7 mg/kg/day **or** 5-25 mg/m²/day in divided doses every 6-12 hours; "Pulse" therapy: 15-30 mg/kg/dose over ≥30 minutes given once daily for 3 days
Status asthmaticus: I.V. (sodium succinate): Loading dose: 2 mg/kg/dose, then 0.5-1 mg/kg/dose every 6 hours for up to 5 days
Acute spinal cord injury: I.V. (sodium succinate): 30 mg/kg over 15 minutes, followed in 45 minutes by a continuous infusion of 5.4 mg/kg/hour for 23 hours
Lupus nephritis: I.V. (sodium succinate): 30 mg/kg over ≥30 minutes every other day for 6 doses
High-dose therapy for acute spinal cord injury: I.V. bolus: 30 mg/kg over 15 minutes, followed 45 minutes later by an infusion of 5.4 mg/kg/hour for 23 hours

Adults:
Anti-inflammatory or immunosuppressive: Oral: 2-60 mg/day in 1-4 divided doses to start, followed by gradual reduction in dosage to the lowest possible level consistent with maintaining an adequate clinical response
I.M. (sodium succinate): 10-80 mg/day once daily
I.M. (acetate): 10-80 mg every 1-2 weeks
I.V. (sodium succinate): 10-40 mg over a period of several minutes and repeated I.V. or I.M. at intervals depending on clinical response; when high dosages are needed, administer 30 mg/kg over a period of ≥30 minutes and may be repeated every 4-6 hours for 48 hours
Status asthmaticus: I.V. (sodium succinate): Loading dose: 2 mg/kg/dose, then 0.5-1 mg/kg/dose every 6 hours for up to 5 days
High-dose therapy for acute spinal cord injury: I.V. bolus: 30 mg/kg over 15 minutes, followed 45 minutes later by an infusion of 5.4 mg/kg/hour for 23 hours
Lupus nephritis: High-dose "pulse" therapy: I.V. (sodium succinate): 1 g/day for 3 days
Aplastic anemia: I.V. (sodium succinate): 1 mg/kg/day or 40 mg/day (whichever dose is higher), for 4 days. After 4 days, change to oral and continue until day 10 or until symptoms of serum sickness resolve, then rapidly reduce over approximately 2 weeks.

Hemodialysis: Slightly dialyzable (5% to 20%); administer dose posthemodialysis
Intra-articular (acetate): Administer every 1-5 weeks
Large joints: 20-80 mg
Small joints: 4-10 mg
Intralesional (acetate): 20-60 mg every 1-5 weeks

**Patient Information** Maintain adequate nutritional intake; consult prescriber for possibility of special dietary instructions. If diabetic, monitor serum glucose closely and notify prescriber of any changes; this medication can alter hypoglycemic requirements. Inform prescriber if you are experiencing unusual stress; dosage may need to be adjusted. You will be susceptible to infection; avoid crowds or infected persons or persons with contagious diseases. You may experience insomnia or nervousness; use caution when driving or engaging in tasks requiring alertness until response to drug is known. Report increased pain, swelling, or redness in area being treated; excessive or sudden weight gain; swelling of extremities; difficulty breathing; muscle pain or weakness; change in menstrual pattern; vision changes; signs of hyperglycemia; signs of infection (eg, fever, chills, mouth sores, perianal itching, vaginal discharge); blackened stool; other persistent side effects; or worsening of condition.

Oral: Take as directed, with food or milk. Take once-a-day dose in the morning. Do not take more than prescribed or discontinue without consulting prescriber.

Intra-articular: Refrain from excessive use of joint following therapy, even if pain is gone.

**Nursing Implications** **Acetate salt should not be given I.V.**

**Dosage Forms**
Injection, as acetate: 20 mg/mL (5 mL, 10 mL); 40 mg/mL (1 mL, 5 mL, 10 mL); 80 mg/mL (1 mL, 5 mL)
Injection, as sodium succinate: 40 mg (1 mL, 3 mL); 125 mg (2 mL, 5 mL); 500 mg (1 mL, 4 mL, 8 mL, 20 mL); 1000 mg (1 mL, 8 mL, 50 mL); 2000 mg (30.6 mL)
Tablet: 2 mg, 4 mg, 8 mg, 16 mg, 24 mg, 32 mg
Tablet, dose pack: 4 mg (21s)

♦ **6-α-Methylprednisolone** *see* Methylprednisolone *on page 359*

♦ **Methylprednisolone Acetate** *see* Methylprednisolone *on page 359*

♦ **Methylprednisolone Sodium Succinate** *see* Methylprednisolone *on page 359*

## Methyltestosterone (meth il tes TOS te rone)

**U.S. Brand Names** Android®; Oreton® Methyl; Testred®; Virilon®

**Pharmacologic Category** Androgen

**Use**

Male: Hypogonadism; delayed puberty; impotence and climacteric symptoms

Female: Palliative treatment of metastatic breast cancer; postpartum breast pain and/or engorgement

**Effects on Mental Status** None reported

**Effects on Psychiatric Treatment** May cause leukopenia; use caution with clozapine and carbamazepine

**Restrictions** C-III

**Pregnancy Risk Factor** X

**Contraindications** Hypersensitivity to methyltestosterone or any component, known or suspected carcinoma of the breast or the prostate, pregnancy

**Warnings/Precautions** Use with extreme caution in patients with liver or kidney disease or serious heart disease; may accelerate bone maturation without producing compensatory gain in linear growth

**Adverse Reactions**

>10%:

Cardiovascular: Edema

Males: Virilism, priapism

Females: Virilism, menstrual problems (amenorrhea), breast soreness

Dermatologic: Acne

1% to 10%:

Males: Prostatic hypertrophy, prostatic carcinoma, impotence, testicular

Females: Hirsutism (increase in pubic hair growth) atrophy

Gastrointestinal: GI irritation, nausea, vomiting

Hepatic: Hepatic dysfunction

<1%: Amenorrhea, cholestatic hepatitis, gynecomastia, hepatic necrosis, hypercalcemia, hypersensitivity reactions, leukopenia, polycythemia

**Overdosage/Toxicology** Signs and symptoms: Abnormal liver function tests

**Drug Interactions** Decreased effect: Oral anticoagulant effect or decrease insulin requirements

**Usual Dosage** Adults (buccal absorption produces twice the androgenic activity of oral tablets):

Male:

Hypogonadism, male climacteric and impotence: Oral: 10-40 mg/day

Androgen deficiency:

Oral: 10-50 mg/day

Buccal: 5-25 mg/day

Postpubertal cryptorchidism: Oral: 30 mg/day

Female:

Breast pain/engorgement:

Oral: 80 mg/day for 3-5 days

Buccal: 40 mg/day for 3-5 days

Breast cancer:

Oral: 50-200 mg/day

Buccal: 25-100 mg/day

**Patient Information** Take as directed; do not discontinue without consulting prescriber. Diabetics should monitor serum glucose closely and notify prescriber of changes; this medication can alter hypoglycemic requirements. You may experience acne, growth of body hair, loss of libido, impotence, or menstrual irregularity (usually reversible); nausea or vomiting (small frequent meals, frequent mouth care, sucking lozenges, or chewing gum may help). Report changes in menstrual pattern; deepening of voice or unusual growth of body hair; fluid retention (swelling of ankles, feet, or hands, difficulty breathing, or sudden weight gain); change in color of urine or stool; yellowing of eyes or skin; unusual bruising or bleeding; or other adverse reactions.

**Nursing Implications** In prepubertal children, perform radiographic examination of the hand and wrist every 6 months to determine the rate of bone maturation and to assess the effect of treatment on the epiphyseal centers

**Dosage Forms**

Capsule: 10 mg

Tablet: 10 mg, 25 mg

Tablet, buccal: 5 mg, 10 mg

## Methysergide (meth i SER jide)

**U.S. Brand Names** Sansert®

**Pharmacologic Category** Ergot Derivative

**Use** Prophylaxis of vascular headache

**Effects on Mental Status** Insomnia is common; may rarely cause drowsiness, euphoria, depression, or confusion

**Effects on Psychiatric Treatment** None reported

**Pregnancy Risk Factor** X

**Contraindications** Peripheral vascular disease, severe arteriosclerosis, pulmonary disease, severe hypertension, phlebitis, serious infections, pregnancy

**Warnings/Precautions** Patients receiving long-term therapy may develop retroperitoneal fibrosis, pleuropulmonary fibrosis and fibrotic thickening of the cardiac valves. Fibrosis occurs rarely when therapy is interrupted for 3-4 weeks every 6 months. Use caution in patients with impairment of renal of hepatic function; some products may contain tartrazine.

**Adverse Reactions**

>10%:

Cardiovascular: Postural hypotension, peripheral ischemia

Central nervous system: Insomnia

Gastrointestinal: Nausea, vomiting, abdominal pain, diarrhea

1% to 10%:

Cardiovascular: Peripheral edema, tachycardia, bradycardia

Dermatologic: Rash

Gastrointestinal: Heartburn

**Overdosage/Toxicology** Signs and symptoms: Hyperactivity, spasms in limbs, impaired mental function, impaired circulation

**Drug Interactions** Beta-blockers may cause peripheral ischemia

**Usual Dosage** Adults: Oral: 4-8 mg/day with meals; if no improvement is noted after 3 weeks, drug is unlikely to be beneficial; must not be given continuously for longer than 6 months, and a drug-free interval of 3-4 weeks must follow each 6-month course

**Patient Information** This drug is meant to prevent migraine headaches, not treat acute attacks. Take as directed; do not take more than recommended and do not discontinue without consulting prescriber (must be discontinued slowly). You may experience weight gain (monitor dietary intake and exercise) or dizziness or vertigo (use caution when driving or engaging in tasks that require alertness until response to drug is known). Small frequent meals may reduce nausea or vomiting. Diarrhea will lessen with use. Report cold, numb, tingling, or painful extremities or leg cramps, chest pain, difficulty breathing or shortness of breath, or pain on urination.

**Dosage Forms** Tablet, as maleate: 2 mg

♦ **Meticorten®** *see* Prednisone *on page 461*

♦ **Metimyd® Ophthalmic** *see* Sulfacetamide Sodium and Prednisolone *on page 523*

## Metipranolol (met i PRAN oh lol)

**Related Information**

Glaucoma Drug Therapy *on page 712*

**U.S. Brand Names** OptiPranolol® Ophthalmic

**Pharmacologic Category** Beta Blocker, Nonselective; Ophthalmic Agent, Antiglaucoma

**Use** Agent for lowering intraocular pressure in patients with chronic open-angle glaucoma

**Effects on Mental Status** None reported

**Effects on Psychiatric Treatment** None reported

**Usual Dosage** Ophthalmic: Adults: Instill 1 drop in the affected eye(s) twice daily

**Dosage Forms** Solution, ophthalmic, as hydrochloride: 0.3% (5 mL, 10 mL)

## Metoclopramide (met oh kloe PRA mide)

**U.S. Brand Names** Maxolon®; Octamide® PFS; Reglan®

**Canadian Brand Names** Apo®-Metoclop; Maxeran®

**Pharmacologic Category** Gastrointestinal Agent, Prokinetic

**Use** Symptomatic treatment of diabetic gastric stasis, gastroesophageal reflux; prevention of nausea associated with chemotherapy or postsurgery and facilitates intubation of the small intestine

**Effects on Mental Status** Drowsiness and restlessness are common; may cause insomnia or depression; drug is a D2 blocker; may cause extrapyramidal symptoms especially when used in high dosages or in the elderly

**Effects on Psychiatric Treatment** Anticholinergics may antagonize metoclopramide's effects; concurrent use with psychotropic may produce additive sedation

**Pregnancy Risk Factor** B

**Contraindications** Hypersensitivity to metoclopramide or any component; GI obstruction, perforation or hemorrhage, pheochromocytoma, history of seizure disorder

**Warnings/Precautions** Use with caution in patients with Parkinson's disease and in patients with a history of mental illness; dosage and/or frequency of administration should be modified in response to degree of renal impairment; extrapyramidal reactions, depression; may exacerbate seizures in seizure patients; to prevent extrapyramidal reactions, patients may be pretreated with diphenhydramine; elderly are more likely to develop dystonic reactions than younger adults; use lowest recommended doses initially

**Adverse Reactions**

>10%:

Central nervous system: Restlessness, drowsiness
Gastrointestinal: Diarrhea
Neuromuscular & skeletal: Weakness

1% to 10%:

Central nervous system: Insomnia, depression
Dermatologic: Rash
Endocrine & metabolic: Breast tenderness, prolactin stimulation
Gastrointestinal: Nausea, xerostomia

<1%: Agitation, anxiety, constipation, extrapyramidal reactions*, fatigue, hypertension or hypotension, methemoglobinemia, tachycardia, tardive dyskinesia

***Note:** A recent study suggests the incidence of extrapyramidal reactions due to metoclopramide may be as high as 34% and the incidence appears more often in the elderly

**Overdosage/Toxicology**

Signs and symptoms: Drowsiness, ataxia, extrapyramidal reactions, seizures, methemoglobinemia (in infants); disorientation, muscle hypertonia, irritability, and agitation are common

Treatment: Metoclopramide often causes extrapyramidal symptoms (eg, dystonic reactions) requiring management with diphenhydramine 1-2 mg/kg (adults) up to a maximum of 50 mg I.M. or I.V. slow push followed by a maintenance dose for 48-72 hours. When these reactions are unresponsive to diphenhydramine, benztropine mesylate I.V. 1-2 mg (adults) may be effective. These agents are generally effective within 2-5 minutes.

**Drug Interactions** CYP1A2 and 2D6 enzyme substrate

Decreased effect: Anticholinergic agents antagonize metoclopramide's actions

Increased toxicity: Opiate analgesics may increase CNS depression

**Usual Dosage**

Children:

Gastroesophageal reflux: Oral: 0.1-0.2 mg/kg/dose up to 4 times/day; efficacy of continuing metoclopramide beyond 12 weeks in reflux has not been determined; total daily dose should not exceed 0.5 mg/kg/day

Gastrointestinal hypomotility (gastroparesis): Oral, I.M., I.V.: 0.1 mg/kg/dose up to 4 times/day, not to exceed 0.5 mg/kg/day

Antiemetic (chemotherapy-induced emesis): I.V.: 1-2 mg/kg 30 minutes before chemotherapy and every 2-4 hours

Facilitate intubation: I.V.:

<6 years: 0.1 mg/kg
6-14 years: 2.5-5 mg

Adults:

Gastroesophageal reflux: Oral: 10-15 mg/dose up to 4 times/day 30 minutes before meals or food and at bedtime; single doses of 20 mg are occasionally needed for provoking situations; efficacy of continuing metoclopramide beyond 12 weeks in reflux has not been determined

Gastrointestinal hypomotility (gastroparesis):

Oral: 10 mg 30 minutes before each meal and at bedtime for 2-8 weeks

I.V. (for severe symptoms): 10 mg over 1-2 minutes; 10 days of I.V. therapy may be necessary for best response

Antiemetic (chemotherapy-induced emesis): I.V.: 1-2 mg/kg 30 minutes before chemotherapy and every 2-4 hours to every 4-6 hours (and usually given with diphenhydramine 25-50 mg I.V./oral)

Postoperative nausea and vomiting: I.M.: 10 mg near end of surgery; 20 mg doses may be used

Facilitate intubation: I.V.: 10 mg

Elderly:

Gastroesophageal reflux: Oral: 5 mg 4 times/day (30 minutes before meals and at bedtime); increase dose to 10 mg 4 times/day if no response at lower dose

Gastrointestinal hypomotility:

Oral: Initial: 5 mg 30 minutes before meals and at bedtime for 2-8 weeks; increase if necessary to 10 mg doses

I.V.: Initiate at 5 mg over 1-2 minutes; increase to 10 mg if necessary

Postoperative nausea and vomiting: I.M.: 5 mg near end of surgery; may repeat dose if necessary

**Dosing adjustment in renal impairment:**

$Cl_{cr}$ 10-40 mL/minute: Administer at 50% of normal dose
$Cl_{cr}$ <10 mL/minute: Administer at 25% of normal dose

Hemodialysis: Not dialyzable (0% to 5%); supplemental dose is not necessary

**Dietary Considerations** Alcohol: Additive CNS effect, avoid use

**Patient Information** Take this drug as prescribed, 30 minutes prior to eating. Do not increase dosage. Do not use alcohol or other CNS depressant or sleeping aids without consulting prescriber. May cause dizziness, drowsiness, or blurred vision; use caution when driving or engaging in tasks that require alertness until response to drug is known. May cause restlessness, anxiety, depression, or insomnia (will reverse when medication is discontinued). Report any CNS changes, involuntary movements, unresolved diarrhea. If diabetic, monitor serum glucose regularly.

**Dosage Forms**

Injection: 5 mg/mL (2 mL, 10 mL, 30 mL, 50 mL, 100 mL)
Solution, oral, concentrated: 10 mg/mL (10 mL, 30 mL)
Syrup, sugar free: 5 mg/5 mL (10 mL, 480 mL)
Tablet: 5 mg, 10 mg

## Metolazone (me TOLE a zone)

**U.S. Brand Names** Mykrox®; Zaroxolyn®

**Pharmacologic Category** Diuretic, Thiazide

**Use** Management of mild to moderate hypertension; treatment of edema in congestive heart failure and nephrotic syndrome, impaired renal function

**Effects on Mental Status** Dizziness is common; may cause drowsiness

**Effects on Psychiatric Treatment** May rarely cause agranulocytosis; use caution with clozapine and carbamazepine; may decrease lithium clearance resulting in an increase in serum lithium levels and potential lithium toxicity; monitor serum lithium levels

**Pregnancy Risk Factor** B (per manufacturer); D (based on expert analysis)

**Contraindications** Hypersensitivity to metolazone or any component, or other thiazides, and sulfonamide derivatives; anuria; hepatic coma; pregnancy

**Warnings/Precautions** Electrolyte disturbances (hypokalemia, hypochloremic alkalosis, hyponatremia) can occur. Use with caution in severe hepatic dysfunction; hepatic encephalopathy can be caused by electrolyte disturbances. Gout can be precipitate in certain patients with a history of gout, a familial predisposition to gout, or chronic renal failure. Cautious use in diabetics; may see a change in glucose control. Hypersensitivity reactions can occur. Can cause SLE exacerbation or activation. Use caution in severe renal impairment. Orthostatic hypotension may occur (potentiated by alcohol, barbiturates, narcotics, other antihypertensive drugs). Mykrox® tablets are not interchangeable with Zaroxolyn® tablets. Use with caution in patients with moderate or high cholesterol concentrations. Photosensitization may occur.

**Adverse Reactions**

1% to 10%:

Cardiovascular: Chest pain (3% with fast-acting product)
Central nervous system: Dizziness (10%), headache (9%)
Endocrine & metabolic: Hypokalemia
Neuromuscular & skeletal: Muscle cramps/spasms (6%)

<1%: Agranulocytosis, anorexia, aplastic anemia, drowsiness, fluid and electrolyte imbalances (hypocalcemia, hypomagnesemia, hyponatremia), hemolytic anemia, hepatitis, hypotension, hyperglycemia, leukopenia, nausea, paresthesia, photosensitivity, polyuria, prerenal azotemia, rarely blood dyscrasias, rash, thrombocytopenia, uremia, vomiting

**Overdosage/Toxicology**

Signs and symptoms: Hypermotility, diuresis, lethargy, confusion, muscle weakness

Treatment: Following GI decontamination, therapy is supportive with I.V. fluids, electrolytes, and I.V. pressors if needed

**Drug Interactions**

Angiotensin-converting enzyme inhibitors: Increased hypotension if aggressively diuresed with a thiazide-type diuretic

Beta-blockers increase hyperglycemic effects in Type 2 diabetes mellitus

Cyclosporine and thiazide- type compounds can increase the risk of gout or renal toxicity; avoid concurrent use

Digoxin toxicity can be exacerbated if a diuretic induces hypokalemia or hypomagnesemia

Lithium toxicity can occur due to a reduced renal excretion of lithium; monitor lithium concentration and adjust as needed

Neuromuscular blocking agents effects may be prolonged; monitor serum potassium and neuromuscular status

NSAIDs can decrease the efficacy of thiazide-type diuretics

**Usual Dosage** Adults: Oral:

Edema: 5-20 mg/dose every 24 hours
Hypertension: 2.5-5 mg/dose every 24 hours
Hypertension (Mykrox®): 0.5 mg/day; if response is not adequate, increase dose to maximum of 1 mg/day
Dialysis: Not dialyzable (0% to 5%) via hemo- or peritoneal dialysis; supplemental dose is not necessary

**Patient Information** Take exactly as directed - with meals. May take early in day to avoid nocturia. Include bananas or orange juice in daily diet but do not take dietary supplements without advice or consultation of prescriber. Do not use alcohol or OTC medication without consulting prescriber. Weigh weekly at the same time, in the same clothes. Report weight gain >5 lb/week. May cause dizziness or weakness (change position slowly when rising from sitting or lying, avoid driving or tasks requiring alertness until response to drug is known). You may experience nausea or loss of appetite (small frequent meals may help), impotence (reversible), constipation (fluids, exercise, dietary fiber may help), photosensitivity (use sunscreen, wear protective clothing and eyewear, and avoid direct sunlight). This medication does not replace other antihypertensive interventions; follow instructions for diet and lifestyle changes. Report flu-like symptoms, headache, joint soreness or weakness, difficulty breathing, skin rash, excessive fatigue, swelling of extremities, or difficulty breathing.

**Nursing Implications** Assess weight, I & O reports daily to determine fluid loss; take blood pressure with patient lying down and standing

(Continued)

## Metolazone *(Continued)*

**Dosage Forms** Tablet:
Zaroxolyn®: 2.5 mg, 5 mg, 10 mg
Mykrox®: 0.5 mg

## Metoprolol (me toe PROE lole)

**Related Information**
Beta-Blockers Comparison Chart *on page 709*

**U.S. Brand Names** Lopressor®; Toprol XL®

**Canadian Brand Names** Apo®-Metoprolol (Type L); Betaloc®; Betaloc® Durules®; Novo-Metoprolol; Nu-Metop

**Pharmacologic Category** Beta Blocker, $Beta_1$ Selective

**Use** Treatment of hypertension and angina pectoris; prevention of myocardial infarction, atrial fibrillation, flutter, symptomatic treatment of hypertrophic subaortic stenosis

**Unlabeled use:** Treatment of ventricular arrhythmias, atrial ectopy, migraine prophylaxis, essential tremor, aggressive behavior

**Effects on Mental Status** Sedation and dizziness are common; may cause depression; may rarely cause insomnia, confusion, amnesia, or nightmares

**Effects on Psychiatric Treatment** Barbiturates may decrease the effects of metoprolol; beta-blockers may increase the effects of psychotropics; monitor clinical status for potential changes

**Pregnancy Risk Factor** C (per manufacturer); D (in second and third trimester, based on expert analysis)

**Contraindications** Hypersensitivity to metoprolol or any component; sinus bradycardia; heart block greater than first degree (except in patients with a functioning artificial pacemaker); cardiogenic shock; uncompensated cardiac failure; pregnancy (2nd and 3rd trimesters)

**Warnings/Precautions** Must use care in compensated heart failure and monitor closely for a worsening of the condition (efficacy has not been established for metoprolol). Avoid abrupt discontinuation in patients with a history of CAD; slowly wean while monitoring for signs and symptoms of ischemia. Use caution in patients with PVD (can aggravate arterial insufficiency). Use caution with concurrent use of beta-blockers and either verapamil or diltiazem; bradycardia or heart block can occur. Avoid concurrent I.V. use of both agents. In general, beta-blockers should be avoided in patients with bronchospastic disease. Metoprolol, with B1 selectivity, should be used cautiously in bronchospastic disease with close monitoring. Use cautiously in diabetics because it can mask prominent hypoglycemic symptoms. Can mask signs of thyrotoxicosis. Can cause fetal harm when administered in pregnancy. Use cautiously in the hepatically impaired. Use care with anesthetic agents which decrease myocardial function.

**Adverse Reactions**

>10%:
- Central nervous system: Fatigue/dizziness (10%)
- Neuromuscular & skeletal: Weakness

1% to 10%:
- Cardiovascular: Bradycardia (3%), arrhythmia, hypotension/reduced peripheral circulation (1%)
- Central nervous system: Mental depression (5%)
- Dermatologic: Pruritus/rash (5%)
- Gastrointestinal: Heartburn (1%), diarrhea (5%), nausea (1%), xerostomia, abdominal pain (1%)
- Respiratory: Wheezing (1%), dyspnea (3%)

<1%: Chest pain, cold extremities, confusion, constipation, decreased sexual activity, headache, heart failure, impotence, insomnia, memory loss, nightmares, Raynaud's phenomenon, stomach discomfort, vomiting

**Overdosage/Toxicology**

Signs and symptoms: Cardiac disturbances, CNS toxicity, bronchospasm, hypoglycemia and hyperkalemia. The most common cardiac symptoms include hypotension and bradycardia; atrioventricular block, intraventricular conduction disturbances, cardiogenic shock, and asystole may occur with severe overdose, especially with membrane-depressant drugs (eg, propranolol); CNS effects include convulsions, coma, and respiratory arrest.

Treatment: Symptomatic treatment of seizures, hypotension, hyperkalemia and hypoglycemia; bradycardia and hypotension resistant to atropine, isoproterenol or pacing, may respond to glucagon; wide QRS defects caused by the membrane-depressant poisoning may respond to hypertonic sodium bicarbonate; repeat-dose charcoal, hemoperfusion, or hemodialysis may be helpful in removal of only those beta-blockers with a small $V_d$, long half-life or low intrinsic clearance (acebutolol, atenolol, nadolol, sotalol)

**Drug Interactions** CYP2D6 enzyme substrate

- Alpha-blockers (prazosin, terazosin): Concurrent use of beta-blockers may increase risk of orthostasis
- Clonidine: Hypertensive crisis after or during withdrawal of either agent
- Drugs which slow AV conduction (digoxin): effects may be additive with beta-blockers
- Fluoxetine may inhibit the metabolism of metoprolol resulting in cardiac toxicity
- Glucagon: Metoprolol may blunt the hyperglycemic action of glucagon
- Hydralazine may enhance the bioavailability of metoprolol
- Insulin and oral hypoglycemics: Metoprolol may mask tachycardia from hypoglycemia
- Metoprolol reduces antipyrine's clearance by 18%
- NSAIDs (ibuprofen, indomethacin, naproxen, piroxicam) may reduce the antihypertensive effects of beta-blockers
- Oral contraceptives may increase the AUC and $C_{max}$ of metoprolol
- Salicylates may reduce the antihypertensive effects of beta-blockers
- Sulfonylureas: Beta-blockers may alter response to hypoglycemic agents
- Verapamil or diltiazem may have synergistic or additive pharmacological effects when taken concurrently with beta-blockers; avoid concurrent I.V. use

**Usual Dosage**

Children: Oral: 1-5 mg/kg/24 hours divided twice daily; allow 3 days between dose adjustments

Adults:
- Oral: 100-450 mg/day in 2-3 divided doses, begin with 50 mg twice daily and increase doses at weekly intervals to desired effect
  - Extended release: Same daily dose administered as a single dose
- I.V.: 5 mg every 2 minutes for 3 doses in early treatment of myocardial infarction; thereafter administer 50 mg orally every 6 hours 15 minutes after last I.V. dose and continue for 48 hours; then administer a maintenance dose of 100 mg twice daily

Elderly: Oral: Initial: 25 mg/day; usual range: 25-300 mg/day

Hemodialysis: Administer dose posthemodialysis or administer 50 mg supplemental dose; supplemental dose is not necessary following peritoneal dialysis

**Dosing adjustment/comments in hepatic disease:** Reduced dose probably necessary

**Patient Information** I.V. use in emergency situations - patient information is included in general instructions.

Oral: Take exactly as directed. Do not increase, decrease, or adjust dosage without consulting prescriber. Take pulse daily, prior to medication and follow prescriber's instruction about holding medication. Do not take with antacids. Do not use alcohol or OTC medications (eg, cold remedies) without consulting prescriber. If diabetic, monitor serum sugars closely (may alter glucose tolerance or mask signs of hypoglycemia). May cause fatigue, dizziness, or postural hypotension; use caution when changing position from lying or sitting to standing, when driving, or when climbing stairs until response to medication is known. May cause alteration in sexual performance (reversible). Report unresolved swelling of extremities, difficulty breathing or new cough, unresolved fatigue, unusual weight gain, unresolved constipation, or unusual muscle weakness.

**Dosage Forms**
Injection, as tartrate: 1 mg/mL (5 mL)
Tablet, as tartrate: 50 mg, 100 mg
Tablet, as succinate [equivalent to tartrate], sustained release: 50 mg, 100 mg, 200 mg


- ♦ **MetroCream™** *see* Metronidazole *on page 362*
- ♦ **Metrodin® Injection** *see* Follitropins *on page 239*
- ♦ **MetroGel® Topical** *see* Metronidazole *on page 362*
- ♦ **MetroGel®-Vaginal** *see* Metronidazole *on page 362*
- ♦ **Metro I.V.® Injection** *see* Metronidazole *on page 362*
- ♦ **MetroLotion®** *see* Metronidazole *on page 362*


## Metronidazole (me troe NI da zole)

**U.S. Brand Names** Flagyl®; Flagyl ER®; MetroCream™; MetroGel® Topical; MetroGel®-Vaginal; Metro I.V.® Injection; MetroLotion®; Noritate® Cream; Protostat® Oral

**Canadian Brand Names** Apo®-Metronidazole; Novo-Nidazol

**Pharmacologic Category** Amebicide; Antibiotic, Topical; Antibiotic, Miscellaneous; Antiprotozoal

**Use** Treatment of susceptible anaerobic bacterial and protozoal infections in the following conditions: amebiasis, symptomatic and asymptomatic trichomoniasis; skin and skin structure infections; CNS infections; intra-abdominal infections; systemic anaerobic infections; topically for the treatment of acne rosacea; treatment of antibiotic-associated pseudomembranous colitis (AAPC), bacterial vaginosis; used in combination with other agents (eg, tetracycline, bismuth subsalicylate, and an $H_2$-antagonist) to treat duodenal ulcer disease due to *Helicobacter pylori*; also used in Crohn's disease and hepatic encephalopathy

**Effects on Mental Status** Dizziness is common; case reports of depression, insomnia, confusion, panic, delusions, hallucinations, exacerbation of schizophrenia

**Effects on Psychiatric Treatment** May rarely cause leukopenia; use caution with clozapine and carbamazepine; may decrease lithium clearance resulting in an increase in serum lithium levels and potential lithium toxicity; monitor serum lithium levels

**Pregnancy Risk Factor** B; May be contraindicated in first trimester

**Contraindications** Hypersensitivity to metronidazole or any component, 1st trimester of pregnancy since found to be carcinogenic in rats

**Warnings/Precautions** Use with caution in patients with liver impairment due to potential accumulation, blood dyscrasias; history of seizures, congestive heart failure, or other sodium retaining states; reduce dosage in patients with severe liver impairment, CNS disease, and severe renal failure ($Cl_{cr}$ <10 mL/minute); if *H. pylori* is not eradicated in patients being treated with metronidazole in a regimen, it should be assumed that metronidazole-resistance has occurred and it should not again be used; seizures and neuropathies have been reported especially with increased doses and chronic treatment; if this occurs, discontinue therapy

**Adverse Reactions**

>10%:

Central nervous system: Dizziness, headache

Gastrointestinal (12%): Nausea, diarrhea, loss of appetite, vomiting

<1%: Ataxia, change in taste sensation, dark urine, disulfiram-type reaction with alcohol, furry tongue, hypersensitivity, leukopenia, metallic taste, neuropathy, pancreatitis, seizures, thrombophlebitis, vaginal candidiasis, xerostomia

**Overdosage/Toxicology**

Signs and symptoms: Nausea, vomiting, ataxia, seizures, peripheral neuropathy

Treatment: Symptomatic and supportive

**Drug Interactions** CYP2C9 enzyme substrate; CYP2C9, 3A3/4, and 3A5-7 enzyme inhibitor

Decreased effect: Phenytoin, phenobarbital may decrease metronidazole half-life

Increased toxicity: Alcohol results in disulfiram-like reactions; metronidazole increases P-T prolongation with warfarin and increases lithium levels/toxicity; cimetidine may increase metronidazole levels

**Usual Dosage**

Neonates: Anaerobic infections: Oral, I.V.:

0-4 weeks: <1200 g: 7.5 mg/kg/dose every 48 hours

Postnatal age <7 days:

1200-2000 g: 7.5 mg/kg/day every 24 hours

>2000 g: 15 mg/kg/day in divided doses every 12 hours

Postnatal age >7 days:

1200-2000 g: 15 mg/kg/day in divided doses every 12 hours

>2000 g: 30 mg/kg/day in divided doses every 12 hours

Infants and Children:

Amebiasis: Oral: 35-50 mg/kg/day in divided doses every 8 hours for 10 days

Trichomoniasis: Oral: 15-30 mg/kg/day in divided doses every 8 hours for 7 days

Anaerobic infections:

Oral: 15-35 mg/kg/day in divided doses every 8 hours

I.V.: 30 mg/kg/day in divided doses every 6 hours

*Clostridium difficile* (antibiotic-associated colitis): Oral: 20 mg/kg/day divided every 6 hours

Maximum dose: 2 g/day

Adults:

Amebiasis: Oral: 500-750 mg every 8 hours for 5-10 days

Trichomoniasis: Oral: 250 mg every 8 hours for 7 days or 2 g as a single dose

Anaerobic infections: Oral, I.V.: 500 mg every 6-8 hours, not to exceed 4 g/day

Antibiotic-associated pseudomembranous colitis: Oral: 250-500 mg 3-4 times/day for 10-14 days

*H. pylori*: 1 capsule with meals and at bedtime for 14 days in combination with other agents (eg, tetracycline, bismuth subsalicylate, and $H_2$-antagonist)

Vaginosis: 1 applicatorful (~37.5 mg metronidazole) intravaginally once or twice daily for 5 days; apply once in morning and evening if using twice daily, if daily, use at bedtime

Elderly: Use lower end of dosing recommendations for adults, do not administer as a single dose

Topical (acne rosacea therapy): Apply and rub a thin film twice daily, morning and evening, to entire affected areas after washing. Significant therapeutic results should be noticed within 3 weeks. Clinical studies have demonstrated continuing improvement through 9 weeks of therapy.

**Dosing adjustment in renal impairment:** $Cl_{cr}$ <10 mL/minute: Administer every 12 hours

Hemodialysis: Extensively removed by hemodialysis and peritoneal dialysis (50% to 100%); administer dose posthemodialysis

Peritoneal dialysis: Dose as for $Cl_{cr}$ <10 mL/minute

Continuous arteriovenous or venovenous hemofiltration (CAVH/CAVHD): Administer usual dose

**Dosing adjustment/comments in hepatic disease:** Unchanged in mild liver disease; reduce dosage in severe liver disease

**Dietary Considerations**

Alcohol: A disulfiram-like reaction characterized by flushing, headache, nausea, vomiting, sweating or tachycardia; patients should be warned to avoid alcohol during and 72 hours after therapy

Food: Peak antibiotic serum concentration lowered and delayed, but total drug absorbed not affected. Take on an empty stomach. Drug may cause GI upset; if GI upset occurs, take with food.

**Patient Information** Take exactly as directed, with meals. Avoid alcohol during and for 24 hours after last dose. With alcohol your may experience severe flushing, headache, nausea, vomiting, or chest and abdominal pain. May discolor urine (brown/black/dark) (normal). You may experience "metallic" taste disturbance or nausea or vomiting (small frequent meals, frequent mouth care, chewing gum, or sucking lozenges may help). Refrain from intercourse or use a barrier contraceptive if being treated for trichomoniasis. Report unresolved or severe fatigue; weakness; fever or chills; mouth or vaginal sores; numbness, tingling, or swelling of extremities; difficulty breathing; or lack of improvement or worsening of condition.

Topical: Wash hands and area before applying and medication thinly. Wash hands after applying. Avoid contact with eyes. Do not cover with occlusive dressing. Report severe skin irritation or if condition does not improve.

**Nursing Implications** No Antabuse®-like reactions have been reported after **topical** application, although metronidazole can be detected in the blood; avoid contact between the drug and aluminum in the infusion set

**Dosage Forms**

Capsule: 375 mg

Gel, topical: 0.75% [7.5 mg/mL] (30 g)

Gel, vaginal: 0.75% (5 g applicator delivering 37.5 mg; 70 g tube)

Injection, ready to use: 5 mg/mL (100 mL)

Powder for injection, as hydrochloride: 500 mg

Tablet: 250 mg, 500 mg

Tablet, extended release: 750 mg

## Metyrosine (me TYE roe seen)

**U.S. Brand Names** Demser®

**Synonyms** AMPT; OGMT

**Pharmacologic Category** Tyrosine Hydroxylase Inhibitor

**Use** Short-term management of pheochromocytoma before surgery, long-term management when surgery is contraindicated or when malignant

**Effects on Mental Status** Drowsiness and extrapyramidal reactions are common; may cause depression, hallucinations, or confusion

**Effects on Psychiatric Treatment** Concurrent use with antipsychotics may increase the risk of extrapyramidal symptoms

**Pregnancy Risk Factor** C

**Contraindications** Hypertension of unknown etiology, known hypersensitivity to metyrosine

**Warnings/Precautions** Maintain fluid volume during and after surgery; use with caution in patients with impaired renal or hepatic function

**Adverse Reactions**

>10%:

Central nervous system: Drowsiness, extrapyramidal symptoms

Gastrointestinal: Diarrhea

1% to 10%:

Endocrine & metabolic: Galactorrhea, edema of the breasts

Gastrointestinal: Nausea, vomiting, xerostomia

Genitourinary: Impotence

Respiratory: Nasal congestion

<1%: Anemia, depression, disorientation, eosinophilia, hallucinations, hematuria, hyperstimulation after withdrawal, lower extremity edema, parkinsonism, urinary problems, urticaria

**Overdosage/Toxicology**

Signs and symptoms: Sedation, fatigue, tremor

Treatment: Reducing dose or discontinuation of therapy usually results in resolution of symptoms

**Drug Interactions** Phenothiazines, haloperidol may potentiate EPS

**Usual Dosage** Children >12 years and Adults: Oral: Initial: 250 mg 4 times/day, increased by 250-500 mg/day up to 4 g/day; maintenance: 2-3 g/day in 4 divided doses; for preoperative preparation, administer optimum effective dosage for 5-7 days

**Dosing adjustment in renal impairment:** Adjustment should be considered

**Dietary Considerations** Alcohol: Additive CNS effect, avoid use

**Patient Information** Take plenty of fluids each day; may cause drowsiness, impair coordination and judgment; notify physician if drooling, tremors, speech difficulty, or diarrhea occurs; avoid alcohol and central nervous system depressants

**Dosage Forms** Capsule: 250 mg

♦ **Mevacor®** *see* Lovastatin *on page 327*

♦ **Mevinolin** *see* Lovastatin *on page 327*

## Mexiletine (MEKS i le teen)

**U.S. Brand Names** Mexitil®

**Pharmacologic Category** Antiarrhythmic Agent, Class I-B

**Use** Management of serious ventricular arrhythmias; suppression of PVCs

**Unlabeled use:** Diabetic neuropathy

**Effects on Mental Status** Dizziness and nervousness are common; may cause confusion and insomnia

(Continued)

## Mexiletine *(Continued)*

**Effects on Psychiatric Treatment** May rarely cause agranulocytosis; use caution with clozapine and carbamazepine; barbiturates may decrease the effects of mexiletine; monitor

**Pregnancy Risk Factor** C

**Contraindications** Hypersensitivity to mexiletine or any component; cardiogenic shock; second- or third-degree AV block (except in patients with a functioning artificial pacemaker)

**Warnings/Precautions** Can be proarrhythmic. May cause acute hepatic injury. Use cautiously in patients with first-degree block, pre-existing sinus node dysfunction, intraventricular conduction delays, significant hepatic dysfunction, hypotension, or severe CHF. Electrolytes disturbances alter response. Alterations in urinary pH may change urinary excretion. Rare hepatic toxicity may occur. Electrolyte abnormalities should be corrected before initiating therapy (can worsen CHF).

**Adverse Reactions**

>10%:
- Central nervous system: Lightheadedness (10.5%), dizziness (20% to 25%), nervousness (5% to 10%), incoordination (10.2%)
- Gastrointestinal: GI distress (41%), nausea/vomiting (40%)
- Neuromuscular & skeletal: Trembling, unsteady gait, tremor (12.6%)

1% to 10%:
- Cardiovascular: Chest pain (2.5% to 7.5%), premature ventricular contractions (1% to 2%), palpitations (4% to 8%)
- Central nervous system: Confusion, headache, insomnia (5% to 7%)
- Dermatologic: Rash (3.8% to 4.2%)
- Gastrointestinal: Constipation or diarrhea (4% to 5%), xerostomia (2.8%), abdominal pain (1.2%)
- Neuromuscular & skeletal: Weakness, numbness of fingers or toes (2% to 4%)
- Ocular: Blurred vision (5% to 7%)
- Otic: Tinnitus (2% to 2.5%)
- Respiratory: Shortness of breath

<1%: Agranulocytosis, diplopia increased LFTs, leukopenia, positive antinuclear antibody, thrombocytopenia

**Overdosage/Toxicology**

Signs and symptoms: Has a narrow therapeutic index and severe toxicity may occur slightly above the therapeutic range, especially with other antiarrhythmic drugs; acute ingestion of twice the daily therapeutic dose is potentially life-threatening; symptoms of overdose includes sedation, confusion, coma, seizures, respiratory arrest and cardiac toxicity (sinus arrest, A-V block, asystole, and hypotension); the QRS and Q-T intervals are usually normal, although they may be prolonged after massive overdose; other effects include dizziness, paresthesias, tremor, ataxia, and GI disturbance.

Treatment: Supportive, using conventional therapies (fluids, positioning, vasopressors, antiarrhythmics, anticonvulsants); sodium bicarbonate may reverse the QRS prolongation, bradyarrhythmias and hypotension; enhanced elimination with dialysis, hemoperfusion or repeat charcoal is not effective.

**Drug Interactions** CYP2D6 enzyme substrate; CYP1A2 enzyme inhibitor

Enzyme inducers (phenobarbital, phenytoin, rifampin) may decrease mexiletine plasma levels

Quinidine may increase mexiletine blood levels

Theophylline blood levels are increased by mexiletine

Urinary alkalinizers (antacids, sodium bicarbonate, acetazolamide) may increase mexiletine blood levels

**Usual Dosage** Adults: Oral: Initial: 200 mg every 8 hours (may load with 400 mg if necessary); adjust dose every 2-3 days; usual dose: 200-300 mg every 8 hours; maximum dose: 1.2 g/day (some patients respond to every 12-hour dosing). Patients with hepatic impairment or CHF may require dose reduction. When switching from another antiarrhythmic, initiate a 200 mg dose 6-12 hours after stopping former agents, 3-6 hours after stopping procainamide.

**Patient Information** Take exactly as directed, with food or antacids, around-the-clock. Do not take additional doses or discontinue without consulting prescriber. Do not change diet without consulting prescriber. You will need regular cardiac checkups and blood tests while taking this medication. You may experience drowsiness or dizziness, numbness, or visual changes (use caution when driving or engaging in tasks requiring alertness until response to drug is known); nausea, vomiting, or heartburn (small frequent meals, frequent mouth care, chewing gum, or sucking lozenges may help); or headaches or sleep disturbances (usually temporary, if persistent consult prescriber). Report chest pain, palpitation, or erratic heartbeat; increased weight or swelling of hands or feet; chills, fever, or persistent sore throat; numbness, weakness, trembling, or unsteady gait; blurred vision or ringing in ears; or difficulty breathing.

**Dosage Forms** Capsule: 150 mg, 200 mg, 250 mg

♦ **Mexitil®** *see* Mexiletine *on page 363*

♦ **Mezlin®** *see* Mezlocillin *on page 364*

## Mezlocillin (mez loe SIL in)

**U.S. Brand Names** Mezlin®

**Pharmacologic Category** Antibiotic, Penicillin

**Use** Treatment of infections caused by susceptible gram-negative aerobic bacilli (*Klebsiella, Proteus, Escherichia coli, Enterobacter, Pseudomonas aeruginosa, Serratia*) involving the skin and skin structure, bone and joint, respiratory tract, urinary tract, gastrointestinal tract, as well as, septicemia

**Effects on Mental Status** May cause dizziness; penicillins reported to cause apprehension, illusions, hallucinations, depersonalization, agitation, encephalopathy, and insomnia

**Effects on Psychiatric Treatment** May cause leukopenia; use caution with clozapine and carbamazepine

**Usual Dosage** I.M., I.V.:

Infants:
- ≤7 days, ≤2000 g: 75 mg/kg every 12 hours
- ≤7 days, >2000 g: Same as above
- >7 days, ≤2000 g: 75 mg/kg every 8 hours
- >7 days, >2000 g: 75 mg/kg every 6 hours

Children: 300 mg/kg/day divided every 4-6 hours; maximum: 24 g/day

Adults: Usual: 3-4 g every 4-6 hours
- Uncomplicated urinary tract infection: 1.5-2 g every 6 hours
- Serious infections: 200-300 mg/kg/day in 4-6 divided doses

**Dosing interval in renal impairment:**
- $Cl_{cr}$ 10-30 mL/minute: Administer every 6-8 hours
- $Cl_{cr}$ <10 mL/minute: Administer every 8 hours

Hemodialysis: Moderately dialyzable (20% to 50%)

**Dosing adjustment in hepatic impairment:** Reduce dose by 50%

**Dosage Forms** Powder for injection, as sodium: 1 g, 2 g, 3 g, 4 g, 20 g

♦ **Miacalcin® Injection** *see* Calcitonin *on page 83*

♦ **Miacalcin® Nasal Spray** *see* Calcitonin *on page 83*

♦ **Micardis®** *see* Telmisartan *on page 532*

♦ **Micatin® Topical [OTC]** *see* Miconazole *on page 364*

## Miconazole (mi KON a zole)

**U.S. Brand Names** Absorbine® Antifungal Foot Powder [OTC]; Breezee® Mist Antifungal [OTC]; Femizol-M® [OTC]; Fungoid® Creme; Fungoid® Tincture; Lotrimin® AF Powder [OTC]; Lotrimin® AF Spray Liquid [OTC]; Lotrimin® AF Spray Powder [OTC]; Maximum Strength Desenex® Antifungal Cream [OTC]; Micatin® Topical [OTC]; Monistat-Derm™ Topical; Monistat i.v.™ Injection; Monistat™ Vaginal; M-Zole® 7 Dual Pack [OTC]; Ony-Clear® Spray; Prescription Strength Desenex® [OTC]; Zeasorb-AF® Powder [OTC]

**Canadian Brand Names** Monazole-7®

**Pharmacologic Category** Antifungal Agent, Parenteral; Antifungal Agent, Topical; Antifungal Agent, Vaginal

**Use**

I.V.: Treatment of severe systemic fungal infections and fungal meningitis that are refractory to standard treatment

Topical: Treatment of vulvovaginal candidiasis and a variety of skin and mucous membrane fungal infections

**Effects on Mental Status** May cause drowsiness

**Effects on Psychiatric Treatment** None reported

**Pregnancy Risk Factor** C

**Contraindications** Hypersensitivity to miconazole, fluconazole, ketoconazole, polyoxyl 35 castor oil, or any component; concomitant administration with cisapride

**Warnings/Precautions** Administer I.V. with caution to patients with hepatic insufficiency; the safety of miconazole in patients <1 year of age has not been established; cardiorespiratory and anaphylaxis have occurred with excessively rapid administration

**Adverse Reactions**

>10%:
- Central nervous system: Fever, chills (10%)
- Dermatologic: Rash, itching, pruritus (21%)
- Gastrointestinal: Anorexia, diarrhea, nausea (18%), vomiting (7%)
- Local: Pain at injection site

1% to 10%: Dermatologic: Rash (9%)

<1%: Anemia, drowsiness, flushing of face or skin, thrombocytopenia

**Overdosage/Toxicology**

Signs and symptoms: Nausea, vomiting, drowsiness

Treatment: Following GI decontamination, supportive care only

**Drug Interactions** CYP3A3/4 enzyme substrate; CYP2C enzyme inhibitor, CYP3A3/4 enzyme inhibitor (moderate), and CYP3A5-7 enzyme inhibitor

Warfarin (increased anticoagulant effect), oral sulfonylureas, amphotericin B (decreased antifungal effect of both agents), phenytoin (levels may be increased)

Increased risk of significant cardiotoxicity with concurrent administration of cisapride - concomitant administration is contraindicated (see interactions associated with ketoconazole)

**Usual Dosage**

Children:
- <1 year: 15-30 mg/kg/day

1-12 years:
I.V.: 20-40 mg/kg/day divided every 8 hours (do not exceed 15 mg/kg/dose)
Topical: Apply twice daily for up to 1 month
Adults:
Topical: Apply twice daily for up to 1 month
I.T.: 20 mg every 1-2 days
I.V.: Initial: 200 mg, then 0.6-3.6 g/day divided every 8 hours for up to 20 weeks
Bladder candidal infections: 200 mg diluted solution instilled in the bladder
Vaginal: Insert contents of 1 applicator of vaginal cream (100 mg) or 100 mg suppository at bedtime for 7 days, or 200 mg suppository at bedtime for 3 days
Hemodialysis: Not dialyzable (0% to 5%)

**Patient Information** Take full course of therapy as directed; do not discontinue without consulting prescriber. Some infections may require long periods of therapy. Practice good hygiene measures to prevent reinfection.

Topical: Wash and dry area before applying medication; apply thinly. Do not get in or near eyes.

Vaginal: Insert high in vagina. Refrain from intercourse during treatment.

If you are diabetic you should test serum glucose regularly at the same time of day. You may experience nausea and vomiting (small, frequent meals may help) or headache, dizziness (use caution when driving). Report unresolved headache, rash, burning, itching, anorexia, unusual fatigue, diarrhea, nausea, or vomiting.

**Nursing Implications** Observe patient closely during first I.V. dose for allergic reactions

**Dosage Forms**
Cream:
Topical, as nitrate: 2% (15 g, 30 g, 56.7 g, 85 g)
Vaginal, as nitrate: 2% (45 g is equivalent to 7 doses)
Dual pack: Vaginal suppositories and external vulvar cream 2%
Injection: 1% [10 mg/mL] (20 mL)
Lotion, as nitrate: 2% (30 mL, 60 mL)
Powder, topical: 2% (45 g, 90 g, 113 g)
Spray, topical: 2% (105 mL)
Suppository, vaginal, as nitrate: 100 mg (7s); 200 mg (3s)
Tincture: 2% with alcohol (7.39 mL, 29.57 mL)


♦ **Micro-K® 10** *see* Potassium Chloride *on page 453*

♦ **Micro-K® 10 Extencaps®** *see* Potassium Chloride *on page 453*

♦ **Micro-K® LS** *see* Potassium Chloride *on page 453*

♦ **Micronase®** *see* Glyburide *on page 252*

♦ **Micronor®** *see* Norethindrone *on page 398*

♦ **Microsulfon®** *see* Sulfadiazine *on page 523*

♦ **Microzide™** *see* Hydrochlorothiazide *on page 271*

♦ **Midamor®** *see* Amiloride *on page 30*


## Midazolam (MID aye zoe lam)

**Related Information**
Benzodiazepines Comparison Chart *on page 708*
Patient Information - Anxiolytics & Sedative Hypnotics (Benzodiazepines) *on page 653*

**Generic Available** No

**U.S. Brand Names** Versed®

**Synonyms** Midazolam Hydrochloride

**Pharmacologic Category** Benzodiazepine

**Use** Preoperative sedation; anxiolysis; amnesia
**Unlabeled use:** Control of agitation

**Restrictions** C-IV

**Pregnancy Risk Factor** D

**Contraindications** Hypersensitivity to this drug or any component of its formulation, including benzyl alcohol (cross-sensitivity with other benzodiazepines may exist); parenteral form is not for intrathecal or epidural injection; narrow-angle glaucoma (not in product labeling, however, benzodiazepines are contraindicated); pregnancy

**Warnings/Precautions** May cause severe respiratory depression, respiratory arrest, or apnea. Use with extreme caution, particularly in noncritical care settings. Appropriate resuscitative equipment and qualified personnel must be available for administration and monitoring. Initial dosing must be cautiously titrated and individualized, particularly in elderly or debilitated patients, patients with hepatic impairment (including alcoholics), or in renal impairment, particularly if other CNS depressants (including opiates) are used concurrently. Initial doses in elderly or debilitated patients should not exceed 2.5 mg. Use with caution in patients with respiratory disease or impaired gag reflex. Use during upper airway procedures may increase risk of hypoventilation. Prolonged responses have been noted following extended administration by continuous infusion (possibly due to metabolite accumulation) or in the presence of drugs which inhibit midazolam metabolism.

May cause hypotension - hemodynamic events are more common in pediatric patients or patients with hemodynamic instability. Hypotension and/or respiratory depression may occur more frequently in patients who have received narcotic analgesics. Use with caution in obese patients, chronic renal failure, and CHF. Parenteral form contains benzyl alcohol - avoid rapid injection in neonates or prolonged infusions. Does not protect against increases in heart rate or blood pressure during intubation. Should not be used in shock, coma, or acute alcohol intoxication. Avoid intra-arterial administration or extravasation of parenteral formulation.

Causes CNS depression (dose-related) resulting in sedation, dizziness, confusion, or ataxia which may impair physical and mental capabilities. Patients must be cautioned about performing tasks which require mental alertness (ie, operating machinery or driving). A minimum of 1 day should elapse after midazolam administration before attempting these tasks. Use with caution in patients receiving other CNS depressants or psychoactive agents. Effects with other sedative drugs or ethanol may be potentiated. Benzodiazepines have been associated with falls and traumatic injury and should be used with extreme caution in patients who are at risk of these events (especially the elderly).

Midazolam causes anterograde amnesia. Paradoxical reactions, including hyperactive or aggressive behavior have been reported with benzodiazepines, particularly in adolescent/pediatric or psychiatric patients. Does not have analgesic, antidepressant, or antipsychotic properties.

Benzodiazepines have been associated with dependence and acute withdrawal symptoms on discontinuation or reduction in dose. Acute withdrawal, including seizures, may be precipitated after administration of flumazenil to patients receiving long-term benzodiazepine therapy.

**Adverse Reactions**
>10%: Respiratory: Decreased tidal volume and/or respiratory rate decrease, apnea
1% to 10%:
Central nervous system: Drowsiness, oversedation, headache
Gastrointestinal: Nausea, vomiting
Local: Pain and local reactions at injection site (severity less than diazepam)
Respiratory: Coughing
Miscellaneous: Physical and psychological dependence with prolonged use, hiccups
<1%: Acid taste, agitation, amnesia, bigeminy, bradycardia, bronchospasm, confusion, dyspnea, emergence delirium, euphoria, excessive salivation, hallucinations, hyperventilation, laryngospasm, PVC, rash, tachycardia, wheezing

**Overdosage/Toxicology**
Signs and symptoms: Respiratory depression, hypotension, coma, stupor, confusion, apnea
Treatment: Treatment for benzodiazepine overdose is supportive. Rarely is mechanical ventilation required. Flumazenil has been shown to selectively block the binding of benzodiazepines to CNS receptors, resulting in a reversal of benzodiazepine-induced CNS depression; respiratory reaction to hypoxia may not be restored

**Drug Interactions** CYP3A3/4 enzyme substrate
CNS depressants: Sedative effects and/or respiratory depression may be additive with CNS depressants; includes ethanol, barbiturates, narcotic analgesics, and other sedative agents; monitor for increased effect. **If narcotics or other CNS depressants are administered concomitantly, the midazolam dose should be reduced by 30% if <65 years of age, or by at least 50% if >65 years of age.**
Enzyme inducers: Metabolism of some benzodiazepines may be increased, decreasing their therapeutic effect; consider using an alternative sedative/hypnotic agent; potential inducers include phenobarbital, phenytoin, carbamazepine, rifampin, and rifabutin
CYP3A3/4 inhibitors: Serum level and/or toxicity of some benzodiazepines may be increased; inhibitors include amiodarone, cimetidine, clarithromycin, erythromycin, delavirdine, diltiazem, dirithromycin, disulfiram, fluoxetine, fluvoxamine, grapefruit juice, indinavir, itraconazole, ketoconazole, nefazodone, nevirapine, propoxyfene, quinupristin-dalfopristin, ritonavir, saquinavir, verapamil, zafirlukast, zileuton; monitor for altered benzodiazepine response. **Use is contraindicated with amprenavir and ritonavir.**
Oral contraceptives: May decrease the clearance of some benzodiazepines (those which undergo oxidative metabolism); monitor for increased benzodiazepine effect
Theophylline: May partially antagonize some of the effects of benzodiazepines; monitor for decreased response; may require higher doses for sedation

**Stability** Stable for 24 hours at room temperature/refrigeration; admixtures do not require protection from light for short-term storage; **compatible** with NS, $D_5W$

Standardized dose for continuous infusion: 100 mg/250 mL $D_5W$ or NS; maximum concentration: 0.5 mg/mL

**Mechanism of Action** Binds to stereospecific benzodiazepine receptors on the postsynaptic GABA neuron at several sites within the central
(Continued)

## Midazolam *(Continued)*

nervous system, including the limbic system, reticular formation. Enhancement of the inhibitory effect of GABA on neuronal excitability results by increased neuronal membrane permeability to chloride ions. This shift in chloride ions results in hyperpolarization (a less excitable state) and stabilization.

**Pharmacodynamics/kinetics**

I.M.:

Onset of sedation: Within 15 minutes

Peak effect: 0.5-1 hour

Duration: 2 hours mean, up to 6 hours

I.V.: Onset of action: Within 1-5 minutes

Absorption: Oral: Rapid

Distribution: $V_d$: 0.8-2.5 L/kg; increased with congestive heart failure (CHF) and chronic renal failure

Protein binding: 95%

Metabolism: Extensively in the liver (microsomally)

Bioavailability: 45% mean

Half-life, elimination: 1-4 hours, increased with cirrhosis, CHF, obesity, elderly

Elimination: As glucuronide conjugated metabolites in urine, ~2% to 10% excreted in feces

**Usual Dosage** The dose of midazolam needs to be individualized based on the patient's age, underlying diseases, and concurrent medications. Decrease dose (by ~30%) if narcotics or other CNS depressants are administered concomitantly. **Personnel and equipment needed for standard respiratory resuscitation should be immediately available during midazolam administration.**

Neonates: Conscious sedation during mechanical ventilation: I.V. continuous infusion: 0.15-1 mcg/kg/minute. Use smallest dose possible; use lower doses (up to 0.5 mcg/kg/minute) for preterm neonates.

Infants <2 months and Children: Status epilepticus refractory to standard therapy: I.V.: Loading dose: 0.15 mg/kg followed by a continuous infusion of 1 mcg/kg/minute; titrate dose upward very 5 minutes until clinical seizure activity is controlled; mean infusion rate required in 24 children was 2.3 mcg/kg/minute with a range of 1-18 mcg/kg/minute

Children:

Preoperative sedation:

I.M.: 0.07-0.08 mg/kg 30-60 minutes presurgery

I.V.: 0.035 mg/kg/dose, repeat over several minutes as required to achieve the desired sedative effect up to a total dose of 0.1-0.2 mg/kg

Conscious sedation during mechanical ventilation: I.V.: Loading dose: 0.05-0.2 mg/kg then follow with initial continuous infusion: 1-2 mcg/kg/minute; titrate to the desired effect; usual range: 0.4-6 mcg/kg/minute

Conscious sedation for procedures:

Oral, Intranasal: 0.2-0.4 mg/kg (maximum: 15 mg) 30-45 minutes before the procedure

I.V.: 0.05 mg/kg 3 minutes before procedure

Adolescents >12 years: I.V.: 0.5 mg every 3-4 minutes until effect achieved

Adults:

Preoperative sedation: I.M.: 0.07-0.08 mg/kg 30-60 minutes presurgery; usual dose: 5 mg

Conscious sedation: I.V.: Initial: 0.5-2 mg slow I.V. over at least 2 minutes; slowly titrate to effect by repeating doses every 2-3 minutes if needed; usual total dose: 2.5-5 mg; use decreased doses in elderly

Healthy Adults <60 years: Some patients respond to doses as low as 1 mg; no more than 2.5 mg should be administered over a period of 2 minutes. Additional doses of midazolam may be administered after a 2-minute waiting period and evaluation of sedation after each dose increment. A total dose >5 mg is generally not needed. If narcotics or other CNS depressants are administered concomitantly, the midazolam dose should be reduced by 30%.

Elderly: I.V.: Conscious sedation: Initial: 0.5 mg slow I.V.; give no more than 1.5 mg in a 2-minute period; if additional titration is needed, give no more than 1 mg over 2 minutes, waiting another 2 or more minutes to evaluate sedative effect; a total dose >3.5 mg is rarely necessary

Sedation in mechanically intubated patients: I.V. continuous infusion: 100 mg in 250 mL $D_5W$ or NS, (if patient is fluid-restricted, may concentrate up to a maximum of 0.5 mg/mL); initial dose: 1 mg/hour; titrate to reach desired level of sedation

Hemodialysis: Supplemental dose is not necessary

Peritoneal dialysis: Significant drug removal is unlikely based on physiochemical characteristics

**Administration** Infuse I.V. doses over 2-3 minutes

**Monitoring Parameters** Respiratory and cardiovascular status, blood pressure, blood pressure monitor required during I.V. administration

**Patient Information** May cause drowsiness; do not drive or operate hazardous machinery until the effects of the drug are gone or until the day after administration

**Nursing Implications** Midazolam is a short-acting benzodiazepine; recovery occurs within 2 hours in most patients, however, may require up to 6 hours in some cases

**Additional Information** Sodium content of 1 mL: 0.14 mEq

**Dosage Forms** Injection, as hydrochloride: 1 mg/mL (2 mL, 5 mL, 10 mL); 5 mg/mL (1 mL, 2 mL, 5 mL, 10 mL)

♦ **Midazolam Hydrochloride** *see* Midazolam *on page 365*

♦ **Midchlor®** *see* Acetaminophen, Isometheptene, and Dichloralphenazone *on page 16*

## Midodrine (MI doe dreen)

**U.S. Brand Names** ProAmatine

**Pharmacologic Category** Alpha$_1$ Agonist

**Use** Treatment of symptomatic orthostatic hypotension

**Unlabeled use:** Management of urinary incontinence

**Effects on Mental Status** May cause anxiety, dizziness, confusion, or insomnia

**Effects on Psychiatric Treatment** None reported

**Pregnancy Risk Factor** C

**Contraindications** Severe organic heart disease, urinary retention, pheochromocytoma, thyrotoxicosis, persistent and significant supine hypertension; hypersensitivity to midodrine or any component; concurrent use of fludrocortisone

**Warnings/Precautions** Only indicated for patients for whom orthostatic hypotension significantly impairs their daily life. Use is not recommended with supine hypertension and caution should be exercised in patients with diabetes, visual problems, urinary retention (reduce initial dose) or hepatic dysfunction; monitor renal and hepatic function prior to and periodically during therapy; safety and efficacy has not been established in children; discontinue and re-evaluate therapy if signs of bradycardia occur.

**Adverse Reactions**

>10%:

Dermatologic: Piloerection (13%), pruritus (12%)

Genitourinary: Urinary urgency, retention, or polyuria, dysuria (up to 13%)

Neuromuscular & skeletal: Paresthesia (18.3%)

1% to 10%:

Cardiovascular: Supine hypertension, (7%) facial flushing

Central nervous system: Confusion, anxiety, dizziness, chills (5%)

Dermatologic: Rash, dry skin (2%)

Gastrointestinal: Xerostomia, nausea, abdominal pain

Neuromuscular & skeletal: Pain (5%)

<1%: Flatulence, flushing, headache, insomnia, leg cramps, visual changes

**Overdosage/Toxicology**

Signs and symptoms: Hypertension, piloerection, urinary retention

Treatment: Symptomatic following gastric decontamination; alpha-sympatholytics and/or dialysis may be helpful

**Drug Interactions** Increased effect: Concomitant fludrocortisone results in hypernatremia or an increase in intraocular pressure and glaucoma; bradycardia may be accentuated with concomitant administration of cardiac glycosides, psychotherapeutics, and beta-blockers; alpha-agonists may increase the pressure effects and alpha-antagonists may negate the effects of midodrine

**Usual Dosage** Adults: Oral: 10 mg 3 times/day during daytime hours (every 3-4 hours) when patient is upright (maximum: 40 mg/day)

**Dosing adjustment in renal impairment:** 2.5 mg 3 times/day, gradually increasing as tolerated

**Patient Information** This drug may relieve positional hypotension; effects must be evaluated regularly. Take prescribed amount 3 times daily (shortly before rising in the morning, at midday, and in late afternoon); do not take after 6 PM or within 4 hours of bedtime or when lying down for any length of time. Follow recommended diet and exercise program. Do not use OTC medications which may affect blood pressure (eg, cough or cold remedies, diet pills, stay-awake medications) without consulting prescriber. You may experience urinary urgency or retention (void before taking or consult prescriber if difficulty persists); or dizziness, drowsiness, or headache (use caution when driving or engaging in tasks that require alertness until response to drug is known). Report skin rash, severe gastric upset or pain, muscle weakness or pain, or other persistent side effects.

**Nursing Implications** Doses may be given in approximately 3- to 4-hour intervals (eg, shortly before or upon rising in the morning, at midday, in the late afternoon not later than 6 PM); avoid dosing after the evening meal or within 4 hours of bedtime; continue therapy only in patients who appear to attain symptomatic improvement during initial treatment; standing systolic blood pressure may be elevated 15-30 mm Hg at 1 hour after a 10 mg dose; some effect may persist for 2-3 hours

**Dosage Forms** Tablet, as hydrochloride: 2.5 mg, 5 mg

♦ **Midol® IB [OTC]** *see* Ibuprofen *on page 280*

♦ **Midol® PM [OTC]** *see* Acetaminophen and Diphenhydramine *on page 15*

- **Midrin®** *see* Acetaminophen, Isometheptene, and Dichloralphenazone *on page 16*

## Miglitol (MIG li tol)

**Related Information**
Hypoglycemic Drugs and Thiazolidinedione Information *on page 714*
**U.S. Brand Names** Glyset™
**Pharmacologic Category** Antidiabetic Agent (Miscellaneous)
**Use**
Noninsulin-dependent diabetes mellitus (NIDDM)
Monotherapy adjunct to diet to improve glycemic control in patients with NIDDM whose hyperglycemia cannot be managed with diet alone
Combination therapy with a sulfonylurea when diet plus either miglitol or a sulfonylurea alone do not result in adequate glycemic control. The effect of miglitol to enhance glycemic control is additive to that of sulfonylureas when used in combination.
**Effects on Mental Status** None reported
**Effects on Psychiatric Treatment** None reported
**Pregnancy Risk Factor** B
**Contraindications** Diabetic ketoacidosis, inflammatory bowel disease, colonic ulceration, partial intestinal obstruction, patients predisposed to intestinal obstruction, chronic intestinal diseases associated with marked disorders of digestion or absorption or with conditions that may deteriorate as a result of increased gas formation in the intestine; hypersensitivity to drug or any of its components
**Warnings/Precautions** GI symptoms are the most common reactions. The incidence of abdominal pain and diarrhea tend to diminish considerably with continued treatment. Long-term clinical trials in diabetic patients with significant renal dysfunction (serum creatinine >2 mg/dL) have not been conducted. Treatment of these patients is not recommended. Because of its mechanism of action, miglitol administered alone should not cause hypoglycemia in the fasting of postprandial state. In combination with a sulfonylurea will cause a further lowering of blood glucose and may increase the hypoglycemic potential of the sulfonylurea.
**Adverse Reactions**
>10%: Gastrointestinal: Flatulence (41.5%), diarrhea (28.7%), abdominal pain (11.7%)
1% to 10%: Dermatologic: Rash
**Overdosage/Toxicology** Signs and symptoms: An overdose of miglitol will not result in hypoglycemia. An overdose may result in transient increases in flatulence, diarrhea, and abdominal discomfort. No serious systemic reactions are expected in the event of an overdose.
**Drug Interactions** Decreased effect:
Miglitol may decrease the absorption and bioavailability of digoxin, propranolol, ranitidine
Digestive enzymes (amylase, pancreatin, charcoal) may reduce the effect of miglitol and should **not** be taken concomitantly
**Usual Dosage** Adults: Oral: 25 mg 3 times/day with the first bite of food at each meal; the dose may be increased to 50 mg 3 times/day after 4-8 weeks; maximum recommended dose: 100 mg 3 times/day

**Dosing adjustment in renal impairment**: Miglitol is primarily excreted by the kidneys; there is little information of miglitol in patients with a $Cl_{cr}$ <25 mL/minute
**Dosing adjustment in hepatic impairment**: No adjustment necessary
**Patient Information** Take this medication exactly as directed, with the first bite of each main meal. Do not change dosage or discontinue without first consulting prescriber. Do not take other medications with or within 2 hours of this medication unless so advised by prescriber. It is important to follow dietary and lifestyle recommendations of prescriber. You will be instructed in signs of hypo-/hyperglycemia by prescriber or diabetic educator. If combining miglitol with other diabetic medication (eg, sulfonylureas, insulin), keep source of glucose (sugar) on hand in case hypoglycemia occurs. You may experience mild side effects during first weeks of therapy (eg, bloating, flatulence, diarrhea, abdominal discomfort); these should diminish over time. Report severe or persistent side effects, fever, extended vomiting or flu, or change in color of urine or stool.
**Dosage Forms** Tablet: 25 mg, 50 mg, 100 mg

- **Migranal®** *see* Ergotamine *on page 200*
- **Migranal® Nasal Spray** *see* Dihydroergotamine *on page 171*
- **Migratine®** *see* Acetaminophen, Isometheptene, and Dichloralphenazone *on page 16*
- **Miles Nervine® Caplets [OTC]** *see* Diphenhydramine *on page 174*
- **Milontin®** *see* Phensuximide *on page 437*
- **Milophene®** *see* Clomiphene *on page 130*

## Milrinone (MIL ri none)

**U.S. Brand Names** Primacor®
**Pharmacologic Category** Phosphodiesterase Enzyme Inhibitor
**Use** Short-term I.V. therapy of congestive heart failure; calcium antagonist intoxication
**Effects on Mental Status** None reported
**Effects on Psychiatric Treatment** None reported
**Usual Dosage** Adults: I.V.: Loading dose: 50 mcg/kg administered over 10 minutes followed by a maintenance dose titrated according to the hemodynamic and clinical response See below:
Minimum: Maintenance dosage:
Dose rate 0.375 mcg/kg/minute; total dose 0.59 mg/kg/24 hours
Standard: Maintenance dosage:
Dose rate 0.500 mcg/kg/minute; total dose 0.77 mg/kg/24 hours
Maximum: Maintenance dosage:
Dose rate 0.750 mcg/kg/minute; total dose 1.13 mg/kg/24 hours

**Dosing adjustment in renal impairment:**
$Cl_{cr}$ 50 mL/minute/1.73 $m^2$: Administer 0.43 mcg/kg/minute.
$Cl_{cr}$ 40 mL/minute/1.73 $m^2$: Administer 0.38 mcg/kg/minute.
$Cl_{cr}$ 30 mL/minute/1.73 $m^2$: Administer 0.33 mcg/kg/minute.
$Cl_{cr}$ 20 mL/minute/1.73 $m^2$: Administer 0.28 mcg/kg/minute.
$Cl_{cr}$ 10 mL/minute/1.73 $m^2$: Administer 0.23 mcg/kg/minute.
$Cl_{cr}$ 5 mL/minute/1.73 $m^2$: Administer 0.2 mcg/kg/minute.
**Dosage Forms** Injection, as lactate: 1 mg/mL (5 mL, 10 mL, 20 mL)

- **Miltown®** *see* Meprobamate *on page 342*
- **Minidyne® [OTC]** *see* Povidone-Iodine *on page 456*
- **Minipress®** *see* Prazosin *on page 459*
- **Minitran™ Patch** *see* Nitroglycerin *on page 397*
- **Minizide®** *see* Prazosin and Polythiazide *on page 459*
- **Minocin® IV Injection** *see* Minocycline *on page 367*
- **Minocin® Oral** *see* Minocycline *on page 367*

## Minocycline (mi noe SYE kleen)

**U.S. Brand Names** Dynacin® Oral; Minocin® IV Injection; Minocin® Oral; Vectrin®
**Canadian Brand Names** Apo®-Minocycline; Syn-Minocycline
**Pharmacologic Category** Antibiotic, Tetracycline Derivative
**Use** Treatment of susceptible bacterial infections of both gram-negative and gram-positive organisms; acne, meningococcal carrier state
**Effects on Mental Status** Reports of memory disturbance, mood stabilizing and antidepressant effects
**Effects on Psychiatric Treatment** Barbiturates and carbamazepine may decrease the effects of tetracyclines; tetracyclines may decrease lithium clearance resulting in an increase in serum lithium levels and potential lithium toxicity; monitor serum lithium levels
**Pregnancy Risk Factor** D
**Contraindications** Hypersensitivity to minocycline, other tetracyclines, or any component; children <8 years of age
**Warnings/Precautions** Should be avoided in renal insufficiency, children ≤8 years of age, pregnant and nursing women; photosensitivity reactions can occur with minocycline
**Adverse Reactions**
>10%: Miscellaneous: Discoloration of teeth in children
1% to 10%:
Dermatologic: Photosensitivity
Gastrointestinal: Nausea, diarrhea
<1%: Abdominal cramps, acute renal failure, anaphylaxis, anorexia, azotemia, bulging fontanels in infants, dermatologic effects, diabetes insipidus syndrome, esophagitis, exfoliative dermatitis, increased intracranial pressure, paresthesia, pericarditis, pigmentation of nails, pruritus, rash, superinfections, vomiting
**Overdosage/Toxicology**
Signs and symptoms: Diabetes insipidus, nausea, anorexia, diarrhea
Treatment: Following GI decontamination, supportive care only; fluid support may be required
**Drug Interactions**
Decreased effect with antacids (aluminum, calcium, zinc, or magnesium), bismuth salts, sodium bicarbonate, barbiturates, carbamazepine, hydantoins; decreased effect of oral contraceptives
Increased effect of warfarin
**Usual Dosage**
Children >8 years: Oral, I.V.: Initial: 4 mg/kg followed by 2 mg/kg/dose every 12 hours
Adults:
Infection: Oral, I.V.: 200 mg stat, 100 mg every 12 hours not to exceed 400 mg/24 hours
Acne: Oral: 50 mg 1-3 times/day
Hemodialysis: Not dialyzable (0% to 5%)
**Patient Information** Take as directed, at regular intervals around-the-clock. May be taken with food or milk. Complete full course of therapy; do not discontinue even if condition is resolved. You may experience sensitivity to sun; avoid sun, use sunblock, or wear protective clothing. Frequent small meals may help reduce nausea, vomiting or diarrhea. If diabetic,
(Continued)

## Minocycline *(Continued)*

drug may cause false tests with Clinitest® urine glucose monitoring; use of glucose oxidase methods (Clinistix®) or serum glucose monitoring is preferable. Report rash or itching, respiratory difficulty, yellowing of skin or eyes, change in color of urine or stool, fever or chills, unusual bruising or bleeding, or unresolved diarrhea.

**Dosage Forms**

Capsule:

As hydrochloride: 50 mg, 100 mg

As hydrochloride (Dynacin®, Vectrin®): 50 mg, 100 mg

Pellet-filled, as hydrochloride (Minocin®): 50 mg, 100 mg

Injection, as hydrochloride (Minocin® IV): 100 mg

Suspension, oral, as hydrochloride (Minocin®)50 mg/5 mL (60 mL)

## Minoxidil (mi NOKS i dil)

**U.S. Brand Names** Loniten®; Rogaine® Extra Strength for Men [OTC]; Rogaine® for Men [OTC]; Rogaine® for Women [OTC]

**Canadian Brand Names** Apo®-Gain; Gen-Minoxidil; Minoxigaine™

**Synonyms** Minoxidilum

**Pharmacologic Category** Topical Skin Product; Vasodilator

**Use** Management of severe hypertension (usually in combination with a diuretic and beta-blocker); treatment of male pattern baldness (alopecia androgenetica)

**Effects on Mental Status** May cause dizziness

**Effects on Psychiatric Treatment** May rarely cause leukopenia; use caution with clozapine and carbamazepine

**Pregnancy Risk Factor** C

**Contraindications** Hypersensitivity to minoxidil or any component; pheochromocytoma; acute MI; dissecting aortic aneurysm

**Warnings/Precautions** Maximum therapeutic doses of a diuretic and two antihypertensives should be used before this drug is ever added. It can cause pericardial effusion, tamponade, or exacerbate angina pectoris. Monitor patients who are receiving guanethidine concurrently (orthostasis can be problematic). May need to add a diuretic to minimize fluid gain and a beta-blocker (if no contraindications) to treat tachycardia. Rapid control of blood pressure can lead to syncope, CVA, MI, ischemia. Hypersensitivity reactions occur rarely. Avoid use for a month after acute MI. Inform patients of hair growth patterns before initiating therapy. May take 1-6 months for hypertrichosis to reverse itself after discontinuation of the drug. Use with caution in patients with pulmonary hypertension, significant renal failure, CHF, or ischemic disease. Renal failure and dialysis patients may require a smaller dose.

**Adverse Reactions**

>10%:

Cardiovascular: EKG changes (60%), tachycardia, congestive heart failure

Dermatologic: Hypertrichosis (commonly occurs within 1-2 months of therapy)

Hematologic: Transient hematocrit/hemoglobin decrease

1% to 10%:

Cardiovascular: Edema (7%)

Endocrine & metabolic: Fluid and electrolyte imbalance

<1%: Angina, breast tenderness, coarsening facial features, dermatologic reactions, dizziness, headache, leukopenia, pericardial effusion tamponade, rashes, Stevens-Johnson syndrome, sunburn, thrombocytopenia, weight gain

**Overdosage/Toxicology**

Signs and symptoms: Hypotension, tachycardia, headache, nausea, dizziness, weakness syncope, warm flushed skin and palpitations; lethargy and ataxia may occur in children

Treatment: Hypotension usually responds to I.V. fluids, Trendelenburg positioning or vasoconstrictor; treatment is primarily supportive and symptomatic

**Drug Interactions**

Antihypertensives: Effects may be additive

Guanethidine can cause severe orthostasis; avoid concurrent use - discontinue 1-3 weeks prior to initiating minoxidil

**Usual Dosage**

Children <12 years: Hypertension: Oral: Initial: 0.1-0.2 mg/kg once daily; maximum: 5 mg/day; increase gradually every 3 days; usual dosage: 0.25-1 mg/kg/day in 1-2 divided doses; maximum: 50 mg/day

Children >12 years and Adults:

Hypertension: Oral: Initial: 5 mg once daily, increase gradually every 3 days; usual dose: 10-40 mg/day in 1-2 divided doses; maximum: 100 mg/day

Alopecia: Topical: Apply twice daily; 4 months of therapy may be necessary for hair growth.

Elderly: Initial: 2.5 mg once daily; increase gradually.

**Note:** Dosage adjustment is needed when added to concomitant therapy.

Dialysis: Supplemental dose is not necessary via hemo- or peritoneal dialysis.

**Patient Information** Topical product must be used every day. Hair growth usually takes 4 months. Notify physician if any of the following occur: Heart rate ≥20 beats per minute over normal; rapid weight gain >5 lb (2 kg); unusual swelling of extremities, face, or abdomen; breathing difficulty, especially when lying down; rise slowly from prolonged lying or sitting; new or aggravated angina symptoms (chest, arm, or shoulder pain); severe indigestion; dizziness, lightheadedness, or fainting; nausea or vomiting may occur. Do not make up for missed doses.

**Nursing Implications** May cause hirsutism or hypertrichosis; observe for fluid retention and orthostatic hypotension

**Dosage Forms**

Solution, topical: 2% [20 mg/metered dose] (60 mL); 5% [50 mg/metered dose] (60 mL)

Tablet: 2.5 mg, 10 mg


- ♦ **Minoxidilum** *see* Minoxidil *on page 368*
- ♦ **Mintezol®** *see* Thiabendazole *on page 541*
- ♦ **Miochol-E®** *see* Acetylcholine *on page 18*
- ♦ **Miostat® Intraocular** *see* Carbachol *on page 90*
- ♦ **Mirapex®** *see* Pramipexole *on page 456*
- ♦ **Mircette™** *see* Ethinyl Estradiol and Desogestrel *on page 211*


## Mirtazapine (mir TAZ a peen)

**Related Information**


Antidepressant Agents Comparison Chart *on page 704*

Clinical Issues in the Use of Antidepressants *on page 627*

Mood Disorders *on page 600*

Patient Information - Antidepressants (Mirtazapine) *on page 645*

Teratogenic Risks of Psychotropic Medications *on page 812*


**Generic Available** No

**U.S. Brand Names** Remeron®

**Pharmacologic Category** Antidepressant, Alpha-2 Antagonist

**Use** Treatment of depression

**Pregnancy Risk Factor** C

**Contraindications** Hypersensitivity to mirtazapine; use of monoamine oxidase inhibitors within 14 days

**Warnings/Precautions** Discontinue immediately if signs and symptoms of neutropenia/agranulocytosis occur. May cause sedation, resulting in impaired performance of tasks requiring alertness (ie, operating machinery or driving). Sedative effects may be additive with other CNS depressants and/or ethanol. The degree of sedation is moderate-high relative to other antidepressants. May worsen psychosis in some patients or precipitate a shift to mania or hypomania in patients with bipolar disease. The risks of orthostatic hypotension or anticholinergic effects are low relative to other antidepressants. The incidence of sexual dysfunction with mirtazapine is generally lower than with SSRIs.

May increase appetite and stimulate weight gain, may increase serum cholesterol and triglyceride levels. Use caution in patients with depression, particularly if suicidal risk may be present. Use caution in patients with a previous seizure disorder or condition predisposing to seizures such as brain damage, alcoholism, or concurrent therapy with other drugs which lower the seizure threshold. Use with caution in patients with hepatic or renal dysfunction and in elderly patients.

**Adverse Reactions**

>10%:

Central nervous system: Somnolence

Endocrine & metabolic: Increased cholesterol

Gastrointestinal: Constipation, xerostomia, increased appetite, weight gain

1% to 10%:

Cardiovascular: Hypertension, vasodilatation, peripheral edema, edema

Central nervous system: Dizziness, abnormal dreams, abnormal thoughts, confusion, malaise

Endocrine & metabolic: Increased triglycerides

Gastrointestinal: Vomiting, anorexia

Genitourinary: Urinary frequency

Neuromuscular & skeletal: Myalgia, back pain, arthralgias, tremor, weakness

Respiratory: Dyspnea

Miscellaneous: Flu-like symptoms, thirst

<1%: Agranulocytosis, dehydration, liver function test increases, lymphadenopathy, neutropenia, orthostatic hypotension, seizures (1 case reported), weight loss

**Overdosage/Toxicology**

Signs and symptoms of overdose include disorientation, drowsiness, impaired memory, and tachycardia

Treatment: No specific antidotes; establish and maintain an airway to ensure adequate oxygenation and ventilation; activated charcoal should be considered in treatment; monitor cardiac and vital signs along with general symptomatic and supportive measures; consider possibility of multiple-drug involvement

**Drug Interactions** CYP1A2, 2C9, 2D6, and 3A3/4 enzyme substrate

Clonidine: Antihypertensive effects of clonidine may be antagonized by mirtazapine (hypertensive urgency has been reported following addition

of mirtazapine to clonidine); in addition, mirtazapine may potentially enhance the hypertensive response associated with abrupt clonidine withdrawal. Avoid this combination; consider an alternative agent.
CNS depressants: Sedative effects may be additive with other CNS depressants; monitor for increased effect; includes barbiturates, benzodiazepines, narcotic analgesics, ethanol and other sedative agents
CYP inhibitors: May increase serum concentrations of mirtazapine; monitor
Enzyme inducers: Metabolism of mirtazapine may be increased; decreasing clinical effect; inducers include barbiturates, carbamazepine, phenytoin, and rifampin
Linezolid: Due to MAO inhibition (see below), this combination should be avoided
MAO inhibitors: Possibly serious or fatal reactions can occur when given with or when given within 14 days of a monoamine oxidase inhibitor
Selegiline: Interaction is less likely than with nonselective MAO inhibitors (see above), but theoretically possible; monitor
Sibutramine: Potential for serotonin syndrome when used in combination

**Mechanism of Action** Mirtazapine is a tetracyclic antidepressant that works by its central presynaptic alpha$_2$-adrenergic antagonist effects, which results in increased release of norepinephrine and serotonin. It is also a potent antagonist of 5HT2 and 5HT3 serotonin receptors and H1 histamine receptors and a moderate peripheral alpha$_1$-adrenergic and muscarinic antagonist; it does not inhibit the reuptake of norepinephrine or serotonin.

**Pharmacodynamics/kinetics**
Protein binding: 85%
Metabolism: Extensive by cytochrome P-450 enzymes in the liver
Bioavailability: 50%
Half-life: 20-40 hours
Time to peak serum concentration: 2 hours
Elimination: Extensive hepatic metabolism via demethylation and hydroxylation, metabolites eliminated primarily renally (75%) and some via the feces (15%); elimination is hampered with renal dysfunction or hepatic dysfunction.

**Usual Dosage** Adults: Oral: Initial: 15 mg nightly, titrate up to 15-45 mg/day with dose increases made no more frequently than every 1-2 weeks; there is an inverse relationship between dose and sedation

**Dietary Considerations** Alcohol: Additive CNS effect, avoid use

**Monitoring Parameters** Patients should be monitored for signs of agranulocytosis or severe neutropenia such as sore throat, stomatitis or other signs of infection or a low WBC; monitor for improvement in clinical signs and symptoms of depression, improvement may be observed within 1-4 weeks after initiating therapy

**Reference Range** Following a 20 mg oral dose, peak serum levels: ~100 ng/mL

**Patient Information** Be aware of the risk of developing agranulocytosis; contact physician if any indication of infection (ie, fever, chills, sore throat, mucous membrane ulceration, and especially flu-like symptoms) occur; may impair judgment, thinking, and particularly motor skills; may impair ability to drive, use machines, or perform tasks requiring alertness; avoid engaging in hazardous activities until certain that therapy does not affect ability to engage in these activities; avoid alcohol consumption

**Additional Information Note:** At least 14 days should elapse between discontinuation of an MAO inhibitor and initiation of therapy with mirtazapine; at least 14 days should be allowed after discontinuing mirtazapine before starting an MAO inhibitor

**Dosage Forms** Tablet: 15 mg, 30 mg

## Misoprostol (mye soe PROST ole)

**U.S. Brand Names** Cytotec®

**Pharmacologic Category** Prostaglandin

**Use** Prevention of NSAID-induced gastric ulcers

**Effects on Mental Status** None reported

**Effects on Psychiatric Treatment** None reported

**Pregnancy Risk Factor** X

**Contraindications** Pregnancy; hypersensitivity to misoprostol or any component

**Warnings/Precautions** Safety and efficacy have not been established in children <18 years of age; use with caution in patients with renal impairment and the elderly; not to be used in pregnant women or women of childbearing potential unless woman is capable of complying with effective contraceptive measures; therapy is normally begun on the second or third day of next normal menstrual period

**Adverse Reactions**
>10%: Gastrointestinal: Diarrhea, abdominal pain
1% to 10%:
Central nervous system: Headache
Gastrointestinal: Constipation, flatulence
<1%: Nausea, uterine stimulation, vaginal bleeding, vomiting

**Overdosage/Toxicology** Signs and symptoms: Sedation, tremor, convulsions, dyspnea, abdominal pain, diarrhea, hypotension, bradycardia

**Drug Interactions** Antacids and food diminish absorption; antacids may enhance diarrhea

**Usual Dosage** Adults: Oral: 200 mcg 4 times/day with food; if not tolerated, may decrease dose to 100 mcg 4 times/day with food or 200 mcg twice daily with food

**Patient Information** Take as directed; continue taking your NSAIDs while taking this medication. Take with meals or after meals to prevent nausea, diarrhea, and flatulence. Avoid using antacids. You may experience increased menstrual pain, or cramping; request analgesics. Report abnormal menstrual periods, spotting (may occur even in postmenstrual women), or severe menstrual bleeding.

**Nursing Implications** Incidence of diarrhea may be lessened by having patient take dose right after meals

**Dosage Forms** Tablet: 100 mcg, 200 mcg

♦ **Mithracin®** *see* Plicamycin *on page 450*

## Mitomycin (mye toe MYE sin)

**U.S. Brand Names** Mutamycin®

**Pharmacologic Category** Antineoplastic Agent, Antibiotic

**Use** Therapy of disseminated adenocarcinoma of stomach or pancreas in combination with other approved chemotherapeutic agents; bladder cancer, colorectal cancer

**Effects on Mental Status** May cause drowsiness

**Effects on Psychiatric Treatment** Myelosuppression is common; avoid with clozapine and carbamazepine

**Usual Dosage** Refer to individual protocols
Children and Adults: I.V.:
Single-agent therapy: 20 mg/m$^2$ every 6-8 weeks
**Note:** Doses >20 mg/m$^2$ have not been shown to be more effective, and are more toxic.
Combination therapy: 10 mg/m$^2$ every 6-8 weeks
Bone marrow transplant:
40-50 mg/m$^2$
2-40 mg/m$^2$/day for 3 days
Total cumulative dose should not exceed 50 mg/m$^2$; see below: **(nadir after prior dose per mm$^3$)**
Leukocytes 4000; platelets >100,000: 100% of prior dose to be given
Leukocytes 3000-3999; platelets 75,000-99,999: 100% of prior dose to be given
Leukocytes 2000-2999; platelets 25,000-74,999: 70% of prior dose to be given
Leukocytes 2000; platelets <25,000: 50% of prior dose to be given
**Dosing adjustment in renal impairment:**
$Cl_{cr}$ <10 mL/minute: Administer 75% of normal dose
**or**
Serum creatinine 1.6-2.4 mg/dL: Administer 50% of the dose
Serum creatinine >2.4 mg/dL: Do not administer
Hemodialysis: Unknown
CAPD effects: Unknown
CAVH effects: Unknown
**Dosing adjustment in hepatic impairment:**
Bilirubin 1.5-3 mg/dL: Administer 50% of the dose
Bilirubin >3.1 mg/dL: Administer 25% of the dose
**or**
Bilirubin >3.0 mg/dL OR hepatitic enzymes >3 times normal: Administer 50% of the dose
Intravesicular instillations for bladder carcinoma: 20-40 mg/dose (1 mg/mL in sterile aqueous solution) instilled into the bladder for 3 hours repeated up to 3 times/week for up to 20 procedures per course

**Dosage Forms** Powder for injection: 5 mg, 20 mg, 40 mg

## Mitotane (MYE toe tane)

**U.S. Brand Names** Lysodren®

**Synonyms** o,p'-DDD

**Pharmacologic Category** Antineoplastic Agent, Miscellaneous

**Use** Treatment of inoperable adrenal cortical carcinoma

**Effects on Mental Status** Dizziness and depression are common; may cause sedation, irritability, or confusion

**Effects on Psychiatric Treatment** May cause myelosuppression; use caution with clozapine and carbamazepine; concurrent use with psychotropics may produce additive sedation

**Pregnancy Risk Factor** C

**Contraindications** Known hypersensitivity to mitotane

**Warnings/Precautions** The U.S. Food and Drug Administration (FDA) currently recommends that procedures for proper handling and disposal of antineoplastic agents be considered. Patients should be hospitalized when mitotane therapy is initiated until a stable dose regimen is established. Discontinue temporarily following trauma or shock since the prime action of mitotane is adrenal suppression; exogenous steroids may be indicated since adrenal function may not start immediately. Administer with care to patients with severe hepatic impairment; observe patients for neurotoxicity with prolonged (2 years) use.
(Continued)

## Mitotane *(Continued)*

**Adverse Reactions**

>10%:

Central nervous system: Vertigo, mental depression, dizziness; all are reversible with discontinuation of the drug and can occur in 15% to 26% of patients

Dermatologic: Rash (15%) which may subside without discontinuation of therapy, hyperpigmentation

Gastrointestinal: 75% to 80% will experience nausea, vomiting, and anorexia; diarrhea can occur in 20% of patients

Ocular: Diplopia, visual disturbances, blurred vision (reversible with discontinuation)

1% to 10%:

Cardiovascular: Orthostatic hypotension

Endocrine & metabolic: Flushing of skin

Genitourinary: Hemorrhagic cystitis

Neuromuscular & skeletal: Myalgia

<1%: Adrenal insufficiency may develop and may require steroid replacement; albuminuria, confusion, fatigue, fever, flushing, headache, hematuria, hypercholesterolemia, hyperpyrexia, hypertension, hypouricemia, irritability, lens opacities, lethargy, mental depression, shortness of breath, somnolence, toxic retinopathy, tremor, weakness, wheezing

Myelosuppressive:

WBC: None

Platelets: None

**Overdosage/Toxicology** Signs and symptoms: Diarrhea, vomiting, numbness of limbs, weakness

**Drug Interactions**

Decreased effect:

Barbiturates, warfarin may be accelerated by induction of the hepatic microsomal enzyme system

Spironolactone has resulted in negation of mitotane's effect

Phenytoin may increase clearance of these drugs by microsomal enzyme stimulation by mitotane

Increased toxicity: CNS depressants may increase CNS depression

**Usual Dosage** Oral:

Children: 0.1-0.5 mg/kg or 1-2 g/day in divided doses increasing gradually to a maximum of 5-7 g/day

Adults: Start at 1-6 g/day in divided doses, then increase incrementally to 8-10 g/day in 3-4 divided doses; dose is changed on basis of side effect with aim of giving as high a dose as tolerated; maximum daily dose: 18 g

**Dosing adjustment in hepatic impairment:** Dose may need to be decreased in patients with liver disease

**Dietary Considerations** Alcohol: Additive CNS effect, avoid use

**Patient Information** Desired effects of this drug may not be seen for 2-3 months. Wear identification that alerts medical personnel that you are taking this drug in event of shock or trauma. Maintain adequate hydration (2-3 L/day of fluids unless instructed to restrict fluid intake) and nutrition. Avoid alcohol or OTC medications unless approved by prescriber. May cause dizziness and vertigo (avoid driving or performing tasks requiring alertness until response to drug is known); nausea, vomiting, or loss of appetite (small frequent meals, frequent mouth care, sucking lozenges, or chewing gum may help); orthostatic hypotension (use caution when rising from sitting or lying position or climbing stairs); muscle aches or pain (if severe, request medication from prescriber). Report severe vomiting or acute loss of appetite, muscular twitching, fever or infection, blood in urine or pain on urinating, or darkening of skin.

**Dosage Forms** Tablet, scored: 500 mg

## Mitoxantrone (mye toe ZAN trone)

**U.S. Brand Names** Novantrone®

**Pharmacologic Category** Antineoplastic Agent, Antibiotic

**Use** Treatment of acute nonlymphocytic leukemia (ANLL) in adults in combination with other agents; very active against various leukemias, lymphoma, and breast cancer, and moderately active against pediatric sarcoma

**Effects on Mental Status** May cause drowsiness

**Effects on Psychiatric Treatment** May cause myelosuppression; use caution with clozapine and carbamazepine

**Usual Dosage** Refer to individual protocols. I.V. (may dilute in $D_5W$ or NS):

ANLL leukemias:

Children ≤2 years: 0.4 mg/kg/day once daily for 3-5 days

Children >2 years and Adults: 12 mg/m²/day once daily for 3 days; acute leukemia in relapse: 8-12 mg/m²/day once daily for 4-5 days

Solid tumors:

Children: 18-20 mg/m² every 3-4 weeks **OR** 5-8 mg/m² every week

Adults: 12-14 mg/m² every 3-4 weeks **OR** 2-4 mg/m²/day for 5 days

Maximum total dose: 80-120 mg/m² in patients with predisposing factor and <160 mg in patients with no predisposing factor

Hemodialysis: Supplemental dose is not necessary

Peritoneal dialysis: Supplemental dose is not necessary

**Dosing adjustment in hepatic impairment:** Official dosage adjustment recommendations have not been established

Moderate dysfunction (bilirubin 1.5-3 mg/dL): Some clinicians recommend a 50% dosage reduction

Severe dysfunction (bilirubin >3.0 mg/dL) have a lower total body clearance and may require a dosage adjustment to 8 mg/m²; some clinicians recommend a dosage reduction to 25% of dose

**Dose modifications based on degree of leukopenia or thrombocytopenia:**

Granulocyte count nadir >2000 cells/mm²; platelet count nadir >150,000 cells/mm²; total bilirubin <1.5 mg/dL: Increase dose by 1 mg/m²

Granulocyte count nadir 1000-2000 cells/mm²; platelet count nadir 75,000-150,000 cells/mm²; total bilirubin <1.5 mg/dL: Maintain same dose

Granulocyte count nadir <1000 cells/mm²; platelet count nadir <75,000 cells/mm²; total bilirubin 1.5-3 mg/dL: Decrease dose by 1 mg/m²

**Dosage Forms** Injection, as base: 2 mg/mL (10 mL, 12.5 mL, 15 mL)

- **Mitran® Oral** *see* Chlordiazepoxide *on page 109*
- **Mitrolan® Chewable Tablet [OTC]** *see* Calcium Polycarbophil *on page 86*
- **Mivacron®** *see* Mivacurium *on page 370*

## Mivacurium (mye va KYOO ree um)

**U.S. Brand Names** Mivacron®

**Pharmacologic Category** Neuromuscular Blocker Agent, Nondepolarizing

**Use** Short-acting nondepolarizing neuromuscular blocking agent; an adjunct to general anesthesia; facilitates endotracheal intubation; provides skeletal muscle relaxation during surgery or mechanical ventilation

**Effects on Mental Status** None reported

**Effects on Psychiatric Treatment** None reported

**Usual Dosage** Continuous infusion requires an infusion pump; dose should be based on ideal body weight

Children 2-12 years (duration of action is shorter and dosage requirements are higher): 200 mcg/kg I.V. bolus; 5-31 mcg/kg/minute I.V. infusion

Adults: Initial: I.V.: 0.15 mg/kg bolus; for prolonged neuromuscular block, infusions of 1-15 mcg/kg/minute are used

**Dosing adjustment in renal impairment:** 150 mcg/kg I.V. bolus; duration of action of blockade: 1.5 times longer in ESRD, may decrease infusion rates by as much as 50%, dependent on degree of renal impairment

**Dosing adjustment in hepatic impairment:** 150 mcg/kg I.V. bolus; duration of blockade: 3 times longer in ESLD, may decrease rate of infusion by as much as 50% in ESLD, dependent on the degree of impairment

**Dosage Forms**

Infusion, as chloride, in $D_5W$: 0.5 mg/mL (50 mL)

Injection, as chloride: 2 mg/mL (5 mL, 10 mL)

- **MJ-13105-1** *see* Bucindolol *on page 74*
- **MK 462** *see* Rizatriptan *on page 498*
- **MK-571** *see* Zafirlukast *on page 589*
- **MK594** *see* Losartan *on page 326*
- **Moban®** *see* Molindone *on page 372*
- **Mobic®** *see* Meloxicam *on page 338*
- **Mobidin®** *see* Magnesium Salicylate *on page 331*

## Modafinil (moe DAF i nil)

**Related Information**

Clinical Issues in the Use of Stimulants *on page 637*

**U.S. Brand Names** Provigil®

**Canadian Brand Names** Alertec®

**Pharmacologic Category** Stimulant

**Use** Improve wakefulness in patients with excessive daytime sleepiness associated with narcolepsy

**Unlabeled use:** ADHD, treatment of fatigue in MS and other disorders

**Restrictions** C-IV

**Pregnancy Risk Factor** C

**Pregnancy/Breast-Feeding Implications** Currently, there are no studies in humans evaluating its teratogenicity. Embryotoxicity of modafinil has been observed in animal models at dosages above those employed therapeutically. As a result, it should be used cautiously during pregnancy and should be used only when the potential risk of drug therapy is outweighed by the drug's benefits. It remains unknown if modafinil is secreted into human milk and, therefore, should be used cautiously in nursing women.

**Contraindications** Hypersensitivity to modafinil or any component

**Warnings/Precautions** History of angina, ischemic EKG changes, left ventricular hypertrophy, or clinically significant mitral valve prolapse in association with CNS stimulant use; caution should be exercised when modafinil is given to patients with a history of psychosis, recent history of myocardial infarction, and because it has not yet been adequately studied in patients with hypertension, periodic monitoring of hypertensive patients receiving modafinil may be appropriate; caution is warranted when operating machinery or driving, although functional impairment has not been demonstrated with modafinil, all CNS-active agents may alter judgment, thinking and/or motor skills. Efficacy of oral contraceptives may be reduced, therefore, use of alternative contraception should be considered.

**Adverse Reactions** Limited to reports that were equal to or greater than placebo-related events:

<10%:

Cardiovascular: Chest pain (2%), hypertension (2%), hypotension (2%), vasodilation (1%), arrhythmia (1%), syncope (1%)

Central nervous system: Headache (50%, compared to 40% with placebo), nervousness (8%), dizziness (5%), depression (4%), anxiety (4%), cataplexy (3%), insomnia (3%), chills (2%), fever (1%), confusion (1%), amnesia (1%), emotional lability (1%), ataxia (1%)

Dermatologic: Dry skin (1%)

Endocrine & metabolic: Hyperglycemia (1%), albuminuria (1%)

Gastrointestinal: Diarrhea (8%), nausea (13%, compared to 4% with placebo), xerostomia (5%), anorexia (5%), vomiting (1%), mouth ulceration (1%), gingivitis (1%)

Genitourinary: Abnormal urine (1%), urinary retention (1%), ejaculatory disturbance (1%)

Hematologic: Eosinophilia (1%)

Hepatic: Abnormal LFTs (3%)

Neuromuscular & skeletal: Paresthesias (3%), dyskinesia (2%), neck pain (2%), hypertonia (2%), neck rigidity (1%), joint disorder (1%), tremor (1%)

Ocular: Amblyopia (2%), abnormal vision (2%)

Respiratory: Pharyngitis (6%), rhinitis (11%, compared to 8% with placebo), lung disorder (4%), dyspnea (2%), asthma (1%), epistaxis (1%)

**Overdosage/Toxicology** Signs and symptoms of an overdose include agitation, irritability, aggressiveness, confusion, nervousness, tremor, sleep disturbance, palpitations, decreased prothrombin time, and slight to moderate elevations of hemodynamic parameters; treatment is symptomatic and supportive, there is no data to suggest the utility of dialysis or urinary pH alteration to enhance elimination; cardiac monitoring is warranted

**Drug Interactions** CYP3A3/4 substrate; CYP2C19 inhibitor; weak inducer of CYP1A2, 2B6, and 3A3/4

CYP2C19 substrates: Serum concentrations of drugs metabolized by this enzyme can be increased, these agents include diazepam, mephenytoin, phenytoin, and propranolol

CYP3A3/4 substrates: May decrease serum concentrations of CYP3A3/4 metabolized drugs such as oral contraceptives, benzodiazepines, and cyclosporine

Enzyme inducers (including phenobarbital, carbamazepine, and rifampin): May result in decreased modafinil levels; there is evidence to suggest that modafinil may induce its own metabolism

Oral contraceptives; serum concentrations may be reduced (enzyme induction); contraceptive failure may result; consider alternative contraceptive measures

Phenytoin: Serum concentrations may be increased by modafinil (enzyme inhibition); modafinil concentrations may be reduced by phenytoin (enzyme induction)

SSRIs: In populations genetically deficient in the CYP2D6 isoenzyme, where CYP2C19 acts as a secondary metabolic pathway, concentrations of selective serotonin reuptake inhibitors may be increased during coadministration

Tricyclic antidepressants: In populations genetically deficient in the CYP2D6 isoenzyme, where CYP2C19 acts as a secondary metabolic pathway, concentrations of tricyclic antidepressants may be increased during coadministration

Warfarin: Serum concentrations/effect may be increased by modafinil

**Mechanism of Action** The exact mechanism of action is unclear, it does not appear to alter the release of dopamine or norepinephrine, it may exert its stimulant effects by decreasing GABA-mediated neurotransmission, although this theory has not yet been fully evaluated; several studies also suggest that an intact central alpha-adrenergic system is required for modafinil's activity; the drug increases high-frequency alpha waves while decreasing both delta and theta wave activity, and these effects are consistent with generalized increases in mental alertness

**Pharmacodynamics/kinetics** Modafinil is a racemic compound (10% *d*-isomer and 90% *l*-isomer at steady state), whose enantiomers have different pharmacokinetics

Distribution: $V_d$: 0.9 L/kg

Protein binding: 60%, mostly to albumin

Metabolism: In the liver; multiple pathways including the cytochrome P-450 system

Half-life: Effective half-life: 15 hours; time to steady-state: 2-4 days

Time to peak serum concentration: 2-4 hours

Elimination: Renal, as metabolites (<10% excreted unchanged)

**Usual Dosage**

Narcolepsy: Initial: 200 mg as a single daily dose in the morning

Doses of 400 mg/day, given as a single dose, have been well tolerated, but there is no consistent evidence that this dose confers additional benefit

**Dosing adjustment in elderly:** Elimination of modafinil and its metabolites may be reduced as a consequence of aging and as a result, lower doses should be considered.

**Dosing adjustment in renal impairment:** Inadequate data to determine safety and efficacy in severe renal impairment

**Dosing adjustment in hepatic impairment:** Dose should be reduced to one-half of that recommended for patients with normal liver function

**Patient Information** Take during the day to avoid insomnia; may cause dependence with prolonged use; patients should be reminded to notify their physician if they become pregnant, intend to become pregnant, or are breast-feeding an infant; patients should be advised that combined use with alcohol has not been studied and that it is prudent to avoid this combination. Patients should notify their physician and/or pharmacist of any concomitant medications they are taking, due to the drug interaction potential this might represent.

**Dosage Forms** Tablet: 100 mg, 200 mg

- **Modane® Bulk [OTC]** *see* Psyllium *on page 479*
- **Modane® Soft [OTC]** *see* Docusate *on page 179*
- **Modicon™** *see* Ethinyl Estradiol and Norethindrone *on page 212*
- **Moduretic®** *see* Amiloride and Hydrochlorothiazide *on page 31*

## Moexipril (mo EKS i pril)

**Related Information**

Angiotensin-Related Agents Comparison Chart *on page 700*

**U.S. Brand Names** Univasc®

**Pharmacologic Category** Angiotensin-Converting Enzyme (ACE) Inhibitors

**Use** Treatment of hypertension, alone or in combination with thiazide diuretics; treatment of left ventricular dysfunction after myocardial infarction

**Effects on Mental Status** May cause drowsiness or dizziness; may rarely cause anxiety or mood changes

**Effects on Psychiatric Treatment** May cause neutropenia; use caution with clozapine and carbamazepine; may decrease lithium clearance resulting in an increase in serum lithium levels and potential lithium toxicity; monitor serum lithium levels

**Pregnancy Risk Factor** C (1st trimester); D (2nd and 3rd trimester)

**Contraindications** Hypersensitivity to moexipril, moexiprilat, or any component; hypersensitivity or allergic reactions or angioedema related to previous treatment with an ACE inhibitor; pregnancy (2nd or 3rd trimester)

**Warnings/Precautions** Anaphylactic reactions can occur. Angioedema can occur at any time during treatment (especially following first dose). Careful blood pressure monitoring with first dose (hypotension can occur especially in volume depleted patients). Dosage adjustment needed in renal impairment. Use with caution in hypovolemia; collagen vascular diseases; valvular stenosis (particularly aortic stenosis); hyperkalemia; or before, during, or immediately after anesthesia. Avoid rapid dosage escalation which may lead to renal insufficiency. Neutropenia/agranulocytosis with myeloid hyperplasia can rarely occur. If patient has renal impairment then a baseline WBC with differential and serum creatinine should be evaluated and monitored closely during the first 3 months of therapy. Hypersensitivity reactions may be seen during hemodialysis with high-flux dialysis membranes (eg, AN69). Deterioration in renal function can occur with initiation. Use with caution in unilateral renal artery stenosis and pre-existing renal insufficiency.

**Adverse Reactions**

1% to 10%:

Central nervous system: Headache, dizziness, fatigue

Dermatologic: Rash, pruritus, alopecia, flushing

Endocrine & metabolic: Hyperkalemia

Gastrointestinal: Diarrhea

Genitourinary: Polyuria

Renal: Oliguria, reversible increases in creatinine or BUN

Respiratory: Nonproductive cough (6%), pharyngitis, upper respiratory infections, rhinitis

Miscellaneous: Flu-like symptoms

<1%: Abdominal pain, abnormal taste, angina, angioedema, anxiety, arrhythmias, arthralgia, bronchospasm, changes in appetite, chest pain, constipation, dyspnea, elevated LFTs, hypercholesterolemia, mood changes, myalgia, myocardial infarction, neutropenia, palpitations, pancreatitis, pemphigus, photosensitivity, peripheral edema, proteinuria, sleep disturbances, symptomatic hypotension, taste disturbance, vomiting, xerostomia

**Overdosage/Toxicology**

Signs and symptoms: Mild hypotension has been the only toxic effect seen with acute overdose; bradycardia may also occur; hyperkalemia occurs even with therapeutic doses, especially in patients with renal insufficiency and those taking NSAIDs

Treatment: Following initiation of essential overdose management, toxic symptom treatment and supportive treatment should be initiated; hypotension usually responds to I.V. fluids or Trendelenburg positioning.

(Continued)

## Moexipril *(Continued)*

**Drug Interactions**

Allopurinol: Potential for allergic reactions increased with moexipril

Alpha$_1$ blockers: Hypotensive effect increased

Aspirin: The effects of ACE inhibitors may be blunted by aspirin administration, particularly at higher dosages

Diuretics: Hypovolemia due to diuretics may precipitate acute hypotensive events or acute renal failure

Insulin: Risk of hypoglycemia may be increased

Lithium: Risk of lithium toxicity may be increased; monitor lithium levels, especially the first 4 weeks of therapy

Mercaptopurine: Risk of neutropenia may be increased

NSAIDs may decrease ACE inhibitor efficacy and/or increase potential to alter renal function

Potassium-sparing diuretics (amiloride, potassium, spironolactone, triamterene): Increased risk of hyperkalemia

Potassium supplements may increase the risk of hyperkalemia

Probenecid: Blood levels of moexipril are increased (may occur with other ACE inhibitors)

Trimethoprim (high dose) may increase the risk of hyperkalemia

**Usual Dosage** Adults: Oral: Initial: 7.5 mg once daily (in patients **not** receiving diuretics), 1 hour prior to a meal **or** 3.75 mg once daily (when combined with thiazide diuretics); maintenance dose: 7.5-30 mg/day in 1 or 2 divided doses 1 hour before meals

**Dosing adjustment in renal impairment:** $Cl_{cr}$ ≤40 mL/minute: Patients may be cautiously placed on 3.75 mg once daily, then upwardly titrated to a maximum of 15 mg/day.

**Patient Information** Take exactly as directed; do not discontinue without consulting prescriber. Take first dose at bedtime. This drug does not eliminate need for diet or exercise regimen as recommended by prescriber. Do not take potassium supplements or salt substitutes containing potassium without consulting prescriber. May cause dizziness, fainting, lightheadedness (use caution when driving or engaging in tasks that require alertness until response to drug is known); postural hypotension (use caution when rising from lying or sitting position or climbing stairs); nausea, vomiting, abdominal pain, dry mouth, or transient loss of appetite (small frequent meals, frequent mouth care, sucking lozenges, or chewing gum may help) - report if these persist. Report chest pain or palpitations; difficulty in breathing or unusual cough; or other persistent adverse reactions.

**Nursing Implications** Observe for symptoms of severe hypotension, especially within the first 2 hours following the initial dose or subsequent increases in dose as well as for signs of hyperkalemia or cough; administer on an empty stomach

**Dosage Forms** Tablet, as hydrochloride: 7.5 mg, 15 mg

## Moexipril and Hydrochlorothiazide

(mo EKS i pril & hye droe klor oh THYE a zide)

**U.S. Brand Names** Uniretic™

**Pharmacologic Category** Antihypertensive Agent, Combination

**Use** Combination therapy for hypertension, however, not indicated for initial treatment of hypertension; replacement therapy in patients receiving separate dosage forms (for patient convenience); when monotherapy with one component fails to achieve desired antihypertensive effect, or when dose-limiting adverse effects limit upward titration of monotherapy

**Effects on Mental Status** May cause drowsiness or dizziness; may rarely cause anxiety or mood changes

**Effects on Psychiatric Treatment** Thiazides and ACEIs may decrease lithium clearance resulting in an increase in serum lithium levels and potential lithium toxicity; monitor serum lithium levels; may cause neutropenia; use caution with clozapine and carbamazepine

**Usual Dosage** Adults: Oral: 7.5-30 mg of moexipril, taken either in a single or divided dose one hour before meals

**Dosage Forms** Tablet: Moexipril hydrochloride 7.5 mg and hydrochlorothiazide 12.5 mg; moexipril hydrochloride 15 mg and hydrochlorothiazide 25 mg

♦ **Moi-Stir® Solution [OTC]** *see* Saliva Substitute *on page 502*

♦ **Moi-Stir® Swabsticks [OTC]** *see* Saliva Substitute *on page 502*

♦ **Moisture® Ophthalmic Drops [OTC]** *see* Artificial Tears *on page 48*

## Molindone (moe LIN done)

**Related Information**

Antipsychotic Agents Comparison Chart *on page 706*

Antipsychotic Medication Guidelines *on page 751*

Clinical Issues in the Use of Antipsychotics *on page 630*

Discontinuation of Psychotropic Drugs - Withdrawal Symptoms and Recommendations *on page 798*

Federal OBRA Regulations Recommended Maximum Doses *on page 756*

Patient Information - Antipsychotics (General) *on page 646*

Schizophrenia *on page 604*

**Generic Available** No

**U.S. Brand Names** Moban®

**Synonyms** Molindone Hydrochloride

**Pharmacologic Category** Antipsychotic Agent, Dihydoindoline

**Use** Management of psychotic disorder

**Pregnancy Risk Factor** C

**Contraindications** Hypersensitivity to molindone or any component (cross reactivity between phenothiazines may occur); severe CNS depression, coma

**Warnings/Precautions** May be sedating, use with caution in disorders where CNS depression is a feature. Use with caution in Parkinson's disease. Caution in patients with hemodynamic instability; bone marrow suppression; predisposition to seizures; subcortical brain damage; severe cardiac, hepatic, renal, or respiratory disease. Esophageal dysmotility and aspiration have been associated with antipsychotic use - use with caution in patients at risk of pneumonia (ie, Alzheimer's disease). Caution in breast cancer or other prolactin-dependent tumors (may elevate prolactin levels). May alter temperature regulation or mask toxicity of other drugs due to antiemetic effects. May alter cardiac conduction; life-threatening arrhythmias have occurred with therapeutic doses of neuroleptics. May cause orthostatic hypotension - use with caution in patients at risk of this effect or those who would tolerate transient hypotensive episodes (cerebrovascular disease, cardiovascular disease, or other medications which may predispose).

May cause anticholinergic effects (confusion, agitation, constipation, dry mouth, blurred vision, urinary retention); therefore, they should be used with caution in patients with decreased gastrointestinal motility, urinary retention, BPH, xerostomia, or visual problems. Conditions which also may be exacerbated by cholinergic blockade include narrow-angle glaucoma (screening is recommended) and worsening of myasthenia gravis. Relative to other neuroleptics, molindone has a low potency of cholinergic blockade.

May cause extrapyramidal reactions, including pseudoparkinsonism, acute dystonic reactions, akathisia, and tardive dyskinesia (risk of these reactions is moderate-high relative to other neuroleptics). May be associated with neuroleptic malignant syndrome (NMS) or pigmentary retinopathy.

**Adverse Reactions**

Cardiovascular: Orthostatic hypotension, tachycardia, arrhythmias

Central nervous system: Extrapyramidal reactions (akathisia, pseudoparkinsonism, dystonia, tardive dyskinesia), mental depression, altered central temperature regulation, sedation, drowsiness, restlessness, anxiety, hyperactivity, euphoria, seizures, neuroleptic malignant syndrome (NMS)

Dermatologic: Pruritus, rash, photosensitivity

Endocrine & metabolic: Change in menstrual periods, edema of breasts, amenorrhea, galactorrhea, gynecomastia

Gastrointestinal: Constipation, xerostomia, nausea, salivation, weight gain, weight loss

Genitourinary: Urinary retention, priapism

Hematologic: Leukopenia, leukocytosis

Ocular: Blurred vision, retinal pigmentation

Miscellaneous: Diaphoresis (decreased)

**Overdosage/Toxicology**

Signs and symptoms: Deep sleep, extrapyramidal symptoms, cardiac arrhythmias, seizures, hypotension

Treatment: Following initiation of essential overdose management, toxic symptom treatment and supportive treatment should be initiated. Hypotension usually responds to I.V. fluids or Trendelenburg positioning. If unresponsive to these measures, the use of a parenteral inotrope may be required (eg, norepinephrine 0.1-0.2 mcg/kg/minute titrated to response). Seizures commonly respond to diazepam (I.V. 5-10 mg bolus in adults every 15 minutes if needed up to a total of 30 mg; I.V. 0.25-0.4 mg/kg/dose up to a total of 10 mg in children) or to phenytoin or phenobarbital. Also critical cardiac arrhythmias often respond to I.V. phenytoin (15 mg/kg up to 1 gram), while other antiarrhythmics can be used. Neuroleptics often cause extrapyramidal symptoms (eg, dystonic reactions) requiring management with diphenhydramine 1-2 mg/kg (adults) up to a maximum of 50 mg I.M. or I.V. slow push followed by a maintenance dose for 48-72 hours. When these reactions are unresponsive to diphenhydramine, benztropine mesylate I.V. 1-2 mg (adults) may be effective. These agents are generally effective within 2-5 minutes.

**Drug Interactions** CYP2D6 enzyme substrate

Aluminum salts: May decrease the absorption of antipsychotics; monitor

Amphetamines: Efficacy may be diminished by antipsychotics; in addition, amphetamines may increase psychotic symptoms; avoid concurrent use

Anticholinergics: May inhibit the therapeutic response to antipsychotics and excess anticholinergic effects may occur; includes benztropine, trihexyphenidyl, biperiden, and drugs with significant anticholinergic activity (TCAs, antihistamines, disopyramide)

Antihypertensives: Concurrent use of antipsychotics with an antihypertensive may produce additive hypotensive effects (particularly orthostasis)

Bromocriptine: Antipsychotics inhibit the ability of bromocriptine to lower serum prolactin concentrations

CNS depressants: Sedative effects may be additive with antipsychotics; monitor for increased effect; includes barbiturates, benzodiazepines, narcotic analgesics, ethanol and other sedative agents

CYP2D6 inhibitors: Metabolism of antipsychotics may be decreased; increasing clinical effect or toxicity; inhibitors include amiodarone, cimetidine, delavirdine, fluoxetine, paroxetine, propafenone, quinidine, and ritonavir; monitor for increased effect/toxicity

Enzyme inducers: May enhance the hepatic metabolism of antipsychotics; larger doses may be required; includes rifampin, rifabutin, barbiturates, phenytoin, and cigarette smoking

Epinephrine: Chlorpromazine (and possibly other low potency antipsychotics) may diminish the pressor effects of epinephrine

Guanethidine and guanadrel: Antihypertensive effects may be inhibited by antipsychotics Levodopa: Antipsychotics may inhibit the antiparkinsonian effect of levodopa; avoid this combination

Lithium: Antipsychotics may produce neurotoxicity with lithium; this is a rare effect

Phenytoin: May reduce serum levels of antipsychotics; antipsychotics may increase phenytoin serum levels

Propranolol: Serum concentrations of antipsychotics may be increased; propranolol also increases antipsychotic concentrations

QTc prolonging agents: Effects on QTc interval may be additive with antipsychotics, increasing the risk of malignant arrhythmias; includes type Ia antiarrhythmics, TCAs, and some quinolone antibiotics (sparfloxacin, moxifloxacin, and gatifloxacin)

Sulfadoxine-pyrimethamine: May increase antipsychotics concentrations

Tricyclic antidepressants: Concurrent use may produce increased toxicity or altered therapeutic response

Trazodone: Antipsychotics and trazodone may produce additive hypotensive effects

Valproic acid: Serum levels may be increased by antipsychotics

**Stability** Protect from light; dispense in amber or opaque vials

**Mechanism of Action** Mechanism of action mimics that of chlorpromazine; however, it produces more extrapyramidal effects and less sedation than chlorpromazine

**Pharmacodynamics/kinetics**

Metabolism: In the liver

Half-life: 1.5 hours

Time to peak serum concentration: Oral: Within 1.5 hours

Elimination: Principally in urine and feces (90% within 24 hours)

**Usual Dosage** Oral:

Children:

3-5 years: 1-2.5 mg/day divided into 4 doses

5-12 years: 0.5-1 mg/kg/day in 4 divided doses

Adults: 50-75 mg/day increase at 3- to 4-day intervals up to 225 mg/day

**Dietary Considerations** Alcohol: Avoid use

**Monitoring Parameters** Monitor blood pressure and pulse rate prior to and during initial therapy evaluate mental status; monitor weight

**Reference Range** Antipsychotic range: 27-69 ng/mL; level of 152 ng/mL seen with rhabdomyolysis

**Test Interactions** ↑ cholesterol (S), glucose, prolactin; ↓ uric acid (S)

**Patient Information** Dry mouth may be helped by sips of water, sugarless gum or hard candy; avoid alcohol; very important to maintain established dosage regimen; photosensitivity to sunlight can occur, do not discontinue abruptly; full effect may not occur for 3-4 weeks; full dosage may be taken at bedtime to avoid daytime sedation; report to physician any involuntary movements or feelings of restlessness

**Nursing Implications** May increase appetite and possibly a craving for sweets; recognize signs of neuroleptic malignant syndrome and tardive dyskinesia

**Additional Information** Coadministration of two or more antipsychotics does not improve clinical response and may increase the potential for adverse effects

**Dosage Forms**

Concentrate, oral, as hydrochloride: 20 mg/mL (120 mL)

Tablet, as hydrochloride: 5 mg, 10 mg, 25 mg, 50 mg, 100 mg

♦ **Molindone Hydrochloride** *see* Molindone *on page 372*

♦ **Mol-Iron® [OTC]** *see* Ferrous Sulfate *on page 223*

♦ **Mollifene® Ear Wax Removing Formula [OTC]** *see* Carbamide Peroxide *on page 92*

## Mometasone (moe MET a sone)

**Related Information**

Corticosteroids Comparison Chart *on page 711*

**U.S. Brand Names** Elocon®; Nasonex®

**Canadian Brand Names** Elocom

**Pharmacologic Category** Corticosteroid, Topical

**Use** Relief of the inflammatory and pruritic manifestations of corticosteroid-responsive dermatoses (medium potency topical corticosteroid)

**Effects on Mental Status** None reported

**Effects on Psychiatric Treatment** None reported

**Pregnancy Risk Factor** C

**Contraindications** Hypersensitivity to mometasone or any component; fungal, viral, or tubercular skin lesions, herpes simplex or zoster

**Warnings/Precautions** Adverse systemic effects may occur when used on large areas of the body, denuded areas, for prolonged periods of time, with an occlusive dressing, and/or in infants or small children

**Adverse Reactions** <1%: Acne, allergic dermatitis, burning, Cushing's syndrome, dryness, folliculitis, growth retardation, HPA suppression, hypertrichosis, hypopigmentation, irritation, itching, maceration of the skin, miliaria, secondary infection skin atrophy, striae

**Drug Interactions** No data reported

**Usual Dosage** Adults: Topical: Apply sparingly to area once daily, do not use occlusive dressings. Therapy should be discontinued when control is achieved; if no improvement is seen, reassessment of diagnosis may be necessary.

**Patient Information** Before applying, gently wash area to reduce risk of infection; apply a thin film to cleansed area and rub in gently and thoroughly until medication vanishes; avoid exposure to sunlight, severe sunburn may occur

**Nursing Implications** For external use only; do not use on open wounds; should not be used in the presence of open or weeping lesions; use sparingly

**Dosage Forms**

Cream: 0.1% (15 g, 45 g)

Lotion: 0.1% (30 mL, 60 mL)

Ointment, topical: 0.1% (15 g, 45 g)

♦ **Monacolin K** *see* Lovastatin *on page 327*

♦ **Monafed®** *see* Guaifenesin *on page 256*

♦ **Monafed® DM** *see* Guaifenesin and Dextromethorphan *on page 257*

♦ **Monistat-Derm™ Topical** *see* Miconazole *on page 364*

♦ **Monistat i.v.™ Injection** *see* Miconazole *on page 364*

♦ **Monistat™ Vaginal** *see* Miconazole *on page 364*

♦ **Monocid®** *see* Cefonicid *on page 99*

♦ **Monoclate-P®** *see* Antihemophilic Factor (Human) *on page 45*

♦ **Monodox® Oral** *see* Doxycycline *on page 186*

♦ **Mono-Gesic®** *see* Salsalate *on page 503*

♦ **Monoket®** *see* Isosorbide Mononitrate *on page 297*

♦ **Mononine®** *see* Factor IX, Purified (Human) *on page 218*

♦ **Monopril®** *see* Fosinopril *on page 241*

## Montelukast (mon te LOO kast)

**U.S. Brand Names** Singulair®

**Pharmacologic Category** Leukotriene Receptor Antagonist

**Use** Prophylaxis and chronic treatment of asthma in adults and children ≥2 years of age

**Effects on Mental Status** May cause dizziness or drowsiness

**Effects on Psychiatric Treatment** Barbiturates may decrease the effects of montelukast; CYP3A3/4 substrate; nefazodone may increase effects

**Pregnancy Risk Factor** B

**Contraindications** Hypersensitivity to any component

**Warnings/Precautions** Montelukast is not indicated for use in the reversal of bronchospasm in acute asthma attacks, including status asthmaticus. Should not be used as monotherapy for the treatment and management of exercise-induced bronchospasm. Advise patients to have appropriate rescue medication available. Appropriate clinical monitoring and caution are recommended when systemic corticosteroid reduction is considered in patients receiving montelukast. Inform phenylketonuric patients that the chewable tablet contains phenylalanine 0.842 mg/5 mg chewable tablet.

In rare cases, patients on therapy with montelukast may present with systemic eosinophilia, sometimes presenting with clinical features of vasculitis consistent with Churg-Strauss syndrome, a condition which is often treated with systemic corticosteroid therapy. See Adverse Reactions.

**Adverse Reactions**

>10%: Central nervous system: Headache

1% to 10%:

Central nervous system: Dizziness, fatigue, fever

Dermatologic: Rash

Gastrointestinal: Dyspepsia, dental pain, gastroenteritis, diarrhea, nausea, abdominal pain

Neuromuscular & skeletal: Weakness

Respiratory: Cough, nasal congestion, laryngitis, pharyngitis

Miscellaneous: Flu-like symptoms, trauma

In rare cases, patients on therapy with montelukast may present with systemic eosinophilia, sometimes presenting with clinical features of vasculitis consistent with Churg-Strauss syndrome, a condition which is often treated with systemic corticosteroid therapy. Physicians should be

(Continued)

## Montelukast *(Continued)*

alert to eosinophilia, vasculitic rash, worsening pulmonary symptoms, cardiac complications, and/or neuropathy presenting in their patients. A casual association between montelukast and these underlying conditions has not been established.

**Overdosage/Toxicology** Treatment: No specific antidote; remove unabsorbed material from the GI tract, employ clinical monitoring and institute supportive therapy if required

**Drug Interactions** CYP2A6, and 2C9, 3A3/4, enzyme substrate

Decreased effect: Phenobarbital, rifampin induce hepatic metabolism and decrease the AUC of montelukast

**Usual Dosage** Oral:

Children:

<2 years: Safety and efficacy have not been established

2-5 years: Chew one 4 mg chewable tablet/day, taken in the evening

6 to 14 years: Chew one 5 mg chewable tablet/day, taken in the evening

Children ≥15 years and Adults: 10 mg/day, taken in the evening

**Dosing adjustment in hepatic impairment**: Mild moderate: No adjustment necessary

**Patient Information** This medication is not for an acute asthmatic attack; in acute attack, follow instructions of prescriber. Do not stop other asthma medication unless advised by prescriber. Take every evening on a continuous basis; do not discontinue even if feeling better (this medication may help reduce incidence of acute attacks). You may experience mild headache (mild analgesic may help); fatigue or dizziness (use caution when driving). Report skin rash or itching, abdominal pain or persistent GI upset, unusual cough or congestion, or worsening of asthmatic condition.

**Dosage Forms**

Tablet, as sodium: 10 mg

Tablet, chewable (cherry), as sodium: 5 mg

♦ **Monurol™** *see* Fosfomycin *on page 241*

♦ **Mood Disorders** *see page 600*

♦ **Mood Stabilizers** *see page 719*

♦ **8-MOP** *see* Methoxsalen *on page 355*

♦ **MoreDophilus® [OTC]** *see Lactobacillus acidophilus* and *Lactobacillus bulgaricus on page 305*

## Moricizine (mor I siz een)

**U.S. Brand Names** Ethmozine®

**Pharmacologic Category** Antiarrhythmic Agent, Class I

**Use** For treatment of ventricular tachycardia and life-threatening ventricular arrhythmias

**Unlabeled use:** PVCs, complete and nonsustained ventricular tachycardia

**Effects on Mental Status** Dizziness is common; may cause sedation or insomnia; may rarely cause anxiety, confusion, amnesia

**Effects on Psychiatric Treatment** Use caution with TCAs may produce Q-T prolongation

**Pregnancy Risk Factor** B

**Contraindications** Hypersensitivity to moricizine or any component; pre-existing second- or third-degree AV block (except in patients with a functioning artificial pacemaker); right bundle branch block when associated with left hemiblock or bifascicular block (unless functional pacemaker in place); cardiogenic shock

**Warnings/Precautions** Can be proarrhythmic; watch for new rhythm disturbances or existing arrhythmias that worsen. Use cautiously in CAD, previous history of MI, CHF, and cardiomegaly. The CAST II trial demonstrated a decreased trend in survival for patients receiving moricizine. Dose-related increases in PR and QRS intervals occur. Use cautiously in patients with pre-existing conduction abnormalities, and significant hepatic impairment. Safety and efficacy have not been established in pediatric patients.

**Adverse Reactions**

>10%: Central nervous system: Dizziness (15%)

1% to 10%:

Cardiovascular: Proarrhythmia, palpitations (5.8%), cardiac death (2% to 5%), EKG abnormalities (1.6%), congestive heart failure (1%)

Central nervous system: Headache (8%), fatigue (6%), insomnia (2% to 5%)

Gastrointestinal: Nausea (3% to 9%), diarrhea (2% to 5%)

Ocular: Blurred vision (2% to 5%)

Respiratory: Dyspnea (6%)

<1%: Anorexia, anxiety, apnea, bitter taste, cardiac chest pain, confusion, diaphoresis, drug fever, dry skin, dyspepsia, flatulence, GI upset, hypo/hypertension, impotence, loss of memory, myocardial infarction, rash, supraventricular arrhythmias, syncope, tinnitus, tremor, urinary incontinence, urinary retention, ventricular tachycardia, vertigo, vomiting

**Overdosage/Toxicology**

Signs and symptoms; Has a narrow therapeutic index and severe toxicity may occur slightly above the therapeutic range, especially if combined with other antiarrhythmic drugs. (Acute single ingestion of twice the daily therapeutic dose is life-threatening). Symptoms of overdose include increases in P-R, QRS, Q-T intervals and amplitude of the T wave, A-V block, bradycardia, hypotension, ventricular arrhythmias (monomorphic or polymorphic ventricular tachycardia), and asystole; other symptoms include dizziness, blurred vision, headache, and GI upset.

Treatment: Supportive, using conventional treatment (fluids, positioning, anticonvulsants, antiarrhythmics). **Note:** Type Ia antiarrhythmic agents should not be used to treat cardiotoxicity caused by type 1c drugs; sodium bicarbonate may reverse QRS prolongation, bradycardia and hypotension; ventricular pacing may be needed.

**Drug Interactions** CYP1A2 inducer

Cimetidine increases moricizine levels by 50%

Digoxin may result in additive prolongation of the PR interval when combined with moricizine (but not rate of second- and third-degree A-V block)

Diltiazem increases moricizine levels resulting in an increased incidence of side effects. Moricizine decreases diltiazem plasma levels and decreases its half-life.

Drugs which may prolong Q-T interval (including cisapride, erythromycin, phenothiazines, cyclic antidepressants, and some quinolones) are contraindicated with Type Ia antiarrhythmics. Moricizine has some Type Ia activity, and caution should be used.

Theophylline levels are decreased by 50% with moricizine due to increased clearance

**Usual Dosage** Adults: Oral: 200-300 mg every 8 hours, adjust dosage at 150 mg/day at 3-day intervals.

Recommendations for transferring patients from other antiarrhythmic agents to Ethmozine®:

When transferred from encainide, propafenone, tocainide, or mexiletine: Start Ethmozine® 8-12 hours after last dose

When transferred from flecainide: Start Ethmozine® 12-24 hours after last dose

When transferred from procainamide: Start Ethmozine® 3-6 hours after last dose

When transferred from quinidine or disopyramide: Start Ethmozine® 6-12 hours after last dose

**Dosing interval in renal or hepatic impairment:** Start at 600 mg/day or less.

**Patient Information** Take exactly as directed; do not take additional doses or discontinue without consulting prescriber. You will need regular cardiac checkups and blood tests while taking this medication. You may experience dizziness or visual changes (use caution when driving or engaging in tasks requiring alertness until response to drug is known); nausea or vomiting (small frequent meals, frequent mouth care, chewing gum, or sucking lozenges may help); or headaches, sleep disturbances, or decreased libido (usually temporary, if persistent consult prescriber). Report chest pain, palpitation, or erratic heartbeat; increased weight or swelling of hands or feet; blurred vision or facial swelling; acute diarrhea; changes in bowel or bladder patterns; or difficulty breathing.

**Nursing Implications** Administering 30 minutes after a meal delays the rate of absorption, resulting in lower peak plasma concentrations

**Dosage Forms** Tablet, as hydrochloride: 200 mg, 250 mg, 300 mg

♦ **Mormon Tea** *see* Ephedra *on page 194*

## Morphine Sulfate (MOR feen SUL fate)

**Related Information**

Hallucinogenic Drugs *on page 713*

Narcotic Agonists Comparison Chart *on page 720*

**U.S. Brand Names** Astramorph™ PF Injection; Duramorph® Injection; Infumorph™ Injection; Kadian™ Capsule; MS Contin® Oral; MSIR® Oral; MS/L®; MS/S®; OMS® Oral; Oramorph SR™ Oral; RMS® Rectal; Roxanol™ Oral; Roxanol Rescudose®; Roxanol SR™ Oral

**Canadian Brand Names** Epimorph®; M-Eslon®; Morphine-HP®; MS-IR®; MST Continus; Statex®

**Pharmacologic Category** Analgesic, Narcotic

**Use** Relief of moderate to severe acute and chronic pain; pain of myocardial infarction; relieves dyspnea of acute left ventricular failure and pulmonary edema; preanesthetic medication

**Effects on Mental Status** Sedation is common; may cause dizziness, restlessness, confusion; may rarely cause insomnia, depression, or hallucinations

**Effects on Psychiatric Treatment** Concurrent use with psychotropics may produce an increase of decrease in morphine's effect; monitor for clinical changes

**Restrictions** C-II

**Pregnancy Risk Factor** B (D if used for prolonged periods or in high doses at term)

**Contraindications** Known hypersensitivity to morphine sulfate; increased intracranial pressure; severe respiratory depression

**Warnings/Precautions** Some preparations contain sulfites which may cause allergic reactions; infants <3 months of age are more susceptible to respiratory depression, use with caution and generally in reduced doses in this age group; use with caution in patients with impaired respiratory function or severe hepatic dysfunction and in patients with hypersensitivity reactions to other phenanthrene derivative opioid agonists (codeine, hydrocodone, hydromorphone, levorphanol, oxycodone, oxymorphone). Morphine shares the toxic potential of opiate agonists and usual precautions of opiate agonist therapy should be observed; may cause hypotension in patients with acute myocardial infarction. Tolerance or drug dependence may result from extended use.

Elderly may be particularly susceptible to the CNS depressant and constipating effects of narcotics

**Adverse Reactions**

Percentage unknown: Antidiuretic hormone release, CNS depression, diaphoresis, drowsiness, flushing, increased intracranial pressure, physical and psychological dependence, sedation

>10%:

Cardiovascular: Palpitations, hypotension, bradycardia

Central nervous system: Dizziness

Gastrointestinal: Nausea, vomiting, constipation, xerostomia

Local: Pain at injection site

Neuromuscular & skeletal: Weakness

Miscellaneous: Histamine release

1% to 10%:

Central nervous system: Restlessness, headache, false feeling of well being, confusion

Gastrointestinal: Anorexia, GI irritation, paralytic ileus

Genitourinary: Decreased urination

Neuromuscular & skeletal: Trembling

Ocular: Vision problems

Respiratory: Respiratory depression, shortness of breath

<1%: Biliary tract spasm, hallucinations, increased intracranial pressure, increased liver function tests, insomnia, mental depression, miosis, muscle rigidity, paradoxical CNS stimulation, peripheral vasodilation, pruritus, urinary tract spasm

**Overdosage/Toxicology**

Signs and symptoms: Respiratory depression, miosis, hypotension, bradycardia, apnea, pulmonary edema

Treatment: Includes support of the patient's airway, establishment of an I.V. line, and administration of naloxone 2 mg I.V. (0.01 mg/kg for children) with repeat administration as necessary up to a total of 10 mg. Primary attention should be directed to ensuring adequate respiratory exchange.

**Drug Interactions** CYP2D6 enzyme substrate

Decreased effect: Phenothiazines may antagonize the analgesic effect of morphine and other opiate agonists

Increased toxicity: CNS depressants, tricyclic antidepressants may potentiate the effects of morphine and other opiate agonists; dextroamphetamine may enhance the analgesic effect of morphine and other opiate agonists

**Usual Dosage** Doses should be titrated to appropriate effect; when changing routes of administration in chronically treated patients, please note that oral doses are approximately one-half as effective as parenteral dose

Infants and Children:

Oral: Tablet and solution (prompt release): 0.2-0.5 mg/kg/dose every 4-6 hours as needed; tablet (controlled release): 0.3-0.6 mg/kg/dose every 12 hours

I.M., I.V., S.C.: 0.1-0.2 mg/kg/dose every 2-4 hours as needed; usual maximum: 15 mg/dose; may initiate at 0.05 mg/kg/dose

I.V., S.C. continuous infusion: Sickle cell or cancer pain: 0.025-2 mg/kg/hour; postoperative pain: 0.01-0.04 mg/kg/hour

Sedation/analgesia for procedures: I.V.: 0.05-0.1 mg/kg 5 minutes before the procedure

Adolescents >12 years: Sedation/analgesia for procedures: I.V.: 3-4 mg and repeat in 5 minutes if necessary

Adults:

Oral: Prompt release: 10-30 mg every 4 hours as needed; controlled release: 15-30 mg every 8-12 hours

I.M., I.V., S.C.: 2.5-20 mg/dose every 2-6 hours as needed; usual: 10 mg/dose every 4 hours as needed

I.V., S.C. continuous infusion: 0.8-10 mg/hour; may increase depending on pain relief/adverse effects; usual range: up to 80 mg/hour

Epidural: Initial: 5 mg in lumbar region; if inadequate pain relief within 1 hour, administer 1-2 mg, maximum dose: 10 mg/24 hours

Intrathecal ($^1/_{10}$ of epidural dose): 0.2-1 mg/dose; repeat doses **not** recommended

Rectal: 10-20 mg every 4 hours

**Dosing adjustment in renal impairment:**

$Cl_{cr}$ 10-50 mL/minute: Administer at 75% of normal dose

$Cl_{cr}$ <10 mL/minute: Administer at 50% of normal dose

**Dosing adjustment/comments in hepatic disease:** Unchanged in mild liver disease; substantial extrahepatic metabolism may occur; excessive sedation may occur in cirrhosis

**Dietary Considerations**

Alcohol: Additive CNS effects, avoid or limit alcohol; watch for sedation

Food:

Glucose may cause hyperglycemia; monitor blood glucose concentrations

Administration of oral morphine solution with food may increase bioavailability (ie, a report of 34% increase in morphine AUC when morphine oral solution followed a high-fat meal). Morphine may cause GI upset. Be consistent when taking morphine with or without meals. Take with food if GI upset.

**Patient Information** If self-administered, use exactly as directed (do not increase dose or frequency); may cause physical and/or psychological dependence. While using this medication, do not use alcohol and other prescription or OTC medications (especially sedatives, tranquilizers, antihistamines, or pain medications) without consulting prescriber. Maintain adequate hydration (2-3 L/day of fluids unless instructed to restrict fluid intake). May cause hypotension, dizziness, drowsiness, impaired coordination, or blurred vision (use caution when driving, climbing stairs, or changing position - rising from sitting or lying to standing, or when engaging in tasks requiring alertness until response to drug is known); loss of appetite, nausea, or vomiting (frequent mouth care, small frequent meals, chewing gum, or sucking lozenges may help); constipation (increased exercise, fluids, or dietary fruit and fiber may help - if constipation remains an unresolved problem, consult prescriber about use of stool softeners). Report chest pain, slow or rapid heartbeat, acute dizziness, or persistent headache; changes in mental status; swelling of extremities or unusual weight gain; changes in urinary elimination or pain on urination; acute headache; back or flank pain or muscle spasms; blurred vision; skin rash; or shortness of breath.

**Nursing Implications** Do not crush controlled release drug product, observe patient for excessive sedation, respiratory depression; implement safety measures, assist with ambulation; use preservative-free solutions for intrathecal or epidural use

**Dosage Forms**

Capsule (MSIR®): 15 mg, 30 mg

Capsule, sustained release (Kadian™): 20 mg, 50 mg, 100 mg

Injection: 0.5 mg/mL (10 mL); 1 mg/mL (10 mL, 30 mL, 60 mL); 2 mg/mL (1 mL, 2 mL, 60 mL); 3 mg/mL (50 mL); 4 mg/mL (1 mL, 2 mL); 5 mg/mL (1 mL, 30 mL); 8 mg/mL (1 mL, 2 mL); 10 mg/mL (1 mL, 2 mL, 10 mL); 15 mg/mL (1 mL, 2 mL, 20 mL); 25 mg/mL (4 mL, 10 mL, 20 mL, 40 mL); 50 mg/mL (10 mL, 20 mL, 40 mL)

Injection:

Preservative free (Astramorph™ PF, Duramorph®): 0.5 mg/mL (2 mL, 10 mL); 1 mg/mL (2 mL, 10 mL); 10 mg/mL (20 mL); 25 mg/mL (20 mL)

I.V. via PCA pump: 1 mg/mL (10 mL, 30 mL, 60 mL); 5 mg/mL (30 mL)

I.V. infusion preparation: 25 mg/mL (4 mL, 10 mL, 20 mL)

Solution, oral: 10 mg/5 mL (5 mL, 10 mL, 100 mL, 120 mL, 500 mL); 20 mg/5 mL (5 mL, 100 mL, 120 mL, 500 mL)

MSIR®: 10 mg/5 mL (5 mL, 120 mL, 500 mL); 20 mg/5 mL (5 mL 120 mL, 500 mL); 20 mg/mL (30 mL, 120 mL)

MS/L®: 100 mg/5 mL (120 mL) 20 mg/5 mL

OMS®: 20 mg/mL (30 mL, 120 mL)

Roxanol™: 10 mg/2.5 mL (2.5 mL); 20 mg/mL (1 mL, 1.5 mL, 30 mL, 120 mL, 240 mL)

Suppository, rectal: 5 mg, 10 mg, 20 mg, 30 mg

MS/S®, RMS®, Roxanol™: 5 mg, 10 mg, 20 mg, 30 mg

Tablet: 15 mg, 30 mg

MSIR®: 15 mg, 30 mg

Controlled release:

MS Contin®: 15 mg, 30 mg, 60 mg, 100 mg, 200 mg

Roxanol™ SR: 30 mg

Soluble: 10 mg, 15 mg, 30 mg

Sustained release (Oramorph SR™): 30 mg, 60 mg, 100 mg


- **Motofen®** *see* Difenoxin and Atropine *on page 168*
- **Motrin®** *see* Ibuprofen *on page 280*
- **Motrin® IB [OTC]** *see* Ibuprofen *on page 280*
- **Motrin® IB Sinus [OTC]** *see* Pseudoephedrine and Ibuprofen *on page 479*
- **Motrin® Migraine Pain [OTC]** *see* Ibuprofen *on page 280*
- **Mouthkote® Solution [OTC]** *see* Saliva Substitute *on page 502*


## Moxifloxacin (mox i FLOKS a sin)

**U.S. Brand Names** Avelox™

**Synonyms** Moxifloxacin Hydrochloride

**Pharmacologic Category** Antibiotic, Quinolone

**Use** Treatment of mild to moderate community-acquired pneumonia, acute bacterial exacerbation of chronic bronchitis, and acute bacterial sinusitis

**Effects on Mental Status** May cause dizziness, insomnia; may rarely produce abnormal thinking, agitation, anorexia, anxiety, asthenia, ataxia, confusion, depersonalization, depression, euphoria, hallucination, hostility, nervousness, panic attacks, paranoia, psychosis, somnolence, or stress

**Effects on Psychiatric Treatment** May have potential to prolong Q-T interval; should avoid in patients with uncorrected hypokalemia, or concurrent administration of other medications known to prolong the Q-T interval (antipsychotics, and tricyclic antidepressants)

**Pregnancy Risk Factor** C

(Continued)

## Moxifloxacin *(Continued)*

**Contraindications** Hypersensitivity to moxifloxacin, other quinolone antibiotics, or any component

**Warnings/Precautions** Use with caution in patients with significant bradycardia or acute myocardial ischemia. Moxifloxacin causes a dose-dependent Q-T prolongation. Coadministration of moxifloxacin with other drugs that also prolong the Q-T interval or induce bradycardia (eg, beta-blockers, amiodarone) should be avoided. Careful consideration should be given in the use of moxifloxacin in patients with cardiovascular disease, particularly in those with conduction abnormalities. Safety and effectiveness in pediatric patients (<18 years of age) have not been established. Experience in immature animals has resulted in permanent arthropathy. Use with caution in individuals at risk of seizures (CNS disorders or concurrent therapy with medications which may lower seizure threshold). Discontinue in patients who experience significant CNS adverse effects (dizziness, hallucinations, suicidal ideation or actions). Not recommended in patients with moderate to severe hepatic insufficiency. Use with caution in diabetes; glucose regulation may be altered.

Severe hypersensitivity reactions, including anaphylaxis, have occurred with quinolone therapy. If an allergic reaction occurs (itching, urticaria, dyspnea or facial edema, loss of consciousness, tingling, cardiovascular collapse) discontinue drug immediately. Prolonged use may result in superinfection; pseudomembranous colitis may occur and should be considered in all patients who present with diarrhea. Tendon inflammation and/or rupture has been reported with other quinolone antibiotics. This has not been reported for moxifloxacin. Discontinue at first sign of tendon inflammation or pain.

**Adverse Reactions**

1% to 10%:

Central nervous system: Dizziness (3%), headache (2%)

Gastrointestinal: Nausea (8%), diarrhea (6%), abdominal pain (2%), vomiting (2%), dyspepsia (1%), taste perversion (1%)

Hepatic: Abnormal liver function test (1%)

<1% (Limited to important or life-threatening symptoms): Asthenia, moniliasis, pain, malaise, allergic reaction, leg pain, back pain, fever, chills, chest pain, palpitation, vasodilation, tachycardia, hypertension, peripheral edema, hypotension, insomnia, nervousness, anxiety, confusion, hallucinations, depersonalization, hypertonia, incoordination, somnolence, tremor, vertigo, paresthesia, dry mouth, constipation, anorexia, stomatitis, gastritis, glossitis, cholestatic jaundice, GGT increased, decreased prothrombin time, increased prothrombin time, thrombocytopenia, eosinophilia, leukopenia, increased amylase, hyperglycemia, hyperlipidemia, increased LDH, arthralgia, myalgia, asthma, dyspnea, increased cough, pneumonia, pharyngitis, rhinitis, sinusitis, tendonitis/tendon rupture, rash, pruritus, sweating, urticaria, dry skin, tinnitus, amblyopia, vaginitis, cystitis, abnormal renal function, Q-T prolongation (see Warnings/Precautions)

**Overdosage/Toxicology** Potential symptoms of overdose may include CNS excitation, seizures, Q-T prolongation, and arrhythmias (including torsade de pointes). Patients should be monitored by continuous EKG in the event of an overdose. Management is supportive and symptomatic. Not removed by dialysis.

**Drug Interactions**

Antineoplastic agents may decrease the absorption of quinolones

Cimetidine, and other $H_2$-antagonists may inhibit renal elimination of quinolones

Digoxin levels may be increased in some patients by quinolones; monitor for increased effect/concentrations

Drugs which prolong Q-T interval (including Class Ia and Class III antiarrhythmics, erythromycin, cisapride, antipsychotics, and cyclic antidepressants) should be avoided with moxifloxacin.

Foscarnet has been associated with an increased risk of seizures with some quinolones

Loop diuretics: Serum levels of some quinolones are increased by loop diuretic administration. May diminish renal excretion

Metal cations (magnesium, aluminum, iron, and zinc) bind quinolones in the gastrointestinal tract and inhibit absorption (by up to 98%). Antacids, electrolyte supplements, sucralfate, quinapril, and some didanosine formulations should be avoided. Moxifloxacin should be administered 4 hours before or 8 hours after these agents.

NSAIDs: The CNS stimulating effect of some quinolones may be enhanced, resulting in neuroexcitation and/or seizures. This effect has not been observed with moxifloxacin.

Probenecid: Blocks renal secretion of quinolones, increasing concentrations

Warfarin: The hypoprothrombinemic effect of warfarin is enhanced by some quinolone antibiotics. No significant effect has been demonstrated for moxifloxacin; however, monitoring of the INR during concurrent therapy is recommended by the manufacturer.

**Usual Dosage** Adults: Oral:

Community acquired pneumonia or acute bacterial sinusitis: 400 mg every 24 hours for 10 days

Chronic bronchitis, acute bacterial exacerbation: 400 mg every 24 hours for 5 days

**Dosage adjustment in renal impairment:** No dosage adjustment is required.

**Dosage adjustment in hepatic impairment:** No dosage adjustment is required in mild to moderate hepatic insufficiency (Child-Pugh Classes A and B). Not recommended in patients with severe hepatic insufficiency.

Elderly: No dosage adjustments are required based on age.

**Patient Information** May be taken with or without food. Drink plenty of fluids. Avoid direct exposure to direct sunlight during therapy and for several days following. Do not take antacids within 4 hours before or 8 hours after dosing. Contact your physician immediately if signs of allergy occur. Contact your physician immediately if signs of tendon inflammation or pain occur. Do not discontinue therapy until your course has been completed. Take a missed dose as soon as possible, unless it is almost time for your next dose. Report immediately any pain, inflammation, or rupture of tendon.

**Dosage Forms** Tablet: 400 mg


- **Moxifloxacin Hydrochloride** *see* Moxifloxacin *on page 375*
- **6-MP** *see* Mercaptopurine *on page 343*
- **M-Prednisol® Injection** *see* Methylprednisolone *on page 359*
- **MS Contin® Oral** *see* Morphine Sulfate *on page 374*
- **MSIR® Oral** *see* Morphine Sulfate *on page 374*
- **MS/L®** *see* Morphine Sulfate *on page 374*
- **MS/S®** *see* Morphine Sulfate *on page 374*
- **MTX** *see* Methotrexate *on page 353*
- **Muco-Fen-DM®** *see* Guaifenesin and Dextromethorphan *on page 257*
- **Muco-Fen-LA®** *see* Guaifenesin *on page 256*
- **Mucomyst®** *see* Acetylcysteine *on page 18*
- **Mucoplex® [OTC]** *see* Vitamin B Complex *on page 586*
- **Mucosil™** *see* Acetylcysteine *on page 18*


## Mupirocin (myoo PEER oh sin)

**U.S. Brand Names** Bactroban®; Bactroban® Nasal

**Pharmacologic Category** Antibiotic, Topical

**Use** Topical treatment of impetigo due to *Staphylococcus aureus*, beta-hemolytic *Streptococcus*, and *S. pyogenes*

**Effects on Mental Status** None reported

**Effects on Psychiatric Treatment** None reported

**Usual Dosage**

Topical: Children and Adults: Apply small amount to affected area 2-5 times/day for 5-14 days

Nasal: In adults (12 years of age and older), approximately one-half of the ointment from the single-use tube should be applied into one nostril and the other half into the other nostril twice daily for 5 days

**Dosage Forms** Ointment, as calcium:

Intranasal: 2% (1 g single use tube)

Topical: 2% (15 g, 30 g)


- **Murine® Ear Drops [OTC]** *see* Carbamide Peroxide *on page 92*
- **Murine® Plus Ophthalmic [OTC]** *see* Tetrahydrozoline *on page 538*
- **Murine® Solution [OTC]** *see* Artificial Tears *on page 48*
- **Murocel® Ophthalmic Solution [OTC]** *see* Artificial Tears *on page 48*
- **Murocoll-2® Ophthalmic** *see* Phenylephrine and Scopolamine *on page 440*


## Muromonab-CD3 (myoo roe MOE nab-see dee three)

**U.S. Brand Names** Orthoclone® OKT3

**Pharmacologic Category** Immunosuppressant Agent

**Use** Treatment of acute allograft rejection in renal transplant patients; treatment of acute hepatic, kidney, and pancreas rejection episodes resistant to conventional treatment. Acute graft-versus-host disease following bone marrow transplantation resistant to conventional treatment.

**Effects on Mental Status** Dizziness is common; may rarely cause sedation, confusion, or hallucinations

**Effects on Psychiatric Treatment** None reported

**Usual Dosage** I.V. (refer to individual protocols):

Children <30 kg: 2.5 mg/day once daily for 7-14 days

Children >30 kg: 5 mg/day once daily for 7-14 days

**OR**

Children <12 years: 0.1 mg/kg/day once daily for 10-14 days

Children ≥12 years and Adults: 5 mg/day once daily for 10-14 days

Hemodialysis: Molecular size of OKT3 is 150,000 daltons; not dialyzed by most standard dialyzers; however, may be dialyzed by high flux dialysis; OKT3 will be removed by plasmapheresis; administer following dialysis treatments

Peritoneal dialysis: Significant drug removal is unlikely based on physiochemical characteristics

**Dosage Forms** Injection: 5 mg/5 mL


- **Muse® Pellet** *see* Alprostadil *on page 27*
- **Muskel Trancopal®** *see* Chlormezanone *on page 111*
- **Mustargen® Hydrochloride** *see* Mechlorethamine *on page 335*
- **Mutamycin®** *see* Mitomycin *on page 369*
- **Myambutol®** *see* Ethambutol *on page 209*
- **Mycelex®** *see* Clotrimazole *on page 135*
- **Mycelex®-7** *see* Clotrimazole *on page 135*
- **Mycelex®-G** *see* Clotrimazole *on page 135*
- **Mycifradin® Sulfate Oral** *see* Neomycin *on page 388*
- **Mycifradin® Sulfate Topical** *see* Neomycin *on page 388*
- **Mycinettes® [OTC]** *see* Benzocaine *on page 61*
- **Mycitracin® Topical [OTC]** *see* Bacitracin, Neomycin, and Polymyxin B *on page 57*
- **Mycobutin®** *see* Rifabutin *on page 492*
- **Mycogen II Topical** *see* Nystatin and Triamcinolone *on page 402*
- **Mycolog®-II Topical** *see* Nystatin and Triamcinolone *on page 402*
- **Myconel® Topical** *see* Nystatin and Triamcinolone *on page 402*


## Mycophenolate (mye koe FEN oh late)

**U.S. Brand Names** CellCept®

**Pharmacologic Category** Immunosuppressant Agent

**Use** Immunosuppressant used with corticosteroids and cyclosporine to prevent organ rejection in patients receiving allogenic renal and cardiac transplants; treatment of rejection in liver transplant patients unable to tolerate tacrolimus or cyclosporine due to neurotoxicity; mild rejection in heart transplant patients; treatment of moderate-severe psoriasis

Intravenous formulation is an alternative dosage form to oral capsules and tablets

**Effects on Mental Status** Dizziness and insomnia are common

**Effects on Psychiatric Treatment** Leukopenia is common; avoid clozapine and carbamazepine

**Pregnancy Risk Factor** C

**Contraindications** Hypersensitivity to mycophenolate mofetil, mycophenolic acid or any ingredient; intravenous is contraindicated in patients who are allergic to polysorbate 80

**Warnings/Precautions** Increased risk for infection and development of lymphoproliferative disorders. Patients should be monitored appropriately and given supportive treatment should these conditions occur. Increased toxicity in patients with renal impairment. Should be used with caution in patients with active peptic ulcer disease.

Because mycophenolate mofetil has demonstrated teratogenic effects in rats and rabbits, tablets should not be crushed and capsules should not be opened or crushed. Avoid inhalation or direct contact with skin or mucous membranes of the powder contained in the capsules. Caution should be exercised in the handling and preparation of solutions of intravenous mycophenolate. Avoid skin contact with the solution. If such contact occurs, wash thoroughly with soap and water, rinse eyes with plain water.

**Adverse Reactions** 1% to 10%: Thrombophlebitis and thrombosis (4%) with intravenous administration

See table.

**Drug Interactions**

Decreased effect: Antacids decrease $C_{max}$ and AUC, **do not administer together**; cholestyramine decreases AUC, **do not administer together**

Increased toxicity: Acyclovir and ganciclovir levels may increase due to competition for tubular secretion of these drugs; probenecid may increase mycophenolate levels due to inhibition of tubular secretion; salicylates: high doses may increase free fraction of mycophenolic acid

**Usual Dosage**

Oral:

Children: 600 mg/m$^2$/dose twice daily; **Note:** Limited information regarding mycophenolate use in pediatric patients is currently available in the literature: 32 pediatric patients (14 underwent living donor and 18 receiving cadaveric donor renal transplants) received mycophenolate 8-30 mg/kg/dose orally twice daily with cyclosporine, prednisone, and Atgam® induction; however, pharmacokinetic studies suggest that doses of mycophenolate adjusted to body surface area resulted in AUCs which better approximated those of adults versus doses adjusted for body weight which resulted in lower AUCs in pediatric patients

Adults: 1 g twice daily within 72 hours of transplant (although 3 g daily has been given in some clinical trials, there was decreased tolerability and no efficacy advantage)

**Dosing adjustment in renal impairment:** Doses >2 g/day are not recommended in these patients because of the possibility for enhanced immunosuppression as well as toxicities

### Adverse Reactions Reported in >10%

| Adverse Reaction | MM 2 g/day | MM 3 g/day |
|---|---|---|
| **Body as a Whole** | | |
| Pain | 33 | 31.2 |
| Abdominal pain | 12.1-24.7 | 11.9-27.6 |
| Fever | 20.4 | 23.3 |
| Headache | 20.1 | 16.1 |
| Infection | 12.7-18.2 | 15.6-20.9 |
| Sepsis | 17.6-20.8 | 17.5-19.7 |
| Asthenia | 13.7 | 16.1 |
| Chest pain | 13.4 | 13.3 |
| Back pain | 11.6 | 12.1 |
| Hypertension | 17.6-32.4 | 16.9-28.2 |
| **Central Nervous System** | | |
| Tremor | 11 | 11.8 |
| Insomnia | 8.9 | 11.8 |
| Dizziness | 5.7 | 11.2 |
| **Dermatologic** | | |
| Acne | 10.1 | 9.7 |
| Rash | 7.7 | 6.4 |
| **Gastrointestinal** | | |
| Diarrhea | 16.4-31 | 18.8-36.1 |
| Constipation | 21.9 | 18.5 |
| Nausea | 19.9 | 23.6 |
| Dyspepsia | 17.6 | 13.6 |
| Vomiting | 12.5 | 13.6 |
| Nausea & vomiting | 10.4 | 9.7 |
| Oral monoliasis | 10.1 | 12.1 |
| **Hemic/Lymphatic** | | |
| Anemia | 25.6 | 25.8 |
| Leukopenia | 11.5-23.2 | 16.3-34.5 |
| Thrombocytopenia | 10.1 | 8.2 |
| Hypochromic anemia | 7.4 | 11.5 |
| Leukocytosis | 7.1 | 10.9 |
| **Metabolic/Nutritional** | | |
| Peripheral edema | 28.6 | 27 |
| Hypercholesterolemia | 12.8 | 8.5 |
| Hypophosphatemia | 12.5 | 15.8 |
| Edema | 12.2 | 11.8 |
| Hypokalemia | 10.1 | 10 |
| Hyperkalemia | 8.9 | 10.3 |
| Hyperglycemia | 8.6 | 12.4 |
| **Respiratory** | | |
| Infection | 15.8-21 | 13.1-23.9 |
| Dyspnea | 15.5 | 17.3 |
| Cough increase | 15.5 | 13.3 |
| Pharyngitis | 9.5 | 11.2 |
| Bronchitis | 8.5 | 11.9 |
| Pneumonia | 3.6 | 10.6 |
| **Urogenital** | | |
| UTI | 37.2-45.5 | 37-44.4 |
| Hematuria | 14 | 12.1 |
| Kidney tubular necrosis | 6.3 | 10 |
| Urinary tract disorder | 6.7 | 10.6 |

**Dosing adjustment in severe chronic renal impairment:** $Cl_{cr}$ <25 mL/minute/1.73 m$^2$: Doses of >1 g administered twice daily should be avoided; patients should also be carefully observed; no dose adjustments are needed in renal transplant patients experiencing delayed graft function postoperatively

Hemodialysis: Not removed; supplemental dose is not necessary

Peritoneal dialysis: Supplemental dose is not necessary

**Dosing adjustment for neutropenia:** ANC <1.3 x 10$^3$/μL: Dosing should be interrupted or the dose reduced, appropriate diagnostic tests performed and patients managed appropriately

**Patient Information** Take as directed, preferably 1 hour before or 2 hours after meals. Do not take within 1 hour before or 2 hours after antacids or cholestyramine medications. Do not alter dose and do not discontinue without consulting prescriber. Maintain adequate hydration (2-3 L/day of fluids unless instructed to restrict fluid intake) during entire course of therapy. You will be susceptible to infection (avoid crowds and people with infections or contagious diseases). If you are diabetic, monitor glucose levels closely (may alter glucose levels). You may experience dizziness or trembling (use caution until response to medication is known); nausea or vomiting (frequent small meals, frequent mouth care may help); diarrhea (boiled milk, yogurt, or buttermilk may help); sores or white plaques in mouth (frequent rinsing of mouth and frequent mouth care may help); or muscle or back pain (mild analgesics may be recommended). Report chest

(Continued)

## Mycophenolate *(Continued)*

pain; acute headache or dizziness; symptoms of respiratory infection, cough, or difficulty breathing; unresolved gastrointestinal effects; fatigue, chills, fever unhealed sores, white plaques in mouth; irritation in genital area or unusual discharge; unusual bruising or bleeding; or other unusual effects related to this medication.

**Dosage Forms**

Capsule, as mofetil: 250 mg
Injection: 500 mg
Suspension, oral, as mofetil: 200 mg/mL (225 mL)
Tablet, film coated: 500 mg


- **Mycostatin®** *see* Nystatin *on page 402*
- **Myco-Triacet® II** *see* Nystatin and Triamcinolone *on page 402*
- **Mydfrin® Ophthalmic Solution** *see* Phenylephrine *on page 439*
- **Mydriacyl®** *see* Tropicamide *on page 574*
- **Mykrox®** *see* Metolazone *on page 361*
- **Mylanta® Gas [OTC]** *see* Simethicone *on page 512*
- **Mylanta® Gelcaps®** *see* Calcium Carbonate and Magnesium Carbonate *on page 85*
- **Mylanta® Liquid [OTC]** *see* Aluminum Hydroxide, Magnesium Hydroxide, and Simethicone *on page 28*
- **Mylanta® Maximum Strength Liquid [OTC]** *see* Aluminum Hydroxide, Magnesium Hydroxide, and Simethicone *on page 28*
- **Myleran®** *see* Busulfan *on page 78*
- **Mylicon® [OTC]** *see* Simethicone *on page 512*
- **Mylosar®** *see* Azacitidine *on page 54*
- **Mylotarg™** *see* Gemtuzumab Ozogamicin *on page 248*
- **Myminic® Expectorant [OTC]** *see* Guaifenesin and Phenylpropanolamine *on page 257*
- **Myotonachol™** *see* Bethanechol *on page 67*
- **Myphetane DC®** *see* Brompheniramine, Phenylpropanolamine, and Codeine *on page 74*
- **Mysoline®** *see* Primidone *on page 462*
- **Mytelase® Caplets®** *see* Ambenonium *on page 29*
- **Mytrex® F Topical** *see* Nystatin and Triamcinolone *on page 402*
- **Mytussin® [OTC]** *see* Guaifenesin *on page 256*
- **Mytussin® AC** *see* Guaifenesin and Codeine *on page 256*
- **Mytussin® DAC** *see* Guaifenesin, Pseudoephedrine, and Codeine *on page 258*
- **Mytussin® DM [OTC]** *see* Guaifenesin and Dextromethorphan *on page 257*
- **M-Zole® 7 Dual Pack [OTC]** *see* Miconazole *on page 364*


## Nabilone (NA bi lone)

**U.S. Brand Names** Cesamet®

**Pharmacologic Category** Antiemetic

**Use** Treatment of nausea and vomiting associated with cancer chemotherapy

**Effects on Mental Status** Dizziness, drowsiness, and euphoria are common; may cause depression; may rarely cause confusion and hallucinations

**Effects on Psychiatric Treatment** Concurrent use with psychotropic may produce additive sedation

**Contraindications** Nausea and vomiting not secondary to cancer chemotherapy

**Warnings/Precautions** Use with caution in the elderly, those with pre-existing CNS depression, or a history of mental illness

**Adverse Reactions**

>10%:
Central nervous system: Dizziness, drowsiness, vertigo, euphoria, clumsiness
Gastrointestinal: Xerostomia

1% to 10%:
Cardiovascular: Orthostatic hypotension
Central nervous system: Ataxia, depression
Ocular: Blurred vision

**Overdosage/Toxicology**

Signs and symptoms: Nausea, vomiting, disorientation, CNS, respiratory depression, dysphoria, euphoria
Treatment: Supportive and symptomatic

**Drug Interactions** CNS depression is potentiated with ethanol

**Usual Dosage** Oral:

Children >4 years:
<18 kg: 0.5 mg twice daily
18-30 kg: 1 mg twice daily
>30 kg: 1 mg 3 times/day

Adults: 1-2 mg twice daily beginning 1-3 hours before chemotherapy is administered and continuing around-the-clock until 1 dose after chemotherapy is completed; maximum daily dose: 6 mg divided in 3 doses

**Patient Information** May cause drowsiness, impair judgment, coordination; avoid alcohol and other CNS depressants; can cause disorientation

**Dosage Forms** Capsule: 1 mg

## Nabumetone (na BYOO me tone)

**Related Information**

Nonsteroidal Anti-inflammatory Agents Comparison Chart *on page 722*

**U.S. Brand Names** Relafen®

**Pharmacologic Category** Nonsteroidal Anti-Inflammatory Agent (NSAID)

**Use** Management of osteoarthritis and rheumatoid arthritis

**Unlabeled use:** Sunburn, mild to moderate pain

**Effects on Mental Status** Dizziness is common; may cause nervousness; may rarely cause insomnia, confusion, depression, or hallucinations

**Effects on Psychiatric Treatment** May rarely cause agranulocytosis; use caution with clozapine and carbamazepine; may decrease lithium clearance resulting in an increase in serum lithium levels and potential lithium toxicity; monitor serum lithium levels

**Pregnancy Risk Factor** C (D if used in third trimester)

**Contraindications** Hypersensitivity to nabumetone; should not be administered to patients with active peptic ulceration and those with severe hepatic impairment or in patients in whom nabumetone, aspirin, or other NSAIDs have induced asthma, urticaria, or other allergic-type reactions; fatal asthmatic reactions have occurred following NSAID administration

**Warnings/Precautions** Elderly patients may sometimes require lower doses; patients with impaired renal function may need a dose reduction; use with caution in patients with severe hepatic impairment; dehydration

**Adverse Reactions**

>10%:
Central nervous system: Dizziness
Dermatologic: Rash
Gastrointestinal: Abdominal cramps, heartburn, indigestion, nausea

1% to 10%:
Central nervous system: Headache, nervousness
Dermatologic: Itching
Endocrine & metabolic: Fluid retention
Gastrointestinal: Vomiting
Otic: Tinnitus

<1%: Acute renal failure, agranulocytosis, allergic rhinitis, anemia, angioedema, arrhythmia, aseptic meningitis, bone marrow suppression, blurred vision, confusion, congestive heart failure, conjunctivitis, cystitis, decreased hearing, drowsiness, dry eyes, epistaxis, erythema multiforme, gastritis, GI ulceration, hallucinations, hemolytic anemia, hepatitis, hot flashes, hypertension, insomnia, leukopenia, mental depression, peripheral neuropathy, polydipsia, polyuria, Stevens-Johnson syndrome, tachycardia, thrombocytopenia, toxic amblyopia, toxic epidermal necrolysis, urticaria

**Drug Interactions**

ACE inhibitors: Effects may be reduced by NSAIDs; use lowest possible dose for shortest duration possible; monitor
Cholestyramine and colestipol: Absorption may be reduced by concurrent administration
Corticosteroids: May increase the risk of GI ulceration; use caution
Cyclosporine: Nephrotoxicity may be increased with concurrent NSAID use; monitor
Hydralazine: Antihypertensive effect may be decreased; avoid concurrent use
Lithium: Serum levels can be increased; avoid concurrent use if possible or monitor lithium levels and adjust dose. When NSAID is stopped, lithium may need adjustment again.
Loop diuretics: Therapeutic effects may be reduced by NSAIDs; avoid
Methotrexate: Toxicity may be increased by concurrent NSAID use; risk is limited in low-dose methotrexate regimens (such as for rheumatoid arthritis); prolonged leucovorin rescue may be required at antineoplastic doses; monitor
Thiazide diuretics: Antihypertensive effects are decreased; avoid concurrent use
Warfarin: INRs may be increased by some NSAIDs. This may depend, in part, on dose and duration; monitor INR closely. Use the lowest dose of NSAIDs possible and for the briefest duration.

**Usual Dosage** Adults: Oral: 1000 mg/day; an additional 500-1000 mg may be needed in some patients to obtain more symptomatic relief; may be administered once or twice daily

**Dosing adjustment in renal impairment:** None necessary; however, adverse effects due to accumulation of inactive metabolites of nabumetone that are renally excreted have not been studied and should be considered

**Dietary Considerations**

Alcohol: May add to irritant action in the stomach, avoid use if possible

Food: Increases the rate but not the extent of oral absorption. Take without regard to meals OR take with food or milk to minimize GI upset.

**Patient Information** Take this medication exactly as directed; do not increase dose without consulting prescriber. Do not crush tablets or break capsules. Take with food or milk to reduce GI distress. Maintain adequate fluid intake (2-3 L/day of fluids unless instructed to restrict fluid intake). Do not use alcohol, aspirin, or aspirin-containing medication, and all other anti-inflammatory medications without consulting prescriber. You may experience drowsiness, dizziness, nervousness, or headache (use caution when driving or engaging in tasks requiring alertness until response to drug is known); anorexia, nausea, vomiting, or heartburn (frequent small meals, frequent oral care, sucking lozenges, or chewing gum may help); fluid retention (weigh yourself weekly and report unusual (3-5 lb/week) weight gain). GI bleeding, ulceration, or perforation can occur with or without pain; discontinue medication and contact prescriber if persistent abdominal pain or cramping, or blood in stool occurs. Report breathlessness, difficulty breathing, or unusual cough; chest pain, rapid heartbeat, palpitations; unusual bruising/bleeding; blood in urine, stool, mouth, or vomitus; swollen extremities; skin rash or itching; acute fatigue; or changes in hearing or ringing in ears.

**Dosage Forms** Tablet: 500 mg, 750 mg


- **NAC** *see* Acetylcysteine *on page 18*
- **N-Acetyl-5-methoxytryptamine** *see* Melatonin *on page 338*
- ***N*-Acetylcysteine** *see* Acetylcysteine *on page 18*
- ***N*-Acetyl-L-cysteine** *see* Acetylcysteine *on page 18*
- **N-Acetyl-P-Aminophenol** *see* Acetaminophen *on page 14*


## Nadolol (nay DOE lole)

**Related Information**

Beta-Blockers Comparison Chart *on page 709*

Special Populations - Mentally Retarded Patients *on page 665*

**U.S. Brand Names** Corgard®

**Canadian Brand Names** Apo®-Nadol; Syn-Nadolol

**Pharmacologic Category** Beta Blocker, Nonselective

**Use** Treatment of hypertension and angina pectoris; prophylaxis of migraine headaches

**Effects on Mental Status** May cause drowsiness, dizziness, depression, insomnia, or confusion

**Effects on Psychiatric Treatment** Barbiturates may decrease the effects of beta-blockers; has been used to treat akathisia; propranolol preferred; concurrent use with antipsychotics may potentiate antihypertensive effect or antipsychotic blood levels; use with MAOIs may cause bradycardia; effects of benzodiazepines may be increased by beta-blockers; monitor for clinical changes

**Pregnancy Risk Factor** C

**Contraindications** Hypersensitivity to nadolol or any component; bronchial asthma; sinus bradycardia; sinus node dysfunction; heart block greater than first degree (except in patients with a functioning artificial pacemaker); cardiogenic shock; uncompensated cardiac failure

**Warnings/Precautions** Administer only with extreme caution in patients with compensated heart failure, monitor for a worsening of the condition. Efficacy in heart failure has not been established for nadolol. Avoid abrupt discontinuation in patients with a history of CAD; slowly wean while monitoring for signs and symptoms of ischemia. Use caution with concurrent use of beta-blockers and either verapamil or diltiazem; bradycardia or heart block can occur. In general, patients with bronchospastic disease should not receive beta-blockers. Nadolol, if used at all, should be used cautiously in bronchospastic disease with close monitoring. Use cautiously in diabetics because it can mask prominent hypoglycemic symptoms. Can mask signs of thyrotoxicosis. Can cause fetal harm when administered in pregnancy. Use cautiously in the renally impaired (dosage adjustments are required). Use care with anesthetic agents which decrease myocardial function.

**Adverse Reactions**

>5%:

Central nervous system: Nightmares

Neuromuscular & skeletal: Paresthesia of toes and fingers

1% to 5%:

Cardiovascular: Bradycardia, reduced peripheral circulation, congestive heart failure, chest pain, orthostatic hypotension, Raynaud's syndrome, edema

Central nervous system: Mental depression, dizziness, drowsiness, vivid dreams, insomnia, lethargy, fatigue (2%), confusion, headache

Dermatologic: Itching, rash

Endocrine & metabolic: Decreased sexual ability

Gastrointestinal: Constipation, vomiting, stomach discomfort, diarrhea, nausea

Genitourinary: Impotence

Hematologic: Thrombocytopenia

Neuromuscular & skeletal: Weakness

Ocular: Dry eyes

Respiratory: Dyspnea, wheezing, nasal congestion

Miscellaneous: Cold extremities

**Overdosage/Toxicology**

Signs and symptoms: Cardiac disturbances, CNS toxicity, bronchospasm, hypoglycemia and hyperkalemia. The most common cardiac symptoms include hypotension and bradycardia; atrioventricular block, intraventricular conduction disturbances, cardiogenic shock, and asystole may occur with severe overdose, especially with membrane-depressant drugs (eg, propranolol); CNS effects include convulsions, coma, and respiratory arrest (commonly seen with propranolol and other membrane-depressant and lipid-soluble drugs).

Treatment: Symptomatic treatment of seizures, hypotension, hyperkalemia, and hypoglycemia; bradycardia and hypotension resistant to atropine, isoproterenol, or pacing may respond to glucagon; wide QRS defects caused by the membrane-depressant poisoning may respond to hypertonic sodium bicarbonate; repeat-dose charcoal, hemoperfusion, or hemodialysis may be helpful in removal of only those beta-blockers with a small $V_d$, long half-life, or low intrinsic clearance (acebutolol, atenolol, nadolol, sotalol)

**Drug Interactions**

Albuterol (and other $beta_2$ agonists): Effects may be blunted by nonspecific beta-blockers

Alpha-blockers (prazosin, terazosin): Concurrent use of beta-blockers may increase risk of orthostasis

Clonidine: Hypertensive crisis after or during withdrawal of either agent

Drugs which slow AV conduction (digoxin): Effects may be additive with beta-blockers

Epinephrine (including local anesthetics with epinephrine): Propranolol may cause hypertension

Glucagon: Nadolol may blunt the hyperglycemic action of glucagon

Insulin and oral hypoglycemics: Nadolol may mask symptoms of hypoglycemia

Nadolol increases antipyrine's half-life

NSAIDs (ibuprofen, indomethacin, naproxen, piroxicam) may reduce the antihypertensive effects of beta-blockers

Salicylates may reduce the antihypertensive effects of beta-blockers

Sulfonylureas: Beta-blockers may alter response to hypoglycemic agents

Verapamil or diltiazem may have synergistic or additive pharmacological effects when taken concurrently with beta-blockers

**Usual Dosage** Oral:

Adults: Initial: 40 mg/day, increase dosage gradually by 40-80 mg increments at 3- to 7-day intervals until optimum clinical response is obtained with profound slowing of heart rate; doses up to 160-240 mg/day in angina and 240-320 mg/day in hypertension may be necessary.

Elderly: Initial: 20 mg/day; increase doses by 20 mg increments at 3- to 7-day intervals; usual dosage range: 20-240 mg/day.

**Dosing adjustment in renal impairment:**

$Cl_{cr}$ 31-40 mL/minute: Administer every 24-36 hours or administer 50% of normal dose.

$Cl_{cr}$ 10-30 mL/minute: Administer every 24-48 hours or administer 50% of normal dose.

$Cl_{cr}$ <10 mL/minute: Administer every 40-60 hours or administer 25% of normal dose.

Hemodialysis: Moderately dialyzable (20% to 50%); administer dose postdialysis or administer 40 mg supplemental dose.

Peritoneal dialysis: Supplemental dose is not necessary.

**Dosing adjustment/comments in hepatic disease:** Reduced dose probably necessary.

**Patient Information** Check pulse daily prior to taking medication. If pulse is <50, hold medication and consult prescriber. Do not adjust dosage without consulting prescriber. May cause dizziness, fatigue, blurred vision; change position slowly (lying/sitting to standing) and use caution when driving or engaging in tasks that require alertness until response to drug is known. Exercise and increasing bulk or fiber in diet may help resolve constipation. If diabetic, monitor serum glucose closely (the drug may mask symptoms of hypoglycemia). Report swelling in feet or legs, difficulty breathing or persistent cough, unresolved fatigue, unusual weight gain >5 lb/week, or unresolved constipation.

**Nursing Implications** Patient's therapeutic response may be evaluated by looking at blood pressure, apical and radial pulses

**Dosage Forms** Tablet: 20 mg, 40 mg, 80 mg, 120 mg, 160 mg

## Nafarelin (NAF a re lin)

**U.S. Brand Names** Synarel®

**Pharmacologic Category** Hormone, Posterior Pituitary; Luteinizing Hormone-Releasing Hormone Analog

**Use** Treatment of endometriosis, including pain and reduction of lesions; treatment of central precocious puberty (gonadotropin-dependent precocious puberty) in children of both sexes

(Continued)

## Nafarelin *(Continued)*

**Effects on Mental Status** Emotional lability is common; may cause insomnia

**Effects on Psychiatric Treatment** None reported

**Pregnancy Risk Factor** X

**Contraindications** Hypersensitivity to GnRH, GnRH-agonist analogs or any components of this product; undiagnosed abnormal vaginal bleeding; pregnancy; lactation

**Warnings/Precautions** Use with caution in patients with risk factors for decreased bone mineral content, nafarelin therapy may pose an additional risk; hypersensitivity reactions occur in 0.2% of the patients; safety and efficacy in children have not been established

**Adverse Reactions**

>10%:

Central nervous system: Headache, emotional lability

Dermatologic: Acne

Endocrine & metabolic: Hot flashes, decreased libido, decreased breast size

Genitourinary: Vaginal dryness

Neuromuscular & skeletal: Myalgia

Respiratory: Nasal irritation

1% to 10%:

Cardiovascular: Edema, chest pain

Central nervous system: Insomnia

Dermatologic: Urticaria, rash, pruritus, seborrhea

Respiratory: Shortness of breath

<1%: Increased libido, weight loss

**Drug Interactions** No data reported

**Usual Dosage**

Endometriosis: Adults: Female: 1 spray (200 mcg) in 1 nostril each morning and the other nostril each evening starting on days 2-4 of menstrual cycle for 6 months

Central precocious puberty: Children: Males/Females: 2 sprays (400 mcg) into each nostril in the morning 2 sprays (400 mcg) into each nostril in the evening. If inadequate suppression, may increase dose to 3 sprays (600 mcg) into alternating nostrils 3 times/day.

**Patient Information** You will begin this treatment between days 2-4 of your regular menstrual cycle. Use as directed - daily at the same time (arising and bedtime), and rotate nostrils. Maintain regular follow-up schedule. You may experience hot flashes, flushing or redness (cold clothes and cool environment may help), decreased or increased libido, emotional lability, weight gain, decreased breast size, or hirsutism. Report any breakthrough bleeding or continuing menstruation or musculoskeletal pain. Do not use a nasal decongestant within 30 minutes after nafarelin.

**Nursing Implications** Do not administer to pregnant or breast-feeding patients; topical nasal decongestant should be used at least 30 minutes after nafarelin use

**Dosage Forms** Solution, nasal, as acetate: 2 mg/mL (10 mL)

♦ **Nafazair® Ophthalmic** *see* Naphazoline *on page 383*

♦ **Nafcil™ Injection** *see* Nafcillin *on page 380*

## Nafcillin (naf SIL in)

**U.S. Brand Names** Nafcil™ Injection; Nallpen® Injection; Unipen® Injection; Unipen® Oral

**Synonyms** Ethoxynaphthamido Penicillin Sodium; Sodium Nafcillin

**Pharmacologic Category** Antibiotic, Penicillin

**Use** Treatment of infections such as osteomyelitis, septicemia, endocarditis, and CNS infections caused by susceptible strains of staphylococci species

**Effects on Mental Status** Penicillins reported to cause apprehension, illusions, hallucinations, depersonalization, agitation, insomnia, and encephalopathy

**Effects on Psychiatric Treatment** May cause neutropenia; use caution with clozapine and carbamazepine

**Pregnancy Risk Factor** B

**Contraindications** Hypersensitivity to nafcillin or any component or penicillins

**Warnings/Precautions** Extravasation of I.V. infusions should be avoided; modification of dosage is necessary in patients with both severe renal and hepatic impairment; elimination rate will be slow in neonates; use with caution in patients with cephalosporin hypersensitivity

**Adverse Reactions** Percentage unknown: Acute interstitial nephritis, diarrhea, fever, hypersensitivity reactions, nausea, neutropenia, oxacillin (less likely to cause phlebitis) is often preferred in pediatric patients, pain, rash, thrombophlebitis

**Overdosage/Toxicology**

Signs and symptoms: Neuromuscular hypersensitivity (agitation, hallucinations, asterixis, encephalopathy, confusion, and seizures) and electrolyte imbalance with potassium or sodium salts, especially in renal failure

Treatment: Hemodialysis may be helpful to aid in the removal of the drug from the blood, otherwise most treatment is supportive or symptom directed

**Drug Interactions**

Decreased effect: Efficacy of oral contraceptives may be reduced; warfarin/anticoagulants

Increased effect: Disulfiram, probenecid may increase penicillin levels

**Usual Dosage**

Neonates:

<2000 g, <7 days: 50 mg/kg/day divided every 12 hours

<2000 g, >7 days: 75 mg/kg/day divided every 8 hours

>2000 g, <7 days: 50 mg/kg/day divided every 8 hours

>2000 g, >7 days: 75 mg/kg/day divided every 6 hours

Children:

Oral: 25-50 mg/kg/day in 4 divided doses

I.M.: 25 mg/kg twice daily

I.V.:

Mild to moderate infections: 50-100 mg/kg/day in divided doses every 6 hours

Severe infections: 100-200 mg/kg/day in divided doses every 4-6 hours

Maximum dose: 12 g/day

Adults:

Oral: 250-500 mg (up to 1 g) every 4-6 hours

I.M.: 500 mg every 4-6 hours

I.V.: 500-2000 mg every 4-6 hours

**Dosing adjustment in renal impairment:** Not necessary

Dialysis: Not dialyzable (0% to 5%) via hemodialysis; supplemental dosage not necessary with hemo- or peritoneal dialysis or continuous arteriovenous or venovenous hemofiltration (CAVH/CAVHD)

**Patient Information** Oral: Take at regular intervals around-the-clock, preferably on and empty stomach with full glass of water. Take complete course of treatment as prescribed. You may experience nausea or vomiting; small frequent meals and good mouth care may help. If diabetic, drug may cause false tests with Clinitest® urine glucose monitoring; use of glucose oxidase methods (Clinistix®) or serum glucose monitoring is preferable. This drug may interfere with oral contraceptives; an alternate form of birth control should be used. Report persistent fever, sore throat, sores in mouth, diarrhea, unusual bleeding or bruising. Report difficulty breathing or skin rash. Notify prescriber if condition does not respond to treatment.

**Nursing Implications**

**Extravasation:** Use cold packs

Hyaluronidase (Wydase®): Add 1 mL NS to 150 unit vial to make 150 units/mL of concentration; mix 0.1 mL of above with 0.9 mL NS in 1 mL syringe to make final concentration = 15 units/mL

**Dosage Forms**

Capsule, as sodium: 250 mg

Powder for injection, as sodium: 500 mg, 1 g, 2 g, 4 g, 10 g

Solution, as sodium: 250 mg/5 mL (100 mL)

Tablet, as sodium: 500 mg

## Naftifine (NAF ti feen)

**U.S. Brand Names** Naftin®

**Pharmacologic Category** Antifungal Agent, Topical

**Use** Topical treatment of tinea cruris (jock itch), tinea corporis (ringworm), and tinea pedis (athlete's foot)

**Effects on Mental Status** None reported

**Effects on Psychiatric Treatment** None reported

**Usual Dosage** Adults: Topical: Apply cream once daily and gel twice daily (morning and evening) for up to 4 weeks

**Dosage Forms**

Cream, as hydrochloride: 1% (15 g, 30 g, 60 g)

Gel, topical, as hydrochloride: 1% (20 g, 40 g, 60 g)

♦ **Naftin®** *see* Naftifine *on page 380*

♦ **$NaHCO_3$** *see* Sodium Bicarbonate *on page 514*

## Nalbuphine (NAL byoo feen)

**Related Information**

Narcotic Agonists Comparison Chart *on page 720*

**U.S. Brand Names** Nubain®

**Pharmacologic Category** Analgesic, Narcotic

**Use** Relief of moderate to severe pain; preoperative analgesia, postoperative and surgical anesthesia, and obstetrical analgesia during labor and delivery

**Effects on Mental Status** Drowsiness is common; may cause dizziness; may rarely cause restlessness, nervousness, confusion, depression, or hallucinations

**Effects on Psychiatric Treatment** Concurrent use with psychotropic may produce additive sedation

**Pregnancy Risk Factor** B (D if used for prolonged periods or in high doses at term)

**Contraindications** Hypersensitivity to nalbuphine or any component, including sulfites

**Warnings/Precautions** Use with caution in patients with recent myocardial infarction, biliary tract surgery, or sulfite sensitivity; may produce respiratory depression; use with caution in women delivering premature infants; use with caution in patients with a history of drug dependence, head trauma or increased intracranial pressure, decreased hepatic or renal function, or pregnancy; tolerance or drug dependence may result from extended use

**Adverse Reactions**

>10%:

Central nervous system: Drowsiness, CNS depression, narcotic withdrawal

Miscellaneous: Histamine release

1% to 10%:

Cardiovascular: Hypotension, flushing

Central nervous system: Dizziness, headache

Dermatologic: Urticaria, rash

Gastrointestinal: Nausea, vomiting, anorexia, xerostomia

Local: Pain at injection site

Neuromuscular & skeletal: Weakness

Respiratory: Pulmonary edema

<1%: Biliary spasm, blurred vision, confusion, decreased urination, hallucinations, hypertension, insomnia, GI irritation, mental depression, nervousness, nightmares, paradoxical CNS stimulation, respiratory depression, restlessness, shortness of breath, tachycardia, toxic megacolon, ureteral spasm

**Overdosage/Toxicology**

Signs and symptoms: CNS depression, respiratory depression, miosis, hypotension, bradycardia

Treatment: Includes support of the patient's airway, establishment of an I.V. line and administration of naloxone 2 mg I.V. (0.01 mg/kg for children) with repeat administration as necessary up to a total of 10 mg.

**Drug Interactions** Increased toxicity: Barbiturate anesthetics may increase CNS depression

**Usual Dosage** I.M., I.V., S.C.:

Children 10 months to 14 years: Premedication: 0.2 mg/kg; maximum: 20 mg/dose

Adults: 10 mg/70 kg every 3-6 hours; maximum single dose: 20 mg; maximum daily dose: 160 mg

**Dosing adjustment/comments in hepatic impairment:** Use with caution and reduce dose

**Dietary Considerations** Alcohol: Additive CNS effects, avoid or limit alcohol; watch for sedation

**Patient Information** If self-administered, use exactly as directed (do not increase dose or frequency); may cause physical and/or psychological dependence. While using this medication, do not use alcohol and other prescription or OTC medications (especially sedatives, tranquilizers, antihistamines, or pain medications) without consulting prescriber. Maintain adequate hydration (2-3 L/day of fluids unless instructed to restrict fluid intake). May cause hypotension, dizziness, drowsiness, impaired coordination, or blurred vision (use caution when driving, climbing stairs, or changing position - rising from sitting or lying to standing, or when engaging in tasks requiring alertness until response to drug is known); loss of appetite, nausea, or vomiting (frequent mouth care, small frequent meals, chewing gum, or sucking lozenges may help); constipation (increased exercise, fluids, or dietary fruit and fiber may help - if constipation remains an unresolved problem, consult prescriber about use of stool softeners). Report chest pain, slow or rapid heartbeat, acute dizziness or persistent headache; changes in mental status; swelling of extremities or unusual weight gain; changes in urinary elimination or pain on urination; acute headache; back or flank pain or muscle spasms; blurred vision; skin rash; or shortness of breath.

**Nursing Implications** Observe patient for excessive sedation, respiratory depression, implement safety measures, assist with ambulation; observe for narcotic withdrawal

**Dosage Forms** Injection, as hydrochloride: 10 mg/mL (1 mL, 10 mL); 20 mg/mL (1 mL, 10 mL)


- ♦ **Naldecol®** *see* Carbinoxamine *on page 92*
- ♦ **Naldecon®** *see* Chlorpheniramine, Phenyltoloxamine, Phenylpropanolamine, and Phenylephrine *on page 116*
- ♦ **Naldecon® DX Adult Liquid [OTC]** *see* Guaifenesin, Phenylpropanolamine, and Dextromethorphan *on page 258*
- ♦ **Naldecon-EX® Children's Syrup [OTC]** *see* Guaifenesin and Phenylpropanolamine *on page 257*
- ♦ **Naldecon® Senior DX [OTC]** *see* Guaifenesin and Dextromethorphan *on page 257*
- ♦ **Naldecon® Senior EX [OTC]** *see* Guaifenesin *on page 256*
- ♦ **Naldelate®** *see* Chlorpheniramine, Phenyltoloxamine, Phenylpropanolamine, and Phenylephrine *on page 116*
- ♦ **Nalfon®** *see* Fenoprofen *on page 221*
- ♦ **Nalgest®** *see* Chlorpheniramine, Phenyltoloxamine, Phenylpropanolamine, and Phenylephrine *on page 116*


## Nalidixic Acid (nal i DIKS ik AS id)

**U.S. Brand Names** NegGram®

**Synonyms** Nalidixinic Acid

**Pharmacologic Category** Antibiotic, Quinolone

**Use** Treatment of urinary tract infections

**Effects on Mental Status** Dizziness and drowsiness are common; may rarely cause confusion or psychosis

**Effects on Psychiatric Treatment** May rarely cause leukopenia; use caution with clozapine and carbamazepine

**Pregnancy Risk Factor** B

**Contraindications** Hypersensitivity to nalidixic acid or any component; infants <3 months of age

**Warnings/Precautions** Use with caution in patients with impaired hepatic or renal function and prepubertal children; has been shown to cause cartilage degeneration in immature animals; may induce hemolysis in patients with G-6-PD deficiency; use caution in patients with seizure disorder. Quinolones have been associated with tendonitis and tendon rupture (discontinue at first signs or symptoms of tendon pain).

**Adverse Reactions**

>10%: Central nervous system: Dizziness, drowsiness, headache

1% to 10%: Gastrointestinal: Nausea, vomiting

<1%: Chills, confusion, convulsions, fever, hepatotoxicity, increased intracranial pressure, leukopenia, malaise, metabolic acidosis, photosensitivity reactions, rash, tendonitis/tendon rupture, thrombocytopenia, toxic psychosis, urticaria, vertigo, visual disturbances

**Overdosage/Toxicology**

Signs and symptoms: Nausea, vomiting, toxic psychosis, convulsions, increased intracranial pressure, metabolic acidosis; severe overdose, intracranial hypertension, increased pressure, and seizures have occurred

Treatment: After GI decontamination, treatment is symptomatic

**Drug Interactions**

Decreased effect with antacids containing magnesium, aluminum, or calcium, sucralfate, metal ions an didanosine; avoid by 2 hours

Increased effect of warfarin

**Usual Dosage** Oral:

Children 3 months to 12 years: 55 mg/kg/day divided every 6 hours; suppressive therapy is 33 mg/kg/day divided every 6 hours

Adults: 1 g 4 times/day for 2 weeks; then suppressive therapy of 500 mg 4 times/day

**Dosing comments in renal impairment:** $Cl_{cr}$ <50 mL/minute: Avoid use

**Patient Information** Avoid undue exposure to direct sunlight or use a sunscreen; take 1 hour before meals, but can take with food to decrease GI upset, finish all medication, do not skip doses; if persistent cough occurs, notify physician. Antacids containing calcium, magnesium or aluminum; sucralfate; minerals; multivitamin with zinc; or didanosine should not be taken within 2 hours of nalidixic acid. Report immediately any pain, inflammation, or rupture of tendon.

**Dosage Forms**

Suspension, oral (raspberry flavor): 250 mg/5 mL (473 mL)

Tablet: 250 mg, 500 mg, 1 g


- ♦ **Nalidixinic Acid** *see* Nalidixic Acid *on page 381*
- ♦ **Nallpen® Injection** *see* Nafcillin *on page 380*
- ♦ ***N*-allylnoroxymorphine Hydrochloride** *see* Naloxone *on page 382*


## Nalmefene (NAL me feen)

**Related Information**

Substance-Related Disorders *on page 609*

**U.S. Brand Names** Revex®

**Pharmacologic Category** Antidote

**Use** Complete or partial reversal of opioid drug effects, including respiratory depression induced by natural or synthetic opioids; reversal of postoperative opioid depression; management of known or suspected opioid overdose

**Pregnancy Risk Factor** B

**Contraindications** Hypersensitivity to nalmefene, naltrexone, or components

**Warnings/Precautions** May induce symptoms of acute withdrawal in opioid-dependent patients; recurrence of respiratory depression is possible if the opioid involved is long-acting; observe patients until there is no reasonable risk of recurrent respiratory depression. Safety and efficacy have not been established in children. Avoid abrupt reversal of opioid effects in patients of high cardiovascular risk or who have received potentially cardiotoxic drugs. Animal studies indicate nalmefene may not completely reverse buprenorphine-induced respiratory depression.

**Adverse Reactions**

>10%: Gastrointestinal: Nausea

1% to 10%:

Cardiovascular: Tachycardia, hypertension, hypotension, vasodilation

Central nervous system: Fever, dizziness, headache, chills

(Continued)

## Nalmefene *(Continued)*

Gastrointestinal: Vomiting

Miscellaneous: Postoperative pain

<1%: Agitation, arrhythmia, bradycardia, confusion, depression, diarrhea, myoclonus, nervousness, pharyngitis, pruritus, somnolence, tremor, urinary retention, xerostomia

**Overdosage/Toxicology** Signs and symptoms: No known symptoms in significant overdose; large doses of opioids administered to overcome a full blockade of opioid antagonists, however, has resulted in adverse respiratory and circulatory reactions

**Drug Interactions**

Flumazenil: May increase the risk of toxicity with flumazenil. An increased risk of seizures has been associated with flumazenil and nalmefene coadministration

Narcotic analgesics: Decreased effect of narcotic analgesics; may precipitate acute withdrawal reaction in physically dependent patients

**Mechanism of Action** As a 6-methylene analog of naltrexone, nalmefene acts as a competitive antagonist at opioid receptor sites, preventing or reversing the respiratory depression, sedation, and hypotension induced by opiates; no pharmacologic activity of its own (eg, opioid agonist activity) has been demonstrated

**Pharmacodynamics/kinetics**

Onset of action: I.M., S.C.: 5-15 minutes

Distribution: $V_d$: 8.6 L/kg; rapid

Protein binding: 45%

Metabolism: Hepatic by glucuronide conjugation to metabolites with little or no activity

Bioavailability: I.M., I.V., S.C.: 100%

$T_{max}$: I.M.: 2.3 hours; I.V.: <2 minutes; S.C.: 1.5 hours

Half-life: 10.8 hours

Time to peak serum concentration: 2.3 hours

Elimination: <5% excreted unchanged in urine, 17% in feces; clearance: 0.8 L/hour/kg

**Usual Dosage**

Reversal of postoperative opioid depression: Blue labeled product (100 mcg/mL): Titrate to reverse the undesired effects of opioids; initial dose for nonopioid dependent patients: 0.25 mcg/kg followed by 0.25 mcg/kg incremental doses at 2- to 5-minute intervals; after a total dose >1 mcg/kg, further therapeutic response is unlikely

Management of known/suspected opioid overdose: Green labeled product (1000 mcg/mL): Initial dose: 0.5 mg/70 kg; may repeat with 1 mg/70 kg in 2-5 minutes; further increase beyond a total dose of 1.5 mg/70 kg will not likely result in improved response and may result in cardiovascular stress and precipitated withdrawal syndrome. (If opioid dependency is suspected, administer a challenge dose of 0.1 mg/70 kg; if no withdrawal symptoms are observed in 2 minutes, the recommended doses can be administered.)

**Dosing adjustment in renal or hepatic impairment:** Not necessary with single uses, however, slow administration (over 60 seconds) of incremental doses is recommended to minimize hypertension and dizziness

**Nursing Implications** Check dosage strength carefully before use to avoid error; monitor patients for signs of withdrawal, especially those physically dependent who are in pain or at high cardiovascular risk

**Additional Information** Proper steps should be used to prevent use of the incorrect dosage strength; the goal of treatment in the postoperative setting is to achieve reversal of excessive opioid effects without inducing a complete reversal and acute pain

If opioid dependence is suspected, nalmefene should only be used in opioid overdose if the likelihood of overdose is high based on history or the clinical presentation of respiratory depression with concurrent pupillary constriction is present

**Dosage Forms** Injection, as hydrochloride: 100 mcg/mL [blue label] (1 mL); 1000 mcg/mL [green label] (2 mL)

---

## Naloxone (nal OKS one)

**Related Information**

Narcotic Agonists Comparison Chart *on page 720*

Special Populations - Elderly *on page 662*

Substance-Related Disorders *on page 609*

**U.S. Brand Names** Narcan® Injection

**Synonyms** *N*-allylnoroxymorphine Hydrochloride; Naloxone Hydrochloride

**Pharmacologic Category** Antidote

**Use**

Complete or partial reversal of opioid depression, including respiratory depression, induced by natural and synthetic opioids, including propoxyphene, methadone, and certain mixed agonist-antagonist analgesics: nalbuphine, pentazocine, and butorphanol

Diagnosis of suspected opioid tolerance or acute opioid overdose

Adjunctive agent to increase blood pressure in the management of septic shock

**Unlabeled use:** PCP and alcohol ingestion

**Pregnancy Risk Factor** B

**Contraindications** Hypersensitivity to naloxone or any component

**Warnings/Precautions** Due to an association between naloxone and acute pulmonary edema, use with caution in patients with cardiovascular disease or in patients receiving medications with potential adverse cardiovascular effects (eg, hypotension, pulmonary edema or arrhythmias). Excessive dosages should be avoided after use of opiates in surgery, because naloxone may cause an increase in blood pressure and reversal of anesthesia; may precipitate withdrawal symptoms in patients addicted to opiates, including pain, hypertension, sweating, agitation, irritability; in neonates: shrill cry, failure to feed. Recurrence of respiratory depression is possible if the opioid involved is long-acting; observe patients until there is no reasonable risk of recurrent respiratory depression.

**Adverse Reactions**

Cardiovascular: Hypertension, hypotension, tachycardia, ventricular arrhythmias, cardiac arrest

Central nervous system: Irritability, anxiety, narcotic withdrawal, restlessness, seizures

Gastrointestinal: Nausea, vomiting, diarrhea

Neuromuscular & skeletal: Tremulousness

Respiratory: Dyspnea, pulmonary edema, runny nose, sneezing

Miscellaneous: Diaphoresis

**Overdosage/Toxicology** Treatment: Naloxone is the drug of choice for respiratory depression that is known or suspected to be caused by an overdose of an opiate or opioid

**Caution:** Naloxone's effects are due to its action on narcotic reversal, not due to any direct effect upon opiate receptors. Therefore, adverse events occur secondarily to reversal (withdrawal) of narcotic analgesia and sedation, which can cause severe reactions.

**Drug Interactions** Narcotic analgesics: Decreased effect of narcotic analgesics; may precipitate acute withdrawal reaction in physically dependent patients

**Stability** Protect from light; stable in 0.9% sodium chloride and $D_5W$ at 4 mcg/mL for 24 hours; do not mix with alkaline solutions

**Mechanism of Action** Pure opioid antagonist that competes and displaces narcotics at opioid receptor sites

**Pharmacodynamics/kinetics**

Onset of effect:

Endotracheal, I.M., S.C.: Within 2-5 minutes

I.V.: Within 2 minutes

Duration: 20-60 minutes; since shorter than that of most opioids, repeated doses are usually needed

Distribution: Crosses the placenta

Metabolism: Primarily by glucuronidation in the liver

Half-life:

Neonates: 1.2-3 hours

Adults: 1-1.5 hours

Elimination: In urine as metabolites

**Usual Dosage** I.M., I.V. (preferred), intratracheal, S.C.:

Postanesthesia narcotic reversal: Infants and Children: 0.01 mg/kg; may repeat every 2-3 minutes as needed based on response

Opiate intoxication:

Birth (including premature infants) to 5 years or <20 kg: 0.1 mg/kg; repeat every 2-3 minutes if needed; may need to repeat doses every 20-60 minutes

>5 years or ≥20 kg: 2 mg/dose; if no response, repeat every 2-3 minutes; may need to repeat doses every 20-60 minutes

Continuous infusion: I.V.: Children and Adults: If continuous infusion is required, calculate dosage/hour based on effective intermittent dose used and duration of adequate response seen, titrate dose 0.04-0.16 mg/kg/hour for 2-5 days in children, up to 0.8 mg/kg/hour in adults; alternatively, continuous infusion utilizes $^2/_3$ of the initial naloxone bolus on an hourly basis; add 10 times this dose to each liter of $D_5W$ and infuse at a rate of 100 mL/hour; $^1/_2$ of the initial bolus dose should be readministered 15 minutes after initiation of the continuous infusion to prevent a drop in naloxone levels; increase infusion rate as needed to assure adequate ventilation

Narcotic overdose: Adults: I.V.: 0.4-2 mg every 2-3 minutes as needed; may need to repeat doses every 20-60 minutes, if no response is observed after 10 mg, question the diagnosis. **Note:** Use 0.1-0.2 mg increments in patients who are opioid dependent and in postoperative patients to avoid large cardiovascular changes.

**Monitoring Parameters** Respiratory rate, heart rate, blood pressure

**Test Interactions** Will not give a false-positive enzymatic urine screen for opiates

**Nursing Implications** The use of neonatal naloxone (0.02 mg/mL) is no longer recommended because unacceptable fluid volumes will result, especially to small neonates; the 0.4 mg/mL preparation is available and can be accurately dosed with appropriately sized syringes (1 mL)

**Additional Information** May contain methyl and propylparabens

**Dosage Forms**

Injection, as hydrochloride: 0.4 mg/mL (1 mL, 2 mL, 10 mL); 1 mg/mL (2 mL, 10 mL)

Injection, neonatal, as hydrochloride: 0.02 mg/mL (2 mL)

♦ **Naloxone Hydrochloride** *see* Naloxone *on page 382*

◆ **Nalspan®** *see* Chlorpheniramine, Phenyltoloxamine, Phenylpropanolamine, and Phenylephrine *on page 116*

## Naltrexone (nal TREKS one)

**Related Information**

Addiction Treatments *on page 772*

Substance-Related Disorders *on page 609*

**U.S. Brand Names** ReVia®

**Pharmacologic Category** Antidote

**Use** Treatment of alcohol dependence; blockade of the effects of exogenously administered opioids

**Pregnancy Risk Factor** C

**Contraindications** Known hypersensitivity to naltrexone; narcotic dependence or current use of opioid analgesics; acute opioid withdrawal; failure to pass Narcan® challenge or positive urine screen for opioids; acute hepatitis or liver failure

**Warnings/Precautions** Dose-related hepatocellular injury is possible; the margin of separation between the apparent safe and hepatotoxic doses appear to be only fivefold or less. May precipitate withdrawal symptoms in patients addicted to opiates, including pain, hypertension, sweating, agitation, irritability; in neonates: shrill cry, failure to feed. Use with caution in patients with hepatic or renal impairment.

Patients who had been treated with naltrexone may respond to lower doses than previously used. This could result in potentially life-threatening opioid intoxication. Patients should be aware that they may be more sensitive to lower doses of opioids after naltrexone treatment is discontinued. Use of naltrexone does not eliminate or diminish withdrawal symptoms.

**Adverse Reactions**

>10%:

Central nervous system: Insomnia, nervousness, headache, low energy

Gastrointestinal: Abdominal cramping, nausea, vomiting

Neuromuscular & skeletal: Arthralgia

1% to 10%:

Central nervous system: Increased energy, feeling down, irritability, dizziness, anxiety, somnolence

Dermatologic: Rash

Endocrine & metabolic: Polydipsia

Gastrointestinal: Diarrhea, constipation

Genitourinary: Delayed ejaculation, impotency

<1%: Bad dreams, blurred vision, confusion, depression, disorientation, edema, fatigue, hallucinations, increased blood pressure, itching rhinorrhea, narcotic withdrawal, nasal congestion, nightmares, palpitations, paranoia, restlessness, sneezing, suicide attempts, tachycardia

**Overdosage/Toxicology** Signs and symptoms: Clonic-tonic convulsions, respiratory failure; patients receiving up to 800 mg/day for 1 week have shown no toxicity; seizures and respiratory failure have been seen in animals

**Drug Interactions**

Narcotic analgesics: Decreased effect of narcotic analgesics; may precipitate acute withdrawal reaction in physically dependent patients; concurrent use is contraindicated

Thioridazine: Lethargy and somnolence have been reported with the combination of naltrexone and thioridazine

**Mechanism of Action** Naltrexone (a pure opioid antagonist) is a cyclopropyl derivative of oxymorphone similar in structure to naloxone and nalorphine (a morphine derivative); it acts as a competitive antagonist at opioid receptor sites

**Pharmacodynamics/kinetics**

Duration of action:

50 mg: 24 hours

100 mg: 48 hours

150 mg: 72 hours

Absorption: Oral: Almost completely

Distribution: $V_d$: 19 L/kg; distributed widely throughout the body but considerable interindividual variation exists

Protein binding: 21%

Metabolism: Undergoes extensive first-pass metabolism to 6-β-naltrexol

Half-life: 4 hours; 6-β-naltrexol: 13 hours

Time to peak serum concentration: Within 60 minutes

Elimination: Principally in urine as metabolites and unchanged drug

**Usual Dosage** Do not give until patient is opioid-free for 7-10 days as determined by urine analysis

Adults: Oral: 25 mg; if no withdrawal signs within 1 hour give another 25 mg; maintenance regimen is flexible, variable and individualized (50 mg/day to 100-150 mg 3 times/week for 12 weeks)

**Dosing cautions in renal/hepatic impairment:** Caution in patients with renal and hepatic impairment. An increase in naltrexone AUC of approximately 5- and 10-fold in patients with compensated or decompensated liver cirrhosis respectively, compared with normal liver function has been reported.

**Monitoring Parameters** For narcotic withdrawal; liver function tests

**Reference Range** Peak plasma naltrexone level after a 100 mg oral dose: 44 μg/L

**Test Interactions** Elevates gonadotropin, serum cortisol

**Patient Information** Will cause narcotic withdrawal; serious overdose can occur after attempts to overcome the blocking effect of naltrexone

**Nursing Implications** Monitor for narcotic withdrawal

**Additional Information** Up to 800 mg/day has been tolerated in adults without an adverse effect

**Dosage Forms** Tablet, as hydrochloride: 50 mg

## Nandrolone (NAN droe lone)

**U.S. Brand Names** Anabolin® Injection; Androlone®-D Injection; Androlone® Injection; Deca-Durabolin® Injection; Hybolin™ Decanoate Injection; Hybolin™ Improved Injection; Neo-Durabolic Injection

**Pharmacologic Category** Androgen

**Use** Control of metastatic breast cancer; management of anemia of renal insufficiency

**Effects on Mental Status** May cause insomnia

**Effects on Psychiatric Treatment** None reported

**Restrictions** C-III

**Usual Dosage** Deep I.M. (into gluteal muscle):

Children 2-13 years: (decanoate): 25-50 mg every 3-4 weeks

Adults:

Male:

Breast cancer (phenpropionate): 50-100 mg/week

Anemia of renal insufficiency (decanoate): 100-200 mg/week

Female: 50-100 mg/week

Breast cancer (phenpropionate): 50-100 mg/week

Anemia of renal insufficiency (decanoate): 50-100 mg/week

**Dosage Forms**

Injection, as phenpropionate, in oil: 25 mg/mL (5 mL); 50 mg/mL (2 mL)

Injection, as decanoate, in oil: 50 mg/mL (1 mL, 2 mL); 100 mg/mL (1 mL, 2 mL); 200 mg/mL (1 mL)

Injection, repository, as decanoate: 50 mg/mL (2 mL); 100 mg/mL (2 mL); 200 mg/mL (2 mL)

## Naphazoline (naf AZ oh leen)

**U.S. Brand Names** AK-Con® Ophthalmic; Albalon® Liquifilm® Ophthalmic; Allerest® Eye Drops [OTC]; Clear Eyes® [OTC]; Comfort® Ophthalmic [OTC]; Degest® 2 Ophthalmic [OTC]; Estivin® II Ophthalmic [OTC]; I-Naphline® Ophthalmic; Nafazair® Ophthalmic; Naphcon Forte® Ophthalmic; Naphcon® Ophthalmic [OTC]; Opcon® Ophthalmic; Privine® Nasal [OTC]; VasoClear® Ophthalmic [OTC]; Vasocon Regular® Ophthalmic

**Canadian Brand Names** Red Away®

**Pharmacologic Category** Alpha$_1$ Agonist; Ophthalmic Agent, Vasoconstrictor

**Use** Topical ocular vasoconstrictor; will temporarily relieve congestion, itching, and minor irritation, and to control hyperemia in patients with superficial corneal vascularity; treatment of nasal congestion; adjunct for sinusitis

**Effects on Mental Status** May cause nervousness or dizziness

**Effects on Psychiatric Treatment** TCAs and MAOIs may potentiate the pressor response of decongestants; monitor for changes in response

**Usual Dosage**

Nasal:

Children:

<6 years: Intranasal: Not recommended (especially infants) due to CNS depression

6-12 years: 1 spray of 0.05% into each nostril every 6 hours if necessary; therapy should not exceed 3-5 days

Children >12 years and Adults: 0.05%, instill 1-2 drops or sprays every 6 hours if needed; therapy should not exceed 3-5 days

Ophthalmic:

Children <6 years: Not recommended for use due to CNS depression (especially in infants)

Children >6 years and Adults: Instill 1-2 drops into conjunctival sac of affected eye(s) every 3-4 hours; therapy generally should not exceed 3-4 days

**Dosage Forms** Solution, as hydrochloride:

Nasal:

Drops: 0.05% (20 mL)

Spray: 0.05% (15 mL)

Ophthalmic: 0.012% (7.5 mL, 30 mL); 0.02% (15 mL); 0.03% (15 mL); 0.1% (15 mL)

## Naphazoline and Antazoline

(naf AZ oh leen & an TAZ oh leen)

**U.S. Brand Names** Albalon-A® Ophthalmic; Antazoline-V® Ophthalmic; Vasocon-A® [OTC] Ophthalmic

**Pharmacologic Category** Ophthalmic Agent, Vasoconstrictor

**Use** Topical ocular congestion, irritation and itching

**Effects on Mental Status** May cause nervousness or dizziness

(Continued)

## Naphazoline and Antazoline *(Continued)*

**Effects on Psychiatric Treatment** TCAs and MAOIs may potentiate the pressor response of decongestants; monitor for changes in response

**Usual Dosage** 1-2 drops every 3-4 hours

**Dosage Forms** Solution: Naphazoline hydrochloride 0.05% and antazoline phosphate 0.5% (15 mL)

## Naphazoline and Pheniramine

(naf AZ oh leen & fen NIR a meen)

**U.S. Brand Names** Naphcon®-A Ophthalmic [OTC]

**Canadian Brand Names** Opcon-A®

**Pharmacologic Category** Ophthalmic Agent, Vasoconstrictor

**Use** Topical ocular vasoconstrictor

**Effects on Mental Status** May cause nervousness or dizziness

**Effects on Psychiatric Treatment** TCAs and MAOIs may potentiate the pressor response of decongestants; monitor for changes in response

**Usual Dosage** 1-2 drops every 3-4 hours

**Dosage Forms** Solution, ophthalmic: Naphazoline hydrochloride 0.025% and pheniramine 0.3% (15 mL)

- **Naphcon®-A Ophthalmic [OTC]** *see* Naphazoline and Pheniramine *on page 384*
- **Naphcon Forte® Ophthalmic** *see* Naphazoline *on page 383*
- **Naphcon® Ophthalmic [OTC]** *see* Naphazoline *on page 383*
- **Naprelan®** *see* Naproxen *on page 384*
- **Naprosyn®** *see* Naproxen *on page 384*

## Naproxen (na PROKS en)

**Related Information**

Nonsteroidal Anti-inflammatory Agents Comparison Chart *on page 722*

**U.S. Brand Names** Aleve® [OTC]; Anaprox®; EC-Naprosyn®; Naprelan®; Naprosyn®

**Canadian Brand Names** Apo®-Naproxen; Naxen®; Novo-Naprox; Nu-Naprox

**Pharmacologic Category** Nonsteroidal Anti-Inflammatory Agent (NSAID)

**Use** Management of inflammatory disease and rheumatoid disorders (including juvenile rheumatoid arthritis); acute gout; mild to moderate pain; dysmenorrhea; fever, migraine headache

**Effects on Mental Status** Dizziness is common; may cause nervousness; may rarely cause drowsiness, confusion, insomnia, depression, or hallucinations

**Effects on Psychiatric Treatment** May rarely cause agranulocytosis; use caution with clozapine and carbamazepine; may decrease lithium clearance resulting in an increase in serum lithium levels and potential lithium toxicity; monitor serum lithium levels

**Pregnancy Risk Factor** B (D if used in the 3rd trimester or near delivery)

**Contraindications** Hypersensitivity to naproxen, aspirin, or other nonsteroidal anti-inflammatory drugs (NSAIDs)

**Warnings/Precautions** Use with caution in patients with GI disease (bleeding or ulcers), cardiovascular disease (CHF, hypertension), dehydration, renal or hepatic impairment, and patients receiving anticoagulants; perform ophthalmologic evaluation for those who develop eye complaints during therapy (blurred vision, diminished vision, changes in color vision, retinal changes); NSAIDs may mask signs/symptoms of infections; photosensitivity reported; elderly are at especially high-risk for adverse effects

**Adverse Reactions**

>10%:

Central nervous system: Dizziness

Dermatologic: Pruritus, rash

Gastrointestinal: Abdominal discomfort, nausea, heartburn, constipation, GI bleeding, ulcers, perforation, indigestion

1% to 10%:

Central nervous system: Headache, nervousness

Dermatologic: Itching

Endocrine & metabolic: Fluid retention

Gastrointestinal: Vomiting

Otic: Tinnitus

<1%: Acute renal failure, agranulocytosis, allergic rhinitis, anemia, angioedema, arrhythmias, aseptic meningitis, blurred vision, bone marrow suppression, confusion, congestive heart failure, conjunctivitis, cystitis, decreased hearing, drowsiness, dry eyes, edema, epistaxis, erythema multiforme, fatigue, gastritis, GI ulceration, hallucinations, hemolytic anemia, hepatitis, hot flashes, hypertension, inhibits platelet aggregation, insomnia, leukopenia, mental depression, peripheral neuropathy, polydipsia, polyuria, prolongs bleeding time, renal dysfunction, shortness of breath, Stevens-Johnson syndrome, tachycardia, thrombocytopenia, toxic amblyopia, toxic epidermal necrolysis, urticaria

**Overdosage/Toxicology**

Signs and symptoms: Drowsiness, heartburn, vomiting, CNS depression, leukocytosis, renal failure

Treatment: Management of a nonsteroidal anti-inflammatory drug (NSAID) intoxication is primarily supportive and symptomatic; fluid therapy is commonly effective in managing the hypotension that may occur following an acute NSAID overdose, except when this is due to an acute blood loss. Seizures tend to be very short-lived and often do not require drug treatment; although, recurrent seizures should be treated with I.V. diazepam; since many of the NSAIDs undergo enterohepatic cycling, multiple doses of charcoal may be needed to reduce the potential for delayed toxicities.

**Drug Interactions** CYP2C8, 2C9, and 2C18 enzyme substrate

ACE inhibitors: Effects may be reduced by NSAIDs; use lowest possible dose for shortest duration possible; monitor

Cholestyramine and colestipol: Absorption may be reduced by concurrent administration

Corticosteroids: May increase the risk of GI ulceration; use caution

Cyclosporine: Nephrotoxicity may be increased with concurrent NSAID use; monitor

CYP2C inhibitors: May increase NSAID concentrations. Inhibitors include amiodarone, cimetidine, fluvoxamine, metronidazole, omeprazole, sulfonamides, valproic acid, and zafirlukast.

Hydralazine: Antihypertensive effect may be decreased; avoid concurrent use

Lithium: Serum levels can be increased; avoid concurrent use if possible or monitor lithium levels and adjust dose. When NSAID is stopped, lithium may need adjustment again.

Loop diuretics: Therapeutic effects may be reduced by NSAIDs; avoid

Methotrexate: Toxicity may be increased by concurrent NSAID use; risk is limited in low-dose methotrexate regimens (such as for rheumatoid arthritis); prolonged leucovorin rescue may be required at antineoplastic doses; monitor

Thiazide diuretics: Antihypertensive effects are decreased; avoid concurrent use

Warfarin: INRs may be increased by some NSAIDs. This may depend, in part, on dose and duration; monitor INR closely. Use the lowest dose of NSAIDs possible and for the briefest duration.

**Usual Dosage** Oral:

Children >2 years:

Fever: 2.5-10 mg/kg/dose; maximum: 10 mg/kg/day

Juvenile arthritis: 10 mg/kg/day in 2 divided doses

Adults:

Rheumatoid arthritis, osteoarthritis, and ankylosing spondylitis: 500-1000 mg/day in 2 divided doses; may increase to 1.5 g/day of naproxen base for limited time period

Mild to moderate pain or dysmenorrhea: Initial: 500 mg, then 250 mg every 6-8 hours; maximum: 1250 mg/day naproxen base

**Dosing adjustment in hepatic impairment:** Reduce dose to 50%

**Dietary Considerations**

Alcohol: Additive impairment of mental alertness and physical coordination, avoid or limit use

Food: Food may decrease the rate but not the extent of oral absorption. Drug may cause GI upset, bleeding, ulceration, perforation; take with food or milk to minimize GI upset.

**Patient Information** Take this medication exactly as directed; do not increase dose without consulting prescriber. Do not crush tablets or break capsules. Take with food or milk to reduce GI distress. Maintain adequate fluid intake (2-3 L/day of fluids unless instructed to restrict fluid intake). Do not use alcohol, aspirin, or aspirin-containing medication, and all other anti-inflammatory medications without consulting prescriber. You may experience drowsiness, dizziness, lightheadedness, or headache (use caution when driving or engaging in tasks requiring alertness until response to drug is known); anorexia, nausea, vomiting, or heartburn (frequent small meals, frequent mouth care, sucking lozenges, or chewing gum may help); fluid retention (weigh yourself weekly and report unusual (3-5 lb/week) weight gain). GI bleeding, ulceration, or perforation can occur with or without pain; discontinue medication and contact prescriber if persistent abdominal pain or cramping, or blood in stool occurs. Report breathlessness, difficulty breathing, or unusual cough; chest pain, rapid heartbeat, palpitations; unusual bruising/bleeding; blood in urine, stool, mouth, or vomitus; swollen extremities; skin rash or itching; acute fatigue; or changes in eyesight (double vision, color changes, blurred vision), hearing, or ringing in ears.

**Dosage Forms**

Suspension, oral: 125 mg/5 mL (15 mL, 30 mL, 480 mL)

Tablet, as sodium:

220 mg (200 mg base)

Anaprox®: 220 mg (200 mg base); 275 mg (250 mg base); 550 mg (500 mg base)

Tablet:

Aleve®: 200 mg

Naprosyn®: 250 mg, 375 mg, 500 mg

Tablet, controlled release (Naprelan®): 375 mg, 500 mg

- **Naqua®** *see* Trichlormethiazide *on page 565*

## Naratriptan (NAR a trip tan)

**U.S. Brand Names** Amerge®
**Synonyms** Naratriptan Hydrochloride
**Pharmacologic Category** Serotonin 5-$HT_{1D}$ Receptor Agonist
**Use** Treatment of acute migraine headache with or without aura
**Effects on Mental Status** May cause drowsiness, dizziness, or fatigue; may rarely cause panic reactions or hallucinations
**Effects on Psychiatric Treatment** SSRIs may cause hyper-reflexia, weakness, or lack of coordination when used with naratriptan; these combinations should be avoided
**Pregnancy Risk Factor** C
**Contraindications** Hypersensitivity to naratriptan or any component; cerebrovascular, peripheral vascular disease (ischemic bowel disease), ischemic heart disease (angina pectoris, history of myocardial infarction, or proven silent ischemia); or in patients with symptoms consistent with ischemic heart disease, coronary artery vasospasm, or Prinzmetal's variant angina; uncontrolled hypertension or patients who have received within 24 hours another 5-HT agonist (sumatriptan, zolmitriptan) or ergotamine-containing product; patients with known risk factors associated with coronary artery disease; patients with severe hepatic or renal disease ($Cl_{cr}$ <15 mL/minute); do not administer naratriptan to patients with hemiplegic or basilar migraine
**Warnings/Precautions** Use only if there is a clear diagnosis of migraine. Patients who are at risk of CAD but have had a satisfactory cardiovascular evaluation may receive naratriptan but with extreme caution (ie, in a physician's office where there are adequate precautions in place to protect the patient). Blood pressure may increase with the administration of naratriptan. Monitor closely, especially with the first administration of the drug. If the patient does not respond to the first dose, re-evaluate the diagnosis of migraine before trying a second dose.
**Adverse Reactions**
1% to 10%:
Central nervous system: Dizziness, drowsiness, malaise/fatigue
Gastrointestinal: Nausea, vomiting
Neuromuscular & skeletal: Paresthesias
Miscellaneous: Pain or pressure in throat or neck
<1% (Limited to important or life-threatening symptoms): allergic reaction, atrial flutter/fibrillation), abnormal bilirubin tests, abnormal liver function tests, bradycardia, convulsions, coronary artery vasospasm, EKG changes (PR prolongation, $QT_c$ prolongation, premature ventricular contractions, eye hemorrhage, glycosuria, hallucinations, heart murmurs, hypercholesterolemia, hyperglycemia, hyperlipidemia, hypertension, hypotension, hypothyroidism, ketonuria, myocardial infarction, palpitations, panic, transient myocardial ischemia, ventricular fibrillation, ventricular tachycardia
**Drug Interactions**
Decreased effect: Smoking increases the clearance of naratriptan
Increased effect/toxicity: Ergot-containing drugs (dihydroergotamine or methysergide) may cause vasospastic reactions when taken with naratriptan. Avoid concomitant use with ergots; separate dose of naratriptan and ergots by at least 24 hours. Oral contraceptives taken with naratriptan reduced the clearance of naratriptan ~30% which may contribute to adverse effects. Selective serotonin reuptake inhibitors (SSRIs) (eg, fluoxetine, fluvoxamine, paroxetine, sertraline) may cause lack of coordination, hyper-reflexia, or weakness and should be avoided when taking naratriptan.
**Usual Dosage**
Adults: Oral: 1-2.5 mg at the onset of headache; it is recommended to use the lowest possible dose to minimize adverse effects. If headache returns or does not fully resolve, the dose may be repeated after 4 hours; do not exceed 5 mg in 24 hours.
Elderly: Not recommended for use in the elderly
**Dosing in renal impairment:**
$Cl_{cr}$: 18-39 mL/minute: Initial: 1 mg; do not exceed 2.5 mg in 24 hours
$Cl_{cr}$: <15 mL/minute: Do not use
**Dosing in hepatic impairment:** Contraindicated in patients with severe liver failure; maximum dose: 2.5 mg in 24 hours for patients with mild or moderate liver failure; recommended starting dose: 1 mg
**Patient Information** This drug is to be used to reduce your migraine, not to prevent or reduce the number of attacks. If headache returns or is not fully resolved, the dose may be repeated after 4 hours. If you have no relief with first dose, do not take a second dose without consulting prescriber. **Do not exceed 5 mg in 24 hours. Do not take within 24 hours of any other migraine medication without first consulting prescriber.** You may experience some dizziness, fatigue, or drowsiness; use caution when driving or engaging in tasks that require alertness until response to drug is known. Frequent mouth care and sucking on lozenges may relieve dry mouth. Report immediately any chest pain, heart throbbing, tightness in throat, skin rash or hives, hallucinations, anxiety, or panic.
**Dosage Forms** Tablet: 1 mg, 2.5 mg


- ♦ **Naratriptan Hydrochloride** *see* Naratriptan *on page 385*
- ♦ **Narcan® Injection** *see* Naloxone *on page 382*
- ♦ **Narcotic Agonists Comparison Chart** *see page 720*
- ♦ **Nardil®** *see* Phenelzine *on page 434*
- ♦ **Nasabid™** *see* Guaifenesin and Pseudoephedrine *on page 257*
- ♦ **Nasacort®** *see* Triamcinolone *on page 563*
- ♦ **Nasacort® AQ** *see* Triamcinolone *on page 563*
- ♦ **Nasahist B®** *see* Brompheniramine *on page 73*
- ♦ **Nasalcrom® Nasal Solution [OTC]** *see* Cromolyn Sodium *on page 142*
- ♦ **Nasalide® Nasal Aerosol** *see* Flunisolide *on page 230*
- ♦ **Nasarel® Nasal Spray** *see* Flunisolide *on page 230*
- ♦ **Nascobal®** *see* Cyanocobalamin *on page 143*
- ♦ **Nasonex®** *see* Mometasone *on page 373*
- ♦ **Natacyn®** *see* Natamycin *on page 385*


## Natamycin (na ta MYE sin)

**U.S. Brand Names** Natacyn®
**Pharmacologic Category** Antifungal Agent, Ophthalmic
**Use** Treatment of blepharitis, conjunctivitis, and keratitis caused by susceptible fungi (*Aspergillus*, *Candida*), *Cephalosporium*, *Curvularia*, *Fusarium*, *Penicillium*, *Microsporum*, *Epidermophyton*, *Blastomyces dermatitidis*, *Coccidioides immitis*, *Cryptococcus neoformans*, *Histoplasma capsulatum*, *Sporothrix schenckii*, and *Trichomonas vaginalis*
**Effects on Mental Status** None reported
**Effects on Psychiatric Treatment** None reported
**Usual Dosage** Adults: Ophthalmic: Instill 1 drop in conjunctival sac every 1-2 hours, after 3-4 days reduce to one drop 6-8 times/day; usual course of therapy is 2-3 weeks.
**Dosage Forms** Suspension, ophthalmic: 5% (15 mL)


- ♦ **Natural/Herbal Products** *see page 746*
- ♦ **Natural Products, Herbals, and Dietary Supplements** *see page 742*
- ♦ **Nature's Tears® Solution [OTC]** *see* Artificial Tears *on page 48*
- ♦ **Naturetin®** *see* Bendroflumethiazide *on page 61*
- ♦ **Navane®** *see* Thiothixene *on page 545*
- ♦ **Navelbine®** *see* Vinorelbine *on page 585*
- ♦ **ND-Stat®** *see* Brompheniramine *on page 73*
- ♦ **Nebcin® Injection** *see* Tobramycin *on page 551*
- ♦ **NebuPent™ Inhalation** *see* Pentamidine *on page 427*
- ♦ **Nectar of the Gods** *see* Garlic *on page 246*


## Nedocromil (ne doe KROE mil)

**Related Information**
Asthma Guidelines *on page 773*
**U.S. Brand Names** Alocril™; Tilade® Inhalation Aerosol
**Canadian Brand Names** Mireze®
**Pharmacologic Category** Antihistamine, Inhalation
**Use** Maintenance therapy in patients with mild to moderate bronchial asthma
**Effects on Mental Status** May cause dizziness or drowsiness
**Effects on Psychiatric Treatment** None reported
**Pregnancy Risk Factor** B
**Contraindications** Hypersensitivity to nedocromil or other ingredients in the preparation
**Warnings/Precautions** Safety and efficacy in children <12 years of age have not been established; if systemic or inhaled steroid therapy is at all reduced, monitor patients carefully; nedocromil is **not** a bronchodilator and, therefore, should not be used for reversal of acute bronchospasm
**Adverse Reactions** 1% to 10%:
Cardiovascular: Chest pain
Central nervous system: Dizziness, dysphonia, headache, fatigue
Dermatologic: Rash
Gastrointestinal: Nausea, vomiting, dyspepsia, diarrhea, abdominal pain, xerostomia, unpleasant taste
Hepatic: Increased ALT
Neuromuscular & skeletal: Arthritis, tremor
Respiratory: Cough, pharyngitis, rhinitis, bronchitis, upper respiratory infection, bronchospasm, increased sputum production
**Usual Dosage**
Inhalation: Children >12 years and Adults: 2 inhalations 4 times/day; may reduce dosage to 2-3 times/day once desired clinical response to initial dose is observed
Ophthalmic: 1-2 drops in each eye
**Patient Information** Do not use during acute bronchospasm. Use exactly as directed; do not use more often than instructed or discontinue without
(Continued)

## Nedocromil *(Continued)*

consulting prescriber. You may experience drowsiness, dizziness, fatigue, especially during early therapy (use caution when driving or engaging in tasks requiring alertness until response to drug is known); dry mouth, nausea, or vomiting (small frequent meals, frequent mouth care, chewing gum, or sucking lozenges may help). Report persistent runny nose, cough, cold symptoms; unresolved gastrointestinal effects; skin rash; joint pain or tremor; or if breathing difficulty persists or worsens.

Use: Review use of inhalator with prescriber or follow package insert for directions. Prime with three activations prior to first use or if unused more than 7 days. Keep inhalator clean and unobstructed. Always rinse mouth and throat after use of inhaler to prevent advantageous infection. If you are also using a steroid bronchodilator, wait 10 minutes before using this aerosol.

**Dosage Forms** Aerosol: 1.75 mg/activation (16.2 g)

♦ **N.E.E.® 1/35** *see* Ethinyl Estradiol and Norethindrone *on page 212*

## Nefazodone (nef AY zoe done)

**Related Information**

Antidepressant Agents Comparison Chart *on page 704*
Anxiety Disorders *on page 606*
Clinical Issues in the Use of Antidepressants *on page 627*
Clinical Issues in the Use of Anxiolytics and Sedative/Hypnotics *on page 634*
Mood Disorders *on page 600*
Patient Information - Antidepressants (Serotonin Blocker) *on page 643*

**Generic Available** No

**U.S. Brand Names** Serzone®

**Synonyms** Nefazodone Hydrochloride

**Pharmacologic Category** Antidepressant, Serotonin Reuptake Inhibitor/Antagonist

**Use** Treatment of depression

**Unlabeled use:** Post-traumatic stress disorder

**Pregnancy Risk Factor** C

**Contraindications** Hypersensitivity to nefazodone or related compounds (phenylpiperazines); concurrent use or use of monoamine oxidase inhibitors within previous 14 days; use in a patient during the acute recovery phase of MI; concurrent use with astemizole, carbamazepine, cisapride, pimozide, or terfenadine; concurrent therapy with triazolam is generally contraindicated (dosage must be reduced by 75%, which often may not be possible with available dosage forms)

**Warnings/Precautions** Nefazodone should not be initiated within 1 week of discontinuing a MAOI. May cause sedation, resulting in impaired performance of tasks requiring alertness (ie, operating machinery or driving). Sedative effects may be additive with other CNS depressants. Does not potentiate ethanol but use is not advised. In particular, triazolobenzodiazepines (alprazolam and triazolam) should be avoided, since the metabolism of these drugs may be impaired. The degree of sedation is low relative to other antidepressants. May worsen psychosis in some patients or precipitate a shift to mania or hypomania in patients with bipolar disease. May increase the risks associated with electroconvulsive therapy. This agent should be discontinued, when possible, prior to elective surgery. Therapy should not be abruptly discontinued in patients receiving high doses for prolonged periods. Rare reports of priapism have occurred. The incidence of sexual dysfunction with nefazodone is generally lower than with SSRIs.

Use with caution in patients at risk of hypotension or in patients where transient hypotensive episodes would be poorly tolerated (cardiovascular disease or cerebrovascular disease). The risk of postural hypotension is low relative to other antidepressants. Use with caution in patients with urinary retention, benign prostatic hypertrophy, narrow-angle glaucoma, xerostomia, visual problems, constipation, or history of bowel obstruction (due to anticholinergic effects). The degree of anticholinergic blockade produced by this agent is very low relative to other cyclic antidepressants.

Use caution in patients with depression, particularly if suicidal risk may be present. Use caution in patients with a previous seizure disorder or condition predisposing to seizures such as brain damage, alcoholism, or concurrent therapy with other drugs which lower the seizure threshold. Use with caution in patients with hepatic or renal dysfunction and in elderly patients. Use with caution in patients with a history of cardiovascular disease (including previous MI, stroke, tachycardia, or conduction abnormalities). However, the risk of conduction abnormalities with this agent is very low relative to other antidepressants.

**Adverse Reactions**

>10%:

Central nervous system: Headache, drowsiness, insomnia, agitation, dizziness
Gastrointestinal: Xerostomia, nausea, constipation
Neuromuscular & skeletal: Weakness

1% to 10%:

Cardiovascular: Postural hypotension
Central nervous system: Lightheadedness, confusion, memory impairment, abnormal dreams, decreased concentration, ataxia
Dermatologic: Pruritus, rash
Gastrointestinal: Vomiting, dyspepsia, diarrhea, increased appetite, thirst, taste perversion
Neuromuscular & skeletal: Arthralgia, paresthesia, tremor
Ocular: Blurred vision, abnormal vision, visual field defect
Respiratory: Cough
Otic: Tinnitus
Miscellaneous: Flu syndrome

<1% or postmarketing case reports: Allergic reaction, AV block, bronchitis, dyspnea, eye pain, hallucinations, hepatic failure, hepatic necrosis, impotence, leukopenia, photosensitivity, priapism, seizures

**Overdosage/Toxicology**

Signs and symptoms: Drowsiness, vomiting, hypotension, tachycardia, incontinence, coma, priapism

Treatment: Following initiation of essential overdose management, toxic symptoms should be treated. Ventricular arrhythmias often respond to lidocaine 1.5 mg/kg bolus followed by 2 mg/minute infusion with concurrent systemic alkalinization (sodium bicarbonate 0.5-2 mEq/kg I.V.). Seizures usually respond to diazepam I.V. boluses (5-10 mg for adults up to 30 mg or 0.25-0.4 mg/kg/dose for children up to 10 mg/dose). If seizures are unresponsive or recur, phenytoin or phenobarbital may be required. Hypotension is best treated by I.V. fluids and by placing the patient in the Trendelenburg position.

**Drug Interactions** CYP3A3/4 enzyme substrate; CYP3A3/4 enzyme inhibitor

Antiarrhythmics: Serum concentrations may be increased due to enzyme inhibition; monitor; includes amiodarone, lidocaine, propafenone, quinidine

Antipsychotics: Serum concentrations of some antipsychotics may be increased by nefazodone due to enzyme inhibition; includes clozapine, haloperidol, mesoridazine, pimozide, quetiapine, and risperidone

Benzodiazepines: Nefazodone inhibits the metabolism of triazolam (decrease dose by 75%) and alprazolam (decrease dose by 50%); triazolam is contraindicated per manufacturer

Buspirone: Concurrent use may result in serotonin syndrome; serum concentrations may be increased due to enzyme inhibition; these combinations are best avoided

Calcium channel blockers: Serum concentrations may be increased due to enzyme inhibition; monitor for increased effect (hypotension)

Carbamazepine: Significantly reduces serum concentrations of nefazodone; coadministration is contraindicated

Cisapride: Nefazodone likely increases cisapride serum concentrations via CYP3A3/4 inhibition; this combination may lead to cardiac arrhythmias and should be avoided

Cyclosporine and tacrolimus: Serum levels and toxicity may be increased by nefazodone; monitor

CYP3A3/4 inhibitors: Serum level and/or toxicity of nefazodone may be increased; inhibitors include amiodarone, cimetidine, clarithromycin, erythromycin, delavirdine, diltiazem, dirithromycin, disulfiram, fluoxetine, fluvoxamine, grapefruit juice, indinavir, itraconazole, ketoconazole, metronidazole, nevirapine, propoxyfene, quinupristin-dalfopristin, ritonavir, saquinavir, verapamil, zafirlukast, zileuton

CYP3A3/4 substrates: Serum concentrations of drugs metabolized by CYP3A3/4 may be elevated by nefazodone; cisapride, pimozide, and triazolam are contraindicated; also see notes on individual drug classes

Digoxin: Serum levels may be increased by nefazodone (modest increases); monitor for digoxin toxicity or increased serum levels

Donepezil: Serum concentrations may be increased due to enzyme inhibition; monitor

HMG CoA reductase inhibitors (statins) have been associated with myositis and rhabdomyolysis when used in combination with nefazodone; this has been associated most strongly with lovastatin and simvastatin

Linezolid: Due to MAO inhibition (see below), this combination should be avoided

MAO inhibitors: Concurrent use may lead to serotonin syndrome; avoid concurrent use or use within 14 days

Meperidine: Combined use theoretically may increase the risk of serotonin syndrome

Methadone: Serum concentrations may be increased due to enzyme inhibition; monitor

Oral contraceptives: Serum concentrations may be increased due to enzyme inhibition; monitor

Pimozide: Serum concentrations may be increased due to enzyme inhibition; may result in life-threatening arrhythmias (also see note on antipsychotics); avoid use

Protease inhibitors: Indinavir, ritonavir saquinavir; serum concentrations may be increased due to enzyme inhibition; monitor

Quinidine: Metabolism is likely to be inhibited by nefazodone; avoid concurrent use

Selegiline: Concurrent use with nefazodone may be associated with a risk of serotonin syndrome, particularly at higher dosages (>10 mg/day)

Serotonin agonists: Theoretically may increase the risk of serotonin syndrome; includes sumatriptan, naratriptan, rizatriptan, and zolmitriptan

Sibutramine: Serum concentrations may be increased by nefazodone; monitor

Sildenafil: Serum concentrations may be increased due to enzyme inhibition; monitor

SSRIs: Combined use of nefazodone with an SSRI may produce serotonin syndrome; in addition, nefazodone may increase serum concentrations of some SSRIs due to enzyme inhibition (fluoxetine and citalopram)

Tricyclic antidepressants: Serum concentrations of some tricyclic antidepressants (amitriptyline, clomipramine) may be increased; monitor for increased effect or toxicity

Venlafaxine: Sertraline may increase the risk of serotonin syndrome

Vinca alkaloids (vincristine, and vinblastine): Serum concentrations may be increased due to enzyme inhibition; may result in increased toxicity

Zolpidem: Serum concentrations may be increased due to enzyme inhibition; monitor

**Mechanism of Action** Inhibits neuronal reuptake of serotonin and norepinephrine; also blocks $5HT_2$ and $alpha_1$ receptors; has no significant affinity for $alpha_2$, beta-adrenergic, 5-HT1A, cholinergic, dopaminergic, or benzodiazepine receptors

**Pharmacodynamics/kinetics**

Onset of effect: Therapeutic effects take at least 2 weeks to appear

Metabolism: In the liver to 3 active metabolites; triazoledione, hydroxynefazodone and m-chlorophenylpiperazine (mCPP)

Half-life: 2-4 hours (parent compound), active metabolites persist longer

Time to peak serum concentration: 1 hour, prolonged in presence of food

Elimination: Primarily as metabolites in urine and secondarily in feces

**Usual Dosage** Oral: Adults: 200 mg/day, administered in two divided doses initially, with a range of 300-600 mg/day in two divided doses thereafter

**Dietary Considerations** Alcohol: Additive CNS effect, avoid use

**Reference Range** Therapeutic plasma levels have not yet been defined

**Patient Information** Take shortly after a meal or light snack; can be given at bedtime dose if drowsiness occurs; optimum effect may take 2-4 weeks to be achieved; avoid alcohol; avoid sudden changes in position

**Nursing Implications** Dosing after meals may decrease lightheadedness and postural hypotension, but may also decrease absorption and therefore effectiveness; use side rails on bed if administered to the elderly; observe patient's activity and compare with admission level; assist with ambulation; sitting and standing blood pressure and pulse

**Additional Information** May cause less sexual dysfunction than other antidepressants; food delays absorption; women and elderly receiving single doses attain significant higher peak concentrations than male volunteers

**Dosage Forms** Tablet, as hydrochloride: 50 mg, 100 mg, 150 mg, 200 mg, 250 mg

◆ **Nefazodone Hydrochloride** *see* Nefazodone *on page 386*

◆ **NegGram®** *see* Nalidixic Acid *on page 381*

## Nelfinavir (nel FIN a veer)

**Related Information**

Protease Inhibitors *on page 724*

**U.S. Brand Names** Viracept®

**Pharmacologic Category** Antiretroviral Agent, Protease Inhibitor

**Use** In combination with other antiretroviral therapy in the treatment of HIV infection

**Effects on Mental Status** May cause dizziness, anxiety, insomnia, difficulty concentrating, depression, and suicidal ideation

**Effects on Psychiatric Treatment** May rarely cause leukopenia; use caution with clozapine and carbamazepine; concurrent use with midazolam and triazolam may produce oversedation; barbiturates and carbamazepine may decrease the effectiveness of nelfinavir

**Pregnancy Risk Factor** B

**Contraindications** Hypersensitivity to nelfinavir or product components; phenylketonuria; concurrent therapy with terfenadine, astemizole, cisapride, triazolam, or midazolam

**Warnings/Precautions** Avoid use of powder in phenylketonurics since contains phenylalanine; use extreme caution when administered to patients with hepatic insufficiency since nelfinavir is metabolized in the liver and excreted predominantly in the feces; avoid use, if possible, with amiodarone, quinidine, ergot derivatives, terfenadine, astemizole, cisapride, triazolam, or midazolam. Concurrent use with some anticonvulsants may significantly limit nelfinavir's effectiveness. Warn patients that redistribution of body fat can occur.

**Adverse Reactions** Protease inhibitors cause dyslipidemia which includes elevated cholesterol and triglycerides and a redistribution of body fat centrally to cause "protease paunch", buffalo hump, facial atrophy, and breast enlargement. These agents also cause hyperglycemia.

>10%: Gastrointestinal: Diarrhea (19%)

1% to 10%:

Central nervous system: Decreased concentration

Dermatologic: Rash

Gastrointestinal: Nausea, flatulence, abdominal pain

Neuromuscular & skeletal: Weakness

<1%: Allergy, anemia, anorexia, anxiety, arthralgia, arthritis, back pain, cramps, depression, dermatitis, diaphoresis, dizziness, dyspepsia, dyspnea, emotional lability, epigastric pain, fever, GI bleeding, headache, hepatitis, hyperkinesia, hyperlipemia, hyperuricemia, hypoglycemia, increased LFTs, insomnia, kidney calculus, leukopenia, malaise, migraine, mouth ulceration, myalgia, myasthenia, myopathy, pancreatitis, paresthesia, pharyngitis, pruritus, rhinitis, seizures, sexual dysfunction, sinusitis, sleep disorder, somnolence, suicide ideation, thrombocytopenia, urticaria, vomiting

**Overdosage/Toxicology** No data available; however, unabsorbed drug should be removed via gastric lavage and activated charcoal; significant symptoms beyond gastrointestinal disturbances is likely following acute overdose; hemodialysis will not be effective due to high protein binding of nelfinavir

**Drug Interactions** CYP3A3/4 enzyme substrate; CYP3A3/4 enzyme inducer; CYP3A3/4 enzyme inhibitor

Increased effect:

Nelfinavir inhibits the metabolism of cisapride and astemizole and should, therefore, not be administered concurrently due to risk of life-threatening cardiac arrhythmias.

A 20% increase in rifabutin plasma AUC has been observed when coadministered with nelfinavir (decrease rifabutin's dose by 50%).

An increase in midazolam and triazolam serum levels may occur resulting in significant oversedation when administered with nelfinavir. These drugs should not be administered together. Use caution with other benzodiazepines.

Amiodarone, quinidine, and ergot alkaloids: Serum levels/toxicity may be increased by nelfinavir - avoid concurrent use.

Indinavir and ritonavir may increase nelfinavir plasma concentrations resulting in potential increases in side effects (the safety of these combinations have not been established).

Nelfinavir increases indinavir concentrations

Decreased effect:

Rifampin decreases nelfinavir's plasma AUC by ~82%; the two drugs should not be administered together.

Ethinyl estradiol concentrations are decreased by nelfinavir.

Oral contraceptives: Serum levels of the hormones in oral contraceptives may decrease significantly with administration of nelfinavir. Patients should use alternative methods of contraceptives during nelfinavir therapy.

Norethindrone concentrations are decreased by nelfinavir.

Phenobarbital, phenytoin, and carbamazepine may decrease serum levels and consequently effectiveness of nelfinavir.

Nelfinavir's effectiveness may be decreased with concomitant nevirapine

**Usual Dosage** Oral:

Children 2-13 years: 20-30 mg/kg 3 times/day with a meal or light snack; if tablets are unable to be taken, use oral powder in small amount of water, milk, formula, or dietary supplements; do not use acidic food/juice or store for >6 hours

Adults: 750 mg 3 times/day with meals

**Dosing adjustment in renal impairment:** No adjustment needed

**Dosing adjustment in hepatic impairment:** Use caution when administering to patients with hepatic impairment since eliminated predominantly by the liver

**Patient Information** This is not a cure for HIV and has not been shown to reduce the risk of transmitting HIV to others. The long-term effects of use are not known. Should be taken as scheduled with food (mix powder with nonacidic, noncitric fluids and do not store reconstituted powder mixture for longer than 6 hours). If you miss a dose, take as soon as possible and return to regular schedule (never take a double dose). Frequent blood tests may be required with prolonged therapy. You may experience nausea and vomiting (small frequent meals, frequent mouth care, sucking lozenges, or chewing gum may help). Report rash; respiratory difficulty; CNS changes (migraine, confusion, suicidal ideation); muscular or skeletal pain, weakness, or tremors; or other adverse reactions. Use appropriate barrier contraceptive measures (as alternative to oral contraceptives) to reduce risk of transmitting infection and potential pregnancy.

**Nursing Implications** If diarrhea occurs, it may be treated with OTC antidiarrheals

**Dosage Forms**

Powder, oral: 50 mg/g (contains 11.2 mg phenylalanine)

Tablet: 250 mg

◆ **Nelova™ 0.5/35E** *see* Ethinyl Estradiol and Norethindrone *on page 212*

◆ **Nelova® 1/50M** *see* Mestranol and Norethindrone *on page 346*

◆ **Nelova™ 10/11** *see* Ethinyl Estradiol and Norethindrone *on page 212*

◆ **Nembutal®** *see* Pentobarbital *on page 428*

◆ **Neo-Calglucon® [OTC]** *see* Calcium Glubionate *on page 85*

◆ **Neo-Cortef®** *see* Neomycin and Hydrocortisone *on page 388*

◆ **NeoDecadron® Ophthalmic** *see* Neomycin and Dexamethasone *on page 388*

◆ **NeoDecadron® Topical** *see* Neomycin and Dexamethasone *on page 388*

- **Neo-Dexameth® Ophthalmic** *see* Neomycin and Dexamethasone *on page 388*
- **Neo-Durabolic Injection** *see* Nandrolone *on page 383*
- **Neo-fradin® Oral** *see* Neomycin *on page 388*
- **Neomixin® Topical [OTC]** *see* Bacitracin, Neomycin, and Polymyxin B *on page 57*


## Neomycin (nee oh MYE sin)

**U.S. Brand Names** Mycifradin® Sulfate Oral; Mycifradin® Sulfate Topical; Neo-fradin® Oral; Neo-Tabs® Oral

**Pharmacologic Category** Ammonium Detoxicant; Antibiotic, Aminoglycoside; Antibiotic, Topical

**Use** Orally to prepare GI tract for surgery; topically to treat minor skin infections; treat diarrhea caused by *E. coli*; adjunct in the treatment of hepatic encephalopathy

**Effects on Mental Status** None reported

**Effects on Psychiatric Treatment** None reported

**Pregnancy Risk Factor** C

**Contraindications** Hypersensitivity to neomycin or any component, or other aminoglycosides; patients with intestinal obstruction

**Warnings/Precautions** Use with caution in patients with renal impairment, pre-existing hearing impairment, neuromuscular disorders; neomycin is more toxic than other aminoglycosides when given parenterally; **do not administer parenterally**; topical neomycin is a contact sensitizer with sensitivity occurring in 5% to 15% of patients treated with the drug; symptoms include itching, reddening, edema, and failure to heal; **do not use as peritoneal lavage** due to significant systemic adsorption of the drug

**Adverse Reactions**

1% to 10%:

Dermatologic: Dermatitis, rash, urticaria, erythema

Local: Burning

Ocular: Contact conjunctivitis

<1%: Diarrhea, nausea, nephrotoxicity, neuromuscular blockade, ototoxicity, vomiting

**Overdosage/Toxicology**

Signs and symptoms (rare due to poor oral bioavailability): Ototoxicity, nephrotoxicity, and neuromuscular toxicity

Treatment: The treatment of choice following a single acute overdose appears to be the maintenance of good urine output of at least 3 mL/kg/hour. Dialysis is of questionable value in the enhancement of aminoglycoside elimination. If required, hemodialysis is preferred over peritoneal dialysis in patients with normal renal function. Chelation with penicillin may be of benefit.

**Drug Interactions**

Decreased effect: May decrease GI absorption of digoxin and methotrexate

Increased effect: Synergistic effects with penicillins

Increased toxicity:

Oral neomycin may potentiate the effects of oral anticoagulants

Increased adverse effects with other neurotoxic, ototoxic, or nephrotoxic drugs

**Usual Dosage**

Children: Oral:

Preoperative intestinal antisepsis: 90 mg/kg/day divided every 4 hours for 2 days; or 25 mg/kg at 1 PM, 2 PM, and 11 PM on the day preceding surgery as an adjunct to mechanical cleansing of the intestine and in combination with erythromycin base

Hepatic coma: 50-100 mg/kg/day in divided doses every 6-8 hours or 2.5-7 g/m$^2$/day divided every 4-6 hours for 5-6 days not to exceed 12 g/day

Children and Adults: Topical: Apply ointment 1-4 times/day; topical solutions containing 0.1% to 1% neomycin have been used for irrigation

Adults: Oral:

Preoperative intestinal antisepsis: 1 g each hour for 4 doses then 1 g every 4 hours for 5 doses; or 1 g at 1 PM, 2 PM, and 11 PM on day preceding surgery as an adjunct to mechanical cleansing of the bowel and oral erythromycin; or 6 g/day divided every 4 hours for 2-3 days

Hepatic coma: 500-2000 mg every 6-8 hours or 4-12 g/day divided every 4-6 hours for 5-6 days

Chronic hepatic insufficiency: 4 g/day for an indefinite period

Hemodialysis: Dialyzable (50% to 100%)

**Patient Information**

Oral: Take as directed. Maintain adequate hydration (2-3 L/day of fluids unless instructed to restrict fluid intake). You may experience nausea or vomiting (small frequent meals, frequent mouth care, sucking lozenges, or chewing gum may help); constipation (exercise, increased fluid or fiber in diet may help, or consult prescriber); or diarrhea (buttermilk, boiled milk, or yogurt may help). Report immediately any change in hearing,; ringing or sense of fullness in ears; persistent diarrhea; changes in voiding patterns; or numbness, tingling, or pain in any extremity.

Topical: Apply a thin film of cream or ointment; do not overuse; report rash, itching, redness, or failure of condition to improve

**Dosage Forms**

Cream, as sulfate: 0.5% (15 g)

Injection, as sulfate: 500 mg

Ointment, topical, as sulfate: 0.5% (15 g, 30 g, 120 g)

Solution, oral, as sulfate: 125 mg/5 mL (480 mL)

Tablet, as sulfate: 500 mg [base 300 mg]

## Neomycin and Dexamethasone

(nee oh MYE sin & deks a METH a sone)

**U.S. Brand Names** AK-Neo-Dex® Ophthalmic; NeoDecadron® Ophthalmic; NeoDecadron® Topical; Neo-Dexameth® Ophthalmic

**Pharmacologic Category** Antibiotic/Corticosteroid, Ophthalmic; Antibiotic/Corticosteroid, Topical

**Use** Treatment of steroid responsive inflammatory conditions of the palpebral and bulbar conjunctiva, lid, cornea, and anterior segment of the globe

**Effects on Mental Status** None reported

**Effects on Psychiatric Treatment** None reported

**Usual Dosage**

Ophthalmic: Instill 1-2 drops in eye(s) every 3-4 hours

Topical: Apply thin coat 3-4 times/day until favorable response is observed, then reduce dose to one application/day

**Dosage Forms**

Cream: Neomycin sulfate 0.5% [5 mg/g] and dexamethasone 0.1% [1 mg/g] (15 g, 30 g)

Ointment, ophthalmic: Neomycin sulfate 0.35% [3.5 mg/g] and dexamethasone 0.05% [0.5 mg/g] (3.5 g)

Solution, ophthalmic: Neomycin sulfate 0.35% [3.5 mg/mL] and dexamethasone 0.1% [1 mg/mL] (5 mL)

## Neomycin and Hydrocortisone

(nee oh MYE sin & hye droe KOR ti sone)

**U.S. Brand Names** Neo-Cortef®

**Pharmacologic Category** Antibiotic/Corticosteroid, Ophthalmic; Antibiotic/Corticosteroid, Topical

**Use** Treatment of susceptible topical bacterial infections with associated inflammation

**Effects on Mental Status** None reported

**Effects on Psychiatric Treatment** None reported

**Usual Dosage** Topical: Apply to area in a thin film 2-4 times/day

**Dosage Forms**

Cream: Neomycin sulfate 0.5% and hydrocortisone 1% (20 g)

Ointment, topical: Neomycin sulfate 0.5% and hydrocortisone 0.5% (20 g); neomycin sulfate 0.5% and hydrocortisone 1% (20 g)

Solution, ophthalmic: Neomycin sulfate 0.5% and hydrocortisone 0.5% (5 mL)

## Neomycin and Polymyxin B

(nee oh MYE sin & pol i MIKS in bee)

**U.S. Brand Names** Neosporin® Cream [OTC]; Neosporin® G.U. Irrigant

**Synonyms** Polymyxin B and Neomycin

**Pharmacologic Category** Antibiotic, Topical

**Use** Short-term as a continuous irrigant or rinse in the urinary bladder to prevent bacteriuria and gram-negative rod septicemia associated with the use of indwelling catheters; to help prevent infection in minor cuts, scrapes, and burns

**Effects on Mental Status** None reported

**Effects on Psychiatric Treatment** None reported

**Pregnancy Risk Factor** C (D G.U. irrigant)

**Contraindications** Hypersensitivity to neomycin or polymyxin B or any component; ophthalmic use for topical cream

**Warnings/Precautions** Use with caution in patients with impaired renal function, infants with diaper rash involving large area of abraded skin, dehydrated patients, burn patients, and patients receiving a high-dose for prolonged periods; topical neomycin is a contact sensitizer; contains methylparaben

**Adverse Reactions** 1% to 10%:

Dermatologic: Contact dermatitis, erythema, rash, urticaria

Genitourinary: Bladder irritation

Local: Burning

Neuromuscular & skeletal: Neuromuscular blockade

Otic: Ototoxicity

Renal: Nephrotoxicity

**Overdosage/Toxicology** Refer to individual monographs

**Drug Interactions** No data reported

**Usual Dosage** Children and Adults:

Bladder irrigation: **Not for injection**; add 1 mL irrigant to 1 liter isotonic saline solution and connect container to the inflow of lumen of 3-way catheter. Continuous irrigant or rinse in the urinary bladder for up to a maximum of 10 days with administration rate adjusted to patient's urine output; usually no more than 1 L of irrigant is used per day.

Topical: Apply cream 1-4 times/day to affected area

**Patient Information** See individual agents

**Dosage Forms**

Cream: Neomycin sulfate 3.5 mg and polymyxin B sulfate 10,000 units per g (0.94 g, 15 g)

Solution, irrigant: Neomycin sulfate 40 mg and polymyxin B sulfate 200,000 units per mL (1 mL, 20 mL)

## Neomycin, Colistin, Hydrocortisone, and Thonzonium

(nee oh MYE sin, koe LIS tin, hye droe KOR ti sone, & thon ZOE nee um)

**U.S. Brand Names** Cortisporin®-TC Otic Suspension

**Pharmacologic Category** Antibiotic/Corticosteroid, Otic

**Use** Treatment of superficial and susceptible bacterial infections of the external auditory canal; for treatment of susceptible bacterial infections of mastoidectomy and fenestration cavities

**Effects on Mental Status** None reported

**Effects on Psychiatric Treatment** None reported

**Usual Dosage** Adults: 5 drops in affected ear 3-4 times/day

**Dosage Forms** Suspension, otic: Neomycin sulfate 3.3 mg, colistin sulfate 3 mg, hydrocortisone acetate 1%, and thonzonium bromide 0.5 mg per mL (10 mL)

## Neomycin, Polymyxin B, and Dexamethasone

(nee oh MYE sin, pol i MIKS in bee, & deks a METH a sone)

**U.S. Brand Names** AK-Trol®; Dexacidin®; Dexasporin®; Maxitrol®

**Pharmacologic Category** Antibiotic/Corticosteroid, Ophthalmic

**Use** Steroid-responsive inflammatory ocular conditions in which a corticosteroid is indicated and where bacterial infection or a risk of bacterial infection exists

**Effects on Mental Status** None reported

**Effects on Psychiatric Treatment** None reported

**Usual Dosage** Children and Adults: Ophthalmic:

Ointment: Place a small amount (~½") in the affected eye 3-4 times/day or apply at bedtime as an adjunct with drops

Solution: Instill 1-2 drops into affected eye(s) every 3-4 hours; in severe disease, drops may be used hourly and tapered to discontinuation

**Dosage Forms** Ophthalmic:

Ointment: Neomycin sulfate 3.5 mg, polymyxin B sulfate 10,000 units and dexamethasone 0.1% per g (3.5 g, 5 g)

Suspension: Neomycin sulfate 3.5 mg, polymyxin B sulfate 10,000 units and dexamethasone 0.1% per mL (5 mL, 10 mL)

## Neomycin, Polymyxin B, and Gramicidin

(nee oh MYE sin, pol i MIKS in bee, & gram i SYE din)

**U.S. Brand Names** AK-Spore® Ophthalmic Solution; Neosporin® Ophthalmic Solution

**Pharmacologic Category** Antibiotic, Ophthalmic

**Use** Treatment of superficial ocular infection, infection prophylaxis in minor skin abrasions

**Effects on Mental Status** None reported

**Effects on Psychiatric Treatment** None reported

**Usual Dosage** Children and Adults: Ophthalmic: Instill 1-2 drops 4-6 times/day or more frequently as required for severe infections

**Dosage Forms** Solution, ophthalmic: Neomycin sulfate 1.75 mg, polymyxin B sulfate 10,000 units, and gramicidin 0.025 mg per mL (2 mL, 10 mL)

## Neomycin, Polymyxin B, and Hydrocortisone

(nee oh MYE sin, pol i MIKS in bee, & hye droe KOR ti sone)

**U.S. Brand Names** AK-Spore® H.C. Ophthalmic Suspension; AK-Spore® H.C. Otic; AntibiOtic® Otic; Cortatrigen® Otic; Cortisporin® Ophthalmic Suspension; Cortisporin® Otic; Cortisporin® Topical Cream; Octicair® Otic; Otic-Care® Otic; Otocort® Otic; Otosporin® Otic; PediOtic® Otic; UAD Otic®

**Pharmacologic Category** Antibiotic/Corticosteroid, Ophthalmic; Antibiotic/Corticosteroid, Otic; Topical Skin Product

**Use** Steroid-responsive inflammatory condition for which a corticosteroid is indicated and where bacterial infection or a risk of bacterial infection exists

**Effects on Mental Status** None reported

**Effects on Psychiatric Treatment** None reported

**Usual Dosage** Duration of use should be limited to 10 days unless otherwise directed by the physician

Otic solution is used **only** for swimmer's ear (infections of external auditory canal)

Otic:

Children: Instill 3 drops into affected ear 3-4 times/day

Adults: Instill 4 drops 3-4 times/day; otic suspension is the preferred otic preparation

Children and Adults:

Ophthalmic: Drops: Instill 1-2 drops 2-4 times/day, or more frequently as required for severe infections; in acute infections, instill 1-2 drops every 15-30 minutes gradually reducing the frequency of administration as the infection is controlled

Topical: Apply a thin layer 1-4 times/day. Therapy should be discontinued when control is achieved; if no improvement is seen, reassessment of diagnosis may be necessary.

**Dosage Forms**

Cream, topical: Neomycin sulfate 5 mg, polymyxin B sulfate 10,000 units, and hydrocortisone 10 mg per mL (7.5 g)

Solution, otic: Neomycin sulfate 5 mg, polymyxin B sulfate 10,000 units, and hydrocortisone 10 mg per mL (10 mL)

Suspension:

Ophthalmic: Neomycin sulfate 5 mg, polymyxin B sulfate 10,000 units, and hydrocortisone 10 mg per mL (7.5 mL)

Otic: Neomycin sulfate 5 mg, polymyxin B sulfate 10,000 units, and hydrocortisone 10 mg per mL (10 mL)

## Neomycin, Polymyxin B, and Prednisolone

(nee oh MYE sin, pol i MIKS in bee, & pred NIS oh lone)

**U.S. Brand Names** Poly-Pred® Ophthalmic Suspension

**Pharmacologic Category** Antibiotic/Corticosteroid, Ophthalmic

**Use** Steroid-responsive inflammatory ocular condition in which bacterial infection or a risk of bacterial ocular infection exists

**Effects on Mental Status** None reported

**Effects on Psychiatric Treatment** None reported

**Usual Dosage** Children and Adults: Ophthalmic: Instill 1-2 drops every 3-4 hours; acute infections may require every 30-minute instillation initially with frequency of administration reduced as the infection is brought under control. To treat the lids: Instill 1-2 drops every 3-4 hours, close the eye and rub the excess on the lids and lid margins.

**Dosage Forms** Suspension, ophthalmic: Neomycin sulfate 0.35%, polymyxin B sulfate 10,000 units, and prednisolone acetate 0.5% per mL (5 mL, 10 mL)


- **Neopap® [OTC]** *see* Acetaminophen *on page 14*
- **Neoral® Oral** *see* Cyclosporine *on page 146*
- **Neosar® Injection** *see* Cyclophosphamide *on page 145*
- **Neosporin® Cream [OTC]** *see* Neomycin and Polymyxin B *on page 388*
- **Neosporin® G.U. Irrigant** *see* Neomycin and Polymyxin B *on page 388*
- **Neosporin® Ophthalmic Ointment** *see* Bacitracin, Neomycin, and Polymyxin B *on page 57*
- **Neosporin® Ophthalmic Solution** *see* Neomycin, Polymyxin B, and Gramicidin *on page 389*
- **Neosporin® Topical Ointment [OTC]** *see* Bacitracin, Neomycin, and Polymyxin B *on page 57*


## Neostigmine (nee oh STIG meen)

**U.S. Brand Names** Prostigmin®

**Pharmacologic Category** Acetylcholinesterase Inhibitor (Central)

**Use** Diagnosis and treatment of myasthenia gravis and prevent and treat postoperative bladder distention and urinary retention; reversal of the effects of nondepolarizing neuromuscular blocking agents after surgery

**Drug Interactions**

Anticholinergics: Effects may be reduced with cholinesterase inhibitors; atropine antagonizes the muscarinic effects of cholinesterase inhibitors

Beta-blockers without ISA: Activity may increase risk of bradycardia

Calcium channel blockers (diltiazem or verapamil): May increase risk of bradycardia

Cholinergic agonists: Effects may be increased with cholinesterase inhibitors

Corticosteroids: May see increased muscle weakness and decreased response to anticholinesterases shortly after onset of corticosteroid therapy in the treatment of myasthenia gravis. Deterioration in muscle strength, including severe muscular depression, has been documented in patients with myasthenia gravis while receiving corticosteroids and anticholinesterases.

Digoxin: Increased risk of bradycardia with concurrent use

Neuromuscular blockers: Depolarizing neuromuscular blocking agents effects may be increased with cholinesterase inhibitors; nondepolarizing agents are antagonized by cholinesterase inhibitors

**Usual Dosage**

Myasthenia gravis: Diagnosis: I.M.:

Children: 0.04 mg/kg as a single dose

Adults: 0.02 mg/kg as a single dose

(Continued)

## Neostigmine *(Continued)*

Myasthenia gravis: Treatment:
Children:
Oral: 2 mg/kg/day divided every 3-4 hours
I.M., I.V., S.C.: 0.01-0.04 mg/kg every 2-4 hours
Adults:
Oral: 15 mg/dose every 3-4 hours up to 375 mg/day maximum
I.M., I.V., S.C.: 0.5-2.5 mg every 1-3 hours up to 10 mg/24 hours maximum
Reversal of nondepolarizing neuromuscular blockade after surgery in conjunction with atropine: I.V.:
Infants: 0.025-0.1 mg/kg/dose
Children: 0.025-0.08 mg/kg/dose
Adults: 0.5-2.5 mg; total dose not to exceed 5 mg
Bladder atony: Adults: I.M., S.C.:
Prevention: 0.25 mg every 4-6 hours for 2-3 days
Treatment: 0.5-1 mg every 3 hours for 5 doses after bladder has emptied
**Dosing adjustment in renal impairment:**
$Cl_{cr}$ 10-50 mL/minute: Administer 50% of normal dose
$Cl_{cr}$ <10 mL/minute: Administer 25% of normal dose

**Dosage Forms**
Injection, as methylsulfate: 0.25 mg/mL (1 mL); 0.5 mg/mL (1 mL, 10 mL); 1 mg/mL (10 mL)
Tablet, as bromide: 15 mg

- **Neo-Synephrine® Nasal Solution [OTC]** *see* Phenylephrine *on page 439*
- **Neo-Synephrine® Ophthalmic Solution** *see* Phenylephrine *on page 439*
- **Neo-Tabs® Oral** *see* Neomycin *on page 388*
- **Neotricin HC® Ophthalmic Ointment** *see* Bacitracin, Neomycin, Polymyxin B, and Hydrocortisone *on page 57*
- **NeoVadrin® [OTC]** *see* Vitamins, Multiple *on page 587*
- **NeoVadrin® B Complex [OTC]** *see* Vitamin B Complex *on page 586*
- **Nephro-Calci® [OTC]** *see* Calcium Carbonate *on page 84*
- **Nephrocaps®** *see* Vitamin B Complex With Vitamin C and Folic Acid *on page 586*
- **Nephro-Fer™ [OTC]** *see* Ferrous Fumarate *on page 223*
- **Nephrox Suspension [OTC]** *see* Aluminum Hydroxide *on page 28*
- **Neptazane®** *see* Methazolamide *on page 351*
- **Nervocaine®** *see* Lidocaine *on page 317*
- **Nestrex®** *see* Pyridoxine *on page 481*

## Netilmicin (ne til MYE sin)

**U.S. Brand Names** Netromycin® Injection
**Pharmacologic Category** Antibiotic, Aminoglycoside
**Use** Short-term treatment of serious or life-threatening infections including septicemia, peritonitis, intra-abdominal abscess, lower respiratory tract infections, urinary tract infections; skin, bone, and joint infections caused by susceptible organisms; active against *Pseudomonas aeruginosa*, *E. coli*, *Proteus*, *Klebsiella*, *Serratia*, *Enterobacter*, *Citrobacter*, and other gram-negative bacilli
**Effects on Mental Status** May cause drowsiness or dizziness
**Effects on Psychiatric Treatment** May rarely cause agranulocytosis; use caution with clozapine and carbamazepine
**Usual Dosage** Individualization is critical because of the low therapeutic index. Use of ideal body weight (IBW) for determining the mg/kg/dose appears to be more accurate than dosing on the basis of total body weight (TBW). In morbid obesity, dosage requirement may best be estimated using a dosing weight of IBW + 0.4 (TBW - IBW). Peak and trough plasma drug levels should be determined, particularly in critically ill patients with serious infections or in disease states known to significantly alter aminoglycoside pharmacokinetics (eg, cystic fibrosis, burns, or major surgery).

I.M., I.V.:
Neonates <6 weeks: 2-3.25 mg/kg/dose every 12 hours
Children 6 weeks to 12 years: 1-2.5 mg/kg/dose every 8 hours
Children >12 years and Adults: 1.5-2 mg/kg/dose every 8-12 hours
Some clinicians suggest a daily dose of 4-7 mg/kg for all patients with normal renal function. This dose is at least as efficacious with similar, if not less, toxicity than conventional dosing.
**Dosing adjustment in renal impairment:** Initial dose:
All patients should receive a loading dose of at least 2 mg/kg (subsequent dosing should be base on serum concentrations)
$Cl_{cr}$ ≥60 mL/minute: Administer every 8 hours
$Cl_{cr}$ 40-60 mL/minute: Administer every 12 hours
$Cl_{cr}$ 20-40 mL/minute: Administer every 24 hours
Continuous arteriovenous or venovenous hemodiafiltration (CAVH) effects: Dose as for $Cl_{cr}$ 10-40 mL/minute and follow levels

**Dosage Forms** Injection, as sulfate: 100 mg/mL (1.5 mL)

- **Netromycin® Injection** *see* Netilmicin *on page 390*
- **Neucalm®** *see* Hydroxyzine *on page 278*
- **Neumega®** *see* Oprelvekin *on page 406*
- **Neupogen®** *see* Filgrastim *on page 225*
- **Neuramate®** *see* Meprobamate *on page 342*
- **Neurontin®** *see* Gabapentin *on page 244*
- **Neut® Injection** *see* Sodium Bicarbonate *on page 514*
- **Neutra-Phos®** *see* Potassium Phosphate and Sodium Phosphate *on page 456*
- **Neutra-Phos®-K** *see* Potassium Phosphate *on page 455*
- **Neutrexin® Injection** *see* Trimetrexate Glucuronate *on page 570*
- **Neutrogena® Acne Mask [OTC]** *see* Benzoyl Peroxide *on page 62*

## Nevirapine (ne VYE ra peen)

**U.S. Brand Names** Viramune®
**Pharmacologic Category** Antiretroviral Agent, Reverse Transcriptase Inhibitor (Non-Nucleoside)
**Use** In combination therapy with other antiretroviral agents for the treatment of HIV-1 in adults
**Effects on Mental Status** None reported
**Effects on Psychiatric Treatment** Neutropenia is common; avoid clozapine and carbamazepine
**Pregnancy Risk Factor** C
**Contraindications** Previous hypersensitivity to nevirapine or its components; concurrent use with oral contraceptives and protease inhibitors (indinavir, nelfinavir, ritonavir, saquinavir)
**Warnings/Precautions** Consider alteration of antiretroviral therapies if disease progression occurs while patients are receiving nevirapine. Resistant HIV virus emerges rapidly and uniformly when nevirapine is administered as monotherapy. Therefore, always administer in combination with at least 1 additional antiretroviral agent. Severe life-threatening skin reactions (eg, Stevens-Johnson syndrome, toxic epidermal necrolysis, hypersensitivity reactions with rash and organ dysfunction) have occurred, usually within 6 weeks. If a severe skin or hypersensitivity reaction (severe rash, rash with fever, blisters, oral lesions, conjunctivitis, facial edema, muscle or joint aches, general malaise and/or hepatic abnormalities) occurs, discontinue nevirapine as soon as possible; mild to moderate alterations in LFTs are not uncommon, however, severe hepatotoxic reactions may occur rarely, and if abnormalities reoccur after temporarily discontinuing therapy, treatment should be permanently halted. Safety and efficacy have not been established in children.
**Adverse Reactions**
>10%:
Central nervous system: Headache (11%), fever (8% to 11%)
Dermatologic: Rash (15% to 20%)
Gastrointestinal: Diarrhea (15% to 20%)
Hematologic: Neutropenia (10% to 11%)
1% to 10%:
Gastrointestinal: Ulcerative stomatitis (4%), nausea, abdominal pain (2%)
Hematologic: Anemia
Hepatic: Hepatitis, increased LFTs (2% to 4%)
Neuromuscular & skeletal: Peripheral neuropathy, paresthesia (2%), myalgia
<1%: Hepatic necrosis, hepatotoxicity, Stevens-Johnson syndrome, thrombocytopenia
**Overdosage/Toxicology** No toxicities have been reported with acute ingestions of large sums of tablets
**Drug Interactions** CYP3A3/4 enzyme substrate; CYP3A3/4 enzyme inducer; CYP3A3/4 enzyme inhibitor
Decreased effect: Rifampin and rifabutin may decrease nevirapine trough concentrations due to induction of CYP3A; since nevirapine may decrease concentrations of protease inhibitors, they should not be administered concomitantly or doses should be increased; nevirapine may decrease the effectiveness of oral contraceptives - suggest alternate method of birth control; decreased effect of ketoconazole
Increased effect/toxicity with cimetidine, macrolides, ketoconazole
Methadone's plasma concentrations may decrease. Monitor for narcotic withdrawal and adjust methadone dose as needed.
**Usual Dosage** Adults: Oral:
Initial: 200 mg once daily for 14 days
Maintenance: 200 mg twice daily (in combination with an additional antiretroviral agent)
**Patient Information** If rash develops stop medicine and contact prescriber
**Nursing Implications** May be given with food, antacids, or didanosine; if a therapy is interrupted for >7 days, the dose should be decreased to the initial regimen and increased after 14 days

**Dosage Forms**
Suspension, oral: 50 mg/5 mL (240 mL)
Tablet: 200 mg

♦ **New Decongestant®** *see* Chlorpheniramine, Phenyltoloxamine, Phenylpropanolamine, and Phenylephrine *on page 116*

♦ **N.G.T.® Topical** *see* Nystatin and Triamcinolone *on page 402*

## Niacin (NYE a sin)

**Related Information**
Lipid-Lowering Agents Comparison Chart *on page 717*

**U.S. Brand Names** Niaspan®; Nicobid® [OTC]; Nicolar® [OTC]; Nicotinex [OTC]; Slo-Niacin® [OTC]

**Synonyms** Nicotinic Acid; Nicotiramide; Vitamin $B_3$

**Pharmacologic Category** Antilipemic Agent (Miscellaneous); Vitamin, Water Soluble

**Use** Adjunctive treatment of hyperlipidemias; peripheral vascular disease and circulatory disorders; treatment of pellagra; dietary supplement

**Effects on Mental Status** May rarely cause dizziness

**Effects on Psychiatric Treatment** None reported

**Pregnancy Risk Factor** A (C if used in doses greater than RDA suggested doses)

**Contraindications** Hypersensitivity to niacin or niacinamide; liver disease; active peptic ulcer; severe hypotension; arterial hemorrhage

**Warnings/Precautions** Use caution in heavy ethanol users, unstable angina or CAD (risk of arrhythmias at high doses), diabetes (interfere with glucose control), renal disease, active gallbladder disease (can exacerbate), gout, or allergies. Avoid large pharmacological amounts in patients with a history of liver disease. Flushing is common and can be attenuated with a gradual increase in dose. Monitor liver function tests.

**Adverse Reactions**
1% to 10%:
- Cardiovascular: Generalized flushing
- Central nervous system: Headache
- Gastrointestinal: Bloating, flatulence, nausea
- Hepatic: Abnormalities of hepatic function tests, jaundice
- Neuromuscular & skeletal: Paresthesia in extremities
- Miscellaneous: Increased sebaceous gland activity, sensation of warmth

<1%: Blurred vision, dizziness, liver damage (dose-related incidence), rash, syncope, tachycardia, vasovagal attacks, wheezing

**Overdosage/Toxicology**
Signs and symptoms: Flushing, GI distress, pruritus; chronic excessive use has been associated with hepatitis
Treatment: Antihistamines may relieve niacin-induced histamine release; otherwise treatment is symptomatic

**Drug Interactions**
Adrenergic blocking agents → additive vasodilating effect and postural hypotension
Aspirin decreases adverse effect of flushing
Lovastatin (and possibly other HMG CoA reductase inhibitors): Increased risk of toxicity (myopathy)
Oral hypoglycemics: Effect may be decreased by niacin
Sulfinpyrazone and probenecid; niacin may inhibit uricosuric effects

**Usual Dosage** Administer I.M., I.V., or S.C. only if oral route is unavailable and use only for vitamin deficiencies (not for hyperlipidemia)

Children: Oral:
- Pellagra: 50-100 mg/dose 3 times/day
- Recommended daily allowances:
  - 0-0.5 years: 5 mg/day
  - 0.5-1 year: 6 mg/day
  - 1-3 years: 9 mg/day
  - 4-6 years: 12 mg/day
  - 7-10 years: 13 mg/day

Children and Adolescents: Oral: Recommended daily allowances:
- Male:
  - 11-14 years: 17 mg/day
  - 15-18 years: 20 mg/day
  - 19-24 years: 19 mg/day
- Female: 11-24 years: 15 mg/day

Adults: Oral:
- Recommended daily allowances:
  - Male: 25-50 years: 19 mg/day; >51 years: 15 mg/day
  - Female: 25-50 years: 15 mg/day; >51 years: 13 mg/day
- Hyperlipidemia: 1.5-6 g/day in 3 divided doses with or after meals using a dosage titration schedule
- Pellagra: 50-100 mg 3-4 times/day, maximum: 500 mg/day
- Niacin deficiency: 10-20 mg/day, maximum: 100 mg/day

**Patient Information** May experience transient cutaneous flushing and sensation of warmth, especially of face and upper body; itching or tingling, and headache may occur, these adverse effects may be decreased by increasing the dose slowly or by taking aspirin or a NSAID 30 minutes to 1 hour prior to taking niacin; may cause GI upset, take with food; if dizziness occurs, avoid sudden changes in posture; report any persistent nausea, vomiting, abdominal pain, dark urine, or pale stools to the physician; do not crush sustained release capsule

**Nursing Implications** Monitor closely for signs of hepatotoxicity and myositis; avoid sudden changes in posture

**Dosage Forms**
Capsule, timed release: 125 mg, 250 mg, 300 mg, 400 mg, 500 mg
Elixir: 50 mg/5 mL (473 mL, 4000 mL)
Injection: 100 mg/mL (30 mL)
Tablet: 25 mg, 50 mg, 100 mg, 250 mg, 500 mg
- Extended release: 500 mg, 750 mg, 1000 mg
- Timed release: 150 mg, 250 mg, 500 mg, 750 mg

## Niacinamide (nye a SIN a mide)

**Pharmacologic Category** Vitamin, Water Soluble

**Use** Prophylaxis and treatment of pellagra

**Effects on Mental Status** None reported

**Effects on Psychiatric Treatment** None reported

**Usual Dosage** Oral:
- Children: Pellagra: 100-300 mg/day in divided doses
- Adults: 50 mg 3-10 times/day
  - Pellagra: 300-500 mg/day
  - Recommended daily allowance: 13-19 mg/day

**Dosage Forms** Tablet: 50 mg, 100 mg, 125 mg, 250 mg, 500 mg

♦ **Niaspan®** *see* Niacin *on page 391*

## Nicardipine (nye KAR de peen)

**Related Information**
Calcium Channel Blocking Agents Comparison Chart *on page 710*

**U.S. Brand Names** Cardene®; Cardene® SR

**Canadian Brand Names** Ridene

**Pharmacologic Category** Calcium Channel Blocker

**Use** Management of essential hypertension

**Effects on Mental Status** Drowsiness and dizziness are common; may rarely cause insomnia

**Effects on Psychiatric Treatment** Concurrent use with propranolol may increase AV nodal effects

**Pregnancy Risk Factor** C

**Contraindications** Hypersensitivity to nicardipine or any component; advanced aortic stenosis

**Warnings/Precautions** Blood pressure lowering should be done at a rate appropriate for the patient's condition. Rapid drops in blood pressure can lead to arterial insufficiency. Use with caution in CAD (can cause increase in angina), CHF (can worsen heart failure symptoms), and pheochromocytoma (limited clinical experience). Peripheral infusion sites (for I.V. therapy) should be changed ever 12 hours. Titrate I.V. dose cautiously in patients with CHF, renal, or hepatic dysfunction. Use the I.V. form cautiously in patients with portal hypertension (can cause increase in hepatic pressure gradient). Safety and efficacy have not been demonstrated in pediatric patients. Abrupt withdrawal may cause rebound angina in patients with CAD.

**Adverse Reactions**
1% to 10%:
- Cardiovascular: Flushing (6% to 10%), palpitations, tachycardia (1% to 3.4%), peripheral edema (7% to 8%), syncope (3% to 4%)
- Central nervous system: Headache (6.4% to 8%), dizziness (4% to 7%), somnolence (4.2% to 6%)
- Gastrointestinal: Nausea (1.9% to 2.2%), abdominal pain (0.8% to 1.5%)
- Neuromuscular & skeletal: Weakness (4.2% to 6%)

<1%: Abnormal dreams, abnormal EKG, constipation, dyspepsia, insomnia, malaise, nocturia, rash, tremor, vomiting, xerostomia

**Overdosage/Toxicology**
Signs and symptoms:

The primary cardiac symptoms of calcium blocker overdose includes hypotension and bradycardia. The hypotension is caused by peripheral vasodilation, myocardial depression, and bradycardia. Bradycardia results from sinus bradycardia, second- or third-degree atrioventricular block, or sinus arrest with junctional rhythm. Intraventricular conduction is usually not affected so QRS duration is normal (verapamil does prolong the P-R interval and bepridil prolongs the Q-T and may cause ventricular arrhythmias, including torsade de pointes).

The noncardiac symptoms include confusion, stupor, nausea, vomiting, metabolic acidosis and hyperglycemia. Following initial gastric decontamination, if possible, repeated calcium administration may promptly reverse the depressed cardiac contractility (but not sinus node depression or peripheral vasodilation); glucagon, epinephrine, and inamrinone may treat refractory hypotension; glucagon and epinephrine also increase the heart rate (outside the U.S., 4-aminopyridine may be available as an antidote); dialysis and hemoperfusion are not effective in enhancing elimination although repeat-dose activated charcoal may serve as an adjunct with sustained-release preparations.

**Drug Interactions** CYP3A3/4 enzyme substrate
(Continued)

## Nicardipine *(Continued)*

Azole antifungals may inhibit the calcium channel blocker's metabolism; avoid this combination. Try an antifungal like terbinafine (if appropriate) or monitor closely for altered effect of the calcium channel blocker.

Calcium may reduce the calcium channel blocker's effects, particularly hypotension

Cyclosporine's serum concentrations are increased by nicardipine; avoid this combination. Use another calcium channel blocker or monitor cyclosporine trough levels and renal function closely

Nafcillin decreases plasma concentration of nicardipine; avoid this combination

Protease inhibitor like amprenavir and ritonavir may increase nicardipine's serum concentration

Rifampin increases the metabolism of the calcium channel blocker; adjust the dose of the calcium channel blocker to maintain efficacy

**Usual Dosage** Adults:

Oral:

Immediate release: Initial: 20 mg 3 times/day; usual: 20-40 mg 3 times/day (allow 3 days between dose increases)

Sustained release: Initial: 30 mg twice daily, titrate up to 60 mg twice daily

I.V. (dilute to 0.1 mg/mL): Initial: 5 mg/hour increased by 2.5 mg/hour every 15 minutes to a maximum of 15 mg/hour

**Dosing adjustment in renal impairment:** Titrate dose beginning with 20 mg 3 times/day (immediate release) or 30 mg twice daily (sustained release).

**Dosing adjustment in hepatic impairment:** Starting dose: 20 mg twice daily (immediate release) with titration.

**Equivalent oral vs I.V. infusion doses:**

20 mg q8h oral, equivalent to 0.5 mg/hour I.V. infusion

30 mg q8h oral, equivalent to 1.2 mg/hour I.V. infusion

40 mg q8h oral, equivalent to 2.2 mg/hour I.V. infusion

**Dietary Considerations** Alcohol: Avoid use

**Patient Information** Take as directed; do not alter dosage regimen or increase, decrease, or discontinue without consulting prescriber. Do not crush or chew tablets or capsules. Take with nonfatty food. Avoid caffeine and alcohol. Consult prescriber before increasing exercise routine (decreased angina does not mean it is safe to increase exercise). Change position slowly to prevent orthostatic events. May cause dizziness or fatigue; use caution when driving or engaging in tasks that require alertness until response to drug is known. Frequent small meals, frequent mouth care, sucking lozenges, or chewing gum may reduce nausea. Report swelling, difficulty breathing or new cough, unresolved fatigue, unusual weight gain, or unresolved dizziness.

**Nursing Implications** Monitor closely for orthostasis; ampuls must be diluted before use; do not crush sustained release product; to assess adequacy of blood pressure response, measure blood pressure 8 hours after dosing

**Dosage Forms**

Caplet: 20 mg, 30 mg

Sustained release: 30 mg, 45 mg, 60 mg

Injection: 2.5 mg/mL (10 mL)

## Nicergoline (nye SER goe leen)

**U.S. Brand Names** Circo-Maren®; Duracebrol®; Ergobel®; Fisifax®; Memoq®; Nicergolyn®; Nicerium®; Sermion®; Varson®

**Pharmacologic Category** Ergot Derivative

**Use** Transient ischemic attacks, cerebrovascular insufficiency, dementia

**Effects on Mental Status** May cause agitation or insomnia

**Effects on Psychiatric Treatment** Potentiates propranolol's cardiac effects

**Contraindications** Hypersensitivity to nicergoline; acute bleeding; recent myocardial infarction; hypertension; pregnancy; breast-feeding; bradycardia; use with alpha- or beta-receptor agonists

**Warnings/Precautions** Use with caution in patients taking anticoagulant agents, antiplatelet agents, antihypertensive agents

**Adverse Reactions**

Cardiovascular: Hypotension, syncope, bradycardia, flushing, sinus bradycardia

Central nervous system: Insomnia, agitation

Dermatologic: Urticaria

Gastrointestinal: Nausea, appetite (increased), diarrhea

Hematologic: Inhibits platelet aggregation

Miscellaneous: Diaphoresis

**Drug Interactions** Enhances cardiac depressive effects of propranolol

**Usual Dosage**

Oral: Initial: 10 mg 3 times/day; maintenance: 5-10 mg 3 times/day (before or during meals)

I.M.: 2-4 mg once or twice daily

I.V.: 4-8 mg diluted in 250 mL of normal saline and given over 30 minutes

**Dosing adjustment in renal impairment**: Reduce dose

♦ **Nicergolyn®** *see* Nicergoline *on page 392*

♦ **Nicerium®** *see* Nicergoline *on page 392*

♦ **N'ice® Vitamin C Drops [OTC]** *see* Ascorbic Acid *on page 48*

♦ **Niclocide®** *see* Niclosamide *on page 392*

## Niclosamide (ni KLOE sa mide)

**U.S. Brand Names** Niclocide®

**Pharmacologic Category** Anthelmintic

**Use** Treatment of intestinal beef and fish tapeworm infections and dwarf tapeworm infections

**Effects on Mental Status** May cause drowsiness or dizziness

**Effects on Psychiatric Treatment** None reported

**Pregnancy Risk Factor** B

**Contraindications** Known hypersensitivity to niclosamide

**Warnings/Precautions** Affects cestodes of the intestine only; it is without effect in cysticercosis

**Adverse Reactions**

1% to 10%:

Central nervous system: Drowsiness, dizziness, headache

Gastrointestinal: Nausea, vomiting, loss of appetite, diarrhea

<1%: Alopecia, backache, bad taste in mouth, constipation, diaphoresis, edema in the arm, fever, oral irritation, palpitations, pruritus ani, rash, rectal bleeding, weakness

**Overdosage/Toxicology**

Signs and symptoms: Nausea, vomiting, anorexia

Treatment: In the event of an overdose, do not administer ipecac; decontaminate with lavage or laxatives

**Drug Interactions** No data reported

**Usual Dosage** Oral:

Beef and fish tapeworm:

Children:

11-34 kg: 1 g (2 tablets) as a single dose

>34 kg: 1.5 g (3 tablets) as a single dose

Adults: 2 g (4 tablets) in a single dose

May require a second course of treatment 7 days later

Dwarf tapeworm:

Children:

11-34 g: 1 g (2 tablets) chewed thoroughly in a single dose the first day, then 500 mg/day (1 tablet) for next 6 days

>34 g: 1.5 g (3 tablets) in a single dose the first day, then 1 g/day for 6 days

Adults: 2 g (4 tablets) in a single daily dose for 7 days

**Patient Information** Chew tablets thoroughly; tablets can be pulverized and mixed with water to form a paste for administration to children; can be taken with food; a mild laxative can be used for constipation

**Nursing Implications** Administer a laxative 2-3 hours after the niclosamide dose if treating *Taenia solium* infections to prevent the development of cysticercosis

**Dosage Forms** Tablet, chewable (vanilla flavor): 500 mg

♦ **Nicobid® [OTC]** *see* Niacin *on page 391*

♦ **Nicoderm® Patch** *see* Nicotine *on page 392*

♦ **Nicolar® [OTC]** *see* Niacin *on page 391*

♦ **Nicorette® DS Gum** *see* Nicotine *on page 392*

♦ **Nicorette® Gum** *see* Nicotine *on page 392*

## Nicotine (nik oh TEEN)

**Related Information**

Addiction Treatments *on page 772*

Substance-Related Disorders *on page 609*

**U.S. Brand Names** Habitrol™ Patch; Nicoderm® Patch; Nicorette® DS Gum; Nicorette® Gum; Nicotrol® NS Nasal Spray; Nicotrol® Patch [OTC]; ProStep® Patch

**Canadian Brand Names** Nicorette®; Nicorette® Plus

**Pharmacologic Category** Smoking Cessation Aid

**Use** Treatment aid to smoking cessation for the relief of nicotine withdrawal symptoms

**Pregnancy Risk Factor** D (transdermal)/X (chewing gum)

**Contraindications** Nonsmokers; patients with a history of hypersensitivity or allergy to nicotine or any components used in the transdermal system; patients who are smoking during the postmyocardial infarction period; pregnant or nursing women; patients with life-threatening arrhythmias, or severe or worsening angina pectoris; active temporomandibular joint disease (gum)

**Warnings/Precautions** Use with caution in oropharyngeal inflammation and in patients with history of esophagitis, peptic ulcer, coronary artery disease, vasospastic disease, angina, hypertension, hyperthyroidism, pheochromocytoma, diabetes, severe renal dysfunction, and hepatic dysfunction. Nicotine is known to be one of the most toxic of all poisons; while the gum is being used to help the patient overcome a health hazard, it also must be considered a hazardous drug vehicle. The inhaler should be used with caution in patients with bronchospastic disease (other forms of nicotine replacement may be preferred).

Nicotine nasal spray: Fatal dose: 40 mg

**Adverse Reactions**

Chewing gum:

>10%:

Cardiovascular: Tachycardia

Central nervous system: Headache (mild)

Gastrointestinal: Nausea, vomiting, indigestion, excessive salivation, belching, increased appetite

Miscellaneous: Mouth or throat soreness, jaw muscle ache, hiccups

1% to 10%:

Central nervous system: Insomnia, dizziness, nervousness

Endocrine & metabolic: Dysmenorrhea

Gastrointestinal: GI distress, eructation

Neuromuscular & skeletal: Muscle pain

Respiratory: Hoarseness

Miscellaneous: Hiccups

<1%: Atrial fibrillation, erythema, hypersensitivity reactions, itching

Transdermal systems:

>10%:

Central nervous system: Insomnia, abnormal dreams

Dermatologic: Pruritus, erythema

Local: Application site reaction

Respiratory: Rhinitis, cough, pharyngitis, sinusitis

1% to 10%:

Cardiovascular: Chest pain

Central nervous system: Dysphoria, anxiety, difficulty concentrating, dizziness, somnolence

Dermatologic: Rash

Gastrointestinal: Diarrhea, dyspepsia, nausea, xerostomia, constipation, anorexia, abdominal pain

Neuromuscular & skeletal: Arthralgia, myalgia

<1%: Atrial fibrillation, hypersensitivity reactions, itching, nervousness, taste perversion, thirst, tremor

**Overdosage/Toxicology**

Signs and symptoms: Nausea, vomiting, abdominal pain, mental confusion, diarrhea, salivation, tachycardia, respiratory and cardiovascular collapse

Treatment: After decontamination is symptomatic and supportive; remove patch, rinse area with water and dry, do not use soap as this may increase absorption

**Drug Interactions** CYP2B6 and 2A6 enzyme substrate; CYP1A2 enzyme inducer

Adenosine: Nicotine increases the hemodynamic and AV blocking effects of adenosine; monitor

Bupropion: Monitor for treatment-emergent hypertension in patients treated with the combination of nicotine patch and bupropion

Cimetidine; May increases nicotine concentrations; therefore, may decrease amount of gum or patches needed

CYP1A2 substrates: May decrease serum concentrations of drugs metabolized by this isoenzyme, including theophylline and tacrine

**Mechanism of Action** Nicotine is one of two naturally-occurring alkaloids which exhibit their primary effects via autonomic ganglia stimulation. The other alkaloid is lobeline which has many actions similar to those of nicotine but is less potent. Nicotine is a potent ganglionic and central nervous system stimulant, the actions of which are mediated via nicotine-specific receptors. Biphasic actions are observed depending upon the dose administered. The main effect of nicotine in small doses is stimulation of all autonomic ganglia; with larger doses, initial stimulation is followed by blockade of transmission. Biphasic effects are also evident in the adrenal medulla; discharge of catecholamines occurs with small doses, whereas prevention of catecholamines release is seen with higher doses as a response to splanchnic nerve stimulation. Stimulation of the central nervous system (CNS) is characterized by tremors and respiratory excitation. However, convulsions may occur with higher doses, along with respiratory failure secondary to both central paralysis and peripheral blockade to respiratory muscles.

**Pharmacodynamics/kinetics** Intranasal nicotine may more closely approximate the time course of plasma nicotine levels observed after cigarette smoking than other dosage forms

Duration of action: Transdermal: 24 hours

Absorption: Transdermal: Slow

Metabolism: In the liver, primarily to cotinine, which is $^1/_5$ as active.

Half-life, elimination: 4 hours

Time to peak serum concentration: Transdermal: 8-9 hours

Elimination: Via the kidneys; renal clearance is pH-dependent

**Usual Dosage**

Gum: Chew 1 piece of gum when urge to smoke, up to 30 pieces/day; most patients require 10-12 pieces of gum/day

Transdermal patch (patients should be advised to completely stop smoking upon initiation of therapy): Apply new patch every 24 hours to nonhairy, clean, dry skin on the upper body or upper outer arm; each patch should be applied to a different site

Initial starting dose: 21 mg/day for 4-8 weeks for most patients

First weaning dose: 14 mg/day for 2-4 weeks

Second weaning dose: 7 mg/day for 2-4 weeks

Initial starting dose for patients <100 pounds, smoke <10 cigarettes/day, have a history of cardiovascular disease: 14 mg/day for 4-8 weeks followed by 7 mg/day for 2-4 weeks

In patients who are receiving >600 mg/day of cimetidine: Decrease to the next lower patch size

Benefits of use of nicotine transdermal patches beyond 3 months have not been demonstrated

Spray: 1-2 sprays/hour; do not exceed more than 5 doses (10 sprays) per hour; each dose (2 sprays) contains 1 mg of nicotine. **Warning:** A dose of 40 mg can cause fatalities.

**Monitoring Parameters** Heart rate and blood pressure periodically during therapy; discontinue therapy if signs of nicotine toxicity occur (eg, severe headache, dizziness, mental confusion, disturbed hearing and vision, abdominal pain; rapid, weak and irregular pulse; salivation, nausea, vomiting, diarrhea, cold sweat, weakness); therapy should be discontinued if rash develops; discontinuation may be considered if other adverse effects of patch occur such as myalgia, arthralgia, abnormal dreams, insomnia, nervousness, dry mouth, sweating

**Reference Range** A serum level of >50 ng/mL associated with toxicity; plasma nicotine level of 13,600 ng/mL associated with fatality; mean plasma level after smoking one cigarette: 5-30 ng//mL; plasma levels of cotinine averaged 0.001 mg/L in children from nonsmoking homes and 0.004 mg/L in children from homes with smoking cohabitants

**Patient Information** Instructions for the proper use of the patch should be given to the patient; notify physician if persistent rash, itching, or burning may occur with the patch; do not smoke while wearing patches chew slowly to avoid jaw ache and to maximize benefit

**Nursing Implications** Patients should be instructed to chew slowly to avoid jaw ache and to maximize benefit; patches cannot be cut; use of an aerosol corticosteroid may diminish local irritation under patches

**Additional Information** Cigarette has 10-25 mg nicotine; use of an aerosol corticosteroid may diminish local irritation under patches

**Dosage Forms**

Patch, transdermal:

Habitrol™: 21 mg/day; 14 mg/day; 7 mg/day (30 systems/box)

Nicoderm®: 21 mg/day; 14 mg/day; 7 mg/day (14 systems/box)

Nicotrol® [OTC]: 15 mg/day (gradually released over 16 hours)

ProStep®: 22 mg/day; 11 mg/day (7 systems/box)

Pieces, chewing gum, as polacrilex: 2 mg/square [OTC] (96 pieces/box); 4 mg/square (96 pieces/box)

Spray, nasal: 0.5 mg/actuation [10 mg/mL - 200 actuations] (10 mL)

- **Nicotinex [OTC]** *see* Niacin *on page 391*
- **Nicotinic Acid** *see* Niacin *on page 391*
- **Nicotiramide** *see* Niacin *on page 391*
- **Nicotrol® NS Nasal Spray** *see* Nicotine *on page 392*
- **Nicotrol® Patch [OTC]** *see* Nicotine *on page 392*
- **Nidrel®** *see* Nitrendipine *on page 396*

## Nifedipine (nye FED i peen)

**Related Information**

Calcium Channel Blocking Agents Comparison Chart *on page 710*

**U.S. Brand Names** Adalat®; Adalat® CC; Procardia®; Procardia XL®

**Canadian Brand Names** Adalat PA®; Apo®-Nifed; Gen-Nifedipine; Novo-Nifedin; Nu-Nifedin

**Synonyms** Nifedipinum

**Pharmacologic Category** Calcium Channel Blocker

**Use** Angina, hypertension (sustained release only), pulmonary hypertension

**Effects on Mental Status** Dizziness is common; may cause nervousness, sedation, or mood changes

**Effects on Psychiatric Treatment** May cause leukopenia; use caution with clozapine and carbamazepine; concurrent use with propranolol may increase AV nodal effects; barbiturates may decrease effects of nifedipine

**Pregnancy Risk Factor** C

**Contraindications** Hypersensitivity to nifedipine or any component; immediately release preparation for treatment of urgent or emergent hypertension; acute MI

**Warnings/Precautions** Blood pressure lowering should be done at a rate appropriate for the patient's condition. Rapid drops in blood pressure can lead to arterial insufficiency. Increased angina and/or MI has occurred with initiation or dosage titration of calcium channel blockers. Use caution in severe aortic stenosis. Use caution in patients with severe hepatic impairment (may need dosage adjustment). Abrupt withdrawal may cause rebound angina in patients with CAD. Use caution in CHF (may cause worsening of symptoms).

**Adverse Reactions**

>10%:

Cardiovascular: Flushing (3% to 25%), peripheral edema (10% to 30%)

Central nervous system: Dizziness/lightheadedness (4% to 27%), giddiness, headache (10% to 23%)

Gastrointestinal: Nausea (3% to 11%), heartburn

(Continued)

## Nifedipine *(Continued)*

Neuromuscular & skeletal: Weakness/jitteriness (≤12%)
Miscellaneous: Heat sensation

1% to 10%:
Cardiovascular: Congestive heart failure (2% to 7%), palpitations (≤7%), hypotension (<5%), myocardial infarction (4% to 7%)
Central nervous system: Nervousness (<7%), mood changes, somnolence(<3%)
Dermatologic: Rash/urticaria (≤3%)
Gastrointestinal: Sore throat, diarrhea (<3%), constipation (~3%), abdominal discomfort/flatulence (≤3%)
Neuromuscular & skeletal: Muscle cramps (<8%), arthritis (≤3%), paresthesia/weakness (<3%)
Respiratory: Dyspnea (≤8%), cough (6%), nasal congestion (≤6%), pulmonary edema (7%)

<1%: Anemia, arthritis with increased ANA, blurred vision, chills, dermatitis, diaphoresis, fever, gingival hyperplasia, joint stiffness, leukopenia, purpura, syncope, tachycardia, thrombocytopenia, transient blindness, urticaria

**Overdosage/Toxicology**
Signs and symptoms:
The primary cardiac symptoms of calcium blocker overdose include hypotension and bradycardia. The hypotension is caused by peripheral vasodilation, myocardial depression, and bradycardia. Bradycardia results from sinus bradycardia, second- or third-degree atrioventricular block, or sinus arrest with junctional rhythm. Intraventricular conduction is usually not affected so QRS duration is normal.
The noncardiac symptoms include confusion, stupor, nausea, vomiting, metabolic acidosis and hyperglycemia. Following initial gastric decontamination, if possible, repeated calcium administration may promptly reverse the depressed cardiac contractility (but not sinus node depression or peripheral vasodilation); glucagon, epinephrine, and inamrinone may treat refractory hypotension; glucagon and epinephrine also increase the heart rate (outside the U.S., 4-aminopyridine may be available as an antidote); dialysis and hemoperfusion are not effective in enhancing elimination although repeat-dose activated charcoal may serve as an adjunct with sustained-release preparations.

**Drug Interactions** CYP3A3/4 and 3A5-7 enzyme substrate
Azole antifungals may inhibit the calcium channel blocker's metabolism; avoid this combination. Try an antifungal like terbinafine (if appropriate) or monitor closely for altered effect of the calcium channel blocker.
Beta-blockers may have increased pharmacokinetic or pharmacodynamic interactions with nifedipine
Calcium may reduce the calcium channel blocker's effects, particularly hypotension
Cimetidine reduced diltiazem's metabolism; consider an alternative $H_2$-antagonist
Cisapride increases nifedipine's effects; monitor blood pressure
Ethanol increased nifedipine's AUC by 53%; watch for a greater hypotensive effect
Grapefruit juice increases the bioavailability of nifedipine; monitor for altered nifedipine effects
Nafcillin decreases plasma concentration of nifedipine; avoid this combination
Phenobarbital reduces the plasma concentration of nifedipine. May require much higher dose of nifedipine
Protease inhibitor like amprenavir and ritonavir may increase nifedipine's serum concentration
Quinidine's serum concentration is reduced and nifedipine's is increased; adjust doses as needed
Rifampin increases the metabolism of the calcium channel blocker; adjust the dose of the calcium channel blocker to maintain efficacy
Tacrolimus's serum concentrations are increased by verapamil; avoid the combination. Use another calcium channel blocker or monitor tacrolimus trough levels and renal function closely.
Vincristine's half-life is increased by nifedipine; monitor closely for vincristine dose adjustment

**Usual Dosage** Oral:
Children: Hypertrophic cardiomyopathy: 0.6-0.9 mg/kg/24 hours in 3-4 divided doses
Adolescents and Adults: (**Note:** When switching from immediate release to sustained release formulations, total daily dose will start the same)
Initial: 10 mg 3 times/day as capsules or 30 mg once daily as sustained release
Usual dose: 10-30 mg 3 times/day as capsules or 30-60 mg once daily as sustained release
Maximum dose: 120-180 mg/day
*Increase sustained release at 7- to 14-day intervals*
Hemodialysis: Supplemental dose is not necessary
Peritoneal dialysis effects: Supplemental dose is not necessary
**Dosing adjustment in hepatic impairment:** Reduce oral dose by 50% to 60% in patients with cirrhosis

**Dietary Considerations**
Alcohol: Avoid use
Melatonin has been reported to decrease the antihypertensive efficacy of nifedipine

**Patient Information** Take as directed; do not alter dosage regimen or increase, decrease, or discontinue without consulting prescriber. Do not crush or chew tablets or capsules. Consult prescriber before increasing exercise routine (decreased angina does not mean it is safe to increase exercise). Change position slowly to prevent orthostatic events. May cause dizziness or fatigue; use caution when driving or engaging in tasks that require alertness until response to drug is known. Maintain good oral care and inspect gums for swelling or redness. May cause frequent urination at night. Report irregular heartbeat, swelling, difficulty breathing or new cough, unresolved fatigue, unusual weight gain, unresolved dizziness or constipation, and swollen or bleeding gums.

**Nursing Implications** May cause some patients to urinate frequently at night; may cause inflamed gums

**Dosage Forms**
Capsule, liquid-filled (Adalat®, Procardia®): 10 mg, 20 mg
Tablet, extended release (Adalat® CC): 30 mg, 60 mg, 90 mg
Tablet, sustained release (Procardia XL®): 30 mg, 60 mg, 90 mg


- ♦ **Nifedipinum** *see* Nifedipine *on page 393*
- ♦ **Niferex® [OTC]** *see* Polysaccharide-Iron Complex *on page 452*
- ♦ **Niferex®-PN** *see* Vitamins, Multiple *on page 587*
- ♦ **Nilandron™** *see* Nilutamide *on page 394*
- ♦ **Nilstat®** *see* Nystatin *on page 402*


## Nilutamide (ni LU ta mide)

**U.S. Brand Names** Nilandron™
**Canadian Brand Names** Anandron®
**Synonyms** RU 23908
**Pharmacologic Category** Antineoplastic Agent, Miscellaneous
**Use** In combination with surgical castration in treatment of metastatic prostatic carcinoma (Stage $D_2$); for maximum benefit, nilutamide treatment must begin on the same day as or on the day after surgical castration
**Effects on Mental Status** Insomnia is common; may cause dizziness or depression
**Effects on Psychiatric Treatment** None reported
**Pregnancy Risk Factor** C
**Contraindications** Severe hepatic impairment; severe respiratory insufficiency; hypersensitivity to nilutamide or any component of this preparation
**Warnings/Precautions** The U.S. Food and Drug Administration (FDA) currently recommends that procedures for proper handling and disposal of antineoplastic agents be considered.

Interstitial pneumonitis has been reported in 2% of patients exposed to nilutamide. Patients typically experienced progressive exertional dyspnea, and possibly cough, chest pain and fever. X-rays showed interstitial or alveolo-interstitial changes. The suggestive signs of pneumonitis most often occurred within the first 3 months of nilutamide treatment.

Hepatitis or marked increases in liver enzymes leading to drug discontinuation occurred in 1% of nilutamide patients. There has been a report of elevated hepatic enzymes followed by death in a 65 year old patient treated with nilutamide.

Foreign postmarketing surveillance has revealed isolated cases of aplastic anemia in which a causal relationship with nilutamide could not be ascertained.

13% to 57% of patients receiving nilutamide reported a delay in adaptation to the dark, ranging from seconds to a few minutes. This effect sometimes does not abate as drug treatment is continued. Caution patients who experience this effect about driving at night or through tunnels. This effect can be alleviated by wearing tinted glasses.

**Adverse Reactions**
>10%:
Central nervous system: Pain, headache, insomnia
Gastrointestinal: Nausea, constipation, anorexia
Genitourinary: Impotence, testicular atrophy, gynecomastia
Endocrine & metabolic: Loss of libido, hot flashes
Neuromuscular & skeletal: Weakness
Ocular: Impaired adaption to dark

1% to 10%:
Cardiovascular: Hypertension
Central nervous system: Flu syndrome, fever, dizziness, depression, hypesthesia
Dermatologic: Alopecia, dry skin, rash
Gastrointestinal: Dyspepsia, vomiting, abdominal pain
Genitourinary: Urinary tract infection, hematuria, urinary tract disorder, nocturia
Ocular: Chromatopsia, impaired adaption to light, abnormal vision
Respiratory: Dyspnea, upper respiratory infection, pneumonia
Miscellaneous: Diaphoresis

**Overdosage/Toxicology**

Signs and symptoms: One case of massive overdosage has been published. A 79-year old man attempted suicide by ingesting 13 g of nilutamide. There were no clinical signs or symptoms or changes in parameters such as transaminases or chest x-ray. Maintenance treatment (150 mg/day) was resumed 30 days later.

Treatment: Management is supportive, dialysis not of benefit; induce vomiting if the patient is alert, general supportive care (including frequent monitoring of the vital signs and close observation of the patient)

**Usual Dosage** Adults: Oral: 6 tablets (50 mg each) once a day for a total daily dose of 300 mg for 30 days followed thereafter by 3 tablets (50 mg each) once a day for a total daily dose of 150 mg

**Dietary Considerations** Food: Can be taken without regard to food

**Patient Information** Take as prescribed; do not change dosing schedule or stop taking without consulting prescriber. Avoid alcohol while taking this medication; may cause severe reaction. Periodic laboratory tests are necessary while taking this medication. You may experience dizziness, confusion, or blurred vision (avoid driving or engaging in tasks that require alertness until response to drug is known); loss of light accommodation (avoid night driving and use caution in poorly lighted or changing light situations); impotence; or loss of libido (discuss with prescriber). Report any decreased respiratory function (eg, dyspnea, increased cough); yellowing of skin or eyes; change in color of urine or stool; unusual bruising or bleeding; chest pain; difficulty or painful voiding.

**Dosage Forms** Tablet: 50 mg

## Nilvadipine (NIL va di peen)

**Synonyms** Nivadipine

**Pharmacologic Category** Calcium Channel Blocker

**Effects on Mental Status** May cause dizziness, sleep disturbances, insomnia

**Effects on Psychiatric Treatment** Concurrent use with psychotropics may produce additive hypotension

**Contraindications** Acute apoplectic stroke; intracranial hemorrhage; raised intracranial pressure

**Adverse Reactions**

Cardiovascular: Flushing, tachycardia, edema, hypotension, ectopy (ventricular), shock, chest pain, angina, palpitations, sinus tachycardia, arrhythmias (ventricular)

Central nervous system: Headache, dizziness, sleep disturbances, insomnia

Gastrointestinal: Nausea

Ocular: Oscillopsia

**Usual Dosage**

Hypertension: 4-16 mg/day; reduce dosage to a maximum dose of 8 mg in patients with cirrhosis or with concomitant use with cimetidine

Cerebrovascular disease: 2-4 mg twice daily

Angina pectoris: 8-16 mg/day

♦ **Nimbex®** *see* Cisatracurium *on page 125*

## Nimodipine (nye MOE di peen)

**U.S. Brand Names** Nimotop®

**Pharmacologic Category** Calcium Channel Blocker

**Use** Spasm following subarachnoid hemorrhage from ruptured intracranial aneurysms in patients who are in good neurological condition postictus

**Effects on Mental Status** May cause dizziness; may rarely cause depression

**Effects on Psychiatric Treatment** None reported

**Pregnancy Risk Factor** C

**Contraindications** Hypersensitivity to nimodipine or any component

**Warnings/Precautions** May cause reductions in blood pressure. Use caution in hepatic impairment. Intestinal pseudo-obstruction and ileus have been reported during the use of nimodipine. Use caution in patients with decreased GI motility of a history of bowel obstruction. Use caution when treating patients with increased intracranial pressure.

**Adverse Reactions**

1% to 10%:

Cardiovascular: Reductions in systemic blood pressure (1.2% to 8.1%)

Central nervous system: Headache (1.4% to 4.1%)

Dermatologic: Rash (0.6% to 2.4%)

Gastrointestinal: Diarrhea (1.7% to 4.2%), abdominal discomfort (2%)

<1%: Acne, bradycardia, depression, dyspnea, edema (0.4% to 1.2%), EKG abnormalities (0.6% to 1.4%), hemorrhage, hepatitis, muscle cramps (0.2% to 1.4%), nausea (0.6% to 1.4%), tachycardia

**Overdosage/Toxicology**

Signs and symptoms:

The primary cardiac symptoms of calcium blocker overdose include hypotension and bradycardia. The hypotension is caused by peripheral vasodilation, myocardial depression, and bradycardia. Bradycardia results from sinus bradycardia, second- or third-degree atrioventricular block, or sinus arrest with junctional rhythm. Intraventricular conduction is usually not affected so QRS duration is normal.

The noncardiac symptoms include confusion, stupor, nausea, vomiting, metabolic acidosis and hyperglycemia. Following initial gastric decontamination, if possible, repeated calcium administration may promptly reverse the depressed cardiac contractility (but not sinus node depression or peripheral vasodilation); glucagon, epinephrine, and inamrinone may treat refractory hypotension; glucagon and epinephrine also increase the heart rate (outside the U.S., 4-aminopyridine may be available as an antidote); dialysis and hemoperfusion are not effective in enhancing elimination although repeat-dose activated charcoal may serve as an adjunct with sustained-release preparations.

**Drug Interactions** CYP3A3/4 enzyme substrate

Antihypertensive agents: Effects may be potentiated by nimodipine

Azole antifungals may inhibit the calcium channel blocker's metabolism; avoid this combination. Try an antifungal like terbinafine (if appropriate) or monitor closely for altered effect of the calcium channel blocker

Calcium may reduce the calcium channel blocker's effects, particularly hypotension

Calcium channel blockers: The effects of other calcium channel blockers may be potentiated by nimodipine

Grapefruit juice increases the bioavailability of nimodipine; monitor for altered nimodipine effects

Protease inhibitor like amprenavir and ritonavir may increase nimodipine's serum concentration

Rifampin increases the metabolism of the calcium channel blocker; adjust the dose of the calcium channel blocker to maintain efficacy

Valproic acid increased nimodipine's serum concentration; monitor altered effect of nimodipine

**Usual Dosage** Adults: Oral: 60 mg every 4 hours for 21 days, start therapy within 96 hours after subarachnoid hemorrhage.

Dialysis: Not removed by hemo- or peritoneal dialysis; supplemental dose is not necessary.

**Dosing adjustment in hepatic impairment:** Reduce dosage to 30 mg every 4 hours in patients with liver failure.

**Patient Information** Take as prescribed, for the length of time prescribed; do not discontinue without consulting prescriber. You may experience headache (if unrelieved, consult prescriber), nausea or vomiting (frequent small meals may help), constipation (increased dietary bulk and fluids may help). Promptly report any chest pain or swelling of hands or feet, respiratory distress, sudden weight gain, or unresolved constipation.

**Nursing Implications** If the capsules cannot be swallowed, the liquid may be removed by making a hole in each end of the capsule with an 18-gauge needle and extracting the contents into a syringe; if given via NG tube, follow with a flush of 30 mL NS

**Dosage Forms** Capsule, liquid-filled: 30 mg

♦ **Nimotop®** *see* Nimodipine *on page 395*

♦ **Nipent™** *see* Pentostatin *on page 430*

♦ **Niprina®** *see* Nitrendipine *on page 396*

## Nisoldipine (NYE sole di peen)

**Related Information**

Calcium Channel Blocking Agents Comparison Chart *on page 710*

**U.S. Brand Names** Sular®

**Pharmacologic Category** Calcium Channel Blocker

**Use** Management of hypertension, alone or in combination with other antihypertensive agents

**Effects on Mental Status** May cause dizziness

**Effects on Psychiatric Treatment** None reported

**Pregnancy Risk Factor** C

**Contraindications** Hypersensitivity to nisoldipine, any component, or other dihydropyridine calcium channel blockers

**Warnings/Precautions** Increased angina and/or myocardial infarction in patients with coronary artery disease. Use with caution in patients with hypotension, congestive heart failure, and hepatic impairment. Blood pressure lowering must be done at a rate appropriate for the patient's condition.

**Adverse Reactions** Percentage unknown: Dizziness, headache, peripheral edema, tachycardia

**Overdosage/Toxicology**

Signs and symptoms:

The primary cardiac symptoms of calcium blocker overdose includes hypotension and bradycardia. The hypotension is caused by peripheral vasodilation, myocardial depression, and bradycardia. Bradycardia results from sinus bradycardia, second- or third-degree atrioventricular block, or sinus arrest with junctional rhythm. Intraventricular conduction is usually not affected so QRS duration is normal.

The noncardiac symptoms include confusion, stupor, nausea, vomiting, metabolic acidosis and hyperglycemia. Following initial gastric decontamination, if possible, repeated calcium administration may promptly reverse the depressed cardiac contractility (but not sinus node depression or peripheral vasodilation); glucagon, epinephrine, and inamrinone may treat refractory hypotension; glucagon and epinephrine also increase the heart rate (outside the U.S., 4-aminopyridine may be

(Continued)

## Nisoldipine *(Continued)*

available as an antidote); dialysis and hemoperfusion are not effective in enhancing elimination although repeat-dose activated charcoal may serve as an adjunct with sustained release preparations.

**Drug Interactions** CYP3A3/4 enzyme substrate

Azole antifungals may inhibit the calcium channel blocker's metabolism; avoid this combination. Try an antifungal like terbinafine (if appropriate) or monitor closely for altered effect of the calcium channel blocker.

Beta-blockers may have increased pharmacokinetic or pharmacodynamic interactions with nisoldipine

Calcium may reduce the calcium channel blocker's effects, particularly hypotension

Cimetidine reduced diltiazem's metabolism; consider an alternative $H_2$-antagonist

Grapefruit juice increases the bioavailability of nisoldipine; monitor for altered nisoldipine effects

Rifampin increases the metabolism of the calcium channel blocker; adjust the dose of the calcium channel blocker to maintain efficacy

Tacrolimus's serum concentrations are increased by nifedipine; avoid the combination. Use another calcium channel blocker or monitor tacrolimus trough levels and renal function closely.

Phenytoin decreases nisoldipine to undetectable levels. Avoid use of any CYP3A4 inducer with nisoldipine.

**Usual Dosage** Adults: Oral: Initial: 20 mg once daily, then increase by 10 mg/week (or longer intervals) to attain adequate control of blood pressure; doses >60 mg once daily are not recommended. A starting dose not exceeding 10 mg/day is recommended for the elderly and those with hepatic impairment.

**Dietary Considerations** Avoid grapefruit products before and after dosing

**Patient Information** Take as prescribed - swallow whole (do not crush or break). May be taken with food but avoid grapefruit products and high fat foods. Do not stop abruptly without consulting prescriber. You may experience headache (if unrelieved, consult prescriber), nausea or vomiting (frequent small meals may help), constipation (increased dietary bulk and fluids may help), depression (should resolve when drug is discontinued). May cause dizziness or drowsiness; use caution when driving or engaging in tasks that require alertness until response to drug is known. Promptly report any chest pain or swelling of hands or feet, respiratory distress, sudden weight gain, or unresolved constipation.

**Nursing Implications** Administer at the same time each day to ensure minimal fluctuation of serum levels

**Dosage Forms** Tablet, extended release: 10 mg, 20 mg, 30 mg, 40 mg

♦ **Nitalapram** *see* Citalopram *on page 126*

♦ **Nitrek® Patch** *see* Nitroglycerin *on page 397*

## Nitrendipine (NYE tren di peen)

**U.S. Brand Names** Bayotensin®; Baypresol®; Baypress®; Deiten®; Gericin®; Nidrel®; Niprina®; Tensogradal®; Trendinol®

**Pharmacologic Category** Calcium Channel Blocker

**Effects on Mental Status** May cause dizziness or fatigue

**Effects on Psychiatric Treatment** Concurrent use with psychotropics may produce additive hypotension

**Contraindications** Hypersensitivity to other calcium channel blocking agents; hypotension; advanced aortic stenosis

**Warnings/Precautions** Reduce dosage in elderly; use with caution in patients with liver insufficiency, digital ischemia, nonobstructive hypertrophic cardiomyopathy, Duchenne muscular dystrophy, or in combination with beta-blocking agents. Blood pressure lowering must be done at a rate appropriate for the patient's clinical condition.

**Adverse Reactions**

Cardiovascular: Flushing, edema, tachycardia, palpitations, sinus tachycardia, vasodilation

Central nervous system: Headache, dizziness, fatigue

Gastrointestinal: Nausea, gingival hyperplasia

Otic: Tinnitus

**Drug Interactions** The following interactions occur with concomitant use

Acebutolol: Increased hypotensive effect

Atenolol: Increased hypotensive effect

Carteolol: Increased hypotensive effect

Digoxin: At nitrendipine doses exceeding 20 mg/day, increased digoxin levels and toxicity can occur

Metoprolol: Increased hypotensive effect

Ranitidine: Decrease in clearance of nitrendipine probably of little clinical significance

**Usual Dosage** 20 mg/day (in patients with liver disease or in the elderly, an initial dose of 10 mg is recommended); maximum dose: 40 mg/day

**Additional Information** Can cause an increase in plasma catecholamine, urinary aldosterone levels, and serum alkaline phosphatase levels; natriuresis and diuresis may also occur on a short-term basis

♦ **Nitro-Bid® I.V. Injection** *see* Nitroglycerin *on page 397*

♦ **Nitro-Bid® Ointment** *see* Nitroglycerin *on page 397*

♦ **Nitrodisc® Patch** *see* Nitroglycerin *on page 397*

♦ **Nitro-Dur® Patch** *see* Nitroglycerin *on page 397*

♦ **Nitrofural** *see* Nitrofurazone *on page 396*

## Nitrofurantoin (nye troe fyoor AN toyn)

**U.S. Brand Names** Furadantin®; Macrobid®; Macrodantin®

**Canadian Brand Names** Apo®-Nitrofurantoin; Nephronex®; Novo-Furan

**Pharmacologic Category** Antibiotic, Miscellaneous

**Use** Prevention and treatment of urinary tract infections caused by susceptible gram-negative and some gram-positive organisms; *Pseudomonas, Serratia*, and most species of *Proteus* are generally resistant to nitrofurantoin

**Effects on Mental Status** May cause drowsiness or dizziness

**Effects on Psychiatric Treatment** Concurrent use with anticholinergic/antiparkinsonian medications may increase the absorption of nitrofurantoin

**Pregnancy Risk Factor** B

**Contraindications** Hypersensitivity to nitrofurantoin or any component; renal impairment; infants <1 month (due to the possibility of hemolytic anemia)

**Warnings/Precautions** Use with caution in patients with G-6-PD deficiency, patients with anemia, vitamin B deficiency, diabetes mellitus or electrolyte abnormalities; therapeutic concentrations of nitrofurantoin are not attained in urine of patients with $Cl_{cr}$ <40 mL/minute (elderly); use with caution if prolonged therapy is anticipated due to possible pulmonary toxicity; acute, subacute, or chronic (usually after 6 months of therapy) pulmonary reactions have been observed in patients treated with nitrofurantoin; if these occur, discontinue therapy; monitor closely for malaise, dyspnea, cough, fever, radiologic evidence of diffuse interstitial pneumonitis or fibrosis

**Adverse Reactions** Percentage unknown: Arthralgia, *C. difficile*-colitis, chest pains, chills, cough, diarrhea, dizziness, drowsiness, dyspnea, exfoliative dermatitis, fatigue, fever, headache, hemolytic anemia, hepatitis, hypersensitivity, increased LFTs, itching, loss of appetite/vomiting/nausea (most common), lupus-like syndrome, numbness, paresthesia, rash, sore throat, stomach upset, weakness

**Overdosage/Toxicology**

Signs and symptoms: Include vomiting

Treatment: Supportive care only

**Drug Interactions**

Decreased effect: Antacids, especially magnesium salts, decrease absorption of nitrofurantoin; nitrofurantoin may antagonize effects of norfloxacin

Increased toxicity: Probenecid (decreases renal excretion of nitrofurantoin); anticholinergic drugs increase absorption of nitrofurantoin

**Usual Dosage** Oral:

Children >1 month: 5-7 mg/kg/day in divided doses every 6 hours; maximum: 400 mg/day

Chronic therapy: 1-2 mg/kg/day in divided doses every 12-24 hours; maximum dose: 100 mg/day

Adults: 50-100 mg/dose every 6 hours

Macrocrystal/monohydrate: 100 mg twice daily

Prophylaxis or chronic therapy: 50-100 mg/dose at bedtime

**Dosing adjustment in renal impairment:** $Cl_{cr}$ <50 mL/minute: Avoid use

Avoid use in hemo and peritoneal dialysis and continuous arteriovenous or venovenous hemofiltration (CAVH/CAVHD)

**Dietary Considerations** Alcohol: Avoid use

**Patient Information** Take per recommended schedule, at regular intervals around-the-clock. Complete full course of therapy; do not skip doses. Maintain adequate hydration (2-3 L/day of fluids unless instructed to restrict fluid intake). Diabetics should consult prescriber if using Clinitest® for glucose testing. Nitrofurantoin may discolor urine dark yellow or brown (normal). You may experience nausea or vomiting or GI upset (small frequent meals, frequent mouth care, sucking lozenges, or chewing gum may help); fatigue, drowsiness, blurred vision (use caution when driving or engaging in tasks that require alertness until response to drug is known). Report chest pains or palpitations; pain on urination or blood in urine; skin rash; muscle weakness, pain, or tremors; excessive fatigue or weakness; other persistent adverse effects; or if condition does not improve.

**Dosage Forms**

Capsule: 50 mg, 100 mg

Capsule:

Macrocrystal: 25 mg, 50 mg, 100 mg

Macrocrystal/monohydrate: 100 mg

Suspension, oral: 25 mg/5 mL (470 mL)

## Nitrofurazone (nye troe FYOOR a zone)

**U.S. Brand Names** Furacin® Topical

**Synonyms** Nitrofural

**Pharmacologic Category** Antibiotic, Topical

**Use** Antibacterial agent in second and third degree burns and skin grafting

**Effects on Mental Status** May cause depression

**Effects on Psychiatric Treatment** None reported

**Pregnancy Risk Factor** C

**Contraindications** Hypersensitivity to nitrofurazone or any component

**Warnings/Precautions** Use with caution in patients with renal impairment and patients with G-6-PD deficiency

**Adverse Reactions** Women should inform their physicians if signs or symptoms of any of the following occur thromboembolic or thrombotic disorders including sudden severe headache or vomiting, disturbance of vision or speech, loss of vision, numbness or weakness in an extremity, sharp or crushing chest pain, calf pain, shortness of breath, severe abdominal pain or mass, mental depression or unusual bleeding

Women should discontinue taking the medication if they suspect they are pregnant or become pregnant. Notify physician if area under dermal patch becomes irritated or a rash develops.

**Drug Interactions** Decreased effect: Sutilains decrease activity of nitrofurazone

**Usual Dosage** Children and Adults: Topical: Apply once daily or every few days to lesion or place on gauze

**Patient Information** Follow specific prescriber instructions for application. Protect skin around treated areas with Vaseline® or zinc ointment. Do not apply to skin around eyes. Report signs of sensitization reaction (eg, swelling, redness, itching, burning).

**Dosage Forms**

Cream: 0.2% (28 g)

Ointment, soluble dressing, topical: 0.2% (28 g, 56 g, 454 g, 480 g)

Solution, topical: 0.2% (480 mL, 4000 mL)

♦ **Nitrogard® Buccal** *see* Nitroglycerin *on page 397*

## Nitroglycerin (nye troe GLI ser in)

**U.S. Brand Names** Deponit® Patch; Minitran™ Patch; Nitrek® Patch; Nitro-Bid® I.V. Injection; Nitro-Bid® Ointment; Nitrodisc® Patch; Nitro-Dur® Patch; Nitrogard® Buccal; Nitroglyn® Oral; Nitrolingual® Translingual Spray; Nitrol® Ointment; Nitrong® Oral Tablet; Nitrostat® Sublingual; Transdermal-NTG® Patch; Transderm-Nitro® Patch; Tridil® Injection

**Synonyms** Glyceryl Trinitrate; Nitroglycerol; NTG

**Pharmacologic Category** Vasodilator

**Use** Treatment of angina pectoris; I.V. for congestive heart failure (especially when associated with acute myocardial infarction); pulmonary hypertension; hypertensive emergencies occurring perioperatively (especially during cardiovascular surgery)

**Effects on Mental Status** May cause dizziness

**Effects on Psychiatric Treatment** None reported, but monitor for hypotension if receiving a psychotropic

**Pregnancy Risk Factor** C

**Contraindications** Hypersensitivity to organic nitrates; hypersensitivity to isosorbide, nitroglycerin, or any component of the product; concurrent use with sildenafil; angle-closure glaucoma (intraocular pressure may be increased); head trauma or cerebral hemorrhage (increase intracranial pressure); severe anemia; allergy to adhesive (transdermal product)

I.V. product: Hypotension; uncorrected hypovolemia; inadequate cerebral circulation; increased intracranial pressure; constrictive pericarditis; pericardial tamponade

**Warnings/Precautions** Severe hypotension can occur. Use with caution in volume depletion, hypotension, and right ventricular infarctions. Paradoxical bradycardia and increased angina pectoris can accompany hypotension. Orthostatic hypotension can also occur. Alcohol can accentuate this. Tolerance does develop to nitrates and appropriate dosing is needed to minimize this (drug-free interval). Safety and efficacy have not been established in pediatric patients. Avoid use of long-acting agents in acute MI or CHF; cannot easily reverse. Nitrate may aggravate angina caused by hypertrophic cardiomyopathy.

**Adverse Reactions**

>10%: Central nervous system: Headache (especially at higher doses, may be recurrent with each daily dose), lightheadedness

1% to 10%:

- Cardiovascular: Reflex tachycardia, hypotension, syncope, angina, rebound hypertension, bradycardia
- Dermatologic: Contact dermatitis, fixed drug eruptions (with ointments or patches)

<1%: Hematologic: Methemoglobinemia (very rare)

**Overdosage/Toxicology**

Signs and symptoms: Hypotension, flushing, syncope, throbbing headache with reflex tachycardia, methemoglobinemia with extremely large overdoses; I.V. overdose may be additionally associated with increased intracranial pressure, confusion, vertigo, palpitation, nausea, vomiting, dyspnea, diaphoresis, heartblock, bradycardia, coma, seizures, and death

Treatment: After gastric decontamination, treatment is supportive and symptomatic; hypotension is treated with positioning, fluids, and careful use of low-dose pressors, if needed; methylene blue may treat methemoglobinemia

**Drug Interactions**

Alteplase (tissue plasminogen activator) has a lesser effect when used with I.V. nitroglycerin; avoid concurrent use

Ergot alkaloids may cause an increase in blood pressure and decrease in antianginal effects; avoid concurrent use

Ethanol can cause hypotension when nitrates are taken 1 hour or more after ethanol ingestion

Heparin's effect may be reduced by I.V. nitroglycerin; may affect only a minority of patients

Sildenafil potentiates the hypotensive effects of nitrates; concurrent use is contraindicated

**Usual Dosage Note:** Hemodynamic and antianginal tolerance often develop within 24-48 hours of continuous nitrate administration

Children: Pulmonary hypertension: Continuous infusion: Start 0.25-0.5 mcg/kg/minute and titrate by 1 mcg/kg/minute at 20- to 60-minute intervals to desired effect; usual dose: 1-3 mcg/kg/minute; maximum: 5 mcg/kg/minute

Adults:

- Buccal: Initial: 1 mg every 3-5 hours while awake (3 times/day); titrate dosage upward if angina occurs with tablet in place
- Oral: 2.5-9 mg 2-4 times/day (up to 26 mg 4 times/day)
- I.V.: 5 mcg/minute, increase by 5 mcg/minute every 3-5 minutes to 20 mcg/minute; if no response at 20 mcg/minute increase by 10 mcg/minute every 3-5 minutes, up to 200 mcg/minute
- Ointment: ½" upon rising and ½" 6 hours later; the dose may be doubled and even doubled again as needed
- Patch, transdermal: Initial: 0.2-0.4 mg/hour, titrate to doses of 0.4-0.8 mg/hour; tolerance is minimized by using a patch-on period of 12-14 hours and patch-off period of 10-12 hours
- Sublingual: 0.2-0.6 mg every 5 minutes for maximum of 3 doses in 15 minutes; may also use prophylactically 5-10 minutes prior to activities which may provoke an attack
- Translingual: 1-2 sprays into mouth under tongue every 3-5 minutes for maximum of 3 doses in 15 minutes, may also be used 5-10 minutes prior to activities which may provoke an attack prophylactically

Hemodialysis: Supplemental dose is not necessary

Peritoneal dialysis: Supplemental dose is not necessary

**May need to use nitrate-free interval (10-12 hours/day) to avoid tolerance development; gradually decrease dose in patients receiving NTG for prolonged period to avoid withdrawal reaction**

**Patient Information**

Oral: Take as directed. Do not chew or swallow sublingual tablets; allow to dissolve under tongue. Do not chew or crush extended release capsules; swallow with 8 oz of water.

Spray. Spray directly on mucous members; do not inhale.

Topical: Spread prescribed amount thinly on applicator; rotate application sites.

Transdermal: Place on hair-free area of skin, rotate sites.

Do not change brands without consulting prescriber. Do not discontinue abruptly. Keep medication in original container, tightly closed. Take medication while sitting down and use caution when changing position (rise from sitting or lying position slowly). May cause dizziness; use caution when driving or engaging in hazardous activities until response to drug is known. If chest pain is unresolved in 15 minutes, seek emergency medical help at once. Report acute headache, rapid heartbeat, unusual restlessness or dizziness, muscular weakness, or blurring vision.

**Nursing Implications** I.V. must be prepared in glass bottles and use special sets intended for nitroglycerin; transdermal patches labeled as mg/hour; do not crush sublingual drug product; NTG infusions should be administered only via a pump that can maintain a constant infusion rate

**Dosage Forms**

Capsule, sustained release: 2.5 mg, 6.5 mg, 9 mg, 13 mg

Injection: 0.5 mg/mL (10 mL); 0.8 mg/mL (10 mL); 5 mg/mL (1 mL, 5 mL, 10 mL, 20 mL); 10 mg/mL (5 mL, 10 mL)

Injection, solution in $D_5W$: 25 mg (250 mL), 50 mg (250 mL, 500 mL), 100 mg (250 mL), 200 mg (500 mL)

Ointment, topical (Nitrol®): 2% [20 mg/g] (30 g, 60 g)

Patch, transdermal, topical: Systems designed to deliver 2.5, 5, 7.5, 10, or 15 mg NTG over 24 hours

Spray, translingual: 0.4 mg/metered spray (13.8 g)

Tablet:

- Buccal, controlled release: 1 mg, 2 mg, 3 mg
- Sublingual (Nitrostat®): 0.3 mg, 0.4 mg, 0.6 mg
- Sustained release: 2.6 mg, 6.5 mg, 9 mg

♦ **Nitroglycerol** *see* Nitroglycerin *on page 397*

♦ **Nitroglyn® Oral** *see* Nitroglycerin *on page 397*

♦ **Nitrolingual® Translingual Spray** *see* Nitroglycerin *on page 397*

♦ **Nitrol® Ointment** *see* Nitroglycerin *on page 397*

♦ **Nitrong® Oral Tablet** *see* Nitroglycerin *on page 397*

♦ **Nitropress®** *see* Nitroprusside *on page 398*

## Nitroprusside (nye troe PRUS ide)

**U.S. Brand Names** Nitropress®
**Pharmacologic Category** Vasodilator
**Use** Management of hypertensive crises; congestive heart failure; used for controlled hypotension to reduce bleeding during surgery
**Effects on Mental Status** May cause restlessness, disorientation, or psychosis
**Effects on Psychiatric Treatment** None reported, but monitor for hypotension if receiving a psychotropic
**Usual Dosage** Administration requires the use of an infusion pump. Average dose: 5 mcg/kg/minute.

Children: Pulmonary hypertension: I.V.: Initial: 1 mcg/kg/minute by continuous I.V. infusion; increase in increments of 1 mcg/kg/minute at intervals of 20-60 minutes; titrating to the desired response; usual dose: 3 mcg/kg/minute, rarely need >4 mcg/kg/minute; maximum: 5 mcg/kg/minute.

Adults: I.V. Initial: 0.3-0.5 mcg/kg/minute; increase in increments of 0.5 mcg/kg/minute, titrating to the desired hemodynamic effect or the appearance of headache or nausea; usual dose: 3 mcg/kg/minute; rarely need >4 mcg/kg/minute; maximum: 10 mcg/kg/minute. When administered by prolonged infusion faster than 2 mcg/kg/minute, cyanide is generated faster than an unaided patient can handle.

**Dosage Forms** Injection, as sodium: 10 mg/mL (5 mL); 25 mg/mL (2 mL)


♦ **Nitrostat® Sublingual** *see* Nitroglycerin *on page 397*

♦ **Nivadipine** *see* Nilvadipine *on page 395*

♦ **Nix™ Creme Rinse** *see* Permethrin *on page 432*


## Nizatidine (ni ZA ti deen)

**U.S. Brand Names** Axid®; Axid® AR [OTC]
**Canadian Brand Names** Apo®-Nizatidine
**Pharmacologic Category** Histamine $H_2$ Antagonist
**Use** Treatment and maintenance of duodenal ulcer; treatment of gastroesophageal reflux disease (GERD); OTC tablet used for the prevention of meal-induced heartburn, acid indigestion, and sour stomach
**Effects on Mental Status** May cause dizziness or drowsiness; may rarely cause insomnia
**Effects on Psychiatric Treatment** May rarely cause agranulocytosis; use caution with clozapine and carbamazepine
**Pregnancy Risk Factor** C
**Contraindications** Hypersensitivity to nizatidine or any component of the preparation; hypersensitivity to other $H_2$-antagonists since a cross-sensitivity has been observed with this class of drugs
**Warnings/Precautions** Use with caution in children <12 years of age; use with caution in patients with liver and renal impairment; dosage modification required in patients with renal impairment
**Adverse Reactions**

1% to 10%:
  Central nervous system: Dizziness, headache
  Gastrointestinal: Constipation, diarrhea

<1%: Abdominal discomfort, acne, agranulocytosis, allergic reaction, anorexia, belching, bradycardia, bronchospasm, drowsiness, dry skin, fatigue, fever, flatulence, hypertension, increased AST/ALT, increased BUN/creatinine, insomnia, neutropenia, palpitations, paresthesia, proteinuria, pruritus, seizures, tachycardia, thrombocytopenia, urticaria, weakness

**Overdosage/Toxicology**

Signs and symptoms: Muscular tremors, vomiting, rapid respiration; $LD_{50}$ ~80 mg/kg
Treatment: Primarily symptomatic and supportive

**Drug Interactions** No data reported
**Usual Dosage** Adults: Oral:

Active duodenal ulcer:
  Treatment: 300 mg at bedtime or 150 mg twice daily
  Maintenance: 150 mg/day

Meal-induced heartburn, acid indigestion, and sour stomach:
  75 mg tablet [OTC] twice daily, 30 to 60 minutes prior to consuming food or beverages

**Dosing adjustment in renal impairment:**
  $Cl_{cr}$ 50-80 mL/minute: Administer 75% of normal dose
  $Cl_{cr}$ 10-50 mL/minute: Administer 50% of normal dose or 150 mg/day for active treatment and 150 mg every other day for maintenance treatment
  $Cl_{cr}$ <10 mL/minute: Administer 25% of normal dose or 150 mg every other day for treatment and 150 mg every 3 days for maintenance treatment

**Patient Information** Take as directed; do not increase dose. It may take several days before you notice relief. If antacids approved by prescriber, take 1 hour between antacid and nizatidine. Avoid OTC medications, especially cold or cough medication and aspirin or anything containing aspirin. Follow ulcer diet as prescriber recommends. May cause drowsiness; use caution when driving or engaging in tasks that require alertness until response to drug is known. Report fever, sore throat, tarry stools, changes in CNS, or muscle or joint pain.
**Nursing Implications** Giving dose at 6 PM may better suppress nocturnal acid secretion than 10 PM
**Dosage Forms**
  Capsule: 150 mg, 300 mg
  Tablet [OTC]: 75 mg


♦ **Nizoral®** *see* Ketoconazole *on page 302*

♦ **Nizoral® A-D Shampoo [OTC]** *see* Ketoconazole *on page 302*

♦ **N-Methylhydrazine** *see* Procarbazine *on page 465*

♦ **Nolamine®** *see* Chlorpheniramine, Phenindamine, and Phenylpropanolamine *on page 115*

♦ **Nolex® LA** *see* Guaifenesin and Phenylpropanolamine *on page 257*

♦ **Nolvadex®** *see* Tamoxifen *on page 530*

♦ **Nonbenzodiazepine Anxiolytics and Hypnotics** *see page 721*


## Nonoxynol 9 (non OKS i nole nine)

**U.S. Brand Names** Because® [OTC]; Delfen® [OTC]; Emko® [OTC]; Encare® [OTC]; Gynol II® [OTC]; Koromex® [OTC]; Ramses® [OTC]; Semicid® [OTC]; Shur-Seal® [OTC]
**Pharmacologic Category** Spermicide
**Use** Spermatocide in contraception
**Effects on Mental Status** None reported
**Effects on Psychiatric Treatment** None reported
**Usual Dosage** Insert into vagina at least 15 minutes before intercourse
**Dosage Forms** Vaginal:
  Cream: 2% (103.5 g)
  Foam: 12.5% (60 g)
  Jelly: 2% (81 g, 126 g)


♦ **Nonsteroidal Anti-inflammatory Agents Comparison Chart** *see page 722*

♦ **No Pain-HP® [OTC]** *see* Capsaicin *on page 89*

♦ **Norco™** *see* Hydrocodone and Acetaminophen *on page 272*

♦ **Nordeoxyguanosine** *see* Ganciclovir *on page 245*

♦ **Nordette®** *see* Ethinyl Estradiol and Levonorgestrel *on page 211*

♦ **Norditropin® Injection** *see* Human Growth Hormone *on page 269*

♦ **Nordryl® Injection** *see* Diphenhydramine *on page 174*

♦ **Nordryl® Oral** *see* Diphenhydramine *on page 174*


## Norepinephrine (nor ep i NEF rin)

**U.S. Brand Names** Levophed® Injection
**Pharmacologic Category** Alpha/Beta Agonist
**Use** Treatment of shock which persists after adequate fluid volume replacement
**Effects on Mental Status** May cause anxiety, dizziness, or insomnia
**Effects on Psychiatric Treatment** Monitor for increased pressor effect when used with TCAs, MAOIs, and antihistamines
**Usual Dosage Administration requires the use of an infusion pump!**

**Note:** Norepinephrine dosage is stated in terms of norepinephrine base and intravenous formulation is norepinephrine bitartrate
  Norepinephrine bitartrate 2 mg = Norepinephrine base 1 mg

Continuous I.V. infusion:
  Children: Initial: 0.05-0.1 mcg/kg/minute; titrate to desired effect; maximum dose: 1-2 mcg/kg/minute
  Adults: Initial: 4 mcg/minute and titrate to desired response; 8-12 mcg/minute is usual range; ACLS dosage range: 0.5-30 mcg/minute

**Dosage Forms** Injection, as bitartrate: 1 mg/mL (4 mL)


♦ **Norethin™ 1/35E** *see* Ethinyl Estradiol and Norethindrone *on page 212*

♦ **Norethin 1/50M** *see* Mestranol and Norethindrone *on page 346*


## Norethindrone (nor eth IN drone)

**U.S. Brand Names** Aygestin®; Micronor®; NOR-QD®
**Synonyms** Norethisterone
**Pharmacologic Category** Contraceptive; Progestin
**Use** Treatment of amenorrhea; abnormal uterine bleeding; endometriosis, oral contraceptive; **higher rate of failure with progestin only contraceptives**
**Effects on Mental Status** May cause insomnia or depression
**Effects on Psychiatric Treatment** None reported
**Contraindications** Hypersensitivity to norethindrone; thromboembolic disorders; severe hepatic disease; breast cancer; undiagnosed vaginal bleeding

**Warnings/Precautions** Use of any progestin during the first 4 months of pregnancy is not recommended. Discontinue if sudden partial or complete loss of vision, proptosis, diplopia, or migraine occur. **There is a higher rate of failure with progestin only contraceptives.** Progestin-induced withdrawal bleeding occurs within 3-7 days after discontinuation of drug. Use with caution in patients with asthma, diabetes, seizure disorder, hyperlipidemias, migraine, cardiac or renal dysfunction, or psychic depression.

**Adverse Reactions**

>10%:

Cardiovascular: Edema

Endocrine & metabolic: Breakthrough bleeding, spotting, changes in menstrual flow, amenorrhea

Gastrointestinal: Anorexia

Local: Pain at injection site

Neuromuscular & skeletal: Weakness

1% to 10%:

Cardiovascular: Edema

Central nervous system: Mental depression, fever, insomnia

Dermatologic: Melasma or chloasma, allergic rash with or without pruritus

Endocrine & metabolic: Increased breast tenderness

Gastrointestinal: Weight gain or loss

Genitourinary: Changes in cervical erosion and secretions

Hepatic: Cholestatic jaundice

**Overdosage/Toxicology** Signs and symptoms: Jaundice, nausea, vomiting

**Drug Interactions** Decreased effect: Aminoglutethimide may decrease effects by increasing hepatic metabolism. Nelfinavir decreases norethindrone concentrations.

**Usual Dosage** Adolescents and Adults: Female: Oral:

Contraception: Progesterone only: Norethindrone 0.35 mg every day of the year starting on first day of menstruation; if one dose is missed take as soon as remembered; then next tablet at regular time; if two doses are missed, take one of the missed doses, discard the other, and take daily dose at usual time; if three doses are missed, use another form of birth control until menses appear or pregnancy is ruled out

Amenorrhea and abnormal uterine bleeding:

Norethindrone: 5-20 mg/day on days 5-25 of menstrual cycle

Acetate salt: 2.5-10 mg on days 5-25 of menstrual cycle

Endometriosis:

Norethindrone: 10 mg/day for 2 weeks; increase at increments of 5 mg/day every 2 weeks until 30 mg/day; continue for 6-9 months or until breakthrough bleeding demands temporary termination

Acetate salt: 5 mg/day for 14 days; increase at increments of 2.5 mg/day every 2 weeks up to 15 mg/day; continue for 6-9 months or until breakthrough bleeding demands temporary termination

**Patient Information** Take according to prescribed schedule. Follow instructions for regular self-breast exam. You may experience dizziness or lightheadedness; use caution when driving or engaging in tasks that require alertness until response to drug is known. Limit intake of caffeine. Avoid high-dose vitamin C, folate, or pyridoxine. You may experience photosensitivity; use sunscreen, wear protective clothing and eyewear, and avoid direct sunlight. You may experience loss of hair (reversible), weight gain or loss. Report sudden severe headache or vomiting, disturbances of vision or speech, sudden blindness, numbness of weakness in an extremity, chest pain, calf pain, respiratory difficulty, depression or acute fatigue, unusual bleeding, spotting, or changes in menstrual flow.

**Dosage Forms**

Tablet: 0.35 mg, 5 mg

Tablet, as acetate: 5 mg


- **Norethindrone and Mestranol** *see* Mestranol and Norethindrone *on page 346*
- **Norethisterone** *see* Norethindrone *on page 398*
- **Norethynodrel and Mestranol** *see* Mestranol and Norethynodrel *on page 346*
- **Norflex™** *see* Orphenadrine *on page 407*


## Norfloxacin (nor FLOKS a sin)

**U.S. Brand Names** Chibroxin™ Ophthalmic; Noroxin® Oral

**Pharmacologic Category** Antibiotic, Quinolone

**Use** Uncomplicated urinary tract infections and cystitis caused by susceptible gram-negative and gram-positive bacteria; sexually transmitted disease (eg, uncomplicated urethral and cervical gonorrhea) caused by *N. gonorrhoeae*; prostatitis due to *E. coli*; ophthalmic solution for conjunctivitis

**Effects on Mental Status** May cause dizziness, drowsiness, or insomnia; quinolones reported to cause restlessness, hallucinations, euphoria, depression, panic, and paranoia

**Effects on Psychiatric Treatment** Inhibits CYP1A2 isoenzyme; use caution with clozapine and other psychotropics; monitor for adverse effects

**Pregnancy Risk Factor** C

**Contraindications** Known hypersensitivity to quinolones

**Warnings/Precautions** Not recommended in children <18 years of age; other quinolones have caused transient arthropathy in children; CNS stimulation may occur which may lead to tremor, restlessness, confusion, and very rarely to hallucinations or convulsive seizures; use with caution in patients with known or suspected CNS disorders; has rarely caused ruptured tendons (discontinue immediately with signs of inflammation or tendon pain)

**Adverse Reactions**

1% to 10%:

Central nervous system: Headache (2.7%), dizziness (1.8%), fatigue

Gastrointestinal: Nausea (2.8%)

<1%: Abdominal pain, acute renal failure, anorexia, back pain, bitter taste, constipation, depression, diarrhea, dyspepsia, erythema, fever, flatulence, GI bleeding, heartburn, hyperhidrosis, increased liver enzymes, increased serum creatinine/BUN, insomnia, loose stools, pruritus, rash, tendonitis/tendon rupture, somnolence, vomiting, weakness, xerostomia

**Overdosage/Toxicology**

Signs and symptoms: Acute renal failure, seizures

Treatment: Following GI decontamination, use supportive measures

**Drug Interactions** CYP1A2 and 3A3/4 enzyme inhibitor

Decreased effect: Decreased absorption with antacids containing aluminum, magnesium, and/or calcium (by up to 98% if given at the same time); decreased serum levels of fluoroquinolones by antineoplastics; nitrofurantoin may antagonize effects of norfloxacin; phenytoin serum levels may be decreased by fluoroquinolones

Increased toxicity/serum levels: Quinolones cause increased levels or toxicity of digoxin, caffeine, warfarin, cyclosporine, and possibly theophylline. Cimetidine and probenecid increase quinolone levels.

**Usual Dosage**

Ophthalmic: Children >1 year and Adults: Instill 1-2 drops in affected eye(s) 4 times/day for up to 7 days

Oral: Adults:

Urinary tract infections: 400 mg twice daily for 3-21 days depending on severity of infection or organism sensitivity; maximum: 800 mg/day

Uncomplicated gonorrhea: 800 mg as a single dose (CDC recommends as an alternative regimen to ciprofloxacin or ofloxacin)

Prostatitis: 400 mg every 12 hours for 4 weeks

**Dosing interval in renal impairment:**

$Cl_{cr}$ 10-30 mL/minute: Administer every 24 hours

$Cl_{cr}$ <10 mL/minute: Do not use

**Patient Information**

Oral: Take per recommended schedule, preferably on empty stomach (1 hour before or 2 hours after meals). Maintain adequate hydration (2-3 L/day of fluids unless instructed to restrict fluid intake). Take complete prescription; do not skip doses. Do not take with antacids. You may experience dizziness, lightheadedness; use caution when driving or engaging in tasks that require alertness until response to drug is known. Small frequent meals and frequent mouth care may reduce nausea or vomiting. You may experience photosensitivity; use sunscreen, wear protective clothing and eyewear, and avoid direct sunlight. Report persistent diarrhea or GI disturbances; excessive sleepiness or agitation; tremors; rash; pain, inflammation, or rupture of tendon; or changes in vision.

Ophthalmic: Tilt head back and instill 1-2 drops in affected eye 4 times a day for length of time prescribed. Do not allow tip of applicator to touch eye or any contaminated surface. Do not wear contact lenses if being treated for a bacterial eye infection.

**Nursing Implications** Hold antacids, sucralfate for 3-4 hours after giving

**Dosage Forms**

Solution, ophthalmic: 0.3% [3 mg/mL] (5 mL)

Tablet: 400 mg


- **Norgesic™** *see* Orphenadrine, Aspirin, and Caffeine *on page 408*
- **Norgesic™ Forte** *see* Orphenadrine, Aspirin, and Caffeine *on page 408*


## Norgestrel (nor JES trel)

**U.S. Brand Names** Ovrette®

**Pharmacologic Category** Contraceptive

**Use** Prevention of pregnancy; **progestin only products have higher risk of failure in contraceptive use**

**Effects on Mental Status** May cause insomnia or depression

**Effects on Psychiatric Treatment** None reported

**Pregnancy Risk Factor** X

**Contraindications** Known hypersensitivity to norgestrel; thromboembolic disorders, severe hepatic disease, breast cancer, undiagnosed vaginal bleeding, pregnancy

**Warnings/Precautions** Discontinue if sudden loss of vision or if diplopia or proptosis occur; use with caution in patients with a history of mental depression; use of any progestin during the first 4 months of pregnancy is not recommended

**Adverse Reactions**

>10%:

Cardiovascular: Edema

(Continued)

## Norgestrel *(Continued)*

Endocrine & metabolic: Breakthrough bleeding, spotting, changes in menstrual flow, amenorrhea
Gastrointestinal: Anorexia
Neuromuscular & skeletal: Weakness

1% to 10%:
Cardiovascular: Embolism, central thrombosis
Central nervous system: Mental depression, fever, insomnia
Dermatologic: Melasma or chloasma, allergic rash with or without pruritus
Endocrine & metabolic: Changes in cervical erosion and secretions, increased breast tenderness
Gastrointestinal: Weight gain or loss
Hepatic: Cholestatic jaundice
Local: Thrombophlebitis

**Overdosage/Toxicology**
Signs and symptoms: Toxicity is unlikely following single exposures of excessive doses
Treatment: Supportive treatment is adequate in most cases

**Drug Interactions** Decreased effect: Aminoglutethimide may decrease effects by increasing hepatic metabolism

**Usual Dosage** Administer daily, starting the first day of menstruation, take 1 tablet at the same time each day, every day of the year. If one dose is missed, take as soon as remembered, then next tablet at regular time; if two doses are missed, take 1 tablet and discard the other, then take daily at usual time; if three doses are missed, use an additional form of birth control until menses or pregnancy is ruled out.

**Patient Information** Take this medicine only as directed; do not take more of it and do not take it for a longer period of time; if you suspect you may have become pregnant, stop taking this medicine; report any loss of vision or vision changes immediately; avoid excessive exposure to sunlight

**Nursing Implications** Patients should receive a copy of the patient labeling

**Dosage Forms** Tablet: 0.075 mg


- **Norinyl® 1+35** *see* Ethinyl Estradiol and Norethindrone *on page 212*
- **Norinyl® 1+50** *see* Mestranol and Norethindrone *on page 346*
- **Noritate® Cream** *see* Metronidazole *on page 362*
- **Normal Human Serum Albumin** *see* Albumin *on page 21*
- **Normal Serum Albumin (Human)** *see* Albumin *on page 21*
- **Normiflo®** *see* Ardeparin *on page 47*
- **Normodyne®** *see* Labetalol *on page 304*
- **Noroxin® Oral** *see* Norfloxacin *on page 399*
- **Norpace®** *see* Disopyramide *on page 177*
- **Norplant® Implant** *see* Levonorgestrel *on page 315*
- **Norpramin®** *see* Desipramine *on page 154*
- **NOR-QD®** *see* Norethindrone *on page 398*


## Nortriptyline (nor TRIP ti leen)

**Related Information**

Antidepressant Agents Comparison Chart *on page 704*
Clinical Issues in the Use of Anxiolytics and Sedative/Hypnotics *on page 634*
Discontinuation of Psychotropic Drugs - Withdrawal Symptoms and Recommendations *on page 798*
Federal OBRA Regulations Recommended Maximum Doses *on page 756*
Mood Disorders *on page 600*
Patient Information - Antidepressants (TCAs) *on page 640*
Pharmacotherapy of Urinary Incontinence *on page 758*
Serum Drug Concentrations Commonly Monitored: Guidelines *on page 759*
Special Populations - Elderly *on page 662*
Substance-Related Disorders *on page 609*


**Generic Available** Yes

**U.S. Brand Names** Aventyl®; Pamelor®

**Canadian Brand Names** Apo®-Nortriptyline

**Synonyms** Nortriptyline Hydrochloride

**Pharmacologic Category** Antidepressant, Tricyclic (Secondary Amine)

**Use** Treatment of symptoms of depression
**Unlabeled use:** Chronic pain, anxiety disorders, enuresis

**Pregnancy Risk Factor** D

**Contraindications** Hypersensitivity to this drug and similar chemical class; use of monoamine oxidase inhibitors within 14 days; use in a patient during the acute recovery phase of MI

**Warnings/Precautions** May cause sedation, resulting in impaired performance of tasks requiring alertness (ie, operating machinery or driving). Sedative effects may be additive with other CNS depressants and/or ethanol. The degree of sedation is low-moderate relative to other antidepressants. May worsen psychosis in some patients or precipitate a shift to mania or hypomania in patients with bipolar disease. May increase the risks associated with electroconvulsive therapy. This agent should be discontinued, when possible, prior to elective surgery. Therapy should not be abruptly discontinued in patients receiving high doses for prolonged periods. May alter glucose regulation - use caution in patients with diabetes.

May cause orthostatic hypotension (risk is low relative to other antidepressants) - use with caution in patients at risk of hypotension or in patients where transient hypotensive episodes would be poorly tolerated (cardiovascular disease or cerebrovascular disease). The degree of anticholinergic blockade produced by this agent is moderate relative to other cyclic antidepressants, however, caution should still be used in patients with urinary retention, benign prostatic hypertrophy, narrow-angle glaucoma, xerostomia, visual problems, constipation, or history of bowel obstruction.

Use caution in patients with depression, particularly if suicidal risk may be present. Use with caution in patients with a history of cardiovascular disease (including previous MI, stroke, tachycardia, or conduction abnormalities). The risk conduction abnormalities with this agent is moderate relative to other antidepressants. Use caution in patients with a previous seizure disorder or condition predisposing to seizures such as brain damage, alcoholism, or concurrent therapy with other drugs which lower the seizure threshold. Use with caution in hyperthyroid patients or those receiving thyroid supplementation. Use with caution in patients with hepatic or renal dysfunction and in elderly patients.

**Adverse Reactions**
Cardiovascular: Postural hypotension, arrhythmias, hypertension, heart block, tachycardia, palpitations, myocardial infarction
Central nervous system: Confusion, delirium, hallucinations, restlessness, insomnia, disorientation, delusions, anxiety, agitation, panic, nightmares, hypomania, exacerbation of psychosis, incoordination, ataxia, extrapyramidal symptoms, seizures
Dermatologic: Alopecia, photosensitivity, rash, petechiae, urticaria, itching
Endocrine & metabolic: Sexual dysfunction, gynecomastia, breast enlargement, galactorrhea, increase or decrease in libido, increase in blood sugar, SIADH
Gastrointestinal: Xerostomia, constipation, vomiting, anorexia, diarrhea, abdominal cramps, black tongue, nausea, unpleasant taste, weight gain or loss
Genitourinary: Urinary retention, delayed micturition, impotence, testicular edema
Hematologic: Rarely agranulocytosis, eosinophilia, purpura, thrombocytopenia
Hepatic: Increased liver enzymes, cholestatic jaundice
Neuromuscular & skeletal: Tremor, numbness, tingling, paresthesias, peripheral neuropathy
Ocular: Blurred vision, eye pain, disturbances in accommodation, mydriasis
Otic: Tinnitus
Miscellaneous: Diaphoresis (excessive), allergic reactions

**Overdosage/Toxicology**
Signs and symptoms: Agitation, confusion, hallucinations, urinary retention, hypothermia, hypotension, seizures, ventricular tachycardia
Treatment: Following initiation of essential overdose management, toxic symptoms should be treated. Ventricular arrhythmias often respond to phenytoin 15-20 mg/kg (adults) with concurrent systemic alkalinization (sodium bicarbonate 0.5-2 mEq/kg I.V.). Arrhythmias unresponsive to this therapy may respond to lidocaine 1 mg/kg I.V. followed by a titrated infusion. Physostigmine (1-2 mg I.V. slowly for adults or 0.5 mg I.V. slowly for children) may be indicated in reversing cardiac arrhythmias that are life-threatening. Seizures usually respond to diazepam I.V. boluses (5-10 mg for adults up to 30 mg or 0.25-0.4 mg/kg/dose for children up to 10 mg/dose). If seizures are unresponsive or recur, phenytoin or phenobarbital may be required.

**Drug Interactions** CYP1A2 and 2D6 enzyme substrate
Altretamine: Concurrent use may cause orthostatic hypertension
Amphetamines: TCAs may enhance the effect of amphetamines; monitor for adverse CV effects
Anticholinergics: Combined use with TCAs may produce additive anticholinergic effects
Antihypertensives: TCAs may inhibit the antihypertensive response to bethanidine, clonidine, debrisoquin, guanadrel, guanethidine, guanabenz, guanfacine; monitor BP; consider alternate antihypertensive agent
Beta-agonists: When combined with TCAs may predispose patients to cardiac arrhythmias
Bupropion: May increase the levels of tricyclic antidepressants; based on limited information; monitor response
Carbamazepine: Tricyclic antidepressants may increase carbamazepine levels; monitor
Cholestyramine and colestipol: May bind TCAs and reduce their absorption; monitor for altered response
Clonidine: Abrupt discontinuation of clonidine may cause hypertensive crisis, amitriptyline may enhance the response

CNS depressants: Sedative effects may be additive with TCAs; monitor for increased effect; includes benzodiazepines, barbiturates, antipsychotics, ethanol and other sedative medications

CYP1A2 inhibitors: Serum levels and/or toxicity of some tricyclic antidepressants may be increased; inhibitors include cimetidine, ciprofloxacin, fluvoxamine, isoniazid, ritonavir, and zileutin

CYP2D6 inhibitors: Serum levels and/or toxicity of some tricyclic antidepressants may be increased; inhibitors include amiodarone, cimetidine, delavirdine, fluoxetine, paroxetine, propafenone, quinidine, and ritonavir; monitor for increased effect/toxicity

Enzyme inducers: May increase the metabolism of TCAs resulting in decreased effect; includes carbamazepine, phenobarbital, phenytoin, and rifampin; monitor for decreased response

Epinephrine (and other direct alpha-agonists): The pressor response to I.V. epinephrine, norepinephrine, and phenylephrine may be enhanced in patients receiving TCAs; this combination is best avoided

Fenfluramine: May increase tricyclic antidepressant levels/effects

Hypoglycemic agents (including insulin): TCAs may enhance the hypoglycemic effects of tolazamide, chlorpropamide, or insulin; monitor for changes in blood glucose levels; reported with chlorpropamide, tolazamide, and insulin

Levodopa: Tricyclic antidepressants may decrease the absorption (bioavailability) of levodopa; rare hypertensive episodes have also been attributed to this combination

Linezolid: Hyperpyrexia, hypertension, tachycardia, confusion, seizures, and **deaths have been reported** with agents which inhibit MAO (serotonin syndrome); this combination should be avoided

Lithium: Concurrent use with a TCA may increase the risk for neurotoxicity

MAO inhibitors: Hyperpyrexia, hypertension, tachycardia, confusion, seizures, and **deaths have been reported** (serotonin syndrome); this combination should be avoided

Methylphenidate: Metabolism of TCAs may be decreased

Phenothiazines: Serum concentrations of some TCAs may be increased; in addition, TCAs may increase concentration of phenothiazines; monitor for altered clinical response

QTc prolonging agents: Concurrent use of tricyclic agents with other drugs which may prolong QTc interval may increase the risk of potentially fatal arrhythmias; includes type Ia and type III antiarrhythmics agents, selected quinolones (sparfloxacin, gatifloxacin, moxifloxacin, grepafloxacin), cisapride, and other agents

Sucralfate: Absorption of tricyclic antidepressants may be reduced with coadministration

Sympathomimetics, indirect-acting: Tricyclic antidepressants may result in a decreased sensitivity to indirect-acting sympathomimetics; includes dopamine and ephedrine; also see interaction with epinephrine (and direct-acting sympathomimetics)

Valproic acid: May increase serum concentrations/adverse effects of some tricyclic antidepressants

Warfarin (and other oral anticoagulants): TCAs may increase the anticoagulant effect in patients stabilized on warfarin; monitor INR

**Stability** Protect from light

**Mechanism of Action** Traditionally believed to increase the synaptic concentration of serotonin and/or norepinephrine in the central nervous system by inhibition of their reuptake by the presynaptic neuronal membrane. However, additional receptor effects have been found including desensitization of adenyl cyclase, down regulation of beta-adrenergic receptors, and down regulation of serotonin receptors.

**Pharmacodynamics/kinetics**

Onset of action: 1-3 weeks

Distribution: $V_d$: 21 L/kg

Protein binding: 93% to 95%

Metabolism: Undergoes significant first-pass metabolism; primarily detoxified in the liver

Half-life: 28-31 hours

Time to peak serum concentration: Oral: Within 7-8.5 hours

Elimination: As metabolites and small amounts of unchanged drug in urine; small amounts of biliary elimination occur

**Usual Dosage** Oral:

Nocturnal enuresis:

Children:

6-7 years (20-25 kg): 10 mg/day

8-11 years (25-35 kg): 10-20 mg/day

>11 years (35-54 kg): 25-35 mg/day

Depression:

Adolescents: 30-50 mg/day in divided doses

Adults: 25 mg 3-4 times/day up to 150 mg/day

Elderly (**Note:** Nortriptyline is one of the best tolerated TCAs in the elderly)

Initial: 10-25 mg at bedtime

Dosage can be increased by 25 mg every 3 days for inpatients and weekly for outpatients if tolerated

Usual maintenance dose: 75 mg as a single bedtime dose, however, lower or higher doses may be required to stay within the therapeutic window

**Dosing adjustment in hepatic impairment:** Lower doses and slower titration dependent on individualization of dosage is recommended

**Dietary Considerations** Alcohol: Additive CNS effect, avoid use

**Monitoring Parameters** Blood pressure and pulse rate (EKG, cardiac monitoring) prior to and during initial therapy in older adults; weight

**Reference Range** Therapeutic: 50-150 ng/mL (SI: 190-570 nmol/L); Toxic: >500 ng/mL (SI: >1900 nmol/L)

**Test Interactions** ↑ glucose

**Patient Information** Avoid alcohol ingestion; do not discontinue medication abruptly; may cause urine to turn blue-green; may cause drowsiness; full effect may not occur for 4-6 weeks; dry mouth may be helped by sips of water, sugarless gum, or hard candy

**Nursing Implications** Evaluate mental status; may increase appetite and possibly a craving for sweets

**Dosage Forms**

Capsule, as hydrochloride: 10 mg, 25 mg, 50 mg, 75 mg

Solution, as hydrochloride: 10 mg/5 mL (473 mL)


- ♦ **Nortriptyline Hydrochloride** *see* Nortriptyline *on page 400*
- ♦ **Norvasc®** *see* Amlodipine *on page 35*
- ♦ **Norvir®** *see* Ritonavir *on page 497*
- ♦ **Norzine®** *see* Thiethylperazine *on page 542*
- ♦ **Nosebleed** *see* Feverfew *on page 224*
- ♦ **Nōstrilla® [OTC]** *see* Oxymetazoline *on page 415*
- ♦ **Nostril® Nasal Solution [OTC]** *see* Phenylephrine *on page 439*
- ♦ **Notézine®, Filarcidan®** *see* Diethylcarbamazine *on page 167*
- ♦ **Novacet® Topical** *see* Sulfur and Sulfacetamide Sodium *on page 527*
- ♦ **Novantrone®** *see* Mitoxantrone *on page 370*
- ♦ **Novocain® Injection** *see* Procaine *on page 465*
- ♦ **Novolin® 70/30** *see* Insulin Preparations *on page 287*
- ♦ **Novolin® L** *see* Insulin Preparations *on page 287*
- ♦ **Novolin® N** *see* Insulin Preparations *on page 287*
- ♦ **Novolin® R** *see* Insulin Preparations *on page 287*
- ♦ **NovoLog™** *see* Insulin Preparations *on page 287*
- ♦ **Novo-Seven®** *see* Factor VIIa, Recombinant *on page 218*
- ♦ **NP-27® [OTC]** *see* Tolnaftate *on page 555*
- ♦ **NPH Iletin® I** *see* Insulin Preparations *on page 287*
- ♦ **NPH-N** *see* Insulin Preparations *on page 287*
- ♦ **NSC 26271** *see* Cyclophosphamide *on page 145*
- ♦ **NTG** *see* Nitroglycerin *on page 397*
- ♦ **NTZ® Long Acting Nasal Solution [OTC]** *see* Oxymetazoline *on page 415*
- ♦ **Nubain®** *see* Nalbuphine *on page 380*
- ♦ **Nucofed®** *see* Guaifenesin, Pseudoephedrine, and Codeine *on page 258*
- ♦ **Nucofed® Pediatric Expectorant** *see* Guaifenesin, Pseudoephedrine, and Codeine *on page 258*
- ♦ **Nucotuss®** *see* Guaifenesin, Pseudoephedrine, and Codeine *on page 258*
- ♦ **Nu-Iron® [OTC]** *see* Polysaccharide-Iron Complex *on page 452*
- ♦ **NuLytely®** *see* Polyethylene Glycol-Electrolyte Solution *on page 451*
- ♦ **Numorphan®** *see* Oxymorphone *on page 415*
- ♦ **Numzitdent® [OTC]** *see* Benzocaine *on page 61*
- ♦ **Numzit Teething® [OTC]** *see* Benzocaine *on page 61*
- ♦ **Nupercainal® [OTC]** *see* Dibucaine *on page 163*
- ♦ **Nuprin® [OTC]** *see* Ibuprofen *on page 280*
- ♦ **Nuromax® Injection** *see* Doxacurium *on page 182*
- ♦ **Nu-Tears® II Solution [OTC]** *see* Artificial Tears *on page 48*
- ♦ **Nu-Tears® Solution [OTC]** *see* Artificial Tears *on page 48*


## Nutmeg

**Pharmacologic Category** Herb

**Use** In folk medicine for delayed menses; stomach complains

**Adverse Reactions**

Cardiovascular: Sinus tachycardia

Dermatologic: Contact dermatitis

**Overdosage/Toxicology** Signs and symptoms: The most prominent effects of significant ingestions appear to be hallucinations, nausea, and profound vomiting; miosis, tachycardia, mydriasis, hypothermia, dry skin, hypotension, and a feeling of impending doom may also be seen; symptoms may be delayed up to 8 hours after ingestion

(Continued)

## Nutmeg *(Continued)*

**Drug Interactions**

Decreased effect of antihypertensives

Increased toxicity with disulfiram (possible seizures, delirium), fluoxetine (and other serotonin active agents), TCAs (cardiovascular instability), meperidine (cardiovascular instability), phenothiazine (hyperpyretic crisis), levodopa, sympathomimetics (hyperpyretic crisis), barbiturates, Rauwolfia alkaloids (eg, reserpine), dextroamphetamine (psychoses), foods containing tyramine (hypertension, headache, seizures); theophylline/caffeine (hyperthermia), cyclobenzaprine (fever/seizures)

Potentiation of hypoglycemia with oral hypoglycemic agents

Serotonin syndrome (shivering, muscle rigidity, salivation, agitation, and hyperthermia) can occur with concomitant administration of venlafaxine and tranylcypromine

**Usual Dosage** It is estimated that 2 tablespoons of ground nutmeg will produce toxicity; however, amounts may vary depending on the content of volatile oil

Toxic dose: 1-3 nutmegs can cause toxic symptoms

**Additional Information** Nutmeg is the seed of *Myristica fragrans*; the spice mace is from the seed coat of *Myristica fragrans*

Family: Myristicaceae

Toxin: Myristicin, elemicin, geraniol

Range: Grows in India, Ceylon, and Grenada

Toxic parts: Volatile oil in seed and seed coat appears to be responsible for pharmacologic effects

- **Nutracort®** *see* Hydrocortisone *on page 273*
- **Nutraplus® Topical [OTC]** *see* Urea *on page 576*
- **Nutropin® AQ Injection** *see* Human Growth Hormone *on page 269*
- **Nutropin® Injection** *see* Human Growth Hormone *on page 269*

## Nystatin (nye STAT in)

**U.S. Brand Names** Mycostatin®; Nilstat®; Nystex®

**Canadian Brand Names** Mestatin®; Nadostine®; Nyaderm; PMS-Nystatin

**Pharmacologic Category** Antifungal Agent, Oral Nonabsorbed; Antifungal Agent, Topical; Antifungal Agent, Vaginal

**Use** Treatment of susceptible cutaneous, mucocutaneous, and oral cavity fungal infections normally caused by the *Candida* species

**Effects on Mental Status** None reported

**Effects on Psychiatric Treatment** None reported

**Pregnancy Risk Factor** B/C (oral)

**Contraindications** Hypersensitivity to nystatin or any component

**Adverse Reactions**

Percentage unknown: Contact dermatitis, Stevens-Johnson syndrome

1% to 10%: Gastrointestinal: Nausea, vomiting, diarrhea, stomach pain

<1%: Hypersensitivity reactions

**Overdosage/Toxicology**

Signs and symptoms: Nausea, vomiting, diarrhea

Treatment: Supportive

**Drug Interactions** No data reported

**Usual Dosage**

Oral candidiasis:

Suspension (swish and swallow orally):

Premature infants: 100,000 units 4 times/day

Infants: 200,000 units 4 times/day or 100,000 units to each side of mouth 4 times/day

Children and Adults: 400,000-600,000 units 4 times/day

Troche: Children and Adults: 200,000-400,000 units 4-5 times/day

Powder for compounding: Children and Adults: 1/8 teaspoon (500,000 units) to equal approximately 1/2 cup of water; give 4 times/day

Mucocutaneous infections: Children and Adults: Topical: Apply 2-3 times/day to affected areas; very moist topical lesions are treated best with powder

Intestinal infections: Adults: Oral tablets: 500,000-1,000,000 units every 8 hours

Vaginal infections: Adults: Vaginal tablets: Insert 1 tablet/day at bedtime for 2 weeks

**Patient Information** Take as directed. Maintain adequate hydration (2-3 L/day of fluids unless instructed to restrict fluid intake). Do not allow medication to come in contact with eyes. Report persistent nausea, vomiting, or diarrhea; or if condition being treated worsens or does not improve.

Oral tablets: Swallow whole; do not crush or chew.

Oral suspension: Shake well before using. Remove dentures, clean mouth (do not replace dentures until after using medications). Swish suspension in mouth for several minutes before swallowing.

Oral troches: Remove dentures, clean mouth (do not replace dentures until after using medication). Allow troche to dissolve in mouth; do not chew or swallow whole.

Topical: Wash and dry area before applying (do not reuse towels without washing, apply clean clothing after use). Report unresolved burning, redness, or swelling in treated areas.

Vaginal tablets: Wash hands before using. Lie down to insert high into vagina at bedtime.

**Dosage Forms**

Cream: 100,000 units/g (15 g, 30 g)

Ointment, topical: 100,000 units/g (15 g, 30 g)

Powder, for preparation of oral suspension: 50 million units, 1 billion units, 2 billion units, 5 billion units

Powder, topical: 100,000 units/g (15 g)

Suspension, oral: 100,000 units/mL (5 mL, 60 mL, 480 mL)

Tablet:

Oral: 500,000 units

Vaginal: 100,000 units (15 and 30/box with applicator)

Troche: 200,000 units

## Nystatin and Triamcinolone

(nye STAT in & trye am SIN oh lone)

**U.S. Brand Names** Mycogen II Topical; Mycolog®-II Topical; Myconel® Topical; Myco-Triacet® II; Mytrex® F Topical; N.G.T.® Topical; Tri-Statin® II Topical

**Pharmacologic Category** Antifungal Agent, Topical; Corticosteroid, Topical

**Use** Treatment of cutaneous candidiasis

**Effects on Mental Status** None reported

**Effects on Psychiatric Treatment** None reported

**Usual Dosage** Children and Adults: Topical: Apply sparingly 2-4 times/day. Therapy should be discontinued when control is achieved; if no improvement is seen, reassessment of diagnosis may be necessary.

**Dosage Forms**

Cream: Nystatin 100,000 units and triamcinolone acetonide 0.1% (1.5 g, 15 g, 30 g, 60 g, 120 g)

Ointment, topical: Nystatin 100,000 units and triamcinolone acetonide 0.1% (15 g, 30 g, 60 g, 120 g)

- **Nystex®** *see* Nystatin *on page 402*
- **Nytol® Oral [OTC]** *see* Diphenhydramine *on page 174*
- **OCL®** *see* Polyethylene Glycol-Electrolyte Solution *on page 451*
- **Octamide® PFS** *see* Metoclopramide *on page 360*
- **Octicair® Otic** *see* Neomycin, Polymyxin B, and Hydrocortisone *on page 389*
- **Octocaine®** *see* Lidocaine *on page 317*

## Octreotide (ok TREE oh tide)

**U.S. Brand Names** Sandostatin®; Sandostatin LAR®

**Pharmacologic Category** Antidiarrheal; Antisecretory Agent; Somatostatin Analog

**Use** Control of symptoms in patients with metastatic carcinoid and vasoactive intestinal peptide-secreting tumors (VIPomas); pancreatic tumors, gastrinoma, secretory diarrhea, acromegaly

**Unlabeled use:** AIDS-associated secretory diarrhea, control of bleeding of esophageal varices, breast cancer, cryptosporidiosis, Cushing's syndrome, insulinomas, small bowel fistulas, postgastrectomy dumping syndrome, chemotherapy-induced diarrhea, graft-versus-host disease (GVHD) induced diarrhea, Zollinger-Ellison syndrome

**Effects on Mental Status** May cause drowsiness, dizziness, or depression; may rarely cause anxiety

**Effects on Psychiatric Treatment** None reported

**Usual Dosage** Adults: S.C.: Initial: 50 mcg 1-2 times/day and titrate dose based on patient tolerance and response

Carcinoid: 100-600 mcg/day in 2-4 divided doses

VIPomas: 200-300 mcg/day in 2-4 divided doses

Diarrhea: Initial: I.V.: 50-100 mcg every 8 hours; increase by 100 mcg/dose at 48-hour intervals; maximum dose: 500 mcg every 8 hours

Esophageal varices bleeding: I.V. bolus: 25-50 mcg followed by continuous I.V. infusion of 25-50 mcg/hour

Acromegaly, carcinoid tumors, and VIPomas (depot injection): Patients must be stabilized on subcutaneous octreotide for at least 2 weeks before switching to the long-acting depot: Upon switch: 20 mg I.M. intragluteally every 4 weeks for 2-3 months, then the dose may be modified based upon response

**Dosage adjustment for acromegaly:** After 3 months of depot injections the dosage may be continued or modified as follows:

GH ≤2.5 ng/mL, IGF-1 is normal, symptoms are controlled: Maintain octreotide LAR® at 20 mg I.M. every 4 weeks

GH >2.5 ng/mL, IGF-1 is elevated, or symptoms: Increase octreotide LAR® to 10 mg I.M. every 4 weeks

GH ≤1 ng/mL, IGF-1 is normal, symptoms controlled: Reduce octreotide LAR® to 10 mg I.M. every 4 weeks

Dosages >40 mg are not recommended

**Dosage adjustment for carcinoid tumors and VIPomas:** After 2 months of depot injections the dosage may be continued or modified as follows:

Increase to 30 mg I.M. every 4 weeks if symptoms are inadequately controlled

Decrease to 10 mg I.M. every 4 weeks, for a trial period, if initially responsive to 20 mg dose

Dosage >30 mg is not recommended

**Dosage Forms**

Injection: 0.05 mg/mL (1 mL); 0.1 mg/mL (1 mL); 0.2 mg/mL (5 mL); 0.5 mg/mL (1 mL); 1 mg/mL (5 mL)

Injection, suspension, depot: 10 mg (5 mL); 20 mg (5 mL); 30 mg (5 mL)


- ♦ **Ocu-Carpine® Ophthalmic** *see* Pilocarpine *on page 445*
- ♦ **OcuClear® Ophthalmic [OTC]** *see* Oxymetazoline *on page 415*
- ♦ **OcuCoat® Ophthalmic Solution [OTC]** *see* Artificial Tears *on page 48*
- ♦ **OcuCoat® PF Ophthalmic Solution [OTC]** *see* Artificial Tears *on page 48*
- ♦ **Ocufen® Ophthalmic** *see* Flurbiprofen *on page 236*
- ♦ **Ocuflox™ Ophthalmic** *see* Ofloxacin *on page 403*
- ♦ **Ocupress® Ophthalmic** *see* Carteolol *on page 95*
- ♦ **Ocusert Pilo-20® Ophthalmic** *see* Pilocarpine *on page 445*
- ♦ **Ocusert Pilo-40® Ophthalmic** *see* Pilocarpine *on page 445*
- ♦ **Ocusulf-10® Ophthalmic** *see* Sulfacetamide *on page 522*
- ♦ **Ocutricin® Topical Ointment** *see* Bacitracin, Neomycin, and Polymyxin B *on page 57*
- ♦ **Ocu-Tropine® Ophthalmic** *see* Atropine *on page 53*


## Ofloxacin (oh FLOKS a sin)

**U.S. Brand Names** Floxin®; Ocuflox™ Ophthalmic

**Pharmacologic Category** Antibiotic, Quinolone

**Use**

Quinolone antibiotic for skin and skin structure, lower respiratory and urinary tract infections and sexually-transmitted diseases. Active against many gram-positive and gram-negative aerobic bacteria.

Ophthalmic: Treatment of superficial ocular infections involving the conjunctiva or cornea due to strains of susceptible organisms

**Effects on Mental Status** May cause drowsiness, dizziness, nervousness, or insomnia; quinolones reported to cause restlessness, hallucinations, euphoria, depression, panic, and paranoia

**Effects on Psychiatric Treatment** Inhibits CYP1A2 isoenzyme; use caution with clozapine and other psychotropics; monitor for adverse effects

**Pregnancy Risk Factor** C

**Contraindications** Hypersensitivity to ofloxacin or other members of the quinolone group such as nalidixic acid, oxolinic acid, cinoxacin, norfloxacin, and ciprofloxacin

**Warnings/Precautions** Use with caution in patients with epilepsy or other CNS diseases which could predispose seizures; use with caution in patients with renal impairment; failure to respond to an ophthalmic antibiotic after 2-3 days may indicate the presence of resistant organisms, or another causative agent; use caution with systemic preparation in children <18 years of age due to association of other quinolones with transient arthropathy; has rarely caused ruptured tendons (discontinue immediately with signs of inflammation or tendon pain)

**Adverse Reactions**

1% to 10%:

Cardiovascular: Chest pain (1% to 3%)

Central nervous system: Headache (1% to 9%), insomnia (3% to 7%), dizziness (1% to 5%), fatigue (1% to 3%), somnolence (1% to 3%), sleep disorders, nervousness (1% to 3%), pyrexia (1% to 3%), pain

Dermatologic: Rash/pruritus (1% to 3%)

Gastrointestinal: Diarrhea (1% to 4%), vomiting (1% to 3%), GI distress, cramps, abdominal cramps (1% to 3%), flatulence (1% to 3%), abnormal taste (1% to 3%), xerostomia (1% to 3%), decreased appetite, nausea (3% to 10%)

Genitourinary: Vaginitis (1% to 3%), external genital pruritus in women

Local: Pain at injection site

Ocular: Superinfection (ophthalmic), photophobia, lacrimation, dry eyes, stinging, visual disturbances (1% to 3%)

Miscellaneous: Trunk pain

<1%: Anxiety, chills, cognitive change, cough, decreased hearing acuity, depression, dream abnormality, edema, euphoria, extremity pain, hallucinations, hepatitis, hypertension, malaise, palpitations, paresthesia, photophobia, photosensitivity, syncope, tendonitis/tendon rupture, thirst, tinnitus, Tourette's syndrome, vasculitis, vasodilation, vertigo, weakness, weight loss

**Overdosage/Toxicology**

Signs and symptoms: Acute renal failure, seizures, nausea, vomiting

Treatment: GI decontamination, if possible, and supportive care; not removed by peritoneal or hemodialysis

**Drug Interactions**

Decreased effect: Decreased absorption with antacids containing aluminum, magnesium, and/or calcium (by up to 98% if given at the same time), iron, vitamins with minerals, mineral supplements, sucralfate, or didanosine; fluoroquinolones may be decreased by antineoplastic agents

Increased toxicity/serum levels: Quinolones cause increased caffeine, warfarin, cyclosporine, procainamide, and possibly theophylline levels. Cimetidine and probenecid increase quinolone levels.

**Usual Dosage**

Children >1 year and Adults: Ophthalmic: Instill 1-2 drops in affected eye(s) every 2-4 hours for the first 2 days, then use 4 times/day for an additional 5 days

Adults:

Lower respiratory tract infection: 400 mg every 12 hours for 10 days

Gonorrhea: 400 mg as a single dose

Cervicitis due to *C. trachomatis* and/or *N. gonorrhoeae*: 300 mg every 12 hours for 7 days

Skin/skin structure: 400 mg every 12 hours for 10 days

Urinary tract infection: 200-400 mg every 12 hours for 3-10 days

Prostatitis: 300 mg every 12 hours for 6 weeks

**Dosing adjustment/interval in renal impairment:** Adults: I.V., Oral:

$Cl_{cr}$ 10-50 mL/minute: Administer 200-400 mg every 24 hours

$Cl_{cr}$ <10 mL/minute: Administer 100-200 mg every 24 hours

Continuous arteriovenous or venovenous hemodiafiltration (CAVH) effects: Administer 300 mg every 24 hours

**Patient Information**

Oral: Take per recommended schedule; complete full course of therapy and do not skip doses. Take on an empty stomach (1 hour before or 2 hours after meals, dairy products, antacids, or other medication). Maintain adequate hydration (2-3 L/day of fluids unless instructed to restrict fluid intake).

Oral/I.V.: You may experience dizziness, lightheadedness (use caution when driving or engaging in tasks that require alertness until response to drug is known); nausea, vomiting, or taste perversion (small frequent meals, frequent mouth care, sucking lozenges, or chewing gum may help); photosensitivity (use sunscreen, wear protective clothing and eyewear, and avoid direct sunlight). Report GI disturbances, CNS changes (excessive sleepiness, agitation, or tremors), skin rash, changes in vision, difficulty breathing, signs of opportunistic infection (sore throat, chills, fever, burning, itching on tendonitis/tendon rupture, urination, vaginal discharge, white plaques in mouth), or worsening of condition.

Ophthalmic: Tilt head back, instill 1-2 drops in affected eye as frequently as prescribed. Do not allow tip of applicator to touch eye or any contaminated surface. You may experience some stinging or burning or a bad taste in you mouth after instillation. Report persistent pain, burning, swelling, or visual disturbances.

**Dosage Forms**

Injection: 200 mg (50 mL); 400 mg (10 mL, 20 mL, 100 mL)

Solution, ophthalmic: 0.3% (5 mL)

Tablet: 200 mg, 300 mg, 400 mg


- ♦ **Ogen® Oral** *see* Estropipate *on page 208*
- ♦ **Ogen® Vaginal** *see* Estropipate *on page 208*
- ♦ **OGMT** *see* Metyrosine *on page 363*


## Olanzapine (oh LAN za peen)

**Related Information**


Antipsychotic Agents Comparison Chart *on page 706*

Antipsychotic Medication Guidelines *on page 751*

Atypical Antipsychotics *on page 707*

Clinical Issues in the Use of Antipsychotics *on page 630*

Discontinuation of Psychotropic Drugs - Withdrawal Symptoms and Recommendations *on page 798*

Patient Information - Antipsychotics (General) *on page 646*

Schizophrenia *on page 604*


**U.S. Brand Names** Zyprexa™; Zyprexa™ Zydis®

**Synonyms** LY170053

**Pharmacologic Category** Antipsychotic Agent, Thienobenzodiaepine

**Use** Treatment of the manifestations of psychotic disorders; short-term treatment of acute mania episodes associated with bipolar I disorder

**Pregnancy Risk Factor** C

**Contraindications** Hypersensitivity to olanzapine or any component

**Warnings/Precautions** Moderate to highly sedating, use with caution in disorders where CNS depression is a feature. Use with caution in Parkinson's disease. Caution in patients with hemodynamic instability; bone marrow suppression; predisposition to seizures; subcortical brain damage; severe cardiac, hepatic, renal, or respiratory disease. Esophageal dysmotility and aspiration have been associated with antipsychotic use - use with caution in patients at risk of pneumonia (ie, Alzheimer's disease). Caution in breast cancer or other prolactin-dependent tumors (may elevate prolactin levels). May alter temperature regulation or mask

(Continued)

## Olanzapine *(Continued)*

toxicity of other drugs due to antiemetic effects. Life-threatening arrhythmias have occurred with therapeutic doses of some neuroleptics. Significant weight gain may occur.

May cause anticholinergic effects (constipation, dry mouth, blurred vision, urinary retention); therefore, they should be used with caution in patients with decreased gastrointestinal motility, urinary retention, BPH, xerostomia, or visual problems. Conditions which also may be exacerbated by cholinergic blockade include narrow-angle glaucoma (screening is recommended) and worsening of myasthenia gravis. Relative to other neuroleptics, olanzapine has a moderate potency of cholinergic blockade.

May cause extrapyramidal reactions, including pseudoparkinsonism, acute dystonic reactions, akathisia, and tardive dyskinesia (risk of these reactions is very low relative to other neuroleptics). May be associated with neuroleptic malignant syndrome (NMS).

**Adverse Reactions**

>10%: Central nervous system: Headache, somnolence, insomnia, agitation, nervousness, hostility, dizziness

1% to 10%:

- Cardiovascular: Postural hypotension, tachycardia, hypotension, peripheral edema
- Central nervous system: Dystonic reactions, parkinsonian events, amnesia, euphoria, stuttering, akathisia, anxiety, personality changes, fever
- Dermatologic: Rash
- Gastrointestinal: Xerostomia, constipation, abdominal pain, weight gain, increased appetite
- Genitourinary: Premenstrual syndrome
- Neuromuscular & skeletal: Arthralgia, neck rigidity, twitching, hypertonia, tremor
- Ocular: Amblyopia
- Respiratory: Rhinitis, cough, pharyngitis

<1%: Neuroleptic malignant syndrome, priapism, seizures, tardive dyskinesia, neutropenia, agranulocytosis

**Overdosage/Toxicology**

Signs and symptoms: Drowsiness and slurred developed in one patient taking 300 mg of olanzapine

Treatment: Supportive; activated charcoal 1 g reduced the $C_{max}$ and AUC by ~60

**Drug Interactions** CYP1A2, 2C19 (minor), and CYP2D6 (minor) enzyme substrate

Activated charcoal: Decreases the $C_{max}$ and AUC of olanzapine by 60%

Antihypertensives: Increased risk of hypotension and orthostatic hypotension with antihypertensives

Clomipramine: When used in combination, clomipramine and olanzapine have been reported to be associated with the development of seizures; limited documentation (case report)

CNS depressants: Sedative effects and may be additive with CNS depressants; includes ethanol, barbiturates, narcotic analgesics, and other sedative agents; monitor for increased effect

CYP1A2 inhibitors: Serum levels may be increased and effect/toxicity increased by CYP1A2 inhibitors; examples include cimetidine, ciprofloxacin, fluvoxamine, isoniazid, and ritonavir

Enzyme inducers: May increase the metabolism of olanzapine resulting in decreased effect; includes carbamazepine, phenobarbital, phenytoin, rifampin, and cigarette smoking; monitor for decreased response

Haloperidol: A case of severe Parkinsonism following the addition of olanzapine to haloperidol therapy has been reported

Levodopa: Antipsychotics may inhibit the antiparkinsonian effect of levodopa; avoid this combination

**Mechanism of Action** Olanzapine is a thienobenzodiazepine neuroleptic; thought to work by antagonizing dopamine and serotonin activities. It is a selective monoaminergic antagonist with high affinity binding to serotonin $5HT2_A$ and $5HT2_C$, dopamine $D_{1-4}$, muscarinic $M_{1-5}$, histamine $H_1$- and $alpha_1$-adrenergic receptor sites. Olanzapine binds weakly to GABA-A, BZD, and beta-adrenergic receptors.

**Pharmacodynamics/kinetics**

Absorption: Well absorbed; not affected by food

Distribution: $V_d$: Extensive, 1000 L

Protein binding, plasma: 93% bound to albumin and $alpha_1$-glycoprotein

Metabolism: Highly metabolized via direct glucuronidation and cytochrome P-450 mediated oxidation

Peak concentrations: ~6 hours

Half-life: 21-54 hours; approximately 1.5 times greater in elderly

Elimination: 57% in urine, 30% feces, 7% excreted unchanged; 40% increase in olanzapine clearance in smokers

Not removed by dialysis

**Usual Dosage**

Schizophrenia: Usual starting dose: 5-10 mg once daily; increase to 10 mg once daily within 5-7 days, thereafter adjust by 5 mg/day at 1-week intervals, up to a maximum of 20 mg/day; doses of 30-50 mg/day have been used

Bipolar mania: Usual starting dose: 10-15 mg once daily; increase by 5 mg/day at intervals of not less than 24 hours; maximum dose: 20 mg/day

**Administration** Orally-disintegrating tablets: Remove from foil blister by peeling back (do not push tablet through the foil); place tablet in mouth immediately upon removal; tablet dissolves rapidly in saliva and may be swallowed with or without liquid

**Test Interactions** Increased ALT, AST, GGT, prolactin, CPK, eosinophils

**Patient Information** Use exactly as directed (do not increase dose or frequency); may cause physical and/or psychological dependence. It may take 2-3 weeks to achieve desired results; do not discontinue without consulting prescriber. Avoid excess alcohol or caffeine and other prescription or OTC medications not approved by prescriber. Maintain adequate hydration (2-3 L/day of fluids unless instructed to restrict fluid intake). You may experience excess drowsiness, restlessness, dizziness, or blurred vision (use caution driving or when engaging in tasks requiring alertness until response to drug is known); or constipation (increased exercise, fluids, or dietary fruit and fiber may help). Report persistent CNS effects (eg, trembling fingers, altered gait or balance, excessive sedation, seizures, unusual movements, anxiety, abnormal thoughts, confusion, personality changes); unresolved constipation or gastrointestinal effects; vision changes; difficulty breathing; unusual cough or flu-like symptoms; or worsening of condition. **Pregnancy/breast-feeding precautions:** Inform prescriber if you are or intend to be pregnant. Do not breast-feed.

Orally-disintegrating tablets: Remove from foil blister by peeling back (do not push tablet through the foil); place tablet in mouth immediately upon removal; tablet dissolves rapidly in saliva and may be swallowed with or without liquid

**Dosage Forms**

Tablet: 2.5 mg, 5 mg, 7.5 mg, 10 mg, 15 mg

Tablet, orally-disintegrating: 5 mg, 10 mg

## Olopatadine (oh LOP ah tah deen)

**U.S. Brand Names** Patanol™

**Pharmacologic Category** Antihistamine; Ophthalmic Agent, Miscellaneous

**Use** Temporary prevention of itching of the eye due to allergic conjunctivitis

**Effects on Mental Status** None reported

**Effects on Psychiatric Treatment** None reported

**Usual Dosage** Adults: Ophthalmic: 1 to 2 drops in affected eye(s) twice daily every 6 to 8 hours

**Dosage Forms** Solution, ophthalmic: 0.1% (5 mL)

## Olsalazine (ole SAL a zeen)

**U.S. Brand Names** Dipentum®

**Pharmacologic Category** 5-Aminosalicylic Acid Derivative

**Use** Maintenance of remission of ulcerative colitis in patients intolerant to sulfasalazine

**Effects on Mental Status** May cause drowsiness or depression

**Effects on Psychiatric Treatment** None reported

**Pregnancy Risk Factor** C

**Contraindications** Hypersensitivity to salicylates

**Warnings/Precautions** Diarrhea is a common adverse effect of olsalazine; use with caution in patients with hypersensitivity to salicylates, sulfasalazine, or mesalamine

**Adverse Reactions**

>10%: Gastrointestinal: Diarrhea, cramps, abdominal pain

1% to 10%:

- Central nervous system: Headache, fatigue, depression
- Dermatologic: Rash, itching
- Gastrointestinal: Nausea, dyspepsia, bloating, anorexia
- Neuromuscular & skeletal: Arthralgia

<1%: Bloody diarrhea, blood dyscrasias, fever, hepatitis

**Overdosage/Toxicology** Signs and symptoms of overdose include decreased motor activity, diarrhea

**Drug Interactions** No data reported

**Usual Dosage** Adults: Oral: 1 g/day in 2 divided doses

**Patient Information** Take as directed, with meals, in evenly divided doses. You may experience flu-like symptoms or muscle pain (a mild analgesic may help); diarrhea (boiled milk or yogurt may help); or nausea or loss of appetite (small frequent meals, frequent mouth care, sucking lozenges, or chewing gum may help). Report persistent diarrhea or abdominal cramping, skin rash or itching, or other adverse reactions.

**Dosage Forms** Capsule, as sodium: 250 mg

## Omeprazole (oh ME pray zol)

**U.S. Brand Names** Prilosec™

**Canadian Brand Names** Losec®

**Pharmacologic Category** Proton Pump Inhibitor

**Use** Short-term (4-8 weeks) treatment of severe erosive esophagitis (grade 2 or above), diagnosed by endoscopy and short-term treatment of symptomatic gastroesophageal reflux disease (GERD) poorly responsive to customary medical treatment; treatment of heartburn and other symptoms associated with GERD; pathological hypersecretory conditions; peptic ulcer disease; gastric ulcer therapy; maintenance of healing of erosive esophagitis; approved for combination use in the eradication of *H. pylori* in patients with active duodenal ulcer.

**Unlabeled use:** Healing NSAID-induced ulcers

**Effects on Mental Status** May cause dizziness; may rarely cause sedation

**Effects on Psychiatric Treatment** May inhibit the metabolism of diazepam; monitor for increased sedation

**Pregnancy Risk Factor** C

**Contraindications** Known hypersensitivity to omeprazole

**Warnings/Precautions** In long-term (2-year) studies in rats, omeprazole produced a dose-related increase in gastric carcinoid tumors. While available endoscopic evaluations and histologic examinations of biopsy specimens from human stomachs have not detected a risk from short-term exposure to omeprazole, further human data on the effect of sustained hypochlorhydria and hypergastrinemia are needed to rule out the possibility of an increased risk for the development of tumors in humans receiving long-term therapy. Bioavailability may be increased in the elderly.

**Adverse Reactions**

1% to 10%:

- Central nervous system: Headache (6.9%), dizziness (1.5%)
- Dermatologic: Rash (1.5%)
- Gastrointestinal: Diarrhea (3%), abdominal pain (2.4%), nausea (2.2%), vomiting (1.5%), constipation (1.1%), taste perversion (<1% to 15%)
- Neuromuscular & skeletal: Weakness (1.1%), back pain (1.1%)
- Respiratory: Upper respiratory infection (1.9%), cough (1.1%)

<1%: Abdominal swelling, abnormal dreams, aggression, agranulocytosis, alopecia, anemia, angina, angioedema, anorexia, anxiety, apathy, benign gastric polyps, bradycardia, confusion, depression, dry mouth, dry skin, elevated serum creatinine, elevated serum transaminases, epistaxis, erythema multiforme, esophageal candidiasis, fatigue, fecal discoloration, fever, flatulence, gastroduodenal carcinoids, glycosuria, gynecomastia, hallucinations, hematuria, hemifacial dysesthesia, hemolytic anemia, hepatic encephalopathy, hepatic failure, hepatic necrosis, hypertension, hypoglycemia, hyponatremia, increased serum alkaline phosphatase, increased sweating, insomnia, interstitial nephritis, irritable colon, jaundice, joint pain, leg pain, leukocytosis, liver disease (hepatocellular, cholestatic, mixed), malaise, microscopic pyuria, mucosal atrophy (tongue), muscle cramps, muscle weakness, myalgia, nervousness, neutropenia, pain, palpitation, pancreatitis, pancytopenia, paresthesia, peripheral edema, pharyngeal pain, proteinuria, pruritus, psychic disturbance, skin inflammation, somnolence, Stevens-Johnson syndrome, tachycardia, testicular pain, thrombocytopenia, tinnitus, toxic epidermal necrolysis, tremor, urinary frequency, urinary tract infection, urticaria, vertigo, weight gain

**Overdosage/Toxicology**

Signs and symptoms of overdose include hypothermia, sedation, convulsions, decreased respiratory rate demonstrated in animals only

Treatment: Supportive; not dialyzable

**Drug Interactions** CYP2C8, 2C9, 2C18, 2C19, and 3A3/4 enzyme substrate; CYP1A2 enzyme inducer; CYP2C19, 2C8, 2C9, and 2C19 enzyme inhibitor, CYP3A3/4 enzyme inhibitor (weak)

Decreased effect: Decreased ketoconazole; decreased itraconazole

Increased toxicity: Diazepam may increase half-life; increased digoxin, increased phenytoin, increased warfarin

**Usual Dosage** Adults: Oral:

- Active duodenal ulcer: 20 mg/day for 4-8 weeks
- GERD or erosive esophagitis: 20 mg/day for 4-8 weeks
- Pathological hypersecretory conditions: 60 mg once daily to start; doses up to 120 mg 3 times/day have been administered; administer daily doses >80 mg in divided doses
- *Helicobacter pylori*: Combination therapy with bismuth subsalicylate, tetracycline, and clarithromycin; or with clarithromycin alone. Adult dose: Oral: 20 mg twice daily
- Gastric ulcers: 40 mg/day for 4-8 weeks

**Patient Information** Take as directed, before eating. Do not crush or chew capsules. You may experience anorexia; small frequent meals may help to maintain adequate nutrition. Report changes in urination or pain on urination, unresolved severe diarrhea, testicular pain, or changes in respiratory status.

**Nursing Implications** Capsule should be swallowed whole; not chewed, crushed, or opened

**Dosage Forms** Capsule, delayed release: 10 mg, 20 mg, 40 mg


- ♦ **Omnicef®** *see* Cefdinir *on page 97*
- ♦ **OmniHIB™** *see Haemophilus* b Conjugate Vaccine *on page 261*
- ♦ **Omnipen®** *see* Ampicillin *on page 42*
- ♦ **Omnipen®-N** *see* Ampicillin *on page 42*
- ♦ **OMS® Oral** *see* Morphine Sulfate *on page 374*
- ♦ **Oncaspar®** *see* Pegaspargase *on page 422*
- ♦ **Oncet®** *see* Hydrocodone and Homatropine *on page 273*
- ♦ **Oncovin® Injection** *see* Vincristine *on page 584*


## Ondansetron (on DAN se tron)

**U.S. Brand Names** Zofran®

**Pharmacologic Category** Selective 5-$HT_3$ Receptor Antagonist

**Use** May be prescribed for patients who are refractory to or have severe adverse reactions to standard antiemetic therapy. Ondansetron may be prescribed for young patients (ie, <45 years of age who are more likely to develop extrapyramidal reactions to high-dose metoclopramide) who are to receive highly emetogenic chemotherapeutic agents as listed:

Ondansetron should not be prescribed for chemotherapeutic agents with a low emetogenic potential (eg, bleomycin, busulfan, cyclophosphamide <1000 mg, etoposide, 5-fluorouracil, vinblastine, vincristine)

**Effects on Mental Status** May cause dizziness

**Effects on Psychiatric Treatment** Barbiturates and carbamazepine may increase the metabolism of ondansetron; monitor for diminished effects

**Pregnancy Risk Factor** B

**Contraindications** Hypersensitivity to ondansetron or any component

**Warnings/Precautions** **Ondansetron should be used on a scheduled basis, not as an "as needed" (PRN) basis,** since data supports the use of this drug in the prevention of nausea and vomiting and not in the rescue of nausea and vomiting. Ondansetron should only be used in the first 24-48 hours of receiving chemotherapy. Data does not support any increased efficacy of ondansetron in delayed nausea and vomiting.

**Adverse Reactions**

>10%:

- Central nervous system: Headache, fever
- Gastrointestinal: Constipation, diarrhea

1% to 10%:

- Central nervous system: Dizziness
- Gastrointestinal: Abdominal cramps, xerostomia
- Hepatic: AST/ALT elevations (5%)
- Neuromuscular & skeletal: Weakness

<1%: Angina, bronchospasm, hypokalemia, lightheadedness, rash, seizures, shortness of breath, tachycardia, transient elevations in serum levels of aminotransferases and bilirubin, wheezing

**Drug Interactions** CYP1A2, 2D6, 2E1, and 3A3/4 enzyme substrate

Decreased effect: Metabolized by the hepatic cytochrome P-450 enzymes; therefore, the drug's clearance and half-life may be changed with concomitant use of cytochrome P-450 inducers (eg, barbiturates, carbamazepine, rifampin, phenytoin, and phenylbutazone)

Increased toxicity: Inhibitors (eg, cimetidine, allopurinol, and disulfiram)

**Usual Dosage**

Chemotherapy-induced emesis: Oral:

- Children 4-11 years: 4 mg 30 minutes before chemotherapy; repeat 4 and 8 hours after initial dose, then 4 mg every 8 hours for 1-2 days after chemotherapy completed
- Children >11 years and Adults: 8 mg every 8 hours for 2 doses beginning 30 minutes before chemotherapy, then 8 mg every 12 hours for 1-2 days after chemotherapy completed
- Total body irradiation: Adults: 8 mg 1-2 hours before each fraction of radiotherapy administered each day
- Single high-dose fraction radiotherapy to abdomen: 8 mg 1-2 hours before irradiation, then 8 mg every 8 hours after first dose for 1-2 days after completion of radiotherapy
- Daily fractionated radiotherapy to abdomen: 8 mg 1-2 hours before irradiation, then 8 mg every 8 hours after first dose for each day of radiotherapy
- Prophylaxis with moderate-emetogenic chemotherapy (not FDA-approved): 8 mg twice daily has been shown to be as effective as doses given 3 times/day

I.V.: Administer either three 0.15 mg/kg doses or a single 32 mg dose; with the 3-dose regimen, the initial dose is given 30 minutes prior to chemotherapy with subsequent doses administered 4 and 8 hours after the first dose. With the single-dose regimen 32 mg is infused over 15 minutes beginning 30 minutes before the start of emetogenic chemotherapy. Dosage should be calculated based on weight:

- Children: Pediatric dosing should follow the manufacturer's guidelines for 0.15 mg/kg/dose administered 30 minutes prior to chemotherapy, 4 and 8 hours after the first dose. While not as yet FDA-approved, literature supports the day's total dose administered as a single dose 30 minutes prior to chemotherapy.
- Adults:
  - >80 kg: 12 mg IVPB
  - 45-80 kg: 8 mg IVPB
  - <45 kg: 0.15 mg/kg/dose IVPB

Postoperative emesis: I.V.:

- Children >2 years: 0.1 mg/kg I.V. slow push; if over 40 kg weight, administer 4 mg IVP over 2-5 minutes (no faster than 30 seconds); give I.V. as s single dose immediately before induction of anesthesia or shortly following procedure if vomiting occurs
- Adults (infuse in not less than 30 seconds, preferably over 2-5 minutes, as undiluted drug): 4 mg as a single dose immediately before induction of anesthesia; or shortly following procedure if vomiting occurs

**Dosing in hepatic impairment:** Maximum daily dose: 8 mg in cirrhotic patients with severe liver disease

(Continued)

## Ondansetron *(Continued)*

**Dietary Considerations**

Food: Increases the extent of absorption. The $C_{max}$ and $T_{max}$ does not change much; take without regard to meals

Potassium: Hypokalemia; monitor potassium serum concentration

**Patient Information** This drug may cause drowsiness; use caution when driving or engaging in tasks that require alertness until response to drug is known. You may experience constipation and headache (request appropriate treatment from prescriber). Do not change position rapidly (rise slowly). Good mouth care and sucking on lozenges may help relieve nausea. Report persistent headache, excessive drowsiness, fever, numbness or tingling, or severe changes in elimination patterns (constipation or diarrhea), chest pain, or palpitations.

**Nursing Implications** First dose should be given 30 minutes prior to beginning chemotherapy

**Dosage Forms**

Injection, as hydrochloride: 2 mg/mL (20 mL); 32 mg (single-dose vials)
Solution, as hydrochloride: 4 mg/5 mL
Tablet, as hydrochloride: 4 mg, 8 mg
Tablet, as hydrochloride, orally disintegrating: 4 mg, 8 mg


- ♦ **Ontak™** *see* Denileukin Diftitox *on page 154*
- ♦ **Ony-Clear® Spray** *see* Miconazole *on page 364*
- ♦ **OP-CCK** *see* Sincalide *on page 513*
- ♦ **Opcon® Ophthalmic** *see* Naphazoline *on page 383*
- ♦ **o,p'-DDD** *see* Mitotane *on page 369*
- ♦ **Operand® [OTC]** *see* Povidone-Iodine *on page 456*
- ♦ **Ophthetic®** *see* Proparacaine *on page 473*


## Opium Alkaloids (OH pee um AL ka loyds)

**Related Information**

Substance-Related Disorders *on page 609*

**U.S. Brand Names** Pantopon®

**Pharmacologic Category** Analgesic, Narcotic

**Use** Relief of severe pain

**Effects on Mental Status** Drowsiness and dizziness are common; may cause nervousness or restlessness; may rarely cause depression or hallucinations

**Effects on Psychiatric Treatment** MAOIs may potentiate the effects of opioids

**Restrictions** C-II

**Pregnancy Risk Factor** B (D if used for prolonged periods or in high doses at term)

**Contraindications** Hypersensitivity to opium alkaloids

**Adverse Reactions**

>10%:

Cardiovascular: Hypotension
Central nervous system: Fatigue, drowsiness, dizziness
Gastrointestinal: Nausea, vomiting
Neuromuscular & skeletal: Weakness

1% to 10%:

Central nervous system: Nervousness, headache, restlessness, malaise, confusion
Gastrointestinal: Stomach cramps, xerostomia, constipation, anorexia, biliary spasm
Genitourinary: Decreased urination, ureteral spasms
Local: Pain at injection site
Respiratory: Troubled breathing, shortness of breath

**Drug Interactions** CNS depressants, MAO inhibitors may potentiate adverse effects

**Usual Dosage** Adults: I.M., S.C.: 5-20 mg every 4-5 hours

**Dosage Forms** Injection: 20 mg/mL (1 mL)

## Opium Tincture (OH pee um TING chur)

**Synonyms** Deodorized Opium Tincture; DTO

**Pharmacologic Category** Analgesic, Narcotic; Antidiarrheal

**Use** Treatment of diarrhea or relief of pain

**Effects on Mental Status** Dizziness and drowsiness are common; may cause restlessness; may rarely cause insomnia or depression

**Effects on Psychiatric Treatment** Concurrent use with psychotropics may alter the analgesic effects of opioids; monitor for altered response

**Restrictions** C-II

**Pregnancy Risk Factor** B (D if used for prolonged periods or in high doses at term)

**Contraindications** Increased intracranial pressure, severe respiratory depression, severe liver or renal insufficiency, known hypersensitivity to morphine sulfate

**Warnings/Precautions** Opium shares the toxic potential of opiate agonists, and usual precautions of opiate agonist therapy should be observed; some preparations contain sulfites which may cause allergic reactions; infants <3 months of age are more susceptible to respiratory depression, use with caution and generally in reduced doses in this age group; this is **not** paregoric, dose accordingly

**Adverse Reactions**

>10%:

Cardiovascular: Palpitations, hypotension, bradycardia
Central nervous system: Drowsiness, dizziness
Neuromuscular & skeletal: Weakness

1% to 10%:

Central nervous system: Restlessness, headache, malaise
Genitourinary: Decreased urination
Miscellaneous: Histamine release

<1%: Anorexia, biliary tract spasm, CNS depression, constipation, increased intracranial pressure, insomnia, mental depression, miosis, nausea, peripheral vasodilation, physical and psychological dependence, respiratory depression, stomach cramps, urinary tract spasm, vomiting

**Overdosage/Toxicology**

Signs and symptoms: Primary attention should be directed to ensuring adequate respiratory exchange; opiate agonist-induced respiratory depression may be reversed with parenteral naloxone hydrochloride

Treatment: Naloxone 2 mg I.V. (0.01 mg/kg for children) with repeat administration as necessary up to a total of 10 mg

**Drug Interactions**

Decreased effect: Phenothiazines may antagonize the analgesic effect of opiate agonists

Increased toxicity: CNS depressants, MAO inhibitors, tricyclic antidepressants may potentiate the effects of opiate agonists; dextroamphetamine may enhance the analgesic effect of opiate agonists

**Usual Dosage** Oral:

Children:

Diarrhea: 0.005-0.01 mL/kg/dose every 3-4 hours for a maximum of 6 doses/24 hours
Analgesia: 0.01-0.02 mL/kg/dose every 3-4 hours

Adults:

Diarrhea: 0.3-1 mL/dose every 2-6 hours to maximum of 6 mL/24 hours
Analgesia: 0.6-1.5 mL/dose every 3-4 hours

**Dietary Considerations** Alcohol: Additive CNS effect, avoid use

**Patient Information** If self-administered, use exactly as directed (do not increase dose or frequency); may cause physical and/or psychological dependence. While using this medication, do not use alcohol and other prescription or OTC medications (especially sedatives, tranquilizers, antihistamines, or pain medications) without consulting prescriber. Maintain adequate hydration (2-3 L/day of fluids unless instructed to restrict fluid intake). May cause hypotension, dizziness, drowsiness, impaired coordination, or blurred vision (use caution when driving, climbing stairs, or changing position - rising from sitting or lying to standing, or when engaging in tasks requiring alertness until response to drug is known); dry mouth (frequent mouth care, small frequent meals, chewing gum, or sucking lozenges may help). Report slow or rapid heartbeat, acute dizziness, or persistent headache; changes in mental status; swelling of extremities or unusual weight gain; changes in urinary elimination or pain on urination; acute headache; trembling or muscle spasms; blurred vision; skin rash; or shortness of breath.

**Dosage Forms** Liquid: 10% [0.6 mL equivalent to morphine 6 mg]

## Oprelvekin (oh PREL ve kin)

**U.S. Brand Names** Neumega®

**Pharmacologic Category** Biological Response Modulator; Human Growth Factor

**Use** Prevention of severe thrombocytopenia and the reduction of the need for platelet transfusions following myelosuppressive chemotherapy in patients with nonmyeloid malignancies who are at high risk of severe thrombocytopenia.

**Effects on Mental Status** Dizziness, insomnia, and fatigue are common

**Effects on Psychiatric Treatment** Anemia is common; use caution with clozapine and carbamazepine

**Usual Dosage** S.C.:

Children: 75-100 mcg/kg once daily for 10-21 days (until postnadir platelet count ≥50,000 cells/μL)

Adults: 50 mcg/kg once daily for 10-21 days (until postnadir platelet count ≥50,000 cells/μL)

**Dosage Forms** Powder for injection, lyophilized: 5 mg


- ♦ **Opticyl®** *see* Tropicamide *on page 574*
- ♦ **Optigene® Ophthalmic [OTC]** *see* Tetrahydrozoline *on page 538*
- ♦ **Optimine®** *see* Azatadine *on page 54*
- ♦ **Optimoist® Solution [OTC]** *see* Saliva Substitute *on page 502*
- ♦ **OptiPranolol® Ophthalmic** *see* Metipranolol *on page 360*
- ♦ **Optivar™** *see* Azelastine *on page 55*
- ♦ **Orabase®-B [OTC]** *see* Benzocaine *on page 61*

- **Orabase® HCA** *see* Hydrocortisone *on page 273*
- **Orabase®-O [OTC]** *see* Benzocaine *on page 61*
- **Orabase® With Benzocaine [OTC]** *see* Benzocaine, Gelatin, Pectin, and Sodium Carboxymethylcellulose *on page 62*
- **Orajel® Brace-Aid Oral Anesthetic [OTC]** *see* Benzocaine *on page 61*
- **Orajel® Maximum Strength [OTC]** *see* Benzocaine *on page 61*
- **Orajel® Mouth-Aid [OTC]** *see* Benzocaine *on page 61*
- **Orajel® Perioseptic [OTC]** *see* Carbamide Peroxide *on page 92*
- **Oramorph SR™ Oral** *see* Morphine Sulfate *on page 374*
- **Orap™** *see* Pimozide *on page 445*
- **Orasept® [OTC]** *see* Benzocaine *on page 61*
- **Orasol® [OTC]** *see* Benzocaine *on page 61*
- **Orasone®** *see* Prednisone *on page 461*
- **Orciprenaline Sulfate** *see* Metaproterenol *on page 347*
- **Ordrine AT® Extended Release Capsule** *see* Caramiphen and Phenylpropanolamine *on page 90*
- **Oretic®** *see* Hydrochlorothiazide *on page 271*
- **Oreton® Methyl** *see* Methyltestosterone *on page 360*
- **Orexin® [OTC]** *see* Vitamin B Complex *on page 586*
- **Organidin® NR** *see* Guaifenesin *on page 256*
- **Orgaran®** *see* Danaparoid *on page 150*
- **Orinase® Diagnostic Injection** *see* Tolbutamide *on page 553*
- **Orinase® Oral** *see* Tolbutamide *on page 553*
- **ORLAAM®** *see* Levomethadyl Acetate Hydrochloride *on page 315*

## Orlistat (OR li stat)

**U.S. Brand Names** Xenical®

**Pharmacologic Category** Lipase Inhibitor

**Use** Management of obesity, including weight loss and weight management when used in conjunction with a reduced-calorie diet; reduce the risk of weight regain after prior weight loss; indicated for obese patients with an initial body mass index (BMI) ≥30 kg/m$^2$ or ≥27 kg/m$^2$ in the presence of other risk factors; see table

**Body Mass Index (BMI), kg/m$^2$**
**Height (feet, inches)**

| Weight (lb) | 5'0" | 5'3" | 5'6" | 5'9" | 6'0" | 6'3" |
|---|---|---|---|---|---|---|
| 140 | 27 | 25 | 23 | 21 | 19 | 18 |
| 150 | 29 | 27 | 24 | 22 | 20 | 19 |
| 160 | 31 | 28 | 26 | 24 | 22 | 20 |
| 170 | 33 | 30 | 28 | 25 | 23 | 21 |
| 180 | 35 | 32 | 29 | 27 | 25 | 23 |
| 190 | 37 | 34 | 31 | 28 | 26 | 24 |
| 200 | 39 | 36 | 32 | 30 | 27 | 25 |
| 210 | 41 | 37 | 34 | 31 | 29 | 26 |
| 220 | 43 | 39 | 36 | 33 | 30 | 28 |
| 230 | 45 | 41 | 37 | 34 | 31 | 29 |
| 240 | 47 | 43 | 39 | 36 | 33 | 30 |
| 250 | 49 | 44 | 40 | 37 | 34 | 31 |

**Pregnancy Risk Factor** B

**Pregnancy/Breast-Feeding Implications** There are no adequate and well-controlled studies of orlistat in pregnant women. Because animal reproductive studies are not always predictive of human response, orlistat is not recommended for use during pregnancy. Teratogenicity studies were conducted in rats and rabbits at doses up to 800 mg/kg/day. Neither study showed embryotoxicity or teratogenicity. This dose is 23 and 47 times the daily human dose calculated on a body surface area basis for rats and rabbits, respectively. It is not know if orlistat is secreted in human milk. Therefore, it should not be taken by nursing women.

**Contraindications** Chronic malabsorption syndrome or cholestasis; hypersensitivity to orlistat or any component

**Warnings/Precautions** Patients should be advised to adhere to dietary guidelines; gastrointestinal adverse events may increase if taken with a diet high in fat (>30% total daily calories from fat). The daily intake of fat should be distributed over three main meals. If taken with any one meal very high in fat, the possibility of gastrointestinal effects increases. Patients should be counseled to take a multivitamin supplement that contains fat-soluble vitamins to ensure adequate nutrition because orlistat has been shown to reduce the absorption of some fat-soluble vitamins and beta-carotene. The supplement should be taken once daily at least 2 hours before or after the administration of orlistat (ie, bedtime). Some patients may develop increased levels of urinary oxalate following treatment; caution should be exercised when prescribing it to patients with a history of hyperoxaluria or calcium oxalate nephrolithiasis. As with any weight-loss agent, the potential exists for misuse in appropriate patient populations (eg, patients with anorexia nervosa or bulimia).

**Adverse Reactions** Percentage unknown: Anxiety, arthritis, back pain, depression, dizziness, dry skin, ear/nose/throat symptoms, fatty/oily stool, fecal incontinence, fecal urgency, flatus with discharge, headache, increased defecation, influenza, joint disorder, myalgia, oily evacuation, oily spotting, otitis, pain of lower extremities, rash, respiratory tract infection, sleep disorder, tendonitis

**Overdosage/Toxicology** Single doses of 800 mg and multiple doses of up to 400 mg 3 times daily for 15 days have been studied in normal weight and obese patients without significant adverse findings; in case of significant overdose, it is recommended that the patient be observed for 24 hours

**Drug Interactions**

Fat-soluble vitamins: Absorption of vitamins A,D,E, and K may be decreased by orlistat (also see note on warfarin)

Nifedipine: Serum levels may be slightly reduced during coadministration of orlistat; monitor

Warfarin: Vitamin K absorption may be decreased when taken with orlistat; because of a potential alteration in vitamin K absorption, patients stabilized on warfarin must be closely monitored; dosage adjustment may be required

**Usual Dosage** 120 mg 3 times/day with each main meal containing fat (during or up to 1 hour after the meal); omit dose if meal is occasionally missed or contains no fat

**Monitoring Parameters** Changes in coagulation parameters

**Patient Information** Patient should be on a nutritionally balanced, reduced-calorie diet that contains approximately 30% of calories from fat; daily intake of fat, carbohydrate, and protein should be distributed over the three main meals

**Dosage Forms** Capsule: 120 mg

- **Ormazine** *see* Chlorpromazine *on page 116*
- **Ornade® Spansule®** *see* Chlorpheniramine and Phenylpropanolamine *on page 114*
- **Ornex® No Drowsiness [OTC]** *see* Acetaminophen and Pseudoephedrine *on page 15*
- **Ornidyl® Injection** *see* Eflornithine *on page 191*

## Orphenadrine (or FEN a dreen)

**Related Information**

Antiparkinsonian Agents Comparison Chart *on page 705*

Patient Information - Agents for Treatment of Extrapyramidal Symptoms *on page 657*

**U.S. Brand Names** Norflex™

**Pharmacologic Category** Anti-Parkinson's Agent (Anticholinergic); Skeletal Muscle Relaxant

**Use** Treatment of muscle spasm associated with acute painful musculoskeletal conditions; supportive therapy in tetanus

**Effects on Mental Status** Drowsiness and dizziness are common; may rarely cause hallucinations

**Effects on Psychiatric Treatment** May rarely cause aplastic anemia; use caution with clozapine and carbamazepine; has been used to treat tardive dyskinesia and augment typical antipsychotics; clozapine is a better option; concurrent use with psychotropics may produce additive sedation

**Pregnancy Risk Factor** C

**Contraindications** Glaucoma, GI obstruction, cardiospasm, myasthenia gravis, hypersensitivity to orphenadrine or any component

**Warnings/Precautions** Use with caution in patients with CHF or cardiac arrhythmias; some products contain sulfites

**Adverse Reactions**

>10%:

- Central nervous system: Drowsiness, dizziness
- Ocular: Blurred vision

1% to 10%:

- Cardiovascular: Flushing of face, tachycardia, syncope
- Dermatologic: Rash
- Gastrointestinal: Nausea, vomiting, constipation
- Genitourinary: Decreased urination
- Neuromuscular & skeletal: Weakness
- Ocular: Nystagmus, increased intraocular pressure
- Respiratory: Nasal congestion

<1%: Aplastic anemia, hallucinations

**Overdosage/Toxicology**

Signs and symptoms: Blurred vision, tachycardia, confusion, seizures, respiratory arrest, dysrhythmias

(Continued)

## Orphenadrine *(Continued)*

Treatment: There is no specific treatment for an antihistamine overdose, however, most of its clinical toxicity is due to anticholinergic effects. Anticholinesterase inhibitors may be useful by reducing acetylcholinesterase. Anticholinesterase inhibitors include physostigmine, neostigmine, pyridostigmine and edrophonium. For anticholinergic overdose with severe life-threatening symptoms, physostigmine 1-2 mg (0.5 or 0.02 mg/kg for children) I.V., slowly may be given to reverse these effects. Lethal dose is 2-3 g; treatment is symptomatic.

**Drug Interactions** CYP2B6, 2D6, and 3A3/4 enzyme substrate; CYP2B6 enzyme inhibitor

**Usual Dosage** Adults:

Oral: 100 mg twice daily

I.M., I.V.: 60 mg every 12 hours

**Dietary Considerations** Alcohol: Additive CNS effect, avoid use

**Patient Information** Take exactly as directed. Do not increase dose or discontinue without consulting prescriber. Do not chew or crush sustained release tablets. Do not use alcohol, prescriptive or OTC antidepressants, sedatives, or pain medications without consulting prescriber. You may experience drowsiness, dizziness, lightheadedness (avoid driving or engaging in tasks requiring alertness until response to drug is known); nausea or vomiting (small, frequent meals, frequent mouth care, or sucking hard candy may help); constipation (increased dietary fluids and fibers or increased exercise may help); or decreased urination (void before taking medication). Report excessive drowsiness or mental agitation, chest pain, skin rash, swelling of mouth/face, difficulty speaking, or vision disturbances.

**Nursing Implications** Do not crush sustained release drug product; raise bed rails, institute safety measures, assist with ambulation

**Dosage Forms**

Injection, as citrate: 30 mg/mL (2 mL, 10 mL)

Tablet, as citrate: 100 mg

Tablet, as citrate, sustained release: 100 mg

## Orphenadrine, Aspirin, and Caffeine

(or FEN a dreen, AS pir in, & KAF een)

**U.S. Brand Names** Norgesic™; Norgesic™ Forte

**Pharmacologic Category** Skeletal Muscle Relaxant

**Use** Relief of discomfort associated with skeletal muscular conditions

**Effects on Mental Status** Drowsiness and dizziness are common; may rarely cause hallucinations

**Effects on Psychiatric Treatment** May rarely cause aplastic anemia; use caution with clozapine and carbamazepine; concurrent use with psychotropics may produce additive sedation

**Usual Dosage** Oral: 1-2 tablets 3-4 times/day

**Dosage Forms**

Tablet: Orphenadrine citrate 25 mg, aspirin 385 mg, and caffeine 30 mg

Tablet: (Norgesic® Forte): Orphenadrine citrate 50 mg, aspirin 770 mg, and caffeine 60 mg

- **Ortho-Cept®** *see* Ethinyl Estradiol and Desogestrel *on page 211*
- **Orthoclone® OKT3** *see* Muromonab-CD3 *on page 376*
- **Ortho-Cyclen®** *see* Ethinyl Estradiol and Norgestimate *on page 212*
- **Ortho® Dienestrol Vaginal** *see* Dienestrol *on page 167*
- **Ortho-Est® Oral** *see* Estropipate *on page 208*
- **Ortho-Novum® 1/35** *see* Ethinyl Estradiol and Norethindrone *on page 212*
- **Ortho-Novum® 1/50** *see* Mestranol and Norethindrone *on page 346*
- **Ortho-Novum® 7/7/7** *see* Ethinyl Estradiol and Norethindrone *on page 212*
- **Ortho-Novum® 10/11** *see* Ethinyl Estradiol and Norethindrone *on page 212*
- **Ortho-Prefest®** *see* Ethinyl Estradiol and Norgestimate *on page 212*
- **Ortho Tri-Cyclen®** *see* Ethinyl Estradiol and Norgestimate *on page 212*
- **Or-Tyl® Injection** *see* Dicyclomine *on page 165*
- **Orudis®** *see* Ketoprofen *on page 302*
- **Orudis® KT [OTC]** *see* Ketoprofen *on page 302*
- **Oruvail®** *see* Ketoprofen *on page 302*
- **Os-Cal® 500 [OTC]** *see* Calcium Carbonate *on page 84*

## Oseltamivir (o sel TAM e veer)

**U.S. Brand Names** Tamiflu™

**Pharmacologic Category** Neuraminidase Inhibitor

**Use** Indicated for the treatment of uncomplicated acute illness due to influenza infection in adults who have been symptomatic for no more than 2 days

**Unlabeled use:** Prophylaxis against influenza A/B infection

**Effects on Mental Status** May cause insomnia

**Effects on Psychiatric Treatment** None reported

**Pregnancy Risk Factor** C

**Contraindications** Hypersensitivity to any components of the product

**Warnings/Precautions** Dosage adjustment is required for creatinine clearance between 10-30 mL/minute, only for Influenza A or B infections; has not been evaluated in prevention of these infections; this medicine is not a substitute for the flu shot. Safe and efficacious use in children (<18 years) has not been established. Also consider primary or concomitant bacterial infections.

**Adverse Reactions**

1% to 10%:

Central nervous system: Insomnia (1.1%), vertigo (1%)

Gastrointestinal: Nausea (10%), vomiting (9%)

<1%: Anemia, humerus fracture, peritonsillar abscess, pneumonia, pseudomembranous colitis, pyrexia, unstable angina

**Overdosage/Toxicology** Single doses of 1000 mg resulted in nausea and vomiting

**Drug Interactions** Cimetidine and amoxicillin have no effect on plasma concentrations. Probenecid increases oseltamivir carboxylate serum concentration by twofold. Dosage adjustments are not required.

**Usual Dosage**

Adults: Oral: 75 mg twice daily initiated within 2 days of onset of symptoms; duration of treatment: 5 days

Prophylaxis (investigational use): 75 mg once daily for duration of exposure period (6 weeks has been used in clinical trials)

**Dosage adjustment in renal impairment:**

$Cl_{cr}$ 10-30 mL/minute: Reduce dose to 75 mg once daily for 5 days

$Cl_{cr}$ <10 mL/minute: Has not been studied

**Dosage adjustment in hepatic impairment:** Has not been evaluated

Elderly: No adjustments required

**Dietary Considerations** Take with or without food; take with food to improve tolerance

**Patient Information** Take within 2 days of flu symptoms (fever, cough, headache, fatigue, muscular weakness, and sore throat). This is not a substitute for the flu shot. Not recommended for pregnant or nursing women. For best results, do not miss doses.

**Nursing Implications** Have patient take with food to decrease the nausea associated with this medicine; administer at breakfast and dinner

**Dosage Forms** Capsule, as phosphate: 75 mg (blister package 10)

- **Osmitrol® Injection** *see* Mannitol *on page 331*
- **Osteocalcin® Injection** *see* Calcitonin *on page 83*
- **Otic-Care® Otic** *see* Neomycin, Polymyxin B, and Hydrocortisone *on page 389*
- **Otobiotic® Otic** *see* Polymyxin B and Hydrocortisone *on page 452*
- **Otocort® Otic** *see* Neomycin, Polymyxin B, and Hydrocortisone *on page 389*
- **Otosporin® Otic** *see* Neomycin, Polymyxin B, and Hydrocortisone *on page 389*
- **Otrivin® Nasal [OTC]** *see* Xylometazoline *on page 589*

## Ouabain (WAH bane)

**Pharmacologic Category** Cardiac Glycoside

**Use** Treatment of congestive heart failure; slows the ventricular rate in tachyarrhythmias such as fibrillation (atrial), flutter (atrial), tachycardia (ventricular), paroxysmal atrial tachycardia, cardiogenic shock; may not be as useful for tachyarrhythmias due to antegrade conduction

**Effects on Mental Status** May cause drowsiness, dizziness, paranoia, or hallucinations

**Effects on Psychiatric Treatment** None reported

**Usual Dosage** Average digitalizing dose: I.V.: 0.03-0.5 g

**Dosage Forms** Injection: 0.25 mg/mL (2 mL)

- **Ovcon® 35** *see* Ethinyl Estradiol and Norethindrone *on page 212*
- **Ovcon® 50** *see* Ethinyl Estradiol and Norethindrone *on page 212*
- **Ovral®** *see* Ethinyl Estradiol and Norgestrel *on page 213*
- **Ovrette®** *see* Norgestrel *on page 399*

## Oxacillin (oks a SIL in)

**U.S. Brand Names** Bactocill®

**Synonyms** Methylphenyl Isoxazolyl Penicillin

**Pharmacologic Category** Antibiotic, Penicillin

**Use** Treatment of infections such as osteomyelitis, septicemia, endocarditis, and CNS infections caused by susceptible strains of *Staphylococcus*

**Effects on Mental Status** Penicillins reported to cause apprehension, illusions, hallucinations, depersonalization, agitation, insomnia, and encephalopathy

**Effects on Psychiatric Treatment** May cause neutropenia; use caution with clozapine and carbamazepine

**Pregnancy Risk Factor** B

**Contraindications** Hypersensitivity to oxacillin or other penicillins or any component

**Warnings/Precautions** Elimination rate will be slow in neonates; modify dosage in patients with renal impairment and in the elderly; use with caution in patients with cephalosporin hypersensitivity

**Adverse Reactions**

1% to 10%: Gastrointestinal: Nausea, diarrhea

<1%: Acute interstitial nephritis, agranulocytosis, eosinophilia, fever, hematuria, hepatotoxicity, increased AST, leukopenia, neutropenia, rash, serum sickness-like reactions, thrombocytopenia, vomiting

**Overdosage/Toxicology**

Signs and symptoms: Neuromuscular hypersensitivity (agitation, hallucinations, asterixis, encephalopathy, confusion, and seizures) and electrolyte imbalance with potassium or sodium salts, especially in renal failure

Treatment: Hemodialysis may be helpful to aid in the removal of the drug from the blood, otherwise most treatment is supportive or symptom directed

**Drug Interactions**

Decreased effect: Efficacy of oral contraceptives may be reduced; effects of penicillins may be impaired by tetracycline

Increased effect: Disulfiram, probenecid may increase penicillin levels, increased effect of anticoagulants are possible with large I.V. doses

**Usual Dosage**

Neonates: I.M., I.V.:
- Postnatal age <7 days:
  - <2000 g: 25 mg/kg/dose every 12 hours
  - >2000 g: 25 mg/kg/dose every 8 hours
- Postnatal age >7 days:
  - <1200 g: 25 mg/kg/dose every 12 hours
  - 1200-2000 g: 30 mg/kg/dose every 8 hours
  - >2000 g: 37.5 mg/kg/dose every 6 hours

Infants and Children:
- Oral: 50-100 mg/kg/day divided every 6 hours
- I.M., I.V.: 150-200 mg/kg/day in divided doses every 6 hours; maximum dose: 12 g/day

Adults:
- Oral: 500-1000 mg every 4-6 hours for at least 5 days
- I.M., I.V.: 250 mg to 2 g/dose every 4-6 hours

**Dosing adjustment in renal impairment:** $Cl_{cr}$ <10 mL/minute: Use lower range of the usual dosage

Hemodialysis: Not dialyzable (0% to 5%)

**Patient Information** Take at regular intervals around-the-clock, preferably on empty stomach with a full glass of water. Take complete course of treatment as prescribed. You may experience nausea or vomiting; small frequent meals and good mouth care may help. If diabetic, drug may cause false tests with Clinitest® urine glucose monitoring; use of glucose oxidase methods (Clinistix®) or serum glucose monitoring is preferable. This drug may interfere with oral contraceptives; an alternate form of birth control should be used. Report persistent fever, sore throat, sores in mouth, diarrhea, unusual bleeding or bruising, difficulty breathing, or skin rash. Notify prescriber if condition does not respond to treatment.

**Dosage Forms**

Capsule, as sodium: 250 mg, 500 mg

Powder:
- For injection, as sodium: 250 mg, 500 mg, 1 g, 2 g, 4 g, 10 g
- For oral solution, as sodium: 250 mg/5 mL (100 mL)

## Oxamniquine (oks AM ni kwin)

**U.S. Brand Names** Vansil™

**Pharmacologic Category** Anthelmintic

**Use** Treatment of all stages of *Schistosoma mansoni* infection

**Effects on Mental Status** Dizziness and drowsiness are common; may cause insomnia or hallucinations

**Effects on Psychiatric Treatment** None reported

**Usual Dosage** Oral:

Children <30 kg: 20 mg/kg in 2 divided doses of 10 mg/kg at 2- to 8-hour intervals

Adults: 12-15 mg/kg as a single dose

**Dosage Forms** Capsule: 250 mg

♦ **Oxandrin®** *see* Oxandrolone *on page 409*

## Oxandrolone (oks AN droe lone)

**U.S. Brand Names** Oxandrin®

**Pharmacologic Category** Androgen

**Use** Adjunctive therapy to promote weight gain after weight loss following extensive surgery, chronic infections, or severe trauma, and in some patients who, without definite pathophysiologic reasons, fail to gain or to maintain normal weight

**Effects on Mental Status** May cause insomnia

**Effects on Psychiatric Treatment** None reported

**Restrictions** C-III

**Pregnancy Risk Factor** X

**Contraindications** Nephrosis, carcinoma of breast or prostate, pregnancy, hypersensitivity to oxandrolone or any component

**Warnings/Precautions** May stunt bone growth in children; anabolic steroids may cause peliosis hepatis, liver cell tumors, and blood lipid changes with increased risk of arteriosclerosis; monitor diabetic patients carefully; use with caution in elderly patients, they may be at greater risk for prostatic hypertrophy; use with caution in patients with cardiac, renal, or hepatic disease or epilepsy

**Adverse Reactions**

**Male:**

Postpubertal:
- >10%:
  - Dermatologic: Acne
  - Endocrine & metabolic: Gynecomastia
  - Genitourinary: Bladder irritability, priapism
- 1% to 10%:
  - Central nervous system: Insomnia, chills
  - Endocrine & metabolic: Decreased libido, hepatic dysfunction
  - Gastrointestinal: Nausea, diarrhea
  - Genitourinary: Prostatic hypertrophy (elderly)
  - Hematologic: Iron deficiency anemia, suppression of clotting factors
- <1%: Hepatic necrosis, hepatocellular carcinoma

Prepubertal:
- >10%:
  - Dermatologic: Acne
  - Endocrine & metabolic: Virilism
- 1% to 10%:
  - Central nervous system: Chills, insomnia,
  - Dermatologic: Hyperpigmentation
  - Gastrointestinal: Diarrhea, nausea
  - Hematologic: Iron deficiency anemia, suppression of clotting factors
- <1%: Hepatic necrosis, hepatocellular carcinoma

**Female:**
- >10%: Endocrine & metabolic: Virilism
- 1% to 10%:
  - Central nervous system: Chills, insomnia
  - Endocrine & metabolic: Hypercalcemia
  - Gastrointestinal: Nausea, diarrhea
  - Hematologic: Iron deficiency anemia, suppression of clotting factors
  - Hepatic: Hepatic dysfunction
- <1%: Hepatic necrosis, hepatocellular carcinoma

**Drug Interactions** Increased toxicity: ACTH, adrenal steroids may increase risk of edema and acne; stanozolol enhances the hypoprothrombinemic effects of oral anticoagulants; enhances the hypoglycemic effects of insulin and sulfonylureas (oral hypoglycemics)

**Usual Dosage**

Children: Total daily dose: ≤0.1 mg/kg **or** ≤0.045 mg/lb

Adults: 2.5 mg 2-4 times/day; however, since the response of individuals to anabolic steroids varies, a daily dose of as little as 2.5 mg or as much as 20 mg may be required to achieve the desired response. A course of therapy of 2-4 weeks is usually adequate. This may be repeated intermittently as needed.

**Dosing adjustment in renal impairment:** Caution is recommended because of the propensity of oxandrolone to cause edema and water retention

**Dosing adjustment in hepatic impairment:** Caution is advised but there are not specific guidelines for dosage reduction

**Patient Information** High protein, high caloric diet is suggested, restrict salt intake; glucose tolerance may be altered in diabetics

**Dosage Forms** Tablet: 2.5 mg

## Oxaprozin (oks a PROE zin)

**Related Information**

Nonsteroidal Anti-inflammatory Agents Comparison Chart *on page 722*

**U.S. Brand Names** Daypro™

**Pharmacologic Category** Nonsteroidal Anti-Inflammatory Agent (NSAID)

**Use** Acute and long-term use in the management of signs and symptoms of osteoarthritis and rheumatoid arthritis

**Effects on Mental Status** Dizziness is common; may cause nervousness; may rarely cause drowsiness, confusion, insomnia, or depression

**Effects on Psychiatric Treatment** May rarely cause agranulocytosis; use caution with clozapine and carbamazepine; may decrease lithium clearance resulting in an increase in serum lithium levels and potential lithium toxicity; monitor serum lithium levels

**Pregnancy Risk Factor** C (D if used in third trimester)

(Continued)

## Oxaprozin *(Continued)*

**Contraindications** Aspirin allergy, 3rd trimester pregnancy or allergy to oxaprozin, history of GI disease, renal or hepatic dysfunction, bleeding disorders, cardiac failure, elderly, debilitated, nursing mothers

**Warnings/Precautions** GI toxicity (bleeding, ulceration, perforation); CNS effects may occur (headaches, confusion, depression); dehydration, hypersensitivity, anaphylactoid reactions (intermittent tolmetin use more often); renal function decline, acute renal insufficiency, interstitial nephritis, dysuria, cystitis, hematuria, nephrotic syndrome, hyperkalemia in acute renal insufficiency, hyponatremia, papillary necrosis, hepatic function impairment; elderly have increased risk for adverse reactions to NSAIDs

**Adverse Reactions**

1% to 10%:

- Central nervous system: CNS inhibition, disturbance of sleep
- Dermatologic: Rash
- Gastrointestinal: Nausea, dyspepsia, abdominal pain, anorexia, flatulence, vomiting
- Genitourinary: Dysuria or frequency

<1%: Acute interstitial nephritis, acute renal failure, agranulocytosis, anaphylaxis, anemia, blurred vision, change in blood pressure, conjunctivitis, decreased menstrual flow, ecchymosis, edema, erythema multiforme, exfoliative dermatitis, hematuria, leukopenia, LFT abnormalities, malaise, nephrotic syndrome, pancreatitis, pancytopenia, peptic ulcer and/or GI bleed, photosensitivity, pruritus, rectal bleeding, renal insufficiency, serum sickness, Stevens-Johnson syndrome, stomatitis, symptoms of upper respiratory infection, thrombocytopenia, urticaria, weakness, weight gain, weight loss

**Overdosage/Toxicology**

Signs and symptoms: Acute renal failure, vomiting, drowsiness, leukocytes

Treatment:

- Management of a nonsteroidal anti-inflammatory drug (NSAID) intoxication is primarily supportive and symptomatic
- Fluid therapy is commonly effective in managing the hypotension that may occur following an acute NSAID overdose, except when this is due to an acute blood loss
- Seizures tend to be very short-lived and often do not require drug treatment. Although, recurrent seizures should be treated with I.V. diazepam
- Since many of the NSAIDs undergo enterohepatic cycling, multiple doses of charcoal may be needed to reduce the potential for delayed toxicities

**Drug Interactions**

- ACE inhibitors: Effects may be reduced by NSAIDs; use lowest possible dose for shortest duration possible; monitor
- Cholestyramine and colestipol: Absorption may be reduced by concurrent administration
- Corticosteroids: May increase the risk of GI ulceration; use caution
- Cyclosporine: Nephrotoxicity may be increased with concurrent NSAID use; monitor
- Hydralazine: Antihypertensive effect may be decreased; avoid concurrent use
- Lithium: Serum levels can be increased; avoid concurrent use if possible or monitor lithium levels and adjust dose. When NSAID is stopped, lithium may need adjustment again.
- Loop diuretics: Therapeutic effects may be reduced by NSAIDs; avoid
- Methotrexate: Toxicity may be increased by concurrent NSAID use; risk is limited in low-dose methotrexate regimens (such as for rheumatoid arthritis); prolonged leucovorin rescue may be required at antineoplastic doses; monitor
- Thiazide diuretics: Antihypertensive effects are decreased; avoid concurrent use
- Warfarin: INRs may be increased by some NSAIDs. This may depend, in part, on dose and duration; monitor INR closely. Use the lowest dose of NSAIDs possible and for the briefest duration.

**Usual Dosage** Adults: Oral (individualize dosage to lowest effective dose to minimize adverse effects):

- Osteoarthritis: 600-1200 mg once daily
- Rheumatoid arthritis: 1200 mg once daily
- Maximum dose: 1800 mg/day or 26 mg/kg (whichever is lower) in divided doses

**Patient Information** Take this medication exactly as directed; do not increase dose without consulting prescriber. Do not crush tablets or break capsules. Take with food or milk to reduce GI distress. Maintain adequate fluid intake (2-3 L/day of fluids unless instructed to restrict fluid intake). Do not use alcohol, aspirin, or aspirin-containing medication, and all other anti-inflammatory medications without consulting prescriber. You may experience drowsiness, dizziness, or nervousness (use caution when driving or engaging in tasks requiring alertness until response to drug is known); anorexia, nausea, vomiting, or heartburn (frequent small meals, frequent mouth care, sucking lozenges, or chewing gum may help). GI bleeding, ulceration, or perforation can occur with or without pain; discontinue medication and contact prescriber if persistent abdominal pain or cramping, or blood in stool occurs. Report vaginal bleeding; breathlessness, difficulty breathing, or unusual cough; chest pain, rapid heartbeat, palpitations; unusual bruising/bleeding; blood in urine, stool, mouth, or vomitus; swollen extremities; skin rash or itching; acute fatigue; or swelling of face, lips, tongue, or throat.

**Dosage Forms** Tablet: 600 mg

## Oxazepam (oks A ze pam)

**Related Information**

- Anxiolytic/Hypnotic Use in Long-Term Care Facilities *on page 754*
- Benzodiazepines Comparison Chart *on page 708*
- Clinical Issues in the Use of Anxiolytics and Sedative/Hypnotics *on page 634*
- Federal OBRA Regulations Recommended Maximum Doses *on page 756*
- Patient Information - Anxiolytics & Sedative Hypnotics (Benzodiazepines) *on page 653*
- Substance-Related Disorders *on page 609*

**Generic Available** Yes

**U.S. Brand Names** Serax®

**Canadian Brand Names** Apo®-Oxazepam; Novo-Oxazepam; Oxpam®; PMS-Oxazepam; Zapex®

**Pharmacologic Category** Benzodiazepine

**Use** Treatment of anxiety and management of alcohol withdrawal

**Unlabeled use:** Anticonvulsant in management of simple partial seizures, hypnotic

**Restrictions** C-IV

**Pregnancy Risk Factor** D

**Contraindications** Hypersensitivity to this drug or any component of its formulation (cross-sensitivity with other benzodiazepines may exist); narrow-angle glaucoma (not in product labeling, however, benzodiazepines are contraindicated); not indicated for use in the treatment of psychosis; pregnancy

**Warnings/Precautions** May cause hypotension (rare) - use with caution in patients with cardiovascular or cerebrovascular disease, or in patients who would not tolerate transient decreases in blood pressure. Serax® 15 contains tartrazine; use is not recommended in pediatric patients <6 years of age; dose has not been established between 6-12 years of age.

Use with caution in elderly or debilitated patients, patients with hepatic disease (including alcoholics), or renal impairment. Use with caution in patients with respiratory disease or impaired gag reflex. Avoid use in patients with sleep apnea.

Causes CNS depression (dose-related) resulting in sedation, dizziness, confusion, or ataxia which may impair physical and mental capabilities. Patients must be cautioned about performing tasks which require mental alertness (ie, operating machinery or driving). Use with caution in patients receiving other CNS depressants or psychoactive agents. Effects with other sedative drugs or ethanol may be potentiated. Benzodiazepines have been associated with falls and traumatic injury and should be used with extreme caution in patients who are at risk of these events (especially the elderly).

Use caution in patients with depression, particularly if suicidal risk may be present. Use with caution in patients with a history of drug dependence. Benzodiazepines have been associated with dependence and acute withdrawal symptoms on discontinuation or reduction in dose. Acute withdrawal, including seizures, may be precipitated after administration of flumazenil to patients receiving long-term benzodiazepine therapy.

Benzodiazepines have been associated with anterograde amnesia. Paradoxical reactions, including hyperactive or aggressive behavior have been reported with benzodiazepines, particularly in adolescent/pediatric or psychiatric patients. Does not have analgesic, antidepressant, or antipsychotic properties.

**Adverse Reactions**

- Cardiovascular: Syncope (rare), edema
- Central nervous system: Drowsiness, ataxia, dizziness, vertigo, memory impairment, headache, paradoxical reactions (excitement, stimulation of effect), lethargy, amnesia, euphoria
- Dermatologic: Rash
- Endocrine & metabolic: Decreased libido, menstrual irregularities
- Genitourinary: Incontinence
- Hematologic: Leukopenia, blood dyscrasias
- Hepatic: Jaundice
- Neuromuscular & skeletal: Dysarthria, tremor, reflex slowing
- Ocular: Blurred vision, diplopia
- Miscellaneous: Drug dependence

**Overdosage/Toxicology**

Signs and symptoms: Somnolence, confusion, coma, hypoactive reflexes, dyspnea, hypotension, slurred speech, impaired coordination

Treatment: Treatment for benzodiazepine overdose is supportive. Rarely is mechanical ventilation required. Flumazenil has been shown to selectively block the binding of benzodiazepines to CNS receptors, resulting in a reversal of benzodiazepine-induced CNS depression but not the respiratory depression due to toxicity.

**Drug Interactions**

CNS depressants: Sedative effects and/or respiratory depression may be additive with CNS depressants; includes ethanol, barbiturates, narcotic analgesics, and other sedative agents; monitor for increased effect

Theophylline: May partially antagonize some of the effects of benzodiazepines; monitor for decreased response; may require higher doses for sedation

**Mechanism of Action** Binds to stereospecific benzodiazepine receptors on the postsynaptic GABA neuron at several sites within the central nervous system, including the limbic system, reticular formation. Enhancement of the inhibitory effect of GABA on neuronal excitability results by increased neuronal membrane permeability to chloride ions. This shift in chloride ions results in hyperpolarization (a less excitable state) and stabilization.

**Pharmacodynamics/kinetics**

Absorption: Oral: Almost completely

Protein binding: 86% to 99%

Metabolism: In the liver to inactive compounds (primarily as glucuronides)

Half-life: 2.8-5.7 hours

Time to peak serum concentration: Within 2-4 hours

Elimination: Excretion of unchanged drug (50%) and metabolites; excreted without need for liver metabolism

**Usual Dosage** Oral:

Children: 1 mg/kg/day has been administered

Adults:

- Anxiety: 10-30 mg 3-4 times/day
- Alcohol withdrawal: 15-30 mg 3-4 times/day
- Hypnotic: 15-30 mg

Hemodialysis: Not dialyzable (0% to 5%)

**Dietary Considerations** Alcohol: Additive CNS effect, avoid use

**Administration** Give orally in divided doses

**Monitoring Parameters** Respiratory and cardiovascular status

**Reference Range** Therapeutic: 0.2-1.4 μg/mL (SI: 0.7-4.9 μmol/L)

**Patient Information** Avoid alcohol and other CNS depressants; avoid activities needing good psychomotor coordination until CNS effects are known; drug may cause physical or psychological dependence; avoid abrupt discontinuation after prolonged use

**Nursing Implications** Provide safety measures (ie, side rails, night light, and call button); remove smoking materials from area; supervise ambulation

**Additional Information** Not intended for management of anxieties and minor distresses associated with everyday life; treatment longer than 4 months should be re-evaluated to determine the patient's need for the drug

**Dosage Forms**

Capsule: 10 mg, 15 mg, 30 mg

Tablet: 15 mg

## Oxcarbazepine (ox car BAZ e peen)

**Related Information**

Anticonvulsants by Seizures Type *on page 703*

**U.S. Brand Names** Trileptal®

**Synonyms** GP 47680

**Pharmacologic Category** Anticonvulsant, Miscellaneous

**Use** Monotherapy or adjunctive therapy in the treatment of partial seizures in adults with epilepsy and as adjunctive therapy in the treatment of partial seizures in children ages 4-16 with epilepsy

**Unlabeled use:** Antimanic

**Pregnancy Risk Factor** C

**Pregnancy/Breast-Feeding Implications** Although many epidemiological studies of congenital anomalies in infants born to women treated with various anticonvulsants during pregnancy have been reported, none of these investigations includes enough women treated with oxcarbazepine to assess possible teratogenic effects of this drug. The frequencies of malformations were not significantly increased among the offspring of pregnant mice treated with 20-46 times the usual human dose of oxcarbazepine. This treatment produced plasma levels in the mice that were at least 6-16 times greater than those that are usually seen in human anticonvulsant therapy. Oxcarbazepine and its active metabolite (MHD) are excreted in human breast milk. A milk-to-plasma concentration ratio of 0.5 was found for both. Because of the potential for serious adverse reactions to oxcarbazepine in nursing infants, a decision should be made whether to discontinue nursing or to discontinue the drug in nursing women.

**Contraindications** Hypersensitivity to oxcarbazepine or any of its components

**Warnings/Precautions** Clinically significant hyponatremia (sodium <125 mmol/L) can develop during oxcarbazepine use. As with all antiepileptic drugs, oxcarbazepine should be withdrawn gradually to minimize the potential of increased seizure frequency. Use of oxcarbazepine has been associated with CNS related adverse events, most significant of these were cognitive symptoms including psychomotor slowing, difficulty with concentration, and speech or language problems, somnolence or fatigue, and coordination abnormalities, including ataxia and gait disturbances.

**Adverse Reactions**

Monotherapy:

>10%:

- Central nervous system: Headache (13% to 31%), dizziness (22% to 28%), somnolence (19%), fatigue (21%)
- Gastrointestinal: Nausea (16% to 22%), vomiting (7% to 15%)
- Ocular: Abnormal vision (4% to 14%), diplopia (12%)

1% to 10%:

- Central nervous system: Anxiety (7%), ataxia (5% to 7%), confusion (7%), nervousness (5% to 7%), insomnia (6%), tremor (4% to 6%), amnesia (4% to 5%), exacerbation of seizures (5%), emotional lability (3%), hypoesthesia (3%), fever (3%), vertigo (3%), abnormal coordination (2% to 4%), speech disorder (2%)
- Cardiovascular: Edema (2%), chest pain (2%)
- Dermatologic: Rash (4%), purpura (2%)
- Endocrine and metabolic: Hyponatremia (5%), hot flashes (2%),
- Gastrointestinal: Diarrhea (7%), dyspepsia (5%), anorexia (5%), abdominal pain (5%), constipation (5%), taste perversion (5%), xerostomia (3%), rectal hemorrhage (2%)
- Genitourinary: Urinary tract infection (5%), urinary frequency (2%), vaginitis (2%)
- Hematologic: Lymphadenopathy (2%)
- Miscellaneous: Viral infection (7%), infection (2%), allergy (2%), thirst (2%), toothache (2%)
- Neuromuscular and skeletal: Back pain (4%)
- Respiratory: Upper respiratory infection (7% to 10%), coughing (5%), epistaxis (4%), sinusitis (4%), bronchitis (3%), pharyngitis (3%)
- Ocular: Nystagmus (2%)
- Otic: Earache (2%), ear infection (2%)

Adjunctive therapy (600-2400 mg/day): Frequencies noted in patients receiving other anticonvulsants

>10%:

- Central nervous system: Headache (26% to 32%), dizziness (26% to 49%), somnolence (20% to 36%), ataxia (9% to 31%), fatigue (12% to 15%), vertigo (6% to 15%)
- Gastrointestinal: Nausea (15% to 29%), vomiting (13% to 36%), abdominal pain (10% to 13%)
- Neuromuscular & skeletal: Abnormal gait (5% to 17%)
- Ocular: Diplopia (14% to 40%), nystagmus (7% to 26%), visual abnormalities (6% to 14%)

1% to 10%:

- Central nervous system: Tremor (3% to 16%), nervousness (2% to 4%), insomnia (2% to 4%), agitation (1% to 2%), incoordination (1% to 3%), confusion (1% to 2%), EEG abnormalities (0% to 2%), abnormal thinking (0% to 4%)
- Cardiovascular: Leg edema (1% to 2%), hypotension (0% to 2%)
- Dermatologic: Acne (1% to 2%)
- Endocrine & metabolic: Hyponatremia (1% to 3%), weight gain (1% to 2%)
- Gastrointestinal: Diarrhea (5% to 7%), dyspepsia (5% to 6%), constipation (2% to 6%), gastritis (1% to 2%)
- Neuromuscular & skeletal: Weakness (3% to 6%), muscle weakness (1% to 2%), sprains and strains (0% to 2%)
- Miscellaneous: Speech disorder (1% to 3%), cranial injury (0% to 2%)
- Ocular: Abnormal accommodation (0% to 2%)
- Respiratory: Rhinitis (2% to 5%)

Pediatrics:

>10%:

- Central nervous system: Headache (31%), somnolence (31%), dizziness (28%), ataxia (13%), fatigue (13%)
- Gastrointestinal: Vomiting (33%), nausea (19%)
- Ocular: Diplopia (17%), visual abnormalities (13%)

1% to 10%:

- Central nervous system: Emotional lability (8%), tremor (6%), speech disorder (3%), impaired concentration (2%), convulsions (2%), vertigo (2%)
- Dermatologic: Bruising (4%)
- Gastrointestinal: Constipation (4%), dyspepsia (2%)
- Miscellaneous: Allergic reaction (2%), increased sweating (3%)
- Neuromuscular and skeletal: Abnormal gait (8%), weakness (2%), involuntary muscle contractions (2%)
- Ocular: Nystagmus (9%)
- Respiratory: Rhinitis (10%), pneumonia (2%)

<1% (all populations): Fever, malaise, chest pain, rigors, weight loss, bradycardia, cardiac failure, cerebral hemorrhage, hypertension, postural hypotension, palpitation, syncope, tachycardia, appetite (increased), cholelithiasis, colitis, duodenal ulcer, dysphagia, enteritis, eructation, esophagitis, flatulence, gastric ulcer, bleeding gums, gingival hyperplasia, hematemesis, rectal hemorrhage, hemorrhoids, hiccups, xerostomia, biliary pain, sialoadenitis, stomatitis, ulcerative stomatitis, leukopenia, thrombocytopenia, increased GGT, hyperglycemia, hypocalcemia, hypoglycemia, hypokalemia, elevation of transaminases, hypertonia, aggressiveness, anxiety, aphasia, aura, aggravated convulsions, delirium, delusion, decreased consciousness, dysphonia, dystonia, euphoria, extrapyramidal symptoms, hemiplegia, hyperkinesia, hyper-

(Continued)

## Oxcarbazepine *(Continued)*

reflexia, hypoesthesia, hypokinesis, hyporeflexia, hypotonia, hysteria, decreased libido, manic reaction, migraine, nervousness, involuntary muscle contractions, nervousness, neuralgia, occulogyric crisis, panic disorder, paralysis, paranoid reaction, personality disorder, psychoses, ptosis, stupor, tetany, asthma, dyspnea, epistaxis, laryngismus, pleurisy, acne, alopecia, angioedema, bruising, contact dermatitis, eczema, rash (facial), flushing, folliculitis, heat rash, hot flashes, photosensitivity, pruritus, psoriasis, purpura, erythematous rash, maculopapular rash, vitiligo, abnormal accommodation, cataracts, conjunctival hemorrhage, ocular edema, hemianopia, mydriasis, otitis externa, photophobia, scotoma, taste perversion, tinnitus, xerophthalmia, dysuria, hematuria, intermenstrual bleeding, leukorrhea, menorrhagia, urinary frequency, renal pain, urinary tract pain, polyuria, priapism, renal calculi, systemic lupus erythematosus.

Rare, severe dermatologic adverse reactions have been reported in postmarketing reports, including Stevens-Johnson syndrome, erythema multiforme, and toxic epidermal necrolysis.

A rare, multiorgan hypersensitivity disorder characterized by rash, fever, lymphadenopathy, abnormal liver function tests, eosinophilia and arthralgia has been described.

**Drug Interactions** CYP2C19 inhibitor; CYP3A4/5 enzyme inducer

Carbamazepine: Oxcarbazepine serum concentrations may be reduced by a mean 40%

Felodipine: Metabolism is increased due to enzyme induction; similar effects may be anticipated with other dihydropyridine calcium channel blockers

Oral contraceptives: Metabolism may be increased due to enzyme induction; use alternative contraceptive measures

Phenobarbital: Levels are increased (average of 14%); oxcarbazepine levels decreases (average of 25%)

Phenytoin levels may be increased (high dosages) by an average of 40%; oxcarbazepine levels may be decreased (by an average of 30%) during concurrent therapy; monitor phenytoin levels

Valproic acid decreases oxcarbazepine levels by an average of 18%

Verapamil's metabolism may be increased due to enzyme induction; verapamil may reduce blood levels of oxcarbazepine's active metabolite (MHD)

**Note:** No evidence of an interaction was noted with erythromycin, cimetidine, dextropropoxyphene, or warfarin

**Mechanism of Action** Pharmacological activity results from both oxcarbazepine and its monohydroxy metabolite (MHD). Precise mechanism of anticonvulsant effect has not been defined. Oxcarbazepine and MHD block voltage sensitive sodium channels, stabilizing hyperexcited neuronal membranes, inhibiting repetitive firing, and decreasing the propagation of synaptic impulses. These actions are believed to prevent the spread of seizures. Oxcarbazepine and MHD also increase potassium conductance and modulate the activity of high-voltage activated calcium channels.

**Pharmacodynamics/kinetics**

Absorption: Completely absorbed and extensively metabolized to its pharmacologically active 10-monohydroxy metabolite (MHD)

Distribution: MHD: $V_d$: 49 L

Protein binding: 40% of MHD is bound to serum proteins

Metabolism: Hepatic, further by conjugation with glucuronic acid.

Half-life: 2 hours (parent), 9 hours (MHD)

Time to peak serum concentration: 2-3 days

Elimination: 95% of the dose appears in the urine, <1% as unchanged oxcarbazepine; fecal (4%)

Dialyzable: Half-life of MHD is prolonged to 19 hours when 300 mg of oxcarbazepine is administered to renally-impaired patients ($Cl_{cr}$ <30 mL/min)

**Usual Dosage**

Children:

Adjunctive therapy: 8-10 mg/kg/day, not to exceed 600 mg/day, given in two divided daily doses. Maintenance dose should be achieved over 2 weeks, and is dependent upon patient weight, according to the following:

20-29 kg: 900 mg/day in 2 divided doses

29.1-39 kg: 1200 mg/day in 2 divided doses

>39 kg: 1800 mg/day in 2 divided doses

Adults:

Adjunctive therapy: Initial: 300 mg twice daily; dose may be increased by as much as 600 mg/day at weekly intervals; recommended daily dose: 1200 mg/day in 2 divided doses

Conversion to monotherapy: Oxcarbazepine 600 mg/day in twice daily divided doses while simultaneously initiating the reduction of the dose of the concomitant antiepileptic drug. The concomitant dosage should be withdrawn over 3-6 weeks, while the maximum dose of oxcarbazepine should be reached in about 2-4 weeks. Recommended daily dose: 2400 mg/day.

Initiation of monotherapy: Oxcarbazepine should be initiated at a dose of 600 mg/day in twice daily divided doses; doses may be titrated upward by 300 mg/day every third day to a final dose of 1200 mg/day given in 2 daily divided doses

**Dosing adjustment in renal impairment:** Therapy should be initiated at one-half the usual starting dose (300 mg/day) and increased slowly to achieve the desired clinical response

**Patient Information** Hormonal contraceptives may be less effective when used with oxcarbazepine; caution should be exercised if alcohol is taken with oxcarbazepine, due to the possible additive sedative effects and that it may cause dizziness and somnolence; therefore, early in therapy be advised not to drive or operate machinery

**Nursing Implications** Inform those patients who have exhibited hypersensitivity reactions to carbamazepine that there is the possibility of cross sensitivity reactions with oxcarbazepine. Inform patients of childbearing age that hormonal contraceptives may be less effective when used with oxcarbazepine. Caution should be exercised if alcohol is taken with oxcarbazepine, due to the possible additive sedative effects. Advise patients that oxcarbazepine may cause dizziness and somnolence and that early in therapy they are advised not to drive or operate machinery.

**Dosage Forms** Tablet: 150 mg, 300 mg, 600 mg

## Oxiconazole (oks i KON a zole)

**U.S. Brand Names** Oxistat®

**Pharmacologic Category** Antifungal Agent, Topical

**Use** Treatment of tinea pedis (athlete's foot), tinea cruris (jock itch), and tinea corporis (ringworm)

**Effects on Mental Status** None reported

**Effects on Psychiatric Treatment** None reported

**Usual Dosage** Children and Adults: Topical: Apply once to twice daily to affected areas for 2 weeks (tinea corporis/tinea cruris) to 1 month (tinea pedis)

**Dosage Forms**

Cream, as nitrate: 1% (15 g, 30 g, 60 g)

Lotion, as nitrate: 1% (30 mL)


- **Oxilapine Succinate** *see* Loxapine *on page 328*
- **Oxistat®** *see* Oxiconazole *on page 412*
- **Oxpentifylline** *see* Pentoxifylline *on page 430*
- **Oxsoralen®** *see* Methoxsalen *on page 355*
- **Oxsoralen-Ultra®** *see* Methoxsalen *on page 355*


## Oxtriphylline (oks TRYE fi lin)

**Pharmacologic Category** Theophylline Derivative

**Use** Bronchodilator in symptomatic treatment of asthma and reversible bronchospasm

**Effects on Mental Status** May cause nervousness or restlessness; may rarely cause insomnia or irritability

**Effects on Psychiatric Treatment** Sedating/calming effects of psychotropics may be counteracted with concurrent use

**Usual Dosage** Oral:

Children 1-9 years: 6.2 mg/kg/dose every 6 hours

Children 9-16 years and Adult smokers: 4.7 mg/kg/dose every 6 hours

Adults: 4.7 mg/kg every 8 hours; sustained release: administer every 12 hours

**Dosage Forms**

Elixir: 100 mg/5 mL (5 mL, 10 mL, 473 mL)

Syrup: 50 mg/5 mL (473 mL)

Tablet: 100 mg, 200 mg

Sustained release: 400 mg, 600 mg


- **Oxtriphylline** *see* Theophylline Salts *on page 539*
- **Oxy-5® Advanced Formula for Sensitive Skin [OTC]** *see* Benzoyl Peroxide *on page 62*
- **Oxy-5® Tinted [OTC]** *see* Benzoyl Peroxide *on page 62*
- **Oxy-10® Advanced Formula for Sensitive Skin [OTC]** *see* Benzoyl Peroxide *on page 62*
- **Oxy 10® Wash [OTC]** *see* Benzoyl Peroxide *on page 62*


## Oxybutynin (oks i BYOO ti nin)

**Related Information**

Clozapine-Induced Side Effects *on page 780*

Pharmacotherapy of Urinary Incontinence *on page 758*

**U.S. Brand Names** Ditropan®

**Canadian Brand Names** Albert® Oxybutynin

**Pharmacologic Category** Antispasmodic Agent, Urinary

**Use** Antispasmodic for neurogenic bladder (urgency, frequency, urge incontinence) and uninhibited bladder

**Effects on Mental Status** Drowsiness is common; may cause insomnia or dizziness

**Effects on Psychiatric Treatment** Concurrent use with psychotropics may produce additive sedation and anticholinergic side effects (dry mouth)

**Pregnancy Risk Factor** B

**Contraindications** Glaucoma, myasthenia gravis, partial or complete GI obstruction, GU obstruction, ulcerative colitis, hypersensitivity to drug or specific component, intestinal atony, megacolon, toxic megacolon

**Warnings/Precautions** Use with caution in patients with urinary tract obstruction, angle-closure glaucoma, hyperthyroidism, reflux esophagitis, heart disease, hepatic or renal disease, prostatic hypertrophy, autonomic neuropathy, ulcerative colitis (may cause ileus and toxic megacolon), hypertension, hiatal hernia. Caution should be used in elderly due to anticholinergic activity (eg, confusion, constipation, blurred vision, and tachycardia).

**Adverse Reactions**

>10%:
- Central nervous system: Drowsiness
- Gastrointestinal: Xerostomia, constipation
- Miscellaneous: Diaphoresis (decreased)

1% to 10%:
- Cardiovascular: Tachycardia, palpitations
- Central nervous system: Dizziness, insomnia, fever, headache
- Dermatologic: Rash
- Endocrine & metabolic: Decreased flow of breast milk, decreased sexual ability, hot flashes
- Gastrointestinal: Nausea, vomiting
- Genitourinary: Urinary hesitancy or retention
- Neuromuscular & skeletal: Weakness
- Ocular: Blurred vision, mydriatic effect

<1%: Allergic reaction, increased intraocular pressure

**Overdosage/Toxicology**

Signs and symptoms: Hypotension, circulatory failure, psychotic behavior, flushing, respiratory failure, paralysis, tremor, irritability, seizures, delirium, hallucinations, coma

Treatment: Symptomatic and supportive treatment; induce emesis or perform gastric lavage followed by charcoal and a cathartic; physostigmine may be required; treat hyperpyrexia with cooling techniques (ice bags, cold applications, alcohol sponges)

**Drug Interactions** Increased toxicity:

Additive sedation with CNS depressants and alcohol

Additive anticholinergic effects with antihistamines and anticholinergic agents

**Usual Dosage** Oral:

Children:
- 1-5 years: 0.2 mg/kg/dose 2-4 times/day
- >5 years: 5 mg twice daily, up to 5 mg 4 times/day maximum

Adults: 5 mg 2-3 times/day up to 5 mg 4 times/day maximum
- Extended release: Initial: 5 mg once daily, may increase in 5-10 mg increments; maximum: 30 mg daily

Elderly: 2.5-5 mg twice daily; increase by 2.5 mg increments every 1-2 days

**Note**: Should be discontinued periodically to determine whether the patient can manage without the drug and to minimize resistance to the drug

**Patient Information** Take prescribed dose preferably on an empty stomach (1 hour before or 2 hours after meals). You may experience dizziness, lightheadedness, or drowsiness (use caution when driving or engaging in tasks requiring alertness until response to drug is known); dry mouth or changes in appetite (small frequent meals, frequent mouth care, sucking lozenges, or chewing gum may help); constipation (frequent exercise or increased dietary fiber, fruit, and fluid or stool softener may help); decreased sexual ability (reversible with discontinuance of drug); decreased sweating (use caution in hot weather, avoid extreme exercise or activity). Report rapid heartbeat, palpitations, or chest pain; difficulty voiding; or vision changes. Swallow extended-release tablets whole, do not chew or crush.

**Nursing Implications** Raise bed rails, institute safety measures, assist with ambulation

**Dosage Forms**
- Syrup, as chloride: 5 mg/5 mL (473 mL)
- Tablet, as chloride: 5 mg
- Tablet, as chloride, extended release: 5 mg, 10 mg

## Oxychlorosene (oks i KLOR oh seen)

**U.S. Brand Names** Clorpactin® WCS-90

**Pharmacologic Category** Antibiotic, Topical

**Use** Treating localized infections

**Effects on Mental Status** None reported

**Effects on Psychiatric Treatment** None reported

**Usual Dosage** Topical (0.1% to 0.5% solutions): Apply by irrigation, instillation, spray, soaks, or wet compresses

**Dosage Forms** Powder for solution, as sodium: 2 g, 5 g

## Oxycodone (oks i KOE done)

**Related Information**

Narcotic Agonists Comparison Chart *on page 720*
Substance-Related Disorders *on page 609*

**U.S. Brand Names** OxyContin®; OxyIR™; Percolone®; Roxicodone™

**Canadian Brand Names** Supeudol®

**Synonyms** Dihydrohydroxycodeinone

**Pharmacologic Category** Analgesic, Narcotic

**Use** Management of moderate to severe pain, normally used in combination with non-narcotic analgesics

**Effects on Mental Status** Drowsiness and dizziness are common; may cause nervousness, restlessness or confusion; may rarely cause depression or hallucinations

**Effects on Psychiatric Treatment** Psychotropics may alter the analgesic effects of opioids; monitor for change in pain relief

**Restrictions** C-II

**Pregnancy Risk Factor** B (D if used for prolonged periods or in high doses at term)

**Contraindications** Hypersensitivity to oxycodone or any component

**Warnings/Precautions** Use with caution in patients with hypersensitivity reactions to other phenanthrene derivative opioid agonists (morphine, hydrocodone, hydromorphone, levorphanol, oxycodone, oxymorphone); respiratory diseases including asthma, emphysema, COPD, or severe liver or renal insufficiency; some preparations contain sulfites which may cause allergic reactions; dextromethorphan has equivalent antitussive activity but has much lower toxicity in accidental overdose; tolerance or drug dependence may result from extended use

**Adverse Reactions**

>10%:
- Cardiovascular: Hypotension
- Central nervous system: Fatigue, drowsiness, dizziness
- Gastrointestinal: Nausea, vomiting
- Neuromuscular & skeletal: Weakness

1% to 10%:
- Central nervous system: Nervousness, headache, restlessness, malaise, confusion
- Gastrointestinal: Anorexia, stomach cramps, xerostomia, constipation, biliary spasm
- Genitourinary: Ureteral spasms, decreased urination
- Local: Pain at injection site
- Respiratory: Dyspnea, shortness of breath

<1%: Hallucinations, histamine release, increased intracranial pressure, mental depression, paradoxical CNS stimulation, paralytic ileus, physical and psychological dependence, skin rash, urticaria

**Overdosage/Toxicology**

Signs and symptoms: CNS depression, respiratory depression, miosis

Treatment: Naloxone 2 mg I.V. (0.01 mg/kg for children) with repeat administration as necessary up to a total of 10 mg

**Drug Interactions** CYP2D6 enzyme substrate

Decreased effect: Phenothiazines may antagonize the analgesic effect of opiate agonists

Increased toxicity: CNS depressants, monoamine oxidase inhibitors, general anesthetics, and tricyclic antidepressants may potentiate the effects of opiate agonists; dextroamphetamine may enhance the analgesic effect of opiate agonists

**Usual Dosage** Oral:

Immediate release:
- Children:
  - 6-12 years: 1.25 mg every 6 hours as needed
  - >12 years: 2.5 mg every 6 hours as needed
- Adults: 5 mg every 6 hours as needed

Controlled release: Adults: 10 mg every 12 hours around-the-clock

**Dosing adjustment in hepatic impairment:** Reduce dosage in patients with severe liver disease

**Dietary Considerations** Alcohol: Additive CNS effect, avoid use

**Patient Information** If self-administered, use exactly as directed (do not increase dose or frequency); may cause physical and/or psychological dependence. While using this medication, do not use alcohol and other prescription or OTC medications (especially sedatives, tranquilizers, antihistamines, or pain medications) without consulting prescriber. Maintain adequate hydration (2-3 L/day of fluids unless instructed to restrict fluid intake). May cause hypotension, dizziness, drowsiness, impaired coordination, or blurred vision (use caution when driving, climbing stairs, or changing position - rising from sitting or lying to standing, or when engaging in tasks requiring alertness until response to drug is known); nausea, vomiting or dry mouth (frequent mouth care, small frequent meals, chewing gum, or sucking lozenges may help); constipation (increased exercise, fluids, or dietary fruit and fiber may help - if constipation remains an unresolved problem, consult prescriber about use of stool softeners). Report persistent dizziness or headache; excessive fatigue or sedation; changes in mental status; changes in urinary elimination or pain on urination; weakness or trembling; blurred vision; or shortness of breath.

**Nursing Implications** Observe patient for excessive sedation, respiratory depression, implement safety measures, assist with ambulation

**Dosage Forms**
- Capsule, as hydrochloride, immediate release (OxyIR™): 5 mg
- Liquid, oral, as hydrochloride: 5 mg/5 mL (500 mL)
- Solution, oral concentrate, as hydrochloride: 20 mg/mL (30 mL)
- Tablet, as hydrochloride: 5 mg

(Continued)

## Oxycodone *(Continued)*

Roxicodone™: 10 mg, 30 mg
Percolone®: 5 mg
Tablet, controlled release, as hydrochloride (OxyContin®): 10 mg, 20 mg, 40 mg, 80 mg

## Oxycodone and Acetaminophen

(oks i KOE done & a seet a MIN oh fen)

**U.S. Brand Names** Endocet®; Percocet® 2.5/325; Percocet® 5/325; Percocet® 7.5/500; Percocet® 10/650; Roxicet® 5/500; Roxilox™; Tylox®

**Canadian Brand Names** Endocet®; Oxycocet; Percocet®-Demi

**Synonyms** Acetaminophen and Oxycodone

**Pharmacologic Category** Analgesic, Narcotic

**Use** Management of moderate to severe pain

**Effects on Mental Status** Drowsiness and fatigue are common. May cause restlessness, nervousness, or confusion; may rarely cause hallucinations, depression, or paradoxical CNS stimulation.

**Effects on Psychiatric Treatment** May see additive sedation with concurrent psychotropic use

**Restrictions** C-II

**Pregnancy Risk Factor** C

**Contraindications** Hypersensitivity to oxycodone, acetaminophen or any component; severe respiratory depression, severe renal or liver insufficiency

**Warnings/Precautions** Use with caution in patients with hypersensitivity reactions to other phenanthrene derivative opioid agonists (morphine, codeine, hydrocodone, hydromorphone, levorphanol, oxymorphone); respiratory diseases including asthma, emphysema, COPD, or severe liver or renal insufficiency; some preparations contain sulfites which may cause allergic reactions; may be habit-forming

Enhanced analgesia has been seen in elderly patients on therapeutic doses of narcotics; duration of action may be increased in the elderly; the elderly may be particularly susceptible to the CNS depressant and constipating effects of narcotics

**Adverse Reactions**

>10%:
- Cardiovascular: Hypotension
- Central nervous system: Fatigue, drowsiness, dizziness
- Gastrointestinal: Nausea, vomiting
- Neuromuscular & skeletal: Weakness

1% to 10%:
- Central nervous system: Nervousness, headache, restlessness, malaise, confusion
- Gastrointestinal: Anorexia, stomach cramps, xerostomia, constipation, biliary spasm
- Genitourinary: Ureteral spasms, decreased urination
- Local: Pain at injection site
- Respiratory: Dyspnea, shortness of breath

**Overdosage/Toxicology**

Symptoms of overdose include hepatic necrosis, transient azotemia, renal tubular necrosis with acute toxicity, anemia, renal damage, and GI disturbances with chronic toxicity

Consult regional poison control center for additional information. Treatment of an overdose includes support of the patient's airway, establishment of an I.V. line and administration of naloxone 2 mg I.V. with repeat administration as necessary. Mucomyst® (acetylcysteine) 140 mg/kg orally (loading) followed by 70 mg/kg (maintenance) every 4 hours for 17 doses. Therapy should be initiated based upon acetaminophen levels that are suggestive of a high probability of hepatotoxic potential.

**Drug Interactions**

Decreased effect: Phenothiazines may antagonize the analgesic effect of opiate agonists

Increased toxicity: CNS depressants, tricyclic antidepressants may potentiate the effects of opiate agonists; dextroamphetamine may enhance the analgesic effect of opiate agonists

**Usual Dosage** Oral (doses should be titrated to appropriate analgesic effects):

Children: Oxycodone: 0.05-0.15 mg/kg/dose to 5 mg/dose (maximum) every 4-6 hours as needed

Adults: 1-2 tablets every 4-6 hours as needed for pain
- Maximum daily dose of acetaminophen: 4 g/day

**Dosing adjustment in hepatic impairment:** Dose should be reduced in patients with severe liver disease

**Dietary Considerations**

Acetaminophen: Refer to acetaminophen monograph

Oxycodone:
- Alcohol: Additive CNS effects; avoid or limit alcohol. Watch for sedation.
- Food: Glucose may cause hyperglycemia; monitor blood glucose concentrations

**Patient Information** See individual agents

**Nursing Implications** Observe patient for excessive sedation, respiratory depression; implement safety measures, assist with ambulation

**Dosage Forms**

Caplet: Oxycodone hydrochloride 5 mg and acetaminophen 500 mg
Capsule: Oxycodone hydrochloride 5 mg and acetaminophen 500 mg
Solution, oral: Oxycodone hydrochloride 5 mg and acetaminophen 325 mg per 5 mL (5 mL, 500 mL)
Tablet: Oxycodone hydrochloride 5 mg and acetaminophen 325 mg

## Oxycodone and Aspirin (oks i KOE done & AS pir in)

**U.S. Brand Names** Codoxy®; Percodan®; Percodan®-Demi; Roxiprin®

**Canadian Brand Names** Endodan®; Oxycodan

**Pharmacologic Category** Analgesic, Narcotic

**Use** Management of moderate to severe pain

**Effects on Mental Status** Drowsiness and fatigue are common. May cause restlessness, nervousness, or confusion; may rarely cause hallucinations, depression, or paradoxical CNS stimulation.

**Effects on Psychiatric Treatment** May see additive sedation with concurrent psychotropic use

**Restrictions** C-II

**Pregnancy Risk Factor** D

**Contraindications** Known hypersensitivity to oxycodone or aspirin; severe respiratory depression

**Warnings/Precautions** Use with caution in patients with hypersensitivity to other phenanthrene derivative opioid agonists (morphine, codeine, hydrocodone, hydromorphone, oxymorphone, levorphanol); children and teenagers should not be given aspirin products if chickenpox or flu symptoms are present; aspirin use has been associated with Reye's syndrome; severe liver or renal insufficiency, pre-existing CNS and depression

Enhanced analgesia has been seen in elderly patients on therapeutic doses of narcotics; duration of action may be increased in the elderly; the elderly may be particularly susceptible to the CNS depressant and constipating effects of narcotics

**Adverse Reactions**

>10%:
- Cardiovascular: Hypotension
- Central nervous system: Fatigue, drowsiness, dizziness
- Gastrointestinal: Nausea, vomiting, heartburn, stomach pains, dyspepsia
- Neuromuscular & skeletal: Weakness

1% to 10%:
- Central nervous system: Nervousness, headache, restlessness, malaise, confusion
- Dermatologic: Rash
- Gastrointestinal: Anorexia, stomach cramps, xerostomia, constipation, biliary spasm, gastrointestinal ulceration
- Genitourinary: Ureteral spasms, decreased urination
- Hematologic: Hemolytic anemia
- Local: Pain at injection site
- Respiratory: Dyspnea, shortness of breath
- Miscellaneous: Anaphylactic shock

**Overdosage/Toxicology**

Symptoms of overdose include CNS and respiratory depression, gastrointestinal cramping, constipation, tinnitus, headache, dizziness, confusion, metabolic acidosis, hyperpyrexia

Consult regional poison control center for additional information. Naloxone 2 mg I.V. (0.01 mg/kg for children) with repeat administration as necessary up to a total of 10 mg

**Drug Interactions**

Decreased effect with phenothiazines

Increased effect/toxicity with CNS depressants, TCAs, dextroamphetamine

**Usual Dosage** Oral (based on oxycodone combined salts):

Children: 0.05-0.15 mg/kg/dose every 4-6 hours as needed; maximum: 5 mg/dose (1 tablet Percodan® or 2 tablets Percodan®-Demi/dose)

Adults: Percodan®: 1 tablet every 6 hours as needed for pain or Percodan®-Demi: 1-2 tablets every 6 hours as needed for pain

**Dosing adjustment in hepatic impairment:** Dose should be reduced in patients with severe liver disease

**Dietary Considerations**

Oxycodone:
- Alcohol: Additive CNS effects; avoid or limit alcohol. Watch for sedation.
- Food: Glucose may cause hyperglycemia; monitor blood glucose concentrations

**Patient Information** See individual agents

**Nursing Implications** Observe patient for excessive sedation, respiratory depression; implement safety measures, assist with ambulation

**Dosage Forms** Tablet:

Percodan®: Oxycodone hydrochloride 4.5 mg, oxycodone terephthalate 0.38 mg, and aspirin 325 mg

Percodan®-Demi: Oxycodone hydrochloride 2.25 mg, oxycodone terephthalate 0.19 mg, and aspirin 325 mg

♦ **OxyContin®** *see* Oxycodone *on page 413*

♦ **Oxydess® II** *see* Dextroamphetamine *on page 159*

♦ **OxyIR™** *see* Oxycodone *on page 413*

## Oxymetazoline (oks i met AZ oh leen)

**U.S. Brand Names** Afrin® Children's Nose Drops [OTC]; Afrin® Sinus [OTC]; Allerest® 12 Hour Nasal Solution [OTC]; Chlorphed®-LA Nasal Solution [OTC]; Dristan® Long Lasting Nasal Solution [OTC]; Duramist® Plus [OTC]; Duration® Nasal Solution [OTC]; Nōstrilla® [OTC]; NTZ® Long Acting Nasal Solution [OTC]; OcuClear® Ophthalmic [OTC]; Sinarest® 12 Hour Nasal Solution; Sinex® Long-Acting [OTC]; Twice-A-Day® Nasal [OTC]; Visine® L.R. Ophthalmic [OTC]; 4-Way® Long Acting Nasal Solution [OTC]

**Pharmacologic Category** Adrenergic Agonist Agent; Vasoconstrictor

**Use**

Adjunctive therapy of middle ear infections, associated with acute or chronic rhinitis, the common cold, sinusitis, hay fever, or other allergies

Ophthalmic: Relief of redness of eye due to minor eye irritations

**Effects on Mental Status** None reported

**Effects on Psychiatric Treatment** May increase toxicity if used with MAO inhibitors (hypertension)

**Usual Dosage** Intranasal (therapy should not exceed 3-5 days):

Children 2-6 years: 0.025% solution: Instill 2-3 drops in each nostril twice daily

Children ≥6 years and Adults: 0.05% solution: Instill 2-3 drops or 2-3 sprays into each nostril twice daily

**Dosage Forms** Solution, nasal:

Drops: 0.05% drops (15 mL, 20 mL)

Drops, pediatric: 0.025% (20 mL)

Spray: 0.05% (15 mL, 30 mL)

## Oxymetholone (oks i METH oh lone)

**U.S. Brand Names** Anadrol®

**Canadian Brand Names** Anapolon®

**Pharmacologic Category** Anabolic Steroid

**Use** Anemias caused by the administration of myelotoxic drugs

**Effects on Mental Status** May cause insomnia

**Effects on Psychiatric Treatment** None reported

**Restrictions** C-III

**Pregnancy Risk Factor** X

**Contraindications** Carcinoma of breast or prostate, nephrosis, pregnancy, hypersensitivity to any component

**Warnings/Precautions** Anabolic steroids may cause peliosis hepatis, liver cell tumors, and blood lipid changes with increased risk of arteriosclerosis; monitor diabetic patients carefully; use with caution in elderly patients, they may be at greater risk for prostatic hypertrophy; use with caution in patients with cardiac, renal, or hepatic disease or epilepsy

**Adverse Reactions**

**Male:**

Postpubertal:

- >10%:
  - Dermatologic: Acne
  - Endocrine & metabolic: Gynecomastia
  - Genitourinary: Bladder irritability, priapism
- 1% to 10%:
  - Central nervous system: Insomnia, chills
  - Endocrine & metabolic: Decreased libido
  - Gastrointestinal: Nausea, diarrhea
  - Genitourinary: Prostatic hypertrophy (elderly)
  - Hematologic: Iron deficiency anemia, suppression of clotting factors
- Hepatic: Hepatic dysfunction
- <1%: Hepatic necrosis, hepatocellular carcinoma

Prepubertal:

- >10%:
  - Dermatologic: Acne
  - Endocrine & metabolic: Virilism
- 1% to 10%:
  - Central nervous system: Chills, insomnia
  - Dermatologic: Hyperpigmentation
  - Gastrointestinal: Diarrhea, nausea
  - Hematologic: Iron deficiency anemia, suppression of clotting factors
- <1%: Hepatic necrosis, hepatocellular carcinoma

**Female:**

- >10%: Endocrine & metabolic: Virilism
- 1% to 10%:
  - Central nervous system: Chills, insomnia
  - Endocrine & metabolic: Hypercalcemia
  - Gastrointestinal: Nausea, diarrhea
  - Hematologic: Iron deficiency anemia, suppression of clotting factors
  - Hepatic: Hepatic dysfunction
- <1%: Hepatic necrosis, hepatocellular carcinoma

**Overdosage/Toxicology** Signs and symptoms: Abnormal liver function test

**Drug Interactions** Increased toxicity: Increased oral anticoagulants, insulin requirements may be decreased

**Usual Dosage** Adults: Erythropoietic effects: Oral: 1-5 mg/kg/day in one daily dose; usual effective dose: 1-2 mg/kg/day; give for a minimum trial of 3-6 months because response may be delayed

**Dosing adjustment in hepatic impairment:**

Mild to moderate impairment: Oxymetholone should be used with caution in patients with liver dysfunction because of it's hepatotoxic potential

Severe impairment: Oxymetholone should **not** be used

**Patient Information** Take as directed; do not exceed recommended dosage. If diabetic, monitor serum glucose closely and notify prescriber of changes; this medication can alter hypoglycemic requirements. You may experience acne, growth of body hair or baldness, deepening of voice, loss of libido, impotence, swelling of breasts, menstrual irregularity, or priapism (most are reversible); drowsiness, dizziness, or blurred vision (use caution driving or engaging in tasks that require alertness until response to drug is known); or nausea or vomiting (small frequent meals and good mouth care may help). Report persistent GI distress or diarrhea; change in color of urine or stool; yellowing of eyes or skin; swelling of ankles, feet, or hands; unusual bruising or bleeding; or other adverse reactions.

**Dosage Forms** Tablet: 50 mg

## Oxymorphone (oks i MOR fone)

**Related Information**

Narcotic Agonists Comparison Chart *on page 720*

**U.S. Brand Names** Numorphan®

**Pharmacologic Category** Analgesic, Narcotic

**Use** Management of moderate to severe pain and preoperatively as a sedative and a supplement to anesthesia

**Effects on Mental Status** Drowsiness and dizziness are common; may cause nervousness, restlessness or confusion; may rarely cause depression or hallucinations

**Effects on Psychiatric Treatment** Psychotropics may alter the analgesic effects of opioids; monitor for change in pain relief

**Restrictions** C-II

**Pregnancy Risk Factor** B (D if used for prolonged periods or in high doses at term)

**Contraindications** Hypersensitivity to oxymorphone or any component, increased intracranial pressure; severe respiratory depression

**Warnings/Precautions** Some preparations contain sulfites which may cause allergic reactions; infants <3 months of age are more susceptible to respiratory depression, use with caution and generally in reduced doses in this age group; use with caution in patients with impaired respiratory function or severe hepatic dysfunction and in patients with hypersensitivity reactions to other phenanthrene derivative opioid agonists (codeine, hydrocodone, hydromorphone, levorphanol, oxycodone, oxymorphone); tolerance or drug dependence may result from extended use

**Adverse Reactions**

- >10%:
  - Cardiovascular: Hypotension
  - Central nervous system: Fatigue, drowsiness, dizziness
  - Gastrointestinal: Nausea, vomiting, constipation
  - Neuromuscular & skeletal: Weakness
  - Miscellaneous: Histamine release
- 1% to 10%:
  - Central nervous system: Nervousness, headache, restlessness, malaise, confusion
  - Gastrointestinal: Anorexia, stomach cramps, xerostomia, biliary spasm
  - Genitourinary: Decreased urination, ureteral spasms
  - Local: Pain at injection site
  - Respiratory: Dyspnea, shortness of breath
- <1%: Hallucinations, histamine release, increased intracranial pressure, mental depression, paradoxical CNS stimulation, paralytic ileus, physical and psychological dependence, rash, urticaria

**Overdosage/Toxicology**

Signs and symptoms: Respiratory depression, miosis, hypotension, bradycardia, apnea, pulmonary edema

Treatment: Includes support of the patient's airway, establishment of an I.V. line and administration of naloxone 2 mg I.V. (0.01 mg/kg for children) with repeat administration as necessary up to a total of 10 mg.

**Drug Interactions**

Decreased effect with phenothiazines

Increased effect/toxicity with CNS depressants, TCAs, dextroamphetamine

**Usual Dosage** Adults:

I.M., S.C.: 0.5 mg initially, 1-1.5 mg every 4-6 hours as needed

I.V.: 0.5 mg initially

Rectal: 5 mg every 4-6 hours

**Dietary Considerations** Alcohol: Additive CNS effect, avoid use

**Patient Information** If self-administered, use exactly as directed (do not increase dose or frequency); may cause physical and/or psychological dependence. While using this medication, do not use alcohol and other prescription or OTC medications (especially sedatives, tranquilizers, antihistamines, or pain medications) without consulting prescriber. Maintain adequate hydration (2-3 L/day of fluids unless instructed to restrict fluid

(Continued)

## Oxymorphone *(Continued)*

intake). May cause hypotension, dizziness, drowsiness, impaired coordination, or blurred vision (use caution when driving, climbing stairs, or changing position - rising from sitting or lying to standing, or when engaging in tasks requiring alertness until response to drug is known); nausea, vomiting or dry mouth (frequent mouth care, small frequent meals, chewing gum, or sucking lozenges may help); constipation (increased exercise, fluids, or dietary fruit and fiber may help - if constipation remains an unresolved problem, consult prescriber about use of stool softeners). Report persistent dizziness or headache; excessive fatigue or sedation; changes in mental status; changes in urinary elimination or pain on urination; weakness or trembling; blurred vision; or shortness of breath.

**Nursing Implications** Observe patient for excessive sedation, respiratory depression, implement safety measures, assist with ambulation

**Dosage Forms**

Injection, as hydrochloride: 1 mg (1 mL); 1.5 mg/mL (1 mL, 10 mL)

Suppository, rectal, as hydrochloride: 5 mg

## Oxyphenbutazone (oks i fen BYOO ta zone)

**Pharmacologic Category** Nonsteroidal Anti-Inflammatory Agent (NSAID)

**Use** Management of inflammatory disorders, as an analgesic in the treatment of mild to moderate pain; acute gouty arthritis

**Effects on Mental Status** Dizziness is common; may cause nervousness; may rarely cause drowsiness, confusion, depression, or hallucinations

**Effects on Psychiatric Treatment** May rarely cause agranulocytosis; use caution with clozapine and carbamazepine; may decrease lithium clearance resulting in an increase in serum lithium levels and potential lithium toxicity; monitor serum lithium levels

**Contraindications** Active GI bleeding; ulcer disease; hypersensitivity to oxyphenbutazone or any component

**Warnings/Precautions** Use with caution in patients with congestive heart failure, hypertension, decreased renal or hepatic function, history of GI disease (bleeding or ulcers), or those receiving anticoagulants; safety and efficacy in children <6 months of age have not yet been established; because of severe hematologic adverse effects, discontinue use if no favorable response is seen

**Adverse Reactions**

>10%:

Central nervous system: Dizziness

Dermatologic: Skin rash

Gastrointestinal: Abdominal cramps, heartburn, indigestion, nausea

1% to 10%:

Central nervous system: Headache, nervousness

Dermatologic: Itching

Endocrine & metabolic: Fluid retention

Gastrointestinal: Vomiting

Otic: Tinnitus

**Overdosage/Toxicology**

Signs and symptoms: Apnea, metabolic acidosis, coma, nystagmus, leukocytosis, renal failure

Treatment: Management of a nonsteroidal anti-inflammatory drug (NSAID) intoxication is primarily supportive and symptomatic. Fluid therapy is commonly effective in managing the hypotension that may occur following an acute NSAID overdose, except when this is due to an acute blood loss. Seizures tend to be very short-lived and often do not require drug treatment. Although, recurrent seizures should be treated with I.V. diazepam. Since many of the NSAIDs undergo enterohepatic cycling, multiple doses of charcoal may be needed to reduce the potential for delayed toxicities.

**Usual Dosage** Adults: Oral:

Rheumatoid arthritis: 100-200 mg 3-4 times/day until desired effect, then reduce dose to not exceeding 400 mg/day

Acute gouty arthritis: Initial: 400 mg then 100 mg every 4 hours until acute attack subsides, not longer than 1 week

**Patient Information** Take with food; may cause dizziness or drowsiness; notify physician and discontinue if persistent sore throat, fatigue, fever, or unusual bleeding or bruising occurs

**Dosage Forms** Tablet: 100 mg

## Oxyphencyclimine (oks i fen SYE kli meen)

**U.S. Brand Names** Daricon®

**Pharmacologic Category** Anticholinergic Agent; Antispasmodic Agent, Gastrointestinal

**Use** Adjunctive treatment of peptic ulcer

**Effects on Mental Status** May cause drowsiness, nervousness, confusion, amnesia, or insomnia

**Effects on Psychiatric Treatment** Concurrent use with psychotropics may alter their clinical effects, but it is not likely to be of significance, however, side effects may be additive especially anticholinergics (drowsiness, dry mouth)

**Pregnancy Risk Factor** C

**Contraindications** Angle-closure glaucoma; obstructive GI tract or uropathy; severe ulcerative colitis; myasthenia gravis; intestinal atony

**Warnings/Precautions** Use with caution in patients with hepatic or renal disease, ulcerative colitis, hyperthyroidism, cardiovascular disease, hypertension, tachycardia, GI obstruction, obstruction of the urinary tract

**Adverse Reactions**

>10%:

Dermatologic: Dry skin

Gastrointestinal: Constipation, dry throat, xerostomia

Respiratory: Dry nose

Miscellaneous: Decreased diaphoresis

1% to 10%:

Dermatologic: Increased sensitivity to light

Gastrointestinal: Dysphagia

**Overdosage/Toxicology**

Signs and symptoms: CNS stimulation followed by depression, confusion, delusions, nonreactive pupils, tachycardia, hypertension; anticholinergic toxicity is caused by strong binding of the drug to cholinergic receptors

Treatment: For anticholinergic overdose with severe life-threatening symptoms, physostigmine 1-2 mg (0.5 or 0.02 mg/kg for children) S.C. or I.V., slowly may be given to reverse these effects

**Drug Interactions** Increased anticholinergic side effects by amantadine; decreased phenothiazines, antiparkinsonian drugs, Haldol® effects

**Usual Dosage** Children >12 years and Adults: Oral: 10 mg twice daily or 5 mg 3 times/day

**Patient Information** May cause drowsiness; avoid alcohol; may impair coordination and judgment may cause blurred vision

**Dosage Forms** Tablet, as hydrochloride: 10 mg

## Oxytetracycline (oks i tet ra SYE kleen)

**U.S. Brand Names** Terramycin® I.M. Injection; Terramycin® Oral

**Pharmacologic Category** Antibiotic, Tetracycline Derivative

**Use** Treatment of susceptible bacterial infections; both gram-positive and gram-negative, as well as, *Rickettsia* and *Mycoplasma* organisms

**Effects on Mental Status** Case reports of tetracyclines report memory disturbances, mood stabilizing and antidepressant effects

**Effects on Psychiatric Treatment** Barbiturates and carbamazepine may decrease the effects of oxytetracycline; may decrease lithium clearance resulting in an increase in serum lithium levels and potential lithium toxicity; monitor serum lithium levels

**Pregnancy Risk Factor** D

**Contraindications** Hypersensitivity to tetracycline or any component

**Warnings/Precautions** Avoid in children ≤8 years of age, pregnant and nursing women; photosensitivity can occur with oxytetracycline

**Adverse Reactions**

>10%: Miscellaneous: Discoloration of teeth and enamel hypoplasia (infants)

1% to 10%:

Dermatologic: Photosensitivity

Gastrointestinal: Nausea, diarrhea

<1%: Abdominal cramps, acute renal failure, anaphylaxis, anorexia, antibiotic-associated pseudomembranous colitis, azotemia, bulging fontanels in infants, candidal superinfection, dermatologic effects, diabetes insipidus syndrome, esophagitis, exfoliative dermatitis, hepatotoxicity, hypersensitivity reactions, increased intracranial pressure, paresthesia, pericarditis, pigmentation of nails, pruritus, pseudotumor cerebri, renal damage, staphylococcal enterocolitis, superinfections, thrombophlebitis, vomiting

**Overdosage/Toxicology**

Signs and symptoms: Nausea, anorexia, diarrhea

Treatment: Following GI decontamination, supportive care only

**Drug Interactions**

Decreased effect with antacids containing aluminum, calcium or magnesium

Iron and bismuth subsalicylate may decrease doxycycline bioavailability

Barbiturates, phenytoin, and carbamazepine decrease doxycycline's half-life

Increased effect of warfarin

**Usual Dosage**

Oral:

Children >8 years: 40-50 mg/kg/day in divided doses every 6 hours (maximum: 2 g/24 hours)

Adults: 250-500 mg/dose every 6-12 hours depending on severity of the infection

I.M.:

Children >8 years: 15-25 mg/kg/day (maximum: 250 mg/dose) in divided doses every 8-12 hours

Adults: 250 mg every 24 hours or 300 mg/day divided every 8-12 hours

Syphilis: 30-40 g in divided doses over 10-15 days

Gonorrhea: 1.5 g, then 500 mg every 6 hours for total of 9 g

Uncomplicated chlamydial infections: 500 mg every 6 hours for 7 days

Severe acne: 1 g/day then decrease to 125-500 mg/day

**Dosing interval in renal impairment:**

$Cl_{cr}$ <10 mL/minute: Administer every 24 hours or avoid use if possible

**Dosing adjustment/comments in hepatic impairment:** Avoid use in patients with severe liver disease

**Patient Information** Take as directed, around-the-clock. Finish all doses; do not skip doses. May take with food to reduce GI upset. Do not take with antacids, iron products, or dairy products. You may be sensitive to sunlight; use sunblock, wear protective clothing, or avoid direct sun. If diabetic, drug may cause false tests with Clinitest® urine glucose monitoring; use of glucose oxidase methods (Clinistix®) or serum glucose monitoring is preferable. Report rash, difficulty breathing, yellowing of skin or eyes, change in color of urine or stool, easy bruising or bleeding, fever, chills, perianal itching, purulent vaginal discharge, white plaques in mouth, or persistent diarrhea.

**Dosage Forms**

Capsule, as hydrochloride: 250 mg

Injection, as hydrochloride, with lidocaine 2%: 5% [50 mg/mL] (2 mL, 10 mL); 12.5% [125 mg/mL] (2 mL)

## Oxytetracycline and Hydrocortisone

(oks i tet ra SYE kleen & hye droe KOR ti sone)

**U.S. Brand Names** Terra-Cortril® Ophthalmic Suspension

**Pharmacologic Category** Antibiotic/Corticosteroid, Ophthalmic

**Use** Treatment of susceptible ophthalmic bacterial infections with associated swelling

**Effects on Mental Status** None reported

**Effects on Psychiatric Treatment** None reported

**Usual Dosage** Ophthalmic: Adults: Instill 1-2 drops in eye(s) every 3-4 hours

**Dosage Forms** Suspension, ophthalmic: Oxytetracycline hydrochloride 0.5% and hydrocortisone 0.5% (5 mL)

## Oxytetracycline and Polymyxin B

(oks i tet ra SYE kleen & pol i MIKS in bee)

**U.S. Brand Names** Terak® Ophthalmic Ointment; Terramycin® Ophthalmic Ointment; Terramycin® w/Polymyxin B Ophthalmic Ointment

**Pharmacologic Category** Antibiotic, Ophthalmic

**Use** Treatment of superficial ocular infections involving the conjunctiva and/or cornea

**Effects on Mental Status** None reported

**Effects on Psychiatric Treatment** None reported

**Usual Dosage** Topical: Apply ½" of ointment onto the lower lid of affected eye 2-4 times/day

**Dosage Forms**

Ointment, ophthalmic/otic: Oxytetracycline hydrochloride 5 mg and polymyxin B 10,000 units per g (3.5 g)

Tablet, vaginal: Oxytetracycline hydrochloride 100 mg and polymyxin B 100,000 units (10s)

## Oxytocin (oks i TOE sin)

**U.S. Brand Names** Pitocin®

**Canadian Brand Names** Toesen®

**Synonyms** Pit

**Pharmacologic Category** Oxytocic Agent

**Use** Induces labor at term; controls postpartum bleeding; nasal preparation used to promote milk letdown in lactating females

**Effects on Mental Status** None reported

**Effects on Psychiatric Treatment** None reported

**Pregnancy Risk Factor** X

**Contraindications** Hypersensitivity to oxytocin or any component; significant cephalopelvic disproportion, unfavorable fetal positions, fetal distress, hypertonic or hyperactive uterus, contraindicated vaginal delivery, prolapse, total placenta previa, and vasa previa

**Warnings/Precautions** To be used for medical rather than elective induction of labor; may produce antidiuretic effect (ie, water intoxication and excess uterine contractions); high doses or hypersensitivity to oxytocin may cause uterine hypertonicity, spasm, tetanic contraction, or rupture of the uterus; severe water intoxication with convulsions, coma, and death is associated with a slow oxytocin infusion over 24 hours

**Adverse Reactions**

Fetal: <1%: Arrhythmias, bradycardia, brain damage, death, hypoxia, intracranial hemorrhage, neonatal jaundice

Maternal: <1%: Anaphylactic reactions, arrhythmias, cardiac arrhythmias, coma, death, fatal afibrinogenemia, hypotension, increased blood loss, increased uterine motility, nausea, pelvic hematoma, postpartum hemorrhage, premature ventricular contractions, seizures, SIADH with hyponatremia, tachycardia, vomiting

**Overdosage/Toxicology**

Signs and symptoms: Tetanic uterine contractions, impaired uterine blood flow, amniotic fluid embolism, uterine rupture, SIADH, seizures

Treatment: Treat SIADH via fluid restriction, diuresis, saline administration, and anticonvulsants, if needed

**Drug Interactions** Sympathomimetic pressor effects may be increased by oxytocin resulting in postpartum hypertension

**Usual Dosage** I.V. administration requires the use of an infusion pump

Adults:

Induction of labor: I.V.: 0.001-0.002 units/minute; increase by 0.001-0.002 units every 15-30 minutes until contraction pattern has been established; maximum dose should not exceed 20 milliunits/minute

Postpartum bleeding:

I.M.: Total dose of 10 units after delivery

I.V.: 10-40 units by I.V. infusion in 1000 mL of intravenous fluid at a rate sufficient to control uterine atony

Promotion of milk letdown: Intranasal: 1 spray or 3 drops in one or both nostrils 2-3 minutes before breast-feeding

**Patient Information**

I.V., I.M.: Generally used in emergency situations; drug teaching should be incorporated in other situational teaching

Intranasal spray: While sitting up, hold bottle upright and squeeze into nostril

**Dosage Forms**

Injection: 10 units/mL (1 mL, 10 mL)

Solution, nasal: 40 units/mL (2 mL, 5 mL)


♦ **Oyst-Cal 500 [OTC]** *see* Calcium Carbonate *on page 84*

♦ **Oystercal® 500** *see* Calcium Carbonate *on page 84*

♦ **P-071** *see* Cetirizine *on page 105*

♦ **Pacerone®** *see* Amiodarone *on page 32*


## Paclitaxel (PAK li taks el)

**U.S. Brand Names** Paxene®; Taxol®

**Pharmacologic Category** Antineoplastic Agent, Natural Source (Plant) Derivative

**Use** Treatment of metastatic carcinoma of the ovary in combination with cisplatin; treatment of metastatic breast cancer; adjuvant treatment of node-positive breast cancer administered sequentially to standard doxorubicin-containing combination therapy

**Effects on Mental Status** None reported

**Effects on Psychiatric Treatment** May cause neutropenia; use caution with clozapine and carbamazepine

**Usual Dosage** Premedication with dexamethasone (20 mg orally or I.V. at 12 and 6 hours **or** 14 and 7 hours before the dose), diphenhydramine (50 mg I.V. 30-60 minutes prior to the dose), and cimetidine, famotidine or ranitidine (I.V. 30-60 minutes prior to the dose) is recommended

Adults: I.V. infusion: Refer to individual protocol

Ovarian carcinoma: 135-175 mg/m² over 1-24 hours administered every 3 weeks

Metastatic breast cancer: Treatment is still undergoing investigation; most protocols have used doses of 175-250 mg/m² over 1-24 hours every 3 weeks

Hemodialysis: Significant drug removal is unlikely based on physiochemical characteristics

Peritoneal dialysis: Significant drug removal is unlikely based on physiochemical characteristics

**Dosage adjustment in hepatic impairment:**

Total bilirubin ≤1.5 mg/dL and AST >2 X normal limits: Total dose <135 mg/m²

Total bilirubin 1.6-3.0 mg/dL: Total dose ≤75 mg/m²

Total bilirubin ≥3.1 mg/dL: Total dose ≤50 mg/m²

**Dosage Forms** Injection: 6 mg/mL (5 mL, 16.7 mL)

## Palivizumab (pah li VIZ u mab)

**U.S. Brand Names** Synagis®

**Pharmacologic Category** Monoclonal Antibody

**Use** Prevention of serious lower respiratory tract disease caused by respiratory syncytial virus (RSV) in pediatric patients at high risk of RSV disease; safety and efficacy were established in infants with bronchopulmonary dysplasia (BPD) and infants with a history of prematurity (≤35 weeks gestational age)

**Effects on Mental Status** May rarely cause nervousness

**Effects on Psychiatric Treatment** May cause anemia; use caution with clozapine and carbamazepine

**Usual Dosage** Children: I.M.: 15 mg/kg of body weight, monthly throughout RSV season (First dose administered prior to commencement of RSV season)

**Dosage Forms** Injection, lyophilized: 100 mg


♦ **Palmetto Scrub** *see* Saw Palmetto *on page 505*

♦ **Palmitate-A® 5000 [OTC]** *see* Vitamin A *on page 585*

♦ **Paludrine®** *see* Proguanil *on page 468*

♦ **Pamelor®** *see* Nortriptyline *on page 400*

## Pamidronate (pa mi DROE nate)

**U.S. Brand Names** Aredia™

**Pharmacologic Category** Antidote; Bisphosphonate Derivative

**Use** Treatment of hypercalcemia associated with malignancy; treatment of osteolytic bone lesions associated with multiple myeloma or metastatic breast cancer; moderate to severe Paget's disease of bone

**Effects on Mental Status** May cause drowsiness

**Effects on Psychiatric Treatment** May rarely cause leukopenia; use caution with clozapine and carbamazepine

**Usual Dosage** Drug must be diluted properly before administration and infused intravenously slowly (over at least 1 hour). Adults: I.V.:

Hypercalcemia of malignancy:

Moderate cancer-related hypercalcemia (corrected serum calcium: 12-13 mg/dL): 60-90 mg given as a slow infusion over 2-24 hours

Severe cancer-related hypercalcemia (corrected serum calcium: >13.5 mg/dL): 90 mg as a slow infusion over 2-24 hours

A period of 7 days should elapse before the use of second course; repeat infusions every 2-3 weeks have been suggested, however, could be administered every 2-3 months according to the degree and of severity of hypercalcemia and/or the type of malignancy

Osteolytic bone lesions with multiple myeloma: 90 mg in 500 mL $D_5W$, 0.45% NaCl or 0.9% NaCl administered over 4 hours on a monthly basis

Osteolytic bone lesions with metastatic breast cancer: 90 mg in 250 mL $D_5W$, 0.45% NaCl or 0.9% NaCl administered over 2 hours, repeated every 3-4 weeks

Paget's disease: 30 mg in 500 mL 0.45% NaCl, 0.9% NaCl or $D_5W$ administered over 4 hours for 3 consecutive days

**Dosing adjustment in renal impairment:** Adjustment is not necessary

**Dosage Forms** Powder for injection, lyophilized, as disodium: 30 mg, 60 mg, 90 mg


- **Pamine®** *see* Methscopolamine *on page 355*
- **Panadol® [OTC]** *see* Acetaminophen *on page 14*
- **Panasal® 5/500** *see* Hydrocodone and Aspirin *on page 272*
- **Panclar®** *see* Deanol *on page 152*
- **Pancrease®** *see* Pancrelipase *on page 418*
- **Pancrease® MT 4** *see* Pancrelipase *on page 418*
- **Pancrease® MT 10** *see* Pancrelipase *on page 418*
- **Pancrease® MT 16** *see* Pancrelipase *on page 418*
- **Pancrease® MT 20** *see* Pancrelipase *on page 418*


## Pancrelipase (pan kre LI pase)

**U.S. Brand Names** Cotazym®; Cotazym-S®; Creon® 10; Creon® 20; Ilozyme®; Ku-Zyme® HP; Pancrease®; Pancrease® MT 4; Pancrease® MT 10; Pancrease® MT 16; Pancrease® MT 20; Protilase®; Ultrase® MT12; Ultrase® MT20; Viokase®; Zymase®

**Synonyms** Lipancreatin

**Pharmacologic Category** Enzyme

**Use** Replacement therapy in symptomatic treatment of malabsorption syndrome caused by pancreatic insufficiency

**Effects on Mental Status** None reported

**Effects on Psychiatric Treatment** None reported

**Pregnancy Risk Factor** C

**Contraindications** Hypersensitivity to pancrelipase or any component, pork protein

**Warnings/Precautions** Pancrelipase is inactivated by acids; use microencapsulated products whenever possible, since these products permit better dissolution of enzymes in the duodenum and protect the enzyme preparations from acid degradation in the stomach

**Adverse Reactions**

1% to 10%: High doses:

Endocrine & metabolic: Hyperuricemia

Gastrointestinal: Nausea, cramps, constipation, diarrhea

Genitourinary: Hyperuricosuria

Ocular: Lacrimation

Respiratory: Sneezing, bronchospasm

<1%: Bronchospasm, irritation of the mouth, rash, shortness of breath

**Overdosage/Toxicology** Signs and symptoms: Diarrhea, other transient intestinal upset, hyperuricosuria, hyperuricemia

**Drug Interactions**

Decreased effect: Calcium carbonate, magnesium hydroxide

Increased effect: $H_2$-antagonists (eg, ranitidine, cimetidine)

**Usual Dosage** Oral:

Powder: Actual dose depends on the digestive requirements of the patient

Children <1 year: Start with 1/8 teaspoonful with feedings

Adults: 0.7 g with meals

Enteric coated microspheres and microtablets: The following dosage recommendations are only an approximation for initial dosages. The actual dosage will depend on the digestive requirements of the individual patient.

Children:

<1 year: 2000 units of lipase with meals

1-6 years: 4000-8000 units of lipase with meals and 4000 units with snacks

7-12 years: 4000-12,000 units of lipase with meals and snacks

Adults: 4000-16,000 units of lipase with meals and with snacks or 1-3 tablets/capsules before or with meals and snacks; in severe deficiencies, dose may be increased to 8 tablets/capsules

Occluded feeding tubes: One tablet of Viokase® crushed with one 325 mg tablet of sodium bicarbonate (to activate the Viokase®) in 5 mL of water can be instilled into the nasogastric tube and clamped for 5 minutes; then, flushed with 50 mL of tap water

**Patient Information** Take before or with meals. Avoid taking with alkaline food. Do not chew, crush, or dissolve delayed release capsules; swallow whole. Do not inhale powder when preparing. You may experience some gastric discomfort. Report unusual joint pain or swelling, respiratory difficulty, or persistent GI upset.

**Dosage Forms**

Capsule:

Cotazym®: Lipase 8000 units, protease 30,000 units, amylase 30,000 units

Ku-Zyme® HP: Lipase 8000 units, protease 30,000 units, amylase 30,000 units

Ultrase® MT12: Lipase 12,000 units, protease 39,000 units, amylase 39,000 units

Ultrase® MT20: Lipase 20,000 units, protease 65,000 units, amylase 65,000 units

Enteric coated microspheres (Pancrease®): Lipase 4000 units, protease 25,000 units, amylase 20,000 units

Enteric coated microtablets:

Pancrease® MT 4: Lipase 4500 units, protease 12,000 units, amylase 12,000 units

Pancrease® MT 10: Lipase 10,000 units, protease 30,000 units, amylase 30,000 units

Pancrease® MT 16: Lipase 16,000 units, protease 48,000 units, amylase 48,000 units

Pancrease® MT 20: Lipase 20,000 units, protease 44,000 units, amylase 56,000 units

Enteric coated spheres:

Cotazym-S®: Lipase 5000 units, protease 20,000 units, amylase 20,000 units

Pancrelipase, Protilase®: Lipase 4000 units, protease 25,000 units, amylase 20,000 units

Zymase®: Lipase 12,000 units, protease 24,000 units, amylase 24,000 units

Delayed release:

Creon® 10: Lipase 10,000 units, protease 37,500 units, amylase 33,200 units

Creon® 20: Lipase 20,000 units, protease 75,000 units, amylase 66,400 units

Powder (Viokase®): Lipase 16,800 units, protease 70,000 units, amylase 70,000 units per 0.7 g

Tablet:

Ilozyme®: Lipase 11,000 units, protease 30,000 units, amylase 30,000 units

Viokase®: Lipase 8000 units, protease 30,000 units, amylase 30,000 units

## Pancuronium (pan kyoo ROE nee um)

**U.S. Brand Names** Pavulon®

**Pharmacologic Category** Neuromuscular Blocker Agent, Nondepolarizing

**Use Drug of choice** for neuromuscular blockade except in patients with renal failure, hepatic failure, or cardiovascular instability; produce skeletal muscle relaxation during surgery after induction of general anesthesia, increase pulmonary compliance during assisted respiration, facilitate endotracheal intubation, preferred muscle relaxant for neonatal cardiac patients, must provide artificial ventilation

**Effects on Mental Status** None reported

**Effects on Psychiatric Treatment** None reported

**Usual Dosage** Based on ideal body weight in obese patients

Infants >1 month, Children, and Adults: I.V.: Initial: 0.04-0.1 mg/kg; maintenance dose: 0.02-0.1 mg/kg/dose every 30 minutes to 3 hours as needed

Continuous I.V. infusions are not recommended due to case reports of prolonged paralysis

**Dosing adjustment in renal impairment:** Elimination half-life is doubled, plasma clearance is reduced and rate of recovery is sometimes much slower

$Cl_{cr}$ 10-50 mL/minute: Administer 50% of normal dose

$Cl_{cr}$ <10 mL/minute: Do not use

**Dosing adjustment/comments in hepatic disease:** Elimination half-life is doubled, plasma clearance is doubled, recovery time is prolonged,

volume of distribution is increased (50%) and results in a slower onset, higher total dosage and prolongation of neuromuscular blockade
Patients with liver disease may develop slow resistance to nondepolarizing muscle relaxant; large doses may be required and problems may arise in antagonism

**Dosage Forms** Injection, as bromide: 1 mg/mL (10 mL); 2 mg/mL (2 mL, 5 mL)

- ♦ **Pandel®** *see* Hydrocortisone *on page 273*
- ♦ **Panhematin®** *see* Hemin *on page 265*
- ♦ **PanOxyl®-AQ** *see* Benzoyl Peroxide *on page 62*
- ♦ **PanOxyl® Bar [OTC]** *see* Benzoyl Peroxide *on page 62*
- ♦ **Panretin®** *see* Alitretinoin *on page 24*
- ♦ **Panthoderm® Cream [OTC]** *see* Dexpanthenol *on page 158*
- ♦ **Pantopon®** *see* Opium Alkaloids *on page 406*

## Pantoprazole (pan TOE pra zole)

**U.S. Brand Names** Protonix®

**Pharmacologic Category** Proton Pump Inhibitor

**Use** Short-term treatment of erosive esophagitis associated with GERD

**Unlabeled use:** Hypersecretory disorders, peptic ulcer disease, active ulcer bleeding with parenterally-administered pantoprazole

**Effects on Mental Status** May cause anxiety or dizziness; may rarely produce confusion, depression, dysarthria, hallucinations, nervousness, or somnolence

**Effects on Psychiatric Treatment** None reported

**Pregnancy Risk Factor** B

**Contraindications** Hypersensitivity to pantoprazole or any component

**Warnings/Precautions** Symptomatic response does not preclude gastric malignancy; not indicated for maintenance therapy; safety and efficacy for use beyond 16 weeks have not been established; safety and efficacy in pediatric patients have not been established

**Adverse Reactions**

1% to 10%:

Cardiovascular: Chest pain
Central nervous system: Pain, migraine, anxiety, dizziness
Endocrine & metabolic: Hyperglycemia (1%), hyperlipidemia
Gastrointestinal: Diarrhea (4%), constipation, dyspepsia, gastroenteritis, nausea, rectal disorder, vomiting
Genitourinary: Urinary frequency, urinary tract infection
Hepatic: Liver function test abnormality increased ALT
Neuromuscular & skeletal: Weakness, back pain, neck pain, arthralgia, hypertonia
Respiratory: Bronchitis, increased cough, dyspnea, pharyngitis, rhinitis, sinusitis, upper respiratory tract infection
Miscellaneous: Flu syndrome, infection

<1%: Rash, allergic reaction, fever, generalized edema, neoplasm, angina pectoris, arrhythmia, congestive heart failure, ECG abnormality, hemorrhage, hypertension, hypotension, myocardial ischemia, palpitation, retinal vascular disorder, syncope, tachycardia, thrombosis, vasodilation, anorexia, aphthous stomatitis, colitis, dry mouth, duodenitis, dysphagia, gastrointestinal carcinoma, gastrointestinal hemorrhage, gastrointestinal moniliasis, gingivitis, glossitis, halitosis, increased appetite, mouth ulceration, oral moniliasis, rectal hemorrhage, stomach ulcer, stomatitis, tongue discoloration, diabetes mellitus, glycosuria, goiter,cholecystitis, cholelithiasis, cholestatic jaundice, hepatitis, increased alkaline phosphatase, increased transaminases, ecchymosis, eosinophilia, anemia, leukocytosis, leukopenia, thrombocytopenia, dehydration, gout, arthritis, bone pain, bursitis, leg cramps, neck rigidity, myalgia, tenosynovitis, confusion, convulsion, depression, dysarthria, hallucinations, hyperkinesia, decreased libido, nervousness, neuralgia, neuritis, paresthesia, decrease reflexes, somnolence, tremor, vertigo, asthma, epistaxis, laryngitis, pneumonia, voice alteration, acne, alopecia, contact dermatitis, dry skin, eczema, fungal dermatitis, herpes simplex, herpes zoster, lichenoid dermatitis, maculopapular rash, pain, pruritus, skin ulcer, sweating, urticaria, abnormal vision, amblyopia, cataract, deafness, diplopia, ear pain, extraocular palsy, glaucoma, otitis externa, taste perversion, tinnitus, albuminuria, balanitis, breast pain, cystitis, dysmenorrhea, dysuria, epididymitis, hematuria, impotence, kidney calculus, kidney pain, nocturia, pyelonephritis, scrotal edema, urethritis, impaired urination, vaginitis, anaphylaxis, angioedema, anterior ischemic optic neuropathy, erythema multiforme, Stevens-Johnson syndrome, toxic epidermal necrolysis, pancreatitis, hypokinesia, speech disorder, increased salivation, vertigo, increased creatinine, hypercholesterolemia, hyperuricemia

**Overdosage/Toxicology** Treatment of an overdose would include appropriate supportive treatment. No adverse events were seen with ingestions of 400 and 600 mg doses. Pantoprazole is not removed by hemodialysis.

**Drug Interactions** CYP2C19 and 3A4 enzyme substrate

Drugs (eg, itraconazole, ketoconazole, and other azole antifungals, ampicillin esters, iron salts) where absorption is determined by an acidic gastric pH, may have decreased absorption when used concurrently. Monitor for change in effectiveness.

**Usual Dosage** Adults: Oral: 40 mg every day for up to 8 weeks; an additional 8 weeks may be used in patients who have not healed after an 8-week course

**Dosage adjustment in renal impairment:** Not required; pantoprazole is not removed by hemodialysis

**Dosage adjustment in hepatic impairment:** Dosage adjustment is not required for mild to moderate impairment. Specific guidelines are not available for patients with severe hepatic impairment.

Elderly: Dosage adjustment not required

**Dietary Considerations** Take with or without food

**Patient Information** Take with or without food. Do not split, chew or crush tablet; take at a similar time every day; inform prescriber if you are or intend to be pregnant; discontinue breast-feeding prior to starting this medicine.

**Nursing Implications** Tablets should be swallowed whole; not chewed, crushed, or split. Do not administer via a nasogastric or feeding tube. Assess other medications the patient may be taking where absorption may be altered by a change in gastric pH (itraconazole, ketoconazole, iron salts, ampicillin esters).

**Dosage Forms** Tablet, enteric coated: 40 mg

## Papaverine (pa PAV er een)

**U.S. Brand Names** Genabid®; Pavabid®; Pavatine®

**Pharmacologic Category** Vasodilator

**Use** Oral: Relief of peripheral and cerebral ischemia associated with arterial spasm and myocardial ischemia complicated by arrhythmias

**Unlabeled use:** Parenteral: Various vascular spasms associated with muscle spasms as in myocardial infarction, angina, peripheral and pulmonary embolism, peripheral vascular disease, angiospastic states, and visceral spasm (ureteral, biliary, and GI colic); testing for impotence

**Effects on Mental Status** May cause drowsiness or dizziness

**Effects on Psychiatric Treatment** May decrease the effects of levodopa

**Pregnancy Risk Factor** C

**Contraindications** Hypersensitivity to papaverine or its components

**Warnings/Precautions** Use with caution in patients with glaucoma; administer I.V. cautiously since apnea and arrhythmias may result; may, in large doses, depress A-V and intraventricular cardiac conduction leading to serious arrhythmias (eg, premature beats, paroxysmal tachycardia); chronic hepatitis noted with jaundice, eosinophilia, and abnormal LFTs

**Adverse Reactions** <1%: Abdominal distress, anorexia, chronic hepatitis, constipation, diarrhea, drowsiness, flushing of the face, headache, hepatic hypersensitivity, lethargy, mild hypertension, nausea, sedation, tachycardias, vertigo

**Overdosage/Toxicology**

Signs and symptoms: Nausea, vomiting weakness, gastric distress, ataxia, drowsiness, nystagmus, diplopia, incoordination, lethargy, and coma with cyanosis, and respiratory depression

Treatment: After gastric decontamination, treatment is supportive with conventional therapy (ie, fluids, positioning and vasopressors for hypotension)

**Drug Interactions** CYP2D6 enzyme substrate

Decreased effect: Papaverine decreases the effects of levodopa
Increased toxicity: Additive effects with CNS depressants

**Usual Dosage** Adults: Oral, sustained release: 150-300 mg every 12 hours; in difficult cases: 150 mg every 8 hours

**Patient Information** Oral: Take as directed; do not alter dosage without consulting prescriber. Do not chew, crush, or dissolve extended release tablets. Avoid alcohol while taking this medication. May cause dizziness, confusion, or blurred vision (avoid driving or engaging in tasks that require alertness until response to drug is known). Increased fiber in diet, exercise, and adequate hydration (2-3 L/day of fluids unless instructed to restrict fluid intake) may help if you experience constipation. Report rapid heartbeat or palpitations, CNS depression, persistent sedation or lethargy, or acute headache.

**Dosage Forms** Capsule, sustained release, as hydrochloride: 150 mg

- ♦ **Parabromdylamine** *see* Brompheniramine *on page 73*
- ♦ **Paracetaldehyde** *see* Paraldehyde *on page 419*
- ♦ **Paracetamol** *see* Acetaminophen *on page 14*
- ♦ **Paraflex®** *see* Chlorzoxazone *on page 120*
- ♦ **Parafon Forte™ DSC** *see* Chlorzoxazone *on page 120*
- ♦ **Paraguay Tea** *see* Maté *on page 333*
- ♦ **Paral®** *see* Paraldehyde *on page 419*

## Paraldehyde (par AL de hyde)

**Related Information**

Anxiolytic/Hypnotic Use in Long-Term Care Facilities *on page 754*

**U.S. Brand Names** Paral®

**Synonyms** Paracetaldehyde

**Pharmacologic Category** Anticonvulsant

(Continued)

## Paraldehyde *(Continued)*

**Use** Treatment of seizures associated with status epilepticus, tetanus, eclampsia, and convulsant drug toxicity

**Unlabeled use:** Delirium tremors, sedative/hypnotic

**Restrictions** C-IV

**Pregnancy Risk Factor** C

**Contraindications** Severe hepatic insufficiency, respiratory disease, GI inflammation or ulceration, disulfiram

**Warnings/Precautions** Use with caution in patients with asthma or other bronchopulmonary disease

**Adverse Reactions**

>10%:

Central nervous system: Drowsiness

Dermatologic: Skin rash

Gastrointestinal: Strong and unpleasant breath, nausea, vomiting, stomach pain, irritation of mucous membrane

Respiratory: Coughing

1% to 10%:

Central nervous system: Clumsiness, dizziness, "hangover effect"

Local: Thrombophlebitis

<1%: Cardiovascular collapse, hepatitis, metabolic acidosis, psychological and physical dependence with prolonged use, pulmonary edema, respiratory depression

**Overdosage/Toxicology**

Signs and symptoms: Hypotension, respiratory depression, metabolic acidosis, pulmonary edema, pulmonary hemorrhage, hemorrhagic gastritis, renal failure; death has occurred with as little as 12-25 mL

Treatment: Metabolic acidosis should be treated with sodium bicarbonate; hemodialysis may be required to treat acidosis and to support renal function

**Drug Interactions**

CNS depressants: Sedative effects and/or respiratory depression may be additive with CNS depressants; includes ethanol, barbiturates, narcotic analgesics, and other sedative agents; monitor for increased effect

Disulfiram: Concurrent use of paraldehyde and disulfiram produces a "disulfiram reaction," this combination is contraindicated

**Stability** Decomposes with exposure to air and light to acetaldehyde which then oxidizes to acetic acid; store in tightly closed containers; protect from light

**Mechanism of Action** Unknown mechanism of action; causes depression of CNS, including the ascending reticular activating system to provide sedation/hypnosis and anticonvulsant activity. Hypnotic activity is rapid, with sleep induction in 10-15 minutes. It has no analgesic properties and may reduce excitement or delirium in the presence of pain.

**Pharmacodynamics/kinetics**

Onset of hypnosis:

Oral: Within 10-15 minutes

I.M.: Within 2-3 minutes

Duration: 6-8 hours

Distribution: Crosses the placenta

Metabolism: ~70% to 80% of a dose metabolized in the liver

Half-life: Adults: 3.5-10 hours

Elimination: Up to 30% excreted as unchanged drug in expired air via the lungs; trace amounts excreted in urine unchanged

**Usual Dosage**

Oral: Dilute in milk or iced fruit juice to mask taste and odor. See table.

**Paraldehyde**

| | Sedative | Hypnotic | Seizures |
|---|---|---|---|
| Adults<br>Oral, rectal | 5-10 mL | 10-30 mL | |
| Children<br>Oral, rectal | 0.15 mL/kg | 0.3 mL/kg | 0.3 mL/kg every 2-4 hours per rectum; maximum dose: 5 mL |

Rectal: Mix paraldehyde 2:1 with oil (cottonseed or olive)

**Dosing adjustment in hepatic impairment:** Dosage may need to be reduced

**Patient Information** Do not attempt tasks requiring psychomotor coordination until the CNS effects by the drug are known; do not drink alcohol; may cause physical and psychological dependence; do not use if solution has a brownish color

**Nursing Implications** Discard unused contents of any container which has been opened for more than 24 hours; do **not** use discolored solution; do **not** use any plastic equipment for administration; parenteral solution may be given orally; should be given in milk or iced fruit juice or dilute to 200 mL with saline

**Additional Information** Do not abruptly discontinue in patients receiving chronic therapy

**Dosage Forms** Liquid, oral or rectal: 1 g/mL (30 mL)

♦ **Paraplatin®** *see* Carboplatin *on page 93*

♦ **Par Decon®** *see* Chlorpheniramine, Phenyltoloxamine, Phenylpropanolamine, and Phenylephrine *on page 116*

♦ **Paredrine®** *see* Hydroxyamphetamine *on page 276*

## Paregoric (par e GOR ik)

**Synonyms** Camphorated Tincture of Opium

**Pharmacologic Category** Analgesic, Narcotic

**Use** Treatment of diarrhea or relief of pain; neonatal opiate withdrawal

**Effects on Mental Status** Drowsiness and dizziness are common; may cause restlessness; may rarely cause insomnia or depression

**Effects on Psychiatric Treatment** Concurrent use with psychotropics may produce additive sedation

**Restrictions** C-III

**Pregnancy Risk Factor** B (D when used long-term or in high doses)

**Contraindications** Hypersensitivity to opium or any component; diarrhea caused by poisoning until the toxic material has been removed

**Warnings/Precautions** Use with caution in patients with respiratory, hepatic or renal dysfunction, severe prostatic hypertrophy, or history of narcotic abuse; opium shares the toxic potential of opiate agonists, and usual precautions of opiate agonist therapy should be observed; some preparations contain sulfites which may cause allergic reactions; infants <3 months of age are more susceptible to respiratory depression, use with caution and generally in reduced doses in this age group; tolerance or drug dependence may result from extended use

**Adverse Reactions**

>10%:

Cardiovascular: Hypotension

Central nervous system: Drowsiness, dizziness

Gastrointestinal: Constipation

Neuromuscular & skeletal: Weakness

1% to 10%:

Central nervous system: Restlessness, headache, malaise

Genitourinary: Ureteral spasms, decreased urination

Miscellaneous: Histamine release

<1%: Anorexia, biliary tract spasm, CNS depression, increased intracranial pressure, increased liver function tests, insomnia, mental depression, miosis, nausea, peripheral vasodilation, physical and psychological dependence, respiratory depression, stomach cramps, urinary tract spasm, vomiting

**Overdosage/Toxicology**

Signs and symptoms: Hypotension, drowsiness, seizures, respiratory depression

Treatment: Naloxone 2 mg I.V. (0.01 mg/kg for children) with repeat administration as necessary up to a total of 10 mg

**Drug Interactions** Increased effect/toxicity with CNS depressants (eg, alcohol, narcotics, benzodiazepines, TCAs, MAO inhibitors, phenothiazine)

**Usual Dosage** Oral:

Neonatal opiate withdrawal: Instill 3-6 drops every 3-6 hours as needed, or initially 0.2 mL every 3 hours; increase dosage by approximately 0.05 mL every 3 hours until withdrawal symptoms are controlled; it is rare to exceed 0.7 mL/dose. Stabilize withdrawal symptoms for 3-5 days, then gradually decrease dosage over a 2- to 4-week period.

Children: 0.25-0.5 mL/kg 1-4 times/day

Adults: 5-10 mL 1-4 times/day

**Dietary Considerations** Alcohol: Additive CNS effect, avoid use

**Patient Information** Take exactly as directed; do not increase dosage. May cause dependence with prolonged or excessive use. Avoid alcohol and all other prescription and OTC that may cause sedation (sleeping medications, some cough/cold remedies, antihistamines, etc). You may experience drowsiness, dizziness, or impaired judgment (use caution when driving or engaging in tasks that require alertness until response to drug is known) or postural hypotension (use caution when rising from sitting or lying position or when climbing stairs). You may experience nausea or loss of appetite (frequent small meals may help) or constipation (a laxative may be necessary). Report unresolved nausea, vomiting, respiratory difficulty (shortness of breath or decreased respirations), chest pain, or palpitations.

**Nursing Implications** Observe patient for excessive sedation, respiratory depression, implement safety measures, assist with ambulation

**Dosage Forms** Liquid: 2 mg morphine equivalent/5 mL [equivalent to 20 mg opium powder] (5 mL, 60 mL, 473 mL, 4000 mL)

♦ **Paremyd® Ophthalmic** *see* Hydroxyamphetamine and Tropicamide *on page 276*

♦ **Parepectolin®** *see* Kaolin and Pectin With Opium *on page 300*

## Paricalcitol (par eh CAL ci tol)

**U.S. Brand Names** Zemplar™

**Pharmacologic Category** Vitamin D Analog

**Use** Prevention and treatment of secondary hyperparathyroidism associated with chronic renal failure. Has been evaluated only in hemodialysis patients.

**Effects on Mental Status** May cause dizziness

**Effects on Psychiatric Treatment** None reported

**Usual Dosage** Adults: I.V.: 0.04-0.1 mcg/kg (2.8-7 mcg) given as a bolus dose no more frequently than every other day at any time during dialysis; doses as high as 0.24 mcg/kg (16.8 mcg) have been administered safely; usually start with 0.04 mcg/kg 3 times/week by I.V. bolus, increased by 0.04 mcg/kg every 2 weeks; the dose of paricalcitol should be adjusted based on serum PTH levels, as follows:

- Same or increasing serum PTH level: Increase paricalcitol dose
- Serum PTH level decreased by <30%: Increase paricalcitol dose
- Serum PTH level decreased by >30% and <60%: Maintain paricalcitol dose
- Serum PTH level decrease by >60%: Decrease paricalcitol dose
- Serum PTH level 1.5-3 times upper limit of normal: Maintain paricalcitol dose

**Dosage Forms** Injection: 5 mcg/mL (1 mL, 2 mL, 5 mL)

♦ **Pariprazole** *see* Rabeprazole *on page 487*

♦ **Parlodel®** *see* Bromocriptine *on page 72*

♦ **Parnate®** *see* Tranylcypromine *on page 559*

## Paromomycin (par oh moe MYE sin)

**U.S. Brand Names** Humatin®

**Pharmacologic Category** Amebicide

**Use** Treatment of acute and chronic intestinal amebiasis; preoperatively to suppress intestinal flora; tapeworm infestations; treatment of *Cryptosporidium*

**Effects on Mental Status** May cause dizziness

**Effects on Psychiatric Treatment** None reported

**Pregnancy Risk Factor** C

**Contraindications** Intestinal obstruction, renal failure, known hypersensitivity to paromomycin or components

**Warnings/Precautions** Use with caution in patients with impaired renal function or possible or proven ulcerative bowel lesions

**Adverse Reactions**

1% to 10%: Gastrointestinal: Diarrhea, abdominal cramps, nausea, vomiting, heartburn

<1%: Eosinophilia, exanthema, headache, ototoxicity, pruritus, rash, secondary enterocolitis, steatorrhea, vertigo

**Overdosage/Toxicology**

Signs and symptoms: Nausea, vomiting, diarrhea

Treatment: Following GI decontamination, care is supportive

**Drug Interactions**

Decreased effect of digoxin, vitamin A, and methotrexate

Increased effect of oral anticoagulants, neuromuscular blockers, and polypeptide antibiotics

**Usual Dosage** Oral:

Intestinal amebiasis: Children and Adults: 25-35 mg/kg/day in 3 divided doses for 5-10 days

*Dientamoeba fragilis*: Children and Adults: 25-30 mg/kg/day in 3 divided doses for 7 days

*Cryptosporidium*: Adults with AIDS: 1.5-2.25 g/day in 3-6 divided doses for 10-14 days (occasionally courses of up to 4-8 weeks may be needed)

Tapeworm (fish, dog, bovine, porcine):
- Children: 11 mg/kg every 15 minutes for 4 doses
- Adults: 1 g every 15 minutes for 4 doses

Hepatic coma: Adults: 4 g/day in 2-4 divided doses for 5-6 days

Dwarf tapeworm: Children and Adults: 45 mg/kg/dose every day for 5-7 days

**Patient Information** Take as directed, for full course of therapy. Do not skip doses. Maintain adequate hydration (2-3 L/day of fluids unless instructed to restrict fluid intake) and nutrition. If GI upset occurs, small frequent meals, frequent mouth care, sucking lozenges, or chewing gum may help. Report unresolved or severe nausea or vomiting, dizziness, ringing in ears, or loss of hearing.

**Dosage Forms** Capsule, as sulfate: 250 mg

## Paroxetine (pa ROKS e teen)

**Related Information**

Antidepressant Agents Comparison Chart *on page 704*
Anxiety Disorders *on page 606*
Clinical Issues in the Use of Antidepressants *on page 627*
Clinical Issues in the Use of Anxiolytics and Sedative/Hypnotics *on page 634*
Discontinuation of Psychotropic Drugs - Withdrawal Symptoms and Recommendations *on page 798*
Mood Disorders *on page 600*
Patient Information - Antidepressants (SSRIs) *on page 639*
Pharmacokinetics of Selective Serotonin-Reuptake Inhibitors (SSRIs) *on page 723*
Special Populations - Elderly *on page 662*

**Generic Available** No

**U.S. Brand Names** Paxil™

**Pharmacologic Category** Antidepressant, Selective Serotonin Reuptake Inhibitor

**Use** Treatment of depression; treatment of panic disorder with or without agoraphobia; obsessive-compulsive disorder; social anxiety disorder (social phobia)

**Unlabeled uses:** May be useful in eating disorders, GAD, premenstrual disorders, impulse control disorders, post-traumatic stress disorder, and vasomotor symptoms of menopause

**Pregnancy Risk Factor** C

**Contraindications** Hypersensitivity to paroxetine; use of MAO inhibitors or within 14 days

**Warnings/Precautions** Potential for severe reaction when used with MAO inhibitors - serotonin syndrome (hyperthermia, muscular rigidity, mental status changes/agitation, autonomic instability) may occur. May precipitate a shift to mania or hypomania in patients with bipolar disease. Has a low potential to impair cognitive or motor performance - caution operating hazardous machinery or driving. Low potential for sedation or anticholinergic effects relative to cyclic antidepressants. Use caution in patients with depression, particularly if suicidal risk may be present. Use caution in patients with a previous seizure disorder or condition predisposing to seizures such as brain damage, alcoholism, or concurrent therapy with other drugs which lower the seizure threshold. Use with caution in patients with hepatic or dysfunction and in elderly patients. May cause hyponatremia/SIADH. Use with caution in patients at risk of bleeding or receiving anticoagulant therapy - may cause impairment in platelet aggregation. Use with caution in patients with renal insufficiency or other concurrent illness (due to limited experience). May cause or exacerbate sexual dysfunction.

**Adverse Reactions**

>10%:
- Central nervous system: Headache, somnolence, dizziness, insomnia
- Gastrointestinal: Nausea, xerostomia, constipation, diarrhea
- Genitourinary: Ejaculatory disturbances
- Neuromuscular & skeletal: Weakness
- Miscellaneous: Diaphoresis

1% to 10%:
- Cardiovascular: Palpitations, vasodilation, postural hypotension
- Central nervous system: Nervousness, anxiety, yawning, abnormal dreams
- Dermatologic: Rash
- Endocrine & metabolic: Decreased libido, delayed ejaculation
- Gastrointestinal: Anorexia, flatulence, vomiting, dyspepsia, taste perversion
- Genitourinary: Urinary frequency, impotence
- Neuromuscular & skeletal: Tremor, paresthesia, myopathy, myalgia

<1%: Acne, akinesia, alopecia, amenorrhea, anemia, arthritis, asthma, bradycardia, bruxism, colitis, ear pain, eye pain, EPS, hypotension, leukopenia, mania, migraine, thirst

**Overdosage/Toxicology**

Signs and symptoms: Nausea, vomiting, drowsiness, sinus tachycardia, and dilated pupils

Treatment: There are no specific antidotes, following attempts at decontamination, treatment is supportive and symptomatic; forced diuresis, dialysis, and hemoperfusion are unlikely to be beneficial

**Drug Interactions** CYP2D6 enzyme substrate (minor); CYP2D6 and 1A2 enzyme inhibitor (weak), and CYP3A3/4 enzyme inhibitor (weak)

Amphetamines: SSRIs may increase the sensitivity to amphetamines, and amphetamines may increase the risk of serotonin syndrome

Buspirone: Combined use with SSRIs may cause serotonin syndrome

Carvedilol: Serum concentrations may be increased; monitor carefully for increased carvedilol effect (hypotension and bradycardia)

Cimetidine: Cimetidine may reduce the first-pass metabolism of paroxetine resulting in elevated paroxetine serum concentrations; consider an alternative $H_2$-antagonist

Clozapine: May increase serum levels of clozapine; monitor for increased effect/toxicity

Cyproheptadine: May inhibit the effects of serotonin reuptake inhibitors; monitor for altered antidepressant response; cyproheptadine acts as a serotonin agonist

Dextromethorphan: Metabolism of dextromethorphan may be inhibited; visual hallucinations occurred; monitor

Haloperidol: Metabolism may be inhibited and cause extrapyramidal symptoms (EPS); monitor patients for EPS if combination is utilized

HMG CoA reductase inhibitors: Metabolism may be inhibited by SSRIs; particularly lovastatin and simvastatin resulting in myositis and rhabdomyolysis; paroxetine appears to have weak interaction with CYP3A3/4, and therefore, appears to have a low risk of this interaction

Lithium: Patients receiving SSRIs and lithium have developed neurotoxicity; if combination is used; monitor for neurotoxicity

Loop diuretics: SSRIs may cause hyponatremia; additive hyponatremic effects may be seen with combined use of a loop diuretic (bumetanide, furosemide, torsemide); monitor for hyponatremia

(Continued)

## Paroxetine *(Continued)*

MAOIs: SSRIs should not be used with nonselective MAOIs (isocarboxazid, phenelzine); fatal reactions have been reported; wait 5 weeks after stopping fluoxetine before starting an MAOI and 2 weeks after stopping an MAOI before starting fluoxetine
Meperidine: Combined use may cause serotonin syndrome; monitor
Nefazodone and trazodone: May increase the risk of serotonin syndrome with SSRIs; monitor
Phenytoin: Metabolism of phenytoin may be inhibited, resulting in phenytoin toxicity; monitor for toxicity (ataxia, confusion, dizziness, nystagmus, involuntary muscle movement)
Selegiline: SSRIs have been reported to cause mania or hypertension when combined with selegiline; this combination is best avoided; concurrent use with SSRIs has also been reported to cause serotonin syndrome; as a MAO-B inhibitor, the risk of serotonin syndrome may be less than with nonselective MAO inhibitors
Serotonin agonists: Theoretically, may increase the risk of serotonin syndrome; includes sumatriptan, naratriptan, rizatriptan, and zolmitriptan
Serotonergic uptake inhibitors: Combined use with other drugs which inhibit the reuptake may cause serotonin syndrome
Sibutramine: May increase the risk of serotonin syndrome with SSRIs; avoid coadministration
Sympathomimetics: May increase the risk of serotonin syndrome with SSRIs
Tramadol: Combined use may cause serotonin syndrome; monitor
Tricyclic antidepressants: The metabolism of tricyclic antidepressants (amitriptyline, desipramine, imipramine, nortriptyline) may be inhibited by SSRIs resulting is elevated serum levels; if combination is warranted, a low dose of TCA (10-25 mg/day) should be utilized
Tryptophan: Combination with tryptophan, a serotonin precursor, may cause agitation and restlessness; this combination is best avoided
Venlafaxine: Sertraline may increase the risk of serotonin syndrome
Warfarin: May alter the hypoprothombinemic response to warfarin; monitor INR
Zolpidem: A case of acute delirium in association with combined therapy has been reported

**Mechanism of Action** Paroxetine is a selective serotonin reuptake inhibitor, chemically unrelated to tricyclic, tetracyclic, or other antidepressants; presumably, the inhibition of serotonin reuptake from brain synapse stimulated serotonin activity in the brain

**Pharmacodynamics/kinetics**
Metabolism: Extensive following absorption by cytochrome P-450 enzymes
Half-life: 21 hours
Elimination: Metabolites are excreted in bile and urine

**Usual Dosage** Adults: Oral:
Depression: 20 mg once daily (maximum: 50 mg/day), preferably in the morning; in elderly, debilitated, or patients with hepatic or renal impairment, start with 10 mg/day (maximum: 40 mg/day); adjust doses at 7-day intervals
Panic disorder and obsessive compulsive disorder: Recommended average daily dose: 40 mg, this dosage should be given after an adequate trial on 20 mg/day and then titrating upward

**Reference Range** Oral doses of 40 mg produced a peak serum level of 26.6 ng/mL

**Test Interactions** ↑ LFTs

**Patient Information** Caution should be used in activities that require alertness like driving or operating machinery; avoid alcoholic beverage intake; notify physician if pregnant or breast feeding

**Nursing Implications** Offer patient sugarless hard candy for dry mouth

**Additional Information** Similar properties to fluvoxamine maleate; buspirone (15-60 mg/day) may be useful in treatment of sexual dysfunction during treatment with a selective serotonin reuptake inhibitor

**Dosage Forms**
Suspension, oral: 10 mg/5 mL
Tablet: 10 mg, 20 mg, 30 mg, 40 mg


- **Partuss® LA** *see* Guaifenesin and Phenylpropanolamine *on page 257*
- **Patanol™** *see* Olopatadine *on page 404*
- **Pathilon®** *see* Tridihexethyl *on page 566*
- **Pathocil®** *see* Dicloxacillin *on page 165*
- **Patient Information - Agents for Treatment of Extrapyramidal Symptoms** *see page 657*
- **Patient Information - Antidepressants (Bupropion)** *see page 641*
- **Patient Information - Antidepressants (MAOIs)** *see page 644*
- **Patient Information - Antidepressants (Mirtazapine)** *see page 645*
- **Patient Information - Antidepressants (Serotonin Blocker)** *see page 643*
- **Patient Information - Antidepressants (SSRIs)** *see page 639*
- **Patient Information - Antidepressants (TCAs)** *see page 640*
- **Patient Information - Antidepressants (Venlafaxine)** *see page 642*
- **Patient Information - Antipsychotics (Clozapine)** *see page 648*
- **Patient Information - Antipsychotics (General)** *see page 646*
- **Patient Information - Anxiolytics & Sedative Hypnotics (Barbiturates)** *see page 654*
- **Patient Information - Anxiolytics & Sedative Hypnotics (Benzodiazepines)** *see page 653*
- **Patient Information - Anxiolytics & Sedative Hypnotics (Buspirone)** *see page 655*
- **Patient Information - Anxiolytics & Sedative Hypnotics (Nonbenzodiazepine Hypnotics)** *see page 656*
- **Patient Information - Mood Stabilizers (Carbamazepine)** *see page 651*
- **Patient Information - Mood Stabilizers (Lithium)** *see page 649*
- **Patient Information - Mood Stabilizers (Valproic Acid)** *see page 650*
- **Patient Information - Stimulants** *see page 652*
- **Pavabid®** *see* Papaverine *on page 419*
- **Pavatine®** *see* Papaverine *on page 419*
- **Pavulon®** *see* Pancuronium *on page 418*
- **Paxene®** *see* Paclitaxel *on page 417*
- **Paxil™** *see* Paroxetine *on page 421*
- **Paxipam®** *see* Halazepam *on page 261*
- **PBZ®** *see* Tripelennamine *on page 572*
- **PBZ-SR®** *see* Tripelennamine *on page 572*
- **PCA** *see* Procainamide *on page 464*
- **PCE® Oral** *see* Erythromycin *on page 200*
- **PCV7** *see* Pneumococcal Conjugate Vaccine, 7-Valent *on page 450*
- **Pectin and Kaolin** *see* Kaolin and Pectin *on page 300*
- **Pedia Care® Oral** *see* Pseudoephedrine *on page 478*
- **Pediacof®** *see* Chlorpheniramine, Phenylephrine, and Codeine *on page 115*
- **Pediapred® Oral** *see* Prednisolone *on page 459*
- **Pediatric ALS Algorithms** *see page 760*
- **Pediatric Triban®** *see* Trimethobenzamide *on page 569*
- **Pediazole®** *see* Erythromycin and Sulfisoxazole *on page 201*
- **Pedi-Boro® [OTC]** *see* Aluminum Sulfate and Calcium Acetate *on page 28*
- **Pedi-Cort V® Creme** *see* Clioquinol and Hydrocortisone *on page 129*
- **PediOtic® Otic** *see* Neomycin, Polymyxin B, and Hydrocortisone *on page 389*
- **Pedituss®** *see* Chlorpheniramine, Phenylephrine, and Codeine *on page 115*
- **PedvaxHIB™** *see Haemophilus* b Conjugate Vaccine *on page 261*


## Pegademase Bovine (peg A de mase BOE vine)

**U.S. Brand Names** Adagen™

**Pharmacologic Category** Enzyme

**Use** Enzyme replacement therapy for adenosine deaminase (ADA) deficiency in patients with severe combined immunodeficiency disease (SCID) who can not benefit from bone marrow transplant; not a cure for SCID, unlike bone marrow transplants, injections must be used the rest of the child's life, therefore is not really an alternative

**Effects on Mental Status** None reported

**Effects on Psychiatric Treatment** None reported

**Usual Dosage** Children: I.M.: Dose given every 7 days, 10 units/kg the first dose, 15 units/kg the second dose, and 20 units/kg the third dose; maintenance dose: 20 units/kg/week is recommended depending on patient's ADA level; maximum single dose: 30 units/kg

**Dosage Forms** Injection: 250 units/mL (1.5 mL)


- **Peganone®** *see* Ethotoin *on page 214*


## Pegaspargase (peg AS par jase)

**U.S. Brand Names** Oncaspar®

**Pharmacologic Category** Antineoplastic Agent, Miscellaneous

**Use** Patients with acute lymphoblastic leukemia (ALL) who require asparaginase in their treatment regimen, but have developed hypersensitivity to the native forms of asparaginase. Use as a single agent should only be undertaken when multiagent chemotherapy is judged to be inappropriate for the patient.

**Effects on Mental Status** Drowsiness is common

**Effects on Psychiatric Treatment** May cause pancytopenia; use caution with clozapine and carbamazepine

**Usual Dosage** Refer to individual protocols; dose must be individualized based upon clinical response and tolerance of the patient

I.M. administration is **preferred** over I.V. administration; I.M. administration may decrease the incidence of hepatotoxicity, coagulopathy, and GI and renal disorders

Children: I.M., I.V.:

Body surface area <0.6 $m^2$: 82.5 international units/kg every 14 days

Body surface area ≥0.6 $m^2$: 2500 international units/$m^2$ every 14 days

Adults: I.M., I.V.: 2500 international units/$m^2$ every 14 days

Hemodialysis: Significant drug removal is unlikely based on physiochemical characteristics

Peritoneal dialysis: Significant drug removal is unlikely based on physiochemical characteristics

**Dosage Forms** Injection, preservative free: 750 units/mL

## Pemirolast (pe MIR oh last)

**U.S. Brand Names** Alamast™

**Pharmacologic Category** Mast Cell Stabilizer; Ophthalmic Agent, Miscellaneous

**Use** Prevent itching of the eye due to allergic conjunctivitis

**Effects on Mental Status** None reported

**Effects on Psychiatric Treatment** None reported

**Usual Dosage** Children >3 years and Adults: 1-2 drops instilled in affected eye(s) 4 times/day

**Dosage Forms** Solution, ophthalmic: 0.1% (10 mL)

## Pemoline (PEM oh leen)

**Related Information**

Clinical Issues in the Use of Stimulants *on page 637*

Patient Information - Stimulants *on page 652*

Stimulant Agents Used for ADHD *on page 728*

**Generic Available** No

**U.S. Brand Names** Cylert®

**Synonyms** Phenylisohydantoin; PIO

**Pharmacologic Category** Stimulant

**Use** Treatment of attention deficit hyperactivity disorder (ADHD) (not first-line)

**Unlabeled use:** Narcolepsy

**Restrictions** C-IV

**Pregnancy Risk Factor** B

**Contraindications** Known hypersensitivity to pemoline or any component; hepatic impairment (including abnormalities on baseline liver function tests); children <6 years of age; Tourette's syndrome

**Warnings/Precautions** Not considered first-line therapy for ADHD due to association with hepatic failure. Signed informed consent following a discussion of risks and benefits must or should be obtained prior to the initiation of therapy. Therapy should be discontinued if a response is not evident after 3 weeks of therapy. Pemoline should not be started in patients with abnormalities in baseline liver function tests, and should be discontinued if clinically significant liver function test abnormalities are revealed at any time during therapy. Use with caution in patients with renal dysfunction or psychosis. In general, stimulant medications should be used with caution in patients with bipolar disorder, diabetes mellitus, cardiovascular disease, seizure disorders, insomnia, porphyria, or hypertension (although pemoline has been demonstrated to have a low potential to elevate blood pressure relative to other stimulants). May exacerbate symptoms of behavior and thought disorder in psychotic patients. Potential for drug dependency exists - avoid abrupt discontinuation in patients who have received for prolonged periods. Stimulant use has been associated with growth suppression, and careful monitoring is recommended.

**Adverse Reactions**

Central nervous system: Insomnia, dizziness, drowsiness, mental depression, increased irritability, seizures, precipitation of Tourette's syndrome, hallucinations, headache, movement disorders

Dermatologic: Rash

Endocrine & metabolic: Suppression of growth in children

Gastrointestinal: Anorexia, weight loss, stomach pain, nausea

Hematologic: Aplastic anemia

Hepatic: Increased liver enzyme (usually reversible upon discontinuation), hepatitis, jaundice, hepatic failure

**Overdosage/Toxicology**

Signs and symptoms: Tachycardia, hallucinations, agitation

Treatment:

There is no specific antidote for intoxication and the bulk of the treatment is supportive

Hyperactivity and agitation usually respond to reduced sensory input or benzodiazepines, however, with extreme agitation haloperidol (2-5 mg I.M. for adults) may be required

Hyperthermia is best treated with external cooling measures, or when severe or unresponsive, muscle paralysis with pancuronium may be needed

**Drug Interactions**

Anticonvulsants: Pemoline may decrease seizure threshold; efficacy of anticonvulsants may be decreased

CNS depressants: Effects may be additive; use caution when pemoline is used with other CNS acting medications

**Mechanism of Action** Blocks the reuptake mechanism of dopaminergic neurons, appears to act at the cerebral cortex and subcortical structures; CNS and respiratory stimulant with weak sympathomimetic effects; actions may be mediated via increase in CNS dopamine

**Pharmacodynamics/kinetics**

Peak effect: 4 hours

Duration: 8 hours

Protein binding: 50%

Metabolism: Partially by the liver

Half-life:

Children: 7-8.6 hours

Adults: 12 hours

Time to peak serum concentration: Oral: Within 2-4 hours

Elimination: In urine; only negligible amounts can be detected in feces

**Usual Dosage** Children ≥6 years: Oral: Initial: 37.5 mg given once daily in the morning, increase by 18.75 mg/day at weekly intervals; usual effective dose range: 56.25-75 mg/day; maximum: 112.5 mg/day; dosage range: 0.5-3 mg/kg/24 hours; significant benefit may not be evident until third or fourth week of administration

**Dosing adjustment/comments in renal impairment:** $Cl_{cr}$ <50 mL/minute: Avoid use

**Dietary Considerations** Alcohol: Additive CNS effect, avoid use

**Monitoring Parameters** Baseline liver enzymes and every 2 weeks thereafter; the labeling for Cylert® has been revised to provide updated recommendations for liver function monitoring and a Patient Information Consent Form

**Reference Range** Therapeutic plasma range: 1-7 μg/mL

**Patient Information** Avoid caffeine; avoid alcoholic beverages; last daily dose should be given several hours before retiring; do not abruptly discontinue; prolonged use may cause dependence

**Nursing Implications** Give medication in the morning

**Additional Information** Treatment of ADHD should include "Drug Holidays" or periodic discontinuation of stimulant medication in order to assess the patient's requirements and to decrease tolerance and limit suppression of linear growth and weight

**Dosage Forms**

Tablet: 18.75 mg, 37.5 mg, 75 mg

Tablet, chewable: 37.5 mg

## Penbutolol (pen BYOO toe lole)

**Related Information**

Beta-Blockers Comparison Chart *on page 709*

**U.S. Brand Names** Levatol®

**Pharmacologic Category** Beta Blocker (with Intrinsic Sympathomimetic Activity)

**Use** Treatment of mild to moderate arterial hypertension

**Effects on Mental Status** May cause dizziness or depression; may rarely cause insomnia, confusion, or nightmares

**Effects on Psychiatric Treatment** Concurrent use with phenothiazines may potentiate hypotensive effects of penbutolol

**Contraindications** Hypersensitivity to penbutolol; uncompensated congestive heart failure; cardiogenic shock; bradycardia or heart block (except in patients with a functioning artificial pacemaker); sinus node dysfunction; asthma; bronchospastic disease; COPD; pulmonary edema; pregnancy (2nd and 3rd trimester)

**Warnings/Precautions** Avoid abrupt discontinuation in patients with a history of CAD; slowly wean while monitoring for signs and symptoms of ischemia. Use caution with concurrent use of beta-blockers and either verapamil or diltiazem; bradycardia or heart block can occur. Use caution in patients with PVD (can aggravate arterial insufficiency). Use cautiously in diabetics because it can mask prominent hypoglycemic symptoms. Can mask signs of thyrotoxicosis. Can cause fetal harm when administered in pregnancy. Use cautiously in the renally impaired (dosage adjustment required). Use care with anesthetic agents which decrease myocardial function. Beta-blockers with intrinsic sympathomimetic activity (including penbutolol) do not appear to be of benefit in congestive heart failure.

**Adverse Reactions** 1% to 10%:

Cardiovascular: Congestive heart failure, arrhythmias

Central nervous system: Mental depression, headache, dizziness

Neuromuscular & skeletal: Back pain, arthralgia

(Continued)

## Penbutolol *(Continued)*

**Overdosage/Toxicology** Treatment: Sympathomimetics (eg, epinephrine or dopamine), glucagon, or a pacemaker can be used to treat toxic bradycardia, asystole, and/or hypotension; initially fluids may be the best treatment for toxic hypotension; patients should remain supine; serum glucose and potassium should be measured; use supportive measures: lavage, syrup of ipecac. I.V. glucose should be administered for hypoglycemia; seizures may be treated with phenytoin or diazepam intravenously; continuous monitoring of blood pressure and EKG is necessary. If PVCs occur, treat with lidocaine or phenytoin; avoid quinidine, procainamide, and disopyramide since these agents further depress myocardial function; bronchospasm can be treated with theophylline or $beta_2$ agonists (epinephrine).

**Drug Interactions**

Albuterol (and other $beta_2$ agonists): Effects may be blunted by nonspecific beta-blockers

Alpha-blockers (prazosin, terazosin): Concurrent use of beta-blockers may increase risk of orthostasis

Clonidine: Hypertensive crisis after or during withdrawal of either agent

Drugs which slow AV conduction (digoxin): Effects may be additive with beta-blockers

Epinephrine (including local anesthetics with epinephrine): Penbutolol may cause hypertension

Glucagon: Penbutolol may blunt the hyperglycemic action

Insulin and oral hypoglycemics: May mask symptoms of hypoglycemia

NSAIDs (ibuprofen, indomethacin, naproxen, piroxicam) may reduce the antihypertensive effects of beta-blockers

Penbutolol masks the tachycardia that usually accompanies insulin-induced hypoglycemia

Salicylates may reduce the antihypertensive effects of beta-blockers

Sulfonylureas: beta-blockers may alter response to hypoglycemic agents

Verapamil or diltiazem may have synergistic or additive pharmacological effects when taken concurrently with beta-blockers

**Usual Dosage** Adults: Oral: Initial: 20 mg once daily, full effect of a 20 or 40 mg dose is seen by the end of a 2-week period, doses of 40-80 mg have been tolerated but have shown little additional antihypertensive effects

**Patient Information** Take exactly as directed. Do not increase, decrease, or adjust dosage without consulting prescriber. Take pulse daily, prior to medication and follow prescriber's instruction about holding medication. Do not take with antacids. Do not use alcohol or OTC medications (eg, cold remedies) without consulting prescriber. If diabetic, monitor serum sugars closely (may alter glucose tolerance or mask signs of hypoglycemia). May cause fatigue, dizziness, or postural hypotension; use caution when changing position from lying or sitting to standing, when driving, or when climbing stairs until response to medication is known. May cause alteration in sexual performance (reversible). Report unresolved swelling of extremities, difficulty breathing or new cough, unresolved fatigue, unusual weight gain, unresolved constipation, or unusual muscle weakness.

**Dosage Forms** Tablet, as sulfate: 20 mg

## Penciclovir (pen SYE kloe veer)

**U.S. Brand Names** Denavir™

**Pharmacologic Category** Antiviral Agent

**Use** Topical treatment of herpes simplex labialis (cold sores); potentially used for Epstein-Barr virus infections

**Effects on Mental Status** None reported

**Effects on Psychiatric Treatment** None reported

**Usual Dosage** Apply cream at the first sign or symptom of cold sore (eg, tingling, swelling); apply every 2 hours during waking hours for 4 days

**Dosage Forms** Cream: 1% [10 mg/g] (2 g)

♦ **Penecort®** *see* Hydrocortisone *on page 273*

♦ **Penetrex™** *see* Enoxacin *on page 193*

## Penicillamine (pen i SIL a meen)

**U.S. Brand Names** Cuprimine®; Depen®

**Synonyms** D-3-Mercaptovaline; β,β-Dimethylcysteine; D-Penicillamine

**Pharmacologic Category** Chelating Agent

**Use** Treatment of Wilson's disease, cystinuria, adjunct in the treatment of rheumatoid arthritis; lead, mercury, copper, and possibly gold poisoning. (**Note:** Oral DMSA is preferable for lead or mercury poisoning); primary biliary cirrhosis; as adjunctive therapy following initial treatment with calcium EDTA or BAL

**Effects on Mental Status** May cause drowsiness

**Effects on Psychiatric Treatment** May cause aplastic anemia; use caution with clozapine and carbamazepine

**Pregnancy Risk Factor** D

**Contraindications** Hypersensitivity to penicillamine or components; renal insufficiency; patients with previous penicillamine-related aplastic anemia or agranulocytosis; concomitant administration with other hematopoietic-depressant drugs (eg, gold, immunosuppressants, antimalarials, phenylbutazone)

**Warnings/Precautions** Cross-sensitivity with penicillin is possible; therefore, should be used cautiously in patients with a history of penicillin allergy. Patients on penicillamine for Wilson's disease or cystinuria should receive pyridoxine supplementation 25 mg/day; once instituted for Wilson's disease or cystinuria, continue treatment on a daily basis; interruptions of even a few days have been followed by hypersensitivity with reinstitution of therapy. Penicillamine has been associated with fatalities due to agranulocytosis, aplastic anemia, thrombocytopenia, Goodpasture's syndrome, and myasthenia gravis; patients should be warned to report promptly any symptoms suggesting toxicity; approximately 33% of patients will experience an allergic reaction; since toxicity may be dose related, it is recommended not to exceed 750 mg/day in elderly.

**Adverse Reactions**

>10%:

Dermatologic: Rash, urticaria, itching (44% to 50%)

Gastrointestinal: Hypogeusia (25% to 33%)

Neuromuscular & skeletal: Arthralgia

1% to 10%:

Cardiovascular: Edema of the face, feet, or lower legs

Central nervous system: Fever, chills

Gastrointestinal: Weight gain, sore throat

Genitourinary: Bloody or cloudy urine

Hematologic: Aplastic or hemolytic anemia, leukopenia (2%), thrombocytopenia (4%)

Miscellaneous: White spots on lips or mouth, positive ANA

<1%: Allergic reactions, anorexia, cholestatic jaundice, coughing, fatigue, hepatitis, increased friability of the skin, iron deficiency, lymphadenopathy, myasthenia gravis syndrome, nausea, nephrotic syndrome, optic neuritis, pancreatitis, pemphigus, SLE-like syndrome, spitting of blood, tinnitus, toxic epidermal necrolysis, vomiting, weakness, wheezing

**Overdosage/Toxicology**

Signs and symptoms: Nausea and vomiting

Treatment: Following GI decontamination, treatment is supportive

**Drug Interactions**

Decreased effect with iron and zinc salts, antacids (magnesium, calcium, aluminum) and food

Decreased effect/levels of digoxin

Increased effect of gold, antimalarials, immunosuppressants, phenylbutazone (hematologic, renal toxicity)

**Usual Dosage** Oral:

Rheumatoid arthritis:

Children: Initial: 3 mg/kg/day (≤250 mg/day) for 3 months, then 6 mg/kg/day (≤500 mg/day) in divided doses twice daily for 3 months to a maximum of 10 mg/kg/day in 3-4 divided doses

Adults: 125-250 mg/day, may increase dose at 1- to 3-month intervals up to 1-1.5 g/day

Wilson's disease (doses titrated to maintain urinary copper excretion >1 mg/day):

Infants <6 months: 250 mg/dose once daily

Children <12 years: 250 mg/dose 2-3 times/day

Adults: 250 mg 4 times/day

Cystinuria:

Children: 30 mg/kg/day in 4 divided doses

Adults: 1-4 g/day in divided doses every 6 hours

Lead poisoning (continue until blood lead level is <60 μg/dL): Children and Adults: 25-35 mg/kg/d, administered in 3-4 divided doses; initiating treatment at 25% of this dose and gradually increasing to the full dose over 2-3 weeks may minimize adverse reactions

Primary biliary cirrhosis: 250 mg/day to start, increase by 250 mg every 2 weeks up to a maintenance dose of 1 g/day, usually given 250 mg 4 times/day

Arsenic poisoning: Children: 100 mg/kg/day in divided doses every 6 hours for 5 days; maximum: 1 g/day

**Dosing adjustment/comments in renal impairment:** $Cl_{cr}$ <50 mL/minute: Avoid use

**Patient Information** Take this medication exactly as directed; do not increase dose without consulting prescriber. Capsules may be opened and contents mixed in 15-30 mL of chilled fruit juice or puree; do not take with milk or milk products. Avoid alcohol or excess intake of vitamin A. It is preferable to take penicillamine on empty stomach (1 hour before or 2 hours after meals). Maintain adequate hydration (2-3 L/day of fluids unless instructed to restrict fluid intake).

Wilson's disease: Avoid chocolate, shellfish, nuts, mushrooms, liver, broccoli, molasses.

Lead poisoning: Decrease dietary calcium.

Cystinuria: Take with large amounts of water.

You may experience anorexia, nausea, vomiting (frequent small meals, frequent mouth care, sucking lozenges, or chewing gum may help). Report persistent fever or chills, unhealed sores, white spots or sores in mouth or vaginal area, extreme fatigue, or signs of infection; breathlessness, difficulty breathing, or unusual cough; unusual bruising/bleeding; blood in urine, stool, mouth, or vomitus; swollen face or extremities; skin rash or itching; muscle pain or cramping; or pain on urination.

**Nursing Implications** For patients who cannot swallow, contents of capsules may be administered in 15-30 mL of chilled puréed fruit or fruit juice; patients should be warned to report promptly any symptoms suggesting toxicity

**Dosage Forms**

Capsule: 125 mg, 250 mg

Tablet: 250 mg

## Penicillin G Benzathine (pen i SIL in jee BENZ a theen)

**U.S. Brand Names** Bicillin® L-A; Permapen®

**Canadian Brand Names** Megacillin® Susp

**Synonyms** Benzathine Benzylpenicillin; Benzathine Penicillin G; Benzylpenicillin Benzathine

**Pharmacologic Category** Antibiotic, Penicillin

**Use** Active against some gram-positive organisms, few gram-negative organisms such as *Neisseria gonorrhoeae*, and some anaerobes and spirochetes; used in the treatment of syphilis; used only for the treatment of mild to moderately severe infections caused by organisms susceptible to low concentrations of penicillin G or for prophylaxis of infections caused by these organisms

**Effects on Mental Status** May rarely cause drowsiness or confusion; penicillins reported to cause apprehension, illusions, hallucinations, depersonalization, agitation, insomnia, and encephalopathy

**Effects on Psychiatric Treatment** None reported

**Pregnancy Risk Factor** B

**Contraindications** Known hypersensitivity to penicillin or any component

**Warnings/Precautions** Use with caution in patients with impaired renal function, seizure disorder, or history of hypersensitivity to other beta-lactams; CDC and AAP do not currently recommend the use of penicillin G benzathine to treat congenital syphilis or neurosyphilis due to reported treatment failures and lack of published clinical data on its efficacy

**Adverse Reactions**

1% to 10%: Local: Pain

<1%: Acute interstitial nephritis, anaphylaxis, confusion, convulsions, drowsiness, electrolyte imbalance, fever, hemolytic anemia, hypersensitivity reactions, Jarisch-Herxheimer reaction, myoclonus, positive Coombs' reaction, rash, thrombophlebitis

**Overdosage/Toxicology**

Signs and symptoms: Neuromuscular hypersensitivity (agitation, hallucinations, asterixis, encephalopathy, confusion, and seizures) and electrolyte imbalance with potassium or sodium salts, especially in renal failure

Treatment: Hemodialysis may be helpful to aid in the removal of the drug from the blood, otherwise most treatment is supportive or symptom directed

**Drug Interactions**

Decreased effect: Tetracyclines may decrease penicillin effectiveness; decreased oral contraceptive effect is possible

Increased effect:

Probenecid may increase penicillin levels

Aminoglycosides → synergistic efficacy; heparin and parenteral penicillins may result in increased bleeding

**Usual Dosage** I.M.: Administer undiluted injection; higher doses result in more sustained rather than higher levels. Use a penicillin G benzathine-penicillin G procaine combination to achieve early peak levels in acute infections.

Infants and Children:

Group A streptococcal upper respiratory infection: 25,000-50,000 units/kg as a single dose; maximum: 1.2 million units

Prophylaxis of recurrent rheumatic fever: 25,000-50,000 units/kg every 3-4 weeks; maximum: 1.2 million units/dose

Early syphilis: 50,000 units/kg as a single injection; maximum: 2.4 million units

Syphilis of more than 1-year duration: 50,000 units/kg every week for 3 doses; maximum: 2.4 million units/dose

Adults:

Group A streptococcal upper respiratory infection: 1.2 million units as a single dose

Prophylaxis of recurrent rheumatic fever: 1.2 million units every 3-4 weeks or 600,000 units twice monthly

Early syphilis: 2.4 million units as a single dose in 2 injection sites

Syphilis of more than 1-year duration: 2.4 million units in 2 injection sites once weekly for 3 doses

Not indicated as single drug therapy for neurosyphilis, but may be given 1 time/week for 3 weeks following I.V. treatment (refer to Penicillin G monograph for dosing)

**Patient Information** Take as directed, for full course of therapy. Maintain adequate hydration (2-3 L/day of fluids unless instructed to restrict fluid intake). If begin treated for sexually transmitted disease, partner will also need to be treated. Small frequent meals, frequent mouth care, sucking lozenges, or chewing gum may reduce nausea or dry mouth. Important to maintain good oral and vaginal hygiene to reduce incidence of opportunistic infection. If diabetic, drug may cause false tests with Clinitest® urine glucose monitoring; use of glucose oxidase methods (Clinistix®) or serum glucose monitoring is preferable. This drug may interfere with oral contraceptives; an alternate form of birth control should be used. Report persistent diarrhea, fever, chills, unhealed sores, bloody urine or stool, muscle pain, mouth sores, or difficulty breathing.

**Dosage Forms** Injection: 300,000 units/mL (10 mL); 600,000 units/mL (1 mL, 2 mL, 4 mL)

## Penicillin G Benzathine and Procaine Combined

(pen i SIL in jee BENZ a theen & PROE kane KOM bined)

**U.S. Brand Names** Bicillin® C-R 900/300 Injection; Bicillin® C-R Injection

**Pharmacologic Category** Antibiotic, Penicillin

**Use** May be used in specific situations in the treatment of streptococcal infections

**Effects on Mental Status** May rarely cause drowsiness or confusion

**Effects on Psychiatric Treatment** None reported

**Usual Dosage** I.M.:

Children:

<30 lb: 600,000 units in a single dose

30-60 lb: 900,000 units to 1.2 million units in a single dose

Children >60 lb and Adults: 2.4 million units in a single dose

**Dosage Forms**

Injection:

300,000 units [150,000 units each of penicillin g benzathine and penicillin g procaine] (10 mL)

600,000 units [300,000 units each penicillin g benzathine and penicillin g procaine] (1 mL)

1,200,000 units [600,000 units each penicillin g benzathine and penicillin g procaine] (2 mL)

2,400,000 units [1,200,000 units each penicillin g benzathine and penicillin g procaine] (4 mL)

Injection: Penicillin g benzathine 900,000 units and penicillin g procaine 300,000 units per dose (2 mL)

## Penicillin G, Parenteral, Aqueous

(pen i SIL in jee, pa REN ter al, AYE kwee us)

**U.S. Brand Names** Pfizerpen®

**Pharmacologic Category** Antibiotic, Penicillin

**Use** Active against some gram-positive organisms, generally not *Staphylococcus aureus*; some gram-negative organisms such as *Neisseria gonorrhoeae*, and some anaerobes and spirochetes

**Effects on Mental Status** May rarely cause drowsiness or confusion

**Effects on Psychiatric Treatment** None reported

**Usual Dosage** I.M., I.V.:

Infants:

>7 days, >2000 g: 100,000 units/kg/day in divided doses every 6 hours

>7 days, <2000 g: 75,000 units/kg/day in divided doses every 8 hours

<7 days, >2000 g: 50,000 units/kg/day in divided doses every 8 hours

<7 days, <2000 g: 50,000 units/kg/day in divided doses every 12 hours

Infants and Children (sodium salt is preferred in children): 100,000-250,000 units/kg/day in divided doses every 4 hours

Severe infections: Up to 400,000 units/kg/day in divided doses every 4 hours; maximum dose: 24 million units/day

Adults: 2-24 million units/day in divided doses every 4 hours depending on sensitivity of the organism and severity of the infection

Congenital syphilis:

Newborns: 50,000 units/kg/day I.V. every 8-12 hours for 10-14 days

Infants: 50,000 units/kg every 4-6 hours for 10-14 days

Disseminated gonococcal infections or gonococcus ophthalmia (if organism proven sensitive): 100,000 units/kg/day in 2 equal doses (4 equal doses/day for infants >1 week)

Gonococcal meningitis: 150,000 units/kg in 2 equal doses (4 doses/day for infants >1 week)

**Dosing interval in renal impairment:**

$Cl_{cr}$ 30-50 mL/minute: Administer every 6 hours

$Cl_{cr}$ 10-30 mL/minute: Administer every 8 hours

$Cl_{cr}$ <10 mL/minute: Administer every 12 hours

Hemodialysis: Moderately dialyzable (20% to 50%)

Continuous arteriovenous or venovenous hemodiafiltration (CAVH) effects: Dose as for $Cl_{cr}$ 10-50 mL/minute

**Dosage Forms**

Penicillin G potassium:

Injection, as sodium: 5 million units

Injection:

Frozen premixed, as potassium: 1 million units, 2 million units, 3 million units

Powder, as potassium: 1 million units, 5 million units, 10 million units, 20 million units

## Penicillin G Procaine (pen i SIL in jee PROE kane)

**U.S. Brand Names** Crysticillin® A.S.; Wycillin®

**Canadian Brand Names** Ayercillin®

(Continued)

## Penicillin G Procaine *(Continued)*

**Pharmacologic Category** Antibiotic, Penicillin

**Use** Moderately severe infections due to *Treponema pallidum* and other penicillin G-sensitive microorganisms that are susceptible to low but prolonged serum penicillin concentrations

**Effects on Mental Status** May rarely cause drowsiness, confusion, or CNS stimulation

**Effects on Psychiatric Treatment** None reported

**Usual Dosage** I.M.:

Children: 25,000-50,000 units/kg/day in divided doses 1-2 times/day; not to exceed 4.8 million units/24 hours

Congenital syphilis: 50,000 units/kg/day for 10-14 days

Adults: 0.6-4.8 million units/day in divided doses every 12-24 hours

Endocarditis caused by susceptible viridans *Streptococcus* (when used in conjunction with an aminoglycoside): 1.2 million units every 6 hours for 2-4 weeks

Neurosyphilis: I.M.: 2-4 million units/day with 500 mg probenecid by mouth 4 times/day for 10-14 days; **penicillin G aqueous I.V. is the preferred agent**

Hemodialysis: Moderately dialyzable (20% to 50%)

**Dosage Forms** Injection, suspension: 300,000 units/mL (10 mL); 500,000 units/mL (1.2 mL); 600,000 units/mL (1 mL, 2 mL, 4 mL)

## Penicillin V Potassium (pen i SIL in vee poe TASS ee um)

**U.S. Brand Names** Beepen-VK®; Betapen®-VK; Pen.Vee® K; Robicillin® VK; Veetids®

**Canadian Brand Names** Apo®-Pen VK; Nadopen-V®; Novo-Pen-VK®; Nu-Pen-VK; PVF® K

**Synonyms** Pen VK; Phenoxymethyl Penicillin

**Pharmacologic Category** Antibiotic, Penicillin

**Use** Treatment of infections caused by susceptible organisms involving the respiratory tract, otitis media, sinusitis, skin, and urinary tract; prophylaxis in rheumatic fever

**Effects on Mental Status** Penicillins reported to cause apprehension, illusions, hallucinations, depersonalization, agitation, insomnia, and encephalopathy

**Effects on Psychiatric Treatment** None reported

**Pregnancy Risk Factor** B

**Contraindications** Known hypersensitivity to penicillin or any component

**Warnings/Precautions** Use with caution in patients with severe renal impairment (modify dosage), history of seizures, or hypersensitivity to cephalosporins

**Adverse Reactions**

>10%: Gastrointestinal: Mild diarrhea, vomiting, nausea, oral candidiasis

<1%: Acute interstitial nephritis, anaphylaxis, convulsions, fever, hemolytic anemia, hypersensitivity reactions, positive Coombs' reaction

**Overdosage/Toxicology**

Signs and symptoms: Neuromuscular hypersensitivity (agitation, hallucinations, asterixis, encephalopathy, confusion, and seizures) and electrolyte imbalance with potassium or sodium salts, especially in renal failure

Treatment: Hemodialysis may be helpful to aid in the removal of the drug from the blood, otherwise most treatment is supportive or symptom directed

**Drug Interactions**

Decreased effect: Tetracyclines may decrease penicillin effectiveness; decreased oral contraceptive effect is possible

Increased effect:

Aminoglycosides may result in synergistic efficacy; heparin and parenteral penicillins may result in increased bleeding

Probenecid may increase penicillin levels

**Usual Dosage** Oral:

Systemic infections:

Children <12 years: 25-50 mg/kg/day in divided doses every 6-8 hours; maximum dose: 3 g/day

Children ≥12 years and Adults: 125-500 mg every 6-8 hours

Prophylaxis of pneumococcal infections:

Children <5 years: 125 mg twice daily

Children ≥5 years and Adults: 250 mg twice daily

Prophylaxis of recurrent rheumatic fever:

Children <5 years: 125 mg twice daily

Children ≥5 years and Adults: 250 mg twice daily

**Dosing interval in renal impairment:** $Cl_{cr}$ <10 mL/minute: Administer 250 mg every 6 hours

**Dietary Considerations** Food: Decreases drug absorption rate; decreases drug serum concentration. Take on an empty stomach 1 hour before or 2 hours after meals.

**Patient Information** Take at regular intervals around-the-clock, preferably on an empty stomach (1 hour before or 2 hours after meals) with 8 oz of water. Take entire prescription; do not skip doses or discontinue without consulting prescriber. Small frequent meals, frequent mouth care, sucking lozenges, or chewing gum may reduce nausea or dry mouth. Important to maintain good oral and vaginal hygiene to reduce incidence of opportunistic infection. If diabetic, drug may cause false tests with Clinitest® urine glucose monitoring; use of glucose oxidase methods (Clinistix®) or serum glucose monitoring is preferable. This drug may interfere with oral contraceptives; an alternate form of birth control should be used. Report persistent diarrhea, fever, chills, unhealed sores, bloody urine or stool, muscle pain, mouth sores, and difficulty breathing.

**Dosage Forms** 250 mg = 400,000 units

Powder for oral solution: 125 mg/5 mL (3 mL, 100 mL, 150 mL, 200 mL); 250 mg/5 mL (100 mL, 150 mL, 200 mL)

Tablet: 125 mg, 250 mg, 500 mg

## Pennyroyal Oil

**Synonyms** *Mentha pulegium*

**Pharmacologic Category** Herb

**Use** Insect repellent; inducing delayed menses; rubefacient; its used primarily by natural health advocates (not FDA approved for stated use); digestive disorders; liver and gallbladder disorders; gout; colds; skin diseases (used externally)

**Adverse Reactions**

Cardiovascular: Hypotension

Central nervous system: Confusion, delirium, agitation, hallucinations (auditory and visual), seizures (within 3 hours)

Endocrine & metabolic: Abortifacient

Gastrointestinal: Nausea, vomiting, abdominal pain

Genitourinary: Menstrual bleeding

Hematologic: Hemolytic anemia, disseminated intravascular coagulation

Hepatic: Hepatic failure, centrilobular necrosis

Renal: Renal failure, hematuria, acute tubular necrosis

Respiratory: Epistaxis

**Overdosage/Toxicology**

Decontamination: Due to aspiration risk, do **not** induce emesis; lavage (within 1 hour) is recommended; activated charcoal (with cathartic) may be useful

Treatment: Supportive therapy; N-acetylcysteine (loading dose: 140 mg/kg, then 70 mg/kg every 4 hours) should be administered within the first few hours postingestion for ingestions >10 mL; benzodiazepines can be used for seizures

**Usual Dosage**

Oil dose used for above purposes: 0.12-0.6 mL

Fatal dose: 15 mL

**Additional Information** Not reviewed by Commission E; mint-like odor; pulegone may deplete glutathione stores in the liver; a yellow oil; hepatotoxicity has occurred after drinking teas from the herb; should not be taken internally; postmortem pulegone and menthofuran levels in a fatality were 18 ng/mL and 1 ng/mL respectively; a menthofuran level of 40 ng/mL obtained 10 hours postingestion associated with mild toxicity

♦ **Pentacarinat® Injection** *see* Pentamidine *on page 427*

## Pentaerythritol Tetranitrate
(pen ta er ITH ri tole te tra NYE trate)

**U.S. Brand Names** Duotrate®; Peritrate®; Peritrate® SA

**Synonyms** PETN

**Pharmacologic Category** Vasodilator

**Use** Possibly effective for the prophylactic long-term management of angina pectoris. **Note:** Not indicated to abort acute anginal episodes.

**Effects on Mental Status** May cause drowsiness

**Effects on Psychiatric Treatment** None reported

**Contraindications** Hypersensitivity to pentaerythritol tetranitrate or other nitrates; severe anemia; angle-closure glaucoma; postural hypotension; cerebral hemorrhage; head trauma

**Warnings/Precautions** Use with caution in patients with hypotension, hypovolemia, or increased intracranial pressure.

**Adverse Reactions**

>10%:

Cardiovascular: Flushing, postural hypotension

Central nervous system: Headache, lightheadedness, dizziness

Neuromuscular & skeletal: Weakness

1% to 10%: Dermatologic: Drug rash, exfoliative dermatitis

**Overdosage/Toxicology**

Signs and symptoms: Hypotension, throbbing headache, palpitations, bloody diarrhea, bradycardia, cyanosis, tissue hypoxia, metabolic acidosis, clonic convulsions, circulatory collapse; formation of methemoglobinemia is dose-related and unusual in normal doses; high levels can cause signs and symptoms of hypoxemia

Treatment: Supportive and symptomatic; keep patient recumbent; elevate legs if needed; hypotension is treated with fluids and alpha-adrenergic pressors if needed

**Drug Interactions**

Alcohol (increased hypotension)

Aspirin (increases serum nitrate concentration)

Calcium channel blockers (increases hypotension)

Heparin's anticoagulant effect may be antagonized

Sildenafil: May cause severe hypotension; use is contraindicated.

**Usual Dosage** Adults: Oral: 10-20 mg 4 times/day up to 40 mg 4 times/day before or after meals and at bedtime; sustained release preparation 80 mg twice daily; use lowest recommended doses in elderly initially; titrations up to 240 mg/day are tolerated, however, headache may occur with increasing doses (reduce dose for a few days; if headache returns or is persistent, an analgesic can be used to treat symptoms)

**Patient Information** Keep tablets in original tightly closed container; do not chew or crush sustained release product

**Dosage Forms**

Capsule: sustained release: 15 mg, 30 mg

Tablet: 10 mg, 20 mg, 40 mg

Tablet, sustained release: 80 mg

- **Pentam-300® Injection** *see* Pentamidine *on page 427*

## Pentamidine (pen TAM i deen)

**U.S. Brand Names** NebuPent™ Inhalation; Pentacarinat® Injection; Pentam-300® Injection

**Synonyms** Pentamidine Isethionate

**Pharmacologic Category** Antibiotic, Miscellaneous

**Use** Treatment and prevention of pneumonia caused by *Pneumocystis carinii*; treatment of trypanosomiasis and visceral leishmaniasis

**Effects on Mental Status** Sedation and dizziness are common; may cause confusion or hallucinations

**Effects on Psychiatric Treatment** May cause leukopenia; use caution with clozapine and carbamazepine

**Pregnancy Risk Factor** C

**Contraindications** Hypersensitivity to pentamidine isethionate or any component (inhalation and injection)

**Warnings/Precautions** Use with caution in patients with diabetes mellitus, renal or hepatic dysfunction; hypertension or hypotension; leukopenia, thrombocytopenia, asthma, hypo/hyperglycemia

**Adverse Reactions** Injection (I); Aerosol (A)

>10%:

Cardiovascular: Chest pain (A - 10% to 23%)

Central nervous system: Fatigue (A - 50% to 70%); dizziness (A - 31% to 47%)

Dermatologic: Rash (31% to 47%)

Endocrine & metabolic: Hyperkalemia

Gastrointestinal: Anorexia (A - 50% to 70%), nausea (A - 10% to 23%)

Local: Local reactions at injection site

Renal: Increased creatinine (I - 23%)

Respiratory: Wheezing (A - 10% to 23%), dyspnea (A - 50% to 70%), coughing (A - 31% to 47%), pharyngitis (10% to 23%)

1% to 10%:

Cardiovascular: Hypotension (I - 4%)

Central nervous system: Confusion/hallucinations (1% to 2%), headache (A - 1% to 5%)

Dermatologic: Rash (I - 3.3%)

Endocrine & metabolic: Hypoglycemia <25 mg/dL (I - 2.4%)

Gastrointestinal: Nausea/anorexia (I - 6%), diarrhea (A - 1% to 5%), vomiting

Hematologic: Severe leukopenia (I - 2.8%), thrombocytopenia <20,000/mm$^3$ (I - 1.7%), anemia (A - 1% to 5%)

Hepatic: Increased LFTs (I - 8.7%)

<1%: Arrhythmias, dizziness (I), extrapulmonary pneumocystosis, fatigue (I), fever, granulocytopenia, hyperglycemia or hypoglycemia, hypocalcemia, hypotension <60 mm Hg systolic (I - 0.9%), irritation of the airway, Jarisch-Herxheimer-like reaction, leukopenia, megaloblastic anemia, mild renal or hepatic injury, pancreatitis, pneumothorax, renal insufficiency, tachycardia

**Overdosage/Toxicology**

Signs and symptoms: Hypotension, hypoglycemia, cardiac arrhythmias

Treatment: Supportive

**Drug Interactions** CYP2C19 enzyme substrate

**Usual Dosage**

Children:

Treatment: I.M., I.V. (I.V. preferred): 4 mg/kg/day once daily for 10-14 days

Prevention:

I.M., I.V.: 4 mg/kg monthly or every 2 weeks

Inhalation (aerosolized pentamidine in children ≥5 years): 300 mg/dose given every 3-4 weeks via Respirgard® II inhaler (8 mg/kg dose has also been used in children <5 years)

Treatment of trypanosomiasis: I.V.: 4 mg/kg/day once daily for 10 days

Adults:

Treatment: I.M., I.V. (I.V. preferred): 4 mg/kg/day once daily for 14-21 days

Prevention: Inhalation: 300 mg every 4 weeks via Respirgard® II nebulizer

Dialysis: Not removed by hemo or peritoneal dialysis or continuous arterio-venous or venovenous hemofiltration (CAVH/CAVHD); supplemental dosage is not necessary

**Dosing adjustment in renal impairment:** Adults: I.V.:

$Cl_{cr}$ 10-50 mL/minute: Administer 4 mg/kg every 24-36 hours

$Cl_{cr}$ <10 mL/minute: Administer 4 mg/kg every 48 hours

**Patient Information** I.V. or I.M. preparations must be given every day. For inhalant use as directed. Prepare solution and nebulizer as directed. Protect medication from light. You will be required to have frequent laboratory tests and blood pressure monitoring while taking this drug. PCP pneumonia may still occur despite pentamidine use. Maintain adequate hydration (2-3 L/day of fluids unless instructed to restrict fluid intake). Frequent mouth care or sucking on lozenges may relieve the metallic taste. Diabetics should check glucose levels frequently. You may experience dizziness or weakness with posture changes; rise or change position slowly. Report unusual confusion or hallucinations, chest pain, unusual bleeding, or rash.

**Nursing Implications** Virtually indetectable amounts are transferred to healthcare personnel during aerosol administration; **do not use NS as a diluent**

**Dosage Forms**

Inhalation, as isethionate: 300 mg

Powder for injection, as isethionate, lyophilized: 300 mg

- **Pentamidine Isethionate** *see* Pentamidine *on page 427*
- **Pentasa® Oral** *see* Mesalamine *on page 344*

## Pentazocine (pen TAZ oh seen)

**Related Information**

Narcotic Agonists Comparison Chart *on page 720*

**U.S. Brand Names** Talwin®; Talwin® NX

**Synonyms** Pentazocine Hydrochloride; Pentazocine Lactate

**Pharmacologic Category** Analgesic, Narcotic

**Use** Relief of moderate to severe pain; has also been used as a sedative prior to surgery and as a supplement to surgical anesthesia

**Effects on Mental Status** Drowsiness and euphoria are common; may cause restlessness or nightmares; may rarely cause confusion, depression, or hallucinations

**Effects on Psychiatric Treatment** Concurrent use with psychotropics may produce additive effects or toxicity; may cause withdrawal in patients currently dependent on narcotics

**Restrictions** C-IV

**Pregnancy Risk Factor** B (D if used for prolonged periods or in high doses at term)

**Contraindications** Hypersensitivity to pentazocine or any component, increased intracranial pressure (unless the patient is mechanically ventilated)

**Warnings/Precautions** Use with caution in seizure-prone patients, acute myocardial infarction, patients undergoing biliary tract surgery, patients with renal and hepatic dysfunction, head trauma, increased intracranial pressure, and patients with a history of prior opioid dependence or abuse; pentazocine may precipitate opiate withdrawal symptoms in patients who have been receiving opiates regularly; injection contains sulfites which may cause allergic reaction; tolerance or drug dependence may result from extended use

**Adverse Reactions**

>10%:

Central nervous system: Euphoria, drowsiness

Gastrointestinal: Nausea, vomiting

Neuromuscular & skeletal: Weakness

1% to 10%:

Cardiovascular: Hypotension

Central nervous system: Malaise, headache, restlessness, nightmares

Dermatologic: Rash

Gastrointestinal: Xerostomia

Genitourinary: Ureteral spasm

Ocular: Blurred vision

Respiratory: Dyspnea

<1%: Antidiuretic hormone release, biliary tract spasm, bradycardia, CNS depression, confusion, constipation, disorientation, GI irritation, hallucinations, histamine release, increased intracranial pressure, insomnia, miosis, palpitations, peripheral vasodilation, physical and psychological dependence, pruritus, sedation, seizures may occur in seizure-prone patients, tissue damage and irritation with I.M./S.C. use, urinary tract spasm

**Overdosage/Toxicology**

Signs and symptoms: Drowsiness, sedation, respiratory depression, coma

Treatment: Naloxone 2 mg I.V. (0.01 mg/kg for children) with repeat administration as necessary up to a total of 10 mg

**Drug Interactions** CYP2D6 enzyme substrate

May potentiate or reduce analgesic effect of opiate agonist, (eg, morphine) depending on patients tolerance to opiates can precipitate withdrawal in narcotic addicts

Increased effect/toxicity with tripelennamine (can be lethal), CNS depressants (phenothiazines, tranquilizers, anxiolytics, sedatives, hypnotics, or alcohol)

(Continued)

## Pentazocine *(Continued)*

**Usual Dosage**

Children: I.M., S.C.:

5-8 years: 15 mg

8-14 years: 30 mg

Children >12 years and Adults: Oral: 50 mg every 3-4 hours; may increase to 100 mg/dose if needed, but should not exceed 600 mg/day

Adults:

I.M., S.C.: 30-60 mg every 3-4 hours, not to exceed total daily dose of 360 mg

I.V.: 30 mg every 3-4 hours

**Dosing adjustment in renal impairment:**

$Cl_{cr}$ 10-50 mL/minute: Administer 75% of normal dose

$Cl_{cr}$ <10 mL/minute: Administer 50% of normal dose

**Dosing adjustment in hepatic impairment:** Reduce dose or avoid use in patients with liver disease

**Dietary Considerations** Alcohol: Additive CNS effect, avoid use

**Patient Information** If self-administered, use exactly as directed (do not increase dose or frequency); may cause physical and/or psychological dependence. While using this medication, do not use alcohol and other prescription or OTC medications (especially sedatives, tranquilizers, antihistamines, or pain medications) without consulting prescriber. Maintain adequate hydration (2-3 L/day of fluids unless instructed to restrict fluid intake). May cause hypotension, dizziness, drowsiness, impaired coordination, or blurred vision (use caution when driving, climbing stairs, or changing position - rising from sitting or lying to standing, or when engaging in tasks requiring alertness until response to drug is known); nausea, vomiting, loss of appetite, or dry mouth (frequent mouth care, small frequent meals, chewing gum, or sucking lozenges may help); constipation (increased exercise, fluids, or dietary fruit and fiber may help - if constipation remains an unresolved problem, consult prescriber about use of stool softeners). Report persistent dizziness or headache; excessive fatigue or sedation; changes in mental status; changes in urinary elimination or pain on urination; weakness or trembling; blurred vision; or shortness of breath.

**Nursing Implications** Observe patient for excessive sedation, respiratory depression, implement safety measures, assist with ambulation; observe for narcotic withdrawal

**Dosage Forms**

Injection, as lactate: 30 mg/mL (1 mL, 1.5 mL, 2 mL, 10 mL)

Tablet: Pentazocine hydrochloride 50 mg and naloxone hydrochloride 0.5 mg

♦ **Pentazocine Hydrochloride** *see* Pentazocine *on page 427*

♦ **Pentazocine Lactate** *see* Pentazocine *on page 427*

## Pentobarbital (pen toe BAR bi tal)

**Related Information**

Anxiolytic/Hypnotic Use in Long-Term Care Facilities *on page 754*

Federal OBRA Regulations Recommended Maximum Doses *on page 756*

Patient Information - Anxiolytics & Sedative Hypnotics (Barbiturates) *on page 654*

Substance-Related Disorders *on page 609*

**Generic Available** Yes

**U.S. Brand Names** Nembutal®

**Synonyms** Pentobarbital Sodium

**Pharmacologic Category** Anticonvulsant, Barbiturate; Barbiturate

**Use** Sedative/hypnotic; preanesthetic; high-dose barbiturate coma for treatment of increased intracranial pressure or status epilepticus unresponsive to other therapy

**Unlabeled use:** Tolerance test during withdrawal of sedative hypnotics

**Restrictions** C-II (capsules, injection); C-III (suppositories)

**Pregnancy Risk Factor** D

**Contraindications** Hypersensitivity to barbiturates or any component of the formulation; marked hepatic impairment; dyspnea or airway obstruction; porphyria

**Warnings/Precautions** Tolerance to hypnotic effect can occur; do not use for >2 weeks to treat insomnia. Potential for drug dependency exists, abrupt cessation may precipitate withdrawal, including status epilepticus in epileptic patients. Do not administer to patients in acute pain. Use caution in elderly, debilitated, renally impaired, hepatic dysfunction, or pediatric patients. May cause paradoxical responses, including agitation and hyperactivity, particularly in acute pain and pediatric patients. Use with caution in patients with depression or suicidal tendencies, or in patients with a history of drug abuse. Tolerance, psychological and physical dependence may occur with prolonged use.

May cause CNS depression, which may impair physical or mental abilities. Patients must cautioned about performing tasks which require mental alertness (ie, operating machinery or driving). Effects with other sedative drugs or ethanol may be potentiated. Use of this agent as a hypnotic in the elderly is not recommended due to its long half-life and potential for physical and psychological dependence.

May cause respiratory depression or hypotension, particularly when administered intravenously. Use with caution in hemodynamically unstable patients or patients with respiratory disease. High doses (loading doses of 15-35 mg/kg given over 1-2 hours) have been utilized to induce pentobarbital coma, but these higher doses often cause hypotension requiring vasopressor therapy.

**Adverse Reactions**

Cardiovascular: Bradycardia, hypotension, syncope

Central nervous system: Drowsiness, lethargy, CNS excitation or depression, impaired judgment, "hangover" effect, confusion, somnolence, agitation, hyperkinesia, ataxia, nervousness, headache, insomnia, nightmares, hallucinations, anxiety, dizziness

Dermatologic: Rash, exfoliative dermatitis, Stevens-Johnson syndrome

Gastrointestinal: Nausea, vomiting, constipation

Hematologic: Agranulocytosis, thrombocytopenia, megaloblastic anemia

Local: Pain at injection site, thrombophlebitis with I.V. use

Renal: Oliguria

Respiratory: Laryngospasm, respiratory depression, apnea (especially with rapid I.V. use), hypoventilation, apnea

Miscellaneous: Gangrene with inadvertent intra-arterial injection

**Overdosage/Toxicology**

Signs and symptoms: Unsteady gait, slurred speech, confusion, jaundice, hypothermia, hypotension, respiratory depression, coma

Treatment: If hypotension occurs, administer I.V. fluids and place the patient in the Trendelenburg position. If unresponsive, an I.V. vasopressor (eg, dopamine, epinephrine) may be required. Forced alkaline diuresis is of no value in the treatment of intoxications with short-acting barbiturates. Charcoal hemoperfusion or hemodialysis may be useful in the harder to treat intoxications, especially in the presence of very high serum barbiturate levels when the patient is in a coma, shock, or renal failure.

**Drug Interactions** Barbiturates are enzyme inducers; patients should be monitored when these drugs are started or stopped for a decreased or increased therapeutic effect respectively

Acetaminophen: Barbiturates may enhance the hepatotoxic potential of acetaminophen overdoses

Antiarrhythmics: Barbiturates may increase the metabolism of antiarrhythmics, decreasing their clinical effect; includes disopyramide, propafenone, and quinidine

Anticonvulsants: Barbiturates may increase the metabolism of anticonvulsants; includes ethosuximide, felbamate (possibly), lamotrigine, phenytoin, tiagabine, topiramate, and zonisamide; does not appear to affect gabapentin or levetiracetam

Antineoplastics: Limited evidence suggests that enzyme-inducing anticonvulsant therapy may reduce the effectiveness of some chemotherapy regimens (specifically in ALL); teniposide and methotrexate may be cleared more rapidly in these patients

Antipsychotics: Barbiturates may enhance the metabolism (decrease the efficacy) of antipsychotics; monitor for altered response; dose adjustment may be needed

Beta-blockers: Metabolism of beta-blockers may be increased and clinical effect decreased; atenolol and nadolol are unlikely to interact given their renal elimination

Calcium channel blockers: Barbiturates may enhance the metabolism of calcium channel blockers, decreasing their clinical effect

Chloramphenicol: Barbiturates may increase the metabolism of chloramphenicol and chloramphenicol may inhibit barbiturate metabolism; monitor for altered response

Cimetidine: Barbiturates may enhance the metabolism of cimetidine, decreasing its clinical effect

CNS depressants: Sedative effects and/or respiratory depression with barbiturates may be additive with other CNS depressants; monitor for increased effect; includes ethanol, sedatives, antidepressants, narcotic analgesics, and benzodiazepines

Corticosteroids: Barbiturates may enhance the metabolism of corticosteroids, decreasing their clinical effect

Cyclosporine: Levels may be decreased by barbiturates; monitor

Doxycycline: Barbiturates may enhance the metabolism of doxycycline, decreasing its clinical effect; higher dosages may be required

Estrogens: Barbiturates may increase the metabolism of estrogens and reduce their efficacy

Felbamate may inhibit the metabolism of barbiturates and barbiturates may increase the metabolism of felbamate

Griseofulvin: Barbiturates may impair the absorption of griseofulvin, and griseofulvin metabolism may be increased by barbiturates, decreasing clinical effect

Guanfacine: Effect may be decreased by barbiturates

Immunosuppressants: Barbiturates may enhance the metabolism of immunosuppressants, decreasing its clinical effect; includes both cyclosporine and tacrolimus

Loop diuretics: Metabolism may be increased and clinical effects decreased; established for furosemide, effect with other loop diuretics not established

MAOIs: Metabolism of barbiturates may be inhibited, increasing clinical effect or toxicity of the barbiturates

Methadone: Barbiturates may enhance the metabolism of methadone resulting in methadone withdrawal
Methoxyflurane: Barbiturates may enhance the nephrotoxic effects of methoxyflurane
Oral contraceptives: Barbiturates may enhance the metabolism of oral contraceptives, decreasing their clinical effect; an alternative method of contraception should be considered
Theophylline: Barbiturates may increase metabolism of theophylline derivatives and decrease their clinical effect
Tricyclic antidepressants: Barbiturates may increase metabolism of tricyclic antidepressants and decrease their clinical effect; sedative effects may be additive
Valproic acid: Metabolism of barbiturates may be inhibited by valproic acid; monitor for excessive sedation; a dose reduction may be needed
Warfarin: Barbiturates inhibit the hypoprothrombinemic effects of oral anticoagulants via increased metabolism; this combination should generally be avoided

**Stability** Protect from freezing; aqueous solutions are not stable, commercially available vehicle (containing propylene glycol) is more stable; low pH may cause precipitate; use only clear solution

**Mechanism of Action** Short-acting barbiturate with sedative, hypnotic, and anticonvulsant properties. Barbiturates depress the sensory cortex, decrease motor activity, alter cerebellar function, and produce drowsiness, sedation, and hypnosis. In high doses, barbiturates exhibit anticonvulsant activity; barbiturates produce dose-dependent respiratory depression.

**Pharmacodynamics/kinetics**
Onset of action:
- Oral, rectal: 15-60 minutes
- I.M.: Within 10-15 minutes
- I.V.: Within 1 minute

Duration:
- Oral, rectal: 1-4 hours
- I.V.: 15 minutes

Distribution: $V_d$:
- Children: 0.8 L/kg
- Adults: 1 L/kg

Protein binding: 35% to 55%
Metabolism: Extensively in liver via hydroxylation and oxidation pathways
Half-life, terminal:
- Children: 25 hours
- Adults, normal: 22 hours; range: 35-50 hours

Elimination: <1% excreted unchanged renally

**Usual Dosage**
Children:
- Sedative: Oral: 2-6 mg/kg/day divided in 3 doses; maximum: 100 mg/day
- Hypnotic: I.M.: 2-6 mg/kg; maximum: 100 mg/dose
- Rectal:
  - 2 months to 1 year (10-20 lb): 30 mg
  - 1-4 years (20-40 lb): 30-60 mg
  - 5-12 years (40-80 lb): 60 mg
  - 12-14 years (80-110 lb): 60-120 mg
  - **or**
  - <4 years: 3-6 mg/kg/dose
  - >4 years: 1.5-3 mg/kg/dose
- Preoperative/preprocedure sedation: ≥6 months:
  - Oral, I.M., rectal: 2-6 mg/kg; maximum: 100 mg/dose
  - I.V.: 1-3 mg/kg to a maximum of 100 mg until asleep
- Children 5-12 years: Conscious sedation prior to a procedure: I.V.: 2 mg/kg 5-10 minutes before procedures, may repeat one time

Adolescents: Conscious sedation: Oral, I.V.: 100 mg prior to a procedure
Adults:
- Hypnotic:
  - Oral: 100-200 mg at bedtime or 20 mg 3-4 times/day for daytime sedation
  - I.M.: 150-200 mg
  - I.V.: Initial: 100 mg, may repeat every 1-3 minutes up to 200-500 mg total dose
- Rectal: 120-200 mg at bedtime
- Preoperative sedation: I.M.: 150-200 mg

Children and Adults: Barbiturate coma in head injury patients: I.V.: Loading dose: 5-10 mg/kg given slowly over 1-2 hours; monitor blood pressure and respiratory rate; Maintenance infusion: Initial: 1 mg/kg/hour; may increase to 2-3 mg/kg/hour; maintain burst suppression on EEG
Tolerance testing: 200 mg every 2 hours until signs of intoxication are exhibited at any time during the 2 hours after the dose; maximum dose: 1000 mg
**Dosing adjustment in hepatic impairment:** Reduce dosage in patients with severe liver dysfunction

**Dietary Considerations** Alcohol: Additive CNS effect, avoid use

**Administration** Pentobarbital may be administered by deep I.M. or slow I.V. injection. I.M.: No more than 5 mL (250 mg) should be injected at any one site because of possible tissue irritation I.V. push doses can be given undiluted, but should be administered no faster than 50 mg/minute; parenteral solutions are highly alkaline; avoid extravasation; avoid rapid I.V. administration >50 mg/minute; avoid intra-arterial injection

**Monitoring Parameters** Respiratory status (for conscious sedation, includes pulse oximetry), cardiovascular status, CNS status; cardiac monitor and blood pressure monitor required

**Reference Range** Therapeutic: Hypnotic: 1-5 µg/mL (SI: 4-22 µmol/L), Coma: 10-50 µg/mL (SI: 88-221 µmol/L); Toxic: >10 µg/mL (SI: >44 µmol/L)

**Test Interactions** ↑ ammonia (B); ↓ bilirubin (S)

**Patient Information** Avoid the use of alcohol and other CNS depressants; avoid driving and other hazardous tasks; avoid abrupt discontinuation; may cause physical and psychological dependence; do not alter dose without notifying physician

**Nursing Implications** Avoid extravasation; institute safety measures to avoid injuries; has many incompatibilities when given I.V.

**Additional Information** Pentobarbital: Nembutal® elixir pentobarbital sodium: Nembutal® capsule, injection, and suppository
Sodium content of 1 mL injection: 5 mg (0.2 mEq)

**Dosage Forms**
- Capsule, as sodium (C-II): 50 mg, 100 mg
- Elixir (C-II): 18.2 mg/5 ml (473 mL, 1000 mL)
- Injection, as sodium (C-II): 50 mg/mL (1 mL, 2 mL, 20 mL, 50 mL)
- Suppository, rectal (C-III): 30 mg, 60 mg, 120 mg, 200 mg

♦ **Pentobarbital Sodium** *see* Pentobarbital *on page 428*

## Pentosan Polysulfate Sodium

(PEN toe san pol i SUL fate SOW dee um)

**U.S. Brand Names** Elmiron®

**Synonyms** PPS

**Pharmacologic Category** Analgesic, Urinary

**Use** Relief of bladder pain or discomfort due to interstitial cystitis

**Effects on Mental Status** May cause dizziness

**Effects on Psychiatric Treatment** May cause anemia and leukopenia; use caution with clozapine and carbamazepine

**Pregnancy Risk Factor** B

**Contraindications** Hypersensitivity to pentosan polysulfate sodium or any component

**Warnings/Precautions** Pentosan polysulfate is a low-molecular weight heparin-like compound with anticoagulant and fibrinolytic effects, therefore, bleeding complications such as ecchymosis, epistaxis and gum bleeding, may occur; patients with the following diseases should be carefully evaluated before initiating therapy: aneurysm, thrombocytopenia, hemophilia, gastrointestinal ulcerations, polyps, diverticula, or hepatic insufficiency; patients undergoing invasive procedures or having signs or symptoms of underlying coagulopathies or other increased risk of bleeding (eg, receiving heparin, warfarin, thrombolytics, or high dose aspirin) should be evaluated for hemorrhage; elevations in transaminases and alopecia can occur

**Adverse Reactions**
1% to 10%:
- Central nervous system: Headache, dizziness
- Dermatologic: Alopecia, rash
- Gastrointestinal: Diarrhea, nausea, dyspepsia, abdominal pain
- Hepatic: Liver function test abnormalities

<1%: Allergic reactions, amblyopia, anemia, anorexia, bleeding, bruising, colitis, conjunctivitis, constipation, dyspnea, epistaxis, esophagitis, flatulence, gastritis, gum bleeding, increased partial thromboplastin time, leukopenia, mouth ulcer, optic neuritis, pharyngitis, photosensitivity, prolonged PT, pruritus, retinal hemorrhage, rhinitis, thrombocytopenia, tinnitus, urticaria, vomiting

**Overdosage/Toxicology**
Signs and symptoms: Drowsiness, lethargy, nausea, vomiting, seizures, paresthesia, headache, dizziness, GI bleeding, cerebral edema, tinnitus, leukocytosis, renal failure
Treatment: Management of a nonsteroidal anti-inflammatory drug (NSAID) intoxication is primarily supportive and symptomatic. Fluid therapy is commonly effective in managing the hypotension that may occur following an acute NSAID overdose, except when this is due to an acute blood loss. Seizures tend to be very short-lived and often do not require drug treatment. Although, recurrent seizures should be treated with I.V. diazepam.

**Drug Interactions** Although there is no information about potential drug interactions, it is expected that pentosan polysulfate sodium would have at least additive anticoagulant effects when administered with anticoagulant drugs such as warfarin or heparin, and possible similar effects when administered with aspirin or thrombolytics

**Usual Dosage** Adults: Oral: 100 mg 3 times/day taken with water 1 hour before or 2 hours after meals

Patients should be evaluated at 3 months and may be continued an additional 3 months if there has been no improvement and if there are no therapy-limiting side effects. **The risks and benefits of continued use beyond 6 months in patients who have not responded is not yet known.**

(Continued)

## Pentosan Polysulfate Sodium *(Continued)*

**Patient Information** Patients should be advised to take the medication as prescribed and no more frequently; tell patients about the slight anticoagulant effects and the potential for increased bleeding; until more is known about drug interactions, carefully monitor the medication profile of patients receiving pentosan polysulfate sodium for drugs that might increase the anticoagulant effects

**Dosage Forms** Capsule: 100 mg

## Pentostatin (PEN toe stat in)

**U.S. Brand Names** Nipent™

**Synonyms** DCF; Deoxycoformycin; 2′-deoxycoformycin

**Pharmacologic Category** Antineoplastic Agent, Antibiotic

**Use** Treatment of adult patients with alpha-interferon-refractory hairy cell leukemia; non-Hodgkin's lymphoma, cutaneous T-cell lymphoma

**Effects on Mental Status** Sedation is common; may cause anxiety, confusion, insomnia, depression

**Effects on Psychiatric Treatment** Leukopenia is common; avoid clozapine and carbamazepine

**Pregnancy Risk Factor** D

**Contraindications** Limited or severely compromised bone marrow reserves (white blood cell count <3000 cells/mm$^3$)

**Warnings/Precautions** The FDA currently recommends that procedures for proper handling and disposal of antineoplastic agents be considered. Pregnant women or women of childbearing age should be apprised of the potential risk to the fetus; use extreme caution in the presence of renal insufficiency; use with caution in patients with signs or symptoms of impaired hepatic function.

**Adverse Reactions**

>10%:

Central nervous system: Headache, neurologic disorder, fever, fatigue, chills, pain
Dermatologic: Rash
Gastrointestinal: Vomiting, nausea, anorexia, diarrhea
Hematologic: Leukopenia, anemia, thrombocytopenia
Hepatic: Hepatic disorder, abnormal LFTs
Neuromuscular & skeletal: Myalgia
Respiratory: Coughing
Miscellaneous: Allergic reaction

1% to 10%:

Cardiovascular: Chest pain, arrhythmia, peripheral edema
Central nervous system: Anxiety, confusion, depression, dizziness, insomnia, lethargy, coma, seizures, malaise
Dermatologic: Dry skin, eczema, pruritus
Gastrointestinal: Constipation, flatulence, stomatitis, weight loss
Genitourinary: Dysuria
Hematologic: Myelosuppression
Hepatic: Liver dysfunction
Local: Thrombophlebitis
Neuromuscular & skeletal: Arthralgia, paresthesia, back pain, weakness
Ocular: Abnormal vision, eye pain, keratoconjunctivitis
Otic: Ear pain
Renal: Renal failure, hematuria
Respiratory: Bronchitis, dyspnea, lung edema, pneumonia
Miscellaneous: Death, opportunistic infections, diaphoresis

**Overdosage/Toxicology**

Signs and symptoms: Severe renal, hepatic, pulmonary, and CNS toxicity
Treatment: Supportive therapy

**Drug Interactions** Increased toxicity: Vidarabine, fludarabine, allopurinol

**Usual Dosage** Refractory hairy cell leukemia: Adults (refer to individual protocols): 4 mg/m$^2$ every other week; I.V. bolus over ≥3-5 minutes in $D_5W$ or NS at concentrations ≥2 mg/mL

**Dosing interval in renal impairment:**

$Cl_{cr}$ <60 mL/minute: Use extreme caution
$Cl_{cr}$ 50-60 mL/minute: 2 mg/m$^2$/dose

**Patient Information** This drug can only be administered by infusion on a specific schedule. Frequent blood tests and monitoring will be necessary. Maintain adequate hydration (2-3 L/day of fluids unless instructed to restrict fluid intake). You may experience nausea and vomiting, diarrhea, or loss of appetite (frequent small meals or frequent mouth care may help or request medication from prescriber); dizziness, weakness, or lethargy (use caution when driving); susceptibility to infections (avoid crowds and exposure to infection). Use frequent oral care with soft toothbrush or cotton swabs to reduce incidence of mouth sores. May cause headache (request medication). Report signs of infection (eg, fever, chills, sore throat, mouth sores, burning urination, perianal itching, or vaginal discharge); unusual bruising or bleeding (tarry stools, blood in urine, stool, or vomitus); vision changes or hearing; muscle tremors, weakness, or pain; CNS changes (eg, hallucinations, confusion, insomnia, seizures); or respiratory difficulty.

**Dosage Forms** Powder for injection: 10 mg/vial

♦ **Pentothal® Sodium** *see* Thiopental *on page 543*

## Pentoxifylline (pen toks I fi leen)

**U.S. Brand Names** Trental®

**Canadian Brand Names** Albert® Pentoxifylline; Apo®-Pentoxifylline SR

**Synonyms** Oxpentifylline

**Pharmacologic Category** Blood Viscosity Reducer Agent

**Use** Symptomatic management of peripheral vascular disease, mainly intermittent claudication

**Unlabeled use:** AIDS patients with increased TNF, CVA, cerebrovascular diseases, diabetic atherosclerosis, diabetic neuropathy, gangrene, hemodialysis shunt thrombosis, vascular impotence, cerebral malaria, septic shock, sickle cell syndromes, and vasculitis

**Effects on Mental Status** May cause dizziness or rarely agitation

**Effects on Psychiatric Treatment** None reported

**Pregnancy Risk Factor** C

**Contraindications** Hypersensitivity to pentoxifylline or any component and other xanthine derivatives; patients with recent cerebral and/or retinal hemorrhage

**Warnings/Precautions** Use with caution in patients with renal impairment

**Adverse Reactions**

1% to 10%:

Central nervous system: Dizziness, headache
Gastrointestinal: Dyspepsia, nausea, vomiting

<1%: Angina, agitation, blurred vision, earache mild hypotension

**Overdosage/Toxicology**

Signs and symptoms: Hypotension, flushing, convulsions, deep sleep, agitation, bradycardia, A-V block
Treatment: Supportive; seizures can be treated with diazepam 5-10 mg (0.25-0.4 mg/kg in children); arrhythmias respond to lidocaine

**Drug Interactions**

Increased effect/toxic potential with cimetidine (increased levels) and other $H_2$-antagonists, warfarin; increased effect of antihypertensives
Increased toxicity with theophylline

**Usual Dosage** Adults: Oral: 400 mg 3 times/day with meals; may reduce to 400 mg twice daily if GI or CNS side effects occur

**Patient Information** Take as prescribed for full length of prescription. This may relieve pain of claudication, but additional therapy may be recommended. You may experience dizziness (use caution when driving); GI upset (small frequent meals may help). Report chest pain, persistent headache, nausea or vomiting.

**Dosage Forms** Tablet, controlled release: 400 mg

♦ **Pen.Vee® K** *see* Penicillin V Potassium *on page 426*

♦ **Pen VK** *see* Penicillin V Potassium *on page 426*

♦ **Pepcid®** *see* Famotidine *on page 218*

♦ **Pepcid® AC Acid Controller [OTC]** *see* Famotidine *on page 218*

♦ **Pepcid RPD™** *see* Famotidine *on page 218*

♦ **Pepto-Bismol® [OTC]** *see* Bismuth *on page 69*

♦ **Pepto® Diarrhea Control [OTC]** *see* Loperamide *on page 324*

♦ **Percocet® 2.5/325** *see* Oxycodone and Acetaminophen *on page 414*

♦ **Percocet® 5/325** *see* Oxycodone and Acetaminophen *on page 414*

♦ **Percocet® 7.5/500** *see* Oxycodone and Acetaminophen *on page 414*

♦ **Percocet® 10/650** *see* Oxycodone and Acetaminophen *on page 414*

♦ **Percodan®** *see* Oxycodone and Aspirin *on page 414*

♦ **Percodan®-Demi** *see* Oxycodone and Aspirin *on page 414*

♦ **Percogesic® [OTC]** *see* Acetaminophen and Phenyltoloxamine *on page 15*

♦ **Percolone®** *see* Oxycodone *on page 413*

♦ **Perdiem® Plain [OTC]** *see* Psyllium *on page 479*

♦ **Perfectoderm® Gel [OTC]** *see* Benzoyl Peroxide *on page 62*

## Pergolide (PER go lide)

**Related Information**

Discontinuation of Psychotropic Drugs - Withdrawal Symptoms and Recommendations *on page 798*

**Generic Available** No

**U.S. Brand Names** Permax®

**Synonyms** Pergolide Mesylate

**Pharmacologic Category** Anti-Parkinson's Agent (Dopamine Agonist); Ergot Derivative

**Use** Adjunctive treatment to levodopa/carbidopa in the management of Parkinson's disease

**Pregnancy Risk Factor** B

**Contraindications** Hypersensitivity to pergolide mesylate or other ergot derivatives

**Warnings/Precautions** Symptomatic hypotension occurs in 10% of patients; use with caution in patients with a history of cardiac arrhythmias, hallucinations, or mental illness

**Adverse Reactions**

>10%:

Central nervous system: Dizziness, somnolence, confusion, hallucinations, dystonia

Gastrointestinal: Nausea, constipation

Neuromuscular & skeletal: Dyskinesia

Respiratory: Rhinitis

1% to 10%:

Cardiovascular: Myocardial infarction, postural hypotension, syncope, arrhythmias, peripheral edema, vasodilation, palpitations, chest pain, hypertension

Central nervous system: Chills, insomnia, anxiety, psychosis, EPS, incoordination

Dermatologic: Rash

Gastrointestinal: Diarrhea, abdominal pain, xerostomia, anorexia, weight gain, dyspepsia, taste perversion

Hematologic: Anemia

Neuromuscular & skeletal: Weakness, myalgia, tremor, NMS (with rapid dose reduction), pain

Ocular: Abnormal vision, diplopia

Respiratory: Dyspnea, epistaxis

Miscellaneous: Flu syndrome, hiccups

**Overdosage/Toxicology**

Signs and symptoms: Vomiting, hypotension, agitation, hallucinations, ventricular extrasystoles, possible seizures; data on overdose is limited;

Treatment: Supportive and may require antiarrhythmias and/or neuroleptics for agitation; hypotension, when unresponsive to I.V. fluids or Trendelenburg positioning, often responds to norepinephrine infusions started at 0.1-0.2 mcg/kg/minute followed by a titrated infusion. If signs of CNS stimulation are present, a neuroleptic may be indicated; antiarrhythmics may be indicated, monitor EKG; activated charcoal is useful to prevent further absorption and to hasten elimination

**Drug Interactions**

Antipsychotics: May diminish the effects of pergolide (due to dopamine antagonism); these combinations should generally be avoided

Entacapone: Fibrotic complications (retroperitoneal or pulmonary fibrosis) have been associated with combinations of entacapone and bromocriptine

Highly protein-bound drugs: May cause displacement/increased effect; use caution with other highly plasma protein bound drugs

Metoclopramide: May diminish the effects of pergolide (due to dopamine antagonism); concurrent therapy should generally be avoided

**Mechanism of Action** Pergolide is a semisynthetic ergot alkaloid similar to bromocriptine but stated to be more potent (10-1000 times) and longer-acting; it is a centrally-active dopamine agonist stimulating both $D_1$ and $D_2$ receptors. Pergolide is believed to exert its therapeutic effect by directly stimulating postsynaptic dopamine receptors in the nigrostriatal system.

**Pharmacodynamics/kinetics**

Absorption: Oral: Well absorbed

Protein binding: Plasma 90%

Metabolism: Extensive in the liver (on first-pass)

Elimination: ~50% excreted in urine and 50% in feces

**Usual Dosage** When adding pergolide to levodopa/carbidopa, the dose of the latter can usually and should be decreased. Patients no longer responsive to bromocriptine may benefit by being switched to pergolide.

Adults: Oral: Start with 0.05 mg/day for 2 days, then increase dosage by 0.1 or 0.15 mg/day every 3 days over next 12 days, increase dose by 0.25 mg/day every 3 days until optimal therapeutic dose is achieved, up to 5 mg/day maximum; usual dosage range: 2-3 mg/day in 3 divided doses

**Monitoring Parameters** Blood pressure (both sitting/supine and standing), symptoms of parkinsonism, dyskinesias, mental status

**Patient Information** May cause hypotension, arise slowly from prolonged sitting or lying; take with food or meals to lessen GI upset, may cause drowsiness and impair judgment and coordination; report any unusual CNS symptoms, palpitations, chest pain, or involuntary movements to physician

**Nursing Implications** Monitor closely for orthostasis and other adverse effects; raise bed rails and institute safety measures; aid patient with ambulation, may cause postural hypotension and drowsiness

**Dosage Forms** Tablet, as mesylate: 0.05 mg, 0.25 mg, 1 mg


♦ **Pergolide Mesylate** *see* Pergolide *on page 430*

♦ **Pergonal®** *see* Menotropins *on page 340*

♦ **Periactin®** *see* Cyproheptadine *on page 148*

♦ **Peridex® Oral Rinse** *see* Chlorhexidine Gluconate *on page 111*


## Perindopril Erbumine (per IN doe pril er BYOO meen)

**Related Information**

Angiotensin-Related Agents Comparison Chart *on page 700*

**U.S. Brand Names** Aceon®

**Pharmacologic Category** Angiotensin-Converting Enzyme (ACE) Inhibitors

**Use** Treatment of stage I or II hypertension and congestive heart failure treatment of left ventricular dysfunction after myocardial infarction

**Effects on Mental Status** May cause dizziness or fatigue; may rarely cause sedation, insomnia, or depression

**Effects on Psychiatric Treatment** May cause neutropenia; use caution with clozapine and carbamazepine; may decrease lithium clearance resulting in an increase in serum lithium levels and potential lithium toxicity; monitor serum lithium levels

**Pregnancy Risk Factor** C (first trimester); D (during 2nd and 3rd trimester)

**Contraindications** Hypersensitivity to perindopril or any component; angioedema related to previous treatment with an ACE inhibitor; bilateral renal artery stenosis; primary hyperaldosteronism; pregnancy (2nd and 3rd trimesters)

**Warnings/Precautions** Anaphylactic reactions can occur. Angioedema can occur at any time during treatment (especially following first dose). Careful blood pressure monitoring with first dose (hypotension can occur especially in volume depleted patients). Dosage adjustment needed in renal impairment. Use with caution in hypovolemia; collagen vascular diseases; valvular stenosis (particularly aortic stenosis); hyperkalemia; or before, during, or immediately after anesthesia. Avoid rapid dosage escalation, which may lead to renal insufficiency. Neutropenia/agranulocytosis with myeloid hyperplasia can rarely occur. If patient has renal impairment then a baseline WBC with differential and serum creatinine should be evaluated and monitored closely during the first 3 months of therapy. Hypersensitivity reactions may be seen during hemodialysis with high-flux dialysis membranes (eg, AN69). Use with caution in unilateral renal artery stenosis and pre-existing renal insufficiency.

**Adverse Reactions**

1% to 10%:

Central nervous system: Headache, dizziness, mood and sleep disorders, fatigue

Dermatologic: Rash, pruritus

Gastrointestinal: Nausea, epigastric pain, diarrhea, vomiting

Neuromuscular & skeletal: Muscle cramps

Respiratory: Cough (incidence is greater in women, 3:1)

<1%: Agranulocytosis for all ACE inhibitors (especially in patients with renal impairment or collagen vascular disease), angioedema, blurred vision, decreases in creatinine clearance in some elderly hypertensive patients or those with chronic renal failure, dry eyes, hyperkalemia, hypotension, impotence, neutropenia (possibly), optic phosphenes, proteinuria, psoriasis, taste disturbances, worsening of renal function in patients with bilateral renal artery stenosis or furosemide therapy

**Overdosage/Toxicology**

Signs and symptoms: Mild hypotension has been the only toxic effect seen with acute overdose. Bradycardia may also occur; hyperkalemia occurs even with therapeutic doses, especially in patients with renal insufficiency and those taking NSAIDs.

Treatment: Following initiation of essential overdose management, toxic symptom treatment and supportive treatment should be initiated. Hypotension usually responds to I.V. fluids or Trendelenburg positioning.

**Drug Interactions**

Alpha$_1$ blockers: Hypotensive effect increased

Aspirin: The effects of ACE inhibitors may be blunted by aspirin administration, particularly at higher dosages

Diuretics: Hypovolemia due to diuretics may precipitate acute hypotensive events or acute renal failure

Insulin: Risk of hypoglycemia may be increased

Lithium: Risk of lithium toxicity may be increased; monitor lithium levels, especially the first 4 weeks of therapy

Mercaptopurine: Risk of neutropenia may be increased

NSAIDs may decrease ACE inhibitor efficacy and/or increase risk of renal effects

Potassium-sparing diuretics (amiloride, spironolactone, triamterene): Increased risk of hyperkalemia

Potassium supplements may increase the risk of hyperkalemia

Trimethoprim (high dose) may increase the risk of hyperkalemia

**Usual Dosage** Adults: Oral:

Congestive heart failure: 4 mg once daily

Hypertension: Initial: 4 mg/day but may be titrated to response; usual range: 4-8 mg/day, maximum: 16 mg/day

**Dosing adjustment in renal impairment:**

$Cl_{cr}$ >60 mL/minute: Administer 4 mg/day.

$Cl_{cr}$ 30-60 mL/minute: Administer 2 mg/day.

$Cl_{cr}$ 15-29 mL/minute: Administer 2 mg every other day.

$Cl_{cr}$ <15 mL/minute: Administer 2 mg on the day of dialysis.

Hemodialysis: Perindopril and its metabolites are dialyzable

**Dosing adjustment in hepatic impairment:** None needed

**Dosing adjustment in geriatric patients:** Due to greater bioavailability and lower renal clearance of the drug in elderly subjects, dose reduction of 50% is recommended.

**Patient Information** This medication does not replace the to need to follow exercise and diet recommendations for hypertension. Take as

(Continued)

## Perindopril Erbumine *(Continued)*

directed; do not miss doses, alter dosage, or discontinue without consulting prescriber. Consult prescriber for appropriate diet. Change position slowly when rising from sitting or lying. May cause transient drowsiness; avoid driving or engaging in tasks that require alertness until response to drug is known. Small frequent meals may help reduce any nausea, vomiting, or epigastric pain. You may experience persistent cough; contact prescriber. Report unusual weight gain or swelling of ankles and hands; persistent fatigue; dry cough; difficulty breathing; palpitations; or swelling of face, eyes, or lips.

**Nursing Implications** A reduction in clinical signs of congestive heart failure (dyspnea, orthopnea, cough) and an improvement in exercise duration are indicative of therapeutic response; a reduction of supine diastolic blood pressure of 10 mm Hg or to 90 mm Hg is indicative of excellent therapeutic response in patients with hypertension; observe for cough, difficulty breathing/swallowing, perioral swelling and signs and symptoms of agranulocytosis; monitor for 6 hours after initial dosing for profound hypotension or first-dose phenomenon

**Dosage Forms** Tablet: 2 mg, 4 mg, 8 mg

- **PerioChip®** *see* Chlorhexidine Gluconate *on page 111*
- **PerioGard®** *see* Chlorhexidine Gluconate *on page 111*
- **Periostat®** *see* Doxycycline *on page 186*
- **Peritrate®** *see* Pentaerythritol Tetranitrate *on page 426*
- **Peritrate® SA** *see* Pentaerythritol Tetranitrate *on page 426*
- **Permapen®** *see* Penicillin G Benzathine *on page 425*
- **Permax®** *see* Pergolide *on page 430*

## Permethrin (per METH rin)

**U.S. Brand Names** Acticin® Cream; Elimite™ Cream; Nix™ Creme Rinse

**Pharmacologic Category** Antiparasitic Agent, Topical; Scabicidal Agent

**Use** Single application treatment of infestation with *Pediculus humanus capitis* (head louse) and its nits or *Sarcoptes scabiei* (scabies); indicated for prophylactic use during epidemics of lice

**Effects on Mental Status** None reported

**Effects on Psychiatric Treatment** None reported

**Pregnancy Risk Factor** B

**Contraindications** Known hypersensitivity to pyrethyroid, pyrethrin, or chrysanthemums; lotion is contraindicated for use in infants <2 months of age

**Warnings/Precautions** Treatment may temporarily exacerbate the symptoms of itching, redness, swelling; for external use only; use during pregnancy only if clearly needed

**Adverse Reactions** 1% to 10%:

Dermatologic: Pruritus, erythema, rash of the scalp

Local: Burning, stinging, tingling, numbness or scalp discomfort, edema

**Drug Interactions** No data reported

**Usual Dosage** Topical:

Head lice: Children >2 months and Adults: After hair has been washed with shampoo, rinsed with water, and towel dried, apply a sufficient volume of topical liquid (lotion or cream rinse) to saturate the hair and scalp. Leave on hair for 10 minutes before rinsing off with water; remove remaining nits; may repeat in 1 week if lice or nits still present.

Scabies: Apply cream from head to toe; leave on for 8-14 hours before washing off with water; for infants, also apply on the hairline, neck, scalp, temple, and forehead; may reapply in 1 week if live mites appear

Permethrin 5% cream was shown to be safe and effective when applied to an infant <1 month of age with neonatal scabies; time of application was limited to 6 hours before rinsing with soap and water

**Patient Information** For external use only. Do not apply to face and avoid contact with eyes or mucous membrane. Clothing and bedding must be washed in hot water or dry cleaned to kill nits. May need to treat all members of household and all sexual contacts concurrently. Wash all combs and brushes with permethrin and thoroughly rinse.

**Administration:**

Cream rinse/lotion: Apply immediately after hair is shampooed, rinsed, and towel-dried. Apply enough to saturate hair and scalp (especially behind ears and on nape of neck). Leave on hair for 10 minutes before rinsing with water. Remove nits with fine-tooth comb. May repeat in 1 week if lice or nits are still present.

Cream: Apply from neck to toes. Bathe to remove drug after 8-14 hours before washing off. Repeat in 7 days if lice or nits are still present. Report if condition persists or infection occurs.

**Dosage Forms**

Cream: 5% (60 g)

Liquid, topical: 1% (60 mL)

- **Permitil® Oral** *see* Fluphenazine *on page 234*
- **Peroxin A5®** *see* Benzoyl Peroxide *on page 62*
- **Peroxin A10®** *see* Benzoyl Peroxide *on page 62*

## Perphenazine (per FEN a zeen)

**Related Information**

Antipsychotic Agents Comparison Chart *on page 706*

Antipsychotic Medication Guidelines *on page 751*

Clinical Issues in the Use of Antipsychotics *on page 630*

Discontinuation of Psychotropic Drugs - Withdrawal Symptoms and Recommendations *on page 798*

Federal OBRA Regulations Recommended Maximum Doses *on page 756*

Patient Information - Antipsychotics (General) *on page 646*

Schizophrenia *on page 604*

**Generic Available** Yes

**U.S. Brand Names** Trilafon®

**Canadian Brand Names** Apo®-Perphenazine; PMS-Perphenazine

**Pharmacologic Category** Antipsychotic Agent, Phenothazine, Piperazine

**Use** Management of manifestations of psychotic disorders; nausea and vomiting

**Pregnancy Risk Factor** C

**Contraindications** Hypersensitivity to perphenazine or any component (cross reactivity between phenothiazines may occur); severe CNS depression, subcortical brain damage, bone marrow suppression, blood dyscrasias, and coma

**Warnings/Precautions** May cause hypotension, particularly with parenteral administration. May be sedating, use with caution in disorders where CNS depression is a feature. Use with caution in Parkinson's disease. Caution in patients with hemodynamic instability; predisposition to seizures; severe cardiac, hepatic, renal, or respiratory disease. Esophageal dysmotility and aspiration have been associated with antipsychotic use - use with caution in patients at risk of pneumonia (ie, Alzheimer's disease). Caution in breast cancer or other prolactin-dependent tumors (may elevate prolactin levels). May alter temperature regulation or mask toxicity of other drugs due to antiemetic effects. May alter cardiac conduction - life-threatening arrhythmias have occurred with therapeutic doses of phenothiazines. May cause orthostatic hypotension - use with caution in patients at risk of this effect or those who would tolerate transient hypotensive episodes (cerebrovascular disease, cardiovascular disease, or other medications which may predispose).

Phenothiazines may cause anticholinergic effects (confusion, agitation, constipation, dry mouth, blurred vision, urinary retention); therefore, they should be used with caution in patients with decreased gastrointestinal motility, urinary retention, BPH, xerostomia, or visual problems. Conditions which also may be exacerbated by cholinergic blockade include narrow-angle glaucoma (screening is recommended) and worsening of myasthenia gravis. Relative to other neuroleptics, perphenazine has a low potency of cholinergic blockade.

May cause extrapyramidal reactions, including pseudoparkinsonism, acute dystonic reactions, akathisia, and tardive dyskinesia (risk of these reactions is moderate-high relative to other neuroleptics). May be associated with neuroleptic malignant syndrome (NMS) or pigmentary retinopathy.

**Adverse Reactions**

Cardiovascular: Hypotension, orthostatic hypotension, hypertension, tachycardia, bradycardia, dizziness, cardiac arrest

Central nervous system: Extrapyramidal signs (pseudoparkinsonism, akathisia, dystonias, tardive dyskinesia), dizziness, cerebral edema, seizures, headache, drowsiness, paradoxical excitement, restlessness, hyperactivity, insomnia, neuroleptic malignant syndrome (NMS), impairment of temperature regulation

Dermatologic: Increased sensitivity to sun, rash, discoloration of skin (blue-gray)

Endocrine & metabolic: Hypoglycemia, hyperglycemia, galactorrhea, lactation, breast enlargement, gynecomastia, menstrual irregularity, amenorrhea, SIADH, changes in libido

Gastrointestinal: Constipation, weight gain, vomiting, stomach pain, nausea, xerostomia, salivation, diarrhea, anorexia, ileus

Genitourinary: Difficulty in urination, ejaculatory disturbances, incontinence, polyuria, ejaculating dysfunction, priapism

Hematologic: Agranulocytosis, leukopenia, eosinophilia, hemolytic anemia, thrombocytopenic purpura, pancytopenia

Hepatic: Cholestatic jaundice, hepatotoxicity

Neuromuscular & skeletal: Tremor

Ocular: Pigmentary retinopathy, blurred vision, cornea and lens changes

Respiratory: Nasal congestion

Miscellaneous: Diaphoresis

**Overdosage/Toxicology**

Signs and symptoms: Deep sleep, dystonia, agitation, coma, abnormal involuntary muscle movements, hypotension, arrhythmias

Treatment:

Following initiation of essential overdose management, toxic symptom treatment and supportive treatment should be initiated

Hypotension usually responds to I.V. fluids or Trendelenburg positioning. If unresponsive to these measures, the use of a parenteral inotrope may be required (eg, norepinephrine 0.1-0.2 mcg/kg/minute titrated to response).

Seizures commonly respond to diazepam (I.V. 5-10 mg bolus in adults every 15 minutes if needed up to a total of 30 mg; I.V. 0.25-0.4 mg/kg/dose up to a total of 10 mg in children) or to phenytoin or phenobarbital

Extrapyramidal symptoms (eg, dystonic reactions) may be managed with diphenhydramine or benztropine mesylate.

**Drug Interactions** CYP2D6 enzyme substrate; CYP2D6 enzyme inhibitor

Aluminum salts: May decrease the absorption of phenothiazines; monitor

Amphetamines: Efficacy may be diminished by antipsychotics; in addition, amphetamines may increase psychotic symptoms; avoid concurrent use

Anticholinergics: May inhibit the therapeutic response to phenothiazines and excess anticholinergic effects may occur; includes benztropine, trihexyphenidyl, biperiden, and drugs with significant anticholinergic activity (TCAs, antihistamines, disopyramide)

Antihypertensives: Concurrent use of phenothiazines with an antihypertensive may produce additive hypotensive effects (particularly orthostasis)

Bromocriptine: Phenothiazines inhibit the ability of bromocriptine to lower serum prolactin concentrations

CNS depressants: Sedative effects may be additive with phenothiazines; monitor for increased effect; includes barbiturates, benzodiazepines, narcotic analgesics, ethanol, and other sedative agents

CYP2D6 inhibitors: Metabolism of phenothiazines may be decreased; increasing clinical effect or toxicity; inhibitors include amiodarone, cimetidine, delavirdine, fluoxetine, paroxetine, propafenone, quinidine, and ritonavir; monitor for increased effect/toxicity

Enzyme inducers: May enhance the hepatic metabolism of phenothiazines; larger doses may be required; includes rifampin, rifabutin, barbiturates, phenytoin, and cigarette smoking

Epinephrine: Chlorpromazine (and possibly other low potency antipsychotics) may diminish the pressor effects of epinephrine

Guanethidine and guanadrel: Antihypertensive effects may be inhibited by phenothiazines

Levodopa: Phenothiazines may inhibit the antiparkinsonian effect of levodopa; avoid this combination

Lithium: Phenothiazines may produce neurotoxicity with lithium; this is a rare effect

Phenytoin: May reduce serum levels of phenothiazines; phenothiazines may increase phenytoin serum levels

Propranolol: Serum concentrations of phenothiazines may be increased; propranolol also increases phenothiazine concentrations

Polypeptide antibiotics: Rare cases of respiratory paralysis have been reported with concurrent use of phenothiazines

QTc prolonging agents: Effects on QTc interval may be additive with phenothiazines, increasing the risk of malignant arrhythmias; includes type Ia antiarrhythmics, TCAs, and some quinolone antibiotics (sparfloxacin, moxifloxacin, and gatifloxacin)

Sulfadoxine-pyrimethamine: May increase phenothiazine concentrations

Tricyclic antidepressants: Concurrent use may produce increased toxicity or altered therapeutic response

Trazodone: Phenothiazines and trazodone may produce additive hypotensive effects

Valproic acid: Serum levels may be increased by phenothiazines

**Stability** Do not mix with beverages containing caffeine (coffee, cola), tannins (tea), or pectinates (apple juice) since physical incompatibility exists; use ~60 mL diluent for each 5 mL of concentrate; protect all dosage forms from light; clear or slightly yellow solutions may be used; should be dispensed in amber or opaque vials/bottles. Solutions may be diluted or mixed with fruit juices or other liquids but must be administered immediately after mixing; do not prepare bulk dilutions or store bulk dilutions.

**Mechanism of Action** Blocks postsynaptic mesolimbic dopaminergic receptors in the brain; exhibits alpha-adrenergic blocking effect and depresses the release of hypothalamic and hypophyseal hormones

**Pharmacodynamics/kinetics**

Absorption: Oral: Well absorbed

Distribution: Crosses the placenta

Metabolism: In the liver

Half-life: 9 hours

Time to peak serum concentration: Within 4-8 hours

Elimination: In urine and bile

**Usual Dosage**

Children:

Psychoses: Oral:

1-6 years: 4-6 mg/day in divided doses

6-12 years: 6 mg/day in divided doses

>12 years: 4-16 mg 2-4 times/day

I.M.: 5 mg every 6 hours

Nausea/vomiting: I.M.: 5 mg every 6 hours

Adults:

Psychoses:

Oral: 4-16 mg 2-4 times/day not to exceed 64 mg/day

I.M.: 5 mg every 6 hours up to 15 mg/day in ambulatory patients and 30 mg/day in hospitalized patients

Nausea/vomiting:

Oral: 8-16 mg/day in divided doses up to 24 mg/day

I.M.: 5-10 mg every 6 hours as necessary up to 15 mg/day in ambulatory patients and 30 mg/day in hospitalized patients

I.V. (severe): 1 mg at 1- to 2-minute intervals up to a total of 5 mg

Hemodialysis: Not dialyzable (0% to 5%)

**Dosing adjustment in hepatic impairment:** Dosage reductions should be considered in patients with liver disease although no specific guidelines are available

**Dietary Considerations** Alcohol: Additive CNS effect, avoid use

**Administration** Dilute oral concentration to at least 2 oz with water, juice, or milk; for I.V. use, injection should be diluted to at least 0.5 mg/mL with NS and given at a rate of 1 mg/minute; observe for tremor and abnormal movements or posturing

**Monitoring Parameters** Cardiac, blood pressure (hypotension when administering I.M. or I.V.); respiratory status

**Reference Range** 2-6 nmol/L

**Test Interactions** ↑ cholesterol (S), glucose; ↓ uric acid (S); false-positive pregnancy test

**Patient Information** May cause drowsiness, impair judgment and coordination; report any feelings of restlessness or any involuntary movements; avoid alcohol and other CNS depressants; do not alter dose or discontinue without consulting physician

**Nursing Implications** Dilute oral concentration to at least 2 oz with water, juice, or milk; for I.V. use, injection should be diluted to at least 0.5 mg/mL with normal saline and given at a rate of 1 mg/minute; monitor for hypotension when administering I.M. or I.V. during the first 3-5 days after initiating therapy or making a dosage adjustment

**Additional Information** Coadministration of two or more antipsychotics does not improve clinical response and may increase the potential for adverse effects

**Dosage Forms**

Concentrate, oral: 16 mg/5 mL (118 mL)

Injection: 5 mg/mL (1 mL)

Tablet: 2 mg, 4 mg, 8 mg, 16 mg

- **Perphenazine and Amitriptyline** *see* Amitriptyline and Perphenazine *on page 34*
- **Persa-Gel®** *see* Benzoyl Peroxide *on page 62*
- **Persantine®** *see* Dipyridamole *on page 176*
- **Personality Disorders** *see page 625*
- **Perspectives on the Safety of Herbal Medicines** *see page 736*
- **Pertussin® CS [OTC]** *see* Dextromethorphan *on page 160*
- **Pertussin® ES [OTC]** *see* Dextromethorphan *on page 160*
- **Pethidine Hydrochloride** *see* Meperidine *on page 341*
- **PETN** *see* Pentaerythritol Tetranitrate *on page 426*
- **Pfizerpen®** *see* Penicillin G, Parenteral, Aqueous *on page 425*
- **$PGE_2$** *see* Dinoprostone *on page 173*
- **$PGF_{2\alpha}$** *see* Dinoprost Tromethamine *on page 174*
- **Phanatuss® Cough Syrup [OTC]** *see* Guaifenesin and Dextromethorphan *on page 257*
- **Pharmacokinetics of Selective Serotonin-Reuptake Inhibitors (SSRIs)** *see page 723*
- **Pharmacotherapy of Urinary Incontinence** *see page 758*
- **Phazyme® [OTC]** *see* Simethicone *on page 512*
- **Phenadex® Senior [OTC]** *see* Guaifenesin and Dextromethorphan *on page 257*
- **Phenahist-TR®** *see* Chlorpheniramine, Phenylephrine, Phenylpropanolamine, and Belladonna Alkaloids *on page 115*
- **Phenameth® DM** *see* Promethazine and Dextromethorphan *on page 471*
- **Phenantoin** *see* Mephenytoin *on page 341*
- **Phenaphen® With Codeine** *see* Acetaminophen and Codeine *on page 14*
- **Phenazine®** *see* Promethazine *on page 470*

## Phenazopyridine (fen az oh PEER i deen)

**U.S. Brand Names** Azo-Standard® [OTC]; Baridium® [OTC]; Prodium™ [OTC]; Pyridiate®; Pyridium®; Urodine®; Urogesic®

**Canadian Brand Names** Phenazo; Pyronium®; Vito Reins®

**Pharmacologic Category** Analgesic, Urinary

**Use** Symptomatic relief of urinary burning, itching, frequency and urgency in association with urinary tract infection or following urologic procedures

**Effects on Mental Status** May cause dizziness

**Effects on Psychiatric Treatment** None reported

**Pregnancy Risk Factor** B

(Continued)

## Phenazopyridine *(Continued)*

**Contraindications** Hypersensitivity to phenazopyridine or any component; kidney or liver disease

**Warnings/Precautions** Does not treat infection, acts only as an analgesic; drug should be discontinued if skin or sclera develop a yellow color; use with caution in patients with renal impairment. Use of this agent in the elderly is limited since accumulation of phenazopyridine can occur in patients with renal insufficiency. It should not be used in patients with a $Cl_{cr}$ <50 mL/minute.

**Adverse Reactions**

1% to 10%:

Central nervous system: Headache, dizziness

Gastrointestinal: Stomach cramps

<1%: Acute renal failure, hemolytic anemia, hepatitis, methemoglobinemia, rash, skin pigmentation, vertigo

**Overdosage/Toxicology**

Signs and symptoms: Methemoglobinemia, hemolytic anemia, skin pigmentation, renal and hepatic impairment

Treatment: Antidote is methylene blue 1-2 mg/kg I.V. for methemoglobinemia

**Drug Interactions** No data reported

**Usual Dosage** Oral:

Children: 12 mg/kg/day in 3 divided doses administered after meals for 2 days

Adults: 100-200 mg 3 times/day after meals for 2 days when used concomitantly with an antibacterial agent

**Dosing interval in renal impairment:**

$Cl_{cr}$ 50-80 mL/minute: Administer every 8-16 hours

$Cl_{cr}$ <50 mL/minute: Avoid use

**Patient Information** Take prescribed dose after meals. May discolor urine (orange/yellow) or feces (orange/red); this is normal but will stain fabric. Report persistent headache, dizziness, or stomach cramping.

**Dosage Forms** Tablet, as hydrochloride:

Azo-Standard®, Prodium™: 95 mg

Baridium®, Geridium®, Pyridiate®, Pyridium®, Urodine®, Urogesic®: 100 mg

Geridium®, Phenazodine®, Pyridium®, Urodine®: 200 mg

♦ **Phenchlor® S.H.A.** *see* Chlorpheniramine, Phenylephrine, Phenylpropanolamine, and Belladonna Alkaloids *on page 115*

## Phencyclidine (fen SYE kli deen)

**Related Information**

Hallucinogenic Drugs *on page 713*

Substance-Related Disorders *on page 609*

**Pharmacologic Category** General Anesthetic

**Effects on Mental Status** May cause paranoia, bizarre or violent behavior, or psychosis

**Effects on Psychiatric Treatment** May counteract the therapeutic effects of the antipsychotics

**Pregnancy/Breast-Feeding Implications** Neonatal irritability, hypertonia, tremors

**Adverse Reactions**

Cardiovascular: Tachycardia, pericardial effusion/pericarditis, sinus tachycardia

Central nervous system: Violent behavior, psychosis, paranoia, hallucinations, ataxia, synesthesia, dysphoria, sympathetic storm

Endocrine & metabolic: Hypoglycemia

Gastrointestinal: Vomiting

Ocular: Nystagmus, lacrimation, mydriasis (miosis in children)

**Overdosage/Toxicology**

Symptoms of overdose: Myoglobinuria, fear, hyperuricemia, mania, delirium, hyperacusis, lacrimation, insomnia, ptosis, hypoglycemia, myopathy, impotence, fasciculations, depression, encephalopathy, hyperthermia, headache, rhabdomyolysis, fever, coma, sweating, respiratory depression, hypothermia, seizures, hypertension, tachycardia, myoclonus

Treatment: Supportive therapy; benzodiazepine for agitation; haloperidol (5 mg I.M.) improves psychotic symptoms; rhabdomyolysis can be treated with I.V. hydration, alkalinization, and mannitol; lorazepam or diazepam can be used to calm and sedate the patient

**Mechanism of Action** Related to ketamine, PCP is an arylcyclohexylamine which stimulates alpha-adrenergic receptors

**Pharmacodynamics/kinetics**

Distribution: $V_d$: 6.2 L/kg

Protein binding: 60% to 70%

Metabolism: Hepatic by oxidative hydroxylation

Half-life: 1 hour (in overdose: 17.6 hours)

Elimination: Renal (33 mL/minute)

**Usual Dosage** Joints are 100-400 mg PCP by weight; tablets are ~5 mg

**Reference Range**

Catatonia and excitation: 20-30 ng/mL

Myoclonus and coma: 30-100 ng/mL

Hypotension, seizures, fatalities: >100 ng/mL

Urinary levels do not correlate with clinical symptoms

In the postmortem state, anatomical site concentration differences (ie, postmortem redistribution) may occur.

**Test Interactions** Adulteration with bleach can cause false-negative urine immunoassays; doxylamine can cause a false-positive urine gas chromatographic result; dextromethorphan or diphenhydramine can give a false-positive on an immunoassay screen; ketamine is not expected to give a positive immunoassay on most systems

♦ **Phendry® Oral [OTC]** *see* Diphenhydramine *on page 174*

## Phenelzine (FEN el zeen)

**Related Information**

Antidepressant Agents Comparison Chart *on page 704*

Clinical Issues in the Use of Antidepressants *on page 627*

Mood Disorders *on page 600*

Patient Information - Antidepressants (MAOIs) *on page 644*

Teratogenic Risks of Psychotropic Medications *on page 812*

**Generic Available** No

**U.S. Brand Names** Nardil®

**Synonyms** Phenelzine Sulfate

**Pharmacologic Category** Antidepressant, Monoamine Oxidase Inhibitor

**Use** Symptomatic treatment of atypical, nonendogenous, or neurotic depression

**Pregnancy Risk Factor** C

**Contraindications** Hypersensitivity to phenelzine; uncontrolled hypertension; pheochromocytoma; hepatic disease; congestive heart failure; concurrent use of sympathomimetics (and related compounds), CNS depressants, ethanol, meperidine, bupropion, buspirone, guanethidine, serotonergic drugs (including SSRIs) - do not use within 5 weeks of fluoxetine discontinuation or 2 weeks of other antidepressant discontinuation; general anesthesia, local vasoconstrictors; spinal anesthesia (hypotension may be exaggerated). Foods with a high content of tyramine, tryptophan, or dopamine, chocolate, or caffeine.

**Warnings/Precautions** Safety in children <16 years of age has not been established; use with caution in patients who are hyperactive, hyperexcitable, or who have glaucoma, hyperthyroidism, suicidal tendencies, or diabetes; avoid use of meperidine within 2 weeks of phenelzine use. Hypertensive crisis may occur with tyramine, tryptophan, or dopamine-containing foods. Should not be used in combination with other antidepressants. Hypotensive effects of antihypertensives (beta-blockers, thiazides) may be exaggerated. Use with caution in depressed patients at risk of suicide. May cause orthostatic hypotension - use with caution in patients with hypotension or patients who would not tolerate transient hypotensive episodes (cardiovascular or cerebrovascular disease) - effects may be additive with other agents which cause orthostasis. Has been associated with activation of hypomania and/or mania in bipolar patients. May worsen psychotic symptoms in some patients. Use with caution in patients at risk of seizures, or in patients receiving other drugs which may lower seizure threshold. Toxic reactions have occurred with dextromethorphan. Discontinue at least 48 hours prior to myelography.

The MAO inhibitors are effective and generally well tolerated by older patients. It is the potential interactions with tyramine or tryptophan-containing foods and other drugs, and their effects on blood pressure that have limited their use.

**Adverse Reactions**

Cardiovascular: Orthostatic hypotension, edema

Central nervous system: Dizziness, headache, drowsiness, sleep disturbances, fatigue, hyper-reflexia, twitching, ataxia, mania

Dermatologic: Rash, pruritus

Endocrine & metabolic: Decreased sexual ability (anorgasmia, ejaculatory disturbances, impotence), hypernatremia, hypermetabolic syndrome

Gastrointestinal: Xerostomia, constipation, weight gain

Genitourinary: Urinary retention

Hematologic: Leukopenia

Hepatic: Hepatitis

Neuromuscular & skeletal: Weakness, tremor, myoclonus

Ocular: Blurred vision, glaucoma

Miscellaneous: Diaphoresis

**Overdosage/Toxicology**

Signs and symptoms: Tachycardia, palpitations, muscle twitching, seizures, insomnia, restlessness, transient hypertension, hypotension, drowsiness, hyperpyrexia, coma

Treatment: Competent supportive care is the most important treatment for an overdose with a monoamine oxidase (MAO) inhibitor. Both hypertension or hypotension can occur with intoxication. Hypotension may respond to I.V. fluids or vasopressors and hypertension usually responds to an alpha-adrenergic blocker. While treating the hypertension, care is warranted to avoid sudden drops in blood pressure, since this may worsen the MAO inhibitor toxicity. Muscle irritability and seizures often respond to diazepam, while hyperthermia is best treated antipyretics and cooling blankets. Cardiac arrhythmias are best treated with phenytoin or procainamide.

**Drug Interactions**

Amphetamines: MAOIs in combination with amphetamines may result in severe hypertensive reaction; these combinations are best avoided

Anorexiants: Concurrent use of anorexiants may result in serotonin syndrome; these combinations are best avoided; includes dexfenfluramine, fenfluramine, or sibutramine

Barbiturates: MAOIs may inhibit the metabolism of barbiturates and prolong their effect

CNS stimulants: MAOIs in combination with stimulants (methylphenidate) may result in severe hypertensive reaction; these combinations are best avoided

Dextromethorphan: Concurrent use of MAOIs may result in serotonin syndrome; these combinations are best avoided

Disulfiram: MAOIs may produce delirium in patients receiving disulfiram; monitor

Guanadrel and guanethidine: MAOIs inhibit the antihypertensive response to guanadrel or guanethidine; use an alternative antihypertensive agent

Hypoglycemic agents: MAOIs may produce hypoglycemia in patients with diabetes; monitor

Levodopa: MAOIs in combination with levodopa may result in hypertensive reactions; monitor

Lithium: MAOIs in combination with lithium have resulted in malignant hyperpyrexia; this combination is best avoided

Meperidine: May cause serotonin syndrome when combined with an MAO inhibitor; avoid this combination

Nefazodone: Concurrent use of MAOIs may result in serotonin syndrome; these combinations are best avoided

Norepinephrine: MAOIs may increase the pressor response of norepinephrine (effect is generally small); monitor

Reserpine: MAOIs in combination with reserpine may result in hypertensive reactions; monitor

Serotonin agonists: Theoretically may increase the risk of serotonin syndrome; includes sumatriptan, naratriptan, rizatriptan, and zolmitriptan

SSRIs: May cause serotonin syndrome when combined with an MAO inhibitor; avoid this combination

Succinylcholine: MAOIs may prolong the muscle relaxation produced by succinylcholine via decreased plasma pseudocholinesterase

Sympathomimetics (indirect-acting): MAOIs in combination with sympathomimetics such as dopamine, metaraminol, phenylephrine, and decongestants (pseudoephedrine) may result in severe hypertensive reaction; these combinations are best avoided

Tramadol: May increase the risk of seizures and serotonin syndrome in patients receiving an MAOI

Trazodone: Concurrent use of MAOIs may result in serotonin syndrome; these combinations are best avoided

Tricyclic antidepressants: May cause serotonin syndrome when combined with an MAO inhibitor; avoid this combination

Tyramine: Foods (eg, cheese) and beverages (eg, ethanol) containing tyramine, should be avoided in patients receiving an MAOI; hypertensive crisis may result

Venlafaxine: Concurrent use of MAOIs may result in serotonin syndrome; these combinations are best avoided

**Stability** Protect from light

**Mechanism of Action** Thought to act by increasing endogenous concentrations of norepinephrine, dopamine, and serotonin through inhibition of the enzyme (monoamine oxidase) responsible for the breakdown of these neurotransmitters

**Pharmacodynamics/kinetics**

Onset of action: Within 2-4 weeks

Absorption: Oral: Well absorbed

Duration: May continue to have a therapeutic effect and interactions 2 weeks after discontinuing therapy

Elimination: In urine primarily as metabolites and unchanged drug

**Usual Dosage** Oral:

Adults: 15 mg 3 times/day; may increase to 60-90 mg/day during early phase of treatment, then reduce to dose for maintenance therapy slowly after maximum benefit is obtained; takes 2-4 weeks for a significant response to occur

Elderly: Initial: 7.5 mg/day; increase by 7.5-15 mg/day every 3-4 days as tolerated; usual therapeutic dose: 15-60 mg/day in 3-4 divided doses

**Dietary Considerations**

Alcohol: Additive CNS effect, avoid use

Food: Avoid tyramine-containing foods

**Monitoring Parameters** Blood pressure, heart rate, diet, weight, mood (if depressive symptoms)

**Reference Range** Inhibition of platelet monoamine oxidase (≥80%) correlates with clinical response

**Test Interactions** ↓ glucose; ↑ serum transaminases

**Patient Information** Avoid tyramine-containing foods: red wine, cheese (except cottage, ricotta, and cream), smoked or pickled fish, beef or chicken liver, dried sausage, fava or broad bean pods, yeast vitamin supplements; do not begin any prescription or OTC medications without consulting your physician or pharmacist; may take as long as 3 weeks to see effects

**Nursing Implications** Watch for postural hypotension; monitor blood pressure carefully, especially at therapy onset or if other CNS drugs or cardiovascular drugs are added; check for dietary and drug restriction

**Additional Information** Pyridoxine deficiency has occurred; symptoms include numbness and edema of hands; may respond to supplementation

The MAO inhibitors are usually reserved for patients who do not tolerate or respond to other antidepressants. The brain activity of monoamine oxidase increases with age and even more so in patients with Alzheimer's disease. Therefore, the MAO inhibitors may have an increased role in patients with Alzheimer's disease who are depressed. Phenelzine is less stimulating than tranylcypromine.

**Dosage Forms** Tablet, as sulfate: 15 mg


- **Phenelzine Sulfate** *see* Phenelzine *on page 434*
- **Phenergan®** *see* Promethazine *on page 470*
- **Phenergan® VC Syrup** *see* Promethazine and Phenylephrine *on page 471*
- **Phenergan® VC With Codeine** *see* Promethazine, Phenylephrine, and Codeine *on page 471*
- **Phenergan® With Codeine** *see* Promethazine and Codeine *on page 471*
- **Phenergan® With Dextromethorphan** *see* Promethazine and Dextromethorphan *on page 471*
- **Phenhist® Expectorant** *see* Guaifenesin, Pseudoephedrine, and Codeine *on page 258*


## Pheniramine, Phenylpropanolamine, and Pyrilamine

(fen EER a meen, fen il proe pa NOLE a meen, & peer IL a meen)

**U.S. Brand Names** Triaminic® Oral Infant Drops

**Pharmacologic Category** Antihistamine/Decongestant Combination

**Use** Symptomatic relief of nasal congestion and postnasal drip as well as allergic rhinitis

**Effects on Mental Status** May cause dizziness, restlessness, anxiety, or insomnia

**Effects on Psychiatric Treatment** Concurrent use with MAOIs may result in hypertensive crisis; avoid combination

**Usual Dosage**

Infants <1 year: Drops: 0.05 mL/kg/dose 4 times/day

Children: Syrup:

- <1 year: 0.4 mL/kg/dose 4 times/day
- 1-6 years: 2.5 mL/dose every 4 hours
- 6-12 years: 5 mL dose every 4 hours

**Dosage Forms** Drops: Pheniramine maleate 10 mg, phenylpropanolamine hydrochloride 20 mg, and pyrilamine maleate 10 mg per mL (15 mL)

## Phenobarbital (fee noe BAR bi tal)

**Related Information**

Anticonvulsants by Seizures Type *on page 703*

Epilepsy Treatment *on page 783*

Patient Information - Anxiolytics & Sedative Hypnotics (Barbiturates) *on page 654*

Serum Drug Concentrations Commonly Monitored: Guidelines *on page 759*

Substance-Related Disorders *on page 609*

**Generic Available** Yes

**U.S. Brand Names** Barbita®; Luminal®; Solfoton®

**Canadian Brand Names** Barbilixir®

**Synonyms** Phenobarbital Sodium; Phenobarbitone; Phenylethylmalonylurea

**Pharmacologic Category** Anticonvulsant, Barbiturate; Barbiturate

**Use** Management of generalized tonic-clonic (grand mal) and partial seizures; sedative

**Unlabeled uses:** Febrile seizures in children; may also be used for prevention and treatment of neonatal hyperbilirubinemia and lowering of bilirubin in chronic cholestasis; neonatal seizures; management of sedative/hypnotic withdrawal

**Restrictions** C-IV

**Pregnancy Risk Factor** D

**Pregnancy/Breast-Feeding Implications**

Clinical effects on the fetus: Crosses the placenta. Cardiac defect reported; hemorrhagic disease of newborn due to fetal vitamin K depletion may occur; may induce maternal folic acid deficiency; withdrawal symptoms observed in infant following delivery. Epilepsy itself, number of medications, genetic factors, or a combination of these probably influence the teratogenicity of anticonvulsant therapy. Benefit:risk ratio usually favors continued use during pregnancy and breast-feeding.

Breast-feeding/Lactation: Crosses into breast milk

(Continued)

## Phenobarbital *(Continued)*

Clinical effects on the infant: Sedation; withdrawal with abrupt weaning reported. American Academy of Pediatrics recommends **use with caution.**

**Contraindications** Hypersensitivity to barbiturates or any component of the formulation; marked hepatic impairment; dyspnea or airway obstruction; porphyria

**Warnings/Precautions** Potential for drug dependency exists, abrupt cessation may precipitate withdrawal, including status epilepticus in epileptic patients. Do not administer to patients in acute pain. Use caution in elderly, debilitated, renally or hepatic dysfunction, and pediatric patients. May cause paradoxical responses, including agitation and hyperactivity, particularly in acute pain and pediatric patients. Use with caution in patients with depression or suicidal tendencies, or in patients with a history of drug abuse. Tolerance, psychological and physical dependence may occur with prolonged use. May cause CNS depression, which may impair physical or mental abilities. Patients must cautioned about performing tasks which require mental alertness (ie, operating machinery or driving). Effects with other sedative drugs or ethanol may be potentiated. May cause respiratory depression or hypotension, particularly when administered intravenously. Use with caution in hemodynamically unstable patients (hypovolemic shock, CHF) or patients with respiratory disease. Due to its long half-life and risk of dependence, phenobarbital is not recommended as a sedative in the elderly. Use has been associated with cognitive deficits in children. Use with caution in patients with hypoadrenalism.

**Adverse Reactions**

Cardiovascular: Bradycardia, hypotension, syncope

Central nervous system: Drowsiness, lethargy, CNS excitation or depression, impaired judgment, "hangover" effect, confusion, somnolence, agitation, hyperkinesia, ataxia, nervousness, headache, insomnia, nightmares, hallucinations, anxiety, dizziness

Dermatologic: Rash, exfoliative dermatitis, Stevens-Johnson syndrome

Gastrointestinal: Nausea, vomiting, constipation

Hematologic: Agranulocytosis, thrombocytopenia, megaloblastic anemia

Local: Pain at injection site, thrombophlebitis with I.V. use

Renal: Oliguria

Respiratory: Laryngospasm, respiratory depression, apnea (especially with rapid I.V. use), hypoventilation, apnea

Miscellaneous: Gangrene with inadvertent intra-arterial injection

**Overdosage/Toxicology**

Signs and symptoms: Unsteady gait, slurred speech, confusion, jaundice, hypothermia, hypotension, respiratory depression, coma

Treatment: If hypotension occurs, administer I.V. fluids and place the patient in the Trendelenburg position. If unresponsive, an I.V. vasopressor (eg, dopamine, epinephrine) may be required.

Repeated oral doses of activated charcoal significantly reduce the half-life of phenobarbital resulting from an enhancement of nonrenal elimination. The usual dose is 0.1-1 g/kg every 4-6 hours for 3-4 days unless the patient has no bowel movement causing the charcoal to remain in the GI tract. Assure adequate hydration and renal function. Urinary alkalinization with I.V. sodium bicarbonate also helps to enhance elimination. Hemodialysis or hemoperfusion is of uncertain value. Patients in stage IV coma due to high serum barbiturate levels may require charcoal hemoperfusion.

**Drug Interactions** CYP1A2, 2C, 3A3/4, and 3A5-7 inducer

**Note:** Barbiturates are enzyme inducers; patients should be monitored when these drugs are started or stopped for a decreased or increased therapeutic effect respectively

Acetaminophen: Barbiturates may enhance the hepatotoxic potential of acetaminophen overdoses

Antiarrhythmics: Barbiturates may increase the metabolism of antiarrhythmics, decreasing their clinical effect; includes disopyramide, propafenone, and quinidine

Anticonvulsants: Barbiturates may increase the metabolism of anticonvulsants; includes ethosuximide, felbamate (possibly), lamotrigine, phenytoin, tiagabine, topiramate, and zonisamide; does not appear to affect gabapentin or levetiracetam

Antineoplastics: Limited evidence suggests that enzyme-inducing anticonvulsant therapy may reduce the effectiveness of some chemotherapy regimens (specifically in ALL); teniposide and methotrexate may be cleared more rapidly in these patients

Antipsychotics: Barbiturates may enhance the metabolism (decrease the efficacy) of antipsychotics; monitor for altered response; dose adjustment may be needed

Beta-blockers: Metabolism of beta-blockers may be increased and clinical effect decreased; atenolol and nadolol are unlikely to interact given their renal elimination

Calcium channel blockers: Barbiturates may enhance the metabolism of calcium channel blockers, decreasing their clinical effect

Chloramphenicol: Barbiturates may increase the metabolism of chloramphenicol and chloramphenicol may inhibit barbiturate metabolism; monitor for altered response

Cimetidine: Barbiturates may enhance the metabolism of cimetidine, decreasing its clinical effect

CNS depressants: Sedative effects and/or respiratory depression with barbiturates may be additive with other CNS depressants; monitor for increased effect; includes ethanol, sedatives, antidepressants, narcotic analgesics, and benzodiazepines

Corticosteroids: Barbiturates may enhance the metabolism of corticosteroids, decreasing their clinical effect

Cyclosporine: Levels may be decreased by barbiturates; monitor

Doxycycline: Barbiturates may enhance the metabolism of doxycycline, decreasing its clinical effect; higher dosages may be required

Estrogens: Barbiturates may increase the metabolism of estrogens and reduce their efficacy

Felbamate may inhibit the metabolism of barbiturates and barbiturates may increase the metabolism of felbamate

Griseofulvin: Barbiturates may impair the absorption of griseofulvin, and griseofulvin metabolism may be increased by barbiturates, decreasing clinical effect

Guanfacine: Effect may be decreased by barbiturates

Immunosuppressants: Barbiturates may enhance the metabolism of immunosuppressants, decreasing its clinical effect; includes both cyclosporine and tacrolimus

Loop diuretics: Metabolism may be increased and clinical effects decreased; established for furosemide, effect with other loop diuretics not established

MAOIs: Metabolism of barbiturates may be inhibited, increasing clinical effect or toxicity of the barbiturates

Methadone: Barbiturates may enhance the metabolism of methadone resulting in methadone withdrawal

Methoxyflurane: Barbiturates may enhance the nephrotoxic effects of methoxyflurane

Oral contraceptives: Barbiturates may enhance the metabolism of oral contraceptives, decreasing their clinical effect; an alternative method of contraception should be considered

Theophylline: Barbiturates may increase metabolism of theophylline derivatives and decrease their clinical effect

Tricyclic antidepressants: Barbiturates may increase metabolism of tricyclic antidepressants and decrease their clinical effect; sedative effects may be additive

Valproic acid: Metabolism of barbiturates may be inhibited by valproic acid; monitor for excessive sedation; a dose reduction may be needed

Warfarin: Barbiturates inhibit the hypoprothrombinemic effects of oral anticoagulants via increased metabolism; this combination should generally be avoided

**Stability** Protect elixir from light; not stable in aqueous solutions; use only clear solutions; do not add to acidic solutions, precipitation may occur; I.V. form is **incompatible** with benzquinamide (in syringe), cephalothin, chlorpromazine, hydralazine, hydrocortisone, hydroxyzine, insulin, levorphanol, meperidine, methadone, morphine, norepinephrine, pentazocine, prochlorperazine, promazine, promethazine, ranitidine (in syringe), vancomycin

**Mechanism of Action** Short-acting barbiturate with sedative, hypnotic, and anticonvulsant properties. Barbiturates depress the sensory cortex, decrease motor activity, alter cerebellar function, and produce drowsiness, sedation, and hypnosis. In high doses, barbiturates exhibit anticonvulsant activity; barbiturates produce dose-dependent respiratory depression.

**Pharmacodynamics/kinetics**

Oral:
- Onset of hypnosis: Within 20-60 minutes
- Duration: 6-10 hours

I.V.:
- Onset of action: Within 5 minutes
- Peak effect: Within 30 minutes
- Duration: 4-10 hours

Absorption: Oral: 70% to 90%

Protein binding: 20% to 45%, decreased in neonates

Metabolism: In the liver via hydroxylation and glucuronide conjugation

Half-life:
- Neonates: 45-500 hours
- Infants: 20-133 hours
- Children: 37-73 hours
- Adults: 53-140 hours

Time to peak serum concentration: Oral: Within 1-6 hours

Elimination: 20% to 50% excreted unchanged in urine

**Usual Dosage**

Children:
- Sedation: Oral: 2 mg/kg 3 times/day
- Hypnotic: I.M., I.V., S.C.: 3-5 mg/kg at bedtime
- Preoperative sedation: Oral, I.M., I.V.: 1-3 mg/kg 1-1.5 hours before procedure

Adults:
- Sedation: Oral, I.M.: 30-120 mg/day in 2-3 divided doses
- Hypnotic: Oral, I.M., I.V., S.C.: 100-320 mg at bedtime
- Preoperative sedation: I.M.: 100-200 mg 1-1.5 hours before procedure

Anticonvulsant: Status epilepticus: **Loading dose:** I.V.:
- Infants and Children: 10-20 mg/kg in a single or divided dose; in select patients may administer additional 5 mg/kg/dose every 15-30 minutes until seizure is controlled or a total dose of 40 mg/kg is reached

Adults: 300-800 mg initially followed by 120-240 mg/dose at 20-minute intervals until seizures are controlled or a total dose of 1-2 g

Anticonvulsant maintenance dose: Oral, I.V.:

Infants: 5-8 mg/kg/day in 1-2 divided doses

Children:

1-5 years: 6-8 mg/kg/day in 1-2 divided doses

5-12 years: 4-6 mg/kg/day in 1-2 divided doses

Children >12 years and Adults: 1-3 mg/kg/day in divided doses or 50-100 mg 2-3 times/day

Withdrawal: Initial daily requirement is determined by substituting phenobarbital 30 mg for every 100 mg pentobarbital used during tolerance testing; then daily requirement is decreased by 10% of initial dose

**Dosing interval in renal impairment:** $Cl_{cr}$ <10 mL/minute: Administer every 12-16 hours

Hemodialysis: Moderately dialyzable (20% to 50%)

**Dosing adjustment/comments in hepatic disease:** Increased side effects may occur in severe liver disease; monitor plasma levels and adjust dose accordingly

**Dietary Considerations**

Alcohol: Additive CNS effect, avoid use

Food:

Protein-deficient diets: Increases duration of action of barbiturates. Should not restrict or delete protein from diet unless discussed with physician. Be consistent with protein intake during therapy with barbiturates.

Fresh fruits containing vitamin C: Displaces drug from binding sites, resulting in increased urinary excretion of barbiturate. Educate patients regarding the potential for a decreased anticonvulsant effect of barbiturates with consumption of foods high in vitamin C.

Vitamin D: Loss in vitamin D due to malabsorption; increase intake of foods rich in vitamin D. Supplementation of vitamin D may be necessary.

**Administration** Avoid rapid I.V. administration >50 mg/minute; avoid intra-arterial injection

**Monitoring Parameters** Phenobarbital serum concentrations, mental status, CBC, LFTs, seizure activity

**Reference Range**

Therapeutic:

Infants and children: 15-30 μg/mL (SI: 65-129 μmol/L)

Adults: 20-40 μg/mL (SI: 86-172 μmol/L)

Toxic: >40 μg/mL (SI: >172 μmol/L)

Toxic concentration: Slowness, ataxia, nystagmus: 35-80 μg/mL (SI: 150-344 μmol/L)

Coma with reflexes: 65-117 μg/mL (SI: 279-502 μmol/L)

Coma without reflexes: >100 μg/mL (SI: >430 μmol/L)

**Test Interactions** ↑ ammonia (B), copper (S), assay interference of LDH, LFTs; ↓ bilirubin (S)

**Patient Information** Avoid use of alcohol and other CNS depressants; avoid driving and other hazardous tasks; avoid abrupt discontinuation; may cause physical and psychological dependence; do not alter dose without notifying physician

**Nursing Implications** Parenteral solutions are highly alkaline; avoid extravasation; institute safety measures to avoid injuries; observe patient for excessive sedation and respiratory depression

**Additional Information** Injectable solutions contain propylene glycol

Sodium content of injection (65 mg, 1 mL): 6 mg (0.3 mEq)

Phenobarbital: Barbita®, Solfoton®

Phenobarbital sodium: Luminal®

**Dosage Forms**

Capsule: 16 mg

Elixir: 15 mg/5 mL (5 mL, 10 mL, 20 mL); 20 mg/5 mL (3.75 mL, 5 mL, 7.5 mL, 120 mL, 473 mL, 946 mL, 4000 mL)

Injection, as sodium: 30 mg/mL (1 mL); 60 mg/mL (1 mL); 65 mg/mL (1 mL); 130 mg/mL (1 mL)

Powder for injection: 120 mg

Tablet: 8 mg, 15 mg, 16 mg, 30 mg, 32 mg, 60 mg, 65 mg, 100 mg

♦ **Phenobarbital Sodium** *see* Phenobarbital *on page 435*

♦ **Phenobarbitone** *see* Phenobarbital *on page 435*

♦ **Phenoxine® [OTC]** *see* Phenylpropanolamine *on page 440*

## Phenoxybenzamine (fen oks ee BEN za meen)

**U.S. Brand Names** Dibenzyline®

**Pharmacologic Category** $Alpha_1$ Blockers

**Use** Symptomatic management of pheochromocytoma; treatment of hypertensive crisis caused by sympathomimetic amines

**Unlabeled use:** Micturition problems associated with neurogenic bladder, functional outlet obstruction, and partial prostate obstruction

**Effects on Mental Status** May cause sedation, confusion, or dizziness

**Effects on Psychiatric Treatment** Concurrent use with low potency antipsychotics, TCAs and MAOIs may produce additive hypotension

**Pregnancy Risk Factor** C

**Contraindications** Conditions in which a fall in blood pressure would be undesirable (eg, shock)

**Warnings/Precautions** Use with caution in patients with renal impairment, cerebral, or coronary arteriosclerosis, can exacerbate symptoms of respiratory tract infections. Because of the risk of adverse effects, avoid the use of this medication in the elderly if possible.

**Adverse Reactions**

>10%:

Cardiovascular: Postural hypotension, tachycardia, syncope

Ocular: Miosis

Respiratory: Nasal congestion

1% to 10%:

Cardiovascular: Shock

Central nervous system: Lethargy, headache, confusion, fatigue

Gastrointestinal: Vomiting, nausea, diarrhea, xerostomia

Genitourinary: Inhibition of ejaculation

Neuromuscular & skeletal: Weakness

**Overdosage/Toxicology**

Signs and symptoms: Hypotension, tachycardia, lethargy, dizziness, shock

Treatment: Hypotension and shock should be treated with fluids and by placing the patient in the Trendelenburg position; only alpha-adrenergic pressors such as norepinephrine should be used; mixed agents such as epinephrine, may cause more hypotension

**Drug Interactions**

Alpha-adrenergic agonists decrease the effect of phenoxybenzamine

Beta-blockers may result in increased toxicity (hypotension, tachycardia)

**Usual Dosage** Oral:

Children: Initial: 0.2 mg/kg (maximum: 10 mg) once daily, increase by 0.2 mg/kg increments; usual maintenance dose: 0.4-1.2 mg/kg/day every 6-8 hours, higher doses may be necessary

Adults: Initial: 10 mg twice daily, increase by 10 mg every other day until optimum dose is achieved; usual range: 20-40 mg 2-3 times/day

**Dietary Considerations** Alcohol: Avoid use

**Patient Information** Avoid alcoholic beverages; if dizziness occurs, avoid sudden changes in posture; may cause nasal congestion and constricted pupils; may inhibit ejaculation; avoid cough, cold or allergy medications containing sympathomimetics

**Nursing Implications** Monitor for orthostasis; assist with ambulation

**Dosage Forms** Capsule, as hydrochloride: 10 mg

♦ **Phenoxymethyl Penicillin** *see* Penicillin V Potassium *on page 426*

## Phensuximide (fen SUKS i mide)

**U.S. Brand Names** Milontin®

**Pharmacologic Category** Anticonvulsant, Succinimide

**Use** Control of absence (petit mal) seizures

**Contraindications** Intermittent porphyria

**Warnings/Precautions** Use with caution in patients with hepatic or renal disease; abrupt withdrawal of the drug may precipitate absence status

**Adverse Reactions**

Central nervous system: Ataxia, drowsiness, sedation, dizziness, lethargy, euphoria, headache, irritability, hyperactivity, fatigue, night terrors, disturbance in sleep, inability to concentrate, aggressiveness, mental depression, paranoid psychosis

Dermatologic: Stevens-Johnson syndrome, SLE, rash, hirsutism

Endocrine & metabolic: Increased libido

Gastrointestinal: Weight loss, gastric upset, cramps, epigastric pain, diarrhea, nausea, vomiting, anorexia, abdominal pain

Genitourinary: Vaginal bleeding, microscopic hematuria

Hematologic: Leukopenia, agranulocytosis, pancytopenia, eosinophilia

Ocular: Myopia

Miscellaneous: Hiccups

**Overdosage/Toxicology**

Signs and symptoms: Acute overdosage can cause CNS depression, ataxia, stupor, coma, hypotension; chronic overdose can cause skin rash, confusion, ataxia, proteinuria, hepatic dysfunction, hematuria

Treatment: Supportive; hemoperfusion and hemodialysis may be useful

**Drug Interactions**

CNS depressants: Sedative effects and/or respiratory depression may be additive with CNS depressants; includes ethanol, benzodiazepines, barbiturates, narcotic analgesics, and other sedative agents; monitor for increased effect

Enzyme inducers: Metabolism of succimides may be increased, decreasing their therapeutic effect; consider using an alternative sedative/hypnotic agent; potential inducers include phenobarbital, phenytoin, carbamazepine, rifampin, and rifabutin

CYP3A3/4 inhibitors: Serum level and/or toxicity of succimides may be increased; inhibitors include amiodarone, cimetidine, clarithromycin, erythromycin, delavirdine, diltiazem, dirithromycin, disulfiram, fluoxetine, fluvoxamine, grapefruit juice, indinavir, itraconazole, ketoconazole, nefazodone, nevirapine, propoxyfene, quinupristin-dalfopristin, ritonavir, saquinavir, verapamil, zafirlukast, zileuton; monitor for altered benzodiazepine response. **Use is contraindicated with amprenavir and ritonavir.**

(Continued)

## Phensuximide *(Continued)*

**Mechanism of Action** Increases the seizure threshold and suppresses paroxysmal spike-and-wave pattern in absence seizures; depresses nerve transmission in the motor cortex

**Pharmacodynamics/kinetics**

Absorption: Oral: Well absorbed

Metabolism: In the liver

Half-life: 5-12 hours

Time to peak serum concentration: Within 1-4 hours

Elimination: In urine as active and inactive metabolites

**Usual Dosage** Children and Adults: Oral: 0.5-1 g 2-3 times/day

**Reference Range** Therapeutic: 40-60 µg/mL (SI: 228-324 µmol/L)

**Test Interactions** ↑ alkaline phosphatase (S); positive Coombs' [direct]; ↓ calcium (S)

**Patient Information** Take with food; do not discontinue abruptly; may cause drowsiness and impair judgment

**Dosage Forms** Capsule: 500 mg

## Phentermine (FEN ter meen)

**Generic Available** Yes

**U.S. Brand Names** Adipex-P®; Fastin®; Ionamin®; Zantryl®

**Synonyms** Phentermine Hydrochloride

**Pharmacologic Category** Anorexiant

**Use** Short-term adjunct in a regimen of weight reduction based on exercise, behavioral modification, and caloric reduction in the management of exogenous obesity for patients with an initial body mass index ≥30 kg/m$^2$ or ≥27 kg/m$^2$ in the presence of other risk factors (diabetes, hypertension); see table

**Body Mass Index (BMI), kg/m$^2$**
**Height (feet, inches)**

| Weight (lb) | 5'0" | 5'3" | 5'6" | 5'9" | 6'0" | 6'3" |
|---|---|---|---|---|---|---|
| 140 | 27 | 25 | 23 | 21 | 19 | 18 |
| 150 | 29 | 27 | 24 | 22 | 20 | 19 |
| 160 | 31 | 28 | 26 | 24 | 22 | 20 |
| 170 | 33 | 30 | 28 | 25 | 23 | 21 |
| 180 | 35 | 32 | 29 | 27 | 25 | 23 |
| 190 | 37 | 34 | 31 | 28 | 26 | 24 |
| 200 | 39 | 36 | 32 | 30 | 27 | 25 |
| 210 | 41 | 37 | 34 | 31 | 29 | 26 |
| 220 | 43 | 39 | 36 | 33 | 30 | 28 |
| 230 | 45 | 41 | 37 | 34 | 31 | 29 |
| 240 | 47 | 43 | 39 | 36 | 33 | 30 |
| 250 | 49 | 44 | 40 | 37 | 34 | 31 |

**Restrictions** C-IV

**Pregnancy Risk Factor** C

**Contraindications** Known hypersensitivity or idiosyncrasy to sympathomimetic amines; patients with advanced arteriosclerosis, symptomatic cardiovascular disease, moderate to severe hypertension (stage II or III), hyperthyroidism, glaucoma, agitated states; patients with a history of drug abuse; use during or within 14 days following MAO inhibitor therapy; stimulant medications are contraindicated for use in children with attention deficit/hyperactivity disorders and concomitant Tourette's syndrome or tics

**Warnings/Precautions** Use with caution in patients with bipolar disorder, diabetes mellitus, cardiovascular disease, seizure disorders, insomnia, porphyria, or mild hypertension (stage I). May exacerbate symptoms of behavior and thought disorder in psychotic patients. Potential for drug dependency exists - avoid abrupt discontinuation in patients who have received for prolonged periods. Use in weight reduction programs only when alternative therapy has been ineffective. Stimulant use has been associated with growth suppression, and careful monitoring is recommended.

Do not use in children <16 years of age. Primary pulmonary hypertension (PPH), a rare and frequently fatal pulmonary disease, has been reported to occur in patients receiving a combination of phentermine and fenfluramine or dexfenfluramine. The possibility of an association between PPH and the use of phentermine alone cannot be ruled out.

**Adverse Reactions**

Cardiovascular: Hypertension, palpitations, tachycardia, primary pulmonary hypertension and/or regurgitant cardiac valvular disease

Central nervous system: Euphoria, insomnia, overstimulation, dizziness, dysphoria, headache, restlessness, psychosis

Dermatologic: Urticaria

Gastrointestinal: Nausea, constipation, xerostomia, unpleasant taste, diarrhea

Endocrine & metabolic: Changes in libido, impotence

Hematologic: Blood dyscrasias

Neuromuscular & skeletal: Tremor

Ocular: Blurred vision

**Overdosage/Toxicology**

Signs and symptoms: Hyperactivity, agitation, hyperthermia, hypertension, seizures

Treatment: There is no specific antidote for phentermine intoxication and the bulk of the treatment is supportive. Hyperactivity and agitation usually respond to reduced sensory input, however with extreme agitation haloperidol (2-5 mg I.M. for adults) may be required. Hyperthermia is best treated with external cooling measures, or when severe or unresponsive, muscle paralysis with pancuronium may be needed. Hypertension is usually transient and generally does not require treatment unless severe. For diastolic blood pressures >110 mm Hg, a nitroprusside infusion should be initiated. Seizures usually respond to diazepam IVP and/or phenytoin maintenance regimens.

**Drug Interactions**

Antihypertensives: Phentermine may decrease the effect of antihypertensive medications

Antipsychotics: Efficacy of anorexiants may be decreased by antipsychotics; in addition, amphetamines or related compounds may induce an increase in psychotic symptoms in some patients

Furazolidine: Amphetamines (and related compounds) may induce hypertensive episodes in patients receiving furazolidone

Guanethidine: Amphetamines (and related compounds) inhibit the antihypertensive response to guanethidine; probably also may occur with guanadrel

Hypoglycemic agents: Dosage may need to be adjusted when phentermine is used in a diabetic receiving a special diet

Linezolid: Due to MAO inhibition (see below), this combination should generally be avoided

MAO inhibitors: Concurrent use may be associated with hypertensive episodes

SSRIs: Concurrent use may be associated with a risk of serotonin syndrome

**Mechanism of Action** Phentermine is structurally similar to dextroamphetamine and is comparable to dextroamphetamine as an appetite suppressant, but is generally associated with a lower incidence and severity of CNS side effects. Phentermine, like other anorexiants, stimulates the hypothalamus to result in decreased appetite; anorexiant effects are most likely mediated via norepinephrine and dopamine metabolism. However, other CNS effects or metabolic effects may be involved.

**Pharmacodynamics/kinetics**

Absorption: Well absorbed; resin absorbed slower and produces more prolonged clinical effects

Half-life: 20 hours

Elimination: Primarily unchanged in urine

**Usual Dosage** Oral:

Children 3-15 years: 5-15 mg/day for 4 weeks

Adults: 8 mg 3 times/day 30 minutes before meals or food or 15-37.5 mg/day before breakfast or 10-14 hours before retiring

**Monitoring Parameters** CNS

**Patient Information** Take during day to avoid insomnia; do not discontinue abruptly, may cause physical and psychological dependence with prolonged use

**Nursing Implications** Dose should not be given in evening or at bedtime

**Dosage Forms**

Capsule, as hydrochloride: 15 mg, 18.75 mg, 30 mg, 37.5 mg

Capsule, resin complex, as hydrochloride: 15 mg, 30 mg

Tablet, as hydrochloride: 8 mg, 37.5 mg

♦ **Phentermine Hydrochloride** *see* Phentermine *on page 438*

## Phentolamine (fen TOLE a meen)

**Related Information**

Substance-Related Disorders *on page 609*

**U.S. Brand Names** Regitine®

**Canadian Brand Names** Rogitine®

**Pharmacologic Category** Alpha$_1$ Blockers

**Use** Diagnosis of pheochromocytoma and treatment of hypertension associated with pheochromocytoma or other caused by excess sympathomimetic amines; as treatment of dermal necrosis after extravasation of drugs with alpha-adrenergic effects (norepinephrine, dopamine, epinephrine, dobutamine)

**Effects on Mental Status** May cause dizziness

**Effects on Psychiatric Treatment** Concurrent use with psychotropics may produce additive hypotension; treatment of choice for hypertensive crisis secondary to MAOIs

**Pregnancy Risk Factor** C

**Contraindications** Hypersensitivity to phentolamine or any component; renal impairment; coronary or cerebral arteriosclerosis

**Warnings/Precautions** Myocardial infarction, cerebrovascular spasm and cerebrovascular occlusion have occurred following administration. Use with caution in patients with gastritis or peptic ulcer, tachycardia, or a history of cardiac arrhythmias.

**Adverse Reactions**

>10%:

Cardiovascular: Hypotension, tachycardia, arrhythmias, reflex tachycardia, anginal pain, orthostatic hypotension

Gastrointestinal: Nausea, vomiting, diarrhea, exacerbation of peptic ulcer, abdominal pain

Respiratory: Nasal congestion

1% to 10%:

Cardiovascular: Flushing of face, syncope

Central nervous system: Dizziness

Neuromuscular & skeletal: Weakness

Respiratory: Nasal congestion

<1%: Myocardial infarction, severe headache

**Overdosage/Toxicology**

Signs and symptoms: Tachycardia, shock, vomiting, dizziness

Treatment: Hypotension and shock should be treated with fluids and by placing the patient in the Trendelenburg position; only alpha-adrenergic pressors such as norepinephrine should be used; mixed agents such as epinephrine, may cause more hypotension. Take care not to cause so much swelling of the extremity or digit that a compartment syndrome occurs.

**Drug Interactions**

Epinephrine, ephedrine: Effects may be decreased

Ethanol: Increased toxicity (disulfiram reaction)

**Usual Dosage**

Treatment of alpha-adrenergic drug extravasation: S.C.:

Children: 0.1-0.2 mg/kg diluted in 10 mL 0.9% sodium chloride infiltrated into area of extravasation within 12 hours

Adults: Infiltrate area with small amount of solution made by diluting 5-10 mg in 10 mL 0.9% sodium chloride within 12 hours of extravasation

If dose is effective, normal skin color should return to the blanched area within 1 hour

Diagnosis of pheochromocytoma: I.M., I.V.:

Children: 0.05-0.1 mg/kg/dose, maximum single dose: 5 mg

Adults: 5 mg

Surgery for pheochromocytoma: Hypertension: I.M., I.V.:

Children: 0.05-0.1 mg/kg/dose given 1-2 hours before procedure; repeat as needed every 2-4 hours until hypertension is controlled; maximum single dose: 5 mg

Adults: 5 mg given 1-2 hours before procedure and repeated as needed every 2-4 hours

Hypertensive crisis: Adults: 5-20 mg

**Patient Information** Immediately report pain at infusion site. Report any dizziness, feelings of faintness, or palpitations. Do not change position rapidly; rise slowly or ask for assistance.

**Nursing Implications** Monitor patient for orthostasis; assist with ambulation

**Dosage Forms** Injection, as mesylate: 5 mg/mL (1 mL)

♦ **Phenylalanine Mustard** *see* Melphalan *on page 339*

## Phenylbutazone (fen il BYOO ta zone)

**U.S. Brand Names** Azolid®; Butazolidin®

**Pharmacologic Category** Nonsteroidal Anti-Inflammatory Agent (NSAID)

**Use** Management of inflammatory disorders, as an analgesic in the treatment of mild to moderate pain and as an antipyretic; I.V. form used as an alternate to surgery in management of patent ductus arteriosus in premature neonates; acute gouty arthritis

**Effects on Mental Status** Dizziness is common; may rarely cause drowsiness, confusion, depression, or hallucinations

**Effects on Psychiatric Treatment** May rarely cause agranulocytosis; use caution with clozapine and carbamazepine; may decrease lithium clearance resulting in an increase in serum lithium levels and potential lithium toxicity; monitor serum lithium levels

**Contraindications** Active gastrointestinal bleeding; ulcer disease; hypersensitivity to phenylbutazone or any component

**Warnings/Precautions** May cause agranulocytosis and aplastic anemia; is not just a simple analgesic; use only when other NSAIDs have failed; use with caution in patients with congestive heart failure, hypertension, decreased renal or hepatic function, history of gastrointestinal disease (bleeding or ulcers), or those receiving anticoagulants; safety and efficacy in children <6 months of age have not yet been established; because of severe hematologic adverse effects, discontinue use if no favorable response is seen

**Adverse Reactions**

Cardiovascular: Tachycardia, hypotension, myocarditis (hypersensitivity), fibrillation (atrial), flutter (atrial), angina, congestive heart failure, myocardial depression, pericardial effusion/pericarditis, sinus tachycardia

Central nervous system: Dizziness, drowsiness, headache, fatigue, seizures, gustatory hallucinations

Dermatologic: Rash, edema, erythema multiforme, toxic epidermal necrolysis

Endocrine & metabolic: Parotitis

Gastrointestinal: Dyspepsia, heartburn, nausea, vomiting, abdominal pain, peptic ulcer, GI bleeding, GI perforation, loss of taste perception, esophagitis

Hematologic: Anemia, platelet inhibition, thrombocytopenia, coagulopathy, leukopenia, neutropenia, agranulocytosis, granulocytopenia, red blood cell aplasia

Hepatic: Hepatitis, granulomatous hepatitis, primary biliary cirrhosis

Ocular: Vision changes

Otic: Ototoxicity, tinnitus

Renal: Renal failure (acute), myoglobinuria, glomerulonephritis

Respiratory: Pulmonary edema

Miscellaneous: Systemic lupus erythematosus (SLE), lymphadenopathy

**Drug Interactions** CYP3A3/4 enzyme inducer; CYP2C9 enzyme inhibitor

**Usual Dosage** Adults: Oral: Initial:

Rheumatoid arthritis: 100-200 mg 3-4 times/day until desired effect, then reduce dose to not exceeding 400 mg/day

Acute gouty arthritis: 400 mg, 100 mg every 4 hours until acute attack subsides, not to continue longer than 1 week

**Dosing adjustment in hepatic impairment:** Should not be administered to patients with liver dysfunction

**Dosage Forms**

Capsule: 100 mg

Tablet: 100 mg

♦ **Phenyldrine® [OTC]** *see* Phenylpropanolamine *on page 440*

## Phenylephrine (fen il EF rin)

**U.S. Brand Names** AK-Dilate® Ophthalmic Solution; AK-Nefrin® Ophthalmic Solution; Alconefrin® Nasal Solution [OTC]; I-Phrine® Ophthalmic Solution; Mydfrin® Ophthalmic Solution; Neo-Synephrine® Nasal Solution [OTC]; Neo-Synephrine® Ophthalmic Solution; Nostril® Nasal Solution [OTC]; Prefrin™ Ophthalmic Solution; Relief® Ophthalmic Solution; Rhinall® Nasal Solution [OTC]; Sinarest® Nasal Solution [OTC]; St. Joseph® Measured Dose Nasal Solution [OTC]; Vicks Sinex® Nasal Solution [OTC]

**Canadian Brand Names** Dionephrine; Novahistine® Decongestant; Prefrin™ Liquifilm®

**Pharmacologic Category** Alpha/Beta Agonist; Ophthalmic Agent, Antiglaucoma; Ophthalmic Agent, Mydriatic

**Use** Treatment of hypotension, vascular failure in shock; as a vasoconstrictor in regional analgesia; symptomatic relief of nasal and nasopharyngeal mucosal congestion; as a mydriatic in ophthalmic procedures and treatment of wide-angle glaucoma; supraventricular tachycardia

**Effects on Mental Status** May cause anxiety or restlessness

**Effects on Psychiatric Treatment** Concurrent use with MAOIs may result in hypertensive crisis; avoid combination

**Pregnancy Risk Factor** C

**Contraindications** Hypersensitivity to phenylephrine, bisulfite (some products contain metabisulfite), or any component; hypertension; ventricular tachycardia

**Warnings/Precautions** Use with caution in the elderly, patients with hyperthyroidism, bradycardia, partial heart block, myocardial disease, or severe CAD. Not a substitute for volume replacement. Avoid hypertension; monitor blood pressure closely and adjust infusion rate. Infuse into a large vein if possible. Watch I.V. site closely. Avoid extravasation. The elderly can be more sensitive to side effects from the nasal decongestant form. Rebound congestion can occur when the drug is discontinued after chronic use.

**Adverse Reactions**

Nasal:

>10%: Burning, rebound congestion, sneezing

1% to 10%: Stinging, dryness

Ophthalmic:

>10%: Transient stinging

1% to 10%:

Central nervous system: Headache, browache

Ocular: Blurred vision, photophobia, lacrimation

Systemic:

>10%: Neuromuscular & skeletal: Tremor

1% to 10%:

Cardiovascular: Peripheral vasoconstriction hypertension, angina, reflex bradycardia, arrhythmias

Central nervous system: Restlessness, excitability

**Overdosage/Toxicology**

Signs and symptoms: Vomiting, hypertension, palpitations, paresthesia, ventricular extrasystoles

Treatment: Supportive; in extreme cases, I.V. phentolamine may be used

**Drug Interactions**

Beta-blockers (nonselective ones) may increase hypertensive effect; avoid concurrent use

Cocaine may cause malignant arrhythmias; avoid concurrent use

Guanethidine can increase the pressor response; be aware of the patient's drug regimen

(Continued)

## Phenylephrine *(Continued)*

Methyldopa can increase the pressor response; be aware of patient's drug regimen

Phenytoin administration during a dopamine infusion may result in hypotension and possibly cardiac arrest; use cautiously

Reserpine increases the pressor response; be aware of patient's drug regimen

TCAs increase the pressor response; be aware of patient's drug regimen

MAO inhibitors potentiate hypertension and hypertensive crisis; avoid concurrent use

**Usual Dosage**

Ophthalmic procedures:
- Infants <1 year: Instill 1 drop of 2.5% 15-30 minutes before procedures
- Children and Adults: Instill 1 drop of 2.5% or 10% solution, may repeat in 10-60 minutes as needed

Nasal decongestant: (therapy should not exceed 5 continuous days)
- Children:
  - 2-6 years: Instill 1 drop every 2-4 hours of 0.125% solution as needed
  - 6-12 years: Instill 1-2 sprays or instill 1-2 drops every 4 hours of 0.25% solution as needed
- Children >12 years and Adults: Instill 1-2 sprays or instill 1-2 drops every 4 hours of 0.25% to 0.5% solution as needed; 1% solution may be used in adult in cases of extreme nasal congestion; do not use nasal solutions more than 3 days

Hypotension/shock:
- Children:
  - I.M., S.C.: 0.1 mg/kg/dose every 1-2 hours as needed (maximum: 5 mg)
  - I.V. bolus: 5-20 mcg/kg/dose every 10-15 minutes as needed
  - I.V. infusion: 0.1-0.5 mcg/kg/minute
- Adults:
  - I.M., S.C.: 2-5 mg/dose every 1-2 hours as needed (initial dose should not exceed 5 mg)
  - I.V. bolus: 0.1-0.5 mg/dose every 10-15 minutes as needed (initial dose should not exceed 0.5 mg)
  - I.V. infusion: 10 mg in 250 mL $D_5W$ or NS (1:25,000 dilution) (40 mcg/mL); start at 100-180 mcg/minute (2-5 mL/minute; 50-90 drops/minute) initially; when blood pressure is stabilized, maintenance rate: 40-60 mcg/minute (20-30 drops/minute)

Paroxysmal supraventricular tachycardia: I.V.:
- Children: 5-10 mcg/kg/dose over 20-30 seconds
- Adults: 0.25-0.5 mg/dose over 20-30 seconds

**Patient Information**

Nasal decongestant: Do not use for more than 5 days in a row. Clear nose as much as possible before use. Tilt head back and instill recommended dose of drops or spray. Do not blow nose for 5-10 minutes. You may experience transient stinging or burning.

Ophthalmic: Open eye, look at ceiling, and instill prescribed amount of solution. Close eye and roll eye in all directions, and apply gentle pressure to inner corner of eye for 1-2 minutes after instillation. Do not let tip of applicator touch eye or contaminate tip of applicator. Temporary stinging or blurred vision may occur. Report persistent pain, burning, double vision, severe headache, or if condition worsens.

**Nursing Implications** May cause necrosis or sloughing tissue if extravasation occurs during I.V. administration or S.C. administration

**Extravasation:** Use phentolamine as antidote; mix 5 mg with 9 mL of NS; inject a small amount of this dilution into extravasated area; blanching should reverse immediately. Monitor site; if blanching should recur, additional injections of phentolamine may be needed.

**Dosage Forms**

Injection, as hydrochloride (Neo-Synephrine®): 1% [10 mg/mL] (1 mL)

Nasal solution, as hydrochloride:
- Drops:
  - Neo-Synephrine®: 0.125% (15 mL)
  - Alconefrin® 12: 0.16% (30 mL)
  - Alconefrin® 25, Neo-Synephrine®, Children's Nostril®, Rhinall®: 0.25% (15 mL, 30 mL, 40 mL)
  - Alconefrin®, Neo-Synephrine®: 0.5% (15 mL, 30 mL)
- Spray:
  - Alconefrin® 25, Neo-Synephrine®, Rhinall®: 0.25% (15 mL, 30 mL, 40 mL)
  - Neo-Synephrine®, Nostril®, Sinex®: 0.5% (15 mL, 30 mL)
  - Neo-Synephrine®: 1% (15 mL)

Ophthalmic solution, as hydrochloride:
- AK-Nefrin®, Prefrin™ Liquifilm®, Relief®: 0.12% (0.3 mL, 15 mL, 20 mL)
- AK-Dilate®, Mydfrin®, Neo-Synephrine®, Phenoptic®: 2.5% (2 mL, 3 mL, 5 mL, 15 mL)
- AK-Dilate®, Neo-Synephrine®, Neo-Synephrine® Viscous: 10% (1 mL, 2 mL, 5 mL, 15 mL)

## Phenylephrine and Scopolamine

(fen il EF rin & skoe POL a meen)

**U.S. Brand Names** Murocoll-2® Ophthalmic

**Pharmacologic Category** Anticholinergic/Adrenergic Agonist

**Use** Mydriasis, cycloplegia, and to break posterior synechiae in iritis

**Effects on Mental Status** None reported

**Effects on Psychiatric Treatment** None reported

**Usual Dosage** Instill 1-2 drops into eye(s); repeat in 5 minutes

**Dosage Forms** Solution, ophthalmic: Phenylephrine hydrochloride 10% and scopolamine hydrobromide 0.3% (7.5 mL)

## Phenylephrine and Zinc Sulfate

(fen il EF rin & zingk SUL fate)

**U.S. Brand Names** Zincfrin® Ophthalmic [OTC]

**Pharmacologic Category** Adrenergic Agonist Agent

**Use** Soothe, moisturize, and remove redness due to minor eye irritation

**Effects on Mental Status** None reported

**Effects on Psychiatric Treatment** None reported

**Usual Dosage** Instill 1-2 drops in eye(s) 2-4 times/day as needed

**Dosage Forms** Solution, ophthalmic: Phenylephrine hydrochloride 0.12% and zinc sulfate 0.25% (15 mL)

♦ **Phenylethylmalonylurea** *see* Phenobarbital *on page 435*

♦ **Phenylfenesin® L.A.** *see* Guaifenesin and Phenylpropanolamine *on page 257*

♦ **Phenylisohydantoin** *see* Pemoline *on page 423*

## Phenylpropanolamine (fen il proe pa NOLE a meen)

**Related Information**

Pharmacotherapy of Urinary Incontinence *on page 758*

**U.S. Brand Names** Acutrim® 16 Hours [OTC]; Acutrim® II, Maximum Strength [OTC]; Acutrim® Late Day [OTC]; Control® [OTC]; Dexatrim® Pre-Meal [OTC]; Maximum Strength Dex-A-Diet® [OTC]; Maximum Strength Dexatrim® [OTC]; Phenoxine® [OTC]; Phenyldrine® [OTC]; Propagest® [OTC]; Unitrol® [OTC]

**Synonyms** *dl*-Norephedrine Hydrochloride; Phenylpropanolamine Hydrochloride; PPA

**Pharmacologic Category** Alpha/Beta Agonist

**Use** Anorexiant; nasal decongestant

**Effects on Mental Status** May cause dizziness, restlessness, anxiety, or insomnia

**Effects on Psychiatric Treatment** Concurrent use with MAOIs may result in hypertensive crisis; avoid combination

**Pregnancy Risk Factor** C

**Contraindications** Known hypersensitivity to drug

**Warnings/Precautions** Use with caution in patients with high blood pressure, tachyarrhythmias, pheochromocytoma, bradycardia, cardiac disease, arteriosclerosis; do not use for more than 3 weeks for weight loss

**Adverse Reactions**

>10%: Cardiovascular: Hypertension, palpitations

1% to 10%:
- Central nervous system: Insomnia, restlessness, dizziness
- Gastrointestinal: Xerostomia, nausea

<1%: Angina, anxiety, arrhythmias, bradycardia, dysuria, nervousness, restlessness, severe headache, tightness in chest

**Overdosage/Toxicology**

Signs and symptoms: Vomiting, hypertension, palpitations, paresthesia, excitation, seizures

Treatment: Supportive; diazepam 5-10 mg I.V. (0.25-0.4 mg/kg for children) may be used for excitation and seizures

**Drug Interactions**

Decreased effect of antihypertensives

Increased effect/toxicity with MAO inhibitors (hypertensive crisis), beta-blockers (increased pressor effects)

**Usual Dosage** Oral:

Children: Decongestant:
- 2-6 years: 6.25 mg every 4 hours
- 6-12 years: 12.5 mg every 4 hours not to exceed 75 mg/day

Adults:
- Decongestant: 25 mg every 4 hours or 50 mg every 8 hours, not to exceed 150 mg/day
- Anorexic: 25 mg 3 times/day 30 minutes before meals or 75 mg (timed release) once daily in the morning
- Precision release: 75 mg after breakfast

**Patient Information** Nasal decongestant: Do not use for longer than recommended (4-5 days in a row). Anorexiant: Do not use for longer than 3 weeks. With timed release form, take early in day; do not chew or crush. Do not use more often, or in greater dose than prescribed. You may experience dizziness or blurred vision (use caution when driving or engaging in tasks requiring alertness until response to drug is known). With nasal use you may experience burning or stinging (this will resolve). Report rapid heartbeat, chest pain, palpitations; persistent vomiting; excessive nervousness, trembling, or insomnia; difficult or painful urination; unresolved burning or stinging (eyes or nose); or acute headache.

**Nursing Implications** Administer dose early in day to prevent insomnia; observe for signs of nervousness, excitability

**Dosage Forms**

Capsule, as hydrochloride: 37.5 mg
Capsule, as hydrochloride, timed release: 25 mg, 75 mg
Tablet, as hydrochloride: 25 mg, 50 mg
Tablet, as hydrochloride:
Precision release: 75 mg
Timed release: 75 mg

♦ **Phenylpropanolamine Hydrochloride** *see* Phenylpropanolamine *on page 440*

## Phenyltoloxamine, Phenylpropanolamine, and Acetaminophen

(fen il tol OKS a meen, fen il proe pa NOLE a meen, & a seet a MIN oh fen)

**U.S. Brand Names** Sinubid®

**Pharmacologic Category** Antihistamine/Decongestant/Analgesic

**Use** Intermittent symptomatic treatment of nasal congestion in sinus or other frontal headache; allergic rhinitis, vasomotor rhinitis, coryza; facial pain and pressure of acute and chronic sinusitis

**Usual Dosage** Oral:

Children 6-12 years: ½ tablet every 12 hours (twice daily)
Adults: 1 tablet every 12 hours (twice daily)

**Dosage Forms** Tablet: Phenyltoloxamine citrate 22 mg, phenylpropanolamine hydrochloride 25 mg, and acetaminophen 325 mg

## Phenyltoloxamine, Phenylpropanolamine, Pyrilamine, and Pheniramine

(fen il tol OKS a meen, fen il proe pa NOLE a meen, peer IL a meen, & fen IR a meen)

**U.S. Brand Names** Poly-Histine-D® Capsule

**Pharmacologic Category** Cold Preparation

**Use** Treatment of nasal congestion

**Usual Dosage** Oral: Adults: One capsule every 8-12 hours

**Dosage Forms** Capsule: Phenyltoloxamine citrate 16 mg, phenylpropanolamine hydrochloride 50 mg, pyrilamine maleate 16 mg, and pheniramine maleate 16 mg

## Phenytoin (FEN i toyn)

**Related Information**

Anticonvulsants by Seizures Type *on page 703*
Serum Drug Concentrations Commonly Monitored: Guidelines *on page 759*

**Generic Available** Yes

**U.S. Brand Names** Dilantin®; Diphenylan Sodium®

**Canadian Brand Names** Tremytoine®

**Synonyms** Diphenylhydantoin; DPH; Phenytoin Sodium; Phenytoin Sodium, Extended; Phenytoin Sodium, Prompt

**Pharmacologic Category** Antiarrhythmic Agent, Class I-B; Anticonvulsant, Hydantoin

**Use** Management of generalized tonic-clonic (grand mal), complex partial seizures; prevention of seizures following head trauma/neurosurgery

**Unlabeled uses:** Ventricular arrhythmias, including those associated with digitalis intoxication, prolonged Q-T interval and surgical repair of congenital heart diseases in children; epidermolysis bullosa

**Pregnancy Risk Factor** D

**Pregnancy/Breast-Feeding Implications**

Clinical effects on the fetus: Crosses the placenta. Cardiac defects and multiple other malformations reported; characteristic pattern of malformations called "fetal hydantoin syndrome"; hemorrhagic disease of newborn due to fetal vitamin K depletion, maternal folic acid deficiency may occur. Epilepsy itself, number of medications, genetic factors, or a combination of these probably influence the teratogenicity of anticonvulsant therapy. Benefit:risk ratio usually favors continued use during pregnancy and breast-feeding.

Breast-feeding/lactation: Crosses into breast milk

Clinical effects on the infant: Methemoglobinemia, drowsiness and decreased sucking reported in 1 case. American Academy of Pediatrics considers **compatible** with breast-feeding.

**Contraindications** Hypersensitivity to phenytoin, other hydantoins, or any component

**Warnings/Precautions** May increase frequency of petit mal seizures; I.V. form may cause hypotension, skin necrosis at I.V. site; avoid I.V. administration in small veins; use with caution in patients with porphyria; discontinue if rash or lymphadenopathy occurs; use with caution in patients with hepatic dysfunction, sinus bradycardia, S-A block, or A-V block; use with caution in elderly or debilitated patients, or in any condition associated with low serum albumin levels, which will increase the free fraction of phenytoin in the serum and, therefore, the pharmacologic response. Sedation, confusional states, or cerebellar dysfunction (loss of motor coordination) may occur at higher total serum concentrations, or at lower total serum concentrations when the free fraction of phenytoin is increased. Abrupt withdrawal may precipitate status epilepticus.

**Adverse Reactions** I.V. effects: Hypotension, bradycardia, cardiac arrhythmias, cardiovascular collapse (especially with rapid I.V. use), venous irritation and pain, thrombophlebitis

**Effects not related to plasma phenytoin concentrations:** Hypertrichosis, gingival hypertrophy, thickening of facial features, carbohydrate intolerance, folic acid deficiency, peripheral neuropathy, vitamin D deficiency, osteomalacia, systemic lupus erythematosus

**Dose-related effects:** Nystagmus, blurred vision, diplopia, ataxia, slurred speech, dizziness, drowsiness, lethargy, coma, rash, fever, nausea, vomiting, gum tenderness, confusion, mood changes, folic acid depletion, osteomalacia, hyperglycemia

**Related to elevated concentrations:**

>20 mcg/mL: Far lateral nystagmus
>30 mcg/mL: 45° lateral gaze nystagmus and ataxia
>40 mcg/mL: Decreased mentation
>100 mcg/mL: Death

Cardiovascular: Hypotension, bradycardia, cardiac arrhythmias, cardiovascular collapse
Central nervous system: Psychiatric changes, slurred speech, dizziness, drowsiness, headache, insomnia
Dermatologic: Rash
Gastrointestinal: Constipation, nausea, vomiting, gingival hyperplasia, enlargement of lips
Hematologic: Leukopenia, thrombocytopenia, agranulocytosis
Hepatic: Hepatitis
Local: Thrombophlebitis
Neuromuscular & skeletal: Tremor, peripheral neuropathy, paresthesia
Ocular: Diplopia, nystagmus, blurred vision
Rarely seen effects: SLE-like syndrome, lymphadenopathy, hepatitis, Stevens-Johnson syndrome, blood dyscrasias, dyskinesias, pseudolymphoma, lymphoma, venous irritation and pain, coarsening of the facial features, hypertrichosis

**Overdosage/Toxicology**

Signs and symptoms: Unsteady gait, slurred speech, confusion, nausea, hypothermia, fever, hypotension, respiratory depression, coma

Treatment: Supportive for hypotension; treat with I.V. fluids and place patient in Trendelenburg position; seizures may be controlled with diazepam 5-10 mg (0.25-0.4 mg/kg in children)

**Drug Interactions** CYP2C9 and 2C19 enzyme substrate; CYP1A2, 3A3/4, and 3A5-7 enzyme inducer

Acetaminophen: Phenytoin may enhance the hepatotoxic potential of acetaminophen overdoses

Acetazolamide: Concurrent use with phenytoin may result in an increased risk of osteomalacia

Acyclovir: May decrease phenytoin serum levels; limited documentation; monitor

Allopurinol: May increase phenytoin serum concentrations; monitor

Antacids: May decrease absorption of phenytoin; separate oral doses by several hours

Antiarrhythmics: Phenytoin may increase the metabolism of antiarrhythmics, decreasing their clinical effect; includes disopyramide, propafenone, and quinidine; amiodarone also may increase phenytoin concentrations (see CYP inhibitors)

Anticonvulsants: Phenytoin may increase the metabolism of anticonvulsants; includes barbiturates, carbamazepine, ethosuximide, felbamate, lamotrigine, tiagabine, topiramate, and zonisamide; does not appear to affect gabapentin or levetiracetam; felbamate and gabapentin may increase phenytoin levels; monitor

Antineoplastics: Several chemotherapeutic agents have been associated with a decrease in serum phenytoin levels; includes cisplatin, bleomycin, carmustine, methotrexate, and vinblastine; monitor phenytoin serum levels. Limited evidence also suggest that enzyme-inducing anticonvulsant therapy may reduce the effectiveness of some chemotherapy regimens (specifically in ALL). Teniposide and methotrexate may be cleared more rapidly in these patients.

Antipsychotics: Phenytoin may enhance the metabolism (decrease the efficacy) of antipsychotics; monitor for altered response; dose adjustment may be needed; also see clozapine (below)

Benzodiazepines: Phenytoin may decrease the serum concentrations of some benzodiazepines; monitor for decreased benzodiazepine effect

Beta-blockers: Metabolism of beta-blockers may be increased and clinical effect decreased; atenolol and nadolol are unlikely to interact given their renal elimination

Calcium channel blockers: Phenytoin may enhance the metabolism of calcium channel blockers, decreasing their clinical effect; nifedipine has been reported to increase phenytoin levels (case report); monitor

Capecitabine: May increase the serum concentrations of phenytoin; monitor

(Continued)

## Phenytoin *(Continued)*

Chloramphenicol: Phenytoin may increase the metabolism of chloramphenicol and chloramphenicol may inhibit phenytoin metabolism; monitor for altered response
Ciprofloxacin: Case reports indicate ciprofloxacin may increase or decrease serum phenytoin concentrations; monitor
Clozapine: May decrease phenytoin serum concentrations; monitor
CNS depressants: Sedative effects may be additive with other CNS depressants; monitor for increased effect; includes ethanol, barbiturates, sedatives, antidepressants, narcotic analgesics, and benzodiazepines
Corticosteroids: Phenytoin may increase the metabolism of corticosteroids, decreasing their clinical effect; also see dexamethasone
Cyclosporine and tacrolimus: Levels may be decreased by phenytoin; monitor
CYP2C8/9 inhibitors: Serum levels and/or toxicity of phenytoin may be increased; inhibitors include amiodarone, cimetidine, fluvoxamine, some NSAIDs, metronidazole, ritonavir, sulfonamides, troglitazone, valproic acid, and zafirlukast; monitor for increased effect/toxicity
CYP2C19 inhibitors: Serum levels of phenytoin may be increased; inhibitors include cimetidine, felbamate, fluconazole, fluoxetine, fluvoxamine, omeprazole, teniposide, tolbutamide, and troglitazone
Dexamethasone: May decrease serum phenytoin due to increased metabolism; monitor
Digoxin: Effects and/or levels of digitalis glycosides may be decreased by phenytoin
Disulfiram: May increase serum phenytoin concentrations; monitor
Dopamine: Phenytoin (I.V.) may increase the effect of dopamine (enhanced hypotension)
Doxycycline: Phenytoin may enhance the metabolism of doxycycline, decreasing its clinical effect; higher dosages may be required
Estrogens: Phenytoin may increase the metabolism of estrogens, decreasing their clinical effect; monitor
Enzyme inducers: The serum levels of phenytoin may be reduced by barbiturates, carbamazepine, chronic ethanol, dexamethasone, and rifampin
Folic acid: Replacement of folic acid has been reported to increase the metabolism of phenytoin, decreasing its serum concentrations and/or increasing seizures
Furosemide: Diuretic effect may be blunted by phenytoin (mechanism unclear); possibly due to decreased furosemide bioavailability
HMG CoA reductase inhibitors: Phenytoin may increase the metabolism of these agents, reducing their clinical effect; monitor
Itraconazole: Phenytoin may decrease the effect of itraconazole
Levodopa: Phenytoin may inhibit the anti-Parkinson effect of levodopa
Lithium: Concurrent use of phenytoin and lithium has resulted in lithium intoxication
Methadone: Phenytoin may enhance the metabolism of methadone resulting in methadone withdrawal
Methylphenidate: May increase serum phenytoin concentrations; monitor
Neuromuscular blocking agents: Duration of effect may be decreased by phenytoin
Omeprazole: May increase serum phenytoin concentrations; monitor
Oral contraceptives: Phenytoin may enhance the metabolism of oral contraceptives, decreasing their clinical effect; an alternative method of contraception should be considered
Phenylbutazone: May increase phenytoin concentrations; monitor and adjust dosage
Primidone: Phenytoin enhances the conversion of primidone to phenobarbital resulting in elevated phenobarbital serum concentrations
Quetiapine: Serum concentrations may be substantially reduced by phenytoin, potentially resulting in a loss of efficacy; limited documentation; monitor
SSRIs: May increase phenytoin serum concentrations; fluoxetine and fluvoxamine are known to inhibit metabolism via CYP enzymes; sertraline and paroxetine have also been shown to increase concentrations in some patients; monitor
Sucralfate: May reduce the GI absorption of phenytoin; monitor
Theophylline: Phenytoin may increase metabolism of theophylline derivatives and decrease their clinical effect; theophylline may also increase phenytoin concentrations
Thyroid hormones (including levothyroxine): Phenytoin may alter the metabolism of thyroid hormones, reducing its effect; there is limited documentation of this interaction, but monitoring should be considered
Ticlopidine: May increase serum phenytoin concentrations and/or toxicity; monitor
Tricyclic antidepressants: Phenytoin may increase metabolism of tricyclic antidepressants and decrease their clinical effect; sedative effects may be additive; tricyclics may also increase phenytoin concentrations
Topiramate: Phenytoin may decrease serum levels of topiramate; topiramate may increase the effect of phenytoin
Trazodone: Serum levels of phenytoin may be increased; limited documentation; monitor
Trimethoprim: May increase serum phenytoin concentrations; monitor
Valproic acid (and sulfisoxazole): May displace phenytoin from binding sites; valproic acid may increase, decrease, or have no effect on phenytoin serum concentrations
Vigabatrin: May reduce phenytoin serum concentrations; monitor
Warfarin: Phenytoin transiently increased the hypothrombinemia response to warfarin initially; this is followed by an inhibition of the hypoprothombinemic response

**Stability**
Phenytoin is stable as long as it remains free of haziness and precipitation
Use only clear solutions; parenteral solution may be used as long as there is no precipitate and it is not hazy, slightly yellowed solution may be used
Refrigeration may cause precipitate, sometimes the precipitate is resolved by allowing the solution to reach room temperature again
Drug may precipitate at a pH <11.5
May dilute with normal saline for I.V. infusion; stability is concentration dependent
Standard diluent: Dose/100 mL NS
Minimum volume: Concentration should be maintained at 1-10 mg/mL secondary to stability problems (stable for 4 hours)
Comments: Maximum rate of infusion: 50 mg/minute

IVPB dose should be administered via an in-line 0.22-5 micron filter because of high potential for precipitation I.V. form is highly **incompatible** with many drugs and solutions such as dextrose in water, some saline solutions, amikacin, bretylium, dobutamine, cephapirin, insulin, levorphanol, lidocaine, meperidine, metaraminol, morphine, norepinephrine, heparin, potassium chloride, vitamin B complex with C

**Mechanism of Action** Stabilizes neuronal membranes and decreases seizure activity by increasing efflux or decreasing influx of sodium ions across cell membranes in the motor cortex during generation of nerve impulses; prolongs effective refractory period and suppresses ventricular pacemaker automaticity, shortens action potential in the heart

**Pharmacodynamics/kinetics**
Absorption: Oral: Slow
Distribution: $V_d$:
Neonates:
Premature: 1-1.2 L/kg
Full-term: 0.8-0.9 L/kg
Infants: 0.7-0.8 L/kg
Children: 0.7 L/kg
Adults: 0.6-0.7 L/kg
Protein binding:
Neonates: Up to 20% free
Infants: Up to 15% free
Adults: 90% to 95%
Others: Increased free fraction (decreased protein binding)
Patients with hyperbilirubinemia, hypoalbuminemia, uremia
Metabolism: Follows dose-dependent capacity-limited (Michaelis-Menten) pharmacokinetics with increased $V_{max}$ in infants >6 months of age and children versus adults
Bioavailability: Dependent upon formulation administered
Time to peak serum concentration (dependent upon formulation administered): Oral:
Extended-release capsule: Within 4-12 hours
Immediate release preparation: Within 2-3 hours
Elimination: Highly variable clearance dependent upon intrinsic hepatic function and dose administered; increased clearance and decreased serum concentrations with febrile illness; <5% excreted unchanged in urine; major metabolite (via oxidation) HPPA undergoes enterohepatic recycling and elimination in urine as glucuronides

| Disease States Resulting in a Decrease in Serum Albumin Concentration | Disease States Resulting in an Apparent Decrease in Affinity of Phenytoin for Serum Albumin |
|---|---|
| Burns | Renal failure |
| Hepatic cirrhosis | Jaundice (severe) |
| Nephrotic syndrome | Other drugs (displacers) |
| Pregnancy | Hyperbilirubinemia (total bilirubin >15 mg/dL) |
| Cystic fibrosis | $Cl_{cr}$ <25 mL/min (unbound fraction is increased two- to threefold in uremia) |

**Usual Dosage**
Status epilepticus: I.V.:
Infants and Children: Loading dose: 15-20 mg/kg in a single or divided dose; maintenance dose: Initial: 5 mg/kg/day in 2 divided doses, usual doses:
6 months to 3 years: 8-10 mg/kg/day
4-6 years: 7.5-9 mg/kg/day
7-9 years: 7-8 mg/kg/day
10-16 years: 6-7 mg/kg/day, some patients may require every 8 hours dosing
Adults: Loading dose: 15-20 mg/kg in a single or divided dose, followed by 100-150 mg/dose at 30-minute intervals up to a maximum of 1500 mg/24 hours; maintenance dose: 300 mg/day or 5-6 mg/kg/day in 3 divided doses or 1-2 divided doses using extended release
Anticonvulsant: Children and Adults: Oral:
Loading dose: 15-20 mg/kg; based on phenytoin serum concentrations and recent dosing history; administer oral loading dose in 3 divided doses given every 2-4 hours to decrease GI adverse effects and to ensure complete oral absorption; maintenance dose: same as I.V.

**Dosing adjustment/comments in renal impairment or hepatic disease:** Safe in usual doses in mild liver disease; clearance may be substantially reduced in cirrhosis and plasma level monitoring with dose adjustment advisable. Free phenytoin levels should be monitored closely.

**Dietary Considerations**

Status epilepticus: I.V.:

Alcohol (acute use): Inhibits metabolism of phenytoin; avoid or limit use; watch for sedation

Alcohol (chronic use): Stimulates metabolism of phenytoin; avoid or limit use

Food:

Folic acid: Low erythrocyte and CSF folate concentrations. Phenytoin may decrease mucosal uptake of folic acid; to avoid folic acid deficiency and megaloblastic anemia, some clinicians recommend giving patients on anticonvulsants prophylactic doses of folic acid and cyanocobalamin.

Calcium: Hypocalcemia has been reported in patients taking prolonged high-dose therapy with an anticonvulsant. Phenytoin may decrease calcium absorption. Monitor calcium serum concentration and for bone disorders (eg, rickets, osteomalacia). Some clinicians have given an additional 4000 units/week of vitamin D (especially in those receiving poor nutrition and getting no sun exposure) to prevent hypocalcemia.

Vitamin D: Phenytoin interferes with vitamin D metabolism and osteomalacia may result; may need to supplement with vitamin D

Glucose: Hyperglycemia and glycosuria may occur in patients receiving high-dose therapy. Monitor blood glucose concentration, especially in patients with impaired renal function.

Tube feedings: Tube feedings decrease phenytoin bioavailability; to avoid decreased serum levels with continuous NG feeds, hold feedings for 2 hours prior to and 2 hours after phenytoin administration, if possible. There is a variety of opinions on how to administer phenytoin with enteral feedings. Be **consistent** throughout therapy.

**Administration**

Phenytoin may be administered by IVP or IVPB administration

I.M. administration is not recommended due to erratic absorption, pain on injection and precipitation of drug at injection site

S.C. administration is not recommended because of the possibility of local tissue damage

The maximum rate of I.V. administration is 50 mg/minute; highly sensitive patients (eg, elderly, patients with pre-existing cardiovascular conditions) should receive phenytoin more slowly (eg, 20 mg/minute)

An in-line 0.22-5 micron filter is recommended for IVPB solutions due to the high potential for precipitation of the solution; avoid extravasation; following I.V. administration, NS should be injected through the same needle or I.V. catheter to prevent irritation

**Monitoring Parameters** Blood pressure, vital signs (with I.V. use), plasma phenytoin level, CBC, liver function tests

**Reference Range**

Therapeutic range:

Total phenytoin: 10-20 µg/mL (children and adults), 8-15 µg/mL (neonates)

Concentrations of 5-10 µg/mL may be therapeutic for some patients but concentrations <5 µg/mL are not likely to be effective

50% of patients show decreased frequency of seizures at concentrations >10 µg/mL

86% of patients show decreased frequency of seizures at concentrations >15 µg/mL

Add another anticonvulsant if satisfactory therapeutic response is not achieved with a phenytoin concentration of 20 µg/mL

Free phenytoin: 1-2.5 µg/mL

Toxic: <30-50 µg/mL (SI: <120-200 µmol/L)

**Lethal**: >100 µg/mL (SI: >400 µmol/L)

**Test Interactions** ↑ glucose, alkaline phosphatase (S); ↓ thyroxine (S), calcium (S)

**Patient Information** Shake oral suspension well prior to each dose; do not change brand or dosage form without consulting physician; do not skip doses, may cause drowsiness, dizziness, ataxia, loss of coordination or judgment; take with food; maintain good oral hygiene

**Adjustment of Serum Concentration in Patients With Renal Failure ($Cl_{cr}$ ≤10 mL/min) (Product Information From Parke-Davis)**

| Measured Total Phenytoin Concentration (mcg/mL) | Patient's Serum Albumin (g/dL) | | | | |
|---|---|---|---|---|---|
| | 4 | 3.5 | 3 | 2.5 | 2 |
| | Adjusted Total Phenytoin Concentration (mcg/mL)* | | | | |
| 5 | 10 | 11 | 13 | 14 | 17 |
| 10 | 20 | 22 | 25 | 29 | 33 |
| 15 | 30 | 33 | 38 | 43 | 50 |

*Adjusted concentration = measured total concentration ÷ [(0.1 x albumin) + 0.1].

**Adjustment of Serum Concentration in Patients With Low Serum Albumin**

| Measured Total Phenytoin Concentration (mcg/mL) | Patient's Serum Albumin (g/dL) | | | |
|---|---|---|---|---|
| | 3.5 | 3 | 2.5 | 2 |
| | Adjusted Total Phenytoin Concentration (mcg/mL)* | | | |
| 5 | 6 | 7 | 8 | 10 |
| 10 | 13 | 14 | 17 | 20 |
| 15 | 19 | 21 | 25 | 30 |

*Adjusted concentration = measured total concentration ÷ [(0.2 x albumin) + 0.1].

**Additional Information**

Phenytoin: Dilantin® chewable tablet and oral suspension

Phenytoin sodium, extended: Dilantin® Kapseal®

Phenytoin sodium, prompt: Diphenylan Sodium® capsule

Sodium content of 1 g injection: 88 mg (3.8 mEq)

**Dosage Forms**

Capsule, as sodium:

Extended: 30 mg, 100 mg

Prompt: 100 mg

Injection, as sodium: 50 mg/mL (2 mL, 5 mL)

Suspension, oral: 30 mg/5 mL (5 mL, 240 mL); 125 mg/5 mL (5 mL, 240 mL)

Tablet, chewable: 50 mg

♦ **Phenytoin Sodium** *see* Phenytoin *on page 441*

♦ **Phenytoin Sodium, Extended** *see* Phenytoin *on page 441*

♦ **Phenytoin Sodium, Prompt** *see* Phenytoin *on page 441*

## Phenytoin With Phenobarbital

(FEN i toyn with fee noe BAR bi tal)

**Pharmacologic Category** Anticonvulsant, Barbiturate; Anticonvulsant, Hydantoin

**Use** Management of generalized tonic-clonic (grand mal), simple partial and complex partial seizures

**Effects on Mental Status** Phenytoin may cause ataxia, slurred speech, dizziness, drowsiness, lethargy, coma, confusion, mood changes, insomnia (dose related); phenobarbital may cause drowsiness, lethargy, CNS excitation or depression, impaired judgment, "hangover" effect, confusion, somnolence, agitation, hyperkinesia, ataxia, nervousness, headache, insomnia, nightmares, hallucinations, anxiety, dizziness

**Effects on Psychiatric Treatment** Both compounds are sedating and produce enzyme induction; concurrent use with psychotropics may produce additive sedation and/or lessened effects of other psychotropic agents; may cause leukopenia, use caution with clozapine and carbamazepine; disulfiram may decrease the metabolism of phenytoin; valproic acid may increase, decrease, or have no effect on phenytoin serum concentrations; phenytoin may increase the metabolism of alprazolam, carbamazepine, clozapine, diazepam, lamotrigine, meperidine, methadone, midazolam, quetiapine, thyroid hormones, triazolam, and valproic acid resulting in decreased levels/effect; concurrent use with lithium has resulted in toxicity

**Usual Dosage** Adults: Oral: Initial:

Rheumatoid arthritis: 100-200 mg 3-4 times/day until desired effect, then reduce dose to not exceeding 400 mg/day

Acute gouty arthritis: 400 mg, 100 mg every 4 hours until acute attack subsides, not to continue longer than 1 week

**Dosage Forms** Capsule: Phenytoin 100 mg and phenobarbital 15 mg; phenytoin 100 mg and phenobarbital 30 mg

♦ **Pherazine® VC w/ Codeine** *see* Promethazine, Phenylephrine, and Codeine *on page 471*

♦ **Pherazine® w/DM** *see* Promethazine and Dextromethorphan *on page 471*

♦ **Pherazine® With Codeine** *see* Promethazine and Codeine *on page 471*

♦ **Phicon® [OTC]** *see* Pramoxine *on page 457*

♦ **Phillips'® Milk of Magnesia [OTC]** *see* Magnesium Hydroxide *on page 330*

♦ **PhosLo®** *see* Calcium Acetate *on page 84*

♦ **Phosphate, Potassium** *see* Potassium Phosphate *on page 455*

♦ **Phospholine Iodide® Ophthalmic** *see* Echothiophate Iodide *on page 189*

♦ **Photofrin®** *see* Porfimer *on page 453*

♦ **Phrenilin®** *see* Butalbital Compound and Acetaminophen *on page 80*

♦ **Phrenilin® Forte** *see* Butalbital Compound and Acetaminophen *on page 80*

♦ **Phyllocontin®** *see* Theophylline Salts *on page 539*

♦ **Phylloquinone** *see* Phytonadione *on page 444*

## Physostigmine (fye zoe STIG meen)

**Related Information**

Clinical Issues in the Use of Antipsychotics *on page 630*
Glaucoma Drug Therapy *on page 712*
Psychiatric Emergencies - Neuroleptic Malignant Syndrome *on page 660*
Special Populations - Elderly *on page 662*

**U.S. Brand Names** Antilirium®

**Synonyms** Eserine Salicylate; Physostigmine Salicylate; Physostigmine Sulfate

**Pharmacologic Category** Acetylcholinesterase Inhibitor (Central); Ophthalmic Agent, Antiglaucoma

**Use** Reverse toxic CNS effects caused by anticholinergic drugs; used as miotic in treatment of glaucoma

**Effects on Mental Status** May cause restlessness, nervousness, or hallucinations

**Effects on Psychiatric Treatment** None reported

**Pregnancy Risk Factor** C

**Contraindications** Hypersensitivity to physostigmine or any component; GI or GU obstruction; physostigmine therapy of drug intoxications should be used with extreme caution in patients with asthma, gangrene, severe cardiovascular disease, or mechanical obstruction of the GI tract or urogenital tract. In these patients, physostigmine should be used only to treat life-threatening conditions.

**Warnings/Precautions** Use with caution in patients with epilepsy, asthma, diabetes, gangrene, cardiovascular disease, bradycardia. Discontinue if excessive salivation or emesis, frequent urination or diarrhea occur. Reduce dosage if excessive sweating or nausea occurs. Administer I.V. slowly or at a controlled rate not faster than 1 mg/minute. Due to the possibility of hypersensitivity or overdose/cholinergic crisis, atropine should be readily available; ointment may delay corneal healing, may cause loss of dark adaptation; not intended as a first-line agent for anticholinergic toxicity or Parkinson's disease.

**Adverse Reactions**

Ophthalmic:
- >10%:
  - Ocular: Lacrimation, marked miosis, blurred vision, eye pain
  - Miscellaneous: Diaphoresis
- 1% to 10%:
  - Central nervous system: Headache, browache
  - Dermatologic: Burning, redness

Systemic:
- >10%:
  - Gastrointestinal: Nausea, salivation, diarrhea, stomach pains
  - Ocular: Lacrimation
  - Miscellaneous: Diaphoresis
- 1% to 10%:
  - Cardiovascular: Palpitations, bradycardia
  - Central nervous system: Restlessness, nervousness, hallucinations, seizures
  - Genitourinary: Frequent urge to urinate
  - Neuromuscular & skeletal: Muscle twitching
  - Ocular: Miosis
  - Respiratory: Dyspnea, bronchospasm, respiratory paralysis, pulmonary edema

**Overdosage/Toxicology**

Signs and symptoms: Muscle weakness, blurred vision, excessive sweating, tearing and salivation, nausea, vomiting, bronchospasm, seizures

Treatment: If physostigmine is used in excess or in the absence of an anticholinergic overdose, patients may manifest signs of cholinergic toxicity. At this point a cholinergic agent (eg, atropine 0.015-0.05 mg/kg) may be necessary.

**Drug Interactions** Increased toxicity: Bethanechol, methacholine, succinylcholine may increase neuromuscular blockade with systemic administration

**Usual Dosage**

Children: Anticholinergic drug overdose: Reserve for life-threatening situations only: I.V.: 0.01-0.03 mg/kg/dose, (maximum: 0.5 mg/minute); may repeat after 5-10 minutes to a maximum total dose of 2 mg or until response occurs or adverse cholinergic effects occur

Adults: Anticholinergic drug overdose:
- I.M., I.V., S.C.: 0.5-2 mg to start, repeat every 20 minutes until response occurs or adverse effect occurs
- Repeat 1-4 mg every 30-60 minutes as life-threatening signs (arrhythmias, seizures, deep coma) recur; maximum I.V. rate: 1 mg/minute

Ophthalmic:
- Ointment: Instill a small quantity to lower fornix up to 3 times/day
- Solution: Instill 1-2 drops into eye(s) up to 4 times/day

**Patient Information** Systemic: Maintain adequate hydration (2-3 L/day of fluids unless instructed to restrict fluid intake). May cause dizziness, drowsiness, or hypotension (rise slowly from sitting or lying position and use caution when driving or climbing stairs); vomiting or loss of appetite (frequent small meals, frequent mouth care, chewing gum, or sucking lozenges may help); or diarrhea (boiled milk, yogurt, or buttermilk may help). Report persistent abdominal discomfort; significantly increased salivation, sweating, tearing, or urination; flushed skin; chest pain or palpitations; acute headache; unresolved diarrhea; excessive fatigue, insomnia, dizziness, or depression; increased muscle, joint, or body pain; vision changes or blurred vision; or shortness of breath or wheezing.

Ophthalmic: For ophthalmic use only. Wash hands before using. Tilt head back and look upward. Put drops of suspension or apply thin ribbon of ointment inside lower eyelid. Close eye and roll eyeball in all directions. Do not blink for 1/2 minute. Apply gentle pressure to inner corner of eye for 30 seconds. Do not use any other eye preparation for at least 10 minutes. Do not touch tip of applicator to eye or contaminate tip of applicator. Do not share medication with anyone else. Wear sunglasses when in sunlight; you may be more sensitive to bright light. Inform prescriber if condition worsens or fails to improve or if you experience eye pain, vision disturbances, or other adverse eye response; excess sweating; urinary frequency; severe headache; or skin rash, redness, or burning.

**Dosage Forms**

Injection, as salicylate: 1 mg/mL (2 mL)
Ointment, ophthalmic, as sulfate: 0.25% (3.5 g, 3.7 g)

♦ **Physostigmine Salicylate** *see* Physostigmine *on page 444*

♦ **Physostigmine Sulfate** *see* Physostigmine *on page 444*

♦ **Phytomenadione** *see* Phytonadione *on page 444*

## Phytonadione (fye toe na DYE one)

**U.S. Brand Names** AquaMEPHYTON® Injection; Konakion® Injection; Mephyton® Oral

**Synonyms** Methylphytyl Napthoquinone; Phylloquinone; Phytomenadione; Vitamin $K_1$

**Pharmacologic Category** Vitamin, Fat Soluble

**Use** Prevention and treatment of hypoprothrombinemia caused by drug-induced or anticoagulant-induced vitamin K deficiency, hemorrhagic disease of the newborn; phytonadione is more effective and is preferred to other vitamin K preparations in the presence of impending hemorrhage; oral absorption depends on the presence of bile salts

**Effects on Mental Status** May rarely cause dizziness

**Effects on Psychiatric Treatment** None reported

**Pregnancy Risk Factor** C

**Contraindications** Hypersensitivity to phytonadione or any component

**Warnings/Precautions** Severe reactions resembling anaphylaxis or hypersensitivity have occurred rarely during or immediately after I.V. administration (even with proper dilution and rate of administration); restrict I.V. administration for emergency use only; ineffective in hereditary hypoprothrombinemia, hypoprothrombinemia caused by severe liver disease; severe hemolytic anemia has been reported rarely in neonates following large doses (10-20 mg) of phytonadione

**Adverse Reactions** <1%: Abnormal taste, anaphylaxis, cyanosis, diaphoresis, dizziness (rarely), dyspnea, GI upset (oral), hemolysis in neonates and in patients with G-6-PD deficiency, hypersensitivity reactions, pain, rarely hypotension, tenderness at injection site, transient flushing reaction

**Drug Interactions** Decreased effect: Warfarin sodium, dicumarol, anisindione effects antagonized by phytonadione; mineral oil may decrease GI absorption of vitamin K

**Usual Dosage** I.V. route should be restricted for emergency use only

Minimum daily requirement: Not well established
- Infants: 1-5 mcg/kg/day
- Adults: 0.03 mcg/kg/day

Hemorrhagic disease of the newborn:
- Prophylaxis: I.M.: 0.5-1 mg within 1 hour of birth
- Treatment: I.M., S.C.: 1-2 mg/dose/day

Oral anticoagulant overdose:
- Infants: I.M., S.C.: 1-2 mg/dose every 4-8 hours
- Children and Adults: Oral, I.M., I.V., S.C.: 2.5-10 mg/dose; rarely up to 25-50 mg has been used; may repeat in 6-8 hours if given by I.M., I.V., S.C. route; may repeat 12-48 hours after oral route

Vitamin K deficiency: Due to drugs, malabsorption or decreased synthesis of vitamin K
- Infants and Children:
  - Oral: 2.5-5 mg/24 hours
  - I.M., I.V.: 1-2 mg/dose as a single dose
- Adults:
  - Oral: 5-25 mg/24 hours
  - I.M., I.V.: 10 mg

**Patient Information** Oral: Take only as directed; do not take more or more often than prescribed. Avoid excessive or increased intake of vitamin K containing food (eg, green leafy vegetables, dairy products, meats) unless recommended by prescriber. Avoid alcohol and any OTC or prescribed medications containing aspirin that are not approved by prescriber. Report bleeding gums; blood in urine, stool, or vomitus; unusual bruising of bleeding; or abdominal cramping.

**Dosage Forms**
Injection:
Aqueous colloidal: 2 mg/mL (0.5 mL); 10 mg/mL (1 mL, 2.5 mL, 5 mL)
Aqueous (I.M. only): 2 mg/mL (0.5 mL); 10 mg/mL (1 mL)
Tablet: 5 mg

♦ **Pilagan® Ophthalmic** *see* Pilocarpine *on page 445*

♦ **Pilocar® Ophthalmic** *see* Pilocarpine *on page 445*

## Pilocarpine (pye loe KAR peen)

**Related Information**
Glaucoma Drug Therapy *on page 712*

**U.S. Brand Names** Adsorbocarpine® Ophthalmic; Akarpine® Ophthalmic; Isopto® Carpine Ophthalmic; Ocu-Carpine® Ophthalmic; Ocusert Pilo-20® Ophthalmic; Ocusert Pilo-40® Ophthalmic; Pilagan® Ophthalmic; Pilocar® Ophthalmic; Pilopine HS® Ophthalmic; Piloptic® Ophthalmic; Pilostat® Ophthalmic; Salagen® Oral

**Canadian Brand Names** Minims® Pilocarpine

**Pharmacologic Category** Cholinergic Agonist; Ophthalmic Agent, Antiglaucoma; Ophthalmic Agent, Miotic

**Use**
Ophthalmic: Management of chronic simple glaucoma, chronic and acute angle-closure glaucoma; counter effects of cycloplegics
Oral: Symptomatic treatment of xerostomia caused by salivary gland hypofunction resulting from radiotherapy for cancer of the head and neck

**Effects on Mental Status** None reported

**Effects on Psychiatric Treatment** Pilocarpine may antagonize the effects of anticholinergics and produce cardiac conduction abnormalities in patients receiving beta-blockers

**Usual Dosage** Adults:
Ophthalmic:
Nitrate solution: Shake well before using; instill 1-2 drops 2-4 times/day
Hydrochloride solution:
Instill 1-2 drops up to 6 times/day; adjust the concentration and frequency as required to control elevated intraocular pressure
To counteract the mydriatic effects of sympathomimetic agents: Instill 1 drop of a 1% solution in the affected eye
Gel: Instill 0.5" ribbon into lower conjunctival sac once daily at bedtime
Ocular systems: Systems are labeled in terms of mean rate of release of pilocarpine over 7 days; begin with 20 mcg/hour at night and adjust based on response
Oral: 5 mg 3 times/day, titration up to 10 mg 3 times/day may be considered for patients who have not responded adequately

**Dosage Forms** Tablet: 5 mg
See table.

**Pilocarpine**

| Dosage Form | Strength % | 1 mL | 2 mL | 15 mL | 30 mL | 3.5 g |
|---|---|---|---|---|---|---|
| Gel | 4 | | | | | x |
| Solution as hydrochloride | 0.25 | | | x | | |
| | 0.5 | | | x | x | |
| | 1 | x | x | x | x | |
| | 2 | x | x | x | x | |
| | 3 | | | x | x | |
| | 4 | x | x | x | x | |
| | 6 | | | x | x | |
| | 8 | | x | | | |
| | 10 | | | x | | |
| Solution as nitrate | 1 | | | x | | |
| | 2 | | | x | | |
| | 4 | | | x | | |

Ocusert® Pilo-20: Releases 20 mcg/hour for 1 week.
Ocusert® Pilo-40: Releases 40 mcg/hour for 1 week.

## Pilocarpine and Epinephrine
(pye loe KAR peen & ep i NEF rin)

**U.S. Brand Names** E-Pilo-x® Ophthalmic; $P_xE_x$® Ophthalmic

**Canadian Brand Names** E-Pilo®

**Pharmacologic Category** Ophthalmic Agent, Antiglaucoma; Ophthalmic Agent, Miotic

**Use** Treatment of glaucoma; counter effect of cycloplegics

**Effects on Mental Status** None reported

**Effects on Psychiatric Treatment** Pilocarpine may antagonize the effects of anticholinergic and produce cardiac conduction abnormalities in patients receiving beta-blockers

**Usual Dosage** Instill 1-2 drops up to 6 times/day

**Dosage Forms** Solution, ophthalmic: Epinephrine bitartrate 1% and pilocarpine hydrochloride 1%, 2%, 3%, 4%, 6% (15 mL)

♦ **Pilopine HS® Ophthalmic** *see* Pilocarpine *on page 445*

♦ **Piloptic® Ophthalmic** *see* Pilocarpine *on page 445*

♦ **Pilostat® Ophthalmic** *see* Pilocarpine *on page 445*

♦ **Pima®** *see* Potassium Iodide *on page 454*

## Pimozide (PI moe zide)

**Related Information**
Antipsychotic Agents Comparison Chart *on page 706*
Antipsychotic Medication Guidelines *on page 751*
Clinical Issues in the Use of Antipsychotics *on page 630*
Discontinuation of Psychotropic Drugs - Withdrawal Symptoms and Recommendations *on page 798*
Patient Information - Antipsychotics (General) *on page 646*
Schizophrenia *on page 604*

**Generic Available** No

**U.S. Brand Names** Orap™

**Pharmacologic Category** Antipsychotic Agent, Diphenylbutylperidine

**Use** Suppression of severe motor and phonic tics in patients with Tourette's disorder who have failed to respond satisfactorily to standard treatment
**Unlabeled use:** Psychosis; reported use in individuals with delusions focused on physical symptoms (ie, preoccupation with parasitic infestation); anorexia nervosa; generalized anxiety; Huntington's chorea

**Pregnancy Risk Factor** C

**Contraindications** Concomitant use of drugs that are inhibitors of CYP3A, see Drug Interactions; avoid grapefruit juice; hypersensitivity to pimozide or any component; severe CNS depression, coma, history of dysrhythmia, prolonged Q-T syndrome, concurrent use of macrolide antibiotics (such as erythromycin or clarithromycin), azole antifungals, simple tics other than Tourette's, protease inhibitors (ie, ritonavir, saquinavir, indinavir, nelfinavir), nefazodone, and zileuton

**Warnings/Precautions** May cause hypotension, use with caution in patients with autonomic instability. Moderately sedating, use with caution in disorders where CNS depression is a feature. Use with caution in Parkinson's disease. Caution in patients with hemodynamic instability; bone marrow suppression; predisposition to seizures; subcortical brain damage; severe cardiac, hepatic, renal, or respiratory disease. Esophageal dysmotility and aspiration have been associated with antipsychotic use - use with caution in patients at risk of pneumonia (ie, Alzheimer's disease). Caution in breast cancer or other prolactin-dependent tumors (may elevate prolactin levels). May alter temperature regulation or mask toxicity of other drugs due to antiemetic effects. May alter cardiac conduction - sudden unexplained deaths have occurred in patients taking high doses (>10 mg). This may be due to prolongation of the Q-T interval predisposing patients to ventricular arrhythmias. May cause orthostatic hypotension - use with caution in patients at risk of this effect or those who would tolerate transient hypotensive episodes (cerebrovascular disease, cardiovascular disease, or other medications which may predispose).

May cause anticholinergic effects (confusion, agitation, constipation, dry mouth, blurred vision, urinary retention); therefore, they should be used with caution in patients with decreased gastrointestinal motility, urinary retention, BPH, xerostomia, or visual problems. Conditions which also may be exacerbated by cholinergic blockade include narrow-angle glaucoma (screening is recommended) and worsening of myasthenia gravis. Relative to neuroleptics, pimozide has a moderate potency of cholinergic blockade.

May cause extrapyramidal reactions, including pseudoparkinsonism, acute dystonic reactions, akathisia, and tardive dyskinesia (risk of these reactions is high relative to other neuroleptics). May be associated with neuroleptic malignant syndrome (NMS) or pigmentary retinopathy.

Avoid grapefruit juice due to potential inhibition of pimozide metabolism

**Adverse Reactions**
Cardiovascular: Swelling of face, tachycardia, orthostatic hypotension, chest pain, hypertension, palpitations, ventricular arrhythmias, Q-T prolongation
Central nervous system: Extrapyramidal signs (akathisia, akinesia, dystonia, pseudoparkinsonism, tardive dyskinesia), drowsiness, NMS, headache, dizziness, excitement
Dermatologic: Rash
Endocrine & metabolic: Edema of breasts, decreased libido
Gastrointestinal: Constipation, xerostomia, weight gain or loss, nausea, salivation, vomiting, anorexia
Genitourinary: Impotence
Hematologic: Blood dyscrasias
Hepatic: Jaundice
Neuromuscular & skeletal: Weakness, tremor
Ocular: Visual disturbance, decreased accommodation, blurred vision
Miscellaneous: Diaphoresis

**Overdosage/Toxicology**
Signs and symptoms: Hypotension, respiratory depression, EKG abnormalities, extrapyramidal symptoms
(Continued)

## Pimozide *(Continued)*

Treatment: Following attempts at decontamination, treatment is supportive and symptomatic. Seizures can be treated with diazepam, phenytoin, or phenobarbital.

**Drug Interactions** CYP3A3/4 enzyme substrate; CYP1A2 (minor)

Aluminum salts: May decrease the absorption of antipsychotics; monitor

Amphetamines: Efficacy may be diminished by antipsychotics; in addition, amphetamines may increase psychotic symptoms; avoid concurrent use

Anticholinergics: May inhibit the therapeutic response to antipsychotics and excess anticholinergic effects may occur; includes benztropine, trihexyphenidyl, biperiden, and drugs with significant anticholinergic activity (TCAs, antihistamines, disopyramide)

Antihypertensives: Concurrent use of antipsychotics with an antihypertensive may produce additive hypotensive effects (particularly orthostasis)

Bromocriptine: Antipsychotics inhibit the ability of bromocriptine to lower serum prolactin concentrations

CNS depressants: Sedative effects may be additive with antipsychotics; monitor for increased effect; includes barbiturates, benzodiazepines, narcotic analgesics, ethanol, and other sedative agents

CYP3A3/4 inhibitors: Serum level and/or toxicity of some benzodiazepines may be increased; inhibitors include amiodarone, cimetidine, clarithromycin, erythromycin, delavirdine, diltiazem, dirithromycin, disulfiram, fluoxetine, fluvoxamine, grapefruit juice, indinavir, itraconazole, ketoconazole, metronidazole, nefazodone, nevirapine, propoxyfene, quinupristin-dalfopristin, ritonavir, saquinavir, verapamil, zafirlukast, zileuton. May cause life-threatening arrhythmias; avoid these combinations.

Enzyme inducers: May enhance the hepatic metabolism of antipsychotics; larger doses may be required; includes rifampin, rifabutin, barbiturates, phenytoin, and cigarette smoking

Epinephrine: Chlorpromazine (and possibly other low potency antipsychotics) may diminish the pressor effects of epinephrine

Guanethidine and guanadrel: Antihypertensive effects may be inhibited by antipsychotics

Levodopa: Antipsychotics may inhibit the antiparkinsonian effect of levodopa; avoid this combination

Lithium: Antipsychotics may produce neurotoxicity with lithium; this is a rare effect

Phenytoin: May reduce serum levels of antipsychotics; antipsychotics may increase phenytoin serum levels

Propranolol: Serum concentrations of antipsychotics may be increased; propranolol also increases antipsychotics concentrations

QTc prolonging agents: Effects on QTc interval may be additive with antipsychotics, increasing the risk of malignant arrhythmias; includes type Ia antiarrhythmics, tricyclic antidepressants, and some quinolone antibiotics (sparfloxacin, moxifloxacin, and gatifloxacin)

Sulfadoxine-pyrimethamine: May increase antipsychotics concentrations

Tricyclic antidepressants: Concurrent use may produce increased toxicity or altered therapeutic response (also see note under QTc prolonging agents)

Trazodone: Antipsychotics and trazodone may produce additive hypotensive effects

Valproic acid: Serum levels may be increased by antipsychotics

**Mechanism of Action** A potent centrally-acting dopamine-receptor antagonist resulting in its characteristic neuroleptic effects

**Pharmacodynamics/kinetics**

Absorption: Oral: 50%

Protein binding: 99%

Metabolism: In the liver with significant first-pass decay

Half-life: 50 hours

Time to peak serum concentration: Within 6-8 hours

Elimination: In urine

**Usual Dosage** Children >12 years and Adults: Oral: Initial: 1-2 mg/day, then increase dosage as needed every other day; range is usually 7-16 mg/day, maximum dose: 20 mg/day or 0.3 mg/kg/day should not be exceeded. **Note:** Sudden unexpected deaths have occurred in patients taking doses >10 mg.

**Dosing adjustment in hepatic impairment:** Reduction of dose is necessary in patients with liver disease

**Reference Range** 3 mg dose produces a plasma level of 3.3 ng/mL

**Test Interactions** ↑ prolactin (S)

**Patient Information** Treatment with pimozide exposes the patient to serious risks; a decision to use pimozide chronically in Tourette's disorder is one that deserves full consideration by the patient (or patient's family) as well as by the treating physician. Because the goal of treatment is symptomatic improvement, the patient's view of the need for treatment and assessment of response are critical in evaluating the impact of therapy and weighing its benefits against the risks.

**Nursing Implications** Must obtain baseline EKG and an EKG with dose increases

**Additional Information** Less sedation but more likely to cause acute extrapyramidal signs than chlorpromazine

**Dosage Forms** Tablet: 2 mg

## Pindolol (PIN doe lole)

**Related Information**

Beta-Blockers Comparison Chart *on page 709*

**Generic Available** No

**U.S. Brand Names** Visken®

**Canadian Brand Names** Apo®-Pindol; Gen-Pindolol; Novo-Pindol; Nu-Pindol; Syn-Pindol®

**Pharmacologic Category** Beta Blocker (with Intrinsic Sympathomimetic Activity)

**Use** Management of hypertension

**Unlabeled uses:** Potential augmenting agent for antidepressants; ventricular arrhythmias/tachycardia, antipsychotic-induced akathisia, situational anxiety; aggressive behavior associated with dementia

**Effects on Mental Status** Insomnia is common; may cause dizziness, fatigue, nervousness, or nightmares; may rarely cause depression or hallucinations

**Effects on Psychiatric Treatment** Has been used as an augmentive agent to the SSRIs for the treatment of depression; barbiturates may decrease the effects of beta-blockers

**Pregnancy Risk Factor** B

**Contraindications** Hypersensitivity to pindolol, beta-blockers or any component; uncompensated congestive heart failure, cardiogenic shock, bradycardia or heart block (2nd or 3rd degree), pulmonary edema, severe hyperactive airway disease (asthma or COPD), Raynaud's disease

**Warnings/Precautions** Administer very cautiously to patients with CHF, asthma, diabetes mellitus, hyperthyroidism. Abrupt withdrawal of the drug should be avoided, drug should be discontinued over 1-2 weeks. Do not use in pregnant or nursing women. May potentiate hypoglycemia in a diabetic patient and mask signs and symptoms. Use with caution in patients with myasthenia gravis or peripheral vascular disease. May cause CNS depression - use caution in patients with a history of psychiatric illness. May potentiate anaphylactic reactions and/or blunt response to epinephrine treatment.

**Adverse Reactions**

1% to 10%:

Cardiovascular: Chest pain (3%), edema (6%)

Central nervous system: Nightmares/vivid dreams (5%), dizziness (9%), insomnia (10%), fatigue (8%), nervousness (7%)

Dermatologic: Rash, itching (4%)

Gastrointestinal: Nausea (5%), abdominal discomfort (4%)

Neuromuscular & skeletal: Weakness (4%), paresthesia (3%), arthralgia (7%), muscle pain (10%)

Respiratory: Dyspnea (5%)

<1%: Bradycardia, CHF, claudication, hypotension, palpitations

Central nervous system: Confusion, mental depression, hallucinations, anxiety (<2%), impotence, thrombocytopenia, dry eyes, wheezing

**Overdosage/Toxicology**

Signs and symptoms: Cardiac disturbances, CNS toxicity, bronchospasm, hypoglycemia and hyperkalemia. The most common cardiac symptoms include hypotension and bradycardia; atrioventricular block, intraventricular conduction disturbances, cardiogenic shock, and asystole may occur with severe overdose, especially with membrane-depressant drugs (eg, propranolol); CNS effects include convulsions, coma, and respiratory arrest is commonly seen with propranolol and other membrane-depressant and lipid-soluble drugs.

Treatment: Includes symptomatic treatment of seizures, hypotension, hyperkalemia and hypoglycemia; bradycardia and hypotension resistant to atropine, isoproterenol or pacing may respond to glucagon; wide QRS defects caused by the membrane-depressant poisoning may respond to hypertonic sodium bicarbonate; repeat-dose charcoal, hemoperfusion, or hemodialysis may be helpful in removal of only those beta-blockers with a small $V_d$, long half-life or low intrinsic clearance (acebutolol, atenolol, nadolol, sotalol).

**Drug Interactions** CYP2D6 enzyme substrate

Albuterol (and other $beta_2$ agonists): Effects may be blunted by nonspecific beta-blockers

Alpha-blockers (prazosin, terazosin): Concurrent use of beta-blockers may increase risk of orthostasis

Clonidine: Hypertensive crisis after or during withdrawal of either agent

CYP2D6 inhibitors: Serum levels and/or toxicity of some beta-blockers may be increased; inhibitors include amiodarone, cimetidine, delavirdine, fluoxetine, paroxetine, propafenone, quinidine, and ritonavir; monitor for increased effect/toxicity

Drugs which slow AV conduction (digoxin): Effects may be additive with beta-blockers

Epinephrine (including local anesthetics with epinephrine): Pindolol may cause hypertension

Glucagon: Pindolol may blunt the hyperglycemic action

Insulin and oral hypoglycemics: May mask symptoms of hypoglycemia

NSAIDs (ibuprofen, indomethacin, naproxen, piroxicam): May reduce the antihypertensive effects of beta-blockers

Salicylates: May reduce the antihypertensive effects of beta-blockers

Sulfonylureas: Beta-blockers may alter response to hypoglycemic agents

Verapamil or diltiazem may have synergistic or additive pharmacological effects when taken concurrently with beta-blockers

**Stability** Protect from light

**Mechanism of Action** Blocks both $beta_1$- and $beta_2$-receptors and has mild intrinsic sympathomimetic activity; pindolol has negative inotropic and chronotropic effects and can significantly slow A-V nodal conduction. Augmentive action of antidepressants thought to be mediated via a serotonin 1A autoreceptor antagonism.

**Pharmacodynamics/kinetics**

Absorption: Oral: Rapid, 50% to 95%

Protein binding: 50%

Metabolism: In the liver (60% to 65%) to conjugates

Half-life: 2.5-4 hours; increased with renal insufficiency, age, and cirrhosis

Time to peak serum concentration: Within 1-2 hours

Elimination: In urine (35% to 50% unchanged drug)

**Usual Dosage** Oral:

Adults:

Hypertension: Initial: 5 mg twice daily, increase as necessary by 10 mg/day every 3-4 weeks; maximum daily dose: 60 mg

Antidepressant augmentation: 2.5 mg 3 times/day

Elderly: Initial: 5 mg once daily, increase as necessary by 5 mg/day every 3-4 weeks

**Dosing adjustment in renal and hepatic impairment:** Reduction is necessary in severely impaired

**Monitoring Parameters** Blood pressure, standing and sitting/supine, pulse, respiratory function

**Patient Information** Adhere to dosage regimen; watch for postural hypotension; abrupt withdrawal of the drug should be avoided; take at the same time each day; may mask diabetes symptoms; do not discontinue medication abruptly; consult pharmacist or physician before taking over-the-counter cold preparations

**Nursing Implications** Evaluate blood pressure, apical and radial pulses; do not discontinue abruptly

**Dosage Forms** Tablet: 5 mg, 10 mg

♦ **Pink Bismuth® [OTC]** *see* Bismuth *on page 69*

♦ **Pin-Rid® [OTC]** *see* Pyrantel Pamoate *on page 480*

♦ **Pin-X® [OTC]** *see* Pyrantel Pamoate *on page 480*

♦ **PIO** *see* Pemoline *on page 423*

## Pioglitazone (pye oh GLI ta zone)

**Related Information**

Hypoglycemic Drugs and Thiazolidinedione Information *on page 714*

**U.S. Brand Names** Actos™

**Pharmacologic Category** Antidiabetic Agent (Thiazolidinedione)

**Use**

Type 2 diabetes, monotherapy: Adjunct to diet and exercise, to improve glycemic control

Type 2 diabetes, combination therapy with sulfonylurea, metformin, or insulin: When diet, exercise, and a single agent alone does not result in adequate glycemic control

**Effects on Mental Status** May cause fatigue

**Effects on Psychiatric Treatment** Weight gain is common; caution with atypical antipsychotics; nefazodone and other CYP3A4 inhibitors may decrease the metabolism of pioglitazone; glucose may need to be checked more frequently

**Pregnancy Risk Factor** C

**Contraindications** Hypersensitivity to pioglitazone or any component of the formulation. Active liver disease (transaminases >2.5 times the upper limit of normal at baseline). Contraindicated in patients who have experienced jaundice during troglitazone therapy.

**Warnings/Precautions** Should not be used in diabetic ketoacidosis. Mechanism requires the presence of insulin, therefore use in type 1 diabetes is not recommended. May potentiate hypoglycemia when used in combination with sulfonylureas or insulin. Use with caution in premenopausal, anovulatory women - may result in a resumption of ovulation, increasing the risk of pregnancy. Use with caution in patients with anemia (may reduce hemoglobin and hematocrit). Use with caution in patients with heart failure or edema - may increase plasma volume and/or increase cardiac hypertrophy. In general, use should be avoided in patients with NYHA class III or IV heart failure. Use with caution in patients with elevated transaminases (AST or ALT) - see Contraindications. Idiosyncratic hepatotoxicity has been reported with another thiazolidinedione agent (troglitazone) - monitoring should include periodic determinations of liver function.

**Adverse Reactions**

>10%:

Endocrine & metabolic: Decreased serum triglycerides, increased HDL cholesterol

Gastrointestinal: Weight gain

Respiratory: Upper respiratory tract infection (13.2%)

1% to 10%:

Cardiovascular: Edema (4.8%)

Central nervous system: Headache (9.1%), fatigue (3.6%)

Endocrine & metabolic: Aggravation of diabetes mellitus (5.1%), hypoglycemia (range 2% to 15% when used in combination with sulfonylureas or insulin)

Hematologic; Anemia (1%)

Neuromuscular & skeletal: Myalgia (5.4%)

Respiratory: Sinusitis (6.3%), pharyngitis (5.1%)

<1%: Elevated CPK, elevated transaminases

In combination trials with sulfonylureas or insulin, the incidence of edema was as high as 15%.

**Overdosage/Toxicology** Experience in overdose is limited; symptoms may include hypoglycemia. Treatment is supportive.

**Drug Interactions** Substrate for cytochrome P-450 isoenzyme 2C8 (CYP2C8) and 3A4 (CYP3A4)

Decreased effect: Effects of oral contraceptives may be decreased, based on data from a related compound. This has not been specifically evaluated for pioglitazone.

Increased effect/toxicity: Ketoconazole (*in vitro*) inhibits metabolism of pioglitazone. Other inhibitors of CYP3A4, including itraconazole, are likely to decrease pioglitazone metabolism. Patients receiving inhibitors of CYP3A4 should have their glycemic control evaluated more frequently.

**Usual Dosage** Adults: Oral:

Monotherapy: Initial: 15-30 mg once daily; if response is inadequate, the dosage may be increased in increments up to 45 mg once daily; maximum recommended dose: 45 mg once daily

Combination therapy:

With sulfonylureas: Initial: 15-30 mg once daily; dose of sulfonylurea should be reduced if the patient reports hypoglycemia

With metformin: Initial: 15-30 mg once daily; it is unlikely that the dose of metformin will need to be reduced due to hypoglycemia

With insulin: Initial: 15-30 mg once daily; dose of insulin should be reduced by 10% to 25% if the patient reports hypoglycemia or if the plasma glucose falls to <100 mg/dL. Doses >30 mg/day have not been evaluated in combination regimens.

A 1-week washout period is recommended in patients with normal liver enzymes who are changed from troglitazone to pioglitazone therapy.

**Dosage adjustment in renal impairment:** No dosage adjustment is required.

**Dosage adjustment in hepatic impairment:** Clearance is significantly lower in hepatic impairment. Therapy should not be initiated if the patient exhibits active liver disease or increased transaminases (>2.5 times the upper limit of normal) at baseline.

Elderly patients: No dosage adjustment is recommended in elderly patients.

**Dietary Considerations** Management of type 2 diabetes should include diet control. Peak concentrations are delayed when administered with food, but the extent of absorption is not affected. Pioglitazone may be taken without regard to meals.

**Administration** Oral: May be taken without regard to meals

**Patient Information** Use exactly as directed (do not increase dose or frequency or discontinue without consulting prescriber). May be taken without regard to meals; avoid alcohol while taking this medication. If dose is missed, take as soon as possible. If dose is missed completely one day, do not double dose the next day. Follow dietary, exercise, and glucose monitoring instructions of prescriber (more frequent monitoring may be advised in periods of stress, trauma, surgery, increased exercise etc). Report respiratory infection, unusual weight gain, aggravation of hyper- or hypoglycemic condition, unusual swelling of extremities, fatigue, yellowing of skin or eyes, dark urine, pale stool, nausea/vomiting, or muscle pain.

**Dosage Forms** Tablet: 15 mg, 30 mg, 45 mg

## Pipecuronium (pi pe kur OH nee um)

**U.S. Brand Names** Arduan®

**Pharmacologic Category** Neuromuscular Blocker Agent, Nondepolarizing

**Use** Adjunct to general anesthesia, to provide skeletal muscle relaxation during surgery and to provide skeletal muscle relaxation for endotracheal intubation; recommended only for procedures anticipated to last 90 minutes or longer

**Effects on Mental Status** None reported

**Effects on Psychiatric Treatment** None reported

**Usual Dosage** I.V.:

Children:

3 months to 1 year: Adult dosage

1-14 years: May be less sensitive to effects

Adults: Dose is individualized based on ideal body weight, ranges are 85-100 mcg/kg initially to a maintenance dose of 5-25 mcg/kg

**Dosing adjustment in renal impairment:**

$Cl_{cr}$ 61-80 mL/minute: 70 mcg/kg

$Cl_{cr}$ 41-60 mL/minute: 55 mcg/kg

$Cl_{cr}$ <40 mL/minute: 50 mcg/kg

(Continued)

## Pipecuronium *(Continued)*

Extended duration should be expected

**Dosage Forms** Injection, as bromide: 10 mg (10 mL)

## Piperacillin (pi PER a sil in)

**U.S. Brand Names** Pipracil®

**Pharmacologic Category** Antibiotic, Penicillin

**Use** Treatment of susceptible infections such as septicemia, acute and chronic respiratory tract infections, skin and soft tissue infections, and urinary tract infections due to susceptible strains of *Pseudomonas, Proteus*, and *Escherichia coli* and *Enterobacter*, active against some streptococci and some anaerobic bacteria

**Effects on Mental Status** May cause drowsiness or confusion; penicillins reported to cause apprehension, illusions, hallucinations, depersonalization, agitation, encephalopathy, and insomnia

**Effects on Psychiatric Treatment** None reported

**Usual Dosage**

Neonates: 100 mg/kg every 12 hours

Infants and Children: I.M., I.V.: 200-300 mg/kg/day in divided doses every 4-6 hours

Higher doses have been used in cystic fibrosis: 350-500 mg/kg/day in divided doses every 4-6 hours

Adults: I.M., I.V.:

Moderate infections (urinary tract infections): 2-3 g/dose every 6-12 hours; maximum: 2 g I.M./site

Serious infections: 3-4 g/dose every 4-6 hours; maximum: 24 g/24 hours

Uncomplicated gonorrhea: 2 g I.M. in a single dose accompanied by 1 g probenecid 30 minutes prior to injection

**Dosing adjustment in renal impairment:** Adults: I.V.:

$Cl_{cr}$ 20-40 mL/minute: Administer 3-4 g every 8 hours

$Cl_{cr}$ <20 mL/minute: Administer 3-4 g every 12 hours

Moderately dialyzable (20% to 50%)

Continuous arteriovenous or venovenous hemodiafiltration (CAVH) effects: Dose as for $Cl_{cr}$ 10-50 mL/minute

**Dosage Forms** Powder for injection, as sodium: 2 g, 3 g, 4 g, 40 g

## Piperacillin and Tazobactam Sodium

(pi PER a sil in & ta zoe BAK tam SOW dee um)

**U.S. Brand Names** Zosyn™

**Pharmacologic Category** Antibiotic, Penicillin

**Use** Treatment of infections of lower respiratory tract, urinary tract, skin and skin structures, gynecologic, bone and joint infections, and septicemia caused by susceptible organisms. Tazobactam expands activity of piperacillin to include beta-lactamase producing strains of *S. aureus, H. influenzae, Bacteroides*, and other gram-negative bacteria.

**Effects on Mental Status** May cause insomnia, dizziness or agitation; may rarely cause confusion; penicillins reported to cause apprehension, illusions, hallucinations, depersonalization, agitation, encephalopathy, and insomnia

**Effects on Psychiatric Treatment** None reported

**Usual Dosage**

Children <12 years: Not recommended due to lack of data

Children >12 years and Adults:

Severe infections: I.V.: Piperacillin/tazobactam 4/0.5 g every 8 hours or 3/0.375 g every 6 hours

Moderate infections: I.M.: Piperacillin/tazobactam 2/0.25 g every 6-8 hours; treatment should be continued for ≥7-10 days depending on severity of disease (Note: I.M. route not FDA-approved)

**Dosing interval in renal impairment:**

$Cl_{cr}$ 20-40 mL/minute: Administer 2/0.25 g every 6 hours

$Cl_{cr}$ <20 mL/minute: Administer 2/0.25 g every 8 hours

Hemodialysis: Administer 2/0.25 g every 8 hours with an additional dose of 0.75 g after each dialysis

Continuous arteriovenous or venovenous hemodiafiltration (CAVH) effects: Dose as for $Cl_{cr}$ 10-50 mL/minute

**Dosage Forms** Injection: Piperacillin sodium 2 g and tazobactam sodium 0.25 g; piperacillin sodium 3 g and tazobactam sodium 0.375 g; piperacillin sodium 4 g and tazobactam sodium 0.5 g (vials at an 8:1 ratio of piperacillin sodium/tazobactam sodium)

## Piperazine (PI per a zeen)

**U.S. Brand Names** Vermizine®

**Pharmacologic Category** Anthelmintic

**Use** Treatment of pinworm and roundworm infections (used as an alternative to first-line agents, mebendazole, or pyrantel pamoate)

**Effects on Mental Status** May cause dizziness

**Effects on Psychiatric Treatment** May cause seizures; use caution with high-dose clozapine

**Pregnancy Risk Factor** B

**Contraindications** Seizure disorders, liver or kidney impairment, hypersensitivity to piperazine or any component

**Warnings/Precautions** Use with caution in patients with anemia or malnutrition; avoid prolonged use especially in children

**Adverse Reactions** <1%: Bronchospasms, diarrhea, dizziness, EEG changes, headache, hemolytic anemia, hypersensitivity reactions, nausea, seizures, vertigo, visual impairment, vomiting, weakness

**Drug Interactions** Pyrantel pamoate (antagonistic mode of action)

**Usual Dosage** Oral:

Pinworms: Children and Adults: 65 mg/kg/day (not to exceed 2.5 g/day) as a single daily dose for 7 days; in severe infections, repeat course after a 1-week interval

Roundworms:

Children: 75 mg/kg/day as a single daily dose for 2 days; maximum: 3.5 g/day

Adults: 3.5 g/day for 2 days (in severe infections, repeat course, after a 1-week interval)

**Patient Information** Take on empty stomach; if severe or persistent headache, loss of balance or coordination, dizziness, vomiting, diarrhea, or rash occurs, contact physician. If used for pinworm infections, all members of the family should be treated.

**Dosage Forms**

Syrup, as citrate: 500 mg/5 mL (473 mL, 4000 mL)

Tablet, as citrate: 250 mg

♦ **Piperazine Estrone Sulfate** *see* Estropipate *on page 208*

♦ ***Piper methysticum*** *see* Kava *on page 301*

## Pipobroman (pi poe BROE man)

**U.S. Brand Names** Vercyte®

**Pharmacologic Category** Antineoplastic Agent, Alkylating Agent

**Use** Treat polycythemia vera; chronic myelocytic leukemia (in patients refractory to busulfan)

**Effects on Mental Status** None reported

**Effects on Psychiatric Treatment** May cause leukopenia; avoid clozapine or carbamazepine

**Pregnancy Risk Factor** D

**Contraindications** Pre-existing bone marrow suppression, hypersensitivity to any component

**Warnings/Precautions** The U.S. Food and Drug Administration (FDA) currently recommends that procedures for proper handling and disposal of antineoplastic agents be considered; bone marrow suppression may not occur for 4 weeks

**Adverse Reactions** 1% to 10%:

Dermatologic: Rash

Gastrointestinal: Vomiting, diarrhea, nausea, abdominal cramps

Hematologic: Leukopenia, thrombocytopenia, anemia

**Overdosage/Toxicology**

Signs and symptoms: Severe marrow suppression

Treatment: Supportive therapy is required

**Usual Dosage** Children >15 years and Adults: Oral:

Polycythemia: 1 mg/kg/day for 30 days; may increase to 1.5-3 mg/kg until hematocrit reduced to 50% to 55%; maintenance: 0.1-0.2 mg/kg/day

Myelocytic leukemia: 1.5-2.5 mg/kg/day until WBC drops to 10,000/$mm^3$ then start maintenance 7-175 mg/day; stop if WBC falls to <3000/$mm^3$ or platelets fall to <150,000/$mm^3$

**Patient Information** Notify physician if nausea, vomiting, diarrhea, or rash become severe or if unusual bleeding or bruising, sore throat, or fatigue occur; contraceptives are recommended during therapy

**Dosage Forms** Tablet: 25 mg

♦ **Pipracil®** *see* Piperacillin *on page 448*

## Pirbuterol (peer BYOO ter ole)

**U.S. Brand Names** Maxair™ Inhalation Aerosol

**Pharmacologic Category** $Beta_2$ Agonist

**Use** Prevention and treatment of reversible bronchospasm including asthma

**Effects on Mental Status** Nervousness and restlessness are common; may cause dizziness; may rarely cause insomnia

**Effects on Psychiatric Treatment** Concurrent use with TCAs and MAOIs may results in increased toxicity; monitor

**Pregnancy Risk Factor** C

**Contraindications** Hypersensitivity to pirbuterol or albuterol

**Warnings/Precautions** Excessive use may result in tolerance; some adverse reactions may occur more frequently in children 2-5 years of age; use with caution in patients with hyperthyroidism, diabetes mellitus; cardiovascular disorders including coronary insufficiency or hypertension or sensitivity to sympathomimetic amines

**Adverse Reactions**

>10%:

Central nervous system: Nervousness, restlessness

Neuromuscular & skeletal: Trembling

1% to 10%:
- Central nervous system: Headache, dizziness
- Gastrointestinal: Taste changes, vomiting, nausea

<1%: Anorexia, arrhythmias, bruising, chest pain, hypertension, insomnia, numbness in hands, paradoxical bronchospasm, weakness

**Overdosage/Toxicology**

Signs and symptoms: Hypertension, tachycardia, angina, hypokalemia

Treatment: In cases of overdose, supportive therapy should be instituted, and prudent use of a cardioselective beta-adrenergic blocker (eg, atenolol or metoprolol) should be considered, keeping in mind the potential for induction of bronchoconstriction in an asthmatic individual. Dialysis has not been shown to be of value in the treatment of an overdose with this agent.

**Drug Interactions**

Decreased effect with beta-blockers

Increased toxicity with other beta agonists, MAO inhibitors, TCAs

**Usual Dosage** Children >12 years and Adults: 2 inhalations every 4-6 hours for prevention; two inhalations at an interval of at least 1-3 minutes, followed by a third inhalation in treatment of bronchospasm, not to exceed 12 inhalations/day

**Patient Information** Use exactly as directed. Do not use more often than recommended. Maintain adequate hydration (2-3 L/day of fluids unless instructed to restrict fluid intake). You may experience nervousness, dizziness, or fatigue (use caution when driving or engaging in tasks requiring alertness until response to drug is known); or dry mouth, stomach upset (frequent small meals, frequent mouth care, chewing gum, or sucking hard candy may help). Report unresolved GI upset; dizziness or fatigue; vision changes; chest pain, rapid heartbeat, or palpitations; nervousness or insomnia; muscle cramping or tremor; or unusual cough.

**Administration:** Self-administered inhalation: Store canister upside down; do not freeze. Shake canister before using. Sit when using medication. Close eyes when administering pirbuterol to avoid spray getting into eyes. Exhale slowly and completely through nose; inhale deeply through mouth while administering aerosol. Hold breath for 1-3 seconds after inhalation. Wait at least 1 full minute between inhalations. Wash mouthpiece between use. If more than one inhalation medication is used, use bronchodilator first and wait 5 minutes between medications.

**Nursing Implications** Before using, the inhaler must be shaken well; assess lung sounds, pulse, and blood pressure before administration and during peak of medication; observe patient for wheezing after administration, if this occurs, call physician

**Dosage Forms**

Aerosol, oral, as acetate: 0.2 mg per actuation (25.6 g)

Aerosol (Autohaler™): 0.2 mg per actuation (2.8 g - 80 inhalations, 14 g - 400 inhalations)

## Piroxicam (peer OKS i kam)

**Related Information**

Nonsteroidal Anti-inflammatory Agents Comparison Chart *on page 722*

**U.S. Brand Names** Feldene®

**Canadian Brand Names** Apo®-Piroxicam; Novo-Piroxicam; Nu-Pirox; Pro-Piroxicam®

**Pharmacologic Category** Nonsteroidal Anti-Inflammatory Agent (NSAID)

**Use** Management of inflammatory disorders; symptomatic treatment of acute and chronic rheumatoid arthritis, osteoarthritis, and ankylosing spondylitis; also used to treat sunburn

**Effects on Mental Status** Dizziness is common; may cause nervousness; may rarely cause drowsiness, confusion, depression, or hallucinations

**Effects on Psychiatric Treatment** May rarely cause agranulocytosis; use caution with clozapine and carbamazepine; may decrease lithium clearance resulting in an increase in serum lithium levels and potential lithium toxicity; monitor serum lithium levels

**Pregnancy Risk Factor** B (D if used in the 3rd trimester)

**Contraindications** Hypersensitivity to piroxicam, any component, aspirin or other nonsteroidal anti-inflammatory drugs (NSAIDs); active GI bleeding

**Warnings/Precautions** Use with caution in patients with impaired cardiac function, dehydration, hypertension, impaired renal function, GI disease (bleeding or ulcers) and patients receiving anticoagulants; elderly have increased risk for adverse reactions to NSAIDs

**Adverse Reactions**

>10%:
- Central nervous system: Dizziness
- Dermatologic: Rash
- Gastrointestinal: Abdominal cramps, heartburn, indigestion, nausea

1% to 10%:
- Central nervous system: Headache, nervousness
- Dermatologic: Itching
- Endocrine & metabolic: Fluid retention
- Gastrointestinal: Vomiting
- Otic: Tinnitus

<1%: Acute renal failure, agranulocytosis, allergic rhinitis, anemia, angioedema, arrhythmias, aseptic meningitis, blurred vision, bone marrow suppression, confusion, congestive heart failure, conjunctivitis, cystitis, decreased hearing, drowsiness, dry eyes, epistaxis, erythema multiforme, gastritis, GI ulceration, hallucinations, hemolytic anemia, hepatitis, hot flashes, hypertension, insomnia, leukopenia, mental depression, peripheral neuropathy, polydipsia, polyuria, shortness of breath, Stevens-Johnson syndrome, tachycardia, thrombocytopenia, toxic amblyopia, toxic epidermal necrolysis, urticaria

**Overdosage/Toxicology**

Signs and symptoms: Nausea, epigastric distress, CNS depression, leukocytosis, renal failure

Treatment: Management of a nonsteroidal anti-inflammatory drug (NSAID) intoxication is primarily supportive and symptomatic. Fluid therapy is commonly effective in managing the hypotension that may occur following an acute NSAID overdose, except when this is due to an acute blood loss.

Seizures tend to be very short-lived and often do not require drug treatment; although, recurrent seizures should be treated with I.V. diazepam

Since many of the NSAIDs undergo enterohepatic cycling, multiple doses of charcoal may be needed to reduce the potential for delayed toxicities

**Drug Interactions** CYP2C9 and 2C18 enzyme substrate

ACE inhibitors: Effects may be reduced by NSAIDs; use lowest possible dose for shortest duration possible; monitor

Cholestyramine and colestipol: Absorption may be reduced by concurrent administration

Corticosteroids: May increase the risk of GI ulceration; use caution

Cyclosporine: Nephrotoxicity may be increased with concurrent NSAID use; monitor

CYP2C9 inhibitors: May increase concentrations; inhibitors include amiodarone, cimetidine, fluvoxamine, metronidazole, omeprazole, sulfonamides, valproic acid, and zafirlukast

Hydralazine: Antihypertensive effect may be decreased; avoid concurrent use

Lithium: Serum levels can be increased; avoid concurrent use if possible or monitor lithium levels and adjust dose. When NSAID is stopped, lithium may need adjustment again.

Loop diuretics: Therapeutic effects may be reduced by NSAIDs; avoid

Methotrexate: Toxicity may be increased by concurrent NSAID use; risk is limited in low-dose methotrexate regimens (such as for rheumatoid arthritis); prolonged leucovorin rescue may be required at antineoplastic doses; monitor

Thiazide diuretics: Antihypertensive effects are decreased; avoid concurrent use

Warfarin: INRs may be increased by some NSAIDs. This may depend, in part, on dose and duration; monitor INR closely. Use the lowest dose of NSAIDs possible and for the briefest duration.

**Usual Dosage** Oral:

Children: 0.2-0.3 mg/kg/day once daily; maximum dose: 15 mg/day

Adults: 10-20 mg/day once daily; although associated with increase in GI adverse effects, doses >20 mg/day have been used (ie, 30-40 mg/day)

**Dosing adjustment in hepatic impairment:** Reduction of dosage is necessary

**Patient Information** Take this medication exactly as directed; do not increase dose without consulting prescriber. Do not crush tablets or break capsules. Take with food or milk to reduce GI distress. Maintain adequate fluid intake (2-3 L/day of fluids unless instructed to restrict fluid intake). Do not use alcohol, aspirin, or aspirin-containing medication, and all other anti-inflammatory medications without consulting prescriber. You may experience drowsiness, dizziness, or nervousness (use caution when driving or engaging in tasks requiring alertness until response to drug is known); anorexia, nausea, vomiting, flatulence, or heartburn (frequent small meals, frequent mouth care, sucking lozenges, or chewing gum may help); fluid retention (weigh yourself weekly and report unusual (3-5 lb/week) weight gain). GI bleeding, ulceration, or perforation can occur with or without pain; discontinue medication and contact prescriber if persistent abdominal pain or cramping, or blood in stool occurs. Report unusual swelling of extremities or unusual weight gain; breathlessness, difficulty breathing, or unusual cough; chest pain, rapid heartbeat, palpitations; unusual bruising/bleeding; blood in urine, stool, mouth, or vomitus; unusual fatigue; changes in urinary pattern (polyuria or anuria); skin rash or itching; or change in hearing or ringing in ears.

**Dosage Forms** Capsule: 10 mg, 20 mg

- ♦ ***p*-Isobutylhydratropic Acid** *see* Ibuprofen *on page 280*
- ♦ **Pit** *see* Oxytocin *on page 417*
- ♦ **Pitocin®** *see* Oxytocin *on page 417*
- ♦ **Pitressin® Injection** *see* Vasopressin *on page 581*

## Pituitary Hormones, Posterior

(pi TOO i tare ee HOR mones, pose TEAR ee or)

**Pharmacologic Category** Hormone, Posterior Pituitary

**Use** Induce peristalsis by directly stimulating smooth muscle contraction to relieve postoperative abdominal distention and abdominal radiographic procedures; to control or prevent enuresis in diabetes insipidus

**Effects on Mental Status** None reported

(Continued)

## Pituitary Hormones, Posterior *(Continued)*

**Effects on Psychiatric Treatment** None reported

**Pregnancy Risk Factor** C

**Contraindications** Cardiac disease; hypertension; epilepsy; not to be used as an oxytocic

**Usual Dosage** Adults: I.M., S.C.: 10 units (usual range: 5-20 units)

**Dosage Forms** Injection: 20 units/mL (1 mL)


- ♦ **Placidyl®** *see* Ethchlorvynol *on page 210*
- ♦ **Plan B™** *see* Levonorgestrel *on page 315*
- ♦ **Plantago Seed** *see* Psyllium *on page 479*
- ♦ **Plantain Seed** *see* Psyllium *on page 479*
- ♦ **Plaquenil®** *see* Hydroxychloroquine *on page 276*
- ♦ **Plasbumin®** *see* Albumin *on page 21*
- ♦ **Platinol®** *see* Cisplatin *on page 126*
- ♦ **Platinol®-AQ** *see* Cisplatin *on page 126*
- ♦ **Plavix®** *see* Clopidogrel *on page 134*
- ♦ **Plendil®** *see* Felodipine *on page 220*
- ♦ **Pletal®** *see* Cilostazol *on page 123*


## Plicamycin (plye kay MYE sin)

**U.S. Brand Names** Mithracin®

**Pharmacologic Category** Antidote; Antineoplastic Agent, Antibiotic

**Use** Malignant testicular tumors, in the treatment of hypercalcemia and hypercalciuria of malignancy not responsive to conventional treatment; Paget's disease

**Effects on Mental Status** May cause drowsiness or depression

**Effects on Psychiatric Treatment** May rarely cause agranulocytosis; use caution with clozapine and carbamazepine

**Usual Dosage** Refer to individual protocols. Dose should be diluted in 1 L of $D_5W$ or NS and administered over 4-6 hours. Dosage should be based on the patient's body weight. If a patient has abnormal fluid retention (ie, edema, hydrothorax or ascites), the patient's ideal weight rather than actual body weight should be used to calculate the dose.

Adults: I.V.:
- Testicular cancer: 25-30 mcg/kg/day for 8-10 days
- Blastic chronic granulocytic leukemia: 25 mcg/kg over 2-4 hours every other day for 3 weeks
- Paget's disease: 15 mcg/kg/day once daily for 10 days
- Hypercalcemia:
  - 25 mcg/kg single dose which may be repeated in 48 hours if no response occurs
  - **OR** 25 mcg/kg/day for 3-4 days
  - **OR** 25-50 mcg/kg/dose every other day for 3-8 doses

**Dosing adjustment in renal impairment:**
- $Cl_{cr}$ 10-50 mL/minute: Decrease dosage to 75% of normal dose
- $Cl_{cr}$ <10 mL/minute: Decrease dosage to 50% of normal dose

Hemodialysis: Unknown

CAPD effects: Unknown

CAVH effects: Unknown

**Dosing in hepatic impairment:** In the treatment of hypercalcemia in patients with hepatic dysfunction: Reduce dose to 12.5 mcg/kg/day

**Dosage Forms** Powder for injection: 2.5 mg

♦ **Pneumococcal 7-Valent Conjugate Vaccine** *see* Pneumococcal Conjugate Vaccine, 7-Valent *on page 450*

## Pneumococcal Conjugate Vaccine, 7-Valent

(noo moe KOK al KON ju gate vak SEEN, seven VA lent)

**U.S. Brand Names** Prevnar™

**Synonyms** Diphtheria $CRM_{197}$ Protein; PCV7; Pneumococcal 7-Valent Conjugate Vaccine

**Pharmacologic Category** Vaccine

**Use** Immunization of infants and toddlers against *Streptococcus pneumoniae* infection caused by serotypes included in the vaccine

American Academy of Pediatrics policy statement: Recommended for all children ≤23 months of age; it is administered concurrently with other recommended vaccines at 2-, 4-, 6-, and 12-15 months. The number of doses required depends upon the age of initiation. All children 24-59 months of age who are at high risk should receive the vaccine (see Usual Dosage).

**High risk (attack rate of invasive pneumococcal disease >150/100,000 cases per year):** Sickle cell disease, congenital or acquired asplenia, or splenic dysfunction, HIV infection

**Presumed high risk (attack rate not calculated):**
- Congenital immune deficiency; Some B- (humoral) or T-lymphocyte deficiencies, complement deficiencies (particularly C1, C2, C3, and C4 deficiencies), or phagycytic disorders (excluding chronic granulomatous disease)
- Chronic cardiac disease (particularly cyanotic congenital heart disease and cardiac failure)
- Chronic pulmonary disease (including asthma treated with high-dose oral corticosteroid therapy)
- Cerebrospinal fluid leaks
- Chronic renal insufficiency, including nephrotic syndrome
- Diseases associated with immunosuppressive therapy or radiation therapy (including malignant neoplasms, leukemias, lymphomas, and Hodgkin's disease) and solid organ transplant (guidelines for use of pneumococcal vaccines for children who have undergone bone marrow transplants are currently under revision)
- Diabetes mellitus

**Moderate risk (attack rate of invasive pneumococcal disease >20/100,000 per year):**
- All children 24-35 months of age
- Children 36-59 months of age attending "out of home" care
- Children 36-59 months of age who are Native American (American Indian or Alaska Native) or are of African American descent

**Effects on Mental Status** Irritability, drowsiness, and restlessness are common

**Effects on Psychiatric Treatment** May lessen the effects of anxiolytics

**Pregnancy Risk Factor** C

**Contraindications** Patients with a hypersensitivity to the vaccine or any component, including diphtheria toxoid; current or recent severe or moderate febrile illness; thrombocytopenia; any contraindication to I.M. injection; not for I.V. use

**Warnings/Precautions** Caution in latex sensitivity. Children with impaired immune responsiveness may have a reduced response to active immunization. Use of the pneumococcal conjugate vaccine does not replace the use of the 23-valent vaccine in children >24 months of age with sickle cell disease, asplenia, HIV infection, chronic illness, or immunocompromise. Safety and efficacy have not been established in children <6 weeks of age. Not for I.V. use.

**Adverse Reactions All serious adverse reactions must be reported to the U.S. Department of Health and Human Services (DHHS) Vaccine Adverse Event Reporting System (VAERS) 1-800-822-7967.**

>10%:
- Central nervous system: Fever, irritability, drowsiness, restlessness
- Dermatologic: Erythema
- Gastrointestinal: Decreased appetite, vomiting, diarrhea
- Local: Induration, tenderness, nodule

1% to 10%: Dermatologic: Rash (0.5% to 1.4%)

**Usual Dosage** Dosing as recommended in the policy statement of the American Academy of Pediatrics: I.M. (0.5 mL each dose):

Previously Unvaccinated Infants and Children:
- 2-6 months: Primary series: Three doses (0.5 mL each dose) at 6- to 8-week intervals; booster dose: 0.5 mL at 12-15 months of age (booster dose given at least 6-8 weeks after the final dose of primary series)
- 7-11 months: Primary series: Two doses (0.5 mL each dose) at 6- to 8-week intervals; booster dose: 0.5 mL at 12-15 months of age (booster dose given at least 6-8 weeks after the final dose of primary series)
- 12-23 months: Primary series: Two doses (0.5 mL each dose) at 6- to 8-week intervals
- ≥24 months: 0.5 mL as a single dose

Dosing recommendations for "High-Risk" Children (see Use):

≤23 months:
- Previous doses: None
  - Recommendation: See dosing above for "Previously Unvaccinated Infants and Children"

24-59 months:
- Previous doses: Four doses PCV7
  - Recommendations: One dose 23PS vaccine at 24 months, at least 6-8 weeks after last dose of PCV7; one dose 23PS vaccine 3-5 years after the first dose of 23PS
- Previous doses: 1-3 doses PCV7
  - Recommendations: One dose PCV7; one dose 23PS vaccine, at least 6-8 weeks after last dose of PCV7; one dose 23PS vaccine 3-5 years after the first dose of 23PS
- Previous doses: One dose 23PS
  - Recommendations: Two doses PCV7 6-8 weeks apart, beginning at least 6-8 weeks after the last dose of 23PS; one dose 23PS vaccine 3-5 years after the first dose of 23PS
- Previous dose: None
  - Recommendations: Two doses PCV7 6-8 weeks apart; one dose 23PS vaccine, at least 6-8 weeks after last dose of PCV7; one dose 23PS vaccine 3-5 years after the first dose of 23PS

**Dosage Forms** Injection; 2 mcg of each saccharide for each of six serotypes and 4 mcg of a seventh serotype; also 20 mcg of CRM197 carrier protein and 0.125 mg of aluminum phosphate adjuvant per 0.5 mL per dose

♦ **Pneumococcal Polysaccharide Vaccine** *see* Pneumococcal Vaccine *on page 451*

## Pneumococcal Vaccine (noo moe KOK al vak SEEN)

**U.S. Brand Names** Pneumovax® 23; Pnu-Imune® 23
**Synonyms** Pneumococcal Polysaccharide Vaccine
**Pharmacologic Category** Vaccine
**Use** Children >2 years of age and adults who are at increased risk of pneumococcal disease and its complications because of underlying health conditions; older adults, including all those ≥65 years of age
**Effects on Mental Status** None reported
**Effects on Psychiatric Treatment** None reported
**Pregnancy Risk Factor** C
**Contraindications** Active infections, Hodgkin's disease patients, <2 years of age, pregnancy, hypersensitivity to pneumococcal vaccine or any component; <10 days prior to or during treatment with immunosuppressive drugs or radiation; (children <5 years of age do not respond satisfactorily to the capsular types of 23 capsular pneumococcal vaccine; the safety of vaccine in pregnant women has not been evaluated; it should not be given during pregnancy unless the risk of infection is high)
**Warnings/Precautions** Epinephrine injection (1:1000) must be immediately available in the case of anaphylaxis; use caution in individuals who have had episodes of pneumococcal infection within the preceding 3 years (pre-existing pneumococcal antibodies may result in increased reactions to vaccine); may cause relapse in patients with stable idiopathic thrombocytopenia purpura
**Adverse Reactions All serious adverse reactions must be reported to the U.S. Department of Health and Human Services (DHHS) Vaccine Adverse Event Reporting System (VAERS) 1-800-822-7967.**
>10%: Local: Induration and soreness at the injection site (~72%) (2-3 days)
<1%: Anaphylaxis, arthralgia, erythema, Guillain-Barré syndrome, low-grade fever, myalgia, paresthesias, rash
**Drug Interactions** Decreased effect with immunosuppressive agents, immunoglobulin, other live vaccines within 1 month
**Usual Dosage** Children >2 years and Adults: I.M., S.C.: 0.5 mL
Revaccination should be considered:
1. If ≥6 years since initial vaccination has elapsed, or
2. In patients who received 14-valent pneumococcal vaccine and are at highest risk (asplenic) for fatal infection or
3. At ≥6 years in patients with nephrotic syndrome, renal failure, or transplant recipients, or
4. 3-5 years in children with nephrotic syndrome, asplenia, or sickle cell disease

**Patient Information** Be aware of adverse effects
**Dosage Forms** Injection: 25 mcg each of 23 polysaccharide isolates/0.5 mL dose (0.5 mL, 1 mL, 5 mL)


- **Pneumomist®** *see* Guaifenesin *on page 256*
- **Pneumovax® 23** *see* Pneumococcal Vaccine *on page 451*
- **Pnu-Imune® 23** *see* Pneumococcal Vaccine *on page 451*
- **Pod-Ben-25®** *see* Podophyllum Resin *on page 451*
- **Podocon-25™** *see* Podophyllum Resin *on page 451*
- **Podofin®** *see* Podophyllum Resin *on page 451*


## Podophyllin and Salicylic Acid
(po DOF fil um & sal i SIL ik AS id)

**U.S. Brand Names** Verrex-C&M®
**Pharmacologic Category** Keratolytic Agent; Topical Skin Product
**Use** Topical treatment of benign growths including external genital and perianal warts, papillomas, fibroids
**Effects on Mental Status** None reported
**Effects on Psychiatric Treatment** None reported
**Usual Dosage** Apply daily with applicator, allow to dry; remove necrotic tissue before each application
**Dosage Forms** Solution, topical: Podophyllum 10% and salicylic acid 30% with penederm 0.5% (7.5 mL)

## Podophyllum Resin (po DOF fil um REZ in)

**U.S. Brand Names** Pod-Ben-25®; Podocon-25™; Podofin®
**Canadian Brand Names** Podofilm®
**Pharmacologic Category** Keratolytic Agent
**Use** Topical treatment of benign growths including external genital and perianal warts, papillomas, fibroids; compound benzoin tincture generally is used as the medium for topical application
**Effects on Mental Status** None reported
**Effects on Psychiatric Treatment** May rarely cause leukopenia, use caution with clozapine and carbamazepine
**Usual Dosage** Topical:
Children and Adults: 10% to 25% solution in compound benzoin tincture; apply drug to dry surface, use 1 drop at a time allowing drying between drops until area is covered; total volume should be limited to <0.5 mL per treatment session
Condylomata acuminatum: 25% solution is applied daily; use a 10% solution when applied to or near mucous membranes
Verrucae: 25% solution is applied 3-5 times/day directly to the wart
**Dosage Forms** Liquid, topical: 25% in benzoin (5 mL, 7.5 mL, 30 mL)


- **Poladex®** *see* Dexchlorpheniramine *on page 158*
- **Polaramine®** *see* Dexchlorpheniramine *on page 158*
- **Polistine®** *see* Carbinoxamine *on page 92*
- **Polocaine®** *see* Mepivacaine *on page 342*
- **Polycillin-N®** *see* Ampicillin *on page 42*
- **Polydine® [OTC]** *see* Povidone-Iodine *on page 456*


## Polyestradiol (pol i es tra DYE ole)

**Pharmacologic Category** Antineoplastic Agent, Miscellaneous; Estrogen Derivative
**Use** Palliative treatment of advanced, inoperable carcinoma of the prostate
**Effects on Mental Status** May rarely cause anxiety, dizziness, or depression
**Effects on Psychiatric Treatment** None reported
**Usual Dosage** Adults: Deep I.M.: 40 mg every 2-4 weeks or less frequently; maximum dose: 80 mg
**Dosage Forms** Powder for injection, as phosphate: 40 mg

## Polyethylene Glycol-Electrolyte Solution
(pol i ETH i leen GLY kol ee LEK troe lite soe LOO shun)

**U.S. Brand Names** Colovage®; CoLyte®; GoLYTELY®; NuLytely®; OCL®
**Canadian Brand Names** Klean-Prep®; Peglyte™
**Synonyms** Electrolyte Lavage Solution
**Pharmacologic Category** Cathartic; Laxative, Bowel Evacuant
**Use** Bowel cleansing prior to GI examination or following toxic ingestion
**Effects on Mental Status** None reported
**Effects on Psychiatric Treatment** Oral medications should not be administered within 1 hour of start of therapy
**Pregnancy Risk Factor** C
**Contraindications** Gastrointestinal obstruction, gastric retention, bowel perforation, toxic colitis, megacolon
**Warnings/Precautions** Safety and efficacy not established in children; do not add flavorings as additional ingredients before use; observe unconscious or semiconscious patients with impaired gag reflex or those who are otherwise prone to regurgitation or aspiration during administration; use with caution in ulcerative colitis, caution against the use of hot loop polypectomy
**Adverse Reactions**
>10%: Gastrointestinal: Nausea, abdominal fullness, bloating
1% to 10%: Gastrointestinal: Abdominal cramps, vomiting, anal irritation
<1%: Rash
**Drug Interactions** Oral medications should not be administered within 1 hour of start of therapy
**Usual Dosage** The recommended dose for adults is 4 L of solution prior to gastrointestinal examination, as ingestion of this dose produces a satisfactory preparation in >95% of patients. Ideally the patient should fast for approximately 3-4 hours prior to administration, but in no case should solid food be given for at least 2 hours before the solution is given. The solution is usually administered orally, but may be given via nasogastric tube to patients who are unwilling or unable to drink the solution.

Children: Oral: 25-40 mL/kg/hour for 4-10 hours
Adults:
Oral: At a rate of 240 mL (8 oz) every 10 minutes, until 4 liters are consumed or the rectal effluent is clear; rapid drinking of each portion is preferred to drinking small amounts continuously
Nasogastric tube: At a rate of 20-30 mL/minute (1.2-1.8 L/hour); the first bowel movement should occur approximately 1 hour after the start of administration
**Dietary Considerations** Ideally the patient should fast for approximately 3-4 hours prior to administration, but in no case should solid food be given for at least 2 hours before the solution is given
**Patient Information** Chilled solution is often more palatable. Produces a watery stool which cleanses the bowel before examination. Prepare solution according to instructions on the bottle. For best results, no solid food should be consumed during the 3- to 4-hour period before drinking solution, but in no case should solid foods be eaten within 2 hours of taking. Drink 240 mL every 10 minutes. Rapid drinking of each portion is better than drinking small amounts continuously. The first bowel movement should occur approximately 1 hour after the start of administration. May experience some abdominal bloating and distention before bowel starts to move. If severe discomfort or distention occurs, stop drinking temporarily or drink each portion at longer intervals until these symptoms disappear. Continue drinking until the watery stool is clear and free of solid matter. (Continued)

## Polyethylene Glycol-Electrolyte Solution *(Continued)*

This usually requires at least 3 L. It is best to drink all of the solutions. Discard any unused portion.

**Nursing Implications** Rapid drinking of each portion is preferred over small amounts continuously; first bowel movement should occur in 1 hour; chilled solution often more palatable; do not add flavorings as additional ingredients before use

**Dosage Forms** Powder, for oral solution: PEG 3350 236 g, sodium sulfate 22.74 g, sodium bicarbonate 6.74 g, sodium chloride 5.86 g and potassium chloride 2.97 g (2000 mL, 4000 mL, 4800 mL, 6000 mL)

♦ **Polygam® S/D** *see* Immune Globulin, Intravenous *on page 284*

## *Polygonum multiflorum*

**Pharmacologic Category** Herb

**Use** Tuberous root (raw or processed) used for vertigo, insomnia, constipation

**Adverse Reactions**

Cardiovascular: Palpitations
Central nervous system: Dizziness, fever
Dermatologic: Erythema, rash, pruritus
Gastrointestinal: Nausea, diarrhea
Hepatic: Hepatitis, jaundice
Ocular: Blurred vision
Respiratory: Tachypnea

**Overdosage/Toxicology** Treatment: Supportive therapy; hepatitis can resolve within 3 weeks upon discontinuation of drug; antihistamines can be used for pruritus

**Drug Interactions**

Hypoglycemic agents: Effects may be altered; monitor glucose
Digoxin: Herb may promote hypokalemia, increasing risk of toxicity

**Additional Information** A climbing evergreen plant native in Japan

♦ **Poly-Histine CS®** *see* Brompheniramine, Phenylpropanolamine, and Codeine *on page 74*

♦ **Poly-Histine-D® Capsule** *see* Phenyltoloxamine, Phenylpropanolamine, Pyrilamine, and Pheniramine *on page 441*

## Polymyxin B (pol i MIKS in bee)

**U.S. Brand Names** Aerosporin® Injection

**Pharmacologic Category** Antibiotic, Irrigation; Antibiotic, Miscellaneous

**Use**

Topical: Wound irrigation and bladder irrigation against *Pseudomonas aeruginosa*; used occasionally for gut decontamination

Parenteral use of polymyxin B has mainly been replaced by less toxic antibiotics; it is reserved for life-threatening infections caused by organisms resistant to the preferred drugs (eg, pseudomonal meningitis - intrathecal administration)

**Effects on Mental Status** May rarely cause irritability, drowsiness, or ataxia

**Effects on Psychiatric Treatment** None reported

**Usual Dosage**

Otic: 1-2 drops, 3-4 times/day; should be used sparingly to avoid accumulation of excess debris

Infants <2 years:
- I.M.: Up to 40,000 units/kg/day divided every 6 hours (not routinely recommended due to pain at injection sites)
- I.V.: Up to 40,000 units/kg/day by continuous I.V. infusion
- Intrathecal: 20,000 units/day for 3-4 days, then 25,000 units every other day for at least 2 weeks after CSF cultures are negative and CSF (glucose) has returned to within normal limits

Children ≥2 years and Adults:
- I.M.: 25,000-30,000 units/kg/day divided every 4-6 hours (not routinely recommended due to pain at injection sites)
- I.V.: 15,000-25,000 units/kg/day divided every 12 hours or by continuous infusion
- Intrathecal: 50,000 units/day for 3-4 days, then every other day for at least 2 weeks after CSF cultures are negative and CSF (glucose) has returned to within normal limits
- Total daily dose should not exceed 2,000,000 units/day
- Bladder irrigation: Continuous irrigant or rinse in the urinary bladder for up to 10 days using 20 mg (equal to 200,000 units) added to 1 L of normal saline; usually no more than 1 L of irrigant is used per day unless urine flow rate is high; administration rate is adjusted to patient's urine output
- Topical irrigation or topical solution: 500,000 units/L of normal saline; topical irrigation should not exceed 2 million units/day in adults
- Gut sterilization: Oral: 15,000-25,000 units/kg/day in divided doses every 6 hours
- *Clostridium difficile* enteritis: Oral: 25,000 units every 6 hours for 10 days

Ophthalmic: A concentration of 0.1% to 0.25% is administered as 1-3 drops every hour, then increasing the interval as response indicates to 1-2 drops 4-6 times/day

**Dosing adjustment/interval in renal impairment:**
- $Cl_{cr}$ 20-50 mL/minute: Administer 75% to 100% of normal dose every 12 hours
- $Cl_{cr}$ 5-20 mL/minute: Administer 50% of normal dose every 12 hours
- $Cl_{cr}$ <5 mL/minute: Administer 15% of normal dose every 12 hours

**Dosage Forms**

Injection: 500,000 units (20 mL)
Solution (otic): 10,000 units of polymyxin B per mL in combination with hydrocortisone 0.5% solution (eg, Otobiotic®)
Suspension (otic): 10,000 units of polymixin B per mL in combination with hydrocortisone 1% and neomycin sulfate 0.5% (eg, PediOtic®)
Also available in a variety of other combination products for ophthalmic and otic use.

## Polymyxin B and Hydrocortisone

(pol i MIKS in bee & hye droe KOR ti sone)

**U.S. Brand Names** Otobiotic® Otic

**Pharmacologic Category** Antibiotic/Corticosteroid, Otic

**Use** Treatment of superficial bacterial infections of external ear canal

**Effects on Mental Status** None reported

**Effects on Psychiatric Treatment** None reported

**Usual Dosage** Instill 4 drops 3-4 times/day

**Dosage Forms** Solution, otic: Polymyxin B sulfate 10,000 units and hydrocortisone 0.5% [5 mg/mL] per mL (10 mL, 15 mL)

♦ **Polymyxin B and Neomycin** *see* Neomycin and Polymyxin B *on page 388*

♦ **Polymyxin E** *see* Colistin *on page 139*

♦ **Poly-Pred® Ophthalmic Suspension** *see* Neomycin, Polymyxin B, and Prednisolone *on page 389*

## Polysaccharide-Iron Complex

(pol i SAK a ride-EYE ern KOM pleks)

**U.S. Brand Names** Hytinic® [OTC]; Niferex® [OTC]; Nu-Iron® [OTC]

**Pharmacologic Category** Iron Salt

**Use** Prevention and treatment of iron deficiency anemias

**Effects on Mental Status** None reported

**Effects on Psychiatric Treatment** Constipation is common, concurrent use with psychotropic may produce additive effects

**Usual Dosage** Oral:

Children: 3 mg/kg 3 times/day
Adults: 200 mg 3-4 times/day

**Dosage Forms**

Capsule: Elemental iron 150 mg
Elixir: Elemental iron 100 mg/5 mL (240 mL)
Tablet: Elemental iron 50 mg

♦ **Polysporin® Ophthalmic** *see* Bacitracin and Polymyxin B *on page 57*

♦ **Polysporin® Topical** *see* Bacitracin and Polymyxin B *on page 57*

## Polythiazide (pol i THYE a zide)

**U.S. Brand Names** Renese®

**Pharmacologic Category** Diuretic, Thiazide

**Use** Adjunctive therapy in treatment of edema and hypertension

**Effects on Mental Status** May cause drowsiness

**Effects on Psychiatric Treatment** May decrease lithium clearance resulting in an increase in serum lithium levels and potential lithium toxicity; monitor serum lithium levels

**Pregnancy Risk Factor** D

**Contraindications** Hypersensitivity to polythiazide or any other sulfonamide-derived drugs; anuria; renal decompensation; pregnancy

**Warnings/Precautions** Avoid in severe renal disease (ineffective). Electrolyte disturbances (hypokalemia, hypochloremic alkalosis, hyponatremia) can occur. Use with caution in severe hepatic dysfunction; hepatic encephalopathy can be caused by electrolyte disturbances. Gout can be precipitate in certain patients with a history of gout, a familial predisposition to gout, or chronic renal failure. Cautious use in diabetics; may see a change in glucose control. Hypersensitivity reactions can occur. Can cause SLE exacerbation or activation. Use with caution in patients with moderate or high cholesterol concentrations. Photosensitization may occur. Correct hypokalemia before initiating therapy.

**Adverse Reactions** 1% to 10%: Hypokalemia

**Overdosage/Toxicology**

Signs and symptoms: Hypermotility, diuresis, lethargy, confusion, muscle weakness
Treatment: Following GI decontamination, therapy is supportive with I.V. fluids, electrolytes, and I.V. pressors if needed

**Drug Interactions**

Angiotensin-converting enzyme inhibitors: Increased hypotension if aggressively diuresed with a thiazide diuretic

Beta-blockers increase hyperglycemic effects in Type 2 diabetes mellitus

Cyclosporine and thiazides can increase the risk of gout or renal toxicity; avoid concurrent use

Digoxin toxicity can be exacerbated if a thiazide induces hypokalemia or hypomagnesemia

Lithium toxicity can occur by reducing renal excretion of lithium; monitor lithium concentration and adjust as needed

Neuromuscular blocking agents can prolong blockade; monitor serum potassium and neuromuscular status

NSAIDs can decrease the efficacy of thiazides reducing the diuretic and antihypertensive effects

**Usual Dosage** Adults: Oral:

Edema: 1-4 mg/day

Hypertension: 2-4 mg/day

**Patient Information** May be taken with food or milk; take early in day to avoid nocturia; take the last dose of multiple doses no later than 6 PM unless instructed otherwise. A few people who take this medication become more sensitive to sunlight and may experience skin rash, redness, itching, or severe sunburn, especially if sun block SPF ≥15 is not used on exposed skin areas.

**Dosage Forms** Tablet: 1 mg, 2 mg, 4 mg

## Polythiazide and Reserpine

(pol i THYE a zide & re SER peen)

**Pharmacologic Category** Antihypertensive Agent, Combination

**Effects on Mental Status** Thiazides may cause drowsiness; reserpine may cause dizziness, headache, nightmares, nervousness, drowsiness, fatigue, mental depression, parkinsonism, dull sensorium, syncope, paradoxical anxiety

**Effects on Psychiatric Treatment** May decrease lithium clearance resulting in an increase in serum lithium levels and potential lithium toxicity; monitor serum lithium levels. Use caution in patients with depression, may lessen the antidepressant effects of antidepressants; may cause hypertensive reaction if used with MAOI, use an alternative antihypertensive agent.


♦ **Ponstel®** *see* Mefenamic Acid *on page 337*

♦ **Pontocaine®** *see* Tetracaine *on page 537*

♦ **Poor Mans Treacle** *see* Garlic *on page 246*

♦ **Poptillo** *see* Ephedra *on page 194*

♦ **Porcelana® [OTC]** *see* Hydroquinone *on page 276*

♦ **Porcelana® Sunscreen [OTC]** *see* Hydroquinone *on page 276*


## Porfimer (POR fi mer)

**U.S. Brand Names** Photofrin®

**Pharmacologic Category** Antineoplastic Agent, Miscellaneous

**Use** Esophageal cancer: Photodynamic therapy (PDT) with porfimer for palliation of patients with completely obstructing esophageal cancer, or of patients with partially obstructing esophageal cancer who cannot be satisfactorily treated with Nd:YAG laser therapy

**Effects on Mental Status** Insomnia is common; may cause anxiety or confusion

**Effects on Psychiatric Treatment** May cause anemia; use caution with clozapine and carbamazepine; concurrent use with psychotropics may increase the risk of photosensitivity reactions

**Usual Dosage** I.V. (refer to individual protocols):

Children: Safety and efficacy have not been established

Adults: I.V.: 2 mg/kg over 3-5 minutes

Photodynamic therapy is a two-stage process requiring administration of both drug and light. The first stage of PDT is the I.V. injection of porfimer. Illumination with laser light 40-50 hours following the injection with porfimer constitutes the second stage of therapy. A second laser light application may be given 90-120 hours after injection, preceded by gentle debridement of residual tumor.

Patients may receive a second course of PDT a minimum of 30 days after the initial therapy; up to three courses of PDT (each separated by a minimum of 30 days) can be given. Before each course of treatment, evaluate patients for the presence of a tracheoesophageal or bronchoesophageal fistula.

**Dosage Forms** Powder for injection, as sodium: 75 mg


♦ **Pork NPH Iletin® II** *see* Insulin Preparations *on page 287*

♦ **Pork Regular Iletin® II** *see* Insulin Preparations *on page 287*

♦ **Posture® [OTC]** *see* Calcium Phosphate, Tribasic *on page 86*

♦ **Potasalan®** *see* Potassium Chloride *on page 453*


## Potassium Bicarbonate and Potassium Citrate, Effervescent

(poe TASS ee um bye KAR bun ate & poe TASS ee um SIT rate, ef er VES ent)

**U.S. Brand Names** Effer-K™; K-Ide®; Klor-con®/EF; K-Lyte®; K-Vescent®

**Pharmacologic Category** Electrolyte Supplement, Oral

**Use** Treatment or prevention of hypokalemia

**Effects on Mental Status** May rarely cause confusion

**Effects on Psychiatric Treatment** None reported

**Usual Dosage** Oral:

Children: 1-4 mEq/kg/24 hours in divided doses as required to maintain normal serum potassium

Adults:

Prevention: 16-24 mEq/day in 2-4 divided doses

Treatment: 40-100 mEq/day in 2-4 divided doses

**Dosage Forms**

Capsule, extended release: 8 mEq, 10 mEq

Powder for oral solution: 15 mEq/packet; 20 mEq/packet; 25 mEq/packet

Tablet, effervescent: 25 mEq, 50 mEq

## Potassium Chloride (poe TASS ee um KLOR ide)

**U.S. Brand Names** Cena-K®; Gen-K®; K+ 10®; Kaochlor®; Kaochlor® SF; Kaon-Cl®; Kaon-Cl-10®; Kay Ciel®; K+ Care®; K-Dur® 10; K-Dur® 20; K-Lease®; K-Lor™; Klor-Con®; Klor-Con® 8; Klor-Con® 10; Klor-Con®/25; Klorvess®; Klotrix®; K-Lyte®/Cl; K-Norm®; K-Tab®; Micro-K® 10; Micro-K® 10 Extencaps®; Micro-K® LS; Potasalan®; Rum-K®; Slow-K®; Ten-K®

**Synonyms** KCl

**Pharmacologic Category** Electrolyte Supplement, Oral

**Use** Treatment or prevention of hypokalemia

**Effects on Mental Status** None reported

**Effects on Psychiatric Treatment** None reported

**Pregnancy Risk Factor** A

**Contraindications** Severe renal impairment, untreated Addison's disease, heat cramps, hyperkalemia, severe tissue trauma; solid oral dosage forms are contraindicated in patients in whom there is a structural, pathological, and/or pharmacologic cause for delay or arrest in passage through the GI tract; an oral liquid potassium preparation should be used in patients with esophageal compression or delayed gastric emptying time

**Warnings/Precautions** Use with caution in patients with cardiac disease, severe renal impairment, hyperkalemia

**Adverse Reactions**

>10%: Gastrointestinal: Diarrhea, nausea, stomach pain, flatulence, vomiting (oral)

1% to 10%:

Cardiovascular: Bradycardia

Endocrine & metabolic: Hyperkalemia

Local: Local tissue necrosis with extravasation, pain at the site of injection

Neuromuscular & skeletal: Weakness

Respiratory: Dyspnea

<1%: Chest pain, arrhythmias, heart block, hypotension, mental confusion, alkalosis, abdominal pain, throat pain, phlebitis, paresthesias, paralysis

**Overdosage/Toxicology**

Symptoms of overdose include muscle weakness, paralysis, peaked T waves, flattened P waves, prolongation of QRS complex, ventricular arrhythmias

Removal of potassium can be accomplished by various means; removal through the GI tract with Kayexalate® administration; by way of the kidney through diuresis, mineralocorticoid administration or increased sodium intake; by hemodialysis or peritoneal dialysis; or by shifting potassium back into the cells by insulin and glucose infusion or sodium bicarbonate; calcium chloride reverses cardiac effects.

**Drug Interactions** Increased effect/levels with potassium-sparing diuretics, salt substitutes, ACE inhibitors

**Usual Dosage** I.V. doses should be incorporated into the patient's maintenance I.V. fluids; intermittent I.V. potassium administration should be reserved for severe depletion situations in patients undergoing EKG monitoring.

Normal daily requirements: Oral, I.V.:

Premature infants: 2-6 mEq/kg/24 hours

Term infants 0-24 hours: 0-2 mEq/kg/24 hours

Infants >24 hours: 1-2 mEq/kg/24 hours

Children: 2-3 mEq/kg/day

Adults: 40-80 mEq/day

Prevention during diuretic therapy: Oral:

Children: 1-2 mEq/kg/day in 1-2 divided doses

Adults: 20-40 mEq/day in 1-2 divided doses

Treatment of hypokalemia: Children:

Oral: 1-2 mEq/kg initially, then as needed based on frequently obtained lab values. If deficits are severe or ongoing losses are great, I.V. route should be considered.

(Continued)

## Potassium Chloride *(Continued)*

I.V.: 1 mEq/kg over 1-2 hours initially, then repeated as needed based on frequently obtained lab values; severe depletion or ongoing losses may require >200% of normal limit needs

I.V. intermittent infusion: Dose should not exceed 1 mEq/kg/hour, or 40 mEq/hour; if it exceeds 0.5 mEq/kg/hour, physician should be at bedside and patient should have continuous EKG monitoring; usual pediatric maximum: 3 mEq/kg/day or 40 mEq/m$^2$/day

Treatment of hypokalemia: Adults:

I.V. intermittent infusion: 5-10 mEq/hour (continuous cardiac monitor recommended for rates >5 mEq/hour), not to exceed 40 mEq/hour; usual adult maximum per 24 hours: 400 mEq/day.

Potassium dosage/rate of infusion guidelines:

Serum potassium >2.5 mEq/L: Maximum infusion rate: 10 mEq/hour; maximum concentration: 40 mEq/L; maximum 24-hour dose: 200 mEq

Serum potassium <2.5 mEq/L: Maximum infusion rate: 40 mEq/hour; maximum concentration: 80 mEq/L; maximum 24-hour dose: 400 mEq

Potassium >2.5 mEq/L:

Oral: 60-80 mEq/day plus additional amounts if needed

I.V.: 10 mEq over 1 hour with additional doses if needed

Potassium <2.5 mEq/L:

Oral: Up to 40-60 mEq initial dose, followed by further doses based on lab values

I.V.: Up to 40 mEq over 1 hour, with doses based on frequent lab monitoring; deficits at a plasma level of 2 mEq/L may be as high as 400-800 mEq of potassium

**Dietary Considerations** Administer with plenty of fluid and/or food because of stomach irritation and discomfort

**Patient Information** Sustained release and wax matrix tablets should be swallowed whole, do not crush or chew; effervescent tablets must be dissolved in water before use; take with food; liquid and granules can be diluted or dissolved in water or juice

**Nursing Implications** Wax matrix tablets must be swallowed and not allowed to dissolve in mouth

**Dosage Forms**

Capsule, controlled release (microcapsulated): 600 mg [8 mEq]; 750 mg [10 mEq]

Micro-K® Extencaps®: 600 mg [8 mEq]

K-Lease®, K-Norm®, Micro-K® 10: 750 mg [10 mEq]

Liquid: 10% [20 mEq/15 mL] (480 mL, 4000 mL); 20% [40 mEq/15 mL] (480 mL, 4000 mL)

Cena-K®, Kaochlor®, Kaochlor® SF, Kay Ciel®, Klorvess®, Potasalan®: 10% [20 mEq/15 mL] (480 mL, 4000 mL)

Rum-K®: 15% [30 mEq/15 mL] (480 mL, 4000 mL)

Cena-K®, Kaon-Cl® 20%: 20% [40 mEq/15 mL]

Crystals for oral suspension, extended release (Micro-K® LS®): 20 mEq per packet

Powder: 20 mEq per packet (30s, 100s)

K+ Care®, K-Lor™: 15 mEq per packet (30s, 100s)

Gen-K®, Kay Ciel®, K+ Care®, K-Lor™, Klor-Con®: 20 mEq per packet (30s, 100s)

K+ Care®, Klor-Con/25®: 25 mEq per packet (30s, 100s)

K-Lyte/Cl®: 25 mEq per dose (30s)

Infusion, concentrate: 0.1 mEq/mL, 0.2 mEq/mL, 0.3 mEq/mL, 0.4 mEq/mL

Injection, concentrate: 1.5 mEq/mL, 2 mEq/mL, 3 mEq/mL

Tablet, controlled release (microencapsulated)

K-Dur® 10, Ten-K®: 750 mg [10 mEq]

K-Dur® 20: 1500 mg [20 mEq]

Tablet, controlled release (wax matrix): 600 mg [8 mEq]; 750 mg [10 mEq]

Kaon-Cl®: 500 mg [6.7 mEq]

Klor-Con® 8, Slow-K®: 600 mg [8 mEq]

K+ 10®, Kaon-Cl-10®, Klor-Con® 10, Klotrix®, K-Tab®: 750 mg [10 mEq]

## Potassium Citrate and Potassium Gluconate

(poe TASS ee um SIT rate & poe TASS ee um GLOO coe nate)

**U.S. Brand Names** Twin-K®

**Pharmacologic Category** Electrolyte Supplement, Oral

**Use** Treatment or prevention of hypokalemia

**Effects on Mental Status** None reported

**Effects on Psychiatric Treatment** None reported

**Usual Dosage** Oral:

Children: 1-4 mEq/kg/24 hours in divided doses as required to maintain normal serum potassium

Adults:

Prevention: 16-24 mEq/day in 2-4 divided doses

Treatment: 40-100 mEq/day in 2-4 divided doses

**Dosage Forms** Solution, oral: 20 mEq/5 mL from potassium citrate 170 mg and potassium gluconate 170 mg per 5 mL

## Potassium Gluconate (poe TASS ee um GLOO coe nate)

**U.S. Brand Names** Kaon®; K-G®

**Pharmacologic Category** Electrolyte Supplement, Oral

**Use** Treatment or prevention of hypokalemia

**Effects on Mental Status** None reported

**Effects on Psychiatric Treatment** None reported

**Pregnancy Risk Factor** A

**Contraindications** Severe renal impairment, untreated Addison's disease, heat cramps, hyperkalemia, severe tissue trauma; solid oral dosage forms are contraindicated in patients in whom there is a structural, pathological, and/or pharmacologic cause for delay or arrest in passage through the GI tract; an oral liquid potassium preparation should be used in patients with esophageal compression or delayed gastric emptying time

**Warnings/Precautions** Use with caution in patients with cardiac disease, severe renal impairment, hyperkalemia; patients must be on a cardiac monitor during intermittent infusions

**Adverse Reactions**

>10%: Gastrointestinal: Diarrhea, nausea, stomach pain, flatulence, vomiting (oral)

1% to 10%:

Cardiovascular: Bradycardia

Endocrine & metabolic: Hyperkalemia

Neuromuscular & skeletal: Weakness

Respiratory: Dyspnea

<1%: Chest pain, mental confusion, alkalosis, throat pain, phlebitis, paresthesias, paralysis

**Overdosage/Toxicology**

Symptoms of overdose include muscle weakness, paralysis, peaked T waves, flattened P waves, prolongation of QRS complex, ventricular arrhythmias

Removal of potassium can be accomplished by various means; removal through the GI tract with Kayexalate® administration; by way of the kidney through diuresis, mineralocorticoid administration or increased sodium intake; by hemodialysis or peritoneal dialysis; or by shifting potassium back into the cells by insulin, glucose infusion, or sodium bicarbonate; calcium chloride reverses cardiac effects

**Drug Interactions** Increased effect/levels with potassium-sparing diuretics, salt substitutes, ACE inhibitors; increased effect of digitalis

**Usual Dosage** Oral (doses listed as mEq of potassium):

Normal daily requirement:

Children: 2-3 mEq/kg/day

Adults: 40-80 mEq/day

Prevention of hypokalemia during diuretic therapy:

Children: 1-2 mEq/kg/day in 1-2 divided doses

Adults: 16-24 mEq/day in 1-2 divided doses

Treatment of hypokalemia:

Children: 2-5 mEq/kg/day in 2-4 divided doses

Adults: 40-100 mEq/day in 2-4 divided doses

**Patient Information** Take with food, water, or fruit juice; swallow tablets whole; do not crush or chew

**Nursing Implications** Do not administer liquid full strength, must be diluted in 2-6 parts of water or juice

**Dosage Forms**

Elixir: 20 mEq/15 mL

K-G®, Kaon®, Kaylixir®: 20 mEq/15 mL

Tablet:

Glu-K®: 2 mEq

Kaon®: 5 mEq

## Potassium Iodide (poe TASS ee um EYE oh dide)

**U.S. Brand Names** Pima®; SSKI®; Thyro-Block®

**Synonyms** KI; Lugol's Solution; Strong Iodine Solution

**Pharmacologic Category** Antithyroid Agent; Cough Preparation; Expectorant

**Use** Facilitate bronchial drainage and cough; reduce thyroid vascularity prior to thyroidectomy and management of thyrotoxic crisis; block thyroidal uptake of radioactive isotopes of iodine in a radiation emergency

**Effects on Mental Status** None reported

**Effects on Psychiatric Treatment** Concurrent use with lithium may produce additive hypothyroid effects

**Pregnancy Risk Factor** D

**Contraindications** Known hypersensitivity to iodine; hyperkalemia, pulmonary tuberculosis, pulmonary edema, bronchitis, impaired renal function

**Warnings/Precautions** Prolonged use can lead to hypothyroidism; cystic fibrosis patients have an exaggerated response; can cause acne flare-ups, can cause dermatitis, some preparations may contain sodium bisulfite (allergy); use with caution in patients with a history of thyroid disease, patients with renal failure, or GI obstruction

**Adverse Reactions** 1% to 10%:

Central nervous system: Fever, headache

Dermatologic: Urticaria, acne, angioedema, cutaneous hemorrhage

Endocrine & metabolic: Goiter with hypothyroidism
Gastrointestinal: Metallic taste, GI upset, soreness of teeth and gums
Hematologic: Eosinophilia, hemorrhage (mucosal)
Neuromuscular & skeletal: Arthralgia
Respiratory: Rhinitis
Miscellaneous: Lymph node enlargement

**Overdosage/Toxicology**

Symptoms of overdose include angioedema, laryngeal edema in patients with hypersensitivity; muscle weakness, paralysis, peaked T waves, flattened P waves, prolongation of QRS complex, ventricular arrhythmias

Removal of potassium can be accomplished by various means; removal through the GI tract with Kayexalate® administration; by way of the kidney through diuresis, mineralocorticoid administration or increased sodium intake; by hemodialysis or peritoneal dialysis; or by shifting potassium back into the cells by insulin and glucose infusion.

**Drug Interactions** Increased toxicity: Lithium → additive hypothyroid effects

**Usual Dosage** Oral:

Adults: RDA: 130 mcg
Expectorant:
Children: 60-250 mg every 6-8 hours; maximum single dose: 500 mg
Adults: 300-650 mg 2-3 times/day
Preoperative thyroidectomy: Children and Adults: 50-250 mg (1-5 drops SSKI®) 3 times/day **or** 0.1-0.3 mL (3-5 drops) of strong iodine (Lugol's solution) 3 times/day; administer for 10 days before surgery
Thyrotoxic crisis:
Infants <1 year: 150-250 mg (3-5 drops SSKI®) 3 times/day
Children and Adults: 300-500 mg (6-10 drops SSKI®) 3 times/day or 1 mL strong iodine (Lugol's solution) 3 times/day
Sporotrichosis:
Initial:
Preschool: 50 mg/dose 3 times/day
Children: 250 mg/dose 3 times/day
Adults: 500 mg/dose 3 times/day
Oral increase 50 mg/dose daily
Maximum dose:
Preschool: 500 mg/dose 3 times/day
Children and Adults: 1-2 g/dose 3 times/day
Continue treatment for 4-6 weeks after lesions have completely healed

**Patient Information** Take after meals. Dilute in 6 oz of water, fruit juice, milk, or broth. Do not chew tablets; swallow whole. Do not exceed recommended dosage. You may experience a metallic taste. Discontinue use and report stomach pain, severe nausea or vomiting, black or tarry stools, or unresolved weakness.

**Nursing Implications** Must be diluted before administration of 240 mL of water, fruit juice, milk, or broth

**Dosage Forms**

Solution, oral:
SSKI®: 1 g/mL (30 mL, 240 mL, 473 mL)
Lugol's solution, strong iodine: 100 mg/mL with iodine 50 mg/mL (120 mL)
Syrup: 325 mg/5 mL
Tablet: 130 mg

## Potassium Phosphate (poe TASS ee um FOS fate)

**U.S. Brand Names** Neutra-Phos®-K

**Synonyms** Phosphate, Potassium

**Pharmacologic Category** Electrolyte Supplement, Oral

**Use** Treatment and prevention of hypophosphatemia or hypokalemia

**Effects on Mental Status** None reported

**Effects on Psychiatric Treatment** None reported

**Pregnancy Risk Factor** C

**Contraindications** Hyperphosphatemia, hyperkalemia, hypocalcemia, hypomagnesemia, renal failure

**Warnings/Precautions** Use with caution in patients with renal insufficiency, cardiac disease, metabolic alkalosis; admixture of phosphate and calcium in I.V. fluids can result in calcium phosphate precipitation

**Adverse Reactions**

>10%: Gastrointestinal: Diarrhea, nausea, stomach pain, flatulence, vomiting
1% to 10%:
Cardiovascular: Bradycardia
Endocrine & metabolic: Hyperkalemia
Neuromuscular & skeletal: Weakness
Respiratory: Dyspnea
<1%: Chest pain, mental confusion, alkalosis, hypocalcemia tetany (with large doses of phosphate), abdominal pain, throat pain, phlebitis, paresthesias, paralysis, acute renal failure

**Overdosage/Toxicology**

Symptoms of overdose include muscle weakness, paralysis, peaked T waves, flattened P waves, prolongation of QRS complex, ventricular arrhythmias, tetany, calcium-phosphate precipitation

Removal of potassium can be accomplished by various means; removal through the GI tract with Kayexalate® administration; by way of the kidney through diuresis, mineralocorticoid administration or increased sodium intake; by hemodialysis or peritoneal dialysis; or by shifting potassium back into the cells by insulin, glucose infusion, or sodium bicarbonate; calcium chloride reverses cardiac effects.

**Drug Interactions**

Decreased effect/levels with aluminum and magnesium-containing antacids or sucralfate which can act as phosphate binders
Increased effect/levels with potassium-sparing diuretics, salt substitutes, or ACE inhibitors; increased effect of digitalis

**Usual Dosage** I.V. doses should be incorporated into the patient's maintenance I.V. fluids; intermittent I.V. infusion should be reserved for severe depletion situations in patients undergoing continuous EKG monitoring. It is difficult to determine total body phosphorus deficit; the following dosages are empiric guidelines:

Normal requirements elemental phosphorus: Oral:
0-6 months: 240 mg
6-12 months: 360 mg
1-10 years: 800 mg
>10 years: 1200 mg
Pregnancy lactation: Additional 400 mg/day
Adults: 800 mg

Treatment: It is difficult to provide concrete guidelines for the treatment of severe hypophosphatemia because the extent of total body deficits and response to therapy are difficult to predict. Aggressive doses of phosphate may result in a transient serum elevation followed by redistribution into intracellular compartments or bone tissue. It is recommended that repletion of severe hypophosphatemia (<1 mg/dL in adults) be done I.V. because large doses of oral phosphate may cause diarrhea and intestinal absorption may be unreliable

**Pediatric I.V. phosphate repletion:**
Children: 0.25-0.5 mmol/kg **administer over 4-6 hours and repeat if symptomatic hypophosphatemia persists**; to assess the need for further phosphate administration, obtain serum inorganic phosphate after administration of the first dose and base further doses on serum levels and clinical status

**Adult I.V. phosphate repletion:**
Initial dose: 0.08 mmol/kg if recent uncomplicated hypophosphatemia
Initial dose: 0.16 mmol/kg if prolonged hypophosphatemia with presumed total body deficits; increase dose by 25% to 50% if patient symptomatic with severe hypophosphatemia
**Do not exceed 0.24 mmol/kg/day; administer over 6 hours by I.V. infusion**

**With orders for I.V. phosphate, there is considerable confusion associated with the use of millimoles (mmol) versus milliequivalents (mEq) to express the phosphate requirement.** Because inorganic phosphate exists as monobasic and dibasic anions, with the mixture of valences dependent on pH, ordering by mEq amounts is unreliable and may lead to large dosing errors. In addition, I.V. phosphate is available in the sodium and potassium salt; therefore, the content of these cations must be considered when ordering phosphate. The most reliable method of ordering I.V. phosphate is by millimoles, then specifying the potassium or sodium salt. For example, an order for 15 mmol of phosphate as potassium phosphate in one liter of normal saline The dosing of phosphate should be 0.2-0.3 mmol/kg with a usual daily requirement of 30-60 mmol/day or 15 mmol of phosphate per liter of TPN or 15 mmol phosphate per 1000 calories of dextrose. Would also provide 22 mEq of potassium.

Maintenance:
I.V. solutions:
Children: 0.5-1.5 mmol/kg/24 hours I.V. or 2-3 mmol/kg/24 hours orally in divided doses
Adults: 15-30 mmol/24 hours I.V. or 50-150 mmol/24 hours orally in divided doses
Oral:
Children <4 years: 1 capsule (250 mg phosphorus/8 mmol) 4 times/day; dilute as instructed
Children >4 years and Adults: 1-2 capsules (250-500 mg phosphorus/8-16 mmol) 4 times/day; dilute as instructed

**Dietary Considerations** Avoid administering with oxalate (berries, nuts, chocolate, beans, celery, tomato) or phytate (bran, whole wheat) containing foods

**Patient Information** Do not swallow the capsule; empty contents of capsule into 75 mL (2.5 oz) of water before taking; take with food to reduce the risk of diarrhea

**Nursing Implications** Capsule must be emptied into 3-4 oz of water before administration

**Dosage Forms**

Oral:
Whole cow's milk per mL: Phosphate 0.29 mmol, Na 0.025 mEq, K 0.035 mEq
Neutra-Phos® capsule, powder concentrate: Elemental phosphorus 250 mg, phosphate 8 mmol, Na 7.1 mEq, K 7.1 mEq
Neutra-Phos®-K capsule, powder: Elemental phosphorus 250 mg, phosphate 8 mmol, K 14.2 mEq
K-Phos® Neutral tablets: Elemental phosphorus 250 mg, phosphate 8 mmol, Na 13 mEq, K 1.1 mEq

(Continued)

## Potassium Phosphate *(Continued)*

K-Phos® MF tablets: Elemental phosphorus 125.6 mg, phosphate 4 mmol, Na 2.9 mEq, K 1.1 mEq
K-Phos® No. 2: Elemental phosphorus 250 mg, phosphate 8 mmol, Na 5.8 mEq, K 2.3 mEq
K-Phos® Original tablets: Elemental phosphorus 114 mg, phosphate 3.6 mmol, K 3.7 mEq
Uro-KP-Neutral® tablets: Elemental phosphorus 250 mg, phosphate 8 mmol, Na 10.8 mEq, K 1.3 mEq
Intravenous: K phosphate, per mL: Phosphate 3 mmol, K 4.4 mEq

## Potassium Phosphate and Sodium Phosphate

(poe TASS ee um FOS fate & SOW dee um FOS fate)

**U.S. Brand Names** K-Phos® Neutral; Neutra-Phos®; Uro-KP-Neutral®

**Synonyms** Sodium Phosphate and Potassium Phosphate

**Pharmacologic Category** Electrolyte Supplement, Oral

**Use** Treatment of conditions associated with excessive renal phosphate loss or inadequate GI absorption of phosphate; to acidify the urine to lower calcium concentrations; to increase the antibacterial activity of methenamine; reduce odor and rash caused by ammonia in urine

**Effects on Mental Status** None reported

**Effects on Psychiatric Treatment** None reported

**Pregnancy Risk Factor** C

**Contraindications** Addison's disease, hyperkalemia, hyperphosphatemia, infected urolithiasis or struvite stone formation, patients with severely impaired renal function

**Warnings/Precautions** Use with caution in patients with renal disease, hyperkalemia, cardiac disease and metabolic alkalosis

**Adverse Reactions**

>10%: Gastrointestinal: Diarrhea, nausea, stomach pain, flatulence, vomiting

1% to 10%:
- Cardiovascular: Bradycardia
- Endocrine & metabolic: Hyperkalemia
- Neuromuscular & skeletal: Weakness
- Respiratory: Dyspnea

<1%: Arrhythmia, chest pain, edema, mental confusion, tetany (with large doses of phosphate), alkalosis, weight gain, throat pain, decreased urine output, phlebitis, paresthesias, paralysis, pain/weakness of extremities, bone pain, arthralgia, acute renal failure, shortness of breath, thirst

**Overdosage/Toxicology**

Symptoms of overdose include muscle weakness, paralysis, peaked T waves, flattened P waves, prolongation of QRS complex, ventricular arrhythmias, tetany, calcium phosphate precipitation

Removal of potassium can be accomplished by various means; removal through the GI tract with Kayexalate® administration; by way of the kidney through diuresis, mineralocorticoid administration or increased sodium intake; by hemodialysis or peritoneal dialysis; or by shifting potassium back into the cells by insulin and glucose infusion; calcium chloride reverses cardiac effects.

**Drug Interactions**

Decreased effect/levels with aluminum and magnesium-containing antacids or sucralfate which can act as phosphate binders

Increased effect/levels with potassium-sparing diuretics or ACE inhibitors; salicylates

**Usual Dosage** All dosage forms to be mixed in 6-8 oz of water prior to administration

Children: 2-3 mmol phosphate/kg/24 hours given 4 times/day **or** 1 capsule 4 times/day

Adults: 1-2 capsules (250-500 mg phosphorus/8-16 mmol) 4 times/day after meals and at bedtime

**Dietary Considerations** Should be administered after meals

**Patient Information** Do not swallow, open capsule and dissolve in 6-8 oz of water; powder packets are to be mixed in 6-8 oz of water; tablets should be crushed and mixed in 6-8 oz of water

**Nursing Implications** Tablets may be crushed and stirred vigorously to speed dissolution

**Dosage Forms** See Potassium Phosphate monograph

## Povidone-Iodine (POE vi done EYE oh dyne)

**U.S. Brand Names** ACU-dyne® [OTC]; Aerodine® [OTC]; Betadine® [OTC]; Betadine® 5% Sterile Ophthalmic Prep Solution; Betagan® [OTC]; Biodine [OTC]; Efodine® [OTC]; Iodex® [OTC]; Iodex-p® [OTC]; Mallisol® [OTC]; Massengill® Medicated Douche w/Cepticin [OTC]; Minidyne® [OTC]; Operand® [OTC]; Polydine® [OTC]; Summer's Eve® Medicated Douche [OTC]; Yeast-Gard® Medicated Douche

**Pharmacologic Category** Antibiotic, Topical; Topical Skin Product

**Use** External antiseptic with broad microbicidal spectrum against bacteria, fungi, viruses, protozoa, and yeasts

**Effects on Mental Status** None reported

**Effects on Psychiatric Treatment** None reported

**Usual Dosage**

Shampoo: Apply 2 teaspoons to hair and scalp, lather and rinse; repeat application 2 times/week until improvement is noted, then shampoo weekly

Topical: Apply as needed for treatment and prevention of susceptible microbial infections

**Dosage Forms**

Aerosol: 5% (88.7 mL, 90 mL)
Antiseptic gauze pads: 10% (3" x 9")
Cleanser:
- Skin: 7.5% (30 mL, 118 mL)
- Skin, foam: 7.5% (170 g)
- Topical: 60 mL, 240 mL

Concentrate, whirlpool: 3,840 mL
Cream: 5% (14 g)
Douche (10%): 0.5 oz/packet (6 packets/box), 240 mL
Foam, topical (10%): 250 g
Gel:
- Lubricating: 5% (5 g)
- Vaginal (10%): 18 g, 90 g

Liquid: 473 mL
Mouthwash (0.5%): 177 mL
Ointment, topical: 10% (0.94 g, 3.8 g, 28 g, 30 g, 454 g); 1 g, 1.2 g, 2.7 g packets
Perineal wash concentrate: 1% (240 mL); 10% (236 mL)
Scrub, surgical: 7.5% (15 mL, 473 mL, 946 mL)
Shampoo: 7.5% (118 mL)
Solution:
- Ophthalmic sterile prep: 5% (50 mL)
- Prep: 30 mL, 60 mL, 240 mL, 473 mL, 1000 mL, 4000 mL
- Swab aid: 1%
- Swabsticks: 4"
- Topical: 10% (15 mL, 30 mL, 120 mL, 237 mL, 473 mL, 480 mL, 1000 mL, 4000 mL)

Suppositories, vaginal: 10%

♦ **PPA** *see* Phenylpropanolamine *on page 440*

♦ **PPD** *see* Tuberculin Purified Protein Derivative *on page 575*

♦ **PPS** *see* Pentosan Polysulfate Sodium *on page 429*

♦ ***P. quinquefolium L.*** *see* Ginseng *on page 249*

## Pralidoxime (pra li DOKS eem)

**U.S. Brand Names** Protopam®

**Pharmacologic Category** Antidote

**Use** Reverse muscle paralysis with toxic exposure to organophosphate anticholinesterase pesticides and chemicals; control of overdose of drugs used to treat myasthenia gravis (ambenonium, neostigmine, pyridostigmine)

**Effects on Mental Status** May cause dizziness or drowsiness

**Effects on Psychiatric Treatment** Avoid with phenothiazines; effects of barbiturates may be increased

**Usual Dosage** Poisoning: I.M. (use in conjunction with atropine; atropine effects should be established before pralidoxime is administered), I.V.:

Children: 20-50 mg/kg/dose; repeat in 1-2 hours if muscle weakness has not been relieved, then at 10- to 12-hour intervals if cholinergic signs recur

Adults: 1-2 g; repeat in 1-2 hours if muscle weakness has not been relieved, then at 10- to 12-hour intervals if cholinergic signs recur

Treatment of acetylcholinesterase inhibitor toxicity: Initial: 1-2 g followed by increments of 250 mg every 5 minutes until response is observed

**Dosing adjustment in renal impairment:** Dose should be reduced

**Dosage Forms**

Injection: 20 mL vial containing 1 g each pralidoxime chloride with one 20 mL ampul diluent, disposable syringe, needle, and alcohol swab
Injection, as chloride: 300 mg/mL (2 mL)

♦ **PrameGel® [OTC]** *see* Pramoxine *on page 457*

## Pramipexole (pra mi PEX ole)

**U.S. Brand Names** Mirapex®

**Pharmacologic Category** Anti-Parkinson's Agent (Dopamine Agonist)

**Use** Treatment of the signs and symptoms of idiopathic Parkinson's Disease;

**Unlabeled use:** Treatment of depression

**Pregnancy Risk Factor** C

**Contraindications** Patients with known hypersensitivity to pramipexole or any of the product's ingredients

**Warnings/Precautions** Caution should be taken in patients with renal insufficiency and in patients with pre-existing dyskinesias. May cause orthostatic hypotension; Parkinson's disease patients appear to have an impaired capacity to respond to a postural challenge. Use with caution in patients at risk of hypotension (such as those receiving antihypertensive drugs) or where transient hypotensive episodes would be poorly tolerated (cardiovascular disease or cerebrovascular disease). Parkinson's patients being treated with dopaminergic agonists ordinarily require careful monitoring for signs and symptoms of postural hypotension, especially during dose escalation, and should be informed of this risk. May cause hallucinations, particularly in older patients. Pathologic degenerative changes were observed in the retinas of albino rats during studies with this agent, but were not observed in the retinas of pigmented rats or in other species. The significance of these data for humans remains uncertain.

Although not reported for pramipexole, other dopaminergic agents have been associated with a syndrome resembling neuroleptic malignant syndrome on withdrawal or significant dosage reduction after long-term use. Dopaminergic agents from the ergot class have also been associated with fibrotic complications, such as retroperitoneum, lungs, and pleura. Episodes of falling asleep during routine daily activities have been reported.

**Adverse Reactions**

>10%:
- Cardiovascular: Postural hypotension
- Central nervous system: Asthenia, dizziness, somnolence, insomnia, hallucinations, abnormal dreams
- Gastrointestinal: Nausea, constipation
- Neuromuscular & skeletal: Weakness, dyskinesia, EPS

1% to 10%:
- Cardiovascular: Edema, postural hypotension, syncope, tachycardia, chest pain
- Central nervous system: Malaise, confusion, amnesia, dystonias, akathisia, thinking abnormalities, myoclonus, hyperesthesia, gait abnormalities, hypertonia, paranoia
- Endocrine & metabolic: Decreased libido
- Gastrointestinal: Anorexia, weight loss, xerostomia
- Genitourinary: Urinary frequency (up to 6%), impotence
- Neuromuscular & skeletal: Muscle twitching, leg cramps, arthritis, bursitis
- Ocular: Vision abnormalities (3%)
- Respiratory: Dyspnea, rhinitis

<1%: Elevated liver transaminase levels

**Drug Interactions**

Antipsychotics: May decrease the efficiency of pramipexole due to dopamine antagonism

Cationic drugs: Drugs secreted by the cationic transport system (diltiazem, triamterene, verapamil, quinidine, quinine, ranitidine) decrease the clearance of pramipexole by ~20%

Cimetidine: May increase serum concentrations; cimetidine in combination with pramipexole produced a 50% increase in AUC and a 40% increase in half-life

Metoclopramide: May decrease the efficiency of pramipexole due to dopamine antagonism

**Mechanism of Action** Pramipexole is a nonergot dopamine agonist with specificity for the $D_2$ subfamily dopamine receptor, and has also been shown to bind to $D_3$ and $D_4$ receptors. By binding to these receptors, it is thought that pramipexole can stimulate dopamine activity on the nerves of the striatum and substantia nigra.

**Pharmacodynamics/kinetics**

Protein binding: 15%

Bioavailability: 90%

Half-life: ~8 hours (12-14 hours in the elderly)

Time to peak serum concentration: Within 2 hours

Elimination: Urine, 90% recovered as unmetabolized drug

**Usual Dosage** Adults: Oral: Initial: 0.375 mg/day given in 3 divided doses, increase gradually by 0.125 mg/dose every 5-7 days; range: 1.5-4.5 mg/day

**Dietary Considerations** Food intake does not affect the extent of drug absorption, although the time to maximal plasma concentration is delayed by 60 minutes when taken with a meal

**Administration** Doses should be titrated gradually in all patients to avoid the onset of intolerable side effects. The dosage should be increased to achieve a maximum therapeutic effect, balanced against the side effects of dyskinesia, hallucinations, somnolence, and dry mouth.

**Monitoring Parameters** Monitor for improvement in symptoms of Parkinson's disease (eg, mentation, behavior, daily living activities, motor examinations), blood pressure, body weight changes, and heart rate

**Patient Information** Ask your physician or pharmacist before taking any other medicine, including over-the-counter products; especially important are other medicines that could make you sleepy such as sleeping pills, tranquilizers, some cold and allergy medicines, narcotic pain killers, or medicines that relax muscles. Avoid alcohol. Use caution in performing activities that require alertness (driving or operating machinery); can cause significant drowsiness.

**Dosage Forms** Tablet: 0.125 mg, 0.25 mg, 1 mg, 1.25 mg, 1.5 mg

♦ **Pramosone®** *see* Pramoxine and Hydrocortisone *on page 457*

## Pramoxine (pra MOKS een)

**U.S. Brand Names** Anusol® Ointment [OTC]; Fleet® Pain Relief [OTC]; Itch-X® [OTC]; Phicon® [OTC]; PrameGel® [OTC]; Prax® [OTC]; ProctoFoam® NS [OTC]; Tronolane® [OTC]

**Pharmacologic Category** Local Anesthetic

**Use** Temporary relief of pain and itching associated with anogenital pruritus or irritation; dermatosis, minor burns, or hemorrhoids

**Effects on Mental Status** None reported

**Effects on Psychiatric Treatment** None reported

**Usual Dosage** Adults: Topical: Apply as directed, usually every 3-4 hours to affected area (maximum adult dose: 200 mg)

**Dosage Forms** Pramoxine hydrochloride:

Aerosol foam (ProctoFoam® NS): 1% (15 g)

Cream:
- Prax®: 1% (30 g, 113.4 g, 454 g)
- Tronolane®: 1% (30 g, 60 g)
- Tronothane® HCl: 1% (28.4 g)

Gel, topical:
- Itch-X®: 1% (35.4 g)
- PrameGel®: 1% (118 g)

Lotion (Prax®): 1% (15 mL, 120 mL, 240 mL)

Ointment (Anusol®): 1% (30 g)

Pads (Fleet® Pain Relief): 1% (100s)

Spray (Itch-X®): 1% (60 mL)

## Pramoxine and Hydrocortisone
(pra MOKS een & hye droe KOR ti sone)

**U.S. Brand Names** Enzone®; Pramosone®; Proctofoam®-HC; Zone-A Forte®

**Pharmacologic Category** Anesthetic/Corticosteroid

**Use** Treatment of severe anorectal or perianal swelling

**Effects on Mental Status** None reported

**Effects on Psychiatric Treatment** None reported

**Usual Dosage** Apply to affected areas 3-4 times/day

**Dosage Forms**

Cream, topical: Pramoxine hydrochloride 1% and hydrocortisone acetate 0.5% (30 g); pramoxine hydrochloride 1% and hydrocortisone acetate 1%

Foam, rectal: Pramoxine hydrochloride 1% and hydrocortisone acetate 1% (10 g)

Lotion, topical: Pramoxine hydrochloride 1% and hydrocortisone 0.25%; pramoxine hydrochloride 1% and hydrocortisone 2.5%; pramoxine hydrochloride 2.5% and hydrocortisone 1% (37.5 mL, 120 mL, 240 mL)

♦ **Prandin™** *see* Repaglinide *on page 490*

♦ **Pravachol®** *see* Pravastatin *on page 457*

## Pravastatin (PRA va stat in)

**Related Information**

Lipid-Lowering Agents Comparison Chart *on page 717*

**U.S. Brand Names** Pravachol®

**Pharmacologic Category** Antilipemic Agent (HMG-CoA Reductase Inhibitor)

**Use**

"Primary prevention" in hypercholesterolemic patients without clinically-evident coronary heart disease to reduce the risk of myocardial infarction, reduce the risk of undergoing myocardial revascularization procedures, reduce the risk of cardiovascular mortality with no increase in death from noncardiovascular causes

"Secondary prevention" in hypercholesterolemic patients with clinically-evident coronary artery disease, including prior myocardial infarction, to slow the progression of coronary atherosclerosis, and reduce the risk of acute coronary events

"Secondary prevention" in patients with previous myocardial infarction, and normal cholesterol levels; to reduce the risk of recurrent myocardial infarction; reduce the risk of undergoing myocardial revascularization procedures; and reduce the risk of stroke or transient ischemic attack (TIA)

Adjunct to diet to reduce elevated total cholesterol, LDL cholesterol, apolipoprotein B (apo-B) and triglyceride levels, and increasing HDL-C in patients with primary hypercholesterolemia and mixed dyslipidemia (Fredrickson types IIa and IIb); Fredrickson type IV, type III (who do not respond adequately to diet)

**Effects on Mental Status** May cause dizziness

**Effects on Psychiatric Treatment** None reported

**Pregnancy Risk Factor** X

**Contraindications** Hypersensitivity to pravastatin or any component; active liver disease; unexplained persistent elevations of serum transaminases; pregnancy

(Continued)

## Pravastatin *(Continued)*

**Warnings/Precautions** Liver function must be monitored by periodic laboratory assessment. Rhabdomyolysis with acute renal failure has occurred with other HMG-CoA reductase inhibitors. Risk is increased with concurrent use of clarithromycin, danazol, diltiazem, fluvoxamine, indinavir, nefazodone, nelfinavir, ritonavir, verapamil, troleandomycin, cyclosporine, fibric acid derivatives, erythromycin, niacin, or azole antifungals. The risk of combining any of these drugs with pravastatin is minimal. Temporarily discontinue in any patient experiencing an acute or serious condition predisposing to renal failure secondary to rhabdomyolysis. Use with caution in patients who consume large amounts of alcohol or have a history of liver disease.

**Adverse Reactions**

1% to 10%:

Central nervous system: Headache, dizziness

Dermatologic: Rash

Gastrointestinal: Flatulence, abdominal cramps, diarrhea, constipation, nausea, dyspepsia, heartburn

Neuromuscular & skeletal: Myalgia, increased CPK

<1%: Abnormal taste, blurred vision, lenticular opacities

**Overdosage/Toxicology**

Signs and symptoms: Very little adverse events

Treatment: Symptomatic

**Drug Interactions** CYP3A3/4 enzyme substrate

Cholestyramine reduces pravastatin absorption; separate administration times by at least 4 hours

Cholestyramine and colestipol (bile acid sequestrants): Cholesterol-lowering effects are additive

Clofibrate and fenofibrate may increase the risk of myopathy and rhabdomyolysis

Colestipol reduces pravastatin absorption

Gemfibrozil: Increased risk of myopathy and rhabdomyolysis

Niacin may increase the risk of myopathy and rhabdomyolysis

**Usual Dosage** Adults: Oral: 10-40 mg once daily at bedtime. **Dosing adjustment in renal impairment:** 10 mg daily.

**Patient Information** Take at bedtime since highest rate of cholesterol synthesis occurs between midnight and 5 AM. Do not change dosage without consulting prescriber. Maintain diet and exercise program as as prescribed. Have periodic ophthalmic exam while taking pravastatin (check for cataracts). You may experience mild GI disturbances (gas, diarrhea, constipation); inform prescriber if these are severe, or if you experience severe muscle pain or tenderness accompanied with malaise, blurred vision, or chest pain.

**Nursing Implications** Liver enzyme elevations may be observed during therapy with pravastatin; diet, weight reduction, and exercise should be attempted prior to therapy with pravastatin

**Dosage Forms** Tablet, as sodium: 10 mg, 20 mg, 40 mg

♦ **Prax® [OTC]** *see* Pramoxine *on page 457*

## Prazepam (PRA ze pam)

**Related Information**

Benzodiazepines Comparison Chart *on page 708*

Federal OBRA Regulations Recommended Maximum Doses *on page 756*

Patient Information - Anxiolytics & Sedative Hypnotics (Benzodiazepines) *on page 653*

**Generic Available** Yes

**U.S. Brand Names** Centrax®

**Pharmacologic Category** Benzodiazepine

**Use** Treatment of anxiety

**Unlabeled use:** Alcohol withdrawal; duodenal ulcer; narcotic addiction; spasticity; partial seizures

**Restrictions** C-IV

**Pregnancy Risk Factor** D

**Contraindications** Hypersensitivity to this drug or any component of its formulation (cross-sensitivity with other benzodiazepines may exist); narrow-angle glaucoma; pregnancy

**Warnings/Precautions** Use with caution in elderly or debilitated patients, patients with hepatic disease (including alcoholics), or renal impairment. Use with caution in patients with respiratory disease, or impaired gag reflex. Avoid use in patients with sleep apnea.

Causes CNS depression (dose-related) resulting in sedation, dizziness, confusion, or ataxia which may impair physical and mental capabilities. Patients must be cautioned about performing tasks which require mental alertness (operating machinery or driving). Use with caution in patients receiving other CNS depressants or psychoactive agents. Effects with other sedative drugs or ethanol may be potentiated. Benzodiazepines have been associated with falls and traumatic injury and should be used with extreme caution in patients who are at risk of these events (especially the elderly).

Use caution in patients with depression, particularly if suicidal risk may be present. Use with caution in patients with a history of drug dependence. Benzodiazepines have been associated with dependence and acute withdrawal symptoms on discontinuation or reduction in dose. Acute withdrawal, including seizures, may be precipitated after administration of flumazenil to patients receiving long-term benzodiazepine therapy.

Benzodiazepines have been associated with anterograde amnesia. Paradoxical reactions, including hyperactive or aggressive behavior have been reported with benzodiazepines, particularly in adolescent/pediatric or psychiatric patients. Does not have analgesic, antidepressant, or antipsychotic properties.

**Adverse Reactions**

Cardiovascular: Hypotension

Central nervous system: Drowsiness, fatigue, impaired coordination, lightheadedness, memory impairment, insomnia, depression, headache, anxiety, confusion, nervousness, syncope, dizziness, akathisia, drowsiness, ataxia, lightheadedness, vivid dreams

Dermatologic: Rash, pruritus

Endocrine & metabolic: Decreased libido, menstrual irregularities

Gastrointestinal: Xerostomia, constipation, diarrhea, decreased salivation, nausea, vomiting, increased or decreased appetite, increased salivation, weight gain or loss

Hematologic: Blood dyscrasias

Neuromuscular & skeletal: Dysarthria, tremor, muscle cramps, rigidity, weakness, reflex slowing

Ocular: Blurred vision, increased lenticular pressure

Otic: Tinnitus

Respiratory: Nasal congestion, hyperventilation

Miscellaneous: Diaphoresis, drug dependence

**Overdosage/Toxicology**

Signs and symptoms: Somnolence, confusion, coma, hypoactive reflexes, dyspnea, hypotension, slurred speech, impaired coordination

Treatment: Treatment for benzodiazepine overdose is supportive. Rarely is mechanical ventilation required. Flumazenil has been shown to selectively block the binding of benzodiazepines to CNS receptors, resulting in a reversal of benzodiazepine-induced CNS depression, but not respiratory depression

**Drug Interactions**

CNS depressants: Sedative effects and/or respiratory depression may be additive with CNS depressants; includes ethanol, barbiturates, narcotic analgesics, and other sedative agents; monitor for increased effect

Enzyme inducers: Metabolism of some benzodiazepines may be increased, decreasing their therapeutic effect; consider using an alternative sedative/hypnotic agent; potential inducers include phenobarbital, phenytoin, carbamazepine, rifampin, and rifabutin

Oral contraceptives: May decrease the clearance of some benzodiazepines (those which undergo oxidative metabolism); monitor for increased benzodiazepine effect

Theophylline: May partially antagonize some of the effects of benzodiazepines; monitor for decreased response; may require higher doses for sedation

**Mechanism of Action** Binds to stereospecific benzodiazepine receptors on the postsynaptic GABA neuron at several sites within the central nervous system, including the limbic system, reticular formation. Enhancement of the inhibitory effect of GABA on neuronal excitability results by increased neuronal membrane permeability to chloride ions. This shift in chloride ions results in hyperpolarization (a less excitable state) and stabilization.

**Pharmacodynamics/kinetics**

Peak action: Within 6 hours

Duration: 48 hours

Metabolism: First-pass hepatic metabolism

Half-life:

Parent drug: 78 minutes

Desmethyldiazepam: 30-100 hours

Elimination: Renal excretion of unchanged drug and primarily N-desmethyldiazepam (active)

**Usual Dosage** Adults: Oral: 30 mg/day in divided doses, may increase gradually to a maximum of 60 mg/day

**Monitoring Parameters** Respiratory and cardiovascular status

**Reference Range** Therapeutic: 50-240 ng/mL (SI: 156-746 nmol/L)

**Patient Information** Avoid alcohol and other CNS depressants; avoid activities needing good psychomotor coordination until CNS effects are known; drug may cause physical or psychological dependence; avoid abrupt discontinuation after prolonged use

**Nursing Implications** Institute safety measures, remove smoking materials from area, supervise ambulation

**Additional Information** Prazepam offers no significant advantage over other benzodiazepines

**Dosage Forms**

Capsule: 5 mg, 10 mg, 20 mg

Tablet: 5 mg, 10 mg

## Praziquantel (pray zi KWON tel)

**U.S. Brand Names** Biltricide®

**Pharmacologic Category** Anthelmintic

**Use** All stages of schistosomiasis caused by all *Schistosoma* species pathogenic to humans; clonorchiasis and opisthorchiasis

**Unlabeled use:** Cysticercosis, flukes, and many intestinal tapeworms

**Effects on Mental Status** May cause dizziness or drowsiness

**Effects on Psychiatric Treatment** None reported

**Pregnancy Risk Factor** B

**Contraindications** Ocular cysticercosis, known hypersensitivity to praziquantel

**Warnings/Precautions** Use caution in patients with severe hepatic disease; patients with cerebral cysticercosis require hospitalization

**Adverse Reactions**

1% to 10%:

- Central nervous system: Dizziness, drowsiness, headache, malaise
- Gastrointestinal: Abdominal pain, loss of appetite, nausea, vomiting
- Miscellaneous: Diaphoresis

<1%: CSF reaction syndrome in patients being treated for neurocysticercosis, diarrhea, fever, itching, rash, urticaria

**Overdosage/Toxicology**

Signs and symptoms: Dizziness, drowsiness, headache, liver function impairment

Treatment: Supportive following GI decontamination; administer fast-acting laxative

**Drug Interactions** Hydantoins may decrease praziquantel levels causing treatment failures

**Usual Dosage** Children >4 years and Adults: Oral:

- Schistosomiasis: 20 mg/kg/dose 2-3 times/day for 1 day at 4- to 6-hour intervals
- Flukes: 25 mg/kg/dose every 8 hours for 1-2 days
- Cysticercosis: 50 mg/kg/day divided every 8 hours for 14 days
- Tapeworms: 10-20 mg/kg as a single dose (25 mg/kg for *Hymenolepis nana*)
- Clonorchiasis/opisthorchiasis: 3 doses of 25 mg/kg as a 1-day treatment

**Patient Information** Take exactly as directed for full course of medication. Tablets may be chewed, swallowed whole, or crushed and mixed with food. Increase dietary intake of fruit juices. All family members and close friends should also be treated. To reduce possibility of reinfection, wash hands and scrub nails carefully with soap and hot water before handling food, before eating, and before and after toileting. Keep hands out of mouth. Disinfect toilet daily and launder bed lines, undergarments, and nightclothes daily with hot water and soap. Do not go barefoot and do not sit directly on grass or ground. May cause dizziness, fainting, lightheadedness (use caution when driving or engaging in tasks that require alertness until response to drug is known); abdominal pain, nausea, or vomiting (frequent small meals, frequent mouth care, sucking lozenges, or chewing gum may help). Report unusual fatigue, persistent dizziness, CNS changes, change in color of urine or stool, or easy bruising or unusual bleeding.

**Nursing Implications** Tablets can be halved or quartered

**Dosage Forms** Tablet, tri-scored: 600 mg

## Prazosin (PRA zoe sin)

**U.S. Brand Names** Minipress®

**Canadian Brand Names** Apo®-Prazo; Novo-Prazin; Nu-Prazo

**Synonyms** Furazosin

**Pharmacologic Category** Alpha$_1$ Blockers

**Use** Treatment of hypertension, severe congestive heart failure (in conjunction with diuretics and cardiac glycosides); reduce mortality in stable post-myocardial patients with left ventricular dysfunction (ejection fraction ≤40%)

**Unlabeled use:** Symptoms of benign prostatic hypertrophy

**Effects on Mental Status** Dizziness is common; may cause drowsiness or nervousness; may rarely cause nightmares

**Effects on Psychiatric Treatment** Concurrent use with low potency antipsychotics and TCAs may increase risk of postural hypotension

**Pregnancy Risk Factor** C

**Contraindications** Hypersensitivity to quinazolines (doxazosin, prazosin, terazosin) or any component

**Warnings/Precautions** Can cause significant orthostatic hypotension and syncope, especially with first dose. Risk is increased at doses > 1 mg, hypovolemia, or in patients receiving concurrent beta-blocker therapy. Anticipate a similar effect if therapy is interrupted for a few days, if dosage is rapidly increased, or if another antihypertensive drug is introduced.

**Adverse Reactions**

>10%: Central nervous system: Dizziness (10.3%), lightheadedness

1% to 10%:

- Cardiovascular: Edema, palpitations (5%)
- Central nervous system: Nervousness, drowsiness (7.6%), headache (7.8%), orthostatic hypotension
- Gastrointestinal: Xerostomia, nausea (5%)
- Genitourinary: Urinary incontinence
- Neuromuscular & skeletal: Weakness (7%)

<1%: Angina, dyspnea, hypothermia, nasal congestion, nightmares, polyuria, priapism, rash, sexual dysfunction

**Overdosage/Toxicology**

Signs and symptoms: Hypotension, drowsiness

Treatment: Hypotension usually responds to I.V. fluids, Trendelenburg positioning or vasoconstrictors; treatment is otherwise supportive and symptomatic

**Drug Interactions**

- ACE inhibitors: Hypotensive effect may be increased
- Beta-blockers: Hypotensive effect may be increased
- Calcium channel blockers: Hypotensive effect may be increased
- NSAIDs may reduce antihypertensive efficacy

**Usual Dosage** Oral:

Children: Initial: 5 mcg/kg/dose (to assess hypotensive effects); usual dosing interval: every 6 hours; increase dosage gradually up to maximum of 25 mcg/kg/dose every 6 hours

Adults:

- CHF, hypertension: Initial: 1 mg/dose 2-3 times/day; usual maintenance dose: 3-15 mg/day in divided doses 2-4 times/day; maximum daily dose: 20 mg
- Hypertensive urgency: 10-20 mg once, may repeat in 30 minutes
- Raynaud's: 0.5-0 mg twice daily
- Benign prostatic hypertrophy: 2 mg twice daily

**Dietary Considerations** Alcohol: Avoid use

**Patient Information** Take as directed (first dose at bedtime). Do not skip dose or discontinue without consulting prescriber. Follow recommended diet and exercise program. Do not use alcohol or OTC medications which may affect blood pressure (eg, cough or cold remedies, diet pills, stay-awake medications) without consulting physician. You may experience drowsiness, dizziness, or impaired judgment (use caution when driving or engaging in tasks that require alertness until response to drug is known); postural hypotension (use caution when rising from sitting or lying position or when climbing stairs); dry mouth or nausea (frequent mouth care or sucking lozenges may help); or urinary incontinence (void before taking medication). Report altered CNS status (eg, fatigue, lethargy, confusion, nervousness); sudden weight gain (weigh yourself in the same clothes at the same time of day once a week); unusual or persistent swelling of ankles, feet, or extremities; palpitations or rapid heartbeat; difficulty breathing; or other persistent side effects.

**Nursing Implications** Syncope may occur (usually within 90 minutes of the initial dose)

**Dosage Forms** Capsule, as hydrochloride: 1 mg, 2 mg, 5 mg

## Prazosin and Polythiazide (PRA zoe sin & pol i THYE a zide)

**U.S. Brand Names** Minizide®

**Pharmacologic Category** Antihypertensive Agent, Combination

**Use** Management of mild to moderate hypertension

**Effects on Mental Status** Dizziness is common; may cause drowsiness or nervousness; may rarely cause nightmares

**Effects on Psychiatric Treatment** Concurrent use with low potency antipsychotics and TCAs may increase risk of postural hypotension; may decrease lithium clearance resulting in an increase in serum lithium levels and potential lithium toxicity; monitor serum lithium levels

**Usual Dosage** Adults: Oral: 1 capsule 2-3 times/day

**Dosage Forms** Capsule:

- 1: Prazosin 1 mg and polythiazide 0.5 mg
- 2: Prazosin 2 mg and polythiazide 0.5 mg
- 5: Prazosin 5 mg and polythiazide 0.5 mg

♦ **Precose®** *see* Acarbose *on page 13*

♦ **Predcor-TBA® Injection** *see* Prednisolone *on page 459*

♦ **Pred Forte® Ophthalmic** *see* Prednisolone *on page 459*

♦ **Pred-G® Ophthalmic** *see* Prednisolone and Gentamicin *on page 460*

♦ **Pred Mild® Ophthalmic** *see* Prednisolone *on page 459*

## Prednicarbate (PRED ni kar bate)

**U.S. Brand Names** Dermatop®

**Pharmacologic Category** Corticosteroid, Topical

**Use** Relief of the inflammatory and pruritic manifestations of corticosteroid-responsive dermatoses (medium potency topical corticosteroid)

**Effects on Mental Status** None reported

**Effects on Psychiatric Treatment** None reported

**Usual Dosage** Adults: Topical: Apply a thin film to affected area twice daily

**Dosage Forms** Cream: 0.1% (15 g, 60 g)

♦ **Prednicen-M®** *see* Prednisone *on page 461*

## Prednisolone (pred NIS oh lone)

**Related Information**

Corticosteroids Comparison Chart *on page 711*

**U.S. Brand Names** AK-Pred® Ophthalmic; Articulose-50® Injection; Delta-Cortef® Oral; Econopred® Ophthalmic; Econopred® Plus Ophthalmic; (Continued)

## Prednisolone *(Continued)*

Inflamase® Forte Ophthalmic; Inflamase® Mild Ophthalmic; Key-Pred® Injection; Key-Pred-SP® Injection; Pediapred® Oral; Predcor-TBA® Injection; Pred Forte® Ophthalmic; Pred Mild® Ophthalmic; Prednisol® TBA Injection; Prelone® Oral

**Canadian Brand Names** Novo-Prednisolone

**Pharmacologic Category** Corticosteroid, Ophthalmic; Corticosteroid, Parenteral

**Use** Treatment of palpebral and bulbar conjunctivitis; corneal injury from chemical, radiation, thermal burns, or foreign body penetration; endocrine disorders, rheumatic disorders, collagen diseases, dermatologic diseases, allergic states, ophthalmic diseases, respiratory diseases, hematologic disorders, neoplastic diseases, edematous states, and gastrointestinal diseases; useful in patients with inability to activate prednisone (liver disease)

**Effects on Mental Status** Nervousness and insomnia are common; may rarely cause delirium, mood swings, euphoria, and hallucinations

**Effects on Psychiatric Treatment** Barbiturates and carbamazepine may decrease corticosteroid effectiveness

**Pregnancy Risk Factor** C

**Contraindications** Acute superficial herpes simplex keratitis; systemic fungal infections; varicella; hypersensitivity to prednisolone or any component

**Warnings/Precautions** Use with caution in patients with hyperthyroidism, cirrhosis, nonspecific ulcerative colitis, hypertension, osteoporosis, thromboembolic tendencies, CHF, convulsive disorders, myasthenia gravis, thrombophlebitis, peptic ulcer, diabetes; acute adrenal insufficiency may occur with abrupt withdrawal after long-term therapy or with stress; young pediatric patients may be more susceptible to adrenal axis suppression from topical therapy. Because of the risk of adverse effects, systemic corticosteroids should be used cautiously in the elderly, in the smallest possible dose, and for the shortest possible time.

**Adverse Reactions**

>10%:
- Central nervous system: Insomnia, nervousness
- Gastrointestinal: Increased appetite, indigestion

1% to 10%:
- Dermatologic: Hirsutism
- Endocrine & metabolic: Diabetes mellitus
- Neuromuscular & skeletal: Arthralgia
- Ocular: Cataracts, glaucoma
- Respiratory: Epistaxis

<1%: Abdominal distention, acne, alkalosis, amenorrhea, bruising, Cushing's syndrome, delirium, edema, euphoria, fractures, glucose intolerance, growth suppression, hallucinations, headache, hyperglycemia, hyperpigmentation, hypersensitivity reactions, hypertension, hypokalemia, mood swings, muscle wasting, muscle weakness, nausea, osteoporosis, pancreatitis, peptic ulcer, pituitary-adrenal axis suppression, pseudotumor cerebri, psychoses, seizures, skin atrophy, sodium and water retention, ulcerative esophagitis, vertigo, vomiting

**Overdosage/Toxicology**

Signs and symptoms: When consumed in excessive quantities for prolonged periods, systemic hypercorticism and adrenal suppression may occur

Treatment: In those cases where systemic hypercorticism and adrenal suppression occur, discontinuation and withdrawal of the corticosteroid should be done judiciously

**Drug Interactions** CYP3A3/4 enzyme substrate; CYP3A3/4 enzyme inducer

Decreased effect:
- Barbiturates, phenytoin, rifampin decrease corticosteroid effectiveness
- Decreases salicylates
- Decreases vaccines
- Decreases toxoids effectiveness

**Usual Dosage** Dose depends upon condition being treated and response of patient; dosage for infants and children should be based on severity of the disease and response of the patient rather than on strict adherence to dosage indicated by age, weight, or body surface area. Consider alternate day therapy for long-term therapy. Discontinuation of long-term therapy requires gradual withdrawal by tapering the dose.

Children:
- Acute asthma:
  - Oral: 1-2 mg/kg/day in divided doses 1-2 times/day for 3-5 days
  - I.V. (sodium phosphate salt): 2-4 mg/kg/day divided 3-4 times/day
- Anti-inflammatory or immunosuppressive dose: Oral, I.V., I.M. (sodium phosphate salt): 0.1-2 mg/kg/day in divided doses 1-4 times/day
- Nephrotic syndrome: Oral:
  - Initial (first 3 episodes): 2 mg/kg/day **or** 60 mg/m²/day (maximum: 80 mg/day) in divided doses 3-4 times/day until urine is protein free for 3 consecutive days (maximum: 28 days); followed by 1-1.5 mg/kg/dose **or** 40 mg/m²/dose given every other day for 4 weeks
  - Maintenance (long-term maintenance dose for frequent relapses): 0.5-1 mg/kg/dose given every other day for 3-6 months

Adults:
- Oral, I.V., I.M. (sodium phosphate salt): 5-60 mg/day
- Multiple sclerosis (sodium phosphate): Oral: 200 mg/day for 1 week followed by 80 mg every other day for 1 month
- Rheumatoid arthritis: Oral: Initial: 5-7.5 mg/day; adjust dose as necessary

Elderly: Use lowest effective dose

**Dosing adjustment in hyperthyroidism:** Prednisolone dose may need to be increased to achieve adequate therapeutic effects

Hemodialysis: Slightly dialyzable (5% to 20%); administer dose posthemodialysis

Peritoneal dialysis: Supplemental dose is not necessary

Intra-articular, intralesional, soft-tissue administration:
- Tebutate salt: 4-40 mg/dose
- Sodium phosphate salt: 2-30 mg/dose

Ophthalmic suspension/solution: Children and Adults: Instill 1-2 drops into conjunctival sac every hour during day, every 2 hours at night until favorable response is obtained, then use 1 drop every 4 hours

**Patient Information** Take exactly as directed; do not increase dose or discontinue abruptly without consulting prescriber. Take oral medication with or after meals. Limit intake of caffeine or stimulants. Prescriber may recommend increased dietary vitamins, minerals, or iron. Diabetics should monitor glucose levels closely (antidiabetic medication may need to be adjusted). Inform prescriber if you are experiencing greater than normal levels of stress (medication may need adjustment). Some forms of this medication may cause GI upset (oral medication may be taken with meals to reduce GI upset; small frequent meals and frequent mouth care may reduce GI upset). You may be more susceptible to infection (avoid crowds and persons with contagious or infective conditions). Report promptly excessive nervousness or sleep disturbances; any signs of infection (sore throat, unhealed injuries); excessive growth of body hair or loss of skin color; changes in vision; excessive or sudden weight gain (>3 lb/week); swelling of face or extremities; difficulty breathing; muscle weakness; change in color of stools (black or tarry) or persistent abdominal pain; or worsening of condition or failure to improve.

Ophthalmic: For ophthalmic use only. Wash hands before using. Tilt head back and look upward. Put drops of suspension or apply thin ribbon of ointment inside lower eyelid. Close eye and roll eyeball in all directions. Do not blink for ½ minute. Apply gentle pressure to inner corner of eye for 30 seconds. Do not use any other eye preparation for at least 10 minutes. Do not touch tip of applicator to eye or contaminate tip of applicator. Do not share medication with anyone else. Wear sunglasses when in sunlight; you may be more sensitive to bright light. Inform prescriber if condition worsens or fails to improve or if you experience eye pain, disturbances of vision, or other adverse eye response.

**Nursing Implications** Do not administer acetate or tebutate salt I.V.

**Dosage Forms**

Injection:
- As acetate (for I.M., intralesional, intra-articular, or soft tissue administration only): 25 mg/mL (10 mL, 30 mL); 50 mg/mL (30 mL)
- As sodium phosphate (for I.M., I.V., intra-articular, intralesional, or soft tissue administration): 20 mg/mL (2 mL, 5 mL, 10 mL)
- As tebutate (for intra-articular, intralesional, soft tissue administration only): 20 mg/mL (1 mL, 5 mL, 10 mL)

Liquid, oral, as sodium phosphate: 5 mg/5 mL (120 mL)

Solution, ophthalmic, as sodium phosphate: 0.125% (5 mL, 10 mL, 15 mL); 1% (5 mL, 10 mL, 15 mL)

Suspension, ophthalmic, as acetate: 0.12% (5 mL, 10 mL); 0.125% (5 mL, 10 mL, 15 mL); 1% (1 mL, 5 mL, 10 mL, 15 mL)

Syrup: 15 mg/5 mL (240 mL)

Tablet: 5 mg

## Prednisolone and Gentamicin

(pred NIS oh lone & jen ta MYE sin)

**U.S. Brand Names** Pred-G® Ophthalmic

**Pharmacologic Category** Antibiotic/Corticosteroid, Ophthalmic

**Use** Treatment of steroid responsive inflammatory conditions and superficial ocular infections due to strains of microorganisms susceptible to gentamicin such as *Staphylococcus*, *E. coli*, *H. influenzae*, *Klebsiella*, *Neisseria*, *Pseudomonas*, *Proteus*, and *Serratia* species

**Effects on Mental Status** None reported

**Effects on Psychiatric Treatment** None reported

**Usual Dosage** Children and Adults: Ophthalmic: 1 drop 2-4 times/day; during the initial 24-48 hours, the dosing frequency may be increased if necessary

**Dosage Forms**

Ointment, ophthalmic: Prednisolone acetate 0.6% and gentamicin sulfate 0.3% (3.5 g)

Suspension, ophthalmic: Prednisolone acetate 1% and gentamicin sulfate 0.3% (2 mL, 5 mL, 10 mL)

♦ **Prednisol® TBA Injection** *see* Prednisolone *on page 459*

## Prednisone (PRED ni sone)

**Related Information**
Anticonvulsants by Seizures Type *on page 703*
Corticosteroids Comparison Chart *on page 711*

**U.S. Brand Names** Deltasone®; Liquid Pred®; Meticorten®; Orasone®; Prednicen-M®

**Canadian Brand Names** Apo®-Prednisone; Jaa-Prednisone®; Novo-Prednisone; Wimpred

**Synonyms** Deltacortisone; Deltadehydrocortisone

**Pharmacologic Category** Corticosteroid, Oral

**Use** Treatment of a variety of diseases including adrenocortical insufficiency, hypercalcemia, rheumatic, and collagen disorders; dermatologic, ocular, respiratory, gastrointestinal, and neoplastic diseases; organ transplantation and a variety of diseases including those of hematologic, allergic, inflammatory, and autoimmune in origin; not available in injectable form, prednisolone must be used

**Unlabeled use:** Prevention of postherpetic neuralgia and relief of acute pain in the early stages

**Effects on Mental Status** Nervousness and insomnia are common; may rarely cause delirium, mood swings, euphoria, and hallucinations

**Effects on Psychiatric Treatment** Barbiturates and carbamazepine may decrease corticosteroid effectiveness

**Pregnancy Risk Factor** B

**Contraindications** Serious infections, except septic shock or tuberculous meningitis; systemic fungal infections; hypersensitivity to prednisone or any component; varicella

**Warnings/Precautions** Withdraw therapy with gradual tapering of dose, may retard bone growth; use with caution in patients with hypothyroidism, cirrhosis, hypertension, congestive heart failure, ulcerative colitis, thromboembolic disorders, and patients at increased risk for peptic ulcer disease. Because of the risk of adverse effects, systemic corticosteroids should be used cautiously in the elderly, in the smallest possible dose, and for the shortest possible time.

**Adverse Reactions**
>10%:
Central nervous system: Insomnia, nervousness
Gastrointestinal: Increased appetite, indigestion
1% to 10%:
Dermatologic: Hirsutism
Endocrine & metabolic: Diabetes mellitus
Ocular: Cataracts, glaucoma
Neuromuscular & skeletal: Arthralgia
Respiratory: Epistaxis
<1%: Abdominal distention, acne, alkalosis, amenorrhea, bruising, Cushing's syndrome, delirium, edema, euphoria, fractures, glucose intolerance, growth suppression, hallucinations, headache, hyperglycemia, hyperpigmentation, hypersensitivity reactions, hypertension, hypokalemia, mood swings, muscle wasting, muscle weakness, osteoporosis, pancreatitis, peptic ulcer, pituitary-adrenal axis suppression, pseudotumor cerebri, psychoses, seizures, skin atrophy, sodium and water retention, ulcerative esophagitis, vertigo, vomiting

**Overdosage/Toxicology**
Signs and symptoms: When consumed in excessive quantities for prolonged periods, systemic hypercorticism and adrenal suppression may occur
Treatment: In those cases where systemic hypercorticism and adrenal suppression occur, discontinuation and withdrawal of the corticosteroid should be done judiciously

**Drug Interactions** CYP3A3/4 enzyme substrate; CYP3A3/4 enzyme inducer
Decreased effect:
Barbiturates, phenytoin, rifampin decrease corticosteroid effectiveness
Decreases salicylates
Decreases vaccines
Decreases toxoids effectiveness

**Usual Dosage** Oral: Dose depends upon condition being treated and response of patient; dosage for infants and children should be based on severity of the disease and response of the patient rather than on strict adherence to dosage indicated by age, weight, or body surface area. Consider alternate day therapy for long-term therapy. Discontinuation of long-term therapy requires gradual withdrawal by tapering the dose.

Children:
Anti-inflammatory or immunosuppressive dose: 0.05-2 mg/kg/day divided 1-4 times/day
Acute asthma: 1-2 mg/kg/day in divided doses 1-2 times/day for 3-5 days
Alternatively (for 3- to 5-day "burst"):
<1 year: 10 mg every 12 hours
1-4 years: 20 mg every 12 hours
5-13 years: 30 mg every 12 hours
>13 years: 40 mg every 12 hours
Asthma long-term therapy (alternative dosing by age):
<1 year: 10 mg every other day
1-4 years: 20 mg every other day
5-13 years: 30 mg every other day
>13 years: 40 mg every other day
Nephrotic syndrome: Initial (first 3 episodes): 2 mg/kg/day **or** 60 mg/m²/day (maximum: 80 mg/day) in divided doses 3-4 times/day until urine is protein free for 3 consecutive days (maximum: 28 days); followed by 1-1.5 mg/kg/dose **or** 40 mg/m²/dose given every other day for 4 weeks
Maintenance dose (long-term maintenance dose for frequent relapses): 0.5-1 mg/kg/dose given every other day for 3-6 months
Children and Adults: Physiologic replacement: 4-5 mg/m²/day
Adults: 5-60 mg/day in divided doses 1-4 times/day
Elderly: Use the lowest effective dose

**Dosing adjustment in hepatic impairment:** Prednisone is inactive and must be metabolized by the liver to prednisolone. This conversion may be impaired in patients with liver disease, however, prednisolone levels are observed to be higher in patients with severe liver failure than in normal patients. Therefore, compensation for the inadequate conversion of prednisone to prednisolone occurs.

**Dosing adjustment in hyperthyroidism:** Prednisone dose may need to be increased to achieve adequate therapeutic effects
Hemodialysis: Supplemental dose is not necessary
Peritoneal dialysis: Supplemental dose is not necessary

**Patient Information** Take exactly as directed. Do not take more than prescribed dose and do not discontinue abruptly; consult prescriber. Take with or after meals. Take once-a-day dose with food in the morning. Limit intake of caffeine or stimulants. Maintain adequate nutrition; consult prescriber for possibility of special dietary recommendations. If diabetic, monitor serum glucose closely and notify prescriber of changes; this medication can alter hypoglycemic requirements. Notify prescriber if you are experiencing higher than normal levels of stress; medication may need adjustment. Periodic ophthalmic examinations will be necessary with long-term use. You will be susceptible to infection; avoid crowds or infected persons or persons with contagious diseases. You may experience insomnia or nervousness; use caution when driving or engaging in tasks requiring alertness until response to drug is known. Report weakness, change in menstrual pattern, vision changes, signs of hyperglycemia, signs of infection (eg, fever, chills, mouth sores, perianal itching, vaginal discharge), other persistent side effects, or worsening of condition.

**Nursing Implications** Withdraw therapy with gradual tapering of dose

**Dosage Forms**
Solution, oral: Concentrate (30% alcohol): 5 mg/mL (30 mL); Nonconcentrate (5% alcohol): 5 mg/5 mL (5 mL, 500 mL)
Syrup: 5 mg/5 mL (120 mL, 240 mL)
Tablet: 1 mg, 2.5 mg, 5 mg, 10 mg, 20 mg, 50 mg


- **Prefrin™ Ophthalmic Solution** *see* Phenylephrine *on page 439*
- **Pregnenedione** *see* Progesterone *on page 468*
- **Pregnyl®** *see* Chorionic Gonadotropin *on page 122*
- **Prelone® Oral** *see* Prednisolone *on page 459*
- **Premarin®** *see* Estrogens, Conjugated *on page 206*
- **Premarin® With Methyltestosterone** *see* Estrogens and Methyltestosterone *on page 206*
- **Premphase™** *see* Estrogens and Medroxyprogesterone *on page 205*
- **Prempro™** *see* Estrogens and Medroxyprogesterone *on page 205*
- **Prepidil® Vaginal Gel** *see* Dinoprostone *on page 173*
- **Prescription Strength Desenex® [OTC]** *see* Miconazole *on page 364*
- **Pre-Sed®** *see* Hexobarbital *on page 267*
- **Pretz-D® [OTC]** *see* Ephedrine *on page 195*
- **Prevacid®** *see* Lansoprazole *on page 307*
- **Prevalite®** *see* Cholestyramine Resin *on page 120*
- **PREVEN™** *see* Ethinyl Estradiol and Levonorgestrel *on page 211*
- **Preveon™** *see* Adefovir *on page 20*
- **Prevnar™** *see* Pneumococcal Conjugate Vaccine, 7-Valent *on page 450*
- **Prevpac™** *see* Lansoprazole, Amoxicillin, and Clarithromycin *on page 308*
- **Priftin®** *see* Rifapentine *on page 494*
- **Prilosec™** *see* Omeprazole *on page 404*
- **Primaclone** *see* Primidone *on page 462*
- **Primacor®** *see* Milrinone *on page 367*


## Primaquine (PRIM a kween)

**Synonyms** Prymaccone

**Pharmacologic Category** Aminoquinoline (Antimalarial)

**Use** Provides radical cure of *P. vivax* or *P. ovale* malaria after a clinical attack has been confirmed by blood smear or serologic titer and postexposure prophylaxis

**Effects on Mental Status** None reported

(Continued)

## Primaquine *(Continued)*

**Effects on Psychiatric Treatment** Contraindicated in patients receiving clozapine or carbamazepine

**Pregnancy Risk Factor** C

**Contraindications** Acutely ill patients who have a tendency to develop granulocytopenia (rheumatoid arthritis, SLE); patients receiving other drugs capable of depressing the bone marrow (eg, quinacrine and primaquine)

**Warnings/Precautions** Use with caution in patients with G-6-PD deficiency, NADH methemoglobin reductase deficiency, acutely ill patients who have a tendency to develop granulocytopenia; patients receiving other drugs capable of depressing the bone marrow; do not exceed recommended dosage

**Adverse Reactions**

>10%:

Gastrointestinal: Abdominal pain, nausea, vomiting

Hematologic: Hemolytic anemia in G-6-PD deficiency

1% to 10%: Hematologic: Methemoglobinemia in NADH-methemoglobin reductase-deficient individuals

<1%: Agranulocytosis, arrhythmias, headache, interference with visual accommodation, leukocytosis, leukopenia, pruritus

**Overdosage/Toxicology**

Signs and symptoms: Abdominal cramps, vomiting, cyanosis, methemoglobinemia (possibly severe), leukopenia, acute hemolytic anemia (often significant), granulocytopenia; with chronic overdose, symptoms include ototoxicity and retinopathy

Treatment: Following GI decontamination, treatment is supportive (fluids, anticonvulsants, blood transfusions, methylene blue if methemoglobinemia severe - 1-2 mg/kg over several minutes)

**Drug Interactions** Quinacrine may potentiate the toxicity of antimalarial compounds which are structurally related to primaquine

**Usual Dosage** Oral:

Children: 0.3 mg base/kg/day once daily for 14 days (not to exceed 15 mg/day) or 0.9 mg base/kg once weekly for 8 weeks not to exceed 45 mg base/week

Adults: 15 mg/day (base) once daily for 14 days or 45 mg base once weekly for 8 weeks

CDC treatment recommendations: Begin therapy during last 2 weeks of, or following a course of, suppression with chloroquine or a comparable drug

**Patient Information** It is important to complete full course of therapy for full effect. May be taken with meals to decrease GI upset and bitter aftertaste. Avoid alcohol. You should have regular ophthalmic exams (every 4-6 months) if using this medication over extended periods. You may experience nausea, vomiting, or loss of appetite (small frequent meals, frequent mouth care, sucking lozenges, or chewing gum may help). Report persistent GI disturbance, chest pain or palpitation, unusual fatigue, easy bruising or bleeding, visual or hearing disturbances, changes in urine (darkening, tinged with red, decreased volume), or any other persistent adverse reactions.

**Dosage Forms** Tablet: 26.3 mg [15 mg base]

♦ **Primaquine and Chloroquine** *see* Chloroquine and Primaquine *on page 111*

♦ **Primatene® Mist [OTC]** *see* Epinephrine *on page 195*

♦ **Primaxin®** *see* Imipenem and Cilastatin *on page 282*

## Primidone (PRI mi done)

**Related Information**

Patient Information - Anxiolytics & Sedative Hypnotics (Barbiturates) *on page 654*

Serum Drug Concentrations Commonly Monitored: Guidelines *on page 759*

**U.S. Brand Names** Mysoline®

**Canadian Brand Names** Apo®-Primidone; Sertan®

**Synonyms** Desoxyphenobarbital; Primaclone

**Pharmacologic Category** Anticonvulsant, Miscellaneous; Barbiturate

**Use** Management of grand mal, psychomotor, and focal seizures

**Unlabeled use:** Benign familial tremor (essential tremor)

**Contraindications** Hypersensitivity to primidone, phenobarbital, or any component; porphyria

**Warnings/Precautions** Use with caution in patients with renal or hepatic impairment, pulmonary insufficiency; abrupt withdrawal may precipitate status epilepticus. Potential for drug dependency exists. Do not administer to patients in acute pain. Use caution in elderly, debilitated, or pediatric patients - may cause paradoxical responses. May cause CNS depression, which may impair physical or mental abilities. Patients must cautioned about performing tasks which require mental alertness (ie, operating machinery or driving). Effects with other sedative drugs or ethanol may be potentiated. Use with caution in patients with depression or suicidal tendencies, or in patients with a history of drug abuse. Tolerance or psychological and physical dependence may occur with prolonged use. Primidone's metabolite, phenobarbital, has been associated with cognitive deficits in children. Use with caution in patients with hypoadrenalism.

**Adverse Reactions**

Central nervous system: Drowsiness, vertigo, ataxia, lethargy, behavior change, fatigue, hyperirritability

Dermatologic: Rash

Gastrointestinal: Nausea, vomiting, anorexia

Genitourinary: Impotence

Hematologic: Agranulocytopenia, agranulocytosis, anemia

Ocular: Diplopia, nystagmus

**Overdosage/Toxicology**

Signs and symptoms: Unsteady gait, slurred speech, confusion, jaundice, hypothermia, fever, hypotension, coma, respiratory arrest

Treatment: Assure adequate hydration and renal function. Urinary alkalinization with I.V. sodium bicarbonate also helps to enhance elimination. Repeated oral doses of activated charcoal significantly reduces the half-life of primidone resulting from an enhancement of nonrenal elimination. The usual dose is 0.1-1 g/kg every 4-6 hours for 3-4 days unless the patient has no bowel movement causing the charcoal to remain in the GI tract. Hemodialysis or hemoperfusion is of uncertain value. Patients in stage IV coma due to high serum drug levels may require charcoal hemoperfusion.

**Drug Interactions Note:** Primidone is metabolically converted to Phenobarbital. Barbiturates are cytochrome P 450 enzyme inducers. Patients should be monitored when these drugs are started or stopped for a decreased or increased therapeutic effect respectively.

Acetaminophen: Barbiturates may enhance the hepatotoxic potential of acetaminophen overdoses

Antiarrhythmics: Barbiturates may increase the metabolism of antiarrhythmics, decreasing their clinical effect; includes disopyramide, propafenone, and quinidine

Anticonvulsants: Barbiturates may increase the metabolism of anticonvulsants; includes ethosuximide, felbamate (possibly), lamotrigine, phenytoin, tiagabine, topiramate, and zonisamide; does not appear to affect gabapentin or levetiracetam

Antineoplastics: Limited evidence suggests that enzyme-inducing anticonvulsant therapy may reduce the effectiveness of some chemotherapy regimens (specifically in ALL); teniposide and methotrexate may be cleared more rapidly in these patients

Antipsychotics: Barbiturates may enhance the metabolism (decrease the efficacy) of antipsychotics; monitor for altered response; dose adjustment may be needed

Beta-blockers: Metabolism of beta-blockers may be increased and clinical effect decreased; atenolol and nadolol are unlikely to interact given their renal elimination

Calcium channel blockers: Barbiturates may enhance the metabolism of calcium channel blockers, decreasing their clinical effect

Chloramphenicol: Barbiturates may increase the metabolism of chloramphenicol and chloramphenicol may inhibit barbiturate metabolism; monitor for altered response

Cimetidine: Barbiturates may enhance the metabolism of cimetidine, decreasing its clinical effect

CNS depressants: Sedative effects and/or respiratory depression with barbiturates may be additive with other CNS depressants; monitor for increased effect. Includes ethanol, sedatives, antidepressants, narcotic analgesics, and benzodiazepines

Corticosteroids: Barbiturates may enhance the metabolism of corticosteroids, decreasing their clinical effect

Cyclosporine: Levels may be decreased by barbiturates; monitor

Doxycycline: Barbiturates may enhance the metabolism of doxycycline, decreasing its clinical effect; higher dosages may be required

Estrogens: Barbiturates may increase the metabolism of estrogens and reduce their efficacy

Felbamate may inhibit the metabolism of barbiturates and barbiturates may increase the metabolism of felbamate

Griseofulvin: Barbiturates may impair the absorption of griseofulvin, and griseofulvin metabolism may be increased by barbiturates, decreasing clinical effect

Guanfacine: Effect may be decreased by barbiturates

Immunosuppressants: Barbiturates may enhance the metabolism of immunosuppressants, decreasing its clinical effect; includes both cyclosporine and tacrolimus

Loop diuretics: Metabolism may be increased and clinical effects decreased; established for furosemide, effect with other loop diuretics not established

MAOIs: Metabolism of barbiturates may be inhibited, increasing clinical effect or toxicity of the barbiturates

Methadone: Barbiturates may enhance the metabolism of methadone resulting in methadone withdrawal

Methoxyflurane: Barbiturates may enhance the nephrotoxic effects of methoxyflurane

Oral contraceptives: Barbiturates may enhance the metabolism of oral contraceptives, decreasing their clinical effect; an alternative method of contraception should be considered

Theophylline: Barbiturates may increase metabolism of theophylline derivatives and decrease their clinical effect

Tricyclic antidepressants: Barbiturates may increase metabolism of tricyclic antidepressants and decrease their clinical effect; sedative effects may be additive
Valproic acid: Metabolism of barbiturates may be inhibited by valproic acid; monitor for excessive sedation; a dose reduction may be needed
Warfarin: Barbiturates inhibit the hypoprothrombinemic effects of oral anticoagulants via increased metabolism; this combination should generally be avoided

**Stability** Protect from light

**Mechanism of Action** Decreases neuron excitability, raises seizure threshold similar to phenobarbital; primidone has two active metabolites, phenobarbital and phenylethylmalonamide (PEMA); PEMA may enhance the activity of phenobarbital

**Pharmacodynamics/kinetics**
Distribution: $V_d$: 2-3 L/kg in adults
Protein binding: 99%
Metabolism: In the liver to phenobarbital (active) and phenylethylmalonamide (PEMA)
Bioavailability: 60% to 80%
Half-life (age dependent):
Primidone: 10-12 hours
PEMA: 16 hours
Phenobarbital: 52-118 hours
Time to peak serum concentration: Oral: Within 4 hours
Elimination: Urinary excretion of both active metabolites and unchanged primidone (15% to 25%)

**Usual Dosage** Oral:
Children <8 years: Initial: 50-125 mg/day given at bedtime; increase by 50-125 mg/day increments every 3-7 days; usual dose: 10-25 mg/kg/day in divided doses 3-4 times/day
Children >8 years and Adults: Initial: 125-250 mg/day at bedtime; increase by 125-250 mg/day every 3-7 days; usual dose: 750-1500 mg/day in divided doses 3-4 times/day with maximum dosage of 2 g/day

**Dosing interval in renal impairment:**
$Cl_{cr}$ 50-80 mL/minute: Administer every 8 hours
$Cl_{cr}$ 10-50 mL/minute: Administer every 8-12 hours
$Cl_{cr}$ <10 mL/minute: Administer every 12-24 hours
Hemodialysis: Moderately dialyzable (20% to 50%); administer dose postdialysis or administer supplemental 30% dose

**Patient Information** May cause drowsiness, impair judgment and coordination; do not abruptly discontinue or change dosage without notifying physician; can take with food to avoid GI upset

**Dosage Forms**
Suspension, oral: 250 mg/5 mL (240 mL)
Tablet: 50 mg, 250 mg


- **Principen®** *see* Ampicillin *on page 42*
- **Prinivil®** *see* Lisinopril *on page 320*
- **Prinzide®** *see* Lisinopril and Hydrochlorothiazide *on page 321*
- **Priscoline®** *see* Tolazoline *on page 553*
- **Privine® Nasal [OTC]** *see* Naphazoline *on page 383*
- **ProAmatine** *see* Midodrine *on page 366*
- **Probalan®** *see* Probenecid *on page 463*
- **Probampacin®** *see* Ampicillin and Probenecid *on page 43*
- **Pro-Banthine®** *see* Propantheline *on page 472*


## Probenecid (proe BEN e sid)

**U.S. Brand Names** Benemid®; Probalan®

**Canadian Brand Names** Benuryl™

**Pharmacologic Category** Uricosuric Agent

**Use** Prevention of gouty arthritis; hyperuricemia; prolongation of beta-lactam effect (ie, serum levels)

**Effects on Mental Status** May cause dizziness

**Effects on Psychiatric Treatment** May rarely cause leukopenia; use caution with clozapine and carbamazepine

**Pregnancy Risk Factor** B

**Contraindications** Hypersensitivity to probenecid or any component; high-dose aspirin therapy; moderate to severe renal impairment; children <2 years of age

**Warnings/Precautions** Use with caution in patients with peptic ulcer; use extreme caution in the use of probenecid with penicillin in patients with renal insufficiency; probenecid may not be effective in patients with a creatinine clearance <30 to 50 mL/minute; may cause exacerbation of acute gouty attack

**Adverse Reactions**
>10%:
Central nervous system: Headache
Gastrointestinal: Anorexia, nausea, vomiting
Neuromuscular & skeletal: Gouty arthritis (acute)

1% to 10%:
Cardiovascular: Flushing of face
Central nervous system: Dizziness
Dermatologic: Rash, itching
Gastrointestinal: Sore gums
Genitourinary: Painful urination
Renal: Renal calculi

<1%: Anaphylaxis, aplastic anemia, hemolytic anemia, hepatic necrosis, leukopenia, nephrotic syndrome, urate nephropathy

**Overdosage/Toxicology**
Signs and symptoms: Nausea, vomiting, tonic-clonic seizures, coma
Treatment: Activated charcoal is especially effective at binding probenecid, for GI decontamination

**Drug Interactions**
Decreased effect:
Salicylates (high dose) may decrease uricosuria
Nitrofurantoin may decrease efficacy
Increased toxicity:
Increases methotrexate toxic potential; combination with diflunisal has resulted in 40% decrease in its clearance and as much as a 65% increase in plasma concentrations due to inhibition of diflunisal metabolism
Probenecid decreases clearance of beta-lactams such as penicillins and cephalosporins; increases levels/toxicity of acyclovir, thiopental, clofibrate, dyphylline, pantothenic acid, benzodiazepines, rifampin, sulfonamide, dapsone, sulfonylureas, and zidovudine
Avoid concomitant use with ketorolac (and other NSAIDs) since its half-life is increased twofold and levels and toxicity are significantly increased
Allopurinol readministration may be beneficial by increasing the uric acid lowering effect
Pharmacologic effects of penicillamine may be attenuated

**Usual Dosage** Oral:
Children:
<2 years: Not recommended
2-14 years: Prolong penicillin serum levels: 25 mg/kg starting dose, then 40 mg/kg/day given 4 times/day
Gonorrhea: <45 kg: 25 mg/kg x 1 (maximum: 1 g/dose) 30 minutes before penicillin, ampicillin or amoxicillin
Adults:
Hyperuricemia with gout: 250 mg twice daily for one week; increase to 250-500 mg/day; may increase by 500 mg/month, if needed, to maximum of 2-3 g/day (dosages may be increased by 500 mg every 6 months if serum urate concentrations are controlled)
Prolong penicillin serum levels: 500 mg 4 times/day
Gonorrhea: 1 g 30 minutes before penicillin, ampicillin, procaine, or amoxicillin
Pelvic inflammatory disease: Cefoxitin 2 g I.M. plus probenecid 1 g orally as a single dose
Neurosyphilis: Aqueous procaine penicillin 2.4 units/day I.M. plus probenecid 500 mg 4 times/day for 10-14 days

**Dosing adjustment in renal impairment:** $Cl_{cr}$ <50 mL/minute: Avoid use

**Dietary Considerations** Food: Drug may cause GI upset; take with food if GI upset. Drink plenty of fluids.

**Patient Information** Take as directed; do not discontinue without consulting prescriber. May take 6-12 months to reduce gouty attacks (attacks may increase in frequency and severity for first few months of therapy). Take with food or antacids or alkaline ash foods (milk, nuts, beets, spinach, turnip greens). Maintain adequate hydration (2-3 L/day of fluids unless instructed to restrict fluid intake). Avoid aspirin, or aspirin-containing substances. Diabetics should use serum glucose monitoring. If you experience severe headache, contact prescriber for medication. You may experience dizziness or lightheadedness (use caution when driving, changing position, or engaging in tasks requiring alertness until response to drug is known); nausea, vomiting, indigestion, or loss of appetite (small frequent meals, frequent mouth care, chewing gum, or sucking lozenges may help). Report skin rash or itching, persistent headache, blood in urine or painful urination, excessive tiredness or easy bruising or bleeding, or sore gums.

**Nursing Implications** An alkaline urine is recommended to avoid crystallization of urates; use of sodium bicarbonate or potassium citrate is suggested until serum uric acid normalizes and tophaceous deposits disappear

**Dosage Forms** Tablet: 500 mg


- **Pro-Bionate® [OTC]** *see Lactobacillus acidophilus* and *Lactobacillus bulgaricus on page 305*


## Probucol (PROE byoo kole)

**Related Information**
Lipid-Lowering Agents Comparison Chart *on page 717*

**Synonyms** Biphenabid

**Pharmacologic Category** Antilipemic Agent (Miscellaneous)

**Use** Adjunct to dietary therapy to decrease elevated serum total and LDL cholesterol concentrations in primary hypercholesterolemia
(Continued)

## Probucol *(Continued)*

**Effects on Mental Status** May cause dizziness

**Effects on Psychiatric Treatment** Concurrent use with phenothiazines, TCAs, or beta-blockers may produce AV block

**Contraindications** Ventricular arrhythmias; hypersensitivity to probucol or any component

**Warnings/Precautions** Avoid use in hypokalemia, hypomagnesemia, severe bradycardia due to intrinsic heart disease, recent or AMI, ischemia or inflammation, and those receiving other cardioactive drugs that prolong the Q-T; serious cardiovascular toxicity (arrhythmias associated with abnormally long Q-T intervals) have been reported; the manufacturer recommends that a baseline EKG be performed and at appropriate intervals during therapy; use with caution in patients with prolonged Q-T intervals

**Adverse Reactions**

>10%:

Cardiovascular: Q-T prolongation, serious arrhythmias

Gastrointestinal: Bloating, diarrhea, stomach pain, nausea, vomiting

1% to 10%: Central nervous system: Dizziness, headache, numbness of extremities

**Overdosage/Toxicology**

Signs and symptoms: Diarrhea, flatulence; probucol is not dialyzable

Treatment: Following GI decontamination, treatment is supportive

**Drug Interactions** Increased toxicity: Drugs that prolong the Q-T interval (eg, tricyclic antidepressants, some antiarrhythmic agents, phenothiazines) or with drugs that affect the atrial rate (eg, beta-adrenergic blocking agents) or that can cause A-V block (eg, digoxin)

**Usual Dosage** Oral:

Children:

<27 kg: 250 mg twice daily with meals

>27 kg: 500 mg twice daily with meals

Adults: 500 mg twice daily administered with the morning and evening meals

**Patient Information** Take with meals; notify physician if diarrhea, abdominal pain, nausea, or vomiting becomes severe or persist

**Dosage Forms** Tablet: 250 mg, 500 mg

## Procainamide (proe kane A mide)

**Related Information**

Serum Drug Concentrations Commonly Monitored: Guidelines *on page 759*

**U.S. Brand Names** Procanbid™; Pronestyl®

**Canadian Brand Names** Apo®-Procainamide

**Synonyms** PCA; Procaine Amide Hydrochloride

**Pharmacologic Category** Antiarrhythmic Agent, Class I-A

**Use** Treatment of ventricular tachycardia, premature ventricular contractions, paroxysmal atrial tachycardia, and atrial fibrillation; prevent recurrence of ventricular tachycardia, paroxysmal supraventricular tachycardia, atrial fibrillation or flutter

**Effects on Mental Status** May cause dizziness, confusion, depression, or hallucinations

**Effects on Psychiatric Treatment** May rarely cause agranulocytosis; use caution with clozapine and carbamazepine; concurrent use with phenothiazines, TCAs, or beta-blockers may produce AV block

**Pregnancy Risk Factor** C

**Contraindications** Hypersensitivity to procaine or other ester-type local anesthetics; complete heart block (except in patients with a functioning artificial pacemaker); second-degree AV block (without a functional pacemaker); various types of hemiblock (without a functional pacemaker); SLE; torsade de pointes; concurrent cisapride use

**Warnings/Precautions** Monitor and adjust dose to prevent QTc prolongation. Watch for proarrhythmic effects. May precipitate or exacerbate CHF. Reduce dosage in renal impairment. May increase ventricular response rate in patients with atrial fibrillation or flutter; control AV conduction before initiating. Correct hypokalemia before initiating therapy. Hypokalemia may worsen toxicity. Use caution in digoxin-induced toxicity (can further depress AV conduction). Reduce dose if first-degree heart block occurs. Use caution with concurrent use of other antiarrhythmics. Avoid use in myasthenia gravis (may worsen condition). Hypersensitivity reactions can occur. Some tablets contain tartrazine; injection may contain bisulfite (allergens).

Potentially fatal blood dyscrasias have occurred with therapeutic doses; close monitoring is recommended during the first 3 months of therapy.

Long-term administration leads to the development of a positive antinuclear antibody (ANA) test in 50% of patients which may result in a drug-induced lupus erythematosus-like syndrome (in 20% to 30% of patients); discontinue procainamide with SLE symptoms and choose an alternative agent

**Adverse Reactions**

>1%:

Dermatologic: Rash

Gastrointestinal: Diarrhea (3% to 4%), nausea, vomiting, GI complaints (3% to 4%)

<1%: Agranulocytosis, arthralgia, confusion, disorientation, dizziness, drug fever, fever, hallucinations, hemolytic anemia, hypotension, lightheadedness, mental depression, myalgia (<0.5%), neutropenia, pleural effusion, positive Coombs' test, Q-T prolongation, second degree heart block, SLE-like syndrome (increased incidence with long-term therapy), tachycardia, thrombocytopenia (0.5%)

**Overdosage/Toxicology**

Signs and symptoms: Has a low toxic:therapeutic ratio and may easily produce fatal intoxication (acute toxic dose: 5 g in adults); symptoms of overdose include sinus bradycardia, sinus node arrest or asystole, P-R, QRS or Q-T interval prolongation, torsade de pointes (polymorphous ventricular tachycardia) and depressed myocardial contractility, which along with alpha-adrenergic or ganglionic blockade, may result in hypotension and pulmonary edema; other effects are seizures, coma, and respiratory arrest.

Treatment: Primarily symptomatic and effects usually respond to conventional therapies (fluids, positioning, vasopressors, anticonvulsants, antiarrhythmics). **Note:** Do not use other type 1a or 1c antiarrhythmic agents to treat ventricular tachycardia; sodium bicarbonate may treat wide QRS intervals or hypotension; markedly impaired conduction or high degree A-V block, unresponsive to bicarbonate, indicates consideration of a pacemaker is needed.

**Drug Interactions**

Amiodarone increases procainamide and NAPA blood levels; consider reducing procainamide dosage by 25% with concurrent use

Cimetidine increases procainamide and NAPA blood concentrations; monitor blood levels closely or use an alternative $H_2$-antagonist

Cisapride and procainamide may increase the risk of malignant arrhythmia; concurrent use is contraindicated

Drugs which may prolong the Q-T interval include amiodarone, amitriptyline, astemizole, bepridil, disopyramide, erythromycin, haloperidol, imipramine, pimozide, quinidine, sotalol, and thioridazine. Effects/toxicity may be increased; use with caution

Neuromuscular blocking agents: Procainamide may potentiate neuromuscular blockade

Ofloxacin may increase procainamide levels due to an inhibition of renal secretion; monitor levels for procainamide closely

Sparfloxacin, gatifloxacin, and moxifloxacin may result in additional prolongation of the Q-T interval; concurrent use is contraindicated

Trimethoprim increases procainamide and NAPA blood levels; closely monitor levels

**Usual Dosage** Must be titrated to patient's response

Children:

Oral: 15-50 mg/kg/24 hours divided every 3-6 hours

I.M.: 50 mg/kg/24 hours divided into doses of $^1/_8$ to $^1/_4$ every 3-6 hours in divided doses until oral therapy is possible

I.V. (infusion requires use of an infusion pump):

Load: 3-6 mg/kg/dose over 5 minutes not to exceed 100 mg/dose; may repeat every 5-10 minutes to maximum of 15 mg/kg/load

Maintenance as continuous I.V. infusion: 20-80 mcg/kg/minute; maximum: 2 g/24 hours

Adults:

Oral: 250-500 mg/dose every 3-6 hours or 500 mg to 1 g every 6 hours sustained release; usual dose: 50 mg/kg/24 hours; maximum: 4 g/24 hours (**Note:** Twice daily dosing approved for Procanbid™)

I.M.: 0.5-1 g every 4-8 hours until oral therapy is possible

I.V. (infusion requires use of an infusion pump): Loading dose: 15-18 mg/kg administered as slow infusion over 25-30 minutes or 100-200 mg/dose repeated every 5 minutes as needed to a total dose of 1 g; maintenance dose: 1-6 mg/minute by continuous infusion

Infusion rate: 2 g/250 mL $D_5W$/NS (I.V. infusion requires use of an infusion pump):

1 mg/minute: 7 mL/hour

2 mg/minute: 15 mL/hour

3 mg/minute: 21 mL/hour

4 mg/minute: 30 mL/hour

5 mg/minute: 38 mL/hour

6 mg/minute: 45 mL/hour

Refractory ventricular fibrillation: 30 mg/minute, up to a total of 17 mg/kg; I.V. maintenance infusion: 1-4 mg/minute; monitor levels and do not exceed 3 mg/minute for >24 hours in adults with renal failure.

ACLS guidelines: I.V.: Infuse 20 mg/minute until arrhythmia is controlled, hypotension occurs, QRS complex widens by 50% of its original width, or total of 17 mg/kg is given.

**Dosing interval in renal impairment:**

$Cl_{cr}$ 10-50 mL/minute: Administer every 6-12 hours.

$Cl_{cr}$ <10 mL/minute: Administer every 8-24 hours.

Dialysis:

Procainamide: Moderately hemodialyzable (20% to 50%): 200 mg supplemental dose posthemodialysis is recommended.

N-acetylprocainamide: Not dialyzable (0% to 5%)

Procainamide/N-acetylprocainamide: Not peritoneal dialyzable (0% to 5%)

Procainamide/N-acetylprocainamide: Replace by blood level during continuous arteriovenous or venovenous hemofiltration (CAVH/CAVHD).

**Dosing adjustment in hepatic impairment:** Reduce dose 50%.

**Patient Information** Oral: Take exactly as directed; do not take additional doses or discontinue without consulting prescriber. You will need regular cardiac checkups and blood tests while taking this medication. You may experience dizziness, lightheadedness, or visual changes (use caution when driving or engaging in tasks requiring alertness until response to drug is known); loss of appetite (small frequent meals, frequent mouth care, chewing gum, or sucking lozenges may help); headaches (prescriber may recommend mild analgesic); or diarrhea (exercise, yogurt, or boiled milk may help - if persistent consult prescriber). Report chest pain, palpitation, or erratic heartbeat; increased weight or swelling of hands or feet; acute diarrhea; or unusual fatigue and tiredness.

**Nursing Implications** Do not crush sustained release drug product

**Dosage Forms**

Capsule, as hydrochloride: 250 mg, 375 mg, 500 mg

Injection, as hydrochloride: 100 mg/mL (10 mL); 500 mg/mL (2 mL)

Tablet, as hydrochloride: 250 mg, 375 mg, 500 mg

Tablet, as hydrochloride, sustained release: 250 mg, 500 mg, 750 mg, 1000 mg

Tablet, as hydrochloride, sustained release (Procanbid™): 500 mg, 1000 mg

## Procaine (PROE kane)

**U.S. Brand Names** Novocain® Injection

**Pharmacologic Category** Local Anesthetic

**Use** Produces spinal anesthesia and epidural and peripheral nerve block by injection and infiltration methods

**Effects on Mental Status** None reported

**Effects on Psychiatric Treatment** If used with a vasoconstrictor, the effects of MAOIs may be enhanced

**Usual Dosage** Dose varies with procedure, desired depth, and duration of anesthesia, desired muscle relaxation, vascularity of tissues, physical condition, and age of patient

**Dosage Forms** Injection, as hydrochloride: 1% [10 mg/mL] (2 mL, 6 mL, 30 mL, 100 mL); 2% [20 mg/mL] (30 mL, 100 mL); 10% (2 mL)

♦ **Procaine Amide Hydrochloride** *see* Procainamide *on page 464*

♦ **Pro-Cal-Sof® [OTC]** *see* Docusate *on page 179*

♦ **Procanbid™** *see* Procainamide *on page 464*

## Procarbazine (proe KAR ba zeen)

**U.S. Brand Names** Matulane®

**Synonyms** Benzmethyzin; N-Methylhydrazine

**Pharmacologic Category** Antineoplastic Agent, Alkylating Agent

**Use** Treatment of Hodgkin's disease, non-Hodgkin's lymphoma, brain tumor, bronchogenic carcinoma

**Effects on Mental Status** Dizziness, nervousness, insomnia, confusion, mania, depression, and hallucinations are common

**Effects on Psychiatric Treatment** May cause myelosuppression; use caution with clozapine and carbamazepine; procarbazine possesses MAOI activity; avoid with antidepressants, narcotics, phenothiazines, and foods containing tyramine

**Pregnancy Risk Factor** D

**Contraindications** Hypersensitivity to procarbazine or any component, or pre-existing bone marrow aplasia, alcohol ingestion

**Warnings/Precautions** The U.S. Food and Drug Administration (FDA) currently recommends that procedures for proper handling and disposal of antineoplastic agents be considered; use with caution in patients with pre-existing renal or hepatic impairment; modify dosage in patients with renal or hepatic impairment, or marrow disorders; reduce dosage with serum creatinine >2 mg/dL or total bilirubin >3 mg/dL; procarbazine possesses MAO inhibitor activity. Procarbazine is a carcinogen which may cause acute leukemia; procarbazine may cause infertility.

**Adverse Reactions**

>10%:

Central nervous system: Mental depression, manic reactions, hallucinations, dizziness, headache, nervousness, insomnia, nightmares, ataxia, disorientation, confusion, seizure, CNS stimulation

Gastrointestinal: Severe nausea and vomiting occur frequently and may be dose-limiting; anorexia, abdominal pain, stomatitis, dysphagia, diarrhea, and constipation; use a nonphenothiazine antiemetic, when possible

Emetic potential: Moderately high (60% to 90%)

Time course of nausea/vomiting: Onset: 24-27 hours; Duration: variable

Hematologic: Thrombocytopenia, hemolytic anemia

Myelosuppressive: May be dose-limiting toxicity; procarbazine should be discontinued if leukocyte count is <4000/mm³ or platelet count <100,000/mm³

WBC: Moderate

Platelets: Moderate

Onset (days): 14

Nadir (days): 21

Recovery (days): 28

Neuromuscular & skeletal: Weakness, paresthesia, neuropathies, decreased reflexes, foot drop, tremors

Ocular: Nystagmus

Respiratory: Pleural effusion, cough

1% to 10%:

Dermatologic: Hyperpigmentation

Hepatic: Hepatotoxicity

Neuromuscular & skeletal: Peripheral neuropathy

<1%: Allergic reactions, alopecia, arthralgia, cessation of menses, dermatitis, diplopia, disulfiram-like reaction, flu-like syndrome, hoarseness, hypersensitivity rash, hypertensive crisis, irritability, jaundice, myalgia, orthostatic hypotension, photophobia, pneumonitis, pruritus, secondary malignancy, somnolence

**Overdosage/Toxicology**

Signs and symptoms: Arthralgia, alopecia, paresthesia, bone marrow suppression, hallucinations, nausea, vomiting, diarrhea, seizures, coma

Treatment: Supportive, adverse effects such as marrow toxicity may begin as late as 2 weeks after exposure

**Drug Interactions** Increased toxicity:

Alcohol has caused a disulfiram-like reaction with procarbazine; may result in headache, respiratory difficulties, nausea, vomiting, sweating, thirst, hypotension, and flushing

Barbiturates, narcotics, phenothiazines, and other CNS depressants can cause somnolence, ataxia, and other symptoms of CNS depression

Procarbazine exhibits weak monoamine oxidase (MAO) inhibitor activity; foods containing high amounts of tyramine should, therefore, be avoided (ie, beer, yogurt, yeast, wine, cheese, pickled herring, chicken liver, and bananas). When a MAO inhibitor is given with food high in tyramine, a hypertensive crisis, intracranial bleeding, and headache have been reported.

Sympathomimetic amines (epinephrine and amphetamines) and antidepressants (tricyclics) should be used cautiously with procarbazine.

**Usual Dosage** Refer to individual protocols. Dose based on patient's ideal weight if the patient is obese or has abnormal fluid retention. Oral:

Children:

BMT aplastic anemia conditioning regimen: 12.5 mg/kg/dose every other day for 4 doses

Hodgkin's disease: MOPP/IC-MOPP regimens: 100 mg/m²/day for 14 days and repeated every 4 weeks

Neuroblastoma and medulloblastoma: Doses as high as 100-200 mg/m²/day once daily have been used

Adults: Initial: 2-4 mg/kg/day in single or divided doses for 7 days then increase dose to 4-6 mg/kg/day until response is obtained or leukocyte count decreased <4000/mm³ or the platelet count decreased <100,000/mm³; maintenance: 1-2 mg/kg/day

In MOPP, 100 mg/m²/day on days 1-14 of a 28-day cycle

**Dosing in renal/hepatic impairment:** Use with caution, may result in increased toxicity

**Dietary Considerations**

Alcohol: Avoid use, including alcohol-containing products

Food: Avoid foods with high tyramine content

**Patient Information** Take as directed. Maintain adequate hydration (2-3 L/day of fluids unless instructed to restrict fluid intake). Avoid aspirin and aspirin-containing substances. Avoid alcohol; may cause acute disulfiram reaction - flushing, headache, acute vomiting, chest and/or abdominal pain. Avoid tyramine-containing foods (aged cheese, chocolate, pickles, aged meat, wine, etc). You may experience mental depression, nervousness, insomnia, nightmares, dizziness, confusion, or lethargy (use caution when driving or engaging in tasks that require alertness until response to drug is known); photosensitivity (use sunscreen, wear protective clothing and eyewear, and avoid direct sunlight). You may experience rash or hair loss (reversible), loss of libido, increased sensitivity to infection (avoid crowds and infected persons). Report persistent fever, chills, sore throat; unusual bleeding; blood in urine, stool (black stool), or vomitus; unresolved depression; mania; hallucinations; nightmares; disorientation; seizures; chest pain or palpitations; or difficulty breathing.

**Dosage Forms** Capsule, as hydrochloride: 50 mg

♦ **Procardia®** *see* Nifedipine *on page 393*

♦ **Procardia XL®** *see* Nifedipine *on page 393*

♦ **Procetofene** *see* Fenofibrate *on page 220*

## Prochlorperazine (proe klor PER a zeen)

**Related Information**

Antipsychotic Medication Guidelines *on page 751*

Clinical Issues in the Use of Antipsychotics *on page 630*

Patient Information - Antipsychotics (General) *on page 646*

**Generic Available** Yes

(Continued)

## Prochlorperazine *(Continued)*

**U.S. Brand Names** Compazine®

**Canadian Brand Names** Nu-Prochlor; PMS-Prochlorperazine; Prorazin®; Stemetil®

**Synonyms** Prochlorperazine Edisylate; Prochlorperazine Maleate

**Pharmacologic Category** Antipsychotic Agent, Phenothazine, Piperazine

**Use** Management of nausea and vomiting; psychosis; anxiety

**Pregnancy Risk Factor** C

**Pregnancy/Breast-Feeding Implications**

Clinical effects on the fetus: Crosses the placenta. Isolated reports of congenital anomalies, however some included exposures to other drugs. Available evidence with use of occasional low doses suggests safe use during pregnancy.

Breast-feeding/lactation: No data available. American Academy of Pediatrics considers **compatible** with breast-feeding.

**Contraindications** Hypersensitivity to prochlorperazine or any component (cross reactivity between phenothiazines may occur); severe CNS depression; coma; bone marrow suppression; should not be used in children <2 years of age or <20 pounds.

**Warnings/Precautions** May be sedating; use with caution in disorders where CNS depression is a feature. May impair physical or mental abilities; patients must cautioned about performing tasks which require mental alertness (ie, operating machinery or driving). Effects with other sedative drugs or ethanol may be potentiated. Avoid use in Reye's syndrome. Use with caution in Parkinson's disease; hemodynamic instability; bone marrow suppression; predisposition to seizures; subcortical brain damage; and in severe cardiac, hepatic, renal or respiratory disease. Caution in breast cancer or other prolactin-dependent tumors (may elevate prolactin levels). May alter temperature regulation or mask toxicity of other drugs due to antiemetic effects. May alter cardiac conduction - life threatening arrhythmias have occurred with therapeutic doses of phenothiazines. May cause orthostatic hypotension; use with caution in patients at risk of hypotension or where transient hypotensive episodes would be poorly tolerated (cardiovascular disease or cerebrovascular disease). Hypotension may occur following administration, particularly when parenteral form is used or in high dosages.

Phenothiazines may cause anticholinergic effects (constipation, dry mouth, blurred vision, urinary retention); therefore, they should be used with caution in patients with decreased gastrointestinal motility, urinary retention, BPH, xerostomia, or visual problems. Conditions which also may be exacerbated by cholinergic blockade include narrow-angle glaucoma (screening is recommended) and worsening of myasthenia gravis. May cause extrapyramidal reactions, including pseudoparkinsonism, acute dystonic reactions, akathisia and tardive dyskinesia. May be associated with neuroleptic malignant syndrome (NMS).

**Adverse Reactions**

Cardiovascular: Hypotension, orthostatic hypotension, hypertension, tachycardia, bradycardia, dizziness, cardiac arrest

Central nervous system: Extrapyramidal signs (pseudoparkinsonism, akathisia, dystonias, tardive dyskinesia), dizziness, cerebral edema, seizures, headache, drowsiness, paradoxical excitement, restlessness, hyperactivity, insomnia, neuroleptic malignant syndrome (NMS), impairment of temperature regulation

Dermatologic: Increased sensitivity to sun, rash, discoloration of skin (blue-gray)

Endocrine & metabolic: Hypoglycemia, hyperglycemia, galactorrhea, lactation, breast enlargement, gynecomastia, menstrual irregularity, amenorrhea, SIADH, changes in libido

Gastrointestinal: Constipation, weight gain, vomiting, stomach pain, nausea, xerostomia, salivation, diarrhea, anorexia, ileus

Genitourinary: Difficulty in urination, ejaculatory disturbances, incontinence, polyuria, ejaculating dysfunction, priapism

Hematologic: Agranulocytosis, leukopenia, eosinophilia, hemolytic anemia, thrombocytopenic purpura, pancytopenia

Hepatic: Cholestatic jaundice, hepatotoxicity

Neuromuscular & skeletal: Tremor

Ocular: Pigmentary retinopathy, blurred vision, cornea and lens changes

Respiratory: Nasal congestion

Miscellaneous: Diaphoresis

**Overdosage/Toxicology**

Signs and symptoms: Deep sleep, coma, extrapyramidal symptoms, abnormal involuntary muscle movements, hypotension

Treatment:

Following initiation of essential overdose management, toxic symptom treatment and supportive treatment should be initiated.

Hypotension usually responds to I.V. fluids or Trendelenburg positioning. If unresponsive to these measures, the use of a parenteral inotrope may be required (eg, norepinephrine 0.1-0.2 mcg/kg/minute titrated to response).

Seizures commonly respond to diazepam (I.V. 5-10 mg bolus in adults every 15 minutes if needed up to a total of 30 mg; I.V. 0.25-0.4 mg/kg/dose up to a total of 10 mg in children) or to phenytoin or phenobarbital.

Also critical cardiac arrhythmias often respond to I.V. phenytoin (15 mg/kg up to 1 gram), while other antiarrhythmics can be used.

Extrapyramidal symptoms (eg, dystonic reactions) may require management with diphenhydramine 1-2 mg/kg (adults) up to a maximum of 50 mg I.M. or I.V. slow push followed by a maintenance dose for 48-72 hours. When these reactions are unresponsive to diphenhydramine, benztropine mesylate I.V. 1-2 mg (adults) may be effective. These agents are generally effective within 2-5 minutes.

**Drug Interactions**

Aluminum salts: May decrease the absorption of phenothiazines; monitor

Amphetamines: Efficacy may be diminished by antipsychotics; in addition, amphetamines may increase psychotic symptoms; avoid concurrent use

Anticholinergics: May inhibit the therapeutic response to phenothiazines and excess anticholinergic effects may occur; includes benztropine, trihexyphenidyl, biperiden, and drugs with significant anticholinergic activity (TCAs, antihistamines, disopyramide)

Antihypertensives: Concurrent use of phenothiazines with an antihypertensive may produce additive hypotensive effects (particularly orthostasis)

Bromocriptine: Phenothiazines inhibit the ability of bromocriptine to lower serum prolactin concentrations

CNS depressants: Sedative effects may be additive with phenothiazines; monitor for increased effect; includes barbiturates, benzodiazepines, narcotic analgesics, ethanol and other sedative agents

CYP2D6 inhibitors: Metabolism of phenothiazines may be decreased, increasing clinical effect or toxicity; inhibitors include amiodarone, cimetidine, delavirdine, fluoxetine, paroxetine, propafenone, quinidine, and ritonavir; monitor for increased effect/toxicity

Enzyme inducers: May enhance the hepatic metabolism of phenothiazines; larger doses may be required; includes rifampin, rifabutin, barbiturates, phenytoin, and cigarette smoking

Epinephrine: Chlorpromazine (and possibly other low potency antipsychotics) may diminish the pressor effects of epinephrine

Guanethidine and guanadrel: Antihypertensive effects may be inhibited by phenothiazines

Levodopa: Phenothiazines may inhibit the antiparkinsonian effect of levodopa; avoid this combination

Lithium: Phenothiazines may produce neurotoxicity with lithium; this is a rare effect

Phenytoin: May reduce serum levels of phenothiazines; phenothiazines may increase phenytoin serum levels

Propranolol: Serum concentrations of phenothiazines may be increased; propranolol also increases phenothiazine concentrations

Polypeptide antibiotics: Rare cases of respiratory paralysis have been reported with concurrent use of phenothiazines

QTc prolonging agents: Effects on QTc interval may be additive with phenothiazines, increasing the risk of malignant arrhythmias; includes type Ia antiarrhythmics, TCAs, and some quinolone antibiotics (sparfloxacin, moxifloxacin, and gatifloxacin)

Sulfadoxine-pyrimethamine: May increase phenothiazine concentrations

Tricyclic antidepressants: Concurrent use may produce increased toxicity or altered therapeutic response

Trazodone: Phenothiazines and trazodone may produce additive hypotensive effects

Valproic acid: Serum levels may be increased by phenothiazines

**Stability** Protect from light; clear or slightly yellow solutions may be used; **incompatible** when mixed with aminophylline, amphotericin B, ampicillin, calcium salts, cephalothin, foscarnet (Y-site), furosemide, hydrocortisone, hydromorphone, methohexital, midazolam, penicillin G, pentobarbital, phenobarbital, thiopental

**Mechanism of Action** Blocks postsynaptic mesolimbic dopaminergic $D_1$ and $D_2$ receptors in the brain, including the medullary chemoreceptor trigger zone; exhibits a strong alpha-adrenergic and anticholinergic blocking effect and depresses the release of hypothalamic and hypophyseal hormones; believed to depress the reticular activating system, thus affecting basal metabolism, body temperature, wakefulness, vasomotor tone and emesis

**Pharmacodynamics/kinetics**

Onset of effect:

- Oral: Within 30-40 minutes
- I.M.: Within 10-20 minutes
- Rectal: Within 60 minutes

Duration: Persists longest with I.M. and oral extended-release doses (12 hours); shortest following rectal and immediate release oral administration (3-4 hours)

Distribution: Crosses the placenta; appears in breast milk

Metabolism: Hepatic

Half-life: 23 hours

Elimination: Primarily by hepatic metabolism

**Usual Dosage**

Antiemetic: Children:

Oral, rectal:

- >10 kg: 0.4 mg/kg/24 hours in 3-4 divided doses; **or**
- 9-14 kg: 2.5 mg every 12-24 hours as needed; maximum: 7.5 mg/day
- 14-18 kg: 2.5 mg every 8-12 hours as needed; maximum: 10 mg/day
- 18-39 kg: 2.5 mg every 8 hours or 5 mg every 12 hours as needed; maximum: 15 mg/day

I.M.: 0.1-0.15 mg/kg/dose; usual: 0.13 mg/kg/dose; change to oral as soon as possible
I.V.: Not recommended in children <10 kg or <2 years
Antiemetic: Adults:
Oral: 5-10 mg 3-4 times/day; usual maximum: 40 mg/day
I.M.: 5-10 mg every 3-4 hours; usual maximum: 40 mg/day
I.V.: 2.5-10 mg; maximum 10 mg/dose or 40 mg/day; may repeat dose every 3-4 hours as needed
Rectal: 25 mg twice daily
Antipsychotic:
Children 2-12 years:
Oral, rectal: 2.5 mg 2-3 times/day; increase dosage as needed to maximum daily dose of 20 mg for 2-5 years and 25 mg for 6-12 years
I.M.: 0.13 mg/kg/dose; change to oral as soon as possible
Adults:
Oral: 5-10 mg 3-4 times/day; doses up to 150 mg/day may be required in some patients for treatment of severe disturbances
I.M.: 10-20 mg every 4-6 hours may be required in some patients for treatment of severe disturbances; change to oral as soon as possible
Dementia behavior (nonpsychotic): Elderly: Initial: 2.5-5 mg 1-2 times/day; increase dose at 4- to 7-day intervals by 2.5-5 mg/day; increase dosing intervals (twice daily, 3 times/day, etc) as necessary to control response or side effects; maximum daily dose should probably not exceed 75 mg in elderly; gradual increases (titration) may prevent some side effects or decrease their severity
Hemodialysis: Not dialyzable (0% to 5%)

**Administration** Prochlorperazine may be administered I.M. or I.V.
I.M. should be administered into the upper outer quadrant of the buttock
I.V. may be administered IVP or IVPB
IVP should be administered at a concentration of 1 mg/mL at a rate of 1 mg/minute

**Monitoring Parameters** CBC with differential and periodic ophthalmic exams (if chronically used)

**Reference Range** Blood level >1 µg/mL associated with toxicity

**Test Interactions** False-positives for phenylketonuria, urinary amylase, uroporphyrins, urobilinogen

**Patient Information** May cause drowsiness, impair judgment and coordination; may cause photosensitivity; avoid excessive sunlight; notify physician of involuntary movements or feelings of restlessness

**Nursing Implications** Avoid skin contact with oral solution or injection, contact dermatitis has occurred; observe for extrapyramidal symptoms

**Additional Information** Not recommended as an antipsychotic due to inferior efficacy compared to other phenothiazines
Prochlorperazine: Compazine® suppository
Prochlorperazine edisylate: Compazine® oral solution and injection
Prochlorperazine maleate: Compazine® capsule and tablet

**Dosage Forms**
Capsule, sustained action, as maleate: 10 mg, 15 mg, 30 mg
Injection, as edisylate: 5 mg/mL (2 mL, 10 mL)
Suppository, rectal: 2.5 mg, 5 mg, 25 mg (12/box)
Syrup, as edisylate: 5 mg/5 mL (120 mL)
Tablet, as maleate: 5 mg, 10 mg, 25 mg


- **Prochlorperazine Edisylate** *see* Prochlorperazine *on page 465*
- **Prochlorperazine Maleate** *see* Prochlorperazine *on page 465*
- **Procort® [OTC]** *see* Hydrocortisone *on page 273*
- **Procrit®** *see* Epoetin Alfa *on page 197*
- **Proctocort™** *see* Hydrocortisone *on page 273*
- **Proctofene** *see* Fenofibrate *on page 220*
- **Proctofoam®-HC** *see* Pramoxine and Hydrocortisone *on page 457*
- **ProctoFoam® NS [OTC]** *see* Pramoxine *on page 457*


## Procyclidine (proe SYE kli deen)

**Related Information**
Antiparkinsonian Agents Comparison Chart *on page 705*
Patient Information - Agents for Treatment of Extrapyramidal Symptoms *on page 657*

**Generic Available** No

**U.S. Brand Names** Kemadrin®

**Canadian Brand Names** PMS-Procyclidine; Procyclid

**Synonyms** Procyclidine Hydrochloride

**Pharmacologic Category** Anticholinergic Agent; Anti-Parkinson's Agent (Anticholinergic)

**Use** Relieves symptoms of parkinsonian syndrome and drug-induced extrapyramidal symptoms

**Pregnancy Risk Factor** C

**Contraindications** Angle-closure glaucoma; safe use in children not established

**Warnings/Precautions** Use with caution in hot weather or during exercise. Elderly patients frequently develop increased sensitivity and require strict dosage regulation - side effects may be more severe in elderly patients with atherosclerotic changes. Use with caution in patients with tachycardia, cardiac arrhythmias, hypertension, hypotension, prostatic hypertrophy (especially in the elderly) or any tendency toward urinary retention, liver or kidney disorders and obstructive disease of the GI or GU tract. When given in large doses or to susceptible patients, may cause weakness and inability to move particular muscle groups.

**Adverse Reactions**
Cardiovascular: Tachycardia, palpitations
Central nervous system: Confusion, drowsiness, headache, loss of memory, fatigue, ataxia, giddiness, lightheadedness
Dermatologic: Dry skin, increased sensitivity to light, rash
Gastrointestinal: Constipation, xerostomia, dry throat, nausea, vomiting, epigastric distress
Genitourinary: Difficult urination
Neuromuscular & skeletal: Weakness
Ocular: Increased intraocular pain, blurred vision, mydriasis
Respiratory: Dry nose
Miscellaneous: Diaphoresis (decreased)

**Overdosage/Toxicology**
Signs and symptoms: Disorientation, hallucinations, delusions, blurred vision, dysphagia, absent bowel sounds, hyperthermia, hypertension, urinary retention; anticholinergic toxicity is caused by strong binding of the drug to cholinergic receptors; anticholinesterase inhibitors reduce acetylcholinesterase, the enzyme that breaks down acetylcholine and thereby allows acetylcholine to accumulate and compete for receptor binding with the offending anticholinergic
Treatment: For anticholinergic overdose with severe life-threatening symptoms, physostigmine 1-2 mg (0.5 or 0.02 mg/kg for children) S.C. or I.V., slowly may be given to reverse these effects.

**Drug Interactions**
Amantadine, rimantadine: Central and/or peripheral anticholinergic syndrome can occur when administered with amantadine or rimantadine
Anticholinergic agents: Central and/or peripheral anticholinergic syndrome can occur when administered with narcotic analgesics, phenothiazines and other antipsychotics (especially with high anticholinergic activity), tricyclic antidepressants, quinidine and some other antiarrhythmics, and antihistamines
Atenolol: Anticholinergics may increase the bioavailability of atenolol (and possibly other beta-blockers); monitor for increased effect
Cholinergic agents: Anticholinergics may antagonize the therapeutic effect of cholinergic agents; includes tacrine and donepezil
Digoxin: Anticholinergics may decrease gastric degradation and increase the amount of digoxin absorbed by delaying gastric emptying
Levodopa: Anticholinergics may increase gastric degradation and decrease the amount of levodopa absorbed by delaying gastric emptying
Neuroleptics: Anticholinergics may antagonize the therapeutic effects of neuroleptics

**Mechanism of Action** Thought to act by blocking excess acetylcholine at cerebral synapses; many of its effects are due to its pharmacologic similarities with atropine; it exerts an antispasmodic effect on smooth muscle, is a potent mydriatic; inhibits salivation

**Pharmacodynamics/kinetics**
Onset of effect: Oral: Within 30-40 minutes
Duration: 4-6 hours

**Usual Dosage** Adults: Oral: 2.5 mg 3 times/day after meals; if tolerated, gradually increase dose, maximum of 20 mg/day if necessary
**Dosing adjustment in hepatic impairment:** Decrease dose to a twice daily dosing regimen

**Monitoring Parameters** Symptoms of EPS or Parkinson's disease, pulse, anticholinergic effects (ie, CNS, bowel and bladder function)

**Patient Information** Take after meals; do not discontinue drug abruptly; notify physician if adverse GI effects, fever or heat intolerance occurs; may cause drowsiness; avoid alcohol; adequate fluid intake or sugar free gum or hard candy may help dry mouth; adequate fluid and exercise may help constipation

**Dosage Forms** Tablet, as hydrochloride: 5 mg


- **Procyclidine Hydrochloride** *see* Procyclidine *on page 467*
- **Prodium™ [OTC]** *see* Phenazopyridine *on page 433*
- **Profasi® HP** *see* Chorionic Gonadotropin *on page 122*
- **Profenal® Ophthalmic** *see* Suprofen *on page 528*
- **Profen II®** *see* Guaifenesin and Phenylpropanolamine *on page 257*
- **Profen II DM®** *see* Guaifenesin, Phenylpropanolamine, and Dextromethorphan *on page 258*
- **Profen LA®** *see* Guaifenesin and Phenylpropanolamine *on page 257*
- **Profilate® OSD** *see* Antihemophilic Factor (Human) *on page 45*
- **Profilate® SD** *see* Antihemophilic Factor (Human) *on page 45*
- **Profilnine® SD** *see* Factor IX Complex (Human) *on page 217*
- **Progestasert®** *see* Progesterone *on page 468*

## Progesterone (proe JES ter one)

**U.S. Brand Names** Crinone™; Progestasert®; Prometrium®

**Canadian Brand Names** PMS-Progesterone; Progesterone Oil

**Synonyms** Pregnenedione; Progestin

**Pharmacologic Category** Progestin

**Use** Intrauterine contraception in women who have had at least 1 child, are in a stable, mutually monogamous relationship, and have no history of pelvic inflammatory disease; amenorrhea; functional uterine bleeding; replacement therapy

Oral: Prevention of endometrial hyperplasia in nonhysterectomized postmenopausal women who are receiving conjugated estrogen tablets; secondary amenorrhea

Intravaginal gel: Part of assisted reproductive technology for infertile women with progesterone deficiency; secondary amenorrhea (8% gel is used in those who fail to respond to 4%)

**Effects on Mental Status** May cause insomnia or depression

**Effects on Psychiatric Treatment** None reported

**Pregnancy Risk Factor** X (manufacturer lists oral capsules as B)

**Contraindications** Hypersensitivity to progesterone or any component; pregnancy; thrombophlebitis; undiagnosed vaginal bleeding; carcinoma of the breast; cerebral apoplexy; severe liver dysfunction; capsules contain peanut oil and are contraindicated in patients with allergy to peanuts

**Warnings/Precautions** Use with caution in patients with impaired liver function, depression, diabetes, and epilepsy. Use of any progestin during the first 4 months of pregnancy is not recommended. Monitor closely for loss of vision, proptosis, diplopia, migraine, and signs or symptoms of embolic disorders. Not a progestin of choice in the elderly for hormonal cycling. Capsules may cause some degree of fluid retention, use with caution in conditions which may be aggravated by this factor, including CHF, renal dysfunction, epilepsy, migraine, or asthma. Patients should be warned that progesterone may cause transient dizziness or drowsiness during initial therapy. Use of progestin treatment may adversely effect carbohydrate and lipid metabolism.

**Adverse Reactions**

**Intrauterine device:**

>10%:

Cardiovascular: Edema

Endocrine & metabolic: Breakthrough bleeding, spotting, changes in menstrual flow, amenorrhea

Gastrointestinal: Anorexia

Neuromuscular & skeletal: Weakness

1% to 10%:

Cardiovascular: Embolism, central thrombosis

Central nervous system: Mental depression, fever, insomnia

Dermatologic: Melasma or chloasma, allergic rash with or without pruritus

Endocrine: Changes in cervical erosion and secretions, increased breast tenderness

Gastrointestinal: Weight gain or loss

Hepatic: Cholestatic jaundice

**Injection (I.M.):**

>10% Local: Pain at injection site

1% to 10%: Local: Thrombophlebitis

**Oral capsules:**

>10%:

Central nervous system: Dizziness (16%)

Endocrine & metabolic: Breast pain (11%)

5% to 10%:

Central nervous system: Headache (10%), fatigue (7%), emotional lability (6%), irritability (5%)

Gastrointestinal: Abdominal pain (10%), abdominal distention (6%)

Neuromuscular & skeletal: Musculoskeletal pain (6%)

Respiratory: Upper respiratory tract infection (5%)

Miscellaneous: Viral infection (7%)

<5% (limited to important or life-threatening symptoms): Dry mouth, accidental injury, chest pain, fever, hypertension, confusion, somnolence, speech disorder, constipation, dyspepsia, gastroenteritis, hemorrhagic rectum, hiatus hernia, vomiting, earache, palpitation, edema, arthritis, leg cramps, hypertonia, muscle disorder, myalgia, angina pectoris, anxiety, impaired concentration, insomnia, personality disorder, leukorrhea, uterine fibroid, vaginal dryness, fungal vaginitis, vaginitis, abscess, herpes simplex, bronchitis, nasal congestion, pharyngitis, pneumonitis, sinusitis, acne, verruca, urinary tract infection, abnormal vision, lymphadenopathy

Other report adverse effects (incidence unspecified): Hepatitis, elevated transaminases, breakthrough bleeding, change in menstrual flow, amenorrhea, weight change, cervical changes, cholestatic jaundice, anaphylactoid reactions, anaphylaxis, rash, pruritus, melasma, chloasma, pyrexia, insomnia, increased sweating, weakness, tooth disorder, anorexia, increased appetite, nervousness, breast enlargement

**Systemic:**

>10%:

Cardiovascular: Swelling of face

Central nervous system: Headache, mood changes, nervousness

Endocrine & metabolic: Amenorrhea, irregular menstrual cycles, menorrhagia, spotting, ovarian enlargement, ovarian cyst formation

Gastrointestinal: Abdominal pain

1% to 10%:

Cardiovascular: Hot flashes

Central nervous system: Dizziness, mental depression, insomnia

Dermatologic: Dermatitis, acne, melasma, loss or gain of body, facial, or scalp hair

Endocrine & metabolic: Hyperglycemia, galactorrhea, breast pain, libido decrease

Gastrointestinal: Nausea, change in appetite, weight gain

Genitourinary: Vaginitis, leukorrhea

Neuromuscular & skeletal: Myalgia

<1% (limited to important or life-threatening symptoms): Aggressive reactions, allergic reaction, asthma, forgetfulness, hot flashes, migraine, thromboembolism, tremor

**Overdosage/Toxicology**

Signs and symptoms: Toxicity is unlikely following single exposures of excessive doses

Treatment: Supportive treatment is adequate in most cases

**Drug Interactions** CYP3A3/4 enzyme substrate; CYP3A3/4 enzyme inducer

Decreased effect: Aminoglutethimide may decrease effect by increasing hepatic metabolism

Increased effect: Ketoconazole may increase the bioavailability of progesterone. Progesterone may increase concentrations of estrogenic compounds during concurrent therapy with conjugated estrogens.

**Usual Dosage** Adults:

Amenorrhea: I.M.: 5-10 mg/day for 6-8 consecutive days

Functional uterine bleeding: I.M.: 5-10 mg/day for 6 doses

Contraception: Female: Intrauterine device: Insert a single system into the uterine cavity; contraceptive effectiveness is retained for 1 year and system must be replaced 1 year after insertion

Replacement therapy: Gel: Administer 90 mg once daily in women who require progesterone supplementation

Oral:

Prevention of endometrial hyperplasia (in postmenopausal women with a uterus who are receiving daily conjugated estrogen tablets): 200 mg as a single daily dose every evening for 12 days sequentially per 28 day cycle.

Amenorrhea: 400 mg every evening for 10 days.

Intravaginal gel:

Partial or complete ovarian failure (assisted reproductive technology): 90 mg (8% gel) intravaginally once daily; if pregnancy is achieved, may continue up to 10-12 weeks

Secondary amenorrhea: 45 mg (4% gel) intravaginally every other day for up to 6 doses; women who fail to respond may be increased to 90 mg (8% gel) every other day for up to 6 doses

**Patient Information** This drug can only be given I.M. on a daily basis for a specific number of days (or inserted vaginally to remain for 1 year as a contraceptive). It is important that you you have an annual physical assessment, Pap smear, and vision assessment while taking this medication. You may experience increased facial hair or loss of head hair (reversible); photosensitivity (use sunscreen, wear protective clothing and eyewear, and avoid direct sunlight); loss of appetite (small frequent meals will help); constipation (increased fluids, exercise, dietary fiber, or stool softeners may help). Diabetics should use accurate serum glucose testing to identify any changes in glucose tolerance. Report immediately pain or muscle soreness; swelling, heat, or redness in calves; shortness of breath; sudden loss of vision; unresolved leg or foot swelling; change in menstrual pattern (unusual bleeding, amenorrhea, breakthrough spotting); breast tenderness that does not go away; acute abdominal cramping; signs of vaginal infection (drainage, pain, itching); or changes in CNS (eg, blurred vision, confusion, acute anxiety, or unresolved depression).

**Nursing Implications** Patients should receive a copy of the patient labeling for the drug; administer deep I.M. only; monitor patient closely for loss of vision, sudden onset of proptosis, diplopia, migraine, and signs and symptoms of embolic disorders

**Dosage Forms**

Capsule: 100 mg

Gel: 4% (45 mg), 8% (90 mg)

Injection, in oil: 50 mg/mL (10 mL)

Intrauterine system, reservoir: 38 mg in silicone fluid

♦ **Progestin** *see* Progesterone *on page 468*

♦ **Proglycem® Oral** *see* Diazoxide *on page 163*

♦ **Prograf®** *see* Tacrolimus *on page 529*

## Proguanil (pro KWA nil)

**U.S. Brand Names** Paludrine®

**Synonyms** Bigumalum

**Pharmacologic Category** Antimalarial Agent

**Use** Malarial prophylaxis (*Plasmodium falciparum* and *vivax*)

**Effects on Mental Status** May cause dizziness

**Effects on Psychiatric Treatment** May cause pancytopenia; use caution with clozapine and carbamazepine

**Warnings/Precautions** Use with caution in pregnancy, renal insufficiency; cross-resistance can occur with other antimalarial agents; hypersensitivity to proguanil

**Adverse Reactions**

Central nervous system: Dizziness

Dermatologic: Urticaria, alopecia (reversible), exanthema, photosensitivity

Gastrointestinal: Anorexia, vomiting, diarrhea, aphthous ulceration

Hematologic: Pancytopenia, megaloblastic anemia, thrombocytopenia, aplastic anemia (1:10,000 patient years), neutropenia

Miscellaneous: Thirst

**Drug Interactions** CYP2C18, 2C19, and 3A3/4 enzyme substrate; CYP2C19 enzyme inhibitor

**Usual Dosage**

Malaria prophylaxis may be used with chloroquine:

Adults: 200 mg/day beginning at least 1 day before entering a malarious region and for 6 weeks after leaving the area; lower dosage in renal failure

Children:

- <1 year: 25 mg once daily
- 1-4 years: 50 mg once daily
- 5-8 years: 100 mg once daily
- 9-14 years: 150 mg once daily
- >14 years: 200 mg once daily

**Dosage Forms** Tablet: 100 mg


♦ **ProHIBiT®** *see Haemophilus* b Conjugate Vaccine *on page 261*

♦ **Proleukin®** *see* Aldesleukin *on page 23*

♦ **Prolixin Decanoate® Injection** *see* Fluphenazine *on page 234*

♦ **Prolixin Enanthate® Injection** *see* Fluphenazine *on page 234*

♦ **Prolixin® Injection** *see* Fluphenazine *on page 234*

♦ **Prolixin® Oral** *see* Fluphenazine *on page 234*

♦ **Proloprim®** *see* Trimethoprim *on page 570*


## Promazine (PROE ma zeen)

**Related Information**


Antipsychotic Agents Comparison Chart *on page 706*

Antipsychotic Medication Guidelines *on page 751*

Clinical Issues in the Use of Antipsychotics *on page 630*

Discontinuation of Psychotropic Drugs - Withdrawal Symptoms and Recommendations *on page 798*

Federal OBRA Regulations Recommended Maximum Doses *on page 756*

Patient Information - Antipsychotics (General) *on page 646*


**Generic Available** Yes: Injection only

**U.S. Brand Names** Sparine®

**Synonyms** Promazine Hydrochloride

**Pharmacologic Category** Antipsychotic Agent, Phenothiazine, Aliphatic

**Use** Management of manifestations of psychotic disorders

**Unlabeled use:** Nausea and vomiting; preoperative sedation

**Pregnancy Risk Factor** C

**Contraindications** Hypersensitivity to promazine or any component (cross reactivity between phenothiazines may occur); severe CNS depression, bone marrow suppression and coma; intra-arterial injection of the parenteral formulation

**Warnings/Precautions** Moderately sedating, use with caution in disorders where CNS depression is a feature. Use with caution in Parkinson's disease. Caution in patients with hemodynamic instability; bone marrow suppression; predisposition to seizures; subcortical brain damage; severe cardiac, hepatic, renal, or respiratory disease. Esophageal dysmotility and aspiration have been associated with antipsychotic use - use with caution in patients at risk of pneumonia (ie, Alzheimer's disease). Caution in breast cancer or other prolactin-dependent tumors (may elevate prolactin levels). May alter temperature regulation or mask toxicity of other drugs due to antiemetic effects. May alter cardiac conduction - life-threatening arrhythmias have occurred with therapeutic doses of phenothiazines. May cause orthostatic hypotension - use with caution in patients at risk of this effect or those who would tolerate transient hypotensive episodes (cerebrovascular disease, cardiovascular disease, or other medications which may predispose).

Phenothiazines may cause anticholinergic effects (confusion, agitation, constipation, dry mouth, blurred vision, urinary retention); therefore, they should be used with caution in patients with decreased gastrointestinal motility, urinary retention, BPH, xerostomia, or visual problems. Conditions which also may be exacerbated by cholinergic blockade include narrow-angle glaucoma (screening is recommended) and worsening of myasthenia gravis. Relative to other neuroleptics, promazine has a high potency of cholinergic blockade.

May cause extrapyramidal reactions, including pseudoparkinsonism, acute dystonic reactions, akathisia, and tardive dyskinesia (risk of these reactions is moderate relative to other neuroleptics). May be associated with neuroleptic malignant syndrome (NMS) or pigmentary retinopathy.

**Adverse Reactions**

Cardiovascular: Postural hypotension, tachycardia, dizziness, nonspecific Q-T changes

Central nervous system: Drowsiness, dystonias, akathisia, pseudoparkinsonism, tardive dyskinesia, neuroleptic malignant syndrome, seizures

Dermatologic: Photosensitivity, dermatitis, skin pigmentation (slate gray)

Endocrine & metabolic: Lactation, breast engorgement, false-positive pregnancy test, amenorrhea, gynecomastia, hyper- or hypoglycemia

Gastrointestinal: Xerostomia, constipation, nausea

Genitourinary: Urinary retention, ejaculatory disorder, impotence

Hematologic: Agranulocytosis, eosinophilia, leukopenia, hemolytic anemia, aplastic anemia, thrombocytopenic purpura

Hepatic: Jaundice

Ocular: Blurred vision, corneal and lenticular changes, epithelial keratopathy, pigmentary retinopathy

**Overdosage/Toxicology**

Signs and symptoms: Deep sleep, coma, extrapyramidal symptoms, abnormal involuntary muscle movements, hypotension

Treatment:

Following initiation of essential overdose management, toxic symptom treatment and supportive treatment should be initiated

Hypotension usually responds to I.V. fluids or Trendelenburg positioning. If unresponsive to these measures, the use of a parenteral inotrope may be required (eg, norepinephrine 0.1-0.2 mcg/kg/minute titrated to response).

Seizures commonly respond to diazepam (I.V. 5-10 mg bolus in adults every 15 minutes if needed up to a total of 30 mg; I.V. 0.25-0.4 mg/kg/dose up to a total of 10 mg in children) or to phenytoin or phenobarbital

Also critical cardiac arrhythmias often respond to I.V. phenytoin (15 mg/kg up to 1 gram), while other antiarrhythmics can be used

Neuroleptics often cause extrapyramidal symptoms (eg, dystonic reactions) requiring management with diphenhydramine 1-2 mg/kg (adults) up to a maximum of 50 mg I.M. or I.V. slow push followed by a maintenance dose for 48-72 hours. When these reactions are unresponsive to diphenhydramine, benztropine mesylate I.V. 1-2 mg (adults) may be effective. These agents are generally effective within 2-5 minutes.

**Drug Interactions**

Aluminum salts: May decrease the absorption of phenothiazines; monitor

Amphetamines: Efficacy may be diminished by antipsychotics; in addition, amphetamines may increase psychotic symptoms; avoid concurrent use

Anticholinergics: May inhibit the therapeutic response to phenothiazines and excess anticholinergic effects may occur; includes benztropine, trihexyphenidyl, biperiden, and drugs with significant anticholinergic activity (TCAs, antihistamines, disopyramide)

Antihypertensives: Concurrent use of phenothiazines with an antihypertensive may produce additive hypotensive effects (particularly orthostasis)

Bromocriptine: Phenothiazines inhibit the ability of bromocriptine to lower serum prolactin concentrations

CNS depressants: Sedative effects may be additive with phenothiazines; monitor for increased effect; includes barbiturates, benzodiazepines, narcotic analgesics, ethanol, and other sedative agents

CYP2D6 inhibitors: Metabolism of phenothiazines may be decreased; increasing clinical effect or toxicity; inhibitors include amiodarone, cimetidine, delavirdine, fluoxetine, paroxetine, propafenone, quinidine, and ritonavir; monitor for increased effect/toxicity

Enzyme inducers: May enhance the hepatic metabolism of phenothiazines; larger doses may be required; includes rifampin, rifabutin, barbiturates, phenytoin, and cigarette smoking

Epinephrine: Chlorpromazine (and possibly other low potency antipsychotics) may diminish the pressor effects of epinephrine

Guanethidine and guanadrel: Antihypertensive effects may be inhibited by phenothiazines

Levodopa: Phenothiazines may inhibit the antiparkinsonian effect of levodopa; avoid this combination

Lithium: Phenothiazines may produce neurotoxicity with lithium; this is a rare effect

Phenytoin: May reduce serum levels of phenothiazines; phenothiazines may increase phenytoin serum levels

Propranolol: Serum concentrations of phenothiazines may be increased; propranolol also increases phenothiazine concentrations

Polypeptide antibiotics: Rare cases of respiratory paralysis have been reported with concurrent use of phenothiazines

QTc prolonging agents: Effects on QTc interval may be additive with phenothiazines, increasing the risk of malignant arrhythmias; includes type Ia antiarrhythmics, TCAs, and some quinolone antibiotics (sparfloxacin, moxifloxacin, and gatifloxacin)

Sulfadoxine-pyrimethamine: May increase phenothiazine concentrations

Tricyclic antidepressants: Concurrent use may produce increased toxicity or altered therapeutic response

Trazodone: Phenothiazines and trazodone may produce additive hypotensive effects

(Continued)

## Promazine *(Continued)*

Valproic acid: Serum levels may be increased by phenothiazines

**Stability** Protect all dosage forms from light, clear or slightly yellow solutions may be used; should be dispensed in amber or opaque vials/bottles. Solutions may be diluted or mixed with fruit juices or other liquids, but must be administered immediately after mixing

Injection: **Incompatible** when mixed with aminophylline, dimenhydrinate, methohexital, nafcillin, penicillin G, pentobarbital, phenobarbital, sodium bicarbonate, thiopental

**Mechanism of Action** Blocks postsynaptic mesolimbic dopaminergic $D_1$ and $D_2$ receptors in the brain; exhibits a strong alpha-adrenergic blocking and anticholinergic effect, depresses the release of hypothalamic and hypophyseal hormones; believed to depress the reticular activating system thus affecting basal metabolism, body temperature, wakefulness, vasomotor tone, and emesis

**Pharmacodynamics/kinetics** The specific pharmacokinetics of promazine are poorly established but probably resemble those of other phenothiazines.

Absorption: Phenothiazines are only partially absorbed; great variability in plasma levels resulting from a given dose

Metabolism: Extensively in the liver

Half-life: Most phenothiazines have long half-lives in the range of 24 hours or more

**Usual Dosage** Oral, I.M.:

Children >12 years: Antipsychotic: 10-25 mg every 4-6 hours

Adults:

Psychosis: 10-200 mg every 4-6 hours not to exceed 1000 mg/day

Antiemetic: 25-50 mg every 4-6 hours as needed

Hemodialysis: Not dialyzable (0% to 5%)

**Administration** I.M. injections should be deep injections; if giving I.V., dilute to at least 25 mg/mL and administer slowly

**Monitoring Parameters** Orthostatic blood pressure, tremors, gait changes, abnormal movement in trunk, neck, buccal area or extremities; monitor target behaviors for which the agent is given; monitor hepatic function (especially if fever with flu-like symptoms)

**Reference Range** Not useful

**Test Interactions** ↑ cholesterol (S), glucose, prolactin; ↓ uric acid (S)

**Patient Information** May cause drowsiness, impair judgment and coordination; may cause photosensitivity; avoid excessive sunlight; notify physician of involuntary movements or feelings of restlessness

**Nursing Implications** I.M. injections should be deep injections; if giving I.V., dilute to at least 25 mg/mL and give slowly; watch for hypotension; protect injection from light

**Additional Information** Coadministration of two or more antipsychotics does not improve clinical response and may increase the potential for adverse effects; not recommended as an antipsychotic due to inferior efficacy compared to other phenothiazines

**Dosage Forms**

Injection, as hydrochloride: 25 mg/mL (10 mL); 50 mg/mL (1 mL, 2 mL, 10 mL)

Tablet, as hydrochloride: 25 mg, 50 mg, 100 mg

♦ **Promazine Hydrochloride** *see* Promazine *on page 469*

♦ **Prometa®** *see* Metaproterenol *on page 347*

## Promethazine (proe METH a zeen)

**Generic Available** Yes

**U.S. Brand Names** Phenazine®; Phenergan®; Prorex®

**Synonyms** Promethazine Hydrochloride

**Pharmacologic Category** Antiemetic

**Use** Symptomatic treatment of various allergic conditions; antiemetic; motion sickness; sedative; analgesic adjunct for control of postoperative pain; anesthetic adjunct

**Pregnancy Risk Factor** C

**Pregnancy/Breast-Feeding Implications**

Clinical effects on the fetus: Crosses the placenta. Possible respiratory depression if drug is administered near time of delivery; behavioral changes, EEG alterations, impaired platelet aggregation reported with use during labor. Available evidence with use of occasional low doses suggests safe use during pregnancy.

Breast-feeding/lactation: No data available; American Academy of Pediatrics makes **no recommendation**

**Contraindications** Hypersensitivity to promethazine or any component (cross reactivity between phenothiazines may occur); severe CNS depression; coma; intra-arterial or subcutaneous injection

**Warnings/Precautions** May be sedating; use with caution in disorders where CNS depression is a feature. May impair physical or mental abilities; patients must cautioned about performing tasks which require mental alertness (ie, operating machinery or driving). Effects with other sedative drugs or ethanol may be potentiated. Avoid use in Reye's syndrome. Use with caution in Parkinson's disease; hemodynamic instability; bone marrow suppression; predisposition to seizures; subcortical brain damage; and in severe cardiac, hepatic, renal, or respiratory disease. Caution in breast cancer or other prolactin-dependent tumors (may elevate prolactin levels). May alter temperature regulation or mask toxicity of other drugs due to antiemetic effects. May alter cardiac conduction - life threatening arrhythmias have occurred with therapeutic doses of phenothiazines. May cause orthostatic hypotension; use with caution in patients at risk of hypotension or where transient hypotensive episodes would be poorly tolerated (cardiovascular disease or cerebrovascular disease).

Phenothiazines may cause anticholinergic effects (constipation, dry mouth, blurred vision, urinary retention); therefore, they should be used with caution in patients with decreased gastrointestinal motility, urinary retention, BPH, xerostomia, or visual problems. Conditions which also may be exacerbated by cholinergic blockade include narrow-angle glaucoma (screening is recommended) and worsening of myasthenia gravis. May cause extrapyramidal reactions, including pseudoparkinsonism, acute dystonic reactions, akathisia, and tardive dyskinesia. May be associated with neuroleptic malignant syndrome (NMS). Ampuls contain sodium metabisulfite.

**Adverse Reactions**

Cardiovascular: Postural hypotension, tachycardia, dizziness, nonspecific Q-T changes

Central nervous system: Drowsiness, dystonias, akathisia, pseudoparkinsonism, tardive dyskinesia, neuroleptic malignant syndrome, seizures

Dermatologic: Photosensitivity, dermatitis, skin pigmentation (slate gray)

Endocrine & metabolic: Lactation, breast engorgement, false-positive pregnancy test, amenorrhea, gynecomastia, hyper- or hypoglycemia

Gastrointestinal: Xerostomia, constipation, nausea

Genitourinary: Urinary retention, ejaculatory disorder, impotence

Hematologic: Agranulocytosis, eosinophilia, leukopenia, hemolytic anemia, aplastic anemia, thrombocytopenic purpura

Hepatic: Jaundice

Ocular: Blurred vision, corneal and lenticular changes, epithelial keratopathy, pigmentary retinopathy

**Overdosage/Toxicology**

Signs and symptoms: CNS depression, respiratory depression, possible CNS stimulation, dry mouth, fixed and dilated pupils, hypotension

Treatment:

Following initiation of essential overdose management, toxic symptom treatment and supportive treatment should be initiated

Hypotension usually responds to I.V. fluids or Trendelenburg positioning. If unresponsive to these measures, norepinephrine 0.1-0.2 mcg/kg/minute titrated to response may be tried.

Seizures commonly respond to diazepam (I.V. 5-10 mg bolus in adults every 15 minutes if needed up to a total of 30 mg; I.V. 0.25-0.4 mg/kg/dose up to a total of 10 mg in children) or to phenytoin or phenobarbital

Also critical cardiac arrhythmias often respond to I.V. phenytoin (15 mg/kg up to 1 gram), while other antiarrhythmics can be used

Neuroleptics often cause extrapyramidal symptoms (eg, dystonic reactions) requiring management with diphenhydramine 1-2 mg/kg (adults) up to a maximum of 50 mg I.M. or I.V. slow push followed by a maintenance dose for 48-72 hours. When these reactions are unresponsive to diphenhydramine, benztropine mesylate I.V. 1-2 mg (adults) may be effective. These agents are generally effective within 2-5 minutes.

**Drug Interactions** CYP2D6 enzyme substrate

Aluminum salts: May decrease the absorption of phenothiazines; monitor

Amphetamines: Efficacy may be diminished by antipsychotics; in addition, amphetamines may increase psychotic symptoms; avoid concurrent use

Anticholinergics: May inhibit the therapeutic response to phenothiazines and excess anticholinergic effects may occur; includes benztropine, trihexyphenidyl, biperiden, and drugs with significant anticholinergic activity (TCAs, antihistamines, disopyramide)

Antihypertensives: Concurrent use of phenothiazines with an antihypertensive may produce additive hypotensive effects (particularly orthostasis)

Bromocriptine: Phenothiazines inhibit the ability of bromocriptine to lower serum prolactin concentrations

CNS depressants: Sedative effects may be additive with phenothiazines; monitor for increased effect; includes barbiturates, benzodiazepines, narcotic analgesics, ethanol, and other sedative agents

CYP2D6 inhibitors: Metabolism of phenothiazines may be decreased; increasing clinical effect or toxicity; inhibitors include amiodarone, cimetidine, delavirdine, fluoxetine, paroxetine, propafenone, quinidine, and ritonavir; monitor for increased effect/toxicity

Enzyme inducers: May enhance the hepatic metabolism of phenothiazines; larger doses may be required; includes rifampin, rifabutin, barbiturates, phenytoin, and cigarette smoking

Epinephrine: Chlorpromazine (and possibly other low potency antipsychotics) may diminish the pressor effects of epinephrine

Guanethidine and guanadrel: Antihypertensive effects may be inhibited by phenothiazines

Levodopa: Phenothiazines may inhibit the antiparkinsonian effect of levodopa; avoid this combination

Lithium: Phenothiazines may produce neurotoxicity with lithium; this is a rare effect

Phenytoin: May reduce serum levels of phenothiazines; phenothiazines may increase phenytoin serum levels

Propranolol: Serum concentrations of phenothiazines may be increased; propranolol also increases phenothiazine concentrations
Polypeptide antibiotics: Rare cases of respiratory paralysis have been reported with concurrent use of phenothiazines
QTc prolonging agents: Effects on QTc interval may be additive with phenothiazines, increasing the risk of malignant arrhythmias; includes type Ia antiarrhythmics, TCAs, and some quinolone antibiotics (sparfloxacin, moxifloxacin, and gatifloxacin)
Sulfadoxine-pyrimethamine: May increase phenothiazine concentrations
Tricyclic antidepressants: Concurrent use may produce increased toxicity or altered therapeutic response
Trazodone: Phenothiazines and trazodone may produce additive hypotensive effects
Valproic acid: Serum levels may be increased by phenothiazines

**Stability** Protect from light and from freezing; **compatible** (when comixed in the same syringe) with atropine, chlorpromazine, diphenhydramine, droperidol, fentanyl, glycopyrrolate, hydromorphone, hydroxyzine hydrochloride, meperidine, midazolam, nalbuphine, pentazocine, prochlorperazine, scopolamine; **incompatible** when mixed with aminophylline, cefoperazone (Y-site), chloramphenicol, dimenhydrinate (same syringe), foscarnet (Y-site), furosemide, heparin, hydrocortisone, methohexital, penicillin G, pentobarbital, phenobarbital, thiopental

**Mechanism of Action** Blocks postsynaptic mesolimbic dopaminergic receptors in the brain; exhibits a strong alpha-adrenergic blocking effect and depresses the release of hypothalamic and hypophyseal hormones; competes with histamine for the $H_1$-receptor; reduces stimuli to the brainstem reticular system

**Pharmacodynamics/kinetics**
Onset of effect: I.V.: Within 20 minutes (3-5 minutes with I.V. injection)
Duration: 2-6 hours
Metabolism: In the liver
Half-life: 16-19 hours
Peak effect: $C_{max}$: 9.04 mg/mL (suppository); 19.3 mg/mL (syrup)
Time to maximum serum concentration: 4.4 hours (syrup); 6.7-8.6 hours (suppositories)
Elimination: Principally as inactive metabolites in urine and in feces

**Usual Dosage**
Children:
Antihistamine: Oral, rectal: 0.1 mg/kg/dose every 6 hours during the day and 0.5 mg/kg/dose at bedtime as needed
Antiemetic: Oral, I.M., I.V., rectal: 0.25-1 mg/kg 4-6 times/day as needed
Motion sickness: Oral, rectal: 0.5 mg/kg/dose 30 minutes to 1 hour before departure, then every 12 hours as needed
Sedation: Oral, I.M., I.V., rectal: 0.5-1 mg/kg/dose every 6 hours as needed
Adults:
Antihistamine (including allergic reactions to blood or plasma):
Oral, rectal: 12.5 mg 3 times/day and 25 mg at bedtime
I.M., I.V.: 25 mg, may repeat in 2 hours when necessary; switch to oral route as soon as feasible
Antiemetic: Oral, I.M., I.V., rectal: 12.5-25 mg every 4 hours as needed
Motion sickness: Oral, rectal: 25 mg 30-60 minutes before departure, then every 12 hours as needed
Sedation: Oral, I.M., I.V., rectal: 25-50 mg/dose
Hemodialysis: Not dialyzable (0% to 5%)

**Administration** Avoid I.V. use; if necessary, may dilute to a maximum concentration of 25 mg/mL and infuse at a maximum rate of 25 mg/minute; rapid I.V. administration may produce a transient fall in blood pressure

**Monitoring Parameters** Relief of symptoms, mental status

**Reference Range** Therapeutic: 11-23 ng/mL; Toxic: >48 ng/mL; Fatal: 156 ng/mL (postmortem)

**Test Interactions** Alters the flare response in intradermal allergen tests

**Patient Information** May cause drowsiness, impair judgment and coordination; may cause photosensitivity; avoid excessive sunlight; notify physician of involuntary movements or feelings of restlessness

**Nursing Implications** Rapid I.V. administration may produce a transient fall in blood pressure, rate of administration should not exceed 25 mg/minute; slow I.V. administration may produce a slightly elevated blood pressure; avoid extravasation since tissue necrosis has occurred with extravasation

**Dosage Forms**
Injection, as hydrochloride: 25 mg/mL (1 mL, 10 mL); 50 mg/mL (1 mL, 10 mL)
Suppository, rectal, as hydrochloride: 12.5 mg, 25 mg, 50 mg
Syrup, as hydrochloride: 6.25 mg/5 mL (5 mL, 120 mL, 240 mL, 480 mL, 4000 mL); 25 mg/5 mL (120 mL, 480 mL, 4000 mL)
Tablet, as hydrochloride: 12.5 mg, 25 mg, 50 mg

## Promethazine and Codeine (proe METH a zeen & KOE deen)

**U.S. Brand Names** Phenergan® With Codeine; Pherazine® With Codeine; Prothazine-DC®

**Pharmacologic Category** Antihistamine/Antitussive

**Use** Temporary relief of coughs and upper respiratory symptoms associated with allergy or the common cold

**Effects on Mental Status** May cause drowsiness

**Effects on Psychiatric Treatment** concurrent use with psychotropics may produce additive sedation

**Restrictions** C-V

**Usual Dosage** Oral (in terms of codeine):
Children: 1-1.5 mg/kg/day every 4 hours as needed; maximum: 30 mg/day
**or**
2-6 years: 1.25-2.5 mL every 4-6 hours or 2.5-5 mg/dose every 4-6 hours as needed; maximum: 30 mg codeine/day
6-12 years: 2.5-5 mL every 4-6 hours as needed or 5-10 mg/dose every 4-6 hours as needed; maximum: 60 mg codeine/day
Adults: 10-20 mg/dose every 4-6 hours as needed; maximum: 120 mg codeine/day; or 5-10 mL every 4-6 hours as needed

**Dosage Forms** Syrup: Promethazine hydrochloride 6.25 mg and codeine phosphate 10 mg per 5 mL (120 mL, 180 mL, 473 mL)

## Promethazine and Dextromethorphan
(proe METH a zeen & deks troe meth OR fan)

**U.S. Brand Names** Phenameth® DM; Phenergan® With Dextromethorphan; Pherazine® w/DM

**Pharmacologic Category** Antihistamine/Antitussive

**Use** Temporary relief of coughs and upper respiratory symptoms associated with allergy or the common cold

**Effects on Mental Status** May cause drowsiness

**Effects on Psychiatric Treatment** Concurrent use with psychotropics may produce additive sedation

**Usual Dosage** Oral:
Children:
2-6 years: 1.25-2.5 mL every 4-6 hours up to 10 mL in 24 hours
6-12 years: 2.5-5 mL every 4-6 hours up to 20 mL in 24 hours
Adults: 5 mL every 4-6 hours up to 30 mL in 24 hours

**Dosage Forms** Syrup: Promethazine hydrochloride 6.25 mg and dextromethorphan hydrobromide 15 mg per 5 mL with alcohol 7% (120 mL, 480 mL, 4000 mL)

## Promethazine and Phenylephrine
(proe METH a zeen & fen il EF rin)

**U.S. Brand Names** Phenergan® VC Syrup; Promethazine VC Plain Syrup; Promethazine VC Syrup; Prometh VC Plain Liquid

**Pharmacologic Category** Antihistamine/Decongestant Combination

**Use** Temporary relief of upper respiratory symptoms associated with allergy or the common cold

**Effects on Mental Status** May cause drowsiness

**Effects on Psychiatric Treatment** Concurrent use with psychotropics may produce additive sedation

**Usual Dosage** Oral:
Children:
2-6 years: 1.25 mL every 4-6 hours, not to exceed 7.5 mL in 24 hours
6-12 years: 2.5 mL every 4-6 hours, not to exceed 15 mL in 24 hours
Children >12 years and Adults: 5 mL every 4-6 hours, not to exceed 30 mL in 24 hours

**Dosage Forms** Liquid: Promethazine hydrochloride 6.25 mg and phenylephrine hydrochloride 5 mg per 5 mL (120 mL, 240 mL, 473 mL)

♦ **Promethazine Hydrochloride** *see* Promethazine *on page 470*

## Promethazine, Phenylephrine, and Codeine
(proe METH a zeen, fen il EF rin, & KOE deen)

**U.S. Brand Names** Phenergan® VC With Codeine; Pherazine® VC w/ Codeine; Promethist® With Codeine; Prometh® VC With Codeine

**Pharmacologic Category** Antihistamine/Decongestant/Antitussive

**Use** Temporary relief of coughs and upper respiratory symptoms including nasal congestion

**Effects on Mental Status** May cause drowsiness

**Effects on Psychiatric Treatment** Concurrent use with psychotropics may produce additive sedation

**Restrictions** C-V

**Usual Dosage** Oral:
Children (expressed in terms of codeine dosage): 1-1.5 mg/kg/day every 4 hours, maximum: 30 mg/day **or**
<2 years: Not recommended
2 to 6 years:
Weight 25 lb: 1.25-2.5 mL every 4-6 hours, not to exceed 6 mL/24 hours
Weight 30 lb: 1.25-2.5 mL every 4-6 hours, not to exceed 7 mL/24 hours
Weight 35 lb: 1.25-2.5 mL every 4-6 hours, not to exceed 8 mL/24 hours
Weight 40 lb: 1.25-2.5 mL every 4-6 hours, not to exceed 9 mL/24 hours
6 to <12 years: 2.5-5 mL every 4-6 hours, not to exceed 15 mL/24 hours
(Continued)

## Promethazine, Phenylephrine, and Codeine *(Continued)*

Adults: 5 mL every 4-6 hours, not to exceed 30 mL/24 hours

**Dosage Forms** Liquid: Promethazine hydrochloride 6.25 mg, phenylephrine hydrochloride 5 mg, and codeine phosphate 10 mg per 5 mL with alcohol 7% (120 mL, 240 mL, 480 mL, 4000 mL)

- **Promethazine VC Plain Syrup** *see* Promethazine and Phenylephrine *on page 471*
- **Promethazine VC Syrup** *see* Promethazine and Phenylephrine *on page 471*
- **Promethist® With Codeine** *see* Promethazine, Phenylephrine, and Codeine *on page 471*
- **Prometh VC Plain Liquid** *see* Promethazine and Phenylephrine *on page 471*
- **Prometh® VC With Codeine** *see* Promethazine, Phenylephrine, and Codeine *on page 471*
- **Prometrium®** *see* Progesterone *on page 468*
- **Pronestyl®** *see* Procainamide *on page 464*
- **Pronto® Shampoo [OTC]** *see* Pyrethrins *on page 480*
- **Propacet®** *see* Propoxyphene and Acetaminophen *on page 474*

## Propafenone (proe pa FEEN one)

**U.S. Brand Names** Rythmol®

**Pharmacologic Category** Antiarrhythmic Agent, Class I-C

**Use** Life-threatening ventricular arrhythmias

**Unlabeled use:** Supraventricular tachycardias, including those patients with Wolff-Parkinson-White syndrome

**Effects on Mental Status** Dizziness and drowsiness are common; may cause anxiety

**Effects on Psychiatric Treatment** May rarely cause agranulocytosis; use caution with clozapine and carbamazepine; use TCAs with caution; may cause Q-T prolongation

**Pregnancy Risk Factor** C

**Contraindications** Hypersensitivity to propafenone or any component; sinoatrial, AV, and intraventricular disorders of impulse generation and/or conduction (except in patients with a functioning artificial pacemaker); sinus bradycardia; cardiogenic shock; uncompensated cardiac failure; hypotension; bronchospastic disorders; uncorrected electrolyte abnormalities

**Warnings/Precautions** Monitor for proarrhythmic events. Patients with bronchospastic disease should generally not receive this drug. Monitor for worsening CHF if patient has underlying condition. Can cause or unmask a variety of conduction disturbances. May alter pacing and sensing thresholds of artificial pacemakers. Administer cautiously in significant hepatic dysfunction.

**Adverse Reactions**

>10%: Central nervous system: Dizziness (6.5%), drowsiness

1% to 10%:

Cardiovascular: A-V block (first (4.5%) and second (1.2%) degree), cardiac conduction disturbances (eg, bundle-branch block (1.2%)), palpitations (2% to 4%), congestive heart failure, angina (1.2%), bradycardia

Central nervous system: Headache (4.5%), anxiety (2%), loss of balance (1.2%)

Gastrointestinal: Abnormal taste (7.3%), constipation (4%), nausea (1.2%), vomiting (2.8%), abdominal pain, dyspepsia, anorexia (1.6%), flatulence (1.2%), diarrhea (1.2%), xerostomia (2%)

Ocular: Blurred vision (2%)

Respiratory: Dyspnea (2%)

<1%: Abnormal speech/vision/dreams, agranulocytosis, arrhythmias (new or worsened) (proarrhythmic effect), bundle-branch block, leukopenia, numbness, paresthesias, thrombocytopenia, (+) ANA titers

**Overdosage/Toxicology**

Signs and symptoms: Has a narrow therapeutic index and severe toxicity may occur slightly above the therapeutic range, especially if combined with other antiarrhythmic drugs. Acute single ingestion of twice the daily therapeutic dose is life-threatening. Symptoms of overdose include increases in P-R, QRS, Q-T intervals and amplitude of the T wave, A-V block, bradycardia, hypotension, ventricular arrhythmias (monomorphic or polymorphic ventricular tachycardia), and asystole; other symptoms include dizziness, blurred vision, headache, and GI upset.

Treatment: Supportive, using conventional treatment (fluids, positioning, anticonvulsants, antiarrhythmics). **Note:** Type Ia antiarrhythmic agents should not be used to treat cardiotoxicity caused by type 1c drugs; sodium bicarbonate may reverse QRS prolongation, bradycardia and hypotension; ventricular pacing may be needed; hemodialysis only of possible benefit for tocainide or flecainide overdose in patients with renal failure.

**Drug Interactions** CYP2D6 substrate/inhibitor, CYP1A2 substrate

Inhibitors of CYP2D6 or CYP1A2 may increase blood levels of propafenone

Amprenavir and ritonavir may increase propafenone levels; concurrent use is contraindicated

Cimetidine increases propafenone blood levels

Digoxin blood levels are increased; monitor for toxicity

Enzyme inducers (phenobarbital, phenytoin, rifabutin, rifampin) may decrease propafenone blood levels

Metoprolol blood levels are increased

Propranolol blood levels are increased

Quinidine increases propafenone blood levels

Theophylline blood levels may be increased

Warfarin blood levels are increased; response may be increased; monitor INR closely

**Usual Dosage** Adults: Oral: 150 mg every 8 hours, increase at 3- to 4-day intervals up to 300 mg every 8 hours. **Note:** Patients who exhibit significant widening of QRS complex or second- or third-degree A-V block may need dose reduction.

**Dosing adjustment in hepatic impairment:** Reduction is necessary.

**Patient Information** Take exactly as directed; do not take additional doses or discontinue without consulting prescriber. You will need regular cardiac checkups and blood tests while taking this medication. You may experience dizziness, drowsiness, or visual changes (use caution when driving or engaging in tasks requiring alertness until response to drug is known); abnormal taste, nausea or vomiting, or loss of appetite (small frequent meals, frequent mouth care, chewing gum, or sucking lozenges may help); headaches (prescriber may recommend mild analgesic); or diarrhea (exercise, yogurt, or boiled milk may help - if persistent consult prescriber). Report chest pain, palpitation, or erratic heartbeat; difficulty breathing, increased weight or swelling of hands or feet; acute persistent diarrhea or constipation; or changes in vision.

**Nursing Implications** Patients should be on a cardiac monitor during initiation of therapy or when dosage is increased; monitor heart sounds and pulses for rate, rhythm and quality

**Dosage Forms** Tablet, as hydrochloride: 150 mg, 225 mg, 300 mg

- **Propagest® [OTC]** *see* Phenylpropanolamine *on page 440*

## Propantheline (proe PAN the leen)

**Related Information**

Pharmacotherapy of Urinary Incontinence *on page 758*

**U.S. Brand Names** Pro-Banthine®

**Pharmacologic Category** Anticholinergic Agent

**Use** Adjunctive treatment of peptic ulcer, irritable bowel syndrome, pancreatitis, ureteral and urinary bladder spasm; reduce duodenal motility during diagnostic radiologic procedures

**Effects on Mental Status** May cause drowsiness, confusion, amnesia, nervousness, or insomnia

**Effects on Psychiatric Treatment** Concurrent use with psychotropics may produce additive sedation or anticholinergic side effects (dry mouth)

**Pregnancy Risk Factor** C

**Contraindications** Narrow-angle glaucoma, known hypersensitivity to propantheline; ulcerative colitis; toxic megacolon; obstructive disease of the GI or urinary tract

**Warnings/Precautions** Use with caution in patients with hyperthyroidism, hepatic, cardiac, or renal disease, hypertension, GI infections, or other endocrine diseases.

**Adverse Reactions**

>10%:

Dermatologic: Dry skin

Gastrointestinal: Constipation, xerostomia, dry throat

Respiratory: Dry nose

Miscellaneous: Diaphoresis (decreased)

1% to 10%: Gastrointestinal: Dysphagia

**Overdosage/Toxicology**

Signs and symptoms: CNS disturbances, flushing, respiratory failure, paralysis, coma, urinary retention, hyperthermia

Treatment: Anticholinergic toxicity is caused by strong binding of the drug to cholinergic receptors. For anticholinergic overdose with severe life-threatening symptoms, physostigmine 1-2 mg (0.5 or 0.02 mg/kg for children) S.C. or I.V., slowly may be given to reverse these effects.

**Drug Interactions**

Decreased effect with antacids (decreased absorption); decreased effect of sustained release dosage forms (decreased absorption)

Increased effect/toxicity with anticholinergics, disopyramide, narcotic analgesics, bretylium, type I antiarrhythmics, antihistamines, phenothiazines, TCAs, corticosteroids (increased IOP), CNS depressants (sedation), adenosine, amiodarone, beta-blockers, amoxapine

**Usual Dosage** Oral:

Antisecretory:

Children: 1-2 mg/kg/day in 3-4 divided doses

Adults: 15 mg 3 times/day before meals or food and 30 mg at bedtime

Elderly: 7.5 mg 3 times/day before meals and at bedtime

Antispasmodic:

Children: 2-3 mg/kg/day in divided doses every 4-6 hours and at bedtime

Adults: 15 mg 3 times/day before meals or food and 30 mg at bedtime

**Patient Information** Take as directed before meals; do not increase dose and do not discontinue without consulting prescriber. Void before taking medication. You may experience constipation (increased dietary fruit, fluids, fiber, and exercise may help). Report chest pain or rapid heartbeat, or excessive and persistent anticholinergic effects (blurred vision, headache, flushing, tachycardia, nervousness, constipation, dizziness, insomnia, mental confusion or excitement, dry mouth, altered taste perception, dysphagia, palpitations, bradycardia, urinary hesitancy or retention, impotence, decreased sweating).

**Dosage Forms** Tablet, as bromide: 7.5 mg, 15 mg

## Proparacaine (proe PAR a kane)

**U.S. Brand Names** AK-Taine®; Alcaine®; I-Paracaine®; Ophthetic®

**Pharmacologic Category** Local Anesthetic

**Use** Anesthesia for tonometry, gonioscopy; suture removal from cornea; removal of corneal foreign body; cataract extraction, glaucoma surgery; short operative procedure involving the cornea and conjunctiva

**Effects on Mental Status** May rarely produce CNS depression

**Effects on Psychiatric Treatment** None reported

**Usual Dosage** Children and Adults:

Ophthalmic surgery: Instill 1 drop of 0.5% solution in eye every 5-10 minutes for 5-7 doses

Tonometry, gonioscopy, suture removal: Instill 1-2 drops of 0.5% solution in eye just prior to procedure

**Dosage Forms** Ophthalmic, solution, as hydrochloride: 0.5% (2 mL, 15 mL)

♦ **Propine® Ophthalmic** *see* Dipivefrin *on page 176*

## Propiomazine (proe pee OH ma zeen)

**U.S. Brand Names** Largon® Injection

**Pharmacologic Category** Antianxiety Agent, Miscellaneous; Antiemetic; Sedative, Miscellaneous

**Use** Relief of restlessness, nausea and apprehension before and during surgery or during labor

**Effects on Mental Status** Dizziness and drowsiness are common; may cause confusion; may rarely cause neuroleptic malignant syndrome

**Effects on Psychiatric Treatment** Propiomazine is a phenothiazine; concurrent use with other psychotropics may produce additive side effects

**Contraindications** Hypersensitivity to propiomazine

**Warnings/Precautions** Do not give S.C. or intra-arterially due to causing of severe irritation and arteriospasm; use with caution in patients with angle-closure glaucoma, severe hepatic, or cardiac disease

**Adverse Reactions**

>10%:

Central nervous system: Dizziness, drowsiness

Gastrointestinal: Xerostomia

1% to 10%:

Cardiovascular: Tachycardia

Central nervous system: Confusion

Dermatologic: Skin rash

Gastrointestinal: Diarrhea, stomach pain

Respiratory: Shortness of breath

**Overdosage/Toxicology**

Signs and symptoms: Deep sleep, coma, extrapyramidal symptoms, abnormal involuntary muscle movements, hypotension

Treatment: Following initiation of essential overdose management, toxic symptom treatment and supportive treatment should be initiated. Hypotension usually responds to I.V. fluids or Trendelenburg positioning; if unresponsive to these measures, the use of a parenteral inotrope may be required (ie, norepinephrine 0.1-0.2 mcg/kg/minute titrated to response). Seizures commonly respond to diazepam (I.V. 5-10 mg bolus in adults every 15 minutes if needed up to a total of 30 mg; I.V. 0.25-0.4 mg/kg/dose up to a total of 10 mg in children) or to phenytoin or phenobarbital. Also critical cardiac arrhythmias often respond to I.V. phenytoin (15 mg/kg up to 1 g), while other antiarrhythmics can be used. Neuroleptics often cause extrapyramidal symptoms (ie, dystonic reactions) requiring management with diphenhydramine 1-2 mg/kg (adults) up to a maximum of 50 mg I.M. or I.V. slow push followed by a maintenance dose for 48-72 hours. When these reactions are unresponsive to diphenhydramine, benztropine mesylate I.V. 1-2 mg (adults) may be effective. These agents are generally effective within 2-5 minutes.

**Drug Interactions** CNS depressants, epinephrine

**Usual Dosage** I.M., I.V.:

Children <27 kg: 0.55-1.1 mg/kg

Adults: 10-40 mg prior to procedure, additional may be repeated at 3-hour intervals

**Dosage Forms** Injection, as hydrochloride: 20 mg/mL (1 mL)

♦ **Proplex® T** *see* Factor IX Complex (Human) *on page 217*

## Propofol (PROE po fole)

**U.S. Brand Names** Diprivan® Injection

**Pharmacologic Category** General Anesthetic

**Use** Induction or maintenance of anesthesia for inpatient or outpatient surgery; may be used (for patients >18 years of age who are intubated and mechanically ventilated) as an alternative to benzodiazepines for the treatment of agitation in the intensive care unit; pain should be treated with analgesic agents, propofol must be titrated separately from the analgesic agent; has demonstrated antiemetic properties in the postoperative setting

**Effects on Mental Status** May cause dizziness

**Effects on Psychiatric Treatment** Concurrent use with psychotropics may produce additive CNS depression and respiratory depression; monitor and adjust dosages as needed

**Pregnancy Risk Factor** B

**Contraindications**

**Absolute contraindications:**

Patients with a hypersensitivity to propofol

Patients with a hypersensitivity to propofol's emulsion which contains soybean oil, egg phosphatide, and glycerol or any of the components

Patients who are not intubated or mechanically ventilated

Patients who are pregnant or nursing: Propofol is not recommended for obstetrics, including cesarian section deliveries. Propofol crosses the placenta and, therefore, may be associated with neonatal depression.

**Relative contraindications:**

Pediatric Intensive Care Unit patients: Safety and efficacy of propofol is not established

Patients with severe cardiac disease (ejection fraction <50%) or respiratory disease - propofol may have more profound adverse cardiovascular responses

Patients with a history of epilepsy or seizures

Patients with increased intracranial pressure or impaired cerebral circulation - substantial decreases in mean arterial pressure and subsequent decreases in cerebral perfusion pressure may occur

Patients with hyperlipidemia as evidenced by increased serum triglyceride levels or serum turbidity

Patients who are hypotensive, hypovolemic, or hemodynamically unstable

**Warnings/Precautions** Use slower rate of induction in the elderly; transient local pain may occur during I.V. injection; perioperative myoclonia has occurred; do not administer with blood or blood products through the same I.V. catheter; not for obstetrics, including cesarean section deliveries. Safety and effectiveness has not been established in children. Abrupt discontinuation prior to weaning or daily wake up assessments should be avoided. Abrupt discontinuation can result in rapid awakening, anxiety, agitation, and resistance to mechanical ventilation; not for use in neurosurgical anesthesia.

**Adverse Reactions**

>10%:

Cardiovascular: Hypotension, intravenous propofol produces a dose-related degree of hypotension and decrease in systemic vascular resistance which is not associated with a significant increase in heart rate or decrease in cardiac output

Local: Pain at injection site occurs at an incidence of 28.5% when administered into smaller veins of hand versus 6% when administered into antecubital veins

Respiratory: Apnea (incidence occurs in 50% to 84% of patients and may be dependent on premedication, speed of administration, dose and presence of hyperventilation and hyperoxia)

1% to 10%:

Anaphylaxis: Several cases of anaphylactic reactions have been reported with propofol

Central nervous system: Dizziness, fever, headache; although propofol has demonstrated anticonvulsant activity, several cases of propofol-induced seizures with opisthotonos have occurred

Gastrointestinal: Nausea, vomiting, abdominal cramps

Respiratory: Cough, apnea

Neuromuscular & skeletal: Twitching

Miscellaneous: Hiccups

**Overdosage/Toxicology**

Signs and symptoms: Hypotension, bradycardia, cardiovascular collapse

Treatment: Symptomatic and supportive; hypotension usually responds to I.V. fluids and/or Trendelenburg positioning; parenteral inotropes may be needed

**Drug Interactions**

Increased toxicity:

Neuromuscular blockers:

Atracurium: Anaphylactoid reactions (including bronchospasm) have been reported in patients who have received concomitant atracurium and propofol

Vecuronium: Propofol may potentiate the neuromuscular blockade of vecuronium

Central nervous system depressants: Additive CNS depression and respiratory depression may necessitate dosage reduction when used

(Continued)

## Propofol *(Continued)*

with: Anesthetics, benzodiazepines, opiates, ethanol, narcotics, phenothiazines

Decreased effect: Theophylline: May antagonize the effect of propofol, requiring dosage increases

**Usual Dosage** Dosage must be individualized based on total body weight and titrated to the desired clinical effect; however, as a general guideline:

No pediatric dose has been established; however, induction for children 1-12 years 2-2.8 mg/kg has been used

Induction: I.V.:

Adults ≤55 years, and/or ASA I or II patients: 2-2.5 mg/kg of body weight (approximately 40 mg every 10 seconds until onset of induction)

Elderly, debilitated, hypovolemic, and/or ASA III or IV patients: 1-1.5 mg/kg of body weight (approximately 20 mg every 10 seconds until onset of induction)

Maintenance: I.V. infusion:

Adults ≤55 years, and/or ASA I or II patients: 0.1-0.2 mg/kg of body weight/minute (6-12 mg/kg of body weight/hour)

Elderly, debilitated, hypovolemic, and/or ASA III or IV patients: 0.05-0.1 mg/kg of body weight/minute (3-6 mg/kg of body weight/hour)

I.V. intermittent: 25-50 mg increments, as needed

ICU sedation: Rapid bolus injection should be avoided. Bolus injection can result in hypotension, oxyhemoglobin desaturation, apnea, airway obstruction, and oxygen desaturation. The preferred route of administration is slow infusion. Doses are based on individual need and titrated to response.

Recommended starting dose: 5 mcg/kg/minute (0.3-0.6 mg/kg/hour) over 5-10 minutes may be used until the desired level of sedation is achieved; infusion rate should be increased by increments of 5-10 mcg/kg/minute (0.3-0.6 mg/kg/hour) until the desired level of sedation is achieved; most adult patients require maintenance rates of 5-50 mcg/kg/minute (0.3-3 mg/kg/hour) or higher

Adjustments in dose can occur at 3- to 5-minute intervals. An 80% reduction in dose should be considered in elderly, debilitated, and ASA III or IV patients. Once sedation is established, the dose should be decreased for the maintenance infusion period and adjusted to response.

**Patient Information** Protect from light; shake well

**Nursing Implications** **Changes urine color to green**; abrupt discontinuation of infusion may result in rapid awakening of the patient associated with anxiety, agitation, and resistance to mechanical ventilation, making weaning from mechanical ventilation difficult; use a light level of sedation throughout the weaning process until 10-15 minutes before extubation; titrate the infusion rate so the patient awakens slowly. Tubing and any unused portions of propofol vials should be discarded after 12 hours.

**Dosage Forms** Injection: 10 mg/mL (20 mL, 50 mL, 100 mL)

## Propoxyphene (proe POKS i feen)

**Related Information**

Narcotic Agonists Comparison Chart *on page 720*

**U.S. Brand Names** Darvon®; Darvon-N®; Dolene®

**Canadian Brand Names** Novo-Propoxyn; 624® Tablets

**Synonyms** Dextropropoxyphene; Propoxyphene Napsylate

**Pharmacologic Category** Analgesic, Narcotic

**Use** Management of mild to moderate pain

**Effects on Mental Status** Dizziness, drowsiness, insomnia, and paradoxical excitement are common; may cause nervousness, restlessness, confusion; may rarely cause depression or hallucinations

**Effects on Psychiatric Treatment** Concurrent use with psychotropics may produce additive sedation as well as increase their serum levels; monitor for altered clinical response or preferably, use a different analgesic

**Restrictions** C-IV

**Pregnancy Risk Factor** C (D if used for prolonged periods)

**Contraindications** Hypersensitivity to propoxyphene or any component

**Warnings/Precautions** Administer with caution in patients dependent on opiates, substitution may result in acute opiate withdrawal symptoms, use with caution in patients with severe renal or hepatic dysfunction; when given in excessive doses, either alone or in combination with other CNS depressants or propoxyphene products, propoxyphene is a major cause of drug-related deaths; **do not exceed recommended dosage**; tolerance or drug dependence may result from extended use

**Adverse Reactions**

Percentage unknown: Increased liver enzymes, may increase LFTs; may decrease glucose, urinary 17-OHCS

>10%:

Cardiovascular: Hypotension

Central nervous system: Dizziness, lightheadedness, sedation, paradoxical excitement and insomnia, fatigue, drowsiness

Gastrointestinal: Nausea, vomiting, constipation

Neuromuscular & skeletal: Weakness

1% to 10%:

Central nervous system: Nervousness, headache, restlessness, malaise, confusion

Gastrointestinal: Anorexia, stomach cramps, xerostomia, biliary spasm

Genitourinary: Decreased urination, ureteral spasms

Respiratory: Dyspnea, shortness of breath

<1%: Histamine release, increased intracranial pressure, mental depression hallucinations, paradoxical CNS stimulation, paralytic ileus, psychologic and physical dependence with prolonged use, rash, urticaria

**Overdosage/Toxicology**

Signs and symptoms: CNS, respiratory depression, hypotension, pulmonary edema, seizures

Treatment: Includes support of the patient's airway; establishment of an I.V. line and administration of naloxone 2 mg I.V. (0.01 mg/kg for children) with repeat administration as necessary up to a total of 10 mg; emesis is not indicated as overdose may cause seizures; charcoal is very effective (>95%) at binding propoxyphene

**Drug Interactions** CYP3A3/4 enzyme inhibitor

Decreased effect with charcoal, cigarette smoking

Increased toxicity: CNS depressants may potentiate pharmacologic effects; propoxyphene may inhibit the metabolism and increase the serum concentrations of carbamazepine, phenobarbital, MAO inhibitors, tricyclic antidepressants, and warfarin

**Usual Dosage** Oral:

Children: Doses for children are not well established; doses of the hydrochloride of 2-3 mg/kg/d divided every 6 hours have been used

Adults:

Hydrochloride: 65 mg every 3-4 hours as needed for pain; maximum: 390 mg/day

Napsylate: 100 mg every 4 hours as needed for pain; maximum: 600 mg/day

**Dosing comments in renal impairment:** $Cl_{cr}$ <10 mL/minute: Avoid use

Hemodialysis: Not dialyzable (0% to 5%)

**Dosing adjustment in hepatic impairment:** Reduced doses should be used

**Dietary Considerations**

Alcohol: Additive CNS effects, avoid or limit alcohol; watch for sedation

Food: May decrease rate of absorption, but may slightly increase bioavailability

Glucose may cause hyperglycemia; monitor blood glucose concentrations

**Patient Information** Take as directed; do not take a larger dose or more often than prescribed. Do not use alcohol, other prescription or OTC sedatives, tranquilizers, antihistamines, or pain medications without consulting prescriber. May cause dizziness, drowsiness, or impaired judgment; avoid driving or engaging in tasks requiring alertness until response to drug is known. If you experience vomiting or loss of appetite, frequent mouth care, small frequent meals, chewing gum, or sucking lozenges may help. Increased fluid intake, exercise, fiber in diet may help with constipation (if unresolved consult prescriber). Report unresolved nausea or vomiting, difficulty breathing or shortness of breath, or unusual weakness.

**Dosage Forms**

Capsule, as hydrochloride: 65 mg

Tablet, as napsylate: 100 mg

## Propoxyphene and Acetaminophen

(proe POKS i feen & a seet a MIN oh fen)

**U.S. Brand Names** Darvocet-N®; Darvocet-N® 100; Propacet®; Wygesic®

**Synonyms** Propoxyphene Hydrochloride and Acetaminophen; Propoxyphene Napsylate and Acetaminophen

**Pharmacologic Category** Analgesic, Narcotic

**Use** Management of mild to moderate pain

**Effects on Mental Status** Dizziness, drowsiness, insomnia, and paradoxical excitement are common; may cause nervousness, restlessness, confusion; may rarely cause depression or hallucinations

**Effects on Psychiatric Treatment** Concurrent use with psychotropics may produce additive sedation as well as increase their serum levels; monitor for altered clinical response or preferably, use a different analgesic

**Restrictions** C-IV

**Contraindications** Hypersensitivity to propoxyphene, acetaminophen, or any component; patients with known G-6-PD deficiency

**Warnings/Precautions** When given in excessive doses, either alone or in combination with other CNS depressants, propoxyphene is a major cause of drug-related deaths; do not exceed recommended dosage; give with caution in patients dependent on opiates, substitution may result in acute opiate withdrawal symptoms

**Drug Interactions** Decreased effect with charcoal, cigarette smoking; increased toxicity with cimetidine, CNS depressants; increased toxicity/effect of carbamazepine, phenobarbital, TCAs, MAO inhibitors, benzodiazepines

**Usual Dosage** Adults: Oral:

Darvocet-N®: 1-2 tablets every 4 hours as needed; maximum: 600 mg propoxyphene napsylate/day

Darvocet-N® 100: 1 tablet every 4 hours as needed; maximum: 600 mg propoxyphene napsylate/day

**Patient Information** See individual agents

**Dosage Forms** Tablet:

Darvocet-N®: Propoxyphene napsylate 50 mg and acetaminophen 325 mg

Darvocet-N® 100: Propoxyphene napsylate 100 mg and acetaminophen 650 mg

Genagesic®, Wygesic®: Propoxyphene hydrochloride 65 mg and acetaminophen 650 mg

## Propoxyphene and Aspirin (proe POKS i feen & AS pir in)

**U.S. Brand Names** Bexophene®; Darvon® Compound-65 Pulvules®

**Canadian Brand Names** Darvon-N® With ASA; Novo-Propoxyn Compound (contains caffeine); Darvon-N® Compound (contains caffeine)

**Pharmacologic Category** Analgesic, Narcotic

**Use** Management of postoperative and mild to moderate pain

**Effects on Mental Status** Dizziness, drowsiness, insomnia, and paradoxical excitement are common; may cause nervousness, restlessness, confusion; may rarely cause depression or hallucinations

**Effects on Psychiatric Treatment** Concurrent use with psychotropics may produce additive sedation as well as increase their serum levels; monitor for altered clinical response or preferably, use a different analgesic

**Restrictions** C-IV

**Usual Dosage** Oral:

Children: Not recommended

Adults: 1-2 capsules every 4 hours as needed

**Dosage Forms**

Capsule: Propoxyphene hydrochloride 65 mg and aspirin 389 mg with caffeine 32.4 mg

Tablet (Darvon-N® with A.S.A.): Propoxyphene napsylate 100 mg and aspirin 325 mg

♦ **Propoxyphene Hydrochloride and Acetaminophen** *see* Propoxyphene and Acetaminophen *on page 474*

♦ **Propoxyphene Napsylate** *see* Propoxyphene *on page 474*

♦ **Propoxyphene Napsylate and Acetaminophen** *see* Propoxyphene and Acetaminophen *on page 474*

## Propranolol (proe PRAN oh lole)

**Related Information**

Beta-Blockers Comparison Chart *on page 709*

Clinical Issues in the Use of Anxiolytics and Sedative/Hypnotics *on page 634*

Clozapine-Induced Side Effects *on page 780*

Impulse Control Disorders *on page 622*

Nonbenzodiazepine Anxiolytics and Hypnotics *on page 721*

Special Populations - Children and Adolescents *on page 663*

Special Populations - Mentally Retarded Patients *on page 665*

**Generic Available** Yes

**U.S. Brand Names** Betachron E-R®; Inderal®; Inderal® LA

**Canadian Brand Names** Apo®-Propranolol; Detensol®; Nu-Propranolol

**Synonyms** Propranolol Hydrochloride

**Pharmacologic Category** Antiarrhythmic Agent, Class II; Beta Blocker, Nonselective

**Use** Management of hypertension; angina pectoris; pheochromocytoma; essential tremor; tetralogy of Fallot cyanotic spells; arrhythmias (such as atrial fibrillation and flutter, A-V nodal re-entrant tachycardias, and catecholamine-induced arrhythmias); prevention of myocardial infarction; migraine headache; symptomatic treatment of hypertrophic subaortic stenosis

**Unlabeled uses:** Tremor due to Parkinson's disease; alcohol withdrawal; aggressive behavior; antipsychotic-induced akathisia; esophageal varices bleeding; anxiety; schizophrenia; acute panic; gastric bleeding in portal hypertension

**Effects on Mental Status** Fatigue and malaise are common and often mistaken for depression; may also cause dizziness, confusion, insomnia, or hallucinations

**Effects on Psychiatric Treatment** Low-dose propranolol is considered by many to be the drug of choice for akathisia; concurrent use with psychotropic drugs may produce additive hypotensive effects; monitor blood pressure

**Pregnancy Risk Factor** C

**Pregnancy/Breast-Feeding Implications**

Clinical effects on the fetus: Crosses the placenta; intrauterine growth retardation (IUGR), hypoglycemia, bradycardia, respiratory depression, hyperbilirubinemia, polycythemia, polydactyly reported. IUGR probably related to maternal hypertension. Preterm labor has been reported. Available evidence suggests safe use during pregnancy and breast-feeding. Monitor breast-fed infant for symptoms of beta-blockade.

Breast-feeding/lactation: Crosses into breast milk. American Academy of Pediatrics considers **compatible** with breast-feeding.

**Contraindications** Hypersensitivity to propranolol, beta-blockers or any component; uncompensated congestive heart failure (unless the failure is due to tachyarrhythmias being treated with propranolol), cardiogenic shock, bradycardia or heart block (2nd or 3rd degree), pulmonary edema, severe hyperactive airway disease (asthma or COPD), Raynaud's disease

**Warnings/Precautions** Administer very cautiously to patients with CHF, 1st-degree AV block, Wolff-Parkinson-White syndrome, asthma, diabetes mellitus, hyperthyroidism. Abrupt withdrawal of the drug should be avoided, drug should be discontinued over 1-2 weeks. Do not use in pregnant or nursing women. May potentiate hypoglycemia in a diabetic patient and mask signs and symptoms. Use with caution in patients with myasthenia gravis, hyperlipidemia, or peripheral vascular disease. May cause CNS depression - use caution in patients with a history of psychiatric illness (although controversial, some evidence suggests risk may be higher than with more polar beta-blockers). May potentiate anaphylactic reactions and/or blunt response to epinephrine treatment. Safety and efficacy of I.V. form have not been established in children.

**Adverse Reactions**

Cardiovascular: Bradycardia, congestive heart failure, reduced peripheral circulation, thrombocytopenia, purpura, chest pain, hypotension, impaired myocardial contractility, worsening of A-V conduction disturbance

Central nervous system: Mental depression, lightheadedness, amnesia, emotional lability, confusion, hallucinations, dizziness, insomnia, fatigue, vivid dreams, lethargy, cold extremities

Dermatologic: Rash, alopecia

Endocrine & metabolic: Hypoglycemia, hyperglycemia

Gastrointestinal: Diarrhea, nausea, vomiting, stomach discomfort, constipation

Genitourinary: Impotence

Hematologic: Agranulocytosis

Neuromuscular & skeletal: Weakness

Respiratory: Wheezing, pharyngitis, bronchospasm

**Overdosage/Toxicology**

Signs and symptoms: Severe hypotension, bradycardia, heart failure and bronchospasm, hypoglycemia

Treatment: Sympathomimetics (eg, epinephrine or dopamine), glucagon, or a pacemaker can be used to treat the toxic bradycardia, asystole, and/or hypotension. Initially, fluids may be the best treatment for hypotension.

**Drug Interactions** CYP1A2, 2C18, 2C19, and 2D6 enzyme substrate

Albuterol (and other $beta_2$-agonists): Effects may be blunted by nonspecific beta-blockers

Alpha-blockers (prazosin, terazosin): Concurrent use of beta-blockers may increase risk of orthostasis

Cimetidine increases the plasma concentration of propranolol and its pharmacodynamic effects may be increased

Clonidine: Hypertensive crisis after or during withdrawal of either agent

CYP1A2 inhibitors: Metabolism of propranolol may be decreased; increasing clinical effect or toxicity; inhibitors include cimetidine, ciprofloxacin, fluvoxamine, isoniazid, ritonavir, and zileutin

CYP2C19 inhibitors: Serum levels of some beta-blockers may be increased; inhibitors include cimetidine, felbamate, fluconazole, fluoxetine, fluvoxamine, omeprazole, teniposide, tolbutamide, and troglitazone

CYP2D6 inhibitors: Serum levels and/or toxicity of some beta-blockers may be increased; inhibitors include amiodarone, cimetidine, delavirdine, fluoxetine, paroxetine, propafenone, quinidine, and ritonavir; monitor for increased effect/toxicity

Drugs which slow AV conduction (digoxin): Effects may be additive with beta-blockers

Epinephrine (including local anesthetics with epinephrine): Propranolol may cause hypertension

Flecainide: Pharmacological activity of both agents may be increased when used concurrently

Fluoxetine may inhibit the metabolism of propranolol, resulting in cardiac toxicity

Glucagon: Propranolol may blunt hyperglycemic action

Haloperidol: Hypotensive effects may be potentiated

Hydralazine: The bioavailability propranolol (rapid release) and hydralazine may be enhanced with concurrent dosing

Insulin: Propranolol inhibits recovery and may cause hypertension and bradycardia following insulin-induced hypoglycemia; also masks the tachycardia that usually accompanies insulin-induced hypoglycemia

NSAIDs (ibuprofen, indomethacin, naproxen, piroxicam) may reduce the antihypertensive effects of beta-blockers

Salicylates may reduce the antihypertensive effects of beta-blockers

Sulfonylureas: Beta-blockers may alter response to hypoglycemic agents

Verapamil or diltiazem may have synergistic or additive pharmacological effects when taken concurrently with beta-blockers; avoid concurrent I.V. use of both

**Stability Compatible** in saline, **incompatible** with $HCO_3^-$; protect injection from light; solutions have maximum stability at pH of 3 and decompose rapidly in alkaline pH; propranolol is stable for 24 hours at room temperature in $D_5W$ or NS

**Mechanism of Action** Nonselective beta-adrenergic blocker (class II antiarrhythmic); competitively blocks response to $beta_1$- and $beta_2$-adrenergic stimulation which results in decreases in heart rate, myocardial contractility, blood pressure, and myocardial oxygen demand

(Continued)

## Propranolol *(Continued)*

**Pharmacodynamics/kinetics**

Onset of beta-blockade: Oral: Within 1-2 hours
Duration: ~6 hours
Distribution: $V_d$: 3.9 L/kg in adults; crosses the placenta; small amounts appear in breast milk
Protein binding:
Newborns: 68%
Adults: 93%
Metabolism: Extensive first-pass effect; metabolized in the liver to active and inactive compounds
Bioavailability: 30% to 40%; oral bioavailability may be increased in Down syndrome children
Half-life:
Neonates and Infants: Possible increased half-life
Children: 3.9-6.4 hours
Adults: 4-6 hours
Elimination: Primarily in urine (96% to 99%)

**Usual Dosage**

Tachyarrhythmias:
Oral:
Children: Initial: 0.5-1 mg/kg/day in divided doses every 6-8 hours; titrate dosage upward every 3-7 days; usual dose: 2-4 mg/kg/day; higher doses may be needed; do not exceed 16 mg/kg/day or 60 mg/day
Adults: 10-30 mg/dose every 6-8 hours
Elderly: Initial: 10 mg twice daily; increase dosage every 3-7 days; usual dosage range: 10-320 mg given in 2 divided doses
I.V.:
Children: 0.01-0.1 mg/kg slow IVP over 10 minutes; maximum dose: 1 mg
Adults: 1 mg/dose slow IVP; repeat every 5 minutes up to a total of 5 mg
Hypertension: Oral:
Children: Initial: 0.5-1 mg/kg/day in divided doses every 6-12 hours; increase gradually every 3-7 days; maximum: 2 mg/kg/24 hours
Adults: Initial: 40 mg twice daily; increase dosage every 3-7 days; usual dose: ≤320 mg divided in 2-3 doses/day; maximum daily dose: 640 mg
Migraine headache prophylaxis: Oral:
Children: 0.6-1.5 mg/kg/day **or**
≤35 kg: 10-20 mg 3 times/day
>35 kg: 20-40 mg 3 times/day
Adults: Initial: 80 mg/day divided every 6-8 hours; increase by 20-40 mg/dose every 3-4 weeks to a maximum of 160-240 mg/day given in divided doses every 6-8 hours; if satisfactory response not achieved within 6 weeks of starting therapy, drug should be withdrawn gradually over several weeks
Tetralogy spells: Children:
Oral: 1-2 mg/kg/day every 6 hours as needed, may increase by 1 mg/kg/day to a maximum of 5 mg/kg/day, or if refractory may increase slowly to a maximum of 10-15 mg/kg/day
I.V.: 0.15-0.25 mg/kg/dose slow IVP; may repeat in 15 minutes
Thyrotoxicosis:
Adolescents and Adults: Oral: 10-40 mg/dose every 6 hours
Adults: I.V.: 1-3 mg/dose slow IVP as a single dose
Adults: Oral:
Angina: 80-320 mg/day in doses divided 2-4 times/day
Pheochromocytoma: 30-60 mg/day in divided doses
Myocardial infarction prophylaxis: 180-240 mg/day in 3-4 divided doses
Hypertrophic subaortic stenosis: 20-40 mg 3-4 times/day
Essential tremor: 40 mg twice daily initially; maintenance doses: usually 120-320 mg/day
Akathisia: 30-120 mg/day in 2-3 divided doses

**Dosing adjustment in renal impairment:**
$Cl_{cr}$ 31-40 mL/minute: Administer every 24-36 hours or administer 50% of normal dose
$Cl_{cr}$ 10-30 mL/minute: Administer every 24-48 hours or administer 50% of normal dose
$Cl_{cr}$ <10 mL/minute: Administer every 40-60 hours or administer 25% of normal dose
Hemodialysis: Not dialyzable (0% to 5%); supplemental dose is not necessary
Peritoneal dialysis: Supplemental dose is not necessary

**Dosing adjustment/comments in hepatic disease:** Marked slowing of heart rate may occur in cirrhosis with conventional doses; low initial dose and regular heart rate monitoring

**Administration** I.V. administration should not exceed 1 mg/minute; I.V. dose much smaller than oral dose

**Monitoring Parameters** Blood pressure, EKG, heart rate, CNS and cardiac effects

**Reference Range** Therapeutic: 50-100 ng/mL (SI: 190-390 nmol/L) at end of dose interval

**Test Interactions** ↑ thyroxine (S)

**Patient Information** Do not discontinue abruptly; notify physician if CHF symptoms become worse; take at the same time each day; may mask diabetes symptoms; sweating will continue

**Nursing Implications** Patient's therapeutic response may be evaluated by looking at blood pressure, apical and radial pulses, fluid I & O, daily weight, respirations, and circulation in extremities before and during therapy

**Additional Information** Not significantly removed by hemodialysis; not indicated for hypertensive emergencies; do not abruptly discontinue therapy, taper dosage gradually over 2 weeks

**Dosage Forms**

Capsule, as hydrochloride, sustained action: 60 mg, 80 mg, 120 mg, 160 mg
Injection, as hydrochloride: 1 mg/mL (1 mL)
Solution, oral, as hydrochloride (strawberry-mint flavor): 4 mg/mL (5 mL, 500 mL); 8 mg/mL (5 mL, 500 mL)
Solution, oral, concentrate, as hydrochloride: 80 mg/mL (30 mL)
Tablet, as hydrochloride: 10 mg, 20 mg, 40 mg, 60 mg, 80 mg, 90 mg

## Propranolol and Hydrochlorothiazide

(proe PRAN oh lole & hye droe klor oh THYE a zide)

**U.S. Brand Names** Inderide®

**Pharmacologic Category** Antihypertensive Agent, Combination

**Use** Management of hypertension

**Effects on Mental Status** Propranolol may cause fatigue and malaise which are commonly mistaken for depression; may also cause dizziness, confusion, insomnia, or hallucinations

**Effects on Psychiatric Treatment** Concurrent use with psychotropic drugs may produce additive hypotensive effects; monitor blood pressure; may decrease lithium clearance resulting in an increase in serum lithium levels and potential lithium toxicity; monitor serum lithium levels

**Usual Dosage** Dose is individualized

**Dosage Forms**

Capsule, long-acting (Inderide® LA):
80/50 Propranolol hydrochloride 80 mg and hydrochlorothiazide 50 mg
120/50 Propranolol hydrochloride 120 mg and hydrochlorothiazide 50 mg
160/50 Propranolol hydrochloride 160 mg and hydrochlorothiazide 50 mg
Tablet (Inderide®):
40/25 Propranolol hydrochloride 40 mg and hydrochlorothiazide 25 mg
80/25 Propranolol hydrochloride 80 mg and hydrochlorothiazide 25 mg


♦ **Propranolol Hydrochloride** *see* Propranolol *on page 475*

♦ **Propulsid®** *see* Cisapride *on page 124*

♦ **2-Propylpentanoic Acid** *see* Valproic Acid and Derivatives *on page 578*


## Propylthiouracil (proe pil thye oh YOOR a sil)

**Canadian Brand Names** Propyl-Thyracil®

**Synonyms** PTU

**Pharmacologic Category** Antithyroid Agent

**Use** Palliative treatment of hyperthyroidism as an adjunct to ameliorate hyperthyroidism in preparation for surgical treatment or radioactive iodine therapy and in the management of thyrotoxic crisis. The use of antithyroid thioamides is as effective in elderly as they are in younger adults; however, the expense, potential adverse effects, and inconvenience (compliance, monitoring) make them undesirable. The use of radioiodine, due to ease of administration and less concern for long-term side effects and reproduction problems, makes it a more appropriate therapy.

**Effects on Mental Status** May cause dizziness or drowsiness

**Effects on Psychiatric Treatment** Leukopenia is common; avoid clozapine and carbamazepine

**Pregnancy Risk Factor** D

**Contraindications** Hypersensitivity to propylthiouracil or any component

**Warnings/Precautions** Use with caution in patients >40 years of age because PTU may cause hypoprothrombinemia and bleeding, use with extreme caution in patients receiving other drugs known to cause agranulocytosis; may cause agranulocytosis, thyroid hyperplasia, thyroid carcinoma (usage >1 year); breast-feeding (enters breast milk)

**Adverse Reactions**

>10%:
Central nervous system: Fever
Dermatologic: Skin rash
Hematologic: Leukopenia
1% to 10%:
Central nervous system: Dizziness
Gastrointestinal: Nausea, vomiting, loss of taste perception, stomach pain
Hematologic: Agranulocytosis
Miscellaneous: SLE-like syndrome

<1%: Alopecia, aplastic anemia, arthralgia, bleeding, cholestatic jaundice, constipation, cutaneous vasculitis, drowsiness, drug fever, edema, exfoliative dermatitis, goiter, headache, hepatitis, nephritis, neuritis, paresthesia, pruritus, swollen salivary glands, thrombocytopenia, urticaria, vertigo, weight gain

**Overdosage/Toxicology**

Signs and symptoms: Nausea, vomiting, epigastric pain, headache, fever, arthralgia, pruritus, edema, pancytopenia, epigastric distress, headache, fever, CNS stimulation or depression

Treatment: Supportive; monitor bone marrow response, forced diuresis, peritoneal and hemodialysis, as well as charcoal hemoperfusion

**Drug Interactions** Increased effect: Increases anticoagulant activity

**Usual Dosage** Oral: Administer in 3 equally divided doses at approximately 8-hour intervals. Adjust dosage to maintain $T_3$, $T_4$, and TSH levels in normal range; elevated $T_3$ may be sole indicator of inadequate treatment. Elevated TSH indicates excessive antithyroid treatment.

Children: Initial: 5-7 mg/kg/day **or** 150-200 mg/m$^2$/day in divided doses every 8 hours

**or**

6-10 years: 50-150 mg/day

>10 years: 150-300 mg/day

Maintenance: Determined by patient response **or** $^1/_3$ to $^2/_3$ of the initial dose in divided doses every 8-12 hours. This usually begins after 2 months on an effective initial dose.

Adults: Initial: 300 mg/day in divided doses every 8 hours. In patients with severe hyperthyroidism, very large goiters, or both, the initial dosage is usually 450 mg/day; an occasional patient will require 600-900 mg/day; maintenance: 100-150 mg/day in divided doses every 8-12 hours

Elderly: Use lower dose recommendations; Initial: 150-300 mg/day

Withdrawal of therapy: Therapy should be withdrawn gradually with evaluation of the patient every 4-6 weeks for the first 3 months then every 3 months for the first year after discontinuation of therapy to detect any reoccurrence of a hyperthyroid state.

**Dosing adjustment in renal impairment:** Adjustment is not necessary

**Patient Information** Take as directed, at the same time each day around-the-clock; do not miss doses or make up missed doses. This drug will need to be taken for an extended period of time to achieve appropriate results. You may experience nausea or vomiting (small frequent meals may help), dizziness or drowsiness (use caution when driving or engaging in tasks that require alertness until response to drug is known). Report rash, fever, unusual bleeding or bruising, unresolved headache, yellowing of eyes or skin, or changes in color of urine or feces, unresolved malaise.

**Dosage Forms** Tablet: 50 mg


- **2-Propylvaleric Acid** *see* Valproic Acid and Derivatives *on page 578*
- **Prorex®** *see* Promethazine *on page 470*
- **Proscar®** *see* Finasteride *on page 226*
- **ProSom™** *see* Estazolam *on page 202*
- **Prostaglandin $E_2$** *see* Dinoprostone *on page 173*
- **Prostaglandin $F_2$ Alpha** *see* Dinoprost Tromethamine *on page 174*
- **ProStep® Patch** *see* Nicotine *on page 392*
- **Prostigmin®** *see* Neostigmine *on page 389*
- **Prostin $E_2$® Vaginal Suppository** *see* Dinoprostone *on page 173*
- **Prostin $F_2$ Alpha®** *see* Dinoprost Tromethamine *on page 174*


## Protamine Sulfate (PROE ta meen SUL fate)

**Pharmacologic Category** Antidote

**Use** Treatment of heparin overdosage; neutralize heparin during surgery or dialysis procedures

**Effects on Mental Status** May cause drowsiness

**Effects on Psychiatric Treatment** None reported

**Usual Dosage** Protamine dosage is determined by the dosage of heparin; 1 mg of protamine neutralizes 90 USP units of heparin (lung) and 115 USP units of heparin (intestinal); maximum dose: 50 mg

In the situation of heparin overdosage, since blood heparin concentrations decrease rapidly **after** administration, adjust the protamine dosage depending upon the duration of time since heparin administration as follows:

| Time Elapsed | Dose of Protamine (mg) to Neutralize 100 units of Heparin |
|---|---|
| Immediate | 1-1.5 |
| 30-60 min | 0.5-0.75 |
| >2 h | 0.25-0.375 |

If heparin administered by deep S.C. injection, use 1-1.5 mg protamine per 100 units heparin; this may be done by a portion of the dose (eg, 25-50 mg) given slowly I.V. followed by the remaining portion as a continuous infusion over 8-16 hours (the expected absorption time of the S.C. heparin dose)

**Dosage Forms** Injection: 10 mg/mL (5 mL, 10 mL, 25 mL)


- **Protease Inhibitors** *see page 724*
- **Prothazine-DC®** *see* Promethazine and Codeine *on page 471*
- **Protilase®** *see* Pancrelipase *on page 418*


## Protirelin (proe TYE re lin)

**U.S. Brand Names** Relefact® TRH Injection; Thypinone® Injection

**Canadian Brand Names** Combantrin®

**Pharmacologic Category** Diagnostic Agent, Thyroid Function

**Use** Adjunct in the diagnostic assessment of thyroid function, and an adjunct to other diagnostic procedures in patients with pituitary or hypothalamic dysfunction; also causes release of prolactin from the pituitary and is used to detect defective control of prolactin secretion

**Effects on Mental Status** Dizziness is common; may cause anxiety

**Effects on Psychiatric Treatment** None reported

**Usual Dosage** I.V.:

Infants and Children <6 years: Experience limited, but doses of 7 mcg/kg have been administered

Children 6-16 years: 7 mcg/kg to a maximum dose of 500 mcg

Adults: 500 mcg (range 200-500 mcg)

**Dosage Forms** Injection: 500 mcg/mL (1 mL)


- **Protonix®** *see* Pantoprazole *on page 419*
- **Protopam®** *see* Pralidoxime *on page 456*
- **Protostat® Oral** *see* Metronidazole *on page 362*


## Protriptyline (proe TRIP ti leen)

**Related Information**


Antidepressant Agents Comparison Chart *on page 704*

Clinical Issues in the Use of Antidepressants *on page 627*

Discontinuation of Psychotropic Drugs - Withdrawal Symptoms and Recommendations *on page 798*

Federal OBRA Regulations Recommended Maximum Doses *on page 756*

Mood Disorders *on page 600*

Patient Information - Antidepressants (TCAs) *on page 640*


**Generic Available** No

**U.S. Brand Names** Vivactil®

**Canadian Brand Names** Triptil®

**Synonyms** Protriptyline Hydrochloride

**Pharmacologic Category** Antidepressant, Tricyclic (Secondary Amine)

**Use** Treatment of depression

**Pregnancy Risk Factor** C

**Contraindications** Hypersensitivity to protriptyline (cross-reactivity to other cyclic antidepressants may occur); use of monoamine oxidase inhibitors within 14 days; use of cisapride; use in a patient during the acute recovery phase of MI

**Warnings/Precautions** May cause sedation, resulting in impaired performance of tasks requiring alertness (ie, operating machinery or driving). Sedative effects may be additive with other CNS depressants and/or ethanol. The degree of sedation is low relative to other antidepressants. May worsen psychosis in some patients or precipitate a shift to mania or hypomania in patients with bipolar disease. In addition, may aggravate aggressive behavior. May increase the risks associated with electroconvulsive therapy. This agent should be discontinued, when possible, prior to elective surgery. Therapy should not be abruptly discontinued in patients receiving high doses for prolonged periods. May alter glucose regulation - use with caution in patients with diabetes.

May cause orthostatic hypotension (risk is moderate relative to other antidepressants) - use with caution in patients at risk of hypotension or in patients where transient hypotensive episodes would be poorly tolerated (cardiovascular disease or cerebrovascular disease). The degree of anticholinergic blockade produced by this agent is moderate relative to other cyclic antidepressants, however, caution should still be used in patients with urinary retention, benign prostatic hypertrophy, narrow-angle glaucoma, xerostomia, visual problems, constipation, or history of bowel obstruction.

Use caution in patients with depression, particularly if suicidal risk may be present. Use with caution in patients with a history of cardiovascular disease (including previous MI, stroke, tachycardia, or conduction abnormalities). The risk conduction abnormalities with this agent is moderate-high relative to other antidepressants. Use caution in patients with a previous seizure disorder or condition predisposing to seizures such as brain damage, alcoholism, or concurrent therapy with other drugs which lower the seizure threshold. Use with caution in hyperthyroid patients or those receiving thyroid supplementation. Use with caution in patients with hepatic or renal dysfunction and in elderly patients.

(Continued)

## Protriptyline *(Continued)*

**Adverse Reactions**

Cardiovascular: Arrhythmias, hypotension, myocardial infarction, stroke, heart block, hypertension, tachycardia, palpitations

Central nervous system: Dizziness, drowsiness, headache, confusion, delirium, hallucinations, restlessness, insomnia, nightmares, fatigue, delusions, anxiety, agitation, hypomania, exacerbation of psychosis, panic, seizures, incoordination, ataxia, EPS

Dermatologic: Alopecia, photosensitivity, rash, petechiae, urticaria, itching

Endocrine & metabolic: Breast enlargement, galactorrhea, SIADH, gynecomastia, increased or decreased libido

Gastrointestinal: Xerostomia, constipation, unpleasant taste, weight gain, increased appetite, nausea, diarrhea, heartburn, vomiting, anorexia, weight loss, trouble with gums, decreased lower esophageal sphincter tone may cause GE reflux

Genitourinary: Difficult urination, impotence, testicular edema

Hematologic: Agranulocytosis, leukopenia, eosinophilia, thrombocytopenia, purpura

Hepatic: Cholestatic jaundice, increased liver enzymes

Neuromuscular & skeletal: Fine muscle tremors, weakness, tremor, numbness, tingling

Ocular: Blurred vision, eye pain, increased intraocular pressure

Otic: Tinnitus

Miscellaneous: Diaphoresis (excessive), allergic reactions

**Overdosage/Toxicology**

Signs and symptoms: Confusion, hallucinations, urinary retention, hypotension, tachycardia, seizures, hyperthermia

Treatment:

Following initiation of essential overdose management, toxic symptoms should be treated

Ventricular arrhythmias often respond to systemic alkalinization (sodium bicarbonate 0.5-2 mEq/kg I.V.). Arrhythmias unresponsive to this therapy may respond to lidocaine 1 mg/kg I.V. followed by a titrated infusion. Physostigmine (1-2 mg I.V. slowly for adults or 0.5 mg I.V. slowly for children) may be indicated in reversing cardiac arrhythmias that are life-threatening.

Seizures usually respond to diazepam I.V. boluses (5-10 mg for adults up to 30 mg or 0.25-0.4 mg/kg/dose for children up to 10 mg/dose). If seizures are unresponsive or recur, phenytoin or phenobarbital may be required.

**Drug Interactions** Metabolism by CYP450 isoenzymes is likely, but not fully characterized. Use caution when combined with inhibitors and inducers of this enzyme system.

Altretamine: Concurrent use may cause orthostatic hypertension

Amphetamines: TCAs may enhance the effect of amphetamines; monitor for adverse CV effects

Anticholinergics: Combined use with TCAs may produce additive anticholinergic effects

Antihypertensives: Cyclic antidepressants may inhibit the antihypertensive response to bethanidine, clonidine, debrisoquin, guanadrel, guanethidine, guanabenz, guanfacine; monitor BP; consider alternate antihypertensive agent

Beta-agonists: When combined with TCAs may predispose patients to cardiac arrhythmias

Bupropion: May increase the levels of tricyclic antidepressants; based on limited information; monitor response

Carbamazepine: Tricyclic antidepressants may increase carbamazepine levels; monitor

Cholestyramine and colestipol: May bind TCAs and reduce their absorption; monitor for altered response

Clonidine: Abrupt discontinuation of clonidine may cause hypertensive crisis, cyclic antidepressants may enhance the response

CNS depressants: Sedative effects may be additive with TCAs; monitor for increased effect; includes benzodiazepines, barbiturates, antipsychotics, ethanol, and other sedative medications

Epinephrine (and other direct alpha-agonists): The pressor response to I.V. epinephrine, norepinephrine, and phenylephrine may be enhanced in patients receiving TCAs; this combination is best avoided

Fenfluramine: May increase tricyclic antidepressant levels/effects

Hypoglycemic agents (including insulin): TCAs may enhance the hypoglycemic effects of tolazamide, chlorpropamide, or insulin; monitor for changes in blood glucose levels; reported with chlorpropamide, tolazamide, and insulin

Levodopa: tricyclic antidepressants may decrease the absorption (bioavailability) of levodopa; rare hypertensive episodes have also been attributed to this combination

Linezolid: Hyperpyrexia, hypertension, tachycardia, confusion, seizures, and **deaths have been reported** with agents which inhibit MAO (serotonin syndrome); this combination should be avoided

Lithium: Concurrent use with a TCA may increase the risk for neurotoxicity

MAO inhibitors: Hyperpyrexia, hypertension, tachycardia, confusion, seizures, and **deaths have been reported** (serotonin syndrome); this combination should be avoided

Methylphenidate: Metabolism of tricyclic antidepressants may be decreased

Phenothiazines: Serum concentrations of some TCAs may be increased; in addition, TCAs may increase concentration of phenothiazines; monitor for altered clinical response

QTc prolonging agents: Concurrent use of tricyclic agents with other drugs which may prolong QTc interval may increase the risk of potentially fatal arrhythmias; includes type Ia and type III antiarrhythmics agents, selected quinolones (sparfloxacin, gatifloxacin, moxifloxacin, grepafloxacin), cisapride, and other agents

Sucralfate: Absorption of tricyclic antidepressants may be reduced with coadministration

Sympathomimetics, indirect-acting: Tricyclic antidepressants may result in a decreased sensitivity to indirect-acting sympathomimetics; includes dopamine and ephedrine; also see interaction with epinephrine (and direct-acting sympathomimetics)

Valproic acid: May increase serum concentrations/adverse effects of some tricyclic antidepressants

Warfarin (and other oral anticoagulants): Tricyclic antidepressants may increase the anticoagulant effect in patients stabilized on warfarin; monitor INR

**Mechanism of Action** Increases the synaptic concentration of serotonin and/or norepinephrine in the central nervous system by inhibition of their reuptake by the presynaptic neuronal membrane

**Pharmacodynamics/kinetics**

Distribution: Crosses the placenta

Protein binding: 92%

Metabolism: Undergoes first-pass metabolism (10% to 25%); extensively metabolized in the liver by N-oxidation, hydroxylation and glucuronidation

Half-life: 54-92 hours, averaging 74 hours

Time to peak serum concentration: Oral: Within 24-30 hours

Elimination: In urine

**Usual Dosage** Oral:

Adolescents: 15-20 mg/day

Adults: 15-60 mg in 3-4 divided doses

Elderly: 15-20 mg/day

**Administration** Make any dosage increase in the morning dose

**Monitoring Parameters** Monitor for cardiac abnormalities in elderly patients receiving doses >20 mg

**Reference Range** Therapeutic: 70-250 ng/mL (SI: 266-950 nmol/L); Toxic: >500 ng/mL (SI: >1900 nmol/L)

**Test Interactions** ↑ glucose

**Patient Information** Avoid unnecessary exposure to sunlight; do not discontinue abruptly; take dose in morning to avoid insomnia

**Nursing Implications** Offer patient sugarless hard candy or gum for dry mouth

**Dosage Forms** Tablet, as hydrochloride: 5 mg, 10 mg


- **Protriptyline Hydrochloride** *see* Protriptyline *on page 477*
- **Protropin® Injection** *see* Human Growth Hormone *on page 269*
- **Proventil®** *see* Albuterol *on page 22*
- **Proventil® HFA** *see* Albuterol *on page 22*
- **Provera® Oral** *see* Medroxyprogesterone *on page 336*
- **Provigil®** *see* Modafinil *on page 370*
- **Proxigel® Oral [OTC]** *see* Carbamide Peroxide *on page 92*
- **Prozac®** *see* Fluoxetine *on page 232*
- **Prymaccone** *see* Primaquine *on page 461*
- **Pseudo-Car® DM** *see* Carbinoxamine, Pseudoephedrine, and Dextromethorphan *on page 92*


## Pseudoephedrine (soo doe e FED rin)

**Related Information**

Pharmacotherapy of Urinary Incontinence *on page 758*

**U.S. Brand Names** Actifed® Allergy Tablet (Day) [OTC]; Afrin® Tablet [OTC]; Cenafed® [OTC]; Children's Silfedrine® [OTC]; Decofed® Syrup [OTC]; Drixoral® Non-Drowsy [OTC]; Efidac/24® [OTC]; Pedia Care® Oral; Sudafed® [OTC]; Sudafed® 12 Hour [OTC]; Triaminic® AM Decongestant Formula [OTC]

**Canadian Brand Names** Balminil® Decongestant; Eltor®; PMS-Pseudoephedrine; Robidrine®

**Synonyms** *d*-Isoephedrine Hydrochloride; Pseudoephedrine Sulfate

**Pharmacologic Category** Alpha/Beta Agonist

**Use** Temporary symptomatic relief of nasal congestion due to common cold, upper respiratory allergies, and sinusitis; also promotes nasal or sinus drainage

**Effects on Mental Status** Dizziness, drowsiness, nervousness, and insomnia are common; may rarely cause hallucinations

**Effects on Psychiatric Treatment** Contraindicated with MAOIs

**Pregnancy Risk Factor** C

**Contraindications** Hypersensitivity to pseudoephedrine or any component; MAO inhibitor therapy

**Warnings/Precautions** Use with caution in patients >60 years of age; administer with caution to patients with hypertension, hyperthyroidism, diabetes mellitus, cardiovascular disease, ischemic heart disease, increased intraocular pressure, or prostatic hypertrophy. Elderly patients are more likely to experience adverse reactions to sympathomimetics. Overdosage may cause hallucinations, seizures, CNS depression, and death.

**Adverse Reactions**

>10%:

Cardiovascular: Tachycardia, palpitations, arrhythmias

Central nervous system: Nervousness, transient stimulation, insomnia, excitability, dizziness, drowsiness

Neuromuscular & skeletal: Tremor

1% to 10%:

Central nervous system: Headache

Neuromuscular & skeletal: Weakness

Miscellaneous: Diaphoresis

<1%: Convulsions, dyspnea, dysuria, hallucinations, nausea, shortness of breath, vomiting

**Overdosage/Toxicology**

Signs and symptoms: Seizures, nausea, vomiting, cardiac arrhythmias, hypertension, agitation

Treatment: There is no specific antidote for pseudoephedrine intoxication; the bulk treatment is supportive. Hyperactivity and agitation usually respond to reduced sensory input; however, with extreme agitation, haloperidol (2-5 mg I.M. for adults) may be required. Hyperthermia is best treated with external cooling measures; or when severe or unresponsive, muscle paralysis with pancuronium may be needed. Hypertension is usually transient and generally does not require treatment unless severe. For diastolic blood pressures >110 mm Hg, a nitroprusside infusion should be initiated. Seizures usually respond to diazepam I.V. and/or phenytoin maintenance regimens.

**Drug Interactions**

Decreased effect of methyldopa, reserpine

Increased toxicity: MAO inhibitors may increase blood pressure effects of pseudoephedrine; propranolol, sympathomimetic agents may increase toxicity

**Usual Dosage** Oral:

Children:

<2 years: 4 mg/kg/day in divided doses every 6 hours

2-5 years: 15 mg every 6 hours; maximum: 60 mg/24 hours

6-12 years: 30 mg every 6 hours; maximum: 120 mg/24 hours

Adults: 30-60 mg every 4-6 hours, sustained release: 120 mg every 12 hours; maximum: 240 mg/24 hours

**Dosing adjustment in renal impairment:** Reduce dose

**Patient Information** Take only as prescribed; do not exceed prescribed dose or frequency. Do not chew or crush timed release capsule. Maintain adequate hydration (2-3 L/day of fluids unless instructed to restrict fluid intake). You may experience nervousness, insomnia, dizziness, or drowsiness (use caution when driving or engaging in tasks requiring alertness until response to drug is known). Report persistent CNS changes (dizziness, sedation, tremor, agitation, or convulsions); difficulty breathing; chest pain, palpitations, or rapid heartbeat; muscle tremor; or lack of improvement or worsening or condition.

**Nursing Implications** Do not crush extended release drug product; elderly patients should be counseled about the proper use of over-the-counter cough and cold preparations

**Dosage Forms**

Capsule: 60 mg

Capsule, timed release, as hydrochloride: 120 mg

Drops, oral, as hydrochloride: 7.5 mg/0.8 mL (15 mL)

Liquid, as hydrochloride: 15 mg/5 mL (120 mL); 30 mg/5 mL (120 mL, 240 mL, 473 mL)

Syrup, as hydrochloride: 15 mg/5 mL (118 mL)

Tablet, as hydrochloride: 30 mg, 60 mg

Tablet:

Timed release, as hydrochloride: 120 mg

Extended release, as sulfate: 120 mg, 240 mg

## Pseudoephedrine and Dextromethorphan

(soo doe e FED rin & deks troe meth OR fan)

**U.S. Brand Names** Drixoral® Cough & Congestion Liquid Caps [OTC]; Vicks® 44D Cough & Head Congestion; Vicks® 44 Non-Drowsy Cold & Cough Liqui-Caps [OTC]

**Pharmacologic Category** Antitussive/Decongestant

**Use** Temporary symptomatic relief of nasal congestion due to common cold, upper respiratory allergies, and sinusitis; also promotes nasal or sinus drainage; symptomatic relief of coughs caused by minor viral upper respiratory tract infections or inhaled irritants; most effective for a chronic nonproductive cough

**Effects on Mental Status** Dizziness, drowsiness, nervousness, and insomnia are common; may rarely cause hallucinations

**Effects on Psychiatric Treatment** Contraindicated with MAOIs

**Usual Dosage** Oral: Adults: One capsule or 5-10 mL every 6 hours

**Dosage Forms**

Capsule: Pseudoephedrine hydrochloride 60 mg and dextromethorphan hydrobromide 30 mg

Liquid: Pseudoephedrine hydrochloride 20 mg and dextromethorphan hydrobromide 10 mg per 5 mL

## Pseudoephedrine and Ibuprofen

(soo doe e FED rin & eye byoo PROE fen)

**U.S. Brand Names** Advil® Cold & Sinus Caplets [OTC]; Dimetapp® Sinus Caplets [OTC]; Dristan® Sinus Caplets [OTC]; Motrin® IB Sinus [OTC]; Sine-Aid® IB [OTC]

**Pharmacologic Category** Decongestant/Analgesic

**Use** Temporary symptomatic relief of nasal congestion due to common cold, upper respiratory allergies, and sinusitis; also promotes nasal or sinus drainage; sinus headaches and pains

**Effects on Mental Status** Dizziness, drowsiness, nervousness, and insomnia are common; may rarely cause hallucinations, insomnia, confusion, or depression

**Effects on Psychiatric Treatment** Contraindicated with MAOIs; may rarely cause agranulocytosis; use caution with clozapine and carbamazepine; may decrease lithium clearance resulting in an increase in serum lithium levels and potential lithium toxicity; monitor serum lithium levels

**Usual Dosage** Oral: Adults: 1-2 caplets every 4-6 hours

**Dosage Forms** Caplet: Pseudoephedrine hydrochloride 30 mg and ibuprofen 200 mg


♦ **Pseudoephedrine Sulfate** *see* Pseudoephedrine *on page 478*

♦ **Pseudo-Gest Plus® Tablet [OTC]** *see* Chlorpheniramine and Pseudoephedrine *on page 114*

♦ **Psorcon™** *see* Diflorasone *on page 168*

♦ **Psychiatric Assessment - General Patient** *see page 598*

♦ **Psychiatric Assessment - Rating Scales** *see page 598*

♦ **Psychiatric Emergencies - Acute Extrapyramidal Syndromes** *see page 660*

♦ **Psychiatric Emergencies - Catatonia** *see page 660*

♦ **Psychiatric Emergencies - Neuroleptic Malignant Syndrome** *see page 660*

♦ **Psychiatric Emergencies - Overdosage** *see page 658*

♦ **Psychiatric Emergencies - Violence** *see page 659*


## Psyllium (SIL i yum)

**Related Information**

Natural Products, Herbals, and Dietary Supplements *on page 742*

Perspectives on the Safety of Herbal Medicines *on page 736*

**U.S. Brand Names** Effer-Syllium® [OTC]; Fiberall® Powder [OTC]; Fiberall® Wafer [OTC]; Hydrocil® [OTC]; Konsyl® [OTC]; Konsyl-D® [OTC]; Metamucil® [OTC]; Metamucil® Instant Mix [OTC]; Modane® Bulk [OTC]; Perdiem® Plain [OTC]; Reguloid® [OTC]; Serutan® [OTC]; Syllact® [OTC]; V-Lax® [OTC]

**Canadian Brand Names** Fibrepur®; Novo-Mucilax; Prodiem® Plain

**Synonyms** Plantago Seed; Plantain Seed; Psyllium Hydrophilic Mucilloid

**Pharmacologic Category** Laxative, Bulk-Producing

**Use** Treatment of chronic atonic or spastic constipation and in constipation associated with rectal disorders; management of irritable bowel syndrome

**Effects on Mental Status** None reported

**Effects on Psychiatric Treatment** None reported

**Pregnancy Risk Factor** B

**Contraindications** Fecal impaction, GI obstruction, hypersensitivity to psyllium or any component

**Warnings/Precautions** May contain aspartame which is metabolized in the GI tract to phenylalanine which is contraindicated in individuals with phenylketonuria; use with caution in patients with esophageal strictures, ulcers, stenosis, or intestinal adhesions; elderly may have insufficient fluid intake which may predispose them to fecal impaction and bowel obstruction.

**Adverse Reactions** 1% to 10%:

Gastrointestinal: Esophageal or bowel obstruction, diarrhea, constipation, abdominal cramps

Respiratory: Bronchospasm

Miscellaneous: Anaphylaxis upon inhalation in susceptible individuals, rhinoconjunctivitis

**Overdosage/Toxicology** Signs and symptoms: Abdominal pain, diarrhea, constipation

**Drug Interactions** Decreased effect of warfarin, digitalis, potassium-sparing diuretics, salicylates, tetracyclines, nitrofurantoin

**Usual Dosage** Oral (administer at least 3 hours before or after drugs):

Children 6-11 years: (Approximately ½ adult dosage) ½ to 1 rounded teaspoonful in 4 oz glass of liquid 1-3 times/day

(Continued)

## Psyllium *(Continued)*

Adults: 1-2 rounded teaspoonfuls or 1-2 packets or 1-2 wafers in 8 oz glass of liquid 1-3 times/day

**Patient Information** Mix in large (8 oz or more) glass of water or juice and drink immediately. Mix carefully; do not inhale powder. Report unresolved or persistent constipation, watery diarrhea, or respiratory difficulty.

**Nursing Implications** Inhalation of psyllium dust may cause sensitivity to psyllium (runny nose, watery eyes, wheezing)

**Dosage Forms**

Granules: 4.03 g per rounded teaspoon (100 g, 250 g); 2.5 g per rounded teaspoon

Powder: Psyllium 50% and dextrose 50% (6.5 g, 325 g, 420 g, 480 g, 500 g)

Powder:

Effervescent: 3 g/dose (270 g, 480 g); 3.4 g/dose (single-dose packets)

Psyllium hydrophilic: 3.4 g per rounded teaspoon (210 g, 300 g, 420 g, 630 g)

Squares, chewable: 1.7 g, 3.4 g

Wafers: 3.4 g


♦ **Psyllium Hydrophilic Mucilloid** *see* Psyllium *on page 479*

♦ **Pteroylglutamic Acid** *see* Folic Acid *on page 239*

♦ ***P. trifolius* L.** *see* Ginseng *on page 249*

♦ **PTU** *see* Propylthiouracil *on page 476*

♦ **Pulmicort® Turbuhaler®** *see* Budesonide *on page 75*

♦ **Pulmozyme®** *see* Dornase Alfa *on page 182*

♦ **Puralube® Tears Solution [OTC]** *see* Artificial Tears *on page 48*

♦ **Purinethol®** *see* Mercaptopurine *on page 343*

♦ **Purple Coneflower** *see* Echinacea *on page 189*

♦ **P-V-Tussin®** *see* Hydrocodone, Phenylephrine, Pyrilamine, Phenindamine, Chlorpheniramine, and Ammonium Chloride *on page 273*

♦ **$P_xE_x$® Ophthalmic** *see* Pilocarpine and Epinephrine *on page 445*


## Pyrantel Pamoate (pi RAN tel PAM oh ate)

**U.S. Brand Names** Antiminth® [OTC]; Pin-Rid® [OTC]; Pin-X® [OTC]; Reese's® Pinworm Medicine [OTC]

**Canadian Brand Names** Combantrin®

**Pharmacologic Category** Anthelmintic

**Use** Treatment of pinworms (*Enterobius vermicularis*), whipworms (*Trichuris trichiura*), roundworms (*Ascaris lumbricoides*), and hookworms (*Ancylostoma duodenale*)

**Effects on Mental Status** May cause dizziness, drowsiness, or insomnia

**Effects on Psychiatric Treatment** None reported

**Pregnancy Risk Factor** C

**Contraindications** Known hypersensitivity to pyrantel pamoate

**Warnings/Precautions** Use with caution in patients with liver impairment, anemia, malnutrition, or pregnancy. Since pinworm infections are easily spread to others, treat all family members in close contact with the patient.

**Adverse Reactions**

1% to 10%: Gastrointestinal: Anorexia, nausea, vomiting, abdominal cramps, diarrhea

<1%: Dizziness, drowsiness, elevated liver enzymes, headache, insomnia, rash, tenesmus, weakness

**Overdosage/Toxicology**

Signs and symptoms: Anorexia, nausea, vomiting, cramps, diarrhea, ataxia

Treatment: Supportive following GI decontamination

**Drug Interactions** Decreased effect with piperazine

**Usual Dosage** Children and Adults (purgation is not required prior to use):

Oral:

Roundworm, pinworm, or trichostrongyliasis: 11 mg/kg administered as a single dose; maximum dose: 1 g. (**Note:** For pinworm infection, dosage should be repeated in 2 weeks and all family members should be treated).

Hookworm: 11 mg/kg administered once daily for 3 days

**Patient Information** May mix drug with milk or fruit juice; strict hygiene is essential to prevent reinfection

**Nursing Implications** Shake well before pouring to assure accurate dosage; protect from light

**Dosage Forms**

Capsule: 180 mg

Liquid: 50 mg/mL (30 mL); 144 mg/mL (30 mL)

Suspension, oral (caramel-currant flavor): 50 mg/mL (60 mL)

## Pyrazinamide (peer a ZIN a mide)

**Canadian Brand Names** PMS-Pyrazinamide; Tebrazid

**Synonyms** Pyrazinoic Acid Amide

**Pharmacologic Category** Antitubercular Agent

**Use** Adjunctive treatment of tuberculosis in combination with other antituberculosis agents

**Effects on Mental Status** May cause drowsiness

**Effects on Psychiatric Treatment** None reported

**Pregnancy Risk Factor** C

**Contraindications** Severe hepatic damage; hypersensitivity to pyrazinamide or any component; acute gout

**Warnings/Precautions** Use with caution in patients with renal failure, chronic gout, diabetes mellitus, or porphyria

**Adverse Reactions**

1% to 10%:

Central nervous system: Malaise

Gastrointestinal: Nausea, vomiting, anorexia

Neuromuscular & skeletal: Arthralgia, myalgia

<1%: Acne, dysuria, fever, gout, hepatotoxicity, interstitial nephritis, itching, photosensitivity, porphyria, rash, thrombocytopenia

**Overdosage/Toxicology**

Signs and symptoms: Gout, gastric upset, hepatic damage (mild)

Treatment: Following GI decontamination is supportive

**Drug Interactions** No data reported

**Usual Dosage** Oral (calculate dose on ideal body weight rather than total body weight): **Note:** A four-drug regimen (isoniazid, rifampin, pyrazinamide, and either streptomycin or ethambutol) is preferred for the initial, empiric treatment of TB. When the drug susceptibility results are available, the regimen should be altered as appropriate.

Children and Adults:

Daily therapy: 15-30 mg/kg/day (maximum: 2 g/day)

Directly observed therapy (DOT): Twice weekly: 50-70 mg/kg (maximum: 4 g)

DOT: 3 times/week: 50-70 mg/kg (maximum: 3 g)

Elderly: Start with a lower daily dose (15 mg/kg) and increase as tolerated

**Dosing adjustment in renal impairment:** $Cl_{cr}$ <50 mL/minute: Avoid use or reduce dose to 12-20 mg/kg/day

**Dosing adjustment in hepatic impairment:** Reduce dose

**Patient Information** Take with food for full length of therapy. Do not miss doses and do not discontinue without consulting prescriber. You will need regular medical follow-up while taking this medication. You may experience nausea or loss of appetite; small frequent meals, frequent mouth care, sucking lozenges, or chewing gum may help. Report unusual fever, unresolved nausea or vomiting, change in color of urine, pale stools, easy bruising or bleeding, blood in urine or difficulty urinating, yellowing of skin or eyes, or extreme joint pain.

**Dosage Forms** Tablet: 500 mg

♦ **Pyrazinoic Acid Amide** *see* Pyrazinamide *on page 480*

## Pyrethrins (pye RE thrins)

**U.S. Brand Names** A-200™ Shampoo [OTC]; Barc™ Liquid [OTC]; End Lice® Liquid [OTC]; Lice-Enz® Shampoo [OTC]; Pronto® Shampoo [OTC]; Pyrinex® Pediculicide Shampoo [OTC]; Pyrinyl II® Liquid [OTC]; Pyrinyl Plus® Shampoo [OTC]; R & C® Shampoo [OTC]; RID® Shampoo [OTC]; Tisit® Blue Gel [OTC]; Tisit® Liquid [OTC]; Tisit® Shampoo [OTC]; Triple X® Liquid [OTC]

**Canadian Brand Names** Lice-Enz®

**Pharmacologic Category** Antiparasitic Agent, Topical; Pediculocide; Shampoo, Pediculocide

**Use** Treatment of *Pediculus humanus* infestations (head lice, body lice, pubic lice and their eggs)

**Effects on Mental Status** None reported

**Effects on Psychiatric Treatment** None reported

**Pregnancy Risk Factor** C

**Contraindications** Known hypersensitivity to pyrethrins, ragweed, or chrysanthemums

**Warnings/Precautions** For external use only; do not use in eyelashes or eyebrows

**Adverse Reactions** 1% to 10%:

Dermatologic: Pruritus

Local: Burning, stinging, irritation with repeat use

**Drug Interactions** No data reported

**Usual Dosage** Application of pyrethrins: Topical:

Apply enough solution to completely wet infested area, including hair

Allow to remain on area for 10 minutes

Wash and rinse with large amounts of warm water

Use fine-toothed comb to remove lice and eggs from hair

Shampoo hair to restore body and luster

Treatment may be repeated if necessary once in a 24-hour period

Repeat treatment in 7-10 days to kill newly hatched lice

**Patient Information** For external use only; avoid touching eyes, mouth, or other mucous membranes; contact physician if irritation occurs or if condition does not improve in 2-3 days

**Dosage Forms**

Gel, topical: 0.3% (30 g)

Liquid, topical: 0.18% (60 mL); 0.2% (60 mL, 120 mL); 0.3% (60 mL, 118 mL, 120 mL, 177 mL, 237 mL, 240 mL)
Shampoo: 0.3% (59 mL, 60 mL, 118 mL, 120 mL, 240 mL); 0.33% (60 mL, 120 mL)

♦ **Pyridiate®** *see* Phenazopyridine *on page 433*

♦ **Pyridium®** *see* Phenazopyridine *on page 433*

## Pyridostigmine (peer id oh STIG meen)

**U.S. Brand Names** Mestinon® Injection; Mestinon® Oral; Regonol® Injection

**Pharmacologic Category** Acetylcholinesterase Inhibitor (Central)

**Use** Symptomatic treatment of myasthenia gravis; also used as an antidote for nondepolarizing neuromuscular blockers; not a cure; patient may develop resistance to the drug

**Effects on Mental Status** May rarely cause dysphoria or drowsiness

**Effects on Psychiatric Treatment** None reported; but mouth watering is common and may be additive to the sialorrhea associated with clozapine therapy

**Pregnancy Risk Factor** C

**Contraindications** Hypersensitivity to pyridostigmine, bromides, or any component; GI or GU obstruction

**Warnings/Precautions** Use with caution in patients with epilepsy, asthma, bradycardia, hyperthyroidism, cardiac arrhythmias, or peptic ulcer; adequate facilities should be available for cardiopulmonary resuscitation when testing and adjusting dose for myasthenia gravis; have atropine and epinephrine ready to treat hypersensitivity reactions; overdosage may result in cholinergic crisis, this must be distinguished from myasthenic crisis; anticholinesterase insensitivity can develop for brief or prolonged periods

**Adverse Reactions**

>10%:
- Gastrointestinal: Diarrhea, nausea, stomach cramps, mouth watering
- Miscellaneous: Diaphoresis (increased)

1% to 10%:
- Genitourinary: Urge to urinate
- Ocular: Small pupils, lacrimation
- Respiratory: Increased bronchial secretions

<1%: A-V block, bradycardia, diplopia, drowsiness, dysphoria, headache, hyper-reactive cholinergic responses, hypersensitivity, laryngospasm, miosis, muscle spasms, respiratory paralysis, seizures, thrombophlebitis, weakness

**Overdosage/Toxicology**

Signs and symptoms: Muscle weakness, blurred vision, excessive sweating, tearing and salivation, nausea, vomiting, diarrhea, hypertension, bradycardia, paralysis

Treatment: Atropine is the treatment of choice for intoxications manifesting with significant muscarinic symptoms. Atropine I.V. 2-4 mg every 3-60 minutes (or 0.04-0.08 mg I.V. every 5-60 minutes if needed for children) should be repeated to control symptoms and then continued as needed for 1-2 days following the acute ingestion.

**Drug Interactions**

Anticholinergics: Effects may be reduced with cholinesterase inhibitors; atropine antagonizes the muscarinic effects of cholinesterase inhibitors

Beta-blockers without ISA: Activity may increase risk of bradycardia

Calcium channel blockers (diltiazem or verapamil): May increase risk of bradycardia

Cholinergic agonists: Effects may be increased with cholinesterase inhibitors

Corticosteroids: May see increased muscle weakness and decreased response to anticholinesterases shortly after onset of corticosteroid therapy in the treatment of myasthenia gravis. Deterioration in muscle strength, including severe muscular depression, has been documented in patients with myasthenia gravis while receiving corticosteroids and anticholinesterases.

Digoxin: Increased risk of bradycardia with concurrent use

Neuromuscular blockers: Depolarizing neuromuscular blocking agents effects may be increased with cholinesterase inhibitors; nondepolarizing agents are antagonized by cholinesterase inhibitors

**Usual Dosage** Normally, sustained release dosage form is used at bedtime for patients who complain of morning weakness

Myasthenia gravis:
- Oral:
  - Children: 7 mg/kg/day in 5-6 divided doses
  - Adults: Initial: 60 mg 3 times/day with maintenance dose ranging from 60 mg to 1.5 g/day; sustained release formulation should be dosed at least every 6 hours (usually 12-24 hours)
- I.M., I.V.:
  - Children: 0.05-0.15 mg/kg/dose (maximum single dose: 10 mg)
  - Adults: 2 mg every 2-3 hours or 1/30 of oral dose

Reversal of nondepolarizing neuromuscular blocker: I.M., I.V.:
- Children: 0.1-0.25 mg/kg/dose preceded by atropine
- Adults: 10-20 mg preceded by atropine

**Patient Information** This drug will not cure myasthenia gravis, but may help reduce symptoms. Use as directed; do not increase dose or discontinue without consulting prescriber. Take extended release tablets at bedtime; do not chew or crush extended release tablets. Maintain adequate hydration (2-3 L/day of fluids unless instructed to restrict fluid intake). May cause dizziness, drowsiness, or hypotension (rise slowly from sitting or lying position and use caution when driving or climbing stairs); vomiting or loss of appetite (frequent small meals, frequent mouth care, chewing gum, or sucking lozenges may help); or diarrhea (boiled milk, yogurt, or buttermilk may help). Report persistent abdominal discomfort; significantly increased salivation, sweating, tearing, or urination; flushed skin; chest pain or palpitations; acute headache; unresolved diarrhea; excessive fatigue, insomnia, dizziness, or depression; increased muscle, joint, or body pain; vision changes or blurred vision; or shortness of breath or wheezing.

**Nursing Implications** Do not crush sustained release drug product; observe for cholinergic reactions, particularly when administered I.V.

**Dosage Forms**

Injection, as bromide: 5 mg/mL (2 mL, 5 mL)
Syrup, as bromide (raspberry flavor): 60 mg/5 mL (480 mL)
Tablet, as bromide: 60 mg
Tablet, as bromide, sustained release: 180 mg

## Pyridoxine (peer i DOKS een)

**U.S. Brand Names** Nestrex®

**Pharmacologic Category** Vitamin, Water Soluble

**Use** Prevents and treats vitamin $B_6$ deficiency, pyridoxine-dependent seizures in infants, adjunct to treatment of acute toxicity from isoniazid, cycloserine, or hydralazine overdose

**Effects on Mental Status** None reported

**Effects on Psychiatric Treatment** May decrease the effects of levodopa and phenobarbital

**Usual Dosage**

Recommended daily allowance (RDA):
- Children:
  - 1-3 years: 0.9 mg
  - 4-6 years: 1.3 mg
  - 7-10 years: 1.6 mg
- Adults:
  - Male: 1.7-2.0 mg
  - Female: 1.4-1.6 mg

Pyridoxine-dependent Infants:
- Oral: 2-100 mg/day
- I.M., I.V., S.C.: 10-100 mg

Dietary deficiency: Oral:
- Children: 5-25 mg/24 hours for 3 weeks, then 1.5-2.5 mg/day in multiple vitamin product
- Adults: 10-20 mg/day for 3 weeks

Drug-induced neuritis (eg, isoniazid, hydralazine, penicillamine, cycloserine): Oral:
- Children:
  - Treatment: 10-50 mg/24 hours
  - Prophylaxis: 1-2 mg/kg/24 hours
- Adults:
  - Treatment: 100-200 mg/24 hours
  - Prophylaxis: 25-100 mg/24 hours

Treatment of seizures and/or coma from acute isoniazid toxicity, a dose of pyridoxine hydrochloride equal to the amount of INH ingested can be given I.M./I.V. in divided doses together with other anticonvulsants; if the amount INH ingested is not known, administer 5 g I.V. pyridoxine

Treatment of acute hydralazine toxicity, a pyridoxine dose of 25 mg/kg in divided doses I.M./I.V. has been used

**Dosage Forms**

Injection, as hydrochloride: 100 mg/mL (10 mL, 30 mL)
Tablet, as hydrochloride: 25 mg, 50 mg, 100 mg
Tablet, as hydrochloride, extended release: 100 mg

## Pyrimethamine (peer i METH a meen)

**U.S. Brand Names** Daraprim®

**Pharmacologic Category** Antimalarial Agent

**Use** Prophylaxis of malaria due to susceptible strains of plasmodia; used in conjunction with quinine and sulfadiazine for the treatment of uncomplicated attacks of chloroquine-resistant *P. falciparum* malaria; used in conjunction with fast-acting schizonticide to initiate transmission control and suppression cure; synergistic combination with sulfonamide in treatment of toxoplasmosis

**Effects on Mental Status** May rarely cause drowsiness, insomnia, or depression

**Effects on Psychiatric Treatment** May cause leukopenia; use caution with clozapine and carbamazepine; mild hepatotoxicity associated with concurrent usage of lorazepam

**Pregnancy Risk Factor** C

(Continued)

## Pyrimethamine *(Continued)*

**Contraindications** Megaloblastic anemia secondary to folate deficiency; known hypersensitivity to pyrimethamine, chloroguanide; resistant malaria

**Warnings/Precautions** When used for more than 3-4 days, it may be advisable to administer leucovorin to prevent hematologic complications; monitor CBC and platelet counts every 2 weeks; use with caution in patients with impaired renal or hepatic function or with possible G-6-PD

**Adverse Reactions**

1% to 10%:

Gastrointestinal: Anorexia, abdominal cramps, vomiting

Hematologic: Megaloblastic anemia, leukopenia, thrombocytopenia, agranulocytosis

<1%: Abnormal skin pigmentation, anaphylaxis, atrophic glossitis, depression, dermatitis, diarrhea, erythema multiforme, fever, insomnia, lightheadedness, malaise, pulmonary eosinophilia, rash, seizures, Stevens-Johnson syndrome, xerostomia

**Overdosage/Toxicology**

Signs and symptoms: Megaloblastic anemia, leukopenia, thrombocytopenia, anorexia, CNS stimulation, seizures, nausea, vomiting, hematemesis

Treatment: Following GI decontamination, leucovorin should be administered in a dosage of 5-15 mg/day I.M., I.V., or oral for 5-7 days or as required to reverse symptoms of folic acid deficiency; diazepam 0.1-0.25 mg/kg can be used to treat seizures

**Drug Interactions**

Decreased effect: Pyrimethamine effectiveness decreased by acid

Increased effect: Sulfonamides (synergy), methotrexate, TMP/SMX may increase the risk of bone marrow suppression; mild hepatotoxicity with lorazepam

**Usual Dosage**

Malaria chemoprophylaxis (for areas where chloroquine-resistant *P. falciparum* exists): Begin prophylaxis 2 weeks before entering endemic area:

Children: 0.5 mg/kg once weekly; not to exceed 25 mg/dose

**or**

Children:

<4 years: 6.25 mg once weekly

4-10 years: 12.5 mg once weekly

Children >10 years and Adults: 25 mg once weekly

Dosage should be continued for all age groups for at least 6-10 weeks after leaving endemic areas

Chloroquine-resistant *P. falciparum* malaria (when used in conjunction with quinine and sulfadiazine):

Children:

<10 kg: 6.25 mg/day once daily for 3 days

10-20 kg: 12.5 mg/day once daily for 3 days

20-40 kg: 25 mg/day once daily for 3 days

Adults: 25 mg twice daily for 3 days

Toxoplasmosis:

Infants for congenital toxoplasmosis: Oral: 1 mg/kg once daily for 6 months with sulfadiazine then every other month with sulfa, alternating with spiramycin.

Children: Loading dose: 2 mg/kg/day divided into 2 equal daily doses for 1-3 days (maximum: 100 mg/day) followed by 1 mg/kg/day divided into 2 doses for 4 weeks; maximum: 25 mg/day

With sulfadiazine or trisulfapyrimidines: 2 mg/kg/day divided every 12 hours for 3 days followed by 1 mg/kg/day once daily or divided twice daily for 4 weeks given with trisulfapyrimidines or sulfadiazine

Adults: 50-75 mg/day together with 1-4 g of a sulfonamide for 1-3 weeks depending on patient's tolerance and response, then reduce dose by 50% and continue for 4-5 weeks **or** 25-50 mg/day for 3-4 weeks

In HIV, life-long suppression is necessary to prevent relapse; leucovorin (5-10 mg/day) is given concurrently

**Patient Information** Take on schedule as directed and take full course of therapy. If used for prophylaxis, begin 2 weeks before traveling to endemic areas, continue during travel period, and for 6-10 weeks following return. Regular blood tests will be necessary during therapy. You may experience GI distress (frequent small meals may help). You may experience dizziness, changes in mentation, insomnia, headache, or visual disturbances (use caution when driving or operating dangerous machinery). Report unresolved nausea or vomiting, anorexia, skin rash, fever, sore throat, unusual bleeding or bruising, yellowing of skin or eyes, and change in color of urine or stool.

**Dosage Forms** Tablet: 25 mg


♦ **Pyrinex® Pediculicide Shampoo [OTC]** *see* Pyrethrins *on page 480*

♦ **Pyrinyl II® Liquid [OTC]** *see* Pyrethrins *on page 480*

♦ **Pyrinyl Plus® Shampoo [OTC]** *see* Pyrethrins *on page 480*


## Quazepam (KWAY ze pam)

**Related Information**


Anxiolytic/Hypnotic Use in Long-Term Care Facilities *on page 754*

Benzodiazepines Comparison Chart *on page 708*

Patient Information - Anxiolytics & Sedative Hypnotics (Benzodiazepines) *on page 653*


**Generic Available** No

**U.S. Brand Names** Doral®

**Pharmacologic Category** Benzodiazepine

**Use** Treatment of insomnia

**Restrictions** C-IV

**Pregnancy Risk Factor** X

**Contraindications** Hypersensitivity to this drug or any component of its formulation (cross-sensitivity with other benzodiazepines may exist); narrow-angle glaucoma (not in product labeling, however, benzodiazepines are contraindicated); pregnancy

**Warnings/Precautions** Should be used only after evaluation of potential causes of sleep disturbance. Failure of sleep disturbance to resolve after 7-10 days may indicate psychiatric or medical illness. A worsening of insomnia or the emergence of new abnormalities of thought or behavior may represent unrecognized psychiatric or medical illness and requires immediate and careful evaluation. Use with caution in elderly or debilitated patients, patients with hepatic disease (including alcoholics), or renal impairment. Use with caution in patients with respiratory disease or impaired gag reflex. Avoid use in patients with sleep apnea.

Causes CNS depression (dose-related) resulting in sedation, dizziness, confusion, or ataxia which may impair physical and mental capabilities. Patients must be cautioned about performing tasks which require mental alertness (operating machinery or driving). Use with caution in patients receiving other CNS depressants or psychoactive agents. Effects with other sedative drugs or ethanol may be potentiated. Benzodiazepines have been associated with falls and traumatic injury and should be used with extreme caution in patients who are at risk of these events (especially the elderly).

Use caution in patients with depression, particularly if suicidal risk may be present. Use with caution in patients with a history of drug dependence. Benzodiazepines have been associated with dependence and acute withdrawal symptoms on discontinuation or reduction in dose. Acute withdrawal, including seizures, may be precipitated after administration of flumazenil to patients receiving long-term benzodiazepine therapy.

Benzodiazepines have been associated with anterograde amnesia. Paradoxical reactions, including hyperactive or aggressive behavior have been reported with benzodiazepines, particularly in adolescent/pediatric or psychiatric patients. Does not have analgesic, antidepressant, or antipsychotic properties.

**Adverse Reactions**

Cardiovascular: Palpitations

Central nervous system: Drowsiness, fatigue, ataxia, memory impairment, anxiety, depression, headache, confusion, nervousness, dizziness, incoordination, hypo- and hyperkinesia, agitation, euphoria, paranoid reaction, nightmares, abnormal thinking

Dermatologic: Dermatitis, pruritus, rash

Endocrine & metabolic: Decreased libido, menstrual irregularities

Gastrointestinal: Xerostomia, constipation, diarrhea, dyspepsia, anorexia, abnormal taste perception, nausea, vomiting, increased or decreased appetite, abdominal pain

Genitourinary: Impotence, incontinence

Hematologic: Blood dyscrasias

Neuromuscular & skeletal: Dysarthria, rigidity, tremor, muscle cramps, reflex slowing

Ocular: Blurred vision

Miscellaneous: Drug dependence

**Overdosage/Toxicology**

Signs and symptoms: Somnolence, confusion, coma, hypoactive reflexes, dyspnea, hypotension, slurred speech, impaired coordination

Treatment:

Treatment for benzodiazepine overdose is supportive; rarely is mechanical ventilation required

Flumazenil has been shown to selectively block the binding of benzodiazepines to CNS receptors, resulting in a reversal of benzodiazepine-induced CNS depression, but not respiratory depression

**Drug Interactions**

CNS depressants: Sedative effects and/or respiratory depression may be additive with CNS depressants; includes ethanol, barbiturates, narcotic analgesics, and other sedative agents; monitor for increased effect

Enzyme inducers: Metabolism of some benzodiazepines may be increased, decreasing their therapeutic effect; consider using an alternative sedative/hypnotic agent; potential inducers include phenobarbital, phenytoin, carbamazepine, rifampin, and rifabutin

Oral contraceptives: May decrease the clearance of some benzodiazepines (those which undergo oxidative metabolism); monitor for increased benzodiazepine effect

Theophylline: May partially antagonize some of the effects of benzodiazepines; monitor for decreased response; may require higher doses for sedation

**Mechanism of Action** Binds to stereospecific benzodiazepine receptors on the postsynaptic GABA neuron at several sites within the central nervous system, including the limbic system, reticular formation. Enhancement of the inhibitory effect of GABA on neuronal excitability results by increased neuronal membrane permeability to chloride ions. This shift in chloride ions results in hyperpolarization (a less excitable state) and stabilization.

**Pharmacodynamics/kinetics**

Absorption: Oral: Rapid
Protein binding: 95%
Metabolism: In the liver to at least one active compound
Half-life:
Parent drug: 25-41 hours
Active metabolite: 40-114 hours

**Usual Dosage** Adults: Oral: Initial: 15 mg at bedtime, in some patients the dose may be reduced to 7.5 mg after a few nights

**Dosing adjustment in hepatic impairment:** Dose reduction may be necessary

**Dietary Considerations** Alcohol: Additive CNS effect, avoid use

**Monitoring Parameters** Respiratory and cardiovascular status

**Reference Range** Mean plasma level of 148 ng/mL 1.5 hours after ingestion of 25 mg

**Patient Information** Avoid alcohol and other CNS depressants; avoid activities needing good psychomotor coordination until CNS effects are known; drug may cause physical or psychological dependence; avoid abrupt discontinuation after prolonged use

**Nursing Implications** Institute safety measures, remove smoking materials from area, supervise ambulation

**Additional Information** More likely than short-acting benzodiazepine to cause daytime sedation and fatigue; is classified as a long-acting benzodiazepine hypnotic (eg, flurazepam), this long duration of action may prevent withdrawal symptoms when therapy is discontinued.

**Dosage Forms** Tablet: 7.5 mg, 15 mg

- **Quelicin® Injection** *see* Succinylcholine *on page 521*
- **Questran®** *see* Cholestyramine Resin *on page 120*
- **Questran® Light** *see* Cholestyramine Resin *on page 120*

## Quetiapine (kwe TYE a peen)

**Related Information**

Antipsychotic Agents Comparison Chart *on page 706*
Antipsychotic Medication Guidelines *on page 751*
Atypical Antipsychotics *on page 707*
Clinical Issues in the Use of Antipsychotics *on page 630*
Discontinuation of Psychotropic Drugs - Withdrawal Symptoms and Recommendations *on page 798*
Patient Information - Antipsychotics (General) *on page 646*
Schizophrenia *on page 604*

**U.S. Brand Names** Seroquel®

**Synonyms** Quetiapine Fumarate

**Pharmacologic Category** Antipsychotic Agent, Dibenzothiazepine

**Use** Treatment of manifestations of psychotic disorders

**Pregnancy Risk Factor** C

**Contraindications** Hypersensitivity to quetiapine or any component; severe CNS depression, bone marrow suppression, blood dyscrasias, severe hepatic disease, coma

**Warnings/Precautions** Has been noted to cause cataracts in animals, although QTP-associated cataracts have not been observed in humans; lens examination on initiation of therapy and every 6 months is recommended. May be sedating, use with caution in disorders where CNS depression is a feature. Use with caution in Parkinson's disease. Caution in patients with hemodynamic instability; prior myocardial infarction or ischemic heart disease; hypercholesterolemia; thyroid disease; predisposition to seizures; subcortical brain damage; hepatic impairment; severe cardiac, renal, or respiratory disease. May alter temperature regulation or mask toxicity of other drugs due to antiemetic effects. May alter cardiac conduction - life-threatening arrhythmias have occurred with therapeutic doses of antipsychotics. May cause orthostatic hypotension - use with caution in patients at risk of this effect or those who would tolerate transient hypotensive episodes (cerebrovascular disease, cardiovascular disease, or other medications which may predispose). Esophageal dysmotility and aspiration have been associated with antipsychotic use - use with caution in patients at risk of pneumonia (ie, Alzheimer's disease).

May cause anticholinergic effects (confusion, agitation, constipation, dry mouth, blurred vision, urinary retention); therefore, they should be used with caution in patients with decreased gastrointestinal motility, urinary retention, BPH, xerostomia, or visual problems. Conditions which also may be exacerbated by cholinergic blockade include narrow-angle glaucoma (screening is recommended) and worsening of myasthenia gravis. Relative to other antipsychotics, quetiapine has a moderate potency of cholinergic blockade. The risk of extrapyramidal symptoms, tardive dyskinesia, and neuroleptic malignant syndrome in association with quetiapine is very low relative to other antipsychotics.

**Adverse Reactions**

>10%:
Central nervous system: Headache, somnolence
Gastrointestinal: Weight gain

1% to 10%:
Cardiovascular: Postural hypotension, tachycardia, palpitations
Central nervous system: Dizziness, hypotension
Dermatologic: Rash
Gastrointestinal: Abdominal pain, constipation, xerostomia, dyspepsia, anorexia
Hematologic: Leukopenia
Neuromuscular & skeletal: Dysarthria, back pain, weakness
Respiratory: Rhinitis, pharyngitis, cough, dyspnea
Miscellaneous: Diaphoresis

<1%: Abnormal dreams, anemia, bradycardia, diabetes, elevated alkaline phosphatase, elevated GGT, epistaxis, hyperlipidemia, hypothyroidism, increased appetite, increased salivation, involuntary movements, leukocytosis, Q-T prolongation, rash, tardive dyskinesia, vertigo

**Drug Interactions** CYP3A4, 2D6 (minor); 2C9 (minor) enzyme substrate

Antihypertensives: Concurrent use with an antihypertensive may produce additive hypotensive effects (particularly orthostasis)

Cimetidine: May decrease quetiapine's clearance by 20%; increasing serum concentrations

CNS depressants: Quetiapine may enhance the sedative effects of other CNS depressants; includes antidepressants, benzodiazepines, barbiturates, ethanol, narcotic analgesics, and other sedative agents; monitor for increased effect

CYP3A3/4 inhibitors: Serum level and/or toxicity of quetiapine may be increased; inhibitors include amiodarone, cimetidine, clarithromycin, erythromycin, delavirdine, diltiazem, dirithromycin, disulfiram, fluoxetine, fluvoxamine, grapefruit juice, indinavir, itraconazole, ketoconazole, metronidazole, nefazodone, nevirapine, propoxyfene, quinupristin-dalfopristin, ritonavir, saquinavir, verapamil, zafirlukast, zileuton; monitor for altered response

Enzyme inducers: May increase the metabolism of quetiapine, reducing serum levels and effect; enzyme inducers include carbamazepine, barbiturates, and rifampin; also see note on phenytoin

Levodopa: Quetiapine may inhibit the antiparkinsonian effect of levodopa; avoid this combination

Lorazepam: Metabolism of lorazepam may be reduced by quetiapine; clearance is reduced 20% in the presence of quetiapine; monitor for increased sedative effect

Phenytoin: Metabolism/clearance of quetiapine may be increased; 5-fold changes have been noted

Thioridazine: May increase clearance of quetiapine, decreasing serum concentrations; clearance may be increased by 65%

**Mechanism of Action** Mechanism of action of quetiapine, as with other antipsychotic drugs, is unknown. However, it has been proposed that this drug's antipsychotic activity is mediated through a combination of dopamine type 2 ($D_2$) and serotonin type 2 ($5HT_2$) antagonism. However, it is an antagonist at multiple neurotransmitter receptors in the brain: serotonin $5HT_{1A}$ and $5HT_2$, dopamine $D_1$ and $D_2$, histamine $H_1$, and adrenergic $alpha_1$- and $alpha_2$-receptors; but appears to have no appreciable affinity at cholinergic muscarinic and benzodiazepine receptors.

Antagonism at receptors other than dopamine and $5HT_2$ with similar receptor affinities may explain some of the other effects of quetiapine. The drug's antagonism of histamine $H_1$-receptors may explain the somnolence observed with it. The drug's antagonism of adrenergic $alpha_1$-receptors may explain the orthostatic hypotension observed with it.

**Pharmacodynamics/kinetics**

Absorption: Accumulation is predictable upon multiple dosing
Distribution: Steady-state concentrations are expected to be achieved within 2 days of dosing; unlikely to interfere with the metabolism of drugs metabolized by cytochrome P-450 enzymes
Metabolism: Both metabolites are pharmacologically inactive
Half-life, mean terminal: ~6 hours
Time to peak plasma concentrations: 1.5 hours
Elimination: Mainly via hepatic metabolism

**Usual Dosage** Adults: Oral: 25-100 mg 2-3 times/day; usual starting dose: 25 mg twice daily and then increased in increments of 25-50 mg 2-3 times/day on the second or third day; by day 4, the dose should be in the range of 300-400 mg/day in 2-3 divided doses. Make further adjustments as needed at intervals of at least 2 days in adjustments of 25-50 mg twice daily. Usual maintenance range: 150-750 mg/day

**Dosing comments in geriatric patients:** 40% lower mean oral clearance of quetiapine in adults >65 years of age; higher plasma levels expected and, therefore, dosage adjustment may be needed; elderly patients usually require 50-200 mg/day

**Dosing comments in hepatic insufficiency:** 30% lower mean oral clearance of quetiapine than normal subjects; higher plasma levels expected in hepatically impaired subjects; dosage adjustment may be needed

**Dietary Considerations** In healthy volunteers, administration of quetiapine with food resulted in an increase in the peak serum concentration and AUC (each by ~15%) compared to the fasting state; can be taken with or without food

**Monitoring Parameters** Patients should have eyes checked every 6 months for cataracts while on this medication

**Test Interactions** ↑ ALT, total cholesterol, triglycerides

(Continued)

## Quetiapine *(Continued)*

**Patient Information** May cause drowsiness, dizziness, and/or headache; might increase risk of cataracts

**Additional Information** Quetiapine has a very low incidence of extrapyramidal symptoms such as restlessness and abnormal movement, and is at least as effective as conventional antipsychotics

**Dosage Forms** Tablet: 25 mg, 100 mg, 200 mg

- ♦ **Quetiapine Fumarate** *see* Quetiapine *on page 483*
- ♦ **Quibron®** *see* Theophylline and Guaifenesin *on page 539*
- ♦ **Quibron®-T** *see* Theophylline Salts *on page 539*
- ♦ **Quibron®-T/SR** *see* Theophylline Salts *on page 539*
- ♦ **Quiess®** *see* Hydroxyzine *on page 278*
- ♦ **Quinaglute® Dura-Tabs®** *see* Quinidine *on page 485*
- ♦ **Quinalan®** *see* Quinidine *on page 485*
- ♦ **Quinalbarbitone Sodium** *see* Secobarbital *on page 507*

## Quinapril (KWIN a pril)

**Related Information**

Angiotensin-Related Agents Comparison Chart *on page 700*

**U.S. Brand Names** Accupril®

**Pharmacologic Category** Angiotensin-Converting Enzyme (ACE) Inhibitors

**Use** Management of hypertension; treatment of congestive heart failure, left ventricular dysfunction after myocardial infarction

**Effects on Mental Status** May cause dizziness or drowsiness; may rarely cause insomnia or depression

**Effects on Psychiatric Treatment** May cause neutropenia; use caution with clozapine and carbamazepine; may decrease lithium clearance resulting in an increase in serum lithium levels and potential lithium toxicity; monitor serum lithium levels

**Pregnancy Risk Factor** C (1st trimester); D (2nd and 3rd trimester)

**Contraindications** Hypersensitivity to quinapril or any component; angioedema related to previous treatment with an ACE inhibitor; bilateral renal artery stenosis; primary hyperaldosteronism; patients with idiopathic or hereditary angioedema; pregnancy (2nd and 3rd trimesters)

**Warnings/Precautions** Anaphylactic reactions can occur. Angioedema can occur at any time during treatment (especially following first dose). Careful blood pressure monitoring with first dose (hypotension can occur especially in volume depleted patients). Dosage adjustment needed in renal impairment. Use with caution in hypovolemia; collagen vascular diseases; valvular stenosis (particularly aortic stenosis); hyperkalemia; or before, during, or immediately after anesthesia. Avoid rapid dosage escalation, which may lead to renal insufficiency. Neutropenia/agranulocytosis with myeloid hyperplasia can rarely occur. If patient has renal impairment, a baseline WBC with differential and serum creatinine should be evaluated and monitored closely during the first 3 months of therapy. Hypersensitivity reactions may be seen during hemodialysis with high-flux dialysis membranes (eg, AN69). Use with caution in unilateral renal artery stenosis and pre-existing renal insufficiency. Deterioration in renal function can occur with initiation.

**Adverse Reactions**

1% to 10%:

Cardiovascular: Hypotension

Central nervous system: Dizziness (3.9%), headache (5.6%), fatigue (2.6%)

Gastrointestinal: Vomiting/nausea (1.4%)

Renal: Increased BUN/serum creatinine (transient)

Respiratory: Upper respiratory symptoms, cough (2%)

<1%: Abdominal pain, angina pectoris, angioedema, anorexia, arthralgia, blurred vision, bone marrow suppression, bronchitis, chest discomfort, constipation, depression, diaphoresis, fever, flatulence, flushing, gout, hepatitis, insomnia, malaise, myocardial infarction, neutropenia, orthostatic hypotension, palpitations, pancreatitis, peripheral edema, pharyngeal pain, pruritus, rhythm disturbances, shoulder pain, sinusitis, somnolence, syncope, tachycardia, urticaria, vasculitis, xerostomia

**Overdosage/Toxicology**

Signs and symptoms: Mild hypotension has been the only toxic effect seen with acute overdose. Bradycardia may also occur; hyperkalemia occurs even with therapeutic doses, especially in patients with renal insufficiency and those taking NSAIDs.

Treatment: Following initiation of essential overdose management, toxic symptom treatment and supportive treatment should be initiated. Hypotension usually responds to I.V. fluids or Trendelenburg positioning.

**Drug Interactions**

Alpha$_1$ blockers: Hypotensive effect increased

Aspirin: The effects of ACE inhibitors may be blunted by aspirin administration, particularly at higher dosages

Diuretics: Hypovolemia due to diuretics may precipitate acute hypotensive events or acute renal failure

Insulin: Risk of hypoglycemia may be increased

Lithium: Risk of lithium toxicity may be increased; monitor lithium levels, especially the first 4 weeks of therapy

Mercaptopurine: Risk of neutropenia may be increased

NSAIDs may decrease ACE inhibitor efficacy and/or increase risk of adverse renal effects

Potassium-sparing diuretics (amiloride, spironolactone, triamterene): Increased risk of hyperkalemia

Potassium supplements may increase the risk of hyperkalemia

Quinolones: Absorption may be decreased by quinapril; separate administration by at least 2-4 hours

Tetracyclines: Absorption may be reduced by quinapril; separate administration by at least 2-4 hours

Trimethoprim (high dose) may increase the risk of hyperkalemia

**Usual Dosage**

Adults: Oral: Initial: 10 mg once daily, adjust according to blood pressure response at peak and trough blood levels; in general, the normal dosage range is 20-80 mg/day for hypertension and 20-40 mg/day for edema in single or divided doses.

Elderly: Initial: 2.5-5 mg/day; increase dosage at increments of 2.5-5 mg at 1- to 2-week intervals.

**Dosing adjustment in renal impairment:**

$Cl_{cr}$ >60 mL/minute: Administer 10 mg/day.

$Cl_{cr}$ 30-60 mL/minute: Administer 5 mg/day.

$Cl_{cr}$ 10-30 mL/minute: Administer 2.5 mg/day.

**Dosing comments in hepatic impairment:** In patients with alcoholic cirrhosis, hydrolysis of quinapril to quinaprilat is impaired; however, the subsequent elimination of quinaprilat is unaltered.

**Patient Information** Take exactly as directed; do not discontinue without consulting prescriber. Take first dose at bedtime. Take all doses on an empty stomach (30 minutes before or 2 hours after meals). This drug does not eliminate need for diet or exercise regimen as recommended by prescriber. May cause dizziness, fainting, lightheadedness (use caution when driving or engaging in tasks requiring alertness until response to drug is known); postural hypotension (use caution when rising from lying or sitting position or climbing stairs); nausea, vomiting, altered taste, abdominal pain, dry mouth, or transient loss of appetite (small frequent meals, frequent mouth care, sucking lozenges, or chewing gum may help) - report if these persist. Report chest pain or palpitations; mouth sores; fever or chills; swelling of extremities; skin rash; numbness, tingling, or pain in muscles; difficulty in breathing or unusual cough; or other persistent adverse reactions.

**Nursing Implications** May cause depression in some patients; discontinue if angioedema of the face, extremities, lips, tongue, or glottis occurs; watch for hypotensive effects within 1-3 hours of first dose or new higher dose

**Dosage Forms** Tablet, as hydrochloride: 5 mg, 10 mg, 20 mg, 40 mg

## Quinestrol (kwin ES trole)

**Pharmacologic Category** Estrogen Derivative

**Use** Atrophic vaginitis; hypogonadism; primary ovarian failure; vasomotor symptoms of menopause; prostatic carcinoma; osteoporosis prophylactic

**Effects on Mental Status** May rarely cause dizziness, anxiety, or depression

**Effects on Psychiatric Treatment** Barbiturates may decrease the effects of estrogens

**Contraindications** Thrombophlebitis; undiagnosed vaginal bleeding; hypersensitivity to quinestrol or any component; known or suspected pregnancy; carcinoma of the breast; estrogen-dependent tumor

**Warnings/Precautions** Use with caution in patients with asthma, seizure disorders, migraine, cardiac, renal or hepatic impairment, cerebrovascular disorders or history of breast cancer, past or present thromboembolic disease, smokers >35 years of age; may cause serious bleeding in women sterilized by endometriosis

**Adverse Reactions**

>10%:

Cardiovascular: Peripheral edema

Endocrine & metabolic: Enlargement of breasts (female and male), breast tenderness

Gastrointestinal: Nausea, anorexia, bloating

1% to 10%:

Central nervous system: Headache

Endocrine & metabolic: Increased libido (female), decreased libido (male)

Gastrointestinal: Vomiting, diarrhea

**Overdosage/Toxicology**

Signs and symptoms: Fluid retention, jaundice, thrombophlebitis, nausea, toxicity is unlikely following single exposures of excessive doses

Treatment: Any treatment following emesis and charcoal administration should be supportive and symptomatic

**Drug Interactions** No significant interactions reported

**Usual Dosage** Adults: Female: Oral: 100 mcg once daily for 7 days; followed by 100 mcg/week beginning 2 weeks after inception of treatment; may increase to 200 mcg/week if necessary

**Dosing comments in hepatic impairment:** Administer with caution

**Patient Information** Patients should inform their physicians if signs or symptoms of any of the following occur: Thromboembolic or thrombotic disorders including sudden severe headache or vomiting, disturbance of vision or speech, loss of vision, numbness or weakness in an extremity, sharp or crushing chest pain, calf pain, shortness of breath, severe abdominal pain or mass, mental depression or unusual bleeding; patients should discontinue taking the medication if they suspect they are pregnant or become pregnant.

**Dosage Forms** Tablet: 100 mcg

## Quinethazone (kwin ETH a zone)

**U.S. Brand Names** Hydromox®

**Pharmacologic Category** Diuretic, Thiazide

**Use** Adjunctive therapy in treatment of edema and hypertension

**Effects on Mental Status** May cause drowsiness

**Effects on Psychiatric Treatment** May rarely cause agranulocytosis; use caution with clozapine and carbamazepine; may decrease lithium clearance resulting in an increase in serum lithium levels and potential lithium toxicity; monitor serum lithium levels

**Pregnancy Risk Factor** D

**Contraindications** Anuria; hypersensitivity to sulfonamide-derived drugs

**Warnings/Precautions** Use with caution in renal disease, hepatic disease, gout, lupus erythematosus, diabetes mellitus; some products may contain tartrazine

**Adverse Reactions** 1% to 10%: Endocrine & metabolic: Hypokalemia

**Overdosage/Toxicology**

Signs and symptoms: Hypermotility, diuresis, lethargy, confusion, muscle weakness

Treatment: Following GI decontamination, therapy is supportive with I.V. fluids, electrolytes, and I.V. pressors if needed

**Drug Interactions**

Decreased effect:

- Thiazides may decrease the effect of anticoagulants, antigout agents, sulfonylureas
- Bile acid sequestrants, methenamine, and NSAIDs may decrease the effect of the thiazides

Increased effect: Thiazides may increase the toxicity of allopurinol, anesthetics, antineoplastics, calcium salts, diazoxide, digitalis, lithium, loop diuretics, methyldopa, nondepolarizing muscle relaxants, vitamin D; amphotericin B and anticholinergics may increase the toxicity of thiazides

**Usual Dosage** Adults: Oral: 50-100 mg once daily; usual maximum: 200 mg/day

**Patient Information** May be taken with food or milk; take early in day to avoid nocturia; take the last dose of multiple doses no later than 6 PM unless instructed otherwise. A few people who take this medication become more sensitive to sunlight and may experience skin rash, redness, itching, or severe sunburn, especially if sun block SPF ≥15 is not used on exposed skin areas.

**Dosage Forms** Tablet: 50 mg

♦ **Quinidex® Extentabs®** *see* Quinidine *on page 485*

## Quinidine (KWIN i deen)

**Related Information**

Serum Drug Concentrations Commonly Monitored: Guidelines *on page 759*

**U.S. Brand Names** Cardioquin®; Quinaglute® Dura-Tabs®; Quinalan®; Quinidex® Extentabs®; Quinora®

**Synonyms** Quinidine Gluconate; Quinidine Polygalacturonate; Quinidine Sulfate

**Pharmacologic Category** Antiarrhythmic Agent, Class I-A

**Use** Prophylaxis after cardioversion of atrial fibrillation and/or flutter to maintain normal sinus rhythm; prevent recurrence of paroxysmal supraventricular tachycardia, paroxysmal A-V junctional rhythm, paroxysmal ventricular tachycardia, paroxysmal atrial fibrillation, and atrial or ventricular premature contractions; has activity against *Plasmodium falciparum* malaria

**Effects on Mental Status** May cause dizziness; may rarely cause confusion or delirium

**Effects on Psychiatric Treatment** May cause anemia; use caution with clozapine and carbamazepine; concurrent use with TCAs may raise serum levels or produce AV block; avoid combination; concurrent use with beta-blockers may increase bradycardia

**Pregnancy Risk Factor** C

**Contraindications** Hypersensitivity to quinidine or any component; thrombocytopenia; thrombocytopenic purpura; myasthenia gravis; heart block greater than first degree; idioventricular conduction delays (except in patients with a functioning artificial pacemaker); those adverse affected by anticholinergic activity; concurrent use of quinolone antibiotics which prolong Q-T interval, cisapride, amprenavir, or ritonavir

**Warnings/Precautions** Monitor and adjust dose to prevent QTc prolongation. Watch for proarrhythmic effects. May precipitate or exacerbate CHF. Reduce dosage in hepatic impairment. In patients with atrial fibrillation or flutter, block the AV node before initiating. Correct hypokalemia before initiating therapy. Hypokalemia may worsen toxicity. Use may cause digoxin-induced toxicity (adjust digoxin's dose). Use caution with concurrent use of other antiarrhythmics. Avoid use in myasthenia gravis (may worsen condition). Hypersensitivity reactions can occur. Can unmask sick sinus syndrome (causes bradycardia). Has been associated with severe hepatotoxic reactions, including granulomatous hepatitis. Hemolysis may occur in patients with G-6-PD (glucose-6-phosphate dehydrogenase) deficiency.

**Adverse Reactions**

>10%: Gastrointestinal: Bitter taste, diarrhea, anorexia, nausea, vomiting, stomach cramping

1% to 10%:

- Cardiovascular: Hypotension, syncope
- Central nervous system: Lightheadedness, severe headache
- Dermatologic: Rash
- Ocular: Blurred vision
- Otic: Tinnitus
- Respiratory: Wheezing

<1%: Anemia, angioedema, blood dyscrasias, bronchospasm, confusion, delirium, fever, heart block, impaired hearing, pneumonitis, respiratory depression, tachycardia, thrombocytopenic purpura, vascular collapse, ventricular fibrillation, vertigo

**Overdosage/Toxicology**

Signs and symptoms: Has a low toxic:therapeutic ratio and may easily produce fatal intoxication (acute toxic dose: 1 g in adults); symptoms of overdose include sinus bradycardia, sinus node arrest or asystole, P-R, QRS or Q-T interval prolongation, torsade de pointes (polymorphous ventricular tachycardia) and depressed myocardial contractility, which along with alpha-adrenergic or ganglionic blockade, may result in hypotension and pulmonary edema; other effects are anticholinergic (dry mouth, dilated pupils, and delirium) as well as seizures, coma and respiratory arrest.

Treatment: Primarily symptomatic and effects usually respond to conventional therapies (fluids, positioning, vasopressors, anticonvulsants, antiarrhythmics). **Note:** Do not use other type 1a or 1c antiarrhythmic agents to treat ventricular tachycardia; sodium bicarbonate may treat wide QRS intervals or hypotension; markedly impaired conduction or high degree A-V block, unresponsive to bicarbonate, indicates consideration of a pacemaker is needed.

**Drug Interactions** CYP3A3/4 substrate/inhibitor, CYP2D6 inhibitor

- Inhibitors of CYP3A3/4 (clarithromycin, erythromycin, itraconazole, ketoconazole, troleandomycin, protease inhibitors) may increase quinidine blood levels
- Amiloride may cause prolonged ventricular conduction leading to arrhythmias
- Amiodarone may increase quinidine blood levels; monitor quinidine levels
- Cimetidine: Increase quinidine blood levels; closely monitor levels or use an alternative $H_2$-antagonist
- Cisapride and quinidine may increase risk of malignant arrhythmias; concurrent use is contraindicated
- Codeine: Analgesic efficacy may be reduced
- Digoxin blood levels may be increased; monitor digoxin blood levels
- Drugs which prolong the Q-T interval include amiodarone, amitriptyline, astemizole, bepridil, disopyramide, erythromycin, haloperidol, imipramine, pimozide, procainamide, sotalol, and thioridazine. Effects may be additive; use with caution
- Enzyme inducers (aminoglutethimide, carbamazepine, phenobarbital, phenytoin, primidone, rifabutin, rifampin) may decrease quinidine blood levels
- Metoprolol: Increased metoprolol blood levels
- Mexiletine blood levels may be increased
- Nifedipine blood levels may be increased by quinidine; nifedipine may decrease quinidine blood levels
- Propafenone blood levels may be increased
- Propranolol blood levels may be increased
- Ritonavir, nelfinavir and amprenavir may increase quinidine levels and toxicity; concurrent use is contraindicated
- Sparfloxacin, gatifloxacin, and moxifloxacin may result in additional prolongation of the Q-T interval; concurrent use is contraindicated
- Timolol blood levels may be increased
- Urinary alkalinizers (antacids, sodium bicarbonate, acetazolamide) increase quinidine blood levels
- Verapamil and diltiazem increase quinidine blood levels
- Warfarin effects may be increased by quinidine; monitor INR closely during addition or withdrawal of quinidine

**Usual Dosage Dosage expressed in terms of the salt: 267 mg of quinidine gluconate = 200 mg of quinidine sulfate.**

Children: Test dose for idiosyncratic reaction (sulfate, oral or gluconate, I.M.): 2 mg/kg or 60 mg/m$^2$

Oral (quinidine sulfate): 15-60 mg/kg/day in 4-5 divided doses or 6 mg/kg every 4-6 hours; usual 30 mg/kg/day or 900 mg/m$^2$/day given in 5 daily doses

(Continued)

## Quinidine *(Continued)*

I.V. **not** recommended (quinidine gluconate): 2-10 mg/kg/dose given at a rate ≤10 mg/minute every 3-6 hours as needed

Adults: Test dose: Oral, I.M.: 200 mg administered several hours before full dosage (to determine possibility of idiosyncratic reaction)

Oral (for malaria):

Sulfate: 100-600 mg/dose every 4-6 hours; begin at 200 mg/dose and titrate to desired effect (maximum daily dose: 3-4 g)

Gluconate: 324-972 mg every 8-12 hours

I.M.: 400 mg/dose every 2-6 hours; initial dose: 600 mg (gluconate)

I.V.: 200-400 mg/dose diluted and given at a rate ≤10 mg/minute; may require as much as 500-750 mg

**Dosing adjustment in renal impairment:** $Cl_{cr}$ <10 mL/minute: Administer 75% of normal dose.

Hemodialysis: Slightly hemodialyzable (5% to 20%); 200 mg supplemental dose posthemodialysis is recommended.

Peritoneal dialysis: Not dialyzable (0% to 5%)

**Dosing adjustment/comments in hepatic impairment:** Larger loading dose may be indicated, reduce maintenance doses by 50% and monitor serum levels closely.

**Patient Information** Take exactly as directed, around-the-clock; do not take additional doses or discontinue without consulting prescriber. Do not crush, chew, or break sustained release capsules. You will need regular cardiac checkups and blood tests while taking this medication. You may experience dizziness, drowsiness, or visual changes (use caution when driving or engaging in tasks requiring alertness until response to drug is known); abnormal taste, nausea or vomiting, or loss of appetite (small frequent meals, frequent mouth care, chewing gum, or sucking lozenges may help); headaches (prescriber may recommend mild analgesic); or diarrhea (exercise, yogurt, or boiled milk may help - if persistent consult prescriber). Report chest pain, palpitation, or erratic heartbeat; difficulty breathing or wheezing; CNS changes (confusion, delirium, fever, consistent dizziness); skin rash; sense of fullness or ringing in ears; or changes in vision.

**Nursing Implications** Do not crush sustained release drug product

**Dosage Forms**

Injection, as gluconate: 80 mg/mL (10 mL)

Tablet, as polygalacturonate: 275 mg

Tablet, as sulfate: 200 mg, 300 mg

Tablet:

Sustained action, as sulfate: 300 mg

Sustained release, as gluconate: 324 mg

- **Quinidine Gluconate** *see* Quinidine *on page 485*
- **Quinidine Polygalacturonate** *see* Quinidine *on page 485*
- **Quinidine Sulfate** *see* Quinidine *on page 485*

## Quinine (KWYE nine)

**U.S. Brand Names** Formula Q®

**Pharmacologic Category** Antimalarial Agent

**Use** In conjunction with other antimalarial agents, suppression or treatment of chloroquine-resistant *P. falciparum* malaria; treatment of *Babesia microti* infection in conjunction with clindamycin; prevention and treatment of nocturnal recumbency leg muscle cramps

**Effects on Mental Status** None reported

**Effects on Psychiatric Treatment** Barbiturates and carbamazepine may decrease serum concentrations of quinine; CYP2D6 inhibitor; may interact with TCAs or beta-blockers; monitor

**Pregnancy Risk Factor** X

**Contraindications** Tinnitus, optic neuritis, G-6-PD deficiency, hypersensitivity to quinine or any component, history of black water fever, and thrombocytopenia with quinine or quinidine

**Warnings/Precautions** Use with caution in patients with cardiac arrhythmias (quinine has quinidine-like activity) and in patients with myasthenia gravis

**Adverse Reactions**

Percentage unknown: Cinchonism (risk of cinchonism is directly related to dose and duration of therapy): Blurred vision, diarrhea, nausea, severe headache, tinnitus, vomiting

<1%: Anginal symptoms, diplopia, epigastric pain, fever, flushing of the skin, hemolysis in G-6-PD deficiency, hepatitis, hypersensitivity reactions, hypoglycemia, impaired hearing, nightblindness, optic atrophy, pruritus, rash, thrombocytopenia

**Overdosage/Toxicology**

Signs and symptoms of mild toxicity include nausea, vomiting, and cinchonism; severe intoxication may cause ataxia, obtundation, convulsions, coma, and respiratory arrest; with massive intoxication quinidine-like cardiotoxicity (hypotension, QRS and Q-T interval prolongation, A-V block, and ventricular arrhythmias) may be fatal; retinal toxicity occurs 9-10 hours after ingestion (blurred vision, impaired color perception, constriction of visual fields and blindness); other toxic effects include hypokalemia, hypoglycemia, hemolysis and congenital malformations when taken during pregnancy.

Treatment: Includes symptomatic therapy with conventional agents (anticonvulsants, fluids, positioning, vasoconstrictors, antiarrhythmias). **Note:** Avoid type 1a and 1c antiarrhythmic drugs; treat cardiotoxicity with sodium bicarbonate; dialysis and hemoperfusion procedures are ineffective in enhancing elimination.

**Drug Interactions** CYP3A3/4 enzyme substrate; CYP3A3/4 enzyme inhibitor

Decreased effect: Phenobarbital, phenytoin, aluminum salt antacids, and rifampin may decrease quinine serum concentrations

Increased toxicity:

To avoid risk of seizures and cardiac arrest, delay mefloquine dosing at least 12 hours after last dose of quinine

Beta-blockers + quinine may increase bradycardia

Quinine may enhance coumarin anticoagulants and potentiate nondepolarizing and depolarizing muscle relaxants

Quinine may inhibit metabolism of astemizole resulting in toxic levels and potentially life-threatening cardiotoxicity

Quinine may increase plasma concentration of digoxin by as much as twofold; closely monitor digoxin concentrations and decrease digoxin dose with initiation of quinine by ½

Verapamil, amiodarone, urinary alkalinizing agents, and cimetidine may increase quinine serum concentrations

**Usual Dosage** Oral:

Children:

Treatment of chloroquine-resistant malaria: 25-30 mg/kg/day in divided doses every 8 hours for 5-7 days in conjunction with another agent

Babesiosis: 25 mg/kg/day divided every 8 hours for 7 days

Adults:

Treatment of chloroquine-resistant malaria: 260-650 mg every 8 hours for 6-12 days in conjunction with another agent

Suppression of malaria: 325 mg twice daily and continued for 6 weeks after exposure

Babesiosis: 650 mg every 6-8 hours for 7 days

Leg cramps: 200-300 mg at bedtime

**Dosing interval/adjustment in renal impairment:**

$Cl_{cr}$ 10-50 mL/minute: Administer every 8-12 hours or 75% of normal dose

$Cl_{cr}$ <10 mL/minute: Administer every 24 hours or 30% to 50% of normal dose

Dialysis: Not removed

Peritoneal dialysis: Dose as for $Cl_{cr}$ <10 mL/min

Continuous arteriovenous or venovenous hemodiafiltration (CAVH) effects: Dose for $Cl_{cr}$ 10-50 mL/minute

**Patient Information** Take on schedule as directed, with full 8 oz of water. Do not chew or crush sustained release tablets. You will need to return for follow-up blood tests. You may experience GI distress (taking medication with food, and frequent small meals may help). You may experience dizziness, changes in mentation, insomnia, headache, or visual disturbances (use caution when driving or engaging in tasks requiring alertness until response to drug is known). May discolor urine (black/brown/dark). Report persistent sore throat, fever, chills, flu-like signs, ringing in ears, vision disturbances, or unusual bruising or bleeding. Seek emergency help for palpitations or chest pain.

**Dosage Forms**

Capsule, as sulfate: 200 mg, 260 mg, 325 mg

Tablet, as sulfate: 260 mg

- **Quinora®** *see* Quinidine *on page 485*
- **Quinsana Plus® [OTC]** *see* Tolnaftate *on page 555*

## Quinupristin and Dalfopristin

(kwi NYOO pris tin & dal FOE pris tin)

**U.S. Brand Names** Synercid®

**Pharmacologic Category** Antibiotic, Streptogramin

**Use** Treatment of serious or life-threatening infections associated with vancomycin-resistant *Enterococcus faecium* bacteremia; treatment of complicated skin and skin structure infections caused by methicillin-susceptible *Staphylococcus aureus* or *Streptococcus pyogenes*

Has been studied in the treatment of a variety of infections caused by *Enterococcus faecium* (not *E. fecalis*) including vancomycin-resistant strains. May also be effective in the treatment of serious infections caused by *Staphylococcus* species including those resistant to methicillin.

**Effects on Mental Status** May rarely cause anxiety, confusion, or insomnia

**Effects on Psychiatric Treatment** May rarely produce pancytopenia; caution with clozapine and carbamazepine

**Usual Dosage**

Adults: I.V.:

Vancomycin-resistant *Enterococcus faecium:* 7.5 mg/kg every 8 hours

Complicated skin and skin structure infection: 7.5 mg/kg every 12 hours

**Dosage adjustment in renal impairment:** No adjustment required in renal failure, hemodialysis, or peritoneal dialysis

**Dosage adjustment in hepatic impairment:** Pharmacokinetic data suggest dosage adjustment may be necessary; however, specific recommendations have not been proposed

Elderly: No dosage adjustment is required

**Dosage Forms** Powder for injection: 500 mg (350 mg dalfopristin and 150 mg quinupristin)

- **R-51619** *see* Cisapride *on page 124*

## Rabeprazole (ra BE pray zole)

**U.S. Brand Names** Aciphex™

**Synonyms** Pariprazole

**Pharmacologic Category** Gastric Acid Secretion Inhibitor

**Use** Short-term (4-8 weeks) treatment and maintenance of erosive or ulcerative gastroesophageal reflux disease (GERD); short-term (up to 4 weeks) treatment of duodenal ulcers; long-term treatment of pathological hypersecretory conditions, including Zollinger-Ellison syndrome. Also, possibly used for *H. pylori* eradication, symptomatic GERD, maintenance of healing of GERD, and maintenance of duodenal ulcer

**Effects on Mental Status** May cause insomnia, anxiety, dizziness, depression, nervousness, somnolence, vertigo, convulsions, abnormal dreams; may rarely cause agitation, amnesia, confusion, extrapyramidal syndrome

**Effects on Psychiatric Treatment** None reported

**Pregnancy Risk Factor** B

**Contraindications** Contraindicated in patients with known hypersensitivity to rabeprazole, substituted benzimidazoles, or to any component of the formulation

**Warnings/Precautions** Severe hepatic impairment; relief of symptoms with rabeprazole does not preclude the presence of a gastric malignancy

**Adverse Reactions**

1% to 10%: Central nervous system: Headache

<1%:

Body as a whole: Weakness, fever, allergic reaction, chills, malaise, chest pain substernal, neck rigidity, photosensitivity reaction

Rare: Abdomen enlarged, face edema, hangover effect

Cardiovascular system: Hypertension, myocardial infarct, electrocardiogram abnormal, migraine, syncope, angina pectoris, bundle branch block, palpitation, sinus bradycardia, tachycardia

Rare: Bradycardia, pulmonary embolus, supraventricular tachycardia

Central nervous system: Insomnia, anxiety, dizziness, depression, nervousness, somnolence, hypertonia, neuralgia, vertigo, convulsions, abnormal dreams, libido decreased, neuropathy, paresthesia, tremor

Rare: Agitation, amnesia, confusion, extrapyramidal syndrome, hyperkinesia

Digestive system: Diarrhea, nausea, abdominal pain, vomiting, dyspepsia, flatulence, constipation, dry mouth, eructation, gastroenteritis, rectal hemorrhage, melena, anorexia, cholelithiasis, mouth ulceration, stomatitis, dysphagia, gingivitis, cholecystitis, increased appetite, abnormal stools, colitis, esophagitis, glossitis, pancreatitis, proctitis

Rare: Bloody diarrhea, cholangitis, duodenitis, gastrointestinal hemorrhage, hepatic encephalopathy, hepatitis, hepatoma, liver fatty deposit, salivary gland enlargement, thirst

Endocrine system: Hyperthyroidism, hypothyroidism

Hemic & lymphatic system: Anemia, ecchymosis, lymphadenopathy, hypochromic anemia

Metabolic & nutritional disorders: Peripheral edema, edema, weight gain, gout, dehydration, weight loss

Neuromuscular & skeletal: Myalgia, arthritis, leg cramps, bone pain, arthrosis, bursitis

Rare: Twitching

Respiratory system: Dyspnea, asthma, epistaxis, laryngitis, hiccups, hyperventilation

Rare: Apnea, hypoventilation

Skin & appendages: Rash, pruritus, sweating, urticaria, alopecia

Rare: Dry skin, herpes zoster, psoriasis, skin discoloration

Special senses: Cataract, amblyopia, glaucoma, dry eyes, abnormal vision, tinnitus, otitis media

Rare: Corneal opacity, blurry vision, diplopia, deafness, eye pain, retinal degeneration, strabismus

Urogenital system: Cystitis, urinary frequency, dysmenorrhea, dysuria, kidney calculus, metrorrhagia, polyuria

Rare: Breast enlargement, hematuria, impotence, leukorrhea, menorrhagia, orchitis, urinary incontinence

**Overdosage/Toxicology** There has been no experience with large overdoses with rabeprazole. Seven reports of accidental overdosage with rabeprazole have been received. The maximum reported overdose was 80 mg. There were no clinical signs of symptoms associated with any reported overdose. Patients with Zollinger-Ellison syndrome have been treated with up to 120 mg/day. No specific antidote for rabeprazole is known. The single oral dose of 2000 mg/kg was not lethal to dogs.

**Drug Interactions** Cytochrome P-450 inhibitor (extremely high concentrations); may alter the absorption of pH-dependent drugs (eg, ketoconazole, digoxin)

**Usual Dosage** Adults >18 years and Elderly:

GERD: 20 mg once daily for 4-8 weeks; maintenance: 20 mg once daily

Duodenal ulcer: 20 mg/day after breakfast for 4 weeks

Hypersecretory conditions: 60 mg once daily; dose may need to be adjusted as necessary. Doses as high as 100 mg and 60 mg twice daily have been used.

**Patient Information** Swallow whole - do not crush, chew, or split tablet; take before eating

**Nursing Implications** Do not crush tablet

**Dosage Forms** Tablet, delayed release (enteric coated): 20 mg

- **Racemic Amphetamine Sulfate** *see* Amphetamine *on page 39*
- **Racemic Epinephrine** *see* Epinephrine *on page 195*
- **Radix** *see* Valerian *on page 577*
- **R-albuterol** *see* Levalbuterol *on page 310*

## Raloxifene (ral OX i feen)

**U.S. Brand Names** Evista®

**Synonyms** Keoxifene Hydrochloride

**Pharmacologic Category** Selective Estrogen Receptor Modulator (SERM)

**Use** Prevention and treatment of osteoporosis in postmenopausal women

**Effects on Mental Status** May cause insomnia or depression

**Effects on Psychiatric Treatment** None reported

**Pregnancy Risk Factor** X

**Contraindications** Pregnancy; prior hypersensitivity to raloxifene; active thromboembolic disorder; not intended for use in premenopausal women

**Warnings/Precautions** History of venous thromboembolism/pulmonary embolism; patients with cardiovascular disease; history of cervical/uterine carcinoma; renal/hepatic insufficiency (however, pharmacokinetic data are lacking); concurrent use of estrogens

**Adverse Reactions** ≥2%:

Cardiovascular: Chest pain

Central nervous system: Migraine, depression, insomnia, fever

Dermatologic: Rash

Endocrine & metabolic: Hot flashes

Gastrointestinal: Nausea, dyspepsia, vomiting, flatulence, gastroenteritis, weight gain

Genitourinary: Vaginitis, urinary tract infection, cystitis, leukorrhea

Neuromuscular & skeletal: Leg cramps, arthralgia, myalgia, arthritis

Respiratory: Sinusitis, pharyngitis, cough, pneumonia, laryngitis

Miscellaneous: Infection, flu syndrome, diaphoresis

**Overdosage/Toxicology**

Signs and symptoms: Incidence of overdose in humans has not been reported. In an 8-week study of postmenopausal women, a dose of raloxifene 600 mg/day was safely tolerated. No mortality was seen after a single oral dose in rats or mice at 810 times the human dose for rats and 405 times the human dose for mice.

Treatment: There is no specific antidote for raloxifene

**Drug Interactions** Decreased effects: Ampicillin and cholestyramine decreases raloxifene absorption

**Usual Dosage** Adults: Female: Oral: 60 mg/day which may be administered any time of the day without regard to meals

**Patient Information** May be taken at any time of day without regard to meals. This medication is given to reduce incidence of osteoporosis; it will not reduce hot flashes or flushing. You may experience flu-like symptoms at beginning of therapy (these may resolve with use). Mild analgesics may reduce joint pain. Rest and cool environment may reduce hot flashes. Report fever; acute migraine; insomnia or emotional depression; unusual weight gain; unresolved gastric distress; urinary infection or vaginal burning or itching; chest pain; or swelling, warmth, or pain in calves.

**Dosage Forms** Tablet, as hydrochloride: 60 mg

## Ramipril (ra MI pril)

**Related Information**

Angiotensin-Related Agents Comparison Chart *on page 700*

**U.S. Brand Names** Altace™

**Pharmacologic Category** Angiotensin-Converting Enzyme (ACE) Inhibitors

**Use** Treatment of hypertension, alone or in combination with thiazide diuretics; treatment of congestive heart failure; treatment of left ventricular dysfunction after myocardial infarction

**Effects on Mental Status** May cause dizziness or drowsiness; may rarely cause nervousness, amnesia, insomnia, or depression

**Effects on Psychiatric Treatment** May cause neutropenia; use caution with clozapine and carbamazepine; may decrease lithium clearance resulting in an increase in serum lithium levels and potential lithium toxicity; monitor serum lithium levels

**Pregnancy Risk Factor** C (1st trimester); D (2nd and 3rd trimester)

**Contraindications** Hypersensitivity to ramipril or any component; angioedema related to previous treatment with an ACE inhibitor; bilateral renal

(Continued)

## Ramipril *(Continued)*

artery stenosis; primary hyperaldosteronism; pregnancy (2nd and 3rd trimesters)

**Warnings/Precautions** Anaphylactic reactions can occur. Angioedema can occur at any time during treatment (especially following first dose). Careful blood pressure monitoring with first dose (hypotension can occur especially in volume depleted patients). Dosage adjustment needed in renal impairment. Use with caution in hypovolemia; collagen vascular diseases; valvular stenosis (particularly aortic stenosis); hyperkalemia; or before, during, or immediately after anesthesia. Avoid rapid dosage escalation, which may lead to renal insufficiency. Neutropenia/agranulocytosis with myeloid hyperplasia can rarely occur. If patient has renal impairment then a baseline WBC with differential and serum creatinine should be evaluated and monitored closely during the first 3 months of therapy. Hypersensitivity reactions may be seen during hemodialysis with high-flux dialysis membranes (eg, AN69). Use with caution in unilateral renal artery stenosis and pre-existing renal insufficiency.

**Adverse Reactions**

>10% Respiratory: Cough (12%)

<1%: Abdominal pain (rarely occurs but may with enzyme changes which suggest pancreatitis), alopecia, amnesia, angioedema rash, angina, anorexia, arrhythmia, arthralgia, arthritis, constipation, convulsions, decreased hemoglobin (rare), depression, dermatitis, diaphoresis diarrhea, dizziness, drowsiness, dysgeusia, dyspepsia, dysphagia, dyspnea, eosinophilia, epistaxis, fatigue, flu-like symptoms, headache, hyperkalemia (small increase in patients with renal dysfunction), hypotension, impotence, increased salivation, insomnia, malaise, muscle cramps, myalgia, myocardial infarction, nausea, nervousness, neuralgia, neuropathy, neutropenia, palpitations, paresthesia, photosensitivity, proteinuria, pruritus, rash, syncope, tinnitus, transient increases BUN/serum creatinine, tremor, vertigo, vomiting, weight gain, xerostomia

**Overdosage/Toxicology**

Signs and symptoms; Mild hypotension has been the only toxic effect seen with acute overdose. Bradycardia may also occur; mild hyperkalemia may occur even with therapeutic doses, especially in patients with renal insufficiency and those taking NSAIDs.

Treatment: Following initiation of essential overdose management, toxic symptom treatment and supportive treatment should be initiated. Hypotension usually responds to I.V. fluids or Trendelenburg positioning.

**Drug Interactions**

Alpha$_1$ blockers: Hypotensive effect increased

Aspirin: The effects of ACE inhibitors may be blunted by aspirin administration, particularly at higher dosages

Diuretics: Hypovolemia due to diuretics may precipitate acute hypotensive events or acute renal failure

Insulin: Risk of hypoglycemia may be increased

Lithium: Risk of lithium toxicity may be increased; monitor lithium levels, especially the first 4 weeks of therapy

Mercaptopurine: Risk of neutropenia may be increased

NSAIDs may decrease ACE inhibitor efficacy and/or increase risk of adverse renal effects

Potassium-sparing diuretics (amiloride, spironolactone, triamterene): Increased risk of hyperkalemia

Potassium supplements may increase the risk of hyperkalemia

Trimethoprim (high dose) may increase the risk of hyperkalemia

**Usual Dosage** Adults: Oral:

Hypertension: 2.5-5 mg once daily, maximum: 20 mg/day

Heart failure postmyocardial infarction: Initial: 2.5 mg twice daily titrated upward, if possible, to 5 mg twice daily.

**Note:** The dose of any concomitant diuretic should be reduced. If the diuretic cannot be discontinued, initiate therapy with 1.25 mg. After the initial dose, the patient should be monitored carefully until blood pressure has stabilized.

**Dosing adjustment in renal impairment:**

$Cl_{cr}$ <40 mL/minute: Administer 25% of normal dose.

Renal failure and hypertension: Administer 1.25 mg once daily, titrated upward as possible.

Renal failure and heart failure: Administer 1.25 mg once daily, increasing to 1.25 mg twice daily up to 2.5 mg twice daily as tolerated.

**Patient Information** Take exactly as directed; do not discontinue without consulting prescriber. Take first dose at bedtime. This drug does not eliminate need for diet or exercise regimen as recommended by prescriber. Do not take potassium supplements or salt substitutes containing potassium without consulting prescriber. May cause dizziness, fainting, lightheadedness (use caution when driving or engaging in tasks requiring alertness until response to drug is known); postural hypotension (use caution when rising from lying or sitting position or climbing stairs); nausea or vomiting (small frequent meals, frequent mouth care, sucking lozenges, or chewing gum may help) - report if these persist. Report chest pain or palpitations; difficulty in breathing or unusual cough; or other persistent adverse reactions.

**Nursing Implications** May cause depression in some patients; discontinue if angioedema of the face, extremities, lips, tongue, or glottis occurs; watch for hypotensive effects within 1-3 hours of first dose or new higher dose; may be mixed in water, apple juice, or applesauce and will remain stable for 48 hours if refrigerated or 24 hours at room temperature

**Dosage Forms** Capsule: 1.25 mg, 2.5 mg, 5 mg, 10 mg

♦ **Ramses® [OTC]** *see* Nonoxynol 9 *on page 398*

## Ranitidine Bismuth Citrate (ra NI ti deen BIZ muth SIT rate)

**U.S. Brand Names** Tritec®

**Synonyms** GR122311X; RBC

**Pharmacologic Category** Histamine $H_2$ Antagonist

**Use** In combination with clarithromycin for the treatment of active duodenal ulcer associated with *H. pylori* infection; not to be used as monotherapy

**Effects on Mental Status** May cause dizziness

**Effects on Psychiatric Treatment** May cause anemia; use caution with clozapine and carbamazepine

**Pregnancy Risk Factor** C

**Contraindications** Hypersensitivity to ranitidine or bismuth compounds or components; acute porphyria

**Warnings/Precautions** Avoid use in patients with $Cl_{cr}$ <25 mL/minute; do not use for maintenance therapy or for >16 weeks/year

**Adverse Reactions**

>1%:

Central nervous system: Headache (14%), dizziness (1% to 2%)

Gastrointestinal: Diarrhea (5%), nausea/vomiting (3%), constipation (2%), abdominal pain, gastric upset (<10%), darkening of the tongue and/or stool (60% to 70%), taste disturbance (11%)

Miscellaneous: Flu-like symptoms (2%)

<1%: Anemia, elevated LFTs, pruritus, rash, thrombocytopenia

**Drug Interactions** See individual monographs

Increased effect: Optimal antimicrobial effects of ranitidine bismuth citrate occur when the drug is taken with food

**Usual Dosage** Adults: Oral: 400 mg twice daily for 4 weeks with clarithromycin 500 mg 2 times/day for first 2 week

**Dosing adjustment in renal impairment:** Not recommended with $Cl_{cr}$ <25 mL/minute

**Dosing adjustment in hepatic impairment:** No dosage change necessary

**Note:** Most patients not eradicated of *H. pylori* following an adequate course of therapy that includes clarithromycin will have clarithromycin-resistant isolates and should be treated with an alternative multiple drug regimen

**Dietary Considerations** May be taken without regard to food

**Patient Information** Take as directed, with food. Do not supplement therapy with OTC medications. This drug may cause darkening of tongue or stool and may change your taste sensation. Report unresolved headache (prescriber may recommend something for relief), dizziness, diarrhea, constipation (prescriber may recommend something for relief), weakness, or loss of appetite.

**Dosage Forms** Tablet: 400 mg (ranitidine 162 mg, trivalent bismuth 128 mg, and citrate 110 mg)

## Ranitidine Hydrochloride (ra NI ti deen hye droe KLOR ide)

**U.S. Brand Names** Zantac®; Zantac® 75 [OTC]

**Canadian Brand Names** Apo®-Ranitidine; Novo-Ranidine; Nu-Ranit

**Pharmacologic Category** Histamine $H_2$ Antagonist

**Use** Short-term treatment of active duodenal ulcers and benign gastric ulcers; long-term prophylaxis of duodenal ulcer and gastric hypersecretory states, gastroesophageal reflux, recurrent postoperative ulcer, upper GI bleeding, prevention of acid-aspiration pneumonitis during surgery, and prevention of stress-induced ulcers; causes fewer interactions than cimetidine

**Effects on Mental Status** May cause drowsiness or dizziness

**Effects on Psychiatric Treatment** May rarely cause agranulocytosis; use caution with clozapine and carbamazepine; concurrent use with diazepam may reduce diazepam's effectiveness

**Pregnancy Risk Factor** B

**Contraindications** Hypersensitivity to ranitidine or any component

**Warnings/Precautions** Use with caution in children <12 years of age; use with caution in patients with liver and renal impairment; dosage modification required in patients with renal impairment; long-term therapy may cause vitamin $B_{12}$ deficiency

**Adverse Reactions**

1% to 10%:

Central nervous system: Dizziness, sedation, malaise, headache, drowsiness

Dermatologic: Rash

Gastrointestinal: Constipation, nausea, vomiting, diarrhea

<1%: Agranulocytosis, arthralgia, bradycardia, bronchospasm, confusion, fever, gynecomastia, hepatitis, neutropenia, tachycardia, thrombocytopenia

**Overdosage/Toxicology**
Signs and symptoms: Muscular tremors, vomiting, rapid respiration, renal failure, CNS depression
Treatment: Primarily symptomatic and supportive

**Drug Interactions** CYP2D6 and 3A3/4 enzyme inhibitor
Decreased effect: Variable effects on warfarin; antacids may decrease absorption of ranitidine; ketoconazole and itraconazole absorptions are decreased; may produce altered serum levels of procainamide and ferrous sulfate; decreased effect of nondepolarizing muscle relaxants, cefpodoxime, cyanocobalamin (decreased absorption), diazepam, oxaprozin
Decreased toxicity of atropine
Increased toxicity of cyclosporine (increased serum creatinine), gentamicin (neuromuscular blockade), glipizide, glyburide, midazolam (increased concentrations), metoprolol, pentoxifylline, phenytoin, quinidine

**Usual Dosage** Giving oral dose at 6 PM may be better than 10 PM bedtime, the highest acid production usually starts at approximately 7 PM, thus giving at 6 PM controls acid secretion better

Children:
Oral: 1.25-2.5 mg/kg/dose every 12 hours; maximum: 300 mg/day
I.M., I.V.: 0.75-1.5 mg/kg/dose every 6-8 hours, maximum daily dose: 400 mg
Continuous infusion: 0.1-0.25 mg/kg/hour (preferred for stress ulcer prophylaxis in patients with concurrent maintenance I.V.s or TPNs)

Adults:
Short-term treatment of ulceration: 150 mg/dose twice daily or 300 mg at bedtime
Prophylaxis of recurrent duodenal ulcer: Oral: 150 mg at bedtime
Gastric hypersecretory conditions:
Oral: 150 mg twice daily, up to 600mg/day
I.M., I.V.: 50 mg/dose every 6-8 hours (dose not to exceed 400 mg/day)
I.V.: 50 mg/dose IVPB every 6-8 hours (dose not to exceed 400 mg/day)

**or**

Continuous I.V. infusion: Initial: 50 mg IVPB, followed by 6.25 mg/hour titrated to gastric pH >4.0 for prophylaxis or >7.0 for treatment; **continuous I.V. infusion is preferred in patients with active bleeding**
Gastric hypersecretory conditions: Doses up to 2.5 mg/kg/hour (220 mg/hour) have been used

**Dosing adjustment in renal impairment:**
$Cl_{cr}$ 10-50 mL/minute: Administer at 75% of normal dose or administer every 18-24 hours
$Cl_{cr}$ <10 mL/minute: Administer at 50% of normal dose or administer every 18-24 hours

Hemodialysis: Slightly dialyzable (5% to 20%)

**Dosing adjustment/comments in hepatic disease**: Unchanged

**Patient Information** Take exactly as directed (at meals and bedtime); do not increase dose - may take several days before you notice relief. If antacids are approved by prescriber, allow 1 hour between antacid and ranitidine. Avoid OTC medications, especially cold or cough medication and aspirin or anything containing aspirin. Follow diet as prescriber recommends. You may experience constipation or diarrhea (request assistance from prescriber); nausea or vomiting (frequent small meals, frequent mouth care, sucking lozenges, or chewing gum may help); impotence or loss of libido (reversible when drug is discontinued); drowsiness, dizziness, or fatigue (use caution when driving or engaging in tasks requiring alertness until response to drug is known). Report skin rash, fever, sore throat, tarry stools, changes in CNS, muscle or joint pain, yellowing of skin or eyes, and change in color of urine or stool.

**Nursing Implications** I.M. solution does not need to be diluted before use; monitor creatinine clearance for renal impairment; observe caution in patients with renal function impairment and hepatic function impairment

**Dosage Forms**
Capsule (GELdose™): 150 mg, 300 mg
Granules, effervescent (EFFERdose™): 150 mg
Infusion, preservative free, in NaCl 0.45%: 1 mg/mL (50 mL)
Injection: 25 mg/mL (2 mL, 10 mL, 40 mL)
Syrup (peppermint flavor): 15 mg/mL (473 mL)
Tablet: 75 mg [OTC]; 150 mg, 300 mg
Tablet, effervescent (EFFERdose™): 150 mg

## Rapacuronium (ra pa kyoo ROE nee um)

**U.S. Brand Names** Raplon™
**Pharmacologic Category** Neuromuscular Blocker Agent, Nondepolarizing
**Use** Adjunct to general anesthesia to facilitate tracheal intubation; to provide skeletal muscle relaxation during surgical procedures; does not relieve pain
**Effects on Mental Status** May rarely produce anxiety and confusion
**Effects on Psychiatric Treatment** May cause hypotension, concurrent use with psychotropics may exacerbate this effect; lithium and beta-blockers may potentiate its effects while carbamazepine may antagonize effects
**Usual Dosage** I.V. (do not administer I.M.):
Children 1 month to 12 years: Initial: 2 mg/kg. Repeat dosing is not recommended in pediatric patients.
Children 13-17 years: Clinicians should consider the physical maturity, height and weight of the patient in determining the dose. Adults (1.5 mg/kg), pediatric (2 mg/kg) and Cesarean section (2.5 mg/kg) dosing recommendations may serve as a general guideline in determining an intubating dose in this age group.
Adults: Tracheal Intubation:
Initial: Short surgical procedures: 1.5 mg/kg; Cesarean section: 2.5 mg/kg
Repeat dosing: Up to three maintenance doses of 0.5 mg/kg, administered at 25% recovery of control T1 may be administered. **Note:** The duration of neuromuscular blockade increases with each additional dose.
Elderly: No dosing adjustment is recommended in geriatric patients
**Dosage Forms** Powder for injection: 100 mg (5 mL); 200 mg (10 mL)

- **Rapamune®** *see* Sirolimus *on page 513*
- **Raplon™** *see* Rapacuronium *on page 489*
- **Raudixin®** *see* Rauwolfia Serpentina *on page 489*
- **Rauverid®** *see* Rauwolfia Serpentina *on page 489*

## Rauwolfia Serpentina (rah WOOL fee a ser pen TEEN ah)

**U.S. Brand Names** Raudixin®; Rauverid®; Wolfina®
**Pharmacologic Category** Rauwolfia Alkaloid
**Use** Mild essential hypertension; relief of agitated psychotic states
**Effects on Mental Status** May cause drowsiness, fatigue, CNS depression
**Effects on Psychiatric Treatment** Use caution in patients with depression; reported usefulness in psychotic agitation
**Usual Dosage** Adults: Oral: 200-400 mg/day in 2 divided doses
**Dosage Forms** Tablet: 50 mg, 100 mg

- **Raxar®** *see* Grepafloxacin (***Voluntarily Withdrawn From Market***) *on page 255*
- **RBC** *see* Ranitidine Bismuth Citrate *on page 488*
- **R & C® Shampoo [OTC]** *see* Pyrethrins *on page 480*
- **Rea-Lo® [OTC]** *see* Urea *on page 576*
- **Rebetron™** *see* Interferon Alfa-2b and Ribavirin Combination Pack *on page 289*
- **Recombinate™** *see* Antihemophilic Factor (Recombinant) *on page 46*
- **Recombivax HB®** *see* Hepatitis B Vaccine *on page 266*
- **Redutemp® [OTC]** *see* Acetaminophen *on page 14*
- **Red Valerian** *see* Valerian *on page 577*
- **Reese's® Pinworm Medicine [OTC]** *see* Pyrantel Pamoate *on page 480*
- **Refludan™** *see* Lepirudin *on page 308*
- **Refresh® Ophthalmic Solution [OTC]** *see* Artificial Tears *on page 48*
- **Refresh® Plus Ophthalmic Solution [OTC]** *see* Artificial Tears *on page 48*
- **Regitine®** *see* Phentolamine *on page 438*
- **Reglan®** *see* Metoclopramide *on page 360*
- **Regonol® Injection** *see* Pyridostigmine *on page 481*
- **Regranex®** *see* Becaplermin *on page 59*
- **Regular (Concentrated) Iletin® II U-500** *see* Insulin Preparations *on page 287*
- **Regular Iletin® I** *see* Insulin Preparations *on page 287*
- **Regular Insulin** *see* Insulin Preparations *on page 287*
- **Regular Purified Pork Insulin** *see* Insulin Preparations *on page 287*
- **Regular Strength Bayer® Enteric 500 Aspirin [OTC]** *see* Aspirin *on page 49*
- **Regulax SS® [OTC]** *see* Docusate *on page 179*
- **Reguloid® [OTC]** *see* Psyllium *on page 479*
- **Relafen®** *see* Nabumetone *on page 378*
- **Relefact® TRH Injection** *see* Protirelin *on page 477*
- **Relenza®** *see* Zanamivir *on page 591*
- **Relief® Ophthalmic Solution** *see* Phenylephrine *on page 439*
- **Remeron®** *see* Mirtazapine *on page 368*

♦ **Remicade™** *see* Infliximab *on page 287*

## Remifentanil (rem i FEN ta nil)

**Related Information**
Narcotic Agonists Comparison Chart *on page 720*

**U.S. Brand Names** Ultiva™

**Synonyms** GI87084B

**Pharmacologic Category** Analgesic, Narcotic

**Use** Analgesic for use during general anesthesia for continued analgesia

**Effects on Mental Status** May cause dizziness or agitation

**Effects on Psychiatric Treatment** None reported

**Pregnancy Risk Factor** C

**Contraindications** Not for intrathecal or epidural administration, due to the presence of glycine in the formulation, it is also contraindicated in patients with a known hypersensitivity to remifentanil, fentanyl or fentanyl analogs; interruption of an infusion will result in offset of effects within 5-10 minutes; the discontinuation of remifentanil infusion should be preceded by the establishment of adequate postoperative analgesia orders, especially for patients in whom postoperative pain is anticipated

**Warnings/Precautions** Remifentanil is not recommended as the sole agent in general anesthesia, because the loss of consciousness cannot be assured and due to the high incidence of apnea, hypotension, tachycardia and muscle rigidity; it should be administered by individuals specifically trained in the use of anesthetic agents and should not be used in diagnostic or therapeutic procedures outside the monitored anesthesia setting; resuscitative and intubation equipment should be readily available

**Adverse Reactions**
>10%: Gastrointestinal: Nausea, vomiting
1% to 10%:
- Cardiovascular: Hypotension, bradycardia, tachycardia, hypertension
- Central nervous system: Dizziness, headache, agitation, fever
- Dermatologic: Pruritus
- Ocular: Visual disturbances
- Respiratory: Respiratory depression, apnea, hypoxia
- Miscellaneous: Shivering, postoperative pain

**Overdosage/Toxicology**
Signs and symptoms: Apnea, chest wall rigidity, seizures, hypoxemia, hypotension and bradycardia
Treatment: Support of patient's airway, establish an I.V. line, administer intravenous fluids and administer naloxone 2 mg I.V. (0.01 mg/kg for children) with repeat administration as needed up to a total of 10 mg; glycopyrrolate or atropine may be useful for the treatment of bradycardia or hypotension

**Drug Interactions** Increased effect with CNS depressants

**Usual Dosage** Adults: I.V. continuous infusion:
During induction: 0.5-1 mcg/kg/minute
During maintenance:
- With nitrous oxide (66%): 0.4 mcg/kg/minute (range: 0.1-2 mcg/kg/min)
- With isoflurane: 0.25 mcg/kg/minute (range: 0.05-2 mcg/kg/min)
- With propofol: 0.25 mcg/kg/minute (range: 0.05-2 mcg/kg/min)

Continuation as an analgesic in immediate postoperative period: 0.1 mcg/kg/minute (range: 0.025-0.2 mcg/kg/min)

**Dosage Forms** Powder for injection, lyophilized: 1 mg/3 mL vial, 2 mg/5 mL vial, 5 mg/10 mL vial

♦ **Reminyl®** *see* Galantamine *on page 244*

♦ **Renagel®** *see* Sevelamer *on page 510*

♦ **Renese®** *see* Polythiazide *on page 452*

♦ **Renoquid®** *see* Sulfacytine *on page 523*

♦ **Renormax®** *see* Spirapril *on page 517*

♦ **Rentamine®** *see* Chlorpheniramine, Ephedrine, Phenylephrine, and Carbetapentane *on page 115*

♦ **ReoPro®** *see* Abciximab *on page 12*

## Repaglinide (re PAG li nide)

**Related Information**
Diabetes Mellitus Treatment *on page 782*
Hypoglycemic Drugs and Thiazolidinedione Information *on page 714*

**U.S. Brand Names** Prandin™

**Pharmacologic Category** Antidiabetic Agent (Miscellaneous)

**Use** Management of noninsulin-dependent diabetes mellitus (type 2)
An adjunct to diet and exercise to lower the blood glucose in patients with type 2 diabetes mellitus whose hyperglycemia cannot be controlled satisfactorily by diet and exercise alone
In combination with metformin to lower blood glucose in patients whose hyperglycemia cannot be controlled by exercise, diet and either agent alone

**Effects on Mental Status** None reported

**Effects on Psychiatric Treatment** Repaglinide is a CYP3A4 substrate; monitor glucose when used with an enzyme inducer (carbamazepine, barbiturates) or an inhibitor (nefazodone, fluvoxamine)

**Pregnancy Risk Factor** C

**Contraindications** Diabetic ketoacidosis, with or without coma (treat with insulin); type 1 diabetes; hypersensitivity to the drug or its inactive ingredients

**Warnings/Precautions** Use with caution in patients with hepatic impairment. All oral hypoglycemic agents are capable of producing hypoglycemia. Proper patient selection, dosage, and instructions to the patients are important to avoid hypoglycemic episodes. It may be necessary to discontinue repaglinide and administer insulin if the patient is exposed to stress (fever, trauma, infection, surgery).

Product labeling states oral hypoglycemic drugs may be associated with an increased cardiovascular mortality as compared to treatment with diet alone or diet plus insulin. Data to support this association are limited, and several studies, including a large prospective trial (UKPDS) have not supported an association.

**Adverse Reactions**
>10%:
- Central nervous system: Headache
- Endocrine & metabolic: Hyperglycemia, hypoglycemia, related symptoms

1% to 10%:
- Cardiovascular: Chest pain
- Gastrointestinal: Nausea, epigastric fullness, heartburn, constipation, diarrhea, anorexia, tooth disorder
- Genitourinary: Urinary tract infection
- Neuromuscular: Arthralgia, back pain, paresthesia
- Miscellaneous: Allergy

**Overdosage/Toxicology**
Signs and symptoms: Severe hypoglycemia, seizures, cerebral damage, tingling of lips and tongue, nausea, yawning, confusion, agitation, tachycardia, sweating, convulsions, stupor, and coma
Treatment: Intoxications are best managed with glucose administration (oral for milder hypoglycemia or by injection in more severe forms) and symptomatic management

**Drug Interactions** CYP3A4 enzyme substrate
Decreased effect: Drugs that induce cytochrome P-450 3A4 may increase metabolism of repaglinide (troglitazone rifampin, barbiturates, carbamazepine). Certain drugs (thiazides, diuretics, corticosteroids, phenothiazines, thyroid products, estrogens, oral contraceptives, phenytoin, nicotinic acid, sympathomimetics, calcium channel blockers, isoniazid) tend to produce hyperglycemia and may lead to loss of glycemic control.
Increased effect: Agents that inhibit cytochrome P-450 3A4 (ketoconazole, miconazole) and antibacterial agents (erythromycin) may increase repaglinide concentrations
Increased toxicity: Since this agent is highly protein bound, the toxic potential is increased when given concomitantly with other highly protein bound drugs (ie, phenylbutazone, oral anticoagulants, hydantoins, salicylates, NSAIDs, sulfonamides) - increase hypoglycemic effect

**Usual Dosage** Adults: Oral: Should be taken within 15 minutes of the meal, but time may vary from immediately preceding the meal to as long as 30 minutes before the meal

Initial: For patients not previously treated or whose Hb $A_{1c}$ is <8%, the starting dose is 0.5 mg. For patients previously treated with blood glucose-lowering agents whose Hb $A_{1c}$ is ≥8%, the initial dose is 1 or 2 mg before each meal.
- Dose adjustment: Determine dosing adjustments by blood glucose response, usually fasting blood glucose. Double the preprandial dose up to 4 mg until satisfactory blood glucose response is achieved. At least 1 week should elapse to assess response after each dose adjustment.
- Dose range: 0.5-4 mg taken with meals. Repaglinide may be dosed preprandial 2, 3 or 4 times/day in response to changes in the patient's meal pattern. Maximum recommended daily dose: 16 mg.

**Patients receiving other oral hypoglycemic agents:** When repaglinide is used to replace therapy with other oral hypoglycemic agents, it may be started the day after the final dose is given. Observe patients carefully for hypoglycemia because of potential overlapping of drug effects. When transferred from longer half-life sulfonylureas (eg, chlorpropamide), close monitoring may be indicated for up to ≥1 week.

**Combination therapy:** If repaglinide monotherapy does not result in adequate glycemic control, metformin may be added. Or, if metformin therapy does not provide adequate control, repaglinide may be added. The starting dose and dose adjustments for combination therapy are the same as repaglinide monotherapy. Carefully adjust the dose of each drug to determine the minimal dose required to achieve the desired pharmacologic effect. Failure to do so could result in an increase in the incidence of hypoglycemic episodes. Use appropriate monitoring of FPG and Hb $A_{1c}$ measurements to ensure that the patient is not subjected to excessive drug exposure or increased probability of secondary drug failure. If glucose is not achieved after a suitable trial of combination therapy, consider discontinuing these drugs and using insulin.

**Dosing adjustment/comments in renal impairment:** Initial dosage adjustment does not appear to be necessary, but make subsequent increases carefully in patients with renal function impairment or renal failure requiring hemodialysis

**Dosing adjustment in hepatic impairment:** Use conservative initial and maintenance doses and avoid use in severe disease

**Dietary Considerations**

Food: When given with food, the AUC of repaglinide is decreased; administer repaglinide before meals

Glucose: Decreases blood glucose concentration. Hypoglycemia may occur. Educate patients how to detect and treat hypoglycemia. Monitor for signs and symptoms of hypoglycemia. Administer glucose if necessary. Evaluate patient's diet and exercise regimen. May need to decrease or discontinue dose of sulfonylurea.

**Patient Information** Take this medication exactly as directed - 3-4 times a day, 15-30 minutes prior to a meal. If you skip a meal (or add an extra meal) skip (or add) a dose for that meal. Do not change dosage or discontinue without first consulting prescriber. It is important to follow dietary and lifestyle recommendations of prescriber. You will be instructed in signs of hypo-/hyperglycemia by prescriber or diabetic educator; be alert for adverse hypoglycemia (tachycardia, profuse perspiration, tingling of lips and tongue, seizures, or change in sensorium) and follow prescriber's instructions for intervention. You may experience mild side effects during first weeks of therapy (eg, headache, diarrhea, constipation, bloating); if these do not diminish, notify prescriber. Increasing dietary fiber or fluids and increasing exercise may reduce constipation (for persistent diarrhea consult prescriber). Mild analgesics may reduce headaches. Frequent mouth care, small frequent meals, chewing gum, sucking lozenges may help reduce nausea, vomiting, or heartburn. Report chest pain, palpitations, or irregular heartbeat; respiratory difficulty or symptoms of upper respiratory infection; urinary tract infection (burning or itching on urination); muscle pain or back pain; or persistent GI problems.

**Nursing Implications** Patients who are anorexic or NPO, may need to have their dose held to avoid hypoglycemia

**Dosage Forms** Tablet : 0.5 mg, 1 mg, 2 mg


- ♦ **Repan®** *see* Butalbital Compound and Acetaminophen *on page 80*
- ♦ **Reposans-10® Oral** *see* Chlordiazepoxide *on page 109*
- ♦ **Repronex™** *see* Menotropins *on page 340*
- ♦ **Requip™** *see* Ropinirole *on page 500*
- ♦ **Resaid®** *see* Chlorpheniramine and Phenylpropanolamine *on page 114*
- ♦ **Rescaps-D® S.R. Capsule** *see* Caramiphen and Phenylpropanolamine *on page 90*
- ♦ **Rescon Liquid [OTC]** *see* Chlorpheniramine and Phenylpropanolamine *on page 114*
- ♦ **Rescriptor®** *see* Delavirdine *on page 153*
- ♦ **Resectisol® Irrigation Solution** *see* Mannitol *on page 331*


## Reserpine (re SER peen)

**Generic Available** Yes

**U.S. Brand Names** Serpalan®

**Canadian Brand Names** Novo-Reserpine

**Synonyms** Reserpinum

**Pharmacologic Category** Rauwolfia Alkaloid

**Use** Management of mild to moderate hypertension

**Unlabeled use:** Management of tardive dyskinesia

**Pregnancy Risk Factor** C

**Contraindications** Hypersensitivity to reserpine or any component; active peptic ulcer disease, ulcerative colitis, history of mental depression (especially with suicidal tendencies); monoamine oxidase (MAO) inhibitors

**Warnings/Precautions** Discontinue reserpine 7 days before electroshock therapy; use with caution in patients with impaired renal function, inflammatory bowel disease, asthma, gallstones, or history of peptic ulcer disease, and the elderly. At high doses, significant mental depression, anxiety, or psychosis may occur (uncommon at dosages <0.25 mg/day). May cause orthostatic hypotension; use with caution in patients at risk of hypotension or in patients where transient hypotensive episodes would be poorly tolerated (cardiovascular disease or cerebrovascular disease). Some products may contain tartrazine.

**Adverse Reactions**

Cardiovascular: Peripheral edema, arrhythmias, bradycardia, chest pain, PVC, hypotension

Central nervous system: Dizziness, headache, nightmares, nervousness, drowsiness, fatigue, mental depression, parkinsonism, dull sensorium, syncope, paradoxical anxiety

Dermatologic: Rash, pruritus, flushing of skin

Gastrointestinal: Anorexia, diarrhea, dry mouth, nausea, vomiting, increased salivation, weight gain, increased gastric acid secretion

Genitourinary: Impotence, decreased libido

Hematologic: Thrombocytopenia purpura

Ocular: Blurred vision

Respiratory: Nasal congestion, dyspnea, epistaxis

**Overdosage/Toxicology**

Signs and symptoms: Hypotension, bradycardia, CNS depression, sedation, coma, hypothermia, miosis, tremors, diarrhea, vomiting

Treatment: Hypotension usually responds to I.V. fluids or Trendelenburg positioning. If unresponsive to these measures, the use of a parenteral inotrope may be required (eg, norepinephrine 0.1-0.2 mcg/kg/minute titrated to response). Anticholinergic agents may be useful in reducing the parkinsonian effects and bradycardia.

**Drug Interactions** MAO inhibitors: Reserpine may cause hypertensive reactions; use an alternative antihypertensive

**Stability** Protect oral dosage forms from light

**Mechanism of Action** Reduces blood pressure via depletion of sympathetic biogenic amines (norepinephrine and dopamine); this also commonly results in sedative effects

**Pharmacodynamics/kinetics**

Onset of antihypertensive effect: Within 3-6 days

Duration: 2-6 weeks

Absorption: Oral: ~40%

Distribution: Crosses the placenta; appears in breast milk

Protein binding: 96%

Metabolism: Extensively in the liver, >90%

Half-life: 50-100 hours

Elimination: Principal excretion in feces (30% to 60%) and small amounts in urine (10%)

**Usual Dosage** Oral (full antihypertensive effects may take as long as 3 weeks):

Children: 0.01-0.02 mg/kg/24 hours divided every 12 hours; maximum dose: 0.25 mg/day (not recommended in children)

Adults:

Hypertension: 0.1-0.25 mg/day in 1-2 doses; initial: 0.5 mg/day for 1-2 weeks; maintenance: reduce to 0.1-0.25 mg/day

Psychiatric: Initial: 0.5 mg/day; usual range: 0.1-1 mg

Elderly: Initial: 0.05 mg once daily, increasing by 0.05 mg every week as necessary

**Dosing adjustment in renal impairment:** $Cl_{cr}$ <10 mL/minute: Avoid use

Dialysis: Not removed by hemo or peritoneal dialysis; supplemental dose is not necessary

**Monitoring Parameters** Blood pressure, standing and sitting/supine

**Test Interactions** ↓ catecholamines (U)

**Patient Information** Take with food or milk; impotency is reversible; notify physician if a weight gain of more than 5 lb has taken place during therapy; may cause drowsiness, impair judgment and coordination

**Nursing Implications** Observe for mental depression and alert family members to report any symptoms

**Additional Information** Adverse effects are usually dose related, mild, and infrequent when administered for the management of hypertension

**Dosage Forms** Tablet: 0.1 mg, 0.25 mg


- ♦ **Reserpinum** *see* Reserpine *on page 491*
- ♦ **Respa-1st®** *see* Guaifenesin and Pseudoephedrine *on page 257*
- ♦ **Respa®-DM** *see* Guaifenesin and Dextromethorphan *on page 257*
- ♦ **Respa-GF®** *see* Guaifenesin *on page 256*
- ♦ **Respaire®-60 SR** *see* Guaifenesin and Pseudoephedrine *on page 257*
- ♦ **Respaire®-120 SR** *see* Guaifenesin and Pseudoephedrine *on page 257*
- ♦ **Respbid®** *see* Theophylline Salts *on page 539*
- ♦ **Restaid®** *see* Doxylamine *on page 186*
- ♦ **Restavit®** *see* Doxylamine *on page 186*
- ♦ **Restoril®** *see* Temazepam *on page 532*
- ♦ **Retavase™** *see* Reteplase *on page 491*


## Reteplase (RE ta plase)

**U.S. Brand Names** Retavase™

**Pharmacologic Category** Thrombolytic Agent

**Use** Management of acute myocardial infarction (AMI); improvement of ventricular function; reduction of the incidence of CHF and the reduction of mortality following AMI

**Effects on Mental Status** None reported

**Effects on Psychiatric Treatment** None reported

**Usual Dosage**

Children: Not recommended

Adults: 10 units I.V. over 2 minutes, followed by a second dose 30 minutes later of 10 units I.V. over 2 minutes

Withhold second dose if serious bleeding or anaphylaxis occurs

**Dosage Forms** Injection: Powder in vials, each vial contains reteplase 10.8 units; supplied with 2 mL diluent (preservative free)


- ♦ **Retin-A™ Micro Topical** *see* Tretinoin, Topical *on page 563*
- ♦ **Retin-A™ Topical** *see* Tretinoin, Topical *on page 563*

## Ribavirin (rye ba VYE rin)

**U.S. Brand Names** Virazole® Aerosol

**Synonyms** RTCA; Tribavirin

**Pharmacologic Category** Antiviral Agent

**Use** Inhalation: Treatment of patients with respiratory syncytial virus (RSV) infections; may also be used in other viral infections including influenza A and B and adenovirus; specially indicated for treatment of severe lower respiratory tract RSV infections in patients with an underlying compromising condition (prematurity, bronchopulmonary dysplasia and other chronic lung conditions, congenital heart disease, immunodeficiency, immunosuppression), and recent transplant recipients

Oral capsules: The combination therapy of oral ribavirin with interferon $alpha_{2b}$, recombinant (Intron® A) injection is indicated for the treatment of chronic hepatitis C in patients with compensated liver disease who have relapsed after alpha interferon therapy.

**Effects on Mental Status** May cause drowsiness or insomnia

**Effects on Psychiatric Treatment** None reported

**Pregnancy Risk Factor** X

**Contraindications** Females of childbearing age; hypersensitivity to ribavirin; patients with autoimmune hepatitis

**Warnings/Precautions** Use with caution in patients requiring assisted ventilation because precipitation of the drug in the respiratory equipment may interfere with safe and effective patient ventilation; monitor carefully in patients with COPD and asthma for deterioration of respiratory function. Ribavirin is potentially mutagenic, tumor-promoting, and gonadotoxic. Anemia has been observed in patients receiving the interferon/ribavirin combination. Severe psychiatric events have also occurred including depression and suicidal behavior during combination therapy; avoid use in patients with a psychiatric history.

**Adverse Reactions**

Inhalation:

1% to 10%:

Central nervous system: Fatigue, headache, insomnia

Gastrointestinal: Nausea, anorexia

Hematologic: Anemia

<1%: Apnea, cardiac arrest, conjunctivitis, digitalis toxicity, hypotension, mild bronchospasm, rash, skin irritation, worsening of respiratory function

**Note:** Incidence of adverse effects in healthcare workers approximate 51% headache; 32% conjunctivitis; 10% to 20% rhinitis, nausea, rash, dizziness, pharyngitis, and lacrimation

Oral: (All adverse reactions are documented while receiving combination therapy with interferon $alpha_{2b}$)

>10%:

Cardiovascular: Chest pain

Central nervous system: Dizziness, headache, fatigue, fever, insomnia, irritability, depression, emotional lability, impaired concentration

Dermatologic: Alopecia, rash, pruritus

Gastrointestinal: Nausea, anorexia, dyspepsia, vomiting

Hematologic: Decreased hemoglobin and WBC

Neuromuscular & skeletal: Myalgia, arthralgia, musculoskeletal pain, weakness, rigors

Respiratory: Dyspnea, sinusitis

Miscellaneous: Flu-like syndrome

1% to 10%:

Central nervous system: Nervousness

Endocrine & metabolic: Thyroid function test abnormalities

Gastrointestinal: Taste perversion

**Drug Interactions** Decreased effect of zidovudine

**Usual Dosage** Infants, Children, and Adults:

Aerosol inhalation: Use with Viratek® small particle aerosol generator (SPAG-2) at a concentration of 20 mg/mL (6 g reconstituted with 300 mL of sterile water without preservatives)

Aerosol only: 12-18 hours/day for 3 days, up to 7 days in length

**Patient Information** Take as directed, for full course of therapy; do not discontinue even if feeling better. Use aerosol device as instructed. Maintain adequate fluid intake and report any swelling of ankles or feet, difficulty breathing, persistent lethargy, acute headache, insomnia, severe nausea or anorexia, confusion, fever, chills, sore throat, easy bruising or bleeding, mouth sores, or worsening of respiratory condition.

**Nursing Implications** Keep accurate I & O record, discard solutions placed in the SPAG-2 unit at least every 24 hours and before adding additional fluid; healthcare workers who are pregnant or who may become pregnant should be advised of the potential risks of exposure and counseled about risk reduction strategies including alternate job responsibilities; ribavirin may adsorb to contact lenses

**Dosage Forms**

Capsule: 200 mg; available only in Rebetron® combination package

Powder for aerosol: 6 g (100 mL)

## Riboflavin (RYE boe flay vin)

**U.S. Brand Names** Riobin®

**Synonyms** Lactoflavin; Vitamin $B_2$; Vitamin G

**Pharmacologic Category** Vitamin, Water Soluble

**Use** Prevent riboflavin deficiency and treat ariboflavinosis

**Effects on Mental Status** None reported

**Effects on Psychiatric Treatment** None reported

**Pregnancy Risk Factor** A (C if dose exceeds RDA recommendation)

**Warnings/Precautions** Riboflavin deficiency often occurs in the presence of other B vitamin deficiencies

**Adverse Reactions** Genitourinary: Discoloration of urine (yellow-orange)

**Drug Interactions** Decreased absorption with probenecid

**Usual Dosage** Oral:

Riboflavin deficiency:

Children: 2.5-10 mg/day in divided doses

Adults: 5-30 mg/day in divided doses

Recommended daily allowance:

Children: 0.4-1.8 mg

Adults: 1.2-1.7 mg

**Patient Information** Take with food. Large doses may cause bright yellow or orange urine.

**Dosage Forms** Tablet: 25 mg, 50 mg, 100 mg



## Rifabutin (rif a BYOO tin)

**U.S. Brand Names** Mycobutin®

**Synonyms** Ansamycin

**Pharmacologic Category** Antibiotic, Miscellaneous; Antitubercular Agent

**Use** Prevention of disseminated *Mycobacterium avium* complex (MAC) in patients with advanced HIV infection; also utilized in multiple drug regimens for treatment of MAC

**Effects on Mental Status** May rarely cause insomnia

**Effects on Psychiatric Treatment** Neutropenia is common; avoid clozapine and carbamazepine; rifabutin is a hepatic enzyme inducer; monitor for altered clinical effects when used concurrently with psychotropics

**Pregnancy Risk Factor** B

**Contraindications** Hypersensitivity to rifabutin or any other rifamycins; rifabutin is contraindicated in patients with a WBC <1000/mm$^3$ or a platelet count <50,000/mm$^3$; concurrent use with ritonavir

**Warnings/Precautions** Rifabutin as a single agent must not be administered to patients with active tuberculosis since its use may lead to the development of tuberculosis that is resistant to both rifabutin and rifampin; rifabutin should be discontinued in patients with AST >500 units/L or if total bilirubin is >3 mg/dL. Use with caution in patients with liver impairment; modification of dosage should be considered in patients with renal impairment.

**Adverse Reactions**

>10%:

Dermatologic: Rash (11%)

Genitourinary: Discolored urine (30%)

Hematologic: Neutropenia (25%), leukopenia (17%)

1% to 10%:

Central nervous system: Headache (3%)

Gastrointestinal: Vomiting/nausea (3%), abdominal pain (4%), diarrhea (3%), anorexia (2%), flatulence (2%), eructation (3%)

Hematologic: Anemia, thrombocytopenia (5%)

Hepatic: Increased AST/ALT (7% to 9%)

Neuromuscular & skeletal: Myalgia

<1%: Chest pain, dyspepsia, fever, insomnia, taste perversion, uveitis

**Overdosage/Toxicology**

Signs and symptoms: Nausea, vomiting, hepatotoxicity, lethargy, CNS depression

Treatment: Supportive; hemodialysis will remove rifabutin, its effect on outcome is unknown

**Drug Interactions** CYP3A3/4 enzyme inducer

Decreased plasma concentration (due to induction of liver enzymes) of verapamil, methadone, digoxin, cyclosporine, corticosteroids, oral anticoagulants, theophylline, barbiturates, chloramphenicol, ketoconazole, oral contraceptives, quinidine, halothane, protease inhibitors, non-nucleoside reverse transcriptase inhibitors, and perhaps clarithromycin

Increased concentration by indinavir; reduce to 1/2 standard dose when used with indinavir

Increased risk of rifabutin-induced hematologic and ocular toxicity (uveitis) with concurrent administration of drug that inhibits CYP-450 enzymes such as protease inhibitors, erythromycin, clarithromycin, ketoconazole, and itraconazole

**Usual Dosage** Oral:

Children: Efficacy and safety of rifabutin have not been established in children; a limited number of HIV-positive children with MAC have been given rifabutin for MAC prophylaxis; doses of 5 mg/kg/day have been useful

Adults: 300 mg once daily; for patients who experience gastrointestinal upset, rifabutin can be administered 150 mg twice daily with food

**Patient Information** May take with food if GI upset occurs. Will discolor urine, stool, saliva, tears, sweat, and other body fluid a red-brown color. Stains on clothing or contact lenses are permanent. Report skin rash, vomiting, fever, chills, flu-like symptoms, dark urine or pale stools, unusual bleeding or bruising, or unusual confusion, depression, or fatigue.

**Dosage Forms** Capsule: 150 mg

♦ **Rifadin® Injection** *see* Rifampin *on page 493*

♦ **Rifadin® Oral** *see* Rifampin *on page 493*

♦ **Rifamate®** *see* Rifampin and Isoniazid *on page 494*

♦ **Rifampicin** *see* Rifampin *on page 493*

## Rifampin (RIF am pin)

**U.S. Brand Names** Rifadin® Injection; Rifadin® Oral; Rimactane® Oral

**Canadian Brand Names** Rifadin®; Rimactane®; Rofact™

**Synonyms** Rifampicin

**Pharmacologic Category** Antibiotic, Miscellaneous; Antitubercular Agent

**Use** Management of active tuberculosis in combination with other agents; eliminate meningococci from asymptomatic carriers; prophylaxis of *Haemophilus influenzae* type b infection; used in combination with other anti-infectives in the treatment of staphylococcal infections

**Effects on Mental Status** May cause drowsiness, dizziness, confusion, behavioral changes, or ataxia; report of cognitive disturbances, delusions, and hallucinations

**Effects on Psychiatric Treatment** May cause leukopenia; use caution with clozapine and carbamazepine; rifampin is a potent hepatic enzyme inducer; monitor for altered clinical effects when used concurrently with psychotropics

**Pregnancy Risk Factor** C

**Contraindications** Hypersensitivity to any rifamycins or any component

**Warnings/Precautions** Use with caution and modify dosage in patients with liver impairment; observe for hyperbilirubinemia; discontinue therapy if this in conjunction with clinical symptoms or any signs of significant hepatocellular damage develop; since rifampin has enzyme-inducing properties, porphyria exacerbation is possible; use with caution in patients with porphyria; do not use for meningococcal disease, only for short-term treatment of asymptomatic carrier states

Monitor for compliance and effects including hypersensitivity, decreased thrombocytopenia in patients on intermittent therapy; urine, feces, saliva, sweat, tears, and CSF may be discolored to red/orange; do not administer I.V. form via I.M. or S.C. routes; restart infusion at another site if extravasation occurs; remove soft contact lenses during therapy since permanent staining may occur; regimens of 600 mg once or twice weekly have been associated with a high incidence of adverse reactions including a flu-like syndrome

**Adverse Reactions**

Percentage unknown: ataxia, behavioral changes, confusion, dizziness, drowsiness, edema headache, eosinophilia, exudative conjunctivitis, flushing, hemolysis, hemolytic anemia, hepatitis (rare), leukopenia, myalgia, numbness, osteomalacia, pemphigoid reaction, pruritus, thrombocytopenia (especially with high-dose therapy), urticaria, visual changes, weakness

1% to 10%:

Dermatologic: Rash (1% to 5%)

Gastrointestinal: (1% to 2%): Epigastric distress, anorexia, nausea, vomiting, diarrhea, cramps, pseudomembranous colitis, pancreatitis

Hepatic: Increased LFTs (up to 14%)

**Overdosage/Toxicology**

Signs and symptoms: Nausea, vomiting, hepatotoxicity, lethargy, CNS depression

Treatment: Supportive

**Drug Interactions** CYP3A3/4 enzyme substrate; CYP1A2, 2C9, 2C18, 2C19, 2D6, 3A3/4, and 3A5-7 enzyme inducer

Decreased effect: Rifampin induces liver enzymes which may decrease the plasma concentration of calcium channel blockers (verapamil, diltiazem, nifedipine), methadone, digitalis, cyclosporine, corticosteroids, oral anticoagulants, haloperidol, theophylline, barbiturates, chloramphenicol, imidazole antifungals, oral or systemic hormonal contraceptives, acetaminophen, benzodiazepines, hydantoins, sulfa drugs, enalapril, beta-blockers, chloramphenicol, clofibrate, dapsone, antiarrhythmics (disopyramide, mexiletine, quinidine, tocainide), diazepam, doxycycline, fluoroquinolones, levothyroxine, nortriptyline, progestins, tacrolimus, zidovudine, protease inhibitors, and non-nucleoside reverse transcriptase inhibitors

Coadministration with INH or halothane may result in additive hepatotoxicity; probenecid and co-trimoxazole may increase rifampin levels while antacids may decrease its absorption

**Usual Dosage** Oral (I.V. infusion dose is the same as for the oral route):

**Tuberculosis therapy:**

**Note:** A four-drug regimen (isoniazid, rifampin, pyrazinamide, and either streptomycin or ethambutol) is preferred for the initial, empiric treatment of TB. When the drug susceptibility results are available, the regimen should be altered as appropriate.

Infants and Children <12 years:

Daily therapy: 10-20 mg/kg/day usually as a single dose (maximum: 600 mg/day)

Directly observed therapy (DOT): Twice weekly: 10-20 mg/kg (maximum: 600 mg); 3 times/week: 10-20 mg/kg (maximum: 600 mg)

Adults:

Daily therapy: 10 mg/kg/day (maximum: 600 mg/day)

Directly observed therapy (DOT): Twice weekly: 10 mg/kg (maximum: 600 mg); 3 times/week: 10 mg/kg (maximum: 600 mg)

***H. influenzae* prophylaxis:**

Infants and Children: 20 mg/kg/day every 24 hours for 4 days, not to exceed 600 mg/dose

Adults: 600 mg every 24 hours for 4 days

**Meningococcal prophylaxis:**

<1 month: 10 mg/kg/day in divided doses every 12 hours for 2 days

Infants and Children: 20 mg/kg/day in divided doses every 12 hours for 2 days

Adults: 600 mg every 12 hours for 2 days

**Nasal carriers of *Staphylococcus aureus*:**

Children: 15 mg/kg/day divided every 12 hours for 5-10 days in combination with other antibiotics

Adults: 600 mg/day for 5-10 days in combination with other antibiotics

**Synergy for *Staphylococcus aureus* infections:** Adults: 300-600 mg twice daily with other antibiotics

**Dosing adjustment in hepatic impairment:** Dose reductions may be necessary to reduce hepatotoxicity

**Dietary Considerations** Food: Rifampin is best taken on an empty stomach since food decreases the extent of absorption

**Patient Information** Take per recommended schedule. Complete full course of therapy; do not skip doses. Take on an empty stomach (1 hour before or 2 hours after meals). Maintain adequate hydration (2-3 L/day of fluids unless instructed to restrict fluid intake). Will discolor urine, stool, saliva, tears, sweat, and other body fluids red-brown. Stains on clothing or contact lenses are permanent. Report persistent vomiting; fever, chill, or flu-like symptoms; unusual bruising or bleeding; or other persistent adverse effects.

**Dosage Forms**

Capsule: 150 mg, 300 mg

Injection: 600 mg

## Rifampin and Isoniazid (RIF am pin & eye soe NYE a zid)

**U.S. Brand Names** Rifamate®

**Pharmacologic Category** Antibiotic, Miscellaneous

**Use** Management of active tuberculosis; see individual monographs for additional information

**Effects on Mental Status** Rifampin may cause drowsiness, dizziness, confusion, behavioral changes, or ataxia; report of cognitive disturbances, delusions, and hallucinations; isoniazid may cause drowsiness or dizziness; may rarely cause depression or psychosis; reports of insomnia, restlessness, disorientation, hallucinations, delusions, obsessive-compulsive symptoms, and exacerbation of schizophrenia

**Effects on Psychiatric Treatment** May cause leukopenia; use caution with clozapine and carbamazepine; rifampin is a potent hepatic enzyme inducer; monitor for altered clinical effects when used concurrently with psychotropics; isoniazid may impair the metabolism of carbamazepine and oxidatively metabolized benzodiazepines; monitor for adverse effects

**Usual Dosage** Oral: 2 capsules/day

**Dosage Forms** Capsule: Rifampin 300 mg and isoniazid 150 mg

## Rifampin, Isoniazid, and Pyrazinamide

(RIF am pin, eye soe NYE a zid, & peer a ZIN a mide)

**U.S. Brand Names** Rifater®

**Pharmacologic Category** Antibiotic, Miscellaneous

**Use** Management of active tuberculosis

**Effects on Mental Status** Rifampin may cause drowsiness, dizziness, confusion, behavioral changes, or ataxia; report of cognitive disturbances, delusions, and hallucinations; isoniazid may cause drowsiness or dizziness; may rarely cause depression or psychosis; reports of insomnia, restlessness, disorientation, hallucinations, delusions, obsessive-compulsive symptoms, and exacerbation of schizophrenia

**Effects on Psychiatric Treatment** May cause leukopenia; use caution with clozapine and carbamazepine; rifampin is a potent hepatic enzyme inducer; monitor for altered clinical effects when used concurrently with psychotropics; isoniazid may impair the metabolism of carbamazepine and oxidatively metabolized benzodiazepines; monitor for adverse effects

**Usual Dosage** Adults: Oral: Patients weighing:

≤44 kg: 4 tablets
45-54 kg: 5 tablets
≥55 kg: 6 tablets
Doses should be administered in a single daily dose

**Dosage Forms** Tablet: Rifampin 120 mg, isoniazid 50 mg, and pyrazinamide 300 mg

## Rifapentine (RIF a pen teen)

**U.S. Brand Names** Priftin®

**Pharmacologic Category** Antitubercular Agent

**Use** Treatment of pulmonary tuberculosis (indication is based on the 6-month follow-up treatment outcome observed in controlled clinical trial). Rifapentine must always be used in conjunction with at least one other antituberculosis drug to which the isolate is susceptible; it may also be necessary to add a third agent (either streptomycin or ethambutol) until susceptibility is known.

**Effects on Mental Status** May cause dizziness or drowsiness; has rarely been associated with aggression

**Effects on Psychiatric Treatment** May cause neutropenia; use caution with clozapine and carbamazepine; rifapentine is an inducer of CYP3A4; monitor of altered clinical effects with barbiturates, benzodiazepines, phenytoin, beta-blockers, haloperidol and TCAs.

**Pregnancy Risk Factor** C

**Contraindications** Patients with a history of hypersensitivity to rifapentine, rifampin, rifabutin, and any rifamycin analog

**Warnings/Precautions** Compliance with dosing regimen is absolutely necessary for successful drug therapy. patients with abnormal liver tests and/or liver disease should only be given rifapentine when absolutely necessary and under strict medical supervision. Monitoring of liver function tests should be carried out prior to therapy and then every 2-4 weeks during therapy if signs of liver disease occur or worsen, rifapentine should be discontinued. Pseudomembranous colitis has been reported to occur with various antibiotics including other rifamycins. If this is suspected, rifapentine should be stopped and the patient treated with specific and supportive treatment. Experience in treating TB in HIV-infected patients is limited.

Rifapentine may produce a red-orange discoloration of body tissues/fluids including skin, teeth, tongue, urine, feces, saliva, sputum, tears, sweat, and cerebral spinal fluid. Contact lenses may become permanently stained. All patients treated with rifapentine should have baseline measurements of liver function tests and enzymes, bilirubin, and a complete blood count. patients should be seen monthly and specifically questioned regarding symptoms associated with adverse reactions. Routine laboratory monitoring in people with normal baseline measurements is generally not necessary.

**Adverse Reactions**

>10%: Endocrine & metabolic: Hyperuricemia (most likely due to pyrazinamide from initiation phase combination therapy)

1% to 10%:

Cardiovascular: Hypertension
Central nervous system: Headache, dizziness
Dermatologic: Rash, pruritus, acne
Gastrointestinal: Anorexia, nausea, vomiting, dyspepsia, diarrhea
Hematologic: Neutropenia, lymphopenia, anemia, leukopenia, thrombocytosis
Hepatic: Increased ALT/AST
Neuromuscular & skeletal: Arthralgia, pain
Renal: Pyuria, proteinuria, hematuria, urinary casts
Respiratory: Hemoptysis

<1%: Aggressive reaction, arthrosis, bilirubinemia, constipation, esophagitis, fatigue, gastritis, gout, hematoma, hepatitis, hyperkalemia, hypovolemia, increased alkaline phosphatase, increased LDH, leukocytosis, neutrophilia, pancreatitis, peripheral edema, purpura, skin discoloration, thrombocytopenia, urticaria

**Overdosage/Toxicology** There is no experience with treatment of acute overdose with rifapentine; experience with other rifamycins suggests that gastric lavage followed by activated charcoal may help adsorb any remaining drug from the GI tract. Hemodialysis or forced diuresis is not expected to enhance elimination of unchanged rifapentine in an overdose.

**Drug Interactions** CYP3A4 and 2C8/9 inducer. Rifapentine may increase the metabolism of coadministered drugs that are metabolized by these enzymes. Enzymes are induced within 4 days after the first dose and returned to baseline 14 days after discontinuation of rifapentine. The magnitude of enzyme induction is dose and frequency dependent. Rifampin has been shown to accelerate the metabolism and may reduce activity of the following drugs (therefore, rifapentine may also do the same): Phenytoin, disopyramide, mexiletine, quinidine, tocainide, chloramphenicol, clarithromycin, dapsone, doxycycline, fluoroquinolones, warfarin, fluconazole, itraconazole, ketoconazole, barbiturates, benzodiazepines, beta-blockers, diltiazem, nifedipine, verapamil, corticosteroids, cardiac glycoside preparations, clofibrate, oral or other systemic hormonal contraceptives, haloperidol, HIV protease inhibitors, sulfonylureas, cyclosporine, tacrolimus, levothyroxine, methadone, progestins, quinine, delavirdine, zidovudine, sildenafil, theophylline, amitriptyline, and nortriptyline.

Rifapentine should be used with extreme caution, if at all, in patients who are also taking protease inhibitors

Patients using oral or other systemic hormonal contraceptives should be advised to change to nonhormonal methods of birth control when receiving concomitant rifapentine.

Rifapentine metabolism is mediated by esterase activity, therefore, there is minimal potential for rifapentine metabolism to be affected by other drug therapy.

**Usual Dosage**

Children: No dosing information available

Adults: **Rifapentine should not be used alone**; initial phase should include a 3- to 4-drug regimen

Intensive phase of short-term therapy: 600 mg (four 150 mg tablets) given weekly (every 72 hours); following the intensive phase, treatment should continue with rifapentine 600 mg once weekly for 4 months in combination with INH or appropriate agent for susceptible organisms

**Dosing adjustment in renal or hepatic impairment:** Unknown

**Dietary Considerations** Food increases AUC and maximum serum concentration by 43% and 44% respectively as compared to fasting conditions

**Patient Information** Best to take on empty stomach (1 hour before or 2 hours after meals); however, may be taken with food if GI upset occurs. Follow recommended dosing schedule exactly; do not increase dose or skip doses. You will need to be monitored on a regular basis while taking this medication. This medication will stain urine, stool, saliva, tears, sweat, and other body fluids a red-brown color. Stains on clothing or contact lenses are permanent. Report vomiting; fever, chills or flu-like symptoms; muscle weakness or unusual fatigue; dark urine, pale stools, or unusual bleeding or bruising; yellowing skin or eyes; skin rash; swelling of extremities; chest pain or palpitations; or persistent gastrointestinal upset.

**Dosage Forms** Tablet, film-coated: 150 mg

♦ **Rifater®** *see* Rifampin, Isoniazid, and Pyrazinamide *on page 494*

♦ **Rilutek®** *see* Riluzole *on page 494*

## Riluzole (RIL yoo zole)

**U.S. Brand Names** Rilutek®

**Synonyms** 2-Amino-6-Trifluoromethoxy-benzothiazole; RP54274

**Pharmacologic Category** Glutamate Inhibitor

**Use** Amyotrophic lateral sclerosis (ALS): Treatment of patients with ALS; riluzole can extend survival or time to tracheostomy

**Effects on Mental Status** None reported

**Effects on Psychiatric Treatment** None reported
**Pregnancy Risk Factor** C
**Contraindications** Severe hypersensitivity reactions to riluzole or any of the tablet components
**Warnings/Precautions** Among 4000 patients given riluzole for ALS, there were 3 cases of marked neutropenia (ANC <500/mm$^3$), all seen within the first 2 months of treatment. Use with caution in patients with concomitant renal insufficiency. Use with caution in patients with current evidence or history of abnormal liver function. Monitor liver chemistries.
**Adverse Reactions** >10%:
Gastrointestinal: Nausea, abdominal pain, constipation
Hepatic: Increased ALT
**Overdosage/Toxicology** Treatment: No specific antidote or treatment information available; treatment should be supportive and directed toward alleviating symptoms
**Drug Interactions** CYP1A2 enzyme substrate
Decreased effect: Drugs that induce CYP 1A2 (eg, cigarette smoke, charbroiled food, rifampin, omeprazole) could increase the rate of riluzole elimination
Increased toxicity: Inhibitors of CYP 1A2 (eg, caffeine, theophylline, amitriptyline, quinolones) could decrease the rate of riluzole elimination
**Usual Dosage** Adults: Oral: 50 mg every 12 hours; no increased benefit can be expected from higher daily doses, but adverse events are increased

**Dosage adjustment in smoking:** Cigarette smoking is known to induce CYP 1A2; patients who smoke cigarettes would be expected to eliminate riluzole faster. There is no information, however, on the effect of, or need for, dosage adjustment in these patients.
**Dosage adjustment in special populations:** Females and Japanese patients may possess a lower metabolic capacity to eliminate riluzole compared with male and Caucasian subjects, respectively
**Dosage adjustment in renal impairment:** Use with caution in patients with concomitant renal insufficiency
**Dosage adjustment in hepatic impairment:** Use with caution in patients with current evidence or history of abnormal liver function indicated by significant abnormalities in serum transaminase, bilirubin or GGT levels. Baseline elevations of several LFTs (especially elevated bilirubin) should preclude use of riluzole.
**Patient Information** This drug will not cure or stop disease but it may slow progression. Take as directed, at the same time each day, preferably on an empty stomach (1 hour before or 2 hours after meals). Avoid alcohol. You may experience increased spasticity, dizziness or sleepiness; use caution when driving or engaging in tasks requiring alertness until response to drug is known. Small frequent meals, frequent mouth care, chewing gum, or sucking lozenges may reduce nausea, vomiting, or anorexia. Report fever; severe vomiting, diarrhea, or constipation; change in color of urine or stool; yellowing of skin or eyes; acute back pain or muscle pain; or worsening of condition.
**Nursing Implications** Warn patients about the potential for dizziness, vertigo or somnolence and advise them not to drive or operate machinery until they have gained sufficient experience on riluzole to gauge whether or not it affects their mental or motor performance adversely. Whether alcohol increases the risk of serious hepatotoxicity with riluzole is unknown; discourage riluzole-treated patients from drinking alcohol in excess.
**Dosage Forms** Tablet: 50 mg

♦ **Rimactane® Oral** *see* Rifampin *on page 493*

## Rimantadine (ri MAN ta deen)

**U.S. Brand Names** Flumadine®
**Synonyms** Rimantadine Hydrochloride
**Pharmacologic Category** Antiviral Agent
**Use** Prophylaxis (adults and children >1 year) and treatment (adults) of influenza A viral infection
**Effects on Mental Status** May cause dizziness, anxiety, confusion, insomnia, restlessness, irritability, or hallucinations
**Effects on Psychiatric Treatment** None reported
**Pregnancy Risk Factor** C
**Contraindications** Hypersensitivity to drugs of the adamantine class, including rimantadine and amantadine
**Warnings/Precautions** Use with caution in patients with renal and hepatic dysfunction; avoid use, if possible, in patients with recurrent and eczematoid dermatitis, uncontrolled psychosis, or severe psychoneurosis. An increase in seizure incidence may occur in patients with seizure disorders; discontinue drug if seizures occur; consider the development of resistance during rimantadine treatment of the index case as likely if failure of rimantadine prophylaxis among family contact occurs and if index case is a child; viruses exhibit cross-resistance between amantadine and rimantadine.
**Adverse Reactions** 1% to 10%:
Cardiovascular: Orthostatic hypotension, edema
Central nervous system: Dizziness (1.9%), confusion, headache (1.4%), insomnia (2.1%), difficulty in concentrating, anxiety (1.3%), restlessness, irritability, hallucinations; incidence of CNS side effects may be less than that associated with amantadine
Gastrointestinal: Nausea (2.8%), vomiting (1.7%), xerostomia (1.5%), abdominal pain (1.4%), anorexia (1.6%)
Genitourinary: Urinary retention
**Overdosage/Toxicology** Signs and symptoms: Agitation, hallucinations, cardiac arrhythmia, death
**Drug Interactions**
Acetaminophen: Reduction in AUC and peak concentration of rimantadine
Aspirin: Peak plasma and AUC concentrations of rimantadine are reduced
Cimetidine: Rimantadine clearance is decreased (~16%)
**Usual Dosage** Oral:
Prophylaxis:
Children <10 years: 5 mg/kg once daily; maximum: 150 mg
Children >10 years and Adults: 100 mg twice daily; decrease to 100 mg/day in elderly or in patients with severe hepatic or renal impairment ($Cl_{cr}$ ≤10 mL/minute)
Treatment: Adults: 100 mg twice daily; decrease to 100 mg/day in elderly or in patients with severe hepatic or renal impairment ($Cl_{cr}$ ≤10 mL/minute)
**Patient Information** Take as directed, for full course of therapy. Use caution when changing position (rising from sitting or lying) until response is known. Report CNS changes (eg, confusion, insomnia, anxiety, restlessness, irritability, hallucinations), difficulty urinating, or severe nausea or vomiting.
**Dosage Forms**
Syrup, as hydrochloride: 50 mg/5 mL (60 mL, 240 mL, 480 mL)
Tablet, as hydrochloride: 100 mg

♦ **Rimantadine Hydrochloride** *see* Rimantadine *on page 495*

## Rimexolone (ri MEKS oh lone)

**U.S. Brand Names** Vexol® Ophthalmic Suspension
**Pharmacologic Category** Corticosteroid, Ophthalmic
**Use** Treatment of inflammation after ocular surgery and the treatment of anterior uveitis
**Effects on Mental Status** None reported
**Effects on Psychiatric Treatment** None reported
**Usual Dosage** Adults: Ophthalmic: Instill 1 drop in conjunctival sac 2-4 times/day up to every 4 hours; may use every 1-2 hours during first 1-2 days
**Dosage Forms** Suspension, ophthalmic: 1% (5 mL, 10 mL)

♦ **Rimso®-50** *see* Dimethyl Sulfoxide *on page 173*

♦ **Riobin®** *see* Riboflavin *on page 492*

♦ **Riopan® [OTC]** *see* Magaldrate *on page 330*

♦ **Riopan Plus® [OTC]** *see* Magaldrate and Simethicone *on page 330*

## Risedronate (ris ED roe nate)

**U.S. Brand Names** Actonel™
**Pharmacologic Category** Bisphosphonate Derivative
**Use** Paget's disease of the bone; treatment and prevention of glucocorticoid-induced osteoporosis; treatment and prevention of osteoporosis in postmenopausal women
**Effects on Mental Status** May cause dizziness
**Effects on Psychiatric Treatment** None reported
**Pregnancy Risk Factor** C
**Contraindications** Hypersensitivity to risedronate, bisphosphonates, or any component; hypocalcemia; abnormalities of the esophagus which delay esophageal emptying such as stricture or achalasia; inability to stand or sit upright for at least 30 minutes
**Warnings/Precautions** Bisphosphonates may cause upper gastrointestinal disorders such as dysphagia, esophageal ulcer, and gastric ulcer. Use caution in patients with renal impairment; hypocalcemia must be corrected before therapy initiation with alendronate; ensure adequate calcium and vitamin D intake, especially for patients with Paget's disease in whom the pretreatment rate of bone turnover may be greatly elevated.
**Adverse Reactions**
>10%:
Dermatological: Rash
Gastrointestinal: Abdominal pain, diarrhea
Neuromuscular & skeletal: Arthralgia
1% to 10%:
Cardiovascular: Chest pain
Central nervous system: Headache, dizziness
Gastrointestinal: Belching, colitis, constipation, nausea
Neuromuscular & skeletal: Bone pain, leg cramps, myasthenia
Respiratory: Bronchitis, rales/rhinitis
(Continued)

## Risedronate *(Continued)*

**Overdosage/Toxicology**

Signs and symptoms: Decreases in serum calcium following substantial overdose may be expected in some patients; signs and symptoms of hypocalcemia may also occur in some of these patients

Treatment: Gastric lavage may remove unabsorbed drug. Administration of milk or antacids to chelate risedronate may be helpful. Standard procedures that are effective for treating hypocalcemia, including I.V. administration of calcium, would be expected to restore physiologic amounts of ionized calcium to relieve signs and symptoms of hypocalcemia.

**Drug Interactions** Decreased effect: Calcium supplements and antacids interfere with the absorption of risedronate

**Usual Dosage** Oral:

Adults (patients should receive supplemental calcium and vitamin D if dietary intake is inadequate):

Paget's disease of bone: 30 mg once daily for 2 months

Treatment and prevention of postmenopausal osteoporosis or glucocorticoid-induced osteoporosis: 5 mg once daily (efficacy for use longer than 1 year has not been established)

Elderly: No dosage adjustment is necessary

**Dosage adjustment in renal impairment:** $Cl_{cr}$ <30 mL/minute: **Not** recommended

**Patient Information** In order to be effective, this drug must be taken exactly as prescribed. Take 30 minutes before first food of the day with 6-8 ounces of water and avoid lying down for 30 minutes after ingestion. You may experience headache (request analgesic); skin rash; or abdominal pain, diarrhea, or constipation (report if persistent). Report unresolved muscle or bone pain or leg cramps; acute abdominal pain; chest pain, palpitations, or swollen extremities; disturbed vision or excessively dry eyes; ringing in the ears; or persistent flu-like symptoms. Also notify healthcare provider if experiencing difficulty swallowing, pain when swallowing, or severe or persistent heartburn.

**Dosage Forms** Tablet, as sodium: 30 mg

♦ **Risperdal®** *see* Risperidone *on page 496*

## Risperidone (ris PER i done)

**Related Information**



**Generic Available** No

**U.S. Brand Names** Risperdal®

**Pharmacologic Category** Antipsychotic Agent, Benzisoxazole

**Use** Management of psychotic disorders (eg, schizophrenia)

**Unlabeled use:** Behavioral symptoms associated with dementia in elderly

**Pregnancy Risk Factor** C

**Contraindications** Hypersensitivity to risperidone or any component of the formulation

**Warnings/Precautions** Low to moderately sedating, use with caution in disorders where CNS depression is a feature. Use with caution in Parkinson's disease. Caution in patients with hemodynamic instability; bone marrow suppression; predisposition to seizures; subcortical brain damage; severe cardiac, hepatic, or respiratory disease. Use with caution in renal dysfunction. Esophageal dysmotility and aspiration have been associated with antipsychotic use - use with caution in patients at risk of aspiration pneumonia (ie, Alzheimer's disease). Caution in breast cancer or other prolactin-dependent tumors (may elevate prolactin levels). May alter temperature regulation or mask toxicity of other drugs due to antiemetic effects. May alter cardiac conduction (low risk relative to other neuroleptics) - life-threatening arrhythmias have occurred with therapeutic doses of neuroleptics. Avoid in patients with Q-T prolongation. Use with caution in elderly patients or in patients who would not tolerate transient hypotensive episodes (cerebrovascular or cardiovascular disease) due to potential for orthostasis.

May cause anticholinergic effects (confusion, agitation, constipation, dry mouth, blurred vision, urinary retention); therefore, they should be used with caution in patients with decreased gastrointestinal motility, urinary retention, BPH, xerostomia, or visual problems. Conditions which also may be exacerbated by cholinergic blockade include narrow-angle glaucoma (screening is recommended) and worsening of myasthenia gravis. Relative to other neuroleptics, risperidone has a low potency of cholinergic blockade.

May cause extrapyramidal reactions, including pseudoparkinsonism, acute dystonic reactions, akathisia, and tardive dyskinesia (risk of these reactions is low relative to other neuroleptics, and is dose-dependent). May be associated with neuroleptic malignant syndrome (NMS) or pigmentary retinopathy.

**Adverse Reactions**

>10%: Central nervous system: Insomnia, agitation, anxiety, headache

1% to 10%:

Cardiovascular: Hypotension (especially orthostatic), tachycardia

Central nervous system: Sedation, dizziness, restlessness, anxiety, extrapyramidal reactions (dose dependent), dystonic reactions, pseudoparkinson, tardive dyskinesia, neuroleptic malignant syndrome, altered central temperature regulation

Dermatologic: Photosensitivity (rare), rash, dry skin

Endocrine & metabolic: Amenorrhea, galactorrhea, gynecomastia, sexual dysfunction

Gastrointestinal: Constipation, GI upset, xerostomia, dyspepsia, vomiting, abdominal pain, nausea, anorexia, weight gain

Genitourinary: Polyuria

Ocular: Abnormal vision

Respiratory: Rhinitis, coughing, sinusitis, pharyngitis, dyspnea

Incidence Unknown: Dysphagia, esophageal dysmotility

**Overdosage/Toxicology**

Signs and symptoms: Drowsiness, sedation, tachycardia, hypotension, extrapyramidal symptoms; one case involved decreased sodium and potassium and prolonged Q-T and widened QRS

Treatment: Establish and maintain airway to ensure adequate oxygenation and ventilation; consider gastric lavage and activated charcoal together with a laxative; monitor cardiovascular status, including EKG to detect arrhythmias; do not treat arrhythmias with disopyramide, procainamide, or quinidine as these potentiate the Q-T prolonging the effects of risperidone; do not use epinephrine or norepinephrine for hypotension as the beta stimulation may worsen this symptom; anticholinergics may be required for severe extrapyramidal side effects

**Drug Interactions** CYP2D6 enzyme substrate and weak inhibitor; CYP3A4 substrate

Antihypertensives: Risperidone may enhance the hypotensive effects of antihypertensive agents

Clozapine: Decreases clearance of risperidone, increasing its serum concentrations

CYP2D6 inhibitors: Metabolism of risperidone may be decreased; increasing clinical effect or toxicity; inhibitors include amiodarone, cimetidine, delavirdine, fluoxetine, paroxetine, propafenone, quinidine, and ritonavir; monitor for increased effect/toxicity

CYP3A3/4 inhibitors: May increase serum concentrations of risperidone; inhibitors include amiodarone, cimetidine, clarithromycin, erythromycin, delavirdine, diltiazem, dirithromycin, disulfiram, fluoxetine, fluvoxamine, grapefruit juice, indinavir, itraconazole, ketoconazole, metronidazole, nefazodone, nevirapine, propoxyfene, quinupristin-dalfopristin, ritonavir, saquinavir, verapamil, zafirlukast, zileuton; monitor for altered response

Enzyme inducers: May increase the metabolism of risperidone, reducing serum levels and effect; enzyme inducers include carbamazepine, barbiturates, phenytoin and rifampin; see note on carbamazepine

Levodopa: At high doses (>6 mg/day), risperidone may inhibit the antiparkinsonian effect of levodopa; avoid this combination when high doses are used

Valproic acid: Generalized edema has been reported as a consequence of concurrent therapy (case report)

**Mechanism of Action** Risperidone is a benzisoxazole derivative, mixed serotonin-dopamine antagonist; binds to 5-$HT_2$-receptors in the CNS and in the periphery with a very high affinity; binds to dopamine-$D_2$ receptors with less affinity. The binding affinity to the dopamine-$D_2$ receptor is 20 times lower than the 5-$HT_2$ affinity. The addition of serotonin antagonism to dopamine antagonism (classic neuroleptic mechanism) is thought to improve negative symptoms of psychoses and reduce the incidence of extrapyramidal side effects. $Alpha_1$, $alpha_2$ adrenergic, and histaminergic receptors are also antagonized with high affinity. Risperidone has low to moderate affinity for 5HTIC, 5HTID, and 5HTIA receptors, weak affinity for $D_1$ and no affinity for muscarinics or $beta_1$ and $beta_2$ receptors

**Pharmacodynamics/kinetics**

Absorption: Oral: Rapid

Metabolism: Extensive by cytochrome P-450

Protein binding: Plasma: 90%

Half-life: 24 hours (risperidone and its active metabolite)

Time to peak: Peak plasma concentrations within 1 hour

**Usual Dosage** Recommended starting dose: 0.5-1 mg twice daily; slowly increase to the optimum range of 3-6 mg/day; daily dosages >10 mg does not appear to confer any additional benefit, and the incidence of extrapyramidal reactions is higher than with lower doses

**Dosing adjustment in elderly patients:** A starting dose of 0.25-1 mg in 1-2 divided doses, and titration should progress slowly. Additional monitoring or renal function and orthostatic blood pressure may be warranted. If once-a-day dosing in the elderly or debilitated patient is considered, a twice daily regimen should be used to titrate to the target dose, and this dose should be maintained for 2-3 days prior to attempts to switch to a once-daily regimen.

**Dosing adjustment in renal, hepatic impairment:** Starting dose of 0.25-0.5 mg twice daily is advisable

**Monitoring Parameters** Monitor for extrapyramidal effects, orthostatic blood pressure changes for 3-5 days after starting or increasing dose

**Reference Range** Peak plasma level: 12 ng/mL within 2 hours of a 1 mg dose

**Test Interactions** Elevation of prolactin level

**Patient Information** May cause drowsiness

**Nursing Implications** Monitor and observe for extrapyramidal effects, orthostatic blood pressure changes for 3-5 days after starting or increasing dose

**Dosage Forms**

Solution, oral: 1 mg/mL
Tablet: 0.25 mg, 0.5 mg, 1 mg
Tablet, scored: 2 mg, 3 mg, 4 mg

♦ **Ritalin®** *see* Methylphenidate *on page 357*

♦ **Ritalin-SR®** *see* Methylphenidate *on page 357*

## Ritodrine (RI toe dreen)

**U.S. Brand Names** Yutopar®

**Pharmacologic Category** Beta$_2$ Agonist

**Use** Inhibits uterine contraction in preterm labor

**Effects on Mental Status** May cause nervousness, restlessness, or anxiety

**Effects on Psychiatric Treatment** None reported

**Usual Dosage** Adults: I.V.: 50-100 mcg/minute; increase by 50 mcg/minute every 10 minutes; continue for 12 hours after contractions have stopped

Hemodialysis: Removed by hemodialysis

**Dosage Forms**

Infusion, in D$_5$W: 0.3 mL (500 mL)
Injection, as hydrochloride: 10 mg/mL (5 mL); 15 mg/mL (10 mL)

## Ritonavir (rye TON a veer)

**Related Information**

Protease Inhibitors *on page 724*

**U.S. Brand Names** Norvir®

**Pharmacologic Category** Antiretroviral Agent, Protease Inhibitor

**Use** In combination with other antiretroviral agents; treatment of HIV infection when therapy is warranted

**Effects on Mental Status** May cause confusion

**Effects on Psychiatric Treatment** Contraindicated with bupropion, clozapine, pimozide, most benzodiazepines, and zolpidem; may use temazepam or lorazepam

**Pregnancy Risk Factor** B

**Contraindications** Patients with known hypersensitivity to ritonavir or any ingredients; concurrent amiodarone, bepridil, flecainide, propafenone, quinidine, astemizole, terfenadine, dihydroergotamine, ergotamine, midazolam, triazolam, cisapride, pimozide

**Warnings/Precautions** Use caution in patients with hepatic insufficiency; safety and efficacy have not been established in children <16 years of age; use caution with benzodiazepines, antiarrhythmics (flecainide, encainide, bepridil, amiodarone, quinidine) and certain analgesics (meperidine, piroxicam, propoxyphene). Use with HMG CoA-reductase inhibitors (lovastatin, simvastatin, atorvastatin, cerivastatin) not recommended.

**Adverse Reactions** Protease inhibitors cause dyslipidemia which includes elevated cholesterol and triglycerides and a redistribution of body fat centrally to cause "protease paunch", buffalo hump, facial atrophy, and breast enlargement. These agents also cause hyperglycemia.

>10%:

Gastrointestinal: Diarrhea, nausea, vomiting, taste perversion
Endocrine & metabolic: Increased triglycerides
Hematologic: Anemia, decreased WBCs
Hepatic: Increased GGT
Neuromuscular & skeletal: Weakness

1% to 10%:

Cardiovascular: Vasodilation
Central nervous system: Fever, headache, malaise, dizziness, insomnia, somnolence, thinking abnormally
Dermatologic: Rash
Endocrine & metabolic: Hyperlipidemia, increased uric acid, increased glucose
Gastrointestinal: Abdominal pain, anorexia, constipation, dyspepsia, flatulence, local throat irritation
Hematologic: Neutropenia, eosinophilia, neutrophilia, prolonged PT, leukocytosis
Hepatic: Increased LFTs
Neuromuscular & skeletal: Increased CPK, myalgia, paresthesia
Respiratory: Pharyngitis
Miscellaneous: Diaphoresis, increased potassium, increased calcium,

**Drug Interactions** CYP1A2, 2A6, 2C9, 2C19, 2E1, and 3A3/4 enzyme substrate, CYP2D6 enzyme substrate (minor); CYP1A2 enzyme inducer; CYP2A6, 2C9, 1A2, 2C19, 2D6, 2E1, and 3A3/4 inhibitor

Increased effect/toxicity:

Amprenavir AUC is increased by ritonavir
Antiarrhythmics (amiodarone, bepridil, flecainide, propafenone, quinidine) toxicity may be greatly increased - concurrent use of ritonavir is contraindicated
Astemizole and terfenadine: Cardiac toxicity (arrhythmia) is increased; concurrent use is contraindicated
Benzodiazepines (clorazepate, diazepam, estazolam, flurazepam midazolam, triazolam) toxicity may be increased;concurrent use of midazolam and triazolam is specifically contraindicated
Cisapride toxicity (arrhythmia) may be increased by ritonavir; concurrent use is contraindicated
Clarithromycin serum concentrations are increased by ritonavir
Desipramine (and possibly other TCAs) serum levels may be increased by ritonavir, requiring dosage adjustment
Ergot alkaloids (dihydroergotamine, ergotamine) toxicity is increased by ritonavir; concurrent use is contraindicated
HMG CoA reductase inhibitors (atorvastatin, cerivastatin, lovastatin, simvastatin) serum concentrations may be increased by ritonavir, increasing the risk of myopathy/rhabdomyolysis
Indinavir serum concentrations are increased by ritonavir
Ketoconazole serum concentrations are increased by ritonavir
Meperidine: Serum concentrations of metabolite (normeperidine) are increased by ritonavir, which may increase the risk of CNS toxicity
Pimozide toxicity is significantly increased by ritonavir; concurrent use is contraindicated
Rifabutin and rifabutin metabolite serum concentrations may be increased by ritonavir; reduce rifabutin dose to 150 mg every other day
Sildenafil serum concentrations may be increased by ritonavir; do not exceed maximum 25 mg in a 48-hour period

Ritonavir may also increase the serum concentrations of the following drugs (dose decrease may be needed): Amprenavir, bupropion, carbamazepine, clonazepam, clorazepate, cyclosporine, dexamethasone, diltiazem, disopyramide, dronabinol, ethosuximide, fluoxetine (and other SSRIs), lidocaine, methamphetamine, metoprolol, mexiletine, nifedipine, nefazodone, perphenazine, prednisone, propoxyphene, quinine, risperidone, tacrolimus, tramadol, thioridazine, timolol, verapamil, zolpidem

Decreased effect:

Ethinyl estradiol serum concentrations may be decreased (may also decrease effectiveness of combo products)
Methadone serum concentrations are decreased by ritonavir
Theophylline serum concentrations may be decreased by ritonavir

In addition, ritonavir may decrease the serum concentrations of the following drugs (dose increase may be needed): Atovaquone, divalproex, lamotrigine, phenytoin, warfarin

**Usual Dosage** Oral:

Children: 250 mg/m$^2$ twice daily; titrate dose upward to 400 mg/m$^2$ twice daily (maximum: 600 mg twice daily)

Adults: 600 mg twice daily; dose escalation tends to avoid nausea that many patients experience upon initiation of full dosing. Escalate the dose as follows: 300 mg twice daily for 1 day, 400 mg twice daily for 2 days, 500 mg twice daily for 1 day, then 600 mg twice daily. Ritonavir may be better tolerated when used in combination with other antiretrovirals by initiating the drug alone and subsequently adding the second agent within 2 weeks.

If used in combination with saquinavir, dose is 400 mg twice daily

**Dosing adjustment in renal impairment:** None necessary

**Dosing adjustment in hepatic impairment:** Not determined; caution advised with severe impairment

**Patient Information** Take with food. Mix liquid formulation with chocolate milk or liquid nutritional supplement. You may experience headache or confusion; if these persist notify prescriber. Diarrhea may be moderate to severe. Notify prescriber if problematic. Report swelling, numbness of tongue, mouth, lips, unresolved vomiting, fever, chills, or extreme fatigue.

**Dosage Forms**

Capsule: 100 mg
Solution: 80 mg/mL (240 mL)

♦ **Rituxan™** *see* Rituximab *on page 497*

## Rituximab (ri TUK si mab)

**U.S. Brand Names** Rituxan™

**Pharmacologic Category** Antineoplastic Agent, Miscellaneous

**Use** Non-Hodgkin's lymphoma: Treatment of patients with relapsed or refractory low-grade or follicular, CD20 positive, B-cell non-Hodgkin's lymphoma

**Effects on Mental Status** May cause dizziness or depression

**Effects on Psychiatric Treatment** Leukopenia is common; avoid concurrent use with clozapine or carbamazepine

**Usual Dosage** Adults: I.V. (refer to individual protocols): **Do not administer I.V. push or bolus** (hypersensitivity reactions may occur). Consider

(Continued)

## Rituximab *(Continued)*

premedication (consisting of acetaminophen and diphenhydramine) before each infusion of rituximab. Premedication may attenuate infusion-related events. Because transient hypotension may occur during infusion, give consideration to withholding antihypertensive medications 12 hours prior to rituximab infusion.

I.V. infusion: 375 mg/m$^2$ once weekly for 4 doses (days 1, 8, 15, and 22).

**Dosage Forms** Injection, preservative free: 100 mg (10 mL); 500 mg (10 mL)

## Rivastigmine (ri va STIG meen)

**U.S. Brand Names** Exelon®

**Synonyms** ENA 713; SDZ ENA 713

**Pharmacologic Category** Acetylcholinesterase Inhibitor (Central)

**Use** Mild to moderate dementia from Alzheimer's disease

**Pregnancy Risk Factor** B

**Pregnancy/Breast-Feeding Implications** There are no adequate studies in pregnant women. Should be used only if the benefit outweighs the potential risk to the fetus. It is unknown if rivastigmine is excreted in human breast milk. There is no indication for use in nursing mothers.

**Contraindications** Hypersensitivity to rivastigmine, other carbamate derivatives, or other components of the formulation

**Warnings/Precautions** Significant nausea, vomiting, anorexia, and weight loss are associated with use; occurs more frequently in women and during the titration phase. Use caution in patients with a history of peptic ulcer disease or concurrent NSAID use. Caution in patients undergoing anesthesia who will receive succinylcholine-type muscle relaxation, patients with sick sinus syndrome, bradycardia or supraventricular conduction conditions, urinary obstruction, seizure disorders, or pulmonary conditions such as asthma or COPD. There are no trials evaluating the safety and efficacy in children.

**Adverse Reactions**

>10%:

Central nervous system: Dizziness (21%), headache (17%)

Gastrointestinal: Nausea (47%), vomiting (31%), diarrhea (19%), anorexia (17%), abdominal pain (13%)

2% to 10%:

Central nervous system: Fatigue (9%), insomnia (9%), confusion (8%), depression (6%), anxiety (5%), malaise (5%), somnolence (5%), hallucinations (4%), aggressiveness (3%)

Cardiovascular: Syncope (3%), hypertension (3%)

Gastrointestinal: Dyspepsia (9%), constipation (5%), flatulence (4%), weight loss (3%), eructation (2%)

Genitourinary: Urinary tract infection (7%)

Neuromuscular & skeletal: Weakness (6%), tremor (4%)

Respiratory: Rhinitis (4%)

Miscellaneous: Increased sweating (4%), flu-like syndrome (3%)

>2% but frequency equal to placebo: Chest pain, peripheral edema, vertigo, back pain, arthralgia, pain, bone fracture, agitation, nervousness, delusion, paranoid reaction, upper respiratory tract infections, infection, coughing, pharyngitis, bronchitis, rash, urinary incontinence.

<2% (Limited to significant or life-threatening; reactions may be at a similar frequency to placebo): Fever, edema, allergy, periorbital or facial edema, hypothermia, hypotension, postural hypotension, cardiac failure, ataxia, convulsions, apraxia, aphasia, dysphonia, hyperkinesia, hypertonia, hypokinesia, migraine, neuralgia, peripheral neuropathy, hypothyroidism, peptic ulcer, gastroesophageal reflux, GI hemorrhage, intestinal obstruction, pancreatitis, colitis, atrial fibrillation, bradycardia, A-V block, bundle branch block, sick sinus syndrome, cardiac arrest, supraventricular tachycardia, tachycardia, abnormal hepatic function, cholecystitis, dehydration, arthritis, angina pectoris, myocardial infarction, epistaxis, hematoma, thrombocytopenia, purpura, delirium, emotional lability, psychosis, anemia, bronchospasm, apnea, rashes (maculopapular, eczema, bullous, exfoliative, psoriaform, erythematous), urticaria, acute renal failure, peripheral ischemia, pulmonary embolism, thrombosis, thrombophlebitis, intracranial hemorrhage, conjunctival hemorrhage, diplopia, glaucoma, lymphadenopathy, leukocytosis.

**Overdosage/Toxicology** In cases of asymptomatic overdoses, rivastigmine should be held for 24 hours. Cholinergic crisis, caused by significant acetylcholinesterase inhibition, is characterized by severe nausea, vomiting, salivation, sweating, bradycardia, hypotension, respiratory depression, collapse, and convulsions. Treatment is supportive and symptomatic. Dialysis would not be helpful.

**Drug Interactions**

Anticholinergics: Effects may be reduced with rivastigmine

Beta-blockers without ISA: Activity may increase risk of bradycardia

Calcium channel blockers (diltiazem or verapamil): may increase risk of bradycardia

Cholinergic agonists: Effects may be increased with rivastigmine

Cigarette use increases the clearance of rivastigmine by 23%

Digoxin: Increased risk of bradycardia with concurrent use

Neuromuscular blockers: Depolarizing neuromuscular blocking agents effects may be increased with rivastigmine

**Stability** Store below 77°F (25°C); store solution in an upright position and protect from freezing

**Mechanism of Action** A deficiency of cortical acetylcholine is thought to account for some of the symptoms of Alzheimer's disease; rivastigmine increases acetylcholine in the central nervous system through reversible inhibition of its hydrolysis by cholinesterase

**Pharmacodynamics/kinetics**

Absorption: Rapid and complete within 1 hour when administered in the fasting state

Distribution: $V_d$: 1.8-2.7 L/kg

Protein binding: 40%

Metabolism: Extensively metabolized by cholinesterase-mediated hydrolysis in the brain. The metabolite undergoes N-demethylation and/or sulfate conjugation in the liver. Cytochrome P-450 minimally involved. Linear kinetics at 3 mg twice daily, but nonlinear at higher doses.

Bioavailability: 40%

Half-life: 1.5 hours

Time to peak: 1 hour

Elimination: 97% recovered in urine as metabolites; 0.4% in feces

**Usual Dosage** Adults: Oral: Initial: 1.5 mg twice daily to start; if dose is tolerated for at least 2 weeks then it may be increased to 3 mg twice daily; increases to 4.5 mg twice daily and 6 mg twice daily should only be attempted after at least 2 weeks at the previous dose; maximum dose: 6 mg twice daily. If adverse events such as nausea, vomiting, abdominal pain, or loss of appetite occur, the patient should be instructed to discontinue treatment for several doses then restart at the same or next lower dosage level; antiemetics have been used to control GI symptoms.

**Dosage adjustment in renal impairment:** Dosage adjustments are not recommended, however, titrate the dose to the individual's tolerance.

**Dosage adjustment in hepatic impairment:** Clearance is significantly reduced in mild to moderately impaired patients. Although dosage adjustments are not recommended, use lowest possible dose and titrate according to individual's tolerance. May consider waiting >2 weeks between dosage adjustments.

Elderly: Clearance is significantly lower in patients older than 60 years of age, but dosage adjustments are not recommended. Titrate dose to individual's tolerance.

**Dietary Considerations** Food delays absorption by 90 minutes, lowers $C_{max}$ by 30% and increases AUC by 30%; avoid concurrent ethanol use

**Monitoring Parameters** Cognitive function at periodic intervals

**Patient Information** Take with meals at breakfast and dinner. Swallow capsule whole. Do not chew, break, or crush capsule. A liquid (solution) is available for patients who cannot swallow capsules. Monitor for nausea, vomiting, loss of appetite, or weight loss; notify healthcare provider if any of these occur. See instructions for use of oral solution. Can swallow solution directly from syringe or mix with water, juice, or soda. Stir well and drink all of mixture within 4 hours of mixing. Do not mix with other liquids. Avoid concurrent ethanol use.

**Dosage Forms**

Capsule: 1.5 mg, 3 mg, 4.5 mg, 6 mg

Solution, oral: 2 mg/mL (120 mL)

## Rizatriptan (rye za TRIP tan)

**U.S. Brand Names** Maxalt®; Maxalt-MLT™

**Synonyms** MK 462

**Pharmacologic Category** Serotonin 5-$HT_{1D}$ Receptor Agonist

**Use** Acute treatment of migraine with or without aura

**Effects on Mental Status** Drowsiness and dizziness are common

**Effects on Psychiatric Treatment** Contraindicated with other serotonin agonists (SSRIs) and MAOIs

**Pregnancy Risk Factor** C

**Contraindications** Prior hypersensitivity to rizatriptan; documented ischemic heart disease or Prinzmetal's angina; uncontrolled hypertension; basilar or hemiplegic migraine; during or within 2 weeks of MAO inhibitors

**Warnings/Precautions** Use only in patients with a clear diagnosis of migraine; use with caution in elderly or patients with hepatic or renal impairment, history of hypersensitivity to sumatriptan or adverse effects from sumatriptan, and in patients at risk of coronary artery disease. Do not use with ergotamines. May increase blood pressure transiently; may cause coronary vasospasm (less than sumatriptan); avoid in patients with signs/symptoms suggestive of reduced arterial flow (ischemic bowel, Raynaud's) which could be exacerbated by vasospasm. Phenylketonurics (tablets contain phenylalanine).

Patients who experience sensations of chest pain/pressure/tightness or symptoms suggestive of angina following dosing should be evaluated for coronary artery disease or Prinzmetal's angina before receiving additional doses.

Caution in dialysis patients or hepatically impaired. Reconsider diagnosis of migraine if no response to initial dose. Long-term effects on vision have not been evaluated.

**Adverse Reactions**

1% to 10%:

Cardiovascular: Systolic/diastolic blood pressure increases (5-10 mm Hg), chest pain (5%)

Central nervous system: Dizziness, drowsiness, fatigue (13% to 30% - dose related)

Dermatologic: Skin flushing

Endocrine & metabolic: Mild increase in growth hormone, hot flashes

Gastrointestinal: Nausea, vomiting, abdominal pain, xerostomia (<5%)

Respiratory: Dyspnea

<1%: Arthralgia, blurred vision, bradycardia, chills, decreased mental activity, diaphoresis, dry eyes, eye pain, facial edema, hangover, heat sensitivity, muscle weakness, myalgia, nasopharyngeal irritation, neck pain/stiffness, neurological/psychiatric abnormalities, palpitation, polyuria, pruritus, syncope, tachycardia, tinnitus

**Drug Interactions**

Use within 24 hours of another selective 5-$HT_1$ agonist or ergot-containing drug should be avoided due to possible additive vasoconstriction

MAO inhibitors and nonselective MAO inhibitors increase concentration of rizatriptan

Propranolol: Plasma concentration of rizatriptan increased 70%

SSRIs: Rarely, concurrent use results in weakness and incoordination; monitor closely

**Usual Dosage** Oral: 5-10 mg, repeat after 2 hours if significant relief is not attained; maximum: 30 mg in a 24-hour period (Use 5 mg dose in patients receiving propranolol with a maximum of 15 mg in 24 hours)

**Dietary Considerations** Food delays the absorption

**Patient Information** Administration of orally disintegrating tablets: Do not open blister pack before using. Open with dry hands. Do not crush, chew, or swallow tablet; allow to dissolve on tongue. Take as prescribed; do not increase dosing schedule. May repeat one time after 2 hours, if first dose is ineffective. Do not ever take more than two doses without consulting prescriber. You may experience dizziness or drowsiness (use caution when driving, climbing stairs, or engaging in tasks requiring alertness until response to drug is known); skin flushing or hot flashes (cool clothes or a cool environment may help); mild abdominal discomfort or nausea or vomiting. Report severe dizziness, acute headache, chest pain or palpitation, stiff or painful neck or facial swelling, muscle weakness or pain, changes in mental acuity, blurred vision, eye pain, or excessive perspiration or urination.

**Dosage Forms** Tablet, as benzoate:

Maxalt®: 5 mg, 10 mg

Maxalt-MLT™ (orally disintegrating): 5 mg, 10 mg


- ♦ **RMS® Rectal** *see* Morphine Sulfate *on page 374*
- ♦ **Robafen® AC** *see* Guaifenesin and Codeine *on page 256*
- ♦ **Robafen® CF [OTC]** *see* Guaifenesin, Phenylpropanolamine, and Dextromethorphan *on page 258*
- ♦ **Robafen DM® [OTC]** *see* Guaifenesin and Dextromethorphan *on page 257*
- ♦ **Robaxin®** *see* Methocarbamol *on page 352*
- ♦ **Robicillin® VK** *see* Penicillin V Potassium *on page 426*
- ♦ **Robinul®** *see* Glycopyrrolate *on page 253*
- ♦ **Robinul® Forte** *see* Glycopyrrolate *on page 253*
- ♦ **Robitussin® [OTC]** *see* Guaifenesin *on page 256*
- ♦ **Robitussin® A-C** *see* Guaifenesin and Codeine *on page 256*
- ♦ **Robitussin-CF® [OTC]** *see* Guaifenesin, Phenylpropanolamine, and Dextromethorphan *on page 258*
- ♦ **Robitussin® Cough Calmers [OTC]** *see* Dextromethorphan *on page 160*
- ♦ **Robitussin®-DAC** *see* Guaifenesin, Pseudoephedrine, and Codeine *on page 258*
- ♦ **Robitussin®-DM [OTC]** *see* Guaifenesin and Dextromethorphan *on page 257*
- ♦ **Robitussin-PE® [OTC]** *see* Guaifenesin and Pseudoephedrine *on page 257*
- ♦ **Robitussin® Pediatric [OTC]** *see* Dextromethorphan *on page 160*
- ♦ **Robitussin® Severe Congestion Liqui-Gels® [OTC]** *see* Guaifenesin and Pseudoephedrine *on page 257*
- ♦ **Rocaltrol®** *see* Calcitriol *on page 83*
- ♦ **Rocephin®** *see* Ceftriaxone *on page 101*


## Rofecoxib (roe fe COX ib)

**Related Information**

Nonsteroidal Anti-inflammatory Agents Comparison Chart *on page 722*

**U.S. Brand Names** Vioxx®

**Pharmacologic Category** Nonsteroidal Anti-Inflammatory Agent (NSAID), Cyclooxygenase 2 Inhibitor

**Use** Relief of the signs and symptoms of osteoarthritis; management of acute pain in adults; treatment of primary dysmenorrhea

**Effects on Mental Status** May cause dizziness; may rarely cause anxiety, depression, decreased mental acuity, hypesthesia, insomnia, somnolence

**Effects on Psychiatric Treatment** May increase serum lithium levels; monitor

**Pregnancy Risk Factor** C (D after 34-weeks gestation or close to delivery)

**Contraindications** Hypersensitivity to rofecoxib or any component, aspirin, or other nonsteroidal anti-inflammatory drugs (NSAIDs)

**Warnings/Precautions** Gastrointestinal irritation, ulceration, bleeding, and perforation may occur with NSAIDs (it is unclear whether rofecoxib is associated with rates of these events which are similar to nonselective NSAIDs). Use with caution in patients with a history of GI disease (bleeding or ulcers), decreased renal function, hepatic disease, congestive heart failure, hypertension, or asthma. Anaphylactoid reactions may occur, even with no prior exposure to rofecoxib.

**Adverse Reactions**

2% to 10%:

Cardiovascular: Peripheral edema (3.7%), hypertension (3.5%)

Central nervous system: Headache (4.7%), dizziness (3%)

Gastrointestinal: Diarrhea (6.5%), nausea (5.2%), heartburn (4.2%), epigastric discomfort (3.8%), dyspepsia (3.5%), abdominal pain (3.4%)

Genitourinary: Urinary tract infection (2.8%)

Neuromuscular & skeletal: Back pain (2.5%), weakness (2.2%)

Respiratory: Upper respiratory infection (8.5%), bronchitis (2.0%), sinusitis (2.7%)

Miscellaneous: Flu-like syndrome (2.9%)

0.1% to 2%:

Cardiovascular: Chest pain, upper extremity edema, atrial fibrillation, bradycardia, arrhythmia, palpitation, tachycardia, venous insufficiency, fluid retention, syncope

Central nervous system: Anxiety, depression, decreased mental acuity, hypesthesia, insomnia, neuropathy, migraine, somnolence, vertigo, fever, pain

Dermatologic: Alopecia, atopic dermatitis, basal cell carcinoma, contact dermatitis, pruritus, rash, erythema, urticaria, dry skin

Endocrine & metabolic: Hypercholesteremia

Gastrointestinal: Reflux, abdominal distension, abdominal tenderness, constipation, dry mouth, esophagitis, flatulence, gastritis, gastroenteritis, hematochezia, hemorrhoids, oral ulceration, dental caries, aphthous stomatitis, weight gain

Genitourinary: Breast mass, cystitis, dysuria, menopausal disorder, nocturia, urinary retention, vaginitis, pelvic pain

Hematologic: Hematoma

Neuromuscular & skeletal: Muscle spasm, sciatica, arthralgia, bursitis, cartilage trauma, joint swelling, muscle cramps, muscle weakness, myalgia, tendonitis, traumatic arthropathy, fracture (wrist), paresthesia

Ocular: Blurred vision, conjunctivitis

Otic: Otic pain, otitis media, tinnitus

Respiratory: Asthma, cough, dyspnea, pneumonia, respiratory infection, pulmonary congestion, rhinitis, epistaxis, laryngitis, dry throat, pharyngitis, tonsillitis, diaphragmatic hernia

Miscellaneous: Allergy, fungal infection, insect bite reaction, viral syndrome, herpes simplex, herpes zoster, increased sweating

<0.1% (limited to severe): Breast cancer, cerebrovascular accident, cholecystitis, colitis, colonic neoplasm, congestive heart failure, deep venous thrombosis, duodenal ulcer, gastrointestinal bleeding, intestinal obstruction, lymphoma, myocardial infarction, pancreatitis, prostatic cancer, transient ischemic attack, unstable angina, urolithiasis

**Overdosage/Toxicology** Symptoms may include epigastric pain, drowsiness, lethargy, nausea, and vomiting. Gastrointestinal bleeding may occur. Rare manifestations include hypertension, respiratory depression, coma, and acute renal failure. Treatment is symptomatic and supportive. Hemodialysis does not remove rofecoxib.

**Drug Interactions**

May be a mild inducer of cytochrome P-450 isoenzyme 3A4 (CYP3A4)

Increased effect: Cimetidine increases AUC of rofecoxib by 23%. Rofecoxib may increase plasma concentrations of methotrexate and lithium. Rofecoxib may be used with low-dose aspirin, however rates of gastrointestinal bleeding may be increased with coadministration. Rofecoxib may increase the INR in patients receiving warfarin and may increase the risk of bleeding complications.

Decreased effects: Efficacy of thiazide diuretics, loop diuretics (furosemide) or ACE inhibitors may be diminished by rofecoxib. Rifampin reduces the serum concentration of rofecoxib by approximately 50%. Antacids may reduce rofecoxib absorption.

**Usual Dosage** Adults: Oral:

Osteoarthritis: 12.5 mg once daily; may be increased to a maximum of 25 mg once daily

Acute pain and management of dysmenorrhea: 50 mg once daily as needed (use for longer than 5 days has not been studied)

**Dosing comment in renal impairment:** Use in advanced renal disease is not recommended

(Continued)

## Rofecoxib *(Continued)*

**Dosing adjustment in hepatic impairment:** No specific dosage adjustment is recommended (AUC may be increased by 69%)

Elderly: No specific adjustment is recommended; however, the AUC in elderly patients may be increased by 34% as compared to younger subjects; use the lowest recommended dose

**Dietary Considerations** Time to peak concentrations are delayed when taken with a high-fat meal, however peak concentration and AUC are unchanged. Rofecoxib may be taken without regard to meals.

**Patient Information** Do not take more than recommended dose. May be taken with food to reduce GI upset. Do not take with antacids. Avoid alcohol, aspirin, and OTC medication unless approved by prescriber. You may experience dizziness, confusion, or blurred vision (avoid driving or engaging in tasks requiring alertness until response to drug is known); anorexia, nausea, vomiting, taste disturbance, gastric distress (small frequent meals, frequent mouth care, sucking lozenges, or chewing gum may help). GI bleeding, ulceration, or perforation can occur with or without pain; it is unclear whether rofecoxib has rates of these events which are similar to nonselective NSAIDs. Stop taking medication and report immediately stomach pain or cramping, unusual bleeding or bruising, or blood in vomitus, stool, or urine. Report persistent insomnia; skin rash; unusual fatigue or easy bruising or bleeding; muscle pain, tremors, or weakness; sudden weight gain; changes in hearing (ringing in ears); changes in vision; changes in urination pattern; or respiratory difficulty.

**Dosage Forms**

Suspension, oral: 12.5 mg/5 mL, 25 mg/5 mL

Tablets: 12.5 mg, 25 mg


- **Roferon-A®** *see* Interferon Alfa-2a *on page 288*
- **Rogaine® Extra Strength for Men [OTC]** *see* Minoxidil *on page 368*
- **Rogaine® for Men [OTC]** *see* Minoxidil *on page 368*
- **Rogaine® for Women [OTC]** *see* Minoxidil *on page 368*
- **Rolaids® [OTC]** *see* Dihydroxyaluminum Sodium Carbonate *on page 172*
- **Rolaids® Calcium Rich [OTC]** *see* Calcium Carbonate *on page 84*
- **Rolatuss® Plain Liquid** *see* Chlorpheniramine and Phenylephrine *on page 114*
- **Romazicon™ Injection** *see* Flumazenil *on page 229*
- **Rondamine-DM® Drops** *see* Carbinoxamine, Pseudoephedrine, and Dextromethorphan *on page 92*
- **Rondec®** *see* Carbinoxamine *on page 92*
- **Rondec®-DM** *see* Carbinoxamine, Pseudoephedrine, and Dextromethorphan *on page 92*
- **Rondec® Drops** *see* Carbinoxamine and Pseudoephedrine *on page 92*
- **Rondec® Filmtab®** *see* Carbinoxamine and Pseudoephedrine *on page 92*
- **Rondec® Syrup** *see* Carbinoxamine and Pseudoephedrine *on page 92*
- **Rondec-TR®** *see* Carbinoxamine and Pseudoephedrine *on page 92*


## Ropinirole (roe PIN i role)

**U.S. Brand Names** Requip™

**Synonyms** Ropinirole Hydrochloride

**Pharmacologic Category** Anti-Parkinson's Agent (Dopamine Agonist)

**Use** Treatment of idiopathic Parkinson's disease; in patients with early Parkinson's disease who were not receiving concomitant levodopa therapy as well as in patients with advanced disease on concomitant levodopa

**Pregnancy Risk Factor** C

**Contraindications** Known hypersensitivity to ropinirole or any component of the formulation

**Warnings/Precautions** Syncope, sometimes associated with bradycardia, was observed in association with ropinirole in both early Parkinson's disease (without L-dopa) patients and advanced Parkinson's disease (with L-dopa) patients. Dopamine agonists appear to impair the systemic regulation of blood pressure resulting in postural hypotension, especially during dose escalation. Parkinson's disease patients appear to have an impaired capacity to respond to a postural challenge; use with caution in patients at risk of hypotension (ie, those receiving antihypertensive drugs) or where transient hypotensive episodes would be poorly tolerated (cardiovascular disease or cerebrovascular disease). Parkinson's patients being treated with dopaminergic agonists ordinarily require careful monitoring for signs and symptoms of postural hypotension, especially during dose escalation, and should be informed of this risk. May cause hallucinations. Use with caution in patients with pre-existing dyskinesia, severe hepatic or renal dysfunction.

Pathologic degenerative changes were observed in the retinas of albino rats during studies with this agent, but were not observed in the retinas of albino mice or in other species. The significance of these data for humans remains uncertain.

Although not reported for ropinirole, other dopaminergic agents have been associated with a syndrome resembling neuroleptic malignant syndrome on withdrawal or significant dosage reduction after long-term use. Dopaminergic agents from the ergot class have also been associated with fibrotic complications, such as retroperitoneum, lungs, and pleura. Patients treated with ropinirole have reported falling asleep while engaging in activities of daily living.

**Adverse Reactions**

Early Parkinson's disease:

Cardiovascular: Syncope, dependent/leg edema, orthostatic symptoms, flushing, chest pain, hypotension, hypertension, tachycardia, palpitations

Central nervous system: Dizziness (40%), somnolence (40%), headache, fatigue, pain, confusion, hallucinations, amnesia, malaise, hypoesthesia, vertigo, yawning

Gastrointestinal: Nausea (60%), dyspepsia, abdominal pain, xerostomia, anorexia, flatulence, vomiting

Genitourinary: Impotence

Neuromuscular & skeletal: Weakness

Ocular: Abnormal vision

Respiratory: Pharyngitis, dyspnea, rhinitis, sinusitis

Miscellaneous: Viral infection, diaphoresis (increased)

Advanced Parkinson's disease (with levodopa):

Cardiovascular: Hypotension (2%), syncope (3%)

Central nervous system: Dizziness (26%), aggravated parkinsonism, somnolence, headache (17%), insomnia, hallucinations, confusion (9%), pain (5%), paresis (3%), amnesia (5%), anxiety (6%), abnormal dreaming (3%)

Gastrointestinal: Nausea (30%), abdominal pain (9%), vomiting (7%), constipation (6%), diarrhea (5%), dysphagia (2%), flatulence (2%), increased salivation (2%), xerostomia, weight loss (2%)

Genitourinary: Urinary tract infections

Neuromuscular & skeletal: Dyskinesias (34%), falls (10%), hypokinesia (5%), paresthesia (5%), tremor (6%), arthralgia (7%), arthritis (3%)

Respiratory: Upper respiratory tract infection

Miscellaneous: Injury, increased diaphoresis (7%), viral infection, increased drug level (7%)

Endocrine & metabolic: Hypoglycemia, increased LDH, hyperphosphatemia, hyperuricemia, diabetes mellitus, hypokalemia, hypercholesterolemia, hyperkalemia, acidosis, hyponatremia, dehydration, hypochloremia

Gastrointestinal: Weight increase

Hepatic: Increased alkaline phosphatase

Neuromuscular & skeletal: Increased CPK

Renal: Elevated BUN, glycosuria

Miscellaneous: Thirst, increased lactate dehydrogenase (LDH)

**Drug Interactions** CYP1A2 enzyme substrate

Antipsychotics: May reduce the effect of ropinirole due to dopamine antagonism

Ciprofloxacin: May inhibit the metabolism of ropinirole; consider using ofloxacin or lomefloxacin; also may occur with enoxacin

CYP1A2 inhibitors: May increase serum concentrations of ropinirole; inhibitors include cimetidine, ciprofloxacin, erythromycin, fluvoxamine, isoniazid, ritonavir, and zileutin

Enzyme inducers: May increase the metabolism or ropinirole, reducing serum concentrations and/or effect; inducers include barbiturates, carbamazepine, phenytoin, rifampin, cigarette smoking, and rifabutin

Estrogens: May reduce the metabolism of ropinirole; dosage adjustments may be needed; clearance may be reduced by 36%

Metoclopramide: May reduce the effect of ropinirole due to dopamine antagonism

**Mechanism of Action** Ropinirole has a high relative *in vitro* specificity and full intrinsic activity at the $D_2$ and $D_3$ dopamine receptor subtypes, binding with higher affinity to $D_3$ than to $D_2$ or $D_4$ receptor subtypes; relevance of $D_3$ receptor binding in Parkinson's disease is unknown. Ropinirole has moderate *in vitro* affinity for opioid receptors. Ropinirole and its metabolites have negligible *in vitro* affinity for dopamine $D_1$, 5-$HT_1$, 5-$HT_2$, benzodiazepine, GABA, muscarinic, alpha$_1$-, alpha$_2$-, and beta-adrenoreceptors. Although precise mechanism of action of ropinirole is unknown, it is believed to be due to stimulation of postsynaptic dopamine $D_2$-type receptors within the caudate-putamen in the brain. Ropinirole caused decreases in systolic and diastolic blood pressure at doses >0.25 mg. The mechanism of ropinirole-induced postural hypotension is believed to be due to D-$_2$-mediated blunting of the noradrenergic response to standing and subsequent decrease in peripheral vascular resistance.

**Pharmacodynamics/kinetics**

Absorption: Not affected by food; $T_{max}$ increased by 2.5 hours when drug taken with a meal; absolute bioavailability was 55%, indicating first-pass effect; relative bioavailability from tablet compared to oral solution is 85%

Distribution: $V_d$: 525 L; removal of drug by hemodialysis is unlikely

Metabolism: Extensively by liver to inactive metabolites; steady-state concentrations are expected to be achieved within 2 days of dosing; CYP1A2 was the major enzyme responsible for metabolism of ropinirole

Half-life, elimination: ~6 hours

Time to peak concentration: ~1-2 hours

**Usual Dosage** Adults: Oral: The dosage should be increased to achieve a maximum therapeutic effect, balanced against the principal side effects of nausea, dizziness, somnolence and dyskinesia

Recommended starting dose is 0.25 mg three times/day; based on individual patient response, the dosage should be titrated with weekly increments as described below:

•Week 1: 0.25 mg 3 times/day; total daily dose: 0.75 mg
•Week 2: 0.5 mg 3 times/day; total daily dose: 1.5 mg
•Week 3: 0.75 mg 3 times/day; total daily dose: 2.25 mg
•Week 4: 1 mg 3 times/day; total daily dose: 3 mg

After week 4, if necessary, daily dosage may be increased by 1.5 mg per day on a weekly basis up to a dose of 9 mg/day, and then by up to 3 mg/day weekly to a total of 24 mg/day

**Test Interactions** ↑ alkaline phosphatase

**Patient Information** Ropinirole can be taken with or without food. Hallucinations can occur and elderly are at a higher risk than younger patients with Parkinson's disease. Postural hypotension may develop with or without symptoms such as dizziness, nausea, syncope, and sometimes sweating. Hypotension and/or orthostatic symptoms may occur more frequently during initial therapy or with an increase in dose at any time. Use caution when rising rapidly after sitting or lying down, especially after having done so for prolonged periods and especially at the initiation of treatment with ropinirole. Because of additive sedative effects and the possibility of falling asleep while engaging in activities of daily living, caution should be used when taking CNS depressants (eg, benzodiazepines, antipsychotics, antidepressants) in combination with ropinirole.

**Additional Information** If therapy with a drug known to be a potent inhibitor of CYP1A2 is stopped or started during treatment with ropinirole, adjustment of ropinirole dose may be required. Ropinirole binds to melanin-containing tissues (ie, eyes, skin) in pigmented rats. After a single dose, long-term retention of drug was demonstrated, with a half-life in the eye of 20 days; not known if ropinirole accumulates in these tissues over time.

**Dosage Forms** Tablet: 0.25 mg, 0.5 mg, 1 mg, 2 mg, 5 mg

♦ **Ropinirole Hydrochloride** *see* Ropinirole *on page 500*

## Rosiglitazone (roe si GLI ta zone)

**Related Information**

Hypoglycemic Drugs and Thiazolidinedione Information *on page 714*

**U.S. Brand Names** Avandia®

**Pharmacologic Category** Antidiabetic Agent (Thiazolidinedione)

**Use**

Type 2 diabetes, monotherapy: Improve glycemic control as an adjunct to diet and exercise

Type 2 diabetes, combination therapy: In combination with metformin or a sulfonylurea when:

- diet, exercise, and metformin or a sulfonylurea alone do not result in adequate glycemic control, **or**
- diet, exercise, and rosiglitazone alone do not result in adequate glycemic control

**Effects on Mental Status** May cause headache and fatigue

**Effects on Psychiatric Treatment** Weight gain is common; caution with atypical antipsychotics

**Pregnancy Risk Factor** C

**Contraindications** Hypersensitivity to rosiglitazone or any component of the formulation; active liver disease (transaminases >2.5 times the upper limit of normal at baseline); contraindicated in patients who experience jaundice during troglitazone therapy.

**Warnings/Precautions** Should not be used in diabetic ketoacidosis. Mechanism requires the presence of insulin, therefore use in type 1 diabetes is not recommended. Use with caution in premenopausal, anovulatory women; may result in resumption of ovulation, increasing the risk of pregnancy. May result in hormonal imbalance; development of menstrual irregularities should prompt reconsideration of therapy. Use with caution in patients with anemia or depressed leukocyte counts (may reduce hemoglobin, hematocrit, and/or WBC). Use with caution in patients with heart failure or edema; may increase in plasma volume and/or increase cardiac hypertrophy. In general, use should be avoided in patients with NYHA class 3 or 4 heart failure. Use with caution in patients with elevated transaminases (AST or ALT); see Contraindications. Idiosyncratic hepatotoxicity has been reported with another thiazolidinedione agent (troglitazone). Monitoring should include periodic determinations of liver function.

**Adverse Reactions**

>10%:

Gastrointestinal: Weight gain

Endocrine and metabolic: Increase in total cholesterol, increased LDL cholesterol, increased HDL cholesterol

1% to 10%:

Cardiovascular: Edema (4.8%)

Central nervous system: Headache (5.9%), fatigue (3.6%)

Endocrine & metabolic: Hyperglycemia (3.9%), hypoglycemia (0.5% to 1.6%)

Gastrointestinal: Diarrhea (2.3%)

Hematologic: Anemia (1.9%)

Neuromuscular & skeletal: Back pain (4%)

Respiratory: Upper respiratory tract infection (9.9%), sinusitis (3.2%)

Miscellaneous: Injury (7.6%)

<1%: Elevated transaminases, increased bilirubin

**Overdosage/Toxicology** Experience in overdose is limited; symptoms may include hypoglycemia; treatment is supportive

**Drug Interactions** Substrate for cytochrome P-450 isoenzyme 2C8 (CYP2C8); minor metabolism by CYP2C9

When rosiglitazone was coadministered with glyburide, metformin, digoxin, warfarin, ethanol, or ranitidine, no significant pharmacokinetic alterations were observed

**Usual Dosage**

Adults: Oral: Initial: 4 mg daily as a single daily dose or in divided doses twice daily. If response is inadequate after 12 weeks of treatment, the dosage may be increased to 8 mg daily as a single daily dose or in divided doses twice daily. In clinical trials, the 4 mg twice-daily regimen resulted in the greatest reduction in fasting plasma glucose and $HbA_{1c}$. (**Note:** Doses >4 mg in combination with sulfonylureas have not been evaluated in clinical trials.)

Changing patients from troglitazone to rosiglitazone: For patients with normal hepatic enzymes who are switched from troglitazone to rosiglitazone, a 1-week washout is recommended before initiating therapy with rosiglitazone.

Elderly: No dosage adjustment is recommended

**Dosage adjustment in renal impairment:** No dosage adjustment is required

**Dosage comment in hepatic impairment:** Clearance is significantly lower in hepatic impairment. Therapy should not be initiated if the patient exhibits active liver disease of increased transaminases (>2.5 times the upper limit of normal) at baseline.

**Dietary Considerations** Management of type 2 diabetes should include diet control. Peak concentrations are lowered by 28% and delayed when administered with food, but these effects are not believed to be clinically significant. Rosiglitazone may be taken without regard to meals.

**Patient Information** May be taken without regard to meals. Follow directions of prescriber. If dose is missed at the usual meal, take it with next meal. Do not double dose if daily dose is missed completely. Monitor urine or serum glucose as recommended by prescriber. More frequent monitoring is required during periods of stress, trauma, surgery, pregnancy, increased activity or exercise. Avoid alcohol. Report chest pain, rapid heartbeat or palpitations, abdominal pain, fever, rash, hypoglycemia reactions, yellowing of skin or eyes, dark urine or light stool, or unusual fatigue or nausea/vomiting.

**Dosage Forms** Tablet: 2 mg, 4 mg

♦ **Rosin Rose** *see* St Johns Wort *on page 519*

♦ **Rowasa® Rectal** *see* Mesalamine *on page 344*

♦ **Roxanol™ Oral** *see* Morphine Sulfate *on page 374*

♦ **Roxanol Rescudose®** *see* Morphine Sulfate *on page 374*

♦ **Roxanol SR™ Oral** *see* Morphine Sulfate *on page 374*

♦ **Roxicet® 5/500** *see* Oxycodone and Acetaminophen *on page 414*

♦ **Roxicodone™** *see* Oxycodone *on page 413*

♦ **Roxilox™** *see* Oxycodone and Acetaminophen *on page 414*

♦ **Roxiprin®** *see* Oxycodone and Aspirin *on page 414*

♦ **RP10248** *see* Sulthiame *on page 527*

♦ **RP54274** *see* Riluzole *on page 494*

♦ **R-Tannamine® Tablet** *see* Chlorpheniramine, Pyrilamine, and Phenylephrine *on page 116*

♦ **R-Tannate® Tablet** *see* Chlorpheniramine, Pyrilamine, and Phenylephrine *on page 116*

♦ **RTCA** *see* Ribavirin *on page 492*

♦ **RU 23908** *see* Nilutamide *on page 394*

♦ **Rubex®** *see* Doxorubicin *on page 185*

## Rue

**Synonyms** Herb-of-Grace; *Ruta gravedens*

**Pharmacologic Category** Herb

**Use** Antispasmodic; abortifacient; emmenagogue; topical insect repellent; earache; toothache; skin inflammation; contraceptive

**Pregnancy Risk Factor** Contraindicated

**Adverse Reactions** Per Commission E:

Dermatologic: Oil can cause contact dermatitis; phototoxic reactions causing dermatoses have been noted

Hepatic: Severe liver damage

Renal: Kidney damage herb contains furans coumarins which have phototoxic and mutagenic actions

(Continued)

## Rue *(Continued)*

Therapeutic dosages can have these effects:
- Central nervous system: Melancholic moods, sleep disorders, fatigue, dizziness
- Neuromuscular & skeletal: Spasms

Juice of fresh leaves can lead to:
- Cardiovascular: Low pulse
- Central nervous system: Fainting, sleepiness
- Endocrine & metabolic: Abortion
- Gastrointestinal: Painful irritations of stomach and intestines, swelling of tongue
- Miscellaneous: Clammy skin

**Overdosage/Toxicology**
Signs and symptoms: Nausea, vomiting, emesis upon ingestion; volatile oil may be an irritant and can cause hepatic and renal abnormalities; topical administration of fresh leaves can cause dermal erythema, blistering, and photosensitization
Fatal dose: ~100 mL of the oil or 4 ounces of fresh leaves
Decontamination:
- Oral: Lavage (within 1 hour)/activated charcoal with cathartic
- Dermal: Wash with soap and water; avoid sunlight

**Additional Information** See Commission E; rue oil is used as an abortifacient; it is a pale yellow oil (density: 0.8) which is not water soluble; the plant (which is native to Europe but found worldwide) is an evergreen shrub which can grow to 2-3 feet with yellow flowers blooming in summer


- ♦ **Rum-K®** *see* Potassium Chloride *on page 453*
- ♦ **Rustic Treacle** *see* Garlic *on page 246*
- ♦ ***Ruta gravedens*** *see* Rue *on page 501*
- ♦ **Ru-Tuss®** *see* Chlorpheniramine, Phenylephrine, Phenylpropanolamine, and Belladonna Alkaloids *on page 115*
- ♦ **Ru-Tuss® DE** *see* Guaifenesin and Pseudoephedrine *on page 257*
- ♦ **Ru-Tuss® Expectorant [OTC]** *see* Guaifenesin, Pseudoephedrine, and Dextromethorphan *on page 259*
- ♦ **Ru-Tuss® Liquid** *see* Chlorpheniramine and Phenylephrine *on page 114*
- ♦ **Ru-Vert-M®** *see* Meclizine *on page 335*
- ♦ **Rymed®** *see* Guaifenesin and Pseudoephedrine *on page 257*
- ♦ **Rymed-TR®** *see* Guaifenesin and Phenylpropanolamine *on page 257*
- ♦ **Ryna-C® Liquid** *see* Chlorpheniramine, Pseudoephedrine, and Codeine *on page 116*
- ♦ **Ryna-CX®** *see* Guaifenesin, Pseudoephedrine, and Codeine *on page 258*
- ♦ **Ryna® Liquid [OTC]** *see* Chlorpheniramine and Pseudoephedrine *on page 114*
- ♦ **Rynatan®** *see* Azatadine and Pseudoephedrine *on page 55*
- ♦ **Rynatan® Pediatric Suspension** *see* Chlorpheniramine, Pyrilamine, and Phenylephrine *on page 116*
- ♦ **Rynatan® Tablet** *see* Chlorpheniramine, Pyrilamine, and Phenylephrine *on page 116*
- ♦ **Rynatuss® Pediatric Suspension** *see* Chlorpheniramine, Ephedrine, Phenylephrine, and Carbetapentane *on page 115*
- ♦ **Rythmol®** *see* Propafenone *on page 472*


## Sabah Vegetable

**Pharmacologic Category** Herb
**Use** Has been used (at a daily dose of 150 g) for weight reduction and vision protection
**Adverse Reactions**
- Cardiovascular: Palpitations, prolonged Q-T interval, torsade de pointes, chest tightness
- Central nervous system: Insomnia, anxiety, fatigue, dizziness
- Dermatologic: Rashes
- Endocrine & metabolic: Hypokalemia
- Gastrointestinal: Anorexia
- Neuromuscular & skeletal: Tremor
- Respiratory: Dyspnea, hypoxia, cough, tachypnea, obstructive lung disease, bronchiolitis obliterans (may all develop after 4 months of use), wheezing and rales may also occur

**Overdosage/Toxicology**
Decontamination: Ipecac (within 30 minutes)/activated charcoal with cathartic is useful
Treatment: Supportive therapy; lorazepam or diazepam 10-20 mg (0.25-0.4 mg/kg for children) is helpful for seizures; I.V. fluids and alpha-adrenergic pressors should be used for hypotension; sodium bicarbonate (1 mEq/kg) is useful to treat acidosis. Multiple dosing of activated charcoal may be useful.

**Additional Information** Not sold in U.S. market; commonly found in Malaysia, Thailand, India, Taiwan; shrub-like plant which can grow up to 1.5 meters high


- ♦ ***Sabal serrulata*** *see* Saw Palmetto *on page 505*
- ♦ ***Sabaslis serrulatae*** *see* Saw Palmetto *on page 505*
- ♦ **Safe Tussin® 30 [OTC]** *see* Guaifenesin and Dextromethorphan *on page 257*
- ♦ **Saizen® Injection** *see* Human Growth Hormone *on page 269*
- ♦ **Salagen® Oral** *see* Pilocarpine *on page 445*
- ♦ **Salbutamol** *see* Albuterol *on page 22*
- ♦ **Saleto-200® [OTC]** *see* Ibuprofen *on page 280*
- ♦ **Saleto-400®** *see* Ibuprofen *on page 280*
- ♦ **Saleto-600®** *see* Ibuprofen *on page 280*
- ♦ **Saleto-800®** *see* Ibuprofen *on page 280*
- ♦ **Salflex®** *see* Salsalate *on page 503*
- ♦ **Salgesic®** *see* Salsalate *on page 503*
- ♦ **Salicylazosulfapyridine** *see* Sulfasalazine *on page 525*


## Salicylic Acid and Propylene Glycol
(sal i SIL ik AS id & PROE pi leen GLYE cole)

**U.S. Brand Names** Keralyt® Gel
**Pharmacologic Category** Keratolytic Agent
**Use** Removal of excessive keratin in hyperkeratotic skin disorders, including various ichthyosis, keratosis palmaris and plantaris and psoriasis; may be used to remove excessive keratin in dorsal and plantar hyperkeratotic lesions
**Effects on Mental Status** None reported
**Effects on Psychiatric Treatment** None reported
**Usual Dosage** Apply to area at night after soaking region for at least 5 minutes to hydrate area, and place under occlusion; medication is washed off in morning
**Dosage Forms** Gel, topical: Salicylic acid 6% and propylene glycol 60% in ethyl alcohol 19.4% with hydroxypropyl methylcellulose and water (30 g)


- ♦ **Salicylsalicylic Acid** *see* Salsalate *on page 503*
- ♦ **Salivart® Solution [OTC]** *see* Saliva Substitute *on page 502*


## Saliva Substitute (sa LYE va SUB stee tute)

**U.S. Brand Names** Entertainer's Secret® Spray [OTC]; Moi-Stir® Solution [OTC]; Moi-Stir® Swabsticks [OTC]; Mouthkote® Solution [OTC]; Optimoist® Solution [OTC]; Salivart® Solution [OTC]; Salix® Lozenge [OTC]
**Pharmacologic Category** Gastrointestinal Agent, Miscellaneous
**Use** Relief of dry mouth and throat in xerostomia
**Effects on Mental Status** None reported
**Effects on Psychiatric Treatment** None reported
**Usual Dosage** Use as needed
**Dosage Forms**
- Lozenge: 100s
- Solution: 60 mL, 75 mL, 120 mL, 180 mL, 240 mL
- Swabstix: 3s


- ♦ **Salix® Lozenge [OTC]** *see* Saliva Substitute *on page 502*


## Salmeterol (sal ME te role)

**U.S. Brand Names** Serevent®
**Synonyms** Salmeterol Xinafoate
**Pharmacologic Category** Beta$_2$ Agonist
**Use** Maintenance treatment of asthma and in prevention of bronchospasm in patients >12 years of age with reversible obstructive airway disease, including patients with symptoms of nocturnal asthma, who require regular treatment with inhaled, short-acting beta$_2$ agonists; prevention of exercise-induced bronchospasm; treatment of COPD-induced bronchospasm
**Effects on Mental Status** May cause nervousness, dizziness, hyperactivity, or insomnia
**Effects on Psychiatric Treatment** Salmeterol is a sympathomimetic; use MAOIs and TCAs with caution
**Pregnancy Risk Factor** C
**Contraindications** Hypersensitivity to salmeterol, adrenergic amines or any ingredients; need for acute bronchodilation; within 2 weeks of MAO inhibitor use
**Warnings/Precautions** Salmeterol is not meant to relieve acute asthmatic symptoms. Acute episodes should be treated with short-acting beta$_2$ agonist. Do not increase the frequency of salmeterol. Cardiovascular effects are not common with salmeterol when used in recommended

doses. All beta agonists may cause elevation in blood pressure, heart rate, and result in excitement (CNS). Use with caution in patients with prostatic hypertrophy, diabetes, cardiovascular disorders, convulsive disorders, thyrotoxicosis, or others who are sensitive to the effects of sympathomimetic amines. Paroxysmal bronchospasm (which can be fatal) has been reported with this and other inhaled agents. If this occurs, discontinue treatment. The elderly may be at greater risk of cardiovascular side effects; safety and efficacy have not been established in children <12 years of age.

**Adverse Reactions**

>10%:

Central nervous system: Headache

Respiratory: Pharyngitis

1% to 10%:

Cardiovascular: Tachycardia, palpitations, elevation or depression of blood pressure, cardiac arrhythmias

Central nervous system: Nervousness, CNS stimulation, hyperactivity, insomnia, malaise, dizziness

Gastrointestinal: GI upset, diarrhea, nausea

Neuromuscular & skeletal: Tremors (may be more common in the elderly), myalgias, back pain, arthralgia

Respiratory: Upper respiratory infection, cough, bronchitis

<1%: Immediate hypersensitivity reactions (rash, urticaria, bronchospasm)

**Overdosage/Toxicology** Treatment: Decontaminate using lavage/activated charcoal. Beta-blockers can be used for hyperadrenergic signs (use with caution in patients with bronchospasm). Prudent use of a cardioselective beta-adrenergic blocker (eg, atenolol or metoprolol); keep in mind the potential for induction of bronchoconstriction in an asthmatic. Dialysis has not been shown to be of value in the treatment of an overdose with this agent.

**Drug Interactions** CYP3A3/4 enzyme substrate

Decreased effect: Beta-adrenergic blockers (eg, propranolol)

Increased toxicity (cardiovascular): MAO inhibitors, tricyclic antidepressants

**Usual Dosage**

Inhalation: 42 mcg (2 puffs) twice daily (12 hours apart) for maintenance and prevention of symptoms of asthma

Prevention of exercise-induced asthma: 42 mcg (2 puffs) 30-60 minutes prior to exercise; additional doses should not be used for 12 hours

COPD: Adults: For maintenance treatment of bronchospasm associated with COPD (including chronic bronchitis and emphysema): 2 inhalations (42 mcg) twice daily (morning and evening - 12 hours apart); do not use a spacer with the inhalation powder

**Patient Information** Use exactly as directed. Do not use more often than recommended (excessive use may result in tolerance, overdose may result in serious adverse effects) and do not discontinue without consulting prescriber. Do not use for acute attacks. Maintain adequate hydration (2-3 L/day of fluids unless instructed to restrict fluid intake). You may experience nervousness, dizziness, or fatigue (use caution when driving or engaging in tasks requiring alertness until response to drug is known); or dry mouth, stomach upset (frequent small meals, frequent mouth care, chewing gum, or sucking hard candy may help). Report unresolved GI upset; dizziness or fatigue; vision changes; chest pain, rapid heartbeat, or palpitations; insomnia; nervousness or hyperactivity; muscle cramping, tremors, or pain; unusual cough; or rash (hypersensitivity).

**Administration:** Self-administered inhalation: Store canister upside down; do not freeze. Shake canister before using. Sit when using medication. Close eyes when administering salmeterol to avoid spray getting into eyes. Exhale slowly and completely through nose; inhale deeply through mouth while administering aerosol. Hold breath for 1-3 seconds after inhalation. Wait at least 1 full minute between inhalations. Wash mouthpiece between use. If more than one inhalation medication is used, use bronchodilator first and wait 5 minutes between medications.

**Nursing Implications** Not to be used for the relief of acute attacks. Monitor lung sounds, pulse, blood pressure. Before using, the inhaler must be shaken well. Observe for wheezing after administration; if this occurs, call physician.

**Dosage Forms**

Aerosol, oral, as xinafoate: 21 mcg/spray [60 inhalations] (6.5 g), [120 inhalations] (13 g)

Inhaler: 25 mcg/metered inhalation

Powder for inhalation, oral (Serevent® Diskus®): 50 mcg [46 mcg/inhalation] (60 doses)

♦ **Salmeterol Xinafoate** *see* Salmeterol *on page 502*

♦ **Salmonine® Injection** *see* Calcitonin *on page 83*

## Salsalate (SAL sa late)

**U.S. Brand Names** Argesic®-SA; Artha-G®; Disalcid®; Marthritic®; Mono-Gesic®; Salflex®; Salgesic®; Salsitab®

**Synonyms** Disalicylic Acid; Salicylsalicylic Acid

**Pharmacologic Category** Salicylate

**Use** Treatment of minor pain or fever; arthritis

**Effects on Mental Status** May cause drowsiness; may rarely cause nervousness or insomnia

**Effects on Psychiatric Treatment** May rarely cause leukopenia; use caution with clozapine and carbamazepine

**Pregnancy Risk Factor** C; D (3rd trimester)

**Contraindications** GI ulcer or bleeding, known hypersensitivity to salsalate

**Warnings/Precautions** Use with caution in patients with platelet and bleeding disorders, renal dysfunction, erosive gastritis, or peptic ulcer disease, dehydration, previous nonreaction does not guarantee future safe taking of medication; do not use aspirin in children <16 years of age for chickenpox or flu symptoms due to the association with Reye's syndrome

**Adverse Reactions**

>10%: Gastrointestinal: Nausea, heartburn, stomach pains, dyspepsia

1% to 10%:

Central nervous system: Fatigue

Dermatologic: Rash

Gastrointestinal: Gastrointestinal ulceration

Hematologic: Hemolytic anemia

Neuromuscular & skeletal: Weakness

Respiratory: Dyspnea

Miscellaneous: Anaphylactic shock

<1%: Bronchospasm, does not appear to inhibit platelet aggregation, hepatotoxicity, impaired renal function, insomnia, iron deficiency anemia, jitters, leukopenia, nervousness, occult bleeding, thrombocytopenia

**Overdosage/Toxicology** Signs and symptoms: Respiratory alkalosis, hyperpnea, tachypnea, tinnitus, headache, hyperpyrexia, metabolic acidosis, hypoglycemia, coma

Treatment: The "Done" nomogram is very helpful for estimating the severity of aspirin poisoning and directing treatment using serum salicylate levels. Treatment can also be based upon symptomatology.

**Salicylates**

| Toxic Symptoms | Treatment |
|---|---|
| Overdose | Induce emesis with ipecac, and/or lavage with saline, followed with activated charcoal |
| Dehydration | I.V. fluids with KCl (no $D_5W$ only) |
| Metabolic acidosis (must be treated) | Sodium bicarbonate |
| Hyperthermia | Cooling blankets or sponge baths |
| Coagulopathy/hemorrhage | Vitamin K I.V. |
| Hypoglycemia (with coma, seizures, or change in mental status) | Dextrose 25 g I.V. |
| Seizures | Diazepam 5-10 mg I.V. |

**Drug Interactions**

Decreased effect with urinary alkalinizers, antacids, corticosteroids; decreased effect of uricosurics, spironolactone; ACE inhibitor effects may be decreased by concurrent therapy with NSAIDs

Increased effect/toxicity of oral anticoagulants, hypoglycemics, methotrexate

**Usual Dosage** Adults: Oral: 3 g/day in 2-3 divided doses

**Dosing comments in renal impairment:** In patients with end-stage renal disease undergoing hemodialysis: 750 mg twice daily with an additional 500 mg after dialysis

**Patient Information** Take this medication exactly as directed; do not increase dose without consulting prescriber. Do not crush tablets or break capsules. Take with food or milk to reduce GI distress. Maintain adequate fluid intake (2-3 L/day of fluids unless instructed to restrict fluid intake). Do not use alcohol, aspirin, or aspirin-containing medication, and all other anti-inflammatory medications without consulting prescriber. You may experience drowsiness (use caution when driving or engaging in tasks requiring alertness until response to drug is known); nausea or heartburn (frequent small meals, frequent mouth care, sucking lozenges, or chewing gum may help). GI bleeding, ulceration, or perforation can occur with or without pain; discontinue medication and contact prescriber if persistent abdominal pain or cramping, or blood in stool occurs. Report breathlessness or difficulty breathing; unusual bruising/bleeding; blood in urine, stool, mouth, or vomitus; unusual fatigue; skin rash or itching; change in urinary pattern; or change in hearing or ringing in ears.

**Dosage Forms**

Capsule: 500 mg

Tablet: 500 mg, 750 mg

♦ **Salsitab®** *see* Salsalate *on page 503*

♦ **Salt Poor Albumin** *see* Albumin *on page 21*

♦ **Saluron®** *see* Hydroflumethiazide *on page 275*

♦ **Salutensin®** *see* Hydroflumethiazide and Reserpine *on page 275*

## SAMe (S-adenosylmethionine)

**Pharmacologic Category** Nutritional Supplement

**Use** Depression; fibromyalgia; Alzheimer's disease; cardiovascular disease; insomnia; liver disease (cirrhosis, cholestasis, hepatitis); osteoarthritis

**Warnings/Precautions** SAMe is not recommended for the treatment of depressive symptoms associated with bipolar disorder since it may cause (Continued)

## SAMe (S-adenosylmethionine) *(Continued)*

mania or hypomania. SAMe has been demonstrated to inhibit platelet aggregation in animal models, and should be used with caution in patients with bleeding tendencies or those on anticoagulant medication.

**Adverse Reactions** Xerostomia, nausea, restless, anxiety, hypomania, mania

**Drug Interactions**

Antidepressants (SSRI and cyclic agents): May potentiate effect and/or toxicity; monitor

Linezolid: Effect/toxicity may be enhanced; avoid concurrent administration

MAO inhibitors: May potentiate activity and/or toxicities; avoid concurrent use

Serotonergic compounds: May increase risk of serotonin syndrome when concurrently; avoid combinations

**Mechanism of Action** S-adenosyl methionine is involved in several primary biochemical pathways. It functions as a methyl donor in synthetic pathways which form nucleic acids (DNA and RNA), proteins, phospholipids, and neurotransmitters. SAMe's role in phospholipid synthesis may influence membrane fluidity. It has also been noted to protect neuronal anoxia and promote myelination of nerve fibers. It is involved in transsulfuration reactions, regulating formation of sulfur-containing amino acids such as cysteine, glutathione, and taurine. Of note, glutathione is an important antioxidant, involved in the detoxification of a number of physiologic and environmental toxins. SAMe is also a cofactor in the synthesis of polyamines, which include spermidine, puescine, and spermine. Polyamines are essential for cellular growth and differentiation by virtue of their effects on gene expression, protein phosphorylation, neuron regeneration, and the DNA repair.

**Usual Dosage** Range: 200-1600 mg/day; adult RDI, ODA, and RDA have not been established; most common dosage: 400 mg/day

**Patient Information** Consult prescriber before combining SAMe with other antidepressants, tryptophan, or 5-HTP

**Additional Information** SAMe is formed from the essential amino acid methionine. It is a cofactor in three important biochemical pathways, and is synthesized throughout the body. Due to the nature and scope of biochemical reactions that it regulates, SAMe has been investigated for its effect on a wide variety of health problems and disease conditions.

**Dosage Forms** Capsule, tablets, and intravenous solution


- ♦ **Sandimmune® Injection** *see* Cyclosporine *on page 146*
- ♦ **Sandimmune® Oral** *see* Cyclosporine *on page 146*
- ♦ **Sandoglobulin®** *see* Immune Globulin, Intravenous *on page 284*
- ♦ **Sandostatin®** *see* Octreotide *on page 402*
- ♦ **Sandostatin LAR®** *see* Octreotide *on page 402*
- ♦ **Sanorex®** *see* Mazindol *on page 334*
- ♦ **Sansert®** *see* Methysergide *on page 360*


## Saquinavir (sa KWIN a veer)

**Related Information**

Protease Inhibitors *on page 724*

**U.S. Brand Names** Fortovase®; Invirase®

**Pharmacologic Category** Antiretroviral Agent, Protease Inhibitor

**Use** Treatment of HIV infection in selected patients; used in combination with at least two other antiretroviral agents

**Effects on Mental Status** May rarely cause confusion or ataxia; report of acute paranoia reaction to saquinavir

**Effects on Psychiatric Treatment** Contraindicated with triazolam and midazolam; barbiturates and carbamazepine may increase the metabolism of saquinavir

**Pregnancy Risk Factor** B

**Contraindications** Hypersensitivity to saquinavir or any components; exposure to direct sunlight without sunscreen or protective clothing; coadministration with terfenadine, cisapride, astemizole, triazolam, midazolam, or ergot derivatives

**Warnings/Precautions** The indication for saquinavir for the treatment of HIV infection is based on changes in surrogate markers. At present, there are no results from controlled clinical trials evaluating its effect on patient survival or the clinical progression of HIV infection (ie, occurrence of opportunistic infections or malignancies); use caution in patients with hepatic insufficiency; safety and efficacy have not been established in children <16 years of age. May exacerbate pre-existing hepatic dysfunction; use with caution in patients with hepatitis B or C and in cirrhosis

**Adverse Reactions** Protease inhibitors cause dyslipidemia which includes elevated cholesterol and triglycerides and a redistribution of body fat centrally to cause "protease paunch", buffalo hump, facial atrophy, and breast enlargement. These agents also cause hyperglycemia.

1% to 10%:

Dermatologic: Rash

Endocrine & metabolic: Hyperglycemia

Gastrointestinal: Diarrhea, abdominal discomfort, nausea, abdominal pain, buccal mucosa ulceration

Neuromuscular & skeletal: Paresthesia, weakness, increased CPK

<1%: Acute myeloblastic leukemia, altered AST/ALT/bilirubin/Hgb, ascites, ataxia, bullous skin eruption, confusion, elevated LFTs, exacerbation of chronic liver disease, headache, hemolytic anemia, hyper- and hypokalemia, hypoglycemia, jaundice, low serum amylase, pain, polyarthritis, portal hypertension, seizures, Stevens-Johnson syndrome, thrombocytopenia, thrombophlebitis, upper quadrant abdominal pain

**Drug Interactions** CYP3A3/4 enzyme substrate; CYP3A3/4 enzyme inhibitor

Decreased effect: Rifampin may decrease saquinavir's plasma levels and AUC by 40% to 80%; other enzyme inducers may induce saquinavir's metabolism (eg, phenobarbital, phenytoin, dexamethasone, carbamazepine); may decrease delavirdine concentrations

Increased effect: Ketoconazole significantly increases plasma levels and AUC of saquinavir; as a known, although not potent inhibitor of the cytochrome P-450 system, saquinavir may decrease the metabolism of terfenadine and astemizole, as well as cisapride, ergot derivatives, midazolam, and triazolam (and result in rare but serious effects including cardiac arrhythmias); other drugs which may have increased adverse effects if coadministered with saquinavir include calcium channel blockers, clindamycin, dapsone, and quinidine. Both clarithromycin and saquinavir levels/effects may be increased with coadministration. Delavirdine may increase concentration; ritonavir may increase AUC >17-fold; concurrent administration of nelfinavir results in increase in nelfinavir (18%) and saquinavir (mean: 392%).

Saquinavir increased serum concentrations of simvastatin and atorvastatin. Use cautiously with HMG-CoA reductase inhibitors. Avoid use with simvastatin.

**Usual Dosage** Adults: Oral:

Fortovase®: Six 200 mg capsules (1200 mg) 3 times/day within 2 hours after a meal in combination with a nucleoside analog

Invirase®: Three 200 mg capsules (600 mg) 3 times/day within 2 hours after a full meal in combination with a nucleoside analog

Dose of either Fortovase® or Invirase® in combination with ritonavir: 400 mg twice daily

**Patient Information** Saquinavir is is not a cure for HIV nor has it been found to reduce transmission of HIV. Take as directed, with food. Diabetics will need to monitor glucose levels frequently while taking this medication; this medication may exacerbate diabetes and hyperglycemia. You may experience headache or confusion; if these persist notify prescriber. You may develop sensitivity to sunlight (wear protective clothing, use sunblock, or avoid direct sunlight); mouth sores (frequent oral care is necessary). Report persistent nausea, vomiting, abdominal pain, or diarrhea; skin rash or irritation; muscles weakness or tremors; easy bruising or bleeding; fever or chills; yellowing of eyes or skin; or dark urine or pale stools.

**Nursing Implications** Observe for signs of opportunistic infections and other illnesses associated with HIV; administer on a full stomach, if possible

**Dosage Forms**

Capsule (hard) as mesylate (Invirase®): 200 mg

Capsule (soft) (Fortovase®): 200 mg


- ♦ **Sarafem™** *see* Fluoxetine *on page 232*


## Sargramostim (sar GRAM oh stim)

**Related Information**

Clinical Issues in the Use of Antipsychotics *on page 630*

Clozapine-Induced Side Effects *on page 780*

**U.S. Brand Names** Leukine™

**Synonyms** GM-CSF; Granulocyte-Macrophage Colony Stimulating Factor; rGM-CSF

**Pharmacologic Category** Colony Stimulating Factor

**Use**

**Myeloid reconstitution after autologous bone marrow transplantation:**

Non-Hodgkin's lymphoma (NHL)

Acute lymphoblastic leukemia (ALL)

Hodgkin's lymphoma

Metastatic breast cancer

**Myeloid reconstitution after allogeneic bone marrow transplantation**

**Peripheral stem cell transplantation**

Metastatic breast cancer

Non-Hodgkin's lymphoma

Hodgkin's lymphoma

Multiple myeloma

**Acute myelogenous leukemia (AML)** following induction chemotherapy in older adults to shorten time to neutrophil recovery and to reduce the incidence of severe and life-threatening infections and infections resulting in death

**Bone marrow transplant (allogeneic or autologous) failure or engraftment delay**

Safety and efficacy of GM-CSF given simultaneously with cytotoxic chemotherapy have not been established. Concurrent treatment may increase myelosuppression.

**Effects on Mental Status** May cause drowsiness

**Effects on Psychiatric Treatment** May be used to treat clozapine-induced agranulocytosis; lithium may potentiate the release of neutrophils; use with caution

**Pregnancy Risk Factor** C

**Contraindications** GM-CSF is contraindicated in the following instances:

Patients with excessive myeloid blasts (>10%) in the bone marrow or peripheral blood

Patients with known hypersensitivity to GM-CSF, yeast-derived products, or any known component of the product

**Warnings/Precautions** Simultaneous administration with cytotoxic chemotherapy or radiotherapy or administration 24 hours preceding or following chemotherapy is recommended. Use with caution in patients with pre-existing cardiac problems, hypoxia, fluid retention, pulmonary infiltrates or congestive heart failure, renal or hepatic impairment.

Rapid increase in peripheral blood counts: If ANC >20,000/mm$^3$ or platelets >500,000/mm$^3$, decrease dose by 50% or discontinue drug (counts will fall to normal within 3-7 days after discontinuing drug)

Growth factor potential: Use with caution with myeloid malignancies. Precaution should be exercised in the usage of GM-CSF in any malignancy with myeloid characteristics. GM-CSF can potentially act as a growth factor for any tumor type, particularly myeloid malignancies. Tumors of nonhematopoietic origin may have surface receptors for GM-CSF.

There is a "first-dose effect" (refer to Adverse Reactions for details) which is rarely seen with the first dose and does not usually occur with subsequent doses.

**Adverse Reactions**

>10%:

"First-dose" effects: Fever, hypotension, tachycardia, rigors, flushing, nausea, vomiting, dyspnea

Central nervous system: Neutropenic fever

Dermatologic: Alopecia

Endocrine & metabolic: Polydipsia

Gastrointestinal: Nausea, vomiting, diarrhea, stomatitis, GI hemorrhage, mucositis

Neuromuscular & skeletal: Bone pain, myalgia

1% to 10%:

Cardiovascular: Chest pain, peripheral edema, capillary leak syndrome

Central nervous system: Headache

Dermatologic: Rash

Endocrine & metabolic: Fluid retention

Gastrointestinal: Anorexia, sore throat, stomatitis, constipation

Hematologic: Leukocytosis

Local: Pain at injection site

Neuromuscular & skeletal: Weakness

Respiratory: Dyspnea, cough

<1%: Anaphylactic reaction, flushing, hypotension, malaise, pericardial effusion, pericarditis, thrombophlebitis, transient supraventricular arrhythmias

**Overdosage/Toxicology**

Signs and symptoms: Dyspnea, malaise, nausea, fever, headache, chills

Treatment: Discontinue drug, wait for levels to fall, monitor CBC, respiratory symptoms, fluid status. Increase WBC; discontinue drug and wait for levels to fall; monitor for pulmonary edema; toxicity of GM-CSF is dose-dependent. Severe reactions such as capillary leak syndrome are seen at higher doses (>15 mcg/kg/day).

**Drug Interactions** Increased toxicity: Lithium, corticosteroids may potentiate myeloproliferative effects

**Usual Dosage**

Children and Adults: I.V. infusion over ≥2 hours or S.C.

Existing clinical data suggest that starting GM-CSF between 24 and 72 hours subsequent to chemotherapy may provide optimal neutrophil recover; continue therapy until the occurrence of an absolute neutrophil count of 10,000/µL after the neutrophil nadir

**The available data suggest that rounding the dose to the nearest vial size may enhance patient convenience and reduce costs without clinical detriment**

**Myeloid reconstitution after peripheral stem cell, allogeneic or autologous bone marrow transplant:** I.V.: 250 mcg/m$^2$/day for 21 days to begin 2-4 hours after the marrow infusion on day 0 of autologous bone marrow transplant or ≥24 hours after chemotherapy or 12 hours after last dose of radiotherapy

If a severe adverse reaction occurs, reduce or temporarily discontinue the dose until the reaction abates

If blast cells appear or progression of the underlying disease occurs, disrupt treatment

Interrupt or reduce the dose by half if ANC is >20,000 cells/mm$^3$

Patients should not receive sargramostim until the postmarrow infusion ANC is <500 cells/mm$^3$

**Neutrophil recovery following chemotherapy in AML:** I.V.: 250 mg/m$^2$/day over a 4-hour period starting ~day 11 or 4 days following the completion of induction chemotherapy, if day 10 bone marrow is hypoblastic with <5% blasts

If a second cycle of chemotherapy is necessary, administer ~4 days after the completion of chemotherapy if the bone marrow is hypoblastic with <5% blasts

Continue sargramostim until ANC is >1500 cells/mm$^3$ for consecutive days or a maximum of 42 days

Discontinue sargramostim immediately if leukemic regrowth occurs

If a severe adverse reaction occurs, reduce the dose by 50% or temporarily discontinue the dose until the reaction abates

**Mobilization of peripheral blood progenitor cells:** I.V.: 250 mcg/m$^2$/day over 24 hours or S.C. once daily

Continue the same dose through the period of PBPC collection

The optimal schedule for PBPC collection has not been established (usually begun by day 5 and performed daily until protocol specified targets are achieved)

If WBC >50,000 cells/mm$^3$, reduce the dose by 50%

If adequate numbers of progenitor cells are not collected, consider other mobilization therapy

**Postperipheral blood progenitor cell transplantation:** I.V.: 250 mcg/m$^2$/day over 24 hours or S.C. once daily beginning immediately following infusion of progenitor cells and continuing until ANC is >1500 for 3 consecutive days is attained

**BMT failure or engraftment delay:** I.V.: 250 mcg/m$^2$/day for 14 days as a 2-hour infusion

The dose can be repeated after 7 days off therapy if engraftment has not occurred

If engraftment still has not occurred, a third course of 500 mcg/m$^2$/day for 14 days may be tried after another 7 days off therapy; if there is still no improvement, it is unlikely that further dose escalation will be beneficial

If a severe adverse reaction occurs, reduce or temporarily discontinue the dose until the reaction abates

If blast cells appear or disease progression occurs, discontinue treatment

**Patient Information** You may experience bone pain (request analgesic), nausea and vomiting (small frequent meals may help), hair loss (reversible). Report fever, chills, unhealed sores, severe bone pain, difficulty breathing, swelling or pain at infusion site. Avoid crowds or exposure to infected persons; you will be susceptible to infection.

**Nursing Implications** Can premedicate with analgesics and antipyretics; control bone pain with non-narcotic analgesics; do not shake solution; when administering GM-CSF subcutaneously, rotate injection sites

**Dosage Forms** Injection: 250 mcg, 500 mcg

♦ **Sarna [OTC]** *see* Camphor, Menthol, and Phenol *on page 87*

♦ ***Sassafras albidum*** *see* Sassafras Oil *on page 505*

## Sassafras Oil

**Synonyms** *Sassafras albidum*

**Pharmacologic Category** Herb

**Use** Banned by FDA in food since 1960; has been used as a mild counterirritant on the skin (ie, for lice or insect bites); should not be ingested

**Adverse Reactions** (Primarily related to sassafras oil and safrole)

Cardiovascular: Tachycardia, flushing, hypotension, sinus tachycardia

Central nervous system: Anxiety, hallucinations, vertigo, aphasia

Dermatologic: Contact dermatitis

Gastrointestinal: Vomiting

Hepatic: Fatty changes of the liver, hepatic necrosis

Ocular: Mydriasis

Miscellaneous: Diaphoresis

Little documentation of adverse effects due to ingestion of herbal tea

**Overdosage/Toxicology**

Decontamination: Emesis (within 30 minutes) can be considered for ingestion >5 mL if airway is protected; activated charcoal with cathartic can be used

Treatment: Supportive therapy; hypotension can be treated with intravenous crystalloid (10-20 mL/kg) and placement in Trendelenburg position; dopamine or norepinephrine can be used for refractory cases

**Usual Dosage** Sassafras tea can contain as much as 200 mg (3 mg/kg) of safrole

Lethal dose: ~5 mL

Toxic dose: 0.66 mg/kg is considered to be toxic to humans based on rodent studies

**Patient Information** Considered unsafe by the FDA

**Additional Information** Not reviewed by Commission E; specific gravity: 1.07; a yellow liquid which may also contain eugenol, pinene, and d-camphor

## Saw Palmetto

**Related Information**

Natural/Herbal Products *on page 746*

(Continued)

## Saw Palmetto *(Continued)*

Natural Products, Herbals, and Dietary Supplements *on page 742*

**Synonyms** Palmetto Scrub; *Sabal serrulata*; *Sabaslis serrulatae*; *Serenoa repens*

**Pharmacologic Category** Herb

**Use** Benign prostatic hyperplasia

**Contraindications** Pregnancy and breast-feeding

**Adverse Reactions**

Central nervous system: Headache
Endocrine & metabolic: Gynecomastia
Gastrointestinal: Stomach problems (in rare cases) per Commission E

**Overdosage/Toxicology**

Signs and symptoms: Diarrhea
Decontamination: Ipecac within 30 minutes or lavage (within 1 hour)/activated charcoal with cathartic

**Usual Dosage** Adults: Dried fruit: 0.5-1 g 3 times/day

**Additional Information** A fan palm plant growing up to 10 feet tall on the southern Atlantic coast; the red or brownish black berries, when ripe, are used in herbal medicine; this product has no effect on PSA or testosterone levels


- **Scalpicin®** *see* Hydrocortisone *on page 273*
- **SCH-29851** *see* Loratadine *on page 324*
- **Sch-33844** *see* Spirapril *on page 517*
- **Schizophrenia** *see page 604*
- **Scopace® Tablet** *see* Scopolamine *on page 506*


## Scopolamine (skoe POL a meen)

**U.S. Brand Names** Isopto® Hyoscine Ophthalmic; Scopace® Tablet; Transderm Scop® Patch

**Synonyms** Hyoscine

**Pharmacologic Category** Anticholinergic Agent

**Use** Preoperative medication to produce amnesia and decrease salivary and respiratory secretions; to produce cycloplegia and mydriasis; treatment of iridocyclitis; prevention of motion sickness; prevention of nausea/vomiting associated with anesthesia or opiate analgesia (patch); symptomatic treatment of postencephalitic parkinsonism and paralysis agitans (oral); inhibits excessive motility and hypertonus of the gastrointestinal tract in such conditions as the irritable colon syndrome, mild dysentery, diverticulitis, pylorospasm, and cardiospasm; it may also prevent motion sickness (oral)

**Effects on Mental Status** May cause drowsiness; may rarely cause confusion or amnesia

**Effects on Psychiatric Treatment** May decrease the effects of levodopa; concurrent use with psychotropics may produce additive sedation of anticholinergic side effects (dry mouth)

**Pregnancy Risk Factor** C

**Contraindications** Hypersensitivity to scopolamine or any component; narrow-angle glaucoma; acute hemorrhage, gastrointestinal or genitourinary obstruction, thyrotoxicosis, tachycardia secondary to cardiac insufficiency, paralytic ileus

**Warnings/Precautions** Use with caution with hepatic or renal impairment since adverse CNS effects occur more often in these patients; use with caution in infants and children since they may be more susceptible to adverse effects of scopolamine; use with caution in patients with GI obstruction; anticholinergic agents are not well tolerated in the elderly and their use should be avoided when possible

**Adverse Reactions**

Ophthalmic:
- >10%: Ocular: Blurred vision, photophobia
- 1% to 10%:
  - Ocular: Local irritation, increased intraocular pressure
  - Respiratory: Congestion
- <1%: Vascular congestion, edema, drowsiness, eczematoid dermatitis, follicular conjunctivitis, exudate

Systemic:
- >10%:
  - Dermatologic: Dry skin
  - Gastrointestinal: Constipation, xerostomia, dry throat
  - Local: Irritation at injection site
  - Respiratory: Dry nose
  - Miscellaneous: Diaphoresis (decreased)
- 1% to 10%:
  - Dermatologic: Increased sensitivity to light
  - Endocrine & metabolic: Decreased flow of breast milk
  - Gastrointestinal: Dysphagia
- <1%: Ataxia, bloated feeling, blurred vision, confusion, drowsiness, dysuria, fatigue, headache, increased intraocular pain, loss of memory, nausea, orthostatic hypotension, palpitations, rash, tachycardia, ventricular fibrillation, vomiting, weakness

**Note:** Systemic adverse effects have been reported following ophthalmic administration

**Overdosage/Toxicology**

Signs and symptoms: Dilated pupils, flushed skin, tachycardia, hypertension, EKG abnormalities, CNS manifestations resemble acute psychosis; CNS depression, circulatory collapse, respiratory failure, and death can occur

Treatment: Pure scopolamine intoxication is extremely rare. However, for a scopolamine overdose with severe life-threatening symptoms, physostigmine 1-2 mg (0.5 or 0.02 mg/kg for children) S.C. or I.V. slowly should be given to reverse the toxic effects.

**Drug Interactions**

Decreased effect of acetaminophen, levodopa, ketoconazole, digoxin, riboflavin, potassium chloride in wax matrix preparations

Increased toxicity: Additive adverse effects with other anticholinergic agents; GI absorption of the following drugs may be affected: acetaminophen, levodopa, ketoconazole, digoxin, riboflavin, potassium chloride wax-matrix preparations

**Usual Dosage**

Preoperatively:
- Children: I.M., S.C.: 6 mcg/kg/dose (maximum: 0.3 mg/dose) or 0.2 mg/m$^2$ may be repeated every 6-8 hours **or** alternatively:
  - 4-7 months: 0.1 mg
  - 7 months to 3 years: 0.15 mg
  - 3-8 years: 0.2 mg
  - 8-12 years: 0.3 mg
- Adults:
  - I.M., I.V., S.C.: 0.3-0.65 mg; may be repeated every 4-6 hours
  - Transdermal patch: Apply 2.5 cm$^2$ patch to hairless area behind ear the night before surgery (the patch should be applied no sooner than 1 hour before surgery for best results)

Motion sickness: Transdermal: Children >12 years and Adults: Apply 1 disc behind the ear at least 4 hours prior to exposure and every 3 days as needed; effective if applied as soon as 2-3 hours before anticipated need, best if 12 hours before

Ophthalmic:
- Refraction:
  - Children: Instill 1 drop of 0.25% to eye(s) twice daily for 2 days before procedure
  - Adults: Instill 1-2 drops of 0.25% to eye(s) 1 hour before procedure
- Iridocyclitis:
  - Children: Instill 1 drop of 0.25% to eye(s) up to 3 times/day
  - Adults: Instill 1-2 drops of 0.25% to eye(s) up to 4 times/day

Oral: 0.4 to 0.8 mg as a range; the dosage may be cautiously increased in parkinsonism and spastic states.

**Patient Information** Take as directed. You may experience drowsiness, confusion, impaired judgment, or vision changes (use caution when driving or engaging in tasks requiring alertness until response to drug is known); dry mouth, nausea, or vomiting (small frequent meals, frequent mouth care, chewing gum, or sucking lozenges may help); orthostatic hypotension (use caution when climbing stairs and when rising from lying or sitting position); constipation (increased exercise, fluid, or dietary fiber may reduce constipation, if not effective consult prescriber); increased sensitivity to heat and decreased perspiration (avoid extremes of heat, reduce exercise in hot weather); decreased milk if breast-feeding. Report hot, dry, flushed skin; blurred vision or vision changes; difficulty swallowing; chest pain, palpitations, or rapid heartbeat; painful or difficult urination; increased confusion, depression, or loss of memory; rapid or difficult respirations; muscle weakness or tremors; or eye pain.

**Administration:** Transdermal: Apply patch behind ear the day before traveling. Wash hands before applying and avoid contact with the eyes. Do not remove for 3 days.

Ophthalmic: Instill as often as recommended. Wash hands before using. Sit or lie down, open eye, look at ceiling, and instill prescribed amount of solution. Do not blink for 30 seconds, close eye and roll eye in all directions, and apply gentle pressure to inner corner of eye for 1-2 minutes. Do not let tip of applicator touch eye or contaminate tip of applicator. Temporary stinging or blurred vision may occur.

**Nursing Implications** Topical disc is programmed to deliver *in vivo* 0.5 mg over 3 days; wash hands before and after applying the disc to avoid drug contact with eyes

**Dosage Forms**

Disc, transdermal: 1.5 mg/disc (4s)
Injection, as hydrobromide: 0.3 mg/mL (1 mL); 0.4 mg/mL (0.5 mL, 1 mL); 0.86 mg/mL (0.5 mL); 1 mg/mL (1 mL)
Solution, ophthalmic, as hydrobromide: 0.25% (5 mL, 15 mL)
Tablet: 0.4 mg


- **Scot-Tussin® [OTC]** *see* Guaifenesin *on page 256*
- **Scot-Tussin DM® Cough Chasers [OTC]** *see* Dextromethorphan *on page 160*
- **Scot-Tussin® Senior Clear [OTC]** *see* Guaifenesin and Dextromethorphan *on page 257*
- **Scury Root, American Coneflower** *see* Echinacea *on page 189*
- **SDZ ENA 713** *see* Rivastigmine *on page 498*

- **Sea Grape** *see* Ephedra *on page 194*
- **Sebizon® Topical Lotion** *see* Sulfacetamide *on page 522*

## Secobarbital (see koe BAR bi tal)

**Related Information**

Anxiolytic/Hypnotic Use in Long-Term Care Facilities *on page 754*

Federal OBRA Regulations Recommended Maximum Doses *on page 756*

Patient Information - Anxiolytics & Sedative Hypnotics (Barbiturates) *on page 654*

**Generic Available** Yes

**U.S. Brand Names** Seconal™ Injection

**Canadian Brand Names** Novo-Secobarb

**Synonyms** Quinalbarbitone Sodium; Secobarbital Sodium

**Pharmacologic Category** Barbiturate

**Use** Preanesthetic agent; short-term treatment of insomnia

**Restrictions** C-II

**Pregnancy Risk Factor** D

**Contraindications** Hypersensitivity to barbiturates or any component of the formulation; marked hepatic impairment; dyspnea or airway obstruction; porphyria

**Warnings/Precautions** Should be used only after evaluation of potential causes of sleep disturbance. Failure of sleep disturbance to resolve after 7-10 days may indicate psychiatric or medical illness. Potential for drug dependency exists, abrupt cessation may precipitate withdrawal, including status epilepticus in epileptic patients. Do not administer to patients in acute pain. Use caution in elderly, debilitated, renally impaired, or pediatric patients. May cause paradoxical responses, including agitation and hyperactivity, particularly in acute pain and pediatric patients. Use with caution in patients with depression or suicidal tendencies, or in patients with a history of drug abuse. Tolerance, psychological and physical dependence may occur with prolonged use. Use with caution in patients with hepatic function impairment. May cause CNS depression, which may impair physical or mental abilities. Patients must cautioned about performing tasks which require mental alertness (ie, operating machinery or driving). Effects with other sedative drugs or ethanol may be potentiated. May cause respiratory depression or hypotension, Use with caution in hemodynamically unstable patients or patients with respiratory disease.

**Adverse Reactions**

>10%:

Central nervous system: Dizziness, lightheadedness, "hangover" effect, drowsiness, CNS depression, fever

Local: Pain at injection site

1% to 10%:

Central nervous system: Confusion, mental depression, unusual excitement, nervousness, faint feeling, headache, insomnia, nightmares

Gastrointestinal: Nausea, vomiting, constipation

<1%: Agranulocytosis, apnea, exfoliative dermatitis, hallucinations, hypotension, laryngospasm, megaloblastic anemia, rash, respiratory depression, Stevens-Johnson syndrome, thrombocytopenia, thrombophlebitis, urticaria

**Overdosage/Toxicology**

Signs and symptoms: Unsteady gait, slurred speech, confusion, jaundice, hypothermia, fever, hypotension, respiratory depression, coma

Treatment: If hypotension occurs, administer I.V. fluids and place the patient in the Trendelenburg position. If unresponsive, an I.V. vasopressor (eg, dopamine, epinephrine) may be required. Charcoal hemoperfusion or hemodialysis may be useful in the harder to treat intoxications, especially in the presence of very high serum barbiturate levels when the patient is in shock, coma, or renal failure. Forced alkaline diuresis is of no value in the treatment of intoxications with short-acting barbiturates.

**Drug Interactions** CYP2C9, 3A3/4, and 3A5-7 enzyme inducer

**Note:** Barbiturates are enzyme inducers; patients should be monitored when these drugs are started or stopped for a decreased or increased therapeutic effect respectively

Acetaminophen: Barbiturates may enhance the hepatotoxic potential of acetaminophen overdoses

Antiarrhythmics: Barbiturates may increase the metabolism of antiarrhythmics, decreasing their clinical effect; includes disopyramide, propafenone, and quinidine

Anticonvulsants: Barbiturates may increase the metabolism of anticonvulsants; includes ethosuximide, felbamate (possibly), lamotrigine, phenytoin, tiagabine, topiramate, and zonisamide; does not appear to affect gabapentin or levetiracetam

Antineoplastics: Limited evidence suggests that enzyme-inducing anticonvulsant therapy may reduce the effectiveness of some chemotherapy regimens (specifically in ALL); teniposide and methotrexate may be cleared more rapidly in these patients

Antipsychotics: Barbiturates may enhance the metabolism (decrease the efficacy) of antipsychotics; monitor for altered response; dose adjustment may be needed

Beta-blockers: Metabolism of beta-blockers may be increased and clinical effect decreased; atenolol and nadolol are unlikely to interact given their renal elimination

Calcium channel blockers: Barbiturates may enhance the metabolism of calcium channel blockers, decreasing their clinical effect

Chloramphenicol: Barbiturates may increase the metabolism of chloramphenicol and chloramphenicol may inhibit barbiturate metabolism; monitor for altered response

Cimetidine: Barbiturates may enhance the metabolism of cimetidine, decreasing its clinical effect

CNS depressants: Sedative effects and/or respiratory depression with barbiturates may be additive with other CNS depressants; monitor for increased effect; includes ethanol, sedatives, antidepressants, narcotic analgesics, and benzodiazepines

Corticosteroids: Barbiturates may enhance the metabolism of corticosteroids, decreasing their clinical effect

Cyclosporine: Levels may be decreased by barbiturates; monitor

Doxycycline: Barbiturates may enhance the metabolism of doxycycline, decreasing its clinical effect; higher dosages may be required

Estrogens: Barbiturates may increase the metabolism of estrogens and reduce their efficacy

Felbamate may inhibit the metabolism of barbiturates and barbiturates may increase the metabolism of felbamate

Griseofulvin: Barbiturates may impair the absorption of griseofulvin, and griseofulvin metabolism may be increased by barbiturates, decreasing clinical effect

Guanfacine: Effect may be decreased by barbiturates

Immunosuppressants: Barbiturates may enhance the metabolism of immunosuppressants, decreasing its clinical effect; includes both cyclosporine and tacrolimus

Loop diuretics: Metabolism may be increased and clinical effects decreased; established for furosemide, effect with other loop diuretics not established

MAOIs: Metabolism of barbiturates may be inhibited, increasing clinical effect or toxicity of the barbiturates

Methadone: Barbiturates may enhance the metabolism of methadone resulting in methadone withdrawal

Methoxyflurane: Barbiturates may enhance the nephrotoxic effects of methoxyflurane

Oral contraceptives: Barbiturates may enhance the metabolism of oral contraceptives, decreasing their clinical effect; an alternative method of contraception should be considered

Theophylline: Barbiturates may increase metabolism of theophylline derivatives and decrease their clinical effect

Tricyclic antidepressants: Barbiturates may increase metabolism of tricyclic antidepressants and decrease their clinical effect; sedative effects may be additive

Valproic acid: Metabolism of barbiturates may be inhibited by valproic acid; monitor for excessive sedation; a dose reduction may be needed

Warfarin: Barbiturates inhibit the hypoprothrombinemic effects of oral anticoagulants via increased metabolism; this combination should generally be avoided

**Stability** Do not shake vial during reconstitution, rotate ampul; aqueous solutions are not stable, reconstitute with aqueous polyethylene glycol; aqueous (sterile water) solutions should be used within 30 minutes; do not use bacteriostatic water for injection or lactated Ringer's. I.V. form is **incompatible** when mixed with benzquinamide (in syringe), cimetidine (same syringe), codeine, erythromycin, glycopyrrolate (same syringe), hydrocortisone, insulin, levorphanol, methadone, norepinephrine, pentazocine, phenytoin, sodium bicarbonate, tetracycline, vancomycin

**Mechanism of Action** Depresses CNS activity by binding to barbiturate site at GABA-receptor complex enhancing GABA activity, depressing reticular activity system; higher doses may be gabamimetic

**Pharmacodynamics/kinetics**

Onset of hypnosis: Oral: 15-30 minutes; I.M.: 7-10 minutes; I.V. injection: 1-3 minutes

Duration: Oral: 3-4 hours with 100 mg dose; I.V.: ~15 minutes

Distribution: 1.5 L/kg; crosses the placenta; appears in breast milk

Protein binding: 45% to 60%

Metabolism: In the liver by microsomal enzyme system

Half-life: 15-40 hours, mean: 28 hours

Time to peak serum concentration: Within 2-4 hours

Elimination: Renally as inactive metabolites and small amounts as unchanged drug

**Usual Dosage** Hypnotic:

Children: I.M.: 3-5 mg/kg/dose; maximum: 100 mg/dose

Adults:

Oral: 100 mg/dose at bedtime; range: 100-200 mg/dose

I.M.: 100-200 mg/dose

I.V.: 50-250 mg/dose

Hemodialysis: Slightly dialyzable (5% to 20%)

**Dietary Considerations** Alcohol: Additive CNS effect, avoid use

**Administration** I.V.: Administer undiluted or diluted with sterile water for injection, normal saline, or Ringer's injection; maximum infusion rate: 50 mg/15 seconds; avoid intra-arterial injection

(Continued)

## Secobarbital *(Continued)*

**Monitoring Parameters** Blood pressure, heart rate, respiratory rate, CNS status

**Reference Range** Therapeutic: 1-2 µg/mL (SI: 4.2-8.4 µmol/L); Toxic: >5 µg/mL (SI: >21 µmol/L)

**Patient Information** Avoid the use of alcohol and other CNS depressants; avoid driving and other hazardous tasks; avoid abrupt discontinuation; may cause physical and psychological dependence; do not alter dose without notifying physician

**Dosage Forms**

Capsule: 100 mg

Injection, as sodium: 50 mg/mL (2 mL)


- ♦ **Secobarbital and Amobarbital** *see* Amobarbital and Secobarbital *on page 36*
- ♦ **Secobarbital Sodium** *see* Secobarbital *on page 507*
- ♦ **Seconal™ Injection** *see* Secobarbital *on page 507*
- ♦ **Secondary Mental Disorders** *see page 616*
- ♦ **Secran®** *see* Vitamins, Multiple *on page 587*
- ♦ **Sectral®** *see* Acebutolol *on page 13*
- ♦ **Sedapap-10®** *see* Butalbital Compound and Acetaminophen *on page 80*
- ♦ **Sedaplus®** *see* Doxylamine *on page 186*


## Selegiline (seh LEDGE ah leen)

**Related Information**

Clinical Issues in the Use of Antidepressants *on page 627*

Patient Information - Antidepressants (MAOIs) *on page 644*

**Generic Available** No

**U.S. Brand Names** Eldepryl®

**Canadian Brand Names** Apo®-Selegiline; Novo-Selegiline

**Synonyms** Deprenyl; L-Deprenyl; Selegiline Hydrochloride

**Pharmacologic Category** Antidepressant, Monoamine Oxidase Inhibitor; Anti-Parkinson's Agent (Monoamine Oxidase Inhibitor)

**Use** Adjunct in the management of parkinsonian patients in which levodopa/carbidopa therapy is deteriorating

**Unlabeled uses:** Early Parkinson's disease; ADHD; negative symptoms of schizophrenia; extrapyramidal symptoms; depression; Alzheimer's disease (studies have shown some improvement in behavioral and cognitive performance)

**Pregnancy Risk Factor** C

**Contraindications** Hypersensitivity to selegiline; concomitant use of meperidine

**Warnings/Precautions** Increased risk of nonselective MAO inhibition occurs with doses >10 mg/day; it is a monoamine oxidase inhibitor type "B", there should not be a problem with tyramine-containing products as long as the typical doses are employed, however, rare reactions have been reported. Use with tricyclic antidepressants and SSRIs has also been associated with rare reactions and should generally be avoided. Addition to levodopa therapy may result in exacerbation of levodopa adverse effects, requiring a reduction in levodopa dosage.

**Adverse Reactions**

Cardiovascular: Orthostatic hypotension, hypertension, arrhythmias, palpitations, angina, tachycardia, peripheral edema, bradycardia, syncope

Central nervous system: Hallucinations, dizziness, confusion, anxiety, depression, drowsiness, behavior/mood changes, dreams/nightmares, fatigue, delusions

Dermatologic: Rash, photosensitivity

Gastrointestinal: Xerostomia, nausea, vomiting, constipation, weight loss, anorexia, diarrhea, heartburn

Genitourinary: Nocturia, prostatic hypertrophy, urinary retention, sexual dysfunction

Neuromuscular & skeletal: Tremor, chorea, loss of balance, restlessness, bradykinesia

Ocular: Blepharospasm, blurred vision

Miscellaneous: Diaphoresis (increased)

**Overdosage/Toxicology**

Signs and symptoms: Tachycardia, palpitations, muscle twitching, seizures

Treatment: Competent supportive care is the most important treatment; both hypertension or hypotension can occur with intoxication. Hypotension may respond to I.V. fluids or vasopressors, and hypertension usually responds to an alpha-adrenergic blocker. While treating the hypertension, care is warranted to avoid sudden drops in blood pressure, since this may worsen the MAO inhibitor toxicity. Muscle irritability and seizures often respond to diazepam, while hyperthermia is best treated antipyretics and cooling blankets. Cardiac arrhythmias are best treated with phenytoin or procainamide.

**Drug Interactions** CYP2D6 enzyme substrate

**Note:** Many drug interactions involving selegiline are theoretical, primarily based on interactions with nonspecific MAOIs; at doses <10 mg/day, the risk of these interactions with selegiline may be very low

Amphetamines: MAOIs in combination with amphetamines may result in severe hypertensive reaction or serotonin syndrome; these combinations are best avoided

Anorexiants: Concurrent use of selegiline (high dose) in combination with CNS stimulants or anorexiants may result in serotonin syndrome; these combinations are best avoided; includes dexfenfluramine, fenfluramine, or sibutramine

Barbiturates: MAOIs may inhibit the metabolism of barbiturates and prolong their effect

CNS stimulants: MAOIs in combination with stimulants (methylphenidate) may result in serotonin syndrome; these combinations are best avoided

CYP2D6 inhibitors: Theoretically, inhibitors may decrease hepatic metabolism of selegiline, increasing serum concentrations; inhibitors include amiodarone, cimetidine, delavirdine, fluoxetine, paroxetine, propafenone, quinidine, and ritonavir; monitor for increased effect/toxicity

Dextromethorphan: Concurrent use of selegiline (high dose) may result in serotonin syndrome; these combinations are best avoided

Disulfiram: MAOIs may produce delirium in patients receiving disulfiram; monitor

Enzyme inducers: May increase the metabolism of selegiline, reducing serum levels and effect; enzyme inducers include carbamazepine, barbiturates, phenytoin, and rifampin

Guanadrel and guanethidine: MAOIs inhibit the antihypertensive response to guanadrel or guanethidine; use an alternative antihypertensive agent

Hypoglycemic agents: MAOIs may produce hypoglycemia in patients with diabetes; monitor

Levodopa: MAOIs in combination with levodopa may result in hypertensive reactions; monitor

Lithium: MAOIs in combination with lithium have resulted in malignant hyperpyrexia; this combination is best avoided

Meperidine: Concurrent use of selegiline (high dose) may result in serotonin syndrome; these combinations are best avoided

Nefazodone: Concurrent use of selegiline (high dose) may result in serotonin syndrome; these combinations are best avoided

Norepinephrine: MAOIs may increase the pressor response of norepinephrine (effect is generally small); monitor

Oral contraceptives: Increased selegiline levels have been noted with concurrent administration; monitor

Reserpine: MAOIs in combination with reserpine may result in hypertensive reactions; monitor

SSRIs: Concurrent use of selegiline with an SSRI may result in mania or hypertension; it is generally best to avoid these combinations

Sympathomimetics (indirect-acting): MAOIs in combination with sympathomimetics such as dopamine, metaraminol, phenylephrine, and decongestants (pseudoephedrine) may result in severe hypertensive reaction; these combinations are best avoided

Succinylcholine: MAOIs may prolong the muscle relaxation produced by succinylcholine via decreased plasma pseudocholinesterase

Tramadol: May increase the risk of seizures and serotonin syndrome in patients receiving an MAOI

Trazodone: Concurrent use of selegiline (high dose) may result in serotonin syndrome; these combinations are best avoided

Tricyclic antidepressants: May cause serotonin syndrome when combined with an MAO inhibitor; avoid this combination

Tyramine: Selegiline (>10 mg/day) in combination with tyramine (cheese, ethanol) may increase the pressor response; avoid high tyramine-containing foods in patients receiving >10 mg/day of selegiline

Venlafaxine: Concurrent use of selegiline (high dose) may result in serotonin syndrome; these combinations are best avoided

**Mechanism of Action** Potent monoamine oxidase (MAO) type-B inhibitor; MAO-B plays a major role in the metabolism of dopamine; selegiline may also increase dopaminergic activity by interfering with dopamine reuptake at the synapse

**Pharmacodynamics/kinetics**

Onset of therapeutic effects: Within 1 hour

Duration: 24-72 hours

Half-life: 10 hours

Metabolism: In the liver to amphetamine and methamphetamine

**Usual Dosage** Oral:

Adults: 5 mg twice daily with breakfast and lunch or 10 mg in the morning

Elderly: Initial: 5 mg in the morning, may increase to a total of 10 mg/day

**Monitoring Parameters** Blood pressure, symptoms of parkinsonism

**Patient Information** Do not exceed daily doses of 10 mg; report to physician any involuntary movements or CNS agitation

**Nursing Implications** Monoamine oxidase inhibitor type "B"; there should **not** be a problem with tyramine-containing products as long as the typical doses are employed

**Additional Information** When adding selegiline to levodopa/carbidopa the dose of the latter can usually be decreased. Studies are investigating the use of selegiline in early Parkinson's disease to slow the progression of the disease.

**Dosage Forms**

Capsule, as hydrochloride (Eldepryl®): 5 mg

Tablet, as hydrochloride: 5 mg

♦ **Selegiline Hydrochloride** *see* Selegiline *on page 508*

- **Semicid® [OTC]** *see* Nonoxynol 9 *on page 398*
- **Semprex®-D** *see* Acrivastine and Pseudoephedrine *on page 19*
- **Senexon® [OTC]** *see* Senna *on page 509*

## Senna

**Related Information**
Herbals That May Alter Metabolism and GI Absorption of Drugs *on page 745*
Laxatives, Classification and Properties *on page 716*
Natural Products, Herbals, and Dietary Supplements *on page 742*
Perspectives on the Safety of Herbal Medicines *on page 736*

**U.S. Brand Names** Black Draught® [OTC]; Senexon® [OTC]; Senna-Gen® [OTC]; Senokot® [OTC]; X-Prep® Liquid [OTC]

**Synonyms** *C. angustifolia*; *Cassia acutifolia*; Senna Alexandria

**Pharmacologic Category** Herb

**Use** Short-term treatment of constipation; evacuate the colon for bowel or rectal examinations

**Contraindications** Per Commission E: Intestinal obstruction, acute intestinal inflammation (eg, Crohn's disease), colitis ulcerosa, appendicitis, abdominal pain of unknown origin, children <12 years, and pregnancy

**Adverse Reactions**
Cardiovascular: Palpitations
Central nervous system: Tetany, dizziness
Dermatologic: Finger clubbing (reversible)
Endocrine & metabolic: Hypokalemia
Gastrointestinal: Vomiting (with fresh plant leaves or pods), diarrhea, abdominal cramping, nausea, melanosis coli (reversible), cachexia
Genitourinary: red discoloration in alkaline urine (yellow-brown in acidic urine)
Hepatic: Hepatitis
Renal: Oliguria, proteinuria
Respiratory: Dyspnea

Per Commission E:
Endocrine & metabolic: Long-term use/abuse can cause electrolyte imbalance
Gastrointestinal: In single incidents, cramp-like discomforts of G.I. tract requiring a reduction in dosage

**Overdosage/Toxicology** Decontamination: Do **not** induce emesis; lavage (within 1 hour)/activated charcoal can be used

**Drug Interactions** Per Commission E: Potentiation of cardiac glycosides (with long-term use) is possible due to loss in potassium; effect on antiarrhythmics is possible; potassium deficiency can be increased by simultaneous application of thiazide diuretics, corticosteroids, and licorice root

**Usual Dosage**
Children: Oral:
>6 years: 10-20 mg/kg/dose at bedtime; maximum daily dose: 872 mg
6-12 years, >27 kg: 1 tablet at bedtime, up to 4 tablets/day **or** ½ teaspoonful of granules (326 mg/tsp) at bedtime (up to 2 teaspoonfuls/day)
Liquid:
2-5 years: 5-10 mL at bedtime
6-15 years: 10-15 mL at bedtime
Suppository: ½ at bedtime
Syrup:
1 month to 1 year: 1.25-2.5 mL at bedtime up to 5 mL/day
1-5 years: 2.5-5 mL at bedtime up to 10 mL/day
5-10 years: 5-10 mL at bedtime up to 20 mL/day
Adults:
Granules (326 mg/teaspoon): 1 teaspoonful at bedtime, not to exceed 2 teaspoonfuls twice daily
Liquid: 15-30 mL with meals and at bedtime
Suppository: 1 at bedtime, may repeat once in 2 hours
Syrup: 2-3 teaspoonfuls at bedtime, not to exceed 30 mL/day
Tablet: 187 mg: 2 tablets at bedtime, not to exceed 8 tablets/day
Tablet: 374 mg: 1 at bedtime, up to 4/day; 600 mg: 2 tablets at bedtime, up to 3 tablets/day

**Patient Information** May discolor urine or feces (yellow, brown, pink, red, or violet); may cause dependence with prolonged or excessive use

**Additional Information** Both leaf and fruits ("pods") are use; avoid prolonged use; may increase potency and toxicity of digitalis; the plant is found in North Africa and India; a low branching shrub with large yellow leaves on the top of the plant are harvested; compatible for breast-feeding; hypersensitivity to the ingredients; contraindications in fecal impaction, bowel obstruction, and abdominal pain

- **Senna Alexandria** *see* Senna *on page 509*
- **Senna-Gen® [OTC]** *see* Senna *on page 509*
- **Senokot® [OTC]** *see* Senna *on page 509*
- **Sensorcaine®** *see* Bupivacaine *on page 76*
- **Sensorcaine®-MPF** *see* Bupivacaine *on page 76*
- **Septa® Topical Ointment [OTC]** *see* Bacitracin, Neomycin, and Polymyxin B *on page 57*
- **Septra®** *see* Co-Trimoxazole *on page 142*
- **Septra® DS** *see* Co-Trimoxazole *on page 142*
- **Ser-Ap-Es®** *see* Hydralazine, Hydrochlorothiazide, and Reserpine *on page 270*
- **Serax®** *see* Oxazepam *on page 410*
- ***Serenoa repens*** *see* Saw Palmetto *on page 505*
- **Serentil®** *see* Mesoridazine *on page 344*
- **Serevent®** *see* Salmeterol *on page 502*
- **Sermion®** *see* Nicergoline *on page 392*
- **Seromycin® Pulvules®** *see* Cycloserine *on page 146*
- **Serophene®** *see* Clomiphene *on page 130*
- **Seroquel®** *see* Quetiapine *on page 483*
- **Serostim® Injection** *see* Human Growth Hormone *on page 269*
- **Serotonin Syndrome** *see page 805*
- **Serpalan®** *see* Reserpine *on page 491*

## Sertraline (SER tra leen)

**Related Information**
Antidepressant Agents Comparison Chart *on page 704*
Clinical Issues in the Use of Antidepressants *on page 627*
Discontinuation of Psychotropic Drugs - Withdrawal Symptoms and Recommendations *on page 798*
Mood Disorders *on page 600*
Patient Information - Antidepressants (SSRIs) *on page 639*
Pharmacokinetics of Selective Serotonin-Reuptake Inhibitors (SSRIs) *on page 723*
Special Populations - Elderly *on page 662*
Teratogenic Risks of Psychotropic Medications *on page 812*

**Generic Available** No

**U.S. Brand Names** Zoloft®

**Synonyms** Sertraline Hydrochloride

**Pharmacologic Category** Antidepressant, Selective Serotonin Reuptake Inhibitor

**Use** Treatment of major depression; obsessive-compulsive disorder; panic disorder; post-traumatic stress disorder

**Unlabeled use:** Eating disorders; anxiety disorders; premenstrual disorders; impulse control disorders

**Pregnancy Risk Factor** C

**Contraindications** Hypersensitivity to sertraline; use of MAO inhibitors within 14 days

**Warnings/Precautions** Potential for severe reaction when used with MAO inhibitors - serotonin syndrome (hyperthermia, muscular rigidity, mental status changes/agitation, autonomic instability) may occur. May precipitate a shift to mania or hypomania in patients with bipolar disease. Has a very low potential to impair cognitive or motor performance. Does not appear to potentiate the effects of alcohol, however, alcohol use is not advised. Use caution in patients with depression, particularly if suicidal risk may be present. Use caution in patients with a previous seizure disorder or condition predisposing to seizures such as brain damage, alcoholism, or concurrent therapy with other drugs which lower the seizure threshold. Use with caution in patients with hepatic or dysfunction and in elderly patients. May cause hyponatremia/SIADH. Use with caution in patients with renal insufficiency or other concurrent illness (due to limited experience). Sertraline acts as a mild uricosuric - use with caution in patients at risk of uric acid nephropathy. Use with caution in patients at risk of bleeding or receiving anticoagulant therapy - may cause impairment in platelet aggregation. Use with caution in patients where weight loss is undesirable. May cause or exacerbate sexual dysfunction.

**Adverse Reactions**
>10%:
Central nervous system: Insomnia, somnolence, dizziness, headache, fatigue
Gastrointestinal: Xerostomia, diarrhea, nausea
Genitourinary: Ejaculatory disturbances
1% to 10%:
Cardiovascular: Palpitations
Central nervous system: Agitation, anxiety, nervousness
Dermatologic: Rash
Endocrine & metabolic: Decreased libido
Gastrointestinal: Constipation, anorexia, dyspepsia, flatulence, vomiting
Genitourinary: Micturition disorders
Neuromuscular & skeletal: Tremors, paresthesia
Ocular: Visual difficulty, abnormal vision
Otic: Tinnitus
Miscellaneous: Diaphoresis (increased)
(Continued)

## Sertraline *(Continued)*

**Overdosage/Toxicology**

Signs and symptoms: Serious toxicity has not yet been reported, monitor cardiovascular, gastrointestinal, and hepatic functions

Treatment: There are no specific antidotes for sertraline overdose; treatment should be aimed first at decontamination, then symptomatic and supportive care

**Drug Interactions** CYP3A3/4 and CYP2D6 (minor) enzyme substrate; CYP2C19 and 3A3/4 enzyme inhibitor; weak inhibitor of CYP1A2 and 2D6.

Amphetamines: SSRIs may increase the sensitivity to amphetamines, and amphetamines may increase the risk of serotonin syndrome

Benzodiazepines: Sertraline may inhibit the metabolism of alprazolam and diazepam resulting in elevated serum levels; monitor for increased sedation and psychomotor impairment

Buspirone: Sertraline inhibits the reuptake of serotonin; combined use with a serotonin agonist (buspirone) may cause serotonin syndrome

Carbamazepine: Sertraline may inhibit the metabolism of carbamazepine resulting in increased carbamazepine levels and toxicity; monitor for altered carbamazepine response

Clozapine: Sertraline may increase serum levels of clozapine; monitor for increased effect/toxicity

Cyclosporine: Sertraline may increase serum levels of cyclosporine (and possibly tacrolimus); monitor

Cyproheptadine: May inhibit the effects of serotonin reuptake inhibitors (fluoxetine); monitor for altered antidepressant response; cyproheptadine acts as a serotonin agonist

Dextromethorphan: Some SSRIs inhibit the metabolism of dextromethorphan; visual hallucinations occurred; monitor for serotonin syndrome

Erythromycin: Serotonin syndrome has been reported when added to sertraline; limited documentation

Haloperidol: Serum concentrations may be increased by sertraline (small increase); monitor

HMG CoA reductase inhibitors: Sertraline may inhibit the metabolism of lovastatin and simvastatin (metabolized by CYP3A3/4) resulting in myositis and rhabdomyolysis; although its inhibition is weak, these combinations are best avoided

Lamotrigine: Toxicity has been reported following the addition of sertraline; monitor

Lithium: Patients receiving SSRIs and lithium have developed neurotoxicity; if combination is used; monitor for neurotoxicity

Loop diuretics: Sertraline may cause hyponatremia; additive hyponatremic effects may be seen with combined use of a loop diuretic (bumetanide, furosemide, torsemide); monitor for hyponatremia

MAOIs: Sertraline should not be used with nonselective MAOIs (isocarboxazid, phenelzine); fatal reactions have been reported; wait 5 weeks after stopping fluoxetine before starting an MAOI and 2 weeks after stopping an MAOI before starting fluoxetine

Meperidine: Concurrent use may result in serotonin syndrome; these combinations are best avoided

Nefazodone: May increase the risk of serotonin syndrome

Phenytoin: Sertraline inhibits the metabolism of phenytoin and may result in phenytoin toxicity; monitor for phenytoin toxicity (ataxia, confusion, dizziness, nystagmus, involuntary muscle movement)

Selegiline: SSRIs have been reported to cause mania or hypertension when combined with selegiline; this combination is best avoided. Concurrent use with SSRIs has been reported to cause serotonin syndrome. As a MAO-B inhibitor, the risk of serotonin syndrome may be less than with nonselective MAO inhibitors.

Serotonin agonists: Theoretically, may increase the risk of serotonin syndrome; includes sumatriptan, naratriptan, rizatriptan, and zolmitriptan

Sibutramine: May increase the risk of serotonin syndrome with SSRIs

SSRIs: Combined use with other drugs which inhibit the reuptake may cause serotonin syndrome

Sympathomimetics: May increase the risk of serotonin syndrome with SSRIs

Tramadol: Sertraline combined with tramadol (serotonergic effects) may cause serotonin syndrome; monitor

Trazodone: Sertraline may inhibit the metabolism of trazodone resulting in increased toxicity; monitor

Tricyclic antidepressants: Sertraline may inhibit the metabolism of tricyclic antidepressants (amitriptyline, desipramine, imipramine, nortriptyline) resulting is elevated serum levels; if combination is warranted, a low dose of TCA (10-25 mg/day) should be utilized

Tryptophan: Sertraline may inhibit the reuptake of serotonin; combination with tryptophan, a serotonin precursor, may cause agitation and restlessness; this combination is best avoided

Venlafaxine: Sertraline may increase the risk of serotonin syndrome

Warfarin: Sertraline may alter the hypoprothombinemic response to warfarin; monitor

Zolpidem: Onset of hypnosis may be shortened in patients receiving sertraline; monitor

**Mechanism of Action** Antidepressant with selective inhibitory effects on presynaptic serotonin (5-HT) reuptake and only very weak effects on norepinephrine and dopamine neuronal uptake

**Pharmacodynamics/kinetics**

Absorption: Slow

Protein binding: High

Metabolism: Extensive

Half-life:

Parent: 24 hours

Metabolites: 66 hours

Elimination: In both urine and feces

**Usual Dosage** Oral:

Adults: Start with 50 mg/day in the morning and increase by 50 mg/day increments every 2-3 days if tolerated to 100 mg/day; additional increases may be necessary; maximum dose: 200 mg/day. If somnolence is noted, administer at bedtime.

Elderly: Start treatment with 25 mg/day in the morning and increase by 25 mg/day increments every 2-3 days if tolerated to 50-100 mg/day; additional increases may be necessary; maximum dose: 200 mg/day

Hemodialysis: Not removed by hemodialysis

**Dosage comments in hepatic impairment:** Sertraline is extensively metabolized by the liver; caution should be used in patients with hepatic impairment

**Monitoring Parameters** Uric acid, liver function, CBC

**Reference Range** 6 hours after doses of 400 mg and 200 mg, peak plasma levels were 253.2 ng/mL and 105.4 ng/mL respectively; plasma levels correlate poorly to clinical presentation; therapeutic clinical trials: 0.03-0.19 mg/L

**Test Interactions** Minor ↑ triglycerides (S); ↑ LFTs, uric acid (S)

**Patient Information** If you are currently on another antidepressant drug, please notify your physician. Although sertraline has not been shown to increase the effects of alcohol, it is recommended that you refrain from drinking while on this medication. If you are pregnant or intend becoming pregnant while on this drug, please alert your physician to this fact.

**Nursing Implications** Offer patient sugarless hard candy for dry mouth

**Additional Information** Buspirone (15-60 mg/day) may be useful in treatment of sexual dysfunction during treatment with a selective serotonin reuptake inhibitor; may exacerbate tics in Tourette's syndrome

**Dosage Forms**

Concentrate, oral: 20 mg/mL (60 mL)

Tablet, as hydrochloride: 25 mg, 50 mg, 100 mg

♦ **Sertraline Hydrochloride** *see* Sertraline *on page 509*

♦ **Serum Drug Concentrations Commonly Monitored: Guidelines** *see page 759*

♦ **Serutan® [OTC]** *see* Psyllium *on page 479*

♦ **Serzone®** *see* Nefazodone *on page 386*

## Sevelamer (se VEL a mer)

**U.S. Brand Names** Renagel®

**Pharmacologic Category** Phosphate Binder

**Use** Reduction of serum phosphorous in patients with end-stage renal disease

**Effects on Mental Status** None reported

**Effects on Psychiatric Treatment** None reported

**Usual Dosage** Adults: Oral: 2-4 capsules 3 times/day with meals; the initial dose may be based on serum phosphorous:

(Phosphorous: Initial Dose)

>6.0 mg/dL and <7.5 mg/dL: 2 capsules 3 times/day

>7.5 mg/dL and <9.0 mg/dL: 3 capsules 3 times/day

≥9.0 mg/dL: 4 capsules 3 times/day

Dosage should be adjusted based on serum phosphorous concentration, with a goal of lowering to <6.0 mg/dL; maximum daily dose studied was 30 capsules/day

**Dosage Forms** Capsule: 403 mg

## Sevoflurane (see voe FLOO rane)

**U.S. Brand Names** Ultane®

**Pharmacologic Category** General Anesthetic

**Use** General induction and maintenance of anesthesia (inhalation)

**Effects on Mental Status** May cause agitation, somnolence, or dizziness

**Effects on Psychiatric Treatment** None reported

**Usual Dosage**

Induction: Usually administered in concentrations of 1.8% to 5% in $N_2O/O_2$. It has also been given via the vital capacity rapid inhalation technique as 4.5% in $N_2O/O_2$

Maintenance: Surgical levels of anesthesia can usually be obtained with concentrations of 0.75% to 3%

**Dosage Forms** Liquid for inhalation: 250 mL

♦ **Shur-Seal® [OTC]** *see* Nonoxynol 9 *on page 398*

## Sibutramine (si BYOO tra meen)

**U.S. Brand Names** Meridia®

**Synonyms** Sibutramine Hydrochloride

**Pharmacologic Category** Anorexiant

**Use** Management of obesity, including weight loss and maintenance of weight loss, and should be used in conjunction with a reduced calorie diet

**Restrictions** CIV; Recommended only for obese patients with a body mass index ≥30 kg/m² or ≥27 kg/m² in the presence of other risk factors such as hypertension, diabetes, and/or dyslipidemia

**Pregnancy Risk Factor** C

**Contraindications** Hypersensitivity to sibutramine or any component; during or within 2 weeks of MAO inhibitors (eg, phenelzine, selegiline) or concomitant centrally-acting appetite suppressants; anorexia nervosa; uncontrolled or poorly controlled hypertension; congestive heart failure; coronary heart disease; conduction disorders (arrhythmias); stroke

**Warnings/Precautions** Use with caution in severe renal impairment or severe hepatic dysfunction, seizure disorder, hypertension, gallstones, narrow-angle glaucoma, nursing mothers, elderly patients. Primary pulmonary hypertension (PPH), a rare and frequently fatal pulmonary disease, has been reported to occur in patients receiving other agents with serotonergic activity which have been used as anorexiants. Although not reported in clinical trials, it is possible that sibutramine may share this potential, and patients should be monitored closely.

**Adverse Reactions**

>10%:

Central nervous system: Insomnia, somnolence, dizziness, headache, fatigue
Gastrointestinal: Xerostomia, diarrhea, nausea
Genitourinary: Ejaculatory disturbances

1% to 10%:

Cardiovascular: Palpitations
Central nervous system: Agitation, anxiety, nervousness
Dermatologic: Rash
Endocrine & metabolic: Decreased libido
Gastrointestinal: Constipation, anorexia, dyspepsia, flatulence, vomiting
Genitourinary: Micturition disorders
Neuromuscular & skeletal: Tremors, paresthesia
Ocular: Visual difficulty, abnormal vision
Otic: Tinnitus
Miscellaneous: Diaphoresis (increased)

**Overdosage/Toxicology** Treatment: There is no specific antidote; treatment should consist of general supportive measures employed in the management of overdosage. Cautious use of beta-blockers to control elevated blood pressure and tachycardia may be indicated; the benefits of forced diuresis and hemodialysis remain unknown.

**Drug Interactions** CYP3A3/4 enzyme substrate

Buspirone: Concurrent use may result in serotonin syndrome; these combinations are best avoided

CNS stimulants: May increase potential for sibutramine-associated cardiovascular complications or serotonergic effects; includes decongestants, centrally-acting weight loss products, amphetamines, and amphetamine-like compounds

CYP3A3/4 inhibitors: Serum level and/or toxicity of sibutramine may be increased; inhibitors include amiodarone, cimetidine, clarithromycin, erythromycin, delavirdine, diltiazem, dirithromycin, disulfiram, fluoxetine, fluvoxamine, grapefruit juice, indinavir, itraconazole, ketoconazole, metronidazole, nefazodone, nevirapine, propoxyfene, quinupristin-dalfopristin, ritonavir, saquinavir, verapamil, zafirlukast, zileuton; monitor for altered response

Dihydroergotamine: Concurrent use may result in serotonin syndrome; these combinations are best avoided

Dextromethorphan: Concurrent use may result in serotonin syndrome; these combinations are best avoided

Lithium: Concurrent use may result in serotonin syndrome; these combinations are best avoided

MAOIs: Sibutramine should not be used with nonselective MAOIs (isocarboxazid, phenelzine) due to a theoretical risk of serotonin syndrome

Meperidine: Concurrent use may result in serotonin syndrome; these combinations are best avoided

Nefazodone: Concurrent use may result in serotonin syndrome; these combinations are best avoided

Serotonergic agents: Concurrent use may result in serotonin syndrome; includes selective serotonin reuptake inhibitors (eg, sumatriptan, lithium, tryptophan), some opioid/analgesics (eg, meperidine, tramadol), and venlafaxine

SSRIs: Combined use with other drugs which inhibit the reuptake (sibutramine) may cause serotonin syndrome; avoid these combinations

Serotonin agonists: Theoretically may increase the risk of serotonin syndrome; includes sumatriptan, naratriptan, rizatriptan, and zolmitriptan

Tramadol: Sertraline combined with tramadol (serotonergic effects) may cause serotonin syndrome; monitor

Trazodone: Sertraline may inhibit the metabolism of trazodone resulting in increased toxicity; monitor

Tricyclic antidepressants: Sertraline may inhibit the metabolism of tricyclic antidepressants (amitriptyline, desipramine, imipramine, nortriptyline) resulting is elevated serum levels; if combination is warranted, a low dose of TCA (10-25 mg/day) should be utilized

Tryptophan: Sertraline may inhibit the reuptake of serotonin; combination with tryptophan, a serotonin precursor, may cause agitation and restlessness; this combination is best avoided

Venlafaxine: Sertraline may increase the risk of serotonin syndrome

**Mechanism of Action** Sibutramine blocks the neuronal uptake of norepinephrine and, to a lesser extent, serotonin and dopamine

**Usual Dosage** Adults ≥16 years: Initial: 10 mg once daily; after 4 weeks may titrate up to 15 mg once daily as needed and tolerated

**Dietary Considerations** Avoid concurrent excess alcohol ingestion; sibutramine, as an appetite suppressant, is the most effective when combined with a low calorie diet and behavior modification counseling

**Monitoring Parameters** Do initial blood pressure and heart rate evaluation and then monitor regularly during therapy. If patient has sustained increases in either blood pressure or pulse rate, consider discontinuing or reducing the dose of the drug.

**Patient Information** Maintain proper medical follow-up and inform physician of any potential concomitant medications including over-the-counter products you are taking, especially weight loss products, antidepressants, antimigraine drugs, decongestants, lithium, tryptophan, antitussives, or ergot derivatives

**Additional Information** Physicians should carefully evaluate patients for history of drug abuse and follow such patients closely, observing them for signs of misuse or abuse (eg, development of tolerance, excessive increases of doses, drug seeking behavior)

**Dosage Forms** Capsule, as hydrochloride: 5 mg, 10 mg, 15 mg


- **Sibutramine Hydrochloride** *see* Sibutramine *on page 511*
- **Siladryl® Oral [OTC]** *see* Diphenhydramine *on page 174*
- **Silafed® Syrup [OTC]** *see* Triprolidine and Pseudoephedrine *on page 572*
- **Silaminic® Cold Syrup [OTC]** *see* Chlorpheniramine and Phenylpropanolamine *on page 114*
- **Silaminic® Expectorant [OTC]** *see* Guaifenesin and Phenylpropanolamine *on page 257*


## Sildenafil (sil DEN a fil)

**U.S. Brand Names** Viagra®

**Pharmacologic Category** Phosphodiesterase Enzyme Inhibitor

**Use** Treatment of erectile dysfunction

**Effects on Mental Status** May cause dizziness

**Effects on Psychiatric Treatment** Useful for psychotropic-induced sexual dysfunction

**Pregnancy Risk Factor** B

**Contraindications** In patients with a known hypersensitivity to any component of the tablet; has been shown to potentiate the hypotensive effects of nitrates, and its administration to patients who are concurrently using organic nitrates in any form is contraindicated

**Warnings/Precautions** There is a degree of cardiac risk associated with sexual activity; therefore, physicians may wish to consider the cardiovascular status of their patients prior to initiating any treatment for erectile dysfunction. Agents for the treatment of erectile dysfunction should be used with caution in patients with anatomical deformation of the penis (angulation, cavernosal fibrosis, or Peyronie's disease), or in patients who have conditions which may predispose them to priapism (sickle cell anemia, multiple myeloma, leukemia).

The safety and efficacy of sildenafil with other treatments for erectile dysfunction have not been studied and are, therefore, not recommended as combination therapy.

A minority of patients with retinitis pigmentosa have generic disorders of retinal phosphodiesterases. There is no safety information on the administration of sildenafil to these patients and sildenafil should be administered with caution.

**Adverse Reactions**

>10%:

Central nervous system: Headache
Cardiovascular: Flushing

1% to 10%:

Central nervous system: Dizziness
Dermatologic: Rash
Gastrointestinal: Dyspepsia, diarrhea
Genitourinary: Urinary tract infection
Ocular: Abnormal vision
Respiratory: Nasal congestion

**Overdosage/Toxicology** Signs and symptoms: In studies with healthy volunteers of single doses up to 800 mg, adverse events were similar to those seen at lower doses but incidence rates were increased

**Drug Interactions** CYP3A3/4 enzyme substrate (major); CYP2C9 enzyme substrate (minor)

(Continued)

## Sildenafil *(Continued)*

Concurrent use of sildenafil and nitroglycerin (or any other nitrate) is contraindicated due to the potential for severe, potentially fatal, hypotensive responses

Increased effect/toxicity: Cimetidine, erythromycin, ketoconazole, itraconazole, mibefradil, nitroglycerin, protease inhibitors. A reduction in sildenafil's dose is recommended when used with ritonavir, a protease inhibitor, (no more than 25 mg per dose; no more than 25 mg in 48 hours).

Decreased effect: Rifampin

**Usual Dosage** Adults: Oral: For most patients, the recommended dose is 50 mg taken as needed, approximately 1 hour before sexual activity. However, sildenafil may be taken anywhere from 30 minutes to 4 hours before sexual activity. Based on effectiveness and tolerance, the dose may be increased to a maximum recommended dose of 100 mg or decreased to 25 mg. The maximum recommended dosing frequency is once daily.

**Dosage adjustment for patients >65 years of age, hepatic impairment (cirrhosis), severe renal impairment (creatinine clearance <30 mL/minute), or concomitant use of potent cytochrome P-450 3A4 inhibitors (erythromycin, ketoconazole, itraconazole):** Higher plasma levels have been associated which may result in increase in efficacy and adverse effects and a starting dose of 25 mg should be considered

**Patient Information** Inform prescriber of all other medications you are taking; serious side effects can result when sildenafil is used with nitrates and some other medications. Do not combine sildenafil with other approaches to treating erectile dysfunction without consulting prescriber. Note that sildenafil provides no protection against sexually transmitted diseases, including HIV. You may experience headache, flushing, or abnormal vision (blurred or increased sensitivity to light); use caution when driving at night or in poorly lit environments. Report immediately acute allergic reactions, chest pain or palpitations, persistent dizziness, sign of urinary tract infection, rash, respiratory difficulties, genital swelling, or other adverse reactions.

**Dosage Forms** Tablet, as citrate: 25 mg, 50 mg, 100 mg

- **Sildicon-E® [OTC]** *see* Guaifenesin and Phenylpropanolamine *on page 257*
- **Silphen® Cough [OTC]** *see* Diphenhydramine *on page 174*
- **Silphen DM® [OTC]** *see* Dextromethorphan *on page 160*
- **Siltussin® [OTC]** *see* Guaifenesin *on page 256*
- **Siltussin-CF® [OTC]** *see* Guaifenesin, Phenylpropanolamine, and Dextromethorphan *on page 258*
- **Siltussin DM® [OTC]** *see* Guaifenesin and Dextromethorphan *on page 257*
- **Silvadene®** *see* Silver Sulfadiazine *on page 512*

## Silver Nitrate (SIL ver NYE trate)

**U.S. Brand Names** Dey-Drop® Ophthalmic Solution

**Pharmacologic Category** Antibiotic, Ophthalmic; Antibiotic, Topical; Cauterizing Agent, Topical; Topical Skin Product, Antibacterial

**Use** Prevention of gonococcal ophthalmia neonatorum; cauterization of wounds and sluggish ulcers, removal of granulation tissue and warts; aseptic prophylaxis of burns

**Effects on Mental Status** None reported

**Effects on Psychiatric Treatment** None reported

**Usual Dosage**

Neonates: Ophthalmic: Instill 2 drops immediately after birth (no later than 1 hour after delivery) into conjunctival sac of each eye as a single dose, allow to sit for ≥30 seconds; do not irrigate eyes following instillation of eye drops

Children and Adults:

Ointment: Apply in an apertured pad on affected area or lesion for approximately 5 days

Sticks: Apply to mucous membranes and other moist skin surfaces only on area to be treated 2-3 times/week for 2-3 weeks

Topical solution: Apply a cotton applicator dipped in solution on the affected area 2-3 times/week for 2-3 weeks

**Dosage Forms**

Applicator sticks: 75% with potassium nitrate 25% (6")

Ointment: 10% (30 g)

Solution:

Ophthalmic: 1% (wax ampuls)

Topical: 10% (30 mL); 25% (30 mL); 50% (30 mL)

## Silver Sulfadiazine (SIL ver sul fa DYE a zeen)

**U.S. Brand Names** Silvadene®; SSD® AF; SSD® Cream; Thermazene®

**Canadian Brand Names** Dermazin™; Flamazine®

**Pharmacologic Category** Antibiotic, Topical

**Use** Prevention and treatment of infection in second and third degree burns

**Effects on Mental Status** None reported

**Effects on Psychiatric Treatment** May cause leukopenia; use caution with clozapine and carbamazepine

**Usual Dosage** Children and Adults: Topical: Apply once or twice daily with a sterile-gloved hand; apply to a thickness of $^1/_{16}$"; burned area should be covered with cream at all times

**Dosage Forms** Cream, topical: 1% [10 mg/g] (20 g, 50 g, 85 g, 400 g, 1000 g)

## Simethicone (sye METH i kone)

**U.S. Brand Names** Degas® [OTC]; Flatulex® [OTC]; Gas Relief®; Gas-X® [OTC]; Maalox® Anti-Gas [OTC]; Mylanta® Gas [OTC]; Mylicon® [OTC]; Phazyme® [OTC]

**Canadian Brand Names** Baby's Own™ Infant Drops; Ovol®

**Synonyms** Activated Dimethicone; Activated Methylpolysiloxane

**Pharmacologic Category** Antiflatulent

**Use** Relieves flatulence and functional gastric bloating, and postoperative gas pains

**Effects on Mental Status** None reported

**Effects on Psychiatric Treatment** None reported

**Pregnancy Risk Factor** C

**Contraindications** Hypersensitivity to simethicone or any component

**Warnings/Precautions** Not recommended for the treatment of infant colic; do not exceed recommended dosing guidelines

**Overdosage/Toxicology** Nontoxic orally

**Drug Interactions** No data reported

**Usual Dosage** Oral:

Infants: 20 mg 4 times/day

Children <12 years: 40 mg 4 times/day

Children >12 years and Adults: 40-120 mg after meals and at bedtime as needed, not to exceed 500 mg/day

**Patient Information** Some tablets may be chewed thoroughly before swallowing, follow with a glass of water

**Dosage Forms**

Capsule: 125 mg

Drops, oral: 40 mg/0.6 mL (30 mL)

Tablet: 50 mg, 60 mg, 95 mg

Tablet, chewable: 40 mg, 80 mg, 125 mg

- **Simron® [OTC]** *see* Ferrous Gluconate *on page 223*
- **Simulect®** *see* Basiliximab *on page 58*

## Simvastatin (SIM va stat in)

**Related Information**

Lipid-Lowering Agents Comparison Chart *on page 717*

**U.S. Brand Names** Zocor®

**Pharmacologic Category** Antilipemic Agent (HMG-CoA Reductase Inhibitor)

**Use**

Adjunct to dietary therapy to decrease elevated serum total and LDL cholesterol, apolipoprotein B (apo-B), and triglyceride levels, and to increase HDL cholesterol in patients with primary hypercholesterolemia (heterozygous, familial and nonfamilial) and mixed dyslipidemia (Fredrickson types IIa and IIb); treatment of homozygous familial hypercholesterolemia; treatment of isolated hypertriglyceridemia (Fredrickson type IV) and type III hyperlipoproteinemia; to reduce the risk of myocardial infarction, stroke, or TIA

**Effects on Mental Status** May cause drowsiness

**Effects on Psychiatric Treatment** Rhabdomyolysis with acute renal failure has occurred; risk is increased with concurrent use of fluvoxamine nefazodone and verapamil

**Pregnancy Risk Factor** X

**Contraindications** Hypersensitivity to simvastatin or any component; acute liver disease; unexplained persistent elevations of serum transaminases; pregnancy

**Warnings/Precautions** Liver function must be monitored by periodic laboratory assessment. Rhabdomyolysis with acute renal failure has occurred. Risk is increased with concurrent use of clarithromycin, danazol, diltiazem, fluvoxamine, indinavir, nefazodone, nelfinavir, ritonavir, verapamil, troleandomycin, cyclosporine, fibric acid derivatives, erythromycin, niacin, or azole antifungals. Weigh the risk versus benefit when combining any of these drugs with simvastatin. Temporarily discontinue in any patient experiencing an acute or serious condition predisposing to renal failure secondary to rhabdomyolysis.

**Adverse Reactions**

1% to 10%:

Central nervous system: Headache (3.5%)

Gastrointestinal: Flatulence (1.9%), abdominal cramps (3.2%), diarrhea (1.9%), constipation (2.3%), nausea/vomiting (1.3%), dyspepsia/heartburn (1.1%)

Neuromuscular & skeletal: Myalgia, weakness (1.6%), increased CPK

Respiratory: Upper respiratory infection (2.1%)

<1%: Abnormal taste, blurred vision, lenticular opacities

**Overdosage/Toxicology**

Signs and symptoms: Very few adverse events

Treatment: Symptomatic

**Drug Interactions** CYP3A3/4 enzyme substrate

Inhibitors of CYP3A3/4 (clarithromycin, cyclosporine, danazol, diltiazem, fluvoxamine, erythromycin, fluconazole, indinavir, itraconazole, ketoconazole, miconazole, nefazodone, nelfinavir, ritonavir, saquinavir, indinavir, amprenavir, troleandomycin, and verapamil) increase simvastatin blood levels; may increase the risk of simvastatin-induced myopathy and rhabdomyolysis.

Cholestyramine reduces absorption of several HMG-CoA reductase inhibitors. Separate administration times by at least 4 hours

Cholestyramine and colestipol (bile acid sequestrants): Cholesterol-lowering effects are additive

Clofibrate and fenofibrate may increase the risk of myopathy and rhabdomyolysis

Gemfibrozil: Increased risk of myopathy and rhabdomyolysis

Grapefruit juice may inhibit metabolism of simvastatin via CYP3A3/4; avoid high dietary intakes of grapefruit juice

Niacin may increase the risk of myopathy and rhabdomyolysis

Warfarin effects (hypoprothrombinemic response) may be increased; monitor INR closely when simvastatin is initiated or discontinued

**Usual Dosage** Oral:

Adults:

Initial: 20 mg once daily in the evening

Patients who require only a moderate reduction of LDL cholesterol may be started at 10 mg

Patients who require a reduction of >45% in low-density lipoprotein (LDL) cholesterol: 40 mg once daily in the evening

Maintenance: Recommended dosage range: 5-80 mg/day as a single dose in the evening; doses should be individualized according to the baseline LDL cholesterol levels, the recommended goal of therapy, and the patient's response.

Adjustments: Should be made at intervals of 4 weeks or more.

Patients with homozygous familial hypercholesteremia: Adults: 40 mg in the evening or 80 mg/day in 3 divided doses of 20 mg, 20 mg, and an evening dose of 40 mg.

Patients who are concomitantly receiving cyclosporine: Initial: 5 mg, should not exceed 10 mg/day.

Patients receiving concomitant fibrates or niacin: Dose should **not** exceed 10 mg/day.

**Dosing adjustment/comments in renal impairment:** Because simvastatin does not undergo significant renal excretion, modification of dose should not be necessary in patients with mild to moderate renal insufficiency.

Severe renal impairment: $Cl_{cr}$ <10 mL/minute: Initial: 5 mg/day with close monitoring.

**Patient Information** Take this medication as directed, with meals, 1 hour prior to or after any other medications. You may experience nausea, flatulence, dyspepsia (small frequent meals may help), headache, muscle or joint pain (will probably lessen with continued use), and light sensitivity (use sunblock and wear protective clothing). Report severe and unresolved gastric upset, any vision changes, changes in color of urine or stool, yellowing of skin or eyes, and any unusual bruising.

**Nursing Implications** Liver enzyme elevations may be observed during simvastatin therapy; combination therapy with other hypolipidemic agents may be required to achieve optimal reductions of LDL cholesterol; diet, weight reduction, and exercise should be attempted to control hypercholesterolemia before the institution of simvastatin therapy

**Dosage Forms** Tablet: 5 mg, 10 mg, 20 mg, 40 mg, 80 mg

- **Sinarest® 12 Hour Nasal Solution** *see* Oxymetazoline *on page 415*
- **Sinarest® Nasal Solution [OTC]** *see* Phenylephrine *on page 439*
- **Sinarest®, No Drowsiness [OTC]** *see* Acetaminophen and Pseudoephedrine *on page 15*

## Sincalide (SIN ka lide)

**U.S. Brand Names** Kinevac®

**Synonyms** C8-CCK; OP-CCK

**Pharmacologic Category** Diagnostic Agent

**Use** Postevacuation cholecystography; gallbladder bile sampling; stimulate pancreatic secretion for analysis

**Effects on Mental Status** May cause dizziness

**Effects on Psychiatric Treatment** None reported

**Pregnancy Risk Factor** B

**Adverse Reactions** 1% to 10%:

Cardiovascular: Flushing

Central nervous system: Dizziness

Gastrointestinal: Nausea, abdominal pain, urge to defecate

**Usual Dosage** Adults: I.V.:

Contraction of gallbladder: 0.02 mcg/kg over 30 seconds to 1 minute, may repeat in 15 minutes a 0.04 mcg/kg dose

Pancreatic function: 0.02 mcg/kg over 30 minutes administered after secretin

**Dosage Forms** Injection: 5 mcg

- **Sine-Aid® IB [OTC]** *see* Pseudoephedrine and Ibuprofen *on page 479*
- **Sine-Aid®, Maximum Strength [OTC]** *see* Acetaminophen and Pseudoephedrine *on page 15*
- **Sinemet®** *see* Levodopa and Carbidopa *on page 313*
- **Sinemet® CR** *see* Levodopa and Carbidopa *on page 313*
- **Sine-Off® Maximum Strength No Drowsiness Formula [OTC]** *see* Acetaminophen and Pseudoephedrine *on page 15*
- **Sinequan® Oral** *see* Doxepin *on page 183*
- **Sinex® Long-Acting [OTC]** *see* Oxymetazoline *on page 415*
- **Singulair®** *see* Montelukast *on page 373*
- **Sinubid®** *see* Phenyltoloxamine, Phenylpropanolamine, and Acetaminophen *on page 441*
- **Sinufed® Timecelles®** *see* Guaifenesin and Pseudoephedrine *on page 257*
- **Sinumist®-SR Capsulets®** *see* Guaifenesin *on page 256*
- **Sinupan®** *see* Guaifenesin and Phenylephrine *on page 257*
- **Sinus Excedrin® Extra Strength [OTC]** *see* Acetaminophen and Pseudoephedrine *on page 15*
- **Sinus-Relief® [OTC]** *see* Acetaminophen and Pseudoephedrine *on page 15*
- **Sinutab® Tablets [OTC]** *see* Acetaminophen, Chlorpheniramine, and Pseudoephedrine *on page 15*
- **Sinutab® Without Drowsiness [OTC]** *see* Acetaminophen and Pseudoephedrine *on page 15*

## Sirolimus (sir OH li mus)

**U.S. Brand Names** Rapamune®

**Pharmacologic Category** Immunosuppressant Agent

**Use** Prophylaxis of organ rejection in patients receiving renal transplants, in combination with cyclosporine and corticosteroids

**Unlabeled use:** Prophylaxis of organ rejection in solid organ transplant patients in combination with tacrolimus and corticosteroids

**Effects on Mental Status** Insomnia is common; may cause anxiety, confusion, depression, emotional lability, and somnolence

**Effects on Psychiatric Treatment** Leukopenia is common; use caution with clozapine and carbamazepine; nefazodone may increase serum levels of sirolimus

**Pregnancy Risk Factor** C

**Contraindications** Hypersensitivity to sirolimus or any component of the formulation

**Warnings/Precautions** Immunosuppressive agents, including sirolimus, increase the risk of infection and may be associated with the development of lymphoma. Only physicians experienced in the management of organ transplant patients should prescribe sirolimus. May increase serum lipids (cholesterol and triglycerides). Use with caution in patients with hyperlipidemia. May decrease GFR and increase serum creatinine. Use caution in patients with renal impairment, or when used concurrently with medications which may alter renal function. Has been associated with an increased risk of lymphocele. Avoid concurrent use of ketoconazole.

**Adverse Reactions** Incidence of many adverse effects are dose related

>20%:

Cardiovascular: Hypertension (39% to 49%), peripheral edema (54% to 64%), edema (16% to 24%), chest pain (16% to 24%)

Central nervous system: Fever (23% to 34%), headache (23% to 34%), pain (24% to 33%), insomnia (13% to 22%)

Dermatologic: Acne (20% to 31%), rash (10% to 20%)

Endocrine & metabolic: Hypercholesterolemia (38% to 46%), hyperkalemia (12% to 17%), hypokalemia (11% to 21%), hypophosphatemia (15% to 23%), hyperlipidemia (38% to 57%)

Gastrointestinal: Abdominal pain (28% to 36%), nausea (25% to 36%), vomiting (19% to 25%), diarrhea (25% to 42%), constipation (28% to 38%), dyspepsia (17% to 25%), weight gain (8% to 21%)

Genitourinary: Urinary tract infection (20% to 33%)

Hematologic: Anemia (23% to 37%), leukopenia (9% to 15%), thrombocytopenia (13% to 40%)

Neuromuscular & skeletal: Arthralgia (25% to 31%), weakness (22% to 40%), back pain (16% to 26%), tremor (21% to 31%)

Renal: Increased serum creatinine (35% to 40%)

Respiratory: Dyspnea (22% to 30%), upper respiratory infection (20% to 26%), pharyngitis (16% to 21%)

3% to 20%:

Cardiovascular: Atrial fibrillation, congestive heart failure, hypervolemia, hypotension, palpitation, peripheral vascular disorder, postural hypotension, syncope, tachycardia, thrombosis, vasodilation

(Continued)

## Sirolimus *(Continued)*

Central nervous system: Chills, malaise, anxiety, confusion, depression, dizziness, emotional lability, hypesthesia, hypotonia, insomnia, neuropathy, somnolence

Dermatologic: Dermatitis (fungal), hirsutism, pruritus, skin hypertrophy, dermal ulcer, ecchymosis, cellulitis

Endocrine & metabolic: Cushing's syndrome, diabetes mellitus, glycosuria, acidosis, dehydration, hypercalcemia, hyperglycemia, hyperphosphatemia, hypocalcemia, hypoglycemia, hypomagnesemia, hyponatremia

Gastrointestinal: Enlarged abdomen, anorexia, dysphagia, eructation, esophagitis, flatulence, gastritis, gastroenteritis, gingivitis, gingival hyperplasia, ileus, mouth ulceration, oral moniliasis, stomatitis, weight loss

Genitourinary: Pelvic pain, scrotal edema, testis disorder, impotence

Hematologic: Leukocytosis, polycythemia, TTP, hemolytic-uremic syndrome, hemorrhage

Hepatic: Abnormal liver function tests, increased alkaline phosphatase, increased LDH, increased transaminases, ascites

Local: Thrombophlebitis

Neuromuscular & skeletal: Increased CPK, arthrosis, bone necrosis, leg cramps, myalgia, osteoporosis, tetany, hypertonia, paresthesia

Ocular: Abnormal vision, cataract, conjunctivitis

Otic: Ear pain, deafness, otitis media, tinnitus

Renal: Increased BUN, increased serum creatinine, albuminuria, bladder pain, dysuria, hematuria, hydronephrosis, kidney pain, tubular necrosis, nocturia, oliguria, pyuria, nephropathy (toxic), urinary frequency, urinary incontinence, urinary retention

Respiratory: Asthma, atelectasis, bronchitis, cough, epistaxis, hypoxia, lung edema, pleural effusion, pneumonia, rhinitis, sinusitis

Miscellaneous: Abscess, facial edema, flu-like syndrome, hernia, infection, lymphadenopathy, lymphocele, peritonitis, sepsis, diaphoresis

**Overdosage/Toxicology** Experience with overdosage has been limited. Dose-limiting toxicities include immune suppression. Reported symptoms of overdose include atrial fibrillation. Treatment is supportive, dialysis is not likely to facilitate removal.

**Drug Interactions** CYP3A4 substrate and P-glycoprotein substrate

Increased effect/toxicity:

Cyclosporine capsules (modified) or cyclosporine oral solution (modified) increase $C_{max}$ and AUC of sirolimus during concurrent therapy, and cyclosporine clearance may be reduced during concurrent therapy. Sirolimus should be taken 4 hours after cyclosporine oral solution (modified) and/or cyclosporine capsules (modified).

Diltiazem and ketoconazole increase serum concentrations or sirolimus; clearance of sirolimus is increased by rifampin

Grapefruit juice may reduce the metabolism of sirolimus, and should not be used to dilute this product

Other inhibitors of CYP3A4 (eg, nefazodone, calcium channel blockers, antifungal agents, macrolide antibiotics, gastrointestinal prokinetic agents, HIV-protease inhibitors) are likely to increase sirolimus concentrations

Decreased effect: Inducers of CYP3A4 (eg, rifampin, phenobarbital, carbamazepine, rifabutin, phenytoin) are likely to decrease serum concentrations of sirolimus

**Usual Dosage** Oral:

Adults ≥40 kg: Loading dose: For *de novo* transplant recipients, a loading dose of 3 times the daily maintenance dose should be administered on day 1 of dosing. Maintenance dose: 2 mg/day. Doses should be taken 4 hours after cyclosporine, and should be taken consistently either with or without food.

Children ≥13 years or Adults <40 kg: Loading dose: 3 mg/m$^2$ (day 1); followed by a maintenance of 1 mg/m$^2$/day.

**Dosage adjustment in renal impairment:** No dosage adjustment is necessary in renal impairment

**Dosage adjustment in hepatic impairment:** Reduce maintenance dose by approximately 33% in hepatic impairment. Loading dose is unchanged.

**Patient Information** Do not get pregnant while taking this medication. Use reliable contraception while on this medication and for 3 months after discontinuation. May be taken with or without food but take medication consistently with respect to meals (always take with food or always take on an empty stomach).

**Dosage Forms** Solution, oral: 1 mg/mL (1 mL, 2 mL, 5mL, 60 mL, 150 mL)


- **Skelaxin®** *see* Metaxalone *on page 348*
- **Skelid®** *see* Tiludronate *on page 549*
- **Sleep Disorders** *see page 620*
- **Sleep-eze 3® Oral [OTC]** *see* Diphenhydramine *on page 174*
- **Sleepinal® [OTC]** *see* Diphenhydramine *on page 174*
- **Sleepwell 2-nite® [OTC]** *see* Diphenhydramine *on page 174*
- **Slim-Mint® [OTC]** *see* Benzocaine *on page 61*
- **Slo-bid™** *see* Theophylline Salts *on page 539*
- **Slo-Niacin® [OTC]** *see* Niacin *on page 391*
- **Slo-Phyllin®** *see* Theophylline Salts *on page 539*
- **Slo-Phyllin® GG** *see* Theophylline and Guaifenesin *on page 539*
- **Slow FE® [OTC]** *see* Ferrous Sulfate *on page 223*
- **Slow-K®** *see* Potassium Chloride *on page 453*
- **Slow-Mag® [OTC]** *see* Magnesium Chloride *on page 330*
- **SMZ-TMP** *see* Co-Trimoxazole *on page 142*
- **Snakeroot** *see* Echinacea *on page 189*
- **Snaplets-EX® [OTC]** *see* Guaifenesin and Phenylpropanolamine *on page 257*
- **Sodium Acid Carbonate** *see* Sodium Bicarbonate *on page 514*


## Sodium Bicarbonate (SOW dee um bye KAR bun ate)

**U.S. Brand Names** Neut® Injection

**Synonyms** Baking Soda; $NaHCO_3$; Sodium Acid Carbonate; Sodium Hydrogen Carbonate

**Pharmacologic Category** Alkalinizing Agent; Antacid; Electrolyte Supplement, Oral; Electrolyte Supplement, Parenteral

**Use** Management of metabolic acidosis; gastric hyperacidity; as an alkalinization agent for the urine; treatment of hyperkalemia

**Effects on Mental Status** None reported

**Effects on Psychiatric Treatment** May decrease serum lithium levels due to increased clearance but overall effect is minimal; does not offer much benefit in lithium overdose; if lithium toxicity is severe, dialysis is the treatment of choice

**Pregnancy Risk Factor** C

**Contraindications** Alkalosis, hypernatremia, severe pulmonary edema, hypocalcemia, unknown abdominal pain

**Warnings/Precautions** Rapid administration in neonates and children <2 years of age has led to hypernatremia, decreased CSF pressure and intracranial hemorrhage. **Use of I.V. $NaHCO_3$ should be reserved for documented metabolic acidosis and for hyperkalemia-induced cardiac arrest.** Routine use in cardiac arrest is not recommended. Avoid extravasation, tissue necrosis can occur due to the hypertonicity of $NaHCO_3$. May cause sodium retention especially if renal function is impaired; not to be used in treatment of peptic ulcer; use with caution in patients with CHF, edema, cirrhosis, or renal failure. Not the antacid of choice for the elderly because of sodium content and potential for systemic alkalosis.

**Adverse Reactions** Percentage unknown: Aggravation of congestive heart failure, belching, cerebral hemorrhage, edema, flatulence (with oral), gastric distension, hypernatremia, hyperosmolality, hypocalcemia, hypokalemia, increased affinity of hemoglobin for oxygen-reduced pH in myocardial tissue necrosis when extravasated; intracranial acidosis, metabolic alkalosis, milk alkali syndrome (especially with renal dysfunction), pulmonary edema, tetany

**Overdosage/Toxicology**

Signs and symptoms: Hypocalcemia, hypokalemia, hypernatremia, seizures

Treatment: Seizures can be treated with diazepam 0.1-0.25 mg/kg; hypernatremia is resolved through the use of diuretics and free water replacement

**Drug Interactions**

Decreased effect/levels of lithium, chlorpropamide, methotrexate, tetracyclines, and salicylates due to urinary alkalinization

Increased toxicity/levels of amphetamines, anorexiants, mecamylamine, ephedrine, pseudoephedrine, flecainide, quinidine, quinine due to urinary alkalinization

**Usual Dosage**

Cardiac arrest: **Routine use of $NaHCO_3$ is not recommended and should be given only after adequate alveolar ventilation has been established and effective cardiac compressions are provided**

Infants and Children: I.V.: 0.5-1 mEq/kg/dose repeated every 10 minutes or as indicated by arterial blood gases; rate of infusion should not exceed 10 mEq/minute; neonates and children <2 years of age should receive 4.2% (0.5 mEq/mL) solution

Adults: I.V.: Initial: 1 mEq/kg/dose one time; maintenance: 0.5 mEq/kg/dose every 10 minutes or as indicated by arterial blood gases

Metabolic acidosis: Dosage should be based on the following formula if blood gases and pH measurements are available:

Infants and Children:

$HCO_3^-$(mEq) = 0.3 x weight (kg) x base deficit (mEq/L) **or**

$HCO_3^-$(mEq) = 0.5 x weight (kg) x [24 - serum $HCO_3^-$ (mEq/L)]

Adults:

$HCO_3^-$(mEq) = 0.2 x weight (kg) x base deficit (mEq/L) **or**

$HCO_3^-$(mEq) = 0.5 x weight (kg) x [24 - serum $HCO_3^-$ (mEq/L)]

If acid-base status is not available: Dose for older Children and Adults: 2-5 mEq/kg I.V. infusion over 4-8 hours; subsequent doses should be based on patient's acid-base status

Chronic renal failure: Oral: Initiate when plasma $HCO_3^-$ <15 mEq/L

Children: 1-3 mEq/kg/day
Adults: Start with 20-36 mEq/day in divided doses, titrate to bicarbonate level of 18-20 mEq/L
Renal tubular acidosis: Oral:
Distal:
Children: 2-3 mEq/kg/day
Adults: 0.5-2 mEq/kg/day in 4-5 divided doses
Proximal: Children: Initial: 5-10 mEq/kg/day; maintenance: Increase as required to maintain serum bicarbonate in the normal range
Urine alkalinization: Oral:
Children: 1-10 mEq (84-840 mg)/kg/day in divided doses every 4-6 hours; dose should be titrated to desired urinary pH
Adults: Initial: 48 mEq (4 g), then 12-24 mEq (1-2 g) every 4 hours; dose should be titrated to desired urinary pH; doses up to 16 g/day (200 mEq) in patients <60 years and 8 g (100 mEq) in patients >60 years
Antacid: Adults: Oral: 325 mg to 2 g 1-4 times/day

**Patient Information** Do not use for chronic gastric acidity. Take as directed. Chew tablets thoroughly and follow with a full glass of water, preferably on an empty stomach (2 hours before or after food). Take at least 2 hours before or after any other medications. Report CNS effects (eg, irritability, confusion); muscle rigidity or tremors; swelling of feet or ankles; difficulty breathing; chest pain or palpitations; respiratory changes; or tarry stools.

**Nursing Implications** Advise patient of milk-alkali syndrome if use is long-term; observe for extravasation when giving I.V.

**Dosage Forms**
Injection: 4% [40 mg/mL = 2.4 mEq/5 mL] (5 mL); 4.2% [42 mg/mL = 5 mEq/10 mL] (10 mL); 7.5% [75 mg/mL = 8.92 mEq/10 mL] (10 mL, 50 mL); 8.4% [84 mg/mL = 10 mEq/10 mL] (10 mL, 50 mL)
Powder: 120 g, 480 g
Tablet: 300 mg [3.6 mEq]; 325 mg [3.8 mEq]; 520 mg [6.3 mEq]; 600 mg [7.3 mEq]; 650 mg [7.6 mEq]

♦ **Sodium Etidronate** *see* Etidronate Disodium *on page 215*

♦ **Sodium Hydrogen Carbonate** *see* Sodium Bicarbonate *on page 514*

## Sodium Hypochlorite Solution

(SOW dee um hye poe KLOR ite soe LOO shun)

**Pharmacologic Category** Disinfectant, Antibacterial (Topical)

**Use** Treatment of athlete's foot (0.5%); wound irrigation (0.5%); disinfect utensils and equipment (5%)

**Effects on Mental Status** None reported

**Effects on Psychiatric Treatment** None reported

**Usual Dosage** Topical irrigation

**Dosage Forms**
Solution: 5% (4000 mL)
Solution (modified Dakin's solution):
Full strength: 0.5% (1000 mL)
Half strength: 0.25% (1000 mL)
Quarter strength: 0.125% (1000 mL)

♦ **Sodium *L*-Triiodothyronine** *see* Liothyronine *on page 319*

♦ **Sodium Nafcillin** *see* Nafcillin *on page 380*

♦ **Sodium P.A.S.** *see* Aminosalicylate Sodium *on page 31*

♦ **Sodium Phosphate and Potassium Phosphate** *see* Potassium Phosphate and Sodium Phosphate *on page 456*

♦ **Sodium Sulamyd® Ophthalmic** *see* Sulfacetamide *on page 522*

## Sodium Thiosulfate (SOW dee um thye oh SUL fate)

**U.S. Brand Names** Tinver® Lotion

**Pharmacologic Category** Antidote

**Use**
Parenteral: Used alone or with sodium nitrite or amyl nitrite in cyanide poisoning or arsenic poisoning; reduce the risk of nephrotoxicity associated with cisplatin therapy
Topical: Treatment of tinea versicolor

**Effects on Mental Status** May cause coma, CNS depression secondary to thiocyanate intoxication, psychosis, or confusion

**Effects on Psychiatric Treatment** CNS depressant effect of psychotropics may be potentiated; monitor

**Usual Dosage**
Cyanide and nitroprusside antidote: I.V.:
Children <25 kg: 50 mg/kg after receiving 4.5-10 mg/kg sodium nitrite; a half dose of each may be repeated if necessary
Children >25 kg and Adults: 12.5 g after 300 mg of sodium nitrite; a half dose of each may be repeated if necessary
Cyanide poisoning: I.V.: Dose should be based on determination as with nitrite, at rate of 2.5-5 mL/minute to maximum of 50 mL.
Variation of sodium nitrate and sodium thiosulfate dose, based on hemoglobin concentration*:
Hemoglobin 7 g/dL:
Initial dose sodium nitrate: 5.8 mg/kg; initial dose 3% sodium nitrate: 0.19 mL/kg; initial dose 25% sodium thiosulfate: 0.95 mL/kg
Hemoglobin 8 g/dL:
Initial dose sodium nitrate: 6.6 mg/kg; initial dose 3% sodium nitrate: 0.22 mL/kg; initial dose 25% sodium thiosulfate: 1.10 mL/kg
Hemoglobin 9 g/dL:
Initial dose sodium nitrate: 7.5 mg/kg; initial dose 3% sodium nitrate: 0.25 mL/kg; initial dose 25% sodium thiosulfate: 1.25 mL/kg
Hemoglobin 10 g/dL:
Initial dose sodium nitrate: 8.3 mg/kg; initial dose 3% sodium nitrate: 0.27 mL/kg; initial dose 25% sodium thiosulfate: 1.35 mL/kg
Hemoglobin 11 g/dL:
Initial dose sodium nitrate: 9.1 mg/kg; initial dose 3% sodium nitrate: 0.30 mL/kg; initial dose 25% sodium thiosulfate: 1.50 mL/kg
Hemoglobin 12 g/dL:
Initial dose sodium nitrate: 10.0 mg/kg; initial dose 3% sodium nitrate: 0.33 mL/kg; initial dose 25% sodium thiosulfate: 1.65 mL/kg
Hemoglobin 13 g/dL:
Initial dose sodium nitrate: 10.8 mg/kg; initial dose 3% sodium nitrate: 0.36 mL/kg; initial dose 25% sodium thiosulfate: 1.80 mL/kg
Hemoglobin 14 g/dL:
Initial dose sodium nitrate: 11.6 mg/kg; initial dose 3% sodium nitrate: 0.39 mL/kg; initial dose 25% sodium thiosulfate: 1.95 mL/kg
*Adapted from Berlin DM Jr, "The Treatment of Cyanide Poisoning in Children," *Pediatrics*, 1970, 46:793.

Cisplatin rescue should be given before or during cisplatin administration: I.V. infusion (in sterile water): 12 g/m$^2$ over 6 hours or 9 g/m$^2$ I.V. push followed by 1.2 g/m$^2$ continuous infusion for 6 hours

Arsenic poisoning: I.V.: 1 mL first day, 2 mL second day, 3 mL third day, 4 mL fourth day, 5 mL on alternate days thereafter

Children and Adults: Topical: 20% to 25% solution: Apply a thin layer to affected areas twice daily

**Dosage Forms**
Injection: 100 mg/mL (10 mL); 250 mg/mL (50 mL)
Lotion: 25% with salicylic acid 1% and isopropyl alcohol 10% (120 mL, 180 mL)

♦ **Solagé™ Topical Solution** *see* Mequinol and Tretinoin *on page 343*

♦ **Solaquin® [OTC]** *see* Hydroquinone *on page 276*

♦ **Solaquin Forte®** *see* Hydroquinone *on page 276*

♦ **Solarcaine® [OTC]** *see* Benzocaine *on page 61*

♦ **Solarcaine® Aloe Extra Burn Relief [OTC]** *see* Lidocaine *on page 317*

♦ **Solfoton®** *see* Phenobarbital *on page 435*

♦ **Solganal®** *see* Aurothioglucose *on page 54*

♦ **Solu-Cortef®** *see* Hydrocortisone *on page 273*

♦ **Solu-Medrol® Injection** *see* Methylprednisolone *on page 359*

♦ **Solurex®** *see* Dexamethasone *on page 157*

♦ **Solurex L.A.®** *see* Dexamethasone *on page 157*

♦ **Soma®** *see* Carisoprodol *on page 94*

♦ **Soma® Compound** *see* Carisoprodol and Aspirin *on page 94*

♦ **Soma® Compound w/Codeine** *see* Carisoprodol, Aspirin, and Codeine *on page 94*

♦ **Sominex® Oral [OTC]** *see* Diphenhydramine *on page 174*

♦ **Somnil®** *see* Doxylamine *on page 186*

♦ **Sonata®** *see* Zaleplon *on page 590*

## Sorbitol (SOR bi tole)

**Related Information**
Laxatives, Classification and Properties *on page 716*

**Pharmacologic Category** Genitourinary Irrigant; Laxative, Miscellaneous

**Use** Genitourinary irrigant in transurethral prostatic resection or other transurethral resection or other transurethral surgical procedures; diuretic; humectant; sweetening agent; hyperosmotic laxative; facilitate the passage of sodium polystyrene sulfonate through the intestinal tract

**Effects on Mental Status** None reported

**Effects on Psychiatric Treatment** None reported

**Contraindications** Anuria

**Warnings/Precautions** Use with caution in patients with severe cardiopulmonary or renal impairment and in patients unable to metabolize sorbitol

**Adverse Reactions** 1% to 10%:
Cardiovascular: Edema
(Continued)

## Sorbitol *(Continued)*

Endocrine & metabolic: Fluid and electrolyte losses, lactic acidosis
Gastrointestinal: Diarrhea, nausea, vomiting, abdominal discomfort, xerostomia

**Overdosage/Toxicology**

Signs and symptoms: Nausea, diarrhea, fluid and electrolyte loss
Treatment: Supportive to ensure fluid and electrolyte balance

**Usual Dosage** Hyperosmotic laxative (as single dose, at infrequent intervals):

Children 2-11 years:
Oral: 2 mL/kg (as 70% solution)
Rectal enema: 30-60 mL as 25% to 30% solution
Children >12 years and Adults:
Oral: 30-150 mL (as 70% solution)
Rectal enema: 120 mL as 25% to 30% solution
Adjunct to sodium polystyrene sulfonate: 15 mL as 70% solution orally until diarrhea occurs (10-20 mL/2 hours) or 20-100 mL as an oral vehicle for the sodium polystyrene sulfonate resin
When administered with charcoal:
Oral:
Children: 4.3 mL/kg of 35% sorbitol with 1 g/kg of activated charcoal
Adults: 4.3 mL/kg of 70% sorbitol with 1 g/kg of activated charcoal every 4 hours until first stool containing charcoal is passed
Topical: 3% to 3.3% as transurethral surgical procedure irrigation

**Patient Information** Cathartic: Use of cathartics on a regular basis will have adverse effects. Increased exercise, increased fluid intake, or increased dietary fruit and fiber may be effective in preventing and resolving constipation.

**Nursing Implications** Do not use unless solution is clear

**Dosage Forms**

Solution: 70%
Solution, genitourinary irrigation: 3% (1500 mL, 3000 mL); 3.3% (2000 mL)

♦ **Sorbitrate®** *see* Isosorbide Dinitrate *on page 296*

♦ **Soriatane™** *see* Acitretin *on page 18*

## Sotalol (SOE ta lole)

**Related Information**

Beta-Blockers Comparison Chart *on page 709*

**U.S. Brand Names** Betapace®; Betapace AF®

**Canadian Brand Names** Sotacor®

**Pharmacologic Category** Antiarrhythmic Agent, Class II; Antiarrhythmic Agent, Class III; Beta Blocker, Beta$_1$ Selective

**Use** Treatment of documented ventricular arrhythmias, such as sustained ventricular tachycardia, that in the judgment of the prescriber are life-threatening

**Effects on Mental Status** Dizziness and drowsiness are common; may cause confusion, anxiety, or depression

**Effects on Psychiatric Treatment** May rarely cause leukopenia; use caution with clozapine and carbamazepine; barbiturates may decrease the effects of beta-blockers; beta-blockers may alter the effects antipsychotics; monitor for altered response

**Pregnancy Risk Factor** B

**Contraindications** Bronchial asthma, sinus bradycardia, second and third degree A-V block (unless a functioning pacemaker is present), congenital or acquired long Q-T syndromes, cardiogenic shock, uncontrolled congestive heart failure, and previous evidence of hypersensitivity to sotalol; concurrent use with sparfloxacin. Betapace AF® is contraindicated in patients with significantly reduced renal filtration ($Cl_{cr}$ <40 mL/minute).

**Warnings/Precautions** Monitor and adjust dose to prevent QTc prolongation. Watch for proarrhythmic effects. Correct electrolyte imbalances before initiating (especially hypokalemia and hyperkalemia). Consider pre-existing conditions such as sick sinus syndrome before initiating. Conduction abnormalities can occur particularly sinus bradycardia. Use cautiously within the first 2 weeks post-MI (experience limited). Administer cautiously in compensated heart failure and monitor for a worsening of the condition. Use caution in patients with PVD (can aggravate arterial insufficiency). Avoid abrupt discontinuation in patients with a history of CAD; slowly wean while monitoring for signs and symptoms of ischemia. Use caution with concurrent use of beta-blockers and either verapamil or diltiazem; bradycardia or heart block can occur. Use cautiously in diabetics because it can mask prominent hypoglycemic symptoms. Can mask signs of thyrotoxicosis. Use cautiously in the renally impaired (dosage adjustment required). Use care with anesthetic agents which decrease myocardial function.

**Adverse Reactions**

>10%:
Cardiovascular: Bradycardia (16%), chest pain (16%), palpitations (14%)
Central nervous system: Fatigue (20%), dizziness (20%)
Neuromuscular & skeletal: Weakness (13%)
Respiratory: Dyspnea (21%)

1% to 10%:
Cardiovascular: Congestive heart failure, reduced peripheral circulation (3%), edema (8%), abnormal EKG (7%), hypotension (6%), proarrhythmia (5%), syncope (5%)
Central nervous system: Mental confusion (6%), anxiety (4%), headache (8%), sleep problems (8%), depression (4%)
Dermatologic: Itching/rash (5%)
Endocrine & metabolic: Decreased sexual ability (3%)
Gastrointestinal: Diarrhea (7%), nausea/vomiting (10%), stomach discomfort (3% to 6%)
Hematologic: Bleeding (2%)
Neuromuscular & skeletal: Paresthesia (4%)
Ocular: Visual problems (5%)
Respiratory: Upper respiratory problems (5% to 8%), asthma (2%)

<1%: Cold extremities, diaphoresis, leukopenia, phlebitis, red/crusted skin, Raynaud's phenomenon, skin necrosis after extravasation

**Overdosage/Toxicology**

Signs and symptoms: Cardiac disturbances, CNS toxicity, bronchospasm, hypoglycemia and hyperkalemia. The most common cardiac symptoms include hypotension and bradycardia; atrioventricular block, intraventricular conduction disturbances, cardiogenic shock, and asystole may occur with severe overdose, especially with membrane-depressant drugs (eg, propranolol); CNS effects include convulsions, coma, and respiratory arrest is commonly seen with propranolol and other membrane-depressant and lipid-soluble drugs.

Treatment: Includes symptomatic treatment of seizures, hypotension, hyperkalemia and hypoglycemia; bradycardia and hypotension resistant to atropine, isoproterenol or pacing may respond to glucagon; wide QRS defects caused by the membrane-depressant poisoning may respond to hypertonic sodium bicarbonate; repeat-dose charcoal, hemoperfusion, or hemodialysis may be helpful in removal of only those beta-blockers with a small $V_d$, long half-life or low intrinsic clearance (acebutolol, atenolol, nadolol, sotalol)

**Drug Interactions**

Antacids (aluminum/magnesium) decrease sotalol blood levels. Separate by 2 hours

Cisapride and sotalol increases malignant arrhythmias; concurrent use is contraindicated

Clonidine: Sotalol may cause rebound hypertension after discontinuation of clonidine

Drugs which prolong the Q-T interval include amiodarone, amitriptyline, astemizole, bepridil, disopyramide, erythromycin, haloperidol, imipramine, quinidine, pimozide, procainamide, and thioridazine; effect/toxicity may be increased; use with caution

Sparfloxacin, gatifloxacin, and moxifloxacin may result in additional prolongation of the Q-T interval; concurrent use is contraindicated

**Usual Dosage** Sotalol should be initiated and doses increased in a hospital with facilities for cardiac rhythm monitoring and assessment. Proarrhythmic events can occur after initiation of therapy and with each upward dosage adjustment.

Children: Oral: The safety and efficacy of sotalol in children have not been established
Supraventricular arrhythmias: 2-4 mg/kg/24 hours was given in 2 equal doses every 12 hours to 18 infants (≤2 months of age). All infants, except one with chaotic atrial tachycardia, were successfully controlled with sotalol. Ten infants discontinued therapy between the ages of 7-18 months when it was no longer necessary. Median duration of treatment was 12.8 months.

Adults: Oral:
Ventricular arrhythmias (Betapace®):
Initial: 80 mg twice daily
Dose may be increased (gradually allowing 2-3 days between dosing increments in order to attain steady-state plasma concentrations and to allow monitoring of Q-T intervals) to 240-320 mg/day.
Most patients respond to a total daily dose of 160-320 mg/day in 2-3 divided doses.
Some patients, with life-threatening refractory ventricular arrhythmias, may require doses as high as 480-640 mg/day; however, these doses should only be prescribed when the potential benefit outweighs the increased of adverse events.

Atrial fibrillation or atrial flutter (Betapace® AF™): Initial: 80 mg twice daily
If the initial dose does not reduce the frequency of relapses of atrial fibrillation/flutter and is tolerated without excessive Q-T prolongation (not >520 msec) after 3 days, the dose may be increased to 120 mg twice daily This may be further increased to 160 mg twice daily if response is inadequate and Q-T prolongation is not excessive.

Elderly: Age does not significantly alter the pharmacokinetics of sotalol, but impaired renal function in elderly patients can increase the terminal half-life, resulting in increased drug accumulation

**Dosage adjustment in renal impairment:** Impaired renal function can increase the terminal half-life, resulting in increased drug accumulation. Sotalol (Betapace AF®) is contraindicated per the manufacturer for treatment of atrial fibrillation/flutter in patients with a $Cl_{cr}$ <40 mL/minute.

Ventricular arrhythmias (Betapace®):
$Cl_{cr}$ >60 mL/minute: Administer every 12 hours
$Cl_{cr}$ 30-60 mL/minute: Administer every 24 hours

$Cl_{cr}$ 10-30 mL/minute: Administer every 36-48 hours
$Cl_{cr}$ <10 mL/minute: Individualize dose
Atrial fibrillation/flutter (Betapace AF®):
$Cl_{cr}$ >60 mL/minute: Administer every 12 hours
$Cl_{cr}$ 40-60 mL/minute: Administer every 24 hours
$Cl_{cr}$ <40 mL/minute: Use is contraindicated
Dialysis: Hemodialysis would be expected to reduce sotalol plasma concentrations because sotalol is not bound to plasma proteins and does not undergo extensive metabolism; administer dose postdialysis or administer supplemental 80 mg dose; peritoneal dialysis does not remove sotalol; supplemental dose is not necessary

**Patient Information** Take exactly as directed; do not take additional doses or discontinue without consulting prescriber. You will need regular cardiac checkups and blood tests while taking this medication. You may experience dizziness, drowsiness, or visual changes (use caution when driving or engaging in tasks requiring alertness until response to drug is known); orthostatic hypotension (use caution when climbing stairs or when changing position - rising from lying or sitting position); abnormal taste, nausea or vomiting, or loss of appetite (small frequent meals, frequent mouth care, chewing gum, or sucking lozenges may help); decreased sexual ability (reversible); or constipation (increased exercise, dietary fiber, fruit, or fluid may help). Report chest pain, palpitation, or erratic heartbeat; difficulty breathing or unusual cough; mental depression or persistent insomnia (hallucinations); or changes in vision.

**Nursing Implications** Initiation of therapy and dose escalation should be done in a hospital with cardiac monitoring; lidocaine and other resuscitative measures should be available

**Dosage Forms** Tablet, as hydrochloride: 80 mg, 120 mg, 160 mg, 240 mg

- **SPA** *see* Albumin *on page 21*
- **Spancap® No. 1** *see* Dextroamphetamine *on page 159*
- **Span-FF® [OTC]** *see* Ferrous Fumarate *on page 223*

## Sparfloxacin (spar FLOKS a sin)

**U.S. Brand Names** Zagam®

**Pharmacologic Category** Antibiotic, Quinolone

**Use** Treatment of adults with community-acquired pneumonia caused by *C. pneumoniae, H. influenzae, H. parainfluenzae, M. catarrhalis, M. pneumoniae* or *S. pneumoniae*; treatment of acute bacterial exacerbations of chronic bronchitis caused by *C. pneumoniae, E. cloacae, H. influenzae, H. parainfluenzae, K. pneumoniae, M. catarrhalis, S. aureus* or *S. pneumoniae*

**Effects on Mental Status** May cause agitation, anxiety, insomnia, or delirium; quinolones reported to cause restlessness, hallucinations, euphoria, depression, panic, and paranoia

**Effects on Psychiatric Treatment** May cause leukopenia; use caution with clozapine and carbamazepine; contraindicated with TCAs and phenothiazines

**Pregnancy Risk Factor** C

**Contraindications** Hypersensitivity to sparfloxacin, any component, or other quinolones; a concurrent administration with drugs which increase the Q-T interval including: amiodarone, bepridil, bretylium,cisapride, disopyramide, furosemide, procainamide, quinidine, sotalol, albuterol, astemizole, chloroquine, cisapride, halofantrine, phenothiazines, prednisone, terfenadine, and tricyclic antidepressants

**Warnings/Precautions** Not recommended in children <18 years of age, other quinolones have caused transient arthropathy in children; CNS stimulation may occur (tremor, restlessness, confusion, and very rarely hallucinations or seizures); use with caution in patients with known or suspected CNS disorder or renal dysfunction; prolonged use may result in superinfection; if an allergic reaction (itching, urticaria, dyspnea, pharyngeal or facial edema, loss of consciousness, tingling, cardiovascular collapse) occurs, discontinue the drug immediately; use caution to avoid possible photosensitivity reactions during and for several days following fluoroquinolone therapy; pseudomembranous colitis may occur and should be considered in patients who present with diarrhea

**Adverse Reactions**
>1%:
Central nervous system: Insomnia, agitation, sleep disorders, anxiety, delirium
Gastrointestinal: Diarrhea, abdominal pain, vomiting
Hematologic: Leukopenia, eosinophilia, anemia
Hepatic: Increased LFTs
<1%: Arthralgia, myalgia, photosensitivity, rash

**Overdosage/Toxicology**
Signs and symptoms: Acute renal failure, seizures
Treatment: GI decontamination and supportive care; not removed by peritoneal or hemodialysis

**Drug Interactions**
Decreased effect: Decreased absorption with antacids containing aluminum, magnesium, and/or calcium, sucralfate, didanosine and by products containing zinc and iron salts when administered concurrently. Take > 4 hours after sparfloxacin. Phenytoin serum levels may be reduced by quinolones; antineoplastic agents may also decrease serum levels of fluoroquinolones
Increased toxicity/serum levels: Quinolones cause increased levels of caffeine, warfarin, cyclosporine, and theophylline (although one study indicates that sparfloxacin may not affect theophylline metabolism), cimetidine and probenecid increase quinolone levels; an increased incidence of seizures may occur with foscarnet. Avoid use with drugs which increase Q-T interval as significant risk of cardiotoxicity may occur. Concurrent use with cisapride is contraindicated.

**Usual Dosage** Adults: Oral:
Loading dose: 2 tablets (400 mg) on day 1
Maintenance: 1 tablet (200 mg) daily for 10 days total therapy (total 11 tablets)
**Dosing adjustment in renal impairment:** $Cl_{cr}$ <50 mL/minute: Administer 400 mg on day 1, then 200 mg every 48 hours for a total of 9 days of therapy (total 6 tablets)

**Patient Information** Take per recommended schedule around-the-clock. Maintain adequate hydration (2-3 L/day of fluids unless instructed to restrict fluid intake). Take complete prescription and do not skip doses; if dose is missed take as soon as possible, do not double doses. Do not take with antacids. You may experience dizziness, lightheadedness, anxiety, insomnia, or confusion; use caution when driving or engaging in tasks that require alertness until response to drug is known. Small frequent meals, frequent mouth care, sucking lozenges, or chewing gum may reduce nausea, vomiting, or taste disturbances. You may experience photosensitivity; use sunscreen, wear protective clothing and eyewear, and avoid direct sunlight. Report palpitations or chest pain; persistent diarrhea or GI disturbances or abdominal pain; muscle tremor or pain; pain, inflammation, or rupture of tendon; yellowing of eyes or skin, easy bruising or bleeding; unusual fatigue; fever, chills, signs of infection; or worsening of condition.

**Dosage Forms** Tablet: 200 mg

- **Sparine®** *see* Promazine *on page 469*
- **Spasmolin®** *see* Hyoscyamine, Atropine, Scopolamine, and Phenobarbital *on page 279*
- **Special Populations - Children and Adolescents** *see page 663*
- **Special Populations - Elderly** *see page 662*
- **Special Populations - Medically Ill Patients** *see page 666*
- **Special Populations - Mentally Retarded Patients** *see page 665*
- **Special Populations - Pregnant and Breast-Feeding Patients** *see page 668*
- **Spec-T® [OTC]** *see* Benzocaine *on page 61*
- **Spectazole™ Topical** *see* Econazole *on page 189*

## Spectinomycin (spek ti noe MYE sin)

**U.S. Brand Names** Trobicin®

**Pharmacologic Category** Antibiotic, Miscellaneous

**Use** Treatment of uncomplicated gonorrhea

**Effects on Mental Status** May cause dizziness

**Effects on Psychiatric Treatment** None reported

**Usual Dosage** I.M.:
Children:
<45 kg: 40 mg/kg/dose 1 time (ceftriaxone preferred)
≥45 kg: See adult dose
Children >8 years who are allergic to PCNS/cephalosporins may be treated with oral tetracycline
Adults:
Uncomplicated urethral endocervical or rectal gonorrhea: 2 g deep I.M. or 4 g where antibiotic resistance is prevalent 1 time; 4 g (10 mL) dose should be given as two 5 mL injections, followed by doxycycline 100 mg twice daily for 7 days
Disseminated gonococcal infection: 2 g every 12 hours
**Dosing adjustment in renal impairment:** None necessary
Hemodialysis: 50% removed by hemodialysis

**Dosage Forms** Powder for injection: 2 g, 4 g

- **Spectrobid®** *see* Bacampicillin *on page 56*

## Spirapril (SPYE ra pril)

**U.S. Brand Names** Renormax®

**Synonyms** Sch-33844

**Pharmacologic Category** Angiotensin-Converting Enzyme (ACE) Inhibitors

**Use** Management of mild to severe hypertension; treatment of left ventricular dysfunction after myocardial infarction

**Effects on Mental Status** May cause dizziness or drowsiness; may rarely cause insomnia or depression

**Effects on Psychiatric Treatment** May cause neutropenia; use caution with clozapine and carbamazepine; may decrease lithium clearance

(Continued)

## Spirapril *(Continued)*

resulting in an increase in serum lithium levels and potential lithium toxicity; monitor serum lithium levels

**Contraindications** Hypersensitivity to spirapril or any component; angioedema or other sensitivity to any ACE inhibitor; bilateral renal artery stenosis; pregnancy (2nd and 3rd trimesters)

**Warnings/Precautions** Anaphylactic reactions can occur. Angioedema can occur at any time during treatment (especially following first dose). Careful blood pressure monitoring with first dose (hypotension can occur especially in volume depleted patients). Dosage adjustment needed in renal impairment. Use with caution in hypovolemia; collagen vascular diseases; valvular stenosis (particularly aortic stenosis); hyperkalemia; or before, during, or immediately after anesthesia. Avoid rapid dosage escalation which may lead to renal insufficiency. Neutropenia/agranulocytosis with myeloid hyperplasia can rarely occur. If patient has renal impairment then a baseline WBC with differential and serum creatinine should be evaluated and monitored closely during the first 3 months of therapy. Hypersensitivity reactions may be seen during hemodialysis with high-flux dialysis membranes (eg, AN69). Deterioration in renal function can occur with initiation. Use with caution in unilateral renal artery stenosis and pre-existing renal insufficiency.

**Adverse Reactions**

Cardiovascular: Hypotension (orthostatic)

Central nervous system: Headache, dizziness, migraine headache (exacerbation of), hypoesthesia

Dermatologic: Skin rash

Gastrointestinal: Nausea, diarrhea, vomiting

Neuromuscular & skeletal: Back pain

Ocular: Conjunctivitis

Respiratory: Cough

**Drug Interactions**

Alpha$_1$ blockers: Hypotensive effect increased

Aspirin and NSAIDs may decrease ACE inhibitor efficacy and/or increase risk of renal effects

Diuretics: Hypovolemia due to diuretics may precipitate acute hypotensive events or acute renal failure

Insulin: Risk of hypoglycemia may be increased

Lithium: Risk of lithium toxicity may be increased; monitor lithium levels, especially the first 4 weeks of therapy

Mercaptopurine: Risk of neutropenia may be increased

Potassium-sparing diuretics (amiloride, potassium, spironolactone, triamterene): Increased risk of hyperkalemia

Potassium supplements may increase the risk of hyperkalemia

Trimethoprim (high dose) may increase the risk of hyperkalemia

**Usual Dosage** Adults: Oral: 12-48 mg once daily

**Dosage Forms** Tablet: 3 mg, 6 mg, 12 mg, 24 mg

## Spironolactone (speer on oh LAK tone)

**U.S. Brand Names** Aldactone®

**Canadian Brand Names** Novo-Spiroton

**Pharmacologic Category** Diuretic, Potassium Sparing

**Use** Management of edema associated with excessive aldosterone excretion; hypertension; primary hyperaldosteronism; hypokalemia; treatment of hirsutism; cirrhosis of liver accompanied by edema or ascites

**Effects on Mental Status** May cause drowsiness, dizziness, nervousness, or confusion

**Effects on Psychiatric Treatment** Has been used to treat lithium-related edema

**Pregnancy Risk Factor** D

**Contraindications** Hypersensitivity to spironolactone or any component; anuria; acute renal insufficiency; significant impairment of renal excretory function; hyperkalemia; pregnancy

**Warnings/Precautions** Avoid potassium supplements, potassium-containing salt substitutes, a diet rich in potassium, or other drugs that can cause hyperkalemia. Monitor for fluid and electrolyte imbalances. Gynecomastia is related to dose and duration of therapy. Diuretic therapy should be carefully used in severe hepatic dysfunction; electrolyte and fluid shifts can cause or exacerbate encephalopathy.

**Adverse Reactions** Percentage unknown: Arrhythmia, ataxia, breast tenderness in females, chills, confusion, cough or hoarseness, decreased sexual ability, deepening of voice in females, diaphoresis, diarrhea, dizziness, drowsiness, dryness of mouth, dyspnea, dysuria, enlargement of breast in males, fever, headache, hyperkalemia, inability to achieve or maintain an erection, increased hair growth in females, increased thirst, lack of energy, lower back or side pain, menstrual changes, nausea, nervousness, numbness or paresthesia in hands/feet/lips, painful urination, shortness of breath, skin rash, stomach cramps, unusual fatigue, vomiting, weakness

**Overdosage/Toxicology**

Signs and symptoms: Drowsiness, confusion, clinical signs of dehydration and electrolyte imbalance, hyperkalemia; ingestion of large amounts of potassium-sparing diuretics, may result in life-threatening hyperkalemia.

Treatment: Hyperkalemia can be treated with I.V. glucose, with concurrent regular insulin; sodium bicarbonate may also be used as a temporary measure. If needed, Kayexalate® oral or rectal solutions in sorbitol may also be used.

**Drug Interactions**

Angiotensin-converting enzyme inhibitors can cause hyperkalemia, especially in patients with renal impairment, potassium-rich diets, or on other drugs causing hyperkalemia; avoid concurrent use or monitor closely

Cholestyramine can cause hyperchloremic acidosis in cirrhotic patients; avoid concurrent use

Digoxin's positive inotropic effect may be reduced; serum levels of digoxin may increased

Mitotane loses its effect; avoid concurrent use

Potassium supplements may increase potassium retention and cause hyperkalemia; avoid concurrent use

Salicylates may interfere with the natriuretic action of spironolactone

**Usual Dosage** Administration with food increases absorption. To reduce delay in onset of effect, a loading dose of 2 or 3 times the daily dose may be administered on the first day of therapy. Oral:

Neonates: Diuretic: 1-3 mg/kg/day divided every 12-24 hours

Children:

Diuretic, hypertension: 1.5-3.5 mg/kg/day **or** 60 mg/m$^2$/day in divided doses every 6-24 hours

Diagnosis of primary aldosteronism: 125-375 mg/m$^2$/day in divided doses

Vaso-occlusive disease: 7.5 mg/kg/day in divided doses twice daily (not FDA approved)

Adults:

Edema, hypertension, hypokalemia: 25-200 mg/day in 1-2 divided doses

Diagnosis of primary aldosteronism: 100-400 mg/day in 1-2 divided doses

Hirsutism in women: 50-200 mg/day in 1-2 divided doses

Elderly: Initial: 25-50 mg/day in 1-2 divided doses, increasing by 25-50 mg every 5 days as needed.

**Dosing interval in renal impairment:**

$Cl_{cr}$ 10-50 mL/minute: Administer every 12-24 hours.

$Cl_{cr}$ <10 mL/minute: Avoid use.

**Patient Information** Take as directed, with meals or milk. This diuretic does not cause potassium loss; avoid excessive potassium intake (eg, salt substitutes, low-salt foods, bananas, nuts). Weigh yourself weekly at the same time, in the same clothes, and report weight loss more than 5 lb/week. You may experience dizziness, drowsiness, headache; use caution when driving or engaging in tasks requiring alertness until response to drug is known. Small frequent meals, frequent mouth care, sucking lozenges, or chewing gum may reduce dry mouth, nausea, or vomiting. You may experience decreased sexual ability (reversible with discontinuing of medication). Report mental confusion; clumsiness; persistent fatigue, chills, numbness, or muscle weakness in hands, feet, or face; acute persistent diarrhea; breast tenderness or increased body hair in females; breast enlargement or inability to achieve erection in males; chest pain, rapid heartbeat or palpitations; or difficulty breathing.

**Nursing Implications** Diuretic effect may be delayed 2-3 days and maximum hypertensive may be delayed 2-3 weeks; monitor I & O ratios and daily weight throughout therapy

**Dosage Forms** Tablet: 25 mg, 50 mg, 100 mg


- ♦ **Sporanox®** *see* Itraconazole *on page 298*
- ♦ **S-P-T** *see* Thyroid *on page 547*
- ♦ **Squaw Tea** *see* Ephedra *on page 194*
- ♦ **SRC® Expectorant** *see* Hydrocodone, Pseudoephedrine, and Guaifenesin *on page 273*
- ♦ **SSD® AF** *see* Silver Sulfadiazine *on page 512*
- ♦ **SSD® Cream** *see* Silver Sulfadiazine *on page 512*
- ♦ **SSKI®** *see* Potassium Iodide *on page 454*
- ♦ **Stadol®** *see* Butorphanol *on page 81*
- ♦ **Stadol® NS** *see* Butorphanol *on page 81*
- ♦ **Stagesic®** *see* Hydrocodone and Acetaminophen *on page 272*
- ♦ **Stahist®** *see* Chlorpheniramine, Phenylephrine, Phenylpropanolamine, and Belladonna Alkaloids *on page 115*


## Stanozolol (stan OH zoe lole)

**U.S. Brand Names** Winstrol®

**Pharmacologic Category** Anabolic Steroid

**Use** Prophylactic use against hereditary angioedema

**Effects on Mental Status** May cause insomnia

**Effects on Psychiatric Treatment** None reported

**Restrictions** C-III

**Pregnancy Risk Factor** X

**Contraindications** Nephrosis, carcinoma of breast or prostate, pregnancy, hypersensitivity to any component

**Warnings/Precautions** May stunt bone growth in children; anabolic steroids may cause peliosis hepatis, liver cell tumors, and blood lipid changes with increased risk of arteriosclerosis; monitor diabetic patients carefully; use with caution in elderly patients, they may be at greater risk for prostatic hypertrophy; use with caution in patients with cardiac, renal, or hepatic disease or epilepsy

**Adverse Reactions**

**Male:**

Postpubertal:

- >10%:
  - Dermatologic: Acne
  - Endocrine & metabolic: Gynecomastia
  - Genitourinary: Bladder irritability, priapism
- 1% to 10%:
  - Central nervous system: Insomnia, chills
  - Endocrine & metabolic: Decreased libido, hepatic dysfunction
  - Gastrointestinal: Nausea, diarrhea
  - Genitourinary: Prostatic hypertrophy (elderly)
  - Hematologic: Iron deficiency anemia, suppression of clotting factors
- <1%: Hepatic necrosis, hepatocellular carcinoma

Prepubertal:

- >10%:
  - Dermatologic: Acne
  - Endocrine & metabolic: Virilism
- 1% to 10%:
  - Central nervous system: Chills, insomnia, factors
  - Dermatologic: Hyperpigmentation
  - Gastrointestinal: Diarrhea, nausea
  - Hematologic: Iron deficiency anemia, suppression of clotting
- <1%: Hepatic necrosis, hepatocellular carcinoma

**Female:**

- >10%: Endocrine & metabolic: Virilism
- 1% to 10%:
  - Central nervous system: Chills, insomnia
  - Endocrine & metabolic: Hypercalcemia
  - Gastrointestinal: Nausea, diarrhea
  - Hematologic: Iron deficiency anemia, suppression of clotting factors
  - Hepatic: Hepatic dysfunction
- <1%: Hepatic necrosis, hepatocellular carcinoma

**Drug Interactions** Increased toxicity: ACTH, adrenal steroids may increase risk of edema and acne; stanozolol enhances the hypoprothrombinemic effects of oral anticoagulants; enhances the hypoglycemic effects of insulin and sulfonylureas (oral hypoglycemics)

**Usual Dosage**

Children: Acute attacks:
- <6 years: 1 mg/day
- 6-12 years: 2 mg/day

Adults: Oral: Initial: 2 mg 3 times/day, may then reduce to a maintenance dose of 2 mg/day or 2 mg every other day after 1-3 months

**Dosing adjustment in hepatic impairment:** Stanozolol is **not** recommended for patients with severe liver dysfunction

**Patient Information** Take as directed; do not exceed recommended dosage. Diabetics should monitor serum glucose closely and notify prescriber of changes; this medication can alter hypoglycemic requirements. You may experience decrease of libido or impotence (usually reversible); nausea, vomiting, or GI distress (frequent small meals, frequent mouth care, chewing gum, or sucking lozenges may help); or diarrhea (buttermilk, boiled milk, yogurt may help). Report persistent GI distress or diarrhea; change in color of urine or stool; unusual bruising, bleeding, or yellowing of eyes or skin; fluid retention (swelling of ankles, feet, or hands, difficulty breathing, or sudden weight gain); unresolved CNS changes (insomnia or chills); menstrual irregularity; excessive growth of body hair; or other adverse reactions.

**Dosage Forms** Tablet: 2 mg


♦ **Staphcillin®** *see* Methicillin *on page 352*

♦ **Staticin® Topical** *see* Erythromycin, Ophthalmic/Topical *on page 202*


## Stavudine (STAV yoo deen)

**U.S. Brand Names** Zerit®

**Synonyms** d4T

**Pharmacologic Category** Antiretroviral Agent, Reverse Transcriptase Inhibitor (Nucleoside)

**Use** Treatment of adults with HIV infection in combination with other antiretroviral agents

**Effects on Mental Status** May cause drowsiness, insomnia, anxiety, or depression

**Effects on Psychiatric Treatment** May cause neutropenia; use caution with clozapine and carbamazepine; concurrent use with lithium may increase the risk of peripheral neuropathy

**Pregnancy Risk Factor** C

**Contraindications** Hypersensitivity to stavudine

**Warnings/Precautions** Use with caution in patients who demonstrate previous hypersensitivity to zidovudine, didanosine, zalcitabine, pre-existing bone marrow suppression, renal insufficiency, or peripheral neuropathy. Peripheral neuropathy may be the dose-limiting side effect. Zidovudine should not be used in combination with stavudine. Potentially fatal lactic acidosis and hepatomegaly have been reported, use with caution in patients at risk of hepatic disease

**Adverse Reactions** All adverse reactions reported below were similar to comparative agent, zidovudine, except for peripheral neuropathy, which was greater for stavudine.

- >10%:
  - Central nervous system: Headache, chills/fever, malaise, insomnia, anxiety, depression, pain
  - Dermatologic: Rash
  - Gastrointestinal: Nausea, vomiting, diarrhea, pancreatitis, abdominal pain
  - Neuromuscular & skeletal: Peripheral neuropathy (15% to 21%)
- 1% to 10%:
  - Hematologic: Neutropenia, thrombocytopenia
  - Hepatic: Increased hepatic transaminases, increased bilirubin
  - Neuromuscular & skeletal: Myalgia, back pain, weakness
- <1%: Anemia, hepatic failure, hepatomegaly, lactic acidosis, pancreatitis

**Drug Interactions** Drugs associated with peripheral neuropathy (chloramphenicol, cisplatin, dapsone, ethionamide, gold, hydralazine, iodoquinol, isoniazid, lithium, metronidazole, nitrofurantoin, pentamidine, phenytoin, ribavirin, vincristine) may increase risk for stavudine peripheral neuropathy

**Usual Dosage** Oral:

Children: 2 mg/kg/day

Adults:
- ≥60 kg: 40 mg every 12 hours
- <60 kg: 30 mg every 12 hours
- Dose may be cut in half if symptoms of peripheral neuropathy occur

**Dosing adjustment in renal impairment:**

- $Cl_{cr}$ >50 mL/minute:
  - ≥60 kg: 40 mg every 12 hours
  - <60 kg: 30 mg every 12 hours
- $Cl_{cr}$ 26-50 mL/minute:
  - ≥60 kg: 20 mg every 12 hours
  - <60 kg: 15 mg every 12 hours
- Hemodialysis:
  - ≥60 kg: 20 mg every 24 hours
  - <60 kg: 15 mg every 24 hours

**Patient Information** This medication does not cure HIV. Use appropriate precautions to prevent transmission to others. Take as directed, around-the-clock, and take for full length of prescription. Maintain adequate hydration (2-3 L/day of fluids unless instructed to restrict fluid intake) and nutrition. Frequent small meals, frequent mouth care, sucking lozenges, or chewing gum may reduce nausea or vomiting. Buttermilk or yogurt may help reduce diarrhea. Report immediately any tingling, unusual pain, or numbness in extremities. Report fever, chills, unusual fatigue or acute depression, acute abdominal or back pain, persistent muscle pain or weakness, or unusual bruising or bleeding.

**Dosage Forms**

Capsule: 15 mg, 20 mg, 30 mg, 40 mg

Powder for oral solution: 1 mg/mL (200 mL)


♦ **St Bartholomew's Tea** *see* Maté *on page 333*

♦ **S-T Cort®** *see* Hydrocortisone *on page 273*

♦ **Stelazine®** *see* Trifluoperazine *on page 566*

♦ **Stilbestrol** *see* Diethylstilbestrol *on page 168*

♦ **Stilphostrol®** *see* Diethylstilbestrol *on page 168*

♦ **Stimate™ Nasal** *see* Desmopressin *on page 156*

♦ **Stimulant Agents Used for ADHD** *see page 728*

♦ **Stinking Rose** *see* Garlic *on page 246*


## St Johns Wort

**Related Information**


Natural/Herbal Products *on page 746*

Natural Products, Herbals, and Dietary Supplements *on page 742*


**Synonyms** Amber Touch-and-Feel; Goatweed; *Hypercium perforatum*; Klamath Weed; Rosin Rose

**Pharmacologic Category** Herb

**Use** Mild to moderate depression; also used traditionally for treatment of stress, anxiety, insomnia; used topically for vitiligo; also a popular drug for AIDS patients due to possible antiretroviral activity; used topically for wound healing

Per Commission E: Psychovegetative disorders, depressive moods, anxiety and/or nervous unrest; oily preparations for dyspeptic complaints; oily preparations externally for treatment of post-therapy of acute and contused injuries, myalgia, first degree burns

(Continued)

## St Johns Wort *(Continued)*

**Contraindications** St. John's wort is contraindicated in pregnancy (based on animal studies); children <2 years of age (not confirmed in animal models, *in vitro* only); endogenous depression

**Warnings/Precautions** Use with caution in individuals taking digoxin (may alter levels of this medication). It is not for use in severe depression. Use with caution in individuals taking other antidepressants. Based on its pharmacological activity, St John's wort may alter the actions of monoamine oxidase (MAO) inhibitors, tricyclic antidepressants, and selective serotonin reuptake inhibitors (SSRIs). May elevate hepatic transaminases (noted animal studies at high doses). May cause photosensitivity (based on animal studies and a human clinical trial). Use with caution in individuals on reserpine (effects may be antagonized by St John's wort). Use with caution in individuals on narcotic medications (based on animal studies, may enhance sedation from these drugs).

May cause drowsiness (mild). Based on pharmacological activity, use with caution while driving or operating machinery. Caution in individuals taking sedative medications (eg, anxiolytics, benzodiazepines). Effects may be additive with other CNS depressants or natural products with sedative properties.

Antidepressant therapy may precipitate a shift to mania or hypomania in individuals with bipolar affective disorder.

St John's wort may induce the cytochrome P-450 enzyme system, although there is conflicting information about this claim. Specifically, data indicates probable interactions between St John's wort and the HIV-1 protease inhibitor indinavir and between St John's wort and the antirejection medication cyclosporine. Additionally, enzyme induction may result in decreased estrogen levels in individuals taking oral contraceptives. While the FDA has issued a public health advisory regarding this issue, the authors recommend considerable caution be exercised before adding St John's wort to any medication regimen containing a CYP3A substrate.

**Adverse Reactions**

Cardiovascular: Sinus tachycardia

Dermatologic: Photosensitization is possible, especially in fair-skinned persons (per Commission E)

Gastrointestinal: Stomach pains, abdominal pain

Miscellaneous: May exacerbate bipolar disorder by causing mania

**Overdosage/Toxicology**

Signs and symptoms: Photosensitivity/rash, drowsiness, fever, tachycardia, pruritus, diarrhea, nausea

Decontamination: Lavage (within 1hour)/activated charcoal with cathartic

**Drug Interactions**

**Note:** St Johns wort has been proposed to be a CYP3A4 inducer; however, some evidence suggests reported drug interactions may result from inhibition of the p-glycoprotein drug transporter

Antidepressants: Avoid use with SSRIs or other antidepressants

Cyclosporine: Effect/levels may be decreased; contraindicated

CYP3A3/4 substrates: Effect levels may be reduced by St Johns wort; avoid concurrent administration or monitor closely for diminished effect; includes oral contraceptives

Digoxin: AUC decreased 25% and trough $C_{max}$ concentration decreased by 33% and 26% respectively after 15 days of concurrent use

Indinavir (and potentially other protease inhibitors): Effects may be decreased; contraindicated

Linezolid: Effect/toxicity may be potentiated; theoretically, serotonin syndrome may result

MAO inhibitors: Effect/toxicity may be potentiated; theoretically, serotonin syndrome may result

**Usual Dosage** Based on hypericin extract content

Oral: 300 mg 3 times daily (not to be used longer than 8 weeks)

Herb: 2-4 g 3 times daily

Liquid extract: 2-4 mL 3 times/day

Tincture: 2-4 mL 3 times/day

Topical: Crushed leaves and flowers are applied to affected area after cleansing with soap and water

Per Commission E: 2-4 g drug (dried herb) or 0.2-1 mg of total hypericin in other forms of drug application

**Additional Information** VIMRxgn is a synthetic hypericin for HIV treatment; leaves and tops of *Hypericum perforatum* plant used in herbal medicine. St Johns wort is a perennial that reaches 2 feet tall with the aroma similar to turpentine; golden yellow flowers bloom in early summer. Young plant is almost as toxic as the mature plant. Hypericin inhibits both type A and type B monoamine oxidase; contraindications in endogenous depression, pregnancy, children <2 years of age (not confirmed in animal models, *in vitro* only).

- **St Joseph® Adult Chewable Aspirin [OTC]** *see* Aspirin *on page 49*
- **St. Joseph® Cough Suppressant [OTC]** *see* Dextromethorphan *on page 160*
- **St. Joseph® Measured Dose Nasal Solution [OTC]** *see* Phenylephrine *on page 439*
- **Streptase®** *see* Streptokinase *on page 520*

## Streptokinase (strep toe KYE nase)

**U.S. Brand Names** Kabikinase®; Streptase®

**Pharmacologic Category** Thrombolytic Agent

**Use** Thrombolytic agent used in treatment of recent severe or massive deep vein thrombosis, pulmonary emboli, myocardial infarction, and occluded arteriovenous cannulas

**Effects on Mental Status** None reported

**Effects on Psychiatric Treatment** None reported

**Usual Dosage** I.V.:

Children: Safety and efficacy have not been not established. Limited studies have used 3500-4000 units/kg over 30 minutes followed by 1000-1500 units/kg/hour.

Clotted catheter: 25,000 units, clamp for 2 hours then aspirate contents and flush with normal saline.

Adults: Antibodies to streptokinase remain for at least 3-6 months after initial dose: Administration requires the use of an infusion pump.

An intradermal skin test of 100 units has been suggested to predict allergic response to streptokinase. If a positive reaction is not seen after 15-20 minutes, a therapeutic dose may be administered.

**Guidelines for acute myocardial infarction** (AMI): 1.5 million units over 60 minutes

Administration:

Dilute two 750,000 unit vials of streptokinase with 5 mL dextrose 5% in water ($D_5W$) each, gently swirl to dissolve.

Add this dose of the 1.5 million units to 150 mL $D_5W$.

This should be infused over 60 minutes; an in-line filter ≥0.45 micron should be used.

Monitor for the first few hours for signs of anaphylaxis or allergic reaction. **Infusion should be slowed if lowering of 25 mm Hg in blood pressure or terminated if asthmatic symptoms appear.**

Begin heparin 5000-10,000 unit bolus followed by 1000 units/hour approximately 3-4 hours after completion of streptokinase infusion or when PTT is <100 seconds.

**Guidelines for acute pulmonary embolism** (APE): 3 million unit dose over 24 hours

Administration:

Dilute four 750,000 unit vials of streptokinase with 5 mL dextrose 5% in water ($D_5W$) each, gently swirl to dissolve.

Add this dose of 3 million units to 250 mL $D_5W$, an in-line filter ≥0.45 micron should be used.

Administer 250,000 units (23 mL) over 30 minutes followed by 100,000 units/hour (9 mL/hour) for 24 hours.

Monitor for the first few hours for signs of anaphylaxis or allergic reaction. **Infusion should be slowed if blood pressure is lowered by 25 mm Hg or if asthmatic symptoms appear.**

Begin heparin 1000 units/hour about 3-4 hours after completion of streptokinase infusion or when PTT is <100 seconds.

Monitor PT, PTT, and fibrinogen levels during therapy.

Thromboses: 250,000 units to start, then 100,000 units/hour for 24-72 hours depending on location.

**Cannula occlusion:** 250,000 units into cannula, clamp for 2 hours, then aspirate contents and flush with normal saline; **NOT RECOMMENDED**

**Dosage Forms** Powder for injection: 250,000 units (5 mL, 6.5 mL); 600,000 units (5 mL); 750,000 units (6 mL, 6.5 mL); 1,500,000 units (6.5 mL, 10 mL, 50 mL)

## Streptomycin (strep toe MYE sin)

**Pharmacologic Category** Antibiotic, Aminoglycoside; Antitubercular Agent

**Use** Part of combination therapy of active tuberculosis; used in combination with other agents for treatment of streptococcal or enterococcal endocarditis, mycobacterial infections, plague, tularemia, and brucellosis

**Effects on Mental Status** May cause drowsiness

**Effects on Psychiatric Treatment** None reported

**Usual Dosage**

Children:

Daily therapy: 20-30 mg/kg/day (maximum: 1 g/day)

Directly observed therapy (DOT): Twice weekly: 25-30 mg/kg (maximum: 1.5 g)

DOT: 3 times/week: 25-30 mg/kg (maximum: 1 g)

Adults:

Daily therapy: 15 mg/kg/day (maximum: 1 g)

Directly observed therapy (DOT): Twice weekly: 25-30 mg/kg (maximum: 1.5 g)

DOT: 3 times/week: 25-30 mg/kg (maximum: 1 g)

Enterococcal endocarditis: 1 g every 12 hours for 2 weeks, 500 mg every 12 hours for 4 weeks in combination with penicillin

Streptococcal endocarditis: 1 g every 12 hours for 1 week, 500 mg every 12 hours for 1 week

Tularemia: 1-2 g/day in divided doses for 7-10 days or until patient is afebrile for 5-7 days

Plague: 2-4 g/day in divided doses until the patient is afebrile for at least 3 days

Elderly: 10 mg/kg/day, not to exceed 750 mg/day; dosing interval should be adjusted for renal function; some authors suggest not to give more than 5 days/week or give as 20-25 mg/kg/dose twice weekly

**Dosing interval in renal impairment:**

$Cl_{cr}$ 10-50 mL/minute: Administer every 24-72 hours

$Cl_{cr}$ <10 mL/minute: Administer every 72-96 hours

Removed by hemo and peritoneal dialysis: Administer dose postdialysis

**Dosage Forms** Injection, as sulfate: 400 mg/mL (2.5 mL)

## Streptozocin (strep toe ZOE sin)

**U.S. Brand Names** Zanosar®

**Pharmacologic Category** Antineoplastic Agent, Alkylating Agent

**Use** Treat metastatic islet cell carcinoma of the pancreas, carcinoid tumor and syndrome, Hodgkin's disease, palliative treatment of colorectal cancer

**Effects on Mental Status** May cause lethargy, confusion, or depression

**Effects on Psychiatric Treatment** May cause leukopenia; use caution with clozapine and carbamazepine; renal dysfunction occurs commonly with streptozocin; will need to monitor and adjust lithium and gabapentin doses

**Usual Dosage** I.V. (refer to individual protocols):

Children and Adults:

Single agent therapy: 1-1.5 g/m² weekly for 6 weeks followed by a 4-week observation period

Combination therapy: 0.5-1 g/m² for 5 consecutive days followed by a 4- to 6-week observation period

**Dosing adjustment in renal impairment:**

$Cl_{cr}$ 10-50 mL/minute: Administer 75% of dose

$Cl_{cr}$ <10 mL/minute: Administer 50% of dose

Hemodialysis: Unknown

CAPD effects: Unknown

CAVH effects: Unknown

**Dosing adjustment in hepatic impairment:** Dose should be decreased in patients with severe liver disease

**Dosage Forms** Injection: 1 g


- **Stresstabs® 600 Advanced Formula Tablets [OTC]** *see* Vitamins, Multiple *on page 587*
- **Stromectol®** *see* Ivermectin *on page 299*
- **Strong Iodine Solution** *see* Potassium Iodide *on page 454*
- **Sublimaze® Injection** *see* Fentanyl *on page 221*
- **Substance-Related Disorders** *see page 609*


## Succimer (SUKS i mer)

**U.S. Brand Names** Chemet®

**Pharmacologic Category** Antidote

**Use** Treatment of lead poisoning in children with blood levels >45 µg/dL. It is not indicated for prophylaxis of lead poisoning in a lead-containing environment. Following oral administration, succimer is generally well tolerated and produces a linear dose-dependent reduction in serum lead concentrations. This agent appears to offer advantages over existing lead chelating agents.

**Effects on Mental Status** May cause drowsiness or dizziness

**Effects on Psychiatric Treatment** None reported

**Usual Dosage** Children and Adults: Oral: 10 mg/kg/dose every 8 hours for an additional 5 days followed by 10 mg/kg/dose every 12 hours for 14 days

**Dosing adjustment in renal/hepatic impairment:** Administer with caution and monitor closely

Concomitant iron therapy has been reported in a small number of children without the formation of a toxic complex with iron (as seen with dimercaprol); courses of therapy may be repeated if indicated by weekly monitoring of blood lead levels; lead levels should be stabilized <15 µg/dL; 2 weeks between courses is recommended unless more timely treatment is indicated by lead levels

**Dosage Forms** Capsule: 100 mg

## Succinylcholine (suks in il KOE leen)

**U.S. Brand Names** Anectine® Chloride Injection; Anectine® Flo-Pack®; Quelicin® Injection

**Synonyms** Succinylcholine Chloride; Suxamethonium Chloride

**Pharmacologic Category** Neuromuscular Blocker Agent, Depolarizing

**Use** Produces skeletal muscle relaxation in procedures of short duration such as endotracheal intubation or endoscopic exams

**Effects on Mental Status** None reported

**Effects on Psychiatric Treatment** MAOIs may prolong the effects of succinylcholine

**Pregnancy Risk Factor** C

**Contraindications** Malignant hyperthermia, myopathies associated with elevated serum creatine phosphokinase (CPK) values, narrow-angle glaucoma, hyperkalemia, penetrating eye injuries, disorders of plasma pseudocholinesterase, hypersensitivity to succinylcholine or any component

**Warnings/Precautions Use in pediatrics and adolescents**; use with caution in patients with pre-existing hyperkalemia, paraplegia, extensive or severe burns, extensive denervation of skeletal muscle because of disease or injury to the CNS or with degenerative or dystrophic neuromuscular disease; may increase vagal tone

**Adverse Reactions**

>10%:

Ocular: Increased intraocular pressure

Miscellaneous: Postoperative stiffness

1% to 10%:

Cardiovascular: Bradycardia, hypotension, cardiac arrhythmias, tachycardia

Gastrointestinal: Intragastric pressure, salivation

<1%: Apnea, bronchospasm, circulatory collapse, erythema, hyperkalemia, hypertension, itching, malignant hyperthermia, myalgia, myoglobinuria, rash

**Causes of prolonged neuromuscular blockade:**

Excessive drug administration

Cumulative drug effect, decreased metabolism/excretion (hepatic and/or renal impairment)

Accumulation of active metabolites

Electrolyte imbalance (hypokalemia, hypocalcemia, hypermagnesemia, hypernatremia)

Hypothermia

Drug interactions

Increased sensitivity to muscle relaxants (eg, neuromuscular disorders such as myasthenia gravis or polymyositis)

**Overdosage/Toxicology**

Signs and symptoms: Respiratory paralysis, cardiac arrest

Treatment: Bradyarrhythmias can often be treated with atropine 0.1 mg (infants); do not treat with anticholinesterase drugs (eg, neostigmine, physostigmine) since this may worsen its toxicity by interfering with its metabolism

**Drug Interactions**

Increased toxicity: Anticholinesterase drugs (neostigmine, physostigmine, or pyridostigmine) in combination with succinylcholine can cause cardiorespiratory collapse; cyclophosphamide, oral contraceptives, lidocaine, thiotepa, pancuronium, lithium, magnesium salts, aprotinin, chloroquine, metoclopramide, terbutaline, and procaine enhance and prolong the effects of succinylcholine

**Prolonged neuromuscular blockade:**

Inhaled anesthetics

Local anesthetics

Calcium channel blockers

Antiarrhythmics (eg, quinidine or procainamide)

Antibiotics (eg, aminoglycosides, tetracyclines, vancomycin, clindamycin)

Immunosuppressants (eg, cyclosporine)

**Usual Dosage** I.M., I.V.:

Small Children: Intermittent: Initial: 2 mg/kg/dose one time; maintenance: 0.3-0.6 mg/kg/dose at intervals of 5-10 minutes as necessary

Older Children and Adolescents: Intermittent: Initial: 1 mg/kg/dose one time; maintenance: 0.3-0.6 mg/kg every 5-10 minutes as needed

Adults: 0.6 mg/kg (range: 0.3-1.1 mg/kg) over 10-30 seconds, up to 150 mg total dose

Maintenance: 0.04-0.07 mg/kg every 5-10 minutes as needed

Continuous infusion: 2.5 mg/minute (or 0.5-10 mg/minute); dilute to concentration of 1-2 mg/mL in $D_5W$ or NS

**Note:** Pretreatment with atropine may reduce occurrence of bradycardia

**Dosing adjustment in hepatic impairment:** Dose should be decreased in patients with severe liver disease

**Patient Information** Refrigerate

**Dosage Forms**

Injection, as chloride: 20 mg/mL (10 mL); 50 mg/mL (10 mL); 100 mg/mL (5 mL, 10 mL, 20 mL)

Powder for injection, as chloride: 100 mg, 500 mg, 1 g


- **Succinylcholine Chloride** *see* Succinylcholine *on page 521*


## Sucralfate (soo KRAL fate)

**U.S. Brand Names** Carafate®

**Canadian Brand Names** Novo-Sucralate; Sulcrate®; Sulcrate® Suspension Plus

**Synonyms** Aluminum Sucrose Sulfate, Basic

**Pharmacologic Category** Gastrointestinal Agent, Miscellaneous

**Use** Short-term management of duodenal ulcers

**Unlabeled use:** Gastric ulcers; maintenance of duodenal ulcers; suspension may be used topically for treatment of stomatitis due to cancer chemotherapy and other causes of esophageal and gastric erosions;

(Continued)

## Sucralfate *(Continued)*

GERD, esophagitis; treatment of NSAID mucosal damage; prevention of stress ulcers; postsclerotherapy for esophageal variceal bleeding

**Effects on Mental Status** May cause drowsiness, dizziness, or insomnia

**Effects on Psychiatric Treatment** None reported

**Pregnancy Risk Factor** B

**Contraindications** Hypersensitivity to sucralfate or any component

**Warnings/Precautions** Successful therapy with sucralfate should not be expected to alter the posthealing frequency of recurrence or the severity of duodenal ulceration; use with caution in patients with chronic renal failure who have an impaired excretion of absorbed aluminum. Because of the potential for sucralfate to alter the absorption of some drugs, separate administration (take other medication 2 hours before sucralfate) should be considered when alterations in bioavailability are believed to be critical

**Adverse Reactions**

1% to 10%: Gastrointestinal: Constipation

<1%: Back pain diarrhea, dizziness, gastric discomfort, indigestion, insomnia, nausea, pruritus, rash, sleepiness, vertigo, vomiting, xerostomia

**Overdosage/Toxicology** Signs and symptoms: Toxicity is minimal, may cause constipation

**Drug Interactions** Decreased effect: Digoxin, phenytoin (hydantoins), warfarin, ketoconazole, quinidine, ciprofloxacin, norfloxacin (quinolones), tetracycline, theophylline; because of the potential for sucralfate to alter the absorption of some drugs, separate administration (take other medications 2 hours before sucralfate) should be considered when alterations in bioavailability are believed to be critical

**Note:** When given with aluminum-containing antacids, may increase serum/body aluminum concentrations (see Warnings/Precautions)

**Usual Dosage** Oral:

Children: Dose not established, doses of 40-80 mg/kg/day divided every 6 hours have been used

Stomatitis: 2.5-5 mL (1 g/10 mL suspension), swish and spit or swish and swallow 4 times/day

Adults:

Stress ulcer prophylaxis: 1 g 4 times/day

Stress ulcer treatment: 1 g every 4 hours

Duodenal ulcer:

Treatment: 1 g 4 times/day on an empty stomach and at bedtime for 4-8 weeks, or alternatively 2 g twice daily; treatment is recommended for 4-8 weeks in adults, the elderly may require 12 weeks

Maintenance: Prophylaxis: 1 g twice daily

Stomatitis: 1 g/10 mL suspension, swish and spit or swish and swallow 4 times/day

**Dosage comment in renal impairment:** Aluminum salt is minimally absorbed (<5%), however, may accumulate in renal failure

**Patient Information** Take recommended dose before meals or on an empty stomach. Take any other medications at least 2 hours before taking sucralfate. Do not take antacids within 30 minutes of taking sucralfate. May cause constipation; increased exercise, increased dietary fiber, fruit or fluids, or mild stool softener may be helpful. If constipation or gastric distress persists, consult prescriber.

**Nursing Implications** Monitor for constipation; administer other medications 2 hours before sucralfate

**Dosage Forms**

Suspension, oral: 1 g/10 mL (420 mL)

Tablet: 1 g

♦ **Sucrets® Cough Calmers [OTC]** *see* Dextromethorphan *on page 160*

♦ **Sudafed® [OTC]** *see* Pseudoephedrine *on page 478*

♦ **Sudafed® 12 Hour [OTC]** *see* Pseudoephedrine *on page 478*

♦ **Sudafed® Cold & Cough Liquid Caps [OTC]** *see* Guaifenesin, Pseudoephedrine, and Dextromethorphan *on page 259*

♦ **Sudafed® Plus Tablet [OTC]** *see* Chlorpheniramine and Pseudoephedrine *on page 114*

♦ **Sudafed® Severe Cold [OTC]** *see* Acetaminophen, Dextromethorphan, and Pseudoephedrine *on page 16*

♦ **Sufenta® Injection** *see* Sufentanil *on page 522*

## Sufentanil (soo FEN ta nil)

**Related Information**

Narcotic Agonists Comparison Chart *on page 720*

**U.S. Brand Names** Sufenta® Injection

**Pharmacologic Category** Analgesic, Narcotic; General Anesthetic

**Use** Analgesic supplement in maintenance of balanced general anesthesia

**Effects on Mental Status** Drowsiness is common; may cause confusion; may rarely cause delirium or depression

**Effects on Psychiatric Treatment** Concurrent use with psychotropics may produce additive sedation

**Restrictions** C-II

**Usual Dosage**

Children <12 years: 10-25 mcg/kg with 100% $O_2$, maintenance: 25-50 mcg as needed

Adults: Dose should be based on body weight. **Note:** In obese patients (ie, >20% above ideal body weight), use lean body weight to determine dosage.

1-2 mcg/kg with $N_2O/O_2$ for endotracheal intubation; maintenance: 10-25 mcg as needed

2-8 mcg/kg with $N_2O/O_2$ more complicated major surgical procedures; maintenance: 10-50 mcg as needed

8-30 mcg/kg with 100% $O_2$ and muscle relaxant produces sleep; at doses ≥8 mcg/kg maintains a deep level of anesthesia; maintenance: 10-50 mcg as needed

**Dosage Forms** Injection, as citrate: 50 mcg/mL (1 mL, 2 mL, 5 mL)

♦ **Sular®** *see* Nisoldipine *on page 395*

♦ **Sulbactam and Ampicillin** *see* Ampicillin and Sulbactam *on page 43*

## Sulconazole (sul KON a zole)

**U.S. Brand Names** Exelderm® Topical

**Pharmacologic Category** Antifungal Agent, Topical

**Use** Treatment of superficial fungal infections of the skin, including tinea cruris (jock itch), tinea corporis (ringworm), tinea versicolor, and possibly tinea pedis (athlete's foot - cream only)

**Effects on Mental Status** None reported

**Effects on Psychiatric Treatment** None reported

**Usual Dosage** Adults: Topical: Apply a small amount to the affected area and gently massage once or twice daily for 3 weeks (tinea cruris, tinea corporis, tinea versicolor) to 4 weeks (tinea pedis).

**Dosage Forms**

Cream, as nitrate: 1% (15 g, 30 g, 60 g)

Solution, as nitrate, topical: 1% (30 mL)

♦ **Sulf-10® Ophthalmic** *see* Sulfacetamide *on page 522*

## Sulfabenzamide, Sulfacetamide, and Sulfathiazole
(sul fa BENZ a mide, sul fa SEE ta mide & sul fa THYE a zole)

**U.S. Brand Names** Femguard®; Gyne-Sulf®; Sulfa-Gyn®; Sulfa-Trip®; Sultrin™; Trysul®; V.V.S.®

**Pharmacologic Category** Antibiotic, Vaginal

**Use** Treatment of *Haemophilus vaginalis* vaginitis

**Effects on Mental Status** None reported

**Effects on Psychiatric Treatment** None reported

**Usual Dosage** Adults:

Cream: Insert one applicatorful in vagina twice daily for 4-6 days; dosage may then be decreased to 1/2 to 1/4 of an applicatorful twice daily

Tablet: Insert one intravaginally twice daily for 10 days

**Dosage Forms**

Cream, vaginal: Sulfabenzamide 3.7%, sulfacetamide 2.86%, and sulfathiazole 3.42% (78 g with applicator, 90 g, 120 g)

Tablet, vaginal: Sulfabenzamide 184 mg, sulfacetamide 143.75 mg, and sulfathiazole 172.5 mg (20 tablets/box with vaginal applicator)

## Sulfacetamide (sul fa SEE ta mide)

**U.S. Brand Names** AK-Sulf® Ophthalmic; Bleph®-10 Ophthalmic; Cetamide® Ophthalmic; Isopto® Cetamide® Ophthalmic; Ocusulf-10® Ophthalmic; Sebizon® Topical Lotion; Sodium Sulamyd® Ophthalmic; Sulf-10® Ophthalmic

**Pharmacologic Category** Antibiotic, Ophthalmic; Antibiotic, Sulfonamide Derivative

**Use** Treatment and prophylaxis of conjunctivitis due to susceptible organisms; corneal ulcers; adjunctive treatment with systemic sulfonamides for therapy of trachoma; topical application in scaling dermatosis (seborrheic); bacterial infections of the skin

**Effects on Mental Status** None reported

**Effects on Psychiatric Treatment** None reported

**Usual Dosage**

Children >2 months and Adults: Ophthalmic:

Ointment: Apply to lower conjunctival sac 1-4 times/day and at bedtime

Solution: Instill 1-3 drops several times daily up to every 2-3 hours in lower conjunctival sac during waking hours and less frequently at night

Children >12 years and Adults: Topical:

Seborrheic dermatitis: Apply at bedtime and allow to remain overnight; in severe cases, may apply twice daily

Secondary cutaneous bacterial infections: Apply 2-4 times/day until infection clears

**Dosage Forms**

Lotion: 10% (59 mL, 85 mL)

Ointment, ophthalmic: 10% (3.5 g)

Solution, ophthalmic: 10% (1 mL, 2 mL, 2.5 mL, 5 mL, 15 mL); 15% (5 mL, 15 mL); 30% (15 mL)

## Sulfacetamide Sodium and Fluorometholone

(sul fa SEE ta mide SOW dee um & flure oh METH oh lone)

**U.S. Brand Names** FML-S® Ophthalmic Suspension
**Pharmacologic Category** Antibiotic/Corticosteroid, Ophthalmic
**Use** Steroid-responsive inflammatory ocular conditions where infection is present or there is a risk of infection
**Effects on Mental Status** None reported
**Effects on Psychiatric Treatment** None reported
**Usual Dosage** Children >2 months and Adults: Ophthalmic: Instill 1-3 drops every 2-3 hours while awake
**Dosage Forms** Suspension, ophthalmic: Sulfacetamide sodium 10% and fluorometholone 0.1% (5 mL, 10 mL)

## Sulfacetamide Sodium and Phenylephrine

(sul fa SEE ta mide SOW dee um & fen il EF rin)

**U.S. Brand Names** Vasosulf® Ophthalmic
**Pharmacologic Category** Antibiotic, Ophthalmic
**Use** Treatment of conjunctivitis, corneal ulcer, and other superficial ocular infections due to susceptible microorganisms; adjunctive in systemic sulfonamide therapy
**Effects on Mental Status** None reported
**Effects on Psychiatric Treatment** None reported
**Usual Dosage** Instill 1 or 2 drops into the lower conjunctival sac(s) every 2 or 3 hours during the day, less often at night
**Dosage Forms** Solution, ophthalmic: Sulfacetamide sodium 15% and phenylephrine hydrochloride 0.125% (5 mL, 15 mL)

## Sulfacetamide Sodium and Prednisolone

(sul fa SEE ta mide SOW dee um & pred NIS oh lone)

**U.S. Brand Names** AK-Cide® Ophthalmic; Blephamide® Ophthalmic; Cetapred® Ophthalmic; Isopto® Cetapred® Ophthalmic; Metimyd® Ophthalmic; Vasocidin® Ophthalmic
**Pharmacologic Category** Antibiotic/Corticosteroid, Ophthalmic
**Use** Steroid-responsive inflammatory ocular conditions where infection is present or there is a risk of infection; ophthalmic suspension may be used as an otic preparation
**Effects on Mental Status** May rarely cause dizziness or psychosis
**Effects on Psychiatric Treatment** None reported
**Usual Dosage** Children >2 months and Adults: Ophthalmic:
Ointment: Apply to lower conjunctival sac 1-4 times/day
Solution: Instill 1-3 drops every 2-3 hours while awake
**Dosage Forms**
Ointment, ophthalmic:
AK-Cide®, Metimyd®, Vasocidin®: Sulfacetamide sodium 10% and prednisolone acetate 0.5% (3.5 g)
Blephamide®: Sulfacetamide sodium 10% and prednisolone acetate 0.2% (3.5 g)
Cetapred®: Sulfacetamide sodium 10% and prednisolone acetate 0.25% (3.5 g)
Suspension, ophthalmic: Sulfacetamide sodium 10% and prednisolone sodium phosphate 0.25% (5 mL)
Suspension, ophthalmic:
AK-Cide®, Metimyd®: Sulfacetamide sodium 10% and prednisolone acetate 0.5% (5 mL)
Blephamide®: Sulfacetamide sodium 10% and prednisolone acetate 0.2% (2.5 mL, 5 mL, 10 mL)
Isopto® Cetapred®: Sulfacetamide sodium 10% and prednisolone acetate 0.25% (5 mL, 15 mL)
Vasocidin®: Sulfacetamide sodium 10% and prednisolone sodium phosphate: 0.25% (5 mL, 10 mL)

♦ **Sulfacet-R® Topical** *see* Sulfur and Sulfacetamide Sodium *on page 527*

## Sulfacytine (sul fa SYE teen)

**U.S. Brand Names** Renoquid®
**Pharmacologic Category** Antibiotic, Sulfonamide Derivative
**Use** Treatment of urinary tract infections
**Effects on Mental Status** Dizziness is common
**Effects on Psychiatric Treatment** Photosensitivity is common; use caution with concurrent psychotropics; may cause granulocytopenia; caution with clozapine and carbamazepine
**Pregnancy Risk Factor** B (D at term)
**Contraindications** Severe renal or hepatic impairment; porphyria; hypersensitivity to sulfacytine; children <14 years of age
**Adverse Reactions**
>10%:
Central nervous system: Fever, dizziness, headache
Dermatologic: Itching, skin rash, photosensitivity
Gastrointestinal: Anorexia, nausea, vomiting, diarrhea
1% to 10%:
Dermatologic: Lyell's syndrome, Stevens-Johnson syndrome
Hematologic: Granulocytopenia, leukopenia, thrombocytopenia, aplastic anemia, hemolytic anemia
Hepatic: Hepatitis
**Overdosage/Toxicology** Signs and symptoms: Drowsiness, dizziness, anorexia, abdominal pain, nausea, vomiting, hemolytic anemia, acidosis, jaundice
**Usual Dosage** Adults: Oral: Initial: 500 mg, then 250 mg every 4 hours for 10 days
**Dosage Forms** Tablet: 250 mg

## Sulfadiazine (sul fa DYE a zeen)

**U.S. Brand Names** Microsulfon®
**Canadian Brand Names** Coptin®
**Pharmacologic Category** Antibiotic, Sulfonamide Derivative
**Use** Treatment of urinary tract infections and nocardiosis, rheumatic fever prophylaxis; adjunctive treatment in toxoplasmosis; uncomplicated attack of malaria
**Effects on Mental Status** Dizziness is common; sulfonamides reported to cause restlessness, irritability, depression, euphoria, disorientation, panic, hallucinations, and delusions
**Effects on Psychiatric Treatment** Photosensitivity is common; use caution with concurrent psychotropics; may cause granulocytopenia; caution with clozapine and carbamazepine
**Pregnancy Risk Factor** B (D at term)
**Contraindications** Porphyria, hypersensitivity to any sulfa drug or any component, pregnancy at term, children <2 months of age unless indicated for the treatment of congenital toxoplasmosis, sunscreens containing PABA, nursing mothers
**Warnings/Precautions** Use with caution in patients with impaired hepatic function or impaired renal function, G-6-PD deficiency; dosage modification required in patients with renal impairment; fluid intake should be maintained ≥1500 mL/day, or administer sodium bicarbonate to keep urine alkaline; more likely to cause crystalluria because it is less soluble than other sulfonamides
**Adverse Reactions**
>10%:
Central nervous system: Fever, dizziness, headache
Dermatologic: Itching, rash, photosensitivity
Gastrointestinal: Anorexia, nausea, vomiting, diarrhea
1% to 10%:
Dermatologic: Lyell's syndrome, Stevens-Johnson syndrome
Hematologic: Granulocytopenia, leukopenia, thrombocytopenia, aplastic anemia, hemolytic anemia
Hepatic: Hepatitis
<1%: Acute nephropathy, crystalluria, hematuria, interstitial nephritis, jaundice, serum sickness-like reactions, thyroid function disturbance
**Overdosage/Toxicology**
Signs and symptoms: Drowsiness, dizziness, anorexia, abdominal pain, nausea, vomiting, hemolytic anemia, acidosis, jaundice, fever, agranulocytosis; doses of as little as 2-5 g/day may produce toxicity; the aniline radical is responsible for hematologic toxicity
Treatment: High volume diuresis may aid in elimination and prevention of renal failure
**Drug Interactions** Decreased effect with PABA or PABA metabolites of drugs (eg, procaine, proparacaine, tetracaine, sunscreens); increased effect of oral anticoagulants and oral hypoglycemic agents
**Usual Dosage** Oral:
Congenital toxoplasmosis:
Newborns and Children <2 months: 100 mg/kg/day divided every 6 hours in conjunction with pyrimethamine 1 mg/kg/day once daily and supplemental folinic acid 5 mg every 3 days for 6 months
Children >2 months: 25-50 mg/kg/dose 4 times/day
Toxoplasmosis:
Children >2 months: Loading dose: 75 mg/kg; maintenance dose: 120-150 mg/kg/day, maximum dose: 6 g/day; divided every 4-6 hours in conjunction with pyrimethamine 2 mg/kg/day divided every 12 hours for 3 days followed by 1 mg/kg/day once daily (maximum: 25 mg/day) with supplemental folinic acid
Adults: 2-4 g/day divided every 4-8 hours in conjunction with pyrimethamine 25 mg/day and with supplemental folinic acid
Prevention of recurrent attacks of rheumatic fever:
>30 kg: 1 g/day
<30 kg: 0.5 g/day
**Patient Information** Take as directed, at regular intervals around-the-clock. Take 1 hour before or 2 hours after meals with full glass of water. Complete full course of therapy even if you are feeling better. Avoid aspirin or aspirin-containing products and avoid large quantities of vitamin C. It is very important to maintain adequate hydration (2-3 L/day of fluids unless instructed to restrict fluid intake) to prevent kidney damage. You may experience dizziness or headache (use caution when driving or engaging in tasks requiring alertness until response to drug is known); photosensitivity (use sunblock, wear protective clothing and eyewear, and avoid direct
(Continued)

## Sulfadiazine *(Continued)*

sunlight); nausea, vomiting, or loss of appetite (small frequent meals, frequent mouth care, sucking lozenges, or chewing gum may help). Report skin rash, persistent diarrhea, persistent or severe sore throat, fever, vaginal itching or discharge, unusual bruising or bleeding, fatigue, persistent headache or abdominal pain, or difficulty breathing.

**Nursing Implications** Maintain adequate hydration and monitor urine output

**Dosage Forms** Tablet: 500 mg

## Sulfadoxine and Pyrimethamine

(sul fa DOKS een & peer i METH a meen)

**U.S. Brand Names** Fansidar®

**Pharmacologic Category** Antimalarial Agent

**Use** Treatment of *Plasmodium falciparum* malaria in patients in whom chloroquine resistance is suspected; malaria prophylaxis for travelers to areas where chloroquine-resistant malaria is endemic

**Effects on Mental Status** Sulfonamides reported to cause restlessness, irritability, depression, euphoria, disorientation, panic, hallucinations, and delusions

**Effects on Psychiatric Treatment** Photosensitivity is common; use caution with concurrent psychotropics; may cause leukopenia; caution with clozapine and carbamazepine

**Pregnancy Risk Factor** C

**Contraindications** Known hypersensitivity to any sulfa drug, pyrimethamine, or any component; porphyria, megaloblastic anemia, severe renal insufficiency; children <2 months of age due to competition with bilirubin for protein binding sites

**Warnings/Precautions** Use with caution in patients with renal or hepatic impairment, patients with possible folate deficiency, and patients with seizure disorders, increased adverse reactions are seen in patients also receiving chloroquine; fatalities associated with sulfonamides, although rare, have occurred due to severe reactions including Stevens-Johnson syndrome, toxic epidermal necrolysis, hepatic necrosis, agranulocytosis, aplastic anemia and other blood dyscrasias; discontinue use at first sign of rash or any sign of adverse reaction; hemolysis occurs in patients with G-6-PD deficiency; leucovorin should be administered to reverse signs and symptoms of folic acid deficiency

**Adverse Reactions**

>10%:

- Central nervous system: Ataxia, seizures, headache
- Dermatologic: Photosensitivity
- Gastrointestinal: Atrophic glossitis, vomiting, gastritis
- Hematologic: Megaloblastic anemia, leukopenia, thrombocytopenia, pancytopenia
- Neuromuscular & skeletal: Tremors
- Miscellaneous: Hypersensitivity

1% to 10%:

- Dermatologic: Stevens-Johnson syndrome
- Hepatic: Hepatitis

<1%: Anorexia, crystalluria, erythema multiforme, glossitis, hepatic necrosis, rash, respiratory failure, thyroid function dysfunction, toxic epidermal necrolysis

**Overdosage/Toxicology**

Signs and symptoms: Anorexia, vomiting, CNS stimulation including seizures, megaloblastic anemia, leukopenia, thrombocytopenia, crystalluria

Treatment: Following GI contamination; leucovorin should be administered in a dosage of 3-9 mg/day for 3 days or as required to reverse symptoms of folic acid deficiency; doses of as little as 2-5 g/day may produce toxicity; the aniline radical is responsible for hematologic toxicity; high volume diuresis may aid in elimination and prevention of renal failure; diazepam can be used to control seizures

**Drug Interactions**

Decreased effect with PABA or PABA metabolites of local anesthetics

Increased toxicity with methotrexate, other sulfonamides, co-trimoxazole

**Usual Dosage** Children and Adults: Oral:

Treatment of acute attack of malaria: A single dose of the following number of Fansidar® tablets is used in sequence with quinine or alone:

- 2-11 months: 1/4 tablet
- 1-3 years: 1/2 tablet
- 4-8 years: 1 tablet
- 9-14 years: 2 tablets
- >14 years: 2-3 tablets

Malaria prophylaxis:

The first dose of Fansidar® should be taken 1-2 days before departure to an endemic area (CDC recommends that therapy be initiated 1-2 weeks before such travel), administration should be continued during the stay and for 4-6 weeks after return. Dose = pyrimethamine 0.5 mg/kg/dose and sulfadoxine 10 mg/kg/dose up to a maximum of 25 mg pyrimethamine and 500 mg sulfadoxine/dose weekly.

- 2-11 months: 1/8 tablet weekly **or** 1/4 tablet once every 2 weeks
- 1-3 years: 1/4 tablet once weekly **or** 1/2 tablet once every 2 weeks
- 4-8 years: 1/2 tablet once weekly **or** 1 tablet once every 2 weeks
- 9-14 years: 3/4 tablet once weekly **or** 1 1/2 tablets once every 2 weeks
- >14 years: 1 tablet once weekly **or** 2 tablets once every 2 weeks

**Patient Information** Begin prophylaxis at least 2 days before departure; drink plenty of fluids; avoid prolonged exposure to the sun; notify physician if rash, sore throat, pallor, or glossitis occurs

**Dosage Forms** Tablet: Sulfadoxine 500 mg and pyrimethamine 25 mg

♦ **Sulfa-Gyn®** *see* Sulfabenzamide, Sulfacetamide, and Sulfathiazole *on page 522*

♦ **Sulfalax® [OTC]** *see* Docusate *on page 179*

## Sulfamethoxazole (sul fa meth OKS a zole)

**U.S. Brand Names** Gantanol®; Urobak®

**Canadian Brand Names** Apo®-Sulfamethoxazole

**Pharmacologic Category** Antibiotic, Sulfonamide Derivative

**Use** Treatment of urinary tract infections, nocardiosis, toxoplasmosis, acute otitis media, and acute exacerbations of chronic bronchitis due to susceptible organisms

**Effects on Mental Status** Dizziness is common; sulfonamides reported to cause restlessness, irritability, depression, euphoria, disorientation, panic, hallucinations, and delusions

**Effects on Psychiatric Treatment** Photosensitivity is common; use caution with concurrent psychotropics; may cause leukopenia; caution with clozapine and carbamazepine

**Pregnancy Risk Factor** B (D at term)

**Contraindications** Porphyria, hypersensitivity to any sulfa drug or any component, pregnancy during 3rd trimester, children <2 months of age unless indicated for the treatment of congenital toxoplasmosis, sunscreens containing PABA

**Warnings/Precautions** Maintain adequate fluid intake to prevent crystalluria; use with caution in patients with renal or hepatic impairment, and patients with G-6-PD deficiency; should not be used for group A beta-hemolytic streptococcal infections

**Adverse Reactions**

>10%:

- Central nervous system: Fever, dizziness, headache
- Dermatologic: Itching, rash, photosensitivity
- Gastrointestinal: Anorexia, nausea, vomiting, diarrhea

1% to 10%:

- Dermatologic: Lyell's syndrome, Stevens-Johnson syndrome
- Hematologic: Granulocytopenia, leukopenia, thrombocytopenia, aplastic anemia, hemolytic anemia
- Hepatic: Hepatitis

<1%: Acute nephropathy, crystalluria, hematuria, interstitial nephritis, jaundice, serum sickness-like reactions, thyroid function disturbance, vasculitis

**Overdosage/Toxicology**

Signs and symptoms: Drowsiness, dizziness, anorexia, abdominal pain, nausea, vomiting, hemolytic anemia, acidosis, jaundice, fever, agranulocytosis; the aniline radical is responsible for hematologic toxicity

Treatment: High volume diuresis may aid in elimination and prevention of renal failure

**Drug Interactions**

Decreased effect with PABA or PABA metabolites of drugs (ie, procaine, proparacaine, tetracaine); cyclosporine levels may be decreased

Increased effect/toxicity of oral anticoagulants, oral hypoglycemic agents, hydantoins, uricosuric agents, methotrexate when administered with sulfonamides

Increased toxicity of sulfonamides with diuretics, indomethacin, methenamine, probenecid, and salicylates

**Usual Dosage** Oral:

Children >2 months: 50-60 mg/kg as single dose followed by 50-60 mg/kg/day divided every 12 hours; maximum: 3 g/24 hours or 75 mg/kg/day

Adults: Initial: 2 g, then 1 g 2-3 times/day; maximum: 3 g/24 hours

**Dosing adjustment/interval in renal impairment:**

- $Cl_{cr}$ 10-50 mL/minute: Administer every 12-24 hours
- $Cl_{cr}$ <10 mL/minute: Administer every 24 hours

Hemodialysis: Moderately dialyzable (20% to 50%)

**Patient Information** Take as directed, at regular intervals around-the-clock. Take 1 hour before or 2 hours after meals with a full glass of water. Take full course of therapy even if you feeling better. Avoid aspirin or aspirin-containing products and avoid large quantities of vitamin C. It is very important to maintain adequate hydration (2-3 L/day of fluids unless instructed to restrict fluid intake) to prevent kidney damage. You may experience dizziness or headache (use caution when driving or engaging in tasks requiring alertness until response to drug is known); photosensitivity (use sunscreen, wear protective clothing and eyewear, and avoid direct sunlight); nausea, vomiting, or loss of appetite (small frequent meals, frequent mouth care, sucking lozenges, or chewing gum may help). Report skin rash, persistent diarrhea, persistent or severe sore throat, fever, vaginal itching or discharge, unusual bruising or bleeding, fatigue, persistent headache or abdominal pain, blackened stool, or difficulty breathing.

**Nursing Implications** Maintain adequate hydration

**Dosage Forms**

Suspension, oral (cherry flavor): 500 mg/5 mL (480 mL)

Tablet: 500 mg

## Sulfamethoxazole and Phenazopyridine

(sul fa meth OKS a zole & fen az oh PEER i deen)

**Pharmacologic Category** Antibiotic, Sulfonamide Derivative

**Use** Treatment of urinary tract infections complicated with pain

**Effects on Mental Status** May cause confusion, depression, and hallucinations; sulfonamides reported to cause restlessness, irritability, euphoria, disorientation, panic, and delusions

**Effects on Psychiatric Treatment** Photosensitivity is common; use caution with concurrent psychotropics; may cause leukopenia; caution with clozapine and carbamazepine

**Pregnancy Risk Factor** B (D at term)

**Contraindications** Porphyria; hypersensitivity to any sulfa drug or any component

**Warnings/Precautions** Fatalities associated with sulfonamides, although rare, have occurred due to severe reactions including Stevens-Johnson syndrome, toxic epidermal necrolysis, hepatic necrosis, agranulocytosis, aplastic anemia, and other blood dyscrasias; discontinue use at first sign of rash or any sign of adverse reaction; adjust dosage in patients with renal impairment

**Adverse Reactions**

Central nervous system: Confusion, depression, hallucinations, ataxia, seizures, fever, kernicterus in neonates

Dermatologic: Rash, erythema multiforme, Stevens-Johnson syndrome, epidermal necrolysis

Gastrointestinal: Nausea, vomiting, glossitis, stomatitis, diarrhea, pseudomembranous colitis

Hematologic: Thrombocytopenia, megaloblastic anemia, granulocytopenia, aplastic anemia, hemolysis (with G-6-PD deficiency)

Hepatic: Serum sickness, hepatitis

Renal & genitourinary: Interstitial nephritis

**Drug Interactions** Warfarin, methotrexate

**Usual Dosage** Oral: 4 tablets to start, then 2 tablets twice daily for up to 2 days, then switch to sulfamethoxazole only

**Patient Information** See individual agents

**Dosage Forms** Tablet: Sulfamethoxazole 500 mg and phenazopyridine 100 mg

♦ **Sulfamethoxazole and Trimethoprim** *see* Co-Trimoxazole *on page 142*

## Sulfanilamide (sul fa NIL a mide)

**U.S. Brand Names** AVC™ Cream; AVC™ Suppository; Vagitrol®

**Pharmacologic Category** Antifungal Agent, Vaginal

**Use** Treatment of vulvovaginitis caused by *Candida albicans*

**Effects on Mental Status** None reported

**Effects on Psychiatric Treatment** None reported

**Usual Dosage** Adults: Female: Insert one applicatorful intravaginally once or twice daily continued through 1 complete menstrual cycle or insert one suppository intravaginally once or twice daily for 30 days

**Dosage Forms**

Cream, vaginal (AVC™, Vagitrol®): 15% [150 mg/g] (120 g with applicator)

Suppository, vaginal (AVC™): 1.05 g (16s)

## Sulfasalazine (sul fa SAL a zeen)

**U.S. Brand Names** Azulfidine® EN-tabs®; Azulfidine® Tablets

**Canadian Brand Names** Apo®-Sulfasalazine; PMS-Sulfasalazine; Salazopyrin®; Salazopyrin EN-Tabs®; S.A.S™

**Synonyms** Salicylazosulfapyridine

**Pharmacologic Category** 5-Aminosalicylic Acid Derivative

**Use** Management of ulcerative colitis; enteric coated tablets are used for for rheumatoid arthritis in patients who inadequately respond to analgesics and NSAIDs

**Effects on Mental Status** Dizziness is common; sulfonamides reported to cause restlessness, irritability, depression, euphoria, disorientation, panic, hallucinations, and delusions

**Effects on Psychiatric Treatment** Photosensitivity is common; use caution with concurrent psychotropics; may cause leukopenia; caution with clozapine and carbamazepine

**Pregnancy Risk Factor** B (D at term)

**Contraindications** Hypersensitivity to sulfasalazine, sulfa drugs, or any component; porphyria, GI or GU obstruction; hypersensitivity to salicylates; children <2 years of age

**Warnings/Precautions** Use with caution in patients with renal impairment; impaired hepatic function or urinary obstruction, blood dyscrasias severe allergies or asthma, or G-6-PD deficiency; may cause folate deficiency (consider providing 1 mg/day folate supplement)

**Adverse Reactions**

>10%:

Central nervous system: Dizziness, headache (33%)

Dermatologic: Photosensitivity

Gastrointestinal: Anorexia, nausea, vomiting, diarrhea (33%)

Genitourinary: Reversible oligospermia (33%)

<3%:

Dermatologic: Urticaria/pruritus (<3%)

Hematologic: Hemolytic anemia (<3%), Heinz body anemia (<3%)

<0.1%: Acute nephropathy, aplastic anemia, crystalluria, granulocytopenia, hematuria, interstitial nephritis, jaundice, leukopenia, Lyell's syndrome, serum sickness-like reactions, Stevens-Johnson syndrome, thrombocytopenia, thyroid function disturbance

**Overdosage/Toxicology**

Signs and symptoms: Drowsiness, dizziness, anorexia, abdominal pain, nausea, vomiting, hemolytic anemia, acidosis, jaundice, fever, agranulocytosis; the aniline radical is responsible for hematologic toxicity

Treatment: High volume diuresis may aid in elimination and prevention of renal failure

**Drug Interactions**

Decreased effect of iron, digoxin, folic acid, and like other sulfa drugs PABA or PABA metabolites of drugs (ie, procaine, proparacaine, tetracaine)

Increased effect of oral anticoagulants, methotrexate, and oral hypoglycemic agents as with other sulfa drugs

**Usual Dosage** Oral:

Children >2 years: Initial: 40-60 mg/kg/day in 3-6 divided doses; maintenance dose: 20-30 mg/kg/day in 4 divided doses

Adults: Initial: 1 g 3-4 times/day, 2 g/day maintenance in divided doses; may initiate therapy with 0.5-1 g/day enteric-coated tablets

**Dosing interval in renal impairment:**

$Cl_{cr}$ 10-30 mL/minute: Administer twice daily

$Cl_{cr}$ <10 mL/minute: Administer once daily

**Dosing adjustment in hepatic impairment:** Avoid use

**Patient Information** Do not crush, chew, or dissolve coated tablets. Shake suspension well before use. Do not take on an empty stomach or with antacids. Maintain adequate hydration (2-3 L/day of fluids unless instructed to restrict fluid intake) to prevent kidney damage. Increased dietary iron may be recommended. You may experience nervousness or dizziness (use caution when driving or engaging in hazardous activities until response to drug is known). You may experience photosensitivity (use sunscreen, wear protective clothing and eyewear, and avoid direct sunlight). Orange-yellow color of urine, sweat, tears is normal and will stain contact lenses and clothing. Report rash, persistent nausea or anorexia, or lack of improvement in symptoms (after 1-2 months).

**Nursing Implications** Drug commonly imparts an orange-yellow discoloration to urine and skin

**Dosage Forms**

Tablet: 500 mg

Tablet, enteric coated: 500 mg

♦ **Sulfatrim®** *see* Co-Trimoxazole *on page 142*

♦ **Sulfa-Trip®** *see* Sulfabenzamide, Sulfacetamide, and Sulfathiazole *on page 522*

## Sulfinpyrazone (sul fin PEER a zone)

**U.S. Brand Names** Anturane®

**Canadian Brand Names** Antazone®; Anturan®; Apo®-Sulfinpyrazone; Novo-Pyrazone; Nu-Sulfinpyrazone

**Pharmacologic Category** Uricosuric Agent

**Use** Treatment of chronic gouty arthritis and intermittent gouty arthritis

**Unlabeled use:** To decrease the incidence of sudden death postmyocardial infarction

**Effects on Mental Status** May cause dizziness

**Effects on Psychiatric Treatment** May cause leukopenia; use caution with clozapine and carbamazepine

**Pregnancy Risk Factor** C (per manufacturer); D (if near term, per expert analysis)

**Contraindications** Active peptic ulcers, hypersensitivity to sulfinpyrazone, phenylbutazone, or other pyrazoles, GI inflammation, blood dyscrasias

**Warnings/Precautions** Safety and efficacy not established in children <18 years of age, use with caution in patients with impaired renal function and urolithiasis

**Adverse Reactions**

1% to 10%: Gastrointestinal: Nausea, vomiting, stomach pain

<1%: Anemia, dermatitis, dizziness, flushing, headache, hepatic necrosis, increased bleeding time (decreased platelet aggregation), leukopenia, nephrotic syndrome, polyuria, rash, uric acid stones

**Overdosage/Toxicology**

Signs and symptoms: Nausea, vomiting, ataxia, respiratory depression, seizures

Treatment: Following GI decontamination, treatment is supportive only

**Drug Interactions** CYP2C and 3A3/4 enzyme inducer; CYP2C9 enzyme inhibitor

(Continued)

## Sulfinpyrazone *(Continued)*

Decreased effect/levels of theophylline, verapamil; decreased uricosuric activity with salicylates, niacins

Increased effect of oral anticoagulants

Risk of acetaminophen hepatotoxicity is increased, but therapeutic effects may be reduced

**Usual Dosage** Adults: Oral: 100-200 mg twice daily; maximum daily dose: 800 mg

**Dosing adjustment in renal impairment:** $Cl_{cr}$ <50 mL/minute: Avoid use

**Patient Information** Take as directed, with meals or antacids and a full glass of water. Avoid aspirin or acetaminophen products and avoid large quantities of vitamin C. It is very important to maintain adequate hydration (2-3 L/day of fluids unless instructed to restrict fluid intake) to prevent kidney damage. You may experience nausea or vomiting (small frequent meals, frequent mouth care, chewing gum, or sucking lozenges may help). Report skin rash, persistent stomach pain, painful urination or bloody urine, unusual bruising or bleeding, fatigue, or yellowing of eyes or skin.

**Dosage Forms**

Capsule: 200 mg

Tablet: 100 mg

## Sulfisoxazole (sul fi SOKS a zole)

**U.S. Brand Names** Gantrisin®

**Canadian Brand Names** Novo-Soxazole; Sulfizole®

**Synonyms** Sulfisoxazole Acetyl; Sulphafurazole

**Pharmacologic Category** Antibiotic, Sulfonamide Derivative

**Use** Treatment of urinary tract infections, otitis media, *Chlamydia*; nocardiosis; treatment of acute pelvic inflammatory disease in prepubertal children; often used in combination with trimethoprim

**Effects on Mental Status** Dizziness is common; sulfonamides reported to cause restlessness, irritability, depression, euphoria, disorientation, panic, hallucinations, and delusions

**Effects on Psychiatric Treatment** Photosensitivity is common; use caution with concurrent psychotropics; may cause leukopenia; caution with clozapine and carbamazepine

**Pregnancy Risk Factor** B (D at term)

**Contraindications** Hypersensitivity to any sulfa drug or any component, porphyria, pregnancy during 3rd trimester, infants <2 months of age (sulfas compete with bilirubin for protein binding sites), patients with urinary obstruction, sunscreens containing PABA

**Warnings/Precautions** Use with caution in patients with G-6-PD deficiency (hemolysis may occur), hepatic or renal impairment; dosage modification required in patients with renal impairment; risk of crystalluria should be considered in patients with impaired renal function

**Adverse Reactions**

>10%:

Central nervous system: Fever, dizziness, headache

Dermatologic: Itching, rash, photosensitivity

Gastrointestinal: Anorexia, nausea, vomiting, diarrhea

1% to 10%:

Dermatologic: Lyell's syndrome, Stevens-Johnson syndrome

Hematologic: Granulocytopenia, leukopenia, thrombocytopenia, aplastic anemia, hemolytic anemia

Hepatic: Hepatitis

<1%: Acute nephropathy, crystalluria, hematuria, interstitial nephritis, jaundice, serum sickness-like reactions, thyroid function disturbance, vasculitis

**Overdosage/Toxicology**

Signs and symptoms: Drowsiness, dizziness, anorexia, abdominal pain, nausea, vomiting, hemolytic anemia, acidosis, jaundice, fever, agranulocytosis; doses of as little as 2-5 g/day may produce toxicity; the aniline radical is responsible for hematologic toxicity

Treatment: High volume diuresis may aid in elimination and prevention of renal failure

**Drug Interactions**

Decreased effect with PABA or PABA metabolites of drugs (ie, procaine, proparacaine, tetracaine); cyclosporine levels may be decreased

Increased effect/toxicity of oral anticoagulants, oral hypoglycemic agents, hydantoins, uricosuric agents, methotrexate when administered with sulfonamides

Increased toxicity of sulfonamides with diuretics, indomethacin, methenamine, probenecid, and salicylates

**Usual Dosage** Not for use in patients <2 months of age:

Children >2 months: Oral: Initial: 75 mg/kg, followed by 120-150 mg/kg/day in divided doses every 4-6 hours; not to exceed 6 g/day

Pelvic inflammatory disease: 100 mg/kg/day in divided doses every 6 hours; used in combination with ceftriaxone

*Chlamydia trachomatis*: 100 mg/kg/day in divided doses every 6 hours

Adults: Oral: Initial: 2-4 g, then 4-8 g/day in divided doses every 4-6 hours

Pelvic inflammatory disease: 500 mg every 6 hours for 21 days; used in combination with ceftriaxone

*Chlamydia trachomatis*: 500 mg every 6 hours for 10 days

**Dosing interval in renal impairment:**

$Cl_{cr}$ 10-50 mL/minute: Administer every 8-12 hours

$Cl_{cr}$ <10 mL/minute: Administer every 12-24 hours

Hemodialysis: >50% removed by hemodialysis

Children and Adults: Ophthalmic:

Solution: Instill 1-2 drops to affected eye every 2-3 hours

Ointment: Apply small amount to affected eye 1-3 times/day and at bedtime

**Patient Information** Take as directed, at regular intervals around-the-clock. Take 1 hour before or 2 hours after meals with a full glass of water. Take full course of therapy even if you are feeling better. Avoid aspirin or aspirin-containing products and avoid large quantities of vitamin C. It is very important to maintain adequate hydration (2-3 L/day of fluids unless instructed to restrict fluid intake) to prevent kidney damage. You may experience dizziness or headache (use caution when driving or engaging in tasks requiring alertness until response to drug is known); photosensitivity (use sunscreen, wear protective clothing and eyewear, and avoid direct sunlight); nausea, vomiting, or loss of appetite (small frequent meals, frequent mouth care, sucking lozenges, or chewing gum may help). Diabetics: Drug may cause false tests with Clinitest® urine glucose monitoring; use of glucose oxidase methods (Clinistix®) or serum glucose monitoring is preferable. Report persistent nausea, vomiting, diarrhea, or abdominal pain; skin rash; persistent or severe sore throat, mouth sores, fever, or vaginal itching or discharge; unusual bruising or bleeding; blackened stool; fatigue; or difficulty breathing.

Ophthalmic: Instill as often as recommended. Wash hands before using. Sit or lie down, open eye, look at ceiling, and instill prescribed amount of solution. Ointment: Pull lower lid down gently and instill thin ribbon of ointment inside lid. Close eye and roll eye in all directions, and apply gentle pressure to inner corner of eye for 1-2 minutes. Do not let tip of applicator touch eye or contaminate tip of applicator. Temporary stinging or blurred vision may occur. Report persistent pain, redness, burning, double vision, severe headache, or respiratory congestion.

**Nursing Implications** Maintain adequate fluid intake

**Dosage Forms**

Solution, ophthalmic, as diolamine: 4% [40 mg/mL] (15 mL)

Suspension, oral, pediatric, as acetyl (raspberry flavor): 500 mg/5 mL (480 mL)

Tablet: 500 mg

♦ **Sulfisoxazole Acetyl** *see* Sulfisoxazole *on page 526*

## Sulfisoxazole and Phenazopyridine
(sul fi SOKS a zole & fen az oh PEER i deen)

**U.S. Brand Names** Azo-Sulfisoxazole

**Pharmacologic Category** Antibiotic, Sulfonamide Derivative; Local Anesthetic

**Use** Treatment of urinary tract infections and nocardiosis

**Effects on Mental Status** Dizziness is common; sulfonamides reported to cause restlessness, irritability, depression, euphoria, disorientation, panic, hallucinations, and delusions

**Effects on Psychiatric Treatment** Photosensitivity is common; use caution with concurrent psychotropics; may cause leukopenia; caution with clozapine and carbamazepine

**Pregnancy Risk Factor** B (D at term)

**Contraindications** Porphyria; hypersensitivity to any sulfa drug or any component; pregnancy at term; children <2 months of age unless indicated for the treatment of congenital toxoplasmosis; sunscreens containing PABA

**Warnings/Precautions** Use with caution in patients with G-6-PD deficiency (hemolysis may occur), hepatic or renal impairment; dosage modification required in patients with renal impairment; risk of crystalluria should be considered in patients with impaired renal function; drug should be discontinued if skin or sclera develop a yellow color

**Adverse Reactions**

>10%:

Central nervous system: Fever, dizziness, headache

Dermatologic: Itching, rash, photosensitivity

Gastrointestinal: Anorexia, nausea, vomiting, diarrhea

1% to 10%:

Dermatologic: Lyell's syndrome, Stevens-Johnson syndrome

Hematologic: Granulocytopenia, leukopenia, thrombocytopenia, aplastic anemia, hemolytic anemia

Hepatic: Hepatitis

**Overdosage/Toxicology**

Signs and symptoms: Methemoglobinemia, skin pigmentation, renal and hepatic impairment, drowsiness, dizziness, anorexia, abdominal pain, nausea, vomiting, hemolytic anemia, acidosis, jaundice, fever, agranulocytosis

Treatment: High volume diuresis may aid in elimination and prevention of renal failure; methylene blue 1-2 mg/kg I.V. is indicated in the symptomatic patient with methemoglobin levels >20% or when even minimal compromise of oxygen-carrying capacity is potentially harmful (eg, anemia, CHF, angina, etc). **Note:** Methylene blue can slightly worsen methemoglobinemia when given in excess amounts; in G-6-PD deficiency, it may cause hemolysis.

**Drug Interactions**

Decreased effect with PABA or PABA metabolites of drugs (ie, procaine, proparacaine, tetracaine); cyclosporine levels may be decreased

Increased effect/toxicity of oral anticoagulants, oral hypoglycemic agents, hydantoins, uricosuric agents, methotrexate when administered with sulfonamides

Increased toxicity of sulfonamides with diuretics, indomethacin, methenamine, probenecid, and salicylates

**Usual Dosage** Adults: Oral: 4-6 tablets to start, then 2 tablets 4 times/day for 2 days, then continue with sulfisoxazole only

**Dosing adjustment/comments in renal impairment:** $Cl_{cr}$ <50 mL/minute: Avoid use of phenazopyridine

**Patient Information** See individual agents

**Dosage Forms** Tablet: Sulfisoxazole 500 mg and phenazopyridine 50 mg

♦ **Sulfonamide Derivatives** *see page 729*

## Sulfur and Sulfacetamide Sodium

(SUL fur & sul fa SEE ta mide SOW dee um)

**U.S. Brand Names** Novacet® Topical; Sulfacet-R® Topical

**Pharmacologic Category** Topical Skin Product

**Use** Aid in the treatment of acne vulgaris, acne rosacea and seborrheic dermatitis

**Effects on Mental Status** None reported

**Effects on Psychiatric Treatment** None reported

**Usual Dosage** Topical: Apply in a thin film 1-3 times/day

**Dosage Forms** Lotion, topical: Sulfur colloid 5% and sulfacetamide sodium 10% (30 mL)

## Sulindac (sul IN dak)

**Related Information**

Nonsteroidal Anti-inflammatory Agents Comparison Chart *on page 722*

**U.S. Brand Names** Clinoril®

**Canadian Brand Names** Apo®-Sulin; Novo-Sundac

**Pharmacologic Category** Nonsteroidal Anti-Inflammatory Agent (NSAID)

**Use** Management of inflammatory disease, rheumatoid disorders; acute gouty arthritis; structurally similar to indomethacin but acts like aspirin; safest NSAID for use in mild renal impairment

**Effects on Mental Status** Dizziness is common; may cause nervousness; may rarely cause drowsiness, confusion, insomnia, hallucinations, or depression

**Effects on Psychiatric Treatment** May rarely cause agranulocytosis; use caution with clozapine and carbamazepine; may decrease lithium clearance (evidence suggest that this effect may be less than with other NSAIDs) resulting in an increase in serum lithium levels and potential lithium toxicity; monitor serum lithium levels

**Pregnancy Risk Factor** B (D in 3rd trimester and at term)

**Contraindications** Hypersensitivity to sulindac, any component, aspirin or other nonsteroidal anti-inflammatory drugs (NSAIDs)

**Warnings/Precautions** Use with caution in patients with peptic ulcer disease, GI bleeding, bleeding abnormalities, dehydration, impaired renal or hepatic function, congestive heart failure, hypertension, and patients receiving anticoagulants

**Adverse Reactions**

>10%:

Central nervous system: Dizziness

Dermatologic: Rash

Gastrointestinal: Abdominal cramps, heartburn, indigestion, nausea

1% to 10%:

Central nervous system: Headache, nervousness

Dermatologic: Itching

Endocrine & metabolic: Fluid retention

Gastrointestinal: Vomiting

Otic: Tinnitus

<1%: Acute renal failure, agranulocytosis, allergic rhinitis, anemia, angioedema, arrhythmias, aseptic meningitis, blurred vision, bone marrow suppression, confusion, congestive heart failure, conjunctivitis, cystitis, decreased hearing, drowsiness, dry eyes, epistaxis, erythema multiforme, gastritis, GI ulceration, hallucinations, hemolytic anemia, hepatitis, hot flashes, hypertension, insomnia, leukopenia, mental depression, peripheral neuropathy, polydipsia, polyuria, shortness of breath, Stevens-Johnson syndrome, tachycardia, thrombocytopenia, toxic amblyopia, toxic epidermal necrolysis, urticaria

**Overdosage/Toxicology**

Signs and symptoms: Dizziness, vomiting, nausea, abdominal pain, hypotension, coma, stupor, metabolic acidosis, leukocytosis, renal failure

Treatment: Management of a nonsteroidal anti-inflammatory drug (NSAID) intoxication is primarily supportive and symptomatic. Fluid therapy is commonly effective in managing the hypotension that may occur following an acute NSAID overdose, except when this is due to an acute blood loss. Seizures tend to be very short-lived and often do not require drug treatment; although, recurrent seizures should be treated with I.V. diazepam.

**Drug Interactions**

ACE inhibitors: Effects may be reduced by NSAIDs; use lowest possible dose for shortest duration possible; monitor

Cholestyramine and colestipol: Absorption may be reduced by concurrent administration

Corticosteroids: May increase the risk of GI ulceration; use caution

Cyclosporine: Nephrotoxicity may be increased with concurrent NSAID use; monitor

Hydralazine: Antihypertensive effect may be decreased; avoid concurrent use

Lithium: Serum levels can be increased; avoid concurrent use if possible or monitor lithium levels and adjust dose. When NSAID is stopped, lithium may need adjustment again.

Loop diuretics: Therapeutic effects may be reduced by NSAIDs; avoid

Methotrexate: Toxicity may be increased by concurrent NSAID use; risk is limited in low-dose methotrexate regimens (such as for rheumatoid arthritis); prolonged leucovorin rescue may be required at antineoplastic doses; monitor

Thiazide diuretics: Antihypertensive effects are decreased; avoid concurrent use

Warfarin: INRs may be increased by some NSAIDs. This may depend, in part, on dose and duration; monitor INR closely. Use the lowest dose of NSAIDs possible and for the briefest duration.

**Usual Dosage** Maximum therapeutic response may not be realized for up to 3 weeks

Oral:

Children: Dose not established

Adults: 150-200 mg twice daily or 300-400 mg once daily; not to exceed 400 mg/day

**Dosing adjustment in hepatic impairment:** Dose reduction is necessary

**Dietary Considerations** Food: May decrease the rate but not the extent of oral absorption. Drug may cause GI upset, bleeding, ulceration, perforation; take with food or milk to minimize GI upset.

**Patient Information** Take this medication exactly as directed; do not increase dose without consulting prescriber. Take with food or milk to reduce GI distress. Maintain adequate fluid intake (2-3 L/day of fluids unless instructed to restrict fluid intake). Do not use alcohol, aspirin, or aspirin-containing medication, and all other anti-inflammatory medications without consulting prescriber. You may experience dizziness, nervousness, or headache (use caution when driving or engaging in tasks requiring alertness until response to drug is known); nausea, vomiting, or heartburn (frequent small meals, frequent mouth care, sucking lozenges, or chewing gum may help); constipation (increased exercise, fluids, or dietary fruit and fiber may help). GI bleeding, ulceration, or perforation can occur with or without pain; discontinue medication and contact prescriber if persistent abdominal pain or cramping, or blood in stool occurs. Report breathlessness or difficulty breathing; unusual bruising/bleeding; blood in urine, stool, mouth, or vomitus; unusual fatigue; skin rash or itching; change in urinary pattern; or change in hearing or ringing in ears.

**Nursing Implications** Observe for edema and fluid retention; monitor blood pressure

**Dosage Forms** Tablet: 150 mg, 200 mg

♦ **Sulphafurazole** *see* Sulfisoxazole *on page 526*

## Sulthiame (sul THYE ame)

**Synonyms** RP10248; Sultiame; Tetrahydro-2-para-sulfamoylphenyl-1,2-thiazine 1,1 dioxide

**Pharmacologic Category** Anticonvulsant, Miscellaneous

**Use** Not available in the U.S.; anticonvulsant agent used for generalized seizures temporal lobe seizures, myoclonic or focal seizures; not useful for absence seizures

**Effects on Mental Status** May cause drowsiness or dizziness

**Effects on Psychiatric Treatment** None reported

**Warnings/Precautions** Use with caution in patients with renal impairment

**Adverse Reactions**

Central nervous system: Headache, lethargy, ataxia, vertigo

Genitourinary: Crystalluria

Neuromuscular & skeletal: Paresthesia

Ocular: Ptosis

Respiratory: Hyperpnea, dyspnea

**Drug Interactions** By inhibiting its metabolism, sulthiamine can raise phenytoin serum levels

**Usual Dosage** Oral:

Children: Initial: 3-5 mg/kg/day; can increase daily dose: 10-15 mg/kg; maximum daily dose: 1.2 g

Adults: Initial: 100 mg twice daily; can be increased to 200 mg 3 times/day

**Dosage Forms**

Suspension: 50 mg/5 mL

Tablets: 50 mg, 200 mg

♦ **Sultiame** *see* Sulthiame *on page 527*

♦ **Sultrin™** *see* Sulfabenzamide, Sulfacetamide, and Sulfathiazole *on page 522*

## Sumatriptan (SOO ma trip tan SUKS i nate)

**U.S. Brand Names** Imitrex®

**Pharmacologic Category** Serotonin 5-$HT_{1D}$ Receptor Agonist

**Use** Acute treatment of migraine with or without aura

Sumatriptan injection: Acute treatment of cluster headache episodes

**Effects on Mental Status** Dizziness is common; may cause drowsiness

**Effects on Psychiatric Treatment** Contraindicated with other serotonin agonists (SSRIs) and MAOIs

**Pregnancy Risk Factor** C

**Contraindications** Intravenous administration; use in patients with ischemic heart disease or Prinzmetal angina, patients with signs or symptoms of ischemic heart disease, uncontrolled HTN; use with ergotamine derivatives (within 24 hours of); use with in 24 hours of another 5-$HT_1$ agonist; concurrent administration or within 2 weeks of discontinuing an MAOI; hypersensitivity to any component; management of hemiplegic or basilar migraine

**Warnings/Precautions**

Sumatriptan is indicated only in patient populations with a clear diagnosis of migraine or cluster headache

Cardiac events (coronary artery vasospasm, transient ischemia, myocardial infarction, ventricular tachycardia/fibrillation, cardiac arrest and death) have been reported with 5-$HT_1$ agonist administration. Significant elevation in blood pressure, including hypertensive crisis, has also been reported on rare occasions in patients with and without a history of hypertension. Vasospasm-related reactions have been reported other than coronary artery vasospasm. Peripheral vascular ischemia and colonic ischemia with abdominal pain and bloody diarrhea have occurred.

**Adverse Reactions**

>10%:
- Central nervous system: Dizziness
- Endocrine & metabolic: Hot flashes
- Local: Injection site reaction
- Neuromuscular & skeletal: Paresthesia

1% to 10%:
- Cardiovascular: Tightness in chest
- Central nervous system: Drowsiness, headache
- Dermatologic: Burning sensation
- Gastrointestinal: Abdominal discomfort, mouth discomfort
- Neuromuscular & skeletal: Myalgia, numbness, weakness, neck pain, jaw discomfort
- Miscellaneous: Diaphoresis

<1%: Dehydration, dysmenorrhea, dyspnea, dysuria, hiccups, polydipsia, rashes, renal calculus, thirst

**Drug Interactions** Increased toxicity: Ergot-containing drugs, MAOIs, SSRIs can lead to symptoms of hyper-reflexia, weakness, and incoordination

**Usual Dosage** Adults:

Oral: 25 mg (taken with fluids); maximum initial recommended dose is 100 mg. If a headache returns or patient has a partial response to the initial dose, additional doses may be taken at intervals of at least 2 hours up to a daily maximum of 200 mg. There is no evidence that an initial dose of 100 mg provides substantially greater relief than 50 mg.

Intranasal: A single dose of 5, 10 or 20 mg administered in one nostril. A 10 mg dose may be achieved by administering a single 5 mg dose in each nostril. If headache returns, the dose maybe be repeated once after 2 hours not to exceed a total daily dose of 40 mg. The safety of treating an average of >4 headaches in a 30-day period has not been established.

S.C.: 6 mg; a second injection may be administered at least 1 hour after the initial dose, but not more than 2 injections in a 24-hour period. If side effects are dose-limiting, lower doses may be used.

**Patient Information** Take at first sign of migraine attack. This drug is to be used to reduce your migraine, not to prevent or reduce number of attacks. Oral: If headache returns or is not fully resolved after first dose, the dose may be repeated after 2 hours. **Do not exceed 200 mg in 24 hours.** S.C.: If headache returns or is not fully resolved after first dose, the dose may be repeated after 1 hour. **Do not exceed two injections in 24 hours. Do not take within 24 hours of any other migraine medication without first consulting prescriber.** You may experience some dizziness (use caution); hot flashes (cool room may help); nausea or vomiting (frequent small meals, frequent mouth care, sucking lozenges, or chewing gum may help); pain at injection site (lasts about 1 hour, will resolve); or excess sweating (will resolve). Report chest tightness or pain; excessive drowsiness; acute abdominal pain; skin rash or burning sensation; muscle weakness, soreness, or numbness; or respiratory difficulty.

**Nursing Implications** Pain at injection site lasts <1 hour

**Dosage Forms**

Injection, as succinate: 12 mg/mL (0.5 mL, 2 mL)

Spray, intranasal, as base: 5 mg (100 µL unit dose spray device), 20 mg (100 µL unit dose spray device)

Tablet, as succinate: 25 mg, 50 mg

♦ **Summer's Eve® Medicated Douche [OTC]** *see* Povidone-Iodine *on page 456*

♦ **Sumycin® Oral** *see* Tetracycline *on page 537*

♦ **Superdophilus® [OTC]** *see Lactobacillus acidophilus* and *Lactobacillus bulgaricus on page 305*

♦ **Supprelin™ Injection** *see* Histrelin *on page 268*

♦ **Suppress® [OTC]** *see* Dextromethorphan *on page 160*

♦ **Suprax®** *see* Cefixime *on page 98*

## Suprofen (soo PROE fen)

**U.S. Brand Names** Profenal® Ophthalmic

**Pharmacologic Category** Nonsteroidal Anti-Inflammatory Agent (NSAID)

**Use** Inhibition of intraoperative miosis

**Effects on Mental Status** None reported

**Effects on Psychiatric Treatment** None reported

**Usual Dosage** Adults: On day of surgery, instill 2 drops in conjunctival sac at 3, 2, and 1 hour prior to surgery; or 2 drops in sac every 4 hours, while awake, the day preceding surgery

**Dosage Forms** Solution, ophthalmic: 1% (2.5 mL)

## Suramin (SUR a min)

**Pharmacologic Category** Antineoplastic Agent, Miscellaneous

**Use** Prostate cancer

**Effects on Mental Status** None reported

**Effects on Psychiatric Treatment** Leukopenia is common; avoid clozapine and carbamazepine

**Usual Dosage** Refer to individual protocols

350 mg/m$^2$/day continuous I.V. infusion for 7 days, then titrated to a plasma level of 250-300 µg/mL for 7 days, repeated after an 8-week interval

Titrate to a plasma level of 300 µg/mL for 14 days, repeat after an 8-week interval

**Dosage adjustment in renal impairment:** Dosage reductions have been suggested for "severe" renal dysfunction; however, specific guidelines have not been published

**Dosage adjustment in hepatic impairment:** Dosage reductions of 50% to 75% have been suggested for "severe" hepatic dysfunction; however, specific guidelines have not been published

**Dosage Forms** Powder for injection: 1 g

♦ **Surbex® [OTC]** *see* Vitamin B Complex *on page 586*

♦ **Surbex-T® Filmtabs® [OTC]** *see* Vitamin B Complex With Vitamin C *on page 586*

♦ **Surbex® With C Filmtabs® [OTC]** *see* Vitamin B Complex With Vitamin C *on page 586*

♦ **Surfak® [OTC]** *see* Docusate *on page 179*

♦ **Surmontil®** *see* Trimipramine *on page 570*

♦ **Survanta®** *see* Beractant *on page 65*

♦ **Sus-Phrine®** *see* Epinephrine *on page 195*

♦ **Sustaire®** *see* Theophylline Salts *on page 539*

♦ **Sustiva™** *see* Efavirenz *on page 190*

♦ **Suxamethonium Chloride** *see* Succinylcholine *on page 521*

♦ **Sweet Root** *see* Licorice *on page 317*

♦ **Syllact® [OTC]** *see* Psyllium *on page 479*

♦ **Symadine®** *see* Amantadine *on page 28*

♦ **Symmetrel®** *see* Amantadine *on page 28*

♦ **Synacol® CF [OTC]** *see* Guaifenesin and Dextromethorphan *on page 257*

♦ **Synacort®** *see* Hydrocortisone *on page 273*

♦ **Synagis®** *see* Palivizumab *on page 417*

♦ **Synalar®** *see* Fluocinolone *on page 231*

♦ **Synalar-HP®** *see* Fluocinolone *on page 231*

♦ **Synalgos®-DC** *see* Dihydrocodeine Compound *on page 170*

♦ **Synarel®** *see* Nafarelin *on page 379*

♦ **Synemol®** *see* Fluocinolone *on page 231*

♦ **Synercid®** *see* Quinupristin and Dalfopristin *on page 486*

- ♦ **Synthroid®** *see* Levothyroxine *on page 316*
- ♦ **Syprine®** *see* Trientine *on page 566*
- ♦ **Syracol-CF® [OTC]** *see* Guaifenesin and Dextromethorphan *on page 257*
- ♦ **$T_3$ Sodium** *see* Liothyronine *on page 319*
- ♦ **$T_3/T_4$ Liotrix** *see* Liotrix *on page 319*
- ♦ **$T_4$** *see* Levothyroxine *on page 316*
- ♦ **Tac™-3** *see* Triamcinolone *on page 563*
- ♦ **Tac™-40** *see* Triamcinolone *on page 563*
- ♦ **Tacaryl®** *see* Methdilazine *on page 351*
- ♦ **TACE®** *see* Chlorotrianisene *on page 113*


## Tacrine (TAK reen)

**Related Information**
Special Populations - Elderly *on page 662*

**Generic Available** No

**U.S. Brand Names** Cognex®

**Synonyms** Tacrine Hydrochloride; Tetrahydroaminoacrine; THA

**Pharmacologic Category** Acetylcholinesterase Inhibitor; Cholinergic Agonist

**Use** Treatment of mild to moderate dementia of the Alzheimer's type

**Pregnancy Risk Factor** C

**Contraindications** Patients previously treated with the drug who developed jaundice; hypersensitivity to tacrine or acridine derivatives

**Warnings/Precautions** The use of tacrine has been associated with elevations in serum transaminases; serum transaminases (specifically ALT) must be monitored throughout therapy; use extreme caution in patients with current evidence of a history of abnormal liver function tests; use caution in patients with urinary tract obstruction (bladder outlet obstruction or prostatic hypertrophy), asthma, and sick-sinus syndrome (tacrine may cause bradycardia). Also, patients with cardiovascular disease, asthma, or peptic ulcer should use cautiously. Use with caution in patients with a history of seizures. May cause nausea, vomiting, or loose stools. Abrupt discontinuation or dosage decrease may worsen cognitive function. May be associated with neutropenia.

**Adverse Reactions**

>10%
- Central nervous system: Headache, dizziness
- Gastrointestinal: Nausea, vomiting, diarrhea
- Miscellaneous: Elevated transaminases

1% to 10%
- Cardiovascular: Flushing
- Central nervous system: Confusion, ataxia, insomnia, somnolence, depression, anxiety, fatigue
- Dermatologic: Rash
- Gastrointestinal: Dyspepsia, anorexia, abdominal pain, flatulence, constipation, weight loss
- Neuromuscular & skeletal: Myalgia, tremor
- Respiratory: Rhinitis

**Overdosage/Toxicology**

Treatment: General supportive measures; can cause a cholinergic crisis characterized by severe nausea, vomiting, salivation, sweating, bradycardia, hypotension, collapse, and convulsions; increased muscle weakness is a possibility and may result in death if respiratory muscles are involved

Tertiary anticholinergics, such as atropine, may be used as an antidote for overdosage. I.V. atropine sulfate titrated to effect is recommended; initial dose of 10-20 mg I.V. with subsequent doses based upon clinical response. Atypical increases in blood pressure and heart rate have been reported with other cholinomimetics when coadministered with quaternary anticholinergics such as glycopyrrolate.

**Drug Interactions** CYP1A2 enzyme substrate; CYP1A2 inhibitor

Anticholinergic agents: Tacrine may antagonize the therapeutic effect of anticholinergic agents (benztropine, trihexphenidyl); a peripherally-acting agent (glycopyrrolate) has been reported to reduce tacrine-associated gastrointestinal complaints

Beta-blockers: Tacrine in combination with beta blockers may produce additive bradycardia

Calcium channel blockers: Tacrine in combination with heartrate lowering calcium channel blockers (diltiazem and verapamil) may produce additive bradycardia

Cholinergic agents: Tacrine in combination with other cholinergic agents (eg, ambenonium, edrophonium, neostigmine, pyridostigmine, bethanechol), will likely produce additive cholinergic effects

CYP1A2 inhibitors: May increase tacrine concentrations; includes cimetidine, ciprofloxacin, isoniazid, fluvoxamine, ritonavir and zileutin; cigarette smoking may also share this effect

Digoxin: Tacrine, in combination with digoxin, may produce additive bradycardia

Levodopa: Tacrine may worsen Parkinson's disease and inhibit the effects of levodopa

Neuromuscular blocking agents (nondepolarizing): Theoretically, tacrine may antagonize the effect of nondepolarizing neuromuscular blocking agents

Succinylcholine: Tacrine may prolong the effect of succinylcholine

Theophylline: Tacrine may inhibit the metabolism of theophylline resulting in elevated plasma levels; dose adjustment will likely be needed

**Mechanism of Action** Centrally-acting cholinesterase inhibitor. It elevates acetylcholine in cerebral cortex by slowing the degradation of acetylcholine.

**Pharmacodynamics/kinetics**
- Peak plasma concentrations: 1-2 hours
- Plasma bound: 55%
- Metabolism: Cytochrome P-450 enzyme system in the liver
- Half-life, elimination: 2-4 hours, steady-state achieved in 24-36 hours

**Usual Dosage** Adults: Initial: 10 mg 4 times/day; may increase by 40 mg/day adjusted every 6 weeks; maximum: 160 mg/day; best administered separate from meal times; see table.

**Dose Adjustment Based Upon Transaminase Elevations**

| ALT | Regimen |
|---|---|
| ≤3 x ULN* | Continue titration |
| >3 to ≤5 x ULN | Decrease dose by 40 mg/day, resume when ALT returns to normal |
| >5 x ULN | Stop treatment, may rechallenge upon return of ALT to normal |

*ULN = upper limit of normal.

Patients with clinical jaundice confirmed by elevated total bilirubin (>3 mg/dL) should not be rechallenged with tacrine

**Monitoring Parameters** ALT (SGPT) levels and other liver enzymes weekly for at least the first 18 weeks, then monitor once every 3 months

**Reference Range** In clinical trials, serum concentrations >20 ng/mL were associated with a much higher risk of development of symptomatic adverse effects

**Test Interactions** ↑ ALT or AST

**Patient Information** Effect of tacrine therapy is thought to depend upon its administration at regular intervals, as directed; possibility of adverse effects such as those occurring in close temporal association with the initiation of treatment or an increase in dose (ie, nausea, vomiting, loose stools, diarrhea) and those with a delayed onset (ie, rash, jaundice, changes in the color of stool); inform physician of the emergence of new events or any increase in the severity of existing adverse effects; abrupt discontinuation of the drug or a large reduction in total daily dose (80 mg/day or more) may cause a decline in cognitive function and behavioral disturbances; unsupervised increases in the dose may also have serious consequences; do not change dose without consulting physician

**Nursing Implications** May require administration with food to avoid GI side effects however food reduces tacrine bioavailability by 30% to 40% so administer 1 hour before meals. Abrupt withdrawal or rapid reduction in dosage may result in worsening of cognitive function.

**Additional Information** Give with food if GI side effects are intolerable; however, this decreases bioavailability

**Dosage Forms** Capsule, as hydrochloride: 10 mg, 20 mg, 30 mg, 40 mg

♦ **Tacrine Hydrochloride** *see* Tacrine *on page 529*

## Tacrolimus (ta KROE li mus)

**U.S. Brand Names** Prograf®

**Synonyms** FK506

**Pharmacologic Category** Immunosuppressant Agent

**Use** Potent immunosuppressive drug used in liver, kidney, heart, lung, small bowel transplant recipients; immunosuppressive drug for peripheral stem cell/bone marrow transplantation

**Effects on Mental Status** Insomnia is common

**Effects on Psychiatric Treatment** Barbiturates and carbamazepine may decrease the effects of tacrolimus

**Pregnancy Risk Factor** C

**Contraindications** Hypersensitivity to tacrolimus or any component; hypersensitivity to HCO-60 polyoxyl 60 hydrogenated castor oil (used in the parenteral dosage formulation) is a contraindication to parenteral tacrolimus therapy

**Warnings/Precautions** Increased susceptibility to infection and the possible development of lymphoma may occur after administration of tacrolimus; it should not be administered simultaneously with cyclosporine; since the pharmacokinetics show great inter- and intrapatient variability over time, monitoring of serum concentrations (trough for oral therapy) is essential to prevent organ rejection and reduce drug-related toxicity; tonic clonic seizures may have been triggered by tacrolimus. Injection contains small volume of ethanol.

**Adverse Reactions**

>10%:
- Cardiovascular: Hypertension, peripheral edema
- Central nervous system: Headache, insomnia, pain, fever

(Continued)

## Tacrolimus *(Continued)*

Dermatologic: Pruritus
Endocrine & metabolic: Hypo-/hyperkalemia, hyperglycemia, hypomagnesemia
Gastrointestinal: Diarrhea, nausea, anorexia, vomiting, abdominal pain
Hematologic: Anemia, leukocytosis
Hepatic: LFT abnormalities, ascites
Neuromuscular & skeletal: Tremors, paresthesias, back pain, weakness
Renal: Nephrotoxicity, increased BUN/creatinine
Respiratory: Pleural effusion, atelectasis, dyspnea
Miscellaneous: Infection

1% to 10%:
Central nervous system: Seizures
Dermatologic: Rash
Endocrine & metabolic: Hyperphosphatemia, hyperuricemia, pancreatitis
Gastrointestinal: Constipation
Genitourinary: Urinary tract infection
Hematologic: Thrombocytopenia
Neuromuscular & skeletal: Myoclonus
Renal: Oliguria

<1%: Anaphylaxis, arthralgia, expressive aphasia, hemolytic uremic syndrome, hypertrophic cardiomyopathy, myalgia, photophobia, secondary malignancy

**Overdosage/Toxicology**
Signs and symptoms: Extensions of pharmacologic activity and listed adverse effects
Treatment: Symptomatic and supportive treatment required, hemodialysis is not effective

**Drug Interactions** CYP3A3/4 enzyme substrate
Decreased effect: Separate administration of antacids and Carafate® from tacrolimus by at least 2 hours
Increased effect: Cyclosporine is associated with synergistic immunosuppression and increased nephrotoxicity
Increased toxicity: Nephrotoxic antibiotics, NSAIDs and amphotericin B potentially increase nephrotoxicity
Drugs which may INCREASE tacrolimus blood levels:
Calcium channel blockers: Diltiazem, nicardipine, verapamil
Antibiotic/antifungal agents: Clotrimazole, erythromycin, fluconazole, itraconazole, ketoconazole
Other drugs: Bromocriptine, cimetidine, clarithromycin, cyclosporine, danazol, methylprednisolone, metoclopramide, grapefruit juice
Drugs which may DECREASE tacrolimus blood levels:
Anticonvulsants: Carbamazepine, phenobarbital, phenytoin
Antibiotics: Rifabutin, rifampin

**Usual Dosage**
Children: Patients without pre-existing renal or hepatic dysfunction have required and tolerated higher doses than adults to achieve similar blood concentrations. It is recommended that therapy be initiated at high end of the recommended adult I.V. and oral dosing ranges.
Oral: 0.3 mg/kg/day divided every 12 hours; children generally require higher maintenance dosages on a mg/kg basis than adults
I.V. continuous infusion: 0.05-0.15 mg/kg/day
Adults:
Oral (usually 3-4 times the I.V. dose): 0.15-0.30 mg/kg/day in two divided doses administered every 12 hours and given 8-12 hours after discontinuation of the I.V. infusion. Lower tacrolimus doses may be sufficient as maintenance therapy.
**Solid organ transplantation:** Oral: 0.15-0.30 mg/kg/day in two divided doses administered every 12 hours; lower tacrolimus doses may be sufficient as maintenance therapy
**Peripheral stem cell/bone marrow transplantation:** Oral (usually ~2-3 times the intravenous dose): 0.06-0.09 mg/kg/day (maximum: 0.12 mg/kg/day) in two divided doses administered every 12 hours and given 8-12 hours after discontinuation of the intravenous infusion; adjust doses based on trough serum concentrations
I.V.:
**Solid organ transplantation:** Initial (given at least 6 hours after transplantation): 0.05-0.10 mg/kg/day; corticosteroid therapy is advised to enhance immunosuppression. Patients should be switched to oral therapy as soon as possible (within 2-3 days).
**Peripheral stem cell/bone marrow transplantation:** Initial: 0.03 mg/kg/day as a continuous intravenous infusion
**Dosing adjustment in renal impairment:** Evidence suggests that lower doses should be used; patients should receive doses at the lowest value of the recommended I.V. and oral dosing ranges; further reductions in dose below these ranges may be required
Tacrolimus therapy should usually be delayed up to 48 hours or longer in patients with postoperative oliguria
Hemodialysis: Not removed by hemodialysis; supplemental dose is not necessary
Peritoneal dialysis: Significant drug removal is unlikely based on physiochemical characteristics
**Dosing adjustment in hepatic impairment:** Use of tacrolimus in liver transplant recipients experiencing post-transplant hepatic impairment may be associated with increased risk of developing renal insufficiency related to high whole blood levels of tacrolimus. The presence of moderate-to-severe hepatic dysfunction (serum bilirubin >2 mg/dL) appears to affect the metabolism of FK506. The half-life of the drug was prolonged and the clearance reduced after I.V. administration. The bioavailability of FK506 was also increased after oral administration. The higher plasma concentrations as determined by ELISA, in patients with severe hepatic dysfunction are probably due to the accumulation of FK506 metabolites of lower activity. These patients should be monitored closely and dosage adjustments should be considered. Some evidence indicates that lower doses could be used in these patients. See the following dosing considerations:
Switch from I.V. to oral therapy: Threefold increase in dose
T-tube clamping: No change in dose
Pediatric patients: About 2 times higher dose compared to adults
Liver dysfunction: Decrease I.V. dose; decrease oral dose
Renal dysfunction: Does not affect kinetics; decrease dose to decrease levels if renal dysfunction is related to the drug
Dialysis: Not removed
Inhibitors of hepatic metabolism: Decrease dose
Inducers of hepatic metabolism: Monitor drug level; increase dose

**Patient Information** Take as directed, preferably 30 minutes hour before or 30 minutes after meals. Do not take within 2 hours before or after antacids. Do not alter dose and do not discontinue without consulting prescriber. Maintain adequate hydration (2-3 L/day of fluids unless instructed to restrict fluid intake) during entire course of therapy. You will be susceptible to infection (avoid crowds and people with infections or contagious diseases). If you are diabetic, monitor glucose levels closely (may alter glucose levels). You may experience nausea, vomiting, loss of appetite (frequent small meals, frequent mouth care may help); diarrhea (boiled milk, yogurt, or buttermilk may help); constipation (increased exercise or dietary fruit, fluid, or fiber may help, if not consult prescriber); muscle or back pain (mild analgesics may be recommended). Report chest pain; acute headache or dizziness; symptoms of respiratory infection, cough, or difficulty breathing; unresolved gastrointestinal effects; fatigue, chills, fever, unhealed sores, white plaques in mouth, irritation in genital area; unusual bruising or bleeding; pain or irritation on urination or change in urinary patterns; rash or skin irritation; or other unusual effects related to this medication.

**Nursing Implications** For I.V. administration, tacrolimus is dispensed in a 50 mL glass container or nonpolyvinyl chloride container; it is intended to be infused over at least 12 hours; polyolefin administration sets should be used

**Dosage Forms**
Capsule: 1 mg, 5 mg
Injection, with alcohol and surfactant: 5 mg/mL (1 mL)


- **Tagamet®** *see* Cimetidine *on page 123*
- **Tagamet® HB [OTC]** *see* Cimetidine *on page 123*
- **Talwin®** *see* Pentazocine *on page 427*
- **Talwin® NX** *see* Pentazocine *on page 427*
- **Tambocor™** *see* Flecainide *on page 227*
- **Tamiflu™** *see* Oseltamivir *on page 408*
- **Tamine® [OTC]** *see* Brompheniramine and Phenylpropanolamine *on page 74*


## Tamoxifen (ta MOKS i fen)

**U.S. Brand Names** Nolvadex®
**Canadian Brand Names** Alpha-Tamoxifen®; Apo®-Tamox; Novo-Tamoxifen; Tamofen®; Tamone®
**Pharmacologic Category** Antineoplastic Agent, Miscellaneous
**Use** Palliative or adjunctive treatment of advanced breast cancer; reduce the incidence of breast cancer in women at high risk (taking into account age, number of first-degree relatives with breast cancer, previous breast biopsies, age at first live birth, age at first menstrual period, and a history of lobular carcinoma *in situ*); reduce the incidence of invasive breast cancer in women with ductal carcinoma *in situ* (DCIS); induction of ovulation; metastatic male breast cancer
**Unlabeled use:** Treatment of mastalgia, gynecomastia, and pancreatic carcinoma. Studies have shown tamoxifen to be effective in the treatment of primary breast cancer in elderly women. Comparative studies with other antineoplastic agents in elderly women with breast cancer had more favorable survival rates with tamoxifen. Initiation of hormone therapy rather than chemotherapy is justified for elderly patients with metastatic breast cancer who are responsive.
**Effects on Mental Status** May cause dizziness, drowsiness, or confusion
**Effects on Psychiatric Treatment** May cause leukopenia; use caution with clozapine and carbamazepine
**Pregnancy Risk Factor** D
**Contraindications** Hypersensitivity to tamoxifen
**Warnings/Precautions** Use with caution in patients with leukopenia, thrombocytopenia, or hyperlipidemias; ovulation may be induced; "hot flashes" may be countered by Bellergal-S® tablets; decreased visual

acuity, retinopathy and corneal changes have been reported with use for more than 1 year at doses above recommended; hypercalcemia in patients with bone metastasis; hepatocellular carcinomas have been reported in animal studies; endometrial hyperplasia and polyps have occurred

**Adverse Reactions**

>10%:

Cardiovascular: Flushing

Dermatologic: Skin rash

Gastrointestinal: Little to mild nausea (10%), vomiting, weight gain

Hematologic: Myelosuppressive: Transient thrombocytopenia occurs in ~24% of patients receiving 10-20 mg/day; platelet counts return to normal within several weeks in spite of continued administration; leukopenia has also been reported and does resolve during continued therapy; anemia has also been reported

WBC: Rare

Platelets: None

Hepatic: Hepatotoxicity

Neuromuscular & skeletal: Increased bone and tumor pain and local disease flare shortly after starting therapy; this will subside rapidly, but patients should be aware of this since many may discontinue the drug due to the side effects

1% to 10%:

Cardiovascular: Thromboembolism: Tamoxifen has been associated with the occurrence of venous thrombosis and pulmonary embolism; arterial thrombosis has also been described in a few case reports

Central nervous system: Lightheadedness, depression, dizziness, headache, lassitude, mental confusion

Dermatologic: Rash

Endocrine & metabolic: Hypercalcemia may occur in patients with bone metastases; galactorrhea and vitamin deficiency, menstrual irregularities

Genitourinary: Vaginal bleeding or discharge, endometriosis, priapism, possible endometrial cancer

Neuromuscular & skeletal: Weakness

Ocular: Ophthalmologic effects (visual acuity changes, cataracts, or retinopathy), corneal opacities

**Overdosage/Toxicology**

Signs and symptoms: Hypercalcemia, edema

Treatment: General supportive care

**Drug Interactions** CYP1A2, 2A6, 2B6, 2C, 2D6, 2E1, and 3A3/4 enzyme substrate

Increased toxicity: Allopurinol results in exacerbation of allopurinol-induced hepatotoxicity; cyclosporine may result in increase in cyclosporine serum levels; warfarin results in significant enhancement of the anticoagulant effects of warfarin

**Usual Dosage** Oral (refer to individual protocols):

Adults:

Breast cancer: Refer to individual protocols

Adjunct to surgery/radiation therapy: 20-40 mg/day; dosages >20 mg/day in divided doses

Females >50 years with positive axillary nodes: 10 mg twice daily

Metastatic: 20-40 mg/day; dosages >20 mg/day in divided doses

Prevention (in high-risk females): 20 mg/day

DCIS: 20 mg once daily

Males: 20 mg/day

Higher dosages (up to 700 mg/day) have been investigated for use in modulation of multidrug resistance (MDR), but are not routinely used in clinical practice

Induction of ovulation: 5-40 mg twice daily for 4 days

**Patient Information** Take as directed, morning and night and maintain adequate hydration (2-3 L/day of fluids unless instructed to restrict fluid intake). You may experience menstrual irregularities, vaginal bleeding, hot flashes, hair loss, loss of libido (these will subside when treatment is completed). Bone pain may indicate a good therapeutic responses (consult prescriber for mild analgesics). For nausea, vomiting small, frequent meals, chewing gum, or sucking lozenges may help. You may experience photosensitivity (use sunscreen, wear protective clothing and eyewear, and avoid direct sunlight). Report unusual bleeding or bruising, severe weakness, sedation, mental changes, swelling or pain in calves, difficulty breathing, or any changes in vision.

**Nursing Implications** Increase of bone pain usually indicates a good therapeutic response

**Dosage Forms** Tablet, as citrate: 10 mg, 20 mg

## Tamsulosin (tam SOO loe sin)

**U.S. Brand Names** Flomax®

**Pharmacologic Category** Alpha$_1$ Blockers

**Use** Treatment of signs and symptoms of benign prostatic hyperplasia (BPH)

**Effects on Mental Status** Dizziness is common; may cause drowsiness or insomnia

**Effects on Psychiatric Treatment** None reported

**Pregnancy Risk Factor** B

**Contraindications** Hypersensitivity to tamsulosin or any component

**Warnings/Precautions** Not intended for use as an antihypertensive drug. May cause orthostasis, syncope or dizziness. Patients should avoid situations where injury may occur as a result of syncope. Rule out prostatic carcinoma before beginning therapy with tamsulosin. Anticipate a similar effect if therapy is interrupted for a few days, if dosage is rapidly increased, or if another antihypertensive drug is introduced.

**Adverse Reactions**

Central nervous system: Headache, dizziness (0.4 mg: 14.9%; 0.8 mg: 17.1%), somnolence (0.4 mg: 3.0%; 0.8 mg: 4.3%), insomnia

Endocrine & metabolic: Decreased libido

Gastrointestinal: Diarrhea, nausea, tooth disorder

Genitourinary: Ejaculation disturbances

Neuromuscular & skeletal: Back pain, chest pain, weakness

Ocular: Amblyopia

Respiratory: Rhinitis, pharyngitis, increased cough, sinusitis

Miscellaneous: Infections, allergic-type reactions such as skin rash, pruritus, angioedema, and urticaria have been reported upon drug rechallenge

**Drug Interactions**

Alpha-adrenergic blockers; should not be used in combination with other alpha-adrenergic blocking agents

Cimetidine resulted in a significant decrease (26%) in the clearance of tamsulosin which resulted in a moderate increase in tamsulosin AUC (44%); therefore, use with caution when used in combination with cimetidine (especially doses >0.4 mg)

Warfarin: Use caution with concomitant administration of warfarin and tamsulosin

No dosage adjustments necessary if administered with atenolol, enalapril, or Procardia XL®

**Usual Dosage** Oral: Adults: 0.4 mg once daily approximately 30 minutes after the same meal each day

**Dietary Considerations** The time to maximum concentration ($T_{max}$) is reached by 4-5 hours under fasting conditions and by 6-7 hours when administered with food. Taking it under fasted conditions results in a 30% increase in bioavailability and 40% to 70% increase in peak concentrations ($C_{max}$) compared to fed conditions.

**Patient Information** Take as directed 30 minutes, after same meal each day. Do not skip dose or discontinue without consulting prescriber. You may experience drowsiness, dizziness, or impaired judgment (use caution when driving or engaging in tasks that require alertness until response to drug is known); postural hypotension (use caution when rising from sitting or lying position or when climbing stairs); nausea (frequent mouth care or sucking lozenges may help); urinary incontinence (void before taking medication); ejaculatory disturbance (reversible, may resolve with continued use); diarrhea (boiled milk or yogurt may help); palpitations or rapid heartbeat; difficulty breathing, unusual cough, or sore throat; or other persistent side effects.

**Dosage Forms** Capsule, as hydrochloride: 0.4 mg


- **Tanac® [OTC]** *see* Benzocaine *on page 61*
- ***Tanacetum parthenium*** *see* Feverfew *on page 224*
- **Tanoral® Tablet** *see* Chlorpheniramine, Pyrilamine, and Phenylephrine *on page 116*
- **Tao®** *see* Troleandomycin *on page 573*
- **Tapazole®** *see* Methimazole *on page 352*
- **Targretin®** *see* Bexarotene *on page 67*
- **Tarka®** *see* Trandolapril and Verapamil *on page 559*
- **Tasmar®** *see* Tolcapone *on page 554*
- **Tavist®** *see* Clemastine *on page 128*
- **Tavist®-1 [OTC]** *see* Clemastine *on page 128*
- **Tavist-D®** *see* Clemastine and Phenylpropanolamine *on page 128*
- **Taxol®** *see* Paclitaxel *on page 417*
- **Taxotere®** *see* Docetaxel *on page 179*


## Tazarotene (taz AR oh teen)

**U.S. Brand Names** Tazorac®

**Pharmacologic Category** Keratolytic Agent

**Use** Topical treatment of facial acne vulgaris; topical treatment of stable plaque psoriasis of up to 20% body surface area involvement

**Effects on Mental Status** None reported

**Effects on Psychiatric Treatment** Use caution with drugs known to cause photosensitivity (psychotropics), effects may be augmented

**Usual Dosage** Children >12 years and Adults: Topical:

Acne: Cleanse the face gently. After the skin is dry, apply a thin film of tazarotene (2 mg/cm$^2$) once daily, in the evening, to the skin where the acne lesions appear. Use enough to cover the entire affected area. Tazarotene was investigated ≤12 weeks during clinical trials for acne.

Psoriasis: Apply tazarotene once daily, in the evening, to psoriatic lesions using enough (2 mg/cm$^2$) to cover only the lesion with a thin film to no

(Continued)

## Tazarotene *(Continued)*

more than 20% of body surface area. If a bath or shower is taken prior to application, dry the skin before applying the gel. Because unaffected skin may be more susceptible to irritation, avoid application of tazarotene to these areas. Tazarotene was investigated for up to 12 months during clinical trials for psoriasis.

**Dosage Forms** Gel, topical: 0.05% (30 g, 100 g), 0.1% (30 g, 100 g)


- **Tazicef®** *see* Ceftazidime *on page 101*
- **Tazidime®** *see* Ceftazidime *on page 101*
- **Tazorac®** *see* Tazarotene *on page 531*
- **3TC** *see* Lamivudine *on page 306*
- **TCN** *see* Tetracycline *on page 537*
- **Tear Drop® Solution [OTC]** *see* Artificial Tears *on page 48*
- **TearGard® Ophthalmic Solution [OTC]** *see* Artificial Tears *on page 48*
- **Teargen® Ophthalmic Solution [OTC]** *see* Artificial Tears *on page 48*
- **Tearisol® Solution [OTC]** *see* Artificial Tears *on page 48*
- **Tears Naturale® Free Solution [OTC]** *see* Artificial Tears *on page 48*
- **Tears Naturale® II Solution [OTC]** *see* Artificial Tears *on page 48*
- **Tears Naturale® Solution [OTC]** *see* Artificial Tears *on page 48*
- **Tears Plus® Solution [OTC]** *see* Artificial Tears *on page 48*
- **Tears Renewed® Solution [OTC]** *see* Artificial Tears *on page 48*
- **Tebamide®** *see* Trimethobenzamide *on page 569*
- **Teczem®** *see* Enalapril and Diltiazem *on page 192*
- **Tedral®** *see* Theophylline, Ephedrine, and Phenobarbital *on page 539*
- **Tegison®** *see* Etretinate *on page 216*
- **Tegopen®** *see* Cloxacillin *on page 136*
- **Tegretol®** *see* Carbamazepine *on page 90*
- **Tegretol®-XR** *see* Carbamazepine *on page 90*
- **Tegrin®-HC [OTC]** *see* Hydrocortisone *on page 273*
- **Telachlor®** *see* Chlorpheniramine *on page 113*
- **Teladar®** *see* Betamethasone *on page 65*
- **Teldrin® [OTC]** *see* Chlorpheniramine *on page 113*


## Telmisartan (tel mi SAR tan)

**Related Information**

Angiotensin-Related Agents Comparison Chart *on page 700*

**U.S. Brand Names** Micardis®

**Pharmacologic Category** Angiotensin II Antagonists

**Use** Treatment of hypertension; may be used alone or in combination with other antihypertensive agents

**Effects on Mental Status** May cause dizziness or fatigue, may rarely cause insomnia, anxiety, nervousness, depression, or sedation

**Effects on Psychiatric Treatment** None reported

**Pregnancy Risk Factor** C (1st trimester); D (2nd and 3rd trimester)

**Contraindications** Hypersensitivity to telmisartan or any component; hypersensitivity to other A-II receptor antagonists; primary hyperaldosteronism; bilateral renal artery stenosis; pregnancy (2nd and 3rd trimesters)

**Warnings/Precautions** Avoid use or use a smaller dose in patients who are volume depleted; correct depletion first. Deterioration in renal function can occur with initiation. Use with caution in unilateral renal artery stenosis and pre-existing renal insufficiency; significant aortic/mitral stenosis. Use with caution in patients who have biliary obstructive disorders or hepatic dysfunction.

**Adverse Reactions**

1% to 10%:

Cardiovascular: Hypertension (1%), chest pain (1%), peripheral edema (1%)

Central nervous system: Headache (1%), dizziness (1%), pain (1%), fatigue (1%)

Gastrointestinal: Diarrhea (3%, compared to 2% with placebo), dyspepsia (1%), nausea (1%), abdominal pain (1%)

Genitourinary: Urinary tract infection (7%, compared to 6% with placebo)

Neuromuscular & skeletal: Back pain (3%, compared to 1% with placebo), myalgia (1%)

Respiratory: Upper respiratory infection (7%, compared to 6% with placebo), sinusitis (3%, compared to 2% with placebo), pharyngitis (1%), cough (1.6%, same as placebo)

Miscellaneous: Flu-like syndrome (1%)

<1%: Abnormal EKG, abnormal vision, allergic reaction, angina, angioedema, anxiety, arthralgias, asthma, bronchitis, cerebrovascular disorder, conjunctivitis, constipation, cystitis, decreased hemoglobin, depression, dermatitis, diabetes mellitus, dry mouth, dyspnea, earache, eczema, elevated liver enzymes, epistaxis, fever, flatulence, flushing, gastroenteritis, gout, hemorrhoids, hypercholesterolemia impotence, increased creatinine/BUN, infection, insomnia, involuntary muscle contractions, leg cramps, malaise, micturition frequency, migraine, nervousness, palpitations, paresthesias, pruritus, rhinitis, rash, somnolence, sweating, tachycardia, tinnitus, toothache, vertigo

**Overdosage/Toxicology** Signs and symptoms of overdose include hypotension, dizziness and tachycardia; treatment is supportive; vagal stimulation may result in bradycardia

**Drug Interactions**

Digoxin levels may be increased

Lithium: Risk of toxicity may be increased by telmisartan; monitor lithium levels

Potassium-sparing diuretics (amiloride, potassium, spironolactone, triamterene): Increased risk of hyperkalemia

Potassium supplements may increase the risk of hyperkalemia

Trimethoprim (high dose) may increase the risk of hyperkalemia

Warfarin serum concentrations may be decreased (not associated with alteration in INR); monitor INR closely

**Usual Dosage** Adults: Oral: Initial: 40 mg once daily; usual maintenance dose range: 20-80 mg/day. Patients with volume depletion should be initiated on the lower dosage with close supervision.

**Dosage adjustment in hepatic impairment:** Supervise patients closely.

**Dietary Considerations** May be administered without regard to food

**Patient Information** Take exactly as directed. Do not miss doses, alter dosage, or discontinue without consulting prescriber. Do not alter salt or potassium intake without consulting prescriber. Monitor blood pressure on a regular basis as recommended by prescriber; at the same time each day. You may experience postural hypotension (change position slowly when rising from sitting or lying, when climbing stairs, or bending over); or transient nervousness, headache, or dizziness (use caution when driving or engaging in tasks requiring alertness until response to drug is known). Report unusual weight gain or swelling of ankles and hands; swelling of face, lips, throat, or tongue; persistent fatigue; dry cough or difficulty breathing; palpitations or chest pain; CNS changes; gastrointestinal disturbances; muscle or bone pain, cramping, or tremors; change in urinary pattern; or changes in hearing or vision.

**Dosage Forms** Tablet: 40 mg, 80 mg

## Temazepam (te MAZ e pam)

**Related Information**

Anxiolytic/Hypnotic Use in Long-Term Care Facilities *on page 754*

Benzodiazepines Comparison Chart *on page 708*

Clinical Issues in the Use of Anxiolytics and Sedative/Hypnotics *on page 634*

Federal OBRA Regulations Recommended Maximum Doses *on page 756*

Patient Information - Anxiolytics & Sedative Hypnotics (Benzodiazepines) *on page 653*

**Generic Available** Yes

**U.S. Brand Names** Restoril®

**Canadian Brand Names** Apo®-Temazepam

**Pharmacologic Category** Benzodiazepine

**Use** Short-term treatment of insomnia

**Unlabeled use:** Treatment of anxiety; adjunct in the treatment of depression; management of panic attacks

**Restrictions** C-IV

**Pregnancy Risk Factor** X

**Contraindications** Hypersensitivity to this drug or any component of its formulation (cross-sensitivity with other benzodiazepines may exist); narrow-angle glaucoma (not in product labeling, however, benzodiazepines are contraindicated); pregnancy

**Warnings/Precautions** Should be used only after evaluation of potential causes of sleep disturbance. Failure of sleep disturbance to resolve after 7-10 days may indicate psychiatric or medical illness. A worsening of insomnia or the emergence of new abnormalities of thought or behavior may represent unrecognized psychiatric or medical illness and requires immediate and careful evaluation.

Use with caution in elderly or debilitated patients, patients with hepatic disease (including alcoholics), or renal impairment. Use with caution in patients with respiratory disease, or impaired gag reflex. Avoid use inpatients with sleep apnea.

Causes CNS depression (dose-related) resulting in sedation, dizziness, confusion, or ataxia which may impair physical and mental capabilities. Patients must be cautioned about performing tasks which require mental alertness (ie, operating machinery or driving). Use with caution in patients receiving other CNS depressants or psychoactive agents. Effects with other sedative drugs or ethanol may be potentiated. Benzodiazepines have been associated with falls and traumatic injury and should be used with extreme caution in patients who are at risk of these events (especially the elderly).

Use caution in patients with depression, particularly if suicidal risk may be present. Use with caution in patients with a history of drug dependence. Benzodiazepines have been associated with dependence and acute withdrawal symptoms on discontinuation or reduction in dose. Acute withdrawal, including seizures, may be precipitated after administration of flumazenil to patients receiving long-term benzodiazepine therapy.

Benzodiazepines have been associated with anterograde amnesia. Paradoxical reactions, including hyperactive or aggressive behavior, have been reported with benzodiazepines, particularly in adolescent/pediatric or psychiatric patients. Does not have analgesic, antidepressant, or antipsychotic properties.

**Adverse Reactions**

1% to 10%:

Central nervous system: Confusion, dizziness, drowsiness, fatigue, anxiety, headache, lethargy, hangover, euphoria, vertigo

Dermatologic: Rash

Endocrine & metabolic: Decreased libido

Gastrointestinal: Diarrhea

Neuromuscular & skeletal: Dysarthria, weakness

Otic: Blurred vision

Miscellaneous: Diaphoresis

<1%: Amnesia, anorexia, ataxia, back pain, blood dyscrasias, drug dependence, increased dreaming, menstrual irregularities, palpitations, paradoxical reactions, reflex slowing, tremor, vomiting

**Overdosage/Toxicology**

Signs and symptoms: Somnolence, confusion, coma, hypoactive reflexes, dyspnea, hypotension, slurred speech, impaired coordination

Treatment: Supportive; rarely is mechanical ventilation required. Flumazenil has been shown to selectively block the binding of benzodiazepines to CNS receptors, resulting in a reversal of benzodiazepine-induced CNS depression.

**Drug Interactions** CYP3A3/4 enzyme substrate

CNS depressants: Sedative effects and/or respiratory depression may be additive with CNS depressants; includes ethanol, barbiturates, narcotic analgesics, and other sedative agents; monitor for increased effect

CYP3A3/4 inhibitors: Serum level and/or toxicity of some benzodiazepines may be increased; inhibitors include amiodarone, cimetidine, clarithromycin, erythromycin, delavirdine, diltiazem, dirithromycin, disulfiram, fluoxetine, fluvoxamine, grapefruit juice, indinavir, itraconazole, ketoconazole, nefazodone, nevirapine, propoxyfene, quinupristin-dalfopristin, ritonavir, saquinavir, verapamil, zafirlukast, zileuton; monitor for altered benzodiazepine response

Enzyme inducers: Metabolism of some benzodiazepines may be increased, decreasing their therapeutic effect; consider using an alternative sedative/hypnotic agent; potential inducers include phenobarbital, phenytoin, carbamazepine, rifampin, and rifabutin

Oral contraceptives: May decrease the clearance of some benzodiazepines (those which undergo oxidative metabolism); monitor for increased benzodiazepine effect

Theophylline: May partially antagonize some of the effects of benzodiazepines; monitor for decreased response; may require higher doses for sedation

**Mechanism of Action** Binds to stereospecific benzodiazepine receptors on the postsynaptic GABA neuron at several sites within the central nervous system, including the limbic system, reticular formation. Enhancement of the inhibitory effect of GABA on neuronal excitability results by increased neuronal membrane permeability to chloride ions. This shift in chloride ions results in hyperpolarization (a less excitable state) and stabilization.

**Pharmacodynamics/kinetics**

Distribution: $V_d$: 1.4

Protein binding: 96%

Metabolism: In the liver (phase II)

Half-life: 9.5-12.4 hours

Time to peak serum concentration: Within 2-3 hours

Elimination: 80% to 90% excreted in urine as inactive metabolites

**Usual Dosage** Adults: Oral: 15-30 mg at bedtime; 15 mg in elderly or debilitated patients

**Dietary Considerations** Alcohol: Additive CNS effect, avoid use

**Monitoring Parameters** Respiratory and cardiovascular status

**Reference Range** Therapeutic: 26 ng/mL after 24 hours

**Patient Information** Avoid alcohol and other CNS depressants; avoid activities needing good psychomotor coordination until CNS effects are known; drug may cause physical or psychological dependence; avoid abrupt discontinuation after prolonged use

**Nursing Implications** Provide safety measures (ie, side rails, night light, and call button); remove smoking materials from area; supervise ambulation

**Additional Information** Abrupt discontinuation after sustained use (generally >10 days) may cause withdrawal symptoms

**Dosage Forms** Capsule: 7.5 mg, 15 mg, 30 mg

♦ **Temazin® Cold Syrup [OTC]** *see* Chlorpheniramine and Phenylpropanolamine *on page 114*

♦ **Temodar®** *see* Temozolomide *on page 533*

♦ **Temovate® Topical** *see* Clobetasol *on page 129*

## Temozolomide (te mo ZOLE oh mide)

**U.S. Brand Names** Temodar®

**Pharmacologic Category** Antineoplastic Agent, Alkylating Agent

**Use** Treatment of adult patients with refractory (first relapse) anaplastic astrocytoma who have experienced disease progression on nitrosourea and procarbazine

**Unlabeled use:** Glioma, first relapse/advanced metastatic malignant melanoma

**Effects on Mental Status** Fatigue, dizziness amnesia and insomnia are common; may cause somnolence, confusion, anxiety, depression

**Effects on Psychiatric Treatment** Myelosuppression is common, use caution with clozapine and carbamazepine; nausea is very common, avoid use with SSRIs

**Pregnancy Risk Factor** D

**Contraindications** History of hypersensitivity reaction to any of its components or in patients who have a hypersensitivity to DTIC (since both drugs are metabolized to MTIC)

**Warnings/Precautions** Prior to dosing, patients must have an absolute neutrophil count (ANC) of ≥1.5 x 10 9/L and a platelet count of ≥100 x 10 9/L. Must have ANC >1,500/µL, platelet count >100,000/µL before starting each cycle. Geriatric patients and women have a higher incidence of myelosuppression. Safety/efficacy in pediatrics not established. Use caution in patients with severe hepatic or renal impairment. The U.S. Food and Drug Administration (FDA) currently recommends that procedures for proper handling and disposal of antineoplastic agents be considered.

**Adverse Reactions** Women and elderly (≥70 years of age) have a higher incidence of grade 4 neutropenia and thrombocytopenia. Nausea, vomiting, fatigue, and hematologic effects are drug-related; it is unclear about the others. Nausea and vomiting easily controlled with antiemetics. Myelosuppression was the dose-limiting event (occurred within first few cycles, not cumulative). Hematologic effects are as follows (all percentages appear as grade 3/4): Anemia (4%), neutropenia (11%), granulocytopenia (14%), and thrombocytopenia (19%). Other grade 3/4 reactions included nausea (10%), vomiting (6%), hemiparesis (6%), headache (6%), weakness (6%), fatigue (4%), and fever (2%).

>10%:

Cardiovascular: Peripheral edema (11%)

Central nervous system: Headache (41%), fatigue (34%), convulsions (23%), hemiparesis (29%), dizziness (19%), fever (11%), coordination abnormality (11%), amnesia (10%), insomnia (10%)

Gastrointestinal: Nausea (53%), vomiting (42%), constipation (33%), diarrhea (16%)

Hematologic: See above in text

Neuromuscular & skeletal: Weakness (13%)

Miscellaneous: Viral infection (11%)

1% to 10%:

Central nervous system: Somnolence (9%), ataxia (8%), confusion (5%), anxiety (7%), depression (6%)

Dermatologic: Rash (8%), pruritus (8%)

Gastrointestinal: Dysphagia (7%), abdominal pain (9%), anorexia (9%), weight gain (5%)

Endocrine and Metabolic: Adrenal hypercorticism (8%), breast pain in females (6%)

Genitourinary: Urinary incontinence (8%), urinary tract infection (8%), micturition increased (6%)

Neuromuscular and Skeletal: Paresthesia (9%), back pain (8%), myalgia (5%)

Ocular: Diplopia (5%), vision abnormality (5%)

Respiratory: Upper respiratory tract infection (8%), pharyngitis (8%), sinusitis (6%), cough (5%)

**Overdosage/Toxicology** Dose-limiting toxicity is hematological. In the event of an overdose, hematological evaluation is necessary. Treatment is supportive.

**Drug Interactions** Although valproic acid reduces the clearance of temozolomide by 5%, the clinical significance of this is unknown

**Usual Dosage** Dosage is adjusted according to nadir neutrophil and platelet counts of previous cycle and counts at the time of the next cycle

Adults: Initial: 150 mg/m$^2$ once daily for 5 consecutive days per 28-day treatment cycle

Measure day 22 ANC and platelets. Measure day 29 ANC and platelets. Based on lowest counts at either day 22 or day 29:

On day 22 or day 29, if ANC <1,000/µL or the platelet count is <50,000/µL, postpone therapy until ANC >1,500/µL and platelet count >100,000/µL. Reduce dose by 50 mg/m$^2$ for subsequent cycle.

If ANC 1,000-1,500/µL or platelets 50,000-100,000/µL, postpone therapy until ANC >1,500/µL and platelet count >100,000/µL; maintain initial dose.

If ANC >1,500/µL (on day 22 and day 29) and platelet count >100,000/µL, increase dose to, or maintain dose at 200 mg/m$^2$/day for 5 for subsequent cycle.

(Continued)

## Temozolomide *(Continued)*

Temozolomide therapy can be continued until disease progression. Treatment could be continued for a maximum of 2 years in the clinical trial, but the optimum duration of therapy is not known.

**Dosage adjustment in renal impairment:** Caution should be used when administered to patients with severe renal impairment ($Cl_{cr}$ <39 mL/minute)

**Dosage adjustment in hepatic impairment:** Caution should be used when administering to patients with severe hepatic impairment

Dosage adjustment in the elderly: Patients ≥70 years of age had a higher incidence of grade 4 neutropenia and thrombocytopenia in the first cycle of therapy than patients <70 years of age

**Dietary Considerations** Food reduces rate and extent of absorption. In addition, the incidence of nausea/vomiting is decreased when the drug is taken on an empty stomach.

**Patient Information** Swallow capsules whole with a glass of water. Take on an empty stomach at similar time each day. If you have nausea and vomiting, contact healthcare provider for medicine to decrease this. Male and female patients who take temozolomide should protect against pregnancy (use effective contraception). Do not breast-feed while on medicine. Blood work necessary on day 22 and day 29 of each cycle to determine when to start next cycle and how much medicine to give.

**Nursing Implications** Capsules should not be opened. Educate patients about most frequent side effects and blood work required.

**Dosage Forms** Capsule: 5 mg, 20 mg, 100 mg, 250 mg

♦ **Tempra® [OTC]** *see* Acetaminophen *on page 14*

## Tenecteplase (ten EK te plase)

**U.S. Brand Names** TNKase™

**Pharmacologic Category** Thrombolytic Agent

**Use** Reduce mortality associated with acute myocardial infarction

**Effects on Mental Status** May cause stroke

**Effects on Psychiatric Treatment** None reported

**Usual Dosage** I.V.:

Adults: Recommended total dose should not exceed 50 mg and is based on patient's weight; administer as a bolus over 5 seconds

If patient's weight:

- <60 kg, dose: 30 mg
- ≥60 to <70 kg, dose: 35 mg
- ≥70 to <80 kg, dose: 40 mg
- ≥80 to <90 kg, dose: 45 mg
- ≥90 kg, dose: 50 mg

All patients received 150-325 mg of aspirin as soon as possible and then daily. Intravenous heparin was initiated as soon as possible and PTT was maintained between 50-70 seconds.

**Dosage adjustment in renal impairment:** No formal recommendations for renal impairment

**Dosage adjustment in hepatic impairment:** Severe hepatic failure is a relative contraindication. Recommendations were not made for mild to moderate hepatic impairment.

Elderly: Although dosage adjustments are not recommended, the elderly have a higher incidence of morbidity and mortality with the use of tenecteplase. The 30-day mortality in the ASSENT-2 trial was 2.5% for patients <65 years, 8.5% for patients 65-74 years, and 16.2% for patients ≥75 years. The intracranial hemorrhage rate was 0.4% for patients <65, 1.6 % for patients 65-74 years, and 1.7 % for patients ≥75. The risks and benefits of use should be weighted carefully in the elderly.

**Dosage Forms** Powder for injection, lyophilized (recombinant): 50 mg

♦ **Tenex®** *see* Guanfacine *on page 260*

## Teniposide (ten i POE side)

**U.S. Brand Names** Vumon Injection

**Pharmacologic Category** Antineoplastic Agent, Miscellaneous

**Use** Treatment of acute lymphocytic leukemia, small cell lung cancer

**Effects on Mental Status** None reported

**Effects on Psychiatric Treatment** Myelosuppression is common; avoid clozapine and carbamazepine

**Usual Dosage** I.V.:

Children: 130 mg/m²/week, increasing to 150 mg/m² after 3 weeks and up to 180 mg/m² after 6 weeks

Adults: 50-180 mg/m² once or twice weekly for 4-6 weeks or 20-60 mg/m²/day for 5 days

Acute lymphoblastic leukemia (ALL): 165 mg/m² twice weekly for 8-9 doses **or** 250 mg/m² weekly for 4-8 weeks

Small cell lung cancer: 80-90 mg/m²/day for 5 days

**Dosage adjustment in renal/hepatic impairment:** Data is insufficient, but dose adjustments may be necessary in patient with significant renal or hepatic impairment

**Dosage adjustment in Down syndrome patients:** Reduce initial dosing; administer the first course at half the usual dose. Patients with both Down syndrome and leukemia may be especially sensitive to myelosuppressive chemotherapy.

**Dosage Forms** Injection: 10 mg/mL (5 mL)

♦ **Ten-K®** *see* Potassium Chloride *on page 453*

♦ **Tenoretic®** *see* Atenolol and Chlorthalidone *on page 51*

♦ **Tenormin®** *see* Atenolol *on page 51*

♦ **Tensilon® Injection** *see* Edrophonium *on page 189*

♦ **Tensogradal®** *see* Nitrendipine *on page 396*

♦ **Tenuate®** *see* Diethylpropion *on page 167*

♦ **Tenuate® Dospan®** *see* Diethylpropion *on page 167*

♦ **Tequin™** *see* Gatifloxacin *on page 246*

♦ **Terak® Ophthalmic Ointment** *see* Oxytetracycline and Polymyxin B *on page 417*

♦ **Teratogenic Risks of Psychotropic Medications** *see page 812*

♦ **Terazol® Vaginal** *see* Terconazole *on page 536*

## Terazosin (ter AY zoe sin)

**Related Information**

Pharmacotherapy of Urinary Incontinence *on page 758*

**U.S. Brand Names** Hytrin®

**Pharmacologic Category** Alpha$_1$ Blockers

**Use** Management of mild to moderate hypertension; alone or in combination with other agents such as diuretics or beta-blockers; benign prostate hypertrophy

**Effects on Mental Status** Dizziness is common; may cause drowsiness or nervousness; may rarely cause insomnia or depression

**Effects on Psychiatric Treatment** None reported

**Pregnancy Risk Factor** C

**Contraindications** Hypersensitivity to quinazolines (doxazosin, prazosin, terazosin) or any component

**Warnings/Precautions** Can cause significant orthostatic hypotension and syncope, especially with first dose. Prostate cancer should be ruled out before starting for BPH. Anticipate a similar effect if therapy is interrupted for a few days, if dosage is rapidly increased, or if another antihypertensive drug is introduced.

**Adverse Reactions**

>10%:

Central nervous system: Dizziness (9% to 19%), headache (5% to 16%)

Neuromuscular & skeletal: Weakness (7.4% to 11.3%)

1% to 10%:

Cardiovascular: Peripheral edema (5.5%), palpitations (0.9% to 4.3%), postural hypotension (0.6% to 3.9%), tachycardia (1.9%)

Central nervous system: Fatigue, nervousness (2.3%)

Gastrointestinal: Xerostomia, nausea (4.4%), vomiting (1%), diarrhea/constipation (1%), abdominal pain (1%), flatulence (1%)

Neuromuscular & skeletal: Paresthesia (2.9%)

Respiratory: Dyspnea (1.7% to 3.1%), nasal congestion (1.9% to 5.9%)

<1%: Angina (~1%), arthritis, blurred vision, bronchospasm, conjunctivitis, decreased libido, depression, epistaxis, flu-like symptoms, insomnia, myalgia, pharyngitis, polyuria, priapism, rash, sexual dysfunction, syncope, tinnitus

**Overdosage/Toxicology**

Signs and symptoms: Hypotension, drowsiness, shock (but very unusual)

Treatment: Hypotension usually responds to I.V. fluids or Trendelenburg positioning; if unresponsive to these measures, the use of a parenteral vasoconstrictor may be required; treatment is primarily supportive and symptomatic

**Drug Interactions**

ACE inhibitors: Hypotensive effect may be increased

Beta-blockers: Hypotensive effect may be increased

Calcium channel blockers: Hypotensive effect may be increased

NSAIDs may reduce antihypertensive efficacy

**Usual Dosage** Adults: Oral:

Hypertension: Initial: 1 mg at bedtime; slowly increase dose to achieve desired blood pressure, up to 20 mg/day; usual dose: 1-5 mg/day

Dosage reduction may be needed when adding a diuretic or other antihypertensive agent; if drug is discontinued for greater than several days, consider beginning with initial dose and retitrate as needed; dosage may be given on a twice daily regimen if response is diminished at 24 hours and hypotensive is observed at 2-4 hours following a dose

Benign prostatic hypertrophy: Initial: 1 mg at bedtime, increasing as needed; most patients require 10 mg day; if no response after 4-6 weeks of 10 mg/day, may increase to 20 mg/day

**Patient Information** Take as directed, at bedtime. Do not skip dose or discontinue without consulting prescriber. Follow recommended diet and exercise program. Do not use alcohol or OTC medications which may affect blood pressure (eg, cough or cold remedies, diet pills, "stay-awake" medications) without consulting physician. You may experience drowsiness, dizziness, or impaired judgment (use caution when driving or engaging in tasks that require alertness until response to drug is known); postural hypotension (use caution when rising from sitting or lying position or when climbing stairs); dry mouth or nausea (frequent mouth care or sucking lozenges may help); urinary incontinence (void before taking medication); or sexual dysfunction (reversible, may resolve with continued use). Report altered CNS status (eg, fatigue, lethargy, confusion, nervousness); sudden weight gain (weigh yourself in the same clothes at the same time of day once a week); unusual or persistent swelling of ankles, feet, or extremities; palpitations or rapid heartbeat; difficulty breathing; muscle weakness; or other persistent side effects.

**Dosage Forms**

Capsule: 1 mg, 2 mg, 5 mg, 10 mg
Tablet: 1 mg, 2 mg, 5 mg, 10 mg

## Terbinafine (TER bin a feen)

**U.S. Brand Names** Lamisil® AT™ Topical; Lamisil® Dermgel; Lamisil® Topical

**Pharmacologic Category** Antifungal Agent, Oral; Antifungal Agent, Topical

**Use** Active against most strains of *Trichophyton mentagrophytes, Trichophyton rubrum*; may be effective for infections of *Microsporum gypseum* and *M. nanum, Trichophyton verrucosum, Epidermophyton floccosum, Candida albicans,* and *Scopulariopsis brevicaulis*

Oral: Onychomycosis of the toenail or fingernail due to susceptible dermatophytes

Topical: Antifungal for the treatment of tinea pedis (athlete's foot), tinea cruris (jock itch), and tinea corporis (ringworm)

**Unlabeled use:** Topical: Cutaneous candidiasis and pityriasis versicolor

**Effects on Mental Status** None reported

**Effects on Psychiatric Treatment** None reported

**Pregnancy Risk Factor** B

**Contraindications** Hypersensitivity to terbinafine, naftifine or any component; pre-existing liver or renal disease (≤50 mL/minute GFR)

**Warnings/Precautions** While rare, the following complications have been reported and may require discontinuation of therapy: Changes in the ocular lens and retina, pancytopenia, neutropenia, Stevens-Johnson syndrome, toxic epidermal necrolysis. Discontinue if symptoms or signs of hepatobiliary dysfunction or cholestatic hepatitis develop. If irritation/sensitivity develop with topical use, discontinue therapy. **Use caution in writing and/or filling prescription/orders. Confusion between Lamictal® (lamotrigine) and Lamisil® (terbinafine) has occurred.**

**Adverse Reactions**

Oral: 1% to 10%:
- Central nervous system: Headache, dizziness, vertigo
- Dermatologic: Rash, pruritus, and alopecia with oral therapy
- Gastrointestinal: Nausea, diarrhea, dyspepsia, abdominal pain, appetite decrease, taste disturbance
- Hematologic: Neutropenia, lymphocytopenia
- Hepatic: Cholestasis, jaundice, hepatitis, liver enzyme elevations
- Ocular: Visual disturbance
- Miscellaneous: Allergic reaction

Topical: 1% to 10%:
- Dermatologic: Pruritus, contact dermatitis, irritation, burning, dryness
- Local: Irritation, stinging

**Overdosage/Toxicology**

Signs and symptoms; No information on human overdosage
Treatment: Symptomatic and supportive treatment is recommended

**Drug Interactions**

Decreased effect: Cyclosporine clearance is increased (~15%) with concomitant terbinafine; rifampin increases terbinafine clearance (100%)

Increased effect: Terbinafine clearance is decreased by cimetidine (33%) and terfenadine (16%); caffeine clearance is decreased by terfenadine (19%)

**Usual Dosage** Adults:

Oral:
- Superficial mycoses: Fingernail: 250 mg/day for up to 6 weeks; toenail: 250 mg/day for 12 weeks; doses may be given in two divided doses
- Systemic mycosis: 250-500 mg/day for up to 16 months

Topical Cream:
- Athlete's foot: Apply to affected area twice daily for at least 1 week, not to exceed 4 weeks
- Ringworm and jock itch: Apply to affected area once or twice daily for at least 1 week, not to exceed 4 weeks

Topical Gel:
- Tinea versicolor, tinea corporis and tinea pedis: Apply to affected area once daily for 7 days

**Dosing adjustment in renal impairment:** Although specific guidelines are not available, dose reduction in significant renal insufficiency (GFR <50 mL/minute) is recommended

**Patient Information** Topical: Avoid contact with eyes, nose, or mouth during treatment with cream; nursing mothers should not use on breast tissue; advise physician if eyes or skin becomes yellow or if irritation, itching, or burning develops. Do not use occlusive dressings concurrent with therapy. Full clinical effect may require several months due to the time required for a new nail to grow.

**Nursing Implications** Patients should not be considered therapeutic failures until they have been symptom-free for 2-4 weeks off following a course of treatment; GI complaints usually subside with continued administration

**Dosage Forms**

Cream: 1% (15 g, 30 g)
Tablet: 250 mg

## Terbutaline (ter BYOO ta leen)

**U.S. Brand Names** Brethaire®; Brethine®; Bricanyl®

**Pharmacologic Category** $Beta_2$ Agonist

**Use** Bronchodilator in reversible airway obstruction and bronchial asthma

**Effects on Mental Status** Restlessness and nervousness are common; may cause dizziness, drowsiness, or insomnia

**Effects on Psychiatric Treatment** Concurrent use with TCAs or MAOIs may increase toxicity

**Pregnancy Risk Factor** B

**Contraindications** Hypersensitivity to terbutaline or any component, cardiac arrhythmias associated with tachycardia, tachycardia caused by digitalis intoxication

**Warnings/Precautions** Excessive or prolonged use may lead to tolerance; paradoxical bronchoconstriction may occur with excessive use; if it occurs, discontinue terbutaline immediately

**Adverse Reactions**

>10%:
- Central nervous system: Nervousness, restlessness
- Neuromuscular & skeletal: Trembling

1% to 10%:
- Cardiovascular: Tachycardia, hypertension
- Central nervous system: Dizziness, drowsiness, headache, insomnia
- Gastrointestinal: Xerostomia, nausea, vomiting, bad taste in mouth
- Neuromuscular & skeletal: Muscle cramps, weakness
- Miscellaneous: Diaphoresis

<1%: Arrhythmias, chest pain, paradoxical bronchospasm

**Overdosage/Toxicology**

Signs and symptoms: Seizures, nausea, vomiting, tachycardia, cardiac dysrhythmias, hypokalemia

Treatment: In cases of overdose, supportive therapy should be instituted; prudent use of a cardioselective beta-adrenergic blocker (eg, atenolol or metoprolol) should be considered, keeping in mind the potential for induction of bronchoconstriction in an asthmatic individual. Dialysis has not been shown to be of value in the treatment of an overdose with this agent.

**Drug Interactions**

Decreased effect with beta-blockers
Increased toxicity with MAO inhibitors, TCAs

**Usual Dosage**

Children <12 years:
- Oral: Initial: 0.05 mg/kg/dose 3 times/day, increased gradually as required; maximum: 0.15 mg/kg/dose 3-4 times/day or a total of 5 mg/24 hours
- S.C.: 0.005-0.01 mg/kg/dose to a maximum of 0.3 mg/dose every 15-20 minutes for 3 doses
- Nebulization: 0.01-0.03 mg/kg/dose every 4-6 hours
- Inhalation: 1-2 inhalations every 4-6 hours

Children >12 years and Adults:
- Oral:
  - 12-15 years: 2.5 mg every 6 hours 3 times/day; not to exceed 7.5 mg in 24 hours
  - >15 years: 5 mg/dose every 6 hours 3 times/day; if side effects occur, reduce dose to 2.5 mg every 6 hours; not to exceed 15 mg in 24 hours
- S.C.: 0.25 mg/dose repeated in 15-30 minutes for one time only; a total dose of 0.5 mg should not be exceeded within a 4-hour period
- Nebulization: 0.01-0.03 mg/kg/dose every 4-6 hours
- Inhalation: 2 inhalations every 4-6 hours; wait 1 minute between inhalations

**Dosing adjustment/comments in renal impairment:**
- $Cl_{cr}$ 10-50 mL/minute: Administer at 50% of normal dose
- $Cl_{cr}$ <10 mL/minute: Avoid use

**Patient Information** Use exactly as directed. Do not use more often than recommended (excessive use may result in tolerance, overdose may result in serious adverse effects) and do not discontinue without consulting prescriber. Maintain adequate hydration (2-3 L/day of fluids unless instructed to restrict fluid intake). You may experience nervousness, dizziness, or fatigue (use caution when driving or engaging in tasks requiring alertness until response to drug is known); or dry mouth, stomach upset (frequent small meals, frequent mouth care, chewing gum, or sucking hard candy may help). Report unresolved GI upset; dizziness or fatigue; vision changes; chest pain, rapid heartbeat, or palpitations; insomnia, nervousness, or hyperactivity; muscle cramping, tremors, or pain; unusual cough; or rash (hypersensitivity).

(Continued)

## Terbutaline *(Continued)*

Preterm labor: Notify prescriber immediately if labor resumes or adverse side effects are noted.

**Administration:** Self-administered inhalation: Store canister upside down; do not freeze. Shake canister before using. Sit when using medication. Close eyes when administering terbutaline to avoid spray getting into eyes. Exhale slowly and completely through nose; inhale deeply through mouth while administering aerosol. Hold breath for 1-3 seconds after inhalation. Wait at least 1 full minute between inhalations. Wash mouthpiece between use. If more than one inhalation medication is used, use bronchodilator first and wait 5 minutes between medications.

**Dosage Forms**
Aerosol, oral, as sulfate: 0.2 mg/actuation (10.5 g)
Injection, as sulfate: 1 mg/mL (1 mL)
Tablet, as sulfate: 2.5 mg, 5 mg

## Terconazole (ter KONE a zole)

**U.S. Brand Names** Terazol® Vaginal
**Pharmacologic Category** Antifungal Agent, Vaginal
**Use** Local treatment of vulvovaginal candidiasis
**Effects on Mental Status** None reported
**Effects on Psychiatric Treatment** None reported
**Usual Dosage** Adults: Female: Insert 1 applicatorful intravaginally at bedtime for 7 consecutive days
**Dosage Forms**
Cream, vaginal: 0.4% (45 g); 0.8% (20 g)
Suppository, vaginal: 80 mg (3s)

## Terpin Hydrate and Codeine
(TER pin HYE drate & KOE deen)

**Synonyms** ETH and C
**Pharmacologic Category** Expectorant
**Use** Symptomatic relief of cough
**Effects on Mental Status** May cause drowsiness
**Effects on Psychiatric Treatment** Concurrent use with SSRIs may result in loss of pain control although evidence for this is not convincing; monitor
**Restrictions** C-V
**Pregnancy Risk Factor** C
**Adverse Reactions**
Central nervous system: Drowsiness
Gastrointestinal: Nausea, vomiting
**Usual Dosage** Based on codeine content
Adults: 10-20 mg/dose every 4-6 hours as needed
Children (not recommended): 1-1.5 mg/kg/24 hours divided every 4 hours; maximum: 30 mg/24 hours
2-6 years: 1.25-2.5 mL every 4-6 hours as needed
6-12 years: 2.5-5 mL every 4-6 hours as needed
**Patient Information** Drink plenty of fluid
**Dosage Forms** Elixir: Terpin hydrate 85 mg and codeine 10 mg per 5 mL with alcohol 42.5%


- **Terra-Cortril® Ophthalmic Suspension** *see* Oxytetracycline and Hydrocortisone *on page 417*
- **Terramycin® I.M. Injection** *see* Oxytetracycline *on page 416*
- **Terramycin® Ophthalmic Ointment** *see* Oxytetracycline and Polymyxin B *on page 417*
- **Terramycin® Oral** *see* Oxytetracycline *on page 416*
- **Terramycin® w/Polymyxin B Ophthalmic Ointment** *see* Oxytetracycline and Polymyxin B *on page 417*
- **Teslac®** *see* Testolactone *on page 536*
- **Tessalon® Perles** *see* Benzonatate *on page 62*
- **Testex®** *see* Testosterone *on page 536*
- **Testoderm® Transdermal System** *see* Testosterone *on page 536*


## Testolactone (tes toe LAK tone)

**U.S. Brand Names** Teslac®
**Pharmacologic Category** Androgen
**Use** Palliative treatment of advanced disseminated breast carcinoma
**Effects on Mental Status** None reported
**Effects on Psychiatric Treatment** None reported
**Restrictions** C-III
**Pregnancy Risk Factor** C
**Contraindications** In men for the treatment of breast cancer; known hypersensitivity to testolactone
**Warnings/Precautions** The U.S. Food and Drug Administration (FDA) currently recommends that procedures for proper handling and disposal of antineoplastic agents be considered. Use with caution in hepatic, renal, or cardiac disease; prolonged use may cause drug-induced hepatic disease; history or porphyria.
**Adverse Reactions** 1% to 10%:
Cardiovascular: Edema
Dermatologic: Maculopapular rash
Endocrine & metabolic: Hypercalcemia,
Gastrointestinal: Anorexia, diarrhea, nausea, edema of the tongue
Neuromuscular & skeletal: Paresthesias, peripheral neuropathies
**Drug Interactions** No data reported
**Usual Dosage** Adults: Female: Oral: 250 mg 4 times/day for at least 3 months; desired response may take as long as 3 months
**Patient Information** Take as directed; do not discontinue without consulting prescriber. Effectiveness of therapy may take several months. Maintain adequate fluid intake (2-3 L/day of fluids unless instructed to restrict fluid intake) and diet and exercise program recommended by prescriber. You may experience nausea or vomiting (small frequent meals, frequent mouth care, sucking lozenges, or chewing gum may help). Report fluid retention (swelling of ankles, feet, or hands; difficulty breathing or sudden weight gain); numbness, tingling, or swelling of fingers, toes, or face; skin rash, redness, or irritation; or other adverse reactions.
**Dosage Forms** Tablet: 50 mg


- **Testopel® Pellet** *see* Testosterone *on page 536*


## Testosterone (tes TOS ter one)

**U.S. Brand Names** Androderm® Transdermal System; AndroGel®; Andro-L.A.® Injection; Andropository® Injection; Delatest® Injection; Delatestryl® Injection; depAndro® Injection; Depotest® Injection; Depo®-Testosterone Injection; Duratest® Injection; Durathate® Injection; Everone® Injection; Histerone® Injection; Testex®; Testoderm® Transdermal System; Testopel® Pellet
**Synonyms** Aqueous Testosterone; Testosterone Cypionate; Testosterone Enanthate; Testosterone Propionate
**Pharmacologic Category** Androgen
**Use** Androgen replacement therapy in the treatment of delayed male puberty; postpartum breast pain and engorgement; inoperable breast cancer; male hypogonadism
**Effects on Mental Status** May cause anxiety, insomnia, aggressive behavior, or depression
**Effects on Psychiatric Treatment** May rarely cause neutropenia; use caution with clozapine and carbamazepine
**Restrictions** C-III
**Pregnancy Risk Factor** X
**Contraindications** Severe renal or cardiac disease, benign prostatic hypertrophy with obstruction, undiagnosed genital bleeding, males with carcinoma of the breast or prostate; hypersensitivity to testosterone or any component; pregnancy
**Warnings/Precautions** Perform radiographic examination of the hand and wrist every 6 months to determine the rate of bone maturation. May accelerate bone maturation without producing compensating gain in linear growth. Has both androgenic and anabolic activity, the anabolic action may enhance hypoglycemia. Prolonged use has been associated with serious hepatic effects (hepatitis, hepatic neoplasms, cholestatic hepatitis, jaundice). May potentiate sleep apnea in some male patients (obesity or chronic lung disease) or exacerbate heart failure due to fluid retention.
**Adverse Reactions**
>10%:
Dermatologic: Acne
Endocrine & metabolic: Menstrual problems (amenorrhea), virilism, breast soreness
Genitourinary: Epididymitis, priapism, bladder irritability
1% to 10%:
Cardiovascular: Flushing, edema
Central nervous system: Excitation, aggressive behavior, sleeplessness, anxiety, mental depression, headache
Dermatologic: Hirsutism (increase in pubic hair growth)
Gastrointestinal: Nausea, vomiting, GI irritation
Genitourinary: Prostatic hypertrophy, prostatic carcinoma, impotence, testicular atrophy
Hepatic: Hepatic dysfunction
<1%: Cholestatic hepatitis, gynecomastia, hepatic necrosis, hypercalcemia, hypersensitivity reactions, hypoglycemia, leukopenia, polycythemia, suppression of clotting factors
**Drug Interactions** CYP3A3/4 and 3A5-7 enzyme substrate
Increased toxicity: Effects of oral anticoagulants may be enhanced
**Usual Dosage**
Children: I.M.:
Male hypogonadism:
Initiation of pubertal growth: 40-50 mg/m$^2$/dose (cypionate or enanthate ester) monthly until the growth rate falls to prepubertal levels

Terminal growth phase: 100 mg/m²/dose (cypionate or enanthate ester) monthly until growth ceases

Maintenance virilizing dose: 100 mg/m²/dose (cypionate or enanthate ester) twice monthly

Delayed puberty: 40-50 mg/m²/dose monthly (cypionate or enanthate ester) for 6 months

Adults: Inoperable breast cancer: I.M.: 200-400 mg every 2-4 weeks

Male: Short-acting formulations: Testosterone Aqueous/Testosterone Propionate (in oil): I.M.:

Androgen replacement therapy: 10-50 mg 2-3 times/week

Male hypogonadism: 40-50 mg/m²/dose monthly until the growth rate falls to prepubertal levels (~5 cm/year); during terminal growth phase: 100 mg/m²/dose monthly until growth ceases; maintenance virilizing dose: 100 mg/m²/dose twice monthly or 50-400 mg/dose every 2-4 weeks

Male: Long-acting formulations: Testosterone enanthate (in oil)/testosterone cypionate (in oil): I.M.:

Male hypogonadism: 50-400 mg every 2-4 weeks

Male with delayed puberty: 50-200 mg every 2-4 weeks for a limited duration

Male ≥18 years: Transdermal: Primary hypogonadism **or** hypogonadotropic hypogonadism:

Testoderm®: Apply 6 mg patch daily to scrotum (if scrotum is inadequate, use a 4 mg daily system)

Testoderm-TSS®: Apply 5 mg patch daily to clean, dry area of skin on the arm, back or upper buttocks. **Do not apply Testoderm-TSS® to the scrotum**

Androderm®: Apply 2 systems nightly to clean, dry area on the back, abdomen, upper arms or thighs for 24 hours for a total of 5 mg/day

AndroGel®: Males >18 years of age: 5 g (to deliver 50 mg of testosterone) applied once daily (preferably in the morning) to clean, dry, intact skin of the shoulder and upper arms and/or abdomen. Upon opening the packet(s), the entire contents should be squeezed into the palm of the hand and immediately applied to the application site(s). Application sites should be allowed to dry for a few minutes prior to dressing. Hands should be washed with soap and water after application. **Do not apply AndroGel® to the genitals**

**Dosing adjustment/comments in hepatic disease:** Reduce dose

**Patient Information** Diabetics should monitor serum glucose closely and notify prescriber of changes; this medication may alter hypoglycemic requirements. You may experience acne, growth of body hair, loss of libido, impotence, or menstrual irregularity (usually reversible); nausea or vomiting (small frequent meals, frequent mouth care, sucking lozenges, or chewing gum may help). Report changes in menstrual pattern; enlarged or painful breasts; deepening of voice or unusual growth of body hair; persistent penile erection; fluid retention (swelling of ankles, feet, or hands, difficulty breathing or sudden weight gain); unresolved changes in CNS (nervousness, chills, insomnia, depression, aggressiveness); altered urinary patterns; change in color of urine or stool; yellowing of eyes or skin; unusual bruising or bleeding; or other persistent adverse reactions.

Topical: Apply to clean, dry scrotal skin. Dry shave scrotal hair for optimal skin contact. Do not use chemical depilatories.

**Nursing Implications** Warm injection to room temperature and shaking vial will help redissolve crystals that have formed after storage; administer by deep I.M. injection into the upper outer quadrant of the gluteus maximus. Transdermal system should be applied on clean, dry, scrotal skin. Dry-shave scrotal hair for optimal skin contact. Do not use chemical depilatories.

**Dosage Forms**

Injection:

Aqueous suspension: 25 mg/mL (10 mL, 30 mL); 50 mg/mL (10 mL, 30 mL); 100 mg/mL (10 mL, 30 mL)

In oil, as cypionate: 100 mg/mL (1 mL, 10 mL); 200 mg/mL (1 mL, 10 mL)

In oil, as enanthate: 100 mg/mL (1 mL, 5 mL, 10 mL); 200 mg/mL (1 mL, 5 mL, 10 mL)

In oil, as propionate: 100 mg/mL (10 mL, 30 mL)

Pellet: 75 mg (1 pellet per vial)

Transdermal system:

Androderm®: 2.5 mg/day; 5 mg/day

Testoderm®: 4 mg/day; 6 mg/day

Testoderm-TTS®: 5 mg/day


♦ **Testosterone Cypionate** *see* Testosterone *on page 536*

♦ **Testosterone Enanthate** *see* Testosterone *on page 536*

♦ **Testosterone Propionate** *see* Testosterone *on page 536*

♦ **Testred®** *see* Methyltestosterone *on page 360*


## Tetracaine (TET ra kane)

**U.S. Brand Names** Pontocaine®

**Canadian Brand Names** Ametop™

**Pharmacologic Category** Local Anesthetic

**Use** Spinal anesthesia; local anesthesia in the eye for various diagnostic and examination purposes; topically applied to nose and throat for various diagnostic procedures; **approximately 10 times more potent than procaine**

**Effects on Mental Status** None reported

**Effects on Psychiatric Treatment** None reported

**Usual Dosage** Maximum adult dose: 50 mg

Children: Safety and efficacy have not been established

Adults:

Ophthalmic (not for prolonged use):

Ointment: Apply ½" to 1" to lower conjunctival fornix

Solution: Instill 1-2 drops

Spinal anesthesia:

High, medium, low, and saddle blocks: 0.2% to 0.3% solution

Prolonged (2-3 hours): 1% solution

Subarachnoid injection: 5-20 mg

Saddle block: 2-5 mg; a 1% solution should be diluted with equal volume of CSF before administration

Topical mucous membranes (2% solution): Apply as needed; dose should not exceed 20 mg

Topical for skin: Ointment/cream: Apply to affected areas as needed

**Dosage Forms**

Cream, as hydrochloride: 1% (28 g)

Injection, as hydrochloride: 1% [10 mg/mL] (2 mL)

Injection, as hydrochloride, with dextrose 6%: 0.2% [2 mg/mL] (2 mL); 0.3% [3 mg/mL] (5 mL)

Ointment, as hydrochloride:

Ophthalmic: 0.5% [5 mg/mL] (3.75 g)

Topical: 0.5% [5 mg/mL] (28 g)

Powder for injection, as hydrochloride: 20 mg

Solution, as hydrochloride:

Ophthalmic: 0.5% [5 mg/mL] (1 mL, 2 mL, 15 mL, 59 mL)

Topical: 2% [20 mg/mL] (30 mL, 118 mL)

## Tetracycline (tet ra SYE kleen)

**U.S. Brand Names** Achromycin® Ophthalmic; Achromycin® Topical; Sumycin® Oral; Topicycline® Topical

**Canadian Brand Names** Apo®-Tetra; Novo-Tetra; Nu-Tetra

**Synonyms** TCN

**Pharmacologic Category** Antibiotic, Ophthalmic; Antibiotic, Tetracycline Derivative; Antibiotic, Topical

**Use** Treatment of susceptible bacterial infections of both gram-positive and gram-negative organisms; also infections due to *Mycoplasma*, *Chlamydia*, and *Rickettsia*; indicated for acne, exacerbations of chronic bronchitis, and treatment of gonorrhea and syphilis in patients that are allergic to penicillin; used concomitantly with metronidazole, bismuth subsalicylate and an $H_2$-antagonist for the treatment of duodenal ulcer disease induced by *H. pylori*

**Effects on Mental Status** None reported

**Effects on Psychiatric Treatment** Tetracycline may decrease lithium clearance resulting in an increase in serum lithium levels and potential lithium toxicity although the clinical significance is likely minimal; monitor serum lithium levels

**Pregnancy Risk Factor** D; B (topical)

**Contraindications** Hypersensitivity to tetracycline or any component; do not administer to children ≤8 years of age

**Warnings/Precautions** Use of tetracyclines during tooth development may cause permanent discoloration of the teeth and enamel, hypoplasia and retardation of skeletal development and bone growth with risk being the greatest for children <4 years and those receiving high doses; use with caution in patients with renal or hepatic impairment (eg, elderly) and in pregnancy; dosage modification required in patients with renal impairment since it may increase BUN as an antianabolic agent; pseudotumor cerebri has been reported with tetracycline use (usually resolves with discontinuation); outdated drug can cause nephropathy; superinfection possible; use protective measure to avoid photosensitivity

**Adverse Reactions**

>10%: Gastrointestinal: Discoloration of teeth and enamel hypoplasia (young children)

1% to 10%:

Dermatologic: Photosensitivity

Gastrointestinal: Nausea, diarrhea

<1%: Abdominal cramps, acute renal failure, anaphylaxis, anorexia, antibiotic-associated pseudomembranous colitis, azotemia, bulging fontanels in infants, candidal superinfection, dermatologic effects, diabetes insipidus syndrome, esophagitis, exfoliative dermatitis, hepatotoxicity, hypersensitivity reactions, increased intracranial pressure, paresthesia, pericarditis, pigmentation of nails, pruritus, pseudotumor cerebri, renal damage, staphylococcal enterocolitis, superinfections, thrombophlebitis, vomiting

**Overdosage/Toxicology**

Signs and symptoms: Nausea, anorexia, diarrhea;

Treatment: Following GI decontamination, supportive care only

**Drug Interactions**

Decreased effect: Calcium-, magnesium-, or aluminum-containing antacids, oral contraceptives, iron, zinc, sodium bicarbonate, penicillins, cimetidine may decrease tetracycline absorption

(Continued)

## Tetracycline *(Continued)*

Although no clinical evidence exists, may bind with bismuth or calcium carbonate, an excipient in bismuth subsalicylate, during treatment for *H. pylori*

Increased toxicity: Methoxyflurane anesthesia when concurrent with tetracycline may cause fatal nephrotoxicity; warfarin with tetracyclines may result in increased anticoagulation; tetracyclines may rarely increase digoxin serum levels

**Usual Dosage**

Children >8 years: Oral: 25-50 mg/kg/day in divided doses every 6 hours

Children >8 years and Adults:

Ophthalmic:

Ointment: Instill every 2-12 hours

Suspension: Instill 1-2 drops 2-4 times/day or more often as needed

Topical: Apply to affected areas 1-4 times/day

Adults: Oral: 250-500 mg/dose every 6 hours

*Helicobacter pylori*: Clinically effective treatment regimens include triple therapy with amoxicillin or tetracycline, metronidazole, and bismuth subsalicylate; amoxicillin, metronidazole, and $H_2$-receptor antagonist; or double therapy with amoxicillin and omeprazole. Adult dose: 850 mg 3 times/day to 500 mg 4 times/day

**Dosing interval in renal impairment:**

$Cl_{cr}$ 50-80 mL/minute: Administer every 8-12 hours

$Cl_{cr}$ 10-50 mL/minute: Administer every 12-24 hours

$Cl_{cr}$ <10 mL/minute: Administer every 24 hours

Dialysis: Slightly dialyzable (5% to 20%) via hemo- and peritoneal dialysis nor via continuous arteriovenous or venovenous hemofiltration (CAVH/CAVHD); no supplemental dosage necessary

**Dosing adjustment in hepatic impairment:** Avoid use or maximum dose is 1 g/day

**Dietary Considerations** Food: Dairy products decrease effect of tetracycline

**Patient Information** Take this medication exactly as directed. Take all of the prescription even if you see an improvement in your condition. Do not use more or more often than recommended.

Oral: Preferable to take on an empty stomach (1 hour before or 2 hours after meals). Take at regularly scheduled times, around-the-clock. Avoid antacids, iron, or dairy products within 2 hours of taking tetracycline. You may experience photosensitivity (use sunscreen, wear protective clothing and eyewear, and avoid direct sunlight); dizziness or lightheadedness (use caution when driving or engaging in tasks requiring alertness until response to drug is known); nausea/vomiting (frequent small meals, frequent mouth care, chewing gum, or sucking lozenges may help). Effect of oral contraceptives may be reduced; use barrier contraception. Report rash or intense itching, yellowing of skin or eyes, fever or chills, blackened stool, vaginal itching or discharge, foul-smelling stools, excessive thirst or urination, acute headache, unresolved diarrhea, difficulty breathing, condition does not improve, or worsening of condition.

Ophthalmic: Sit down, tilt head back, instill solution or drops inside lower eyelid, and roll eyeball in all directions. Close eye and apply gentle pressure to inner corner of eye for 30 seconds. Do not touch tip of applicator to eye or any contaminated surface. May experience temporary stinging or blurred vision. Inform prescriber if condition worsens or does not improve in 3-4 days.

Topical: Wash area and pat dry (unless contraindicated). Avoid getting in mouth or eyes. You may experience temporary stinging or burning which will resolve quickly. Treated skin may turn yellow; this will wash off. May stain clothing (permanent). Report rash. Inform prescriber if condition worsens or does not improve in a few days.

**Dosage Forms**

Capsule, as hydrochloride: 100 mg, 250 mg, 500 mg

Ointment:

Ophthalmic: 1% [10 mg/mL] (3.5 g)

Topical, as hydrochloride: 3% [30 mg/mL] (14.2 g, 30 g)

Solution, topical: 2.2 mg/mL (70 mL)

Suspension:

Ophthalmic: 1% [10 mg/mL] (0.5 mL, 1 mL, 4 mL)

Oral, as hydrochloride: 125 mg/5 mL (60 mL, 480 mL)

Tablet, as hydrochloride: 250 mg, 500 mg


♦ **Tetrahydro-2-para-sulfamoylphenyl-1,2-thiazine 1,1 dioxide** *see* Sulthiame *on page 527*

♦ **Tetrahydroaminoacrine** *see* Tacrine *on page 529*

♦ **Tetrahydrocannabinol** *see* Dronabinol *on page 187*


## Tetrahydrozoline (tet ra hye DROZ a leen)

**U.S. Brand Names** Collyrium Fresh® Ophthalmic [OTC]; Eyesine® Ophthalmic [OTC]; Geneye® Ophthalmic [OTC]; Mallazine® Eye Drops [OTC]; Murine® Plus Ophthalmic [OTC]; Optigene® Ophthalmic [OTC]; Tetrasine® Extra Ophthalmic [OTC]; Tetrasine® Ophthalmic [OTC]; Tyzine® Nasal; Visine® Extra Ophthalmic [OTC]

**Pharmacologic Category** Adrenergic Agonist Agent; Ophthalmic Agent, Vasoconstrictor

**Use** Symptomatic relief of nasal congestion and conjunctival congestion

**Effects on Mental Status** None reported

**Effects on Psychiatric Treatment** MAO inhibitors can cause an exaggerated adrenergic response if taken concurrently or within 21 days of discontinuing MAO inhibitor; beta-blockers can cause hypertensive episodes and increased risk of intracranial hemorrhage

**Usual Dosage**

Nasal congestion: Intranasal:

Children 2-6 years: Instill 2-3 drops of 0.05% solution every 4-6 hours as needed, no more frequent than every 3 hours

Children >6 years and Adults: Instill 2-4 drops or 3-4 sprays of 0.1% solution every 3-4 hours as needed, no more frequent than every 3 hours

Conjunctival congestion: Ophthalmic: Adults: Instill 1-2 drops in each eye 2-4 times/day

**Dosage Forms** Solution, as hydrochloride:

Nasal: 0.05% (15 mL), 0.1% (30 mL, 473 mL)

Ophthalmic: 0.05% (15 mL)


♦ **Tetrasine® Extra Ophthalmic [OTC]** *see* Tetrahydrozoline *on page 538*

♦ **Tetrasine® Ophthalmic [OTC]** *see* Tetrahydrozoline *on page 538*

♦ ***Teucrium chamaedrys*** *see* Germander *on page 249*

♦ **Teveten®** *see* Eprosartan *on page 198*

♦ **TG** *see* Thioguanine *on page 542*

♦ **6-TG** *see* Thioguanine *on page 542*

♦ **T-Gen®** *see* Trimethobenzamide *on page 569*

♦ **T-Gesic®** *see* Hydrocodone and Acetaminophen *on page 272*

♦ **THA** *see* Tacrine *on page 529*


## Thalidomide (tha LI doe mide)

**U.S. Brand Names** Contergan®; Distaval®; Kevadon®; Thalomid®

**Pharmacologic Category** Immunosuppressant Agent

**Use** Treatment of erythema nodosum leprosum

**Orphan status:** Crohn's disease

**Unlabeled use:** Treatment or prevention of graft-versus-host reactions after bone marrow transplantation; in aphthous ulceration in HIV-positive patients; Langerhans cell histiocytosis, Behçet's syndrome; hypnotic agent; also may be effective in rheumatoid arthritis, discoid lupus, and erythema multiforme; useful in type 2 lepra reactions, but not type 1; can assist in healing mouth ulcers in AIDS patients; Crohn's disease, renal cell carcinoma, multiple myeloma, myeloma, Waldenström's macroglobulinemia

**Effects on Mental Status** Sedation is common; may cause dizziness, nervousness, insomnia or agitation

**Effects on Psychiatric Treatment** May cause leukopenia; use caution with clozapine and carbamazepine; concurrent use with other psychotropics may produce additive sedation

**Restrictions** Thalidomide is approved for marketing only under a special distribution program. This program, called the "System for Thalidomide Education and Prescribing Safety" (STEPS), has been approved by the FDA. Prescribing and dispensing of thalidomide is restricted to prescribers and pharmacists registered with the program.

**Pregnancy Risk Factor** X

**Contraindications** Pregnancy or women in childbearing years, neuropathy (peripheral), thalidomide hypersensitivity

**Warnings/Precautions** Liver, hepatic, neurological disorders, constipation, congestive heart failure, hypertension

**Adverse Reactions** Percentage unknown: Alopecia, amenorrhea, clonus, constipation, dizziness, edema, fever, headache, irritability, lethargy, leukopenia, myoclonus, nausea, pruritus, sensory neuropathy (peripheral) (after prolonged therapy due to neuronal degeneration), sexual dysfunction, sinus tachycardia, tachycardia, vomiting, xerostomia

**Drug Interactions** Other medications known to cause peripheral neuropathy should be used with caution in patients receiving thalidomide; thalidomide may enhance the sedative activity of other drugs such as ethanol, barbiturates, reserpine, and chlorpromazine

**Usual Dosage**

Leprosy: Up to 400 mg/day; usual maintenance dose: 50-100 mg/day

Behçet's syndrome: 100-400 mg/day

Graft-vs-host reactions:

Children: 3 mg/kg 4 times/day

Adults: 100-1600 mg/day; usual initial dose: 200 mg 4 times/day for use up to 700 days

AIDS-related aphthous stomatitis: 200 mg twice daily for 5 days, then 200 mg/day for up to 8 weeks

Discoid lupus erythematosus: 100-400 mg/day; maintenance dose: 25-50 mg

**Patient Information** You will be given oral and written instructions about the necessity of using two methods of contraception and and the necessity of keeping return visits for pregnancy testing. You may experience sleepiness, dizziness, lack of concentration (use caution when driving, climbing stairs, or engaging in tasks requiring alertness until response to drug is known); nausea or vomiting or loss of appetite (small frequent meals, frequent mouth care, chewing gum, or sucking lozenges may help); constipation or diarrhea; oral thrush (frequent mouth care is necessary); sexual dysfunction (reversible). Report any of the above if persistent or severe. Report chest pain or palpitations or swelling of extremities; back, neck, or muscle pain or stiffness; skin rash or eruptions; increased nervousness, anxiety, or insomnia; or any other symptom of adverse reactions.

**Dosage Forms** Capsule: 50 mg (boxes contain 6 prescription packs of 14 capsules each)


- **Thalitone®** *see* Chlorthalidone *on page 119*
- **Thalomid®** *see* Thalidomide *on page 538*
- **THAM-E® Injection** *see* Tromethamine *on page 574*
- **THAM® Injection** *see* Tromethamine *on page 574*
- **THC** *see* Dronabinol *on page 187*
- **Theo-24®** *see* Theophylline Salts *on page 539*
- **Theobid®** *see* Theophylline Salts *on page 539*
- **Theochron®** *see* Theophylline Salts *on page 539*
- **Theoclear® L.A.** *see* Theophylline Salts *on page 539*
- **Theo-Dur®** *see* Theophylline Salts *on page 539*
- **Theo-Dur® Sprinkle** *see* Theophylline Salts *on page 539*
- **Theolair™** *see* Theophylline Salts *on page 539*
- **Theon®** *see* Theophylline Salts *on page 539*
- **Theophylline** *see* Theophylline Salts *on page 539*


## Theophylline and Guaifenesin

(thee OF i lin & gwye FEN e sin)

**U.S. Brand Names** Bronchial®; Glycerol-T®; Quibron®; Slo-Phyllin® GG

**Pharmacologic Category** Theophylline Derivative

**Use** Symptomatic treatment of bronchospasm associated with bronchial asthma, chronic bronchitis and pulmonary emphysema

**Effects on Mental Status** May cause nervousness, agitation, restlessness, insomnia, or dizziness

**Effects on Psychiatric Treatment** Barbiturates and carbamazepine may decrease serum levels while disulfiram, propranolol and fluvoxamine may raise theophylline levels

**Usual Dosage** Adults: Oral: 16 mg/kg/day or 400 mg theophylline/day, in divided doses, every 6-8 hours

**Dosage Forms**

Capsule: Theophylline 150 mg and guaifenesin 90 mg; theophylline 300 mg and guaifenesin 180 mg

Elixir: Theophylline 150 mg and guaifenesin 90 mg per 15 mL (480 mL)

## Theophylline, Ephedrine, and Hydroxyzine

(thee OF i lin, e FED rin, & hye DROKS i zeen)

**U.S. Brand Names** Hydrophed®; Marax®

**Pharmacologic Category** Theophylline Derivative

**Use** Possibly effective for controlling bronchospastic disorders

**Effects on Mental Status** May cause nervousness, agitation, restlessness, anxiety, insomnia, or dizziness

**Effects on Psychiatric Treatment** Barbiturates and carbamazepine may decrease serum levels while disulfiram, propranolol and fluvoxamine may raise theophylline levels; use with MAOIs may produce hypertensive crisis; avoid combination; concurrent use with psychotropics may produce additive anticholinergic effects

**Usual Dosage**

Children:

2-5 years: 1/2 tablet 2-4 times/day or 2.5 mL 3-4 times/day

>5 years: 1/2 tablet 2-4 times/day or 5 mL 3-4 times/day

Adults: 1 tablet 2-4 times/day

**Dosage Forms**

Syrup, dye free: Theophylline 32.5 mg, ephedrine 6.25 mg, and hydroxyzine 2.5 mg per 5 mL

Tablet: Theophylline 130 mg, ephedrine 25 mg, and hydroxyzine 10 mg

## Theophylline, Ephedrine, and Phenobarbital

(thee OF i lin, e FED rin, & fee noe BAR bi tal)

**U.S. Brand Names** Tedral®

**Pharmacologic Category** Theophylline Derivative

**Use** Prevention and symptomatic treatment of bronchial asthma; relief of asthmatic bronchitis and other bronchospastic disorders

**Effects on Mental Status** May cause nervousness, agitation, restlessness, anxiety, insomnia, or dizziness

**Effects on Psychiatric Treatment** Carbamazepine may decrease serum levels while disulfiram, propranolol and fluvoxamine may raise theophylline levels; use with MAOIs may produce hypertensive crisis; avoid combination; concurrent use with psychotropics may produce additive anticholinergic effects

**Usual Dosage**

Children >60 lb: 1 tablet or 5 mL every 4 hours

Adults: 1-2 tablets or 10-20 mL every 4 hours

**Dosage Forms**

Suspension: Theophylline 65 mg, ephedrine sulfate 12 mg, and phenobarbital 4 mg per 5 mL

Tablet: Theophylline 118 mg, ephedrine sulfate 25 mg, and phenobarbital 11 mg; theophylline 130 mg, ephedrine sulfate 24 mg, and phenobarbital 8 mg

## Theophylline Salts (thee OFF i lin salts)

**Related Information**

Serum Drug Concentrations Commonly Monitored: Guidelines *on page 759*

**U.S. Brand Names** Aerolate®; Aerolate III®; Aerolate JR®; Aerolate SR®; Aminophyllin™; Aquaphyllin®; Asmalix®; Bronkodyl®; Choledyl®; Constant-T®; Duraphyl™; Elixophyllin®; Elixophyllin® SR; LaBID®; Phyllocontin®; Quibron®-T; Quibron®-T/SR; Respbid®; Slo-bid™; Slo-Phyllin®; Sustaire®; Theo-24®; Theobid®; Theochron®; Theoclear® L.A.; Theo-Dur®; Theo-Dur® Sprinkle; Theolair™; Theon®; Theospan®-SR; Theovent®; Truphylline®

**Synonyms** Aminophylline; Choline Theophyllinate; Ethylenediamine; Oxtriphylline; Theophylline

**Pharmacologic Category** Theophylline Derivative

**Use** Bronchodilator in reversible airway obstruction due to asthma, chronic bronchitis, and emphysema; for neonatal apnea/bradycardia

**Effects on Mental Status** May cause nervousness, dizziness, agitation, or insomnia

**Effects on Psychiatric Treatment** Barbiturates and carbamazepine may decrease theophylline levels; propranolol and disulfiram may increase theophylline levels

**Pregnancy Risk Factor** C

**Contraindications** Uncontrolled arrhythmias, hyperthyroidism, peptic ulcers, uncontrolled seizure disorders, hypersensitivity to xanthines or any component

**Warnings/Precautions** Use with caution in patients with peptic ulcer, hyperthyroidism, hypertension, tachyarrhythmias, and patients with compromised cardiac function; do not inject I.V. solution faster than 25 mg/minute; elderly, acutely ill, and patients with severe respiratory problems, pulmonary edema, or liver dysfunction are at greater risk of toxicity because of reduced drug clearance

Although there is a great intersubject variability for half-lives of methylxanthines (2-10 hours), elderly as a group have slower hepatic clearance. Therefore, use lower initial doses and monitor closely for response and adverse reactions. Additionally, elderly are at greater risk for toxicity due to concomitant disease (eg, CHF, arrhythmias), and drug use (eg, cimetidine, ciprofloxacin, etc).

**Adverse Reactions** See table.

| Theophylline Serum Levels (mcg/mL)* | Adverse Reactions |
|---|---|
| 15-25 | GI upset, diarrhea, N/V, abdominal pain, nervousness, headache, insomnia, agitation, dizziness, muscle cramp, tremor |
| 25-35 | Tachycardia, occasional PVC |
| >35 | Ventricular tachycardia, frequent PVC, seizure |

*Adverse effects do not necessarily occur according to serum levels. Arrhythmia and seizure can occur without seeing the other adverse effects.

**Uncommon at serum theophylline concentrations ≤20 mcg/mL**

1% to 10%:

Cardiovascular: Tachycardia

Central nervous system: Nervousness, restlessness

Gastrointestinal: Nausea, vomiting

<1%: Allergic reactions, gastric irritation, insomnia, irritability, rash, seizures, tremor

**Overdosage/Toxicology**

Signs and symptoms: Tachycardia, extrasystoles, nausea, vomiting, anorexia, tonic-clonic seizures, insomnia, circulatory failure; agitation, irritability, headache

Treatment: If seizures have not occurred, induce vomiting; ipecac syrup is preferred. Do not induce emesis in the presence of impaired consciousness. Repeated doses of charcoal have been shown to be effective in enhancing the total body clearance of theophylline. Do not repeat charcoal doses if an ileus is present. Charcoal hemoperfusion may be considered if the serum theophylline level exceed 40 mcg/mL, the patient

(Continued)

## Theophylline Salts *(Continued)*

is unable to tolerate repeat oral charcoal administrations, or if severe toxic symptoms are present. Clearance with hemoperfusion is better than clearance from hemodialysis. Administer a cathartic, especially if sustained release agents were used. Phenobarbital administered prophylactically may prevent seizures.

**Drug Interactions** CYP1A2 and 3A3/4 enzyme substrate, CYP2E enzyme substrate (minor)

Decreased effect/increased toxicity: Changes in diet may affect the elimination of theophylline; charcoal-broiled foods may increase elimination, reducing half-life by 50%; see table for factors affecting serum levels.

### Factors Reported to Affect Theophylline Serum Levels

| Decreased Theophylline Level | Increased Theophylline Level |
|---|---|
| Aminoglutethimide | Allopurinol (>600 mg/d) |
| Barbiturates | Beta-blockers |
| Carbamazepine | Calcium channel blockers |
| Charcoal | Carbamazepine |
| High protein/low carbohydrate diet | CHF |
| Hydantoins | Cimetidine |
| Isoniazid | Ciprofloxacin |
| I.V. isoproterenol | Cor pulmonale |
| Ketoconazole | Corticosteroids |
| Loop diuretics | Disulfiram |
| Phenobarbital | Ephedrine |
| Phenytoin | Erythromycin |
| Rifampin | Fever/viral illness |
| Smoking (cigarettes, marijuana) | Hepatic cirrhosis |
| Sulfinpyrazone | Influenza virus vaccine |
| Sympathomimetics | Interferon |
| | Isoniazid |
| | Loop diuretics |
| | Macrolides |
| | Mexiletine |
| | Oral contraceptives |
| | Propranolol |
| | Quinolones |
| | Thiabendazole |
| | Thyroid hormones |
| | Troleandomycin |

**Usual Dosage** Use ideal body weight for obese patients

Neonates:

**Apnea of prematurity:** Oral, I.V.: Loading dose: 4 mg/kg (theophylline); 5 mg/kg (aminophylline)

There appears to be a delay in theophylline elimination in infants <1 year of age, especially neonates; both the initial dose and maintenance dosage should be conservative

I.V.: Initial: Maintenance infusion rates:

Neonates:

≤24 days: 0.08 mg/kg/hour theophylline

>24 days: 0.12 mg/kg/hour theophylline

Infants 6-52 weeks: 0.008 (age in weeks) + 0.21 mg/kg/hour theophylline

Children >1 year and Adults:

**Treatment of acute bronchospasm**: I.V.: Loading dose (in patients not currently receiving aminophylline or theophylline): 6 mg/kg (based on aminophylline) given I.V. over 20-30 minutes; administration rate should not exceed 25 mg/minute (aminophylline). See table.

**Approximate I.V. maintenance dosages are based upon continuous infusions**; bolus dosing (often used in children <6 months of age) may be determined by multiplying the hourly infusion rate by 24 hours and dividing by the desired number of doses/day; see table.

Dosage should be adjusted according to serum level measurements during the first 12- to 24-hour period; see table.

### Maintenance Dose for Acute Symptoms

| Population Group | Oral Theophylline (mg/kg/day) | I.V. Aminophylline |
|---|---|---|
| Premature infant or newborn - 6 wk (for apnea/bradycardia) | 4 | 5 mg/kg/day |
| 6 wk - 6 mo | 10 | 12 mg/kg/day or continuous I.V. infusion* |
| Infants 6 mo - 1 y | 12-18 | 15 mg/kg/day or continuous I.V. infusion* |
| Children 1-9 y | 20-24 | 1 mg/kg/h |
| Children 9-12 y, and adolescent daily smokers of cigarettes or marijuana, and otherwise healthy adult smokers <50 y | 16 | 0.9 mg/kg/h |
| Adolescents 12-16 y (nonsmokers) | 13 | 0.7 mg/kg/h |
| Otherwise healthy nonsmoking adults (including elderly patients) | 10 (not to exceed 900 mg/day) | 0.5 mg/kg/h |
| Cardiac decompensation, cor pulmonale and/or liver dysfunction | 5 (not to exceed 400 mg/day) | 0.25 mg/kg/h |

*For continuous I.V. infusion divide total daily dose by 24 = mg/kg/h.

### Approximate I.V. Theophylline Dosage for Treatment of Acute Bronchospasm

| Group | Dosage for Next 12 h* | Dosage After 12 h* |
|---|---|---|
| Infants 6 wk - 6 mo | 0.5 mg/kg/h | |
| Children 6 mo - 1 y | 0.6-0.7 mg/kg/h | |
| Children 1-9 y | 0.95 mg/kg/h (1.2 mg/kg/h) | 0.79 mg/kg/h (1 mg/kg/h) |
| Children 9-16 y and young adult smokers | 0.79 mg/kg/h (1 mg/kg/h) | 0.63 mg/kg/h (0.8 mg/kg/h) |
| Healthy, nonsmoking adults | 0.55 mg/kg/h (0.7 mg/kg/h) | 0.39 mg/kg/h (0.5 mg/kg/h) |
| Older patients and patients with cor pulmonale | 0.47 mg/kg/h (0.6 mg/kg/h) | 0.24 mg/kg/h (0.3 mg/kg/h) |
| Patients with congestive heart failure or liver failure | 0.39 mg/kg/h (0.5 mg/kg/h) | 0.08-0.16 mg/kg/h (0.1-0.2 mg/kg/h) |

*Equivalent hydrous aminophylline dosage indicated in parentheses.

### Dosage Adjustment After Serum Theophylline Measurement

| Serum Theophylline | | Guidelines |
|---|---|---|
| Within normal limits | 10-20 mcg/mL | Maintain dosage if tolerated. Recheck serum theophylline concentration at 6- to 12-month intervals.* |
| Too high | 20-25 mcg/mL | Decrease doses by about 10%. Recheck serum theophylline concentration after 3 days and then at 6- to 12-month intervals.* |
| | 25-30 mcg/mL | Skip next dose and decrease subsequent doses by about 25%. Recheck serum theophylline. |
| | >30 mcg/mL | Skip next 2 doses and decrease subsequent doses by 50%. Recheck serum theophylline. |
| Too low | 7.5-10 mcg/mL | Increase dose by about 25%.† Recheck serum theophylline concentration after 3 days and then at 6- to 12-month intervals.* |
| | 5-7.5 mcg/mL | Increase dose by about 25% to the nearest dose increment† and recheck serum theophylline for guidance in further dosage adjustment (another increase will probably be needed, but this provides a safety check). |

*Finer adjustments in dosage may be needed for some patients.

†Dividing the daily dose into 3 doses administered at 8-hour intervals may be indicated if symptoms occur repeatedly at the end of a dosing interval.

From Weinberger M and Hendeles L, "Practical Guide to UsingTheophylline," *J Resp Dis*, 1981,2:12-27.

**Oral theophylline:** Initial dosage recommendation: Loading dose (to achieve a serum level of about 10 mcg/mL; loading doses should be given using a rapidly absorbed oral product **not** a sustained release product):

If no theophylline has been administered in the previous 24 hours: 4-6 mg/kg theophylline

If theophylline has been administered in the previous 24 hours: administer $^1/_2$ loading dose or 2-3 mg/kg theophylline can be given in emergencies when serum levels are not available

On the average, for every 1 mg/kg theophylline given, blood levels will rise 2 mcg/mL

Ideally, defer the loading dose if a serum theophylline concentration can be obtained rapidly. However, if this is not possible, exercise clinical judgment. If the patient is not experiencing theophylline toxicity, this is unlikely to result in dangerous adverse effects.

### Oral Theophylline Dosage for Bronchial Asthma*

| Age | Initial 3 Days | Second 3 Days | Steady-State Maintenance |
|---|---|---|---|
| <1 y | 0.2 x (age in weeks) + 5 | | 0.3 x (age in weeks) + 8 |
| 1-9 y | 16 up to a maximum of 400 mg/24 h | 20 | 22 |
| 9-12 y | 16 up to a maximum of 400 mg/24 h | 16 up to a maximum of 600 mg/24 h | 20 up to a maximum of 800 mg/24 h |
| 12-16 y | 16 up to a maximum of 400 mg/24 h | 16 up to a maximum of 600 mg/24 h | 18 up to a maximum of 900 mg/24 h |
| Adults | 400 mg/24 h | 600 mg/24 h | 900 mg/24 h |

*Dose in mg/kg/24 hours of theophylline.

**Increasing dose:** The dosage may be increased in approximately 25% increments at 2- to 3-day intervals so long as the drug is tolerated or until the maximum dose is reached

**Maintenance dose:** In newborns and infants, a fast-release oral product can be used. The total daily dose can be divided every 12 hours in newborns and every 6-8 hours in infants. In children and healthy adults, a slow-release product can be used. The total daily dose can be divided every 8-12 hours.

These recommendations, based on mean clearance rates for age or risk factors, were calculated to achieve a serum level of 10 mcg/mL (5 mcg/mL for newborns with apnea/bradycardia)

Dosage should be adjusted according to serum level

**Oral oxtriphylline:**

Children 1-9 years: 6.2 mg/kg/dose every 6 hours

Children 9-16 years and Adult smokers: 4.7 mg/kg/dose every 6 hours

Adult nonsmokers: 4.7 mg/kg/dose every 8 hours

Dose should be further adjusted based on serum levels

**Dosing adjustment/comments in hepatic disease:** Higher incidence of toxic effects including seizures in cirrhosis; plasma levels should be monitored closely during long-term administration in cirrhosis and during acute hepatitis, with dose adjustment as necessary

Hemodialysis: Administer dose posthemodialysis or administer supplemental 50% dose

Peritoneal dialysis: Supplemental dose is not necessary

Continuous arteriovenous or venovenous hemodiafiltration (CAVH/CAVHD) effects: Supplemental dose is not necessary

**Patient Information** Oral preparations should be taken with a full glass of water; capsule forms may be opened and sprinkled on soft foods; do not chew beads; notify physician if nausea, vomiting, severe GI pain, restlessness, or irregular heartbeat occurs; do not drink or eat large quantities of caffeine-containing beverages or food (colas, coffee, chocolate); remain in bed for 15-20 minutes after inserting suppository; do not chew or crush enteric coated or sustained release products; take at regular intervals; notify physician if insomnia, nervousness, irritability, palpitations, seizures occur; do not change brands or doses without consulting physician

**Nursing Implications** Do not crush sustained release drug products; do not crush enteric coated drug product; encourage patient to drink adequate fluids (2 L/day) to decrease mucous viscosity

**Dosage Forms**

Aminophylline (79% theophylline):

- Injection: 25 mg/mL (10 mL, 20 mL); 250 mg (equivalent to 187 mg theophylline) per 10 mL; 500 mg (equivalent to 394 mg theophylline) per 20 mL
- Liquid, oral: 105 mg (equivalent to 90 mg theophylline) per 5 mL (240 mL, 500 mL)
- Suppository, rectal: 250 mg (equivalent to 198 mg theophylline); 500 mg (equivalent to 395 mg theophylline)
- Tablet: 100 mg (equivalent to 79 mg theophylline); 200 mg (equivalent to 158 mg theophylline)
- Tablet, controlled release: 225 mg (equivalent to 178 mg theophylline)

Oxtriphylline (64% theophylline):

- Elixir: 100 mg (equivalent to 64 mg theophylline)/5 mL (5 mL, 10 mL, 473 mL)
- Syrup: 50 mg (equivalent to 32 mg theophylline)/5 mL (473 mL)
- Tablet: 100 mg (equivalent to 64 mg theophylline); 200 mg (equivalent to 127 mg theophylline)
- Tablet, sustained release: 400 mg (equivalent to 254 mg theophylline); 600 mg (equivalent to 382 mg theophylline)

Theophylline:

- Capsule:
  - Immediate release: 100 mg, 200 mg
  - Sustained release (8-12 hours): 50 mg, 60 mg, 65 mg, 75 mg, 100 mg, 125 mg, 130 mg, 200 mg, 250 mg, 260 mg, 300 mg
  - Timed release (12 hours): 50 mg, 75 mg, 125 mg, 130 mg, 200 mg, 250 mg, 260 mg
  - Timed release (24 hours): 100 mg, 200 mg, 300 mg
- Injection: Theophylline in 5% dextrose: 200 mg/container (50 mL, 100 mL); 400 mg/container (100 mL, 250 mL, 500 mL, 1000 mL); 800 mg/container (250 mL, 500 mL, 1000 mL)
- Elixir, oral: 80 mg/15 mL (15 mL, 30 mL, 500 mL, 4000 mL)
- Solution, oral: 80 mg/15 mL (15 mL, 18.75 mL, 30 mL, 120 mL, 500 mL, 4000 mL); 150 mg/15 mL (480 mL)
- Syrup, oral: 80 mg/15 mL (5 mL, 15 mL, 30 mL, 120 mL, 500 mL, 4000 mL); 150 mg/15 mL (480 mL)
- Tablet:
  - Immediate release: 100 mg, 125 mg, 200 mg, 250 mg, 300 mg
  - Timed release (8-12 hours): 100 mg, 200 mg, 250 mg, 300 mg, 500 mg
  - Timed release (8-24 hours): 100 mg, 200 mg, 300 mg, 450 mg
  - Timed release (12-24 hours): 100 mg, 200 mg, 300 mg
  - Timed release (24 hours): 400 mg

♦ **Theospan®-SR** *see* Theophylline Salts *on page 539*

♦ **Theovent®** *see* Theophylline Salts *on page 539*

♦ **Therabid® [OTC]** *see* Vitamins, Multiple *on page 587*

♦ **Thera-Combex® H-P Kapseals® [OTC]** *see* Vitamin B Complex With Vitamin C *on page 586*

♦ **TheraCys®** *see* BCG Vaccine *on page 58*

♦ **Theraflu® Non-Drowsy Formula Maximum Strength [OTC]** *see* Acetaminophen, Dextromethorphan, and Pseudoephedrine *on page 16*

♦ **Theragran® [OTC]** *see* Vitamins, Multiple *on page 587*

♦ **Theragran® Hematinic®** *see* Vitamins, Multiple *on page 587*

♦ **Theragran® Liquid [OTC]** *see* Vitamins, Multiple *on page 587*

♦ **Theragran-M® [OTC]** *see* Vitamins, Multiple *on page 587*

♦ **Thera-Hist® Syrup [OTC]** *see* Chlorpheniramine and Phenylpropanolamine *on page 114*

♦ **Thermazene®** *see* Silver Sulfadiazine *on page 512*

♦ **Theroxide® Wash [OTC]** *see* Benzoyl Peroxide *on page 62*

## Thiabendazole (thye a BEN da zole)

**U.S. Brand Names** Mintezol®

**Synonyms** Tiabendazole

**Pharmacologic Category** Anthelmintic

**Use** Treatment of strongyloidiasis, cutaneous larva migrans, visceral larva migrans, dracunculiasis, trichinosis, and mixed helminthic infections

**Effects on Mental Status** May cause drowsiness, dizziness, hallucinations, or delirium

**Effects on Psychiatric Treatment** May rarely cause leukopenia; use caution with clozapine and carbamazepine

**Pregnancy Risk Factor** C

**Contraindications** Known hypersensitivity to thiabendazole

**Warnings/Precautions** Use with caution in patients with renal or hepatic impairment, malnutrition or anemia, or dehydration

**Adverse Reactions**

>10%:

- Central nervous system: Seizures, hallucinations, delirium, dizziness, drowsiness, headache
- Gastrointestinal: Anorexia, diarrhea, nausea, vomiting, drying of mucous membranes
- Neuromuscular & skeletal: Numbness
- Otic: Tinnitus

1% to 10%: Dermatologic: Rash, Stevens-Johnson syndrome

<1%: Blurred or yellow vision, chills, hepatotoxicity, hypersensitivity reactions, leukopenia, lymphadenopathy, malodor of urine, nephrotoxicity

**Overdosage/Toxicology**

Signs and symptoms of overdose include altered mental status, visual problems

Treatment: Supportive care only following GI decontamination

**Drug Interactions** Increased levels of theophylline and other xanthines

**Usual Dosage** Purgation is not required prior to use; drinking of fruit juice aids in expulsion of worms by removing the mucous to which the intestinal tapeworms attach themselves.

Children and Adults: Oral: 50 mg/kg/day divided every 12 hours (if >68 kg: 1.5 g/dose); maximum dose: 3 g/day

- Strongyloidiasis, ascariasis, uncinariasis, trichuriasis: For 2 consecutive days
- Cutaneous larva migrans: For 2-5 consecutive days
- Visceral larva migrans: For 5-7 consecutive days
- Trichinosis: For 2-4 consecutive days
- Dracunculosis: 50-75 mg/kg/day divided every 12 hours for 3 days

**Dosing comments in renal/hepatic impairment:** Use with caution

**Patient Information** Take exactly as directed for full course of medication. Tablets may be chewed, swallowed whole, or crushed and mixed with food. Increase dietary intake of fruit juices. All family members and close friends should also be treated. To reduce possibility of reinfection, wash hands and scrub nails carefully with soap and hot water before handling food, before eating, and before and after toileting. Keep hands out of mouth. Disinfect toilet daily and launder bed lines, undergarments, and nightclothes daily with hot water and soap. Do not go barefoot and do not sit directly on grass or ground. May cause dizziness, fainting, lightheadedness (use caution when driving or engaging in tasks requiring alertness until response to drug is known); abdominal pain, nausea, dry mouth, or vomiting (frequent small meals, frequent mouth care, sucking lozenges, or chewing gum may help). Report skin rash or itching, unresolved diarrhea or vomiting, CNS changes (hallucinations, delirium, acute headache), change in color of urine or stool, or easy bruising or unusual bleeding.

**Dosage Forms**

Suspension, oral: 500 mg/5 mL (120 mL)

Tablet, chewable (orange flavor): 500 mg

♦ **Thiamazole** *see* Methimazole *on page 352*

♦ **Thiamilate®** *see* Thiamine *on page 542*

## Thiamine (THYE a min)

**Related Information**
Substance-Related Disorders *on page 609*
**U.S. Brand Names** Thiamilate®
**Canadian Brand Names** Betaxin®; Bewon®
**Synonyms** Aneurine Hydrochloride; Thiamine Hydrochloride; Thiaminium Chloride Hydrochloride; Vitamin $B_1$
**Pharmacologic Category** Vitamin, Water Soluble
**Use** Treatment of thiamine deficiency including beriberi, Wernicke's encephalopathy syndrome, and peripheral neuritis associated with pellagra, alcoholic patients with altered sensorium; various genetic metabolic disorders
**Effects on Mental Status** None reported
**Effects on Psychiatric Treatment** None reported
**Pregnancy Risk Factor** A (C if dose exceeds RDA recommendation)
**Contraindications** Hypersensitivity to thiamine or any component
**Warnings/Precautions** Use with caution with parenteral route (especially I.V.) of administration
**Adverse Reactions** <1%: Angioedema, cardiovascular collapse and death, paresthesia, rash, warmth
**Drug Interactions** Neuromuscular blocking agents; high carbohydrate diets or I.V. dextrose solutions increase thiamine requirement
**Usual Dosage**
Recommended daily allowance:
- <6 months: 0.3 mg
- 6 months to 1 year: 0.4 mg
- 1-3 years: 0.7 mg
- 4-6 years: 0.9 mg
- 7-10 years: 1 mg
- 11-14 years: 1.1-1.3 mg
- >14 years: 1-1.5 mg

Thiamine deficiency (beriberi):
- Children: 10-25 mg/dose I.M. or I.V. daily (if critically ill), or 10-50 mg/dose orally every day for 2 weeks, then 5-10 mg/dose orally daily for 1 month
- Adults: 5-30 mg/dose I.M. or I.V. 3 times/day (if critically ill); then orally 5-30 mg/day in single or divided doses 3 times/day for 1 month

Wernicke's encephalopathy: Adults: Initial: 100 mg I.V., then 50-100 mg/day I.M. or I.V. until consuming a regular, balanced diet
Dietary supplement (depends on caloric or carbohydrate content of the diet):
- Infants: 0.3-0.5 mg/day
- Children: 0.5-1 mg/day
- Adults: 1-2 mg/day
- **Note:** The above doses can be found in multivitamin preparations

Metabolic disorders: Oral: Adults: 10-20 mg/day (dosages up to 4 g/day in divided doses have been used)
**Patient Information** Take exactly as directed; do not discontinue without consulting prescriber (deficiency state can occur in as little as 3 weeks). Follow dietary instructions (dietary sources include legumes, pork, beef, whole grains, yeast, fresh vegetables).
**Nursing Implications** Single vitamin deficiency is rare; look for other deficiencies
**Dosage Forms**
Injection, as hydrochloride: 100 mg/mL (1 mL, 2 mL, 10 mL, 30 mL); 200 mg/mL (30 mL)
Tablet, as hydrochloride: 50 mg, 100 mg, 250 mg, 500 mg
Tablet, as hydrochloride, enteric coated: 20 mg

♦ **Thiamine Hydrochloride** *see* Thiamine *on page 542*

♦ **Thiaminium Chloride Hydrochloride** *see* Thiamine *on page 542*

## Thiamphenicol (thye am FEN i kole)

**Pharmacologic Category** Antibiotic, Miscellaneous
**Use** Gonorrhea, chancroid, *Gardnerella vaginalis*, vaginitis
**Effects on Mental Status** May cause drowsiness or dizziness
**Effects on Psychiatric Treatment** May cause myelosuppression; use caution with clozapine and carbamazepine
**Contraindications** Hypersensitivity to thiamphenicol; bone marrow depression; pregnancy
**Warnings/Precautions** Use with caution if other myelosuppressive drugs are given; reduce dose if multiple doses are required for renal failure and in elderly
**Adverse Reactions** Dose-dependent reversible myelosuppression is more frequent than with chloramphenicol; not seen after single-dose use
Central nervous system: Headache, drowsiness, dizziness, polyneuropathy
Dermatologic: Pruritus
Gastrointestinal: Epigastric pain, abdominal pain, nausea, vomiting
Neuromuscular & skeletal: Neuropathy (peripheral) with long-term use
Ocular: Optic neuritis
**Usual Dosage**
Oral: Single dose of 2.5 g (for uncomplicated gonorrhea) or 500 mg 3 times/day for 6 days
I.M.:
- Children: 25-30 mg/kg/day
- Adults: 1-3 g/day

I.V.: 750 mg to 1 g 3 times/day

## Thiethylperazine (thye eth il PER a zeen)

**U.S. Brand Names** Norzine®; Torecan®
**Pharmacologic Category** Antiemetic
**Use** Relief of nausea and vomiting
**Unlabeled use:** Treatment of vertigo
**Effects on Mental Status** Drowsiness and dizziness are common; may cause confusion and extrapyramidal symptoms
**Effects on Psychiatric Treatment** May rarely cause agranulocytosis, caution with clozapine and carbamazepine. Adverse effects may be increased with concurrent use of CNS depressants (ethanol), lithium, TCAs, and MAO inhibitors
**Usual Dosage** Children >12 years and Adults:
Oral, I.M., rectal: 10 mg 1-3 times/day as needed
I.V. and S.C. routes of administration are not recommended
Hemodialysis: Not dialyzable (0% to 5%)
**Dosing comments in hepatic impairment:** Use with caution
**Dosage Forms**
Injection, as maleate: 5 mg/mL (2 mL)
Suppository, rectal, as maleate: 10 mg
Tablet, as maleate: 10 mg

## Thioguanine (thye oh GWAH neen)

**Synonyms** 2-Amino-6-Mercaptopurine; TG; 6-TG; 6-Thioguanine; Tioguanine
**Pharmacologic Category** Antineoplastic Agent, Antimetabolite
**Use** Remission induction, consolidation, and maintenance therapy of acute myelogenous (nonlymphocytic) leukemia; treatment of chronic myelogenous leukemia and granulocytic leukemia
**Effects on Mental Status** None reported
**Effects on Psychiatric Treatment** Myelosuppression is common; avoid clozapine and carbamazepine
**Pregnancy Risk Factor** D
**Contraindications** History of previous therapy resistance with either thioguanine or mercaptopurine (there is usually complete cross resistance between these two); hypersensitivity to thioguanine or any component
**Warnings/Precautions** The U.S. Food and Drug Administration (FDA) currently recommends that procedures for proper handling and disposal of antineoplastic agents be considered. Use with caution and reduce dose of thioguanine in patients with renal or hepatic impairment; thioguanine is potentially carcinogenic and teratogenic; myelosuppression may be delayed.
**Adverse Reactions**
>10%:
- Hematologic: Myelosuppressive:
  - WBC: Moderate
  - Platelets: Moderate
  - Onset (days): 7-10
  - Nadir (days): 14
  - Recovery (days): 21

1% to 10%:
- Dermatologic: Skin rash
- Endocrine & metabolic: Hyperuricemia
- Gastrointestinal: Mild nausea or vomiting, anorexia, stomatitis, diarrhea
  - Emetic potential: Low (<10%)
- Neuromuscular & skeletal: Unsteady gait

<1%: Hepatitis, jaundice, neurotoxicity, photosensitivity, veno-occlusive hepatic disease
**Overdosage/Toxicology**
Signs and symptoms: Bone marrow suppression, nausea, vomiting, malaise, hypertension, sweating
Treatment: Supportive; dialysis is not useful
**Drug Interactions** Increased toxicity:
Allopurinol can be used in full doses with 6 TG unlike 6-MP
Busulfan → hepatotoxicity and esophageal varices
**Usual Dosage** Total daily dose can be given at one time; offers little advantage over mercaptopurine; is sometimes ordered as 6-thioguanine, with 6 being part of the drug name and not a unit or strength
Oral (refer to individual protocols):
- Infants and Children <3 years: Combination drug therapy for acute nonlymphocytic leukemia: 3.3 mg/kg/day in divided doses twice daily for 4 days
- Children and Adults: 2-3 mg/kg/day calculated to nearest 20 mg or 75-200 mg/m$^2$/day in 1-2 divided doses for 5-7 days or until remission is attained

**Dosing comments in renal or hepatic impairment:** Reduce dose

**Patient Information** You may experience nausea and vomiting, diarrhea, or loss of appetite (frequent small meals may help/request medication) or weakness or lethargy (use caution when driving or engaging in tasks requiring alertness until response to drug is known). Use good oral care to reduce incidence of mouth sores. Maintain adequate hydration (2-3 L/day of fluids unless instructed to restrict fluid intake). May cause headache (request medication). Report signs or symptoms of infection (eg, fever, chills, sore throat, burning urination, fatigue), bleeding (eg, tarry stools, easy bruising), vision changes, unresolved mouth sores, nausea or vomiting, CNS changes (hallucinations), or respiratory difficulty. Avoid crowds or exposure to infected persons; you will be susceptible to infection.

**Dosage Forms** Tablet, scored: 40 mg

♦ **6-Thioguanine** *see* Thioguanine *on page 542*

♦ **Thiola™** *see* Tiopronin *on page 550*

## Thiopental (thye oh PEN tal)

**Related Information**

Patient Information - Anxiolytics & Sedative Hypnotics (Barbiturates) *on page 654*

**Generic Available** No

**U.S. Brand Names** Pentothal® Sodium

**Synonyms** Thiopental Sodium

**Pharmacologic Category** Anticonvulsant, Barbiturate; Barbiturate; General Anesthetic

**Use** Induction of anesthesia; adjunct for intubation in head injury patients; control of convulsive states; treatment of elevated intracranial pressure

**Restrictions** C-III

**Pregnancy Risk Factor** C

**Contraindications** Hypersensitivity to barbiturates or any component of the formulation; status asthmaticus; severe cardiovascular disease; porphyria; inflammatory bowel disease or lower gastrointestinal neoplasm (rectal gel); should not be administered by intra-arterial injection

**Warnings/Precautions** Laryngospasm or bronchospasms may occur; use with extreme caution in patients with reactive airway diseases (asthma or COPD). Use with caution when the hypnotic may be prolonged or potentiated (excessive premedication, Addison's disease, hepatic or renal dysfunction, myxedema, increased blood urea, severe anemia, or myasthenia gravis). Potential for drug dependency exists, abrupt cessation may precipitate withdrawal, including status epilepticus in epileptic patients. Do not administer to patients in acute pain. Use caution in patients with unstable aneurysms, cardiovascular disease, renally impairment, or hepatic disease. Use caution in elderly, debilitated, or pediatric patients. May cause paradoxical responses, including agitation and hyperactivity, particularly in acute pain and pediatric patients. Use with caution in patients with depression or suicidal tendencies, or in patients with a history of drug abuse. Tolerance, psychological and physical dependence may occur with prolonged use. May cause CNS depression, which may impair physical or mental abilities. Patients must cautioned about performing tasks which require mental alertness (ie, operating machinery or driving). Effects with other sedative drugs or ethanol may be potentiated. May cause respiratory depression or hypotension, particularly when administered intravenously. Use with caution in hemodynamically unstable patients (hypotension or shock) or patients with respiratory disease. Repeated dosing or continuous infusions may cause cumulative effects. Extravasation or intra-arterial injection causes necrosis due to pH of 10.6, ensure patient has intravenous access.

**Adverse Reactions**

Cardiovascular: Bradycardia, hypotension, syncope

Central nervous system: Drowsiness, lethargy, CNS excitation or depression, impaired judgment, "hangover" effect, confusion, somnolence, agitation, hyperkinesia, ataxia, nervousness, headache, insomnia, nightmares, hallucinations, anxiety, dizziness

Dermatologic: Rash, exfoliative dermatitis, Stevens-Johnson syndrome

Hematologic: Agranulocytosis, thrombocytopenia, megaloblastic anemia

Local: Pain at injection site, thrombophlebitis with I.V. use

Gastrointestinal: Nausea, vomiting, constipation

Renal: Oliguria

Respiratory: Laryngospasm, respiratory depression, apnea (especially with rapid I.V. use), hypoventilation, apnea

Miscellaneous: Gangrene with inadvertent intra-arterial injection

**Overdosage/Toxicology**

Signs and symptoms: Respiratory depression, hypotension, shock

Treatment: Hypotension should respond to I.V. fluids and placement of patient in Trendelenburg position; if necessary, pressors such as norepinephrine may be used; patient may require ventilatory support

**Drug Interactions** Barbiturates are enzyme inducers; patients should be monitored when these drugs are started or stopped for a decreased or increased therapeutic effect respectively. However, thiopental is generally not used for prolonged periods, so the potential for induction is minimal.

Acetaminophen: Barbiturates may enhance the hepatotoxic potential of acetaminophen overdoses

Antiarrhythmics: Barbiturates may increase the metabolism of antiarrhythmics, decreasing their clinical effect; includes disopyramide, propafenone, and quinidine

Anticonvulsants: Barbiturates may increase the metabolism of anticonvulsants; includes ethosuximide, felbamate (possibly), lamotrigine, phenytoin, tiagabine, topiramate, and zonisamide; does not appear to affect gabapentin or levetiracetam

Antineoplastics: Limited evidence suggests that enzyme-inducing anticonvulsant therapy may reduce the effectiveness of some chemotherapy regimens (specifically in ALL); teniposide and methotrexate may be cleared more rapidly in these patients

Antipsychotics: Barbiturates may enhance the metabolism (decrease the efficacy) of antipsychotics; monitor for altered response; dose adjustment may be needed

Beta-blockers: Metabolism of beta-blockers may be increased and clinical effect decreased; atenolol and nadolol are unlikely to interact given their renal elimination

Calcium channel blockers: Barbiturates may enhance the metabolism of calcium channel blockers, decreasing their clinical effect

Chloramphenicol: Barbiturates may increase the metabolism of chloramphenicol and chloramphenicol may inhibit barbiturate metabolism; monitor for altered response

Cimetidine: Barbiturates may enhance the metabolism of cimetidine, decreasing its clinical effect

CNS depressants: Sedative effects and/or respiratory depression with barbiturates may be additive with other CNS depressants; monitor for increased effect; includes ethanol, sedatives, antidepressants, narcotic analgesics, and benzodiazepines

Corticosteroids: Barbiturates may enhance the metabolism of corticosteroids, decreasing their clinical effect

Cyclosporine: Levels may be decreased by barbiturates; monitor

Immunosuppressants: Barbiturates may enhance the metabolism of immunosuppressants, decreasing its clinical effect; includes both cyclosporine and tacrolimus

Doxycycline: Barbiturates may enhance the metabolism of doxycycline, decreasing its clinical effect; higher dosages may be required

Estrogens: Barbiturates may increase the metabolism of estrogens and reduce their efficacy

Felbamate may inhibit the metabolism of barbiturates and barbiturates may increase the metabolism of felbamate

Griseofulvin: Barbiturates may impair the absorption of griseofulvin, and griseofulvin metabolism may be increased by barbiturates, decreasing clinical effect

Guanfacine: Effect may be decreased by barbiturates

Loop diuretics: Metabolism may be increased and clinical effects decreased; established for furosemide, effect with other loop diuretics not established

MAOIs: Metabolism of barbiturates may be inhibited, increasing clinical effect or toxicity of the barbiturates

Methadone: Barbiturates may enhance the metabolism of methadone resulting in methadone withdrawal

Methoxyflurane: Barbiturates may enhance the nephrotoxic effects of methoxyflurane

Oral contraceptives: Barbiturates may enhance the metabolism of oral contraceptives, decreasing their clinical effect; an alternative method of contraception should be considered

Theophylline: Barbiturates may increase metabolism of theophylline derivatives and decrease their clinical effect

Tricyclic antidepressants: Barbiturates may increase metabolism of tricyclic antidepressants and decrease their clinical effect; sedative effects may be additive

Valproic acid: Metabolism of barbiturates may be inhibited by valproic acid; monitor for excessive sedation; a dose reduction may be needed

Warfarin: Barbiturates inhibit the hypoprothrombinemic effects of oral anticoagulants via increased metabolism; this combination should generally be avoided

**Stability** Reconstituted solutions remain stable for 3 days at room temperature and 7 days when refrigerated; solutions are alkaline and **incompatible** with drugs with acidic pH, such as succinylcholine, atropine sulfate, etc. I.V. form is **incompatible** when mixed with amikacin, codeine, dimenhydrinate, diphenhydramine, hydromorphone, insulin, levorphanol, meperidine, metaraminol, morphine, norepinephrine, penicillin G, prochlorperazine, succinylcholine, tetracycline, benzquinamide, chlorpromazine, glycopyrrolate

**Mechanism of Action** Short-acting barbiturate with sedative, hypnotic, and anticonvulsant properties. Barbiturates depress the sensory cortex, decrease motor activity, alter cerebellar function, and produce drowsiness, sedation, and hypnosis. In high doses, barbiturates exhibit anticonvulsant activity; barbiturates produce dose-dependent respiratory depression.

**Pharmacodynamics/kinetics**

Onset of action: I.V.: Anesthesia occurs in 30-60 seconds

Duration: 5-30 minutes

Distribution: $V_d$: 1.4 L/kg

Protein binding: 72% to 86%

Metabolism: In the liver primarily to inactive metabolites but pentobarbital is also formed

(Continued)

## Thiopental *(Continued)*

Half-life: 3-11.5 hours, decreased in children vs adults

**Usual Dosage** I.V.:

Induction anesthesia:
- Infants: 5-8 mg/kg
- Children 1-12 years: 5-6 mg/kg
- Adults: 3-5 mg/kg

Maintenance anesthesia:
- Children: 1 mg/kg as needed
- Adults: 25-100 mg as needed

Increased intracranial pressure: Children and Adults: 1.5-5 mg/kg/dose; repeat as needed to control intracranial pressure

Seizures:
- Children: 2-3 mg/kg/dose, repeat as needed
- Adults: 75-250 mg/dose, repeat as needed

**Rectal administration:** (Patient should be NPO for no less than 3 hours prior to administration)

**Suggested initial doses of thiopental rectal suspension are:**
- <3 months: 15 mg/kg/dose
- >3 months: 25 mg/kg/dose

**Note:** The age of a premature infant should be adjusted to reflect the age that the infant would have been if full-term (eg, an infant, now age 4 months, who was 2 months premature should be considered to be a 2-month old infant).

Doses should be rounded downward to the nearest 50 mg increment to allow for accurate measurement of the dose

Inactive or debilitated patients and patients recently medicated with other sedatives, (eg, chloral hydrate, meperidine, chlorpromazine, and promethazine), may require smaller doses than usual

**If the patient is not sedated within 15-20 minutes, a single repeat dose of thiopental can be given. The single repeat doses are:**
- <3 months: <7.5 mg/kg/dose
- >3 months: 15 mg/kg/dose

Adults weighing >90 kg should not receive >3 g as a total dose (initial plus repeat doses)

Children weighing >34 kg should not receive >1 g as a total dose (initial plus repeat doses)

Neither adults nor children should receive more than one course of thiopental rectal suspension (initial dose plus repeat dose) per 24-hour period

**Dosing adjustment in renal impairment:** $Cl_{cr}$ <10 mL/minute: Administer at 75% of normal dose

**Note:** Accumulation may occur with chronic dosing due to lipid solubility; prolonged recovery may result from redistribution of thiopental from fat stores

**Monitoring Parameters** Respiratory rate, heart rate, blood pressure

**Reference Range** Therapeutic: Hypnotic: 1-5 μg/mL (SI: 4.1-20.7 μmol/L); Coma: 30-100 μg/mL (SI: 124-413 μmol/L); Anesthesia: 7-130 μg/mL (SI: 29-536 μmol/L); Toxic: >10 μg/mL (SI: >41 μmol/L)

**Test Interactions** ↑ potassium (S)

**Nursing Implications** Monitor vital signs every 3-5 minutes; monitor for respiratory distress; place patient in Sim's position if vomiting, to prevent from aspirating vomitus; avoid extravasation, necrosis may occur

**Additional Information** Sodium content of 1 g (injection) : 86.8 mg (3.8 mEq)

**Dosage Forms**
- Injection, as sodium: 250 mg, 400 mg, 500 mg, 1 g, 2.5 g, 5 g
- Suspension, rectal, as sodium: 400 mg/g (2 g)

♦ **Thiopental Sodium** *see* Thiopental *on page 543*

♦ **Thioplex®** *see* Thiotepa *on page 545*

## Thioridazine (thye oh RID a zeen)

**Related Information**

Antipsychotic Agents Comparison Chart *on page 706*
Antipsychotic Medication Guidelines *on page 751*
Clinical Issues in the Use of Antipsychotics *on page 630*
Discontinuation of Psychotropic Drugs - Withdrawal Symptoms and Recommendations *on page 798*
Federal OBRA Regulations Recommended Maximum Doses *on page 756*
Liquid Compatibility With Antipsychotics and Mood Stabilizers *on page 718*
Patient Information - Antipsychotics (General) *on page 646*
Schizophrenia *on page 604*

**Generic Available** Yes

**U.S. Brand Names** Mellaril®; Mellaril-S®

**Canadian Brand Names** Apo®-Thioridazine; Novo-Ridazine; PMS-Thioridazine

**Synonyms** Thioridazine Hydrochloride

**Pharmacologic Category** Antipsychotic Agent, Phenothazine, Piperidine

**Use** Management of schizophrenic patients who fail to respond adequately to treatment with other antipsychotic drugs, either because of insufficient effectiveness or the inability to achieve an effective dose due to intolerable adverse effects from these drugs

**Pregnancy Risk Factor** C

**Contraindications** In combination with other drugs that are known to prolong the QTc interval and in patients with congenital long Q-T syndrome or a history of cardiac arrhythmias; drugs that inhibit the metabolism of thioridazine (fluoxetine, paroxetine, fluvoxamine, propranolol, pindolol); patients known to have a genetic defect leading to reduced levels of activity of CYP2D6; hypersensitivity to thioridazine or any component (cross reactivity between phenothiazines may occur); severe CNS depression, circulatory collapse, severe hypotension, bone marrow suppression, blood dyscrasias, coma

**Warnings/Precautions** Highly sedating, use with caution in disorders where CNS depression is a feature. Use with caution in Parkinson's disease. Caution in patients with hemodynamic instability; bone marrow suppression; predisposition to seizures; subcortical brain damage; severe cardiac, hepatic, renal, or respiratory disease. Esophageal dysmotility and aspiration have been associated with antipsychotic use - use with caution in patients at risk of pneumonia (ie, Alzheimer's disease). Caution in breast cancer or other prolactin-dependent tumors (may elevate prolactin levels). May alter temperature regulation or mask toxicity of other drugs due to antiemetic effects. Thioridazine has dose-related effects on ventricular repolarization leading to QTc prolongation, a potentially life-threatening effect. Therefore, it should be reserved for patients with schizophrenia who have failed to respond to adequate levels of other antipsychotic drugs. May cause orthostatic hypotension - use with caution in patients at risk of this effect or those who would tolerate transient hypotensive episodes (cerebrovascular disease, cardiovascular disease, or other medications which may predispose).

Phenothiazines may cause anticholinergic effects (confusion, agitation, constipation, dry mouth, blurred vision, urinary retention); therefore, they should be used with caution in patients with decreased gastrointestinal motility, urinary retention, BPH, xerostomia, or visual problems. Conditions which also may be exacerbated by cholinergic blockade include narrow-angle glaucoma (screening is recommended) and worsening of myasthenia gravis. Relative to other neuroleptics, thioridazine has a high potency of cholinergic blockade.

May cause extrapyramidal reactions, including pseudoparkinsonism, acute dystonic reactions, akathisia, and tardive dyskinesia (risk of these reactions is low relative to other neuroleptics). May be associated with neuroleptic malignant syndrome (NMS). Doses exceeding recommended doses may cause pigmentary retinopathy.

**Adverse Reactions**

Cardiovascular: Hypotension, orthostatic hypotension, peripheral edema, EKG changes

Central nervous system: EPS (pseudoparkinsonism, akathisia, dystonias, tardive dyskinesia), dizziness, drowsiness, neuroleptic malignant syndrome (NMS), impairment of temperature regulation, lowering of seizures threshold

Dermatologic: Increased sensitivity to sun, rash, discoloration of skin (blue-gray)

Endocrine & metabolic: Changes in menstrual cycle, changes in libido, breast pain, galactorrhea, amenorrhea

Gastrointestinal: Constipation, weight gain, nausea, vomiting, stomach pain, xerostomia, nausea, vomiting, diarrhea

Genitourinary: Difficulty in urination, ejaculatory disturbances, urinary retention, priapism

Hematologic: Agranulocytosis, leukopenia

Hepatic: Cholestatic jaundice, hepatotoxicity

Neuromuscular & skeletal: Tremor, seizure

Ocular: Pigmentary retinopathy, blurred vision, cornea and lens changes

Respiratory: Nasal congestion

**Overdosage/Toxicology**

Signs and symptoms: Deep sleep, coma, extrapyramidal symptoms, abnormal involuntary muscle movements, hypotension, arrhythmias

Treatment:

Following initiation of essential overdose management, toxic symptom treatment and supportive treatment should be initiated

Hypotension usually responds to I.V. fluids or Trendelenburg positioning. If unresponsive to these measures, the use of a parenteral inotrope may be required (eg, norepinephrine 0.1-0.2 mcg/kg/minute titrated to response); do not use epinephrine or dopamine.

Seizures commonly respond to diazepam (I.V. 5-10 mg bolus in adults every 15 minutes if needed up to a total of 30 mg; I.V. 0.25-0.4 mg/kg/dose up to a total of 10 mg in children) or to phenytoin. Avoid barbiturates; may potentiate respiratory depression.

Neuroleptics often cause extrapyramidal symptoms (eg, dystonic reactions) requiring management with diphenhydramine 1-2 mg/kg (adults) up to a maximum of 50 mg I.M. or I.V. slow push followed by a maintenance dose for 48-72 hours. Alternatively, benztropine mesylate I.V. 1-2 mg (adults) may be effective. These agents are generally effective within 2-5 minutes.

**Drug Interactions** CYP1A2 and 2D6 enzyme substrate; CYP2D6 enzyme inhibitor

Aluminum salts: May decrease the absorption of phenothiazines; monitor

Amphetamines: Efficacy may be diminished by antipsychotics; in addition, amphetamines may increase psychotic symptoms; avoid concurrent use

Anticholinergics: May inhibit the therapeutic response to phenothiazines and excess anticholinergic effects may occur; includes benztropine, trihexyphenidyl, biperiden, and drugs with significant anticholinergic activity (TCAs, antihistamines, disopyramide)

Antihypertensives: Concurrent use of phenothiazines with an antihypertensive may produce additive hypotensive effects (particularly orthostasis)

Beta-blockers: May increase the risk of arrhythmia; propranolol and pindolol are **contraindicated**

Bromocriptine: Phenothiazines inhibit the ability of bromocriptine to lower serum prolactin concentrations

Carvedilol: Serum concentrations may be increased, leading to hypotension and bradycardia; avoid concurrent use

CNS depressants: Sedative effects may be additive with phenothiazines; monitor for increased effect; includes barbiturates, benzodiazepines, narcotic analgesics, ethanol, and other sedative agents

CYP2D6 inhibitors: Metabolism of phenothiazines may be decreased; increasing clinical effect or toxicity. Inhibitors include amiodarone, cimetidine, delavirdine, fluoxetine, paroxetine, propafenone, quinidine, and ritonavir; monitor for increased effect/toxicity. Thioridazine is contraindicated with inhibitors of this enzyme, including fluoxetine and paroxetine.

Enzyme inducers: May enhance the hepatic metabolism of phenothiazines; larger doses may be required; includes rifampin, rifabutin, barbiturates, phenytoin, and cigarette smoking

Epinephrine: Chlorpromazine (and possibly other low potency antipsychotics) may diminish the pressor effects of epinephrine

Guanethidine and guanadrel: Antihypertensive effects may be inhibited by phenothiazines

Levodopa: Phenothiazines may inhibit the antiparkinsonian effect of levodopa; avoid this combination

Lithium: Phenothiazines may produce neurotoxicity with lithium; this is a rare effect

Phenytoin: May reduce serum levels of phenothiazines; phenothiazines may increase phenytoin serum levels

Polypeptide antibiotics: Rare cases of respiratory paralysis have been reported with concurrent use of phenothiazines

Potassium depleting agents: May increase the risk of serious arrhythmias with thioridazine; includes many diuretics, aminoglycosides, and amphotericin; monitor serum potassium closely

Propranolol: Serum concentrations of phenothiazines may be increased; propranolol also increases phenothiazine concentrations

QTc prolonging agents: Effects on QTc interval may be additive with phenothiazines, increasing the risk of malignant arrhythmias; includes type Ia antiarrhythmics, TCAs, and some quinolone antibiotics (sparfloxacin, moxifloxacin and gatifloxacin). **These agents are contraindicated with thioridazine.**

Sulfadoxine-pyrimethamine: May increase phenothiazine concentrations

Trazodone: Phenothiazines and trazodone may produce additive hypotensive effects

Tricyclic antidepressants: Concurrent use may produce increased toxicity or altered therapeutic response

Valproic acid: Serum levels may be increased by phenothiazines

**Stability** Protect all dosage forms from light

**Mechanism of Action** Blocks postsynaptic mesolimbic dopaminergic receptors in the brain; exhibits a strong alpha-adrenergic blocking effect and depresses the release of hypothalamic and hypophyseal hormones

**Pharmacodynamics/kinetics**

Duration of action: 4-5 days

Half-life: 21-25 hours

Time to peak serum concentration: Within 1 hour

**Usual Dosage** Oral:

Children >2 years: Range: 0.5-3 mg/kg/day in 2-3 divided doses; usual: 1 mg/kg/day; maximum: 3 mg/kg/day

Behavior problems: Initial: 10 mg 2-3 times/day, increase gradually

Severe psychoses: Initial: 25 mg 2-3 times/day, increase gradually

Adults:

Psychoses: Initial: 50-100 mg 3 times/day with gradual increments as needed and tolerated; maximum: 800 mg/day in 2-4 divided doses; if >65 years, initial dose: 10 mg 3 times/day

Depressive disorders, dementia: Initial: 25 mg 3 times/day; maintenance dose: 20-200 mg/day

Hemodialysis: Not dialyzable (0% to 5%)

**Dietary Considerations** Alcohol: Additive CNS effect, avoid use

**Administration** Dilute oral concentrate with water or juice before administration

**Monitoring Parameters** Baseline EKG, serum potassium; do not initiate if QTc >450 msec

**Reference Range** Therapeutic: 1.0-1.5 µg/mL (SI: 2.7-4.1 µmol/L); Toxic: >1 mg/mL; Lethal: 2-8 mg/dL

**Test Interactions** False-positives for phenylketonuria, urinary amylase, uroporphyrins, urobilinogen

**Patient Information** Oral concentrate must be diluted in 2-4 oz of liquid (water, fruit juice, carbonated drinks, milk, or pudding); do not take antacid within 1 hour of taking drug; avoid excess sun exposure; may cause drowsiness, restlessness, avoid alcohol and other CNS depressants; do not alter dosage or discontinue without consulting physician; yearly eye exams are necessary; might discolor urine (pink or reddish brown)

**Nursing Implications** Avoid skin contact with oral suspension or solution; may cause contact dermatitis

**Additional Information**

Thioridazine: Mellaril-S® oral suspension

Thioridazine hydrochloride: Mellaril® oral solution and tablet

**Dosage Forms**

Concentrate, as hydrochloride, oral: 30 mg/mL (120 mL); 100 mg/mL (3.4 mL, 120 mL)

Suspension, as hydrochloride, oral: 25 mg/5 mL (480 mL); 100 mg/5 mL (480 mL)

Tablet, as hydrochloride: 10 mg, 15 mg, 25 mg, 50 mg, 100 mg, 150 mg, 200 mg

♦ **Thioridazine Hydrochloride** see Thioridazine *on page 544*

## Thiotepa (thye oh TEP a)

**U.S. Brand Names** Thioplex®

**Pharmacologic Category** Antineoplastic Agent, Alkylating Agent

**Use** Treatment of superficial tumors of the bladder; palliative treatment of adenocarcinoma of breast or ovary; lymphomas and sarcomas; controlling intracavitary effusions caused by metastatic tumors; I.T. use: CNS leukemia/lymphoma

**Effects on Mental Status** May cause dizziness

**Effects on Psychiatric Treatment** Myelosuppression is common; avoid clozapine and carbamazepine; barbiturates may increase clearance of thiotepa

**Usual Dosage** Refer to individual protocols; dosing must be based on the clinical and hematologic response of the patient

Children: Sarcomas: I.V.: 25-65 mg/m$^2$ as a single dose every 21 days

Adults:

I.M., I.V., S.C.: 30-60 mg/m$^2$ once per week

I.V. doses of 0.3-0.4 mg/kg by rapid I.V. administration every 1-4 weeks, or 0.2 mg/kg or 6-8 mg/m$^2$/day for 4-5 days every 2-4 weeks

High-dose therapy for bone marrow transplant: I.V.: 500 mg/m$^2$; up to 900 mg/m$^2$

I.M. doses of 15-30 mg in various schedules have been given

Intracavitary: 0.6-0.8 mg/kg

Intrapericardial dose: Usually 15-30 mg

**Dosing comments/adjustment in renal impairment:** Use with extreme caution, reduced dose may be warranted. Less than 3% of alkylating species are detected in the urine in 24 hours.

Intrathecal: Doses of 1-10 mg/m$^2$ administered 1-2 times/week in concentrations of 1 mg/mL diluted with preservative-free sterile water for injection

Intravesical: Used for treatment of carcinoma of the bladder; patients should be dehydrated for 8-12 hours prior to treatment; instill 60 mg (in 30-60 mL of NS) into the bladder and retain for a minimum of 2 hours. Patient should be positioned every 15 minutes for maximal area exposure. Instillations usually once a week for 4 weeks. Monitor for bone marrow suppression.

Intratumor: Use a 22-gauge needle to inject thiotepa directly into the tumor. Initial dose: 0.6-0.8 mg/kg (diluted to 10 mg/mL) are used every 1-4 weeks; maintenance dose: 0.07-0.8 mg/kg are administered at 1- to 4-week intervals

Ophthalmic: 0.05% solution in LR has been instilled into the eye every 3 hours for 6-8 weeks for the prevention of pterygium recurrence

**Dosage Forms** Powder for injection: 15 mg

## Thiothixene (thye oh THIKS een)

**Related Information**

Antipsychotic Agents Comparison Chart *on page 706*

Antipsychotic Medication Guidelines *on page 751*

Clinical Issues in the Use of Antipsychotics *on page 630*

Discontinuation of Psychotropic Drugs - Withdrawal Symptoms and Recommendations *on page 798*

Federal OBRA Regulations Recommended Maximum Doses *on page 756*

Liquid Compatibility With Antipsychotics and Mood Stabilizers *on page 718*

Patient Information - Antipsychotics (General) *on page 646*

Schizophrenia *on page 604*

**Generic Available** Yes

**U.S. Brand Names** Navane®

**Synonyms** Tiotixene

**Pharmacologic Category** Antipsychotic Agent, Thioxanthene Derivative

**Use** Management of psychotic disorders

**Pregnancy Risk Factor** C

(Continued)

## Thiothixene *(Continued)*

**Contraindications** Hypersensitivity to thiothixene or any component; severe CNS depression, circulatory collapse, blood dyscrasias, coma

**Warnings/Precautions** May be sedating, use with caution in disorders where CNS depression is a feature. Use with caution in Parkinson's disease. Caution in patients with hemodynamic instability; predisposition to seizures; subcortical brain damage; bone marrow suppression; severe cardiac, hepatic, renal, or respiratory disease. Esophageal dysmotility and aspiration have been associated with antipsychotic use - use with caution in patients at risk of pneumonia (ie, Alzheimer's disease). Caution in breast cancer or other prolactin-dependent tumors (may elevate prolactin levels). May alter temperature regulation or mask toxicity of other drugs due to antiemetic effects. May alter cardiac conduction - life-threatening arrhythmias have occurred with therapeutic doses of neuroleptics. May cause orthostatic hypotension - use with caution in patients at risk of this effect or those who would tolerate transient hypotensive episodes (cerebrovascular disease, cardiovascular disease, or other medications which may predispose).

Phenothiazines may cause anticholinergic effects (confusion, agitation, constipation, dry mouth, blurred vision, urinary retention); therefore, they should be used with caution in patients with decreased gastrointestinal motility, urinary retention, BPH, xerostomia, or visual problems. Conditions which also may be exacerbated by cholinergic blockade include narrow-angle glaucoma (screening is recommended) and worsening of myasthenia gravis. Relative to other neuroleptics, thiothixene has a low potency of cholinergic blockade.

May cause extrapyramidal reactions, including pseudoparkinsonism, acute dystonic reactions, akathisia, and tardive dyskinesia (risk of these reactions is high relative to other neuroleptics). May be associated with neuroleptic malignant syndrome (NMS) or pigmentary retinopathy.

**Adverse Reactions**

Cardiovascular: Hypotension, tachycardia, syncope, nonspecific EKG changes

Central nervous system: Extrapyramidal signs (pseudoparkinsonism, akathisia, dystonias, lightheadedness, tardive dyskinesia), dizziness, drowsiness, restlessness, agitation, insomnia

Dermatologic: Discoloration of skin (blue-gray), rash, pruritus, urticaria, photosensitivity

Endocrine & metabolic: Changes in menstrual cycle, changes in libido, breast pain, galactorrhea, lactation, amenorrhea, gynecomastia, hyperglycemia, hypoglycemia

Gastrointestinal: Weight gain, nausea, vomiting, stomach pain, constipation, xerostomia, increased salivation

Genitourinary: Difficulty in urination, ejaculatory disturbances, impotence

Hematologic: Leukopenia, leukocytes

Neuromuscular & skeletal: Tremors

Ocular: Pigmentary retinopathy, blurred vision

Respiratory: Nasal congestion

Miscellaneous: Diaphoresis

**Overdosage/Toxicology**

Signs and symptoms: Muscle twitching, drowsiness, dizziness, rigidity, tremor, hypotension, cardiac arrhythmias

Treatment:

Following initiation of essential overdose management, toxic symptom treatment and supportive treatment should be initiated

Hypotension usually responds to I.V. fluids or Trendelenburg positioning. If unresponsive to these measures, the use of a parenteral inotrope may be required (eg, norepinephrine 0.1-0.2 mcg/kg/minute titrated to response).

Seizures commonly respond to diazepam (I.V. 5-10 mg bolus in adults every 15 minutes if needed up to a total of 30 mg; I.V. 0.25-0.4 mg/kg/dose up to a total of 10 mg in children) or to phenytoin or phenobarbital.

Neuroleptics often cause extrapyramidal symptoms (eg, dystonic reactions) requiring management with diphenhydramine 1-2 mg/kg (adults) up to a maximum of 50 mg I.M. or I.V. slow push followed by a maintenance dose for 48-72 hours. When these reactions are unresponsive to diphenhydramine, benztropine mesylate I.V. 1-2 mg (adults) may be effective. These agents are generally effective within 2-5 minutes.

**Drug Interactions** CYP1A2 enzyme substrate

Aluminum salts: May decrease the absorption of antipsychotics; monitor

Amphetamines: Efficacy may be diminished by antipsychotics; in addition, amphetamines may increase psychotic symptoms; avoid concurrent use

Anticholinergics: May inhibit the therapeutic response to antipsychotics and excess anticholinergic effects may occur; includes benztropine, trihexyphenidyl, biperiden, and drugs with significant anticholinergic activity (TCAs, antihistamines, disopyramide)

Antihypertensives: Concurrent use of antipsychotics with an antihypertensive may produce additive hypotensive effects (particularly orthostasis)

Bromocriptine: Antipsychotics inhibit the ability of bromocriptine to lower serum prolactin concentrations

CNS depressants: Sedative effects may be additive with antipsychotics; monitor for increased effect; includes barbiturates, benzodiazepines, narcotic analgesics, ethanol, and other sedative agents

CYP1A2 inhibitors: Serum levels may be increased; inhibitors include cimetidine, ciprofloxacin, fluvoxamine, isoniazid, ritonavir, and zileutin

Enzyme inducers: May enhance the hepatic metabolism of antipsychotics; larger doses may be required; includes rifampin, rifabutin, barbiturates, phenytoin, and cigarette smoking

Epinephrine: Chlorpromazine (and possibly other low potency antipsychotics) may diminish the pressor effects of epinephrine

Guanethidine and guanadrel: Antihypertensive effects may be inhibited by antipsychotics

Levodopa: Antipsychotics may inhibit the antiparkinsonian effect of levodopa; avoid this combination

Lithium: Antipsychotics may produce neurotoxicity with lithium; this is a rare effect

Phenytoin: May reduce serum levels of antipsychotics; antipsychotics may increase phenytoin serum levels

Propranolol: Serum concentrations of antipsychotics may be increased; propranolol also increases antipsychotics concentrations

QTc prolonging agents: Effects on QTc interval may be additive with antipsychotics, increasing the risk of malignant arrhythmias; includes type Ia antiarrhythmics, TCAs, and some quinolone antibiotics (sparfloxacin, moxifloxacin, and gatifloxacin)

Sulfadoxine-pyrimethamine: May increase antipsychotics concentrations

Trazodone: Antipsychotics and trazodone may produce additive hypotensive effects

Tricyclic antidepressants: Concurrent use may produce increased toxicity or altered therapeutic response

Valproic acid: Serum levels may be increased by antipsychotics

**Stability** Refrigerate

**Mechanism of Action** Elicits antipsychotic activity by postsynaptic blockade of CNS dopamine receptors resulting in inhibition of dopamine-mediated effects; also has alpha-adrenergic blocking activity

**Pharmacodynamics/kinetics**

Metabolism: Extensive in the liver

Half-life: >24 hours with chronic use

**Usual Dosage**

Children <12 years: Oral: 0.25 mg/kg/24 hours in divided doses (dose not well established)

Children >12 years and Adults: Mild to moderate psychosis:

Oral: 2 mg 3 times/day, up to 20-30 mg/day; more severe psychosis: Initial: 5 mg 2 times/day, may increase gradually, if necessary; maximum: 60 mg/day

I.M.: 4 mg 2-4 times/day, increase dose gradually; usual: 16-20 mg/day; maximum: 30 mg/day; change to oral dose as soon as able

Rapid tranquilization of the agitated patient (administered every 30-60 minutes):

Oral: 5-10 mg

I.M.: 10-20 mg

Average total dose for tranquilization: 15-30 mg

Hemodialysis: Not dialyzable (0% to 5%)

**Dietary Considerations** Alcohol: Additive CNS effect, avoid use

**Administration** I.M. dose is 4-10 times the activity of oral dose

**Monitoring Parameters** Orthostatic blood pressures; tremors, gait changes, abnormal movement in trunk, neck, buccal area or extremities; monitor target behaviors for which the agent is given

**Reference Range** Serum concentration: 2-57 ng/mL; concentrations do not always correspond to response and are controversial; dose to response for efficacy and safety

**Test Interactions** ↑ cholesterol (S), glucose; ↓ uric acid (S); may cause false-positive pregnancy test, ↑ serum transaminases and alkaline phosphatase

**Patient Information** May cause drowsiness, restlessness, avoid alcohol and other CNS depressants; do not alter dosage or discontinue without consulting physician

**Nursing Implications** Store injection in the refrigerator; observe for extrapyramidal effects; concentrate should be mixed in juice before administration

**Additional Information** Coadministration of two or more antipsychotics does not improve clinical response and may increase the potential for adverse effects

**Dosage Forms**

Capsule: 1 mg, 2 mg, 5 mg, 10 mg, 20 mg

Concentrate, oral, as hydrochloride: 5 mg/mL (30 mL, 120 mL)

Injection, as hydrochloride: 2 mg/mL (2 mL)

Powder for injection, as hydrochloride: 5 mg/mL (2 mL)


- **Thorazine®** *see* Chlorpromazine *on page 116*
- **Thrombate III®** *see* Antithrombin III *on page 46*
- **Thypinone® Injection** *see* Protirelin *on page 477*
- **Thyrar®** *see* Thyroid *on page 547*
- **Thyro-Block®** *see* Potassium Iodide *on page 454*

## Thyroid (THYE royd)

**U.S. Brand Names** Armour® Thyroid; S-P-T; Thyrar®; Thyroid Strong®

**Synonyms** Desiccated Thyroid; Thyroid Extract; Thyroid USP

**Pharmacologic Category** Thyroid Product

**Use** Replacement or supplemental therapy in hypothyroidism; pituitary TSH suppressants (thyroid nodules, thyroiditis, multinodular goiter, thyroid cancer), thyrotoxicosis, diagnostic suppression tests

**Effects on Mental Status** May cause nervousness or insomnia

**Effects on Psychiatric Treatment** Use to augment antidepressants and treat lithium-induced hypothyroidism

**Contraindications** Recent myocardial infarction or thyrotoxicosis uncomplicated by hypothyroidism uncorrected adrenal insufficiency; hypersensitivity to beef or pork or any constituent

**Warnings/Precautions** Ineffective for weight reduction. High doses may produce serious or even life-threatening toxic effects particularly when used with some anorectic drugs. Use cautiously in patients with pre-existing cardiovascular disease (angina, CHD), elderly since they may be more likely to have compromised cardiovascular function. Chronic hypothyroidism predisposes patients to coronary artery disease. Desiccated thyroid contains variable amounts of $T_3$, $T_4$, and other triiodothyronine compounds which are more likely to cause cardiac signs or symptoms due to fluctuating levels. Should avoid use in the elderly for this reason. Drug of choice is levothyroxine in the minds of many clinicians.

**Adverse Reactions** <1%: Abdominal cramps, alopecia, ataxia, cardiac arrhythmias, changes in menstrual cycle, chest pain, constipation, diaphoresis, diarrhea, excessive bone loss with overtreatment (excess thyroid replacement), fever, hand tremors, headache, heat intolerance, increased appetite, insomnia, myalgia, nervousness, palpitations, shortness of breath, tachycardia, tremor, vomiting, weight loss

**Overdosage/Toxicology**

Signs and symptoms: Chronic excessive use results in signs and symptoms of hyperthyroidism, weight loss, nervousness, sweating, tachycardia, insomnia, heat intolerance, palpitations, vomiting, psychosis, fever, seizures, angina, arrhythmias, and CHF in those predisposed

Treatment: Reduce dose or temporarily discontinue therapy; normal hypothalamic-pituitary-thyroid axis will return to normal in 6-8 weeks; serum $T_4$ levels do not correlate well with toxicity. In massive acute ingestion, reduce GI absorption, administer general supportive care; treat CHF with digitalis glycosides; excessive adrenergic activity (tachycardia) require propranolol 1-3 mg I.V. over 10 minutes or 80-160 mg orally/day; fever may be treated with acetaminophen.

**Drug Interactions**

Decreased effect:
- Beta-blocker effect is decreased when patients become euthyroid
- Thyroid hormones increase the therapeutic need for oral hypoglycemics or insulin
- Estrogens increase TBG, thereby decreasing effect of thyroid replacement
- Cholestyramine and colestipol decrease the effect of orally administered thyroid replacement
- Serum digitalis concentrations are reduced in hyperthyroidism or when hypothyroid patients are converted to a euthyroid state
- Theophylline levels decrease when hypothyroid patients converted to a euthyroid state

Increased toxicity: Thyroid may potentiate the hypoprothrombinemic effect of oral anticoagulants

**Usual Dosage** Oral:

Children: Recommended pediatric dosage for congenital hypothyroidism:
- 0-6 months: 15-30 mg/day; 4.8-6 mg/kg/day
- 6-12 months: 30-45 mg/day; 3.6-4.8 mg/kg/day
- 1-5 years: 45-60 mg/day; 3-3.6 mg/kg/day
- 6-12 years: 60-90 mg/day; 2.4-3 mg/kg/day
- >12 years: >90 mg/day; 1.2-1.8 mg/kg/day

Adults: Initial: 15-30 mg; increase with 15 mg increments every 2-4 weeks; use 15 mg in patients with cardiovascular disease or myxedema. Maintenance dose: Usually 60-120 mg/day; monitor TSH and clinical symptoms.

Thyroid cancer: Requires larger amounts than replacement therapy

**Patient Information** Thyroid replacement therapy is generally for life. Take as directed, in the morning before breakfast. Do not change brands and do not discontinue without consulting prescriber. Consult prescriber if drastically increasing or decreasing intake of goitrogenic food (eg, asparagus, cabbage, peas, turnip greens, broccoli, spinach, Brussels sprouts, lettuce, soybeans). Report chest pain, rapid heart rate, palpitations, heat intolerance, excessive sweating, increased nervousness, agitation, or lethargy.

**Dosage Forms**

Capsule, pork source in soybean oil (S-P-T): 60 mg, 120 mg, 180 mg, 300 mg

Tablet:
- Armour® Thyroid: 15 mg, 30 mg, 60 mg, 90 mg, 120 mg, 180 mg, 240 mg, 300 mg
- Thyrar® (bovine source): 30 mg, 60 mg, 120 mg
- Thyroid Strong® (60 mg is equivalent to 90 mg thyroid USP):
  - Regular: 30 mg, 60 mg, 120 mg
  - Sugar coated: 30 mg, 60 mg, 120 mg, 180 mg
- Thyroid USP: 15 mg, 30 mg, 60 mg, 120 mg, 180 mg, 300 mg


- ♦ **Thyroid Extract** *see* Thyroid *on page 547*
- ♦ **Thyroid Strong®** *see* Thyroid *on page 547*
- ♦ **Thyroid USP** *see* Thyroid *on page 547*
- ♦ **Thyrolar®** *see* Liotrix *on page 319*
- ♦ **Tiabendazole** *see* Thiabendazole *on page 541*


## Tiagabine (tye AJ a bene)

**Related Information**

Anticonvulsants by Seizures Type *on page 703*

**U.S. Brand Names** Gabitril®

**Pharmacologic Category** Anticonvulsant, Miscellaneous

**Use** Adjunctive therapy in adults and children ≥12 years of age in the treatment of partial seizures

**Unlabeled use:** Bipolar disorder

**Pregnancy Risk Factor** C

**Contraindications** Hypersensitivity to tiagabine or any of its ingredients

**Warnings/Precautions** Anticonvulsants should not be discontinued abruptly because of the possibility of increasing seizure frequency; tiagabine should be withdrawn gradually to minimize the potential of increased seizure frequency, unless safety concerns require a more rapid withdrawal. Rarely, nonconvulsive status epilepticus has been reported following abrupt discontinuation or dosage reduction.

Use with caution in patients with hepatic impairment. Experience in patients not receiving enzyme-inducing drugs has been limited - caution should be used in treating any patient who is not receiving one of these medications. Weakness, sedation, and confusion may occur with tiagabine use. Patients must cautioned about performing tasks which require mental alertness (ie, operating machinery or driving). Effects with other sedative drugs or ethanol may be potentiated. May cause potentially serious rash, including Stevens-Johnson syndrome.

**Adverse Reactions**

>10%:
- Central nervous system: Dizziness, somnolence
- Gastrointestinal: Nausea
- Neuromuscular & skeletal: Weakness

1% to 10%:
- Central nervous system: Nervousness, difficulty with concentration, insomnia, ataxia, confusion, speech disorder, depression, emotional lability, abnormal gait, hostility
- Dermatologic: Rash, pruritus
- Gastrointestinal: Diarrhea, vomiting, increased appetite
- Neuromuscular & skeletal: Tremor, paresthesia
- Respiratory: Pharyngitis, cough
- Ocular: Nystagmus
- Otic: Hearing impairment

**Drug Interactions** CYP2D6 and 3A3/4 enzyme substrate

CNS depressants: Sedative effects may be additive with other CNS depressants; monitor for increased effect; includes ethanol, sedatives, antidepressants, narcotic analgesics, other anticonvulsants, and benzodiazepines

CYP2D6 inhibitors: Serum levels and/or toxicity of tiagabine may be increased; inhibitors include amiodarone, cimetidine, delavirdine, fluoxetine, paroxetine, propafenone, quinidine, and ritonavir; monitor for increased effect/toxicity

CYP3A3/4 inhibitors: Serum level and/or toxicity of tiagabine may be increased; inhibitors include amiodarone, cimetidine, clarithromycin, erythromycin, delavirdine, diltiazem, dirithromycin, disulfiram, fluoxetine, fluvoxamine, grapefruit juice, indinavir, itraconazole, ketoconazole, nevirapine, propoxyfene, quinupristin-dalfopristin, ritonavir, saquinavir, verapamil, zafirlukast, zileuton; monitor for altered effects

Enzyme inducers: May increase the metabolism of tiagabine resulting in decreased effect. Primidone, phenobarbital, phenytoin, and carbamazepine increase tiagabine clearance by 60%

Valproate: Increased free tiagabine concentrations by 40%

**Mechanism of Action** The exact mechanism by which tiagabine exerts antiseizure activity is not definitively known; however, *in vitro* experiments demonstrate that it enhances the activity of gamma aminobutyric acid (GABA), the major neuroinhibitory transmitter in the nervous system; it is thought that binding to the GABA uptake carrier inhibits the uptake of GABA into presynaptic neurons, allowing an increased amount of GABA to be available to postsynaptic neurons; based on *in vitro* studies, tiagabine does not inhibit the uptake of dopamine, norepinephrine, serotonin, glutamate, or choline

**Pharmacodynamics/kinetics**

Absorption: Rapid (within 1 hour); food prolongs absorption

Protein binding: 96%

Half-life: 6.7 hours

(Continued)

## Tiagabine *(Continued)*

**Usual Dosage** Children >12 years and Adults: Oral: Starting dose: 4 mg once daily; the total daily dose may be increased in 4 mg increments beginning the second week of therapy; thereafter, the daily dose may be increased by 4-8 mg/day until clinical response is achieved, up to a maximum of 32 mg/day; the total daily dose at higher levels should be given in divided doses, 2-4 times/day

**Monitoring Parameters** A reduction in seizure frequency is indicative of therapeutic response to tiagabine in patients with partial seizures; complete blood counts, renal function tests, liver function tests, and routine blood chemistry should be monitored periodically during therapy

**Reference Range** Maximal plasma level after a 24 mg/dose: 552 ng/mL

**Patient Information** Use exactly as directed by mouth with food, usually beginning at 4 mg once daily, and usually in addition to other antiepilepsy drugs. The dose will be increased based on age and medial condition, up to 2-4 times/day. Do not interrupt or discontinue treatment without consulting your physician or pharmacist. If told to stop this medication, it should be discontinued gradually.

**Dosage Forms** Tablet: 2 mg, 4 mg, 12 mg, 16 mg, 20 mg

♦ **Tiamate®** *see* Diltiazem *on page 172*

♦ **Tiazac™** *see* Diltiazem *on page 172*

♦ **Ticar®** *see* Ticarcillin *on page 548*

## Ticarcillin (tye kar SIL in)

**U.S. Brand Names** Ticar®

**Pharmacologic Category** Antibiotic, Penicillin

**Use** Treatment of susceptible infections such as septicemia, acute and chronic respiratory tract infections, skin and soft tissue infections, and urinary tract infections due to susceptible strains of *Pseudomonas*, and other gram-negative bacteria

**Effects on Mental Status** May cause drowsiness or confusion; penicillins reported to cause apprehension, illusions, hallucinations, depersonalization, agitation, insomnia, and encephalopathy

**Effects on Psychiatric Treatment** None reported

**Usual Dosage** Ticarcillin is generally given I.V., I.M. injection is only for the treatment of uncomplicated urinary tract infections and dose should not exceed 2 g/injection when administered I.M.

Neonates: I.M., I.V.:
- Postnatal age <7 days:
  - <2000 g: 75 mg/kg/dose every 12 hours
  - >2000 g: 75 mg/kg/dose every 8 hours
- Postnatal age >7 days:
  - <1200 g: 75 mg/kg/dose every 12 hours
  - 1200-2000 g: 75 mg/kg/dose every 8 hours
  - >2000 g: 75 mg/kg/dose every 6 hours

Infants and Children:
- Systemic infections: I.V.: 200-300 mg/kg/day in divided doses every 4-6 hours
- Urinary tract infections: I.M., I.V.: 50-100 mg/kg/day in divided doses every 6-8 hours
- Maximum dose: 24 g/day

Adults: I.M., I.V.: 1-4 g every 4-6 hours, usual dose: 3 g I.V. every 4-6 hours

**Dosing adjustment in renal impairment:** Adults:
- $Cl_{cr}$ 30-60 mL/minute: 2 g every 4 hours or 3 g every 8 hours
- $Cl_{cr}$ 10-30 mL/minute: 2 g every 8 hours or 3 g every 12 hours
- $Cl_{cr}$ <10 mL/minute: 2 g every 12 hours

Moderately dialyzable (20% to 50%)

Continuous arteriovenous or venovenous hemodiafiltration (CAVH) effects: Dose as for $Cl_{cr}$ 10-50 mL/minute

**Dosage Forms** Powder for injection, as disodium: 1 g, 3 g, 6 g, 20 g, 30 g

## Ticarcillin and Clavulanate Potassium
(tye kar SIL in & klav yoo LAN ate poe TASS ee um)

**U.S. Brand Names** Timentin®

**Pharmacologic Category** Antibiotic, Penicillin

**Use** Treatment of infections of lower respiratory tract, urinary tract, skin and skin structures, bone and joint, and septicemia caused by susceptible organisms. Clavulanate expands activity of ticarcillin to include beta-lactamase producing strains of *S. aureus, H. influenzae, Bacteroides* species, and some other gram-negative bacilli

**Effects on Mental Status** May cause drowsiness or confusion; penicillins reported to cause apprehension, illusions, hallucinations, depersonalization, agitation, insomnia, and encephalopathy

**Effects on Psychiatric Treatment** None reported

**Usual Dosage** I.V.:
- Children and Adults <60 kg: 200-300 mg of ticarcillin component/kg/day in divided doses every 4-6 hours
- Children >60 kg and Adults: 3.1 g (ticarcillin 3 g plus clavulanic acid 0.1 g) every 4-6 hours; maximum: 24 g/day
- Urinary tract infections: 3.1 g every 6-8 hours

**Dosing adjustment in renal impairment:**
- $Cl_{cr}$ 30-60 mL/minute: Administer 2 g every 4 hours or 3.1 g every 8 hours
- $Cl_{cr}$ 10-30 mL/minute: Administer 2 g every 8 hours or 3.1 g every 12 hours
- $Cl_{cr}$ <10 mL/minute: Administer 2 g every 12 hours

Moderately dialyzable (20% to 50%)

Continuous arteriovenous or venovenous hemodiafiltration (CAVH) effects: Dose as for $Cl_{cr}$ 10-50 mL/minute

**Dosage Forms**

Infusion, premixed (frozen): Ticarcillin disodium 3 g and clavulanate potassium 0.1 g (100 mL)

Powder for injection: Ticarcillin disodium 3 g and clavulanate potassium 0.1 g (3.1 g, 31 g)

♦ **TICE® BCG** *see* BCG Vaccine *on page 58*

♦ **Ticlid®** *see* Ticlopidine *on page 548*

## Ticlopidine (tye KLOE pi deen)

**U.S. Brand Names** Ticlid®

**Pharmacologic Category** Antiplatelet Agent

**Use** Platelet aggregation inhibitor that reduces the risk of thrombotic stroke in patients who have had a stroke or stroke precursors. Should be reserved for patients who are intolerant or allergic to aspirin therapy or who have failed aspirin therapy.

**Unlabeled use:** Protection of aortocoronary bypass grafts, diabetic microangiopathy, ischemic heart disease, prevention of postoperative DVT, reduction of graft loss following renal transplant

**Effects on Mental Status** None reported

**Effects on Psychiatric Treatment** May cause neutropenia; use caution with clozapine and carbamazepine

**Pregnancy Risk Factor** B

**Contraindications** Hypersensitivity to ticlopidine or any component; active pathological bleeding such as PUD or intracranial hemorrhage; severe liver dysfunction; hematopoietic disorders (neutropenia, thrombocytopenia, a past history of either TTP or aplastic anemia)

**Warnings/Precautions** Use with caution in patients who may be at risk of increased bleeding. Consider discontinuing 10-14 days before elective surgery. Use caution in mixing with other antiplatelet drugs. Use with caution in patients with severe liver disease (experience is limited). May cause life-threatening hematological adverse reactions, including neutropenia/agranulocytosis, thrombocytopenia purpura, and aplastic anemia. Monitor for signs and symptoms of neutropenia including WBC count. Discontinue if the absolute neutrophil count falls to <1200/mm$^3$ or if the platelet count falls to <80,000/mm$^3$.

**Adverse Reactions** As with all drugs which may affect hemostasis, bleeding is associated with ticlopidine. Hemorrhage may occur at virtually any site. Risk is dependent on multiple variables, including the use of multiple agents which alter hemostasis and patient susceptibility.

>10%: Gastrointestinal: Diarrhea (12.5%)

1% to 10%: Central nervous system: Dizziness (1.1%)
- Dermatologic: Rash (5.1%), purpura (2.2%), pruritus (1.3%)
- Gastrointestinal: Nausea (7%), dyspepsia (7%), gastrointestinal pain (3.7%), vomiting (1.9%), flatulence (1.5%), anorexia (1%)
- Hematologic: Neutropenia (2.4%)
- Hepatic: Abnormal liver function test (1%)

<1% (Limited to important or life-threatening symptoms): Thrombotic thrombocytopenic purpura (TTP), thrombocytopenia (immune), agranulocytosis, eosinophilia, pancytopenia, thrombocytosis, bone marrow suppression, gastrointestinal bleeding, ecchymosis, epistaxis, hematuria, menorrhagia, conjunctival bleeding, leukemia, intracranial bleeding (rare), urticaria, exfoliative dermatitis, Stevens-Johnson syndrome, erythema multiforme, maculopapular rash, erythema nodosum, headache, weakness, pain, tinnitus, hemolytic anemia, aplastic anemia, hepatitis, jaundice, hepatic necrosis, hepatic failure, peptic ulcer, renal failure, nephrotic syndrome, hyponatremia, vasculitis, sepsis, pneumonitis (allergic), angioedema, anaphylaxis, positive ANA, systemic lupus erythematosus, peripheral neuropathy, serum sickness, arthropathy, myositis

Case reports: Chronic diarrhea, increase in serum creatinine, bronchiolitis obliterans-organized pneumonia

**Overdosage/Toxicology**

Signs and symptoms: Ataxia, seizures, vomiting, abdominal pain, hematologic abnormalities; specific treatments are lacking; after decontamination

Treatment: Symptomatic and supportive

**Drug Interactions** CYP2C19 inhibitor; CYP1A2 inhibitor

Antacids reduce absorption of ticlopidine (~18%).

Anticoagulants or other antiplatelet agents may increase the risk of bleeding; use with caution.

Carbamazepine blood levels may be increased by ticlopidine.

Cimetidine increases ticlopidine levels.

Cyclosporine blood levels may be reduced by ticlopidine.

Digoxin blood levels may be decreased by ticlopidine.
Phenytoin blood levels may be increased by ticlopidine.
Theophylline blood levels may be increased by ticlopidine.

**Usual Dosage** Adults: Oral: 1 tablet twice daily with food

**Patient Information** Take exact dosage prescribed, with food. Do not use aspirin or aspirin-containing medications and OTC medications without consulting prescriber. You may experience easy bleeding or bruising (use soft toothbrush or cotton swabs and frequent mouth care, use electric razor, avoid sharp knives or scissors). Report unusual bleeding or bruising or persistent fever or sore throat; blood in urine, stool, or vomitus; delayed healing of any wounds; skin rash; yellowing of skin or eyes; changes in color of urine of stool; pain or burning on urination; respiratory difficulty; or skin rash.

**Dosage Forms** Tablet, as hydrochloride: 250 mg

♦ **Ticon®** *see* Trimethobenzamide *on page 569*

♦ **Tigan®** *see* Trimethobenzamide *on page 569*

♦ **Tikosyn™** *see* Dofetilide *on page 180*

♦ **Tilade® Inhalation Aerosol** *see* Nedocromil *on page 005*

## Tiludronate (tye LOO droe nate)

**U.S. Brand Names** Skelid®

**Pharmacologic Category** Bisphosphonate Derivative

**Use** Treatment of Paget's disease of the bone (1) who have a level of serum alkaline phosphatase (SAP) at least twice the upper limit of normal, (2) or who are symptomatic, (3) or who are at risk for future complications of their disease

**Effects on Mental Status** May cause dizziness, anxiety, or nervousness

**Effects on Psychiatric Treatment** None reported

**Pregnancy Risk Factor** C

**Contraindications** Hypersensitivity to biphosphonates or any component of the product

**Warnings/Precautions** Not recommended in patients with severe renal impairment ($Cl_{cr}$ <30 mL/minute). Use with caution in patients with active upper GI problems (eg, dysphagia, symptomatic esophageal diseases, gastritis, duodenitis, ulcers).

**Adverse Reactions** 1% to 10%:
- Cardiovascular: Flushing
- Central nervous system: Vertigo, involuntary muscle contractions, anxiety, nervousness
- Dermatologic: Pruritus, increased sweating, Stevens-Johnson type syndrome (rare)
- Gastrointestinal: Xerostomia, gastritis
- Genitourinary: Urinary tract infection
- Neuromuscular & skeletal: Weakness, pathological fracture
- Respiratory: Bronchitis
- Miscellaneous: Increased diaphoresis

**Overdosage/Toxicology**
Signs and symptoms: Hypocalcemia is a potential consequence of tiludronate overdose
Treatment: No specific information on overdose treatment is available; dialysis would not be beneficial. Standard medical practices may be used to manage renal insufficiency or hypocalcemia, if signs of these occur.

**Drug Interactions**
Decreased effect:
- Calcium supplements, antacids interfere with the bioavailability (decreased 60%) when administered 1 hour before tiludronate
- Aspirin decreases the bioavailability of tiludronate by up to 50% when taken 2 hours after tiludronate

Increased effect/toxicity: Indomethacin increases the bioavailability of tiludronate two- to fourfold

**Usual Dosage** Tiludronate should be taken with 6-8 oz of plain water and not taken within 2 hours of food
Adults: Oral: 400 mg (2 tablets of tiludronic acid) daily for a period of 3 months; allow an interval of 3 months to assess response
**Dosing adjustment in renal impairment:** $Cl_{cr}$ <30 mL/minute: **Not recommended**
**Dosing adjustment in hepatic impairment:** Adjustment is not necessary

**Dietary Considerations** In single-dose studies, the bioavailability of tiludronate was reduced by 90% when an oral dose was administered with, or 2 hours after, a standard breakfast compared to the same dose administered after an overnight fast and 4 hours before a standard breakfast; therefore, do not take within 2 hours of food

**Patient Information** In order to be effective this drug must be taken exactly as prescribed: Take 2 hours before or 2 hours after meals, aspirin, indomethacin, or calcium, magnesium, or aluminum containing medications such as antacids. Take with 6-8 oz. of water. Do not remove medication from foil strip until ready to be used. You may experience mild skin rash; abdominal pain, diarrhea, or constipation (report if persistent). Report unresolved muscle or bone pain or leg cramps; acute abdominal pain; chest pain, palpitations, or swollen extremities; disturbed vision or excessively dry eyes; ringing in the ears; persistent rash or skin disorder; unusual weakness or increased perspiration.

**Dosage Forms** Tablet, as disodium: 240 mg [tiludronic acid 200 mg]; dosage is expressed in terms of tiludronic acid.

♦ **Timentin®** *see* Ticarcillin and Clavulanate Potassium *on page 548*

## Timolol (TYE moe lole)

**Related Information**
Beta-Blockers Comparison Chart *on page 709*
Glaucoma Drug Therapy *on page 712*

**U.S. Brand Names** Betimol® Ophthalmic; Blocadren® Oral; Timoptic® Ophthalmic; Timoptic® Ophthalmic in OcuDose®; Timoptic-XE® Ophthalmic

**Canadian Brand Names** Apo®-Timol; Apo®-Timop; Gen-Timolol; Novo-Timol; Nu-Timolol

**Synonyms** Timolol Hemihydrate; Timolol Maleate

**Pharmacologic Category** Beta Blocker, Nonselective; Ophthalmic Agent, Antiglaucoma

**Use** Ophthalmic dosage form used to treat elevated intraocular pressure such as glaucoma or ocular hypertension; oral dosage form used for treatment of hypertension and angina, to reduce mortality following myocardial infarction, and for prophylaxis of migraine

**Effects on Mental Status** May cause dizziness or fatigue; may rarely cause anxiety, depression, or hallucinations

**Effects on Psychiatric Treatment** Barbiturates and carbamazepine may decrease the effects of beta-blockers

**Pregnancy Risk Factor** C (per manufacturer); D (in second or third trimester, based on expert analysis)

**Contraindications** Hypersensitivity to timolol or any component; sinus bradycardia; sinus node dysfunction; heart block greater than first degree (except in patients with a functioning artificial pacemaker); cardiogenic shock; uncompensated cardiac failure; bronchospastic disease; pregnancy (2nd and 3rd trimesters)

**Warnings/Precautions** Administer cautiously in compensated heart failure and monitor for a worsening of the condition. Avoid abrupt discontinuation in patients with a history of CAD; slowly wean while monitoring for signs and symptoms of ischemia. Use caution with concurrent use of beta-blockers and either verapamil or diltiazem; bradycardia or heart block can occur. Beta-blockers can aggravate symptoms in patients with PVD. Patients with bronchospastic disease should generally not receive beta-blockers - monitor closely if used in patients with potential risk of bronchospasm. Use cautiously in diabetics because it can mask prominent hypoglycemic symptoms. Can mask signs of thyrotoxicosis. Can cause fetal harm when administered in pregnancy. Use cautiously in severe renal impairment: marked hypotension can occur in patients maintained on hemodialysis. Use care with anesthetic agents which decrease myocardial function. Can worsen myasthenia gravis. Similar reactions found with systemic administration may occur with topical administration.

**Adverse Reactions**
Ophthalmic:
- 1% to 10%:
  - Dermatologic: Alopecia
  - Ocular: Burning, stinging of eyes
- <1%: Blepharitis, conjunctivitis, keratitis, rash, vision disturbances

Oral:
- >10%: Endocrine & metabolic: Decreased sexual ability
- 1% to 10%:
  - Cardiovascular: Bradycardia, arrhythmia, reduced peripheral circulation
  - Central nervous system: Dizziness, fatigue
  - Dermatologic: Itching
  - Neuromuscular & skeletal: Weakness
  - Ocular: Burning eyes, stinging of eyes
  - Respiratory: Dyspnea
- <1%: Anxiety, chest pain, congestive heart failure, diarrhea, dry sore eyes, hallucinations, mental depression, nausea, nightmares, numbness in toes and fingers, skin rash, stomach discomfort, vomiting

**Overdosage/Toxicology**
Signs and symptoms: Cardiac disturbances, CNS toxicity, bronchospasm, hypoglycemia and hyperkalemia. The most common cardiac symptoms include hypotension and bradycardia; atrioventricular block, intraventricular conduction disturbances, cardiogenic shock, and asystole may occur with severe overdose, especially with membrane-depressant drugs (eg, propranolol); CNS effects include convulsions, coma, and respiratory arrest is commonly seen with propranolol and other membrane-depressant and lipid-soluble drugs.
Treatment: Symptomatic treatment of seizures, hypotension, hyperkalemia and hypoglycemia; bradycardia and hypotension resistant to atropine, isoproterenol or pacing may respond to glucagon; wide QRS defects caused by the membrane-depressant poisoning may respond to hypertonic sodium bicarbonate; repeat-dose charcoal, hemoperfusion, or hemodialysis may be helpful in removal of only those beta-blockers with
(Continued)

## Timolol *(Continued)*

a small $V_d$, long half-life or low intrinsic clearance (acebutolol, atenolol, nadolol, sotalol).

**Drug Interactions** CYP2D6 enzyme substrate

Albuterol (and other $beta_2$ agonists): Effects may be blunted by nonspecific beta-blockers

Alpha-blockers (prazosin, terazosin): Concurrent use of beta-blockers may increase risk of orthostasis

Clonidine: Hypertensive crisis after or during withdrawal of either agent (not reported with timolol ophthalmic solution)

Drugs which slow AV conduction (digoxin): Effects may be additive with beta-blockers

Epinephrine (including local anesthetics with epinephrine): Timolol may cause hypertension

Glucagon: Timolol may blunt hyperglycemic action

Insulin and oral hypoglycemics: May mask symptoms of hypoglycemia

NSAIDs (ibuprofen, indomethacin, naproxen, piroxicam) may reduce the antihypertensive effects of beta-blockers

Salicylates may reduce the antihypertensive effects of beta-blockers

Sulfonylureas: Beta-blockers may alter response to hypoglycemic agents

Verapamil or diltiazem may have synergistic or additive pharmacological effects when taken concurrently with beta-blockers

**Usual Dosage**

Children and Adults: Ophthalmic: Initial: 0.25% solution, instill 1 drop twice daily; increase to 0.5% solution if response not adequate; decrease to 1 drop/day if controlled; do not exceed 1 drop twice daily of 0.5% solution

Adults: Oral:

Hypertension: Initial: 10 mg twice daily, increase gradually every 7 days, usual dosage: 20-40 mg/day in 2 divided doses; maximum: 60 mg/day

Prevention of myocardial infarction: 10 mg twice daily initiated within 1-4 weeks after infarction

Migraine headache: Initial: 10 mg twice daily, increase to maximum of 30 mg/day

**Patient Information**

Oral: Take exact dose prescribed; do not increase, decrease, or discontinue dosage without consulting prescriber. Take at the same time each day. Does not replace recommended diet or exercise program. If diabetic, monitor serum glucose closely. May cause postural hypotension (use caution when rising from sitting or lying position or climbing stairs); dizziness, drowsiness, or blurred vision (use caution when driving or engaging in tasks requiring alertness until response to drug is known); decreased sexual ability (reversible); or nausea or vomiting (small frequent meals or frequent mouth care may help). Report swelling of extremities, respiratory difficulty, or new cough; weight gain (>3 lb/week); unresolved diarrhea or vomiting; or cold blue extremities.

Ophthalmic: For ophthalmic use only. Apply prescribed amount as often as directed. Wash hands before using and do not touch tip of applicator to eye or contaminate tip of applicator. Tilt head back and look upward. Gently pull down lower lid and put drop(s) inside lower eyelid at inner corner. Close eye and roll eyeball in all directions. Do not blink for $^1/_2$ minute. Apply gentle pressure to inner corner of eye for 30 seconds. Wipe away excess from skin around eye. Do not use any other eye preparation for at least 10 minutes. Do not share medication with anyone else. Temporary stinging or blurred vision may occur. Immediately report any adverse cardiac or CNS effects (usually signifies overdose). Report persistent eye pain, redness, burning, watering, dryness, double vision, puffiness around eye, vision disturbances, other adverse eye response, worsening of condition or lack of improvement. Inform prescriber if you are or intend to be pregnant. Consult prescriber if breast-feeding.

**Nursing Implications** Monitor for systemic effect of beta-blockade even when administering ophthalmic product

**Dosage Forms**

Gel, as maleate, ophthalmic (Timoptic-XE®): 0.25% (2.5 mL, 5 mL); 0.5% (2.5 mL, 5 mL)

Solution, as hemihydrate, ophthalmic (Betimol®): 0.25% (2.5 mL, 5 mL, 10 mL, 15 mL); 0.5% (2.5 mL, 5 mL, 10 mL, 15 mL)

Solution, as maleate, ophthalmic (Timoptic®): 0.25% (2.5 mL, 5 mL, 10 mL, 15 mL); 0.5% (2.5 mL, 5 mL, 10 mL, 15 mL)

Solution, as maleate, ophthalmic, preservative free, single use (Timoptic® OcuDose®): 0.25%, 0.5%

Tablet, as maleate, (Blocadren®): 5 mg, 10 mg, 20 mg


♦ **Timolol Hemihydrate** *see* Timolol *on page 549*

♦ **Timolol Maleate** *see* Timolol *on page 549*

♦ **Timoptic® Ophthalmic** *see* Timolol *on page 549*

♦ **Timoptic® Ophthalmic in OcuDose®** *see* Timolol *on page 549*

♦ **Timoptic-XE® Ophthalmic** *see* Timolol *on page 549*

♦ **Tinactin® [OTC]** *see* Tolnaftate *on page 555*

♦ **Tinactin® for Jock Itch [OTC]** *see* Tolnaftate *on page 555*

♦ **Tine Test** *see* Tuberculin Purified Protein Derivative *on page 575*

♦ **Tine Test PPD** *see* Tuberculin Purified Protein Derivative *on page 575*

♦ **Ting® [OTC]** *see* Tolnaftate *on page 555*

♦ **Tinver® Lotion** *see* Sodium Thiosulfate *on page 515*


## Tinzaparin (tin ZA pa rin)

**U.S. Brand Names** Innohep®

**Pharmacologic Category** Low Molecular Weight Heparin

**Use** Treatment of acute symptomatic deep vein thrombosis, with or without pulmonary embolism, in conjunction with warfarin sodium

**Effects on Mental Status** May cause insomnia, confusion, or dizziness

**Effects on Psychiatric Treatment** May rarely cause agranulocytosis; use caution with clozapine and carbamazepine

**Usual Dosage** S.C.:

Adults: 175 anti-Xa int. units/kg of body weight once daily. Warfarin sodium should be started when appropriate. Administer tinzaparin for at least 6 days and until patient is adequately anticoagulated with warfarin.

Note: To calculate the volume of solution to administer per dose: Volume to be administered (mL) = patient weight (kg) x 0.00875 mL/kg (may be rounded off to the nearest 0.05 mL)

Elderly: No significant differences in safety or response were seen when used in patients ≥65 years of age. However, increased sensitivity to tinzaparin in elderly patients may be possible due to a decline in renal function.

**Dosage adjustment in renal impairment:** Patients with severe renal impairment had a 24% decrease in clearance, use with caution.

**Dosage adjustment in hepatic impairment:** No specific dosage adjustment has been recommended.

**Dosage Forms** Vial: 20,000 anti-Xa int. units/mL (2 mL)

## Tioconazole (tye oh KONE a zole)

**U.S. Brand Names** Vagistat®-1 Vaginal [OTC]

**Pharmacologic Category** Antifungal Agent, Vaginal

**Use** Local treatment of vulvovaginal candidiasis

**Effects on Mental Status** None reported

**Effects on Psychiatric Treatment** None reported

**Usual Dosage** Adults: Vaginal: Insert 1 applicatorful in vagina, just prior to bedtime, as a single dose; therapy may extend to 7 days

**Dosage Forms** Cream, vaginal: 6.5% with applicator (4.6 g)

♦ **Tioguanine** *see* Thioguanine *on page 542*

## Tiopronin (tye oh PROE nin)

**U.S. Brand Names** Thiola™

**Pharmacologic Category** Urinary Tract Product

**Use** Prevention of kidney stone (cystine) formation in patients with severe homozygous cystinuric who have urinary cystine >500 mg/day who are resistant to treatment with high fluid intake, alkali, and diet modification, or who have had adverse reactions to penicillamine

**Effects on Mental Status** None reported

**Effects on Psychiatric Treatment** None reported

**Pregnancy Risk Factor** C

**Usual Dosage** Adults: Initial dose is 800 mg/day, average dose is 1000 mg/day

**Patient Information** Take on an empty stomach (1 hour before or 2 hours after meals) with a full glass of water. Maintain adequate hydration (2-3 L/day). You may experience night voiding (normal); nausea or vomiting (frequent small meals, frequent mouth care, or sucking on lozenges may help); or diarrhea (buttermilk or yogurt may help). Report promptly any unusual bruising or bleeding fatigue, abdominal pain, or acute headache, yellowing of skin or eyes, swelling of extremities, increased weight (>5 lb/week), respiratory difficulty, pain on urination, or cloudy or bloody urine. Inform prescriber if you are pregnant. Do not breast-feed.

**Dosage Forms** Tablet: 100 mg

♦ **Tiotixene** *see* Thiothixene *on page 545*

## Tirofiban (tye roe FYE ban)

**U.S. Brand Names** Aggrastat®

**Pharmacologic Category** Antiplatelet Agent

**Use** In combination with heparin, is indicated for the treatment of acute coronary syndrome, including patients who are to be managed medically and those undergoing PTCA or atherectomy. In this setting, it has been shown to decrease the rate of a combined endpoint of death, new myocardial infarction or refractory ischemia/repeat cardiac procedure.

**Effects on Mental Status** May cause dizziness

**Effects on Psychiatric Treatment** Contraindicated in patients with a recent stroke (within 30 days)

**Usual Dosage** Adults: I.V.: Initial rate of 0.4 mcg/kg/minute for 30 minutes and then continued at 0.1 mcg/kg/minute; dosing should be continued through angiography and for 12-24 hours after angioplasty or atherectomy.

**Dosage Forms** Injection: 50 mcg/mL (500 mL); 250 mcg/mL (50 mL)


- **Tisit® Blue Gel [OTC]** *see* Pyrethrins *on page 480*
- **Tisit® Liquid [OTC]** *see* Pyrethrins *on page 480*
- **Tisit® Shampoo [OTC]** *see* Pyrethrins *on page 480*
- **Titralac® Plus Liquid [OTC]** *see* Calcium Carbonate and Simethicone *on page 85*


## Tizanidine (tye ZAN i deen)

**U.S. Brand Names** Zanaflex®

**Pharmacologic Category** $Alpha_2$ Agonist

**Use** Skeletal muscle relaxant used for treatment of muscle spasticity; although not approved for these indications it has been shown to be effective for tension headaches, low back pain and trigeminal neuralgia in a limited number of trials

**Effects on Mental Status** Drowsiness is common; may cause dizziness, anxiety, nervousness, or insomnia; may rarely cause psychosis

**Effects on Psychiatric Treatment** Concurrent use with psychotropics may produce additive sedation and dry mouth

**Pregnancy Risk Factor** C

**Contraindications** Previous hypersensitivity to tizanidine

**Warnings/Precautions** Reduce dose in patients with liver or renal disease; use with caution in patients with hypotension or cardiac disease. Tizanidine clearance is reduced by more than 50% in elderly patients with renal insufficiency ($Cl_{cr}$ <25 mL/minute) compared to healthy elderly subjects; this may lead to a longer duration of effects and, therefore, should be used with caution in renally impaired patients.

**Adverse Reactions**

>10%:
- Cardiovascular: Hypotension
- Central nervous system: Sedation, daytime drowsiness, somnolence
- Gastrointestinal: Xerostomia

1% to 10%:
- Cardiovascular: Bradycardia, syncope
- Central nervous system: Fatigue, dizziness, anxiety, nervousness, insomnia
- Dermatologic: Pruritus, skin rash
- Gastrointestinal: Nausea, vomiting, dyspepsia, constipation, diarrhea
- Hepatic: Elevation of liver enzymes
- Neuromuscular & skeletal: Muscle weakness, tremor

<1%: Delusions, hepatic failure, palpitations, psychotic-like symptoms, ventricular extrasystoles, visual hallucinations

**Overdosage/Toxicology**

Signs and symptoms: Dry mouth, bradycardia, hypotension

Treatment: Lavage (within 2 hours of ingestion) with activated charcoal; benzodiazepines for seizure control; atropine can be given for treatment of bradycardia; flumazenil has been used to reverse coma successfully; forced diuresis is not helpful; multiple dosing of activated charcoal may be helpful. Following attempts to enhance drug elimination, hypotension should be treated with I.V. fluids and/or Trendelenburg positioning.

**Drug Interactions**

Increased effect: Oral contraceptives

Increased toxicity: Additive hypotensive effects may be seen with diuretics, other alpha adrenergic agonists, or antihypertensives; CNS depression with alcohol, baclofen or other CNS depressants

**Usual Dosage**

Adults: 2-4 mg 3 times/day
- Usual initial dose: 4 mg, may increase by 2-4 mg as needed for satisfactory reduction of muscle tone every 6-8 hours to a maximum of three doses in any 24 hour period
- Maximum dose: 36 mg/day

**Dosing adjustment in renal/hepatic impairment:** May require dose reductions or less frequent dosing

**Patient Information** Take exactly as directed; do not miss doses. Do not use alcohol and prescription or OTC medications that may cause sedation (eg, antidepressants, anxiolytics, sleep medications, etc) without consulting prescriber. Change position slowly when rising from sitting or lying. May cause transient drowsiness, dizziness; avoid driving or engaging in tasks that require alertness until response to drug is known. Small frequent meals may help reduce any nausea or vomiting; frequent mouth care or sucking on lozenges may help reduce dry mouth. Report unusual weight gain or swelling of ankles and hands, yellowing of skin or eyes, fever, unusual bruising, extreme fatigue, rash, palpitations or chest pain. Consult prescriber if breast-feeding.

**Dosage Forms** Tablet: 4 mg


- **TMP** *see* Trimethoprim *on page 570*
- **TMP-SMZ** *see* Co-Trimoxazole *on page 142*
- **TNKase™** *see* Tenecteplase *on page 534*
- **TobraDex® Ophthalmic** *see* Tobramycin and Dexamethasone *on page 552*


## Tobramycin (toe bra MYE sin)

**Related Information**

Serum Drug Concentrations Commonly Monitored: Guidelines *on page 759*

**U.S. Brand Names** AKTob® Ophthalmic; Nebcin® Injection; Tobrex® Ophthalmic

**Pharmacologic Category** Antibiotic, Aminoglycoside; Antibiotic, Ophthalmic

**Use** Treatment of documented or suspected infections caused by susceptible gram-negative bacilli including *Pseudomonas aeruginosa*; topically used to treat superficial ophthalmic infections caused by susceptible bacteria. Tobramycin solution for inhalation is indicated for the management of cystic fibrosis patients (>6 years of age) with *Pseudomonas aeruginosa*.

**Effects on Mental Status** May cause drowsiness

**Effects on Psychiatric Treatment** None reported

**Pregnancy Risk Factor** C

**Contraindications** Hypersensitivity to tobramycin or other aminoglycosides or components

**Warnings/Precautions** Use with caution in patients with renal impairment; pre-existing auditory or vestibular impairment; and in patients with neuromuscular disorders; dosage modification required in patients with impaired renal function; (I.M. & I.V.) Aminoglycosides are associated with significant nephrotoxicity or ototoxicity; the ototoxicity is directly proportional to the amount of drug given and the duration of treatment; tinnitus or vertigo are indications of vestibular injury; ototoxicity is often irreversible; renal damage is usually reversible

**Adverse Reactions**

1% to 10%:
- Renal: Nephrotoxicity
- Neuromuscular & skeletal: Neurotoxicity (neuromuscular blockade)
- Otic: Ototoxicity (auditory), ototoxicity (vestibular)

<1%: Anemia, arthralgia, drowsiness, drug fever, dyspnea, edema of the eyelid, eosinophilia, headache, hypotension, itching eyes, keratitis, lacrimation, nausea, paresthesia, rash, tremor, vomiting, weakness

**Overdosage/Toxicology**

Signs and symptoms: Ototoxicity, nephrotoxicity, and neuromuscular toxicity

Treatment: The treatment of choice following a single acute overdose appears to be the maintenance of good urine output of at least 3 mL/kg/hour. Dialysis is of questionable value in the enhancement of aminoglycoside elimination. If required, hemodialysis is preferred over peritoneal dialysis in patients with normal renal function. Careful hydration may be all that is required to promote diuresis and therefore the enhancement of the drug's elimination. Chelation with penicillins is investigational.

**Drug Interactions**

Increased effect: Extended spectrum penicillins (synergistic)

Increased toxicity:
- Neuromuscular blockers increase neuromuscular blockade
- Amphotericin B, cephalosporins, loop diuretics, and vancomycin may increase risk of nephrotoxicity

**Usual Dosage** Individualization is critical because of the low therapeutic index

**Use of ideal body weight (IBW) for determining the mg/kg/dose appears to be more accurate than dosing on the basis of total body weight (TBW)**

In morbid obesity, dosage requirement may best be estimated using a dosing weight of IBW + 0.4 (TBW - IBW)

Initial and periodic peak and trough plasma drug levels should be determined, particularly in critically ill patients with serious infections or in disease states known to significantly alter aminoglycoside pharmacokinetics (eg, cystic fibrosis, burns, or major surgery). Two to three serum level measurements should be obtained after the initial dose to measure the half-life in order to determine the frequency of subsequent doses.

Once daily dosing: Higher peak serum drug concentration to MIC ratios, demonstrated aminoglycoside postantibiotic effect, decreased renal cortex drug uptake, and improved cost-time efficiency are supportive reasons for the use of once daily dosing regimens for aminoglycosides. Current research indicates these regimens to be as effective for nonlife-threatening infections, with no higher incidence of nephrotoxicity, than those requiring multiple daily doses. Doses are determined by calculating the entire day's dose via usual multiple dose calculation techniques and administering this quantity as a single dose. Doses are then adjusted to maintain mean serum concentrations above the MIC(s) of the causative organism(s). (Example: 2.5-5 mg/kg as a single dose; expected $Cp_{max}$: 10-20 mcg/mL and $Cp_{min}$: <1 mcg/mL). Further research is needed for universal recommendation in all patient populations and gram-negative disease; exceptions may include those with known high clearance (eg, children, patients with cystic fibrosis, or burns who may require shorter dosage intervals) and patients with renal function impairment for whom longer than conventional dosage intervals are usually required.

(Continued)

## Tobramycin *(Continued)*

Some clinicians suggest a daily dose of 4-7 mg/kg for all patients with normal renal function. This dose is at least as efficacious with similar, if not less, toxicity than conventional dosing.

Infants and Children <5 years: I.M., I.V.: 2.5 mg/kg/dose every 8 hours
Children >5 years: 1.5-2.5 mg/kg/dose every 8 hours
**Note:** Some patients may require larger or more frequent doses if serum levels document the need (ie, cystic fibrosis or febrile granulocytopenic patients).
Adults: I.M., I.V.:
Severe life-threatening infections: 2-2.5 mg/kg/dose
Urinary tract infection: 1.5 mg/kg/dose
Synergy (for gram-positive infections): 1 mg/kg/dose
Children and Adults: Ophthalmic: Instill 1-2 drops of solution every 4 hours; apply ointment 2-3 times/day; for severe infections apply ointment every 3-4 hours, or solution 2 drops every 30-60 minutes initially, then reduce to less frequent intervals
Inhalation:
Standard aerosolized tobramycin:
Children: 40-80 mg 2-3 times/day
Adults: 60-80 mg 3 times/day
High-dose regimen: Children ≥6 years and Adults: 300 mg every 12 hours (do not administer doses less than 6 hours apart); administer in repeated cycles of 28 days on drug followed by 28 days off drug

**Dosing interval in renal impairment:**
$Cl_{cr}$ ≥60 mL/minute: Administer every 8 hours
$Cl_{cr}$ 40-60 mL/minute: Administer every 12 hours
$Cl_{cr}$ 20-40 mL/minute: Administer every 24 hours
$Cl_{cr}$ 10-20 mL/minute: Administer every 48 hours
$Cl_{cr}$ <10 mL/minute: Administer every 72 hours
Hemodialysis: Dialyzable; 30% removal of aminoglycosides occurs during 4 hours of HD - administer dose after dialysis and follow levels
Continuous arteriovenous or venovenous hemofiltration (CAVH/CAVHD): Dose as for $Cl_{cr}$ of 10-40 mL/minute and follow levels
Administration in CAPD fluid:
Gram-negative infection: 4-8 mg/L (4-8 mcg/mL) of CAPD fluid
Gram-positive infection (ie, synergy): 3-4 mg/L (3-4 mcg/mL) of CAPD fluid
Administration IVPB/I.M.: Dose as for $Cl_{cr}$ <10 mL/minute and follow levels

**Dosing adjustment/comments in hepatic disease:** Monitor plasma concentrations

**Dietary Considerations** Calcium, magnesium, potassium: Renal wasting may cause hypocalcemia, hypomagnesemia, and/or hypokalemia

**Patient Information**
Systemic: Maintain adequate hydration (2-3 L/day of fluids unless instructed to restrict fluid intake). Report decreased urine output, swelling of extremities, difficulty breathing, vaginal itching or discharge, rash, diarrhea, oral thrush, unhealed wounds, dizziness, change in hearing acuity or ringing in ears, or worsening of condition.
Ophthalmic: Use as frequently as recommended; do not overuse. Sit down, tilt head back, instill solution or drops inside lower eyelid, and roll eyeball in all directions. Close eye and apply gentle pressure to inner corner of eye for 30 seconds. Do not touch tip of applicator to eye or any contaminated surface. May experience temporary stinging or blurred vision. Do not use any other eye preparation for 10 minutes. Inform prescriber if condition worsens or does not improve in 3-4 days.

**Nursing Implications** Eye solutions: Allow 5 minutes between application of "multiple-drop" therapy; obtain drug levels after the third dose; peak levels are drawn 30 minutes after the end of a 30-minute infusion or 1 hour after initiation of infusion or I.M. injection; the trough is drawn just before the next dose; administer penicillins or cephalosporins at least 1 hour apart from tobramycin

**Dosage Forms**
Injection, as sulfate (Nebcin®): 10 mg/mL (2 mL); 40 mg/mL (1.5 mL, 2 mL)
Ointment, ophthalmic (Tobrex®): 0.3% (3.5 g)
Powder for injection (Nebcin®): 40 mg/mL (1.2 g vials)
Solution, inhalation (TOBI™): 60 mg/mL (5 mL)
Solution, ophthalmic: 0.3% (5 mL)
AKTob®, Tobrex®: 0.3% (5 mL)

## Tobramycin and Dexamethasone
(toe bra MYE sin & deks a METH a sone)

**U.S. Brand Names** TobraDex® Ophthalmic

**Pharmacologic Category** Antibiotic/Corticosteroid, Ophthalmic

**Use** Treatment of external ocular infection caused by susceptible gram-negative bacteria and steroid responsive inflammatory conditions of the palpebral and bulbar conjunctiva, lid, cornea, and anterior segment of the globe

**Effects on Mental Status** None reported

**Effects on Psychiatric Treatment** None reported

**Usual Dosage** Children and Adults: Ophthalmic: Instill 1-2 drops of solution every 4 hours; apply ointment 2-3 times/day; for severe infections apply ointment every 3-4 hours, or solution 2 drops every 30-60 minutes initially, then reduce to less frequent intervals

**Dosage Forms**
Ointment, ophthalmic: Tobramycin 0.3% and dexamethasone 0.1% (3.5 g)
Suspension, ophthalmic: Tobramycin 0.3% and dexamethasone 0.1% (2.5 mL, 5 mL)

♦ **Tobrex® Ophthalmic** *see* Tobramycin *on page 551*

## Tocainide (toe KAY nide)

**U.S. Brand Names** Tonocard®

**Pharmacologic Category** Antiarrhythmic Agent, Class I-B

**Use** Suppress and prevent symptomatic life-threatening ventricular arrhythmias
**Unlabeled use:** Trigeminal neuralgia

**Effects on Mental Status** Dizziness is common; may cause nervousness or confusion

**Effects on Psychiatric Treatment** May cause agranulocytosis; use caution with clozapine and carbamazepine; barbiturates may decrease the serum levels of tocainide

**Pregnancy Risk Factor** C

**Contraindications** Hypersensitivity to tocainide, any component, or to any local anesthetics of the amide type; second- or third-degree heart block (except in patients with a functioning artificial pacemaker)

**Warnings/Precautions** Watch for proarrhythmic effects. Correct electrolyte imbalances before initiating (especially hypokalemia and hyperkalemia). Use cautiously in heart failure. Adjust dose in patients with significant renal or hepatic impairment. Bone marrow depression can rarely occur during the first 3 months of therapy.

**Adverse Reactions**
>10%:
Central nervous system: Dizziness (8% to 15%)
Gastrointestinal: Nausea (14% to 15%)
1% to 10%:
Cardiovascular: Tachycardia (3%), bradycardia/angina/palpitations (0.5% to 1.8%)
Central nervous system: Nervousness (0.5% to 1.5%), confusion (2% to 3%)
Dermatologic: Rash (0.5% to 8.4%)
Gastrointestinal: Vomiting, diarrhea (4% to 5%), anorexia (1% to 2%)
Neuromuscular & skeletal: Paresthesia (3.5% to 9%), tremor (2.9% to 8.4%)
Ocular: Blurred vision (~1.5%)
<1%: Agranulocytosis, anemia, ataxia, diaphoresis, leukopenia, neutropenia, respiratory arrest

**Overdosage/Toxicology**
Signs and symptoms: Has a narrow therapeutic index and severe toxicity may occur slightly above the therapeutic range, especially with other antiarrhythmic drugs; and acute ingestion of twice the daily therapeutic dose is potentially life-threatening; symptoms of overdose include sedation, confusion, coma, seizures, respiratory arrest and cardiac toxicity (sinus arrest, A-V block, asystole, and hypotension); the QRS and Q-T intervals are usually normal, although they may be prolonged after massive overdose; other effects include dizziness, paresthesias, tremor, ataxia, and GI disturbance.
Treatment: Supportive, using conventional therapies (fluids, positioning, vasopressors, antiarrhythmics, anticonvulsants); sodium bicarbonate may reverse the QRS prolongation (if present), bradyarrhythmias, and hypotension; enhanced elimination with dialysis, hemoperfusion or repeat charcoal is not effective.

**Drug Interactions**
Rifampin may reduce tocainide blood levels
Urinary alkalinizers (antacids, sodium bicarbonate, acetazolamide) may increase tocainide blood levels

**Usual Dosage** Adults: Oral: 1200-1800 mg/day in 3 divided doses, up to 2400 mg/day

**Dosing adjustment in renal impairment:** $Cl_{cr}$ <30 mL/minute: Administer 50% of normal dose or 600 mg once daily.
Hemodialysis: Moderately dialyzable (20% to 50%)
**Dosing adjustment in hepatic impairment:** Maximum daily dose: 1200 mg

**Patient Information** Take exactly as directed, with food. If dose is missed, take as soon as possible, do not double next dose. Do not discontinue without consulting prescriber. You will need regular cardiac checkups while taking this medication. You may experience dizziness, nervousness, or visual changes (use caution when driving or engaging in tasks requiring alertness until response to drug is known); nausea or vomiting, or loss of appetite (frequent small meals, frequent mouth care, chewing gum, or sucking lozenges may help); mild muscle discomfort (analgesics may be recommended). Report chest pain, palpitations, or erratic heartbeat; difficulty breathing or unusual cough; mental confusion or depression; muscle tremor, weakness, or pain; or changes in vision.

**Nursing Implications** Monitor for tremor; titration of dosing and initiation of therapy require cardiac monitoring

**Dosage Forms** Tablet, as hydrochloride: 400 mg, 600 mg

♦ **Tofranil®** *see* Imipramine *on page 282*

♦ **Tofranil-PM®** *see* Imipramine *on page 282*

## Tolazamide (tole AZ a mide)

**Related Information**
Hypoglycemic Drugs and Thiazolidinedione Information *on page 714*

**U.S. Brand Names** Tolinase®

**Pharmacologic Category** Antidiabetic Agent (Sulfonylurea)

**Use** Adjunct to diet for the management of mild to moderately severe, stable, noninsulin-dependent (type 2) diabetes mellitus

**Effects on Mental Status** Dizziness is common

**Effects on Psychiatric Treatment** May cause agranulocytosis; use caution with clozapine and carbamazepine; concurrent use with psychotropics may produce alterations in serum glucose concentrations; monitor glucose; clinical manifestation of hypoglycemia may be blocked by beta-blockers

**Pregnancy Risk Factor** D

**Contraindications** Type 1 diabetes therapy (IDDM), hypersensitivity to sulfonylureas, diabetes complicated by ketoacidosis

**Warnings/Precautions** False-positive response has been reported in patients with liver disease, idiopathic hypoglycemia of infancy, severe malnutrition, acute pancreatitis, renal dysfunction. Transferring a patient from one sulfonylurea to another does not require a priming dose; doses >1000 mg/day normally do not improve diabetic control. Has not been studied in older patients; however, except for drug interactions, it appears to have a safe profile and decline in renal function does not affect its pharmacokinetics. How "tightly" an elderly patient's blood glucose should be controlled is controversial; however, a fasting blood sugar <150 mg/dL is now an acceptable end point. Such a decision should be based on the patient's functional and cognitive status, how well they recognize hypoglycemic or hyperglycemic symptoms, and how to respond to them and their other disease states.

Product labeling states oral hypoglycemic drugs may be associated with an increased cardiovascular mortality as compared to treatment with diet alone or diet plus insulin. Data to support this association are limited, and several studies, including a large prospective trial (UKPDS) have not supported an association.

**Adverse Reactions**

>10%:
- Central nervous system: Headache, dizziness
- Gastrointestinal: Anorexia, nausea, vomiting, diarrhea, constipation, heartburn, epigastric fullness

1% to 10%: Dermatologic: Rash, urticaria, photosensitivity

<1%: Agranulocytosis, aplastic anemia, bone marrow suppression, cholestatic jaundice, diuretic effect, hemolytic anemia, hypoglycemia, thrombocytopenia

**Overdosage/Toxicology**
Signs and symptoms: Low blood sugar, tingling of lips and tongue, nausea, yawning, confusion, agitation, tachycardia, sweating, convulsions, stupor, and coma
Treatment: Intoxications with sulfonylureas can cause hypoglycemia and are best managed with glucose administration (oral for milder hypoglycemia or by injection in more severe forms)

**Drug Interactions** Increased toxicity: Monitor patient closely; large number of drugs interact with sulfonylureas including salicylates, anticoagulants, $H_2$-antagonists, TCAs, MAO inhibitors, beta-blockers, thiazides

**Usual Dosage** Oral (doses >1000 mg/day normally do not improve diabetic control):

Adults:
- Initial: 100-250 mg/day with breakfast or the first main meal of the day
  - Fasting blood sugar <200 mg/dL: 100 mg/day
  - Fasting blood sugar >200 mg/dL: 250 mg/day
  - Patient is malnourished, underweight, elderly, or not eating properly: 100 mg/day
- Adjust dose in increments of 100-250 mg/day at weekly intervals to response. If >500 mg/day is required, give in divided doses twice daily; maximum daily dose: 1 g (doses >1 g/day are not likely to improve control)
- **Conversion from insulin → tolazamide**
  - 10 units day = 100 mg/day
  - 20-40 units/day = 250 mg/day
  - >40 units/day = 250 mg/day and 50% of insulin dose
- Doses >500 mg/day should be given in 2 divided doses

**Dosing adjustment in renal impairment:** Conservative initial and maintenance doses are recommended because tolazamide is metabolized to active metabolites, which are eliminated in the urine

**Dosing comments in hepatic impairment:** Conservative initial and maintenance doses and careful monitoring of blood glucose are recommended

**Dietary Considerations** Alcohol: Avoid use

**Patient Information** This medication is used to control diabetes; it is not a cure. Other components of the treatment plan are important: follow prescribed diet, medication, and exercise regimen. Take exactly as directed; at the same time each day. Do not change dose or discontinue without consulting prescriber. Avoid alcohol while taking this medication; could cause severe reaction. Inform prescriber of all other prescription or OTC medications you are taking; do not introduce new medication without consulting prescriber. Do not take other medication within 2 hours of this medication unless so advised by prescriber. If you experience hypoglycemic reaction, contact prescriber immediately; maintain regular dietary intake and exercise routine and always carry quick source of sugar with you. You may be more sensitive to sunlight (use sunscreen, wear protective clothing and eyewear, and avoid direct sunlight). You may experience side effects during first weeks of therapy (headache, nausea, diarrhea, constipation, anorexia); consult prescriber if these persist. Report severe or persistent side effects, extended vomiting or flu-like symptoms, skin rash, easy bruising or bleeding, or change in color of urine or stool.

**Nursing Implications** Patients who are anorexic or NPO may need to have their dose held to avoid hypoglycemia

**Dosage Forms** Tablet: 100 mg, 250 mg, 500 mg

## Tolazoline (tole AZ oh leen)

**U.S. Brand Names** Priscoline®

**Pharmacologic Category** Vasodilator

**Use** Treatment of persistent pulmonary vasoconstriction and hypertension of the newborn (persistent fetal circulation), peripheral vasospastic disorders

**Effects on Mental Status** None reported

**Effects on Psychiatric Treatment** May cause agranulocytosis, caution with clozapine and carbamazepine; use with alcohol may produce "disulfiram reaction"

**Usual Dosage**

Neonates: Initial: I.V.: 1-2 mg/kg over 10-15 minutes via scalp vein or upper extremity; maintenance: 1-2 mg/kg/hour; use lower maintenance doses in patients with decreased renal function. Also used in neonates for acute vasospasm "cath toes" at 0.25 mg/kg/hour (no load); maximum dose: 6-8 mg/kg/hour.

**Dosing interval in renal impairment in newborns:** Urine output <0.9 mL/kg/hour: Decrease dose to 0.08 mg/kg/hour for every 1 mg/kg of loading dose

Adults: Peripheral vasospastic disorder: I.M., I.V., S.C.: 10-50 mg 4 times/day

**Dosage Forms** Injection, as hydrochloride: 25 mg/mL (4 mL)

## Tolbutamide (tole BYOO ta mide)

**Related Information**
Hypoglycemic Drugs and Thiazolidinedione Information *on page 714*

**U.S. Brand Names** Orinase® Diagnostic Injection; Orinase® Oral

**Canadian Brand Names** Apo®-Tolbutamide; Mobenol®; Novo-Butamide

**Pharmacologic Category** Antidiabetic Agent (Sulfonylurea)

**Use** Adjunct to diet for the management of mild to moderately severe, stable, noninsulin-dependent (type 2) diabetes mellitus

**Effects on Mental Status** Dizziness is common

**Effects on Psychiatric Treatment** May cause agranulocytosis; use caution with clozapine and carbamazepine; concurrent use with psychotropics may produce alterations in serum glucose concentrations; monitor glucose; clinical manifestation of hypoglycemia may be blocked by beta-blockers

**Pregnancy Risk Factor** D

**Contraindications** Diabetes complicated by ketoacidosis, therapy of IDDM, hypersensitivity to sulfonylureas

**Warnings/Precautions** False-positive response has been reported in patients with liver disease, idiopathic hypoglycemia of infancy, severe malnutrition, acute pancreatitis. Because of its low potency and short duration, it is a useful agent in the elderly if drug interactions can be avoided. How "tightly" an elderly patient's blood glucose should be controlled is controversial; however, a fasting blood sugar <150 mg/dL is now an acceptable end point. Such a decision should be based on the patient's functional and cognitive status, how well they recognize hypoglycemic or hyperglycemic symptoms, and how to respond to them and their other disease states.

Product labeling states oral hypoglycemic drugs may be associated with an increased cardiovascular mortality as compared to treatment with diet alone or diet plus insulin. Data to support this association are limited, and several studies, including a large prospective trial (UKPDS) have not supported an association.

**Adverse Reactions**

>10%:
- Central nervous system: Headache, dizziness
- Gastrointestinal: Constipation, diarrhea, heartburn, anorexia, epigastric fullness

1% to 10%: Dermatologic: Rash, urticaria, photosensitivity

(Continued)

## Tolbutamide *(Continued)*

<1%: Agranulocytosis, aplastic anemia, bone marrow suppression, cholestatic jaundice, disulfiram-type reactions, hemolytic anemia, hypersensitivity reaction, hypoglycemia, leukopenia, SIADH, thrombocytopenia, thrombophlebitis, tinnitus, venospasm

**Overdosage/Toxicology**

Signs and symptoms: Low blood sugar, tingling of lips and tongue, nausea, yawning, confusion, agitation, tachycardia, sweating, convulsions, stupor, and coma

Treatment: I.V. glucose (12.5-25 g), epinephrine for anaphylaxis

**Drug Interactions** CYP2C8, 2C9, 2C18, and 2C19 enzyme substrate; CYP2C19 enzyme inhibitor

Increased effects with salicylates, probenecid, MAO inhibitors, chloramphenicol, insulin, phenylbutazone, antidepressants, metformin, $H_2$-antagonists, and others

Decreased effects:

Hypoglycemic effects may be decreased by beta-blockers, cholestyramine, hydantoins, thiazides, rifampin, and others

Ethanol may decrease the half-life of tolbutamide

**Usual Dosage** Divided doses may increase gastrointestinal side effects

Adults:

Oral: Initial: 1-2 g/day as a single dose in the morning or in divided doses throughout the day. Total doses may be taken in the morning; however, divided doses may allow increased gastrointestinal tolerance. Maintenance dose: 0.25-3 g/day; however, a maintenance dose >2 g/day is seldom required.

I.V. bolus: 1 g over 2-3 minutes

Elderly: Oral: Initial: 250 mg 1-3 times/day; usual: 500-2000 mg; maximum: 3 g/day

**Dosing adjustment in renal impairment:** Adjustment is not necessary

Hemodialysis: Not dialyzable (0% to 5%)

**Dosing adjustment in hepatic impairment:** Reduction of dose may be necessary in patients with impaired liver function

**Dietary Considerations** Alcohol: Avoid use

**Patient Information** This medication is used to control diabetes; it is not a cure. Other components of treatment plan are important: follow prescribed diet, medication, and exercise regimen. Take exactly as directed; at the same time each day. Do not change dose or discontinue without consulting prescriber. Avoid alcohol while taking this medication; could cause severe reaction. Inform prescriber of all other prescription or OTC medications you are taking; do not introduce new medication without consulting prescriber. Do not take other medication within 2 hours of this medication unless so advised by prescriber. If you experience hypoglycemic reaction, contact prescriber immediately. Maintain regular dietary intake and exercise routine and always carry quick source of sugar with you. You may be more sensitive to sunlight (use sunscreen, wear protective clothing and eyewear, and avoid direct sunlight). You may experience side effects during first weeks of therapy (headache, nausea, diarrhea, constipation, anorexia); consult prescriber is these persist. Report severe or persistent side effects, extended vomiting or flu-like symptoms, skin rash, easy bruising or bleeding, or change in color of urine or stool.

**Nursing Implications** Patients who are anorexic or NPO may need to have their dose held to avoid hypoglycemia

**Dosage Forms**

Injection, diagnostic, as sodium: 1 g (20 mL)

Tablet: 250 mg, 500 mg

## Tolcapone (TOLE ka pone)

**U.S. Brand Names** Tasmar®

**Pharmacologic Category** Anti-Parkinson's Agent (COMT Inhibitor)

**Use** Adjunct to levodopa and carbidopa for the treatment of signs and symptoms of idiopathic Parkinson's disease

**Pregnancy Risk Factor** C

**Pregnancy/Breast-Feeding Implications** Tolcapone should be used during pregnancy only if the potential benefit justifies the potential risk to the fetus. In animal studies, tolcapone was excreted into maternal rat milk; it is not known whether tolcapone is excreted in human milk. Caution should be taken when tolcapone is administered to nursing women.

**Contraindications** Hypersensitivity to tolcapone or any component

**Warnings/Precautions** Due to reports of fatal liver injury associated with use of this drug, the manufacturer is advising that tolcapone be reserved for use only in patients who do not have severe movement abnormalities and who do not respond to or who are not appropriate candidates for other available treatments. Use with caution in patients with pre-existing dyskinesias, hepatic impairment, or severe renal impairment. May cause orthostatic hypotension; Parkinson's disease patients appear to have an impaired capacity to respond to a postural challenge; use with caution in patients at risk of hypotension (such as those receiving antihypertensive drugs) or where transient hypotensive episodes would be poorly tolerated (cardiovascular disease or cerebrovascular disease). Parkinson's patients being treated with dopaminergic agonists ordinarily require careful monitoring for signs and symptoms of postural hypotension, especially during dose escalation, and should be informed of this risk. May cause hallucinations, which may improve with reduction in levodopa therapy. Use with caution in patients with lower gastrointestinal disease or an increased risk of dehydration - tolcapone has been associated with delayed development of diarrhea (onset after 2-12 weeks).

It is not recommended that patients receive tolcapone concomitantly with nonselective MAO inhibitors (see Drug Interactions). Selegiline is a selective MAO-B inhibitor and can be taken with tolcapone.

Although not reported for tolcapone, other dopaminergic agents have been associated with a syndrome resembling neuroleptic malignant syndrome on withdrawal or significant dosage reduction after long-term use. Dopaminergic agents from the ergot class have also been associated with fibrotic complications, such as retroperitoneum, lungs, and pleura.

**Adverse Reactions**

>10%:

Cardiovascular: Orthostatic hypotension

Central nervous system: Sleep disorder, excessive dreaming, somnolence, headache

Gastrointestinal: Nausea, diarrhea, anorexia

Neuromuscular & skeletal: Dyskinesia, dystonia, muscle cramps

1% to 10%:

Central nervous system: Hallucinations, fatigue, loss of balance, hyperkinesia

Gastrointestinal: Vomiting, constipation, xerostomia, abdominal pain, flatulence, dyspepsia

Genitourinary: Urine discoloration

Neuromuscular & skeletal: Paresthesia, stiffness

Miscellaneous: Diaphoresis (increased)

**Overdosage/Toxicology**

Signs and symptoms include nausea, vomiting, and dizziness, particularly in combination with levodopa/carbidopa

Treatment: Hospitalization and general supportive care; hemodialysis is unlikely to be effective

**Drug Interactions** CYP3A4 and CYP2A6 enzyme substrate

CYP3A3/4 inhibitors: Serum level and/or toxicity of tolcapone may be increased; inhibitors include amiodarone, cimetidine, clarithromycin, erythromycin, delavirdine, diltiazem, dirithromycin, disulfiram, fluoxetine, fluvoxamine, grapefruit juice, indinavir, itraconazole, ketoconazole, nevirapine, propoxyfene, quinupristin-dalfopristin, ritonavir, saquinavir, verapamil, zafirlukast, zileuton; monitor for altered effects

Substrates of COMT: COMT inhibition could slow the metabolism of methyldopa, dobutamine, apomorphine, and isoproterenol

**Mechanism of Action** Tolcapone is a selective and reversible inhibitor of catechol-o-methyltransferase (COMT)

**Pharmacodynamics/kinetics**

Absorption: Rapid with $T_{max}$ at 2 hours

Distribution: $V_d$: 9 L

Protein binding: 99.9%

Metabolism: Tolcapone is almost completely metabolized prior to excretion; the main metabolic pathway is glucuronidation; the glucuronide conjugate is inactive. Tolcapone is hydroxylated and subsequently oxidized via CYP3A4 and CYP2A6.

Bioavailability: 65% (empty stomach), 45% to 55% (with food)

Half-life: 2-3 hours

**Usual Dosage** Adults: Oral: Initial: 100-200 mg 3 times/day; levodopa therapy may need to be decreased upon initiation of tolcapone

**Dosage Forms** Tablet: 100 mg, 200 mg

♦ **Tolectin®** *see* Tolmetin *on page 554*

♦ **Tolectin® DS** *see* Tolmetin *on page 554*

♦ **Tolinase®** *see* Tolazamide *on page 553*

## Tolmetin (TOLE met in)

**Related Information**

Nonsteroidal Anti-inflammatory Agents Comparison Chart *on page 722*

**U.S. Brand Names** Tolectin®; Tolectin® DS

**Canadian Brand Names** Novo-Tolmetin

**Pharmacologic Category** Nonsteroidal Anti-Inflammatory Agent (NSAID)

**Use** Treatment of rheumatoid arthritis and osteoarthritis, juvenile rheumatoid arthritis

**Effects on Mental Status** Dizziness is common; may cause nervousness; may rarely cause drowsiness, confusion, insomnia, hallucinations, or depression

**Effects on Psychiatric Treatment** May rarely cause agranulocytosis; use caution with clozapine and carbamazepine; may decrease lithium clearance resulting in an increase in serum lithium levels and potential lithium toxicity; monitor serum lithium levels

**Pregnancy Risk Factor** C (D if used in the 3rd trimester or near delivery)

**Contraindications** Known hypersensitivity to tolmetin or any component, aspirin, or other nonsteroidal anti-inflammatory drugs (NSAIDs)

**Warnings/Precautions** Use with caution in patients with upper GI disease, impaired renal function, congestive heart failure, dehydration, hypertension, and patients receiving anticoagulants; if GI upset occurs with tolmetin, take with antacids other than sodium bicarbonate

**Adverse Reactions**

>10%:

Central nervous system: Dizziness

Dermatologic: Rash

Gastrointestinal: Abdominal cramps, heartburn, indigestion, nausea

1% to 10%:

Central nervous system: Headache, nervousness

Dermatologic: Itching

Endocrine & metabolic: Fluid retention

Gastrointestinal: Vomiting

Otic: Tinnitus

<1%: Acute renal failure, agranulocytosis, allergic rhinitis, anemia, angioedema, arrhythmias, aseptic meningitis, blurred vision, bone marrow suppression, confusion, congestive heart failure, conjunctivitis, cystitis, decreased hearing, drowsiness, dry eyes, epistaxis, erythema multiforme, gastritis, GI ulceration, hallucinations, hemolytic anemia, hepatitis, hot flashes, hypertension, insomnia, leukopenia, mental depression, peripheral neuropathy, polydipsia, polyuria, shortness of breath, Stevens-Johnson syndrome, tachycardia, thrombocytopenia, toxic amblyopia, toxic epidermal necrolysis, urticaria

**Overdosage/Toxicology**

Signs and symptoms: Lethargy, mental confusion, dizziness, leukocytosis, renal failure

Treatment: Management of a nonsteroidal anti-inflammatory drug (NSAID) intoxication is primarily supportive and symptomatic. Fluid therapy is commonly effective in managing the hypotension that may occur following an acute NSAID overdose, except when this is due to an acute blood loss. Seizures tend to be very short-lived and often do not require drug treatment; although, recurrent seizures should be treated with I.V. diazepam. Since many of the NSAID undergo enterohepatic cycling, multiple doses of charcoal may be needed to reduce the potential for delayed toxicities.

**Drug Interactions**

ACE inhibitors: Effects may be reduced by NSAIDs; use lowest possible dose for shortest duration possible; monitor

Cholestyramine and colestipol: Absorption may be reduced by concurrent administration

Corticosteroids: May increase the risk of GI ulceration; use caution

Cyclosporine: Nephrotoxicity may be increased with concurrent NSAID use; monitor

Hydralazine: Antihypertensive effect may be decreased; avoid concurrent use

Lithium: Serum levels can be increased; avoid concurrent use if possible or monitor lithium levels and adjust dose. When NSAID is stopped, lithium may need adjustment again.

Loop diuretics: Therapeutic effects may be reduced by NSAIDs; avoid

Methotrexate: Toxicity may be increased by concurrent NSAID use; risk is limited in low-dose methotrexate regimens (such as for rheumatoid arthritis); prolonged leucovorin rescue may be required at antineoplastic doses; monitor

Thiazide diuretics: Antihypertensive effects are decreased; avoid concurrent use

Warfarin: INRs may be increased by some NSAIDs. This may depend, in part, on dose and duration; monitor INR closely. Use the lowest dose of NSAIDs possible and for the briefest duration.

**Usual Dosage** Oral:

Children ≥2 years:

Anti-inflammatory: Initial: 20 mg/kg/day in 3 divided doses, then 15-30 mg/kg/day in 3 divided doses

Analgesic: 5-7 mg/kg/dose every 6-8 hours

Adults: 400 mg 3 times/day; usual dose: 600 mg to 1.8 g/day; maximum: 2 g/day

**Patient Information** Take this medication exactly as directed; do not increase dose without consulting prescriber. Do not crush tablets or break capsules. Take with food or milk to reduce GI distress. Maintain adequate fluid intake (2-3 L/day of fluids unless instructed to restrict fluid intake). Do not use alcohol, aspirin, or aspirin-containing medication, and all other anti-inflammatory medications without consulting prescriber. You may experience dizziness, nervousness, or headache (use caution when driving or engaging in tasks requiring alertness until response to drug is known); nausea, vomiting, or heartburn (frequent small meals, frequent mouth care, sucking lozenges, or chewing gum may help); constipation (increased exercise, fluids, or dietary fruit and fiber may help). GI bleeding, ulceration, or perforation can occur with or without pain; discontinue medication and contact prescriber if persistent abdominal pain or cramping, or blood in stool occurs. Report chest pain or palpitations; breathlessness or difficulty breathing; unusual bruising/bleeding; blood in urine, stool, mouth, or vomitus; unusual fatigue; skin rash or itching; unusual weight gain or swelling of extremities; change in urinary pattern; or change in vision or hearing or ringing in ears.

**Dosage Forms**

Capsule, as sodium (Tolectin® DS): 400 mg

Tablet, as sodium (Tolectin®): 200 mg, 600 mg

## Tolnaftate (tole NAF tate)

**U.S. Brand Names** Absorbine® Antifungal [OTC]; Absorbine® Jock Itch [OTC]; Absorbine Jr.® Antifungal [OTC]; Aftate® for Athlete's Foot [OTC]; Aftate® for Jock Itch [OTC]; Blis-To-Sol® [OTC]; Breezee® Mist Antifungal [OTC]; Dr Scholl's Athlete's Foot [OTC]; Dr Scholl's Maximum Strength Tritin [OTC]; Genaspor® [OTC]; NP-27® [OTC]; Quinsana Plus® [OTC]; Tinactin® [OTC]; Tinactin® for Jock Itch [OTC]; Ting® [OTC]; Zeasorb-AF® Powder [OTC]

**Canadian Brand Names** Pitrex®

**Pharmacologic Category** Antifungal Agent, Topical

**Use** Treatment of tinea pedis, tinea cruris, tinea corporis, tinea manuum, tinea versicolor infections

**Effects on Mental Status** None reported

**Effects on Psychiatric Treatment** None reported

**Usual Dosage** Children and Adults: Topical: Wash and dry affected area; apply 1-3 drops of solution or a small amount of cream or powder and rub into the affected areas 2-3 times/day for 2-4 weeks

**Dosage Forms**

Aerosol, topical:

Liquid: 1% (59.2 mL, 90 mL, 120 mL)

Powder: 1% (56.7 g, 100 g, 105 g, 150 g)

Cream: 1% (15 g, 30 g)

Gel, topical: 1% (15 g)

Powder, topical: 1% (45 g, 90 g)

Solution, topical: 1% (10 mL)

## Tolterodine (tole TER oh dine)

**U.S. Brand Names** Detrol™

**Pharmacologic Category** Anticholinergic Agent

**Use** Treatment of patients with an overactive bladder with symptoms of urinary frequency, urgency, or urge incontinence

**Effects on Mental Status** May cause drowsiness, dizziness, or nervousness

**Effects on Psychiatric Treatment** Fluoxetine and likely paroxetine increase the serum concentration of tolterodine

**Pregnancy Risk Factor** C

**Contraindications** Urinary retention or gastric retention; uncontrolled narrow-angle glaucoma; demonstrated hypersensitivity to tolterodine or ingredients

**Warnings/Precautions** Caution in patients with bladder flow obstruction, pyloric stenosis or other GI obstruction, narrow-angle glaucoma (controlled), reduced hepatic/renal function

**Adverse Reactions**

>10%: Central nervous system: Headache

1% to 10%:

Cardiovascular: Chest pain, hypertension (1.5%)

Central nervous system: Vertigo (8.6%), nervousness (1.1%), somnolence (3.0%)

Dermatologic: Pruritus (1.3%), rash (1.9%), dry skin (1.7%)

Gastrointestinal: Abdominal pain (7.6%), constipation (6.5%), diarrhea (4.0%), dyspepsia (5.9%), flatulence (1.3%), nausea (4.2%), vomiting (1.7%), weight gain (1.5%)

Genitourinary: Dysuria (2.5%), polyuria (1.1%), urinary retention (1.7%), urinary tract infection (5.5%)

Neuromuscular & skeletal: Back pain, falling (1.3%), paresthesia (1.1%)

Ocular: Vision abnormalities (4.7%), dry eyes (3.8%)

Respiratory: Bronchitis (2.1%), cough (2.1%), pharyngitis (1.5%), rhinitis (1.1%), sinusitis (1.1%), upper respiratory infection (5.9%)

Miscellaneous: Flu-like symptoms (4.4%), infection (2.1%)

**Overdosage/Toxicology** Overdosage with tolterodine can potentially result in severe central anticholinergic effects and should be treated accordingly. EKG monitoring is recommended in the event of overdosage.

**Drug Interactions** CYP3A3/4 substrate; CYP2D6 substrate

Increased toxicity: Macrolide antibiotics/azole antifungal agents may inhibit the metabolism of tolterodine. Doses of tolterodine >1 mg twice daily should not be exceeded.

Fluoxetine, which inhibits cytochrome P-450 2D6, increases concentration 4.8 times. Other drugs which inhibit this isoenzyme may also interact. Studies with inhibitors of cytochrome isoenzyme 3A4 have not been performed.

**Usual Dosage** Adults: Oral: Initial: 2 mg twice daily; the dose may be lowered to 1 mg twice daily based on individual response and tolerability

Dosing adjustment in patients concurrently taking cytochrome P-450 3A4 inhibitors: 1 mg twice daily

**Dosing adjustment in renal impairment:** Use with caution

**Dosing adjustment in hepatic impairment:** Administer 1 mg twice daily

**Dietary Considerations** Food increases bioavailability (~53% increase)

**Patient Information** Take as directed, preferably with food. You may experience headache (a mild analgesic may help); dizziness, nervousness, or sleepiness (use caution when driving, climbing stairs, or engaging in tasks requiring alertness until response to drug is known); abdominal (Continued)

## Tolterodine *(Continued)*

discomfort, diarrhea, constipation, nausea or vomiting (small frequent meals, increased exercise, adequate fluid intake may help). Report back pain, muscle spasms, alteration in gait, or numbness of extremities; unresolved or persistent constipation, diarrhea, or vomiting; or symptoms of upper respiratory infection or flu. Report immediately any chest pain or palpitations; difficulty urinating or pain on urination.

**Dosage Forms** Tablet, as tartrate: 1 mg, 2 mg

- **Tolu-Sed® DM [OTC]** *see* Guaifenesin and Dextromethorphan *on page 257*
- **Tonga** *see* Kava *on page 301*
- **Tonocard®** *see* Tocainide *on page 552*
- **Topamax®** *see* Topiramate *on page 556*
- **Topamax® Sprinkle** *see* Topiramate *on page 556*
- **Topicort®** *see* Desoximetasone *on page 156*
- **Topicort®-LP** *see* Desoximetasone *on page 156*
- **Topicycline® Topical** *see* Tetracycline *on page 537*

## Topiramate (toe PYE ra mate)

**Related Information**

Anticonvulsants by Seizures Type *on page 703*
Mood Disorders *on page 600*
Mood Stabilizers *on page 719*

**U.S. Brand Names** Topamax®; Topamax® Sprinkle

**Pharmacologic Category** Anticonvulsant, Miscellaneous

**Use** Adjunctive therapy for partial onset seizures in adults and pediatric patients (ages 2-16 years); adjunct therapy of primary generalized tonic-clonic seizures

**Unlabeled use:** Bipolar disorder

**Orphan drug:** Topiramate has also been granted orphan drug status for the treatment of Lennox-Gastaut syndrome

**Pregnancy Risk Factor** C

**Pregnancy/Breast-Feeding Implications** Breast-feeding/lactation: In studies of rats topiramate has been shown to be secreted in milk; however, it has not been studied in humans

**Contraindications** Hypersensitivity to topiramate or any component

**Warnings/Precautions** Avoid abrupt withdrawal of topiramate therapy, it should be withdrawn slowly to minimize the potential of increased seizure frequency. The risk of kidney stones is about 2-4 times that of the untreated population, the risk of this event may be reduced by increasing fluid intake. Use cautiously in patients with hepatic or renal impairment, during pregnancy, or in nursing mothers. May cause paresthesias. Sedation, psychomotor slowing, confusion, and mood disturbances may occur with topiramate use. Patients must cautioned about performing tasks which require mental alertness (ie, operating machinery or driving). Effects with other sedative drugs or ethanol may be potentiated.

**Adverse Reactions**

>10%:

Central nervous system: Dizziness, ataxia, somnolence, psychomotor slowing, nervousness, memory difficulties, speech problems
Gastrointestinal: Nausea
Neuromuscular & skeletal: Paresthesia, tremor
Ocular: Nystagmus, diplopia, abnormal vision
Respiratory: Upper respiratory infections

1% to 10%:

Cardiovascular: Chest pain, edema
Central nervous system: Language problems, abnormal coordination, confusion, depression, difficulty concentrating, hypoesthesia
Endocrine & metabolic: Hot flashes
Gastrointestinal: Dyspepsia, abdominal pain, anorexia, constipation, xerostomia, gingivitis, weight loss
Neuromuscular & skeletal: Myalgia, weakness, back pain, leg pain, rigors
Otic: Decreased hearing
Renal: Nephrolithiasis
Respiratory: Pharyngitis, sinusitis, epistaxis
Miscellaneous: Flu-like symptoms

**Overdosage/Toxicology** Treatment: Activated charcoal has not been shown to adsorb topiramate and is, therefore, not recommended; hemodialysis can remove drug, however, most cases do not require removal and instead is best treated with supportive measures

**Drug Interactions** CYP2C19 enzyme substrate; CYP2C19 enzyme inhibitor

Carbamazepine: May reduce topiramate levels 40%
Carbonic anhydrase inhibitors: Coadministration with other carbonic anhydrase inhibitors may increase the chance of nephrolithiasis; includes acetazolamide
CNS depressants: Sedative effects may be additive with topiramate; monitor for increased effect; includes barbiturates, benzodiazepines, narcotic analgesics, ethanol, and other sedative agents
CYP2C19 inhibitors: Serum levels of topiramate may be increased; inhibitors include cimetidine, felbamate, fluconazole, fluoxetine, fluvoxamine, omeprazole, teniposide, tolbutamide, and troglitazone
Digoxin: Blood levels are decreased when coadministered with topiramate
Estrogens: Blood levels are decreased when coadministered with topiramate, this may lead to a loss of efficacy
Oral contraceptives: See estrogens; alternative contraceptive measures should be used
Phenytoin: May decrease topiramate levels by as much as 48%; topiramate may increase phenytoin concentration by 25%
Valproic acid: May reduce topiramate levels by 14%; topiramate may decrease valproic acid concentration by 11%

**Mechanism of Action** Mechanism is not fully understood, it is thought to decrease seizure frequency by blocking sodium channels in neurons, enhancing GABA activity and by blocking glutamate activity

**Pharmacodynamics/kinetics**

Absorption: Good; unaffected by food
Protein binding: 13% to 17%
Metabolism: Minimal, less than 5% of metabolites are active
Bioavailability: 80%
Half-life: Mean: 21 hours in adults
Time to peak serum concentration: ~2-4 hours
Elimination: Primarily eliminated unchanged in the urine
Dialyzable: ~30%

**Usual Dosage**

Adults: Initial: 25-50 mg/day; titrate in increments of 25-50 mg per week until an effective daily dose is reached; the daily dose may be increased by 25 mg at weekly intervals for the first 4 weeks; thereafter, the daily dose may be increased by 25-50 mg weekly to an effective daily dose (usually at least 400 mg); usual maximum dose: 1600 mg/day

**Note:** A more rapid titration schedule has been previously recommended (ie, 50 mg/week), and may be attempted in some clinical situations; however, this may reduce the patient's ability to tolerate topiramate.

Children 2-16 years: Partial seizures (adjunctive therapy): Initial dose titration should begin at 25 mg (or less, based on a range of 1-3 mg/kg/day) nightly for the first week. Dosage may be increased in increments of 1-3 mg/kg/day (administered in two divided doses) at 1- or 2-week intervals to a total daily dose of 5-9 mg/kg/day.

**Dosing adjustment in renal impairment:** $Cl_{cr}$ <70 mL/minute: Administer 50% dose and titrate more slowly

**Dosing adjustment in hepatic impairment:** Clearance may be minimally reduced

**Additional Information** May be associated with weight loss in some patients

**Dosage Forms**

Capsule (Topamax® Sprinkles): 15 mg, 25 mg
Tablet: 25 mg, 100 mg, 200 mg

- **Toposar® Injection** *see* Etoposide *on page 216*

## Topotecan (toe poe TEE kan)

**U.S. Brand Names** Hycamtin™

**Pharmacologic Category** Antineoplastic Agent, Natural Source (Plant) Derivative

**Use** Treatment of metastatic carcinoma of the ovary after failure of initial or subsequent chemotherapy; second-line treatment of small cell lung cancer

**Unlabeled use:** Under investigation for the treatment of nonsmall cell lung cancer, sarcoma (pediatrics)

**Effects on Mental Status** None reported

**Effects on Psychiatric Treatment** May cause myelosuppression; use caution with clozapine and carbamazepine

**Usual Dosage** Refer to individual protocols

Adults:

Metastatic ovarian cancer and small cell lung cancer: IVPB: 1.5 mg/m$^2$/day for 5 days; repeated every 21 days (neutrophil count should be >1500/mm$^3$ and platelet count should be >100,000/mm$^3$)

Dosage adjustment for hematological effects: If neutrophil count <1500/mm$^3$, reduce dose by 0.25 mg/m$^2$/day for 5 days for next cycle

**Dosing adjustment in renal impairment:**

$Cl_{cr}$ 20-39 mL/minute: Administer 50% of normal dose
$Cl_{cr}$ <20 mL/minute: Do not use, insufficient data available

Hemodialysis: Supplemental dose is not necessary
CAPD effects: Unknown
CAVH effects: Unknown

**Dosing adjustment in hepatic impairment:** Bilirubin 1.5-10 mg/dL: Adjustment is not necessary

**Dosage Forms** Powder for injection, as hydrochloride, lyophilized: 4 mg (base)

- **Toprol XL®** *see* Metoprolol *on page 362*
- **Toradol® Injection** *see* Ketorolac Tromethamine *on page 303*
- **Toradol® Oral** *see* Ketorolac Tromethamine *on page 303*
- **Torecan®** *see* Thiethylperazine *on page 542*

## Toremifene (TORE em i feen)

**U.S. Brand Names** Fareston®

**Synonyms** Toremifene Citrate

**Pharmacologic Category** Antineoplastic Agent, Miscellaneous

**Use** Treatment of metastatic breast cancer in postmenopausal women with estrogen-receptor (ER) positive or ER unknown tumors

**Effects on Mental Status** Dizziness, anxiety, irritability, insomnia, and depression are common

**Effects on Psychiatric Treatment** None reported

**Pregnancy Risk Factor** D

**Contraindications** Hypersensitivity to toremifene

**Warnings/Precautions** Hypercalcemia and tumor flare have been reported in some breast cancer patients with bone metastases during the first weeks of treatment. Tumor flare is a syndrome of diffuse musculoskeletal pain and erythema with increased size of tumor lesions that later regress. It is often accompanied by hypercalcemia. Tumor flare does not imply treatment failure or represent tumor progression. Institute appropriate measures if hypercalcemia occurs, and if severe, discontinue treatment. Drugs that decrease renal calcium excretion (eg, thiazide diuretics) may increase the risk of hypercalcemia in patients receiving toremifene.

Patients with a history of thromboembolic disease should generally not be treated with toremifene

**Adverse Reactions**

>10%:

- Endocrine & metabolic: Vaginal discharge, hot flashes
- Gastrointestinal: Nausea, vomiting
- Miscellaneous: Diaphoresis

1% to 10%:

- Cardiovascular: Thromboembolism: Tamoxifen has been associated with the occurrence of venous thrombosis and pulmonary embolism; arterial thrombosis has also been described in a few case reports; cardiac failure, myocardial infarction, edema
- Central nervous system: Dizziness
- Endocrine & metabolic: Hypercalcemia may occur in patients with bone metastases; galactorrhea and vitamin deficiency, menstrual irregularities
- Genitourinary: Vaginal bleeding or discharge, endometriosis, priapism, possible endometrial cancer
- Ocular: Ophthalmologic effects (visual acuity changes, cataracts, or retinopathy), corneal opacities, dry eyes

**Overdosage/Toxicology**

Signs and symptoms: Theoretically, overdose may be manifested as an increase of antiestrogenic effects such as hot flashes; estrogenic effects such as vaginal bleeding; or nervous system disorders such as vertigo, dizziness, ataxia and nausea

Treatment: No specific antidote exists and treatment is symptomatic

**Drug Interactions** CYP3A3/4 enzyme substrate

Decreased effect: CYP3A4 enzyme inducers: Phenobarbital, phenytoin and carbamazepine increase the rate of toremifene metabolism and lower the steady state concentration in serum

Increased toxicity:

- CYP3A4-6 enzyme inhibitors (ketoconazole, erythromycin) inhibit the metabolism of toremifene
- Warfarin results in significant enhancement of the anticoagulant effects of warfarin; has been speculated that a decrease in antitumor effect of tamoxifen may also occur due to alterations in the percentage of active tamoxifen metabolites

**Usual Dosage** Refer to individual protocols

Adults: Oral: 60 mg once daily, generally continued until disease progression is observed

**Dosage adjustment in renal impairment:** No dosage adjustment necessary

**Dosage adjustment in hepatic impairment:** Toremifene is extensively metabolized in the liver and dosage adjustments may be indicated in patients with liver disease; however, no specific guidelines have been developed

**Patient Information** Take as directed, without regard to food. You may experience an initial "flare" of this disease (increased bone pain and hot flashes) which will subside with continued use. You may experience nausea, vomiting, or loss of appetite (frequent mouth care, frequent small meals, chewing gum, or sucking lozenges may help); dizziness (use caution when driving, climbing stairs, or engaging in tasks requiring alertness until response to drug is known); or loss of hair (will grow back). Report vomiting that occurs immediately after taking medication; chest pain, palpitations or swollen extremities; vaginal bleeding, hot flashes, or excessive perspiration; chest pain, unusual coughing, or difficulty breathing; or any changes in vision or dry eyes.

**Nursing Implications** Increase of bone pain usually indicates a good therapeutic response

**Dosage Forms** Tablet, as citrate: 60 mg

♦ **Toremifene Citrate** *see* Toremifene *on page 557*

♦ **Tornalate®** *see* Bitolterol *on page 70*

## Torsemide (TOR se mide)

**U.S. Brand Names** Demadex®

**Synonyms** AC-4464

**Pharmacologic Category** Diuretic, Loop

**Use** Management of edema associated with congestive heart failure and hepatic or renal disease; used alone or in combination with antihypertensives in treatment of hypertension; I.V. form is indicated when rapid onset is desired

**Effects on Mental Status** May cause dizziness

**Effects on Psychiatric Treatment** May cause agranulocytosis; use caution with clozapine and carbamazepine; may decrease lithium clearance resulting in an increase in serum lithium levels and potential lithium toxicity, however, this is much more common and significant with the thiazide diuretics; monitor serum lithium levels; concurrent use with chloral hydrate may produce hot flashes and hypertension

**Pregnancy Risk Factor** B

**Contraindications** Hypersensitivity to torsemide, any component, or any sulfonylureas; anuria

**Warnings/Precautions** Adjust dose to avoid dehydration. In cirrhosis, avoid electrolyte and acid/base imbalances that might lead to hepatic encephalopathy. Ototoxicity is associated with rapid I.V. administration of other loop diuretics and has been seen with oral torsemide. Do not administer intravenously in less than 2 minutes; single doses should not exceed 200 mg. Hypersensitivity reactions can rarely occur. Monitor fluid status and renal function in an attempt to prevent oliguria, azotemia, and reversible increases in BUN and creatinine. Close medical supervision of aggressive diuresis is required. Monitor closely for electrolyte imbalances particularly hypokalemia and correct when necessary. Coadministration with antihypertensives may increase the risk of hypotension. Use caution in patients with known hypersensitivity to sulfonamides or thiazides (due to possible cross-sensitivity); avoid in patients with history of severe reactions.

**Adverse Reactions**

>10%: Cardiovascular: Orthostatic hypotension

1% to 10%:

- Central nervous system: Headache, dizziness, vertigo, pain
- Dermatologic: Photosensitivity, urticaria
- Endocrine & metabolic: Electrolyte imbalance, dehydration, hyperuricemia
- Gastrointestinal: Diarrhea, loss of appetite, stomach cramps
- Ocular: Blurred vision

<1%: Agranulocytosis, anemia, gout, hepatic dysfunction, interstitial nephritis, leukopenia, nausea, nephrocalcinosis, ototoxicity, pancreatitis, prerenal azotemia, rash, redness at injection site, thrombocytopenia

**Overdosage/Toxicology**

Signs and symptoms: Electrolyte depletion, volume depletion, hypotension, dehydration, circulatory collapse; electrolyte depletion may be manifested by weakness, dizziness, mental confusion, anorexia, lethargy, vomiting, and cramps

Treatment: Following GI decontamination, treatment is supportive; hypotension responds to fluids and Trendelenburg position

**Drug Interactions** CYP2C9 enzyme substrate

- ACE inhibitors: Hypotensive effects and/or renal effects are potentiated by hypovolemia
- Aminoglycosides: Ototoxicity may be increased
- Anticoagulant activity is enhanced
- Antidiabetic agents: Glucose tolerance may be decreased
- Antihypertensive agents: Effects may be enhanced
- Beta-blockers: Plasma concentrations of beta-blockers may be increased with torsemide
- Chloral hydrate: Transient diaphoresis, hot flashes, hypertension may occur
- Cisplatin: Ototoxicity may be increased
- Digitalis: Arrhythmias may occur with diuretic-induced electrolyte disturbances
- Enzyme inducers (phenytoin, phenobarbital, carbamazepine) theoretically may reduce efficacy of torsemide
- Lithium: Plasma concentrations of lithium may be increased; monitor lithium levels
- NSAIDs: Torsemide efficacy may be decreased
- Probenecid: Torsemide action may be reduced
- Salicylates: Diuretic action may be impaired in patients with cirrhosis and ascites
- Thiazides: Synergistic effects may result

**Usual Dosage** Adults: Oral, I.V.:

- Congestive heart failure: 10-20 mg once daily; may increase gradually for chronic treatment by doubling dose until the diuretic response is apparent (for acute treatment, I.V. dose may be repeated every 2 hours with double the dose as needed)
- Chronic renal failure: 20 mg once daily; increase as described above
- Hepatic cirrhosis: 5-10 mg once daily with an aldosterone antagonist or a potassium-sparing diuretic; increase as described above

(Continued)

## Torsemide *(Continued)*

Hypertension: 5 mg once daily; increase to 10 mg after 4-6 weeks if an adequate hypotensive response is not apparent; if still not effective, an additional antihypertensive agent may be added

**Patient Information** Take recommended dosage with food or milk at the same time each day (preferably not in the evening to avoid sleep interruption). Do not miss doses, alter dosage, or discontinue without consulting prescriber. Include orange juice or bananas (or other potassium-rich foods) in daily diet; do not take potassium supplements without consulting prescriber. Do not use alcohol or OTC medications without consulting prescriber. You may experience postural hypotension; change position slowly when rising from sitting or lying. May cause transient drowsiness, blurred vision, or dizziness; avoid driving or engaging in tasks that require alertness until response to drug is known. You may have reduced tolerance to heat (avoid strenuous activity in hot weather or excessively hot showers). Increased exercise and increased dietary fiber, fruit, and fluids may reduce constipation. Report unusual weight gain or loss (>5 lb/week), swelling of ankles and hands, persistent fatigue, unresolved constipation or diarrhea, weakness, fatigue, dizziness, vomiting, cramps, change in hearing, or chest pain or palpitations.

**Dosage Forms**

Injection: 10 mg/mL (2 mL, 5 mL)

Tablet: 5 mg, 10 mg, 20 mg, 100 mg


- ♦ **Toscal®** *see* Carbinoxamine *on page 92*
- ♦ **Totacillin®** *see* Ampicillin *on page 42*
- ♦ **Totacillin®-N** *see* Ampicillin *on page 42*
- ♦ **Touro Ex®** *see* Guaifenesin *on page 256*
- ♦ **Touro LA®** *see* Guaifenesin and Pseudoephedrine *on page 257*
- ♦ **Toxidromes** *see page 793*
- ♦ **Tracrium®** *see* Atracurium *on page 53*


## Tramadol (TRA ma dole)

**U.S. Brand Names** Ultram®

**Pharmacologic Category** Analgesic, Non-narcotic

**Use** Relief of moderate to moderately severe medical pain

**Effects on Mental Status** May cause dizziness, drowsiness, or restlessness

**Effects on Psychiatric Treatment** Contraindicated with opioid-dependent patients, MAOIs, psychotropics; carbamazepine may decrease the effects of tramadol; concurrent use with MAOIs and TCAs may produce seizures; tramadol has MAOI activity and should be used cautiously with other antidepressants

**Pregnancy Risk Factor** C

**Contraindications** Previous hypersensitivity to tramadol, opioids, or any components; opioid-dependent patients; acute intoxication with alcohol, hypnotics, centrally-acting analgesics, opioids, or psychotropic drugs

**Warnings/Precautions** Should be used only with extreme caution in patients receiving MAO inhibitors. Use with caution and reduce dosage when administered to patients receiving other CNS depressants. An increased risk of seizures may occur in patients receiving serotonin reuptake inhibitors (SSRIs or anorectics), tricyclic antidepressants, other cyclic compounds, (including cyclobenzaprine, promethazine), neuroleptics, MAO inhibitors, or drugs which may lower seizure threshold. Patients with a history of seizures, or with a risk of seizures (head trauma, metabolic disorders, CNS infection, or malignancy, or during alcohol/drug withdrawal) are also at increased risk.

Elderly patients and patients with chronic respiratory disorders may be at greater risk of adverse events. Use with caution in patients with increased intracranial pressure or head injury. Use tramadol with caution and reduce dosage in patients with liver disease or renal dysfunction and in patients with myxedema, hypothyroidism, or hypoadrenalism. Not recommended during pregnancy or in nursing mothers. Tolerance or drug dependence may result from extended use; abrupt discontinuation should be avoided.

**Adverse Reactions**

>1%:

Central nervous system: Dizziness, headache, somnolence, stimulation, restlessness

Gastrointestinal: Nausea, diarrhea, constipation, vomiting, dyspepsia

Neuromuscular & skeletal: Weakness

Miscellaneous: Diaphoresis

<1%: Palpitations, respiratory depression, seizures, suicidal tendency

**Overdosage/Toxicology**

Signs and symptoms: CNS and respiratory depression, gastrointestinal cramping, constipation

Treatment: Naloxone 2 mg I.V. (0.01 mg/kg children) with repeat administration as needed up to 18 mg

**Drug Interactions** CYP2D6 enzyme substrate

Decreased effects: Carbamazepine (decreases half-life by 33% to 50%)

Increased toxicity:

Amphetamines may increase the risk of seizures with tramadol

Cimetidine increases the half-life of tramadol by 20% to 25%

SSRIs may increase the risk of seizures with tramadol

Tricyclic antidepressants may increase the risk of seizures

MAOIs may increases the risk of seizures

Naloxone may increase the risk of seizures in tramadol overdose

Neuroleptic agents may increase the risk of tramadol-associated seizures and may have additive CNS depressant effects

Opioids may increase the risk of seizures, and may have additive CNS depressant effects

Quinidine (and other inhibitors of CYP2D6) may increase the tramadol serum concentrations

**Usual Dosage** Adults: Oral: 50-100 mg every 4-6 hours, not to exceed 400 mg/day

Initiation of low dose followed by titration in increments of 50 mg/day every 3 days to effective dose (not >400 mg/day) may minimize dizziness and vertigo

**Patient Information** If self-administered, use exactly as directed (do not increase dose or frequency); may cause physical and/or psychological dependence. Take with food or milk. While using this medication, do not use alcohol and other prescription or OTC medications (especially pain medications, sedatives, antihistamines, or cough preparations) without consulting prescriber. Maintain adequate hydration (2-3 L/day of fluids unless instructed to restrict fluid intake). You may experience drowsiness, dizziness, or blurred vision (use caution when driving or engaging in tasks requiring alertness until response to drug is known); nausea, vomiting, or loss of appetite (small frequent meals, frequent mouth care, chewing gum, or sucking lozenges may help); constipation (increased exercise, fluids, or dietary fruit and fiber may help). Report severe unresolved constipation; difficulty breathing or shortness of breath; excessive sedation or increased insomnia and restlessness; changes in urinary pattern or menstrual pattern; muscle weakness or tremors; or chest pain or palpitations.

**Dosage Forms** Tablet, as hydrochloride: 50 mg


- ♦ **Trancopal®** *see* Chlormezanone *on page 111*
- ♦ **Trandate®** *see* Labetalol *on page 304*


## Trandolapril (tran DOE la pril)

**Related Information**

Angiotensin-Related Agents Comparison Chart *on page 700*

**U.S. Brand Names** Mavik®

**Pharmacologic Category** Angiotensin-Converting Enzyme (ACE) Inhibitors

**Use** Management of hypertension alone or in combination with other antihypertensive agents; treatment of left ventricular dysfunction after myocardial infarction

**Unlabeled use:** As a class, ACE inhibitors are recommended in the treatment of systolic congestive heart failure

**Effects on Mental Status** May cause dizziness, drowsiness, nervousness, or insomnia

**Effects on Psychiatric Treatment** May cause neutropenia; use caution with clozapine and carbamazepine; may decrease lithium clearance resulting in an increase in serum lithium levels and potential lithium toxicity; monitor serum lithium levels; concurrent use with low potency antipsychotics and TCAs may produce additive hypotensive effects

**Pregnancy Risk Factor** C (1st trimester); D (2nd and 3rd trimesters)

**Contraindications** Hypersensitivity to trandolapril or any component; history of angioedema related to previous treatment with an ACE inhibitor; bilateral renal artery stenosis; primary hyperaldosteronism; pregnancy (2nd and 3rd trimesters)

**Warnings/Precautions** Anaphylactic reactions can occur. Angioedema can occur at any time during treatment (especially following first dose). Careful blood pressure monitoring with first dose (hypotension can occur especially in volume depleted patients). Dosage adjustment needed in severe renal dysfunction ($Cl_{cr}$ <30 mL/minute) or in hepatic cirrhosis. Use with caution in hypovolemia; collagen vascular diseases; valvular stenosis (particularly aortic stenosis); hyperkalemia; or before, during, or immediately after anesthesia. Avoid rapid dosage escalation, which may lead to renal insufficiency. Neutropenia/agranulocytosis with myeloid hyperplasia can rarely occur with captopril (another ACE inhibitor). If patient has renal impairment then a baseline WBC with differential and serum creatinine should be evaluated and monitored closely during the first 3 months of therapy. Use with caution in unilateral renal artery stenosis and pre-existing renal insufficiency.

**Adverse Reactions**

1% to 10%:

Cardiovascular: Chest pain, hypotension, syncope

Central nervous system: Fatigue

Gastrointestinal: Dyspepsia

Neuromuscular & skeletal: Myalgia

Respiratory: Cough (1.9% to 35%)

≤1%: Abdominal pain, angioedema, anxiety, constipation, decreased libido, diarrhea, dyspnea, flushing, impotence, insomnia, muscle cramps, palpitations, pancreatitis, paresthesia, pruritus, rash, sleep disturbances, upper respiratory infection, urinary tract infection, vertigo, vomiting

**Overdosage/Toxicology**

Signs and symptoms: Hypertension, vertigo, dizziness

Treatment: Following initiation of essential overdose management, toxic symptom treatment and supportive treatment should be initiated. Hypotension usually responds to I.V. fluids or Trendelenburg positioning. If unresponsive to these measures, the use of a parenteral inotrope may be required (eg, norepinephrine 0.1-0.2 mcg/kg/minute titrated to response). Seizures commonly respond to diazepam (I.V. 5-10 mg bolus in adults every 15 minutes if needed up to a total of 30 mg) or to phenytoin or phenobarbital.

**Drug Interactions**

Alpha$_1$ blockers: Hypotensive effect increased

Aspirin: The effects of ACE inhibitors may be blunted by aspirin administration, particularly at higher dosages

Diuretics: Hypovolemia due to diuretics may precipitate acute hypotensive events or acute renal failure

Insulin: Risk of hypoglycemia may be increased

Lithium: Risk of lithium toxicity may be increased; monitor lithium levels, especially the first 4 weeks of therapy

Mercaptopurine: Risk of neutropenia may be increased

NSAIDs may decrease ACE inhibitor efficacy and/or increase adverse renal effects

Potassium-sparing diuretics (amiloride, potassium, spironolactone, triamterene): Increased risk of hyperkalemia

Potassium supplements may increase the risk of hyperkalemia

Trimethoprim (high dose) may increase the risk of hyperkalemia

**Usual Dosage** Adults: Oral:

Hypertension: Initial dose in patients not receiving a diuretic: 1 mg/day (2 mg/day in black patients). Adjust dosage according to the blood pressure response. Make dosage adjustments at intervals of ≥1 week. Most patients have required dosages of 2-4 mg/day. There is a little experience with doses >8 mg/day. Patients inadequately treated with once daily dosing at 4 mg may be treated with twice daily dosing. If blood pressure is not adequately controlled with trandolapril monotherapy, a diuretic may be added.

Heart failure postmyocardial infarction or left ventricular dysfunction postmyocardial infarction: Initial: 1 mg/day; titrate patients (as tolerated) towards the target dose of 4 mg/day. If a 4 mg dose is not tolerated, patients can continue therapy with the greatest tolerated dose.

**Dosing adjustment in renal impairment:** $Cl_{cr}$ ≤30 mL/minute: Recommended starting dose: 0.5 mg/day.

**Dosing adjustment in hepatic impairment:** Cirrhosis: Recommended starting dose: 0.5 mg/day.

**Patient Information** Take exactly as directed; do not discontinue without consulting prescriber. Take first dose at bedtime. This drug does not eliminate need for diet or exercise regimen as recommended by prescriber. May cause dizziness, fainting, lightheadedness (use caution when driving or engaging in tasks requiring alertness until response to drug is known); diarrhea (buttermilk, boiled milk, yogurt may help). Report chest pain or palpitations; swelling of extremities, mouth or tongue; skin rash; difficulty in breathing or unusual cough; or other persistent adverse reactions.

**Nursing Implications** May cause depression in some patients; discontinue if angioedema of the face, extremities, lips, tongue, or glottis occurs; watch for hypotensive effects within 1-3 hours of first dose or new higher dose

**Dosage Forms** Tablet: 1 mg, 2 mg, 4 mg

## Trandolapril and Verapamil (tran DOE la pril & ver AP a mil)

**U.S. Brand Names** Tarka®

**Pharmacologic Category** Antihypertensive Agent, Combination

**Use** Combination drug for the treatment of hypertension, however, not indicated for initial treatment of hypertension; replacement therapy in patients receiving separate dosage forms (for patient convenience); when monotherapy with one component fails to achieve desired antihypertensive effect, or when dose-limiting adverse effects limit upward titration of monotherapy

**Effects on Mental Status** May cause dizziness, drowsiness, nervousness, or insomnia

**Effects on Psychiatric Treatment** May cause neutropenia; use caution with clozapine and carbamazepine; may decrease lithium clearance resulting in an increase in serum lithium levels and potential lithium toxicity; monitor serum lithium levels; concurrent use with low potency antipsychotics and TCAs may produce additive hypotensive effects; barbiturates may decrease verapamil serum concentrations; verapamil may increase carbamazepine serum concentrations

**Usual Dosage** Dose is individualized

**Dosage Forms** Tablet:

Trandolapril 1 mg and verapamil hydrochloride 240 mg
Trandolapril 2 mg and verapamil hydrochloride 180 mg
Trandolapril 2 mg and verapamil hydrochloride 240 mg
Trandolapril 4 mg and verapamil hydrochloride 240 mg

## Tranexamic Acid (tran eks AM ik AS id)

**U.S. Brand Names** Cyklokapron®

**Pharmacologic Category** Antihemophilic Agent

**Use** Short-term use (2-8 days) in hemophilia patients during and following tooth extraction to reduce or prevent hemorrhage, has also been used as an alternative to aminocaproic acid for subarachnoid hemorrhage

**Effects on Mental Status** None reported

**Effects on Psychiatric Treatment** None reported

**Pregnancy Risk Factor** B

**Contraindications** Acquired defective color vision, active intravascular clotting

**Warnings/Precautions** Dosage modification required in patients with renal impairment; ophthalmic exam before and during therapy required if patient is treated beyond several days; caution in patients with cardiovascular, renal, or cerebrovascular disease; when used for subarachnoid hemorrhage, ischemic complications may occur

**Adverse Reactions**

>10%: Gastrointestinal: Nausea, diarrhea, vomiting

1% to 10%:

Cardiovascular: Hypotension, thrombosis

Ocular: Blurred vision

<1%: Unusual menstrual discomfort

**Drug Interactions** Chlorpromazine (may increase cerebral vasospasm and ischemia)

**Usual Dosage** Children and Adults: I.V.: 10 mg/kg immediately before surgery, then 25 mg/kg/dose orally 3-4 times/day for 2-8 days

Alternatively:

Oral: 25 mg/kg 3-4 times/day beginning 1 day prior to surgery

I.V.: 10 mg/kg 3-4 times/day in patients who are unable to take oral

**Dosing adjustment/interval in renal impairment:**

$Cl_{cr}$ 50-80 mL/minute: Administer 50% of normal dose or 10 mg/kg twice daily I.V. or 15 mg/kg twice daily orally

$Cl_{cr}$ 10-50 mL/minute: Administer 25% of normal dose or 10 mg/kg/day I.V. or 15 mg/kg/day orally

$Cl_{cr}$ <10 mL/minute: Administer 10% of normal dose or 10 mg/kg/dose every 48 hours I.V. or 15 mg/kg/dose every 48 hours orally

**Patient Information** Report any signs of bleeding or myopathy, changes in vision; GI upset usually disappears when dose is reduced

**Nursing Implications** Dosage modification required in patients with renal impairment

**Dosage Forms**

Injection: 100 mg/mL (10 mL)

Tablet: 500 mg

♦ **Transamine Sulphate** *see* Tranylcypromine *on page 559*

♦ **Transdermal-NTG® Patch** *see* Nitroglycerin *on page 397*

♦ **Transderm-Nitro® Patch** *see* Nitroglycerin *on page 397*

♦ **Transderm Scop® Patch** *see* Scopolamine *on page 506*

♦ **Tranxene®** *see* Clorazepate *on page 134*

## Tranylcypromine (tran il SIP roe meen)

**Related Information**

Antidepressant Agents Comparison Chart *on page 704*
Clinical Issues in the Use of Antidepressants *on page 627*
Mood Disorders *on page 600*
Patient Information - Antidepressants (MAOIs) *on page 644*
Teratogenic Risks of Psychotropic Medications *on page 812*

**Generic Available** No

**U.S. Brand Names** Parnate®

**Synonyms** Transamine Sulphate; Tranylcypromine Sulfate

**Pharmacologic Category** Antidepressant, Monoamine Oxidase Inhibitor

**Use** Treatment of major depressive episode without melancholia

**Unlabeled use:** Post-traumatic stress disorder

**Pregnancy Risk Factor** C

**Contraindications** Hypersensitivity to tranylcypromine; uncontrolled hypertension; pheochromocytoma; hepatic or renal disease; cerebrovascular defect; cardiovascular disease; concurrent use of sympathomimetics (and related compounds), CNS depressants, ethanol, meperidine, bupropion, buspirone, guanethidine, and serotonergic drugs (including SSRIs) - do not use within 5 weeks of fluoxetine discontinuation or 2 weeks of other antidepressant discontinuation; general anesthesia, local vasoconstrictors; spinal anesthesia (hypotension may be exaggerated). Foods which are high in tyramine, tryptophan, or dopamine, chocolate, or caffeine.

**Warnings/Precautions** Safety in children <16 years of age has not been established; use with caution in patients who are hyperactive, hyperexcitable, or who have glaucoma, suicidal tendencies, hyperthyroidism, or diabetes; avoid use of meperidine within 2 weeks of phenelzine use. Toxic reactions have occurred with dextromethorphan. Hypertensive crisis may occur with tyramine, tryptophan, or dopamine-containing foods. Should not be used in combination with other antidepressants. Hypotensive effects of (Continued)

## Tranylcypromine *(Continued)*

antihypertensives (beta-blockers, thiazides) may be exaggerated. Use with caution in depressed patients at risk of suicide. May cause orthostatic hypotension (especially at dosages >30 mg/day) - use with caution in patients with hypotension or patients who would not tolerate transient hypotensive episodes - effects may be additive when used with other agents known to cause orthostasis (phenothiazines). Has been associated with activation of hypomania and/or mania in bipolar patients. May worsen psychotic symptoms in some patients. Use with caution in patients at risk of seizures, or in patients receiving other drugs which may lower seizure threshold. Discontinue at least 48 hours prior to myelography. Use with caution in patients receiving disulfiram. Use with caution in patients with renal impairment.

The MAO inhibitors are effective and generally well tolerated by older patients. It is the potential interactions with tyramine or tryptophan-containing foods and other drugs, and their effects on blood pressure that have limited their use.

**Adverse Reactions**

Cardiovascular: Orthostatic hypotension, edema

Central nervous system: Dizziness, headache, drowsiness, sleep disturbances, fatigue, hyper-reflexia, twitching, ataxia, mania

Dermatologic: Rash, pruritus

Endocrine & metabolic: Sexual dysfunction (anorgasmia, ejaculatory disturbances, impotence), hypernatremia, hypermetabolic syndrome

Gastrointestinal: Xerostomia, constipation, weight gain

Genitourinary: Urinary retention

Hematologic: Leukopenia

Hepatic: Hepatitis

Neuromuscular & skeletal: Weakness, tremor, myoclonus

Ocular: Blurred vision, glaucoma

Miscellaneous: diaphoresis

**Overdosage/Toxicology**

Signs and symptoms: Tachycardia, palpitations, muscle twitching, seizures, insomnia, transient hypotension, hypertension, hyperpyrexia, coma

Treatment: Competent supportive care is the most important treatment for an overdose with a monoamine oxidase (MAO) inhibitor. Both hypertension or hypotension can occur with intoxication. Hypotension may respond to I.V. fluids or vasopressors, and hypertension usually responds to an alpha-adrenergic blocker. While treating the hypertension, care is warranted to avoid sudden drops in blood pressure, since this may worsen the MAO inhibitor toxicity. Muscle irritability and seizures often respond to diazepam, while hyperthermia is best treated antipyretics and cooling blankets. Cardiac arrhythmias are best treated with phenytoin or procainamide.

**Drug Interactions** CYP2A6 and 2C19 enzyme inhibitor

Amphetamines: MAOIs in combination with amphetamines may result in severe hypertensive reaction; these combinations are best avoided

Anorexiants: Concurrent use of anorexiants may result in serotonin syndrome; these combinations are best avoided; includes dexfenfluramine, fenfluramine, or sibutramine

Barbiturates: MAOIs may inhibit the metabolism of barbiturates and prolong their effect

CNS stimulants: MAOIs in combination with stimulants (methylphenidate) may result in severe hypertensive reaction; these combinations are best avoided

Dextromethorphan: Concurrent use of MAOIs may result in serotonin syndrome; these combinations are best avoided

Disulfiram: MAOIs may produce delirium in patients receiving disulfiram; monitor

Guanadrel and guanethidine: MAOIs inhibit the antihypertensive response to guanadrel or guanethidine; use an alternative antihypertensive agent

Hypoglycemic agents: MAOIs may produce hypoglycemia in patients with diabetes; monitor

Levodopa: MAOIs in combination with levodopa may result in hypertensive reactions; monitor

Lithium: MAOIs in combination with lithium have resulted in malignant hyperpyrexia; this combination is best avoided

Meperidine: May cause serotonin syndrome when combined with an MAO inhibitor; avoid this combination

Nefazodone: Concurrent use of MAOIs may result in serotonin syndrome; these combinations are best avoided

Norepinephrine: MAOIs may increase the pressor response of norepinephrine (effect is generally small); monitor

Reserpine: MAOIs in combination with reserpine may result in hypertensive reactions; monitor

Serotonin agonists: Theoretically may increase the risk of serotonin syndrome; includes sumatriptan, naratriptan, rizatriptan, and zolmitriptan

SSRIs: May cause serotonin syndrome when combined with an MAO inhibitor; avoid this combination

Succinylcholine: MAOIs may prolong the muscle relaxation produced by succinylcholine via decreased plasma pseudocholinesterase

Sympathomimetics (indirect-acting): MAOIs in combination with sympathomimetics such as dopamine, metaraminol, phenylephrine, and decongestants (pseudoephedrine) may result in severe hypertensive reaction; these combinations are best avoided

Tramadol: May increase the risk of seizures and serotonin syndrome in patients receiving an MAOI

Trazodone: Concurrent use of MAOIs may result in serotonin syndrome; these combinations are best avoided

Tricyclic antidepressants: May cause serotonin syndrome when combined with an MAO inhibitor; avoid this combination

Tyramine: Foods (eg, cheese) and beverages (eg, ethanol) containing tyramine, should be avoided in patients receiving an MAOI; hypertensive crisis may result

Venlafaxine: Concurrent use of MAOIs may result in serotonin syndrome; these combinations are best avoided

**Mechanism of Action** Thought to act by increasing endogenous concentrations of epinephrine, norepinephrine, dopamine and serotonin through inhibition of the enzyme (monoamine oxidase) responsible for the breakdown of these neurotransmitters

**Pharmacodynamics/kinetics**

Onset of action: 2-3 weeks are required of continued dosing to obtain full therapeutic effect

Half-life: 90-190 minutes

Time to peak serum concentration: Within 2 hours

Elimination: In urine

**Usual Dosage** Adults: Oral: 10 mg twice daily, increase by 10 mg increments at 1- to 3-week intervals; maximum: 60 mg/day

**Dosing comments in hepatic impairment:** Use with care and monitor plasma levels and patient response closely

**Dietary Considerations**

Alcohol: Avoid use

Food: Avoid tyramine-containing foods

**Monitoring Parameters** Blood pressure, blood glucose

**Reference Range** Inhibition of platelet monoamine oxidase (≥80%) correlated with clinical response

**Test Interactions** ↓ glucose

**Patient Information** Tablets may be crushed; avoid alcohol; do not discontinue abruptly; avoid foods high in tyramine (eg, aged cheeses, Chianti wine, raisins, liver, bananas, chocolate, yogurt, sour cream); discuss list of drugs and foods to avoid with pharmacist or physician; arise slowly from prolonged sitting or lying

**Nursing Implications** Assist with ambulation during initiation of therapy; monitor blood pressure closely, patients should be cautioned against eating foods high in tyramine or tryptophan (cheese, wine, beer, pickled herring, dry sausage)

**Additional Information** Has a more rapid onset of therapeutic effect than other MAO inhibitors, but causes more severe hypertensive reactions

**Dosage Forms** Tablet, as sulfate: 10 mg

♦ **Tranylcypromine Sulfate** *see* Tranylcypromine *on page 559*

## Trastuzumab (tras TU zoo mab)

**U.S. Brand Names** Herceptin®

**Pharmacologic Category** Monoclonal Antibody

**Use**

Single agent for the treatment of patients with metastatic breast cancer whose tumors overexpress the HER2/neu protein and who have received one or more chemotherapy regimens for their metastatic disease

Combination therapy with paclitaxel for the treatment of patients with metastatic breast cancer whose tumors overexpress the HER2/neu protein and who have not received chemotherapy for their metastatic disease

**Note:** HER2/neu protein overexpression or amplification has been noted in ovarian, gastric, colorectal, endometrial, lung, bladder, prostate, and salivary gland tumors. It is not yet known whether trastuzumab may be effective in these other carcinomas which overexpress HER2/neu protein.

**Effects on Mental Status** Insomnia and dizziness are common; may cause depression

**Effects on Psychiatric Treatment** None reported

**Usual Dosage** I.V. infusion:

Adults:

Initial loading dose: 4 mg/kg intravenous infusion over 90 minutes

Maintenance dose: 2 mg/kg intravenous infusion over 90 minutes (can be administered over 30 minutes if prior infusions are well tolerated) weekly until disease progression

**Dosing adjustment in renal impairment:** Data suggest that the disposition of trastuzumab is not altered based on age or serum creatinine (up to 2 mg/dL); however, no formal interaction studies have been performed

**Dosing adjustment in hepatic impairment:** No data is currently available

**Dosage Forms** Injection: Vial, 440 mg, with vial of bacteriostatic water for injection

♦ **Trasylol®** *see* Aprotinin *on page 47*

## Trazodone (TRAZ oh done)

**Related Information**

Antidepressant Agents Comparison Chart *on page 704*
Clinical Issues in the Use of Antidepressants *on page 627*
Clinical Issues in the Use of Anxiolytics and Sedative/Hypnotics *on page 634*
Federal OBRA Regulations Recommended Maximum Doses *on page 756*
Patient Information - Antidepressants (Serotonin Blocker) *on page 643*
Secondary Mental Disorders *on page 616*
Sleep Disorders *on page 620*
Special Populations - Elderly *on page 662*
Teratogenic Risks of Psychotropic Medications *on page 812*

**Generic Available** Yes

**U.S. Brand Names** Desyrel®

**Synonyms** Trazodone Hydrochloride

**Pharmacologic Category** Antidepressant, Serotonin Reuptake Inhibitor/ Antagonist

**Use** Treatment of depression

**Unlabeled uses:** Potential augmenting agent for antidepressants, hypnotic

**Pregnancy Risk Factor** C

**Contraindications** Hypersensitivity to trazodone or any component of the formulation

**Warnings/Precautions** Priapism, including cases resulting in permanent dysfunction, has occurred with the use of trazodone. Not recommended for use in a patient during the acute recovery phase of MI. Trazodone should be initiated with caution in patients who are receiving concurrent or recent therapy with a MAOI. May cause sedation, resulting in impaired performance of tasks requiring alertness (ie, operating machinery or driving). Sedative effects may be additive with other CNS depressants and ethanol. The degree of sedation is very high relative to other antidepressants. May worsen psychosis in some patients or precipitate a shift to mania or hypomania in patients with bipolar disease. May increase the risks associated with electroconvulsive therapy. This agent should be discontinued, when possible, prior to elective surgery. Therapy should not be abruptly discontinued in patients receiving high doses for prolonged periods.

Use with caution in patients at risk of hypotension or in patients where transient hypotensive episodes would be poorly tolerated (cardiovascular disease or cerebrovascular disease). The risk of postural hypotension is high relative to other antidepressants. Use caution in patients with depression, particularly if suicidal risk may be present. Use caution in patients with a previous seizure disorder or condition predisposing to seizures such as brain damage, alcoholism, or concurrent therapy with other drugs which lower the seizure threshold. Use with caution in patients with hepatic or renal dysfunction and in elderly patients. Use with caution in patients with a history of cardiovascular disease (including previous MI, stroke, tachycardia, or conduction abnormalities). However, the risk of conduction abnormalities with this agent is low relative to other antidepressants.

**Adverse Reactions**

>10%:
- Central nervous system: Dizziness, headache, sedation
- Gastrointestinal: Nausea, xerostomia

1% to 10%:
- Cardiovascular: Syncope, hypertension, hypotension, edema
- Central nervous system: Confusion, decreased concentration, fatigue, incoordination
- Gastrointestinal: Diarrhea, constipation, weight gain or loss
- Neuromuscular & skeletal: Tremor, myalgia
- Ocular: Blurred vision
- Respiratory: Nasal congestion

<1%: Agitation, bradycardia, extrapyramidal reactions, hepatitis, priapism, rash, seizures, tachycardia, urinary retention

**Overdosage/Toxicology**

Signs and symptoms: Drowsiness, vomiting, hypotension, tachycardia, incontinence, coma, priapism

Treatment:
- Following initiation of essential overdose management, toxic symptoms should be treated
- Ventricular arrhythmias often respond to lidocaine 1.5 mg/kg bolus followed by 2 mg/minute infusion with concurrent systemic alkalinization (sodium bicarbonate 0.5-2 mEq/kg I.V.)
- Seizures usually respond to diazepam I.V. boluses (5-10 mg for adults up to 30 mg or 0.25-0.4 mg/kg/dose for children up to 10 mg/dose). If seizures are unresponsive or recur, phenytoin or phenobarbital may be required.
- Hypotension is best treated by I.V. fluids and by placing the patient in the Trendelenburg position.

**Drug Interactions** CYP2D6 and 3A3/4 enzyme substrate

Antipsychotics: Trazodone, in combination with other psychotropics (low potency antipsychotics), may result in additional hypotension (isolated case reports); monitor

Buspirone: Serotonergic effects may be additive (limited documentation); monitor

CNS depressants: Sedative effects may be additive with CNS depressants. Includes ethanol, barbiturates, benzodiazepines, narcotic analgesics, and other sedative agents; monitor for increased effect

CYP2D6 inhibitors: Metabolism of trazodone may be decreased; increasing clinical effect or toxicity; inhibitors include amiodarone, cimetidine, delavirdine, fluoxetine, paroxetine, propafenone, quinidine, and ritonavir; monitor for increased effect/toxicity

CYP3A3/4 inhibitors: Serum level and/or toxicity of trazodone may be increased; inhibitors include amiodarone, cimetidine, clarithromycin, erythromycin, delavirdine, diltiazem, dirithromycin, disulfiram, fluoxetine, fluvoxamine, grapefruit juice, indinavir, itraconazole, ketoconazole, metronidazole, nefazodone, nevirapine, propoxyfene, quinupristin-dalfopristin, ritonavir, saquinavir, verapamil, zafirlukast, zileuton; monitor for altered response

Enzyme inducers: May enhance the hepatic metabolism of trazodone; larger doses may be required; inducers include carbamazepine, rifampin, rifabutin, barbiturates, phenytoin, and cigarette smoking

Linezolid: Due to MAO inhibition (see below), this combination should be avoided

MAO inhibitors: Concurrent use may lead to serotonin syndrome; avoid concurrent use or use within 14 days

Meperidine: Combined use, theoretically, may increase the risk of serotonin syndrome

Serotonin agonists: Theoretically, may increase the risk of serotonin syndrome; includes sumatriptan, naratriptan, rizatriptan, and zolmitriptan

SSRIs: Combined use of trazodone with an SSRI may, theoretically, increase the risk of serotonin syndrome; in addition, some SSRIs may inhibit the metabolism of trazodone resulting in elevated plasma levels and increased sedation; includes fluoxetine and fluvoxamine (see CYP inhibition); low doses of trazodone appear to represent little risk

Venlafaxine: Sertraline may increase the risk of serotonin syndrome

**Mechanism of Action** Inhibits reuptake of serotonin, causes adrenoreceptor subsensitivity, and induces significant changes in 5HT presynaptic receptor adrenoreceptors. Trazodone also significantly blocks histamine (H1) and alpha$_1$ adrenergic receptors.

**Pharmacodynamics/kinetics**

Onset of effect: Therapeutic effects take 1-3 weeks to appear

Protein binding: 85% to 95%

Metabolism: In the liver by hydroxylation, pyridine ring splitting, oxidation, and N-oxidation

Half-life: 7-8 hours, 2 compartment kinetics

Time to peak serum concentration: Within 30-100 minutes, prolonged in the presence of food (up to 2.5 hours)

Elimination: Primarily in urine and secondarily in feces

**Usual Dosage** Oral: Therapeutic effects may take up to 4 weeks to occur; therapy is normally maintained for several months after optimum response is reached to prevent recurrence of depression

Children 6-18 years: Initial: 1.5-2 mg/kg/day in divided doses; increase gradually every 3-4 days as needed; maximum: 6 mg/kg/day in 3 divided doses

Adolescents: Initial: 25-50 mg/day; increase to 100-150 mg/day in divided doses

Adults: Initial: 150 mg/day in 3 divided doses (may increase by 50 mg/day every 3-7 days); maximum: 600 mg/day

Elderly: 25-50 mg at bedtime with 25-50 mg/day dose increase every 3 days for inpatients and weekly for outpatients, if tolerated; usual dose: 75-150 mg/day

**Dietary Considerations** Alcohol: Avoid use

**Monitoring Parameters** EKG for at least 4 hours

**Reference Range** Therapeutic: 0.5-2.5 μg/mL (SI: 1-6 μmol/L)

**Patient Information** Take shortly after a meal or light snack, can be given as bedtime dose if drowsiness occurs; avoid alcohol; be aware of possible photosensitivity reaction; report any prolonged or painful erection

**Nursing Implications** Dosing after meals may decrease lightheadedness and postural hypotension; use side rails on bed if administered to the elderly; observe patient's activity and compare with admission level; assist with ambulation; sitting and standing blood pressure and pulse

**Additional Information** Therapeutic effects may take up to 4 weeks to occur; therapy is normally maintained for several months after optimum response is reached to prevent recurrence of depression

**Dosage Forms** Tablet, as hydrochloride: 50 mg, 100 mg, 150 mg, 300 mg


- **Trazodone Hydrochloride** *see* Trazodone *on page 561*
- **Trecator®-SC** *see* Ethionamide *on page 213*
- **Trelstar™ Depot** *see* Triptorelin *on page 572*
- **Trendinol®** *see* Nitrendipine *on page 396*
- **Trental®** *see* Pentoxifylline *on page 430*


## Tretinoin, Oral (TRET i noyn, oral)

**U.S. Brand Names** Vesanoid®

**Synonyms** All-*trans*-Retinoic Acid

**Pharmacologic Category** Antineoplastic Agent, Miscellaneous

(Continued)

## Tretinoin, Oral *(Continued)*

**Use** Acute promyelocytic leukemia (APL): Induction of remission in patients with APL, French American British (FAB) classification M3 (including the M3 variant), characterized by the presence of the t(15;17) translocation or the presence of the PML/RARα gene who are refractory to or who have relapsed from anthracycline chemotherapy, or for whom anthracycline-based chemotherapy is contraindicated. Tretinoin is for the induction of remission only. All patients should receive an accepted form of remission consolidation or maintenance therapy for APL after completion of induction therapy with tretinoin.

**Effects on Mental Status** Dizziness, anxiety, insomnia, depression, and confusion are common; may cause agitation, hallucinations, or cognitive impairment; may rarely cause mood changes

**Effects on Psychiatric Treatment** None reported

**Pregnancy Risk Factor** D

**Contraindications** Sensitivity to parabens, vitamin A, or other retinoids

**Warnings/Precautions** Patients with acute promyelocytic leukemia (APL) are at high risk and can have severe adverse reactions to tretinoin. Administer under the supervision of a physician who is experienced in the management of patients with acute leukemia and in a facility with laboratory and supportive services sufficient to monitor drug tolerance and to protect and maintain a patient compromised by drug toxicity, including respiratory compromise.

About 25% of patients with APL, who have been treated with tretinoin, have experienced a syndrome called the retinoic acid-APL (RA-APL) syndrome which is characterized by fever, dyspnea, weight gain, radiographic pulmonary infiltrates and pleural or pericardial effusions. This syndrome has occasionally been accompanied by impaired myocardial contractility and episodic hypotension. It has been observed with or without concomitant leukocytosis. Endotracheal intubation and mechanical ventilation have been required in some cases due to progressive hypoxemia, and several patients have expired with multiorgan failure. The syndrome usually occurs during the first month of treatment, with some cases reported following the first dose.

Management of the syndrome has not been defined, but high-dose steroids given at the first suspicion of RA-APL syndrome appear to reduce morbidity and mortality. At the first signs suggestive of the syndrome, immediately initiate high-dose steroids (dexamethasone 10 mg I.V.) every 12 hours for 3 days or until resolution of symptoms, regardless of the leukocyte count. The majority of patients do not require termination of tretinoin therapy during treatment of the RA-APL syndrome.

During treatment, ~40% of patients will develop rapidly evolving leukocytosis. Rapidly evolving leukocytosis is associated with a higher risk of life-threatening complications.

If signs and symptoms of the RA-APL syndrome are present together with leukocytosis, initiate treatment with high-dose steroids immediately. Consider adding full-dose chemotherapy (including an anthracycline, if not contraindicated) to the tretinoin therapy on day 1 or 2 for patients presenting with a WBC count of >5 x $10^9$/L or immediately, for patients presenting with a WBC count of <5 x $10^9$/L, if the WBC count reaches ≥6 x $10^9$/L by day 5, or ≥10 x $10^9$/L by day 10 or ≥15 x $10^9$/L by day 28.

**Not to be used in women of childbearing potential** unless the woman is capable of complying with effective contraceptive measures; therapy is normally begun on the second or third day of next normal menstrual period; two reliable methods of effective contraception must be used during therapy and for 1 month after discontinuation of therapy, unless abstinence is the chosen method. Within one week prior to the institution of tretinoin therapy, the patient should have blood or urine collected for a serum or urine pregnancy test with a sensitivity of at least 50 mIU/L. When possible, delay tretinoin therapy until a negative result from this test is obtained. When a delay is not possible, place the patient on two reliable forms of contraception. Repeat pregnancy testing and contraception counseling monthly throughout the period of treatment.

Initiation of therapy with tretinoin may be based on the morphological diagnosis of APL. Confirm the diagnosis of APL by detection of the t(15;17) genetic marker by cytogenetic studies. If these are negative, PML/RARα fusion should be sought using molecular diagnostic techniques. The response rate of other AML subtypes to tretinoin has not been demonstrated.

Retinoids have been associated with pseudotumor cerebri (benign intracranial hypertension), especially in children. Early signs and symptoms include papilledema, headache, nausea, vomiting and visual disturbances.

Up to 60% of patients experienced hypercholesterolemia or hypertriglyceridemia, which were reversible upon completion of treatment.

Elevated liver function test results occur in 50% to 60% of patients during treatment. Carefully monitor liver function test results during treatment and give consideration to a temporary withdrawal of tretinoin if test results reach >5 times the upper limit of normal.

**Adverse Reactions** Virtually all patients experience some drug-related toxicity, especially headache, fever, weakness and fatigue. These adverse effects are seldom permanent or irreversible nor do they usually require therapy interruption

>10%:
- Cardiovascular: Arrhythmias, flushing, hypotension, hypertension, peripheral edema, chest discomfort, edema
- Central nervous system: Dizziness, anxiety, insomnia, depression, confusion, malaise, pain
- Dermatologic: Burning, redness, cheilitis, inflammation of lips, dry skin, pruritus, photosensitivity
- Endocrine & metabolic: Increased serum concentration of triglycerides
- Gastrointestinal: GI hemorrhage, abdominal pain, other GI disorders, diarrhea, constipation, dyspepsia, abdominal distention, weight gain or loss, xerostomia
- Hematologic: Hemorrhage, disseminated intravascular coagulation
- Local: Phlebitis, injection site reactions
- Neuromuscular & skeletal: Bone pain, arthralgia, myalgia, paresthesia
- Ocular: Itching of eye
- Renal: Renal insufficiency
- Respiratory: Upper respiratory tract disorders, dyspnea, respiratory insufficiency, pleural effusion, pneumonia, rales, expiratory wheezing, dry nose
- Miscellaneous: Infections, shivering

1% to 10%:
- Cardiovascular: Cardiac failure, cardiac arrest, myocardial infarction, enlarged heart, heart murmur, ischemia, stroke, myocarditis, pericarditis, pulmonary hypertension, secondary cardiomyopathy, cerebral hemorrhage, pallor
- Central nervous system: Intracranial hypertension, agitation, hallucination, agnosia, aphasia, cerebellar edema, cerebellar disorders, convulsions, coma, CNS depression, encephalopathy, hypotaxia, no light reflex, neurologic reaction, spinal cord disorder, unconsciousness, dementia, forgetfulness, somnolence, slow speech, hypothermia
- Dermatologic: Skin peeling on hands or soles of feet, rash, cellulitis
- Endocrine & metabolic: Fluid imbalance, acidosis
- Gastrointestinal: Hepatosplenomegaly, ulcer
- Genitourinary: Dysuria, polyuria, enlarged prostate
- Hepatic: Ascites, hepatitis
- Neuromuscular & skeletal: Tremor, leg weakness, hyporeflexia, dysarthria, facial paralysis, hemiplegia, flank pain, asterixis, abnormal gait
- Ocular: Dry eyes, photophobia
- Renal: Acute renal failure, renal tubular necrosis
- Respiratory: Lower respiratory tract disorders, pulmonary infiltration, bronchial asthma, pulmonary/larynx edema, unspecified pulmonary disease
- Miscellaneous: Face edema, lymph disorders

<1%: Alopecia, anorexia, bleeding of gums, cataracts, conjunctivitis, corneal opacities, decrease in hemoglobin and hematocrit, hyperuricemia, increase in erythrocyte sedimentation rate, inflammatory bowel syndrome, mood changes, nausea, optic neuritis, pseudomotor cerebri, vomiting

**Overdosage/Toxicology** Signs and symptoms: Transient headache, facial flushing, cheilosis, abdominal pain, dizziness and ataxia; all signs and symptoms have been transient and have resolved without apparent residual effects

**Drug Interactions** CYP3A3/4 enzyme substrate

Metabolized by the hepatic cytochrome P-450 system; therefore, all drugs that induce or inhibit this system would be expected to interact with tretinoin CYP2C9 substrate

Increased toxicity: Ketoconazole increases the mean plasma AUC of tretinoin

**Usual Dosage** Oral:

Children: There are limited clinical data on the pediatric use of tretinoin. Of 15 pediatric patients (age range: 1-16 years) treated with tretinoin, the incidence of complete remission was 67%. Safety and efficacy in pediatric patients <1 year of age have not been established. Some pediatric patients experience severe headache and pseudotumor cerebri, requiring analgesic treatment and lumbar puncture for relief. Increased caution is recommended. Consider dose reduction in children experiencing serious or intolerable toxicity; however, the efficacy and safety of tretinoin at doses <45 mg/m²/day have not been evaluated.

Adults: 45 mg/m²/day administered as two evenly divided doses until complete remission is documented. Discontinue therapy 30 days after achievement of complete remission or after 90 days of treatment, whichever occurs first. If after initiation of treatment the presence of the t(15;17) translocation is not confirmed by cytogenetics or by polymerase chain reaction studies and the patient has not responded to tretinoin, consider alternative therapy.

**Note:** Tretinoin is for the induction of remission only. Optimal consolidation or maintenance regimens have not been determined. All patients should therefore receive a standard consolidation or maintenance chemotherapy regimen for APL after induction therapy with tretinoin unless otherwise contraindicated.

**Dietary Considerations** Absorption of retinoids has been shown to be enhanced when taken with food

**Patient Information** Take with food. Do not crush, chew, or dissolve capsules. You will need frequent blood tests while taking this medication. Maintain adequate hydration (2-3 L/day of fluids unless instructed to restrict fluid intake), avoid alcohol and foods containing vitamin A, and foods with high fat content. You may experience lethargy, dizziness, visual changes, confusion, anxiety (avoid driving or engaging in tasks requiring alertness until response to drug is known). For nausea and vomiting, loss of appetite, or dry mouth small, frequent meals, chewing gum, or sucking lozenges may help. You may experience photosensitivity (use sunscreen, wear protective clothing and eyewear, and avoid direct sunlight). You may experience dry, itchy, skin, and dry or irritated eyes (avoid contact lenses). Report persistent vomiting or diarrhea, difficulty breathing, unusual bleeding or bruising, acute GI pain, bone pain, or vision changes immediately.

**Dosage Forms** Capsule: 10 mg

## Tretinoin, Topical (TRET i noyn, TOP i kal)

**U.S. Brand Names** Avita®; Retin-A™ Micro Topical; Retin-A™ Topical

**Canadian Brand Names** Retisol-A®; Stieva-A®; Stieva-A® Forte

**Pharmacologic Category** Retinoic Acid Derivative

**Use** Treatment of acne vulgaris, photodamaged skin, and some skin cancers

**Effects on Mental Status** None reported

**Effects on Psychiatric Treatment** None reported

**Usual Dosage** Children >12 years and Adults: Topical: Begin therapy with a weaker formulation of tretinoin (0.025% cream or 0.01% gel) and increase the concentration as tolerated; apply once daily before retiring or on alternate days; if stinging or irritation develop, decrease frequency of application

**Dosage Forms**

Cream:
- Retin-A™: 0.025% (20 g, 45 g); 0.05% (20 g, 45 g); 0.1% (20 g, 45 g)
- Avita®: 0.025% (20 g, 45 g)
- Renova™: 0.05% emollient cream

Gel, topical:
- Retin-A™: 0.01% (15 g, 45 g); 0.025% (15 g, 45 g)
- Retin-A™ Micro: 0.1% (20 g, 45 g)

Liquid, topical (Retin-A™): 0.05% (28 mL)

♦ **Triacet™** *see* Triamcinolone *on page 563*

♦ **Triacetyloleandomycin** *see* Troleandomycin *on page 573*

♦ **Triacin-C®** *see* Triprolidine, Pseudoephedrine, and Codeine *on page 572*

♦ **Triam-A®** *see* Triamcinolone *on page 563*

## Triamcinolone (trye am SIN oh lone)

**Related Information**

Asthma Guidelines *on page 773*
Corticosteroids Comparison Chart *on page 711*

**U.S. Brand Names** Amcort®; Aristocort®; Aristocort® A; Aristocort® Forte; Aristocort® Intralesional; Aristospan® Intra-Articular; Aristospan® Intralesional; Atolone®; Azmacort™; Delta-Tritex®; Flutex®; Kenacort®; Kenaject-40®; Kenalog®; Kenalog-10®; Kenalog-40®; Kenalog® H; Kenalog® in Orabase®; Kenonel®; Nasacort®; Nasacort® AQ; Tac™-3; Tac™-40; Triacet™; Triam-A®; Triam Forte®; Triderm®; Tri-Kort®; Trilog®; Trilone®; Tri-Nasal® Spray; Tristoject®

**Synonyms** Triamcinolone Acetonide, Aerosol; Triamcinolone Acetonide, Parenteral; Triamcinolone Diacetate, Oral; Triamcinolone Diacetate, Parenteral; Triamcinolone Hexacetonide; Triamcinolone, Oral

**Pharmacologic Category** Corticosteroid, Adrenal; Corticosteroid, Oral Inhaler; Corticosteroid, Nasal; Corticosteroid, Parenteral

**Use**

Inhalation: Control of bronchial asthma and related bronchospastic conditions.

Intranasal: Management of seasonal and perennial allergic rhinitis in patients ≥12 years of age

Systemic: Adrenocortical insufficiency, rheumatic disorders, allergic states, respiratory diseases, systemic lupus erythematosus, and other diseases requiring anti-inflammatory or immunosuppressive effects

Topical: Inflammatory dermatoses responsive to steroids

**Effects on Mental Status** Nervousness and insomnia are common; may cause drowsiness, delirium, euphoria, hallucinations, or mood swings

**Effects on Psychiatric Treatment** Barbiturates may increase the metabolism of triamcinolone

**Pregnancy Risk Factor** C

**Contraindications** Known hypersensitivity to triamcinolone; systemic fungal infections; serious infections (except septic shock or tuberculous meningitis); primary treatment of status asthmaticus

**Warnings/Precautions** Fatalities have occurred due to adrenal insufficiency in asthmatic patients during and after transfer from systemic corticosteroids to aerosol steroids; several months may be required for recovery from this syndrome; during this period, aerosol steroids do **not** provide the increased systemic steroid requirement needed to treat patients having trauma, surgery or infections; avoid using higher than recommended dose

Use with caution in patients with hypothyroidism, cirrhosis, nonspecific ulcerative colitis and patients at increased risk for peptic ulcer disease; do not use occlusive dressings on weeping or exudative lesions and general caution with occlusive dressings should be observed; discontinue if skin irritation or contact dermatitis should occur; do not use in patients with decreased skin circulation; avoid the use of high potency steroids on the face

Because of the risk of adverse effects, systemic corticosteroids should be used cautiously in the elderly, in the smallest possible dose, and for the shortest possible time. Azmacort™ (metered dose inhaler) comes with its own spacer device attached and may be easier to use in older patients. Controlled clinical studies have shown that inhaled and intranasal corticosteroids may cause a reduction in growth velocity in pediatric patients. Growth velocity provides a means of comparing the rate of growth among children of the same age.

In studies involving inhaled corticosteroids, the average reduction in growth velocity was approximately 1 cm (about 1/3 of an inch) per year. It appears that the reduction is related to dose and how long the child takes the drug.

FDA's Pulmonary and Allergy Drugs and Metabolic and Endocrine Drugs advisory committees discussed this issue at a July 1998 meeting. They recommended that the agency develop class-wide labeling to inform healthcare providers so they would understand this potential side effect and monitor growth routinely in pediatric patients who are treated with inhaled corticosteroids, intranasal corticosteroids or both.

Long-term effects of this reduction in growth velocity on final adult height are unknown. Likewise, it also has not yet been determined whether patients' growth will "catch up" if treatment in discontinued. Drug manufacturers will continue to monitor these drugs to learn more about long-term effects. Children are prescribed inhaled corticosteroids to treat asthma. Intranasal corticosteroids are generally used to prevent and treat allergy-related nasal symptoms.

Patients are advised not to stop using their inhaled or intranasal corticosteroids without first speaking to their healthcare providers about the benefits of these drugs compared to their risks.

**Adverse Reactions**

>10%:
- Central nervous system: Insomnia, nervousness
- Gastrointestinal: Increased appetite, indigestion

1% to 10%:
- Ocular: Cataracts
- Endocrine & metabolic: Diabetes mellitus, hirsutism
- Neuromuscular & skeletal: Arthralgia
- Respiratory: Epistaxis

<1%: Abdominal distention, acne, amenorrhea, bone growth suppression, bruising, burning, cough, Cushing's syndrome, delirium, dry throat, euphoria, fatigue, hallucinations, headache, hoarseness, hyperglycemia, hyperpigmentation, hypersensitivity reactions, hypertrichosis, hypopigmentation, itching, mood swings, muscle wasting, oral candidiasis, osteoporosis, pancreatitis, peptic ulcer, seizures, skin atrophy, sodium and water retention, ulcerative esophagitis, wheezing, xerostomia

**Overdosage/Toxicology**

Signs and symptoms: When consumed in excessive quantities, systemic hypercorticism and adrenal suppression may occur

Treatment: In those cases where hypercorticism and adrenal suppression occur, discontinuation and withdrawal of the corticosteroid should be done judiciously

**Drug Interactions** CYP3A3/4 inducer

Decreased effect: Barbiturates, phenytoin, rifampin ↑ metabolism of triamcinolone; vaccine and toxoid effects may be reduced

Increased toxicity: Salicylates may increase risk of GI ulceration

**Usual Dosage** In general, single I.M. dose of 4-7 times oral dose will control patient from 4-7 days up to 3-4 weeks

Children 6-12 years:
- Oral inhalation: 1-2 inhalations 3-4 times/day, not to exceed 12 inhalations/day
- I.M. (acetonide or hexacetonide): 0.03-0.2 mg/kg at 1- to 7-day intervals
- Intra-articular, intrabursal, or tendon-sheath injection: 2.5-15 mg, repeated as needed

Children >12 years and Adults:
- Intranasal: 2 sprays in each nostril once daily; may increase after 4-7 days up to 4 sprays once daily or 1 spray 4 times/day in each nostril
- Topical: Apply a thin film 2-3 times/day. Therapy should be discontinued when control is achieved; if no improvement is seen, reassessment of diagnosis may be necessary.
- Oral: 4-48 mg/day
- Oral inhalation: 2 inhalations 3-4 times/day, not to exceed 16 inhalations/day

**I.M.: Systemic:** Children >12 years and Adults:
- Acetonide: 60 mg (usual dose); additional 20-100 mg doses (usual: 40-80 mg) may be given when signs and symptoms recur, best at 6-week intervals to minimize HPA suppression
- Diacetate: Using 40 mg/mL suspension: 40 mg once weekly

(Continued)

## Triamcinolone *(Continued)*

**I.M.: Site-specific injection:** Children >12 years and Adults:

**Acetonide:**

Intra-articular, intrasynovial, or soft tissue: Using 10 mg/mL or 40 mg/mL: Large joints: 15-40 mg; small joints: 2.5-10 mg; amount depends on location, size of joints, and degree of inflammation; repeat when signs and symptoms recur

Intralesional or sublesional: Using 10 mg/mL: 1 mg per injection site, may be repeated 1 or more times weekly depending upon patient's response; may use multiple injections if they are >1 cm apart (maximum: 30 mg at any one time)

Tendon sheath: 2.5-10 mg

**Diacetate:**

Intra-articular, intrasynovial, or soft tissue: Using 25 mg/mL or 40 mg/mL: 2-40 mg; amount depends on location, size of joint or area, and degree of inflammation; may be repeated at 1- to 8-week intervals; large joints often require 25 mg, while smaller joints may require 2-5 mg

Intralesional or sublesional: Using 25 mg/mL: 5-40 mg; amount depends on size, location, and type of lesion; in general, no more than 12.5 mg per injection site or 25 mg per lesion should be used

**Hexacetonide:**

Intra-articular: Large joints: 10-20 mg; small joints: 2-6 mg

Intralesional or sublesional: Up to 0.5 mg per square inch of affected area

**Patient Information** Take exactly as directed; do not increase dose or discontinue abruptly without consulting prescriber. Take oral medication with or after meals. Limit intake of caffeine or stimulants. Prescriber may recommend increased dietary vitamins, minerals, or iron. Diabetics should monitor glucose levels closely (antidiabetic medication may need to be adjusted). Inform prescriber if you are experiencing greater than normal levels of stress (medication may need adjustment). Some forms of this medication may cause GI upset (oral medication may be taken with meals to reduce GI upset; small frequent meals and frequent mouth care may reduce GI upset). You may be more susceptible to infection (avoid crowds and persons with contagious or infective conditions). Report promptly excessive nervousness or sleep disturbances; any signs of infection (sore throat, unhealed injuries); excessive growth of body hair or loss of skin color; changes in vision; excessive or sudden weight gain (>3 lb/week); swelling of face or extremities; difficulty breathing; muscle weakness; change in color of stools (black or tarry) or persistent abdominal pain; or worsening of condition or failure to improve.

Topical: For external use only. Not for eyes or mucous membranes or open wounds. Apply in very thin layer to occlusive dressing. Apply dressing to area being treated. Avoid prolonged or excessive use around sensitive tissues, genital, or rectal areas. Inform prescriber if condition worsens (swelling, redness, irritation, pain, open sores) or fails to improve.

Aerosol: Not for use during acute asthmatic attack. Follow directions that accompany product. Rinse mouth and throat after use to prevent candidiasis. Do not use intranasal product if you have a nasal infection, nasal injury, or recent nasal surgery. If using two products, consult prescriber in which order to use the two products. Inform prescriber if condition worsens or does not improve.

Nasal spray: Shake gently before use. Use at regular intervals, no more frequently than directed. Report unusual cough or spasm; persistent nasal bleeding, burning, or irritation; or worsening of condition.

**Nursing Implications** Once daily doses should be given in the morning; evaluate clinical response and mental status; may mask signs and symptoms of infection; inject I.M. dose deep in large muscle mass, avoid deltoid; avoid S.C. dose; a thin film is effective topically and avoid topical application on the face; do not occlude area unless directed

**Dosage Forms**

Aerosol:

Oral inhalation: 100 mcg/metered spray (20 g)

Topical, as acetonide: 0.2 mg/2 second spray (23 g, 63 g)

Cream, as acetonide: 0.025% (15 g, 30 g, 60 g, 80 g, 120 g, 240 g); 0.1% (15 g, 20 g, 30 g, 60 g, 80 g, 90 g, 120 g, 240 g); 0.5% (15 g, 20 g, 30 g, 120 g, 240 g)

Injection, as acetonide: 3 mg/mL (5 mL); 10 mg/mL (5 mL); 40 mg/mL (1 mL, 5 mL, 10 mL)

Injection, as diacetate: 25 mg/mL (5 mL); 40 mg/mL (1 mL, 5 mL)

Injection, as hexacetonide: 5 mg/mL (5 mL); 20 mg/mL (1 mL, 5 mL)

Lotion, as acetonide: 0.025% (60 mL); 0.1% (15 mL, 60 mL)

Ointment, topical, as acetonide: 0.025% (15 g, 28 g, 30 g, 57 g, 80 g, 113 g, 240 g); 0.1% (15 g, 28 g, 57 g, 60 g, 80 g, 113 g, 240 g, 454 g); 0.5% (15 g, 28 g, 57 g, 113 g, 240 g)

Spray, intranasal acetonide: 55 mcg per actuation (100 sprays/canister) (15 mg canister)

Syrup: 4 mg/5 mL (120 mL)

Tablet: 1 mg, 2 mg, 4 mg, 8 mg

- **Triamcinolone Acetonide, Aerosol** *see* Triamcinolone *on page 563*
- **Triamcinolone Acetonide, Parenteral** *see* Triamcinolone *on page 563*
- **Triamcinolone Diacetate, Oral** *see* Triamcinolone *on page 563*
- **Triamcinolone Diacetate, Parenteral** *see* Triamcinolone *on page 563*
- **Triamcinolone Hexacetonide** *see* Triamcinolone *on page 563*
- **Triamcinolone, Oral** *see* Triamcinolone *on page 563*
- **Triam Forte®** *see* Triamcinolone *on page 563*
- **Triaminic® Allergy Tablet [OTC]** *see* Chlorpheniramine and Phenylpropanolamine *on page 114*
- **Triaminic® AM Decongestant Formula [OTC]** *see* Pseudoephedrine *on page 478*
- **Triaminic® Cold Tablet [OTC]** *see* Chlorpheniramine and Phenylpropanolamine *on page 114*
- **Triaminic® Expectorant [OTC]** *see* Guaifenesin and Phenylpropanolamine *on page 257*
- **Triaminicol® Multi-Symptom Cold Syrup [OTC]** *see* Chlorpheniramine, Phenylpropanolamine, and Dextromethorphan *on page 116*
- **Triaminic® Oral Infant Drops** *see* Pheniramine, Phenylpropanolamine, and Pyrilamine *on page 435*
- **Triaminic® Syrup [OTC]** *see* Chlorpheniramine and Phenylpropanolamine *on page 114*

## Triamterene (trye AM ter een)

**U.S. Brand Names** Dyrenium®

**Pharmacologic Category** Diuretic, Potassium Sparing

**Use** Alone or in combination with other diuretics to treat edema and hypertension; decreases potassium excretion caused by kaliuretic diuretics

**Effects on Mental Status** May cause drowsiness or dizziness

**Effects on Psychiatric Treatment** Triamterene may increase the side effects of amantadine (dizziness, nausea, dry mouth) necessitating a decrease in dosage; monitor

**Pregnancy Risk Factor** B (per manufacturer); D (Based on expert analysis)

**Contraindications** Hypersensitivity to triamterene or any component; patients receiving other potassium-sparing diuretics; anuria; severe hepatic disease; hyperkalemia or history of hyperkalemia; severe or progressive renal disease; pregnancy

**Warnings/Precautions** Avoid potassium supplements, potassium-containing salt substitutes, a diet rich in potassium, or other drugs that can cause hyperkalemia. Monitor for fluid and electrolyte imbalances. Diuretic therapy should be carefully used in severe hepatic dysfunction; electrolyte and fluid shifts can cause or exacerbate encephalopathy. Use cautiously in patients with history of kidney stones and diabetes. Can cause photosensitivity.

**Adverse Reactions**

1% to 10%:

Cardiovascular: Hypotension, edema, congestive heart failure, bradycardia

Central nervous system: Dizziness, headache, fatigue

Dermatologic: Rash

Gastrointestinal: Constipation, nausea

Respiratory: Dyspnea

<1%: Dehydration, flushing, gynecomastia, hyperkalemia, hyperchloremic hyponatremia, inability to achieve or maintain an erection, metabolic acidosis, postmenopausal bleeding

**Overdosage/Toxicology**

Signs and symptoms: Drowsiness, confusion, clinical signs of dehydration, electrolyte imbalance, and hypotension; chronic or acute ingestion of large amounts of potassium-sparing diuretics, may result in life-threatening hyperkalemia especially with decreased renal function

Treatment: If the EKG shows no widening of the QRS or an arrhythmia, discontinue triamterene and any potassium supplement and substitute a thiazide. Consider Kayexalate® to increase potassium excretion. If an abnormal cardiac status is obvious, treat with calcium or sodium bicarbonates as needed, pacing dialysis and/or Kayexalate®. Infusions of glucose and insulin are also useful.

**Drug Interactions**

Angiotensin-converting enzyme inhibitors can cause hyperkalemia, especially in patients with renal impairment, potassium-rich diets, or on other drugs causing hyperkalemia; avoid concurrent use or monitor closely

Potassium supplements may further increase potassium retention and cause hyperkalemia; avoid concurrent use

**Usual Dosage** Adults: Oral: 100-300 mg/day in 1-2 divided doses; maximum dose: 300 mg/day

**Dosing comments in renal impairment:** $Cl_{cr}$ <10 mL/minute: Avoid use.

**Dosing adjustment in hepatic impairment:** Dose reduction is recommended in patients with cirrhosis.

**Patient Information** Take as directed, preferably after meals. This diuretic does not cause potassium loss; avoid excessive potassium intake (eg, salt substitutes, low-salt foods, bananas, nuts). Weigh yourself daily at the same time, in the same clothes, and report weight loss greater than 5 lb/week. Urine may appear blue (normal). You may experience dizziness, drowsiness, headache (use caution when driving or engaging in tasks requiring alertness until response to drug is known); nausea (small frequent meals, frequent mouth care, sucking lozenges, or chewing gum may help); decreased sexual ability (reversible with discontinuing of medication); or postural hypotension (change position slowly when rising from sitting or lying). Report persistent fatigue, muscle weakness, paresthesia, confusion, anorexia, headaches, lethargy, hyper-reflexia, seizures, swelling of extremities or respiratory difficulty (eg, chest pain, rapid heartbeat or palpitations).

**Nursing Implications** Observe for hyperkalemia; assess weight and I & O daily to determine weight loss; if ordered once daily, dose should be given in the morning

**Dosage Forms** Capsule: 50 mg, 100 mg

♦ **Triapin®** *see* Butalbital Compound and Acetaminophen *on page 80*

♦ **Triavil®** *see* Amitriptyline and Perphenazine *on page 34*

## Triazolam (trye AY zoe lam)

**Related Information**

Anxiolytic/Hypnotic Use in Long-Term Care Facilities *on page 754*
Benzodiazepines Comparison Chart *on page 708*
Clinical Issues in the Use of Anxiolytics and Sedative/Hypnotics *on page 634*
Federal OBRA Regulations Recommended Maximum Doses *on page 756*
Patient Information - Anxiolytics & Sedative Hypnotics (Benzodiazepines) *on page 653*

**Generic Available** Yes

**U.S. Brand Names** Halcion®

**Canadian Brand Names** Apo®-Triazo; Gen-Triazolam; Novo-Triolam; Nu-Triazo

**Pharmacologic Category** Benzodiazepine

**Use** Short-term treatment of insomnia

**Restrictions** C-IV

**Pregnancy Risk Factor** X

**Contraindications** Hypersensitivity to this drug or any component of its formulation (cross-sensitivity with other benzodiazepines may exist); concurrent therapy with CYP3A4 inhibitors (such as ketoconazole, itraconazole, and nefazodone); pregnancy

**Warnings/Precautions** Should be used only after evaluation of potential causes of sleep disturbance. Failure of sleep disturbance to resolve after 7-10 days may indicate psychiatric or medical illness. A worsening of insomnia or the emergence of new abnormalities of thought or behavior may represent unrecognized psychiatric or medical illness and requires immediate and careful evaluation.

An increase in daytime anxiety may occur after as few as 10 days of continuous use, which may be related to withdrawal reaction in some patients. Anterograde amnesia may occur at a higher rate with triazolam than with other benzodiazepines. Use with caution in elderly or debilitated patients, patients with hepatic disease (including alcoholics), or renal impairment. Use with caution in patients with respiratory disease or impaired gag reflex. Avoid use in patients with sleep apnea.

Causes CNS depression (dose-related) resulting in sedation, dizziness, confusion, or ataxia which may impair physical and mental capabilities. Patients must be cautioned about performing tasks which require mental alertness (ie, operating machinery or driving). Use with caution in patients receiving other CNS depressants or psychoactive agents. Effects with other sedative drugs or ethanol may be potentiated. Benzodiazepines have been associated with falls and traumatic injury and should be used with extreme caution in patients who are at risk of these events (especially the elderly).

Use caution in patients with depression, particularly if suicidal risk may be present. Use with caution in patients with a history of drug dependence. Benzodiazepines have been associated with dependence and acute withdrawal symptoms on discontinuation or reduction in dose. Acute withdrawal, including seizures, may be precipitated after administration of flumazenil to patients receiving long-term benzodiazepine therapy.

Paradoxical reactions, including hyperactive or aggressive behavior have been reported with benzodiazepines, particularly in adolescent/pediatric or psychiatric patients. Does not have analgesic, antidepressant, or antipsychotic properties.

**Adverse Reactions**

>10%: Central nervous system: Drowsiness, anteriograde amnesia

1% to 10%:

Central nervous system: Headache, dizziness, nervousness, lightheadedness, ataxia

Gastrointestinal: Nausea, vomiting

<1%: Cramps, confusion, depression, euphoria, fatigue, memory impairment, pain, tachycardia, visual disturbance

**Overdosage/Toxicology**

Signs and symptoms: Somnolence, confusion, coma, diminished reflexes, dyspnea, and hypotension

Treatment: Supportive; rarely is mechanical ventilation required. Flumazenil has been shown to selectively block the binding of benzodiazepines to CNS receptors, resulting in a reversal of benzodiazepine-induced CNS depression but not always respiratory depression

**Drug Interactions** CYP3A3/4 and 3A5-7 enzyme substrate

CNS depressants: Sedative effects and/or respiratory depression may be additive with CNS depressants; includes ethanol, barbiturates, narcotic analgesics, and other sedative agents; monitor for increased effect

CYP3A3/4 inhibitors: Serum level and/or toxicity of some benzodiazepines may be increased; inhibitors include amiodarone, cimetidine, clarithromycin, erythromycin, delavirdine, diltiazem, dirithromycin, disulfiram, fluoxetine, fluvoxamine, grapefruit juice, indinavir, itraconazole, ketoconazole, nefazodone, nevirapine, propoxyfene, quinupristin-dalfopristin, ritonavir, saquinavir, verapamil, zafirlukast, zileuton; monitor for altered benzodiazepine response

Enzyme inducers: Metabolism of some benzodiazepines may be increased, decreasing their therapeutic effect; consider using an alternative sedative/hypnotic agent; potential inducers include phenobarbital, phenytoin, carbamazepine, rifampin, and rifabutin

Oral contraceptives: May decrease the clearance of some benzodiazepines (those which undergo oxidative metabolism); monitor for increased benzodiazepine effect

Theophylline: May partially antagonize some of the effects of benzodiazepines; monitor for decreased response; may require higher doses for sedation

**Mechanism of Action** Binds to stereospecific benzodiazepine receptors on the postsynaptic GABA neuron at several sites within the central nervous system, including the limbic system, reticular formation. Enhancement of the inhibitory effect of GABA on neuronal excitability results by increased neuronal membrane permeability to chloride ions. This shift in chloride ions results in hyperpolarization (a less excitable state) and stabilization.

**Pharmacodynamics/kinetics**

Onset of hypnotic effect: Within 15-30 minutes
Duration: 6-7 hours
Distribution: $V_d$: 0.8-1.8 L/kg
Protein binding: 89%
Metabolism: Extensively in the liver
Half-life: 1.7-5 hours
Elimination: In urine as unchanged drug and metabolites

**Usual Dosage** Onset of action is rapid, patient should be in bed when taking medication

Oral:

Children <18 years: Dosage not established
Adults: 0.125-0.25 mg at bedtime

**Dosing adjustment/comments in hepatic impairment:** Reduce dose or avoid use in cirrhosis

**Dietary Considerations** Alcohol: Additive CNS effect, avoid use

**Monitoring Parameters** Respiratory and cardiovascular status

**Reference Range** Fatalities associated with postmortem levels >47 nmol/L

**Patient Information** Avoid alcohol and other CNS depressants; avoid activities needing good psychomotor coordination until CNS effects are known; drug may cause physical or psychological dependence; avoid abrupt discontinuation after prolonged use

**Nursing Implications** Patients may require assistance with ambulation; lower doses in the elderly are usually effective; institute safety measures

**Additional Information** Onset of action is rapid, patient should be in bed when taking medication; prescription should be written for 7-10 days and should not be prescribed in quantities exceeding a 1-month supply

**Dosage Forms** Tablet: 0.125 mg, 0.25 mg

♦ **Triban®** *see* Trimethobenzamide *on page 569*

♦ **Tribavirin** *see* Ribavirin *on page 492*

## Trichlormethiazide (trye klor meth EYE a zide)

**U.S. Brand Names** Metahydrin®; Naqua®

**Pharmacologic Category** Diuretic, Thiazide

**Use** Management of mild to moderate hypertension; treatment of edema in congestive heart failure and nephrotic syndrome

**Effects on Mental Status** None reported

**Effects on Psychiatric Treatment** May decrease lithium clearance resulting in an increase in serum lithium levels and potential lithium toxicity; monitor serum lithium levels; may cause photosensitivity; use caution with concurrent psychotropics; use sunblock or wear protective clothing

**Pregnancy Risk Factor** D

**Contraindications** Hypersensitivity to trichlormethiazide, thiazides, or sulfonamide-derived drugs; anuria; renal decompensation; pregnancy

**Warnings/Precautions** Avoid in severe renal disease (ineffective). Electrolyte disturbances (hypokalemia, hypochloremic alkalosis, hyponatremia) can occur. Use with caution in severe hepatic dysfunction; hepatic encephalopathy can be caused by electrolyte disturbances. Gout can be precipitate in certain patients with a history of gout, a familial predisposition to gout, or chronic renal failure. Cautious use in diabetics; may see a change in glucose control. Hypersensitivity reactions can occur. Can cause SLE exacerbation or activation. Use with caution in patients with moderate or

(Continued)

## Trichlormethiazide *(Continued)*

high cholesterol concentrations. Photosensitization may occur. Correct hypokalemia before initiating therapy.

**Adverse Reactions**

1% to 10%:

Endocrine & metabolic: Hypokalemia

Respiratory: Dyspnea (<5%)

<1%: Fluid and electrolyte imbalances (hypocalcemia, hypomagnesemia, hyponatremia), hyperglycemia, hypotension, lichenoid dermatitis, photosensitivity, prerenal azotemia, rarely blood dyscrasias

**Overdosage/Toxicology**

Signs and symptoms: Hypotension, dizziness, electrolyte abnormalities, lethargy, confusion, muscle weakness

Treatment: Following GI decontamination, therapy is supportive with I.V. fluids, electrolytes, and I.V. pressors if needed; dialysis is unlikely to be effective

**Drug Interactions**

Angiotensin-converting enzyme inhibitors: Increased hypotension if aggressively diuresed with a thiazide diuretic

Beta-blockers increase hyperglycemic effects in Type 2 diabetes mellitus

Cyclosporine and thiazides can increase the risk of gout or renal toxicity; avoid concurrent use

Digoxin toxicity can be exacerbated if a thiazide induces hypokalemia or hypomagnesemia

Lithium toxicity can occur by reducing renal excretion of lithium; monitor lithium concentration and adjust as needed

Neuromuscular blocking agents can prolong blockade; monitor serum potassium and neuromuscular status

NSAIDs can decrease the efficacy of thiazides reducing the diuretic and antihypertensive effects

**Usual Dosage** Adults: Oral: 1-4 mg/day; initially doses may be given twice daily.

**Dosing adjustment in renal impairment:** Reduced dosage is necessary.

**Patient Information** May be taken with food or milk; take early in day to avoid nocturia; take the last dose of multiple doses no later than 6 PM unless instructed otherwise. A few people who take this medication become more sensitive to sunlight and may experience skin rash, redness, itching, or severe sunburn, especially if sun block SPF ≥15 is not used on exposed skin areas.

**Nursing Implications** Assess weight, I & O reports daily to determine fluid loss; take blood pressure with patient lying down and standing

**Dosage Forms** Tablet: 2 mg, 4 mg

♦ **Trichloroacetaldehyde Monohydrate** *see* Chloral Hydrate *on page 107*

♦ **Tri-Clear® Expectorant [OTC]** *see* Guaifenesin and Phenylpropanolamine *on page 257*

♦ **TriCor™** *see* Fenofibrate *on page 220*

♦ **Triderm®** *see* Triamcinolone *on page 563*

## Tridihexethyl (trye dye heks ETH il)

**U.S. Brand Names** Pathilon®

**Synonyms** Tridihexethyl Chloride

**Pharmacologic Category** Anticholinergic Agent; Antispasmodic Agent, Gastrointestinal

**Use** Adjunctive therapy in peptic ulcer treatment

**Effects on Mental Status** May rarely cause drowsiness, confusion, nervousness, amnesia, or insomnia

**Effects on Psychiatric Treatment** Concurrent use with psychotropics may produce additive sedation or dry mouth

**Pregnancy Risk Factor** C

**Contraindications** Glaucoma; obstructive uropathy (ie, bladder neck obstruction secondary to prostatic hypertrophy); obstructive disorders of GI tract (ie, achalasia, paralytic ileus, pyloroduodenal stenosis); intestinal atony (elderly or debilitated patients); acute hemorrhage with unstable cardiovascular status; ulcerative colitis that is severe or complicated by toxic megacolon; myasthenia gravis

**Warnings/Precautions** Use with caution in patients with hyperthyroidism, hepatic, cardiac, or renal disease, hypertension, GI infections, or other endocrine diseases

**Adverse Reactions**

>10%:

Dermatologic: Dry skin

Gastrointestinal: Constipation, xerostomia, dry throat

Respiratory: Dry nose

Miscellaneous: Decreased diaphoresis

1% to 10%: Gastrointestinal: Dysphagia

**Overdosage/Toxicology**

Signs and symptoms: CNS disturbances, flushing, respiratory failure, paralysis, coma, urinary retention, hyperthermia; anticholinergic toxicity is caused by strong binding of the drug to cholinergic receptors

Treatment: Overdose with severe life-threatening symptoms, physostigmine 1-2 mg (0.5 or 0.02 mg/kg for children) S.C. or I.V., slowly may be given to reverse these effects

**Drug Interactions** Potassium chloride wax-matrix preparations

**Usual Dosage** Adults: Oral: 1-2 tablets 3-4 times/day before meals and 2 tablets at bedtime

**Patient Information** Take 30 minutes before meals and at bedtime; maintain good oral hygiene habits, because lack of saliva may increase chance of cavities; observe caution while driving or performing other tasks requiring alertness, as drug may cause drowsiness, dizziness, or blurred vision; notify physician if skin rash, flushing or eye pain occurs; or if difficulty in urinating, constipation, or sensitivity to light becomes severe or persists

**Dosage Forms** Tablet, as chloride: 25 mg

♦ **Tridihexethyl Chloride** *see* Tridihexethyl *on page 566*

♦ **Tridil® Injection** *see* Nitroglycerin *on page 397*

♦ **Tridione®** *see* Trimethadione *on page 569*

## Trientine (TRYE en teen)

**U.S. Brand Names** Syprine®

**Pharmacologic Category** Chelating Agent

**Use** Treatment of Wilson's disease in patients intolerant to penicillamine

**Effects on Mental Status** May cause drowsiness

**Effects on Psychiatric Treatment** None reported

**Usual Dosage** Oral (administer on an empty stomach):

Children <12 years: 500-750 mg/day in divided doses 2-4 times/day; maximum: 1.5 g/day

Adults: 750-1250 mg/day in divided doses 2-4 times/day; maximum dose: 2 g/day

**Dosage Forms** Capsule, as hydrochloride: 250 mg

## Triethanolamine Polypeptide Oleate-Condensate

(trye eth a NOLE a meen pol i PEP tide OH lee ate-KON den sate)

**U.S. Brand Names** Cerumenex® Otic

**Pharmacologic Category** Otic Agent, Cerumenolytic

**Use** Removal of ear wax (cerumen)

**Effects on Mental Status** None reported

**Effects on Psychiatric Treatment** None reported

**Usual Dosage** Children and Adults: Otic: Fill ear canal, insert cotton plug; allow to remain 15-30 minutes; flush ear with lukewarm water as a single treatment; if a second application is needed for unusually hard impactions, repeat the procedure

**Dosage Forms** Solution, otic: 6 mL, 12 mL

♦ **Trifed-C®** *see* Triprolidine, Pseudoephedrine, and Codeine *on page 572*

## Trifluoperazine (trye floo oh PER a zeen)

**Related Information**

Antipsychotic Agents Comparison Chart *on page 706*

Antipsychotic Medication Guidelines *on page 751*

Clinical Issues in the Use of Antipsychotics *on page 630*

Discontinuation of Psychotropic Drugs - Withdrawal Symptoms and Recommendations *on page 798*

Federal OBRA Regulations Recommended Maximum Doses *on page 756*

Liquid Compatibility With Antipsychotics and Mood Stabilizers *on page 718*

Patient Information - Antipsychotics (General) *on page 646*

Schizophrenia *on page 604*

**Generic Available** Yes

**U.S. Brand Names** Stelazine®

**Synonyms** Trifluoperazine Hydrochloride

**Pharmacologic Category** Antipsychotic Agent, Phenothazine, Piperazine

**Use** Management of psychotic disorders and generalized nonpsychotic anxiety

**Pregnancy Risk Factor** C

**Contraindications** Hypersensitivity to trifluoperazine or any component (cross reactivity between phenothiazines may occur); severe CNS depression, bone marrow suppression, blood dyscrasias, severe hepatic disease, coma

**Warnings/Precautions** May result in hypotension, particularly after I.M. administration. May be sedating, use with caution in disorders where CNS depression is a feature. Use with caution in Parkinson's disease. Caution in patients with hemodynamic instability; predisposition to seizures; subcortical brain damage; hepatic impairment; severe cardiac, renal, or respiratory disease. Esophageal dysmotility and aspiration have been associated with antipsychotic use - use with caution in patients at risk of pneumonia (ie, Alzheimer's disease). Caution in breast cancer or other prolactin-dependent tumors (may elevate prolactin levels). May alter temperature regulation or mask toxicity of other drugs due to antiemetic effects. May alter cardiac conduction - life-threatening arrhythmias have occurred with therapeutic doses of phenothiazines. May cause orthostatic hypotension - use with caution in patients at risk of this effect or those who would tolerate transient hypotensive episodes (cerebrovascular disease, cardiovascular disease or other medications which may predispose).

Phenothiazines may cause anticholinergic effects (confusion, agitation, constipation, dry mouth, blurred vision, urinary retention); therefore, they should be used with caution in patients with decreased gastrointestinal motility, urinary retention, BPH, xerostomia, or visual problems. Conditions which also may be exacerbated by cholinergic blockade include narrow-angle glaucoma (screening is recommended) and worsening of myasthenia gravis. Relative to other antipsychotics, trifluoperazine has a low potency of cholinergic blockade.

May cause extrapyramidal reactions, including pseudoparkinsonism, acute dystonic reactions, akathisia, and tardive dyskinesia (risk of these reactions is high relative to other neuroleptics). May be associated with neuroleptic malignant syndrome (NMS) or pigmentary retinopathy.

**Adverse Reactions**

Cardiovascular: Hypotension, orthostatic hypotension, cardiac arrest
Central nervous system: Extrapyramidal signs (pseudoparkinsonism, akathisia, dystonias, tardive dyskinesia), dizziness, headache, neuroleptic malignant syndrome (NMS), impairment of temperature regulation, lowering of seizures threshold
Dermatologic: Increased sensitivity to sun, rash, discoloration of skin (blue-gray)
Endocrine & metabolic: Changes in menstrual cycle, changes in libido, breast pain, hyperglycemia, hypoglycemia, gynecomastia, lactation, galactorrhea
Gastrointestinal: Constipation, weight gain, nausea, vomiting, stomach pain, xerostomia
Genitourinary: Difficulty in urination, ejaculatory disturbances, urinary retention, priapism
Hematologic: Agranulocytosis, leukopenia, pancytopenia, thrombocytopenic purpura, eosinophilia, hemolytic anemia, aplastic anemia
Hepatic: Cholestatic jaundice, hepatotoxicity
Neuromuscular & skeletal: Tremor
Ocular: Pigmentary retinopathy, cornea and lens changes
Respiratory: Nasal congestion

**Overdosage/Toxicology**

Signs and symptoms: Deep sleep, coma, extrapyramidal symptoms, abnormal involuntary muscle movements, hypo- or hypertension, cardiac arrhythmias
Treatment:
Following initiation of essential overdose management, toxic symptom treatment and supportive treatment should be initiated
Hypotension usually responds to I.V. fluids or Trendelenburg positioning. If unresponsive to these measures, the use of a parenteral inotrope may be required (eg, norepinephrine 0.1-0.2 mcg/kg/minute titrated to response).
Seizures commonly respond to diazepam (I.V. 5-10 mg bolus in adults every 15 minutes if needed up to a total of 30 mg; I.V. 0.25-0.4 mg/kg/dose up to a total of 10 mg in children) or to phenytoin or phenobarbital
Neuroleptics often cause extrapyramidal symptoms (eg, dystonic reactions) requiring management with diphenhydramine 1-2 mg/kg (adults) up to a maximum of 50 mg I.M. or I.V. slow push followed by a maintenance dose for 48-72 hours or benztropine mesylate I.V. 1-2 mg (adults). These agents are generally effective within 2-5 minutes.
Cardiac arrhythmias are treated with lidocaine 1-2 mg/kg bolus followed by a maintenance infusion

**Drug Interactions** CYP1A2 enzyme substrate

Aluminum salts: May decrease the absorption of phenothiazines; monitor
Amphetamines: Efficacy may be diminished by antipsychotics; in addition, amphetamines may increase psychotic symptoms; avoid concurrent use
Anticholinergics: May inhibit the therapeutic response to phenothiazines and excess anticholinergic effects may occur; includes benztropine, trihexyphenidyl, biperiden, and drugs with significant anticholinergic activity (TCAs, antihistamines, disopyramide)
Antihypertensives: Concurrent use of phenothiazines with an antihypertensive may produce additive hypotensive effects (particularly orthostasis)
Bromocriptine: Phenothiazines inhibit the ability of bromocriptine to lower serum prolactin concentrations
CNS depressants: Sedative effects may be additive with phenothiazines; monitor for increased effect; includes barbiturates, benzodiazepines, narcotic analgesics, ethanol, and other sedative agents
CYP1A2 inhibitors: Serum concentrations may be increased due to decreased metabolism; includes cimetidine, ciprofloxacin, fluvoxamine, isoniazid, ritonavir, and zileutin
Enzyme inducers: May enhance the hepatic metabolism of phenothiazines; larger doses may be required; includes rifampin, rifabutin, barbiturates, phenytoin, and cigarette smoking
Epinephrine: Chlorpromazine (and possibly other low potency antipsychotics) may diminish the pressor effects of epinephrine
Guanethidine and guanadrel: Antihypertensive effects may be inhibited by phenothiazines
Levodopa: Phenothiazines may inhibit the antiparkinsonian effect of levodopa; avoid this combination
Lithium: Phenothiazines may produce neurotoxicity with lithium; this is a rare effect
Phenytoin: May reduce serum levels of phenothiazines; phenothiazines may increase phenytoin serum levels
Polypeptide antibiotics: Rare cases of respiratory paralysis have been reported with concurrent use of phenothiazines
Propranolol: Serum concentrations of phenothiazines may be increased; propranolol also increases phenothiazine concentrations
QTc prolonging agents: Effects on QTc interval may be additive with phenothiazines, increasing the risk of malignant arrhythmias; includes type Ia antiarrhythmics, TCAs, and some quinolone antibiotics (sparfloxacin, moxifloxacin, and gatifloxacin)
Sulfadoxine-pyrimethamine: May increase phenothiazine concentrations
Trazodone: Phenothiazines and trazodone may produce additive hypotensive effects
Tricyclic antidepressants: Concurrent use may produce increased toxicity or altered therapeutic response
Valproic acid: Serum levels may be increased by phenothiazines

**Stability** Store injection at room temperature; protect from heat and from freezing; use only clear or slightly yellow solutions

**Mechanism of Action** Blocks postsynaptic mesolimbic dopaminergic receptors in the brain; exhibits alpha-adrenergic blocking effect and depresses the release of hypothalamic and hypophyseal hormones

**Pharmacodynamics/kinetics**

Metabolism: Extensive in the liver
Half-life: >24 hours with chronic use

**Usual Dosage**

Children 6-12 years: Psychoses:
Oral: Hospitalized or well supervised patients: Initial: 1 mg 1-2 times/day, gradually increase until symptoms are controlled or adverse effects become troublesome; maximum: 15 mg/day
I.M.: 1 mg twice daily
Adults:
Psychoses:
Outpatients: Oral: 1-2 mg twice daily
Hospitalized or well supervised patients: Initial: 2-5 mg twice daily with optimum response in the 15-20 mg/day range; do not exceed 40 mg/day
I.M.: 1-2 mg every 4-6 hours as needed up to 10 mg/24 hours maximum
Nonpsychotic anxiety: Oral: 1-2 mg twice daily; maximum: 6 mg/day; therapy for anxiety should not exceed 12 weeks; do not exceed 6 mg/day for longer than 12 weeks when treating anxiety; agitation, jitteriness, or insomnia may be confused with original neurotic or psychotic symptoms
Hemodialysis: Not dialyzable (0% to 5%)

**Administration** Administer I.M. injection deep in upper outer quadrant of buttock

**Monitoring Parameters** Mental status, blood pressure

**Reference Range** Therapeutic response and blood levels have not been established

**Test Interactions** ↑ cholesterol (S), glucose; ↓ uric acid (S); false-positive pregnancy test

**Patient Information** This drug usually requires several weeks for a full therapeutic response to be seen. Avoid excessive exposure to sunlight tanning lamps; concentrate must be diluted in 2-4 oz of liquid (water, carbonated drinks, fruit juices, tomato juice, milk, or pudding); wash hands if undiluted concentrate is spilled on skin to prevent contact dermatosis.

**Nursing Implications** Watch for hypotension when administering I.M. or I.V.; observe for extrapyramidal effects

**Additional Information** Do not exceed 6 mg/day for longer than 12 weeks when treating anxiety; agitation, jitteriness, or insomnia may be confused with original neurotic or psychotic symptoms

**Dosage Forms**

Concentrate, oral, as hydrochloride: 10 mg/mL (60 mL)
Injection, as hydrochloride: 2 mg/mL (10 mL)
Tablet, as hydrochloride: 1 mg, 2 mg, 5 mg, 10 mg

♦ **Trifluoperazine Hydrochloride** *see* Trifluoperazine *on page 566*

## Triflupromazine (trye floo PROE ma zeen)

**Related Information**

Antipsychotic Medication Guidelines *on page 751*
Clinical Issues in the Use of Antipsychotics *on page 630*
Federal OBRA Regulations Recommended Maximum Doses *on page 756*
Patient Information - Antipsychotics (General) *on page 646*

**Generic Available** No

**U.S. Brand Names** Vesprin®

**Synonyms** Triflupromazine Hydrochloride

**Pharmacologic Category** Antipsychotic Agent, Phenothiazine, Aliphatic

**Use** Treatment of psychoses; vomiting

(Continued)

## Triflupromazine *(Continued)*

**Unlabeled uses:** Pain; hiccups

**Pregnancy Risk Factor** C

**Contraindications** Hypersensitivity to triflupromazine or any component, cross-sensitivity with other phenothiazines may exist; angle-closure glaucoma; bone marrow depression; severe liver or cardiac disease

**Warnings/Precautions** Safety and efficacy have not been established in children <2.5 years of age; watch for hypotension when administering I.M. or I.V.; use with caution in patients with cardiovascular disease or seizures; benefits of therapy must be weighed against risks of therapy; use caution with CNS depression and severe liver or cardiac disease; avoid use in children and adolescents with suspected Reye's syndrome

**Adverse Reactions**

Cardiovascular: Hypotension, tachycardia, syncope, peripheral edema, Q-T prolongation

Central nervous system: Neuroleptic malignant syndrome, extrapyramidal signs (dystonia, akathisia, pseudoparkinsonism, tardive dyskinesia), sedation, dizziness, drowsiness, insomnia, anxiety, depression, headache, seizures, NMS hyperpyrexia

Dermatologic: Photosensitivity, dermatitis, urticaria

Endocrine & metabolic: Syndrome of inappropriate antidiuretic hormone, galactorrhea, gynecomastia, hyperglycemia, hypoglycemia, breast engorgement, lactation, mastalgia

Gastrointestinal: Xerostomia, weight gain

Hematologic: Agranulocytosis, leukopenia, eosinophilia, thrombocytopenia, aplastic anemia, hemolytic anemia

Hepatic: Jaundice

Neuromuscular & skeletal: Weakness

Ocular: Nystagmus, blurred vision, keratopathy, lacrimation, pigment deposition

**Drug Interactions**

Aluminum salts: May decrease the absorption of phenothiazines; monitor

Amphetamines: Efficacy may be diminished by antipsychotics; in addition, amphetamines may increase psychotic symptoms; avoid concurrent use

Anticholinergics: May inhibit the therapeutic response to phenothiazines and excess anticholinergic effects may occur; includes benztropine, trihexyphenidyl, biperiden, and drugs with significant anticholinergic activity (TCAs, antihistamines, disopyramide)

Antihypertensives: Concurrent use of phenothiazines with an antihypertensive may produce additive hypotensive effects (particularly orthostasis)

Bromocriptine: Phenothiazines inhibit the ability of bromocriptine to lower serum prolactin concentrations

CNS depressants: Sedative effects may be additive with phenothiazines; monitor for increased effect; includes barbiturates, benzodiazepines, narcotic analgesics, ethanol, and other sedative agents

CYP inhibitors: Metabolism of phenothiazines may be decreased, increasing clinical effect or toxicity; monitor for increased effect/toxicity

Enzyme inducers: May enhance the hepatic metabolism of phenothiazines; larger doses may be required; includes rifampin, rifabutin, barbiturates, phenytoin, and cigarette smoking

Epinephrine: Chlorpromazine (and possibly other low potency antipsychotics) may diminish the pressor effects of epinephrine

Guanethidine and guanadrel: Antihypertensive effects may be inhibited by phenothiazines

Levodopa: Phenothiazines may inhibit the antiparkinsonian effect of levodopa; avoid this combination

Lithium: Phenothiazines may produce neurotoxicity with lithium; this is a rare effect

Phenytoin: May reduce serum levels of phenothiazines; phenothiazines may increase phenytoin serum levels

Polypeptide antibiotics: Rare cases of respiratory paralysis have been reported with concurrent use of phenothiazines

Propranolol: Serum concentrations of phenothiazines may be increased; propranolol also increases phenothiazine concentrations

QTc prolonging agents: Effects on QTc interval may be additive with phenothiazines, increasing the risk of malignant arrhythmias; includes type Ia antiarrhythmics, TCAs, and some quinolone antibiotics (sparfloxacin, moxifloxacin, and gatifloxacin)

Sulfadoxine-pyrimethamine: May increase phenothiazine concentrations

Trazodone: Phenothiazines and trazodone may produce additive hypotensive effects

Tricyclic antidepressants: Concurrent use may produce increased toxicity or altered therapeutic response

Valproic acid: Serum levels may be increased by phenothiazines

**Mechanism of Action** The sites of action appear to be the reticular activity system of the midbrain, limbic system, hypothalamus, globus pallidus, and corpus striatum. Postsynaptic, adrenergic, dopaminergic, and serotonergic receptors are blocked.

**Usual Dosage**

Children: I.M.: 0.2-0.25 mg/kg

Adults:

I.M.: 5-15 mg every 4 hours

I.V.: 1 mg

**Monitoring Parameters** Monitor EKG for 24 hours

**Reference Range** Therapeutic: 0.002-0.0600 mg/L

**Test Interactions** Increases cholesterol (S), glucose; decreases uric acid (S)

**Dosage Forms** Injection, as hydrochloride: 20 mg/mL (1 mL)

♦ **Triflupromazine Hydrochloride** *see* Triflupromazine *on page 567*

## Trifluridine (trye FLURE i deen)

**U.S. Brand Names** Viroptic® Ophthalmic

**Pharmacologic Category** Antiviral Agent, Ophthalmic

**Use** Treatment of primary keratoconjunctivitis and recurrent epithelial keratitis caused by herpes simplex virus types I and II

**Effects on Mental Status** None reported

**Effects on Psychiatric Treatment** None reported

**Usual Dosage** Adults: Instill 1 drop into affected eye every 2 hours while awake, to a maximum of 9 drops/day, until re-epithelialization of corneal ulcer occurs; then use 1 drop every 4 hours for another 7 days; do **not** exceed 21 days of treatment; if improvement has not taken place in 7-14 days, consider another form of therapy

**Dosage Forms** Solution, ophthalmic: 1% (7.5 mL)

♦ **Trihexy®** *see* Trihexyphenidyl *on page 568*

## Trihexyphenidyl (trye heks ee FEN i dil)

**Related Information**

Agents for Treatment of Extrapyramidal Symptoms *on page 638*

Antiparkinsonian Agents Comparison Chart *on page 705*

Discontinuation of Psychotropic Drugs - Withdrawal Symptoms and Recommendations *on page 798*

Patient Information - Agents for Treatment of Extrapyramidal Symptoms *on page 657*

**Generic Available** Yes: Tablet

**U.S. Brand Names** Artane®; Trihexy®

**Canadian Brand Names** Apo®-Trihex; Novo-Hexidyl; PMS-Trihexyphenidyl; Trihexyphen®

**Synonyms** Benzhexol Hydrochloride; Trihexyphenidyl Hydrochloride

**Pharmacologic Category** Anticholinergic Agent; Anti-Parkinson's Agent (Anticholinergic)

**Use** Adjunctive treatment of Parkinson's disease; treatment of drug-induced extrapyramidal effects

**Pregnancy Risk Factor** C

**Contraindications** Hypersensitivity to trihexyphenidyl or any component; patients with narrow-angle glaucoma; pyloric or duodenal obstruction, stenosing peptic ulcers; bladder neck obstructions; achalasia; myasthenia gravis

**Warnings/Precautions** Use with caution in hot weather or during exercise. Elderly patients require strict dosage regulation. Use with caution in patients with tachycardia, cardiac arrhythmias, hypertension, hypotension, prostatic hypertrophy or any tendency toward urinary retention, liver or kidney disorders, and obstructive disease of the GI or GU tract. May exacerbate mental symptoms when used to treat extrapyramidal reactions. When given in large doses or to susceptible patients, may cause weakness. Does not improve symptoms of tardive dyskinesias.

**Adverse Reactions**

Cardiovascular: Tachycardia

Central nervous system: Confusion, agitation, euphoria, drowsiness, headache, dizziness, nervousness, delusions, hallucinations, paranoia

Dermatologic: Dry skin, increased sensitivity to light, rash

Gastrointestinal: Constipation, xerostomia, dry throat, ileus, nausea, vomiting, parotitis

Genitourinary: Urinary retention

Neuromuscular & skeletal: Weakness

Ocular: Blurred vision, mydriasis, increase in intraocular pressure, glaucoma

Respiratory: Dry nose

Miscellaneous: Diaphoresis (decreased)

**Overdosage/Toxicology**

Signs and symptoms: Blurred vision, urinary retention, tachycardia; anticholinergic toxicity is caused by strong binding of the drug to cholinergic receptors; anticholinesterase inhibitors reduce acetylcholinesterase

Treatment: For anticholinergic overdose with severe life-threatening symptoms, physostigmine 1-2 mg (0.5 or 0.02 mg/kg for children) S.C. or I.V., slowly may be given to reverse these effects

**Drug Interactions**

Amantadine, rimantadine: Central and/or peripheral anticholinergic syndrome can occur when administered with amantadine or rimantadine

Anticholinergic agents: Central and/or peripheral anticholinergic syndrome can occur when administered with narcotic analgesics, phenothiazines and other antipsychotics (especially with high anticholinergic activity), tricyclic antidepressants, quinidine and some other antiarrhythmics, and antihistamines

Atenolol: Anticholinergics may increase the bioavailability of atenolol (and possibly other beta-blockers); monitor for increased effect

Cholinergic agents: Anticholinergics may antagonize the therapeutic effect of cholinergic agents: Includes tacrine, and donepezil

Digoxin: Anticholinergics may decrease gastric degradation and increase the amount of digoxin absorbed by delaying gastric emptying

Levodopa: Anticholinergics may increase gastric degradation and decrease the amount of levodopa absorbed by delaying gastric emptying

Neuroleptics: Anticholinergics may antagonize the therapeutic effects of neuroleptics

**Mechanism of Action** Exerts a direct inhibitory effect on the parasympathetic nervous system. It also has a relaxing effect on smooth musculature; exerted both directly on the muscle itself and indirectly through parasympathetic nervous system (inhibitory effect)

**Pharmacodynamics/kinetics**

Peak effect: Within 1 hour

Half-life: 3.3-4.1 hours

Time to peak serum concentration: Within 1-1.5 hours

Elimination: Primarily in urine

**Usual Dosage** Adults: Oral: Initial: 1-2 mg/day, increase by 2 mg increments at intervals of 3-5 days; usual dose: 5-15 mg/day in 3-4 divided doses

**Dietary Considerations** Alcohol: Additive CNS effect, avoid use

**Monitoring Parameters** IOP monitoring and gonioscopic evaluations should be performed periodically

**Patient Information** Take after meals or with food if GI upset occurs; do not discontinue drug abruptly; notify physician if adverse GI effects, rapid or pounding heartbeat, confusion, eye pain, rash, fever or heat intolerance occurs. Observe caution when performing hazardous tasks or those that require alertness such as driving, as may cause drowsiness. Avoid alcohol and other CNS depressants. May cause dry mouth - adequate fluid intake or hard sugar free candy may relieve. Difficult urination or constipation may occur - notify physician if effects persist; may increase susceptibility to heat stroke.

**Nursing Implications** Tolerated best if given in 2-3 daily doses and with food; high doses may be divided into 4 doses, at meal times and at bedtime; patients may be switched to sustained-action capsules when stabilized on conventional dosage forms

**Additional Information** Incidence and severity of side effects are dose related; patients may be switched to sustained-action capsules when stabilized on conventional dosage forms

**Dosage Forms**

Capsule, as hydrochloride, sustained release: 5 mg

Elixir, as hydrochloride: 2 mg/5 mL (480 mL)

Tablet, as hydrochloride: 2 mg, 5 mg


- **Trihexyphenidyl Hydrochloride** *see* Trihexyphenidyl *on page 568*
- **TRIKOF-D®** *see* Guaifenesin, Phenylpropanolamine, and Dextromethorphan *on page 258*
- **Tri-Kort®** *see* Triamcinolone *on page 563*
- **Trilafon®** *see* Perphenazine *on page 432*
- **Trileptal®** *see* Oxcarbazepine *on page 411*
- **Tri-Levlen®** *see* Ethinyl Estradiol and Levonorgestrel *on page 211*
- **Trilisate®** *see* Choline Magnesium Trisalicylate *on page 121*
- **Trilog®** *see* Triamcinolone *on page 563*
- **Trilone®** *see* Triamcinolone *on page 563*
- **Trimazide®** *see* Trimethobenzamide *on page 569*


## Trimethadione (trye meth a DYE one)

**U.S. Brand Names** Tridione®

**Synonyms** Troxidone

**Pharmacologic Category** Anticonvulsant, Oxazolidinedione

**Use** Control absence (petit mal) seizures refractory to other drugs

**Contraindications** Hypersensitivity to trimethadione

**Warnings/Precautions** May cause severe blood dyscrasias; use with caution in patients with renal and hepatic impairment, SLE, myasthenia gravis, or intermittent porphyria; do not abruptly discontinue medication

**Adverse Reactions**

Central nervous system: Drowsiness, hiccups

Dermatologic: Alopecia, exfoliative dermatitis, rash

Endocrine & metabolic: Porphyria

Gastrointestinal: Anorexia, vomiting, stomach upset, abdominal pain, weight loss

Hematologic: Aplastic anemia, agranulocytosis, thrombocytopenia,

Hepatic: Hepatitis, jaundice

Neuromuscular & skeletal: Myasthenia gravis-like syndrome

Ocular: Diplopia, photophobia, hemeralopia, nystagmus, scotomata

Renal: Nephrosis, proteinuria

Miscellaneous: Lupus

**Overdosage/Toxicology**

Signs and symptoms: Nausea, drowsiness, ataxia, coma

Treatment: General supportive care is required; urine alkalinization can increase elimination of active metabolites

**Drug Interactions**

Acetylcholinesterase inhibitors: May reduce the antimyasthenic effects of these agents (limited documentation); monitor

CNS depressants: Sedative effects may be additive with other CNS depressants; monitor for increased effect; includes ethanol, sedatives, antidepressants, narcotic analgesics, other anticonvulsants, and benzodiazepines

**Mechanism of Action** An oxazolidinedione with anticonvulsant sedative properties; elevates the cortical and basal seizure thresholds, and reduces the synaptic response to low frequency impulses

**Pharmacodynamics/kinetics**

Metabolism: Metabolized in the liver by microsomal enzymes to dimethadione (active)

Half-life:

Parent drug: 12-24 hours

Dimethadione: 6-13 days

Time to peak serum concentration: Within 30-120 minutes

Elimination: In the urine (3% as unchanged drug)

**Usual Dosage** Oral:

Children: Initial: 25-50 mg/kg/24 hours in 3-4 equally divided doses every 6-8 hours

Adults: Initial: 900 mg/day in 3-4 equally divided doses, increase by 300 mg/day at weekly intervals until therapeutic results or toxic symptoms appear

**Dosing interval in renal impairment:**

$Cl_{cr}$ 10-50 mL/minute: Administer every 8-12 hours

$Cl_{cr}$ <10 mL/minute: Administer every 12-24 hours

**Test Interactions** ↑ alkaline phosphatase (S); ↓ calcium (S)

**Patient Information** Blood test monitoring must be performed periodically, notify physician of persistent or severe fatigue, sore throat, fever, rash, unusual bleeding or bruising; may take with food, may cause drowsiness, impair judgment and coordination, and blurred vision; visual disturbances are normally controlled by reduction of dose

**Nursing Implications** Institute safety measures, assist with ambulation, observe for visual disturbances

**Dosage Forms**

Capsule: 300 mg

Solution: 40 mg/mL (473 mL)

Tablet, chewable: 150 mg

## Trimethobenzamide (trye meth oh BEN za mide)

**U.S. Brand Names** Arrestin®; Pediatric Triban®; Tebamide®; T-Gen®; Ticon®; Tigan®; Triban®; Trimazide®

**Pharmacologic Category** Anticholinergic Agent; Antiemetic

**Use** Control of nausea and vomiting (especially for long-term antiemetic therapy); less effective than phenothiazines but may be associated with fewer side effects

**Effects on Mental Status** Drowsiness is common; may cause dizziness; may rarely cause depression

**Effects on Psychiatric Treatment** Concurrent use with psychotropics may produce additive sedation

**Pregnancy Risk Factor** C

**Contraindications** Hypersensitivity to trimethobenzamide, benzocaine, or any component; injection contraindicated in children and suppositories are contraindicated in premature infants or neonates

**Warnings/Precautions** May mask emesis due to Reye's syndrome or mimic CNS effects of Reye's syndrome in patients with emesis of other etiologies; use in patients with acute vomiting should be avoided

**Adverse Reactions**

>10%: Central nervous system: Drowsiness

1% to 10%:

Cardiovascular: Hypotension

Central nervous system: Dizziness, headache

Gastrointestinal: Diarrhea

Neuromuscular & skeletal: Muscle cramps

<1%: Blood dyscrasias, convulsions, hepatic impairment, hypersensitivity skin reactions, mental depression, opisthotonus

**Overdosage/Toxicology**

Signs and symptoms: Hypotension, seizures, CNS depression, cardiac arrhythmias, disorientation, confusion

Treatment: Following initiation of essential overdose management, toxic symptom treatment and supportive treatment should be initiated. Hypotension usually responds to I.V. fluids or Trendelenburg positioning. If unresponsive to these measures, the use of a parenteral inotrope may be required (eg, norepinephrine 0.1-0.2 mcg/kg/minute titrated to response). Seizures commonly respond to diazepam (I.V. 5-10 mg bolus in adults every 15 minutes, if needed, up to a total of 30 mg; I.V. 0.25-0.4 mg/kg/dose up to a total of 10 mg in children) or to phenytoin or phenobarbital. Critical cardiac arrhythmias often respond to lidocaine 1-2 mg/kg bolus followed by a maintenance infusion. Extrapyramidal symptoms (eg, dystonic reactions) may be managed with diphenhydramine 1-2 mg/kg (adults) up to a maximum of 50 mg I.M. or I.V. slow push followed by

(Continued)

## Trimethobenzamide *(Continued)*

a maintenance dose for 48-72 hours. When these reactions are unresponsive to diphenhydramine, benztropine mesylate I.V. 1-2 mg (adults) may be effective. These agents are generally effective within 2-5 minutes.

**Drug Interactions** Antagonism of oral anticoagulants may occur

**Usual Dosage** Rectal use is contraindicated in neonates and premature infants

Children:

Rectal: <14 kg: 100 mg 3-4 times/day

Oral, rectal: 14-40 kg: 100-200 mg 3-4 times/day

Adults:

Oral: 250 mg 3-4 times/day

I.M., rectal: 200 mg 3-4 times/day

**Patient Information** Take as directed before meals; do not increase dose and do not discontinue without consulting prescriber. You may experience drowsiness or blurred vision (use caution when driving or engaging in tasks that require alertness until response to drug is known) or diarrhea (buttermilk or yogurt may help). Report chest pain or palpitations, persistent dizziness or blurred vision, or CNS changes (disorientation, depression, confusion).

**Nursing Implications** Use only clear solution; observe for extrapyramidal and anticholinergic effects

**Dosage Forms**

Capsule, as hydrochloride: 100 mg, 250 mg

Injection, as hydrochloride: 100 mg/mL (2 mL, 20 mL)

Suppository, rectal, as hydrochloride: 100 mg, 200 mg

## Trimethoprim (trye METH oh prim)

**U.S. Brand Names** Proloprim®; Trimpex®

**Synonyms** TMP

**Pharmacologic Category** Antibiotic, Miscellaneous

**Use** Treatment of urinary tract infections due to susceptible strains of *E. coli, P. mirabilis, K. pneumoniae, Enterobacter* sp and coagulase-negative *Staphylococcus* including *S. saprophyticus*; acute otitis media in children; acute exacerbations of chronic bronchitis in adults; in combination with other agents for treatment of toxoplasmosis, *Pneumocystis carinii*; treatment of superficial ocular infections involving the conjunctiva and cornea

**Effects on Mental Status** None reported

**Effects on Psychiatric Treatment** May cause neutropenia; use caution with clozapine and carbamazepine

**Pregnancy Risk Factor** C

**Contraindications** Hypersensitivity to trimethoprim or any component, megaloblastic anemia due to folate deficiency

**Warnings/Precautions** Use with caution in patients with impaired renal or hepatic function or with possible folate deficiency

**Adverse Reactions**

1% to 10%:

Dermatologic: Rash (3% to 7%), pruritus

Hematologic: Megaloblastic anemia (with chronic high doses)

<1%: Cholestatic jaundice, elevated BUN/serum creatinine, epigastric distress, exfoliative dermatitis, fever, hyperkalemia, increased LFTs, leukopenia, nausea, neutropenia, thrombocytopenia, vomiting

**Overdosage/Toxicology**

Signs and symptoms: Nausea, vomiting, confusion, dizziness; chronic overdose results in bone marrow suppression

Treatment: Supportive following GI decontamination; treatment of chronic overdose is use of oral leucovorin 5-15 mg/day

**Drug Interactions** Increased effect/toxicity/levels of phenytoin; increased myelosuppression with methotrexate; may increase levels of digoxin

**Usual Dosage** Oral:

Children: 4 mg/kg/day in divided doses every 12 hours

Adults: 100 mg every 12 hours or 200 mg every 24 hours; in the treatment of *Pneumocystis carinii* pneumonia; dose may be as high as 15-20 mg/kg/day in 3-4 divided doses

**Dosing interval in renal impairment:** $Cl_{cr}$ 15-30 mL/minute: Administer 50 mg every 12 hours

Hemodialysis: Moderately dialyzable (20% to 50%)

**Patient Information** Take per recommended schedule. Complete full course of therapy; do not skip doses. Do not chew or crush tablets; swallow whole with milk or food. Maintain adequate hydration (2-3 L/day of fluids unless instructed to restrict fluid intake). You may experience nausea, vomiting, or GI upset (small frequent meals, frequent mouth care, sucking lozenges, or chewing gum may help). Report skin rash, redness, or irritation; feelings of acute fatigue or weakness; unusual bleeding or bruising; or other persistent adverse effects.

**Dosage Forms** Tablet: 100 mg, 200 mg

- **Trimethoprim and Sulfamethoxazole** *see* Co-Trimoxazole *on page 142*
- **Trimethylpsoralen** *see* Trioxsalen *on page 571*

## Trimetrexate Glucuronate

(tri me TREKS ate gloo KYOOR oh nate)

**U.S. Brand Names** Neutrexin® Injection

**Pharmacologic Category** Antineoplastic Agent, Miscellaneous

**Use** Alternative therapy for the treatment of moderate-to-severe *Pneumocystis carinii* pneumonia (PCP) in immunocompromised patients, including patients with acquired immunodeficiency syndrome (AIDS), who are intolerant of, or are refractory to, co-trimoxazole therapy or for whom co-trimoxazole and pentamidine are contraindicated. **Concurrent folinic acid (leucovorin) must always be administered.**

**Effects on Mental Status** None reported

**Effects on Psychiatric Treatment** May cause neutropenia; use caution with clozapine and carbamazepine

**Usual Dosage** Adults: I.V.: 45 mg/m$^2$ once daily over 60 minutes for 21 days; it is necessary to reduce the dose in patients with liver dysfunction, although no specific recommendations exist; concurrent folinic acid 20 mg/m$^2$ every 6 hours orally or I.V. for 24 days

**Dosage Forms** Powder for injection: 25 mg

## Trimipramine (trye MI pra meen)

**Related Information**

Antidepressant Agents Comparison Chart *on page 704*

Clinical Issues in the Use of Antidepressants *on page 627*

Discontinuation of Psychotropic Drugs - Withdrawal Symptoms and Recommendations *on page 798*

Federal OBRA Regulations Recommended Maximum Doses *on page 756*

Mood Disorders *on page 600*

Patient Information - Antidepressants (TCAs) *on page 640*

Teratogenic Risks of Psychotropic Medications *on page 812*

**Generic Available** Yes

**U.S. Brand Names** Surmontil®

**Canadian Brand Names** Apo®-Trimip; Novo-Tripramine; Nu-Trimipramine; Rhotrimine®

**Synonyms** Trimipramine Maleate

**Pharmacologic Category** Antidepressant, Tricyclic (Tertiary Amine)

**Use** Treatment of depression

**Pregnancy Risk Factor** C

**Contraindications** Hypersensitivity to this drug or other dibenzodiazepines; use of monoamine oxidase inhibitors within 14 days; use in a patient during the acute recovery phase of MI

**Warnings/Precautions** Often causes sedation, resulting in impaired performance of tasks requiring alertness (ie, operating machinery or driving). Sedative effects may be additive with other CNS depressants and/or ethanol. The degree of sedation is very high relative to other antidepressants. May worsen psychosis in some patients or precipitate a shift to mania or hypomania in patients with bipolar disease. May increase the risks associated with electroconvulsive therapy. This agent should be discontinued, when possible, prior to elective surgery. Therapy should not be abruptly discontinued in patients receiving high doses for prolonged periods. Use with caution in patients with hepatic or renal dysfunction and in elderly patients.

May cause orthostatic hypotension (risk is high relative to other antidepressants) - use with caution in patients at risk of hypotension or in patients where transient hypotensive episodes would be poorly tolerated (cardiovascular disease or cerebrovascular disease). The degree of anticholinergic blockade produced by this agent is very high relative to other cyclic antidepressants - use caution in patients with urinary retention, benign prostatic hypertrophy, narrow-angle glaucoma, xerostomia, visual problems, constipation, or history of bowel obstruction. May cause alteration in glucose regulation - use with caution in patients with diabetes.

Use caution in patients with depression, particularly if suicidal risk may be present. Use with caution in patients with a history of cardiovascular disease (including previous MI, stroke, tachycardia, or conduction abnormalities). The risk conduction abnormalities with this agent is high relative to other antidepressants. Use caution in patients with a previous seizure disorder or condition predisposing to seizures such as brain damage, alcoholism, or concurrent therapy with other drugs which lower the seizure threshold. Use with caution in hyperthyroid patients or those receiving thyroid supplementation.

**Adverse Reactions**

Cardiovascular: Arrhythmias, hypotension, hypertension, tachycardia, palpitations, heart block, stroke, myocardial infarction

Central nervous system: Headache, exacerbation of psychosis, confusion, delirium, hallucinations, nervousness, restlessness, delusions, agitation, insomnia, nightmares, anxiety, seizures

Dermatologic: Photosensitivity, rash, petechiae, itching

Endocrine & metabolic: Sexual dysfunction, breast enlargement, galactorrhea, SIADH

Gastrointestinal: Xerostomia, constipation, increased appetite, nausea, unpleasant taste, weight gain, diarrhea, heartburn, vomiting, anorexia,

trouble with gums, decreased lower esophageal sphincter tone may cause GE reflux
Genitourinary: Difficult urination, urinary retention, testicular edema
Hematologic: Agranulocytosis, eosinophilia, purpura, thrombocytopenia
Hepatic: Cholestatic jaundice, increased liver enzymes
Neuromuscular & skeletal: Tremors, numbness, tingling, paresthesia, incoordination, ataxia, peripheral neuropathy, extrapyramidal symptoms
Ocular: Blurred vision, eye pain, disturbances in accommodation, mydriasis, increased intraocular pressure
Otic: Tinnitus
Miscellaneous: Allergic reactions

**Overdosage/Toxicology**
Signs and symptoms: Agitation, confusion, hallucinations, urinary retention, hypothermia, hypotension, tachycardia, cardiac arrhythmias
Treatment:
Following initiation of essential overdose management, toxic symptoms should be treated
Ventricular arrhythmias often respond to systemic alkalinization (sodium bicarbonate 0.5-2 mEq/kg I.V.). Arrhythmias unresponsive to this therapy may respond to lidocaine 1 mg/kg I.V. followed by a titrated infusion. Physostigmine (1-2 mg I.V. slowly for adults or 0.5 mg I.V. slowly for children) may be indicated in reversing cardiac arrhythmias that are life-threatening.
Seizures usually respond to diazepam I.V. boluses (5-10 mg for adults up to 30 mg or 0.25-0.4 mg/kg/dose for children up to 10 mg/dose). If seizures are unresponsive or recur, phenytoin or phenobarbital may be required.

**Drug Interactions** CYP2D6 enzyme substrate
Altretamine: Concurrent use may cause orthostatic hypertension
Amphetamines: TCAs may enhance the effect of amphetamines; monitor for adverse CV effects
Anticholinergics: Combined use with TCAs may produce additive anticholinergic effects
Antihypertensives: TCAs may inhibit the antihypertensive response to bethanidine, clonidine, debrisoquin, guanadrel, guanethidine, guanabenz, guanfacine; monitor BP; consider alternate antihypertensive agent
Beta-agonists: When combined with TCAs may predispose patients to cardiac arrhythmias
Bupropion: May increase the levels of tricyclic antidepressants; based on limited information; monitor response
Carbamazepine: Tricyclic antidepressants may increase carbamazepine levels; monitor
Cholestyramine and colestipol: May bind TCAs and reduce their absorption; monitor for altered response
Clonidine: Abrupt discontinuation of clonidine may cause hypertensive crisis, amitriptyline may enhance the response (also see note on antihypertensives)
CNS depressants: Sedative effects may be additive with TCAs; monitor for increased effect; includes benzodiazepines, barbiturates, antipsychotics, ethanol, and other sedative medications
CYP2D6 inhibitors: Serum levels and/or toxicity of some tricyclic antidepressants may be increased; inhibitors include amiodarone, cimetidine, delavirdine, fluoxetine, paroxetine, propafenone, quinidine, and ritonavir; monitor for increased effect/toxicity
Enzyme inducers: May increase the metabolism of TCAs resulting in decreased effect; includes carbamazepine, phenobarbital, phenytoin, and rifampin; monitor for decreased response
Epinephrine (and other direct alpha-agonists): The pressor response to I.V. epinephrine, norepinephrine, and phenylephrine may be enhanced in patients receiving TCAs; this combination is best avoided
Fenfluramine: May increase tricyclic antidepressant levels/effects
Hypoglycemic agents (including insulin): TCAs may enhance the hypoglycemic effects of tolazamide, chlorpropamide, or insulin; monitor for changes in blood glucose levels; reported with chlorpropamide, tolazamide, and insulin
Levodopa: Tricyclic antidepressants may decrease the absorption (bioavailability) of levodopa; rare hypertensive episodes have also been attributed to this combination
Linezolid: Hyperpyrexia, hypertension, tachycardia, confusion, seizures, and **deaths have been reported** with agents which inhibit MAO (serotonin syndrome); this combination should be avoided
Lithium: Concurrent use with a TCA may increase the risk for neurotoxicity
MAO Inhibitors: Hyperpyrexia, hypertension, tachycardia, confusion, seizures, and **deaths have been reported** (serotonin syndrome); this combination should be avoided
Methylphenidate: Metabolism of TCAs may be decreased
Phenothiazines: Serum concentrations of some TCAs may be increased; in addition, TCAs may increase concentration of phenothiazines; monitor for altered clinical response
QTc prolonging agents: Concurrent use of tricyclic agents with other drugs which may prolong QTc interval may increase the risk of potentially fatal arrhythmias; includes type Ia and type III antiarrhythmics agents, selected quinolones (sparfloxacin, gatifloxacin, moxifloxacin, grepafloxacin), cisapride, and other agents
Sucralfate: Absorption of tricyclic antidepressants may be reduced with coadministration
Sympathomimetics, indirect-acting: Tricyclic antidepressants may result in a decreased sensitivity to indirect-acting sympathomimetics; includes dopamine and ephedrine; also see interaction with epinephrine (and direct-acting sympathomimetics)
Valproic acid: May increase serum concentrations/adverse effects of some tricyclic antidepressants
Warfarin (and other oral anticoagulants): TCAs may increase the anticoagulant effect in patients stabilized on warfarin; monitor INR

**Stability** Solutions stable at a pH of 4-5; turns yellowish or reddish on exposure to light. Slight discoloration does not affect potency; marked discoloration is associated with loss of potency. Capsules stable for 3 years following date of manufacture.

**Mechanism of Action** Increases the synaptic concentration of serotonin and/or norepinephrine in the central nervous system by inhibition of their reuptake by the presynaptic neuronal membrane

**Pharmacodynamics/kinetics**
Therapeutic plasma levels: Oral: Occurs within 6 hours
Protein binding: 95%
Metabolism: Undergoes significant first-pass metabolism; metabolized in the liver
Half-life: 20-26 hours
Elimination: In urine

**Usual Dosage** Adults: Oral: 50-150 mg/day as a single bedtime dose up to a maximum of 200 mg/day outpatient and 300 mg/day inpatient

**Dietary Considerations** Alcohol: Avoid use

**Monitoring Parameters** Blood pressure and pulse rate prior to and during initial therapy; evaluate mental status; monitor weight; EKG in older adults

**Reference Range** An oral dose of 50 mg yields a peak serum level of 260 nmol/L

**Test Interactions** ↑ glucose

**Patient Information** Avoid unnecessary exposure to sunlight; avoid alcohol ingestion; do not discontinue medication abruptly; may cause urine to turn blue-green; may cause drowsiness; can use sugarless gum or hard candy for dry mouth; full effect may not occur for 4-6 weeks

**Nursing Implications** May increase appetite; may cause drowsiness, raise bed rails, institute safety precautions

**Additional Information** May cause alterations in bleeding time

**Dosage Forms** Capsule, as maleate: 25 mg, 50 mg, 100 mg


- **Trimipramine Maleate** *see* Trimipramine *on page 570*
- **Trimox®** *see* Amoxicillin *on page 38*
- **Trimpex®** *see* Trimethoprim *on page 570*
- **Trinalin®** *see* Azatadine and Pseudoephedrine *on page 55*
- **Tri-Nasal® Spray** *see* Triamcinolone *on page 563*
- **Tri-Nefrin® Extra Strength Tablet [OTC]** *see* Chlorpheniramine and Phenylpropanolamine *on page 114*
- **Tri-Norinyl®** *see* Ethinyl Estradiol and Norethindrone *on page 212*
- **Triofed® Syrup [OTC]** *see* Triprolidine and Pseudoephedrine *on page 572*
- **Triostat™ Injection** *see* Liothyronine *on page 319*
- **Triotann® Tablet** *see* Chlorpheniramine, Pyrilamine, and Phenylephrine *on page 116*


## Trioxsalen (trye OKS a len)

**U.S. Brand Names** Trisoralen®

**Synonyms** Trimethylpsoralen

**Pharmacologic Category** Psoralen

**Use** In conjunction with controlled exposure to ultraviolet light or sunlight for repigmentation of idiopathic vitiligo; increasing tolerance to sunlight with albinism; enhance pigmentation

**Effects on Mental Status** May cause dizziness, nervousness, insomnia, or depression

**Effects on Psychiatric Treatment** None reported

**Pregnancy Risk Factor** C

**Contraindications** Hypersensitivity to psoralens, melanoma, a history of melanoma, or other diseases associated with photosensitivity; porphyria, acute lupus erythematosus; patients <12 years of age

**Warnings/Precautions** Serious burns from UVA or sunlight can occur if dosage or exposure schedules are exceeded; patients must wear protective eye wear to prevent cataracts; use with caution in patients with severe hepatic or cardiovascular disease

**Adverse Reactions**
>10%:
Dermatologic: Itching
Gastrointestinal: Nausea
1% to 10%:
Central nervous system: Dizziness, headache, mental depression, insomnia, nervousness
Dermatologic: Severe burns from excessive sunlight or ultraviolet exposure

(Continued)

## Trioxsalen *(Continued)*

Gastrointestinal: Gastric discomfort

**Drug Interactions** No data reported

**Usual Dosage** Children >12 years and Adults: Oral: 10 mg/day as a single dose, 2-4 hours before controlled exposure to UVA (for 15-35 minutes) or sunlight; do not continue for longer than 14 days

**Patient Information** This medication is used in conjunction with specific ultraviolet treatment. Follow prescriber's directions exactly for oral medication which can be taken with food or milk to reduce nausea. Avoid use of any other skin treatments unless approved by prescriber. You must wear protective eyewear during treatments. Control exposure to direct sunlight as per prescriber's instructions. If sunlight cannot be avoided, use sunblock (consult prescriber for specific SPF level), wear protective clothing, and wraparound protective eyewear. Consult prescriber immediately if burning, blistering, or skin irritation occur.

**Dosage Forms** Tablet: 5 mg

## Tripelennamine (tri pel EN a meen)

**U.S. Brand Names** PBZ®; PBZ-SR®

**Synonyms** Tripelennamine Citrate; Tripelennamine Hydrochloride

**Pharmacologic Category** Antihistamine

**Use** Perennial and seasonal allergic rhinitis and other allergic symptoms including urticaria

**Effects on Mental Status** Drowsiness is common; may cause nervousness or dizziness; may rarely cause insomnia, depression, or paradoxical excitement

**Effects on Psychiatric Treatment** Concurrent use with psychotropics may produce additive sedation

**Pregnancy Risk Factor** B

**Contraindications** Hypersensitivity to tripelennamine or any component

**Warnings/Precautions** Use with caution in patients with narrow-angle glaucoma, bladder neck obstruction, symptomatic prostate hypertrophy, asthmatic attacks, and stenosing peptic ulcer

**Adverse Reactions**

>10%:
- Central nervous system: Slight to moderate drowsiness
- Respiratory: Thickening of bronchial secretions

1% to 10%:
- Central nervous system: Headache, fatigue, nervousness, dizziness
- Gastrointestinal: Appetite increase, weight gain, nausea, diarrhea, abdominal pain, xerostomia
- Neuromuscular & skeletal: Arthralgia
- Respiratory: Pharyngitis

<1%: Angioedema, blurred vision, bronchospasm, depression, edema, epistaxis, hepatitis, hypotension, insomnia, myalgia, palpitations, paradoxical excitement, paresthesia, photosensitivity, rash, sedation, tremor, urinary retention

**Overdosage/Toxicology**

Signs and symptoms: CNS stimulation or depression; flushed skin, mydriasis, ataxia, athetosis, dry mouth

Treatment: There is no specific treatment for an antihistamine overdose, however, most of its clinical toxicity is due to anticholinergic effects. For anticholinergic overdose with severe life-threatening symptoms, physostigmine 1-2 mg (0.5 or 0.02 mg/kg for children) I.V., slowly may be given to reverse these effects.

**Drug Interactions** Increased effect/toxicity with alcohol, CNS depressants, MAO inhibitors

**Usual Dosage** Oral:

Infants and Children: 5 mg/kg/day in 4-6 divided doses, up to 300 mg/day maximum

Adults: 25-50 mg every 4-6 hours, extended release tablets 100 mg morning and evening up to 100 mg every 8 hours

**Dietary Considerations** Alcohol: Additive CNS effect, avoid use

**Patient Information** Take as directed; do not exceed recommended dose. Avoid use of other depressants, alcohol, or sleep-inducing medications unless approved by prescriber. You may experience drowsiness or dizziness (use caution when driving or engaging in tasks requiring alertness until response to drug is known); or dry mouth, nausea, or abdominal discomfort (frequent small meals, frequent mouth care, chewing gum, or sucking hard candy may help). Report persistent dizziness, sedation, or agitation; chest pain, rapid heartbeat, or palpitations; difficulty breathing; changes in urinary pattern; yellowing of skin or eyes; dark urine or pale stool; or lack of improvement or worsening or condition.

**Nursing Implications** Raise bed rails, institute safety measures, assist with ambulation

**Dosage Forms**

Elixir, as citrate: 37.5 mg/5 mL [equivalent to 25 mg hydrochloride] (473 mL)

Tablet, as hydrochloride: 25 mg, 50 mg

Tablet, extended release, as hydrochloride: 100 mg

♦ **Tripelennamine Citrate** *see* Tripelennamine *on page 572*

♦ **Tripelennamine Hydrochloride** *see* Tripelennamine *on page 572*

♦ **Triphasil®** *see* Ethinyl Estradiol and Levonorgestrel *on page 211*

♦ **Tri-Phen-Chlor®** *see* Chlorpheniramine, Phenyltoloxamine, Phenylpropanolamine, and Phenylephrine *on page 116*

♦ **Triphenyl® Expectorant [OTC]** *see* Guaifenesin and Phenylpropanolamine *on page 257*

♦ **Triphenyl® Syrup [OTC]** *see* Chlorpheniramine and Phenylpropanolamine *on page 114*

♦ **Triple Antibiotic® Topical** *see* Bacitracin, Neomycin, and Polymyxin B *on page 57*

♦ **Triple X® Liquid [OTC]** *see* Pyrethrins *on page 480*

♦ **Triposed® Syrup [OTC]** *see* Triprolidine and Pseudoephedrine *on page 572*

♦ **Triposed® Tablet [OTC]** *see* Triprolidine and Pseudoephedrine *on page 572*

## Triprolidine and Pseudoephedrine

(trye PROE li deen & soo doe e FED rin)

**U.S. Brand Names** Actagen® Syrup [OTC]; Actagen® Tablet [OTC]; Allercon® Tablet [OTC]; Allerfrin® Syrup [OTC]; Allerfrin® Tablet [OTC]; Allerphed Syrup [OTC]; Aprodine® Syrup [OTC]; Aprodine® Tablet [OTC]; Cenafed® Plus Tablet [OTC]; Genac® Tablet [OTC]; Silafed® Syrup [OTC]; Triofed® Syrup [OTC]; Triposed® Syrup [OTC]; Triposed® Tablet [OTC]

**Pharmacologic Category** Alpha/Beta Agonist; Antihistamine

**Use** Temporary relief of nasal congestion, decongest sinus openings, running nose, sneezing, itching of nose or throat and itchy, watery eyes due to common cold, hay fever, or other upper respiratory allergies

**Effects on Mental Status** Drowsiness, nervousness, and insomnia are common; may cause dizziness; may rarely cause depression, hallucinations, or paradoxical excitement

**Effects on Psychiatric Treatment** Contraindicated with MAOIs; concurrent use with psychotropics may produce additive sedation

**Usual Dosage** Oral:

Children:
- Syrup:
  - 4 months to 2 years: 1.25 mL 3-4 times/day
  - 2-4 years: 2.5 mL 3-4 times/day
  - 4-6 years: 3.75 mL 3-4 times/day
  - 6-12 years: 5 mL every 4-6 hours; do not exceed 4 doses in 24 hours
- Tablet: 1/2 every 4-6 hours; do not exceed 4 doses in 24 hours

Children >12 years and Adults:
- Syrup: 10 mL every 4-6 hours; do not exceed 4 doses in 24 hours
- Tablet: 1 every 4-6 hours; do not exceed 4 doses in 24 hours

**Dosage Forms**

Capsule: Triprolidine hydrochloride 2.5 mg and pseudoephedrine hydrochloride 60 mg

Capsule, extended release: Triprolidine hydrochloride 5 mg and pseudoephedrine hydrochloride 120 mg

Syrup: Triprolidine hydrochloride 1.25 mg and pseudoephedrine hydrochloride 30 mg per 5 mL

Tablet: Triprolidine hydrochloride 2.5 mg and pseudoephedrine hydrochloride 60 mg

## Triprolidine, Pseudoephedrine, and Codeine

(trye PROE li deen, soo doe e FED rin, & KOE deen)

**U.S. Brand Names** Actagen-C®; Allerfrin® w/Codeine; Aprodine® w/C; Triacin-C®; Trifed-C®

**Pharmacologic Category** Antihistamine/Decongestant/Antitussive

**Use** Symptomatic relief of cough

**Effects on Mental Status** Drowsiness, nervousness, and insomnia are common; may cause dizziness; may rarely cause depression, hallucinations, or paradoxical excitement

**Effects on Psychiatric Treatment** May see increased toxicity with MAO inhibitors (hypertensive crisis), sympathomimetics, CNS depressants, alcohol (sedation)

**Restrictions** C-V

**Usual Dosage** Oral:

Children:
- 2-6 years: 2.5 mL 4 times/day
- 7-12 years: 5 mL 4 times/day

Children >12 years and Adults: 10 mL 4 times/day

**Dosage Forms** Syrup: Triprolidine hydrochloride 1.25 mg, pseudoephedrine hydrochloride 30 mg, and codeine phosphate 10 mg per 5 mL with alcohol 4.3%

♦ **TripTone® Caplets® [OTC]** *see* Dimenhydrinate *on page 173*

## Triptorelin (trip toe REL in)

**U.S. Brand Names** Trelstar™ Depot

**Pharmacologic Category** Luteinizing Hormone-Releasing Hormone Analog

**Use** Palliative treatment of advanced prostate cancer as an alternative to orchiectomy or estrogen administration

**Effects on Mental Status** May cause insomnia, fatigue, emotional lability, or dizziness

**Effects on Psychiatric Treatment** Contraindicated with dopamine antagonists

**Usual Dosage** I.M.: Adults: 3.75 mg once monthly

**Dosage adjustment in renal impairment:** No specific recommendations are made

**Dosage adjustment in hepatic impairment:** No specific recommendations are made

**Dosage Forms** Powder for injection, depot: 3.75 mg


♦ **Trisoralen®** *see* Trioxsalen *on page 571*

♦ **Tri-Statin® II Topical** *see* Nystatin and Triamcinolone *on page 402*

♦ **Tristoject®** *see* Triamcinolone *on page 563*

♦ **Tri-Tannate Plus®** *see* Chlorpheniramine, Ephedrine, Phenylephrine, and Carbetapentane *on page 115*

♦ **Tri-Tannate® Tablet** *see* Chlorpheniramine, Pyrilamine, and Phenylephrine *on page 116*

♦ **Tritec®** *see* Ranitidine Bismuth Citrate *on page 488*

♦ **Trobicin®** *see* Spectinomycin *on page 517*

♦ **Trocaine® [OTC]** *see* Benzocaine *on page 61*

♦ **Trocal® [OTC]** *see* Dextromethorphan *on page 160*


## Troglitazone (TROE gli to zone)

**U.S. Brand Names** Rezulin®

**Synonyms** CS-045

**Pharmacologic Category** Antidiabetic Agent (Thiazolidinedione)

**Use** Troglitazone is indicated for the following:

To improve glycemic control in patients with type 2 diabetes mellitus as an adjunct to diet and exercise in combination (and not substituted for):

- sulfonylureas in patients who are not adequately controlled with a sulfonylurea alone, or
- a sulfonylurea together with metformin for patients who are not adequately controlled with the combination of a sulfonylurea and metformin or
- insulin in patients who are not adequately controlled with insulin alone

Troglitazone is not indicated as initial therapy or monotherapy in patients with type 2 diabetes

**Effects on Mental Status** May cause dizziness

**Effects on Psychiatric Treatment** None reported

**Pregnancy Risk Factor** B

**Contraindications** Hypersensitivity to troglitazone or any component

**Warnings/Precautions** Patients with New York Heart Association (NYHA) Class III and IV cardiac status were not studied during clinical trials. Heart enlargement without microscopic changes has been observed in rodents at exposures exceeding 14 times the AUC of the 400 mg human dose. Caution is advised during the administration of troglitazone to patients with NYHA Class III or IV cardiac status.

Because of rare cases of severe hepatotoxicity that have occurred in patients treated with Rezulin®, the manufacturer and the FDA have agreed that troglitazone will not be indicated as initial single-agent therapy in patients with type 2 diabetes mellitus. A total of 150 adverse event reports postmarketing have been reported to the FDA including 3 deaths from liver failure linked to the use of troglitazone. Approximately 600,000 patients in the U.S. and 200,000 patients in Japan have been treated with troglitazone.

Patients on troglitazone who develop jaundice or whose laboratory results indicate liver injury should stop taking the drug. Approximately 2% of patients can expect to stop taking the drug because of elevated liver enzymes.

Because of its mechanism of action, troglitazone is active only in the presence of insulin. Therefore, do not use in type 1 diabetes or for the treatment of diabetic ketoacidosis.

Patients receiving troglitazone in combination with insulin may be at risk for hypoglycemia, and a reduction in the dose of insulin may be necessary.

Across all clinical studies, hemoglobin declined by 3% to 4% in troglitazone-treated patients compared with 1% to 2% with placebo. White blood cell counts also declined slightly in troglitazone-treated patients compared with those treated with placebo. These changes occurred within the first 4-8 weeks of therapy. Levels stabilized and remained unchanged for ≤2 years of continuing therapy. These changes may be due to the dilutional effects of increased plasma volume and have not been associated with any significant hematologic clinical effects. **The FDA, in conjunction with the manufacturer of Rezulin® (troglitazone) has elected to withdraw Rezulin® (troglitazone) from the market. The FDA based its decision on a review of recent safety data concerning Rezulin® and two similar drugs, rosiglitazone (Avandia®) and pioglitazone (Actos™). This review demonstrated that Rezulin is associated with more hepatotoxicity than the other two drugs. Both Avandia® and Actos™, approved in the past year, appear to offer the same benefits as Rezulin® without the same risk.**

**Adverse Reactions**

>10%:

Central nervous system: Headache, pain

Miscellaneous: Infection

1% to 10%:

Cardiovascular: Peripheral edema

Central nervous system: Dizziness

Gastrointestinal: Nausea, diarrhea, pharyngitis

Genitourinary: Urinary tract infection

Neuromuscular & skeletal: Neck pain, weakness

Respiratory: Rhinitis

**Drug Interactions** CYP3A3/4 enzyme substrate; CYP3A3/4 enzyme inducer; CYP2C9, 2C19, and 3A3/4 enzyme inhibitor

Decreased effects:

Cholestyramine: Concomitant administration of cholestyramine with troglitazone reduces the absorption of troglitazone by 70%; COADMINISTRATION OF CHOLESTYRAMINE AND TROGLITAZONE IS NOT RECOMMENDED.

Oral contraceptives: Administration of troglitazone with an oral contraceptive containing ethinyl estradiol and norethindrone reduced the plasma concentrations of both by 30%. These changes could result in loss of contraception.

Terfenadine: Coadministration of troglitazone with terfenadine decreases plasma concentrations of terfenadine and its active metabolite by 50% to 70% and may reduce the effectiveness of terfenadine

Increased toxicity:

Sulfonylureas (glyburide): Coadministration of troglitazone with glyburide may further decrease plasma glucose levels

**Usual Dosage** Oral (take with meals):

Adults:

Combination therapy with insulin: Continue the current insulin dose upon initiation of troglitazone therapy

Initiate therapy at 200 mg once daily in patients on insulin therapy. For patients not responding adequately, increase the dose after 2-4 weeks. The usual dose is 400 mg/day; maximum recommended dose: 600 mg/day.

It is recommended that the insulin dose be decreased by 10% to 25% when fasting plasma glucose concentrations decrease to <120 mg/dL in patients receiving concomitant insulin and troglitazone. Individualize further adjustments based on glucose-lowering response.

Combination therapy with metformin and sulfonylureas: 400 mg once daily

Elderly: Steady-state pharmacokinetics of troglitazone and metabolites in healthy elderly subjects were comparable to those seen in young adults

**Dosing adjustment/comments in renal impairment:** Dose adjustment is not necessary

**Dosing adjustment in hepatic impairment:** Troglitazone should **not** be initiated if the patient exhibits clinical evidence of active liver disease or increased serum transaminase levels (ALT >1.5 times the upper limit of normal).

**Patient Information** Take with meals. Follow directions of prescriber. If dose is missed at the usual meal, take it with next meal. Do not double dose if daily dose is missed completely. Monitor urine or serum glucose as recommended by prescriber. More frequent monitoring is required during periods of stress, trauma, surgery, pregnancy, increased activity or exercise. Avoid alcohol. Report chest pain, rapid heartbeat or palpitations, abdominal pain, fever, rash, hypoglycemia reactions, yellowing of skin or eyes, dark urine or light stool, or unusual fatigue or nausea/vomiting.

**Nursing Implications** Patients who are NPO may need to have their dose held to avoid hypoglycemia

**Dosage Forms** Tablet: 200 mg, 400 mg

## Troleandomycin (troe lee an doe MYE sin)

**U.S. Brand Names** Tao®

**Synonyms** Triacetyloleandomycin

**Pharmacologic Category** Antibiotic, Macrolide

**Use** Adjunct in the treatment of corticosteroid-dependent asthma due to its steroid-sparing properties; antibiotic with spectrum of activity similar to erythromycin

**Effects on Mental Status** Macrolides reported to cause nightmares, confusion, anxiety, or mood lability

**Effects on Psychiatric Treatment** Contraindicated with pimozide; concurrent use with carbamazepine or triazolam may produce additive toxicity; monitor

**Pregnancy Risk Factor** C

**Contraindications** Hypersensitivity to troleandomycin, other macrolides, or any component; concurrent use with cisapride

(Continued)

## Troleandomycin *(Continued)*

**Warnings/Precautions** Use with caution in patients with impaired hepatic function; chronic hepatitis may occur in patients with long or repetitive courses

**Adverse Reactions**

>10%: Gastrointestinal: Abdominal cramping and discomfort (dose-related)

1% to 10%:

Dermatologic: Urticaria, rashes

Gastrointestinal: Nausea, vomiting, diarrhea

<1%: Cholestatic jaundice, rectal burning

**Overdosage/Toxicology**

Signs and symptoms: Nausea, vomiting, diarrhea, hearing loss

Treatment: Following GI decontamination, treatment is supportive

**Drug Interactions** CYP3A3/4 enzyme substrate; CYP3A3/4 and 3A5-7 enzyme inhibitor

Increased effect/toxicity/levels of carbamazepine, ergot alkaloids, methylprednisolone, oral contraceptives, theophylline, and triazolam; contraindicated with terfenadine, astemizole, cisapride, and pimozide due to decreased metabolism of this agent and resultant risk of cardiac arrhythmias and death

**Usual Dosage** Oral:

Children 7-13 years: 25-40 mg/kg/day divided every 6 hours (125-250 mg every 6 hours)

Adjunct in corticosteroid-dependent asthma: 14 mg/kg/day in divided doses every 6-12 hours not to exceed 250 mg every 6 hours; dose is tapered to once daily then alternate day dosing

Adults: 250-500 mg 4 times/day

**Patient Information** Complete full course of therapy; notify physician if persistent or severe abdominal pain, nausea, vomiting, jaundice, darkened urine, or fever occurs

**Dosage Forms** Capsule: 250 mg

## Tromethamine (troe METH a meen)

**U.S. Brand Names** THAM-E® Injection; THAM® Injection

**Pharmacologic Category** Alkalinizing Agent

**Use** Correction of metabolic acidosis associated with cardiac bypass surgery or cardiac arrest; to correct excess acidity of stored blood that is preserved with acid citrate dextrose; to prime the pump-oxygenator during cardiac bypass surgery; indicated in infants needing alkalinization after receiving maximum sodium bicarbonate (8-10 mEq/kg/24 hours); (advantage of Tham® is that it alkalinizes without increasing $pCO_2$ and sodium)

**Effects on Mental Status** None reported

**Effects on Psychiatric Treatment** None reported

**Usual Dosage** Dose depends on buffer base deficit; when deficit is known: tromethamine (mL of 0.3 M solution) = body weight (kg) x base deficit (mEq/L); when base deficit is not known: 3-6 mL/kg/dose I.V. (1-2 mEq/kg/dose)

Metabolic acidosis with cardiac arrest:

I.V.: 3.5-6 mL/kg (1-2 mEq/kg/dose) into large peripheral vein; 500-1000 mL if needed in adults

I.V. continuous drip: Infuse slowly by syringe pump over 3-6 hours

Acidosis associated with cardiac bypass surgery: Average dose: 9 mL/kg (2.7 mEq/kg); 500 mL is adequate for most adults; maximum dose: 500 mg/kg in ≤1 hour

Excess acidity of acid citrate dextrose priming blood: 14-70 mL of 0.3 molar solution added to each 500 mL of blood

**Dosing comments in renal impairment:** Use with caution and monitor for hyperkalemia and EKG

**Dosage Forms** Injection:

THAM®: 18 g [0.3 molar] (500 mL)

THAM-E®: 36 g with sodium 30 mEq, potassium 5 mEq, and chloride 35 mEq (1000 mL)

♦ **Tronolane® [OTC]** *see* Pramoxine *on page 457*

♦ **Tropicacyl®** *see* Tropicamide *on page 574*

## Tropicamide (troe PIK a mide)

**U.S. Brand Names** Mydriacyl®; Opticyl®; Tropicacyl®

**Canadian Brand Names** Diotrope

**Pharmacologic Category** Ophthalmic Agent, Mydriatic

**Use** Short-acting mydriatic used in diagnostic procedures; as well as preoperatively and postoperatively; treatment of some cases of acute iritis, iridocyclitis, and keratitis

**Effects on Mental Status** May cause drowsiness

**Effects on Psychiatric Treatment** None reported

**Usual Dosage** Children and Adults (individuals with heavily pigmented eyes may require larger doses):

Cycloplegia: Instill 1-2 drops (1%); may repeat in 5 minutes

Exam must be performed within 30 minutes after the repeat dose; if the patient is not examined within 20-30 minutes, instill an additional drop

Mydriasis: Instill 1-2 drops (0.5%) 15-20 minutes before exam; may repeat every 30 minutes as needed

**Dosage Forms** Solution, ophthalmic: 0.5% (2 mL, 15 mL); 1% (2 mL, 3 mL, 15 mL)

## Trovafloxacin (TROE va flox a sin)

**U.S. Brand Names** Trovan™

**Synonyms** CP-99,219-27; Trovafloxacin Mesylate

**Pharmacologic Category** Antibiotic, Quinolone

**Use Should be used only in life- or limb-threatening infections**

Treatment of nosocomial pneumonia, community-acquired pneumonia, complicated intra-abdominal infections, gynecologic/pelvic infections, complicated skin and skin structure infections

**Effects on Mental Status** May cause dizziness; quinolones reported to cause restlessness, hallucinations, euphoria, depression, panic, and paranoia

**Effects on Psychiatric Treatment** None reported

**Pregnancy Risk Factor** C

**Contraindications** History of hypersensitivity to trovafloxacin, alatrofloxacin, quinolone antimicrobial agents or any other components of these products

**Warnings/Precautions** For use only in serious life- or limb-threatening infections. Initiation of therapy must occur in an inpatient healthcare facility. May alter GI flora resulting in pseudomembranous colitis due to *Clostridium difficile*; use with caution in patients with seizure disorders or severe cerebral atherosclerosis; discontinue if skin rash or pain, inflammation, or rupture of a tendon; photosensitivity; CNS stimulation may occur which may lead to tremor, restlessness, confusion, hallucinations, paranoia, depression, nightmares, insomnia, or lightheadedness. Hepatic reactions have resulted in death. Risk of hepatotoxicity is increased if therapy exceeds 14 days.

**Adverse Reactions Note:** Fatalities have occurred in patients developing hepatic necrosis

<10%:

Central nervous system: Dizziness, lightheadedness, headache

Dermatologic: Rash, pruritus

Gastrointestinal: Nausea, vomiting, diarrhea, abdominal pain

Genitourinary: Vaginitis

Hepatic: Increased LFTs

Local: Injection site reaction, pain, or inflammation

<1%: Anaphylaxis, hepatic necrosis, pancreatitis, Stevens-Johnson syndrome

**Overdosage/Toxicology** Treatment: Empty the stomach by vomiting or gastric lavage. Observe carefully and give symptomatic and supportive treatment; maintain adequate hydration.

**Drug Interactions** Decreased effect of oral trovafloxacin:

Antacids containing magnesium or aluminum, sucralfate, citric acid buffered with sodium citrate, and metal cations: Administer oral trovafloxacin doses at least 2 hours before or 2 hours after

Morphine: Administer I.V. morphine at least 2 hours after oral trovafloxacin in the fasting state and at least 4 hours after oral trovafloxacin when taken with food

**Usual Dosage** Adults:

Nosocomial pneumonia: I.V.: 300 mg single dose followed by 200 mg/day orally for a total duration of 10-14 days

Community-acquired pneumonia: Oral, I.V.: 200 mg/day for 7-14 days

Complicated intra-abdominal infections, including postsurgical infections/gynecologic and pelvic infections: I.V.: 300 mg as a single dose followed by 200 mg/day orally for a total duration of 7-14 days

Skin and skin structure infections, complicated, including diabetic foot infections: Oral, I.V.: 200 mg/day for 10-14 days

**Dosage adjustment in renal impairment:** No adjustment is necessary

**Dosage adjustment for hemodialysis:** None required; trovafloxacin not sufficiently removed by hemodialysis

**Dosage adjustment in hepatic impairment:**

Mild to moderate cirrhosis:

Initial dose for normal hepatic function: 300 mg I.V.; 200 mg I.V. or oral; 100 mg oral

Reduced dose: 200 mg I.V.; 100 mg I.V. or oral; 100 mg oral

Severe cirrhosis: No data available

**Dietary Considerations** Dairy products such as milk and yogurt reduce the absorption of oral trovafloxacin - avoid concurrent use. The bioavailability may also be decreased by enteral feedings.

**Patient Information** Take per recommended schedule; complete full course of therapy and do not skip doses. Take on an empty stomach (1 hour before or 2 hours after meals, dairy products, antacids, or other medication). Dizziness may be reduced if taken at bedtime with food. Maintain adequate hydration (2-3 L/day of fluids unless instructed to restrict fluid intake). You may experience dizziness or lightheadedness (use caution when driving or engaging in tasks that require alertness until response to drug is known); nausea or GI upset (small frequent meals, frequent mouth care, sucking lozenges, or chewing gum may help). Report CNS disturbances (hallucinations, gait disturbances); chest pain or palpitations; persistent GI disturbances; signs of opportunistic infection (sore throat, chills, fever, burning, itching on urination, vaginal discharge, white plaques in mouth); tendon pain, swelling, or redness; difficulty breathing, or worsening of condition.

**Dosage Forms**

Injection, as mesylate (alatrofloxacin): 5 mg/mL (40 mL, 60 mL)
Tablet, as mesylate (trovafloxacin): 100 mg, 200 mg

## Trovafloxacin/Azithromycin Compliance Pak

(TROE va flox a sin/az ith roe MYE sin com PLY ance pak)

**U.S. Brand Names** Trovan™/Zithromax™ Compliance Pack
**Pharmacologic Category** Antibiotic, Oxazolidinone; Antibiotic, Macrolide; Antibiotic, Quinolone
**Effects on Mental Status** May cause dizziness; quinolones reported to cause restlessness, hallucinations, euphoria, depression, panic, and paranoia; macrolides have been reported to cause nightmares, confusion, anxiety, and mood lability
**Effects on Psychiatric Treatment** Contraindicated with pimozide; may increase concentration of bromocriptine, carbamazepine and triazolam
**Dosage Forms** Compliance Pak: Oral suspension (Zithromax™) 1 g and tablet (Trovan™) 100 mg


- **Trovafloxacin Mesylate** *see* Trovafloxacin *on page 574*
- **Trovan™** *see* Trovafloxacin *on page 574*
- **Trovan™/Zithromax™ Compliance Pack** *see* Trovafloxacin/Azithromycin Compliance Pak *on page 575*
- **Troxidone** *see* Trimethadione *on page 569*
- **Truphylline®** *see* Theophylline Salts *on page 539*
- **Trusopt®** *see* Dorzolamide *on page 182*
- **Trysul®** *see* Sulfabenzamide, Sulfacetamide, and Sulfathiazole *on page 522*
- **TST** *see* Tuberculin Purified Protein Derivative *on page 575*
- **T-Stat® Topical** *see* Erythromycin, Ophthalmic/Topical *on page 202*


## Tuberculin Purified Protein Derivative

(too BER kyoo lin PURE eh fide PRO teen dah RIV ah tiv)

**U.S. Brand Names** Aplisol®; Aplitest®; Tine Test PPD; Tubersol®
**Synonyms** Mantoux; PPD; Tine Test; TST; Tuberculin Skin Test
**Pharmacologic Category** Diagnostic Agent, Skin Test
**Use** Skin test in diagnosis of tuberculosis, cell-mediated immunodeficiencies
**Effects on Mental Status** None reported
**Effects on Psychiatric Treatment** None reported
**Pregnancy Risk Factor** C
**Contraindications** 250 TU strength should not be used for initial testing
**Warnings/Precautions** Do not administer I.V. or S.C.; epinephrine (1:1000) should be available to treat possible allergic reactions
**Adverse Reactions** 1% to 10%:

Dermatologic: Ulceration, necrosis, vesiculation
Local: Pain at injection site

**Drug Interactions** Decreased effect: Reaction may be suppressed in patients receiving systemic corticosteroids, aminocaproic acid, or within 4-6 weeks following immunization with live or inactivated viral vaccines
**Usual Dosage** Children and Adults: Intradermal: 0.1 mL about 4" below elbow; use 1/4" to 1/2" or 26- or 27-gauge needle; significant reactions are ≥5 mm in diameter

Interpretation of induration of tuberculin skin test injections: Positive: ≥10 mm; inconclusive: 5-9 mm; negative: <5 mm

Interpretation of induration of Tine test injections: Positive: >2 mm and vesiculation present; inconclusive: <2 mm (give patient Mantoux test of 5 TU/0.1 mL - base decisions on results of Mantoux test); negative: <2 mm or erythema of any size (no need for retesting unless person is a contact of a patient with tuberculosis or there is clinical evidence suggestive of the disease)

**Patient Information** Return to physician for reaction interpretation at 48-72 hours
**Nursing Implications** Test dose: 0.1 mL intracutaneously; store in refrigerator; examine site at 48-72 hours after administration; whenever tuberculin is administered, a record should be made of the administration technique (Mantoux method, disposable multiple-puncture device), tuberculin used (OT or PPD), manufacturer and lot number of tuberculin used, date of administration, date of test reading, and the size of the reaction in millimeters (mm).
**Dosage Forms** Injection:

First test strength: 1 TU/0.1 mL (1 mL)
Intermediate test strength: 5 TU/0.1 mL (1 mL, 5 mL, 10 mL)
Second test strength: 250 TU/0.1 mL (1 mL)
Tine: 5 TU each test


- **Tuberculin Skin Test** *see* Tuberculin Purified Protein Derivative *on page 575*
- **Tubersol®** *see* Tuberculin Purified Protein Derivative *on page 575*


## Tubocurarine (too boe kyoor AR een)

**Pharmacologic Category** Neuromuscular Blocker Agent, Nondepolarizing; Skeletal Muscle Relaxant
**Use** Adjunct to anesthesia to induce skeletal muscle relaxation
**Effects on Mental Status** None reported
**Effects on Psychiatric Treatment** None reported
**Usual Dosage** I.V.:

Children and Adults: 0.2-0.4 mg/kg as a single dose; maintenance: 0.04-0.2 mg/kg/dose as needed to maintain paralysis

Alternative adult dose: 6-9 mg once daily, then 3-4.5 mg as needed to maintain paralysis

**Dosing adjustment/comments in renal impairment:** May accumulate with multiple doses and reductions in subsequent doses is recommended

$Cl_{cr}$ 50-80 mL/minute: Administer 75% of normal dose
$Cl_{cr}$ 10-50 mL/minute: Administer 50% of normal dose
$Cl_{cr}$ <10 mL/minute: Avoid use

**Dosing comments in hepatic impairment:** Larger doses may be necessary

**Dosage Forms** Injection, as chloride: 3 mg/mL [3 units/mL] (5 mL, 10 mL, 20 mL)


- **Tuinal®** *see* Amobarbital and Secobarbital *on page 36*
- **Tumeric Root** *see* Golden Seal *on page 254*
- **Tums® [OTC]** *see* Calcium Carbonate *on page 84*
- **Tums® E-X Extra Strength Tablet [OTC]** *see* Calcium Carbonate *on page 84*
- **Tums® Extra Strength Liquid [OTC]** *see* Calcium Carbonate *on page 84*
- **Tusibron® [OTC]** *see* Guaifenesin *on page 256*
- **Tusibron-DM® [OTC]** *see* Guaifenesin and Dextromethorphan *on page 257*
- **Tussafed®** *see* Carbinoxamine *on page 92*
- **Tussafed® Drops** *see* Carbinoxamine, Pseudoephedrine, and Dextromethorphan *on page 92*
- **Tussafin® Expectorant** *see* Hydrocodone, Pseudoephedrine, and Guaifenesin *on page 273*
- **Tuss-Allergine® Modified T.D. Capsule** *see* Caramiphen and Phenylpropanolamine *on page 90*
- **Tussar® SF Syrup** *see* Guaifenesin, Pseudoephedrine, and Codeine *on page 258*
- **Tuss-DM® [OTC]** *see* Guaifenesin and Dextromethorphan *on page 257*
- **Tuss-Genade® Modified Capsule** *see* Caramiphen and Phenylpropanolamine *on page 90*
- **Tussigon®** *see* Hydrocodone and Homatropine *on page 273*
- **Tussionex®** *see* Hydrocodone and Chlorpheniramine *on page 272*
- **Tussi-Organidin® DM NR** *see* Guaifenesin and Dextromethorphan *on page 257*
- **Tussi-Organidin® NR** *see* Guaifenesin and Codeine *on page 256*
- **Tuss-LA®** *see* Guaifenesin and Pseudoephedrine *on page 257*
- **Tussogest® Extended Release Capsule** *see* Caramiphen and Phenylpropanolamine *on page 90*
- **Tusstat® Syrup** *see* Diphenhydramine *on page 174*
- **Twice-A-Day® Nasal [OTC]** *see* Oxymetazoline *on page 415*
- **Twilite® Oral [OTC]** *see* Diphenhydramine *on page 174*
- **Twin-K®** *see* Potassium Citrate and Potassium Gluconate *on page 454*
- **Two-Dyne®** *see* Butalbital Compound and Acetaminophen *on page 80*
- **Tylenol® [OTC]** *see* Acetaminophen *on page 14*
- **Tylenol® Cold Effervescent Medication Tablet [OTC]** *see* Chlorpheniramine, Phenylpropanolamine, and Acetaminophen *on page 116*
- **Tylenol® Cold No Drowsiness [OTC]** *see* Acetaminophen, Dextromethorphan, and Pseudoephedrine *on page 16*
- **Tylenol® Extended Relief [OTC]** *see* Acetaminophen *on page 14*
- **Tylenol® Flu Maximum Strength [OTC]** *see* Acetaminophen, Dextromethorphan, and Pseudoephedrine *on page 16*
- **Tylenol® Sinus, Maximum Strength [OTC]** *see* Acetaminophen and Pseudoephedrine *on page 15*

## Uracil Mustard (YOOR a sil MUS tard)

**Pharmacologic Category** Antineoplastic Agent, Alkylating Agent

**Use** Palliative treatment in symptomatic chronic lymphocytic leukemia; non-Hodgkin's lymphomas, chronic myelocytic leukemia, mycosis fungoides, thrombocytosis, polycythemia vera, ovarian carcinoma

**Effects on Mental Status** May cause nervousness or depression

**Effects on Psychiatric Treatment** Myelosuppression is common; avoid clozapine and carbamazepine

**Pregnancy Risk Factor** X

**Contraindications** Severe leukopenia, thrombocytopenia, aplastic anemia; in patients whose bone marrow is infiltrated with malignant cells; hypersensitivity to any component; pregnancy

**Warnings/Precautions** The U.S. Food and Drug Administration (FDA) currently recommends that procedures for proper handling and disposal of antineoplastic agents be considered. Impaired kidney or liver function. The drug should be discontinued if intractable vomiting or diarrhea, precipitous falls in leukocyte or platelet count, or myocardial ischemia occurs. Use with caution in patients who have had high-dose pelvic radiation or previous use of alkylating agents. Patient should be hospitalized during initial course of therapy; may impair fertility in men and women; use with caution in patients with pre-existing marrow suppression.

**Adverse Reactions**

>10%:
- Gastrointestinal: Nausea, vomiting, diarrhea
- Hematologic: Myelosuppressive; leukopenia and thrombocytopenia nadir: 2-4 weeks, anemia

1% to 10%:
- Central nervous system: Mental depression, nervousness
- Dermatologic: Hyperpigmentation, alopecia
- Endocrine & metabolic: Hyperuricemia

<1%: Hepatotoxicity, pruritus, stomatitis

**Overdosage/Toxicology**
- Signs and symptoms: Diarrhea, vomiting, severe marrow suppression
- Treatment: No specific antidote to marrow toxicity is available

**Usual Dosage** Oral (do not administer until 2-3 weeks after maximum effect of any previous x-ray or cytotoxic drug therapy of the bone marrow is obtained):
- Children: 0.3 mg/kg in a single weekly dose for 4 weeks
- Adults: 0.15 mg/kg in a single weekly dose for 4 weeks
  - Thrombocytosis: 1-2 mg/day for 14 days

**Patient Information** This drug may take weeks or months for effectiveness to become apparent. Do not discontinue without consulting prescriber. Maintain adequate hydration (2-3 L/day of fluids unless instructed to restrict fluid intake). For nausea or vomiting, loss of appetite, or dry mouth, small frequent meals, chewing gum, or sucking lozenges may help. You may experience hair loss (reversible); diarrhea (if persistent, consult prescriber); nervousness, irritability, shakiness, amenorrhea, altered sperm production (usually reversible). Report persistent nausea or vomiting, fever, sore throat, chills, unusual bleeding or bruising, consistent feelings of tiredness or weakness, or yellowing of skin or eyes.

**Dosage Forms** Capsule: 1 mg

## Urea (yoor EE a)

**U.S. Brand Names** Amino-Cerv™ Vaginal Cream; Aquacare® Topical [OTC]; Carmol® Topical [OTC]; Gormel® Creme [OTC]; Lanaphilic® Topical [OTC]; Nutraplus® Topical [OTC]; Rea-Lo® [OTC]; Ultra Mide® Topical; Ureacin®-20 Topical [OTC]; Ureaphil® Injection

**Canadian Brand Names** Onyvul®; Uremol™; Urisec®; Velvelan®

**Synonyms** Carbamide

**Pharmacologic Category** Diuretic, Osmotic; Keratolytic Agent; Topical Skin Product

**Use** Reduces intracranial pressure and intraocular pressure; topically promotes hydration and removal of excess keratin in hyperkeratotic conditions and dry skin; mild cervicitis

**Effects on Mental Status** None reported

**Effects on Psychiatric Treatment** May decrease serum lithium levels but overall effect is minimal; do not use for lithium toxicity/overdose; if overdose is associated with severe clinical manifestations, dialysis is the treatment of choice

**Pregnancy Risk Factor** C

**Contraindications** Severely impaired renal function, hepatic failure; active intracranial bleeding, sickle cell anemia, topical use in viral skin disease

**Warnings/Precautions** Urea should not be used near the eyes; use with caution if applied to face, broken, or inflamed skin; use with caution in patients with mild hepatic or renal impairment

**Adverse Reactions** 1% to 10%:
- Central nervous system: Headache
- Endocrine & metabolic: Electrolyte imbalance
- Gastrointestinal: Nausea, vomiting
- Local: Transient stinging, local irritation, tissue necrosis from extravasation of I.V. preparation

**Overdosage/Toxicology**
- Signs and symptoms: Increased BUN, decreased renal function
- Treatment: Supportive

**Drug Interactions** Decreased effect/toxicity/levels of lithium

**Usual Dosage**
- Children: I.V. slow infusion:
  - ≤2 years: 0.1-0.5 g/kg
  - >2 years: 0.5-1.5 g/kg
- Adults:
  - I.V. infusion: 1-1.5 g/kg by slow infusion (1-2½ hours); maximum: 120 g/24 hours
  - Topical: Apply 1-3 times/day
  - Vaginal: Insert 1 applicatorful in vagina at bedtime for 2-4 weeks

**Patient Information**

Topical: For external use only. Best effect is obtained when applied to skin while still wet or moist after washing or bathing. Do not apply to broken, inflamed, or infected skin. Do not use near eyes. Report skin redness, irritation, or worsening of condition.

Vaginal: Wash hands before using. Insert full applicator into vagina gently and expel cream at bedtime. Wash applicator with soap and water following use. Remain lying down for 30 minutes following administration. Report if condition worsens or does not improve.

**Nursing Implications** Do not infuse into leg veins; injection dosage form may be used orally, mix with carbonated beverages, jelly or jam, to mask unpleasant flavor

**Dosage Forms**
- Cream:
  - Topical: 2% [20 mg/mL] (75 g); 10% [100 mg/mL] (75 g, 90 g, 454 g); 20% [200 mg/mL] (45 g, 75 g, 90 g, 454 g); 30% [300 mg/mL] (60 g, 454 g); 40% (30 g)
  - Vaginal: 8.34% [83.4 mg/g] (82.5 g)
- Injection: 40 g/150 mL

Lotion: 2% (240 mL); 10% (180 mL, 240 mL, 480 mL); 15% (120 mL, 480 mL); 25% (180 mL)

- **Ureacin®-20 Topical [OTC]** *see* Urea *on page 576*
- **Ureaphil® Injection** *see* Urea *on page 576*
- **Urecholine®** *see* Bethanechol *on page 67*
- **Urex®** *see* Methenamine *on page 351*
- **Urispas®** *see* Flavoxate *on page 226*
- **Urobak®** *see* Sulfamethoxazole *on page 524*
- **Urodine®** *see* Phenazopyridine *on page 433*
- **Urogesic®** *see* Phenazopyridine *on page 433*

## Urokinase (yoor oh KIN ase)

**U.S. Brand Names** Abbokinase® Injection

**Pharmacologic Category** Thrombolytic Agent

**Use** Thrombolytic agent used in treatment of recent severe or massive deep vein thrombosis, pulmonary emboli, myocardial infarction, and occluded I.V. or dialysis cannulas; more expensive than streptokinase; not useful on thrombi over 1 week old

**Effects on Mental Status** None reported

**Effects on Psychiatric Treatment** None reported

**Usual Dosage**

Children and Adults: Deep vein thrombosis: I.V.: Loading: 4400 units/kg over 10 minutes, then 4400 units/kg/hour for 12 hours

Adults:

Myocardial infarction: Intracoronary: 750,000 units over 2 hours (6000 units/minute over up to 2 hours)

Occluded I.V. catheters:

5000 units (use only Abbokinase® Open Cath) in each lumen over 1-2 minutes, leave in lumen for 1-4 hours, then aspirate; may repeat with 10,000 units in each lumen if 5000 units fails to clear the catheter; **do not infuse into the patient**; volume to instill into catheter is equal to the volume of the catheter

I.V. infusion: 200 units/kg/hour in each lumen for 12-48 hours at a rate of at least 20 mL/hour

Dialysis patients: 5000 units is administered in each lumen over 1-2 minutes; leave urokinase in lumen for 1-2 days, then aspirate

Clot lysis (large vessel thrombi): Loading: I.V.: 4400 units/kg over 10 minutes, increase to 6000 units/kg/hour; maintenance: 4400-6000 units/kg/hour adjusted to achieve clot lysis or patency of affected vessel; doses up to 50,000 units/kg/hour have been used. **Note:** Therapy should be initiated as soon as possible after diagnosis of thrombi and continued until clot is dissolved (usually 24-72 hours).

Acute pulmonary embolism: Three treatment alternatives: 3 million unit dosage

Alternative 1: 12-hour infusion: 4400 units/kg (2000 units/lb) bolus over 10 minutes followed by 4400 units/kg/hour (2000 units/lb); begin heparin 1000 units/hour approximately 3-4 hours after completion of urokinase infusion or when PTT is <100 seconds

Alternative 2: 2-hour infusion: 1 million unit bolus over 10 minutes followed by 2 million units over 110 minutes; begin heparin 1000 units/hour approximately 3-4 hours after completion of urokinase infusion or when PTT is <100 seconds

Alternative 3: Bolus dose only: 15,000 units/kg over 10 minutes; begin heparin 1000 units/hour approximately 3-4 hours after completion of urokinase infusion or when PTT is <100 seconds

**Dosage Forms**

Powder for injection: 250,000 units (5 mL)

Powder for injection, catheter clear: 5000 units (1 mL)

- **Uro-KP-Neutral®** *see* Potassium Phosphate and Sodium Phosphate *on page 456*
- **Ursodeoxycholic Acid** *see* Ursodiol *on page 577*

## Ursodiol (ER soe dye ole)

**U.S. Brand Names** Actigall™

**Synonyms** Ursodeoxycholic Acid

**Pharmacologic Category** Gallstone Dissolution Agent

**Use** Gallbladder stone dissolution

**Effects on Mental Status** May cause drowsiness

**Effects on Psychiatric Treatment** None reported

**Pregnancy Risk Factor** B

**Contraindications** Not to be used with cholesterol, radiopaque, bile pigment stones, or stones >20 mm in diameter; allergy to bile acids

**Warnings/Precautions** Gallbladder stone dissolution may take several months of therapy; complete dissolution may not occur and recurrence of stones within 5 years has been observed in 50% of patients; use with caution in patients with a nonvisualizing gallbladder and those with chronic liver disease; not recommended for children

**Adverse Reactions**

1% to 10%: Gastrointestinal: Diarrhea

<1%: Abdominal pain, biliary pain, constipation, dyspepsia, fatigue, headache, metallic taste, nausea, pruritus, rash, vomiting

**Overdosage/Toxicology**

Signs and symptoms: Diarrhea

Treatment: No specific therapy for diarrhea and for overdose

**Drug Interactions** Decreased effect with aluminum-containing antacids, cholestyramine, colestipol, clofibrate, oral contraceptives (estrogens)

**Usual Dosage** Adults: Oral: 8-10 mg/kg/day in 2-3 divided doses; use beyond 24 months is not established; obtain ultrasound images at 6-month intervals for the first year of therapy; 30% of patients have stone recurrence after dissolution

**Patient Information** Frequent blood work will be necessary to follow drug effects. Drug will need to be taken for 1-3 months after stone is dissolved. Stones may recur. Report any persistent nausea, vomiting, abdominal pain, or yellowing of skin or eyes.

**Dosage Forms** Capsule: 300 mg

- **Vagifem®** *see* Estradiol *on page 203*
- **Vagistat®-1 Vaginal [OTC]** *see* Tioconazole *on page 550*
- **Vagitrol®** *see* Sulfanilamide *on page 525*
- **Valaciclovir** *see* Valacyclovir *on page 577*

## Valacyclovir (val ay SYE kloe veer)

**U.S. Brand Names** Valtrex®

**Synonyms** Valaciclovir

**Pharmacologic Category** Antiviral Agent, Ophthalmic

**Use** Treatment of herpes zoster (shingles) in immunocompetent patients; episodic treatment or prophylaxis of recurrent genital herpes in immunocompetent patients; for first episode genital herpes

**Effects on Mental Status** May cause dizziness

**Effects on Psychiatric Treatment** None reported

**Pregnancy Risk Factor** B

**Contraindications** Hypersensitivity to the drug or any component

**Warnings/Precautions** Thrombotic thrombocytopenic purpura/hemolytic uremic syndrome has occurred in immunocompromised patients; use caution and adjust the dose in elderly patients or those with renal insufficiency; safety and efficacy in children have not been established

**Adverse Reactions**

>10%:

Central nervous system: Headache (13% to 17%)

Gastrointestinal: Nausea (8% to 16%)

1% to 10%:

Central nervous system: Dizziness (2% to 4%)

Dermatologic: Pruritus

Gastrointestinal: Diarrhea (4% to 5%), constipation (1% to 5%), abdominal pain (2% to 3%), anorexia (≤3%), vomiting (≤7%)

Neuromuscular & skeletal: Weakness (2% to 4%)

Ocular: Photophobia

**Overdosage/Toxicology**

Signs and symptoms: Precipitation in the renal tubules may occur

Treatment: Includes hemodialysis, especially if compromised renal function develops

**Drug Interactions** Decreased toxicity: Cimetidine and/or probenecid has decreased the rate but not the extent of valacyclovir conversion to acyclovir

**Usual Dosage** Oral: Adults:

Shingles: 1 g 3 times/day for 7 days

Genital herpes:

Episodic treatment: 500 mg twice daily for 5 days

Prophylaxis: 500-1000 mg once daily

**Dosing interval in renal impairment:**

$Cl_{cr}$ 30-49 mL/minute: 1 g every 12 hours

$Cl_{cr}$ 10-29 mL/minute: 1 g every 24 hours

$Cl_{cr}$ <10 mL/minute: 500 mg every 24 hours

Hemodialysis: 33% removed during 4-hour session

**Patient Information** Begin use as soon as possible following development of signs of herpes zoster. Take with plenty of fluids. May take without regard to meals.

**Nursing Implications** Observe for CNS changes; avoid dehydration; begin therapy at the earliest sign of zoster infection (within 48 hours of the rash)

**Dosage Forms** Caplets: 500 mg

## Valerian

**Related Information**

Natural/Herbal Products *on page 746*

Natural Products, Herbals, and Dietary Supplements *on page 742*

Perspectives on the Safety of Herbal Medicines *on page 736*

**Synonyms** Radix; Red Valerian; *Valeriana edulis*; *Valeriana wallichi*

(Continued)

## Valerian *(Continued)*

**Pharmacologic Category** Herb

**Use** Herbal medicine use as a sleep-promoting agent and minor tranquilizer (similar to benzodiazepines); used in anxiety, panic attacks, intestinal cramps, headaches

Per Commission E: Restlessness, sleep disorders based on nervous conditions

**Adverse Reactions**

Cardiovascular: Cardiac disturbances (unspecified)
Central nervous system: Lightheadedness, restlessness, fatigue
Gastrointestinal: Nausea
Neuromuscular & skeletal: Tremor
Ocular: Blurred vision

**Overdosage/Toxicology**

Signs and symptoms: Headache, blurred vision, fine tremor, fatigue, mydriasis, abdominal cramping; intravenous exposure can cause hypotension, lethargy, hypophosphatemia, hypocalcemia, hypokalemia, and piloerection. Contact with the plant can cause contact dermatitis. Hepatotoxicity (probably due to an idiosyncratic hypersensitivity) has been noted.

Decontamination: Lavage (within 1 hour)/activated charcoal with cathartic

Treatment: Supportive therapy; hypotension can be treated with I.V. crystalloid therapy

**Drug Interactions** CNS depressants: Potentiation of effect by valerian is possible; no effect noted in some studies with ethanol

**Usual Dosage** Adults:

Sedative: 1-3 g (1-3 mL of tincture)
Sleep aid: 1-3 mL of tincture at bedtime
Dried root: 0.3-1 g

**Additional Information** *Valeriana officinalis* is a perennial plant that can reach 5 feet in height with tiny white or pink flowers. It is found in Europe, Canada, and Northern U.S. Preparations may contain multiple components.


- ***Valeriana edulis*** *see* Valerian *on page 577*
- ***Valeriana wallichi*** *see* Valerian *on page 577*
- **Valertest No.1® Injection** *see* Estradiol and Testosterone *on page 205*
- **Valisone®** *see* Betamethasone *on page 65*
- **Valpin® 50** *see* Anisotropine *on page 45*
- **Valproate Semisodium** *see* Valproic Acid and Derivatives *on page 578*
- **Valproate Sodium** *see* Valproic Acid and Derivatives *on page 578*
- **Valproic Acid** *see* Valproic Acid and Derivatives *on page 578*


## Valproic Acid and Derivatives

(val PROE ik AS id & dah RIV ah tives)

**Related Information**


Anticonvulsants by Seizures Type *on page 703*
Clinical Issues in the Use of Mood Stabilizers *on page 632*
Clozapine-Induced Side Effects *on page 780*
Epilepsy Treatment *on page 783*
Impulse Control Disorders *on page 622*
Liquid Compatibility With Antipsychotics and Mood Stabilizers *on page 718*
Mood Disorders *on page 600*
Mood Stabilizers *on page 719*
Patient Information - Mood Stabilizers (Valproic Acid) *on page 650*
Serum Drug Concentrations Commonly Monitored: Guidelines *on page 759*
Special Populations - Children and Adolescents *on page 663*
Special Populations - Elderly *on page 662*
Special Populations - Mentally Retarded Patients *on page 665*
Special Populations - Pregnant and Breast-Feeding Patients *on page 668*


**Generic Available** Yes

**U.S. Brand Names** Depacon™; Depakene®; Depakote® Delayed Release; Depakote® ER

**Canadian Brand Names** Deproic

**Synonyms** Dipropylacetic Acid; Divalproex Sodium; DPA; 2-Propylpentanoic Acid; 2-Propylvaleric Acid; Valproate Semisodium; Valproate Sodium; Valproic Acid

**Pharmacologic Category** Anticonvulsant, Miscellaneous

**Use**

Mania associated with bipolar disorder (Depakote®)

Migraine prophylaxis (Depakote®, Depakote® ER)

Monotherapy and adjunctive therapy in the treatment of patients with complex partial seizures that occur either in isolation or in association with other types of seizures (Depacon™, Depakote®)

Sole and adjunctive therapy of simple and complex absence seizures (Depacon™, Depakene®, Depakote®)

Adjunctively in patients with multiple seizure types that include absence seizures (Depacon™, Depakene®)

**Unlabeled use:** Behavior disorders in Alzheimer's disease

**Pregnancy Risk Factor** D

**Pregnancy/Breast-Feeding Implications**

Clinical effects on the fetus: Crosses the placenta. Neural tube, cardiac, facial (characteristic pattern of dysmorphic facial features), skeletal, multiple other defects reported. Epilepsy itself, number of medications, genetic factors, or a combination of these probably influence the teratogenicity of anticonvulsant therapy. Risk of neural tube defects with use during first 30 days of pregnancy warrants discontinuation prior to pregnancy and through this period if possible.

Breast-feeding/lactation: Crosses into breast milk. American Academy of Pediatrics considers **compatible** with breast-feeding.

**Contraindications** Hypersensitivity to valproic acid or derivatives or any component; hepatic dysfunction

**Warnings/Precautions** Hepatic failure resulting in fatalities has occurred in patients; children <2 years of age are at considerable risk; other risk factors include organic brain disease, mental retardation with severe seizure disorders, congenital metabolic disorders, and patients on multiple anticonvulsants. Hepatotoxicity has been reported after 3 days to 6 months of therapy. Monitor patients closely for appearance of malaise, weakness, facial edema, anorexia, jaundice, and vomiting; may cause severe thrombocytopenia, inhibition of platelet aggregation and bleeding; tremors may indicate overdosage; use with caution in patients receiving other anticonvulsants.

Cases of life-threatening pancreatitis, occurring at the start of therapy or following years of use, have been reported in adults and children. Some cases have been hemorrhagic with rapid progression of initial symptoms to death.

*In vitro* studies have suggested valproate stimulates the replication of HIV and CMV viruses under experimental conditions. The clinical consequence of this is unknown, but should be considered when monitoring affected patients.

Anticonvulsants should not be discontinued abruptly because of the possibility of increasing seizure frequency; valproate should be withdrawn gradually to minimize the potential of increased seizure frequency, unless safety concerns require a more rapid withdrawal. Concomitant use with clonazepam may induce absence status.

Hyperammonemia may occur, even in the absence of overt liver function abnormalities. Asymptomatic elevations require continued surveillance; symptomatic elevations should prompt modification or discontinuation of valproate therapy. CNS depression may occur with valproate use. Patients must be cautioned about performing tasks which require mental alertness (operating machinery or driving). Effects with other sedative drugs or ethanol may be potentiated.

**Adverse Reactions**

**Adverse reactions reported when used as monotherapy for complex partial seizures:**

>10%:

Central nervous system: Somnolence (18% to 30%), dizziness (13% to 18%), insomnia (9% to 15%), nervousness (7% to 11%)
Dermatologic: Alopecia (13% to 24%)
Gastrointestinal: Nausea (26% to 34%), diarrhea (19% to 23%), vomiting (15% to 23%), abdominal pain (9% to 12%), dyspepsia (10% to 11%), anorexia (4% to 11%)
Hematologic: Thrombocytopenia (1% to 24%)
Neuromuscular & skeletal: Tremor (19% to 57%), weakness (10% to 21%)
Respiratory: Respiratory tract infection (13% to 20%), pharyngitis (2% to 8%), dyspnea (1% to 5%)

1% to 10%

Cardiovascular: Hypertension, palpitation, peripheral edema (3% to 8%), tachycardia, chest pain
Central nervous system: Amnesia (4% to 7%), abnormal dreams, anxiety, confusion, depression (4% to 5%), malaise, personality disorder
Dermatologic: Bruising (4% to 5%), dry skin, petechia, pruritus, rash
Endocrine & metabolic: Amenorrhea, dysmenorrhea
Gastrointestinal: Eructation, flatulence, hematemesis, increased appetite, pancreatitis, periodontal abscess, taste perversion, weight gain (4% to 9%)
Genitourinary: Urinary frequency, urinary incontinence, vaginitis
Hepatic: Increased AST and ALT
Neuromuscular & skeletal: Abnormal gait, arthralgia, back pain, hypertonia, incoordination, leg cramps, myalgia, myasthenia, paresthesia, twitching
Ocular: Amblyopia/blurred vision (4% to 8%), abnormal vision, nystagmus (1% to 7%)
Otic: Deafness, otitis media, tinnitus (1% to 7%)
Respiratory: Epistaxis, increased cough, pneumonia, sinusitis

**Additional adverse effects:**

Cardiovascular: Bradycardia
Central nervous system: Aggression, ataxia, behavioral deterioration, cerebral atrophy (reversible), dementia, emotional upset, encephalopathy (rare), fever, hallucinations, headache, hostility, hyperactivity, hypesthesia, incoordination, Parkinsonism, psychosis, vertigo

Dermatologic: Cutaneous vasculitis, erythema multiforme, photosensitivity, Stevens-Johnson syndrome, toxic epidermal necrolysis (rare)

Endocrine & metabolic: Breast enlargement, galactorrhea, hyperammonemia, hyponatremia, inappropriate ADH secretion, irregular menses, parotid gland swelling, polycystic ovary disease (rare), abnormal thyroid function tests

Genitourinary: Enuresis, urinary tract infection

Hematologic: Anemia, aplastic anemia, bone marrow suppression, eosinophilia, hematoma formation, hemorrhage, hypofibrinogenemia, intermittent porphyria, leukopenia, lymphocytosis, macrocytosis, pancytopenia

Hepatic: Increased bilirubin

Neuromuscular & skeletal: Asterixis, bone pain, dysarthria

Ocular: Diplopia, "spots before the eyes"

Renal: Fanconi-like syndrome (rare, in children)

Miscellaneous: Anaphylaxis, decreased carnitine, hyperglycinemia, lupus

Case reports: Life-threatening pancreatitis (2 cases out of 2416 patients), occurring at the start of therapy or following years of use, has been reported in adults and children. Some cases have been hemorrhagic with rapid progression of initial symptoms to death. Cases have also been reported upon rechallenge.

**Overdosage/Toxicology**

Signs and symptoms: Coma, deep sleep, motor restlessness, visual hallucinations

Treatment: Supportive treatment is necessary; naloxone has been used to reverse CNS depressant effects, but may block action of other anticonvulsants

In an overdose situation, the fraction of unbound valproate is high and hemodialysis or tandem hemodialysis plus hemoperfusion may lead to significant removal of the drug.

**Drug Interactions** CYP2C19 enzyme substrate; CYP2C9 and 2D6 enzyme inhibitor; weak CYP3A3/4 enzyme inhibitor

Acyclovir: Serum levels of valproate may be reduced; monitor

Carbamazepine: Valproic acid may increase, decrease, or have no effect on carbamazepine levels; valproic acid may increase serum concentrations of carbamazepine - epoxide (active metabolite); carbamazepine may induce the metabolism of carbamazepine; monitor

Cholestyramine: Cholestyramine (and possibly colestipol) may bind valproic acid in GI tract; monitor

Clonazepam: Absence seizures have been reported in patients receiving valproic acid and clonazepam

Clozapine: Valproic acid may displace clozapine from protein binding site resulting in decreased clozapine serum concentrations

CYP2C18/19 inhibitors: May increase serum concentrations of valproic acid; inhibitors include cimetidine, felbamate, fluoxetine, fluvoxamine, monitor

Diazepam: Valproic acid may increase serum concentrations; monitor

Enzyme inducers: Carbamazepine, lamotrigine, and phenytoin may induce the metabolism of valproic acid; monitor

Isoniazid: May decrease valproic acid metabolism (limited documentation)

Lamotrigine: Valproic acid inhibits the metabolism of lamotrigine; combination therapy has been proposed to increase the risk of toxic epidermal necrolysis; monitor

Macrolide antibiotics: May decrease valproic acid metabolism (limited documentation); includes clarithromycin, erythromycin, troleandomycin; monitor

Nimodipine: Valproic acid appears to inhibit the metabolism of nimodipine; monitor for increased effect

Phenobarbital: Valproic acid appears to inhibit the metabolism of phenobarbital; monitor for increased effect

Phenothiazines: Chlorpromazine may increase valproic acid concentrations. Other phenothiazines may share this effect; monitor

Phenytoin: Valproic acid may increase, decrease, or have no effect on phenytoin levels

Risperidone: A case report of generalized edema occurred during combination therapy

Salicylates: May displace valproic acid from plasma proteins, leading to acute toxicity

Tricyclic antidepressants: Valproate may increase serum concentrations and/or toxicity of tricyclic antidepressants

**Stability** Injection is physically compatible and chemically stable in $D_5W$, NS, and LR for at least 24 hours when stored in glass or PVC; store vials at room temperature 15°C to 30°C (59°F to 86°F)

**Mechanism of Action** Causes increased availability of gamma-aminobutyric acid (GABA), an inhibitory neurotransmitter, to brain neurons or may enhance the action of GABA or mimic its action at postsynaptic receptor sites

**Pharmacodynamics/kinetics**

Distribution: Total valproate: 11 L/1.73 $m^2$; free valproate 92 L/1.73 $m^2$

Protein binding: 80% to 90% (dose dependent)

Metabolism: Extensively in the liver; glucuronide conjugation and mitochondrial beta-oxidation

Bioavailability: Extended release: 90% of I.V. dose, 81% to 90% of delayed release dose

Half-life (increased in neonates and patients with liver disease): Children: 4-14 hours; Adults: 8-17 hours

Time to peak serum concentration: Within 1-4 hours; 3-5 hours after divalproex (enteric coated)

Elimination: Urine (30% to 50% as glucuronide conjugate, 3% unchanged)

**Usual Dosage**

Seizures:

Children >10 years and Adults:

Oral: Initial: 10-15 mg/kg/day in 1-3 divided doses; increase by 5-10 mg/kg/day at weekly intervals until therapeutic levels are achieved; maintenance: 30-60 mg/kg/day in 2-3 divided doses. Adult usual dose: 1000-2500 mg/day

Children receiving more than one anticonvulsant (ie, polytherapy) may require doses up to 100 mg/kg/day in 3-4 divided doses

I.V.: Administer as a 60-minute infusion (≤20 mg/minute) with the same frequency as oral products; switch patient to oral products as soon as possible

Rectal: Dilute syrup 1:1 with water for use as a retention enema; loading dose: 17-20 mg/kg one time; maintenance: 10-15 mg/kg/dose every 8 hours

Mania: Adults: Oral: 750 mg/day in divided doses; dose should be adjusted as rapidly as possible to desired clinical effect; a loading dose of 20 mg/kg may be used; maximum recommended dosage: 60 mg/kg/day

Migraine prophylaxis: Adults: Oral:

Extended release tablets: 500 mg once daily for 7 days, then increase to 1000 mg once daily; adjust dose based on patient response; usual dosage range 500-1000 mg/day

Delayed release tablets: 250 mg twice a day; adjust dose based on patient response, up to 1000 mg/day

Elderly: Elimination is decreased in the elderly. Studies of elderly patients with dementia show a high incidence of somnolence. In some patients, this was associated with weight loss. Starting doses should be lower and increases should be slow, with careful monitoring of nutritional intake and dehydration. Safety and efficacy for use in patients >65 years have not been studied for migraine prophylaxis.

**Dosing adjustment in renal impairment:** A 27% reduction in clearance of unbound valproate is seen in patients with $Cl_{cr}$ <10 mL/minute. Hemodialysis reduces valproate concentrations by 20%, therefore no dose adjustment is needed in patients with renal failure. Protein binding is reduced, monitoring only total valproate concentrations may be misleading.

**Dosing adjustment/comments in hepatic impairment:** Reduce dose. Clearance is decreased with liver impairment. Hepatic disease is also associated with increased albumin concentrations and 2-to 2.6-fold increase in the unbound fraction. Free concentrations of valproate may be elevated while total concentrations appear normal.

**Dietary Considerations**

Alcohol: Additive CNS depression, avoid or limit alcohol

Food:

Valproic acid may cause GI upset; take with large amount of water or food to decrease GI upset. May need to split doses to avoid GI upset.

Food may delay but does not affect the extent of absorption

Coated particles of divalproex sodium may be mixed with semisolid food (eg, applesauce or pudding) in patients having difficulty swallowing; particles should be swallowed and not chewed

Valproate sodium oral solution will generate valproic acid in carbonated beverages and may cause mouth and throat irritation; do not mix valproate sodium oral solution with carbonated beverages

Milk: No effect on absorption; may take with milk

Sodium: SIADH and water intoxication; monitor fluid status. May need to restrict fluid.

**Administration** Depakote® ER: Swallow whole, do not crush or chew. Patients who need dose adjustments smaller than 500 mg/day for migraine prophylaxis should be changed to Depakote® delayed release tablets. Sprinkle capsules may be swallowed whole or open cap and sprinkle on small amount (1 teaspoonful) of soft food and use immediately (do not store or chew).

**Monitoring Parameters** Liver enzymes, CBC with platelets

**Reference Range** Therapeutic: 50-100 μg/mL (SI: 350-690 μmol/L); Toxic: >200 μg/mL (SI: >1390 μmol/L). Seizure control may improve at levels over 100 μg/mL (SI: 690 μmol/L), but toxicity may occur at levels of 100-150 μg/mL (SI: 690-1040 μmol/L). Bipolar disorder: 50-125 μg/mL; risk of toxicity increases at levels >125 μg/mL.

**Test Interactions** False-positive result for urine ketones

**Patient Information** When used to treat generalized seizures, patient instructions are determined by patient's condition and ability to understand.

Oral: Take as directed; do not alter dose or timing of medication. Do not increase dose or take more than recommended. Do not crush or chew capsule or enteric-coated pill. While using this medication, do not use alcohol and other prescription or OTC medications (especially pain medications, sedatives, antihistamines, or hypnotics) without consulting prescriber. Maintain adequate hydration (2-3 L/day of fluids unless instructed to restrict fluid intake). Diabetics should monitor serum glucose closely (valproic acid will alter results of urine ketones). Report alterations

(Continued)

## Valproic Acid and Derivatives *(Continued)*

in menstrual cycle; abdominal cramps, unresolved diarrhea, vomiting, or constipation; skin rash; unusual bruising or bleeding; blood in urine, stool or vomitus; malaise; weakness; facial swelling; yellowing of skin or eyes; excessive sedation; or restlessness.

Do not get pregnant while taking this medication; use appropriate barrier contraceptive measures

**Nursing Implications** Do not crush enteric coated drug product or capsule; do not crush or chew delayed or extended release gelatin capsules or tablets

**Additional Information** Sodium content of valproate sodium syrup (5 mL): 23 mg (1 mEq)

Divalproex sodium: Depakote®
Valproate sodium: Depakene® syrup
Valproic acid: Depakene® capsule

**Dosage Forms**

Capsule, sprinkle, as divalproex sodium (Depakote® Sprinkle®): 125 mg
Capsule, as valproic acid (Depakene®): 250 mg
Injection, as sodium valproate (Depacon™): 100 mg/mL (5 mL)
Syrup, as sodium valproate (Depakene®): 250 mg/5 mL (5 mL, 50 mL, 480 mL)
Tablet, delayed release, as divalproex sodium (Depakote®): 125 mg, 250 mg, 500 mg
Tablet, extended release, as divalproex sodium (Depakote® ER): 500 mg

## Valrubicin (val ru BYE cin)

**U.S. Brand Names** Valstar™

**Pharmacologic Category** Antineoplastic Agent, Antibiotic

**Use** Intravesical therapy of BCG-refractory carcinoma *in situ* of the urinary bladder

**Effects on Mental Status** May cause dizziness or drowsiness

**Effects on Psychiatric Treatment** None reported

**Usual Dosage** Adults: Intravesical: 800 mg once weekly for 6 weeks

**Dosing adjustment in renal impairment:** No specific adjustment recommended

**Dosing adjustment in hepatic impairment:** No specific adjustment recommended

**Dosage Forms** Injection: 200 mg/5mL

## Valsartan (val SAR tan)

**Related Information**

Angiotensin-Related Agents Comparison Chart *on page 700*

**U.S. Brand Names** Diovan™

**Pharmacologic Category** Angiotensin II Antagonists

**Use** Alone or in combination with other antihypertensive agents in treating essential hypertension; may have an advantage over losartan due to minimal metabolism requirements and consequent use in mild to moderate hepatic impairment

**Effects on Mental Status** May cause dizziness or drowsiness

**Effects on Psychiatric Treatment** May rarely cause neutropenia; use caution with clozapine and carbamazepine; barbiturates and carbamazepine may increase the metabolism of valsartan

**Pregnancy Risk Factor** C (1st trimester); D (2nd and 3rd trimesters)

**Contraindications** Hypersensitivity to valsartan or any component; hypersensitivity to other A-II receptor antagonists; primary hyperaldosteronism; bilateral renal artery stenosis; pregnancy (2nd and 3rd trimesters)

**Warnings/Precautions** Avoid use or use a smaller dose in patients who are volume depleted; correct depletion first. Deterioration in renal function can occur with initiation. Use with caution in unilateral renal artery stenosis and pre-existing renal insufficiency; significant aortic/mitral stenosis. Use caution in patients with severe renal impairment or significant hepatic dysfunction.

**Adverse Reactions** Similar incidence to placebo; independent of race, age, and gender

>1%:
- Central nervous system: Headache, dizziness, drowsiness, ataxia
- Endocrine & metabolic: Decreased libido
- Gastrointestinal: Diarrhea, abdominal pain, nausea, abnormal taste
- Genitourinary: Polyuria
- Hematologic: Neutropenia
- Hepatic: Increased LFTs
- Neuromuscular & skeletal: Arthralgia
- Respiratory: Cough, upper respiratory infection, rhinitis, sinusitis, pharyngitis

<1%: Anemia, increased creatinine

**Overdosage/Toxicology**

Signs and symptoms: Only mild toxicity (hypotension, bradycardia, hyperkalemia) has been reported with large overdoses (up to 5 g of captopril and 300 mg of enalapril); no fatalities have been reported

Treatment: Symptomatic (eg, fluids)

**Drug Interactions**

Lithium: Risk of toxicity may be increased by valsartan; monitor lithium levels
Potassium-sparing diuretics (amiloride, potassium, spironolactone, triamterene): Increased risk of hyperkalemia
Potassium supplements may increase the risk of hyperkalemia
Trimethoprim (high dose) may increase the risk of hyperkalemia

**Usual Dosage** Adults: 80 mg/day; may be increased to 160 mg if needed (maximal effects observed in 4-6 weeks).

**Dosing adjustment in renal impairment:** No dosage adjustment necessary if $Cl_{cr}$ >10 mL/minute.

**Dosing adjustment in hepatic impairment** (mild - moderate): ≤80 mg/day

Dialysis: Not significantly removed

**Patient Information** Take exactly as directed; do not discontinue without consulting prescriber. Take first dose at bedtime. This drug does not eliminate need for diet or exercise regimen as recommended by prescriber. May cause dizziness, fainting, lightheadedness (use caution when driving or engaging in tasks requiring alertness until response to drug is known); mild hypotension use caution when changing position (rising from sitting or lying position) until response to therapy is established; decreased libido (will resolve). Report chest pain or palpitations; unrelenting headache; swelling of extremities, face, or tongue; muscle weakness or pain; difficulty in breathing or unusual cough; flu-like symptoms; or other persistent adverse reactions.

**Dosage Forms** Capsule: 80 mg, 160 mg

## Valsartan and Hydrochlorothiazide

(val SAR tan & hye droe klor oh THYE a zide)

**U.S. Brand Names** Diovan HCTZ®

**Pharmacologic Category** Antihypertensive Agent, Combination

**Use** Treatment of hypertension

**Effects on Mental Status** May cause dizziness or drowsiness

**Effects on Psychiatric Treatment** May rarely cause neutropenia; use caution with clozapine and carbamazepine; barbiturates and carbamazepine may increase the metabolism of valsartan; may decrease lithium clearance resulting in an increase in serum lithium levels and potential lithium toxicity; monitor serum lithium levels

**Usual Dosage** Adults: Oral: Dose is individualized

**Dosage Forms** Tablet: Valsartan 80 mg and hydrochlorothiazide 12.5 mg; valsartan 160 mg and hydrochlorothiazide 12.5 mg

♦ **Valstar™** *see* Valrubicin *on page 580*

♦ **Valtrex®** *see* Valacyclovir *on page 577*

♦ **Vamate®** *see* Hydroxyzine *on page 278*

♦ **Vancenase® AQ Inhaler** *see* Beclomethasone *on page 59*

♦ **Vancenase® Nasal Inhaler** *see* Beclomethasone *on page 59*

♦ **Vanceril® Oral Inhaler** *see* Beclomethasone *on page 59*

♦ **Vancocin®** *see* Vancomycin *on page 580*

♦ **Vancoled®** *see* Vancomycin *on page 580*

## Vancomycin (van koe MYE sin)

**Related Information**

Serum Drug Concentrations Commonly Monitored: Guidelines *on page 759*

**U.S. Brand Names** Lyphocin®; Vancocin®; Vancoled®

**Canadian Brand Names** Vancocin® CP

**Pharmacologic Category** Antibiotic, Miscellaneous

**Use** Treatment of patients with infections caused by staphylococcal species and streptococcal species; used orally for staphylococcal enterocolitis or for antibiotic-associated pseudomembranous colitis produced by *C. difficile*

**Effects on Mental Status** None reported

**Effects on Psychiatric Treatment** May cause neutropenia; use caution with clozapine and carbamazepine

**Pregnancy Risk Factor** C

**Contraindications** Hypersensitivity to vancomycin or any component; avoid in patients with previous severe hearing loss

**Warnings/Precautions** Use with caution in patients with renal impairment or those receiving other nephrotoxic or ototoxic drugs; dosage modification required in patients with impaired renal function (especially elderly)

**Adverse Reactions**

Oral:

>10%: Gastrointestinal: Bitter taste, nausea, vomiting

1% to 10%:
- Central nervous system: Chills, drug fever
- Hematologic: Eosinophilia

<1%: Interstitial nephritis, ototoxicity, renal failure, thrombocytopenia, vasculitis

Parenteral:
>10%:
Cardiovascular: Hypotension accompanied by flushing
Dermatologic: Erythematous rash on face and upper body (red neck or red man syndrome - infusion rate related)
1% to 10%:
Central nervous system: Chills, drug fever
Dermatologic: Rash
Hematologic: Eosinophilia, reversible neutropenia
<1%: Ototoxicity (especially with large doses), renal failure (especially with renal dysfunction or pre-existing hearing loss) Stevens-Johnson syndrome, thrombocytopenia, vasculitis

**Overdosage/Toxicology**
Signs and symptoms: Ototoxicity, nephrotoxicity
Treatment: There is no specific therapy for an overdosage with vancomycin. Care is symptomatic and supportive in nature. Peritoneal filtration and hemofiltration (not dialysis) have been shown to reduce the serum concentration of vancomycin; high flux dialysis may remove up to 25%.

**Drug Interactions** Increased toxicity: Anesthetic agents; other ototoxic or nephrotoxic agents

**Usual Dosage** Initial dosage recommendation: I.V.:
Neonates:
Postnatal age ≤7 days:
<1200 g: 15 mg/kg/dose every 24 hours
1200-2000 g: 10 mg/kg/dose every 12 hours
>2000 g: 15 mg/kg/dose every 12 hours
Postnatal age >7 days:
<1200 g: 15 mg/kg/dose every 24 hours
≥1200 g: 10 mg/kg/dose divided every 8 hours
Infants >1 month and Children:
40 mg/kg/day in divided doses every 6 hours
Prophylaxis for bacterial endocarditis:
Dental, oral, or upper respiratory tract surgery: 20 mg/kg 1 hour prior to the procedure
GI/GU procedure: 20 mg/kg plus gentamicin 2 mg/kg 1 hour prior to surgery
Infants >1 month and Children with staphylococcal central nervous system infection: 60 mg/kg/day in divided doses every 6 hours
Adults:
With normal renal function: 1 g **or** 10-15 mg/kg/dose every 12 hours
Prophylaxis for bacterial endocarditis:
Dental, oral, or upper respiratory tract surgery: 1 g 1 hour before surgery
GI/GU procedure: 1 g plus 1.5 mg/kg gentamicin 1 hour prior to surgery
**Dosing interval in renal impairment (vancomycin levels should be monitored in patients with any renal impairment):**
$Cl_{cr}$ >60 mL/minute: Start with 1 g or 10-15 mg/kg/dose every 12 hours
$Cl_{cr}$ 40-60 mL/minute: Start with 1 g or 10-15 mg/kg/dose every 24 hours
$Cl_{cr}$ <40 mL/minute: Will need longer intervals; determine by serum concentration monitoring
Hemodialysis: Not dialyzable (0% to 5%); generally not removed; exception minimal-moderate removal by some of the newer high-flux filters; dose may need to be administered more frequently; monitor serum concentrations
Continuous ambulatory peritoneal dialysis (CAPD): Not significantly removed; administration via CAPD fluid: 15-30 mg/L (15-30 mcg/mL) of CAPD fluid
Continuous arteriovenous hemofiltration: Dose as for $Cl_{cr}$ 10-40 mL/minute
**Antibiotic lock technique (for catheter infections):** 2 mg/mL in SWI/NS or $D_5W$; instill 3-5 mL into catheter port as a flush solution instead of heparin lock (**Note:** Do not mix with any other solutions)
**Intrathecal:** Vancomycin is available as a powder for injection and may be diluted to 1-5 mg/mL concentration in preservative-free 0.9% sodium chloride for administration into the CSF
Neonates: 5-10 mg/day
Children: 5-20 mg/day
Adults: Up to 20 mg/day
Oral: Pseudomembranous colitis produced by *C. difficile*:
Neonates: 10 mg/kg/day in divided doses
Children: 40 mg/kg/day in divided doses, added to fluids
Adults: 125 mg 4 times/day for 10 days

**Patient Information**
Oral: Take per recommended schedule. Complete full course of therapy; do not skip doses. Maintain adequate hydration (2-3 L/day of fluids unless instructed to restrict fluid intake). You may experience nausea, vomiting, or GI upset (small frequent meals, frequent mouth care, sucking lozenges, or chewing gum may help).
Oral or I.V.: Report chills or pain at infusion site, skin rash or redness, decrease in urine output, chest pain or palpitations, persistent GI disturbances, signs of opportunistic infection (sore throat, chills, fever, burning, itching on urination, vaginal discharge, white plaques in mouth), difficulty breathing, changes in hearing or fullness in ears, or worsening of condition.

**Nursing Implications** Obtain drug levels after the third dose unless otherwise directed; peaks are drawn 1 hour after the completion of a 1- to 2-hour infusion; troughs are obtained just before the next dose; slow I.V. infusion rate if maculopapular rash appears on face, neck, trunk, and upper extremities (Red man reaction)

**Dosage Forms**
Capsule, as hydrochloride: 125 mg, 250 mg
Powder for oral solution, as hydrochloride: 1 g, 10 g
Powder for injection, as hydrochloride: 500 mg, 1 g, 2 g, 5 g, 10 g


- ♦ **Vaniqa™ Cream** *see* Eflornithine *on page 191*
- ♦ **Vanoxide® [OTC]** *see* Benzoyl Peroxide *on page 62*
- ♦ **Vanoxide-HC®** *see* Benzoyl Peroxide and Hydrocortisone *on page 62*
- ♦ **Vansil™** *see* Oxamniquine *on page 409*
- ♦ **Vantin®** *see* Cefpodoxime *on page 100*
- ♦ **Varson®** *see* Nicergoline *on page 392*
- ♦ **Vascor®** *see* Bepridil *on page 64*
- ♦ **Vaseretic® 10-25** *see* Enalapril and Hydrochlorothiazide *on page 192*
- ♦ **Vasocidin® Ophthalmic** *see* Sulfacetamide Sodium and Prednisolone *on page 523*
- ♦ **VasoClear® Ophthalmic [OTC]** *see* Naphazoline *on page 383*
- ♦ **Vasocon-A® [OTC] Ophthalmic** *see* Naphazoline and Antazoline *on page 383*
- ♦ **Vasocon Regular® Ophthalmic** *see* Naphazoline *on page 383*
- ♦ **Vasodilan®** *see* Isoxsuprine *on page 298*


## Vasopressin (vay soe PRES in)

**U.S. Brand Names** Pitressin® Injection
**Canadian Brand Names** Pressyn®
**Synonyms** ADH; Antidiuretic Hormone; 8-Arginine Vasopressin; Vasopressin Tannate
**Pharmacologic Category** Antidiuretic Hormone Analog; Hormone, Posterior Pituitary
**Use** Treatment of diabetes insipidus; prevention and treatment of postoperative abdominal distention; differential diagnosis of diabetes insipidus
**Unlabeled use:** Adjunct in the treatment of GI hemorrhage and esophageal varices
**Effects on Mental Status** May cause dizziness
**Effects on Psychiatric Treatment** May be somewhat useful as a treatment for lithium-induced diabetes insipidus; HCTZ and amiloride are more effective, less expensive options
**Pregnancy Risk Factor** B
**Contraindications** Hypersensitivity to vasopressin or any component
**Warnings/Precautions** Use with caution in patients with seizure disorders, migraine, asthma, vascular disease, renal disease, cardiac disease; chronic nephritis with nitrogen retention. Goiter with cardiac complications, arteriosclerosis; I.V. infiltration may lead to severe vasoconstriction and localized tissue necrosis; also, gangrene of extremities, tongue, and ischemic colitis. Elderly patients should be cautioned not to increase their fluid intake beyond that sufficient to satisfy their thirst in order to avoid water intoxication and hyponatremia; under experimental conditions, the elderly have shown to have a decreased responsiveness to vasopressin with respect to its effects on water homeostasis

**Adverse Reactions**
1% to 10%:
Cardiovascular: Increased blood pressure, bradycardia, arrhythmias, venous thrombosis, vasoconstriction with higher doses, angina
Central nervous system: Pounding in the head, fever, vertigo
Dermatologic: Urticaria, circumoral pallor
Gastrointestinal: Flatulence, abdominal cramps, nausea, vomiting
Neuromuscular & skeletal: Tremor
Miscellaneous: Diaphoresis
<1%: Allergic reaction, myocardial infarction, water intoxication

**Overdosage/Toxicology**
Signs and symptoms: Drowsiness, weight gain, confusion, listlessness, water intoxication
Treatment: Water intoxication requires withdrawal of the drug; severe intoxication may require osmotic diuresis and loop diuretics

**Drug Interactions**
Decreased effect: Lithium, epinephrine, demeclocycline, heparin, and alcohol block antidiuretic activity to varying degrees
Increased effect: Chlorpropamide, phenformin, urea and fludrocortisone potentiate antidiuretic response

**Usual Dosage**
Diabetes insipidus (highly variable dosage; titrated based on serum and urine sodium and osmolality in addition to fluid balance and urine output):
I.M., S.C.:
Children: 2.5-10 units 2-4 times/day as needed
Adults: 5-10 units 2-4 times/day as needed (dosage range 5-60 units/day)

(Continued)

## Vasopressin *(Continued)*

Continuous I.V. infusion: Children and Adults: 0.5 milliunit/kg/hour (0.0005 unit/kg/hour); double dosage as needed every 30 minutes to a maximum of 0.01 unit/kg/hour

Intranasal: Administer on cotton pledget or nasal spray

Abdominal distention (aqueous): Adults: I.M.: 5 mg stat, 10 mg every 3-4 hours

GI hemorrhage: I.V. infusion: Dilute aqueous in NS or $D_5W$ to 0.1-1 unit/mL

Children: Initial: 0.002-0.005 units/kg/minute; titrate dose as needed; maximum: 0.01 unit/kg/minute; continue at same dosage (if bleeding stops) for 12 hours, then taper off over 24-48 hours

Adults: Initial: 0.2-0.4 unit/minute, then titrate dose as needed, if bleeding stops; continue at same dose for 12 hours, taper off over 24-48 hours

**Dosing adjustment in hepatic impairment:** Some patients respond to much lower doses with cirrhosis

**Patient Information** Side effects such as abdominal cramps and nausea may be reduced by drinking a glass of water with each dose. Avoid alcohol use.

**Nursing Implications** Watch for signs of I.V. infiltration and gangrene; elderly patients should be cautioned not to increase their fluid intake beyond that sufficient to satisfy their thirst in order to avoid water intoxication and hyponatremia; under experimental conditions, the elderly have shown to have a decreased responsiveness to vasopressin with respect to its effects on water homeostasis

**Dosage Forms** Injection, aqueous: 20 pressor units/mL (0.5 mL, 1 mL)

- **Vasopressin Tannate** *see* Vasopressin *on page 581*
- **Vasosulf® Ophthalmic** *see* Sulfacetamide Sodium and Phenylephrine *on page 523*
- **Vasotec®** *see* Enalapril *on page 191*
- **Vasotec® I.V.** *see* Enalapril *on page 191*
- **Vasoxyl®** *see* Methoxamine *on page 355*
- **V-Dec-M®** *see* Guaifenesin and Pseudoephedrine *on page 257*
- **Vectrin®** *see* Minocycline *on page 367*
- **Veetids®** *see* Penicillin V Potassium *on page 426*
- **Vegetable arsenic** *see* Colchicine *on page 138*
- **Velban®** *see* Vinblastine *on page 584*
- **Velosef®** *see* Cephradine *on page 104*
- **Velosulin® BR Human (Buffered)** *see* Insulin Preparations *on page 287*
- **Velosulin® Human** *see* Insulin Preparations *on page 287*

## Venlafaxine (VEN la faks een)

**Related Information**

Antidepressant Agents Comparison Chart *on page 704*
Anxiety Disorders *on page 606*
Clinical Issues in the Use of Antidepressants *on page 627*
Mood Disorders *on page 600*
Patient Information - Antidepressants (Venlafaxine) *on page 642*
Special Populations - Elderly *on page 662*

**Generic Available** No

**U.S. Brand Names** Effexor®; Effexor® XR

**Pharmacologic Category** Antidepressant, Serotonin/Norepinephrine Reuptake Inhibitor

**Use** Treatment of depression; generalized anxiety disorder (GAD)

**Unlabeled use:** Obsessive-compulsive disorder, chronic fatigue syndrome

**Pregnancy Risk Factor** C

**Contraindications** Hypersensitivity to venlafaxine; use of monoamine oxidase inhibitors within 14 days; should not initiate MAOI within 7 days of discontinuing venlafaxine

**Warnings/Precautions** May cause sustained increase in blood pressure; may cause increase in anxiety, nervousness, insomnia; may cause weight loss (use with caution in patients where weight loss is undesirable). May worsen psychosis in some patients or precipitate a shift to mania or hypomania in patients with bipolar disease. May increase the risks associated with electroconvulsive therapy. Use caution in patients with depression, particularly if suicidal risk may be present. The risks of cognitive or motor impairment, as well as the potential for anticholinergic effects are very low. May cause or exacerbate sexual dysfunction. Abrupt discontinuation or dosage reduction after extended (>6 weeks) therapy may lead to agitation, dysphoria, nervousness, anxiety, and other symptoms. When discontinuing therapy, dosage should be tapered gradually over at least a 2-week period. Use caution in patients with increased intraocular pressure or at risk of acute narrow-angle glaucoma.

**Adverse Reactions**

≥10%:

Central nervous system: Headache, somnolence, dizziness, insomnia, nervousness

Gastrointestinal: Nausea, xerostomia, constipation, anorexia

Genitourinary: Abnormal ejaculation

Neuromuscular & skeletal: Weakness

Miscellaneous: Diaphoresis

1% to 10%:

Cardiovascular: Hypertension, sinus tachycardia, postural hypotension, vasodilation

Central nervous system: Anxiety, abnormal dreams, agitation, confusion, abnormal thinking, yawning

Dermatologic: Rash, pruritus

Endocrine & metabolic: Decreased libido

Gastrointestinal: Weight loss, vomiting, diarrhea, dyspepsia, flatulence, taste perversion

Genitourinary: Impotence, urinary retention

Neuromuscular & skeletal: Tremor, hypertonia, paresthesia

Ocular: Blurred vision, mydriasis

Otic: Tinnitus

**Overdosage/Toxicology**

Symptoms of overdose include somnolence and occasionally EKG changes (Q-T prolongation, QRS prolongation, bundle branch block), tachycardia, bradycardia, seizures, vertigo, (rare coma); deaths have been reported

Most overdoses resolve with only supportive treatment. Use of activated charcoal, inductions of emesis, or gastric lavage should be considered for acute ingestion; forced diuresis, dialysis, and hemoperfusion not effective due to large volume of distribution

**Drug Interactions** CYP2D6, 2E1, and 3A3/4 enzyme substrate; CYP2D6 enzyme inhibitor (weak)

Buspirone: Concurrent use may result in serotonin syndrome; these combinations are best avoided

CYP2D6 inhibitors: Serum levels and/or toxicity venlafaxine may be increased; inhibitors include amiodarone, cimetidine, delavirdine, fluoxetine, paroxetine, propafenone, quinidine, and ritonavir; monitor for increased effect/toxicity

CYP2E1 inhibitors: Serum levels and/or toxicity venlafaxine may be increased; inhibitors include disulfiram, metronidazole, and ritonavir

CYP3A3/4 inhibitors: Serum level and/or toxicity of venlafaxine may be increased; inhibitors include amiodarone, cimetidine, clarithromycin, erythromycin, delavirdine, diltiazem, dirithromycin, disulfiram, fluoxetine, fluvoxamine, grapefruit juice, indinavir, itraconazole, ketoconazole, metronidazole, nefazodone, nevirapine, propoxyfene, quinupristin-dalfopristin, ritonavir, saquinavir, verapamil, zafirlukast, zileuton; monitor for altered response

Enzyme inducers: May increase the metabolism of venlafaxine, reducing its effectiveness; inducers include phenytoin, carbamazepine, phenobarbital, and rifampin

MAOIs: Serotonin syndrome may result when venlafaxine is used in combination or within 2 weeks of an MAOI; these combinations should be avoided

Meperidine: Concurrent use may increase risk of serotonin syndrome

Methylphenidate: Neuroleptic malignant syndrome (NMS) has been reported in a patient receiving methylphenidate and venlafaxine

Mirtazapine: Concurrent use may increase risk of serotonin syndrome

Nefazodone: Concurrent use may increase risk of serotonin syndrome; in addition, nefazodone may inhibit the metabolism of venlafaxine

Selegiline: Concurrent use may predispose to serotonin syndrome

Serotonin agonists: Theoretically, may increase the risk of serotonin syndrome; includes sumatriptan, naratriptan, rizatriptan, and zolmitriptan

Sibutramine: Concurrent use may increase risk of serotonin syndrome

SSRIs: Concurrent use may increase risk of serotonin syndrome

Trazodone: Concurrent use may increase risk of serotonin syndrome

Tricyclic antidepressants: Concurrent use may increase risk of serotonin syndrome

Venlafaxine: Venlafaxine may decrease serum concentrations of indinavir; clinical significance unknown

**Mechanism of Action** Venlafaxine and its active metabolite o-desmethylvenlafaxine (ODV) are potent inhibitors of neuronal serotonin and norepinephrine reuptake and weak inhibitors of dopamine reuptake; causes beta-receptor down regulation and reduces adenylcyclase coupled beta-adrenergic systems in the brain

**Pharmacodynamics/kinetics**

Absorption: Oral: 92% to 100%

Protein binding: Bound to human plasma 27% to 30%; steady-state achieved within 3 days of multiple dose therapy

Metabolism: In the liver by cytochrome P-450 enzyme system to active metabolite, O-desmyethyl-venlafaxine (ODV)

Half-life: 3-7 hours (venlafaxine) and 11-13 hours (ODV)

Time to peak: 1-2 hours

Elimination: Primarily by renal route

**Usual Dosage** Adults: Oral:

Immediate-release tablets: 75 mg/day, administered in 2 or 3 divided doses, taken with food; dose may be increased in 75 mg/day increments at intervals of at least 4 days, up to 225-375 mg/day

Extended-release capsules: 75 mg once daily taken with food; for some new patients, it may be desirable to start at 37.5 mg/day for 4-7 days before increasing to 75 mg once daily; dose may be increased by up to

75 mg/day increments every 4 days as tolerated, up to a maximum of 225 mg/day

**Dosing adjustment in renal impairment:** $Cl_{cr}$ 10-70 mL/minute: Decrease dose by 25%; decrease total daily dose by 50% if dialysis patients; dialysis patients should receive dosing after completion of dialysis

**Dosing adjustment in moderate hepatic impairment:** Reduce total daily dosage by 50%

**Dietary Considerations**

Alcohol: Additive CNS effect, avoid use

Food: May be taken without regard to food

**Monitoring Parameters** Blood pressure should be regularly monitored, especially in patients with a high baseline blood pressure

**Reference Range** Peak serum level of 163 ng/mL (325 ng/mL of ODV metabolite) obtained after a 150 mg oral dose

**Test Interactions** Venlafaxine was associated with a mean increase of 3 mg/dL of serum cholesterol; ↑ thyroid, uric acid, glucose, potassium, AST

**Patient Information** Avoid use of alcohol; use caution when operating hazardous machinery

**Nursing Implications** Causes mean increase in heart rate of 4 beats/minute; may be taken without regard to food; tapering to minimize symptoms of discontinuation is recommended when the drug is discontinued; tapering should be over a 2-week period if the patient has received it longer than 6 weeks

**Dosage Forms**

Capsule, extended release: 37.5 mg, 75 mg, 150 mg

Tablet: 25 mg, 37.5 mg, 50 mg, 75 mg, 100 mg


- **Venoglobulin®-I** *see* Immune Globulin, Intravenous *on page 284*
- **Venoglobulin®-S** *see* Immune Globulin, Intravenous *on page 284*
- **Ventolin®** *see* Albuterol *on page 22*
- **Ventolin® Rotocaps®** *see* Albuterol *on page 22*
- **VePesid® Injection** *see* Etoposide *on page 216*
- **VePesid® Oral** *see* Etoposide *on page 216*


## Verapamil (ver AP a mil)

**Related Information**

Calcium Channel Blocking Agents Comparison Chart *on page 710*

**U.S. Brand Names** Calan®; Calan® SR; Covera-HS®; Isoptin®; Isoptin® SR; Verelan®

**Canadian Brand Names** Apo®-Verap; Novo-Veramil; Nu-Verap

**Synonyms** Iproveratril Hydrochloride

**Pharmacologic Category** Antiarrhythmic Agent, Class IV; Calcium Channel Blocker

**Use** Orally for treatment of angina pectoris (vasospastic, chronic stable, unstable) and hypertension; I.V. for supraventricular tachyarrhythmias (PSVT, atrial fibrillation, atrial flutter)

**Effects on Mental Status** May cause drowsiness or dizziness

**Effects on Psychiatric Treatment** Barbiturates may decrease verapamil serum concentrations; verapamil may increase carbamazepine serum concentrations; concurrent use with lithium may cause an increase or decrease in serum lithium concentrations; monitor; verapamil has been used to treat bipolar disorder, mania

**Pregnancy Risk Factor** C

**Contraindications** Hypersensitivity to verapamil or any component; severe; left ventricular dysfunction; hypotension (systolic pressure <90 mm Hg) or cardiogenic shock; sick sinus syndrome (except in patients with a functioning artificial pacemaker); second- or third-degree AV block (except in patients with a functioning artificial pacemaker); atrial flutter or fibrillation and an accessory bypass tract (WPW, Lown-Ganoang-Levine syndrome); pregnancy

**Warnings/Precautions** Avoid use in heart failure; can exacerbate condition. Can cause hypotension. Rare increases in liver function tests can be observed. Can cause first-degree AV block or sinus bradycardia. Other conduction abnormalities are rare. Use caution when using verapamil together with a beta-blocker. Avoid use of I.V. verapamil with an I.V. beta-blocker; can result in asystole. Avoid use in patients with hypertrophic cardiomyopathy (IHSS). Use with caution in patients with attenuated neuromuscular transmission. Adjust the dose in severe renal dysfunction and hepatic dysfunction. Verapamil significantly increases digoxin serum concentrations (adjust digoxin's dose).

**Adverse Reactions** O (oral); I.V. (intravenous):

1% to 10%:

Cardiovascular: Bradycardia; first, second, or third degree A-V block; congestive heart failure (1.8%), hypotension (O - 2.5%; I.V. - 1.5%), peripheral edema (2.1%)

Central nervous system: Dizziness/lightheadedness (O - 3.5%; I.V. - 1.2%), fatigue, headache (O - 2.2%; I.V. - 1.2%)

Dermatologic: Rash (1.2%)

Gastrointestinal: Constipation (7.3%), nausea (O - 2.7%; I.V. - 0.9%)

Neuromuscular & skeletal: Weakness

<1%: Chest pain, flushing, galactorrhea, gingival hyperplasia hypotension (excessive), tachycardia

**Overdosage/Toxicology**

Signs and symptoms:

The primary cardiac symptoms of calcium blocker overdose includes hypotension and bradycardia. The hypotension is caused by peripheral vasodilation, myocardial depression, and bradycardia. Bradycardia results from sinus bradycardia, second- or third-degree atrioventricular block, or sinus arrest with junctional rhythm. Intraventricular conduction is usually not affected so QRS duration is normal (verapamil does prolong the P-R interval and bepridil prolongs the Q-T and may cause ventricular arrhythmias, including torsade de pointes).

The noncardiac symptoms include confusion, stupor, nausea, vomiting, metabolic acidosis and hyperglycemia. Following initial gastric decontamination, if possible, repeated calcium administration may promptly reverse the depressed cardiac contractility (but not sinus node depression or peripheral vasodilation); glucagon, epinephrine, and inamrinone may treat refractory hypotension; glucagon and epinephrine also increase the heart rate (outside the U.S., 4-aminopyridine may be available as an antidote); dialysis and hemoperfusion are not effective in enhancing elimination although repeat-dose activated charcoal may serve as an adjunct with sustained-release preparations.

**Drug Interactions** CYP3A3/4 and 1A2 enzyme substrate; CYP3A3/4 inhibitor

Alfentanil's plasma concentration is increased; fentanyl and sufentanil may be affected similarly

Amiodarone use may lead to bradycardia and decreased cardiac output; monitor closely if using together

Aspirin and concurrent verapamil use may increase bleeding times; monitor closely, especially if on other antiplatelet agents or anticoagulants

Azole antifungals may inhibit the calcium channel blocker's metabolism; avoid this combination. Try an antifungal like terbinafine (if appropriate) or monitor closely for altered effect of the calcium channel blocker.

Barbiturates reduce the plasma concentration of verapamil; may require much higher dose of verapamil

Beta-blockers may have increased pharmacodynamic interactions with verapamil (see Warnings/Precautions)

Buspirone's serum concentration may increase; may require dosage adjustment

Calcium may reduce the calcium channel blocker's effects, particularly hypotension

Carbamazepine's serum concentration is increased and toxicity may result; avoid this combination

Cimetidine reduced verapamil's metabolism; consider an alternative $H_2$-antagonist

Cyclosporine's serum concentrations are increased by verapamil; avoid this combination; use another calcium channel blocker or monitor cyclosporine trough levels and renal function closely

Digoxin's serum concentration is increased; reduce digoxin's dose when adding verapamil

Doxorubicin's clearance was reduced; monitor for altered doxorubicin's effect

Erythromycin may increase verapamil's effects; monitor altered verapamil effect

Ethanol's effects may be increased by verapamil; reduce ethanol consumption

Flecainide may have additive negative effects on conduction and inotropy

HMG CoA reductase inhibitors (atorvastatin, cerivastatin, lovastatin, simvastatin): Serum concentration will likely be increased; consider pravastatin/fluvastatin or a dihydropyridine calcium channel blocker.

Lithium neurotoxicity may result when verapamil is added; monitor lithium levels

Midazolam's plasma concentration is increased by verapamil; monitor for prolonged CNS depression

Nafcillin decreases plasma concentration of verapamil; avoid this combination

Nondepolarizing muscle relaxant's neuromuscular blockade is prolonged. Monitor closely

Prazosin's serum concentration increases; monitor blood pressure

Quinidine's serum concentration is increased; adjust quinidine's dose as necessary

Rifampin increases the metabolism of calcium channel blockers; adjust the dose of the calcium channel blocker to maintain efficacy

Tacrolimus's serum concentrations are increased by verapamil; avoid the combination. Use another calcium channel blocker or monitor tacrolimus trough levels and renal function closely.

Theophylline's serum concentration may be increased by verapamil; those at increased risk include children and cigarette smokers

**Usual Dosage**

Children: SVT:

I.V.:

<1 year: 0.1-0.2 mg/kg over 2 minutes; repeat every 30 minutes as needed

(Continued)

## Verapamil *(Continued)*

1-15 years: 0.1-0.3 mg/kg over 2 minutes; maximum: 5 mg/dose, may repeat dose in 15 minutes if adequate response not achieved; maximum for second dose: 10 mg/dose

Oral (dose not well established):

1-5 years: 4-8 mg/kg/day in 3 divided doses **or** 40-80 mg every 8 hours

>5 years: 80 mg every 6-8 hours

Adults:

SVT: I.V.: 5-10 mg (approximately 0.075-0.15 mg/kg); second dose of 10 mg (~0.15 mg/kg) may be given 15-30 minutes after the initial dose if patient tolerates, but does not respond to initial dose.

Angina: Oral: Initial dose: 80-120 mg 3 times/day (elderly or small stature: 40 mg 3 times/day); range: 240-480 mg/day in 3-4 divided doses

Hypertension: Oral: 80 mg 3 times/day or 240 mg/day (sustained release); range: 240-480 mg/day; 120 mg/day in the elderly or small patients (no evidence of additional benefit in doses >360 mg/day).

**Note:** One time per day dosing is recommended at bedtime with Covera-HS®.

**Dosing adjustment in renal impairment:** $Cl_{cr}$ <10 mL/minute: Administer at 50% to 75% of normal dose.

Dialysis: Not dialyzable (0% to 5 %) via hemo- or peritoneal dialysis; supplemental dose is not necessary.

**Dosing adjustment/comments in hepatic disease:** Reduce dose in cirrhosis, reduce dose to 20% to 50% of normal and monitor EKG.

**Patient Information** Oral: Take as directed, around-the-clock. Do not alter dosage or discontinue therapy without consulting prescriber. Do not crush or chew extended release form. Avoid (or limit) alcohol and caffeine. You may experience dizziness or lightheadedness (use caution when driving or engaging in tasks requiring alertness until response to drug is known); nausea or vomiting (small frequent meals, frequent mouth care, chewing gum, or sucking lozenges may help); constipation (increased exercise, dietary fiber, fruit, or fluids may help); diarrhea (buttermilk, boiled milk, or yogurt may help). Report chest pain, palpitations, or irregular heartbeat; unusual cough, difficulty breathing, or swelling of extremities (feet/ankles); muscle tremors or weakness; confusion or acute lethargy; or skin irritation or rash.

**Nursing Implications** Do not crush sustained release drug product

**Dosage Forms**

Capsule, as hydrochloride, sustained release (Verelan®): 120 mg, 180 mg, 240 mg, 360 mg

Injection, as hydrochloride: 2.5 mg/mL (2 mL, 4 mL)

Isoptin®: 2.5 mg/mL (2 mL, 4 mL)

Tablet, as hydrochloride: 40 mg, 80 mg, 120 mg

Calan®, Isoptin®: 40 mg, 80 mg, 120 mg

Tablet, as hydrochloride, sustained release: 180 mg, 240 mg

Calan® SR, Isoptin® SR: 120 mg, 180 mg, 240 mg

Covera-HS®: 180 mg, 240 mg

- **Vercyte®** *see* Pipobroman *on page 448*
- **Verdiana®** *see* Deslanoside *on page 156*
- **Verelan®** *see* Verapamil *on page 583*
- **Vergon® [OTC]** *see* Meclizine *on page 335*
- **Vermizine®** *see* Piperazine *on page 448*
- **Vermox®** *see* Mebendazole *on page 334*
- **Verr-Canth™** *see* Cantharidin *on page 87*
- **Verrex-C&M®** *see* Podophyllin and Salicylic Acid *on page 451*
- **Versacaps®** *see* Guaifenesin and Pseudoephedrine *on page 257*
- **Versed®** *see* Midazolam *on page 365*
- **Vesanoid®** *see* Tretinoin, Oral *on page 561*
- **Vesprin®** *see* Triflupromazine *on page 567*
- **Vexol® Ophthalmic Suspension** *see* Rimexolone *on page 495*
- **Viagra®** *see* Sildenafil *on page 511*
- **Vibramycin® Injection** *see* Doxycycline *on page 186*
- **Vibramycin® Oral** *see* Doxycycline *on page 186*
- **Vibra-Tabs®** *see* Doxycycline *on page 186*
- **Vicks® 44D Cough & Head Congestion** *see* Pseudoephedrine and Dextromethorphan *on page 479*
- **Vicks® 44E [OTC]** *see* Guaifenesin and Dextromethorphan *on page 257*
- **Vicks® 44 Non-Drowsy Cold & Cough Liqui-Caps [OTC]** *see* Pseudoephedrine and Dextromethorphan *on page 479*
- **Vicks Children's Chloraseptic® [OTC]** *see* Benzocaine *on page 61*
- **Vicks Chloraseptic® Sore Throat [OTC]** *see* Benzocaine *on page 61*
- **Vicks® DayQuil® Allergy Relief 4 Hour Tablet [OTC]** *see* Brompheniramine and Phenylpropanolamine *on page 74*
- **Vicks® DayQuil® Sinus Pressure & Congestion Relief [OTC]** *see* Guaifenesin and Phenylpropanolamine *on page 257*
- **Vicks Formula 44® [OTC]** *see* Dextromethorphan *on page 160*
- **Vicks Formula 44® Pediatric Formula [OTC]** *see* Dextromethorphan *on page 160*
- **Vicks® Pediatric Formula 44E [OTC]** *see* Guaifenesin and Dextromethorphan *on page 257*
- **Vicks Sinex® Nasal Solution [OTC]** *see* Phenylephrine *on page 439*
- **Vicodin®** *see* Hydrocodone and Acetaminophen *on page 272*
- **Vicodin® ES** *see* Hydrocodone and Acetaminophen *on page 272*
- **Vicodin® HP** *see* Hydrocodone and Acetaminophen *on page 272*
- **Vicon-C® [OTC]** *see* Vitamin B Complex With Vitamin C *on page 586*
- **Vicon Forte®** *see* Vitamins, Multiple *on page 587*
- **Vicon® Plus [OTC]** *see* Vitamins, Multiple *on page 587*
- **Vicoprofen®** *see* Hydrocodone and Ibuprofen *on page 273*

## Vidarabine (vye DARE a been)

**U.S. Brand Names** Vira-A® Ophthalmic

**Pharmacologic Category** Antiviral Agent, Ophthalmic

**Use** Treatment of acute keratoconjunctivitis and epithelial keratitis due to herpes simplex virus type 1 and 2; superficial keratitis caused by herpes simplex virus

**Effects on Mental Status** None reported

**Effects on Psychiatric Treatment** None reported

**Usual Dosage** Children and Adults: Ophthalmic: Keratoconjunctivitis: Instill ½" of ointment in lower conjunctival sac 5 times/day every 3 hours while awake until complete re-epithelialization has occurred, then twice daily for an additional 7 days

**Dosage Forms** Ointment, ophthalmic, as monohydrate: 3% [30 mg/mL = 28 mg/mL base] (3.5 g)

- **Videx®** *see* Didanosine *on page 166*

## Vinblastine (vin BLAS teen)

**U.S. Brand Names** Alkaban-AQ®; Velban®

**Pharmacologic Category** Antineoplastic Agent, Natural Source (Plant) Derivative

**Use** Treatment of Hodgkin's and non-Hodgkin's lymphoma, testicular, lung, head and neck, breast, and renal carcinomas, Mycosis fungoides, Kaposi's sarcoma, histiocytosis, choriocarcinoma, and idiopathic thrombocytopenic purpura

**Effects on Mental Status** May cause depression

**Effects on Psychiatric Treatment** Bone marrow suppression is common; use caution with clozapine and carbamazepine

**Usual Dosage** Refer to individual protocols. Varies depending upon clinical and hematological response. Give at intervals of at least 14 days and only after leukocyte count has returned to at least 4000/mm$^3$; maintenance therapy should be titrated according to leukocyte count. Dosage should be reduced in patients with recent exposure to radiation therapy or chemotherapy; single doses in these patients should not exceed 5.5 mg/m$^2$.

Children and Adults: I.V.: 4-20 mg/m$^2$ (0.1-0.5 mg/kg) every 7-10 days **or** 5-day continuous infusion of 1.5-2 mg/m$^2$/day **or** 0.1-0.5 mg/kg/week

**Dosing adjustment in hepatic impairment:**

Serum bilirubin 1.5-3.0 mg/dL or AST 60-180 units: Administer 50% of normal dose

Serum bilirubin 3.0-5.0 mg/dL: Administer 25% of dose

Serum bilirubin >5.0 mg/dL or AST >180 units: Omit dose

**Dosage Forms**

Injection, as sulfate: 1 mg/mL (10 mL)

Powder for injection, as sulfate: 10 mg

- **Vincasar® PFS™ Injection** *see* Vincristine *on page 584*

## Vincristine (vin KRIS teen)

**U.S. Brand Names** Oncovin® Injection; Vincasar® PFS™ Injection

**Pharmacologic Category** Antineoplastic Agent, Natural Source (Plant) Derivative

**Use** Treatment of leukemias, Hodgkin's disease, non-Hodgkin's lymphomas, Wilms' tumor, neuroblastoma, rhabdomyosarcoma

**Effects on Mental Status** May cause sedation, confusion, depression, or insomnia

**Effects on Psychiatric Treatment** May cause myelosuppression; use caution with clozapine and carbamazepine

**Usual Dosage** Refer to individual protocols as dosages vary with protocol used; adjustments are made depending upon clinical and hematological response and upon adverse reactions

Children ≤10 kg or BSA <1 m$^2$: Initial therapy: 0.05 mg/kg once weekly then titrate dose; maximum single dose: 2 mg

Children >10 kg or BSA ≥1 m$^2$: 1-2 mg/m$^2$, may repeat once weekly for 3-6 weeks; maximum single dose: 2 mg

Neuroblastoma: I.V. continuous infusion with doxorubicin: 1 mg/m$^2$/day for 72 hours

Adults: I.V.: 0.4-1.4 mg/m$^2$ (up to 2 mg maximum in most patients); may repeat every week

**Dosing adjustment in hepatic impairment:**

Serum bilirubin 1.5-3.0 mg/dL or AST 60-180 units: Administer 50% of normal dose

Serum bilirubin 3.0-5.0 mg/dL: Administer 25% of dose

Serum bilirubin >5.0 mg/dL or AST >180 units: Omit dose

The average total dose per course of treatment should be around 2-2.5 mg; some recommend capping the dose at 2 mg maximum to reduce toxicity; however, it is felt that this measure can reduce the efficacy of the drug

**Dosage Forms** Injection, as sulfate: 1 mg/mL (1 mL, 2 mL, 5 mL)

## Vindesine (VIN de seen)

**Pharmacologic Category** Antineoplastic Agent, Natural Source (Plant) Derivative

**Use** Management of acute lymphocytic leukemia, chronic myelogenous leukemia, breast, head and neck and lung cancers, and lymphomas (Hodgkin's and non-Hodgkin's)

**Effects on Mental Status** Drowsiness is common

**Effects on Psychiatric Treatment** Leukopenia is common; avoid clozapine and carbamazepine

**Usual Dosage** Refer to individual protocols

3-4 mg/m$^2$/week

1-2 mg/m$^2$ days 1 and 2 every 2 weeks

1-2 mg/m$^2$ days 1-5 (continuous infusion) every 2-4 weeks

1-2 mg/m$^2$ days 1-5 every 3-4 weeks

**Dosage adjustment in hepatic impairment:** Dosage reductions of 50% to 75% have been suggested for "severe" hepatic dysfunction; however, specific guidelines have not been published

**Dosage Forms** Powder for injection: 5 mg

## Vinorelbine (vi NOR el been)

**U.S. Brand Names** Navelbine®

**Pharmacologic Category** Antineoplastic Agent, Natural Source (Plant) Derivative

**Use** Treatment of nonsmall cell lung cancer (as a single agent or in combination with cisplatin)

**Unlabeled use:** Breast cancer, ovarian carcinoma (cisplatin-resistant), Hodgkin's disease

**Effects on Mental Status** May cause drowsiness

**Effects on Psychiatric Treatment** Bone marrow suppression is common; avoid clozapine and carbamazepine

**Usual Dosage** Refer to individual protocols; varies depending upon clinical and hematological response

Adults: I.V.: 30 mg/m$^2$ every 7 days

**Dosage adjustment in hematological toxicity**: Granulocyte counts should be ≥1000 cells/mm$^3$ prior to the administration of vinorelbine. Adjustments in the dosage of vinorelbine should be based on granulocyte counts obtained on the day of treatment as follows:

Granulocytes ≥1500 cells/mm$^3$ on day of treatment: Administer 30 mg/m$^2$

Granulocytes 1000-1499 cells/mm$^3$ on day of treatment: Administer 15 mg/m$^2$

Granulocytes <1000 cells/mm$^3$ on day of treatment: Do not administer. Repeat granulocyte count in one week; if 3 consecutive doses are held because granulocyte count is <1000 cells/mm$^3$, discontinue vinorelbine

For patients who, during treatment, have experienced fever and/or sepsis while granulocytopenic or had 2 consecutive weekly doses held due to granulocytopenia, subsequent doses of vinorelbine should be:

22.5 mg/m$^2$ for granulocytes ≥1500 cells/mm$^3$

11.25 mg/m$^2$ for granulocytes 1000-1499 cells/mm$^3$

**Dosage adjustment in renal impairment:** No dose adjustments are required for renal insufficiency. If moderate or severe neurotoxicity develops, discontinue vinorelbine.

**Dosing adjustment in hepatic impairment:** Vinorelbine should be administered with caution in patients with hepatic insufficiency. In patients who develop hyperbilirubinemia during treatment with vinorelbine, the dose should be adjusted for total bilirubin as follows:

Serum bilirubin ≤2 mg/dL: Administer 30 mg/m$^2$

Serum bilirubin 2.1-3 mg/dL: Administer 15 mg/m$^2$

Serum bilirubin >3 mg/dL: Administer 7.5 mg/m$^2$

**Dosing adjustment in patients with concurrent hematologic toxicity and hepatic impairment:** Administer the lower doses determined from the above recommendations

**Dosage Forms** Injection, as tartrate: 10 mg/mL (1 mL, 5 mL)


♦ **Vioform® [OTC]** *see* Clioquinol *on page 129*

♦ **Viokase®** *see* Pancrelipase *on page 418*

♦ **Viosterol** *see* Ergocalciferol *on page 198*

♦ **Vioxx®** *see* Rofecoxib *on page 499*

♦ **Vira-A® Ophthalmic** *see* Vidarabine *on page 584*

♦ **Viracept®** *see* Nelfinavir *on page 387*

♦ **Viramune®** *see* Nevirapine *on page 390*

♦ **Virazole® Aerosol** *see* Ribavirin *on page 492*

♦ **Virilon®** *see* Methyltestosterone *on page 360*

♦ **Viroptic® Ophthalmic** *see* Trifluridine *on page 568*

♦ **Viscoat®** *see* Chondroitin Sulfate-Sodium Hyaluronate *on page 122*

♦ **Visine® Extra Ophthalmic [OTC]** *see* Tetrahydrozoline *on page 538*

♦ **Visine® L.R. Ophthalmic [OTC]** *see* Oxymetazoline *on page 415*

♦ **Visken®** *see* Pindolol *on page 446*

♦ **Vistacon-50®** *see* Hydroxyzine *on page 278*

♦ **Vistaquel®** *see* Hydroxyzine *on page 278*

♦ **Vistaril®** *see* Hydroxyzine *on page 278*

♦ **Vistazine®** *see* Hydroxyzine *on page 278*

♦ **Vistide®** *see* Cidofovir *on page 122*

♦ **Vita-C® [OTC]** *see* Ascorbic Acid *on page 48*

♦ **VitaCarn® Oral** *see* Levocarnitine *on page 312*


## Vitamin A (VYE ta min aye)

**U.S. Brand Names** Aquasol A®; Del-Vi-A®; Palmitate-A® 5000 [OTC]

**Pharmacologic Category** Vitamin, Fat Soluble

**Use** Treatment and prevention of vitamin A deficiency

**Effects on Mental Status** None reported

**Effects on Psychiatric Treatment** None reported

**Usual Dosage**

RDA:

<1 year: 375 mcg

1-3 years: 400 mcg

4-6 years: 500 mcg*

7-10 years: 700 mcg*

>10 years: 800-1000 mcg*

Male: 1000 mcg

Female: 800 mcg

* mcg retinol equivalent (0.3 mcg retinol = 1 unit vitamin A)

Vitamin A supplementation in measles (recommendation of the World Health Organization): Children: Oral: Administer as a single dose; repeat the next day and at 4 weeks for children with ophthalmologic evidence of vitamin A deficiency:

6 months to 1 year: 100,000 units

>1 year: 200,000 units

**Note:** Use of vitamin A in measles is recommended only for patients 6 months to 2 years of age hospitalized with measles and its complications **or** patients >6 months of age who have any of the following risk factors and who are not already receiving vitamin A: immunodeficiency, ophthalmologic evidence of vitamin A deficiency including night blindness, Bitot's spots or evidence of xerophthalmia, impaired intestinal absorption, moderate to severe malnutrition including that associated with eating disorders, or recent immigration from areas where high mortality rates from measles have been observed

**Note:** Monitor patients closely; dosages >25,000 units/kg have been associated with toxicity

Severe deficiency with xerophthalmia: Oral:

Children 1-8 years: 5000-10,000 units/kg/day for 5 days or until recovery occurs

Children >8 years and Adults: 500,000 units/day for 3 days, then 50,000 units/day for 14 days, then 10,000-20,000 units/day for 2 months

Deficiency (without corneal changes): Oral:

Infants <1 year: 100,000 units every 4-6 months

Children 1-8 years: 200,000 units every 4-6 months

Children >8 years and Adults: 100,000 units/day for 3 days then 50,000 units/day for 14 days

Malabsorption syndrome (prophylaxis): Children >8 years and Adults: Oral: 10,000-50,000 units/day of water miscible product

Dietary supplement: Oral:

Infants up to 6 months: 1500 units/day

Children:

6 months to 3 years: 1500-2000 units/day

4-6 years: 2500 units/day

7-10 years: 3300-3500 units/day

Children >10 years and Adults: 4000-5000 units/day

**Dosage Forms**

Capsule: 10,000 units [OTC], 25,000 units, 50,000 units

(Continued)

## Vitamin A *(Continued)*

Drops, oral (water miscible) [OTC]: 5000 units/0.1 mL (30 mL)
Injection: 50,000 units/mL (2 mL)
Tablet [OTC]: 5000 units

## Vitamin A and Vitamin D (VYE ta min aye & VYE ta min dee)

**U.S. Brand Names** A and D™ Ointment [OTC]
**Pharmacologic Category** Topical Skin Product
**Use** Temporary relief of discomfort due to chapped skin, diaper rash, minor burns, abrasions, as well as irritations associated with ostomy skin care
**Effects on Mental Status** None reported
**Effects on Psychiatric Treatment** None reported
**Usual Dosage** Topical: Apply locally with gentle massage as needed
**Dosage Forms** Ointment, topical: In a lanolin-petrolatum base (60 g)

♦ **Vitamin $B_1$** *see* Thiamine *on page 542*

♦ **Vitamin $B_2$** *see* Riboflavin *on page 492*

♦ **Vitamin $B_3$** *see* Niacin *on page 391*

♦ **Vitamin $B_{12}$** *see* Cyanocobalamin *on page 143*

## Vitamin B Complex (VYE ta min bee KOM pleks)

**U.S. Brand Names** Apatate® [OTC]; Gevrabon® [OTC]; Lederplex® [OTC]; Lipovite® [OTC]; Mega B® [OTC]; Megaton™ [OTC]; Mucoplex® [OTC]; NeoVadrin® B Complex [OTC]; Orexin® [OTC]; Surbex® [OTC]
**Pharmacologic Category** Vitamin, Water Soluble
**Use** Supportive nutritional supplementation in conditions in which water-soluble vitamins are required like GI disorders, chronic alcoholism, pregnancy, severe burns, and recovery from surgery
**Effects on Mental Status** None reported
**Effects on Psychiatric Treatment** None reported
**Usual Dosage** Dosage is usually 1 tablet or capsule/day; please refer to package insert
**Dosage Forms**
Capsule
Solution: 5 mL, 360 mL

## Vitamin B Complex With Vitamin C
(VYE ta min bee KOM pleks with VYE ta min see)

**U.S. Brand Names** Allbee® With C [OTC]; Surbex-T® Filmtabs® [OTC]; Surbex® With C Filmtabs® [OTC]; Thera-Combex® H-P Kapseals® [OTC]; Vicon-C® [OTC]
**Pharmacologic Category** Vitamin, Water Soluble
**Use** Supportive nutritional supplementation in conditions in which water-soluble vitamins are required like GI disorders, chronic alcoholism, pregnancy, severe burns, and recovery from surgery
**Effects on Mental Status** None reported
**Effects on Psychiatric Treatment** None reported
**Usual Dosage** Adults: Oral: 1 every day
**Dosage Forms** Actual vitamin content may vary slightly depending on product used
Tablet/capsule: Vitamin $B_1$ 10-15 mg, vitamin $B_2$ 10 mg, vitamin $B_3$ 100 mg, vitamin $B_5$ 20 mg, vitamin $B_6$ 2-5 mg, vitamin $B_{12}$ 6-10 mg, vitamin C 300-500 mg

## Vitamin B Complex With Vitamin C and Folic Acid
(VYE ta min bee KOM pleks with VYE ta min see & FOE lik AS id)

**U.S. Brand Names** Berocca®; Nephrocaps®
**Pharmacologic Category** Vitamin, Water Soluble
**Use** Supportive nutritional supplementation in conditions in which water-soluble vitamins are required like GI disorders, chronic alcoholism, pregnancy, severe burns, and recovery from surgery
**Effects on Mental Status** None reported
**Effects on Psychiatric Treatment** None reported
**Usual Dosage** Adults: Oral: 1 every day
**Dosage Forms** Capsule

♦ **Vitamin $D_2$** *see* Ergocalciferol *on page 198*

## Vitamin E (VYE ta min ee)

**Generic Available** Yes
**U.S. Brand Names** Amino-Opti-E® [OTC]; Aquasol E® [OTC]; E-Complex-600® [OTC]; E-Vitamin® [OTC]; Vita-Plus® E Softgels® [OTC]; Vitec® [OTC]; Vite E® Creme [OTC]
**Synonyms** *d*-Alpha Tocopherol; *dl*-Alpha Tocopherol
**Pharmacologic Category** Vitamin, Fat Soluble
**Use** Prevention and treatment hemolytic anemia secondary to vitamin E deficiency, dietary supplement
**Unlabeled uses:** To reduce the risk of bronchopulmonary dysplasia or retrolental fibroplasia in infants exposed to high concentrations of oxygen; prevention and treatment of tardive dyskinesia and Alzheimer's disease
**Effects on Mental Status** May rarely cause drowsiness
**Effects on Psychiatric Treatment** Used to prevent or treat tardive dyskinesia and Alzheimer's disease
**Pregnancy Risk Factor** A (C if dose exceeds RDA recommendation)
**Contraindications** Hypersensitivity to vitamin E or any component; I.V. route
**Warnings/Precautions** May induce vitamin K deficiency; necrotizing enterocolitis has been associated with oral administration of large dosages (eg, >200 units/day) of a hyperosmolar vitamin E preparation in low birth weight infants
**Adverse Reactions** <1%: Blurred vision, contact dermatitis with topical preparation, diarrhea, fatigue, gonadal dysfunction, headache, intestinal cramps, nausea, weakness
**Drug Interactions**
Cholestyramine (and colestipol): May reduce absorption of vitamin E
Iron: Vitamin E may impair the hematologic response to iron in children with iron-deficiency anemia; monitor
Orlistat: May reduce absorption of vitamin E
Warfarin: Vitamin E may alter the effect of vitamin K actions on clotting factors resulting in an increase hypoprothrombinemic response to warfarin; monitor
**Stability** Protect from light
**Mechanism of Action** Prevents oxidation of vitamin A and C; protects polyunsaturated fatty acids in membranes from attack by free radicals and protects red blood cells against hemolysis
**Pharmacodynamics/kinetics**
Absorption: Oral: Depends upon the presence of bile; absorption is reduced in conditions of malabsorption, in low birth weight premature infants, and as dosage increases; water miscible preparations are better absorbed than oil preparations
Distribution: Distributes to all body tissues, especially adipose tissue, where it is stored
Metabolism: In the liver to glucuronides
Elimination: In feces and bile
**Usual Dosage** One unit of vitamin E = 1 mg *dl*-alpha-tocopherol acetate.
Oral:
Vitamin E deficiency:
Children (with malabsorption syndrome): 1 unit/kg/day of water miscible vitamin E (to raise plasma tocopherol concentrations to the normal range within 2 months and to maintain normal plasma concentrations)
Adults: 60-75 units/day
Prevention of vitamin E deficiency: Adults: 30 units/day
Prevention of retinopathy of prematurity or BPD secondary to $O_2$ therapy: (American Academy of Pediatrics considers this use investigational and routine use is not recommended):
Retinopathy prophylaxis: 15-30 units/kg/day to maintain plasma levels between 1.5-2 μg/mL (may need as high as 100 units/kg/day)
Cystic fibrosis, beta-thalassemia, sickle cell anemia may require higher daily maintenance doses:
Cystic fibrosis: 100-400 units/day
Beta-thalassemia: 750 units/day
Sickle cell: 450 units/day
Alzheimer's disease: 1000 units twice daily
Tardive dyskinesia: 1600 units/day
Recommended daily allowance:
Premature infants ≤3 months: 17 mg (25 units)
Infants:
≤6 months: 3 mg (4.5 units)
6-12 months: 4 mg (6 units)
Children:
1-3 years: 6 mg (9 units)
4-10 years: 7 mg (10.5 units)
Children >11 years and Adults:
Male: 10 mg (15 units)
Female: 8 mg (12 units)
Topical: Apply a thin layer over affected area
**Reference Range** Therapeutic: 0.8-1.5 mg/dL (SI: 19-35 μmol/L), some method variation
**Patient Information** Drops can be placed directly in the mouth or mixed with cereal, fruit juice, or other food; take only the prescribed dose. Vitamin E toxicity appears as blurred vision, diarrhea, dizziness, flu-like symptoms, nausea, headache; swallow capsules whole, do not crush or chew
**Additional Information** 1 mg dl-alpha tocopheryl acetate = 1 IU
**Dosage Forms**
Capsule: 100 units, 200 units, 330 mg, 400 units, 500 units, 600 units, 1000 units
Capsule, water miscible: 73.5 mg, 147 mg, 165 mg, 330 mg, 400 units
Cream: 50 mg/g (15 g, 30 g, 60 g, 75 g, 120 g, 454 g)
Drops, oral: 50 mg/mL (12 mL, 30 mL)

Liquid, topical: 10 mL, 15 mL, 30 mL, 60 mL
Lotion: 120 mL
Oil: 15 mL, 30 mL, 60 mL
Ointment, topical: 30 mg/g (45 g, 60 g)
Tablet: 200 units, 400 units

- **Vitamin G** *see* Riboflavin *on page 492*
- **Vitamin $K_1$** *see* Phytonadione *on page 444*

## Vitamins, Multiple (VYE ta mins, MUL ti pul)

**U.S. Brand Names** Becotin® Pulvules®; Cefol® Filmtab®; Eldercaps® [OTC]; NeoVadrin® [OTC]; Niferex®-PN; Secran®; Stresstabs® 600 Advanced Formula Tablets [OTC]; Therabid® [OTC]; Theragran® [OTC]; Theragran® Hematinic®; Theragran® Liquid [OTC]; Theragran-M® [OTC]; Unicap® [OTC]; Vicon Forte®; Vicon® Plus [OTC]
**Pharmacologic Category** Vitamin
**Use** Dietary supplement
**Effects on Mental Status** None reported
**Effects on Psychiatric Treatment** None reported
**Usual Dosage**
Infants 1.5-3 kg: I.V.: 3.25 mL/24 hours (M.V.I.® Pediatric)
Children:
Oral:
≤2 years: Drops: 1 mL/day (premature infants may get 0.5-1 mL/day)
>2 years: Chew 1 tablet/day
≥4 years: 5 mL/day liquid
I.V.: >3 kg and <11 years: 5 mL/24 hours (M.V.I.® Pediatric)
Adults:
Oral: 1 tablet/day or 5 mL/day liquid
I.V.: >11 years: 5 mL of vials 1 and 2 (M.V.I.®-12)/one TPN bag/day
I.V. solutions: 10 mL/24 hours (M.V.I.®-12)
**Dosage Forms**
Theragran® (content per 5 mL, liquid):
A 10,000 IU, D 400 IU, C 200 mg, $B_1$ 10 mg, $B_2$ 10 mg, $B_3$ 100 mg, $B_6$ 4.1 mg, $B_{12}$ 5 mcg, $B_5$ 21.4 mg
Vi-Daylin® (content per 1 mL, drops):
A 1500 IU, D 400 IU, E 4.1 IU, C 35 mg, $B_1$ 0.5 mg, $B_2$ 0.6 mg, $B_3$ 8 mg, $B_6$ 0.4 mg, $B_{12}$ 1.5 mcg, alcohol <0.5%
Vi-Daylin® Iron (content per 1 mL):
A 1500 IU, D 400 IU, E 4.1 IU, C 35 mg, $B_1$ 0.5 mg, $B_2$ 0.6 mg, $B_3$ 8 mg, $B_6$ 0.4 mg, Fe 10 mg
Albee® with C (content per tablet):
C 300 mg, $B_1$ 15 mg, $B_2$ 10.2 mg, $B_6$ 5 mg, niacinamide 50 mg, pantothenic acid 10 mg
Vitamin B complex (content per tablet):
FA 400 mcg, $B_1$ 1.5 mg, $B_2$ 1.7 mg, $B_6$ 2 mg, $B_{12}$ 6 mcg, niacinamide 20 mg
Hexavitamin (content per cap/tab):
A 5000 IU, D 400 IU, C 75 mg, $B_1$ 2 mg, $B_2$ 3 mg, $B_3$ 20 mg
Iberet-Folic-500® (content per tablet):
C 500 mg, FA 0.8 mg, $B_1$ 6 mg, $B_2$ 6 mg, $B_3$ 30 mg, $B_6$ 5 mg, $B_{12}$ 25 mcg, $B_5$ 10 mg, Fe 105 mg
Stuartnatal® 1+1 (content per tablet):
A 4000 IU, D 400 IU, E 11 IU, C 120 mg, FA 1 mg, $B_1$ 1.5 mg, $B_2$ 3 mg, $B_3$ 20 mg, $B_6$ 10 mg, $B_{12}$ 12 mcg, Cu, Zn 25 mg, Fe 65 mg, Ca 200 mg
Theragran-M® (content per tablet):
A 5000 IU, D 400 IU, E 30 IU, C 90 mg, FA 0.4 mg, $B_1$ 3 mg, $B_2$ 3.4 mg, $B_3$ 30 mg, $B_6$ 3 mg, $B_{12}$ 9 mcg, Cl, Cr, I, K, $B_5$ 10 mg, Mg, Mn, Mo, P, Se, Zn 15 mg, Fe 27 mg, biotin 30 mcg, beta-carotene 1250 IU
Vi-Daylin® (content per tablet):
A 2500 IU, D 400 IU, E 15 IU, C 60 mg, FA 0.3 mg, $B_1$ 1.05 mg, $B_2$ 1.2 mg, $B_3$ 13.5 mg, $B_6$ 1.05 mg, $B_{12}$ 4.5 mcg
M.V.I.®-12 injection (content per 5 mL):
A 3300 IU, D 200 IU, E 10 IU, C 100 mg, FA 0.4 mg, $B_1$ 3 mg, $B_2$ 3.6 mg, $B_3$ 40 mg, $B_6$ 4 mg, $B_{12}$ 5 mcg, $B_5$ 15 mg, biotin 60 mcg
M.V.I.® pediatric powder (content per 5 mL):
A 2300 IU, D 400 IU, E 7 IU, C 80 mg, FA 0.14 mg, $B_1$ 1.2 mg, $B_2$ 1.4 mg, $B_3$ 17 mg, $B_6$ 1 mg, $B_{12}$ 1 mcg, $B_5$ 5 mg, biotin 20 mcg, vitamin K 200 mcg

- **Vita-Plus® E Softgels® [OTC]** *see* Vitamin E *on page 586*
- **Vitec® [OTC]** *see* Vitamin E *on page 586*
- **Vite E® Creme [OTC]** *see* Vitamin E *on page 586*
- ***Vitex agnus-castus*** *see* Chaste Tree *on page 107*
- **Vitrasert®** *see* Ganciclovir *on page 245*
- **Vivactil®** *see* Protriptyline *on page 477*
- **Viva-Drops® Solution [OTC]** *see* Artificial Tears *on page 48*
- **Vivelle® Transdermal** *see* Estradiol *on page 203*
- **V-Lax® [OTC]** *see* Psyllium *on page 479*
- **Volmax®** *see* Albuterol *on page 22*
- **Voltaren® Ophthalmic** *see* Diclofenac *on page 163*
- **Voltaren® Oral** *see* Diclofenac *on page 163*
- **Voltaren®-XR Oral** *see* Diclofenac *on page 163*
- **Vontrol®** *see* Diphenidol *on page 175*
- **Vumon Injection** *see* Teniposide *on page 534*
- **V.V.S.®** *see* Sulfabenzamide, Sulfacetamide, and Sulfathiazole *on page 522*
- **Vytone® Topical** *see* Iodoquinol and Hydrocortisone *on page 291*

## Warfarin (WAR far in)

**U.S. Brand Names** Coumadin®
**Canadian Brand Names** Warfilone®
**Pharmacologic Category** Anticoagulant, Coumarin Derivative
**Use** Prophylaxis and treatment of venous thrombosis, pulmonary embolism and thromboembolic disorders; atrial fibrillation with risk of embolism and as an adjunct in the prophylaxis of systemic embolism after myocardial infarction
**Unlabeled use:** Prevention of recurrent transient ischemic attacks and to reduce risk of recurrent myocardial infarction
**Effects on Mental Status** None reported
**Effects on Psychiatric Treatment** May cause leukopenia; use caution with clozapine and carbamazepine; barbiturates and carbamazepine may decrease the anticoagulant effect of warfarin; chloral hydrate, alcohol, disulfiram, and SSRIs may enhance the anticoagulant effect
**Pregnancy Risk Factor** D
**Contraindications** Hypersensitivity to warfarin or any component of the product; pregnancy; hemorrhagic tendencies; hemophilia; thrombocytopenia purpura; leukemia; recent or potential surgery of the eye or CNS; major regional lumbar block anesthesia or surgery resulting in large, open surfaces; patients bleeding from the GI, respiratory, or GU tract; threatened abortion; aneurysm; ascorbic acid deficiency; history of bleeding diathesis; prostatectomy; continuous tube drainage of the small intestine; polyarthritis; diverticulitis; emaciation; malnutrition; cerebrovascular hemorrhage; eclampsia/pre-eclampsia; blood dyscrasias; severe uncontrolled or malignant hypertension; severe hepatic disease; pericarditis or pericardial effusion; subacute bacterial endocarditis; visceral carcinoma; following spinal puncture and other diagnostic or therapeutic procedures with potential for significant bleeding; history of warfarin-induced necrosis; an unreliable, noncompliant patient; alcoholism; patient who has a history of falls or is a significant fall risk
**Warnings/Precautions** Cautious use in severe renal disease, although has been used. Hemorrhage is the most serious risk. Have patient report any signs or symptoms of bleeding or any falls or accidents immediately. Patient must also report any new or discontinued medications, herbal or alternative products used, significant changes in smoking or eating habits. Necrosis or gangrene of the skin and other tissues can rarely occur due to early hypercoagulability. "Purple toes syndrome," due to cholesterol microembolization, may rarely occur (often after several weeks of therapy). Women may be at risk of developing ovarian hemorrhage at the time of ovulation. Use with caution in traumas, infection (antibiotics and fever may alter affects), renal insufficiency, prolonged dietary insufficiencies (vitamin K deficiency), moderate-severe hypertension, polycythemia vera, vasculitis, open wound, active TB, history of PUD, anaphylactic disorders, indwelling catheters, severe diabetes, and menstruating and postpartum women. Use with caution in protein C deficiency. The elderly may be more sensitive. Use care in selection of patients appropriate for this treatment. Ensure patient cooperation especially from the alcoholic, illicit drug user, demented, or psychotic patient.
**Adverse Reactions**
1% to 10%:
Dermatologic: Skin lesions, alopecia, skin necrosis
Gastrointestinal: Anorexia, nausea, vomiting, stomach cramps, diarrhea
Hematologic: Hemorrhage, leukopenia, unrecognized bleeding sites (eg, colon cancer) may be uncovered by anticoagulation
Respiratory: Hemoptysis
<1%: Agranulocytosis, anorexia, discolored toes (blue or purple), fever, hepatotoxicity, mouth ulcers, rash, renal damage
**Overdosage/Toxicology** See table on next page.
Signs and symptoms: Internal or external hemorrhage, hematuria
Treatment: Avoid emesis and lavage to avoid the possible trauma and incidental bleeding. When overdose occurs, the drug should be immediately discontinued and vitamin $K_1$ (phytonadione) may be administered 1-5 mg I.V. for children or up to 25 mg I.V. for adults. When hemorrhaging occurs, fresh frozen plasma transfusions can help control bleeding by replacing clotting factors. In urgent bleeding, prothrombin complex concentrates may be needed.
**Drug Interactions** CYP1A2 enzyme substrate (minor), CYP2C8, 2C9, 2C18, 2C19, and 3A3/4 enzyme substrate; CYP2C9 enzyme inhibitor
**Decreased anticoagulant effects:** (Decreased anticoagulant effect may occur when these drugs are administered with oral anticoagulants.)
(Continued)

## Warfarin *(Continued)*

Induction of enzymes: Barbiturates, carbamazepine, glutethimide, griseofulvin, nafcillin, phenytoin, rifampin

Increased procoagulant factors: Estrogens, oral contraceptives, vitamin K (including nutritional supplements)

Decreased drug absorption: Aluminum hydroxide, cholestyramine*, colestipol*

Other: Ethchlorvynol, griseofulvin, spironolactone**, sucralfate

*Cholestyramine and colestipol may increase the anticoagulant effect by binding vitamin K in the gut; yet, the decreased drug absorption appears to be of more concern.

**Diuretic-induced hemoconcentration with subsequent concentration of clotting factors has been reported to decrease the effects of oral anticoagulants.

**Increased bleeding tendency:** (Use of these agents with oral anticoagulants may increase the chances of hemorrhage.)

Inhibit platelet aggregation: Cephalosporins, dipyridamole, indomethacin, oxyphenbutazone, penicillin (parenteral), phenylbutazone, salicylates, sulfinpyrazone

Inhibit procoagulant factors: Antimetabolites, quinidine, quinine, salicylates

Ulcerogenic drugs: Adrenal corticosteroids, indomethacin, oxyphenbutazone, phenylbutazone, potassium products, salicylates

**Enhanced anticoagulant effects:**

Decrease Vitamin K: Oral antibiotics can increase or decrease INR. Check INR 3 days after patient begins antibiotics to see the INR value and adjust the warfarin dose accordingly.

Displace anticoagulant: Chloral hydrate, clofibrate, diazoxide, ethacrynic acid, miconazole, nalidixic acid, phenylbutazone, salicylates, sulfonamides, sulfonylureas

Inhibit Metabolism: Alcohol (acute ingestion)*, allopurinol, amiodarone, azole antibiotics, chloramphenicol, chlorpropamide, cimetidine, ciprofloxacin, co-trimoxazole, disulfiram, flutamide, isoniazid, metronidazole, norfloxacin, ofloxacin, omeprazole, phenylbutazone, phenytoin, propafenone, propoxyphene, quinidine, sulfinpyrazone, sulfonamides, tamoxifen, tolbutamide, zafirlukast, zileuton

Other: Acetaminophen, anabolic steroids, capecitabine, celecoxib, clarithromycin, clofibrate, danazol, erythromycin, gemfibrozil, glucagon, influenza vaccine, propranolol, propylthiouracil, ranitidine, rofecoxib, SSRIs, sulindac, tetracycline, thyroid drugs, vitamin E (≥400 int. units)

*The hypoprothrombinemic effect of oral anticoagulants has been reported to be both increased and decreased during chronic and excessive alcohol ingestion. Data are insufficient to predict the direction of this interaction in alcoholic patients.

| INR | Patient Situation | Action |
|---|---|---|
| >3 and ≤6 | No bleeding or need for rapid reversal (ie, no need for surgery) | Omit next few warfarin doses and restart at lower dose when INR ≤3.0 |
| >6 and <10.0 | No bleeding but in need of rapid reversal for surgery | Stop warfarin and give phytonadione 0.5-1 mg I.V.; repeat 0.5 mg phytonadione I.V. if INR >3 after 24 hours; restart warfarin at a lower dose |
| >10.0 and <20.0 | No bleeding | Stop warfarin, give phytonadione 3-5 mg I.V.; check INR every 6-12 hours; repeat phytonadione if needed; reassess need and dose of warfarin |
| >20.0 | Serious bleeding or warfarin overdose | Stop warfarin, give phytonadione 10 mg I.V.; check INR every 6 hours, if needed, repeat phytonadione every 12 hours and give plasma transfusion or factor concentrate; consider giving heparin if warfarin still indicated |

**Usual Dosage**

Oral:

Infants and Children: 0.05-0.34 mg/kg/day; infants <12 months of age may require doses at or near the high end of this range; consistent anticoagulation may be difficult to maintain in children <5 years of age

Adults: 5-15 mg/day for 2-5 days, then adjust dose according to results of prothrombin time; usual maintenance dose ranges from 2-10 mg/day

I.V. (administer as a slow bolus injection): 2-5 mg/day

**Dosing adjustment/comments in hepatic disease:** Monitor effect at usual doses; the response to oral anticoagulants may be markedly enhanced in obstructive jaundice (due to reduced vitamin K absorption) and also in hepatitis and cirrhosis (due to decreased production of vitamin K-dependent clotting factors); prothrombin index should be closely monitored

**Dietary Considerations**

Alcohol: Chronic use of alcohol inhibits warfarin metabolism; avoid or limit use

Food:

Vitamin K: Foods high in vitamin K (eg, beef liver, pork liver, green tea and leafy green vegetables) inhibit anticoagulant effect. Do not change dietary habits once stabilized on warfarin therapy; a balanced diet with a consistent intake of vitamin K is essential; avoid large amounts of alfalfa, asparagus, broccoli, Brussels sprouts, cabbage, cauliflower, green teas, kale, lettuce, spinach, turnip greens, watercress. It is recommended that the diet contain a CONSISTENT vitamin K content of 70-140 mcg/day. Check with physician before changing diet.

Vitamin E: May increase warfarin effect; do not change dietary habits or vitamin supplements once stabilized on warfarin therapy

**Patient Information** Take exactly as directed; if dose is missed, take as soon as possible. Do not double doses. Do not take any medication your prescriber is not aware of and follow diet and activity as recommended by prescriber. You may have a tendency to bleed easily while taking this drug; brush teeth with soft brush, floss with waxed floss, use electric razor, and avoid scissors or sharp knives and potentially harmful activities. You may experience nausea or vomiting (small frequent meals, frequent mouth care, sucking lozenges, or chewing gum may help). May discolor urine or stool. Report skin rash or irritation, unusual fever, persistent nausea or GI upset, unusual bleeding or bruising (bleeding gums, nosebleed, blood in urine, dark stool, bloody emesis), pain in joints or back, swelling or pain at injection site.

**Nursing Implications** Should not be given in close proximity to other drugs because absorption may be decreased. Administer warfarin at least 1-2 hours prior to, or 6 hours after, cholestyramine or sucralfate, because cholestyramine or sucralfate may bind warfarin and decrease its total absorption; avoid all I.M. injections.

**Dosage Forms**

Powder for injection, as sodium, lyophilized: 2 mg, 5 mg

Tablet, as sodium: 1 mg, 2 mg, 2.5 mg, 3 mg, 4 mg, 5 mg, 6 mg, 7.5 mg, 10 mg

- **4-Way® Long Acting Nasal Solution [OTC]** *see* Oxymetazoline *on page 415*
- **Welchol™** *see* Colesevelam *on page 139*
- **Wellbutrin®** *see* Bupropion *on page 77*
- **Wellbutrin SR®** *see* Bupropion *on page 77*
- **Wellcovorin®** *see* Leucovorin *on page 309*
- **Westcort®** *see* Hydrocortisone *on page 273*
- **Whitehorn** *see* Hawthorn *on page 264*
- **Whitfield's Ointment [OTC]** *see* Benzoic Acid and Salicylic Acid *on page 62*
- **Wigraine®** *see* Ergotamine *on page 200*
- **Wild Quinine** *see* Feverfew *on page 224*
- **40 Winks® [OTC]** *see* Diphenhydramine *on page 174*
- **Winstrol®** *see* Stanozolol *on page 518*
- **Wolfina®** *see* Rauwolfia Serpentina *on page 489*

## Wormwood

**Synonyms** Absinthe; *Artemisia absinthium*; Green Ginger

**Pharmacologic Category** Herb

**Use** Homeopathic medicine, used as an anthelmintic, bitter tonic, hair tonic, sedative, flavoring agent (in vermouth)

Per Commission E: Loss of appetite, dyspepsia, biliary dyskinesia

**Adverse Reactions** Vomiting, stomach cramps, intestinal cramps, dizziness, CNS disturbances, headache

**Overdosage/Toxicology**

Signs and symptoms: Headache, vertigo, thirst, vomiting, giddiness, paranoia, tremors, diarrhea, diaphoresis, color vision disturbance, psychosis, seizures (>15 g ingestion), visual hallucinations, euphoria, coma, respiratory depression, contact dermatitis (from flowers), dysphoria, delirium, mania, anorexia, memory impairment

Decontamination: Lavage (within 1 hour)/activated charcoal with cathartic

Treatment: Supportive therapy; seizures can be managed with a benzodiazepine or barbiturate; psychiatric abnormalities can be managed with a benzodiazepine or neuroleptic agent

**Usual Dosage** Tea: 2-3 g/day

**Patient Information** Considered unsafe; avoid long-term use

**Additional Information** Not popular in the U.S.; taste threshold (Absinthin): 1 part in 70,000: A shrub with small green-yellow flowers from July through September. Grows naturally in Europe but found in Northeastern and North Central U.S. Wormwood extract has been used in absinth, an emerald green bitter liquor banned in Europe and U.S. Absinth has been thought to cause Vincent van Gogh's psychosis. The tea uses dried leaves and flowering tops.

Per Commission E: In toxic doses, thujone, the active component of the oil, acts as a convulsant poison. Thus, essential oil must not be used except in combinations.

- **Wyamine® Sulfate Injection** *see* Mephentermine *on page 341*
- **Wycillin®** *see* Penicillin G Procaine *on page 425*
- **Wydase® Injection** *see* Hyaluronidase *on page 269*

- ♦ **Wygesic®** *see* Propoxyphene and Acetaminophen *on page 474*
- ♦ **Wymox®** *see* Amoxicillin *on page 38*
- ♦ **Wytensin®** *see* Guanabenz *on page 259*
- ♦ **Xalatan®** *see* Latanoprost *on page 308*
- ♦ **Xanax®** *see* Alprazolam *on page 26*
- ♦ **Xeloda®** *see* Capecitabine *on page 87*
- ♦ **Xenical®** *see* Orlistat *on page 407*
- ♦ **Xopenex™** *see* Levalbuterol *on page 310*
- ♦ **X-Prep® Liquid [OTC]** *see* Senna *on page 509*
- ♦ **Xylocaine®** *see* Lidocaine *on page 317*


## Xylometazoline (zye loe met AZ oh leen)

**U.S. Brand Names** Otrivin® Nasal [OTC]

**Pharmacologic Category** Ophthalmic Agent, Vasoconstrictor

**Use** Symptomatic relief of nasal and nasopharyngeal mucosal congestion

**Effects on Mental Status** May cause drowsiness or dizziness

**Effects on Psychiatric Treatment** None reported

**Usual Dosage**

Children 2-12 years: Instill 2-3 drops (0.05%) in each nostril every 8-10 hours

Children >12 years and Adults: Instill 2-3 drops or sprays (0.1%) in each nostril every 8-10 hours

**Dosage Forms** Solution, nasal, as hydrochloride: 0.05% [0.5 mg/mL] (20 mL); 0.1% [1 mg/mL] (15 mL, 20 mL)


- ♦ **Yeast-Gard® Medicated Douche** *see* Povidone-Iodine *on page 456*
- ♦ **Yellow Indian Paint** *see* Golden Seal *on page 254*
- ♦ **Yellow Mercuric Oxide** *see* Mercuric Oxide *on page 343*
- ♦ **Yellow Root** *see* Golden Seal *on page 254*
- ♦ **Yocon®** *see* Yohimbine *on page 589*
- ♦ **Yodoxin®** *see* Iodoquinol *on page 291*


## Yohimbine (yo HIM bine)

**U.S. Brand Names** Aphrodyne™; Dayto Himbin®; Yocon®; Yohimex™

**Synonyms** *Corynanthe yohimbe*; Yohimbine Hydrochloride

**Pharmacologic Category** Miscellaneous Product

**Use Unlabeled uses:** Treat SSRI-induced sexual dysfunction; weight loss; impotence; sympathicolytic and mydriatic; may have activity as an aphrodisiac

**Effects on Mental Status** May cause anxiety, irritability, dizziness, insomnia, mania, panic attacks, and psychosis

**Effects on Psychiatric Treatment** May cause neutropenia; use caution with clozapine and carbamazepine; antidepressant should not be used with yohimbine; has been used to treat SSRI-induced sexual dysfunction

**Contraindications** Renal disease, hypersensitivity to yohimbine

**Warnings/Precautions** Do not use in pregnancy; do not use in children; not for use in geriatric, psychiatric, or cardio-renal patients with a history of gastric or duodenal ulcer; generally not for use in females. Should not be used in kidney disease or psychiatric disorders; can cause high blood pressure and anxiety, tachycardia, nausea, or vomiting.

**Adverse Reactions**

Cardiovascular: Tachycardia, hypertension, hypotension (orthostatic), flushing

Central nervous system: Anxiety, mania, hallucinations, irritability, dizziness, psychosis, insomnia, headache, panic attacks

Gastrointestinal: Nausea, vomiting, anorexia, salivation

Neuromuscular & skeletal: Tremors

Miscellaneous: Antidiuretic action, diaphoresis

**Drug Interactions** CYP2D6 and 3A3/4 enzyme substrate; CYP2D6 enzyme inhibitor

Antihypertensives: Effect of antihypertensives may be reduced by yohimbine

CNS active agents: Caution with other CNS acting drugs

CYP3A3/4 inhibitors: Serum level and/or toxicity of yohimbine may be increased; inhibitors include amiodarone, cimetidine, clarithromycin, erythromycin, delavirdine, diltiazem, dirithromycin, disulfiram, fluoxetine, fluvoxamine, grapefruit juice, indinavir, itraconazole, ketoconazole, metronidazole, nefazodone, nevirapine, propoxyfene, quinupristin-dalfopristin, ritonavir, saquinavir, verapamil, zafirlukast, zileuton; monitor for altered response

Linezolid: Due to MAO inhibition (see below), combinations with this agent should generally be avoided

MAO inhibitors: Theoretically may increase toxicity or adverse effects

**Mechanism of Action** Derived from the bark of the yohimbe tree (*Corynanthe yohimbe*), this indole alkaloid produces a presynaptic alpha$_2$-adrenergic blockade. Peripheral autonomic effect is to increase cholinergic and decrease adrenergic activity; yohimbine exerts a stimulating effect on the mood and a mild antidiuretic effect.

**Pharmacodynamics/kinetics**

Duration of action: Usually 3-4 hours, but may last 36 hours

Absorption: Oral: 33%

Distribution: $V_d$: 0.3-3 L/kg

Half-life: 0.6 hours

**Usual Dosage** Adults: Oral:

Male erectile impotence: 5.4 mg tablet 3 times/day have been used. If side effects occur, reduce to $^1/_2$ tablet (2.7 mg) 3 times/day followed by gradual increases to 1 tablet 3 times/day. Results of therapy >10 weeks are not known.

Orthostatic hypotension: Doses of 12.5 mg/day have been utilized; however, more research is necessary

**Reference Range** After a 10 mg oral dose, peak plasma yohimbine level achieved was ~75 µg/L after 45 minutes

**Patient Information** Considered unsafe

**Additional Information** Also a street drug of abuse that can be smoked; has a bitter taste; dissociative state may resemble phencyclidine intoxication

**Dosage Forms** Tablet, as hydrochloride: 5.4 mg


- ♦ **Yohimbine Hydrochloride** *see* Yohimbine *on page 589*
- ♦ **Yohimex™** *see* Yohimbine *on page 589*
- ♦ **Yutopar®** *see* Ritodrine *on page 497*
- ♦ **Zaditor™** *see* Ketotifen *on page 304*


## Zafirlukast (za FIR loo kast)

**U.S. Brand Names** Accolate®

**Synonyms** ICI 204, 219; MK-571

**Pharmacologic Category** Leukotriene Receptor Antagonist

**Use** Prophylaxis and chronic treatment of asthma in adults and children ≥7 years of age

**Effects on Mental Status** May cause dizziness

**Effects on Psychiatric Treatment** None reported

**Pregnancy Risk Factor** B

**Contraindications** Hypersensitivity to zafirlukast or any of its inactive ingredients

**Warnings/Precautions** The clearance of zafirlukast is reduced in patients with stable alcoholic cirrhosis such that the $C_{max}$ and AUC are approximately 50% to 60% greater than those of normal adults.

Zafirlukast is not indicated for use in the reversal of bronchospasm in acute asthma attacks, including status asthmaticus. Therapy with zafirlukast can be continued during acute exacerbations of asthma.

An increased proportion of zafirlukast patients >55 years old reported infections as compared to placebo-treated patients. these infections were mostly mild or moderate in intensity and predominantly affected the respiratory tract. Infections occurred equally in both sexes, were dose-proportional to total milligrams of zafirlukast exposure and were associated with coadministration of inhaled corticosteroids.

Although the frequency of hepatic transaminase elevations was comparable between zafirlukast and placebo-treated patients, a single case of symptomatic hepatitis and hyperbilirubinemia, without other attributable cause, occurred in patient who had received 40 mg/day of zafirlukast for 100 days. In this patient, the liver enzymes returned to normal within 3 months of stopping zafirlukast.

**Adverse Reactions**

>10%: Central nervous system: Headache (12.9%)

1% to 10%:

Central nervous system: Dizziness, pain, fever

Gastrointestinal: Nausea, diarrhea, abdominal pain, vomiting, dyspepsia

Neuromuscular & skeletal: Myalgia, weakness

**Overdosage/Toxicology**

Signs and symptoms: There is no experience to date with zafirlukast overdose in humans

Treatment: Supportive treatment measures

**Drug Interactions** CYP2C9 enzyme substrate; CYP2C9 and 3A3/4 enzyme inhibitor

Decreased effect:

Erythromycin: Coadministration of a single dose of zafirlukast with erythromycin to steady state results in decreased mean plasma levels of zafirlukast by 40% due to a decrease in zafirlukast bioavailability.

Terfenadine: Coadministration of zafirlukast with terfenadine to steady state results in a decrease in the mean $C_{max}$ (66%) and AUC (54%) of zafirlukast. No effect of zafirlukast on terfenadine plasma concentrations or EKG parameters was seen.

Theophylline: Coadministration of zafirlukast at steady state with a single dose of liquid theophylline preparations results in decreased mean plasma levels of zafirlukast by 30%, but no effects on plasma theophylline levels were observed.

Increased effect: Aspirin: Coadministration of zafirlukast with aspirin results in mean increased plasma levels of zafirlukast by 45%

(Continued)

## Zafirlukast *(Continued)*

Increased toxicity: Warfarin: Coadministration of zafirlukast with warfarin results in a clinically significant increase in prothrombin time (PT). Closely monitor prothrombin times of patients on oral warfarin anticoagulant therapy and zafirlukast, and adjust anticoagulant dose accordingly.

**Usual Dosage** Oral:

Children <7 years: Safety and effectiveness has not been established

Children 7-11 years: 10 mg twice daily

Adults: 20 mg twice daily

Elderly: The mean dose (mg/kg) normalized AUC and $C_{max}$ increase and plasma clearance decreases with increasing age. In patients >65 years of age, there is an 2-3 fold greater $C_{max}$ and AUC compared to younger adults.

**Dosing adjustment in renal impairment:** There are no apparent differences in the pharmacokinetics between renally impaired patients and normal subjects.

**Dosing adjustment in hepatic impairment:** In patients with hepatic impairment (ie, biopsy-proven cirrhosis), there is a 50% to 60% greater $C_{max}$ and AUC compared to normal subjects.

**Patient Information** Do not use during acute bronchospasm. Take regularly as prescribed, even during symptom-free periods. Do not take more than recommended or discontinue use without consulting prescriber. Do not stop taking other antiasthmatic medications unless instructed by prescriber. Avoid aspirin or aspirin-containing medications unless approved by prescriber. You may experience headache, drowsiness, dizziness, or blurred vision (use caution when driving or engaging in tasks requiring alertness until response to drug is known); gastric upset, nausea, or vomiting (small frequent meals, frequent mouth care, chewing gum, or sucking lozenges may help). Report persistent CNS or GI symptoms; muscle or back pain; weakness, fever, chills; yellowing of skin or eyes; dark urine, or pale stool; skin rash; or worsening of condition.

**Dosage Forms** Tablet: 10 mg, 20 mg

♦ **Zagam®** *see* Sparfloxacin *on page 517*

## Zalcitabine (zal SITE a been)

**U.S. Brand Names** Hivid®

**Synonyms** ddC; Dideoxycytidine

**Pharmacologic Category** Antiretroviral Agent, Reverse Transcriptase Inhibitor (Nucleoside)

**Use** In combination with at least two other antiretrovirals in the treatment of patients with HIV infection; it is not recommended that zalcitabine be given in combination with didanosine, stavudine, or lamivudine due to overlapping toxicities, virologic interactions, or lack of clinical data

**Effects on Mental Status** Drowsiness is common; may cause dizziness

**Effects on Psychiatric Treatment** May cause granulocytopenia; use caution with clozapine; concurrent use with disulfiram can enhance peripheral neuropathy; avoid combination

**Pregnancy Risk Factor** C

**Contraindications** Hypersensitivity to zalcitabine or any component

**Warnings/Precautions** Careful monitoring of pancreatic enzymes and liver function tests in patients with a history of pancreatitis, increased amylase, those on parenteral nutrition or with a history of ethanol abuse; discontinue use immediately if pancreatitis is suspected; lactic acidosis and severe hepatomegaly and failure have rarely occurred with zalcitabine resulting in fatality (stop treatment if lactic acidosis or hepatotoxicity occur); some cases may possibly be related to underlying hepatitis B; use with caution in patients on digitalis, or with congestive heart failure, renal failure, or hyperphosphatemia; zalcitabine can cause severe peripheral neuropathy; avoid use, if possible, in patients with pre-existing neuropathy or at risk of developing neuropathy. Risk factors include $CD_4$ counts <50 cells/mm$^3$, diabetes mellitus, weight loss, other drugs known to cause peripheral neuropathy.

**Adverse Reactions**

>10%:

Central nervous system: Fever (5% to 17%), malaise (2% to 13%)

Neuromuscular & skeletal: Peripheral neuropathy (28.3%)

1% to 10%:

Central nervous system: Headache (2.1%), dizziness (1.1%), fatigue (3.8%), seizures (1.3%)

Endocrine & metabolic: Hypoglycemia (1.8% to 6.3%), hyponatremia (3.5%), hyperglycemia (1% to 6%)

Hematologic: Anemia (occurs as early as 2-4 weeks), granulocytopenia (usually after 6-8 weeks)

Dermatologic: Rash (2% to 11%), pruritus (3% to 5%)

Gastrointestinal: Nausea (3%), dysphagia (1% to 4%), anorexia (3.9%), abdominal pain (3% to 8%), vomiting (1% to 3%), diarrhea (0.4% to 9.5%), weight loss, oral ulcers (3% to 7%), increased amylase (3% to 8%)

Hepatic: Abnormal hepatic function (8.9%), hyperbilirubinemia (2% to 5%)

Neuromuscular & skeletal: Myalgia (1% to 6%), foot pain

Respiratory: Pharyngitis (1.8%), cough (6.3%), nasal discharge (3.5%)

<1%: Atrial fibrillation, chest pain, constipation, edema, epistaxis, heart racing, hepatitis, hepatic failure, hepatomegaly, hypertension, hypocalcemia, jaundice, myositis, night sweats, pain, palpitations, pancreatitis, syncope, tachycardia, weakness

**Overdosage/Toxicology**

Signs and symptoms: Delayed peripheral neurotoxicity; following oral decontamination

Treatment: Supportive

**Drug Interactions**

Decreased effect: Magnesium/aluminum-containing antacids and metoclopramide may reduce zalcitabine absorption

Increased toxicity:

Amphotericin, foscarnet, cimetidine, probenecid, and aminoglycosides may potentiate the risk of developing peripheral neuropathy or other toxicities associated with zalcitabine by interfering with the renal elimination of zalcitabine

Other drugs associated with peripheral neuropathy which should be avoided, if possible, include chloramphenicol, cisplatin, dapsone, disulfiram, ethionamide, glutethimide, didanosine, gold, hydralazine, iodoquinol, isoniazid, metronidazole, nitrofurantoin, phenytoin, ribavirin, and vincristine

It is not recommended that zalcitabine be given in combination with didanosine, stavudine, or lamivudine due to overlapping toxicities, virologic interactions, or lack of clinical data

Doxorubicin (*in vitro*) decreases zalcitabine phosphorylation; clinical relevance unknown.

**Usual Dosage** Oral:

Children <13 years: Safety and efficacy have not been established

Adults: Daily dose: 0.75 mg every 8 hours

**Dosing adjustment in renal impairment:** Adults:

$Cl_{cr}$ 10-40 mL/minute: 0.75 mg every 12 hours

$Cl_{cr}$ <10 mL/minute: 0.75 mg every 24 hours

Moderately dialyzable (20% to 50%)

**Dietary Considerations** Food: Extent and rate of absorption may be decreased with food

**Patient Information** Zalcitabine is not a cure for AIDS, nor has it been found to reduce transmission of AIDS. Take as directed, preferably on an empty stomach (1 hour before or 2 hours after meals). Take around-the-clock; do not take with other medications. You may experience headache or insomnia; if these persist notify prescriber. Report chest pain, palpitations, or rapid heartbeat; swelling of extremities; weight gain or loss >5 lb/week; signs of infection (eg, fever, chills, sore throat, burning urination, fatigue); unusual bleeding (eg, tarry stools, easy bruising, or blood in stool, urine, or mouth); pain, tingling, or numbness of toes or fingers; skin rash or irritation; or muscles weakness or tremors.

**Dosage Forms** Tablet: 0.375 mg, 0.75 mg

## Zaleplon (ZAL e plon)

**Related Information**

Anxiolytic/Hypnotic Use in Long-Term Care Facilities *on page 754*

Clinical Issues in the Use of Anxiolytics and Sedative/Hypnotics *on page 634*

Nonbenzodiazepine Anxiolytics and Hypnotics *on page 721*

Patient Information - Anxiolytics & Sedative Hypnotics (Nonbenzodiazepine Hypnotics) *on page 656*

**U.S. Brand Names** Sonata®

**Pharmacologic Category** Hypnotic, Nonbenzodiazepine

**Use** Short-term treatment of insomnia

**Pregnancy Risk Factor** C

**Contraindications** Known hypersensitivity to zaleplon or any component

**Warnings/Precautions** Symptomatic treatment of insomnia should be initiated only after careful evaluation of potential causes of sleep disturbance. Failure of sleep disturbance to resolve after 7-10 days may indicate psychiatric and/or medical illness.

Use with caution in patients with depression, particularly if suicidal risk may be present. Use with caution in patients with a history of drug dependence. Abrupt discontinuance may lead to withdrawal symptoms. May impair physical and mental capabilities. Patients must be cautioned about performing tasks which require mental alertness (operating machinery or driving). Use with caution in patients receiving other CNS depressants or psychoactive medications. Effects with other sedative drugs or ethanol may be potentiated.

use with caution in the elderly, those with compromised respiratory function, or renal and hepatic impairment. Because of the rapid onset of action, zaleplon should be administered immediately prior to bedtime or after the patient has gone to bed and is having difficulty falling asleep.

**Adverse Reactions** 1% to 10%:

Central nervous system: Amnesia, anxiety, depersonalization, dizziness, hallucinations, hypesthesia, somnolence, vertigo, malaise, depression, lightheadedness, impaired coordination

Cardiovascular: Peripheral edema

Dermatologic: Photosensitivity reaction, rash, pruritus

Gastrointestinal: Abdominal pain, anorexia, colitis, dyspepsia, nausea, constipation, xerostomia

Genitourinary: Dysmenorrhea
Neuromuscular & skeletal: Paresthesia, tremor, myalgia, weakness
Ocular: Abnormal vision, eye pain
Otic: Hyperacusis
Miscellaneous: Parosmia

**Overdosage/Toxicology** Symptoms include CNS depression, ranging from drowsiness to coma. Mild overdose is associated with drowsiness, confusion, and lethargy. Serious case may result in ataxia, respiratory depression, hypotension, hypotonia, coma, and rarely death. Treatment is supportive.

**Drug Interactions** CYP3A4 substrate (minor metabolic pathway)
Antipsychotics: Zaleplon potentiates the CNS effects of thioridazine (and potentially other antipsychotics)
Cimetidine: May increase zaleplon levels by decreasing its metabolism; cimetidine inhibits both aldehyde oxidase and CYP3A4 leading to an 85% increase in $C_{max}$ and AUC of zaleplon; use 5 mg zaleplon as starting dose in patients receiving cimetidine
CNS depressants: Sedative effects may be additive with phenothiazines; monitor for increased effect; includes barbiturates, benzodiazepines, narcotic analgesics, ethanol, and other sedative agents
CYP3A3/4 inhibitors: Serum level and/or toxicity of zaleplon may be increased; inhibitors include amiodarone, cimetidine, clarithromycin, erythromycin, delavirdine, diltiazem, dirithromycin, disulfiram, fluoxetine, fluvoxamine, grapefruit juice, indinavir, itraconazole, ketoconazole, metronidazole, nefazodone, nevirapine, propoxyfene, quinupristin-dalfopristin, ritonavir, saquinavir, verapamil, zafirlukast, zileuton; monitor for altered response
Enzyme inducers: May increase the metabolism of zaleplon, reducing its effectiveness; inducers include phenytoin, carbamazepine, phenobarbital, and rifampin; rifampin decreased AUC by 80%; consider an alternative hypnotic
Tricyclic antidepressants: Zaleplon potentiates the CNS effects of imipramine (and potentially other TCAs)

**Mechanism of Action** Zaleplon is unrelated to benzodiazepines, barbiturates, or other hypnotics. However, it interacts with the benzodiazepine GABA receptor complex. Nonclinical studies have shown that it binds selectively to the brain omega-1 receptor situated on the alpha subunit of the GABA-A receptor complex.

**Pharmacodynamics/kinetics**
Onset: Rapid
Peak effect: Within 1 hour
Duration: 6-8 hours
Absorption: Rapid and almost complete
Distribution: $V_d$: 1.4 L/kg
Protein binding: 60% ± 15%
Metabolism: Extensively metabolized with <1% of dose excreted unchanged in urine. Primarily metabolized by aldehyde oxidase to form 5-oxo-zaleplon and to a lesser extent by CYP3A4 to desethylzaleplon. All metabolites are pharmacologically inactive. Oral dose plasma clearance: 3 L/hour/kg
Bioavailability: 30%
Half-life: 1 hour
Time to peak serum concentration: 1 hour
Elimination: In urine as metabolites

**Usual Dosage**
Adults: Oral: 10 mg at bedtime (range: 5-20 mg)
Elderly: 5 mg at bedtime
**Dosage adjustment in renal impairment:** No adjustment for mild to moderate renal impairment; use in severe renal impairment has not been adequately studied
**Dosage adjustment in hepatic impairment:** Mild to moderate impairment: 5 mg; not recommended for use in patients with severe hepatic impairment

**Dietary Considerations** High fat meal prolonged absorption; delayed $t_{max}$ by 2 hours, and reduced $C_{max}$ by 35%

**Administration** Immediately before bedtime or when the patient is in bed and cannot fall asleep

**Patient Information** May cause drowsiness, dizziness, or lightheadedness. Avoid alcohol and other CNS depressants. Consult prescriber before taking any prescription or OTC medication. Do not operate machinery or drive while taking this medication. Dose should be taken immediately before bedtime or when you are in bed and cannot fall asleep.

**Additional Information** Prescription quantities should not exceed a 1-month supply

**Dosage Forms** Capsule: 5 mg, 10 mg

♦ **Zanaflex®** *see* Tizanidine *on page 551*

## Zanamivir (za NA mi veer)

**U.S. Brand Names** Relenza®

**Pharmacologic Category** Antiviral Agent

**Use** Treatment of uncomplicated acute illness due to influenza virus in adults and adolescents ≥7 years of age. Treatment should only be initiated in patients who have been symptomatic for no more than 2 days.

**Effects on Mental Status** May cause dizziness; may rarely cause drowsiness

**Effects on Psychiatric Treatment** None reported

**Pregnancy Risk Factor** C

**Contraindications** Hypersensitivity to zanamivir or any component of the formulation

**Warnings/Precautions** Patients must be instructed in the use of the delivery system. No data are available to support the use of this drug in patients who begin treatment after 48 hours of symptoms, as a prophylactic treatment for influenza, or in patients with significant underlying medical conditions. Not recommended for use in patients with underlying respiratory disease, such as asthma or COPD, due to lack of efficacy and risk of serious adverse effects. Bronchospasm, decreased lung function, and other serious adverse reactions, including those with fatal outcomes, have been reported. For a patient with an underlying airway disease where a medical decision has been made to use zanamivir, a fast-acting bronchodilator should be made available, and used prior to each dose. Not a substitute for the flu shot. Consider primary or concomitant bacterial infections.

**Adverse Reactions** Most adverse reactions occurred at a frequency which was equal to the control (lactose vehicle)
>1.5%:
Central nervous system: Headache (2%), dizziness (2%)
Gastrointestinal: Nausea (3%), diarrhea (3% adults, 2% children), vomiting (1% adults, 2% children)
Respiratory: Sinusitis (3%), bronchitis (2%), cough (2%), other nasal signs and symptoms (2%), infection (ear, nose, and throat; 2% adults, 5% children)
<1.5%: Malaise, fatigue, fever, abdominal pain, myalgia, arthralgia, and urticaria
In addition, the following adverse reactions have been reported during postmarketing use: Allergic or allergic-like reaction (including oropharyngeal edema), arrhythmias, syncope, seizures, bronchospasm, dyspnea, rash (including serious cutaneous reactions)

**Overdosage/Toxicology** Information is limited, and symptoms appear similar to reported adverse events from clinical studies

**Drug Interactions** No clinically significant pharmacokinetic interactions are predicted

**Usual Dosage** Adolescents ≥12 years and Adults: 2 Inhalations: (10 mg total) twice daily for 5 days. Two doses should be taken on the first day of dosing, regardless of interval, while doses should be spaced by approximately 12 hours on subsequent days.

**Administration** Inhalation: Must be used with Diskhaler® delivery device. Patients who are scheduled to use an inhaled bronchodilator should use their bronchodilator prior to zanamivir.

**Patient Information** Use delivery device exactly as directed; complete full 5-day regimen, even if symptoms improve sooner. If you have asthma or COPD you may be at risk for bronchospasm; see prescriber for appropriate bronchodilator before using zanamivir. Stop using this medication and contact your physician if you experience shortness of breath, increased wheezing, or other signs of bronchospasm. You may experience dizziness or headache (use caution when driving or engaging in hazardous tasks until response to drug is known). Report unresolved diarrhea, vomiting, or nausea; acute fever or muscle pain; or other acute and persistent adverse effects.

**Additional Information** Majority of patients included in clinical trials were infected with influenza A, however a number of patients with influenza B infections were also enrolled. Patients with lower temperature or less severe symptoms appeared to derive less benefit from therapy. No consistent treatment benefit was demonstrated in patients with chronic underlying medical conditions.

**Dosage Forms** Powder, for inhalation (Rotadisk®): 5 mg per blister

♦ **Zanosar®** *see* Streptozocin *on page 521*

♦ **Zantac®** *see* Ranitidine Hydrochloride *on page 488*

♦ **Zantac® 75 [OTC]** *see* Ranitidine Hydrochloride *on page 488*

♦ **Zantryl®** *see* Phentermine *on page 438*

♦ **Zarontin®** *see* Ethosuximide *on page 213*

♦ **Zaroxolyn®** *see* Metolazone *on page 361*

♦ **Zeasorb-AF® Powder [OTC]** *see* Tolnaftate *on page 555*

♦ **Zeasorb-AF® Powder [OTC]** *see* Miconazole *on page 364*

♦ **Zebeta®** *see* Bisoprolol *on page 70*

♦ **Zefazone®** *see* Cefmetazole *on page 99*

♦ **Zeldox®** *see* Ziprasidone *on page 593*

♦ **Zemplar™** *see* Paricalcitol *on page 420*

♦ **Zenapax®** *see* Daclizumab *on page 149*

♦ **Zephrex®** *see* Guaifenesin and Pseudoephedrine *on page 257*

♦ **Zephrex LA®** *see* Guaifenesin and Pseudoephedrine *on page 257*

♦ **Zerit®** *see* Stavudine *on page 519*

♦ **Zestoretic®** *see* Lisinopril and Hydrochlorothiazide *on page 321*

♦ **Zestril®** *see* Lisinopril *on page 320*

♦ **Ziac™** *see* Bisoprolol and Hydrochlorothiazide *on page 70*

♦ **Ziagen™** *see* Abacavir *on page 12*

## Zidovudine (zye DOE vyoo deen)

**U.S. Brand Names** Retrovir®

**Canadian Brand Names** Apo®-Zidovudine; Novo-AZT

**Synonyms** Azidothymidine; AZT; Compound S

**Pharmacologic Category** Antiretroviral Agent, Reverse Transcriptase Inhibitor (Nucleoside)

**Use** Management of patients with HIV infections in combination with at least two other antiretroviral agents; for prevention of maternal/fetal HIV transmission as monotherapy

**Effects on Mental Status** May cause drowsiness, dizziness, or insomnia; may rarely cause confusion or mania

**Effects on Psychiatric Treatment** Granulocytopenia is common; avoid clozapine and carbamazepine; valproic acid may decrease the clearance of zidovudine

**Pregnancy Risk Factor** C

**Contraindications** Life-threatening hypersensitivity to zidovudine or any component

**Warnings/Precautions** Often associated with hematologic toxicity including granulocytopenia and severe anemia requiring transfusions; zidovudine has been shown to be carcinogenic in rats and mice

**Adverse Reactions**

>10%:

Central nervous system: Severe headache (42%), fever (16%)

Dermatologic: Rash (17%)

Gastrointestinal: Nausea (46% to 61%), anorexia (11%), diarrhea (17%), pain (20%), vomiting (6% to 25%)

Hematologic: Anemia (23% in children), leukopenia, granulocytopenia (39% in children)

Neuromuscular & skeletal: Weakness (19%)

1% to 10%:

Central nervous system: Malaise (8%), dizziness (6%), insomnia (5%), somnolence (8%)

Dermatologic: Hyperpigmentation of nails (bluish-brown)

Gastrointestinal: Dyspepsia (5%)

Hematologic: Changes in platelet count

Neuromuscular & skeletal: Paresthesia (6%)

<1%: Bone marrow suppression, cholestatic jaundice, confusion, granulocytopenia, hepatotoxicity, mania, myopathy, neurotoxicity, pancytopenia, seizures, tenderness, thrombocytopenia

**Overdosage/Toxicology**

Signs and symptoms: Nausea, vomiting, ataxia, granulocytopenia

Treatment: Erythropoietin, thymidine, and cyanocobalamin have been used experimentally to treat zidovudine-induced hematopoietic toxicity, yet none are presently specified as the agent of choice. Treatment is supportive.

**Drug Interactions**

Decreased effect: Acetaminophen may decrease AUC of zidovudine as can the rifamycins

Increased toxicity: Coadministration with drugs that are nephrotoxic (amphotericin B), cytotoxic (flucytosine, Adriamycin®, vincristine, vinblastine, doxorubicin, interferon), inhibit glucuronidation or excretion (acetaminophen, cimetidine, indomethacin, lorazepam, probenecid, aspirin), or interfere with RBC/WBC number or function (acyclovir, ganciclovir, pentamidine, dapsone); although the AUC was unaffected, the rate of absorption and peak plasma concentrations were increased significantly when zidovudine was administered with clarithromycin (n=18); valproic acid increased AZT's AUC by 80% and decreased clearance by 38% (believed due to inhibition first pass metabolism); fluconazole may increase zidovudine's AUC and half-life, concomitant interferon alfa may increase hematologic toxicities and phenytoin, trimethoprim, and interferon beta-1b may increase zidovudine levels

**Usual Dosage**

Prevention of maternal-fetal HIV transmission:

Neonatal: Oral: 2 mg/kg/dose every 6 hours for 6 weeks beginning 8-12 hours after birth; infants unable to receive oral dosing may receive 1.5 mg/kg I.V. infused over 30 minutes every 6 hours

Maternal (>14 weeks gestation): Oral: 100 mg 5 times/day until the start of labor; during labor and delivery, administer zidovudine I.V. at 2 mg/kg over 1 hour followed by a continuous I.V. infusion of 1 mg/kg/hour until the umbilical cord is clamped

Children 3 months to 12 years for HIV infection:

Oral: 160 mg/m$^2$/dose every 8 hours; dosage range: 90 mg/m$^2$/dose to 180 mg/m$^2$/dose every 6-8 hours; some Working Group members use a dose of 180 mg/m$^2$ every 12 hours when using in drug combinations with other antiretroviral compounds, but data on this dosing in children is limited

I.V. continuous infusion: 20 mg/m$^2$/hour

I.V. intermittent infusion: 120 mg/m$^2$/dose every 6 hours

Adults:

Oral: 300 mg twice daily or 200 mg 3 times/day

I.V.: 1-2 mg/kg/dose (infused over 1 hour) administered every 4 hours around-the-clock (6 doses/day)

Prevention of HIV following needlesticks: 200 mg 3 times/day plus lamivudine 150 mg twice daily; a protease inhibitor (eg, indinavir) may be added for high risk exposures; begin therapy within 2 hours of exposure if possible

**Patients should receive I.V. therapy only until oral therapy can be administered**

**Dosing interval in renal impairment:** $Cl_{cr}$ <10 mL/minute: May require minor dose adjustment

Hemodialysis: At least partially removed by hemo- and peritoneal dialysis; administer dose after hemodialysis or administer 100 mg supplemental dose; during CAPD, dose as for $Cl_{cr}$ <10 mL/minute

Continuous arteriovenous or venovenous hemodiafiltration (CAVH) effects: Administer 100 mg every 8 hours

**Dosing adjustment in hepatic impairment:** Reduce dose by 50% or double dosing interval in patients with cirrhosis

**Dietary Considerations** Food: Administration with a fatty meal decreased zidovudine's AUC and peak plasma concentration

**Patient Information** Zidovudine is not a cure for AIDS, nor has it been found to reduce transmission of AIDS. Take as directed, preferably on an empty stomach (1 hour before or 2 hours after meals). Take around-the-clock; do not take with other medications. Take precautions to avoid transmission to others. You may experience headache or insomnia; if these persist notify prescriber. Report unresolved nausea or vomiting; signs of infection (eg, fever, chills, sore throat, burning urination, flu-like symptoms, fatigue); unusual bleeding (eg, tarry stools, easy bruising, or blood in stool, urine, or mouth); pain, tingling, or numbness of toes or fingers; skin rash or irritation; or muscles weakness or tremors.

**Dosage Forms**

Capsule: 100 mg

Injection: 10 mg/mL (20 mL)

Syrup (strawberry flavor): 50 mg/5 mL (240 mL)

Tablet: 300 mg

## Zidovudine and Lamivudine
(zye DOE vyoo deen & la MI vyoo deen)

**U.S. Brand Names** Combivir™

**Pharmacologic Category** Antiretroviral Agent, Reverse Transcriptase Inhibitor (Non-Nucleoside); Antiretroviral Agent, Reverse Transcriptase Inhibitor (Nucleoside)

**Effects on Mental Status** Dizziness, insomnia, sedation are common; may cause depression. May rarely cause confusion or mania

**Effects on Psychiatric Treatment** Leukopenia and granulocytopenia are common; caution with clozapine and carbamazepine. Increased toxicity may result if used concurrently with drugs that inhibit glucuronidation or excretion (lorazepam). Valproic acid increased zidovudine's AUC by 80% and decreased clearance by 38%.

**Dosage Forms** Tablet: Zidovudine 300 mg and lamivudine 150 mg

♦ **Zilactin®-B Medicated [OTC]** *see* Benzocaine *on page 61*

♦ **Zilactin-L® [OTC]** *see* Lidocaine *on page 317*

## Zileuton (zye LOO ton)

**U.S. Brand Names** Zyflo™

**Synonyms** A-64077

**Pharmacologic Category** 5-Lipoxygenase Inhibitor

**Use** Prophylaxis and chronic treatment of asthma in adults and children ≥12 years of age

**Effects on Mental Status** May cause dizziness, drowsiness, insomnia, or nervousness

**Effects on Psychiatric Treatment** Concurrent use with propranolol may enhance beta-blocker activity

**Pregnancy Risk Factor** C

**Contraindications** Active liver disease or transaminase elevations greater than or equal to three times the upper limit of normal (≥3 x ULN), hypersensitivity to zileuton or any of its active ingredients

**Warnings/Precautions** Elevations of one or more liver function tests may occur during therapy. These laboratory abnormalities may progress, remain unchanged or resolve with continued therapy. Use with caution in patients who consume substantial quantities of alcohol or have a past history of liver disease. Zileuton is not indicated for use in the reversal of bronchospasm in acute asthma attacks, including status asthmaticus. Zileuton can be continued during acute exacerbations of asthma.

**Adverse Reactions**

>10%:

Central nervous system: Headache (24.6%)

Hepatic: Increased ALT (12%)

1% to 10%:

Cardiovascular: Chest pain

Central nervous system: Pain, dizziness, fever, insomnia, malaise, nervousness, somnolence
Gastrointestinal: Dyspepsia, nausea, abdominal pain, constipation, flatulence
Hematologic: Low white blood cell count
Neuromuscular & skeletal: Myalgia, arthralgia, weakness
Ocular: Conjunctivitis

**Overdosage/Toxicology**
Signs and symptoms: Human experience is limited. Oral minimum lethal doses in mice and rats were 500-1000 and 300-1000 mg/kg, respectively (providing >3 and 9 times the systemic exposure achieved at the maximum recommended human daily oral dose, respectively). No deaths occurred, but nephritis was reported in dogs at an oral dose of 1000 mg/kg.
Treatment: Symptomatic; institute supportive measures as required. If indicated, achieve elimination of unabsorbed drug by emesis or gastric lavage; observe usual precautions to maintain the airway. Zileuton is **not** removed by dialysis.

**Drug Interactions** CYP1A2, 2C9, and 3A3/4 enzyme substrate; CYP1A2 and 3A3/4 inhibitor
Increased toxicity:
Propranolol: Doubling of propranolol AUC and consequent increased beta-blocker activity
Terfenadine: Decrease in clearance of terfenadine leading to increase in AUC
Theophylline: Doubling of serum theophylline concentrations - reduce theophylline dose and monitor serum theophylline concentrations closely.
Warfarin: Clinically significant increases in prothrombin time (PT) - monitor PT closely

**Usual Dosage** Oral:
Adults: 600 mg 4 times/day with meals and at bedtime
Elderly: Zileuton pharmacokinetics were similar in healthy elderly subjects (>65 years) compared with healthy younger adults (18-40 years)
**Dosing adjustment in renal impairment:** Dosing adjustment is not necessary in renal impairment or renal failure (even during dialysis)
**Dosing adjustment in hepatic impairment:** Contraindicated in patients with active liver disease

**Patient Information** This medication is not for an acute asthmatic attack; in acute attack, follow instructions of prescriber. Do not stop other asthma medication unless advised by prescriber. Take with meals and at bedtime on a continuous bases; do not discontinue even if feeling better (this medication may help reduce incidence of acute attacks). Avoid alcohol and other medications unless approved by your prescriber. You may experience mild headache (mild analgesic may help); fatigue or dizziness (use caution when driving); or nausea or heartburn (small frequent meals, frequent mouth care, sucking lozenges, or chewing gum may help). Report persistent headache, chest pain, rapid heartbeat, or palpitations; skin rash or itching; unusual bleeding (eg, tarry stools, easy bruising, or blood in stool, urine, or mouth); skin rash or irritation; muscle weakness or tremors; redness, irritation, or infections of the eye; or worsening of asthmatic condition.

**Dosage Forms** Tablet: 600 mg

♦ **Zinacef® Injection** *see* Cefuroxime *on page 102*

♦ **Zincfrin® Ophthalmic [OTC]** *see* Phenylephrine and Zinc Sulfate *on page 440*

## Zinc Gelatin (zingk JEL ah tin)

**U.S. Brand Names** Gelucast®
**Pharmacologic Category** Topical Skin Product
**Use** As a protectant and to support varicosities and similar lesions of the lower limbs
**Effects on Mental Status** None reported
**Effects on Psychiatric Treatment** None reported
**Usual Dosage** Apply externally as an occlusive boot
**Dosage Forms** Bandage: 3" x 10 yards, 4" x 10 yards

## Zinc Oxide (zingk OKS ide)

**Synonyms** Base Ointment; Lassar's Zinc Paste
**Pharmacologic Category** Topical Skin Product
**Use** Protective coating for mild skin irritations and abrasions, soothing and protective ointment to promote healing of chapped skin, diaper rash
**Effects on Mental Status** None reported
**Effects on Psychiatric Treatment** None reported
**Contraindications** Hypersensitivity to zinc oxide or any component
**Warnings/Precautions** Do not use in eyes; for external use only
**Adverse Reactions** 1% to 10%: Local: Skin sensitivity, irritation
**Usual Dosage** Infants, Children, and Adults: Topical: Apply as required for affected areas several times daily
**Patient Information** If irritation develops, discontinue use and consult a physician; paste is easily removed with mineral oil; for external use only; do not use in the eyes
**Dosage Forms**
Ointment, topical: 20% in white ointment (480 g)
Paste, topical: 25% in white petrolatum (480 g)

♦ **Zinecard®** *see* Dexrazoxane *on page 159*

♦ ***Zingiber officinale*** *see* Ginger *on page 249*

## Ziprasidone (zi PRAY si done)

**U.S. Brand Names** Zeldox®
**Pharmacologic Category** Antipsychotic Agent, Benzothiazolylpiperazine
**Use Unlabeled use:** Psychosis
**Adverse Reactions**
>10%: Central nervous system: Somnolence
1% to 10%:
Central nervous system: Dizziness
Gastrointestinal: Nausea, constipation, dyspepsia, diarrhea
Neuromuscular & skeletal: Akathisia, asthenia, EPS
Respiratory: Coryzal symptoms

**Drug Interactions**
Carbamazepine: AUC of ziprasidone decreased by 36% and $C_{max}$ decreased by 27% with concurrent administration; the clinical significance of this decrease is unknown; monitor
Ketoconazole: AUC and $C_{max}$ increased by 33% and 34% respectively, with concurrent administration; the clinical significance of this decrease is unknown; monitor

**Mechanism of Action** The exact mechanism of action is unknown. However, *in vitro* radioligand studies show that ziprasidone has high affinity for D2, 5HT2A, 5HT1A, 5HT2C and 5HT1D, moderate affinity for alpha-1 adrenergic and histamine H1 receptors, and low affinity for alpha-2 adrenergic, beta adrenergic, 5HT3, 5HT4, cholinergic, mu, sigma, or benzodiazepine receptors. Ziprasidone moderately inhibits the reuptake of serotonin and norepinephrine.

**Pharmacodynamics/kinetics**
Protein binding: >99%
Metabolism: Linear, CYP3A4; no active metabolites
Bioavailability: 59%
Half-life: 4-5 hours (10 mg and 40 mg); 8-10 hours (80 mg and 120 mg)
Time to peak: 6-8 hours

**Usual Dosage** Adults and Elderly: Oral: 40-160 mg/day given in 2 divided doses
Dosing adjustment in renal/hepatic impairment: None
**Dietary Considerations** Administration with food increases absorption by 100%
**Monitoring Parameters** Mental status
**Test Interactions** Increased cholesterol, triglycerides, and eosinophils
**Additional Information NOTE:** This is a preliminary monograph; consult full prescribing information when it becomes available

♦ **Ziriton®** *see* Carbinoxamine *on page 92*

♦ **Zithromax™** *see* Azithromycin *on page 55*

♦ **Zocor®** *see* Simvastatin *on page 512*

♦ **Zofran®** *see* Ondansetron *on page 405*

♦ **Zoladex® Implant** *see* Goserelin *on page 254*

♦ **Zolicef®** *see* Cefazolin *on page 97*

## Zolmitriptan (zohl mi TRIP tan)

**U.S. Brand Names** Zomig®
**Synonyms** 311C90
**Pharmacologic Category** Serotonin 5-$HT_{1D}$ Receptor Agonist
**Use** Acute treatment of migraine with or without auras
**Effects on Mental Status** Dizziness is common, may cause drowsiness
**Effects on Psychiatric Treatment** Contraindicated with other serotonin agonists (SSRIs) and MAOIs
**Pregnancy Risk Factor** C
**Contraindications**
Use in patients with ischemic heart disease or Prinzmetal angina, patients with signs or symptoms of ischemic heart disease, uncontrolled hypertension; use in patients with symptomatic Wolff-Parkinson-White syndrome or arrhythmias associated with other cardiac accessory conduction pathway disorders
Use with ergotamine derivatives (within 24 hours of); use within 24 hours of another 5-$HT_1$ agonist; concurrent administration or within 2 weeks of discontinuing an MAOI; hypersensitivity to any component; management of hemiplegic or basilar migraine

**Warnings/Precautions** Zolmitriptan is indicated only in patient populations with a clear diagnosis of migraine. Cardiac events (coronary artery
(Continued)

## Zolmitriptan *(Continued)*

vasospasm, transient ischemia, myocardial infarction, ventricular tachycardia/fibrillation, cardiac arrest, and death) have been reported with 5-$HT_1$ agonist administration. Significant elevation in blood pressure, including hypertensive crisis, has also been reported on rare occasions in patients with and without a history of hypertension. Vasospasm-related reactions have been reported other than coronary artery vasospasm. Peripheral vascular ischemia and colonic ischemia with abdominal pain and bloody diarrhea have occurred. Use with caution in patients with hepatic impairment.

**Adverse Reactions**

>10%:

Central nervous system: Dizziness
Endocrine & metabolic: Hot flashes
Neuromuscular & skeletal: Paresthesia

1% to 10%:

Cardiovascular: Tightness in chest
Central nervous system: Drowsiness, headache
Dermatologic: Burning sensation
Gastrointestinal: Abdominal discomfort, mouth discomfort
Neuromuscular & skeletal: Myalgia, numbness, weakness, neck pain, jaw discomfort
Miscellaneous: Diaphoresis

<1%: Dehydration, dysmenorrhea, dyspnea, dysuria, hiccups, polydipsia, rashes, renal calculus, thirst

**Drug Interactions** Increased toxicity: Ergot-containing drugs, MAOIs, cimetidine, oral contraceptives, SSRIs

**Usual Dosage** Adults:

Oral: Initial recommended dose: 2.5 mg or lower (achieved by manually breaking a 2.5 mg tablet in half). If the headache returns, the dose may be repeated after 2 hours, not to exceed 10 mg within a 24-hour period. Response is greater following the 2.5 or 5 mg dose compared with 1 mg, with little added benefit and increased side effects associated with the 5 mg dose.

**Dosage adjustment in hepatic impairment:** Administer with caution in patients with liver disease, generally using doses <2.5 mg. Patients with moderate-to-severe hepatic impairment may have decreased clearance of zolmitriptan, and significant elevation in blood pressure was observed in some patients.

**Patient Information** This drug is to be used to reduce your migraine, not to prevent or reduce number of attacks. If first dose brings relief, second dose may be taken anytime after 2 hours if migraine returns. If you have no relief with first dose, do not take a second dose without consulting prescriber. Do not exceed 10 mg in 24 hours. You may experience some dizziness or drowsiness; use caution when driving or engaging in tasks requiring alertness until response to drug is known. Frequent mouth care and sucking on lozenges may relieve dry mouth. Report immediately any chest pain, heart throbbing or tightness in throat; swelling of eyelids, face, or lips; skin rash or hives; easy bruising; blood in urine, stool, or vomitus; pain or itching with urination; or pain, warmth, or numbness in extremities.

**Dosage Forms** Tablet: 2.5 mg, 5 mg

♦ **Zoloft®** *see* Sertraline *on page 509*

## Zolpidem (zole PI dem)

**Related Information**

Anxiolytic/Hypnotic Use in Long-Term Care Facilities *on page 754*
Clinical Issues in the Use of Anxiolytics and Sedative/Hypnotics *on page 634*
Nonbenzodiazepine Anxiolytics and Hypnotics *on page 721*
Patient Information - Anxiolytics & Sedative Hypnotics (Nonbenzodiazepine Hypnotics) *on page 656*
Secondary Mental Disorders *on page 616*
Sleep Disorders *on page 620*
Special Populations - Elderly *on page 662*

**Generic Available** No

**U.S. Brand Names** Ambien™

**Synonyms** Zolpidem Tartrate

**Pharmacologic Category** Hypnotic, Nonbenzodiazepine

**Use** Short-term treatment of insomnia

**Restrictions** C-IV

**Pregnancy Risk Factor** B

**Contraindications** Known hypersensitivity to zolpidem

**Warnings/Precautions** Should be used only after evaluation of potential causes of sleep disturbance. Failure of sleep disturbance to resolve after 7-10 days may indicate psychiatric or medical illness. Use with caution in patients with depression. Behavioral changes have been associated with sedative-hypnotics. Causes CNS depression, which may impair physical and mental capabilities. Effects with other sedative drugs or ethanol may be potentiated. Closely monitor elderly or debilitated patients for impaired cognitive or motor performance; not recommended for use in children <18 years of age. Avoid use in patients with sleep apnea or a history of sedative-hypnotic abuse.

**Adverse Reactions** 1% to 10%:

Cardiovascular: Palpitations
Central nervous system: Headache, drowsiness, dizziness, lethargy, lightheadedness, depression, abnormal dreams, amnesia
Dermatologic: Rash
Gastrointestinal: Nausea, diarrhea, xerostomia, constipation
Respiratory: Sinusitis, pharyngitis

**Overdosage/Toxicology**

Signs and symptoms: Coma
Treatment: Supportive; rarely is mechanical ventilation required. Flumazenil has been shown to selectively block the binding of benzodiazepines to CNS receptors, resulting in a reversal of benzodiazepine-induced CNS depression but not always respiratory depression

**Drug Interactions** CYP3A3/4 enzyme substrate

Antipsychotics: Sedative effects may be additive with antipsychotics, including phenothiazines; monitor for increased effect
CNS depressants: Sedative effects may be additive with other CNS depressants; monitor for increased effect; includes barbiturates, benzodiazepines, narcotic analgesics, ethanol, and other sedative agents
CYP3A3/4 inhibitors: Serum level and/or toxicity of zolpidem may be increased; inhibitors include amiodarone, cimetidine, clarithromycin, erythromycin, delavirdine, diltiazem, dirithromycin, disulfiram, fluoxetine, fluvoxamine, grapefruit juice, indinavir, itraconazole, ketoconazole, metronidazole, nefazodone, nevirapine, propoxyfene, quinupristin-dalfopristin, ritonavir, saquinavir, verapamil, zafirlukast, zileuton; monitor for increased response
Enzyme inducers: May increase the metabolism of zolpidem, reducing its effectiveness; inducers include phenytoin, carbamazepine, phenobarbital, and rifampin
SSRIs: Sertraline and fluoxetine (to a lesser extent) have been demonstrated to increase zaleplon levels; pharmacodynamic effects were not significantly changed; monitor

**Mechanism of Action** Structurally dissimilar to benzodiazepine, however, has much or all of its actions explained by its effects on benzodiazepine (BZD) receptors, especially the omega-1 receptor (with a high affinity ratio of the alpha 1/alpha 5 subunits); retains hypnotic and much of the anxiolytic properties of the BZD, but has reduced effects on skeletal muscle and seizure threshold.

**Pharmacodynamics/kinetics**

Onset of action: 30 minutes
Duration: 6-8 hours
Absorption: Rapid
Distribution: Very low amounts secreted into breast milk
Protein binding: 92%
Metabolism: Hepatic to inactive metabolites
Half-life: 2-2.6 hours, in cirrhosis increased to 9.9 hours

**Usual Dosage** Duration of therapy should be limited to 7-10 days

Adults: Oral: 10 mg immediately before bedtime; maximum dose: 10 mg
Elderly: 5 mg immediately before bedtime
Hemodialysis: Not dialyzable
**Dosing adjustment in hepatic impairment:** Decrease dose to 5 mg

**Dietary Considerations** Alcohol: Additive CNS effect, avoid useo

**Administration** Ingest immediately before bedtime due to rapid onset of action

**Monitoring Parameters** Daytime alertness; respiratory and cardiac status

**Reference Range** 80-150 ng/mL

**Test Interactions** ↑ ALT

**Patient Information** Avoid alcohol and other CNS depressants while taking this medication

**Nursing Implications** Patients may require assistance with ambulation; lower doses in the elderly are usually effective; institute safety measures

**Additional Information** Causes less disturbances in sleep stages as compared to benzodiazepines; time spent in sleep stages 3 and 4 are maintained; decreases sleep latency. Should not be prescribed in quantities exceeding a 1-month supply.

**Dosage Forms** Tablet, as tartrate: 5 mg, 10 mg

♦ **Zolpidem Tartrate** *see* Zolpidem *on page 594*
♦ **Zomig®** *see* Zolmitriptan *on page 593*
♦ **Zonalon® Topical Cream** *see* Doxepin *on page 183*
♦ **Zone-A Forte®** *see* Pramoxine and Hydrocortisone *on page 457*
♦ **Zonegran™** *see* Zonisamide *on page 594*

## Zonisamide (zoe NIS a mide)

**U.S. Brand Names** Zonegran™

**Pharmacologic Category** Anticonvulsant, Miscellaneous

**Use** Adjunct treatment of partial seizures in adults with epilepsy

**Pregnancy Risk Factor** C

**Pregnancy/Breast-Feeding Implications** Fetal abnormalities and death have been reported in animals, however, there are no studies in pregnant women. It is not known if zonisamide is excreted in human milk. Use during pregnancy/lactation only if the potential benefits outweigh the potential risks.

**Contraindications** Hypersensitivity to sulfonamides or zonisamide

**Warnings/Precautions** Rare, but potentially fatal sulfonamide reactions have occurred following the use of zonisamide. These reactions include Stevens-Johnson syndrome and toxic epidermal necrolysis, usually appearing within 2-16 weeks of drug initiation. Discontinue zonisamide if rash develops. Decreased sweating and hyperthermia requiring hospitalization have been reported in children. The safety and efficacy in children <16 years of age has not been established. Discontinue zonisamide in patients who develop acute renal failure or a significant sustained increase in creatinine/BUN concentration. Kidney stones have been reported. Use cautiously in patients with renal or hepatic dysfunction. Do not use if estimated $Cl_{cr}$ <50 mL/minute. Significant CNS effects include psychiatric symptoms, psychomotor slowing, and fatigue or somnolence. Fatigue and somnolence occur within the first month of treatment, most commonly at doses of 300-500 mg/day. Abrupt withdrawal may precipitate seizures; discontinue or reduce doses gradually.

**Adverse Reactions** Adjunctive Therapy: Frequencies noted in patients receiving other anticonvulsants:

>10%:

Central nervous system: Somnolence (17%), dizziness (13%)

Gastrointestinal: Anorexia (13%)

1% to 10%:

Central nervous system: Headache (10%), agitation/irritability (9%), fatigue (8%), tiredness (7%), ataxia (6%), confusion (6%), decreased concentration (6%), memory impairment (6%), depression (6%), insomnia (6%), speech disorders (5%), mental slowing (4%), anxiety (3%), nervousness (2%), schizophrenic/schizophreniform behavior (2%), difficulty in verbal expression (2%), status epilepticus (1%)

Dermatologic: Rash (3%), bruising (2%)

Gastrointestinal: Nausea (9%), abdominal pain (6%), diarrhea (5%), dyspepsia (3%), weight loss (3%), constipation (2%), dry mouth (2%), taste perversion (2%)

Neuromuscular & skeletal: Paresthesia (4%)

Ocular: Diplopia (6%), nystagmus (4%)

Respiratory: Rhinitis (2%)

Miscellaneous: Flu-like syndrome (4%)

Additional adverse effects have been reported as frequent (occur in at least 1:100 patients), infrequent (occur in 1:100 to 1:1000 patients), or rare (occur in less than 1:1000 patients):

Frequent: Tremor, convulsion, hyperesthesia, incoordination, pruritus, vomiting, weakness, abnormal gait, accidental injury, amblyopia, tinnitus, pharyngitis, increased cough

Infrequent: Flank pain, malaise, abnormal dreams, vertigo, movement disorder, hypotonia, euphoria, chest pain, facial edema, palpitations, tachycardia, vascular insufficiency, hypotension, hypertension, syncope, bradycardia, peripheral edema, edema, cerebrovascular accident, maculopapular rash, acne, alopecia, dry skin, eczema, urticaria, hirsutism, pustular rash, vesiculobullous rash, dehydration, decreased libido, amenorrhea, flatulence, gingivitis, gum hyperplasia, gastritis, gastroenteritis, stomatitis, glossitis, melena, ulcerative stomatitis, gastroduodenal ulcer, dysphagia, weight gain, urinary frequency, dysuria, urinary incontinence, impotence, urinary retention, urinary urgency, polyuria, nocturia, rectal hemorrhage, gum hemorrhage, leukopenia, anemia, cholelithiasis, thrombophlebitis, neck rigidity, leg cramps, myalgia, myasthenia, arthralgia, arthritis, hypertonia, neuropathy, twitching, hyperkinesia, dysarthria, peripheral neuritis, paresthesia, increased reflexes, allergic reaction, lymphadenopathy, immunodeficiency, thirst, sweating, parosmia, conjunctivitis, visual field defect, glaucoma, deafness, hematuria, dyspnea

Rare: Dystonia, encephalopathy, atrial fibrillation, heart failure, ventricular extrasystoles, petechia, hypoglycemia, hyponatremia, gynecomastia, mastitis, menorrhagia, cholangitis, hematemesis, colitis, duodenitis, esophagitis, fecal incontinence, mouth ulceration, enuresis, bladder pain, bladder calculus, thrombocytopenia, microcytic anemia, cholecystitis, cholestatic jaundice, increased AST (SGOT), increased ALT (SGPT), circumoral paresthesia, dyskinesia, facial paralysis, hypokinesia, myoclonus, lupus erythematosus, increased lactic dehydrogenase, oculogyric crisis, photophobia, iritis, albuminuria, pulmonary embolus, apnea, hemoptysis

Case Reports: Stevens-Johnson syndrome, toxic epidermal necrolysis, aplastic anemia, agranulocytosis, kidney stones, increased BUN, increased serum creatinine, increased serum alkaline phosphatase

**Overdosage/Toxicology** No specific antidotes are available; experience with doses >800 mg/day is limited. Emesis or gastric lavage, with airway protection, should be done following a recent overdose. General supportive care and close observation are indicated. Renal dialysis may not be effective due to low protein binding (40%).

**Drug Interactions** CYP3A3/4 enzyme substrate

**Note:** Zonisamide did NOT affect steady state levels of carbamazepine, phenytoin, or valproate; zonisamide half-life is decreased by carbamazepine, phenytoin, phenobarbital, and valproate

Cimetidine: Single dose zonisamide levels were not altered by cimetidine

CNS depressants: Sedative effects may be additive with other CNS depressants; monitor for increased effect; includes barbiturates, benzodiazepines, narcotic analgesics, ethanol, and other sedative agents

CYP3A3/4 inhibitors: Serum level and/or toxicity of zonisamide may be increased; inhibitors include amiodarone, cimetidine, clarithromycin, erythromycin, delavirdine, diltiazem, dirithromycin, disulfiram, fluoxetine, fluvoxamine, grapefruit juice, indinavir, itraconazole, ketoconazole, metronidazole, nefazodone, nevirapine, propoxyfene, quinupristin-dalfopristin, ritonavir, saquinavir, verapamil, zafirlukast, zileuton; monitor for increased response

Enzyme inducers: May increase the metabolism of zonisamide, reducing its effectiveness; inducers include phenytoin, carbamazepine, phenobarbital, and rifampin

**Stability** Store at controlled room temperature 25°C (77°F). Protect from moisture and light

**Mechanism of Action** The exact mechanism of action is not known. May stabilize neuronal membranes and suppress neuronal hypersynchronization through action at sodium and calcium channels. Does not affect GABA activity.

**Pharmacodynamics/kinetics**

Distribution: $V_d$: 1.45 L/kg

Protein binding: 40%

Metabolism: Hepatic (CYP3A4), forms N-acetyl zonisamide and 2-sulfamoylacetyl phenol (SMAP)

Half-life: 63 hours

Time to peak: 2-6 hours

Elimination: Urine, 62% (35% as parent drug, 65% as metabolites); feces, 3%

**Usual Dosage**

Children >16 years and Adults: Oral: For the adjunctive treatment of partial seizures, initial dose is 100 mg/day. Dose may be increased to 200 mg/day after 2 weeks. Further dosage increases to 300 mg and 400 mg/day can then be made with a minimum of 2 weeks between adjustments, in order to reach steady state at each dosage level. Doses of up to 600 mg/day have been studied, however, there is no evidence of increased response with doses above 400 mg/day.

**Dosage adjustment in renal/hepatic impairment:** Slower titration and frequent monitoring are indicated in patients with renal or hepatic disease. Do not use if $Cl_{cr}$ <50 mL/minute.

Elderly: Data from clinical trials is insufficient for patients over 65. Begin dosing at the low end of the dosing range.

**Dietary Considerations** May be taken with or without food

**Administration** Capsules should be swallowed whole; dose may be given once or twice daily; doses of 300 mg/day and higher are associated with increased side effects; steady state levels are reached in 14 days

**Monitoring Parameters** Monitor BUN and serum creatinine

**Patient Information** May cause drowsiness, especially at higher doses. Do not drive a car or operate other complex machinery until effects on performance can be determined. Avoid alcohol and other CNS depressants. Contact healthcare provider immediately if seizures worsen or for any of the following symptoms: skin rash; sudden back pain, abdominal pain, blood in the urine; fever, sore throat, oral ulcers, or easy bruising. Contact healthcare provider before becoming pregnant or breast-feeding. Swallow capsules whole, do not bite or break. It is important to drink 6-8 glasses of water each day while using this medication. Do not stop taking this or other seizure medications without talking to your healthcare professional first.

**Dosage Forms** Capsule: 100 mg


- **ZORprin®** *see* Aspirin *on page 49*
- **Zostrix® [OTC]** *see* Capsaicin *on page 89*
- **Zostrix®-HP [OTC]** *see* Capsaicin *on page 89*
- **Zosyn™** *see* Piperacillin and Tazobactam Sodium *on page 448*
- **Zovia®** *see* Estradiol and Ethynodiol Diacetate *on page 204*
- **Zovirax®** *see* Acyclovir *on page 19*
- **Zyban™** *see* Bupropion *on page 77*
- **Zydone®** *see* Hydrocodone and Acetaminophen *on page 272*
- **Zyflo™** *see* Zileuton *on page 592*
- **Zyloprim®** *see* Allopurinol *on page 24*
- **Zymase®** *see* Pancrelipase *on page 418*
- **Zyprexa™** *see* Olanzapine *on page 403*
- **Zyprexa™ Zydis®** *see* Olanzapine *on page 403*
- **Zyrtec®** *see* Cetirizine *on page 105*
- **Zyvox™** *see* Linezolid *on page 318*

# PSYCHIATRIC SPECIAL TOPICS/ISSUES

## TABLE OF CONTENTS

# PSYCHIATRIC ASSESSMENT

## GENERAL PATIENT ASSESSMENT

Evaluation of a patient with a psychiatric disorder is similar to other medical assessments. The evaluation should include a comprehensive medical and psychiatric history including family psychiatric history, medication, allergies, and review of systems. Collateral history from family members is often crucial in furnishing information that the patient may be unable to provide. History of response to previous treatment is essential in cases where pharmacologic therapy is to be initiated. Basic physical evaluations include physical/neurologic exam and laboratory testing including blood chemistries, blood counts, endocrine, hepatic, and other specialized evaluations as indicated. Imaging or lumbar puncture may be indicated in some cases for ruling out neurological or medical diagnoses.

An outline of components of the comprehensive psychiatric assessment is described below.

1. History of present illness: Include patient's age, sex, race, past psychiatric diagnosis, and current presenting problems including duration and history of onset
2. Past psychiatric history: Include previous psychiatric diagnoses, treatments, hospitalizations, and drug therapies
3. Family psychiatric history: Include history of alcoholism, substance abuse, and any suspected psychiatric disorders
4. Past/current medical history: Include all medical/neurologic disorders, treatments, hospitalizations, surgeries, and medications. For women, obtain gynecological history including last menstrual period (rule out pregnancy).
5. Allergies
6. Developmental history: Include birth history, childhood history (including query for childhood abuse), educational level, and significant traumatic events (eg, loss of parent)
7. Social history: Include marital status, employment history, and level of impairment associated with psychiatric disorder
8. Substance abuse history
9. Review of systems
10. Laboratory data as needed
11. Other specialized studies: EEG, MRI, CT, etc as needed
12. Physical exam (unless done recently, should be obtained; required for acute mental status change)
13. Mental status exam: Includes:
    - A. General impression: Appearance, state of self care, eye contact, etc
    - B. Speech: Note rate, rhythm, coherence
    - C. Affect
    - D. Cognition: Include gross awareness of person, place, time, concentration, memory, and recall; may require specialized testing if impairment exists
    - E. Mood
    - F. Risk assessment: Include potential risk of harm to self or others
    - G. Perceptual disturbances, such as hallucinations
    - H. Thought form: Assess for loosening of associations, formal thought disorder
    - I. Thought content: Include delusions/paranoia
    - J. Insight: Include determination of patient appreciation of the disorder, its impairing effects, and awareness of risk to self or others
    - K. Judgment: In particular judgment based on patient's current status
    - L. Psychometric testing as needed
    - M. Differential diagnosis and preliminary diagnosis
    - N. Treatment plan: Include pharmacotherapy, psychotherapy, additional referrals (eg, marital therapy), nutritional counseling, substance abuse treatment, psychosocial rehabilitation, and other interventions as needed

Most components of the assessment may be done at first patient visit, or shortly thereafter, although some, such as psychometric testing or specialized studies such as EEG, may require more time. Most importantly, the psychiatric diagnosis (and attendant treatments) should not be considered fixed and unchangeable as additional later obtained history may shed insight onto diagnosis (eg, previous "highs" which may clarify a diagnosis of bipolar illness). In acute clinical situations, treatments may be initiated before diagnosis is completely clear, as in the case of the agitated, psychotic patient who is prescribed antipsychotic medication as a full diagnostic assessment is underway.

## PSYCHIATRIC RATING SCALES

Because mental health practitioners have not generally had availability of biologic markers to assess psychiatric illness, a variety of rating instruments, or rating scales, have been developed to assess presence or severity of psychiatric disorders. Rating scales are used in psychiatry to quantify a variety of aspects of mental disorders. These may include symptoms or behaviors which are externally observable such as agitation or hyperactivity, or reported symptoms such as depressed mood. Scales may be focused on specific disorders such as depression or applied widely to multiple disorders such as the Global Assessment of Functioning Scale (GAF) used in the DSM-IV. Rating scales assist both clinicians and clinical researchers in specifying clinical observations, and may be particularly useful when a clinical assessment of change over time is required (eg, evaluation of extrapyramidal symptoms associated with long-term antipsychotic medication use). The best scales are those which have been demonstrated to be reliable and valid in assessing clinical status among large groups of patients. The following table lists some of the most commonly used scales in psychiatry, the types of disorders the scale is used in, and comments on scale administration.

| Scale Name | Target Disorder | Comments |
|---|---|---|
| Brief Psychiatric Rating Scale (BPRS)[1] | Schizophrenia/psychosis | Rater administered; multiple versions exist |
| Positive and Negative Symptom Scale (PANSS)[2] | Schizophrenia | Rater administered; BPRS may be extracted from PANSS |
| Hamilton Depression Scale (HAM-D)[3] | Depression | Rater administered, probably is the most commonly used depression scale; multiple versions |
| Montgomery Asberg Depression Rating Scale (MADRS)[4] | Depression | Rater administered |
| Beck Depression Inventory (BDI)[5] | Depression | Self administered scale |
| Zung Self Rating Scale for Depression[6] | Depression | Self administered scale |
| Young Mania Rating Scale (YMRS)[7] | Bipolar disorder | Rater administered |
| Hamilton Anxiety Scale (HAM-A)[8] | Anxiety disorders | Rater administered; multiple versions; heavily focused on somatic symptoms |
| Yale Brown Obsessive-Compulsive Scale (YBOC)[9] | Obsessive-compulsive disorder | Rater administered |
| Global Assessment of Functioning (GAF)[10] | All psychiatric disorders | Rater administered; single item score, assess functional level; in DSM-IV |
| Clinical Global Impressions (CGI)[11] | All psychiatric disorders | Rater administered; assess severity of illness; single item score |
| Abnormal Involuntary Movement Scale (AIMS)[12] | Neurological symptoms/ extrapyramidal symptoms | Rater administered; most commonly used to assess extrapyramidal symptoms associated with psychotropic medication |
| Mini-Mental State Examination (MMSE)[13] | Dementia | Rater administered; grades cognitive status of patients with cognitive impairment |

1. Overall JE and Gorham DR, "The Brief Psychiatric Rating Scale," *Psychological Reports (BPRS)*, 1962, 10:799-812.
2. Kay SR, Fiszbein A, and Opler LA, "The Positive and Negative Syndrome Scale (PANSS) for Schizophrenia," *Schizophr Bull*, 1987, 13(2):261-76.
3. Hamilton M, "A Rating Scale for Depression," *J Neurol Neurosurg Psychiatry*, 1960, 23:56-62.
4. Montgomery SA and Asberg M, "A New Depression Scale Designed to be Sensitive to Change," *Br J Psychiatry*, 1979, 134:382-9.
5. Beck AT, Ward CH, Mendelson M, et al, "An Inventory for Measuring Depression," *Arch Gen Psychiatry*, 1961, 4:561-71.
6. Zung WWK, "A Self-Rating Depression Scale," *Arch Gen Psychiatry*, 1965, 12:63-70.
7. Young RC, Biggs JT, Ziegler VE, et al, "A Rating Scale for Mania: Reliability, Validity, and Sensitivity," *Br J Psychiatry*, 1978, 133:429-35.
8. Hamilton M, "The Assessment of Anxiety States by Rating," *Br J Med*, 1959, 32:56-62.
9. Goodman WK, Price LH, Rasmussen SA, et al, "The Yale-Brown Obsessive Compulsive Scale. I. Development, Use, and Reliability," *Arch Gen Psychiatry*, 1989, 46(11):1006-11.
10. Endicott J, Spitzer RL, Fleiss JL, et al, "The Global Assessment Scale: A Procedure for Measuring Overall Severity of Psychiatric Disturbance," *Arch Gen Psychiatry*, 1976, 33(6):766-71.
11 & 12. Guy W, "Clinical Global Impressions," in Early Clinical Drug Evaluation Unit (ECDEU): Assessment Manual for Psychopharmacology (Revised), Washington DC, United States Department of Health, Education, and Welfare, 1976 (CGI and AIMS).
13. Folstein MF, Folstein SE, and McHugh PR, "Mini-Mental State: A Practical Method for Grading the Cognitive State of Patients for the Clinician," *J Psychiatr Res*, 1975, 12(3):189-98.

# MOOD DISORDERS

Mood disorders are pathological affective states, primarily divided into depressive disorders and bipolar disorders. Major depression, or unipolar depression, is a common disorder with a lifetime prevalence of 15%. Women are nearly twice as likely to develop major depression as men. Bipolar disorder is seen in approximately 1% of the population, with an equal gender distribution. Mean age of onset for major depression is in the mid 20s, while bipolar disorder usually presents between the ages of 20-40 (mean age 32 years). Both major depression and bipolar disorder tend to be chronic, with a tendency for relapse. However, patients with major depression generally have a better prognosis than those with bipolar disorder. Up to one third of individuals with bipolar disorder have some degree of chronic symptoms, and fairly severe functional impairment. The etiology of mood disorders is not clear. Biological studies have strongly suggested that abnormalities in biogenic amines are associated with some mood-disordered states. The neurotransmitter/biogenic amines, norepinephrine and serotonin, have been the most well studied. Antidepressant drugs, which clearly improve mood state, work by normalizing levels of norepinephrine and serotonin, among other effects. As with other major psychiatric disorders, mood disorders, particularly bipolar disorder, appear to have a genetic basis. The concordance rate for bipolar I disorder in monozygotic twins has been reported to range from 30% to 90%.

## CLINICAL PRESENTATION

### UNIPOLAR MOOD DISORDER

Major depressive disorder, or unipolar mood disorder is characterized by persistent depressed mood or anhedonia, and presence of a variety of other symptoms including significant weight change, sleep disturbance, psychomotor agitation or retardation, decreased energy, feelings of worthlessness or inappropriate guilt, diminished concentration, and thoughts of death. Symptoms may fluctuate in severity, and present in some individuals with a diurnal pattern, usually of greatest severity in the morning, and subsequent improvement as the day progresses. Depression is perceived by the patient as distressing, and is associated with impairments in work or social functioning. Severely depressed individuals may have psychotic features in addition to depressive symptoms. Another subgroup of depressed patients present atypically with increased sleep, increased appetite, and weight gain.

Depressed individuals are at particular risk for suicide, with 10% to 15% of depressed patients eventually committing suicide. Those with psychotic depression may be at greater risk for suicide. Careful monitoring of suicide risk is essential in all phases of treatment of the depressed individual.

Anxiety frequently coexists with depressive symptoms, and the depressed individual may present to care providers with numerous somatic complaints, including headaches, shortness of breath, and chronic fatigue. Substance abuse is not uncommon in depressed individuals, and symptoms of chronic alcohol abuse may be difficult to separate from depressive symptoms.

Depression in the elderly is more common than in younger populations, with prevalence rates up to 40% in some older adult populations. Depression in elderly individuals is often undiagnosed, as patients may report anhedonia as a primary symptom, rather than frankly depressed mood, as well as presenting a variety of somatic complaints. Cognitive impairment associated with major depression, which has been described as pseudo-dementia, may lead to substantial functional impairment.

### BIPOLAR DISORDER

Bipolar disorder is characterized by the presence of at least one manic episode, defined as a period of abnormal, persistently elevated, expansive, or irritable mood. Additional symptoms present during a manic episode include grandiose or inappropriately inflated self-esteem, diminished sleep, excessive/pressured speech, racing thoughts, distractibility, agitation, and involvement in activities that may lead to risk or negative consequences, such as excessive spending, substance abuse, or sexual promiscuity. Although patients frequently deny illness, manic symptoms are associated with severe impairments in functional status. Risk of harm to self or others may occur during manic episodes as patients may behave impulsively, and with poor insight. Many severely manic patients exhibit frank psychotic symptoms and hospitalization is often indicated for safe management of the acute stage of mania.

### SCHIZOAFFECTIVE DISORDER

Schizoaffective disorder is a complex and poorly understood clinical entity. In schizoaffective disorder, a prominent, chronic, mood disorder is concurrent with the active phase of schizophrenia. Mood symptoms are present for a substantial portion of the total duration of the illness. Long-term studies have found that a large number of individuals initially diagnosed with schizoaffective disorder are found to more accurately fulfill diagnostic criteria for either bipolar disorder or for schizophrenia on long-term follow-up. Drug treatment of schizoaffective disorder has not been well studied. In common clinical practice, individuals with schizoaffective disorder, bipolar subtype, are often managed with mood stabilizing medication such as lithium or valproate plus an antipsychotic. Individuals with schizoaffective disorder, depressed type, are often treated with the combination of antidepressant and antipsychotic medications. Clozapine appears to show promise in the treatment of schizoaffective disorder, and recently it has been suggested that the atypical antipsychotics may be particularly useful in management of serious mood disorders. The atypical antipsychotic medication, olanzapine, has recently received an FDA-approved indication for bipolar mania.

## GENERAL TREATMENT RECOMMENDATIONS

### PSYCHOTHERAPY AND COMBINED THERAPY

Psychotherapy is an essential component of the treatment of mood disorders. Most studies suggest that combined psychotherapy and medication management are the most effective treatment for major depressive disorder. There are many types of effective psychotherapies for mood disorders, and psychotherapeutic approaches should be tailored to the individual patient's needs and abilities. Cognitive behavioral therapy (CBT) and interpersonal therapy (IT) are the psychotherapeutic treatments that have the best documented efficacy in the literature for the treatment of major depressive disorder. Significant advances in developments of biologic therapies for the treatment of mood disorders over the last decade have changed the management of mood disorders. Aggressive use of the drug therapies may improve outcome, as it is known that prophylactic drug treatment in major depression lowers rate of relapse. A greater recognition and understanding of mood disorders by both the public and physicians, including primary care providers, suggests promise in improving quality of life for individuals with mood disorders.

### ECT

Electroconvulsive therapy (ECT) is a clearly proven, effective intervention for the treatment of depression. ECT is particularly efficacious in cases of psychotic depression. The exact mechanism of action of ECT remains unclear. Due to the stigma associated with ECT, this procedure is often administered only to those depressed patients who are unable to take antidepressant medication, or those who have failed previous trials of antidepressant medication.

Patients and families of patients undergoing ECT should be instructed regarding the risks and benefits of ECT in depression, and signed, informed consent should be obtained from the patient or guardian. Requirements for documentation of informed consent for ECT may vary geographically.

The process of administering ECT is the following: The patient receives an anticholinergic medication (eg, atropine), a quick-acting anesthetic, and a muscle relaxant (eg, succinylcholine). As the general anesthetic takes effect, the patient requires artificial ventilation. ECT is often administered in recovery room-type settings. The patient receives a brief electrical stimulus via electrodes applied to the scalp, which results in a brief seizure (40-60 seconds). The muscle relaxant administered prior to ECT prevents muscular seizure activity. Monitoring of seizure activity in the brain may occur via electroencephalogram (EEG) monitoring, or alternatively, the physician may prevent muscle relaxation of one distal extremity via placing a blood pressure cuff on the extremity, and monitoring seizure activity of the distal limb. ECT is usually administered 2-3 times weekly, for a total of 5-12 treatments. Recovery is complete by the completion of the course of ECT in treatment responders. An antidepressant medication is generally prescribed in the 6-12 months after ECT to prevent relapse. Some clinicians advise maintenance antidepressant therapy for even longer periods after ECT. Occasionally, maintenance ECT (eg, 1 treatment monthly) is used.

## UNIPOLAR MOOD DISORDER DRUG TREATMENTS

Effective treatments of depression have been available for the past four decades. Recovery from major depressive episode is clearly accelerated with antidepressant therapy, while risk of serious negative sequelae such as suicide or suicide attempt, is reduced in treated depression. The greatest challenge in treating major depression in the general population remains under-recognition and undertreatment of depression. Many patients with depression do not seek professional treatment for their mood disorder, and patients seen in primary care settings are not always adequately treated for depressive illness. See Antidepressant Agents *on page 704*. The main classes of antidepressant medications follow.

1. Tricyclic antidepressants and related compounds (eg, nortriptyline) are effective drugs introduced in the 1950s whose use has been reduced over the last decade due to the appearance of newer, widely used antidepressant drugs
2. Serotonin-selective reuptake inhibitors (SSRIs) (eg, fluoxetine) introduced in the U.S. in the 1980s and used very widely due to their good efficacy, ease of use, and good tolerability
3. Dopamine reuptake blocking compounds (eg, bupropion)
4. Selective serotonin-norepinephrine uptake inhibitors (eg, venlafaxine)
5. 5-$HT_2$ antagonists (eg, nefazodone)
6. Alpha-adrenoceptor antagonist (eg, mirtazapine)
7. Monoamine oxidase inhibitors (MAOIs) (eg, phenelzine) which may be particularly effective in refractory depression, but impose dietary restrictions during use, and have more potentially severe adverse reactions

Antidepressant drugs appear to be approximately equally efficacious in the treatment of major depression, with no one drug or class offering clearly superior efficacy in mood disorders. However, individual patients may respond preferentially to one drug as opposed to another. Selection of antidepressant drug is thus usually based on previous history of drug response (if available), and drug side effect profile. A general overview of antidepressant drugs is discussed in Clinical Issues in the Use of Antidepressants *on page 627*. Unfortunately, at this time, there remain a fairly substantial number of depressed individuals who do not respond to an initial trial of antidepressant drugs. In addition, time to treatment response generally requires 4-6 weeks, and may require up to 8-12 weeks. Antidepressant drugs should generally be initiated slowly, and in low dosages except for SSRI medication, some of which may be administered once daily with little or no dosage titration required (eg, fluoxetine 20 mg/day). For medications that are likely to be sedating (eg, tricyclic compounds, nefazodone), prescribing the bulk of dosing at bedtime is often helpful in eliminating excessive daytime sedation, and in improving nighttime sleep. Special populations, such as the elderly or those with multiple medical conditions, may require reduced dosage of medication. Currently, many clinicians prescribe SSRI medications, or another novel antidepressant (eg, nefazodone or venlafaxine) as first-line treatment due to their relatively benign side effect profile compared to older antidepressant drugs (eg, tricyclic antidepressants). Use of concomitant psychotropics that increase sedation, orthostasis, or drug-drug interactions should be avoided if possible, although many clinicians advocate judicious use of sedative/hypnotic medication in the early treatment of major depression in an effort to restore sleep and manage agitation or anxiety while waiting for full antidepressant medication response. Once full antidepressant response is achieved, the clinician should continue antidepressant medication for at least 6-12 months. For patients with severe, recurrent depression, particularly those with suicidal behavior associated with severe depression, even longer term therapy (prophylactic treatment) may be indicated. Most clinicians also currently advocate continuing the same dosage of antidepressant medication during maintenance treatment, as in the acute phase of treatment. When antidepressant medication is discontinued, it should be done as a slow taper over several weeks, to minimize withdrawal reactions (see Discontinuation of Drugs *on page 798*).

For patients who do not respond to initial trial of antidepressant trial, the clinician is faced with the choice of augmenting antidepressant medication or switching drugs. For partial responder patients, adding another antidepressant (eg, add low-dose tricyclic antidepressant to SSRI), or an augmenting agent such as lithium (usually at dosages of 300-1500 mg/day), or thyroid hormone cytomel ($T_3$) up to 50 mcg/day or levothroid ($T_4$) up to 200 mcg/day may be successful. Some clinicians utilize stimulant drugs as antidepressant agents (eg, methylphenidate 5-20 mg/day) for treatment of refractory illness, particularly in individuals where rapid response is critical (eg, medically ill individuals with severely depleted nutritional status). For nonresponders, switching to another antidepressant drug is usually indicated. When switching to an alternative drug, most clinicians choose an antidepressant medication from a new class, as opposed to initiating a medication from the same class as the failed drug. Clinicians must be aware of the need for washout periods when switching to and from MAOI drugs, as discussed in the section on antidepressant medications (see discussion of antidepressants *on page 627*). Individuals with severe, treatment refractory illness may require judicious, appropriate use of multiple antidepressant/augmenting agents, "rational polypharmacy". As with all psychotropic agents, clinicians should attempt to utilize lowest effective medication dosage, and continuously assess for tolerance and effectiveness of drug regimen. Finally, for patients who are nonresponsive to medication, or who are at physical risk due to depressive symptoms, electroconvulsive therapy (ECT) should be considered.

## BIPOLAR DISORDER DRUG TREATMENTS

The goal in pharmacologic treatment of bipolar disorder is complete remission of symptoms with return to premorbid level of functioning. The cornerstone of drug treatment is mood stabilizing medication. Because bipolar disorder is a chronic, often relapsing condition, long-term maintenance or prophylaxis treatment with mood stabilizing medication is almost always indicated. Many clinicians recommend life-time prophylaxis, however, this view must be balanced with patient preference and history of the individual patient. The two most commonly used mood stabilizers are lithium and valproate (see Clinical Issues in the Use of Mood Stabilizers *on page 632*). Lithium has the strongest evidence for efficacy in prophylaxis of mood episodes in bipolar disorder, due to the long duration of availability in clinical settings. There is limited evidence for the efficacy of carbamazepine in the maintenance phase of bipolar disorder, in spite of the fact that it is widely used by practitioners. There are no published trials of valproate in the maintenance phase, but results of open trials suggest good efficacy. Data on maintenance use of other novel agents such as gabapentin and lamotrigine is still extremely limited.

Regular follow-up with the patient during prophylaxis phase is extremely important. Choice of mood stabilizing medication should be based upon patient history and clinical status. Both lithium and valproate have proven efficacy as first-line agents. Valproate may be particularly efficacious in lithium nonresponders, individuals with rapid cycling mania, and those with concurrent substance abuse. Carbamazepine may be particularly useful for individuals with neurological dysfunction. Patients having a good history of drug response to a particular agent are likely to have a repeat good response with the same agent. During the maintenance visits, medication levels and adverse effects should be reviewed. Patient education is more likely to be effective during periods of clinical stability, and efforts should be made to engage families of patients. The clinician should continuously assess for recurrence of polarity (highs or lows), particularly depressive symptoms, which may be more insidious and less readily obvious.

If patients present with acute mania, clinicians should ensure that mood stabilizing medication is either initiated or dosing optimized for patients already on mood stabilizers. Patients with "break-through" mania on one mood stabilizer, should be switched to another mood stabilizer or have another mood stabilizer added to the existing regimen. Any concurrent antidepressant medication should be discontinued. Patients with acute manic episodes may require hospitalization for protection of self or others. Since mood stabilizers often require several weeks to elicit a clinical response, a patient having psychotic features, agitation, or disruptive behavior, may require adjunctive medication. Adjunctive medications include benzodiazepines or antipsychotic medications. Use of benzodiazepines as adjuncts to mood stabilizers are highly effective in acute management of symptoms. A short-acting agent available in injectable form, such as lorazepam 1-2 mg given 3-4 times/day as needed, is useful in controlling agitation. For outpatients, smaller doses, such as 0.5-2 mg 2-4 times/day, may be effective. Benzodiazepine is usually required only for the initial 1-3 weeks as the acute manic episode resolves. Benzodiazepines should be slowly tapered in individuals who have been receiving regular dosing of benzodiazepines (see Clinical Issues in the Use of Anxiolytics and Sedative/Hypnotics *on page 634*). For severely agitated patients, or those with psychotic symptoms, consideration should be given to the use of adjunct antipsychotic medication. Newer atypical antipsychotics are generally preferred in comparison to conventional neuroleptics in the acute management of manic psychosis, due to their diminished risk of acute extrapyramidal side effects and probable greater efficacy. The atypical antipsychotic medication, olanzapine, has FDA approval for the treatment of bipolar mania.

If there is minimal or no response after 3 weeks of treatment with a mood stabilizer at a therapeutic serum level, a different mood stabilizer should be started, and the first agent tapered. Partial responders should have a second mood stabilizer added. Combination treatment of multiple mood stabilizers may be required in patients who are resistant to monotherapy. ECT has proven efficacy in manic psychosis (see previous discussion on ECT in General Treatment Recommendations in this chapter).

Clozapine appears to have a particular efficacy in treatment - refractory bipolar disorder, however, due to the risk of agranulocytosis, clozapine should be reserved for refractory patients. Other agents that appear to have benefit in some patients with bipolar disorder include thyroid hormones, benzodiazepines (eg, clonazepam), and calcium channel blockers. Finally, novel anticonvulsants such as lamotrigine and topiramate are likely to be used more in the future, as more data becomes available.

Patients with bipolar disorder may develop depressive episodes potentially associated with severe functional impairment, and increased risk of suicide. Lithium is known to be effective in bipolar depression, and may have synergistic antidepressant effects in combination with anticonvulsant mood stabilizers. Patients on carbamazepine or valproate who have persistent depressive symptoms, in spite of therapeutic anticonvulsant levels, should be considered for a trial of lithium augmentation before antidepressant medication therapy is started. Preliminary data suggest that the novel anticonvulsant lamotrigine, may be useful in management of bipolar depression. In all cases of mood stabilizer therapy, care should be taken to optimize dosing and/or blood levels. Antidepressant medication should be used cautiously as there are numerous reports in the literature documenting the potential for "switching" patients into mania or rapid cycling. Most standard antidepressant drugs appear to be equally efficacious in bipolar depression, and choice of agent should be based upon patient past history and current clinical status. The monoamine oxidase inhibitors (MAOIs) may be particularly beneficial in bipolar depression, however, their safety profile severely limits their usefulness. Tricyclic antidepressants may be more likely to induce mania or accelerate the natural course of bipolar disorder and should be used with caution in patients with bipolar disorder. Bupropion, venlafaxine, and SSRI antidepressants may be less likely to induce mania in individuals with bipolar disorder. As in unipolar depression, therapeutic antidepressant response may require up to 6 weeks or longer. Unlike cases of unipolar depression, antidepressant medication should be tapered and discontinued in bipolar patients within 6-12 weeks after resolution of the depressive episode. Although most bipolar individuals fare better with periodic use of antidepressant medication as clinical condition warrants, there does appear to be a subgroup of chronically depressed individuals with bipolar illness who require long-term antidepressant therapy. This decision should be based upon a careful review of longitudinal history of mood episodes and medication response. As with unipolar depression, augmenting agents may be useful in achieving antidepressant response. These include lithium, thyroid hormone, stimulants, and dopaminergic agents such as bromocriptine. Alternative nonpharmacologic interventions include bright light therapy and ECT.

# SCHIZOPHRENIA

Schizophrenia, present in approximately 1% of the world's population, characteristically has its onset in late teenage and young adult years, although a late onset form also exists. Men and women are affected in equal proportions, although clinical outcome, particularly in the premenopausal years, is generally better for women. The course of the illness is often persistent, with functional deficits due to both the acute psychotic symptoms and impairments in attention, motivation, and social interactions. The etiology of schizophrenia is not known, although family aggregation, twin, and adoption studies have pointed in the direction of a genetic association. Over the past 30 years, researchers have explored the effects of antipsychotic medications to investigate neurotransmitter theories of schizophrenia. Most focused study has been on the neurotransmitter dopamine, however, the involvement of other neurotransmitters such as serotonin, GABA, and norepinephrine have been increasingly identified. Other investigators have explored immunologic and viral etiologies of schizophrenia.

## CLINICAL PRESENTATION

There is no clinical symptom which is diagnostic for schizophrenia. Psychotic symptoms seen in schizophrenia may also be seen in a variety of psychiatric and neurologic disorders including serious mood disorders, encephalopathic states, and neurodegenerative illnesses. The Diagnostic and Statistical Manual (DSM-IV) *on page 671* outlines the subtypes of schizophrenia: paranoid, disorganized, catatonic, and residual types. The DSM-IV subtypes do not specifically predict prognosis. Characteristic symptoms of schizophrenia include the positive symptoms of hallucinations, delusions, and thought disorder, and the negative symptoms of impairments in motivation and attention, flattened effect, and social avoidance. To fulfill diagnostic criteria according to DSM-IV, individuals must have symptoms for a minimum of 6 months.

Patients with schizophrenia not uncommonly present with suicidal behaviors or may commit suicide. Approximately 50% of patients with schizophrenia have a lifetime history of suicide attempt, and approximately 10% to 15% die by suicide. It is essential for clinicians treating chronically psychotic patients to be alert to the possibility of suicidal behaviors, and to monitor suicide risk. Additionally, families and other caregivers need to be educated regarding suicide and suicide risk.

An important factor in clinical presentation of schizophrenia is awareness of comorbid conditions, particularly substance abuse, and comorbid medical illness. It has been estimated that 50% of individuals with schizophrenia may have comorbid substance abuse or dependence. In addition to complicating symptom presentation, prognosis for individuals with schizophrenia and concomitant substance abuse is generally poorer than for individuals with schizophrenia who have no concomitant substance abuse. Patients with comorbid medical illness and schizophrenia are frequently underdiagnosed or misdiagnosed, with physical symptoms often mistakenly attributed to psychiatric illness. It is known that individuals with schizophrenia have greater mortality from medical illness and accidents than the general population. It is important for health providers treating patients with schizophrenia to ensure that basic preventative health measures (eg, nutrition education and cholesterol screening, smoking cessation counseling, etc) are offered and implemented, and that underlying medical illness is appropriately managed (eg, monitoring for compliance with antihypertensive medication).

## GENERAL TREATMENT RECOMMENDATIONS

The cornerstone of treatment for schizophrenia is antipsychotic medications. The first specific antipsychotic drug, chlorpromazine, was introduced in the 1950s, and for many years, subsequently introduced antipsychotic medications, "typical antipsychotic", were drugs that primarily block dopamine activity. Potency of a typical antipsychotic drug is defined by a drug's dopamine-blocking ($D_2$) properties, with high-potency typical antipsychotic drugs characterized by compounds such as haloperidol or fluphenazine and low-potency typical antipsychotic drugs characterized by compounds such as chlorpromazine and thioridazine. Over the last 15 years, there has been substantial activity in the area of pharmacologic treatment of schizophrenia. A newer group of antipsychotic medications have been introduced, called "atypical" because they reduce symptoms of psychosis while causing minimal to no neurologic side effects. The newer antipsychotic drugs appear to have significant activity on nondopaminergic systems such as the serotonergic system.

In initiating treatment of the symptoms of schizophrenia, the clinician is faced with the choice of selection of a specific antipsychotic medication. Overall, the antipsychotics are generally safe, well tolerated, and nonaddictive. Among the typical antipsychotic medications, there is no one agent that demonstrates overall superior efficacy. The atypical antipsychotic compound, clozapine, has superior efficacy in treatment-refractory illness, but its benefits must be weighed against it potential adverse effects and difficulty of use. Selection of a specific antipsychotic drug is usually determined by matching side effect profile with clinical status of the patient. Patients who have a history of good response to one particular antipsychotic medication are likely to have a good response again to that particular drug, and patients will often prefer one particular antipsychotic over another. Patient preference should be incorporated into the treatment plan if possible, as this will increase compliance with the pharmacotherapy. Most current treatment guidelines for management of schizophrenia advocate use of atypical medications as first-line treatment. Exceptions to this include stable patients who have had good response to conventional antipsychotics without major side effects, patients who require I.M. medications, for the acute management of aggressive/violent patients, and for patients who require depot (long-acting injectable) antipsychotic medications. For the acute treatment of agitated or violent patients with schizophrenia, many clinicians give an oral or intramuscular dose of a high-potency antipsychotic (eg, haloperidol 2-5 mg). Peak plasma concentration is reached in approximately 30 minutes after intramuscular administration. The atypical antipsychotics risperidone, olanzapine, and quetiapine may only be given orally. The antipsychotics are generally well absorbed with peak plasma levels occurring 2-4 hours after drug ingestion. Oral drug should be initially administered for most medication in divided doses (eg, haloperidol 2-5 mg bid) until steady state is achieved. This occurs during the first week of treatment, after which medication may be given once daily for most antipsychotic medications. Single bedtime dosing minimizes daytime sedation and eases compliance. Maximum drug effect will generally occur over 4-6 weeks. Individual patients will vary in what is lowest effective dosage for management of symptoms, and the amount of antipsychotic medication prescribed must be titrated to the patient's unique clinical situation. If the patient is initially agitated or combative, the clinician may add a benzodiazepine such as lorazepam (1-2 mg) or diazepam (5 mg) to the antipsychotic regimen. The benzodiazepine may be given in a divided dose schedule during the initial days/weeks of treatment, or cautiously on an "as needed" basis, dependent on patient age and clinical status. An anticholinergic drug may be administered in patients who develop extrapyramidal side effects (EPS). Some clinicians prescribe prophylactic anticholinergic drugs in patients with a history of EPS or those patients at high risk for EPS symptoms. Agents for Treatment of Extrapyramidal Symptoms *on page 638* describes the clinical use of anticholinergic agents. Monitoring for tardive dyskinesia should continue for as long as patients receive antipsychotic medication. Assessment should be done at least every 4 months with conventional antipsychotic medications every 6 months for atypical antipsychotics, and every 9 months for clozapine. A commonly used test for EPS in clinical settings is the Abnormal Involuntary Movement Scale (AIMS) (see Psychiatric Assessment - Rating Scales *on page 598*).

Once the individual with schizophrenia has had symptom stabilization, treatment moves from the acute phase to maintenance treatment. Over 75% of individuals with schizophrenia will relapse within the first year, if antipsychotic medication is discontinued after acute stabilization of illness. Once symptoms are stabilized, the clinician may elect to continue oral medication or to initiate long-acting depot antipsychotic. If possible, the depot should be used for patients on a typical antipsychotic as it allows for lower, more reliable dosing with less variability in blood levels and is associated with improved outcomes. Depot preparations are particularly helpful in situations where compliance with antipsychotic medication is a problem. Only haloperidol, usually given I.M. every 4 weeks, and fluphenazine, usually given I.M. every 2 weeks, are available in depot forms.

The introduction of newer, "atypical" antipsychotics has markedly changed the management of schizophrenic illness over the last decade. Clozapine, the first atypical antipsychotic available in the U.S., is the only antipsychotic agent which has clearly demonstrated superior efficacy in treatment refractory schizophrenia. Because of the approximately 1% incidence of agranulocytosis associated with clozapine therapy, and the need for continued blood monitoring, clozapine therapy is reserved for the patient with severe treatment refractory or treatment intolerant illness. Clozapine and the other more recently available atypical antipsychotic medications are associated with less extrapyramidal side effects compared to typical antipsychotic agents. Additionally, the atypical antipsychotic agents may have unique efficacy on the negative and cognitive symptoms of schizophrenia.

Although pharmacotherapy is essential in the treatment of schizophrenia, it cannot optimize outcome without concurrent psychosocial treatments. This includes psychotherapy, education of patients and families, and psychosocial rehabilitation. Patient education should emphasize schizophrenia as a "no fault" brain disorder. There is a greater emphasis in today's managed care settings for more treatment to occur in ambulatory care environments, and less emphasis on the inpatient environments traditionally seen in the past for treatment of schizophrenia. Coordination of care which includes multiple professional care providers including primary care physician, psychiatrist, nonphysician therapists, and case managers is crucial to optimize outcome. Finally, good communication between patient, family, and the various care providers is essential.

# ANXIETY DISORDERS

Anxiety is a sensation experienced at times by all individuals consisting of cognitive, physical, and behavioral symptoms. Cognitive symptoms include feelings of fear or worry, and a sense of uncertainty. Physical symptoms, varying in intensity, may include, hyperventilation; tachycardia or chest pain; GI symptoms such as nausea, diarrhea; "butterflies in the stomach"; or a variety of other physical symptoms such as urinary frequency, sweating, chills, or dry mouth. Behavioral symptoms include insomnia, restlessness, poor attention, and exaggerated startle reflex. These symptoms are perceived as unpleasant by the individual. When anxiety and its attendant symptoms are experienced inappropriately based upon intensity or frequency, it is considered pathological. These are the anxiety disorders. DSM-IV includes the following illnesses under anxiety disorders: Panic disorder, agoraphobia, specific and social phobias, generalized anxiety disorder, post-traumatic stress disorder, and obsessive-compulsive disorder. Additionally, anxiety disorders may be present due to substances use, or due to general medical conditions. Psychosocial aspects of stress response appear to be important in the development of anxiety disorders, and many psychotherapeutic interventions address this issue. Although the biological basis of anxiety disorders has not been clearly established, a number of studies suggest that neurotransmitter abnormalities, particularly involving norepinephrine, serotonin, and gamma-aminobutyric acid (GABA) are also important in anxiety disorders. Additional work in neuro-imaging and genetics suggests possible anatomic and genetic foci.

## CLINICAL PRESENTATION

### PANIC DISORDER

Panic disorder, which may occur with or without agoraphobia, is a relatively common psychiatric illness which may be chronic and may lead to severe functional impairment. Panic disorder has a life-time prevalence of approximately 2%, occurs most often in women, and has onset usually when individuals are in their 20s. Individuals experience recurrent panic attacks which may occur unexpectedly. Panic attack symptoms consist of intense fear or discomfort, and may also include shortness of breath, feeling of choking, paresthesia, tachycardia, palpitations, trembling, flushing or chill, GI symptoms, feeling of depersonalization, or fear of death or going crazy. Panic attacks are usually brief, peaking in approximately 10 minutes and usually lasting no more than 1 hour. Approximately 33% of patients develop agoraphobia, a fear and avoidance of situations from which it would be difficult to escape in the event of a panic attack. Women with panic disorder are more likely to have comorbid conditions/treatment refractory illness compared to men.

### AGORAPHOBIA

Agoraphobia is a fear and avoidance of situations in which it is perceived that management of a panic attack would be difficult, complicated, or embarrassing. Typical situations avoided might include using public transportation, traveling on bridges or tunnels, going to unfamiliar environments, or far from home. In extreme cases, individuals may become house-bound in their efforts to avoid situations that may precipitate anxiety. Severe forms of the illness are grossly disabling. As with other anxiety disorders, better treatment outcome is associated with lesser degree of symptoms and shorter duration of illness. Although agoraphobia may occur on its own, the majority of individuals with agoraphobia also have panic disorder and/or other anxiety disorders.

### SPECIFIC AND SOCIAL PHOBIAS

Specific phobias are persistent, excessive fears of specific objects or situations. Examples include fear of heights, fear of air travel, or fear of some types of animals or insects. Specific phobia is the most common mental disorder among women and the second most common among men (substance-abuse disorders are first). The fear is perceived by the individual as uncomfortable and unreasonable. Unlike panic disorder, the anxiety is not random or unexpected and is directly related to the stimulus or situation.

Social phobia, which affects up to 13% of the population, is characterized by a persistent, extreme fear of social situations. Examples include generalized fear of situations such as eating or drinking in public, using public restrooms, or may be more performance-related such as speaking in public. Social phobia usually begins in adolescence and may restrict or limit social or occupational development.

### POST-TRAUMATIC STRESS DISORDER

Post-traumatic stress disorder (PTSD) is a pathological stress response to what is perceived by the individual as a catastrophic stressor. Examples of catastrophic stressors include physical or sexual assault, witnessing violence, experiencing natural disasters such as a flood or earthquake, and combat experiences. The lifetime prevalence of PTSD is approximately 1% to 3% of the general population, but may be considerably higher in high-risk subgroups such as Vietnam veterans, where PTSD is seen in up to 30% of individuals. Primary clinical features of PTSD are 1) distressing re-experiencing of the event in the form of intrusive recollections, dreams, feelings, or physiologic response; 2) persistent avoidance of stimuli associated with the trauma and numbing or general responsiveness; and 3) persistent symptoms of hyperarousal such as insomnia, irritability, exaggerated startle response, and hypervigilance. PTSD does not develop in all individuals exposed to traumatic events. Clinical features such as premorbid personality, social supports, psychiatric history, and nature of the trauma affect individual stress response and determine vulnerability to PTSD. PTSD may develop months to years after the individual trauma and can occur at any age. Symptoms that persist beyond 3 months are termed chronic PTSD.

### OBSESSIVE-COMPULSIVE DISORDER

Obsessive-compulsive disorder (OCD) is characterized by obsession or compulsions that are distressing, disabling, and time and energy consuming. An obsession is a recurrent and intrusive thought, feeling, or idea such as belief that one is dirty or contaminated. A compulsion is a conscious, recurrent thought or behavior such as checking to see if lights are off or handwashing. Life-time prevalence of OCD is approximately 2% to 3% of the general population. OCD is equally common in men and women, with an onset generally in adolescence for males and in early adulthood for females. Childhood OCD may also occur. OCD may be a very disabling disorder with the most common obsession being fear of contamination with subsequent washing behaviors. OCD symptoms often have onset after a stressful event such as death of a close family member. Up to 50% of OCD patients have symptoms of depression, and suicide risk must be closely assessed. Course of OCD is often long and fluctuating, with up to 40% of individuals having persistent serious symptomatology.

### GENERALIZED ANXIETY DISORDER

Generalized anxiety disorder (GAD) is a common condition, affecting up to 5% of the population. It is characterized by a generalized anxiety, autonomic hyperactivity, muscular tension, and hypervigilance. Symptoms interfere with a variety of life functions. Most patients with GAD do not seek psychiatric help, but may alternately seek assistance from a variety of medical practitioners for somatic symptoms such as chronic diarrhea or insomnia. Women are twice as likely to experience GAD as men, and onset of the illness usually occurs by early adulthood. As with other anxiety disorders, comorbidity with other psychiatric disorders, particularly depression, is relatively common.

## GENERAL TREATMENT RECOMMENDATIONS

### PANIC DISORDER AND AGORAPHOBIA

As agoraphobia usually co-exists with panic disorder, therapy for both disorders is discussed together. Psychiatric management consists of a comprehensive regimen of interventions. Specific components include appropriate diagnostic assessment including evaluation of functional impairment and identification of target symptoms for treatment. The mental health provider must establish a good therapeutic alliance while monitoring the patient's psychiatric status in addition to providing the appropriate patient and family education. In many instances, due to the frequently somatic nature of the illness the mental health provider must work with a variety of nonpsychiatric healthcare providers in order to optimize outcome. Psychosocial interventions, such as psychotherapy have traditionally been crucial in management of panic disorder. Cognitive behavioral therapy (CBT), a symptom-oriented psychotherapeutic approach, has been the best studied of the psychosocial treatments of panic disorder. Primary components of CBT include patient education, symptom monitoring, breathing retraining, cognitive reinterpretation of bodily sensations, and exposure to anxiety cues. Medications from several classes have also been seen to be effective in panic disorder, although, no one agent is clearly proven to be most effective for panic disorder. Potentially beneficial medications include the SSRI antidepressants (eg, paroxetine 40 mg/day), tricyclic antidepressants (eg, imipramine 150 mg/day), benzodiazepines (eg, alprazolam 4-10 mg/day), and novel antidepressants such as venlafaxine or nefazodone. Many clinicians use SSRI antidepressants as first-line agents. Monoamine oxidase inhibitors may be useful for refractory illness. Other miscellaneous second or third line agents that may prove beneficial in some patients include anticonvulsants, such as carbamazepine, and calcium channel blockers. Determination of optimum pharmacotherapy must be based on drug side effect profile and patient clinical status. Treatment should continue for at least 12 months after symptom stabilization, although it appears that many patients may require maintenance treatment for much longer periods.

### SPECIFIC AND SOCIAL PHOBIAS

Treatment of specific phobias most commonly involves exposure therapy, a type of behavioral therapy. The patient becomes desensitized to the phobic stimulus during a series of gradual exposures to the feared object/stimulus. Psychotherapy also involves having the patient deal with the anxiety in a variety of alternative ways, such as controlled breathing, self-relaxation, and cognitive restructuring. Best outcome is usually achieved with highly motivated patients without other comorbid anxiety illness. Use of beta-blocking agents may also benefit some patients.

Social phobia is generally best managed with a combination of psychotherapy and pharmacotherapy. Effective psychotherapy may include cognitive-behavioral therapy (see previous discussion on the treatment of panic disorder earlier in this chapter), desensitization, or other cognitive approaches. Effective drug treatments include beta-blockers such as atenolol (particularly for performance situations), benzodiazepines such as alprazolam, and monoamine oxidase inhibitors such as phenelzine. SSRI antidepressants are also used by some clinicians.

### POST-TRAUMATIC STRESS DISORDER

Most clinicians advocate a combination of psychotherapy and pharmacotherapy for PTSD. Psychotherapeutic interventions include exposure therapy, cognitive therapy, and anxiety management. More controversial therapies include hypnosis and eye movement desensitization and reprocessing (EMDR). In some patients, reconstruction of the traumatic event with subsequent catharsis and abreaction may be helpful, although in other patients this may be experienced as overwhelming and counter-therapeutic. Psychotherapeutic approaches must be carefully tailored to the individual patient. Drug therapies which appear to be most beneficial include SSRI antidepressants, tricyclic antidepressants, other novel antidepressants such as nefazodone and venlafaxine, anticonvulsants, and clonidine. Use of benzodiazepines may help symptoms of anxiety, but should be used cautiously due to possible comorbid substance abuse in some patients, and likelihood of withdrawal symptoms upon drug discontinuation. Although antipsychotic medications are used in some clinical settings, in general their use should be minimized due to risk of long-term neuroleptic related adverse effects in this population.

### OBSESSIVE-COMPULSIVE DISORDER

Although a number of varying psychotherapies have been reported to be useful in management of obsessive-compulsive disorder (OCD), behavior therapy has been best studied, and is believed to be the most effective psychotherapy for OCD by many clinicians. The effectiveness of pharmacotherapy in OCD is also well-established. Most clinicians advocate treatment with an SSRI antidepressant or with clomipramine as first line treatment for OCD. SSRI dosage for OCD is generally higher than that used for the treatment of major depression, (eg, fluoxetine 60-80 mg/day). Clomipramine is usually begun at a dosage of 25-50 mg at bedtime and increased as tolerated up to a maximum of 250 mg/day. If response to SSRI or clomipramine is suboptimal, clinicians may augment or switch to other

## ANXIETY DISORDERS *(Continued)*

agents including lithium, benzodiazepine (particularly clonazepam), or buspirone. Refractory patients may respond to MAOI antidepressants, particularly phenelzine. Judicious use of antipsychotic agents may benefit severe illness. ECT has been reported to be successful in some severely ill patients, and finally, neurosurgery (cingulotomy, capsulotomy), remains an option for severe, intractable OCD.

### GENERALIZED ANXIETY DISORDER

The primary treatment modalities for generalized anxiety disorder (GAD) are psychotherapy and pharmacotherapies. Psychotherapy may be cognitive-behavioral, insight-oriented, or supportive. In general, pharmacotherapy should not be initiated until at least some efforts have been made to reduce anxiety symptoms with psychotherapeutic approaches. The drug treatments most commonly used for GAD are buspirone, benzodiazepines, and antidepressants. Due to the chronic nature of GAD, use of a nonpotentially addicting drug is preferable. The novel antidepressant, venlafaxine XR, has recently been FDA approved for the treatment of GAD. Finally, the clinician must be aware of the potential for comorbid psychiatric illness in GAD patients, particularly mood disorders, and treat these as appropriate.

# SUBSTANCE-RELATED DISORDERS

Substance-related disorders are conditions in which an individual uses/abuses a substance, leading to maladaptive behaviors and symptoms. In DSM-IV, substance-related disorders are further grouped into substance dependence and substance abuse. Substance abuse refers to a maladaptive pattern of substance use leading to clinically significant impairment or distress, manifested by at least one symptom that interferes with life functioning within a 12-month period. Diagnostic criteria for substance dependence requires at least three of the following within a 12-month period: development of tolerance to the substance, withdrawal symptoms, persistent desire/unsuccessful attempts to stop the substance, ingestion of larger amounts of substance than was intended, diminished life functioning, and persistent substance use in the phase of physical or psychological problems. Substance abuse and substance dependence are enormous societal problems. In the United States, the lifetime prevalence of substance abuse or dependence in adults is over 15%. Substance abuse prevalence is greatest among individuals 18-25 years of age. Substance abuse is also more common in men compared to women, and in urban residents compared to rural residents.

Over 50% of individuals with substance-related disorders have comorbid psychiatric disorders. The term "dual diagnosis" usually refers to individuals with concomitant substance abuse and psychiatric diagnosis. Comorbid psychiatric diagnoses, common in individuals who abuse substances, include major depression, personality disorder, particularly antisocial personality, anxiety disorders, and dysthymia. Genetic studies involving twins, adoptees, and siblings raised separately, have suggested good evidence for familial patterns in alcohol abuse. Genetic patterns with other substances of abuse have not been well demonstrated.

## CLINICAL PRESENTATION

Substance abuse can manifest in a variety of formats dependent on substance used, pattern of use, and presence of comorbid illness. Commonly abused substances include alcohol, stimulant compounds (eg, cocaine and amphetamines), sedatives/hypnotic drugs (eg, barbiturates and benzodiazepines), opioids (eg, morphine, codeine), hallucinogens (eg, d-lysergic acid diethylamide/LSD), inhalants (eg, nitrous oxide), and synthesized compounds such as the "designer drugs", and marijuana.

Alcohol is by far the most commonly abused substance, particularly in older adult individuals with substance abuse. In the U.S., 13.8% of all adults have alcohol abuse or dependence at some point in their lives. Individuals who abuse alcohol may present with alcohol intoxication characterized by behavioral changes including expansive mood, social withdrawal, mood lability, irritability, and/or aggression. Physical/neurological symptoms such as diminished concentration, attention, and coordination may lead to falls and injury. Impulsivity and impairments in judgment and insight are associated with violence or accidents. Twenty-five percent of all suicides occur when individuals are intoxicated. Blood alcohol level closely approximates level of intoxication. In many communities, blood alcohol levels ≥80-100 mg/dL are considered unsafe and illegal for the operation of a motor vehicle. As alcohol is a short-acting sedative, in individuals with alcohol dependence, alcohol withdrawal begins 4-12 hours after the last drink. Clinical presentation includes tremor, tachycardia, hypertension, anxiety, and sweating. Symptoms continue over the next 1-2 days, and may last up to 4-5 days. Some individuals may experience alcohol withdrawal seizures. Approximately 5% of individuals experience life-threatening withdrawal symptoms with delirium, termed delirium tremens "DTs". Patients with chronic alcohol abuse may present with acute alcoholic encephalopathy (Wernicke's syndrome) or a persistent amnestic syndrome (Korsakoff's syndrome) which may be irreversible.

Stimulant drugs include cocaine and the synthesized amphetamine compounds. Cocaine is an extremely addictive substance which is classified as a narcotic. Cocaine is used medically as a local anesthetic, particularly for ear, nose, and throat procedures. Although cocaine use appears to have generally decreased over the last decade in the United States, it remains an important public health hazard. A recent report from the Substance Abuse and Mental Health Services Administration notes that 500,000 individuals abuse cocaine weekly. In 1990, there were about 80,000 cocaine-related emergency room visits in the United States. Crack cocaine is an alkaloid or freebase cocaine available in crystalline chunk form. This may be smoked to produce a rapid "high". The behavioral effects of cocaine are experienced almost immediately after drug administration (seconds to minutes) by intranasal, intravenous, or inhalation routes. Individuals become euphoric, talkative, and alert, possibly progressing to irritability, aggressiveness, agitation, and paranoia with frank psychotic symptoms. Physical symptoms of intoxication include hypertension, tachycardia, hyperthermia, and possibly cardiac arrhythmia, stroke, or seizures. As behavioral effects are generally short-lived, individuals using cocaine often repeatedly self-administer the drug. After cessation of cocaine use, individuals may experience a withdrawal syndrome of dysphoria, irritability, agitation, and severe drug craving.

Amphetamines and related compounds are synthesized sympathomimetic agents, used in medical settings to treat attention-deficit disorders, narcolepsy, and depression in some patients. Up to 1% of the U.S. population may abuse these types of stimulants. The acute behavioral and physical effects resemble those described for cocaine, as does the withdrawal syndrome "crash". The smokable free-based form of methamphetamine ("ice") may last ten times as long as effects of crack cocaine. As with cocaine withdrawal, individuals may be particularly prone to drug seeking, depression, and suicide.

Sedative/hypnotic drugs are agents which are central nervous system depressants. These include barbiturates, drugs such as chloral hydrate and meprobamate, and benzodiazepines, Drugs of this type are used to treat a variety of disorders in medical settings (see Clinical Issues in the Use of Anxiolytics and Sedative/Hypnotics *on page 634*) including anxiety, sleep disturbances, and agitation. In medical settings, the benzodiazepines have replaced other sedative/hypnotics due to their safety and effectiveness profile. Behavioral effects of sedative hypnotics include drowsiness, sleep, and decrease in agitation or anxiety. Physical symptoms include hypotension, impairments in coordination/balance, slurred speech,

## SUBSTANCE-RELATED DISORDERS *(Continued)*

severe CNS depression, and respiratory depression. Individuals may become tolerant to the drug, requiring progressively larger doses for the same effect, and cross-tolerance to other CNS depressants including alcohol often develops. Heightened toxicity may occur when sedative/hypnotic drugs are used concurrently or with alcohol. Because of the wide use of sedative/hypnotic agents in medical settings, some patients may become tolerant to the effects of the drugs, and self-initiate a pattern of increasing drug use/abuse. Patients who have developed dependence on sedative/hypnotics will experience a withdrawal reaction upon abrupt discontinuation of the drug. This is characterized by anxiety, restlessness, and GI disturbance in the early phases (first day of symptoms) which may progress to hypotension, tachycardia, tremor, and agitation. Seizures and delirium may occur. Period of time from last drug dose until withdrawal symptom appearance varies depending on the active drug duration. This may be lengthy for long-acting drugs with active metabolites such as diazepam (up to 1 week) or brief (10-12 hours) with short-acting barbiturates.

Opioids refer to compounds derived from natural opium alkaloids (eg, opium and morphine), or synthesized compounds which have mechanisms of action similar to opium (eg, heroin, meperidine, and methadone). Heroin is not legally available in the United States, however, it is the most commonly abused opioid. Heroin is a dangerous drug, with 45% of all drug-related deaths in 1993 due to heroin. Synthetic opioids, called narcotics, have wide medical use in pain management of numerous disorders. Tolerance to opioid drugs develops quickly, and thus abuse potential with this class of drugs is high. Acute behavioral effects include euphoria, sedation, and anorexia, while physical effects include constipation, pupillary constriction, emesis, and respiratory depression. Physical dependence often occurs within a week of receiving regular drug dosing. In addition to the risks associated with opioid intoxication and dependence, individuals that abuse intravenous opioid drugs, usually heroin, are at particular risk for transmission of human immunodeficiency virus (HIV) and hepatitis. These illnesses may be transmitted via shared needle use or sexual practices associated with a drug addiction lifestyle. Opioid overdosages are not uncommon due to the variable tolerance of individuals, difficulty in determining street drug purity, and the fact that depression and suicide are often seen in opioid-abusing populations. Physical symptoms of overdosage are respiratory depression, hypothermia, pupillary constriction, and coma. Opioid withdrawal syndromes occur when a physically dependent individual abruptly ceases drug use. Symptoms include anxiety, diaphoresis, yawning, and rhinorrhea. Later, patients experience pupil dilation, tremor, muscle cramping, agitation, goosebumps, autonomic instability, and GI disturbance. Electrolyte imbalance may occur with GI disturbance and dehydration. Withdrawal symptoms may last 1-2 weeks depending on the drug of abuse.

Hallucinogens, also referred to as psychedelics or psychotomimetics, are agents that lead to hallucinations/illusions and enhanced awareness of consciousness. The group includes d-lysergic acid diethylamide (LSD), psilocybin, and mescaline. Hallucinogens may be natural or synthetic compounds which have no medical use in the United States. All have high abuse potential. Although hallucinogen use was more common in the 1960s, hallucinogen use in the U.S. population has been relatively stable over the last decade. Acute behavioral effects include hallucinations, paranoia, grandiosity, and perceptual changes such as depersonalization and slowing of time. Physical effects include tachycardia, hypertension, hyperpyrexia, and pupillary dilation. Most acute effects resolve over 8-12 hours, however, acute panic reactions during intoxication and flashbacks (spontaneous recurrences of drug-induced effects) may persist for months to years, while individuals with vulnerability to serious mental illness may exhibit persistent postintoxication psychosis. Tolerance develops quickly to behavioral effects of hallucinogens, however, there appears to be no physical dependence or withdrawal syndrome.

Inhalants are volatile gas compounds which produce CNS intoxication. Most commonly abused inhalants include glue and paint thinners (toluene), aerosols (nitrous oxide), and cleaning solutions (carbon tetrachloride). Inhalants are most commonly abused by the young, particularly teenage boys. Methods of administration include inhaling gases from a solvent soaked rag or breathing from a bag in which solvent has been placed. Aerosols may be directly inhaled. Acute behavioral effects occur within minutes and generally last up to 1 hour. These include euphoria, light-headedness, and disinhibition. Larger doses produce agitation, ataxia, and possibly arrhythmias and seizures. Headaches may occur several hours after use, as well as irritation of nasal mucosa and conjunctivitis. Tolerance develops quickly and withdrawal symptoms of tremulousness, tachycardia, agitation, and seizures have been reported when chronic users abruptly discontinue inhalant use. Chronic inhalant abuse may be associated with neurological deficit such as encephalopathy, parkinsonism, or cerebellar ataxia.

Miscellaneous synthesized compounds include "designer drugs" such as 3,4-methylene-dioxy methamphetamine (MDMA or Ecstasy), 3,4-methylene-dioxy amphetamine (MDEA or Eve), and the veterinary tranquilizer phencyclidine (PCP or "Angel Dust").

The designer drugs are illegal compounds with no current medical use in the United States. Acute behavioral effects include euphoria and increased sociability. Physical effects may include cardiac arrhythmias and CNS neuronal damage. The designer drug l-methyl-4-proprionoxy-4-phenyl pyridine (MPPP) is associated with a parkinsonian syndrome in some users.

PCP has been used on the streets since the 1960s. Currently, there is no human medical use for PCP in the United States. The drug is still abused with some degree of frequency in urban populations, but more often is taken as an adulterant in marijuana, heroin, or LSD. PCP is usually smoked with rapid onset of behavioral effects. These include agitation, psychosis, and violent behavior. Physical symptoms include nystagmus, drooling, tachycardia, muscle rigidity, and ataxia. Up to 66% of PCP-intoxicated individuals who present to emergency rooms are agitated and violent, often requiring seclusion, restraint, and pharmacologic management of severely disruptive behavior.

Cannabis, or marijuana, abuse has declined in the U.S. population over the last two decades, although it is estimated that up to 5% of the U.S. population are current users. Marijuana is usually smoked with little development of drug tolerance. The active component is 9-tetrahydrocannibinol from the marijuana (Indian hemp) plant. Drug effects occur within 30 minutes, with behavioral symptoms of well-being and relaxation. Short-term memory and concentration may be impaired. Physical symptoms include increased heart rate, increased appetite, incoordination, and conjunctival redness. Occasionally, individuals may experience acute panic, confusion/disorientation or "flashbacks" as may be seen with hallucinogens. Chronic heavy marijuana use has been associated with an amotivational syndrome characterized by decreased attention span, diminished ambition, distractibility, and impairments in social interactions.

Nicotine dependence and nicotine withdrawal are classified in DSM-IV as psychiatric disorders. Nicotine dependence/withdrawal can occur with all forms of tobacco use including smoking of cigarettes, pipes, and cigars, as well as chewing tobacco and snuff. Smoking has been described as the most important preventable cause of disease, with 45% of smokers dying eventually of tobacco-induced disorders. Smoking is estimated to be responsible for 20% of all deaths in the U.S. and is associated with numerous medical illness, including lung, mouth, and other cancers, emphysema, cardiovascular disease, and peptic ulcer disease. Smoking has also been associated with maternal/fetal complications. Most of the tobacco-induced disorders appear to be due to carcinogens and carbon monoxide in tobacco smoke, although nicotine itself may also cause health problems.

Most individuals who use tobacco in the U.S. are cigarette smokers. Mean age of smoking initiation is approximately 15 years. Within a few years of daily smoking, most smokers develop dependence, with most smokers averaging about 20 cigarettes daily. Among older adult smokers, it is estimated that up to 87% are dependent on nicotine. When an individual who is dependent on nicotine stops or reduces nicotine intake, they typically experience withdrawal symptoms within 24 hours. Symptoms may include depressed mood, insomnia, irritability, anxiety, restlessness, diminished concentration, and lowered heart rate. Appetite may be increased, with weight gain (usually 2-3 kg) often occurring during the first few months after smoking cessation. Individuals who use/abuse alcohol and those with mood disorders or attention-deficit disorders are more likely to be smokers. Smoking may also affect blood levels of psychiatric medications, for example, smoking decreases haloperidol and clozapine levels by 30%.

## GENERAL TREATMENT RECOMMENDATIONS

Individuals with substance abuse are often both physically and psychologically impaired. Management and treatment of substance abuse can be divided in the main areas of:

1. Treatment of acute intoxication/overdose
2. Treatment of withdrawal
3. General treatments for psychological addiction/rehabilitation

Additionally, individuals who abuse substances frequently have comorbid psychiatric disorders which affect final outcome. Proper diagnosis and treatment of comorbid psychiatric disorders improve outcome in nearly all cases.

Psychosocial treatments include inpatient care (now increasingly rare in today's managed care settings), outpatient therapies which may be in individual or group settings, and self-help residential treatment programs (therapeutic communities).

Numerous studies have demonstrated that psychotherapy added to pharmacologic management promotes abstinence better than pharmacologic management alone.

## ALCOHOL

### INTOXICATION/OVERDOSE

Alcohol intoxication may be severe with extreme usage, potentially leading to respiratory depression, coma, and death. These individuals require close monitoring in an intensive care setting. An idiosyncratic reaction of severe behavioral symptoms occurring after relatively low level alcohol ingestion has been reported. Symptomatic support with environmental protection, and possibly the addition of low-dose antipsychotic medication, may be beneficial in these individuals (eg, haloperidol 1-2 mg orally or I.M.).

### WITHDRAWAL

Benzodiazepines are the most effective treatment for alcohol withdrawal. For tremor and mild agitation, an oral benzodiazepine such as lorazepam 1-2 mg every 4-6 hours is generally effective. Individuals with more severe agitation or hallucinations may require I.M. or I.V. medication. Individuals with DTs should be in closely observed medical settings (hospitalized) and must receive maintenance benzodiazepine treatment (eg, diazepam 0.15 mg/kg at 2.5 mg/minute) until behavior and autonomic symptoms (tachycardia, hypertension) stabilize. Dosage should then be titrated as clinically indicated. Most cases of DTs may be avoided if treated with oral or I.M. benzodiazepines when the patient is in the early alcohol withdrawal phase. Vital signs should be closely monitored as an index of severity of withdrawal. A supportive, nonthreatening and therapeutic environment is helpful as patients with alcohol withdrawal are often frightened and severely anxious. Treatment with benzodiazepines may be decreased in both dosage and frequency over the next several days as withdrawal symptoms resolve.

Acute alcoholic encephalopathy (Wernicke's syndrome) should be managed with thiamine 50 mg/day I.M. or 100 mg/day orally for 1-2 weeks. The chronic amnestic syndrome associated with long-term alcohol abuse (Korsakoff's syndrome) may improve with thiamine 100 mg/day continued for 6-12 months although most patients have limited cognitive recovery. Antipsychotics are generally best avoided in alcohol withdrawal as they may lower seizure threshold. However, in cases of failure of benzodiazepines to control paranoid behavioral symptoms or hallucinations, judicious use of antipsychotic medication may be helpful.

### GENERAL TREATMENTS

Most clinicians agree that complete abstinence from alcohol is the cornerstone of successful alcohol abuse treatment. Psychotherapy which focuses on drinking behavior and alternative behaviors is generally the most effective intervention. This includes individual, group, marital, and family therapies. Self-help groups such as Alcoholics Anonymous (AA) may be extremely helpful.

Specific biologic interventions that may be adjunctive in promoting alcohol abstinence are disulfiram, naltrexone, and some psychotropic drugs. Disulfiram competitively inhibits the enzyme aldehyde dehydrogenase, so that

## SUBSTANCE-RELATED DISORDERS *(Continued)*

subsequent alcohol ingestion leads to serum acetaldehyde accumulation and resultant symptoms of flushing, feeling overheated, nausea, and general malaise. Dizziness, palpitations, and hypotension may occur. Symptoms generally persist for 30-60 minutes and may be useful in motivated, healthy patients in assisting with abstinence. Disulfiram must be taken daily, generally in the morning, and is usually prescribed at a dosage of 125-250 mg/day. Although some individuals benefit from the addition of disulfiram to an alcohol treatment regimen, its use must be weighed against the medical risks (severe hypotension, hypocalcemia, respiratory depression) if the individual continues to drink while on disulfiram.

Naltrexone, a narcotic antagonist, may also be a useful adjunct as part of an alcohol treatment regimen. Naltrexone at doses of 50 mg/day may reduce drinking in recovering alcoholics. Adverse effects may include hypertension, GI disturbance, and sedation. Rarely, liver functioning may become impaired, and hepatic screening and monitoring should be done concurrently.

Additional psychotropic medications that have been reported to be useful in alcohol treatment include antidepressants such as serotonin reuptake inhibitors and dopamine agonists. Additionally, treatment of existing comorbid psychiatric disorders such as major depression, bipolar disorder, or post-traumatic stress disorder (PTSD) will usually substantially improve outcome.

### COCAINE

#### INTOXICATION/OVERDOSE

The symptoms of cocaine intoxication are similar to alcohol. In cases of high-dose use or when intravenous route has been used, symptoms may be severe, including extreme anxiety, paranoia, and hallucinations. Severe hypertension, hyperthermia, and arrhythmias may occur. Management of autonomic hyperarousal may benefit from benzodiazepines. Phentolamine may be beneficial in hypertensive crisis. Other supportive measures include close monitoring of vital signs, maintenance of fluid status, and ambient cooling for hyperthermia.

#### WITHDRAWAL

Cocaine withdrawal symptoms generally are managed supportively with no specific identified pharmacologic treatments. Intense cocaine cravings may lead individuals to self-medicate with cocaine or other illicit substances.

#### GENERAL TREATMENT

As with alcohol and other drugs of abuse, abstinence from cocaine is essential in maintaining successful treatment. Psychotherapy has been proven to be helpful while some pharmacotherapies (desipramine, amantadine) have suggested efficacy in some individuals with reduced cocaine craving, dysphoria, and drug use. Comorbid psychiatric illness should be treated as needed to optimize outcome.

### OPIOIDS

#### INTOXICATION/OVERDOSE

Most individuals with self-induced opioid intoxication (as with other types of illicit substance intoxication) do not present for treatment unless distressing physical or behavioral symptoms occur. Overdosage situations, however, are relatively common among chronic opioid drug abusers. Anoxia, coma, and death may occur unless intervention treatment is initiated. Initial measures include airway protection, vital sign monitoring, and administration of naloxone, an opiate antagonist. Naloxone may be given at a dose of 0.4-2 mg I.V. and should reverse overdose symptoms within 2 minutes. Dosage may be repeated twice more at 5-minute intervals, if necessary. Treating clinicians should also be alert to the possibility of concomitant substance overdose (eg, barbiturates) or medical conditions that may contribute to respiratory depression (eg, traumatic head injury). Patients with good response to naloxone may require repeated dosing over the next several hours as duration of action of naloxone generally does not exceed 4 hours. Care should be taken when using naloxone to guard against precipitating a withdrawal reaction in opioid-dependent patients.

#### WITHDRAWAL

Withdrawal symptoms occur within 6-12 hours after ingestion of last drug dose in opioid-dependent persons. Treatment of opioid dependence involves management of primarily acute physical symptoms in the acute phase. For acute phase withdrawal (detoxification), the synthetic opioid methadone has been used successfully by many clinicians who treat substance abuse disorders. In patients who begin to exhibit signs and symptoms of opioid withdrawal (hypertension, tachycardia, sweating, lacrimation, rhinorrhea), methadone 1 mg orally is given as needed over the next 24 hours for a maximum of 10-40 mg over the first day of detoxification treatment. Once maintenance dosage requirements are determined (total methadone dose required to contain symptoms over the first 24 hours of detoxification), this dose can be given for an additional 2 days, then a slow daily taper initiated until the individual is to be maintained off opioid drugs.

Some clinicians use the nonopioid antihypertensive clonidine to treat symptoms of acute opioid withdrawal. Clonidine may be used alone or concurrently with methadone. For acute detoxification, clonidine 0.4-2 mg/day may be used. Due to its antihypertensive properties, pulse and blood pressure must be closely monitored. Some patients experience excessive sedation with clonidine, which may be moderated by dosage adjustments.

An alternative compound, buprenorphine, a partial opioid antagonist, may be useful in acute detoxification situations. Like methadone, dosage should be customized to the individual and tapered and eventually discontinued as tolerated.

#### GENERAL TREATMENT

Treatment of chronic opioid dependence involves both treatment of physical withdrawal symptoms, plus psychological dependence on the drug. Psychosocial and psychotherapeutic treatments are essential in promoting the lifestyle changes needed to prevent relapse.

Methadone maintenance has proven efficacy in some groups of opioid abusers. As with acute phase treatment, chronic methadone treatment dosage/format must be tailored to the individual. Usual daily oral dosage ranges from 40-120 mg/day. Generally, patients must come to the clinic daily (usually morning) to receive methadone. Other interventions involved in clinic treatment may include counseling, urine drug testing, vocational rehabilitation, etc. When used successfully, methadone maintenance reduces illegal drug use, and reduces the medical, legal, and societal ramifications associated with the illicit drug culture.

L-α-acetyl methadol (LAMM) is a long-acting opioid that has been successfully used to treat chronic opioid dependence. LAMM can be dosed at 30-80 mg 3 times/week and may eliminate the need for daily clinic visits, as is required for most methadone programs.

An alternative strategy in managing long-term opioid abuse treatment is the use of opioid antagonists. Naltrexone, a long-acting (72 hours) antagonist, blocks the euphoric effects of opioids, and may be taken 3 times/week at dosages of 100-150 mg. Theoretically, the use of naltrexone discourages persons from opioid use as it eliminates the subsequent CNS effects. Naltrexone works best with highly motivated individuals with good psychosocial support as there are no physical incentives (withdrawal symptoms) to continue taking opioid antagonist on a long-term basis.

## SEDATIVE/HYPNOTIC ABUSE TREATMENT

### INTOXICATION/OVERDOSAGE

Severity of symptoms of sedative-hypnotic intoxication depends on drugs used, route administered, and tolerance of the individual to the drug. Sequelae of overdose are greatly worsened when alcohol or multiple sedative/hypnotics are combined. Respiratory depression is the major danger and successful management includes respiratory and cardiac support. Margin of safety in benzodiazepine overdose is much greater compared to barbiturate overdose where unintentional lethal dosing is not uncommon. In addition to standard supportive measures (vital sign monitoring, gastric lavage, hospitalization, etc), patients with overdose should be closely assessed for suicide risk and intent.

### WITHDRAWAL

As with toxicity, severity of withdrawal symptoms is dependent on a variety of clinical factors including duration of drug use (usually maintenance of 1 month or longer for dependence to develop) and tolerance of the individual. Withdrawal of sedative-hypnotic is generally managed by either 1) gradual reduction of sedative substance, or 2) substitution with a long-acting benzodiazepine or phenobarbital with subsequent taper and eventual discontinuation.

Gradual discontinuation from sedative-hypnotic is best accomplished with motivated patients in settings with good psychosocial supports. The rate of drug taper should be tailored to the individual, with slower titrations generally being most successful.

For benzodiazepine-dependent patients, substitution of an equivalent dose of long-acting benzodiazepine (eg, clonazepam) with gradual downward titration will promote reduction of withdrawal effects over time. As with other addiction treatments, concurrent psychosocial treatments will optimize clinical outcome.

For barbiturate-dependent individuals, the clinician should attempt to determine the patient's daily dose of barbiturates and stabilize withdrawal symptoms with the barbiturate. As many individuals who abuse sedative-hypnotics may be unreliable in providing accurate daily use information, the clinician may elect to assess barbiturate tolerance with a challenge dose of the short-acting barbiturate pentobarbital. This should be done in hospital settings. The patient undergoing sedative withdrawal is given 200 mg of pentobarbital and observed for resolution of withdrawal symptoms and mild intoxication. Patients in whom this occurs may then be maintained on pentobarbital 100-200 mg every 6 hours. Patients who are not intoxicated on the initial challenge dose of 200 mg are given an additional 100 mg pentobarbital every 2 hours (for a maximum of 500 mg) until mild toxicity develops. Maintenance pentobarbital dose is then determined based on total amount of barbiturate needed to cause mild intoxication. Once stabilization is achieved, the clinician can then taper the dose by 10% daily. Alternatively, phenobarbital, a long-acting barbiturate, may be substituted for pentobarbital. Phenobarbital has the advantages of less frequent dosing, fewer fluctuations in blood level, and anticonvulsant activity. The equivalent dosing of phenobarbital is 30-100 mg of a short-acting barbiturate such as pentobarbital.

### GENERAL TREATMENT

Psychotherapeutic interventions appear to be the most effective long-term treatments in sedation/hypnotic abuse.

## STIMULANTS

### INTOXICATION/OVERDOSAGE

Intoxication/overdose management involves reducing autonomic hyperactivity (tachycardia, hypertension) and managing CNS symptoms (agitation, psychosis/delirium, or seizures). Supportive measures such as appropriate hydration, vital sign monitoring, and cooling for hyperthermia are indicated.

Anxiolytics or antipsychotics may be useful on a short-term basis, and a supportive, low-stimulation environment will reduce CNS irritability. Some clinicians advocate promotion of rapid excretion of the drug by acidification of the urine with ammonium chloride 500 mg 4 times/day.

### STIMULANT WITHDRAWAL

Amphetamine withdrawal is generally treated supportively. The judicious use of antipsychotic medication may be of benefit to patients with post-amphetamine psychosis.

### GENERAL TREATMENT

Psychotherapeutic interventions appear to be the most effective long-term treatment.

## HALLUCINOGENS

### INTOXICATION

Individuals who experience toxic delirium, panic reactions, or psychosis associated with hallucinogens require a supportive environment (low stimulation with supervision) and may benefit from judicious dosing of anxiolytics (eg, diazepam 5-10 mg orally).

### WITHDRAWAL

Physical dependence and withdrawal symptoms have not been reported.

### GENERAL TREATMENT

Psychotherapeutic interventions appear to be the most effective in long-term treatment.

## INHALANTS

### INTOXICATION

CNS effects of intoxication usually resolve within minutes to hours of inhalant use. Toxic effects depend on the solvent used and may require emergency treatment for arrhythmias or CNS hyperactivity (seizures). Some agents produce renal damage and renal functioning should be monitored. Intoxication treatment is generally supportive.

### WITHDRAWAL

Withdrawal reactions occur rarely as most inhalant use is relatively short-lived. Symptoms that may occur are generally treated supportively with concurrent psychosocial interventions.

### GENERAL TREATMENT

Psychotherapeutic interventions are generally most effective. Due to the young age of most patients, family therapy is often also indicated.

## SYNTHESIZED COMPOUNDS

### INTOXICATION/OVERDOSAGE

PCP toxicity is best managed in a low-stimulation, secure environment. Benzodiazepines and careful use of antipsychotic medication may be helpful for the severe agitation/aggression sometimes seen in PCP intoxication. Some clinicians advocate promoting rapid drug excretion with ammonium chloride or ascorbic acid. Most PCP toxic reactions resolve within 1-3 days, but behavioral symptoms may persist for 2 weeks or more.

In acute intoxication situations, MDMA has been associated with cardiac arrhythmias suggesting a need for close intensive medical monitoring. Additionally, some designer drugs may contain contaminants which have been associated with chronic neurologic damage.

### WITHDRAWAL

Physical dependence on PCP generally does not occur, although psychological dependence may be associated with drug craving and relapse.

### GENERAL TREATMENT

Psychotherapeutic interventions are generally most effective in the long term. Little is known about long-term treatment of designer drug abuse.

## MARIJUANA

### INTOXICATION

The incidence of acute adverse reactions to marijuana is quite low. In rare cases, individuals may experience acute panic, toxic delirium, or flashbacks. These generally remit spontaneously within 12-48 hours. Management may include anxiolytics of antipsychotics if behavioral symptoms are severe.

### WITHDRAWAL

Tolerance generally does not develop to marijuana, although heavy daily users may experience withdrawal symptoms of insomnia, irritability, tremor, and nausea. There is no recognized withdrawal regimen.

### GENERAL TREATMENT

As with other substance abuse disorders, individuals should receive psychosocial rehabilitation and there should be assessment and treatment of any coexisting psychiatric disorders.

## NICOTINE

### INTOXICATION/OVERDOSE

Nicotine intoxication from tobacco use is rare. Excess nicotine from nicotine replacement therapies used in smoking cessation (ie, nicotine gum) may occasionally cause adverse effects such as nausea, headaches, or cardiac abnormalities.

### WITHDRAWAL

Withdrawal symptoms begin within a few hours and generally peak 24-48 hours after smoking cessation. Most symptoms last for approximately 1 month, although craving can persist for 6 weeks or longer. Smoking cessation is associated with slowing on EEG, and decline in metabolic rate, including mean heart rate decline of 8 beats/minute. Blood levels of some antidepressants (eg, clomipramine, desipramine, doxepin, imipramine, and nortriptyline) may increase as may some antipsychotic medications (eg, clozapine, fluphenazine, haloperidol) and some anxiolytics (eg, oxazepam, desmethyldiazepam).

The most successful treatment of nicotine withdrawal frequently includes both psychosocial and pharmacological interventions. Patients must generally be committed to quitting, and most clinicians advocate abrupt cessation of tobacco rather than gradual reduction. Approximately 33% of adults who smoke make an attempt to stop smoking each year. Relapse is common, particularly among those who attempt to quit smoking on their own without formal treatment. Approximately 50% of smokers eventually quit, although individuals with histories of anxiety or mood disorders or of schizophrenia are less likely to stop smoking. Most smokers require 5-7 attempts at smoking cessation before they eventually quit for good. Psychosocial treatments include behavior therapies (relapse prevention, relaxation, stimulus control among other techniques), education (group or individual), and hypnosis. Pharmacotherapies include nicotine replacement therapy, nicotine antagonists, agents that mimic nicotine effects, aversive therapies, and symptomatic management. Nicotine replacement therapy and antidepressants for symptomatic management are among the most commonly utilized pharmacologic measures.

Nicotine replacement provides the nicotine-dependent patient with nicotine in a form that is not associated with the carcinogenic elements in tobacco. Nicotine gum, transdermal nicotine patches, nicotine nasal spray, and nicotine inhalers are available for smoking cessation. Nicotine gum, now available over-the-counter, consists of 2-4 mg of nicotine in a polacrilex resin designed to be slowly chewed for 20-30 minutes. Nicotine absorption peaks 30 minutes after initiation of gum use. Most common adverse effects are GI complaints (nausea, anorexia) and headache. Although nicotine replacement has been used for relief of withdrawal symptoms, some patients utilize these therapies long-term.

Nicotine patches consist of nicotine impregnated into an adhesive patch for transdermal application. Patches are applied daily each morning upon quitting smoking with starting dosages of 21-22 mg/24-hour patch and 15 mg/16-hour patch. Patients should not smoke cigarettes while on patches as nicotine toxicity may occur. Typical treatment duration is 6-8 weeks. The nicotine inhaler contains a replaceable component that delivers nicotine in inhaled air. Unlike cigarettes which deliver nicotine directly into the arterial blood in the lungs, the inhaler delivers nicotine into the buccal mucosa.

In addition to nicotine replacement, some antidepressants (bupropion, doxepin, and desipramine) have been shown to improve the chances of nicotine abstinence. Sustained-release bupropion hydrochloride has been approved by the FDA for smoking cessation. In addition to reducing nicotine withdrawal symptoms, bupropion S-R may diminish weight gain. Some clinicians utilize both bupropion and nicotine replacement concurrently.

Other pharmacologic therapies that have been reported to be potentially useful in the management of tobacco cessation include nicotine antagonists (eg, mecamylamine) and aversive treatments such as silver acetate gum, although efficacy of these agents are not proven. Some clinicians utilize clonidine at dosages of 0.1-0.4 mg/day for nicotine withdrawal in individuals who fail or are unable to tolerate other symptomatic treatment or nicotine replacement.

## GENERAL TREATMENT

A widely used intervention for practitioners in general medical settings for smoking cessation is the "4 As" strategy of the National Cancer Institute. This consists of the following:

1. **Ask** and record smoking status. In several surveys, only about 50% of physicians asked patients about their tobacco use.
2. **Advise** to stop. Direct recommendation from a physician produces quit rates of 7% to 10%.
3. **Assist** the patient in addressing cessation. Identifying a quit date may assist in obtaining commitment to quit. Patients who are unable or unwilling to commit to quitting may benefit from educational materials at this time.
4. **Arrange** follow-up. This should occur within 3 days as the first several days after quitting are a critical period in relapse risk.

Most pharmacotherapies are primarily utilized during the initial period of quitting tobacco use. Psychological treatments/lifestyle changes while also utilized during nicotine withdrawal, must also become long-term interventions. Although biologic treatments do not require concurrent psychological therapies, best outcome is usually associated with combined treatment.

# SECONDARY MENTAL DISORDERS

Secondary mental disorders make up a group of mental disorders with distinctive symptoms which are primarily a result of brain dysfunction detectable by current methods of clinical, laboratory, or tissue pathology assessment. Traditionally, these were identified as "organic brain disorders", illnesses with an identified physical pathology (eg, brain tumor or stroke). These were separated from "functional" illnesses in which there was traditionally no identified causative physical factor (eg, schizophrenia or depression). In DSM-IV, this nomenclature has been eliminated as it is now recognized that the so called functional disorders also appear to have an organic basis, although this may not be easily identified by current methods of biological assessment. The concept of secondary mental disorders is a useful way of delineating a group of mental disorders in which medical diagnosis and treatment play an important management role. This separation, while clinically practical, does not suggest that primary mental disorders, such as schizophrenia or depression, do not have an organic basis. In DSM-IV, secondary mental disorders include delirium, dementia, amnestic disorders, and the mental disorders due to a general medical condition.

## CLINICAL PRESENTATION

The following table describes common characteristics of secondary mental disorders. A delirium is characterized by a disturbance of consciousness and change in cognition that develops over a short period of time. The disturbance is not due to a dementia, and generally tends to fluctuate over the course of a day. There is an association between the delirium presentation and patient history, physical examination, or laboratory tests which indicate that the behavioral symptoms are a result of a general medical condition or response to a substance. The individual is often disoriented, with memory and attention impairment. Perceptual disturbances such as illusions may be present. There are often acute physical symptoms associated with the underlying disorder such as tachycardia, hyper- or hypotension, fever, etc. Children, elderly, and those individuals with other medical illness are generally most likely to develop delirium. In most cases, symptoms quickly resolve with the resolution of the underlying medical disorder.

A dementia is a condition with multiple cognitive deficits including memory impairment. Dementias may be due to the direct effects of a medical condition (eg, Alzheimer's disease), the effects of a substance (eg, alcohol), or a combination of etiologies (eg, stroke and Alzheimer's disease). Dementias have multiple cognitive impairments including memory deficit, and may include aphasia, apraxia, agnosia, or a disturbance in executive functioning. The cognitive deficits are associated with a significant decrease in level of life functioning. Onset is usually gradual and progressive in dementia, but may have sudden onset in cases of traumatic injury. Physical symptoms of dementia are dependent on the underlying associated disorder, but are usually more subtle than the acute physical symptoms seen in delirium. Dementias are particularly common in the elderly with increases in prevalence occurring particularly after age 75. It is estimated that 2% to 4% of the population 65 years of age have Alzheimer's dementia, the most common type of dementing illness. Course of illness in dementia is often permanent and irreversible, although up to 15% of dementias may be reversible if appropriate medical management is initiated. It is estimated that by the year 2030, approximately 20% of the U.S. population will be older than 65 years of age, and management of dementing illness will become an increasingly important healthcare issue.

Amnestic disorders are characterized by memory impairment in the absence of significant cognitive impairment. Amnesia is most commonly found with alcohol use disorders and with head injury, although there are multiple causes, including vitamin deficiency, hypoglycemia, viral infection, or hypoxia. Individuals with amnestic disorders have impaired ability to learn new information, and impaired ability to recall previously remembered knowledge. Onset of symptoms may be sudden, as with trauma or gradual as with nutritional deficiencies. Course of illness is dependent on underlying etiology with reversible illness occurring in some situations (eg, postepilepsy amnesia), or permanent in other clinical scenarios (eg, posthead trauma).

DSM-IV has introduced the term "due to a general medical condition" to describe those mental disorders for which, based upon available clinical data, the physician believes the behavioral symptoms are caused by a nonpsychiatric medical condition. The behavioral manifestations of mental conditions due to a general medical condition vary widely. They are defined based upon symptoms, so that a patient may be diagnosed with a disorder such as anxiety or personality disorder, with the specifier that the illness is due to an identified medical disorder. Types of mental disorders which may be secondary to a general medical condition include cognitive disorders such as dementia, psychotic disorders, anxiety and mood disorders, sleep disorders, and sexual disorders. There are multiple general medical conditions that may be associated with mental disturbance. Some of the most common include seizure disorders, trauma, tumors, neurological illness, metabolic illness, infections, and substances. Course and outcome of disorders due to a general medical condition are largely dependent upon type and management of the underlying medical disorder.

**Common Characteristics of Secondary Mental Disorders**

| | |
|---|---|
| Age of Affected Individual | Any age, elderly are particularly vulnerable |
| Medical History | Significant medical history, trauma history, substance abuse, etc |
| Psychiatric History | None |
| Onset, Clinical Course | Acute or subacute fluctuating course |
| Physical Symptoms | Hypertension, tachycardia, diaphoresis, pupillary changes, fever, autonomic instability, etc |
| Neurological Symptoms | Exhibits neurological symptoms (ataxia, aphasia, etc) |
| Mental Status Examination | Fluctuating level of consciousness; labile psychomotor status; intermittent agitation; hallucinations of nonauditory type (eg, tactile) |
| Cognitive Status | Impaired, may be chronic or labile; memory impairment |
| Drug Treatment Response | Generally suboptimal response to standard psychopharmacological treatments |
| Optimal Management | Treat/manage underlying disorder; symptomatically manage behavioral manifestations as needed |

## GENERAL TREATMENT RECOMMENDATIONS

General treatment of secondary mental disorders involves four primary interventions. These are summarized as follows:

1. Immediately ensure that the patient is placed in a safe and supportive environment. This may involve hospitalization in an acute setting, such as an intensive care unit, or other close observation medical settings. Some individuals may be best managed in psychiatric settings, such as an acute psychiatric unit or geropsychiatric unit. Determination of optimal care setting is based upon patient needs (eg, availability of vital sign monitoring, I.V. support, laboratory testing, etc) and patient behaviors (eg, agitation or aggressive behavior). New onset conditions generally require continuous monitoring.

2. Identify acute medical illness. A medical and psychiatric history should be taken, and a comprehensive physical/neurological exam should be performed. The mental status examination should be completed (see General Patient Assessment *on page 598*). Basic medical laboratory studies should be run, including electrolytes, complete blood count with differential, thyroid function tests, serologic test for syphilis, HIV testing, drug screen, and pregnancy testing in women of child-bearing age. Based upon the clinical situation, the treating physician may elect to obtain additional laboratory testing, such as $B_{12}$, folate, screening for autoimmune disorders, or cerebrospinal fluid examination. An EKG should be done, with more rigorous cardiac monitoring as indicated. Brain imaging such as head CT or MRI should be done in new onset illness.

3. Optimize treatment for medical illness. Biologic treatments for underlying medical illness should be initiated promptly. Often, diagnosis may not be entirely clear at onset of illness, and the differential diagnosis may consist of a variety of medical disorders. Incoming data from diagnostic testing (eg, blood cultures or brain imaging) should be followed up to clarify diagnosis and appropriate treatment. Patients may be able to tolerate less intensive medical settings as illness improves, but it should be remembered that behavioral manifestations of secondary mental disorders are often labile, and care should be taken to provide appropriate supervision and monitoring until symptoms are truly stabilized. Finally, it must be recognized that there may be comorbid conditions such as alcoholism and accompanying head trauma which will require different treatments.

4. Provide appropriate management of behavioral symptoms. Although many individuals with secondary mental disorders will require psychotropic medication to manage behavioral symptoms, there are a variety of nonpharmacologic measures that should be initiated to optimize patient safety and comfort. These nonpharmacologic efforts will often minimize need for psychotropic drug treatments. Appropriate measures may include use of highly visible reality links such as name tags on staff and on patient rooms in hospital or nursing home settings, use of calendars and clocks to assist in orientation, and identifying pictures on bathrooms and eating areas. There should be availability for quiet time alone or with families, and a safe enclosed outdoor area may be helpful for more long-term settings. A home-like setting is ideal, and there should be adequate, appropriate lighting. The person with secondary mental disorders may require assistance to varying degree with basic activities of daily living (ADLs) such as help with walking, eating, dressing, bathing, or toileting. It is particularly important to assess amount of assistance required for ADLs when determining optimum patient residential setting. A variety of basic services may be available as in home services or in assisted-living situations. Patients with secondary mental disorder may not consistently appreciate symptoms or functional impairment, and should be assessed for safety and competency in such areas as meal preparation, handling of personal finances, and basic housekeeping as clinically warranted.

Patients with secondary mental disorders may require psychotropic medication to manage behavioral symptoms. Drug treatments should generally be based upon symptom manifestation, as there are no specific pharmacologic treatments for secondary mental disorders (aside from treatment of the underlying disorder). In treating individuals with secondary mental disorders, medication dosage should be low, and very slowly titrated. Often, patients will be more intolerant to medication side effects, compared to physically healthy populations. Additionally, individuals with secondary mental illness are often being treated with other nonpsychotropic medication, and risk of drug-drug interactions is generally increased. Symptoms that generally require treatment most acutely are agitation and psychosis. Antipsychotic medication in low doses (eg, risperidone 0.5 mg daily or twice daily) may be beneficial for both psychosis and agitation. Individuals with secondary mental disorders may be particularly prone to adverse side effects from drug anticholinergic activity. Agitation may also respond to a variety of alternative medications such as mood stabilizers (eg, carbamazepine) or anxiolytics (eg, buspirone). Benzodiazepines, while effective in managing

## SECONDARY MENTAL DISORDERS *(Continued)*

agitation, should be used cautiously as there may be associated hypotension, sedation, and risk or falls. Individuals with secondary mental disorders may also experience mood disorder symptoms (both unipolar and bipolar), anxiety disorders, or sleep disturbance. For mood disorders, clinicians should select antidepressant agents with least potential for drug-drug interactions. This is usually an SSRI, although other novel antidepressants and the tricyclic compounds have been reported to be effective also. Cardiac status may be a concern with the TCA antidepressants, and these should be used cautiously. Anxiety may respond to buspirone or low-dose benzodiazepines (eg, lorazepam 0.25-0.5 mg). Secondary bipolar disorder may respond particularly well to anticonvulsant mood stabilizers. Sleep disturbance may be a problem for patients with secondary mental disorders. Effective medications that may be beneficial include zolpidem (5 mg orally) or trazodone (25 mg orally). Some individuals who primarily report insomnia, may in fact suffer from depression, and should be treated accordingly. Once the behavioral symptoms have stabilized on medication, all efforts should be made to titrate dosage downward and determine lowest effective dosage. In transient medical conditions, patients frequently do not require long-term psychotropic drug treatment. In chronic secondary medical conditions, such as dementia, individuals may require long-term psychotropic drug therapy. Modification of drug regimen to optimize patient comfort and compliance, such as dosing the bulk of drug at bedtime, should be considered as needed.

# EATING DISORDERS

Eating disorders are characterized by severe disturbances in eating behavior. The primary disorders are anorexia nervosa and bulimia nervosa. Both of these disorders have increased in prevalence over the last two decades. Prevalence of anorexia is approximately 0.5%, and is most common in industrialized countries where there is an abundance of food, and where physical attractiveness among women is equated with being thin. Mean age of onset for anorexia is 17 years. In anorexia, individuals do not maintain a minimally normal body weight. Bulimia is characterized by repeated episodes of binge eating followed by inappropriate measures to lose weight, such as self-induced vomiting, laxative abuse, fasting, or excessive exercising. Bulimia has a slightly later mean age of onset compared to anorexia, and has a prevalence of approximately 1% to 2%. Eating disorders are more commonly seen in females than in males. Weight preoccupation and extreme self-assessment of weight/shape are the primary symptoms of both anorexia and bulimia and many patients demonstrate a mixture of both anorexic and bulimic features.

## CLINICAL PRESENTATION

Individuals with anorexia expend an inordinate amount of effort focused upon losing weight and maintaining low body weight. Most behavior occurs in secret and individuals may refuse to eat in public or with family members. Individuals severely restrict food intake, and generally avoid intake of high calorie or high fat foods. They may become preoccupied with preparing elaborate meals for others, but will eat little themselves. When confronted with their abnormal eating patterns, many individuals will deny the problem. If weight loss becomes severe, individuals develop physical symptoms such as hypothermia, hypotension, bradycardia, amenorrhea, growth failure, and osteoporosis. Electrolyte abnormalities and cardiac arrhythmias put patients with anorexia at substantial medical risk. Individuals may also exhibit purging behaviors such as self-induced vomiting or laxative abuse that may further endanger physical health. During the course of the illness, over 50% of patients meet criteria for major depression. There is also a high prevalence of obsessive-compulsive disorder in patients with anorexia.

Individuals with bulimia exhibit recurrent episodes of binge eating and compensatory maladaptive behavior to minimize effects of the binge. Self-induced vomiting is common, as is laxative abuse. Unlike individuals with anorexia, patients with bulimia usually are of normal body weight. Individuals may appear sociable and assertive, but are generally lacking in self-esteem, and are greatly concerned about how they appear to others. Unlike individuals with anorexia who have diminished sexual activity, individuals with bulimia are often sexually active. Medical complications of bulimia are usually related to the binging and purging behaviors, and include electrolyte abnormalities, GI disturbances, and dental problems due to tooth enamel erosion. As with anorexia, existence of comorbid mood disorder is common.

## GENERAL TREATMENT RECOMMENDATIONS

Treatment for eating disorders is generally multidimensional and includes psychotherapy, pharmacotherapy, nutritional counseling, medical monitoring, and family therapy. A thorough medical assessment and psychiatric evaluation is essential to delineate acute and subacute medical problems, such as electrolyte imbalance, and to screen for the presence of comorbid psychiatric disorders. In situations of profound weight loss and medical instability, hospitalization may be indicated. This is much more common with anorexia than with bulimia. Psychotherapeutic approaches are usually cognitive-behavioral, although interpersonal and psychodynamic therapies may also be used and a variety of psychotherapeutic approaches may be combined. Pharmacotherapy may be used as an adjunct to psychotherapy in both anorexia and bulimia. In anorexia, first-line agents are usually a SSRI antidepressant or a TCA antidepressant. Drug treatments should be compatible with the medical status of the patient. Some clinicians do not recommend using antidepressants in acute treatment for severely malnourished patients, but prefer waiting to initiate these agents after some weight has been gained. Patients with anorexia who do not respond to SSRI or TCA antidepressants may benefit from anxiolytics or MAOIs. In some cases, antipsychotic medication or ECT may be of benefit. In bulimia, SSRI medication has been reported to be useful, at similar or slightly higher than might me used for the treatment of depression. Other drug treatments that may be of benefit include TCA antidepressants, MAOIs, or lithium. Bupropion is contraindicated as there have been reports of seizures with bulimic patients. Estrogen replacement is sometimes used in anorexia nervosa patients with chronic amenorrhea to reduce calcium loss and future osteoporosis. However, data supporting the effectiveness of this is not entirely consistent.

# SLEEP DISORDERS

Sleep disorders are classified mainly into 1) primary sleep disorders and 2) other sleep disorders which are secondary to either another mental disorder, a general medical condition, or a substance. The primary sleep disorders are believed to arise from abnormalities in the sleep-wake cycle. Primary sleep disorders may be further subdivided into dyssomnias characterized by abnormalities in amount, quality, or timing of sleep, and parasomnias characterized by pathological behaviors or physical symptoms occurring in association with sleep. While sleep disorders secondary to other conditions often resolve with resolution of the underlying disorder, primary sleep disorders are usually the main focus of treatment in clinical settings. The dyssomnias include primary insomnia, primary hypersomnia, narcolepsy, breathing-related sleep disorder (includes sleep apnea), and circadian rhythm sleep disorder. Insomnia is the most common sleep complaint, with between 15% to 20% of the population reporting insomnia, and 10% reporting the use of sleeping pills. Insomnia is most commonly found among women, the elderly, and individuals from lower socioeconomic groups, and may cause discomfort and substantial functional impairment. The parasomnias include nightmare disorder, sleep terror disorder, and sleepwalking. The parasomnias involve activation of the autonomic nervous system, motor system, or cognitive activity during sleep.

## CLINICAL PRESENTATION

### DYSSOMNIAS

Insomnia is difficulty in initiating or maintaining sleep, and may be short-term or chronic. Short-term insomnia is most often related to anxiety, for example anticipation of a serious life change, and usually resolves when anxiety lessens. Individuals with chronic insomnia most often report not being able to fall asleep, although individuals may also complain of frequent night-time awakening. Time of onset of primary insomnia is usually young adulthood or middle age, and course varies widely depending upon multiple clinical variables.

Hypersomnia is excessive daytime sleepiness (somnolence) and excessive amounts of sleep in the absence of other medical causes. Sleep/wake schedule and sleep efficiency in these individuals is normal, and there appears to be a familial pattern. The sleep abnormality must persist for at least 1 month to fulfill criteria for the illness. Individuals with hypersomnia may fall asleep at inappropriate time during the day. Narcolepsy is characterized by repeated sudden episodes of sleep (sleep attacks), cataplexy (sudden loss of muscle tone), and repeated onset of rapid eye movement (REM) sleep into the sleep/awake transition period. Some individuals with narcolepsy experience daytime sleepiness between sleep attacks. Night-time sleep is often fragmented with reports of vivid dreams, and frequent complaint of insomnia. Polysomnography (recording of EEG activity, electro-oculographic activity, and electromyographic activity during sleep) is usually abnormal. Narcolepsy is seen in approximately 0.1% of the population, affects both genders equally, and has a mean time of onset in adolescence or young adulthood.

Breathing-related sleep disorder is characterized by sleep disturbance due to breathing abnormalities during sleep. Obstructive sleep apnea is the most common pathology. The airway is occluded by excess tissue, or poor tone of pharyngeal muscles. Patients may snore loudly, snort, or partially awaken multiple times during the course of the night. In sleep apnea there are repetitive episodes of diminished or absent respiration during sleep, leading to reduced blood oxygenation, fall in blood pH, and pulmonary hypertension. Apneic periods may last 10 seconds. Serious cardiorespiratory problems may occur in untreated apnea. The use of polysomnography and recording of respiration and airflow can be used to clarify diagnosis in suspected sleep apnea.

Circadian rhythm sleep disorder involves a mismatch between desired and actual sleep patterns. Examples are jet lag and shift work sleep abnormalities. In these situations, individual's circadian rhythms (sleep/wake cycles) are inappropriate for expected environmental norms. Jet lag usually disappears spontaneously, while shift work sleep abnormalities may persist until work schedule is stabilized.

### PARASOMNIAS

Nightmares, occurring periodically in up to 50% of the adult population, are vivid, distressing dreams from which the individual awakens in a state of fear or anxiety. Nightmares occur during REM sleep, and are largely self-limited.

Sleep terror is an awakening during the early part of the night while in deep non-REM sleep. Individuals typically scream or cry loudly, sit up in bed, and sometimes awaken. Autonomic symptoms of tachycardia, tachypnea, and sweating are usually present. Generally, individuals return to sleep, and the episode is forgotten by morning with no dream recall. Sleepwalking may follow the sleep terror. Night terrors are particularly common in children with boys more commonly affected than girls. Mean age of onset is between ages 4 and 12 years, frequently with spontaneous resolution during adolescence. The disorder has a familial tendency, and has some association with temporal lobe epilepsy when night terrors begin during the teenage years or young adulthood.

Sleepwalking, or somnambulism, is characterized by repeated episodes of complex motor behavior such as walking during deep non-REM sleep. Patients may leave their beds and may perform such acts as dressing, using the toilet, eating, or talking. Most behaviors are routine and of low complexity. During the episode the individual remains asleep, with reduced alertness and responsiveness, a blank stare, and relative disregard of efforts to communicate with them by others. Usually the person returns to bed and has no subsequent memory of the sleepwalking. Like sleep terrors, the disorder usually begins in childhood, tends to run in families, and affects boys more often than girls. Sleepwalking is potentially dangerous due to the possibility of accidental injury. Sleepwalking generally resolves during adolescence, but may continue into adulthood.

## GENERAL TREATMENT RECOMMENDATIONS

Clinicians treating sleep disorders should attempt to determine the cause of the disorder before initiating treatment. Secondary sleep disorders generally are best managed by treating the underlying disorder. A detailed sleep history, including time sleep begins, time of awakening, and assessment of quality of sleep including episodes of awakening, can assist in diagnostic clarification and treatment planning. Spouses or family members can often furnish information on behaviors such as snoring or motor activity. Additional factors that need to be evaluated include current stressors, medications or substance use, psychiatric history, and environmental factors that may affect sleep (for example, shift work). Behavioral strategies that promote good "sleep hygiene", such as regular sleep/wake schedule, moderate exercise, avoidance of alcohol or stimulating substances, such as caffeine, and a regular schedule of activities that allow the individual to prepare for sleep may effectively manage sleep problems.

If behavioral management is not effective, the clinician may consider pharmacotherapy. For insomnia, benzodiazepines and the related compounds, zolpidem and zaleplon, are the safest and most effective hypnotic agents. Ideally, use of these medications is short-term. Other medications that may be used for insomnia include sedating antidepressants such as TCAs or trazodone, as well as antihistamines (eg, diphenhydramine). Barbiturates and related compounds should be used cautiously, if at all, as they are more likely to be associated with addiction and adverse effects without significantly increasing effectiveness.

Pharmacotherapy for hypersomnia includes the SSRI antidepressants and stimulants such as amphetamines.

Management of narcolepsy includes a regimen of daytime naps, unlike insomnia, where daytime naps are to be avoided. As with hypersomnia, individuals with narcolepsy may benefit from stimulant medications such as methylphenidate.

Sleep apnea treatment often responds well to nasal continuous positive airway pressure (NCPAP) which maintains an unobstructed airway. Additional measures include weight loss and surgical procedures, such as nasal surgery to promote an open airway. Benzodiazepines, alcohol, and other sedative medications should be avoided in apneic patients, as this reduces respiration and may critically worsen apnea.

Management of the parasomnias is generally supportive, with no specific pharmacologic treatments. Measures to reduce sleep deprivation and stress may reduce frequency and intensity of parasomnias. Occasionally, drugs that suppress REM sleep, such as TCA antidepressants, may be prescribed for nightmares.

# IMPULSE CONTROL DISORDERS

Impulse-control disorders are characterized by the failure to resist an impulse, drive, or temptation to perform an act that presents potential risk of harm to self or others. Disorders included in this category in the DSM-IV are intermittent explosive disorder, kleptomania, pyromania, pathological gambling, and trichotillomania. Additional not otherwise specified impulse control disorders include a variety of impulse control issues such as compulsive shopping and compulsive sexual behavior. Generally, before committing the potentially harmful act, the individual feels an increasing sense of tension or arousal, and while committing the act, feels relief, pleasure, or gratification. Immediately after the act, the individuals may feel remorseful or guilty. The exact cause of impulse-control disorders is not clear, although there appears to be an interaction of psychodynamic, biological, and psychosocial factors that are associated with the disorders. Possible organic factors include abnormalities in specific brain regions such as the limbic system. There have been reports of abnormalities in the serotonin system associated with violence, suicide, and impulse-control disorders. Psychosocial factors associated with impulse control disorders include early exposure to domestic violence, alcoholism and drug abuse, and antisocial personality.

## CLINICAL PRESENTATION

**Intermittent explosive disorder** is the occurrence of episodes of aggressive impulses that result in serious assaultive behaviors or destruction of property. The severity of aggressiveness greatly exceeds the precipitating stressor or provocation. Individuals with intermittent explosive disorder have a high incidence of hyperactivity, subtle neurological abnormalities, and nonspecific electroencephalogram (EEG) abnormalities. Men are more likely to be affected than women, and the disorder usually begins in late adolescence/young adulthood.

**Kleptomania** is recurrent failure to resist impulses to steal objects that are not needed for personal use or monetary value. Stolen objects are often hidden or given away and may be of minor monetary value. The stealing is a solitary and unplanned activity, and the individuals frequently feel guilty or remorseful after the theft. Kleptomania is more common among women than men, although the disorder is generally rare, occurring in less than 5% of shoplifters. Kleptomania should be differentiated from stealing for the gain of the object. For individuals with kleptomania, the act of stealing is the goal, rather than the stolen object. Kleptomania is often associated with mood disorders and with eating disorders, particularly bulimia.

**Pyromania** is characterized by deliberate fire setting. Individuals have excitement or arousal before the act and relief or gratification when causing the fire or participating in the aftermath. The fire setting is not done for monetary gain (in contrast with arson) or to express anger or revenge, but rather, reflects an attraction to fire and its related components such as firefighting equipment. Individuals with pyromania tend to have higher prevalence of alcoholism, borderline or low IQ, and chronic personal stress.

**Pathological gambling** is characterized by recurrent gambling that causes interpersonal, domestic, and vocational impairments. Individuals with pathological gambling may be preoccupied with gambling, and like individuals with substance abuse disorders, may have repeated unsuccessful attempts to control or stop the gambling behaviors. The gambling may be a way of escaping from problems or uncomfortable mood states, and individuals may lie or steal to hide or support the gambling behaviors. Pathological gambling may be seen in 1% to 3% of the adult population, and typically begins in adolescence. Approximately 66% of pathological gamblers are male. Women with pathological gambling are more likely to have comorbid major depression.

**Trichotillomania** is characterized by the recurrent pulling out of an individual's own hair to the extent that noticeable hair loss is evident. Most hair is pulled from the head, although axillary, pubic, or other body hair may be pulled on rarer occasions. As with other impulse-control disorders, individuals feel a sense of anxiety or tension prior to committing the act (hair pulling in this case), and immediate relief or gratification when committing the act. Trichotillomania is more common in women than men, and onset is usually in childhood or adolescence. Stressful events may exacerbate hair pulling behavior, although individuals may also pull their hair when in a state of relaxation (eg, watching television). Scalp or body/facial hair in individuals with trichotillomania is characteristically abnormal. There may be short or broken hairs, with damaged follicles intermixed with normal, long hairs. There is generally no abnormality of the scalp or skin.

## GENERAL TREATMENT RECOMMENDATIONS

Treatment for **intermittent explosive disorder** often involves a combination of psychotherapy and medication therapy. Use of psychotropic agents may be helpful in reducing severity of explosive episodes. Treating clinicians must emphasize limit setting, and the safety of the patient and others. Many clinicians use anticonvulsants in treating episodically violent patients, in particular carbamazepine or valproate. Lithium has been reported to reduce aggressive episodes as has buspirone, and the SSRI antidepressants. Benzodiazepines should be used with caution in this population, as there may be a resultant paradoxical dyscontrol syndrome. In most patients, severity of violent episodes decreases during middle age.

Little is known about optimum treatments of **kleptomania**, and most of the literature has focused on psychotherapeutic interventions. As kleptomania tends to be a chronic disorder, long-term psychotherapy appears to be helpful. As with most psychotherapeutic interventions, individuals who are motivated to change generally respond best. There have been reports that the SSRI antidepressants may be useful in kleptomania.

As with kleptomania, little has been published on the treatment of **pyromania**. Behavioral therapy has been reported to be useful in some cases. Individuals often incur legal problems when they are caught setting fires, and their acts may cause tremendous personal injury or property damage. Adults with pyromania often present particular challenges in treatment as they may be unable or unwilling to take responsibility for their actions.

Treatment for **pathological gambling** is generally similar to the addiction model seen with alcohol abuse. Gamblers Anonymous (GA), a self-help group similar to Alcoholics Anonymous (AA), is helpful for motivated individuals. As with alcoholism, gamblers who are unwilling to engage in treatment generally will continue destructive gambling behaviors. As with other impulse control disorders, clinicians must be vigilant regarding presence of comorbid psychiatric illness, particularly depression and anxiety disorders, and treat these aggressively.

Individuals with **trichotillomania** often come to psychiatric attention when hair loss becomes severe. They may be referred from a dermatologist or internist when medical causes of alopecia have been ruled out. Many clinicians use the SSRI antidepressants as first line treatment for trichotillomania. Other drugs that may be useful include lithium and anxiolytics such as hydroxyzine. Atypical antipsychotics may be useful in individuals who do not respond to SSRIs, as may the typical antipsychotic drug pimozide. Clinicians should closely assess for comorbid psychiatric illness, such as mood disorders.

# ATTENTION-DEFICIT HYPERACTIVITY DISORDER

Attention-deficit/hyperactivity disorder (ADHD) is characterized by persistent inattention and/or hyperactivity that is age inappropriate. ADHD occurs in approximately 3% to 5% of grade-school age children, and is more commonly seen in boys than girls. Although the cause of ADHD is not clear, there does appear to be some familiar trend for the disorders. It is believed that ADHD may involve subtle brain injury during fetal or perinatal development, as soft neurological findings are often present. Brain imaging with individuals with ADHD is usually normal. There has been a recent increase in attention to the persistence of ADHD in adults, and pharmacologic treatment of the adult with ADHD has become substantially more common in clinical settings over the last 5 years. Prognosis for ADHD is variable, with poorer outcomes associated with chaotic or disruptive family situations, and with comorbid substance abuse.

## CLINICAL PRESENTATION

Symptoms of inattention in ADHD may include careless mistakes in school work or other activities, difficulty in sustaining attention in work or play activity, inability to listen or follow instructions, difficulty in organizing tasks or activities, easy distractibility, and forgetfulness. Symptoms of hyperactivity-impulsivity in ADHD may include excessive physical activity, inability to sit still when required, rapid/excessive talking, feelings of restlessness, intruding on or interrupting others, and impatient to allow others to finish speaking or complete an activity. Individuals with ADHD must have symptoms that caused impairment before 7 years of age, and there must be evidence of clinically significant school, work, or social impairment. Aggression or oppositional behavior is not uncommon. Many individuals are not diagnosed until hyperactive behavior and inattention begins to lead to problems at school. ADHD frequently remits during adolescence/early adulthood with hyperactivity symptoms improving most readily. Approximately 15% to 20% of children with ADHD continue to experience symptoms into adulthood. In older children, and in adults, the symptoms of motor hyperactivity become markedly less obvious, and hyperactivity may be manifested more as "fidgetiness" or subjective restlessness. Older children or adults with ADHD often exhibit disruptive interpersonal relationships due to their impulsivity and irritability, and adults may be unable to tolerate jobs or leisure activities that involve sitting for long periods, or tasks that require long periods of focused concentration. Comorbid psychiatric illness risk is increased in individuals with ADHD, particularly for mood disorders, substance abuse disorders, and personality disorders.

## GENERAL TREATMENT RECOMMENDATIONS

Treatment of ADHD generally involves a combination of psychotherapy and pharmacotherapy. The Children and Adolescents section in Special Populations *on page 663* further describes management of ADHD in child patients. Overall, the stimulant drugs are considered to be first-line treatment for ADHD by many clinicians. Other drugs which have been reported to be useful include TCA antidepressants, clonidine, and the MAOI antidepressants. Psychotherapeutic interventions for children must involve the family and school. In management of adult patients with ADHD, some clinicians utilize stimulants, although attention must be paid to the abuse potential of these drugs. Antidepressants are less problematic with adults than with children, as there is a greatly enhanced literature base on the use of antidepressants in adults compared to children. Comorbid psychiatric illness should be assessed and aggressively treated. Psychotherapy should be continued with adults, and may involve couples or family therapy.

# PERSONALITY DISORDERS

Personality consists of the behavioral and psychological traits/patterns manifested by an individual. Personality disorders occur when those traits and patterns deviate markedly from the expectations of an individual's culture, are inflexible, and cause impairment or distress. Individuals with personality disorders exhibit a maladaptive way of coping with their environment. Personality disorders have an onset which can be traced back to at least adolescence or early adulthood. In DSM-IV, personality disorder diagnoses are made on Axis II, as opposed to other disorders such as schizophrenia or bipolar disorder, which are classified on Axis I.

## CLINICAL PRESENTATION

The personality disorders are grouped into three separate clusters in DSM-IV. Cluster A includes the psychotic-like disorders which are more common in the biological relatives of schizophrenic individuals than among nonpsychotic control groups. This cluster includes paranoid personality disorder, schizoid personality disorder, and schizotypal personality. Schizotypal personality appears to have a greater genetic linkage to schizophrenia compared to paranoid and schizoid personality disorders, and occurs in approximately 3% of the general population. Individuals with schizotypal personality disorder have a chronic pattern of social and interpersonal impairment characterized by diminished capacity for interpersonal relationships, cognitive/perceptual distortions, and eccentric behavior. This has been described as an "attenuated" schizophrenia presentation. Individuals with schizoid personality disorder exhibit a pattern of chronic social withdrawal. The disorder may be more common in men than in women, and individuals may appear quite functional if they have occupations that allow them to remain secure and somewhat isolated. Individuals with paranoid personality disorder manifest a persistent pattern of distrust and suspiciousness of others. The prevalence of the disorder has been reported to be 0.5% to 2.5% of the general population. When stressed, individuals with paranoid personality disorder may exhibit frankly psychotic episodes, although these are usually brief in duration (<1 day).

Cluster B personality disorders are composed of a dramatic/emotional group of disorders, including antisocial personality disorder, borderline personality disorder, histrionic personality disorder, and narcissistic personality disorder. Individuals with antisocial personality disorder have a persistent pattern of disregard for, and violation of the rights of others. Terms that are used at times to describe these individuals include psychopathic or "sociopathic". The disorder cannot be diagnosed before the age of 18 years. Antisocial personality disorder tends to be associated with urban settings and low socioeconomic status, and is more common in men than in women. Individuals may engage in such behaviors as theft, violence, and use of illegal substances. Antisocial personality is seen in approximately 3% of men, and 1% of women. As expected, prevalence is much higher in prison or felon populations. Individuals with borderline personality disorder experience a chronic pattern of impulsiveness, unstable mood and self image, and chaotic interpersonal relationships. Borderline personality disorder is more common in women than in men, and occurs in approximately 1% to 2% of the population. Individuals may exhibit such self-injurious behavior as extreme spending, promiscuity, substance abuse, or binge eating. Individuals may also experience self-mutilating behavior such as wrist cutting or self-burning. Borderline personality disorder may be seen in up to 10% of acute psychiatric hospital admission, and may occur in 10% to 30% of individuals seeking psychiatric treatment. Suicide attempts, or suicidal behaviors, may be seen in the clinical presentation of up to 70% of acutely hospitalized individuals with borderline personality disorder. Individuals with histrionic personality disorder show excessive emotionality and attention seeking. Other characteristic features of histrionic personality may include rapidly shifting emotions, theatricality, and inappropriate, sexually seductive behavior. Histrionic personality disorder is seen in approximately 2% of the population, and appears to be more often diagnosed in women than in men. Individuals with narcissistic personality disorder exhibit an exaggerated sense of self-importance and need for admiration. Narcissistic personality occurs in <1% of the population, and may occur more often in men than in women.

Cluster C personality disorders all have an anxiety/fearfulness component, and include avoidant personality disorder, dependent personality disorder, and obsessive-compulsive disorder. Individuals with avoidant personality disorder experience chronic social inhibition associated with feelings of inadequacy and fear of rejection. Individuals often appear anxious and socially inept, usually reluctant to take any personal risks or attempt new activities due to fear of failure or rejection. Avoidant personality is seen in <1% of the population. There appears to be an increased risk of social phobia in individuals with avoidant personality disorder. Dependent personality disorder is among the most frequently reported personality disorder in mental health clinics, and is more commonly seen in women than in men. Characteristic features are a persistent pattern of dependent, clinging, and submissive behavior. Individuals may be unable to make everyday decisions on their own or feel helpless and uncomfortable when alone. Occupational functioning is often impaired, as individuals may be unable to handle positions of authority, and risk for comorbid mood disorder is increased when the individual suffers loss of support from others. Individuals with obsessive-compulsive disorder have preoccupation with orderliness and control, at the expense of flexibility and efficiency. These individuals may be preoccupied with details, rules, etc, and often become preoccupied with perfectionism. Obsessive-compulsive personality disorder is seen in approximately 1% of the population, and is more common in men than in women.

## GENERAL TREATMENT RECOMMENDATIONS

Overall, personality disorders do not respond greatly to medication treatment, and many clinicians primarily recommend psychotherapeutic interventions for personality disorders. The exceptions to this are specific target symptoms that may severely affect functioning such as aggression, severe mood lability, or paranoid behaviors.

Additionally, individuals with personality disorders may require psychotropic therapy when comorbid psychiatric conditions occur, such as mood disorders. These should be treated aggressively, as most individuals with personality disorders exhibit worsening of maladaptive coping when stressed or when suffering from acute comorbid psychiatric conditions.

## PERSONALITY DISORDERS *(Continued)*

Cluster A, the psychotic-like disorders, may require pharmacologic treatment for severely paranoid behavior or frankly psychotic symptoms. Small doses of antipsychotics may be beneficial in these individuals. Other medication interventions that have been reported to be useful are lithium (in paranoid personality), antidepressants (schizoid personality), and stimulants (schizoid personality). Anxiolytics (eg, lorazepam) may be helpful in the short-term management of anxiety or agitation.

Cluster B, the dramatic/emotional disorders, may frequently come to the attention of the mental health practitioner. The cluster B illness, which has received the most study in the area of psychopharmacology recently, is borderline personality disorder. Many clinicians advocate the use of antidepressants, particularly the SSRI antidepressants, as first-line treatment for dysphoric mood and impulsivity seen in borderline personality. The relatively benign side-effect profile and relative low potential for toxic overdose make the SSRI antidepressants particularly attractive for this group of patients. There is also a fairly substantial database on the effectiveness of low-dose antipsychotic medication to treat some of the more psychotic-like symptoms (paranoia, depersonalization, referential thinking) sometimes seen in borderline personality. Antipsychotics should generally not be tried before other medications that have less potential for long-term adverse effects such as tardive dyskinesia. The newer, atypical antipsychotic compounds may offer benefit in individuals with borderline personality disorder, although this has not been well studied. Other psychotropic medications that may be of benefit with individuals with borderline personality disorder include lithium and anticonvulsants such as carbamazepine. Benzodiazepines should be used with caution in this population as the potential for misuse/abuse is relatively great. Pharmacotherapy for antisocial personality disorder, narcissistic personality disorder, and histrionic personality disorder has been less well studied. Drugs that have been reported to have some efficacy in some patients are generally focused on a few target symptoms, such as emotional lability in narcissistic personality (lithium), and violence/aggression in antisocial personality (anticonvulsant). As with borderline personality disorder, benzodiazepines or other compounds with addiction potential should be used with extreme caution.

Individuals with cluster C personality disorders may benefit from pharmacotherapies focused at specific target symptoms. Patients with dependent or avoidant personalities may exhibit severe anxiety or depressive symptoms that are responsive to anxiolytics or to antidepressants such as TCA or SSRI compounds. Beta-blockers have been reported to be useful in some individuals with somatic anxiety symptoms. Individuals with severe obsessive-compulsive personality disorder may benefit from similar medications used to treat obsessive-compulsive disorder (see Anxiety Disorders *on page 606*). These may include antidepressants, particularly the SSRI class, and clomipramine. Anxiolytic medications such as benzodiazepines may be beneficial for the short-term management of anxiety/agitation.

# ANTIDEPRESSANTS

The choice of antidepressant medications available to clinicians has expanded greatly over the past decade. See Antidepressant Agents *on page 704*. Major classes of antidepressant medications available in the U.S. include:

1. Tricyclic (TCA) and related compounds
2. Selective serotonin reuptake inhibitors (SSRIs)
3. Dopamine-reuptake blocking compounds
4. Selective serotonin-norepinephrine reuptake inhibitors
5. Serotonin (5-$HT_2$) antagonists
6. Alpha-adrenoceptor antagonist
7. Monoamine oxidase inhibitors (MAOIs)

There are a variety of additional compounds currently being investigated that are likely to be added to the available pharmacologic treatment for depression.

Additionally, some antidepressant medications have been found to be useful in other illnesses, such as anxiety disorders including panic and obsessive-compulsive disorder, and other disorders such as eating disorders and nicotine dependence.

## SPECIFIC CLASSES OF ANTIDEPRESSANTS

### TRICYCLIC (TCA) AND RELATED COMPOUNDS

The TCAs have been available in the United States for the last four decades. The Antidepressant Agents table *on page 704* identifies all TCAs and related compounds available in the U.S. All of these drugs are indicated for the treatment of major depression, except for clomipramine which is FDA-approved for the treatment of obsessive-compulsive disorder. The TCAs and related compounds work primarily via serotonin and norepinephrine reuptake blockade. Additionally, antihistaminic, antiadrenergic, and anticholinergic effects are seen to a varying degree. TCAs and related compounds all have primary hepatic metabolism. Selection of TCA agents is based primarily on the patient's prior history of antidepressant response, and on drug side effect profile. All TCAs appear to be equally efficacious in the treatment of depression; however, as is common in clinical settings, individual patients may respond well to one TCA and not respond to another. Over the last 10 years, TCAs have dropped from being first-line treatment for depression to become second-line agents. This has been due to the relatively greater difficulty of use (need for titration) and the more problematic side effect profile compared to SSRI antidepressant agents. Antidepressant response to TCAs and related compounds generally requires 4-6 weeks, but response may take up to 8-12 weeks in some medication responders. TCAs may be more effective than some other antidepressant classes such as SSRIs in the treatment of severe, melancholic depression.

Nortriptyline and desipramine have become among the most popular TCA-type agents due to their relatively benign side effect profile among their drug class and the possibility of reliable blood levels. Most common adverse effects of TCAs include sedation/somnolence, anticholinergic side effects (eg, dry mouth, blurred vision, constipation, and urinary retention), weight gain, and cardiovascular effects (eg, orthostasis and risk for cardiac arrhythmias). As a general rule, it is advisable to start with low doses of the TCAs and titrate upwards as tolerated using blood levels, if available, to assist in optimizing clinical response. Elderly patients and those with cardiac disease or cardiac risk factors should have a baseline EKG prior to beginning TCA treatment. Elderly patients, or those with slowed metabolism due to medical illness or cytochrome P-450 isoenzyme deficiency, generally need lower and slower drug dosing (see Cytochrome P-450 and Drug Interactions *on page 730*). Side effects are usually best minimized by slow drug titration to optimize adverse effect tolerance, prescription of a larger proportion of daily drug dosing at bedtime once steady state is achieved, and use of lowest effective drug dosage. Plasma TCA levels, drawn 12 hours after last drug dose in a patient who has achieved medication steady state, may assist in determining lowest effective drug dosage. There appears to be a therapeutic window for nortriptyline (50-150 mg/mL).

Once antidepressant response has been achieved, the TCA should be continued for 6-12 months at full dosage. When the decision is made to discontinue the TCA, the drug should be slowly tapered in order to minimize TCA withdrawal symptoms (ie, nausea, vomiting, sweating, and headache). See Discontinuation of Drugs *on page 798*.

The TCAs have a relatively narrow therapeutic index, and toxicity may occur with relatively small overdoses. There is no antidote to TCA overdose, and supportive measures include close cardiac monitoring/support.

### SELECTIVE SEROTONIN REUPTAKE INHIBITORS (SSRIs)

The SSRIs, available in the U.S. for nearly a decade, have become extremely popular due to their effectiveness in the treatment of depression, their relatively benign side effect/safety profile, and their general ease of use with minimal titration required. The table *on page 704* lists the SSRIs available in the United States. SSRIs may be more effective than TCAs in the treatment of atypical depression. Fluvoxamine, fluoxetine, sertraline, and paroxetine are all additionally indicated for the treatment of obsessive-compulsive disorder. Sertraline and paroxetine are indicated for panic disorder. Paroxetine has an indication for social phobia and fluoxetine has indications for eating disorder and premenstrual disorder. Sertraline has an indication for post-traumatic stress disorder. SSRIs may also be useful in personality disorders, disorders of impulse control, and premenstrual dysphoria.

The mechanism of action of SSRIs is primarily a selective inhibition of 5-HT reuptake. In comparison with TCAs, there is relatively weak adrenergic, histaminic, or muscarinic activity. SSRIs are hepatically metabolized. Both fluoxetine and sertraline have active metabolites, however, this generally is clinically significant only for fluoxetine where half-life of the active metabolite, norfluoxetine, is approximately 1 week.

Most common side effects of SSRIs are GI disturbances (including nausea, vomiting, and diarrhea), CNS symptoms (eg, agitation, anxiety, insomnia), and sexual dysfunction including decreased libido and impotence. GI complaints often resolve after the first month of therapy and may be minimized by taking SSRI medication with/after meals. Although some patients experience weight loss when SSRIs are initiated, weight gain may occur with long-term use of SSRIs. CNS symptoms may be minimized by prescribing all SSRI medication before noon. Additional

## ANTIDEPRESSANTS *(Continued)*

sedative/hypnotic medication at bedtime, such as trazodone 50 mg at bedtime may be helpful. Sexual dysfunction, seen in up to 50% to 80% of patients on SSRIs, is often associated with medication noncompliance in patients on SSRI maintenance therapy. Clinicians must carefully assess for SSRI-related sexual dysfunction and modify antidepressant treatment accordingly in order to prevent medication noncompliance.

Initiation of SSRIs is generally fairly straightforward with minimal titration required. Dosing for nondepression indications may be higher than for the treatment of depression (eg, fluoxetine 60-80 mg/day for OCD treatment). SSRI overdose is generally less of a problem in clinical settings compared to TCAs due to the wide therapeutic index of the SSRIs. As SSRIs inhibit cytochrome P-450 isoenzymes, SSRIs may be associated with increased blood levels of other drugs metabolized by these enzymes. One of the most common clinical issues in this respect is elevated TCA blood levels when prescribing SSRIs and TCAs concurrently. Adverse effects may be minimized by decreasing TCA dosage, monitoring of TCA levels, if available, and EKG monitoring. As with TCAs, SSRIs should not be used concurrently with MAOIs.

SSRIs should be continued at full therapeutic dosage for 6-12 months after resolution of depression, and dosing should be slowly tapered (over several weeks) when the decision is made to discontinue antidepressants. The exception to tapered discontinuation is fluoxetine, where abrupt discontinuation is less problematic due to the long drug half-life. Fluoxetine for premenstrual disorder (PMDD) is marketed under a different trade name than fluoxetine for depression.

### DOPAMINE-REUPTAKE BLOCKING COMPOUNDS

The only dopamine-reuptake blocking compound available in the U.S. is bupropion. Bupropion acts by blocking the reuptake of dopamine. Bupropion has a generally wide therapeutic index with less medical risk in overdose compared to TCAs. Side effect profile for bupropion is relatively benign, and bupropion has been reported to improve SSRI-associated sexual dysfunction. Reports of seizures in some patients, particularly those with bulimia, suggest that a history of seizure disorder or eating disorder may be a relative contraindication for the use of bupropion. Seizure risk may be minimized by slow drug titration and prescribing no more than 150 mg of bupropion in a single dosage.

Bupropion SR is indicated for use in smoking cessation and is marketed under a different trade name than bupropion prescribed for depression.

### SELECTIVE SEROTONIN-NOREPINEPHRINE REUPTAKE INHIBITORS

The only selective serotonin-norepinephrine reuptake inhibitor available in the U.S. is venlafaxine, introduced in 1994. Venlafaxine adds norepinephrine reuptake blockade to serotonin reuptake blockade, and is hepatically metabolized. Venlafaxine may have particular efficacy in severely ill, melancholic, depressed patients. Venlafaxine has also recently received an FDA indication for the treatment of generalized anxiety disorder (GAD).

Most common adverse effects for venlafaxine include nausea, sedation, and sexual dysfunction. Five percent to 10% of patients may experience dose-dependent hypertension secondary to venlafaxine therapy. Patients being started on venlafaxine therapy should have regular, close blood pressure monitoring. Elevations in blood pressure may be more problematic when venlafaxine is used concurrently with cimetidine. Slow titration of venlafaxine at drug initiation will minimize adverse effects such as nausea and somnolence. Strategy for time lines of maintenance treatment and discontinuation are similar to short-acting SSRIs.

### SEROTONIN (5-HT$_2$) ANTAGONISTS

Trazodone and nefazodone are the two drugs of this class available in the U.S. This class of drugs is believed to work by 5-HT$_2$ antagonism and modest inhibition of serotonin and norepinephrine reuptake presynaptically. Both drugs are effective antidepressants which also have anxiolytic properties although trazodone is not often used for monotherapy as an antidepressant by most clinicians. However, low-dose trazodone has been used as a sedative/hypnotic for many years in clinical settings, often as an alternative to benzodiazepines in patients with substance abuse histories. Nefazodone is generally less sedating than trazodone and is generally used for its antidepressant and anxiolytic properties. Both trazodone and nefazodone have fairly robust alpha-adrenergic activity. Most common adverse effects of both agents include orthostasis, sedation, and GI distress. Sexual adverse effects are uncommon. Trazodone has been infrequently associated with priapism in males, and patients should be educated regarding need to seek acute treatment if priapism occurs.

Sedation may be minimized by giving the majority of medication at bedtime. Due to the wide therapeutic index of both nefazodone and trazodone, overdose is a lesser clinical concern compared to TCAs.

### ALPHA-ADRENOCEPTOR ANTAGONISTS

Mirtazapine introduced in 1996, is the only agent of this class available in the U.S. Mirtazapine appears to act via central alpha$_2$-receptor antagonism with indirect norepinephrine and serotonin agonism. Mirtazapine appears to be an effective, well-tolerated antidepressant. Most common adverse effects include sedation and dry mouth. Rare cases of severe neutropenia (1.1 per thousand patients) have been reported. Fifteen percent of patients may experience increase in cholesterol/triglycerides. Mirtazapine may be particularly efficacious in severely depressed patients and those with depression characterized by prominent anxiety symptoms.

### MONOAMINE OXIDASE INHIBITORS (MAOIs)

MAOIs, the first specific antidepressant medications available, are currently reserved for use in refractory depression. Although MAOIs are clearly effective agents and appear to offer particular efficacy in severely depressed or atypical depressed patients, their side effect profile and food/drug and drug/drug interactions restrict their use in general clinical practice. The Antidepressant Agents table *on page 704* lists the MAOIs available in the U.S.

The most common side effects associated with MAOIs include orthostatic hypotension, sleep abnormalities, and sexual dysfunction. The most serious side effect is hypertensive crisis, potentially leading to cerebrovascular accident or serotonin syndromes characterized by acute change in mental status, fever, autonomic instability, and possible coma/death. MAOIs prevent the normal degradation of amines such as tyramine. A variety of high tyramine foods (see Tyramine Content of Foods *on page 813*) are associated with potential for MAOI hypertensive crisis. Avoidance of these foods by patients receiving MAOIs markedly reduces risk of hypertensive crisis. Serotonin syndrome appears to be associated with increased central 5-HT activity. The syndrome may be precipitated by concurrent use of MAOIs and medications that increase serotonin, including other antidepressant agents. After MAOI discontinuation, it takes 2 weeks for monoamine oxidase recovery. Other antidepressants should generally not be started until after the 2-week "washout" period off MAOIs is completed. Washout required in switching from other antidepressant to an MAOI varies from 1 week (after TCA, nefazodone, trazodone therapy) to 5-6 weeks (after fluoxetine therapy).

Development of elevation in blood pressure, particularly associated with severe headache, is a medical emergency and should be monitored and treated in acute medical settings.

Patients on MAOIs should be educated regarding risks/benefits of their medication and should be able to communicate their antidepressant regimen to their other medical practitioners. Sympathomimetics used in anesthetics (eg, meperidine and epinephrine), may be associated with severe drug interactions, and MAOIs are often discontinued prior to surgical procedures.

# ANTIPSYCHOTICS

All current FDA-approved antipsychotic medications are effective treatments for psychotic symptoms; however, individual patients may respond well to one antipsychotic drug and not another. Choice of antipsychotic is, thus, based upon individual patient response and drug side effect profile. The atypical antipsychotic agent, clozapine, offers superior efficacy in treatment refractory schizophrenia, and the atypical antipsychotics available in the U.S., clozapine, olanzapine, risperidone, and quetiapine, may offer particular benefit for negative symptoms of schizophrenia. The Antipsychotic Agents table *on page 706* lists antipsychotic drugs available in the U.S. Side effects of antipsychotic drugs can be divided into neurological and non-neurological effects.

As a general rule, neurological effects are primarily associated with high-potency traditional antipsychotics; while non-neurologic effects, usually a result of nondopamine receptor interactions, are more associated with lower-potency typical antipsychotic agents, and the atypical antipsychotic agents to a varying degree.

Neurological adverse effects are mainly associated with dopaminergic blockade in the nigrostriatum. Various types of extrapyramidal symptoms (EPS), both acute and chronic may occur. Major acute extrapyramidal syndromes are acute dystonias, drug-induced parkinsonism, and akathisia. Management of the acute syndromes are more fully described in the section on Psychiatric Emergencies - Acute EPS *on page 660*. Acute EPS is significantly more likely to occur with conventional antipsychotic medications compared to atypical antipsychotic compounds. Tardive dyskinesia (TD) is a chronic, potentially irreversible abnormal movement disorder associated with long-term use of antipsychotic medication. Movements may be choreiform, tonic, or athetotic and most commonly involve the face and mouth. Those at greater risk for developing TD are those on prolonged antipsychotic therapy, those older than 50 years of age, and those with diabetes or primary affective disorder. TD prevalence estimates for neuroleptic-treated patients range from 10% to 15% in young patients, 12% to 25% in "chronic" patients, and 25% to 45% of "state hospital" patients. There is no definitive treatment for TD, although studies show reduced symptoms when treated with clozapine. A small number of cases remit with discontinuation of antipsychotic medication; however, many cases are permanent. Risk for TD development is best reduced by careful use of the lowest possible effective dose of antipsychotic medication and careful reassessment of treatment needs. Individuals on maintenance antipsychotic medication should have regular, periodic assessment for involuntary movements (at least 2-3 times/year). The Abnormal Involuntary Movement Scale (AIMS *on page 598*) is a widely used assessment tool. A key point in long-term antipsychotic therapy is education of patients and families regarding risks and benefits of therapy including TD in particular. Clozapine is the only antipsychotic that does not appear to cause TD. Current data on the newer atypical antipsychotics suggests a greatly reduced risk of TD, compared to typical agents, however, insufficient data exists to clearly assess TD risk with other atypical antipsychotics.

Non-neurologic side effects, except for endocrine changes, are generally a result of activity on receptors other than dopamine. Sedation is perhaps the most common non-neurologic side effect associated with antipsychotic medication. It is most often seen with low-potency typical antipsychotic medication (chlorpromazine, thioridazine), and with clozapine. Sedation appears to be due to histaminergic and adrenergic blockade. Daytime sedation can be reduced by prescribing all, or the majority of antipsychotic medication dosing at bedtime. Occasionally, psychostimulants (methylphenidate) are used to counteract persistent sedation.

Orthostatic hypotension may occur with any antipsychotic, but like sedation, is most often associated with low-potency typical agents and with some of the atypical antipsychotics. Orthostasis is most problematic during treatment initiation, and tolerance usually develops. Elderly patients and those on multiple psychotropic medications are particularly prone to develop orthostasis. Management consists of modification of medication regimen to reduce additive orthostatic effects (eg, antihypertensive medication dosage reduction and dosage reduction of concomitant sedating/hypotension-inducing psychotropic medications), increasing fluid intake, close vital sign monitoring, and patient education in minimizing effects of orthostasis (eg, arising slowly from a supine position).

The typical antipsychotic, thioridazine, is now indicated only for schizophrenic patients who fail to show an acceptable response to other antipsychotic drugs due to warnings concerning $QT_c$ interval prolongation in a dose-related manner. Patients on thioridazine should have EKG assessments periodically, as well as monitoring of serum potassium levels. Thioridazine has not been demonstrated to be efficacious in treatment refractory schizophrenia.

Anticholinergic side effects may be manifested both peripherally and centrally. Peripheral effects include dry mouth, blurred vision, mydriasis, constipation, and urinary retention. These symptoms are particularly problematic in older patients who are most likely to experience anticholinergic effects, and who are most likely to have functional or medical sequelae as a result of anticholinergic effects. Individuals with narrow-angle glaucoma may have worsening of glaucoma, and should have frequent ophthalmologic monitoring. As anticholinergic effects are greatest with low-potency antipsychotics, switching to a higher-potency agent or the addition of amantadine in place of anticholinergic antiparkinsonian agents may be helpful in controlling anticholinergic effects. Central anticholinergic toxicity is rare when antipsychotics are used alone at therapeutic doses. Anticholinergic toxicity is more likely to occur as a result of anticholinergic medication prescribed for neurologic side effects of antipsychotics. Anticholinergic delirium is characterized by change in consciousness, agitation, mydriasis, urinary retention, tachycardia, and fever. Seizures, shock, and arrhythmias can occur. Moderate to severe cases may be managed with physostigmine 1 mg I.M./I.V. repeated as needed every 30 minutes, while milder cases respond to supportive therapy and prompt discontinuation of anticholinergic drugs.

Some endocrine effects of antipsychotic medication are related to dopamine antagonism and hyperprolactinemia. Gynecomastia or galactorrhea may occur, as may a false-positive pregnancy test, and secondary amenorrhea in women. These effects are most likely to occur with typical antipsychotics and least likely to occur with atypical antipsychotic agents particularly clozapine, olanzapine, and quetiapine.

Sexual dysfunction, such as diminished libido, may occur in both men and women, while men may experience retrograde ejaculation. Amantadine can be beneficial for some patients with endocrine adverse effects.

Skin changes are seen occasionally with antipsychotic drugs, particularly photosensitivity reactions. Severe sunburn may result from exposure to bright sunlight in patients on antipsychotics, and patients should be instructed to wear sunscreen and have appropriate sun protection when outdoors. Prolonged use of chlorpromazine has been associated with unusual blue-gray discoloration of sun-exposed skin.

Weight gain can occur with all antipsychotic compounds, both typical and atypical, although is generally less problematic with high-potency typical antipsychotics, and the atypical antipsychotic, risperidone. Careful attention to diet and nutrition while on medication may greatly minimize weight gain.

Ophthalmological side effects may be seen, particularly with chronic high-dose chlorpromazine therapy, and to a lesser extent with thiothixene. Patients develop brownish, granular deposits in the anterior lens and posterior cornea, although these deposits do not impair vision. In animal studies, dogs given high doses of quetiapine developed cataracts. Although subsequent human studies found no causative association between quetiapine therapy and cataract development, the product package insert for quetiapine recommends eye exams for cataract screening twice yearly for patients on quetiapine therapy. Thioridazine may cause a retinopathy similar to retinitis pigmentosa when used in doses >800 mg/day. This may proceed to blindness even after thioridazine discontinuation. Retinopathy is unlikely at daily doses <800 mg.

Agranulocytosis occurs in approximately 0.01% to 0.1% of patients on conventional antipsychotics. It is seen in approximately 0.3% to 1% of patients on clozapine. The newer atypical antipsychotics, risperidone, olanzapine, and quetiapine do not have significant associations with blood dyscrasias. Agranulocytosis risk is greatest during the first 6 months of antipsychotic treatment. The exact etiology of drug-induced agranulocytosis is not clear. With clozapine, female gender and increasing age appear to be risk factors for drug-induced neutropenia and agranulocytosis. Patients of Jewish descent with haplotype HLA-B38, DR4, DQ W3 may also be at increased risk. Risk of agranulocytosis is not dose-dependent. The recommendations for blood monitoring while on clozapine are changed to weekly monitoring for the first 6 months of therapy, and monitoring every other week thereafter for as long as clozapine is received, and up to 4 weeks after clozapine discontinuation. If WBC drops, clozapine must be promptly discontinued. Granulocyte colony-stimulating factor may speed recovery of clozapine-induced agranulocytosis. Individuals with a history of clozapine-induced agranulocytosis should generally not be rechallenged with clozapine. The other newer atypical antipsychotic medications may be an option for these individuals if they have not already been tried.

# MOOD STABILIZERS

Mood stabilizers are agents that are effective in decreasing or preventing the manic and depressive episodes of bipolar and related disorders. See Mood Stabilizers table in the Appendix *on page 719*. Lithium carbonate was the first recognized mood stabilizer, and for many years was the only drug with an FDA-approved indication for mood stabilization. In 1995, valproate was FDA approved as an antimanic agent in the anticonvulsant class. Currently, these are the two drugs most commonly used by clinicians as mood stabilizers, although a variety of compounds, primarily anticonvulsants, are used in clinical settings to manage bipolar and related disorders.

## LITHIUM

Lithium salts were recognized as beneficial for psychiatric disorders in the 1940s, and there is a very large body of literature on the use of lithium in clinical settings. It is known that lithium both effectively treats acute mania, and reduces recurrences of mania and depression in serious mood disorder. Lithium has acute depressant effect and may potentiate other antidepressant medications.

Lithium is also used in a variety of other disorders, particularly where decreasing irritability or aggression is a goal. This includes rage/aggression in post-traumatic stress disorder and episodic violent behavior in patients with mental retardation, organic brain syndromes, and personality disorders.

The mechanism of action of lithium is not clearly understood. Multiple neurotransmitter systems are affected including serotonergic, noradrenergic, and dopaminergic systems.

Lithium is not metabolized in the liver. It is eliminated unchanged in the urine. Blood levels are affected by disease of the kidney or renal changes associated with aging. In spite of its rather narrow therapeutic index, most patients readily tolerate lithium if there is strict adherence to maintenance of therapeutic blood levels of the drug. In the management of acute mania, blood levels of 0.7-1.5 mEq/L are appropriate, while levels of 0.7-1.2 mEq/L are appropriate for maintenance treatment of bipolar disorder. It is important to remember to "treat the patient, not the blood level." An example of this is the elderly patient who has good therapeutic response on low doses of lithium while becoming toxic on so-called "therapeutic" lithium blood levels.

Most clinicians begin lithium dosing at 300 mg 2-4 times/day in young patients, and check serial lithium levels during the first weeks of therapy. Dosage is then gradually titrated dependent on optimal clinical response and on blood levels. Elderly patients, or those with renal impairment are likely to require smaller doses.

Most common adverse effects of lithium therapy include tremor, polydipsia with associated polyuria, changes in mentation characterized by difficulty concentrating and remembering, elevated white blood cell count, hypothyroidism, weight gain, GI disturbances, EKG changes, and rarely, renal impairment. Lithium tremor may respond to the addition of a beta-blocker (eg, propranolol 10 mg 3 times/day). Cardiac, renal, and endocrine status should be monitored by regular EKG, kidney function, and thyroid function testing. Lithium has been associated with cardiac birth defect (Ebstein's anomaly) when used during pregnancy, and this should be avoided in pregnancy, if possible. Blood levels should be drawn approximately 12 hours after last dose after steady-state levels (after about 1 week of treatment) are achieved. Alternatively, some clinicians advocate a "loading dose" of lithium with serial blood levels over the next 24-36 hours and subsequent determination of final lithium dosage.

Response to lithium in acute mania generally takes approximately 1-2 weeks. If no response occurs after 3-4 weeks with therapeutic blood levels, the patient is determined to be a lithium nonresponder and alternative or adjunctive drug therapies should be explored. After resolution of the acute mood episode, after daily dosing stability is achieved, lithium dosing may be changed to a twice daily schedule. Alternatively, if the total daily dose is ≤1500 mg/day, lithium may be given as a single daily dose, if tolerated. Some clinicians advocate once daily dosing in an effort to increase ease with compliance. Lithium levels should be checked at least every 3 months once the patient is stable. Kidney functioning and thyroid functioning as well as routine EKG monitoring should be done periodically (every 6-12 months) for patients on long-term lithium therapy.

## ANTICONVULSANTS

Anticonvulsant medications have become increasingly important in the management of bipolar and related disorders. The Mood Stabilizer table *on page 719* lists the anticonvulsants commonly used in clinical settings for serious mood disorders.

Carbamazepine was the first widely used anticonvulsant for the management of bipolar and related disorders, although the drug does not have an approved indication as a mood stabilizer. Nevertheless, there are a large number of studies that document its efficacy in psychiatric illness. For the most part, carbamazepine is used as a second-line treatment in bipolar disorder, for patients who either fail or cannot tolerate lithium or valproate. Often carbamazepine is utilized as "add-on" therapy, although it may be highly effective as monotherapy in some bipolar patients.

The most common adverse effects of carbamazepine are sedation, orthostasis, and GI disturbances. Rarely, agranulocytosis or aplastic anemia may occur. Frequent blood monitoring was widely advocated in the past, particularly during initiation of carbamazepine therapy. However, in current common clinical practice, regular, frequent blood monitoring while on carbamazepine therapy is not often implemented, particularly during the maintenance phase of treatment.

Carbamazepine is a liver enzyme inducer, and thus blood levels may be expected to decrease during the first month of therapy as auto-induction takes place. Carbamazepine may decrease plasma concentrations of other concomitantly used psychotropics. Patients should be monitored for potential changes in psychiatric symptomatology.

Valproate is an anticonvulsant that received an FDA antimania indication in 1995. It is utilized in controlling mood episodes in cyclical affective disorders, and may have particular benefit in rapid-cycling patients, lithium nonresponders, and bipolar individuals with substance abuse. Manic phases of illness generally respond better than depressive phases. Valproate may be given in loading doses, with rapid titration over a few days, in addition to a gradual, slower titration. As with lithium, blood levels may be used to assist in optimum clinical management. In acute mania, serum levels of 50-125 mcg/mL appear to be associated with best response. As with lithium and carbamazepine, use of valproate with other mood stabilizers is common. Although there may be an increase in carbamazepine level and decrease in valproate level when valproate and carbamazepine are used concurrently, this is generally not a clinically significant interaction. Most common adverse effects of valproate include sedation, GI disturbance, tremor, and weight gain. Use of enteric coated forms of valproate may reduce GI distress, while prescribing a greater portion of the drug at bedtime generally reduces daytime sedation. More serious side effects are severe hepatotoxicity, usually seen only in children, and also, rarely, hematological disturbance with decreased platelets. Severe, life-threatening pancreatitis has been reported rarely, and a warning concerning abdominal symptoms has recently been added to the manufacturer's package insert. Periodic monitoring of liver function tests and platelet levels may be checked, particularly when serum valproate levels are already being drawn. As with the other anticonvulsants, valproate should be avoided during pregnancy as it has been associated with neural tube birth defects.

Lamotrigine, an anticonvulsant, was recently approved in the United States for management of partial seizures. Current studies are examining efficacy in bipolar disorder, and there have been a number of clinical reports suggesting benefit in bipolar illness. The drug is being increasingly used in clinical psychiatric settings. Most common adverse effects are hypotension, sedation, GI distress, and rash. In rare cases, rash is severe with toxic epidermal necrosis or Stevens-Johnson syndrome. Risk of rash may be minimized by slow dose titration and dosage reduction when used concurrently with valproate. Higher dosages of lamotrigine are generally needed when lamotrigine and carbamazepine are used concurrently and lower dosages of lamotrigine are needed when valproate is used concurrently.

Gabapentin is a novel anticonvulsant approved in 1994 as an antiepileptic. Unlike the other anticonvulsants previously described, gabapentin does not undergo significant hepatic metabolism. Gabapentin is eliminated by the kidneys. Although most research data does not strongly support efficacy of gabapentin in bipolar illness, this is another novel anticonvulsant which is often used in clinical settings. Most common adverse effects associated with gabapentin include sedation, orthostasis, and GI disturbances.

Topiramate is an anticonvulsant compound which has been reported to be beneficial in acute mania. There may also be some efficacy in rapid cycling bipolar disorder, although data is still very preliminary. Unlike other anticonvulsants, topiramate may be associated with weight loss.

## OTHER AGENTS USED FOR MOOD STABILIZATION

Other agents which have demonstrated efficacy in some patients with bipolar and related disorders include antipsychotic medications, benzodiazepines (particularly clonazepam and lorazepam), thyroid compounds, and calcium channel blockers. Clozapine has been reported to be particularly efficacious in treatment of refractory bipolar disorder, and the newer atypical antipsychotics (eg, olanzapine, risperidone, and quetiapine) may have a unique role in management of bipolar and related disorders.

# ANXIOLYTICS & SEDATIVE/HYPNOTICS

The treatment of anxiety and related disorders and the treatment of sleep disturbances frequently involve medications of the same type/class, although clinical indications and medication dosing patterns may be quite different. Most anxiolytic medications have sedative properties with higher doses being used for insomnia and lower doses being used for anxiety. Clinical presentation of anxiety and related disorders are described in Anxiety Disorders *on page 606*. Insomnia is a common problem that may be seen in up to 33% of adults. Approximately 10% of adults report chronic insomnia. Insomnia frequently occurs in a variety of psychiatric conditions, including depressive disorders, anxiety disorders, schizophrenia, and dementias. In general, optimum treatment of anxiety or insomnia associated with a psychiatric condition involves treatment of the underlying condition with appropriate medications (eg, antidepressant therapy for major depression). As the psychiatric condition improves, insomnia and anxiety improve concurrently with other psychiatric symptoms. Many clinicians may augment primary psychiatric medication treatment with sedative/hypnotic or anxiolytic medications as symptoms stabilize, particularly in the early phases of treatment.

## BENZODIAZEPINES

Anxiolytics are the most commonly prescribed psychotropic medications, with approximately 80% of prescriptions being written by nonpsychiatrist physicians. The most frequently prescribed drug class for anxiety and insomnia are the benzodiazepines. Benzodiazepines are used in approximately 10% of the population annually. Benzodiazepines with FDA-approved anxiety indications in the United States include diazepam, alprazolam, chlordiazepoxide, clorazepate, lorazepam, halazepam, oxazepam, and prazepam. Benzodiazepine with FDA-approved insomnia indications in the U.S. include flurazepam, temazepam, triazolam, quazepam, and estazolam.

Additionally, clonazepam and diazepam have FDA indications for seizures and the rapid-acting benzodiazepine, midazolam, has an indication for anesthesia induction and preoperative sedation.

In psychiatric settings, benzodiazepines may be effective in anxiety disorders such as panic and agoraphobia, in depression, and in alcohol withdrawal.

All benzodiazepines are DEA Schedule IV controlled substances (see Controlled Substances *on page 796*. In short-term use, therapeutic doses of benzodiazepines are associated with substantial clinical benefit, and minimal toxicity and dependence. Long-term use may be associated with tolerance to CNS effects, cognitive impairment in the elderly, and withdrawal symptoms if stopped abruptly. However, the benzodiazepines, lorazepam, alprazolam, and clonazepam, may be used and well tolerated in maintenance treatment for panic disorder. Maintenance benzodiazepine treatment with alprazolam or clonazepam may also improve social phobia. The Benzodiazepines Comparison Chart *on page 708* lists benzodiazepines available in the U.S. along with their dosage ranges, relative potencies, onset of action time, and elimination half-life. Benzodiazepines are believed to act at least in part, on $\gamma$-aminobutyric acid (GABA) receptors in various brain regions. The benzodiazepine antagonist, flumazenil, reverses sedative effects of benzodiazepines and may be of use in benzodiazepine overdose.

When considering the use of a benzodiazepine medication, clinicians should carefully assess psychiatric differential diagnosis. For example, anxiety symptoms of major depression may be best treated with antidepressants plus judicious, transient benzodiazepine augmentation during the initial 4-6 weeks of drug therapy. Nonmedication treatment interventions, such as appropriate sleep hygiene and avoidance of stimulants, such as caffeine, may eliminate or reduce the need for benzodiazepine treatment. Finally, patients with histories of alcohol or other substance abuse should generally not receive benzodiazepines.

When initiating a benzodiazepine, patients should be educated regarding adverse effects, including risk of driving and other activities requiring good attention/motor coordination and the need to avoid concomitant alcohol use. Clinicians and patients must plan medication supply to avoid sudden discontinuation of maintenance benzodiazepine therapy.

Most benzodiazepines are well absorbed upon oral administration, although ingested food or aluminum-containing antacids may delay gastric absorption of benzodiazepines. Some benzodiazepines are available in I.M. or I.V. formulations.

Fast-acting benzodiazepines are used when rapid sedative effect is required, such as initial insomnia, drug withdrawal syndromes, or severe situational anxiety. Due to the brief nature of panic attacks, PRN rapid-acting benzodiazepines are of limited benefit. Long-acting or slow-acting benzodiazepines are used when maintenance anxiolytic activity is required.

Anxiolytic and hypnotic benzodiazepines are divided into four structural subgroups: 2-keto compounds (diazepam, chlordiazepoxide, flurazepam, prazepam, clorazepate, halazepam, and clonazepam), 3-hydroxy compounds (oxazepam, lorazepam, temazepam), triazolo compounds (triazolam, alprazolam, and adinazolam), and a trifluoroethyl compound (quazepam). The 2-keto compounds and quazepam are oxidized in the liver, and have relatively long half-lives (20-60 hours). Active metabolites may extend half-life. Quazepam also has a half-life of 40 hours.

The 3-hydroxy compounds are directly conjugated in the liver with no active metabolites and have a shorter half-life (8-14 hours). The triazolo compounds, also oxidized, have limited active metabolites with generally short half-lives (2-14 hours). Onset and duration of benzodiazepine activity is also influenced by drug lipophilic and hydrophilic properties. Highly lipophilic compounds such as diazepam are associated with rapid CNS effects, while less lipophilic compounds such as lorazepam may be associated with less rapid but more sustained CNS effects. Speed of drug distribution is particularly crucial to consider when benzodiazepines are dosed as a single dose or in sporadic dosing as opposed to maintenance dosing.

Selection of a benzodiazepine for sedative/hypnotic use is generally based on distribution and elimination half-life, route of administration, and patient clinical history as the benzodiazepines appear to have comparable efficacy when prescribed in equipotent doses.

Dosing of benzodiazepines is dependent on the disorder being treated. In treatment of panic disorder, alprazolam is approved in dosages of up to 10 mg/day, although many clinicians prescribe in the order of 2-4 mg/day in divided doses (3-4 times/day). In generalized anxiety disorder, 15-20 mg/day of diazepam (maximum: 40 mg/day) may be used. Starting dosage of benzodiazepines in anxiety disorders should be low (eg, alprazolam 1.5 mg/day with lower dosages in the elderly). When benzodiazepines are used on a PRN basis for situational anxiety, dosing is generally lower (lorazepam 0.5-1 mg PRN). Single bedtime dosages of benzodiazepines (eg, temazepam 15-30 mg orally at bedtime) may be effective. When maintenance benzodiazepines are discontinued, they should be slowly tapered (over 8-12 weeks) in order to avoid withdrawal symptoms of anxiety, tremor, autonomic arousal, and GI disturbance. Abrupt withdrawal from short-acting benzodiazepines (eg, alprazolam) has been associated with psychosis and seizures. Drug tapering and discontinuation may be better tolerated by patients when long-acting benzodiazepines (eg, clonazepam) are used.

Benzodiazepines are generally well tolerated with the majority of effects on the CNS. Effects on heart rate, blood pressure, and cardiac output are generally minimal. Risk of dependence is relatively low in populations without substance abuse while patients with alcohol abuse histories and those with personality disorders are at significantly greater risk of benzodiazepine abuse and dependence.

Excessive sedation is the most common adverse effect seen with benzodiazepines, with more pronounced effects in the elderly. Other CNS side effects include muscle weakness, ataxia, motor incoordination, cognitive impairment, and anterograde amnesia. CNS effects are dose-dependent and may be minimized by utilizing lowest effective dosages, slow dose titration, and careful monitoring of CNS status, particularly in high risk groups such as the elderly or those patients on concomitant psychotropic medications which may be associated with CNS depression. Although benzodiazepines generally have minimal effect on respiration, all anxiolytic/hypnotic agents should be used with caution in patients with pulmonary disease.

## BUSPIRONE

Buspirone is a non-benzodiazepine with an approved indication for the treatment of generalized anxiety. Buspirone is nonsedating, nonaddictive, and has no anticonvulsive activity. Buspirone is well tolerated by patients with comorbid medical illness as it does not cause cognitive slowing, motor incoordination, or CNS depression. Buspirone starting dose is 7.5 mg twice daily with an average therapeutic dosage of 20-40 mg/day. Many clinicians do not use buspirone due to belief that antianxiety effects of buspirone are often unacceptable to patients who have previously (effectively) been treated with benzodiazepines. Buspirone requires 2-4 weeks for full antianxiety effect, and does not treat benzodiazepine withdrawal symptoms. Buspirone is not effective as a hypnotic, nor is it useful for panic disorder.

## ANTIDEPRESSANTS

A number of antidepressants also produce important anti-anxiety effects. SSRIs are effective in obsessive-compulsive disorder (OCD) with demonstrated efficacy for paroxetine, fluoxetine, sertraline, and fluvoxamine. Management of OCD generally requires higher doses than for management of depression (eg, fluoxetine 60 mg/day), although lower dosages may be effective in some patients. The tricyclic antidepressant, clomipramine, is effective in OCD, although TCA-related adverse effects may limit its use. The novel antidepressant, nefazodone, appears to have antidepressant and anxiolytic properties.

Panic disorder may improve with SSRIs (eg, paroxetine used at similar dosages recommended for the management of major depression). Patients with panic disorder may require lower initial dosages and slower dose titration of antidepressant in order to avoid paradoxical activation in the early phases of therapy. The TCA antidepressants, imipramine and clomipramine, may also be beneficial in panic disorder. MAOI antidepressants may be effective in panic disorder, although potential side effects generally severely restrict their use.

Social phobia may be treated with SSRI or MAOI antidepressants at dosages similar to those recommended for treatment of major depression. SSRI class antidepressants also have an increasingly important role in the treatment of other anxiety disorders such as generalized anxiety and post-traumatic stress disorder.

Finally, antidepressants with sedating properties, particularly TCAs (eg, nortriptyline 25 mg orally at bedtime) and trazodone are used in low dosages by some clinicians for their hypnotic effects.

## BETA-BLOCKERS

Beta-adrenergic blocking agents may be beneficial in acute situational types of social phobia with the specific medications of propranolol, atenolol, nadolol, and metoprolol reported to be useful in this disorder. There are limited reports of usefulness of beta-blockers in GAD and PTSD. Propranolol is the beta-blocker most studied in the U.S. for anxiety disorder, although currently there is no FDA-approved indication for beta-blockers as anxiolytics. Mechanism of action of beta-blockers in anxiety is believed to be peripherally mediated. For treatment of acute situational anxiety, single doses of propranolol 10-60 mg taken 1-2 hours before the stressful event may be effective. For GAD and PTSD, maintenance doses of 80-160 mg/day may be useful. Unfortunately, the association of adverse effects with propranolol in anxiety disorders appears to be 25% to 40%, significantly higher than that seen when propranolol is used for other disorders. Reactions include dizziness, insomnia, and cardiac arrhythmias. Beta-blockers should be used very cautiously in patients with cardiac disease, baseline bradycardia, diabetes, peptic ulcer disease, or reactive pulmonary conditions such as asthma. Beta-blockers are not effective as hypnotics.

## ZOLPIDEM

Zolpidem is an imidazopyridine with an FDA-approved indication as a hypnotic. Zolpidem is a FDA schedule IV drug (see Controlled Substances *on page 796*) which is not used as an anxiolytic. It does not appear to have anticonvulsant activity. Zolpidem is rapidly absorbed from the GI tract with peak serum plasma occurring within 2 hours. Elimination half-life is 2-5 hours. Adverse effects associated with zolpidem include dizziness, headache, GI disturbance, and daytime drowsiness. Recommended dosing is 10 mg at bedtime for most patients, although 5 mg at bedtime is better suited to elderly patients or those with

## ANXIOLYTICS & SEDATIVE/HYPNOTICS *(Continued)*

concomitant medical illness. As with all hypnotics, transient, rather than long-term use, is recommended.

### ZALEPLON

Zaleplon is a nonbenzodiazepine hypnotic from the pyrazolipyrimidine class. Zaleplon is a hypnotic in the FDA schedule IV drug class, which should not be used as an anxiolytic. Zaleplon does not appear to have anticonvulsant activity. Zaleplon is rapidly absorbed from the GI tract after oral administration ($t_{max}$ = 1 hour). Drug ingestion after a high-fat/heavy meal may delay peak absorption time by as much as 2 hours.

Zaleplon is then cleared rapidly, with mean half-life of approximately one hour. Because of the rapid onset of action of zaleplon, it should be ingested immediately prior to going to bed, or after the patient has gone to bed and has experienced difficulty falling asleep.

Adverse effects associated with the use of zaleplon include somnolence, amnesia, and dizziness. Most adverse effects appear to be dosage-dependent. Recommended dosage of zaleplon is 10 mg for nonelderly patients. Elderly patients and those with comorbid medical illness should be started started at a dose of 5 mg. As with all hypnotics, transient, rather than long-term, use is recommended.

### BARBITURATES

Use of barbiturates as either anxiolytics or sedative/hypnotics has been largely replaced by benzodiazepines which tend to be at least as equally efficacious for sedative/antianxiety effects while presenting less risk for abuse potential and less development of tolerance to antianxiety effects. Additionally, overdose of barbiturates is likely to be associated with more serious sequelae than benzodiazepine overdose. Amobarbital sodium is used rarely for grossly agitated patients (50-150 mg I.M.); however, in most cases I.M. lorazepam (1-2 mg) is generally safer and equally efficacious.

### ANTIHISTAMINES

Sedating antihistamines (eg, diphenhydramine and hydroxyzine) may be used as hypnotics and as mild anxiolytics for patients in whom benzodiazepines are to be avoided (eg, those with history of alcohol abuse). Diphenhydramine 50 mg orally at bedtime frequently may improve sleep of psychiatric patients with insomnia. If diphenhydramine 50 mg is not successful in improving insomnia, an alternative agent should be tried as higher doses are likely to cause anticholinergic adverse effects without improving sleep. Elderly individuals may be particularly prone to problematic anticholinergic adverse effects.

### CHLORAL HYDRATE

Chloral hydrate is a nonbenzodiazepine hypnotic which is hepatically metabolized and which is occasionally used in clinical practice. Chloral hydrate is sedating and has potential for tolerance development. Paradoxical reactions of disorientation and agitation may occur rarely in elderly patients. Usual dosage of chloral hydrate is 500-2000 mg for sleep. Physical dependence may occur, but is uncommon.

### MELATONIN

Melatonin is a naturally occurring hormone produced by the pineal gland. Melatonin production and sales are not FDA regulated currently as it is generally sold as a "dietary supplement." Commercial preparations may be synthetic or prepared from the porcine pineal gland. There have been a limited number of controlled trials suggesting that melatonin may promote or normalize sleep. Dosages ranged from 0.3-100 mg. Given the small amount of literature data and unregulated manufacture of melatonin, the effectiveness, safety, and potential risk of this compound is still unclear.

# STIMULANTS

Currently available stimulant drugs in the U.S. which are used for psychiatric disorders are methylphenidate, D-amphetamine, pemoline, and modafinil. Modafinil is a nonamphetamine stimulant to improve wakefulness in patients with excessive daytime sleepiness associated with narcolepsy. Stimulants appear to have both dopaminergic and noradrenergic activity. D-amphetamine and methylphenidate have abuse potential, and are FDA Class II drugs while pemoline has less abuse potential, and is classified as FDA schedule IV (see Controlled Substances *on page 796*). Physical effects include hypertension, tachycardia, and diminished sleep and appetite.

Pemoline and amphetamine stimulants are FDA approved for attention deficit hyperactivity disorder (ADHD) and narcolepsy. More than 66% of children with ADHD improve on stimulants. Adverse effects may include activation in some children, and potential growth inhibition. A substantial number of children with ADHD have spontaneous resolution of symptoms during adolescence (see Children and Adolescents in Special Populations *on page 663*). However, some individuals continue to exhibit symptoms into adulthood. Stimulants may be of benefit in adult ADHD patients, although abuse potential is a clear risk. The behavioral effects of the stimulants in ADHD are to improve attention and decrease restlessness/hyperactivity.

Although amphetamine stimulants do not have an FDA indication for the treatment of depression, they may clearly be useful for treatment refractory illness. The advantage of stimulant medication in the management of depression is rapid onset of improvement in responders (hours to days). This is particularly useful in medically compromised patients where severe depression interferes with nutrition and/or medical care (eg, patients with HIV). D-amphetamine (5-40 mg/day) or methylphenidate (10-80 mg/day) may be used. While pemoline has the lowest abuse potential among the stimulants, there have been cases of acute liver failure associated with its use. Regular hepatic monitoring (every other week) is recommended by the manufacturer for as long as pemoline is utilized.

# AGENTS FOR TREATMENT OF EXTRAPYRAMIDAL SYMPTOMS

A variety of agents exist for treatment of extrapyramidal symptoms (EPS) associated with the use of antipsychotic agents. See the Antiparkinsonian Agents Comparison Chart *on page 705*. These include anticholinergic agents, dopaminergic agents, levodopa, beta-blockers, clonidine, and benzodiazepines. Ideally, prevention of EPS should be attempted with lowest effective dosing of conventional antipsychotics or use of the newer atypical antipsychotics.

Anticholinergic drugs may be used to treat all forms of acute EPS and are generally considered first-line agents for these drug-induced syndromes. Anticholinergic agents are believed to work by normalizing the dopaminergic-cholinergic balance in the corpus striatum although a clear understanding of exactly how this may occur remains lacking.

Anticholinergic medication should begin with benztropine 1-2 mg/day or an equivalent dosage of an alternative anticholinergic. For severe, painful, or potentially dangerous EPS, such as dysarthria or laryngospasm, anticholinergic medication may be given I.V. or I.M. I.V. anticholinergic (eg, benztropine 2 mg or diphenhydramine 50 mg) relieves EPS within 2-3 minutes, while I.M. administration requires 15-30 minutes for symptom relief. Individuals with a history of acute EPS should be given prophylactic anticholinergic medication. Additionally, clinicians may consider prophylactic anticholinergic medication for individuals with high risk for EPS (eg, young males on higher doses of high-potency conventional antipsychotic).

Geriatric patients generally require lower doses of anticholinergic drug. Adverse effects associated with anticholinergic medication include constipation, urinary retention, tachycardia, and blurred vision. Intraocular pressure may be increased, posing some danger for patients with narrow-angle glaucoma. In addition, some individuals, particularly elderly patients, may develop a delirium-like presentation associated with anticholinergics that is characterized by disorientation, hallucinations, behavioral lability, and cognitive impairment. Occasionally, patients may abuse anticholinergics.

Patients on anticholinergic medication should be reassessed on a regular basis to determine continued need for medication. A significant number of patients on antipsychotic medication exhibit spontaneous reduction or resolution of EPS during continued antipsychotic medication therapy, particularly during the first 3 months of treatment. Therefore, after this time period, one should consider tapering anticholinergic agent.

Dopaminergic agents, such as amantadine and levodopa, have also been reported to be useful in management of EPS. Amantadine has been reported to be beneficial in acute dystonia, akathisia, and drug-induced parkinsonism. As with anticholinergics, amantadine is believed to work by normalizing dopamine-acetylcholine balance in the striatum. Dosing of 100-400 mg/day in a once or twice daily pattern is usually used. Adverse effects with amantadine include orthostasis, peripheral edema, and a skin reaction called livedo reticularis (venous marbleization of the skin, usually lower extremities). Also, worsening of psychosis or delirium have been reported. Generally, amantadine should only be utilized after failure of anticholinergic agents. Levodopa is far less commonly used due to concern regarding worsening of psychotic illness.

Beta-blocking drugs (eg, propranolol, atenolol, pindolol) may be useful in EPS. Beta-blockers appear to be most effective in treating akathisia. Patients on beta-blockers may experience hypotension or bradycardia, thus, blood pressure and pulse should be monitored during initial drug titration.

Clonidine is another agent that may be effective in akathisia. Usual dosage for akathisia is 0.2-0.8 mg/day. As with beta-blockers, hypotension may occur, and blood pressure should be monitored during initial titration. Clonidine should generally be tried after failure of beta-blockers to control akathisia.

Benzodiazepines may also be useful in improving symptoms of dystonia and akathisia, although they are generally less effective than anticholinergic medications. Lorazepam, clonazepam, and diazepam have been most often utilized, generally at dosages of diazepam ≤40 mg/day, or its equivalent.

# ANTIDEPRESSANT MEDICATIONS

## SELECTIVE SEROTONIN REUPTAKE INHIBITORS (SSRIs)

### TYPE OF MEDICATION:

Antidepressant medication, selective serotonin reuptake inhibitor (SSRI)

### MEDICATIONS IN THIS GROUP

Citalopram (Celexa®) *on page 126*

Fluoxetine (Prozac® - depression; Sarafem™ - premenstrual disorder) *on page 232*

Fluvoxamine (Luvox®) *on page 237*

Paroxetine (Paxil®) *on page 421*

Sertraline (Zoloft®) *on page 509*

### THIS MEDICATION IS USED FOR:

Treatment of depression; may also be used for obsessive-compulsive disorder and other anxiety disorders (eg, post-traumatic stress disorder), eating disorders, premenstrual dysphoric disorder, and addiction disorders. Usual duration of treatment is at least 1 year; may be used indefinitely for severe or relapsing depressive or related conditions.

### DIRECTIONS BEFORE TAKING THIS MEDICATION

Tell your healthcare provider (HCP) if any of the following circumstances apply to you:

1. You are pregnant, intending to become pregnant, or are breast-feeding.
2. You have any medication allergies.
3. You are using any prescription medications or over-the-counter medications; remember to include any medications prescribed by your dentist and any herbal or natural products.
4. You have any medical problems.
5. You have had any problems with this medication in the past.

### INSTRUCTIONS ON APPROPRIATE USE OF THIS MEDICATION

- Take this medication exactly as recommended by your HCP. Do not take more or less than recommended dosage. Talk with your HCP concerning what you ought to do about missed doses of medication should this occur.
- Know the name, spelling, and milligram dosage amount of your medication. This may be written down on a card kept in your wallet or purse. This information is extremely important should you become suddenly ill or are involved in an emergency situation.
- Always try to take this medication at the same time of day. SSRIs are usually taken 1-2 times daily.
- SSRI antidepressants are generally best tolerated if taken with or shortly after food. This may minimize any potential digestive system upset.
- Store medication in a clean, dry place at room temperature, away from children.

### PRECAUTIONS

- Improvement in energy level and sleep/appetite may occur during the first week, while depressive symptoms may take up to 4-6 weeks to improve. Do not abruptly stop medication as there may be a drug withdrawal reaction.
- This medication may add to the effects of alcohol or other drugs.
- Do not use alcohol or street drugs while on this medication.
- If this medication makes you sleepy or drowsy, do not operate a machine or motor vehicle as this may be dangerous.
- Tell your HCP immediately if you become pregnant while on this medication.
- Do not take any new or additional prescription or over-the-counter medications without discussing them with your HCP. This includes herbal and natural products.
- Do not take SSRI antidepressant medications if you have taken a monoamine oxidase inhibitor (MAOI) within the past 2 weeks. This may be associated with potentially life-threatening high blood pressure.
- Prozac® and Sarafem™ are the same medication (fluoxetine) sold under different brand names for different disorders. Discuss all your medications with your healthcare provider to ensure that you are only taking one prescription of fluoxetine at a time.

### COMMON SIDE EFFECTS

All drugs are associated with side effects. Most side effects are mild, and often may improve over time. Discuss side effects of this medication with your HCP prior to starting therapy, including how you should contact your HCP if side effects occur. The following side effects are more common and should be discussed with your HCP.

- Drowsiness
- Decreased appetite/weight loss/weight gain
- Decrease in sexual function
- Nausea or digestive system upset
- Dry mouth

More rare side effects include agitation, anxiety, or other physical symptoms such as rash, itching, or muscle twitching. Report these symptoms immediately to your HCP. Other side effects not listed may occur in some individuals. If these occur, report them to your HCP.

# TRICYCLIC ANTIDEPRESSANTS (TCA) AND RELATED MEDICATIONS

## TYPE OF MEDICATION:

Antidepressant medication, cyclic/tricyclic class

## MEDICATIONS IN THIS GROUP

Amitriptyline (Elavil®, Enovil®) *on page 33*

Amoxapine (Asendin®) *on page 37*

Clomipramine (Anafranil®) *on page 131*

Desipramine (Norpramin®) *on page 154*

Doxepin (Adapin®, Sinequan®) *on page 183*

Imipramine (Janamine®, Tofranil®) *on page 282*

Maprotiline (Ludiomil®) *on page 332*

Nortriptyline (Aventyl®, Pamelor®) *on page 400*

Protriptyline (Vivactil®) *on page 477*

Trimipramine (Surmontil®) *on page 570*

## THIS MEDICATION IS USED FOR:

Treatment of depression; may also be used for some anxiety disorders such as obsessive-compulsive disorder, panic disorder, and post-traumatic stress disorder as well as eating disorders, chronic pain conditions, and enuresis (bedwetting) in children. Usual duration of the treatment for depression and anxiety disorders is at least 1 year, although may be used indefinitely for severe or relapsing depressive or related conditions.

## DIRECTIONS BEFORE TAKING THIS MEDICATION

Tell your healthcare provider (HCP) if any of the following circumstances apply to you:

1. You are pregnant, intending to become pregnant, or are breast-feeding.
2. You have any medication allergies.
3. You are using any prescription medications or over-the-counter medications; remember to include any medications prescribed by your dentist and any herbal or natural products.
4. You have any medical problems.
5. You have had any problems with this medication in the past.

## INSTRUCTIONS ON APPROPRIATE USE OF THIS MEDICATION

- Take this medication exactly as recommended by your HCP. Do not take more or less than recommended dosage. Talk with your HCP concerning what you ought to do about missed doses of medication should this occur.
- Know the name, spelling, and milligram dosage amount of your medication. This may be written down on a card kept in your wallet or purse. This information is extremely important should you become suddenly ill or are involved in an emergency situation.
- Always try to take this medication at the same time of day. TCAs are usually taken 1-2 times daily, frequently with a larger proportion of medication at bedtime.
- Store medication in a clean, dry place at room temperature, away from children.

## PRECAUTIONS

- Improvement in energy level and sleep/appetite may occur during the first week, while depressive symptoms may take up to 4-6 weeks to improve. Do not abruptly stop medication as there may be a drug withdrawal reaction.
- TCAs may cause drowsiness or sleepiness. If this medication makes you sleepy or drowsy, do not operate a dangerous machine or motor vehicle as this may be hazardous.
- Dizziness or light-headedness may occur, particularly when getting up quickly from a seated or lying down position. Getting up slowly may help.
- Dry mouth may occur; sucking on sugarless candy or chewing gum may help.
- This medication may add to the effects of alcohol or "street" drugs.
- Do not use alcohol or "street" drugs while on this medication.
- Tell your HCP immediately if you become pregnant while on this medication.
- Do not take any new or additional prescription or over-the-counter medications without discussing them with your HCP. This includes herbal and natural products.

## COMMON SIDE EFFECTS

All drugs are associated with side effects. Most side effects are mild, and often may improve over time. Discuss side effects of this medication with your HCP prior to starting therapy, including how you should contact your HCP if side effects occur. The following side effects are more common with TCAs and should be discussed with your HCP.

- Drowsiness/sleepiness/fatigue
- Dizziness
- Dry mouth
- Constipation
- Increased appetite/weight gain
- Headache
- Blurred vision
- Unpleasant metallic taste in mouth

More rare side effects include irregular heart beat or fainting, confusion, twitching, seizures, problems in urination, skin rash, or yellowing of eyes or skin. Report these symptoms immediately to your HCP. Other side effects not listed may occur in some individuals. If these occur, report them to your HCP.

# BUPROPION

## TYPE OF MEDICATION:

Antidepressant medication, dopamine-reuptake inhibitor

## MEDICATIONS IN THIS GROUP

Bupropion (Wellbutrin® - depression; Zyban® - smoking cessation) *on page 77* is the only medication in this group available in the U.S.

## THIS MEDICATION IS USED FOR:

Treatment of depression and to help in stopping smoking.

## DIRECTIONS BEFORE TAKING THIS MEDICATION

Tell your healthcare provider (HCP) if any of the following circumstances apply to you:

1. You are pregnant, intending to become pregnant, or are breast-feeding.
2. You have any medication allergies.
3. You are using any prescription medications or over-the-counter medications; remember to include any medications prescribed by your dentist and any herbal or natural products.
4. You have any medical problems.
5. You have had any problems with this medication in the past.
6. You have or have had an eating disorder such as bulimia or anorexia.
7. You have a seizure disorder or have ever had a seizure disorder (convulsion).

## INSTRUCTIONS ON APPROPRIATE USE OF THIS MEDICATION

- Take this medication exactly as recommended by your HCP. Do not take more or less than recommended dosage. Talk with your HCP concerning what you ought to do about missed doses of medication should this occur.
- Know the name, spelling, and milligram dosage amount of your medication. This may be written down on a card kept in your wallet or purse. This information is extremely important should you become suddenly ill or are involved in an emergency situation.
- Always try to take this medication at the same time of day. Bupropion is generally prescribed 2-3 times/day. A slow-release (SR) form is also available to be taken 1-2 times/day.
- Store medication in a clean, dry place at room temperature, away from children.

## PRECAUTIONS

- Improvement in energy level and sleep/appetite may occur during the first week, while depressive symptoms may take up to 4-6 weeks to improve. Do not abruptly stop medication as there may be a drug withdrawal reaction.
- This medication may add to the effects of alcohol or other drugs.
- Do not use alcohol or "street" drugs while on this medication.
- If this medication makes you sleepy or drowsy, do not operate heavy machinery or a motor vehicle as this may be hazardous.
- Tell your HCP immediately if you become pregnant while on this medication.
- Do not take any new or additional prescription or over-the-counter medications without discussing them with your HCP. This includes herbal and natural products.
- Dizziness or light-headedness may occur, particularly when getting up quickly from a seated or lying down position. Getting up slowly may help.
- Do not take bupropion if you have taken a monoamine oxidase inhibitor (MAOI) within the past 2 weeks; this may be associated with potentially life-threatening high blood pressure.
- Bupropion is sold under different brand names for different uses. Discuss all your medications with your HCP so that you only take one prescription of bupropion at a time.

## COMMON SIDE EFFECTS

All drugs are associated with side effects. Most side effects are mild, and often may improve over time. Discuss side effects of this medication with your HCP prior to starting therapy, including how you should contact your HCP if side effects occur. The following side effects are more common with bupropion and should be discussed with your HCP.

- Agitation/anxiety
- Nausea, constipation, loss of appetite
- Trembling/shaking
- Dizziness
- Sleepiness
- Transient weight loss

More rare side effects include seizures, confusion, headache, or skin rash. Report these symptoms immediately to your HCP. Other side effects not listed may occur in some individuals. If these occur, report them to your HCP.

# VENLAFAXINE

### TYPE OF MEDICATION:

Antidepressant, selective serotonin-norepinephrine reuptake inhibitor

### MEDICATIONS IN THIS GROUP

Venlafaxine (Effexor®) *on page 582* is the only medication in this group available in the U.S.

### THIS MEDICATION IS USED FOR:

Treatment of depression and anxiety

### DIRECTIONS BEFORE TAKING THIS MEDICATION

Tell your healthcare provider (HCP) if any of the following circumstances apply to you:

1. You are pregnant, intending to become pregnant, or are breast-feeding.
2. You have any medication allergies.
3. You are using any prescription medications or over-the-counter medications; remember to include any medications prescribed by your dentist and any herbal or natural products.
4. You have any medical problem.
5. You have had any problems with this medication in the past.

### INSTRUCTIONS ON APPROPRIATE USE OF THIS MEDICATION

- Take this medication exactly as recommended by your HCP. Do not take more or less than recommended dosage. Talk with your HCP concerning what you ought to do about missed doses of medication should this occur.
- Know the name, spelling, and milligram dosage amount of your medication. This may be written down on a card kept in your wallet or purse. This information is extremely important should you become suddenly ill or are involved in an emergency situation.
- Always try to take this medication at the same time of day. Venlafaxine is generally prescribed 1-3 times/day. A slow-acting formulation is available which is prescribed once daily.
- Store medication in a clean, dry place at room temperature, away from children.

### PRECAUTIONS

- Improvement in energy level and sleep/appetite may occur during the first week, while depressive symptoms may take up to 4-6 weeks to improve. Do not abruptly stop medication as there may be a drug withdrawal reaction.
- This medication may add to the effects of alcohol or other drugs.
- Do not use alcohol or "street" drugs while on this medication.
- If this medication makes you sleepy or drowsy, do not operate heavy machinery or a motor vehicle as this may be hazardous.
- Tell your HCP immediately if you become pregnant while on this medication.
- Do not take any new or additional prescription or over-the-counter medications without discussing them with your HCP. This includes herbal and natural products.
- Dizziness or light-headedness may occur, particularly when getting up quickly from a seated or lying down position. Getting up slowly may help.
- Venlafaxine may be associated with increases in blood pressure, even in individuals who do not have high blood pressure to begin with. Your blood pressure should be monitored during the initial period when you begin to take venlafaxine.

### COMMON SIDE EFFECTS

All drugs are associated with side effects. Most side effects are mild, and often may improve over time. Discuss side effects of this medication with your HCP prior to starting therapy, including how you should contact your HCP if side effects occur. The following side effects are more common with venlafaxine and should be discussed with your HCP.

- Nausea
- Dizziness
- Dry mouth
- Anxiety or difficulty sleeping
- Headache
- Sleepiness
- Constipation
- Abnormal ejaculation or abnormal orgasm
- Blurred vision

More rare side effects include irregular heart beat, confusion, difficulty urinating, skin rash, seizures. Report these symptoms immediately to your HCP. Other side effects not listed may occur in some individuals. If these occur, report them to your HCP.

# SEROTONIN BLOCKER

**TYPE OF MEDICATION:**

Antidepressant medication, serotonin antagonist

**MEDICATIONS IN THIS GROUP**

Nefazodone (Serzone®) *on page 386*

Trazodone (Desyrel®) *on page 561*

**THIS MEDICATION IS USED FOR:**

Treatment of depression; also used in anxiety disorders such as post-traumatic stress disorder. Trazodone is sometimes used as a sleep inducer.

**DIRECTIONS BEFORE TAKING THIS MEDICATION**

Tell your healthcare provider (HCP) if any of the following circumstances apply to you:

1. You are pregnant, intending to become pregnant, or are breast-feeding.
2. You have any medication allergies.
3. You are using any prescription medications or over-the-counter medications; remember to include any medications prescribed by your dentist and any herbal or natural products.
4. You have any medical problems.
5. You have had any problems with this medication in the past.

**INSTRUCTIONS ON APPROPRIATE USE OF THIS MEDICATION**

- Take this medication exactly as recommended by your HCP. Do not take more or less than recommended dosage. Talk with your HCP concerning what you ought to do about missed doses of medication should this occur.
- Know the name, spelling, and milligram dosage amount of your medication. This may be written down on a card kept in your wallet or purse. This information is extremely important should you become suddenly ill or are involved in an emergency situation.
- Always try to take this medication at the same time of day. Serotonin blockers are generally prescribed 2-3 times/day.
- Store medication in a clean, dry place at room temperature, away from children.

**PRECAUTIONS**

- Improvement in energy level and sleep/appetite may occur during the first week, while depressive symptoms may take up to 4-6 weeks to improve. Do not abruptly stop medication as there may be a drug withdrawal reaction.
- This medication may add to the effects of alcohol or other drugs.
- Do not use alcohol or "street" drugs while on this medication.
- If this medication makes you sleepy or drowsy, do not operate heavy machinery or a motor vehicle as this may be hazardous.
- Tell your HCP immediately if you become pregnant while on this medication.
- Do not take any new or additional prescription or over-the-counter medications without discussing them with your HCP. This includes herbal and natural products.
- Dizziness or light-headedness may occur, particularly when getting up quickly from a seated or lying down position. Getting up slowly may help.
- Do not take nefazodone if you have taken a monoamine oxidase inhibitor (MAOI) within the past 2 weeks; this may be associated with potentially life-threatening high blood pressure.
- Nefazodone should not be taken if you are on the following medications:
  - Cisapride (Propulsid®) *on page 124* for gastrointestinal problems
  - Pimozide (Orap®) *on page 445* for psychological problems of tics in children/adolescents

**COMMON SIDE EFFECTS**

All drugs are associated with side effects. Most side effects are mild, and often may improve over time. Discuss side effects of this medication with your HCP prior to starting therapy, including how you should contact your HCP if side effects occur. The following side effects are more common with this group of antidepressants and should be discussed with your HCP:

- Sleepiness
- Dry mouth
- Blurred vision
- Dizziness
- Constipation
- Nausea

More rare side effects include irregular heartbeat (with trazodone), painful, prolonged erection (with trazodone), confusion, or headache. Report these symptoms immediately to your HCP. Other side effects not listed may occur in some individuals. If these occur, report them to your HCP.

**ANTIDEPRESSANT MEDICATIONS** *(Continued)*

# MONOAMINE OXIDASE INHIBITORS (MAOIs)

**TYPE OF MEDICATION:**

Antidepressant medication, monoamine oxidase inhibitor

**MEDICATIONS IN THIS GROUP**

Isocarboxazid (Marplan®) *on page 294*
Phenelzine (Nardil®) *on page 434*
Selegiline (Eldepryl®) *on page 508*
Tranylcypromine (Parnate®) *on page 559*

**THIS MEDICATION IS USED FOR:**

Treatment of depression; also used in the treatment of anxiety disorders (eg, obsessive-compulsive disorders), and sometimes used to treat severe sleep disorders

**DIRECTIONS BEFORE TAKING THIS MEDICATION**

Tell your healthcare provider (HCP) if any of the following circumstances apply to you:

1. You are pregnant, intending to become pregnant, or are breast-feeding.
2. You have any medication allergies.
3. You are using any prescription medications or over-the-counter medications; remember to include any medications prescribed by your dentist and any herbal or natural products.
4. You have any medical problems.
5. You have had any problems with this medication in the past.

**INSTRUCTIONS ON APPROPRIATE USE OF THIS MEDICATION**

- Take this medication exactly as recommended by your HCP. Do not take more or less than recommended dosage. Talk with your HCP concerning what you ought to do about missed doses of medication should this occur.
- Know the name, spelling, and milligram dosage amount of your medication. This may be written down on a card kept in your wallet or purse. This information is extremely important should you become suddenly ill or are involved in an emergency situation.
- Always try to take this medication at the same time of day. MAOIs are generally prescribed twice daily.
- Store medication in a clean, dry place at room temperature, away from children.

**PRECAUTIONS**

- Improvement in energy level and sleep/appetite may occur during the first week, while depressive symptoms may take up to 4-6 weeks to improve. Do not abruptly stop medication as there may be a drug withdrawal reaction.
- If this medication makes you sleepy or drowsy, do not operate heavy machinery or a motor vehicle as this may be hazardous.
- Tell your HCP immediately if you become pregnant while on this medication.
- Do not take any new or additional prescription or over-the-counter medications without discussing them with your HCP. This includes herbal and natural products.
- Dizziness or light-headedness may occur, particularly when getting up quickly from a seated or lying down position. Getting up slowly may help.
- MAOIs can cause very dangerous reactions (life-threatening high blood pressure) with certain foods, drinks, or medications. These include:
  - Foods that are fermented or aged (eg, smoked or pickled meats, sauerkraut or other pickled fruits or vegetables)
  - Aged cheeses, yogurt, sour cream, tofu
  - Meat tenderizers or soy sauce
  - Some types of red wine, beer (including nonalcoholic), champagne
  - Tea, coffee, cola
  - Chocolate
  - Nuts
  - Narcotics (eg, codeine or other painkillers)
  - Cold preparations (eg, antihistamines, cough syrups, nasal spray)
  - Medications to induce sleep
  - Stimulant medications (eg, some diet pills)
  - Yeast or dietary supplements
- If you need to have any surgery or dental procedure, notify your HCP or dentist that you are taking an MAOI or have taken an MAOI within the past 2 weeks.
- After stopping an MAOI, you must adhere to all the above precautions and instructions for at least 2 weeks, as there may be enough MAOI in your body to interact with certain foods, drinks, or medications.

**COMMON SIDE EFFECTS**

All drugs are associated with side effects. Most side effects are mild, and often may improve over time. Discuss side effects of this medication with your HCP prior to starting therapy, including how you should contact your HCP if side effects occur. The following side effects are more common with MAOIs and should be discussed with your HCP.

- Drowsiness
- Mild/moderate headache
- Mild/moderate agitation
- Dry mouth
- Dizziness
- Blurred vision
- Gastrointestinal problems (eg, nausea, constipation)
- Shakiness or trembling

More rare side effects include severe headache, skin rash, fever, or sore throat. Symptoms of potentially life-threatening high blood pressure (hypertensive crisis) include chest pain, increased sweating, enlarged pupils, eye sensitivity to light, severe headache and sore neck. Report any of these symptoms immediately to your HCP. Other side effects not listed may occur in some individuals. If these occur, report them to your HCP.

# MIRTAZAPINE

## TYPE OF MEDICATION:

Antidepressant medication, alpha-adrenoceptor antagonist

## MEDICATIONS IN THIS GROUP

Mirtazapine (Remeron®) *on page 368* is the only medication in this group available in the U.S.

## THIS MEDICATION IS USED FOR:

Treatment of depression

## DIRECTIONS BEFORE TAKING THIS MEDICATION

Tell your healthcare provider (HCP) if any of the following circumstances apply to you:

1. You are pregnant, intending to become pregnant, or are breast-feeding.
2. You have any medication allergies.
3. You are using any prescription medications or over-the-counter medications; remember to include any medications prescribed by your dentist and any herbal or natural products.
4. You have any medical problems.
5. You have had any problems with this medication in the past.
6. You have ever had a disorder of low red blood cell count (anemia) or low white blood cell count (neutropenia).

## INSTRUCTIONS ON APPROPRIATE USE OF THIS MEDICATION

- Take this medication exactly as recommended by your HCP. Do not take more or less than recommended dosage. Talk with your HCP concerning what you ought to do about missed doses of medication should this occur.
- Know the name, spelling, and milligram dosage amount of your medication. This may be written down on a card kept in your wallet or purse. This information is extremely important should you become suddenly ill or are involved in an emergency situation.
- Always try to take this medication at the same time of day. Mirtazapine is generally prescribed once daily.
- Store medication in a clean, dry place at room temperature, away from children.

## PRECAUTIONS

- Improvement in energy level and sleep/appetite may occur during the first week, while depressive symptoms may take up to 4-6 weeks to improve. Do not abruptly stop medication as there may be a drug withdrawal reaction.
- This medication may add to the effects of alcohol or other drugs.
- Do not use alcohol or "street" drugs while on this medication.
- If this medication makes you sleepy or drowsy, do not operate heavy machinery or a motor vehicle as this may be hazardous.
- Tell your HCP immediately if you become pregnant while on this medication.
- Do not take any new or additional prescription or over-the-counter medications without discussing them with your HCP. This includes herbal and natural products.
- Dizziness or light-headedness may occur, particularly when getting up quickly from a seated or lying down position. Getting up slowly may help.
- Do not take mirtazapine if you have taken a monoamine oxidase inhibitor (MAOI) within the past 2 weeks; this may be associated with potentially life-threatening high blood pressure.

## COMMON SIDE EFFECTS

All drugs are associated with side effects. Most side effects are mild, and often may improve over time. Discuss side effects of this medication with your HCP prior to starting therapy, including how you should contact your HCP if side effects occur. The following side effects are more common with mirtazapine and should be discussed with your HCP.

- Dry mouth
- Constipation
- Dizziness
- Tiredness
- Increased appetite/weight gain

More rare side effects include seizures, confusion, headache, or fever. Report these symptoms immediately to your HCP. Other side effects not listed may occur in some individuals. If these occur, report them to your HCP.

# ANTIPSYCHOTIC MEDICATIONS

## GENERAL

### TYPE OF MEDICATION:

Antipsychotic medication, typical group and atypical group

### MEDICATIONS IN THIS GROUP

Typical medications in this group include:

**Typical:**

Acetophenazine *on page 17*
Chlorpromazine (Ormazine®, Thorazine®) *on page 116*
Chlorprothixene (Trilafon®) *on page 118*
Droperidol (Inapsine®) *on page 187*
Fluphenazine (Permitil®, Prolixin®) *on page 234*
Haloperidol (Haldol®) *on page 263*
Loxapine (Loxitane®) *on page 328*
Mesoridazine (Serentil®) *on page 344*
Molindone (Moban®) *on page 372* (typical)
Perphenazine (Trilafon®) *on page 432*
Pimozide (Orap®) *on page 445*
Prochlorperazine (Compazine®) *on page 465*
Promazine (Sparine®) *on page 469*
Thioridazine (Mellaril®) *on page 544*
Thiothixene (Navane®) *on page 545*
Trifluoperazine (Stelazine®) *on page 566*

**Atypical:**

Clozapine (Clozaril®) *on page 136*
Olanzapine (Zyprexa®) *on page 403*
Quetiapine (Seroquel®) *on page 483*
Risperidone (Risperdal®) *on page 496*

### THIS MEDICATION IS USED FOR:

Treatment of psychosis which may be seen in a variety of mental disorders such as schizophrenia, manic-depressive disorder, and dementia. Other uses of antipsychotic medications include tic disorders (Tourette's disorder) or severe aggressive or impulsive conditions.

### DIRECTIONS BEFORE TAKING THIS MEDICATION

Tell your healthcare provider (HCP) if any of the following circumstances apply to you:

1. You are pregnant, intending to become pregnant, or are breast-feeding.
2. You have any medication allergies.
3. You are using any prescription medications or over-the-counter medications; remember to include any medications prescribed by your dentist and any herbal or natural products.
4. You have any medical problems.
5. You have had any problems with this medication in the past.
6. You have ever had neuroleptic malignant syndrome in the past with antipsychotic medications.

### INSTRUCTIONS ON APPROPRIATE USE OF THIS MEDICATION

- Take this medication exactly as recommended by your HCP. Do not take more or less than recommended dosage. Talk with your HCP concerning what you ought to do about missed doses of medication should this occur.
- Know the name, spelling, and milligram dosage amount of your medication. This may be written down on a card kept in your wallet or purse. This information is extremely important should you become suddenly ill or are involved in an emergency situation.
- Always try to take this medication at the same time of day. Antipsychotic medications are usually taken as tablets, 1-2 times/day. Alternatively, your HCP may prescribe antipsychotic medications in other forms which include:
  1. Short-acting injectable medications to treat symptoms quickly
  2. Liquid form for ease of swallowing
  3. Long-acting injectable medications usually given once or twice monthly to minimize missed doses. Currently no atypical antipsychotic medications are available in either short- or long-acting injectable forms.
- Store medication in a clean, dry place at room temperature, away from children.

### PRECAUTIONS

- Full effect of antipsychotic medication may take 6 weeks or longer to occur. Do not abruptly stop medication as there may be a drug withdrawal reaction.
- This medication may add to the effects of alcohol or other drugs.
- Do not use alcohol or "street" drugs while on this medication.
- If this medication makes you sleepy or drowsy, do not operate heavy machinery or a motor vehicle as this may be hazardous.
- Tell your HCP immediately if you become pregnant while on this medication.
- Do not take any new or additional prescription or over-the-counter medications without discussing them with your HCP. This includes natural and herbal products.
- Dizziness or light-headedness may occur, particularly when getting up quickly from a seated or lying down position. Getting up slowly may help.
- Avoid extreme heat (eg, saunas) or activities that may lead to becoming overheated as some antipsychotic medications disturb the body's ability to self-regulate body temperature.
- Avoid direct, prolonged sun exposure and take appropriate sun precautions (eg, sun screen, protective clothing/headgear) as antipsychotic medications may increase risk of severe sunburn/reactivity to the sun.
- Minimize cigarette smoking, as this may alter blood levels of antipsychotic medication in the body.

### COMMON SIDE EFFECTS

All drugs are associated with side effects. Most side effects are mild, and often may improve over time. Discuss side effects of this medication with your HCP prior to starting therapy, including how you should contact your HCP if side effects occur. The following side effects are more common with antipsychotic medications and should be discussed with your HCP.

- Muscle spasm, shaking, muscle stiffness, or restlessness (extrapyramidal symptoms). These are more common with typical antipsychotic medications and may be improved or resolved with the use of agents to treat extrapyramidal symptoms. Risk of extrapyramidal symptoms are greater with typical antipsychotic medications and less with atypical antipsychotic medications.
- Tiredness
- Dizziness
- Dry mouth
- Blurred vision
- Weight gain (generally more common with atypical antipsychotic medications)
- Breast enlargement, menstrual irregularities (generally more common with typical antipsychotic medications)
- Constipation
- Involuntary body movements (tardive dyskinesia), usually of the lips, tongue, and face. May also involve arms, legs, or trunk. These usually only occur after long-term use of antipsychotic medication (months to years). Risk of tardive dyskinesia appears to be greater with typical antipsychotic medications and less with atypical antipsychotic medications.

More rare side effects include seizures, confusion, skin rash, changes in the eyes/decreased vision, fast or irregular heartbeat, liver damage, or yellowing of skin or eyes. If you experience fever, sweating, muscle stiffness, you may have a very serious medical condition called neuroleptic malignant syndrome. Report any of these symptoms to your HCP immediately. Other side effects not listed may occur in some individuals. If these occur, report them to your HCP.

## ANTIPSYCHOTIC MEDICATIONS *(Continued)*

# CLOZAPINE

### TYPE OF MEDICATION:

Antipsychotic medication, atypical group

### MEDICATIONS IN THIS GROUP

Clozapine (Clozaril® and others) *on page 136* is the only medication approved by the FDA for treatment-resistant schizophrenia

### THIS MEDICATION IS USED FOR:

Treatment-resistant schizophrenia; also used sometimes for severe manic-depressive illness, other severe psychotic conditions, and severe aggressive behavior. Due to the need for regular blood tests (every 1-2 weeks) and potential for serious side effects, clozapine therapy is generally reserved for situations where other medications have been ineffective.

### DIRECTIONS BEFORE TAKING THIS MEDICATION

Tell your healthcare provider (HCP) if any of the following circumstances apply to you:

1. You are pregnant, intending to become pregnant, or are breast-feeding.
2. You have any medication allergies.
3. You are using any prescription medications or over-the-counter medications; remember to include any medications prescribed by your dentist and any herbal or natural products.
4. You have any medical problems.
5. You have had any problems with this medication in the past.
6. You have ever had a disorder of low blood cell count (anemia) or low white blood cell count (neutropenia)
7. You have ever had a seizure or a seizure disorder.

### INSTRUCTIONS ON APPROPRIATE USE OF THIS MEDICATION

- Take this medication exactly as recommended by your HCP. Do not take more or less than recommended dosage. Talk with your HCP concerning what you ought to do about missed doses of medication should this occur.
- Know the name, spelling, and milligram dosage amount of your medication. This may be written down on a card kept in your wallet or purse. This information is extremely important should you become suddenly ill or are involved in an emergency situation.
- Always try to take this medication at the same time of day. Clozapine is generally prescribed twice daily.
- Store medication in a clean, dry place at room temperature, away from children.

### PRECAUTIONS

- Full effect of antipsychotic medications may take 6 weeks or longer to occur. Do not abruptly stop medication as there may be a drug withdrawal reaction.
- This medication may add to the effects of alcohol or other drugs.
- Do not use alcohol or "street" drugs while on this medication.
- If this medication makes you sleepy or drowsy, do not operate heavy machinery or a motor vehicle as this may be hazardous.
- Tell your HCP immediately if you become pregnant while on this medication.
- Do not take any new or additional prescription or over-the-counter medications without discussing them with your HCP. This includes natural and herbal products.
- Dizziness or light-headedness may occur, particularly when getting up quickly from a seated or lying down position. Getting up slowly may help.
- In rare cases (less than 1% of patients) clozapine has been associated with a decrease in white blood cells, which are used by the body to fight infection. In order to closely follow white blood cell levels, your HCP will order a blood test once weekly during the first 6 months of clozapine therapy. If there are no blood count abnormalities after 6 months, blood checks are reduced to once every 2 weeks. These will continue indefinitely, as long as you are on clozapine. After stopping clozapine, the blood checks should continue for 4 additional weeks.

### COMMON SIDE EFFECTS

All drugs are associated with side effects. Most side effects are mild, and often may improve over time. Discuss side effects of this medication with your HCP prior to starting therapy, including how you should contact your HCP if side effects occur. The following side effects are common with clozapine and should be discussed with your HCP.

- Tiredness
- Dizziness
- Dry mouth or drooling
- Constipation
- Weight gain
- Blurred vision

More rare side effects include seizures, confusion, fast or irregular heartbeat, skin rash, or liver damage. If you experience fever, sweating, muscle stiffness, you may have a serious medical condition called neuroleptic malignant syndrome. Report any of these symptoms immediately to your HCP. Other side effects not listed may occur in some individuals. If these occur, report them to your HCP.

# MEDICATIONS TO STABILIZE MOOD

## LITHIUM

### TYPE OF MEDICATION:

Mood stabilizer

### MEDICATIONS IN THIS GROUP

Typical medications in this group include:

Lithium (Lithobid®, generic formulations) *on page 321*

### THIS MEDICATION IS USED FOR:

Treatment of manic-depressive (bipolar) disorder; also used sometimes in the treatment of depression, post-traumatic stress disorder, severe aggressive behaviors, and personality disorders.

### DIRECTIONS BEFORE TAKING THIS MEDICATION

Tell your healthcare provider (HCP) if any of the following circumstances apply to you:

1. You are pregnant, intending to become pregnant, or are breast-feeding
2. You have any medication allergies
3. You are using any prescription medications or over-the-counter medications; remember to include any medications prescribed by your dentist and any herbal or natural products.
4. You have any medical problems
5. You have had any problems with this medication in the past

### INSTRUCTIONS ON APPROPRIATE USE OF THIS MEDICATION

- Improvement in mood stability (mood "leveling out") may require 1-3 weeks. Do not abruptly stop medication as there may be a drug withdrawal reaction.
- Know the name, spelling, and milligram dosage amount of your medication. This may be written down on a card kept in your wallet or purse. This information is extremely important should you become suddenly ill or are involved in an emergency situation.
- Always try to take this medication at the same time of day. Lithium is generally prescribed twice daily. Your HCP will check blood level of lithium to determine the most appropriate dosage for you. Lithium blood levels are usually done in the morning. On the morning of your lithium blood level test, wait to take your morning dose of lithium until **after** the blood test.
- Store medication in a clean, dry place at room temperature, away from children.

### PRECAUTIONS

- Improvement in mood stability (mood "leveling out") may require 1-3 weeks. Do not abruptly stop medication as there may be a drug withdrawal reaction.
- This medication may add to the effects of alcohol or other drugs.
- Do not use alcohol or "street" drugs while on this medication.
- If this medication makes you sleepy or drowsy, do not operate heavy machinery or a motor vehicle as this may be hazardous.
- Tell your HCP immediately if you become pregnant while on this medication.
- Do not take any new or additional prescription or over-the-counter medications without discussing them with your HCP. This includes herbal or natural products.
- Dizziness or light-headedness may occur, particularly when getting up quickly from a seated or lying down position. Getting up slowly may help.
- Excessive heat or exercise in hot weather may cause extreme sweating and dehydration. This, in the presence of taking lithium may cause serious problems with blood pressure or heart functioning. Avoid circumstances of extreme heat or physical activity that can lead to dehydration/body fluid imbalance.
- Do not take diuretic medications ("water pills") while on lithium without consulting your HCP.
- Avoid excessive amount of caffeine-containing drinks such as coffee and cola.

### COMMON SIDE EFFECTS

All drugs are associated with side effects. Most side effects are mild, and often may improve over time. Discuss side effects of this medication with your HCP prior to starting therapy, including how you should contact your HCP if side effects occur. The following side effects are more common with lithium and should be discussed with your HCP.

- Increased thirst
- Frequent urination
- Tiredness
- Muscle tremor or shakiness
- Weight gain
- Skin changes (eg, rashes)
- Nausea

More rare side effects include problems in coordination or balance, severe muscle tremor, diarrhea, confusion, slurred speech, rapid heart rate or irregular pulse, blurred vision, severe weakness, severe rash, and neck swelling (goiter). Report these symptoms immediately to your HCP. Your HCP may use a blood test to check for lithium overdose (lithium toxicity) as well as any physical or neurological examinations. Other side effects not listed may occur in some individuals. If these occur, report them to your HCP.

## MEDICATIONS TO STABILIZE MOOD *(Continued)*

# VALPROIC ACID (valproate, divalproex)

### TYPE OF MEDICATION:

Mood stabilizer, anticonvulsant type

### MEDICATIONS IN THIS GROUP

Valproate (Depakote®, and others) *on page 578* is the only mood stabilizer in the anticonvulsant group which is FDA approved as an agent to treat mania in bipolar disorder

### THIS MEDICATION IS USED FOR:

Treatment of bipolar disorder; also FDA approved to treat seizures

### DIRECTIONS BEFORE TAKING THIS MEDICATION

Tell your healthcare provider (HCP) if any of the following circumstances apply to you:

1. You are pregnant, intending to become pregnant, or are breast-feeding
2. You have any medication allergies
3. You are using any prescription medications or over-the-counter medications; remember to include any medications prescribed by your dentist and any herbal or natural products
4. You have any medical problems
5. You have had any problems with this medication in the past

### INSTRUCTIONS ON APPROPRIATE USE OF THIS MEDICATION

- Take this medication exactly as recommended by your HCP. Do not take more or less than recommended dosage. Talk with your HCP concerning what you ought to do about missed doses of medication should this occur.
- Know the name, spelling, and milligram dosage amount of your medication. This may be written down on a card kept in your wallet or purse. This information is extremely important should you become suddenly ill or are involved in an emergency situation.
- Always try to take this medication at the same time of day. Valproate is usually taken 2-3 times/day. Your HCP will determine the appropriate dosage of valproate for you by checking valproate blood levels periodically.
- Store medication in a clean, dry place at room temperature, away from children.

### PRECAUTIONS

- Improvement in mood stability (mood "leveling out") may require 1-3 weeks. Do not abruptly stop medication as there may be a drug withdrawal reaction.
- This medication may add to the effects of alcohol or other drugs.
- Do not use alcohol or "street" drugs while on this medication.
- If this medication makes you sleepy or drowsy, do not operate heavy machinery or a motor vehicle as this may be hazardous.
- Tell your HCP immediately if you become pregnant while on this medication.
- Do not take any new or additional prescription or over-the-counter medications without discussing them with your HCP. This includes herbal or natural products.
- Dizziness or light-headedness may occur, particularly when getting up quickly from a seated or lying down position. Getting up slowly may help.

### COMMON SIDE EFFECTS

All drugs are associated with side effects. Most side effects are mild, and often may improve over time. Discuss side effects of this medication with your HCP prior to starting therapy, including how you should contact your HCP if side effects occur. The following side effects are common with valproate and should be discussed with your HCP.

- Tiredness
- Nausea, abdominal cramping (mild)
- Hand/arm trembling
- Weight change (usually gain)
- Menstrual period changes
- Blurred vision
- Unsteadiness

More rare side effects include severe nausea/abdominal cramping, severe fatigue, easy bruising/bleeding, severe dizziness, soreness of mouth or gums, eye rolling/abnormal movements. Report these symptoms immediately to your HCP. Your HCP may use a blood test to check for valproate overdose (toxicity) as well as any physical or neurological examinations. Other side effects not listed may occur in some individuals. If these occur, report them to your HCP.

# CARBAMAZEPINE

## TYPE OF MEDICATION:

Anticonvulsant, used in psychiatry as a mood stabilizer

## MEDICATIONS IN THIS GROUP

Carbamazepine (Tegretol®, generic formulations) *on page 90* is not approved by the FDA as a mood stabilizer but has been widely used in this capacity by physicians for many years.

## THIS MEDICATION IS USED FOR:

Treatment of manic-depressive (bipolar) disorder, seizure disorder, post-traumatic stress disorder, chronic pain, and severe aggressive behavior.

## DIRECTIONS BEFORE TAKING THIS MEDICATION

Tell your healthcare provider (HCP) if any of the following circumstances apply to you:

1. You are pregnant, intending to become pregnant, or are breast-feeding
2. You have any medication allergies
3. You are using any prescription medications or over-the-counter medications; remember to include any medications prescribed by your dentist and any herbal or natural products
4. You have any medical problems
5. You have had any problems with this medication in the past
6. You have ever had a disorder of low red blood cell count (anemia) or low white blood cell count (neutropenia)

## INSTRUCTIONS ON APPROPRIATE USE OF THIS MEDICATION

- Take this medication exactly as recommended by your HCP. Do not take more or less than recommended dosage. Talk with your HCP concerning what you ought to do about missed doses of medication should this occur.
- Know the name, spelling, and milligram dosage amount of your medication. This may be written down on a card kept in your wallet or purse. This information is extremely important should you become suddenly ill or are involved in an emergency situation.
- Always try to take this medication at the same time of day. Carbamazepine is usually taken 2-3 times/day. Your HCP will determine the appropriate dosage of carbamazepine for you by checking carbamazepine blood levels periodically.
- Store medication in a clean, dry place at room temperature, away from children.

## PRECAUTIONS

- Improvement in mood stability (mood "leveling out") may require 1-3 weeks. Do not abruptly stop medication as there may be a drug withdrawal reaction.
- This medication may add to the effects of alcohol or other drugs.
- Do not use alcohol or "street" drugs while on this medication.
- If this medication makes you sleepy or drowsy, do not operate heavy machinery or a motor vehicle as this may be hazardous.
- Tell your HCP immediately if you become pregnant while on this medication.
- Do not take any new or additional prescription or over-the-counter medications without discussing them with your HCP. This includes herbal or natural products.
- Dizziness or light-headedness may occur, particularly when getting up quickly from a seated or lying down position. Getting up slowly may help.
- In rare cases, carbamazepine may be associated with a decrease in white blood cells, the cells in a person's blood which fight infection. For this reason, your HCP may decide to order a blood test periodically to screen for blood abnormalities.

## COMMON SIDE EFFECTS

All drugs are associated with side effects. Most side effects are mild, and often may improve over time. Discuss side effects of this medication with your HCP prior to starting therapy, including how you should contact your HCP if side effects occur. The following side effects are common with carbamazepine and should be discussed with your HCP.

- Tiredness
- Dizziness
- Blurred vision
- Muscle incoordination
- Dry mouth
- Weight gain
- Nausea

More rare side effects include confusion, severe nausea, severe fatigue, easy bruising or bleeding, gum or mouth soreness, skin rash. Report these symptoms immediately to your HCP. Your HCP may use a blood test to check for carbamazepine overdose (toxicity) as well as any physical or neurological examinations. Other side effects not listed may occur in some individuals. If these occur, report them to your HCP.

# STIMULANTS

## TYPE OF MEDICATION:

Stimulant

## MEDICATIONS IN THIS GROUP

Typical medications in this group include:

Dextroamphetamine (Dexedrine®, Oxydess®, Spancap®) *on page 159*

Methylphenidate (Ritalin®) *on page 357*

Modafinil (Provigil®) *on page 370*

Pemoline (Cylert®) *on page 423*

## THIS MEDICATION IS USED FOR:

Pemoline and amphetamine compounds: Treatment of attention deficit hyperactivity disorder (ADHD), primarily in children, for some types of depressive illness, for some sleep disorders, and in Parkinson's disease

Modafinil (Provigil®): Treatment of daytime sleepiness due to narcolepsy

## DIRECTIONS BEFORE TAKING THIS MEDICATION

Tell your healthcare provider (HCP) if any of the following circumstances apply to you:

1. You are pregnant, intending to become pregnant, or are breast-feeding
2. You have any medication allergies
3. You are using any prescription medications or over-the-counter medications; remember to include any medications prescribed by your dentist and any herbal or natural products
4. You have any medical problems
5. You have had any problems with this medication in the past

## INSTRUCTIONS ON APPROPRIATE USE OF THIS MEDICATION

- Know the name, spelling, and milligram dosage amount of your medication. This may be written down on a card kept in your wallet or purse. This information is extremely important should you become suddenly ill or are involved in an emergency situation.
- Always try to take this medication at the same time of day. Stimulants are generally given 1-2 times daily. Some stimulants are available in short-acting and slow-release (SR) forms.
- Store medication in a clean, dry place at room temperature, away from children.

## PRECAUTIONS

- Improvement in attention span and restless in ADHD may require up to 3 weeks to improve.
- This medication may add to the effects of alcohol or other drugs.
- Do not use alcohol or "street" drugs while on this medication.
- If this medication makes you sleepy or drowsy, do not operate heavy machinery or a motor vehicle as this may be hazardous.
- Tell your HCP immediately if you become pregnant while on this medication.
- Do not take any new or additional prescription or over-the-counter medications without discussing them with your HCP. This includes any herbal or natural products.
- Dizziness or light-headedness may occur, particularly when getting up quickly from a seated or lying down position. Getting up slowly may help.
- All stimulant drugs have potential for addiction. Pemoline is generally less likely to become a drug of abuse compared to methylphenidate and dextroamphetamine. All medications should be used responsibly and exactly as prescribed. Care should be taken that they are not used by anyone except the individual for whom they are prescribed.
- Liver damage has been reported in rare cases with pemoline. Tell your HCP if you have ever had liver disease before beginning to take pemoline.

## COMMON SIDE EFFECTS

All drugs are associated with side effects. Most side effects are mild, and often may improve over time. Discuss side effects of this medication with your HCP prior to starting therapy, including how you should contact your HCP if side effects occur. The following side effects are more common with stimulants and should be discussed with your HCP.

- Decreased sleep
- Decreased appetite and weight
- Anxiousness
- Increased pulse rate and blood pressure
- Headache
- Nausea
- Blurred vision

More rare side effects include muscle twitching, severe headache, extreme increase in pulse rate, severe agitation, elevated mood, or skin rash. Report these symptoms immediately to your HCP. Other side effects not listed may occur in some individuals. If these occur, report them to your HCP.

# ANXIOLYTICS & SEDATIVE HYPNOTICS

## BENZODIAZEPINES

### TYPE OF MEDICATION:

Anxiolytic, sedative/hypnotic

### MEDICATIONS IN THIS GROUP

Typical medications in this group include:

Alprazolam (Xanax®) *on page 26*
Chlordiazepoxide (Libritabs®, Librium®, Mitran®, Reposans®) *on page 109*
Clonazepam (Klonopin®) *on page 132*
Clorazepate (Gen-XENE®, Tranxene®) *on page 134*
Diazepam (Diastat®, Diazemuls®, Emulsified Dizac®, Emulsified Valium®) *on page 161*
Estazolam (ProSom®) *on page 202*
Flurazepam (Dalmane®) *on page 235*
Halazepam (Paxipam®) *on page 261*
Lorazepam (Ativan®) *on page 325*
Midazolam (Versed®) *on page 365*
Oxazepam (Serax®) *on page 410*
Quazepam (Doral®) *on page 482*
Temazepam (Restoril®) *on page 532*
Triazolam (Halcion®) *on page 565*

### THIS MEDICATION IS USED FOR:

Treatment of insomnia, anxiety/agitation, panic disorder, and alcohol withdrawal. Frequently prescribed with other psychiatric medications, such as antidepressants.

### DIRECTIONS BEFORE TAKING THIS MEDICATION

Tell your healthcare provider (HCP) if any of the following circumstances apply to you:

1. You are pregnant, intending to become pregnant, or are breast-feeding.
2. You have any medication allergies.
3. You are using any prescription medications or over-the-counter medications; remember to include any medications prescribed by your dentist and any herbal or natural products.
4. You have any medical problems.
5. You have had any problems with this medication in the past.
6. You have ever been addicted to or abused alcohol or any other drugs, especially benzodiazepines.

### INSTRUCTIONS ON APPROPRIATE USE OF THIS MEDICATION

- Take this medication exactly as recommended by your HCP. Do not take more or less than recommended dosage. Talk with your HCP concerning what you ought to do about missed doses of medication should this occur.
- Know the name, spelling, and milligram dosage amount of your medication. This may be written down on a card kept in your wallet or purse. This information is extremely important should you become suddenly ill or are involved in an emergency situation.
- Benzodiazepines may be prescribed to be taken on a regular basis, either at bedtime or several times daily. In some cases, benzodiazepines are prescribed to be taken on as "as needed" basis.
- Store medication in a clean, dry place at room temperature, away from children.

### PRECAUTIONS

- Benzodiazepines may be habit-forming. Do not exceed prescribed dosage, or take medication for a longer period than is prescribed. Do not abruptly stop medication as there may be a drug withdrawal reaction
- This medication may add to the effects of alcohol or other drugs.
- Do not use alcohol or "street" drugs while on this medication.
- If this medication makes you sleepy or drowsy, do not operate heavy machinery or a motor vehicle as this may be hazardous.
- Tell your HCP immediately if you become pregnant while on this medication.
- Do not take any new or additional prescription or over-the-counter medications without discussing them with your HCP. This includes natural and herbal products.
- Dizziness or light-headedness may occur, particularly when getting up quickly from a seated or lying down position. Getting up slowly may help.
- Coffee or other caffeine-containing beverages may counteract the effects of benzodiazepines. Limiting the amount of caffeine-containing beverages consumed will avoid this problem.

### COMMON SIDE EFFECTS

All drugs are associated with side effects. Most side effects are mild, and often may improve over time. Discuss side effects of this medication with your HCP prior to starting therapy, including how you should contact your HCP if side effects occur. The following side effects are more common with benzodiazepine medications and should be discussed with your HCP.

- Drowsiness
- Muscle weakness or problems with muscle coordination
- Forgetfulness or difficulty concentrating
- Slurred speech
- Dizziness

More rare side effects include severe drowsiness or clumsiness, confusion, agitation or excitement, severe dizziness, skin rash, slowed heart rate. Report these symptoms immediately to your HCP. Other side effects not listed may occur in some individuals. If these occur, report them to your HCP.

# BARBITURATES

### TYPE OF MEDICATION:

Anxiolytic, sedative/hypnotic

### MEDICATIONS IN THIS GROUP

Typical medications in this group include:

Amobarbital (Amytal®) *on page 35*
Amobarbital and Secobarbital (Tuinal®) *on page 36*
Butabarbital Sodium (Butalan®, Buticaps®, Butisol®) *on page 79*
Mephobarbital (Mebaral®) *on page 342*
Pentobarbital (Nembutal®) *on page 428*
Phenobarbital (Barbita®, Luminal®, Solfoton®) *on page 435*
Primidone (Mysoline®) *on page 462*
Secobarbital (Seconal®) *on page 507*
Thiopental (Pentothal®) *on page 543*

### THIS MEDICATION IS USED FOR:

Treatment of insomnia, anxiety/agitation. Generally reserved for situations where other medications have been ineffective.

### DIRECTIONS BEFORE TAKING THIS MEDICATION

Tell your healthcare provider (HCP) if any of the following circumstances apply to you:

1. You are pregnant, intending to become pregnant, or are breast-feeding.
2. You have any medication allergies.
3. You are using any prescription medications or over-the-counter medications; remember to include any medications prescribed by your dentist and any herbal or natural products.
4. You have any medical problems.
5. You have had any problems with this medication in the past.
6. You have ever been addicted to or abused alcohol or any other drugs, especially barbiturates.

### INSTRUCTIONS ON APPROPRIATE USE OF THIS MEDICATION

- Take this medication exactly as recommended by your HCP. Do not take more or less than recommended dosage. Talk with your HCP concerning what you ought to do about missed doses of medication should this occur.
- Know the name, spelling, and milligram dosage amount of your medication. This may be written down on a card kept in your wallet or purse. This information is extremely important should you become suddenly ill or are involved in an emergency situation.
- Barbiturates may be prescribed to be taken on a regular basis, either at bedtime or several times daily. In some cases, barbiturates are prescribed to be taken on as "as needed" basis.
- Store medication in a clean, dry place at room temperature, away from children.

### PRECAUTIONS

- Barbiturates may be habit-forming. Do not exceed prescribed dosage, or take medication for a longer period than is prescribed. Do not abruptly stop medication as there may be a drug withdrawal reaction
- This medication may add to the effects of alcohol or other drugs.
- Do not use alcohol or "street" drugs while on this medication.
- If this medication makes you sleepy or drowsy, do not operate heavy machinery or a motor vehicle as this may be hazardous.
- Tell your HCP immediately if you become pregnant while on this medication.
- Do not take any new or additional prescription or over-the-counter medications without discussing them with your HCP. This includes natural and herbal products.
- Dizziness or light-headedness may occur, particularly when getting up quickly from a seated or lying down position. Getting up slowly may help.
- Coffee or other caffeine-containing beverages may counteract the effects of barbiturates. Limiting the amount of caffeine-containing beverages consumed will avoid this problem.

### COMMON SIDE EFFECTS

All drugs are associated with side effects. Most side effects are mild, and often may improve over time. Discuss side effects of this medication with your HCP prior to starting therapy, including how you should contact your HCP if side effects occur. The following side effects are more common with barbiturate medications and should be discussed with your HCP.

- Drowsiness
- Muscle weakness or problems with muscle coordination
- Forgetfulness or difficulty concentrating
- Slurred speech
- Dizziness

More rare side effects include severe drowsiness or clumsiness, confusion, agitation or excitement, severe dizziness, skin rash, slowed heart rate. Report these symptoms immediately to your HCP. Other side effects not listed may occur in some individuals. If these occur, report them to your HCP.

# BUSPIRONE

### TYPE OF MEDICATION:

Anxiolytic (antianxiety medication)

### MEDICATIONS IN THIS GROUP

Buspirone (Buspar®) *on page 78* is the only medication in this group available in the U.S.

### THIS MEDICATION IS USED FOR:

Treatment of generalized anxiety. Also used sometimes to treat premenstrual syndrome and to treat agitation, especially in older people.

### DIRECTIONS BEFORE TAKING THIS MEDICATION

Tell your healthcare provider (HCP) if any of the following circumstances apply to you:

1. You are pregnant, intending to become pregnant, or are breast-feeding.
2. You have any medication allergies.
3. You are using any prescription medications or over-the-counter medications; remember to include any medications prescribed by your dentist and any herbal or natural products.
4. You have any medical problems.
5. You have had any problems with this medication in the past.

### INSTRUCTIONS ON APPROPRIATE USE OF THIS MEDICATION

- Take this medication exactly as recommended by your HCP. Do not take more or less than recommended dosage. Talk with your HCP concerning what you ought to do about missed doses of medication should this occur.
- Know the name, spelling, and milligram dosage amount of your medication. This may be written down on a card kept in your wallet or purse. This information is extremely important should you become suddenly ill or are involved in an emergency situation.
- Always try to take this medication at the same time of day. Buspirone is generally prescribed twice daily.
- Store medication in a clean, dry place at room temperature, away from children.

### PRECAUTIONS

- This medication may add to the effects of alcohol or other drugs.
- Do not use alcohol or "street" drugs while on this medication.
- If this medication makes you sleepy or drowsy, do not operate heavy machinery or a motor vehicle as this may be hazardous.
- Tell your HCP immediately if you become pregnant while on this medication.
- Do not take any new or additional prescription or over-the-counter medications without discussing them with your HCP. This includes natural and herbal products.
- Dizziness or light-headedness may occur, particularly when getting up quickly from a seated or lying down position. Getting up slowly may help.

### COMMON SIDE EFFECTS

All drugs are associated with side effects. Most side effects are mild, and often may improve over time. Discuss side effects of this medication with your HCP prior to starting therapy, including how you should contact your HCP if side effects occur. The following side effects are more common with buspirone and should be discussed with your HCP.

- Dizziness
- Headache
- Nausea
- Drowsiness

More rare side effects include severe drowsiness or dizziness, confusion, chest pain, fast heart rate, fever, weakness, or skin rash. Report these symptoms immediately to your HCP. Other side effects not listed may occur in some individuals. If these occur, report them to your HCP.

# NONBENZODIAZEPINE HYPNOTICS

**TYPE OF MEDICATION:**

Sedative/hypnotic

**MEDICATIONS IN THIS GROUP**

Zaleplon (Sonata®) *on page 590*

Zolpidem (Ambien®) *on page 594*

**THIS MEDICATION IS USED FOR:**

Treatment of insomnia

**DIRECTIONS BEFORE TAKING THIS MEDICATION**

Tell your healthcare provider (HCP) if any of the following circumstances apply to you:

1. You are pregnant, intending to become pregnant, or are breast-feeding.
2. You have any medication allergies.
3. You are using any prescription medications or over-the-counter medications; remember to include any medications prescribed by your dentist and any herbal or natural products.
4. You have any medical problems.
5. You have had any problems with this medication in the past.

**INSTRUCTIONS ON APPROPRIATE USE OF THIS MEDICATION**

- Take this medication exactly as recommended by your HCP. Do not take more or less than recommended dosage. Talk with your HCP concerning what you ought to do about missed doses of medication should this occur.
- Know the name, spelling, and milligram dosage amount of your medication. This may be written down on a card kept in your wallet or purse. This information is extremely important should you become suddenly ill or are involved in an emergency situation.
- Always try to take this medication at the same time of day. Zolpidem and zaleplon are generally prescribed at bedtime. Zaleplon may be taken after going to bed and experiencing difficulty falling asleep.
- Store medication in a clean, dry place at room temperature, away from children.

**PRECAUTIONS**

- This medication may add to the effects of alcohol or other drugs.
- Do not use alcohol or "street" drugs while on this medication.
- If this medication makes you sleepy or drowsy, do not operate heavy machinery or a motor vehicle as this may be hazardous.
- Tell your HCP immediately if you become pregnant while on this medication.
- Do not take any new or additional prescription or over-the-counter medications without discussing them with your HCP. This includes natural and herbal products.
- Dizziness or light-headedness may occur, particularly when getting up quickly from a seated or lying down position. Getting up slowly may help.

**COMMON SIDE EFFECTS**

All drugs are associated with side effects. Most side effects are mild, and often may improve over time. Discuss side effects of this medication with your HCP prior to starting therapy, including how you should contact your HCP if side effects occur. The following side effects are more common with zaleplon and zolpidem and should be discussed with your HCP.

- Drowsiness
- Dizziness
- Lightheadedness
- Difficulty with coordination

More rare side effects include severe dizziness or drowsiness, confusion, vomiting, shakiness, and memory loss. Report these symptoms immediately to your HCP. Other side effects not listed may occur in some individuals. If these occur, report them to your HCP.

# AGENTS FOR TREATMENT OF EXTRAPYRAMIDAL SYMPTOMS
## (Anti-EPS Medications)

### TYPE OF MEDICATION:

Agent for the treatment of extrapyramidal symptoms

### MEDICATIONS IN THIS GROUP

Typical medications in this group include:

Amantadine (Symadine®, Symmetrel®) *on page 28*
Benztropine (Cogentin®) *on page 63*
Biperiden (Akineton®) *on page 68*
Diphenhydramine (various trade names) *on page 174*
Ethopropazine
Orphenadrine (Norflex®) *on page 407*
Procyclidine (Kemadrin®) *on page 467*
Trihexyphenidyl (Artane®, Trihexy®) *on page 568*

### THIS MEDICATION IS USED FOR:

Treatment of abnormal body movements caused by antipsychotic medications; also used to treat the symptoms of Parkinson's disease.

### DIRECTIONS BEFORE TAKING THIS MEDICATION

Tell your healthcare provider (HCP) if any of the following circumstances apply to you:

1. You are pregnant, intending to become pregnant, or are breast-feeding
2. You have any medication allergies
3. You are using any prescription medications or over-the-counter medications; remember to include any medications prescribed by your dentist and any herbal or natural products
4. You have any medical problems
5. You have had any problems with this medication in the past

### INSTRUCTIONS ON APPROPRIATE USE OF THIS MEDICATION

- Know the name, spelling, and milligram dosage amount of your medication. This may be written down on a card kept in your wallet or purse. This information is extremely important should you become suddenly ill or are involved in an emergency situation.
- Always try to take this medication at the same time of day. Anti-EPS medications are generally prescribed 2-3 times/day. Medications may be given in rapidly acting injectable forms, or as a tablet or liquid. In some cases, your HCP may recommend that you take this medication only "as needed."
- Store medication in a clean, dry place at room temperature, away from children.

### PRECAUTIONS

- Anti-EPS agents may work within a few minutes for injectable forms, and oral tablets may take up to several hours for full effectiveness. Your HCP may prescribe anti-EPS medications to be taken on a regular basis if abnormal body movements related to antipsychotic medication are a continuing problem for you.
- This medication may add to the effects of alcohol or other drugs.
- Do not use alcohol or "street" drugs while on this medication.
- If this medication makes you sleepy or drowsy, do not operate heavy machinery or a motor vehicle as this may be hazardous.
- Tell your HCP immediately if you become pregnant while on this medication.
- Do not take any new or additional prescription or over-the-counter medications without discussing them with your HCP.
- Dizziness or light-headedness may occur, particularly when getting up quickly from a seated or lying down position. Getting up slowly may help.
- Avoid extreme heat (eg, saunas) or activities that may lead to becoming overheated. Some individuals experience decreased ability for their body to tolerate high temperatures while on anti-EPS medications.

### COMMON SIDE EFFECTS

All drugs are associated with side effects. Most side effects are mild, and often may improve over time. Discuss side effects of this medication with your HCP prior to starting therapy, including how you should contact your HCP if side effects occur. The following side effects are more common with EPS medications and should be discussed with your HCP.

- Tiredness
- Dizziness
- Blurred vision
- Dry mouth
- Constipation
- Nausea

More rare side effects include rapid heart rate, confusion, severe dizziness or fatigue, inability to urinate, small pupils of the eyes, or muscle cramping. Report these symptoms immediately to your HCP. Other side effects not listed may occur in some individuals. If these occur, report them to your HCP.

# PSYCHIATRIC EMERGENCIES

## OVERDOSAGE

Drug overdosage may be seen in a variety of clinical settings with almost any drug (see Toxidromes *on page 793*). In both psychiatric and medical settings, suicide attempts or gestures, as well as accidental overdoses, may occur. Medication toxicity in elderly individuals or those who are medically compromised may easily occur as these individuals are more intolerant to medication and risk of adverse effects from medications are greater compared to younger and healthier populations. Manifestation of drug overdose varies widely, dependent upon type and amount of drug ingested, drug pharmacokinetics, and patient clinical status. Initial management of drug overdosage involves medical assessment and stabilization of the patient. In many instances, this is best delivered in full medical support situations, such as an emergency room or intensive care unit. Basic procedures for drug overdose include the following:

1. Assess need for respiratory/cardiac support, intubate if necessary.
2. Establish I.V. access with large bore catheter, draw blood for basic screening, including toxicology testing. Maintain fluid support as needed. Drug-induced seizure management may be initiated intravenously (may use diazepam) if indicated. Arrhythmias managed as needed.
3. Administer opiate antagonist (naloxone 0.4-2 mg) if there is possibility of opioid overdose. Give I.V. thiamine (100 mg) when giving glucose to patients who may be thiamine deficient (eg, alcoholic individuals). Give I.V. glucose (50-100 mL of 50% glucose) if hypoglycemia is a possibility. Naloxone, thiamine, and glucose are given by many clinicians in emergency settings if the patient history is unknown, as the benefits of quickly reversing adverse clinical status generally outweigh any risks of administering these interventions.
4. Induce vomiting or implement gastric lavage. Syrup of ipecac (30 mL) will induce vomiting in conscious patients, although ipecac should not be given to patients who have lost gag reflex, who are so sedated they may aspirate while vomiting, or those who have ingested caustic agents such as acids, alkalies, or other compounds in which vomiting is contraindicated. In gastric lavage, the stomach is emptied via repeated administration and subsequent draining with saline or water delivered via a large-bore nasogastric tube.
5. Optimize speed of elimination of toxin with activated charcoal (50-100 mg in saline solution) orally or via nasogastric tube. Charcoal may be given repeatedly in some overdose states. Many clinicians also administer cathartics (eg, sorbitol 75 mg in a 35% to 70% solution). Hemodialysis may be an option for some drug overdosage (eg, lithium).

The following information lists specific clinical considerations with the major classes of psychotropic medications.

### ANTIPSYCHOTICS

Antipsychotic overdosages are generally less problematic compared to toxic states seen with drugs such as TCA antidepressants and with sedatives. In overdosage with antipsychotic drugs, individuals may experience hypotension, hypothermia, and respiratory failure. Basic supportive procedures, as described above, should be implemented. Extrapyramidal effects may occur, particularly with high potency typical agents (eg, haloperidol). Dystonic reactions can be managed with I.V. anticholinergics (eg, diphenhydramine 50 mg). Anticholinergic effects may be associated with cardiac abnormalities seen on EKG as prolonged Q-T interval. Cardiac monitoring is indicated in individuals with EKG abnormalities due to overdose. Hemodialysis is ineffective.

### ANTIDEPRESSANTS

Depressed patients may use antidepressant medication in suicide attempts. TCA antidepressants are the most common antidepressants to cause serious medical outcome in overdose, generally due to uncontrolled arrhythmias. Serious overdose has become less of an issue in recent years with the preponderant use of SSRI and other novel antidepressant drugs for the management of depression. General management of TCA overdose includes basic assessment/stabilization as described above. Cardiac monitoring should be implemented. Charcoal lavage may help speed drug elimination while appropriate fluid support will offset TCA adrenergic blockade. Physostigmine (1 mg) may be administered for severe anticholinergic symptoms and clinicians should be alert to the possibility of seizure development. In overdose with MAOIs there is risk of arrhythmia and cardiovascular collapse associated with rhabdomyolysis and renal failure. In addition to basic supportive measures, there may be indication for antihypertensives and sedatives, such as benzodiazepine, for CNS stimulation associated with MAOI overdose. Overdose with bupropion may be associated with seizures, and benzodiazepines or anticonvulsants may be utilized along with basic supportive measures. The SSRI and other novel antidepressants are generally less problematic in overdose situations than the older antidepressants. Patients may present with GI distress, sedation, or agitation. Basic supportive measures, including gastric lavage, should be used as needed. SSRI antidepressants may be associated with a toxic state called serotonin syndrome when combined with some other psychotropic medications, particularly MAOIs. Serotonin syndrome is characterized by tremor, autonomic instability, mental clouding, rhabdomyolysis, and possibly coma (see Serotonin Syndrome *on page 805*). Management involves basic supportive measures and discontinuation of causative medications. Cooling measures, such as cooling blankets, may be used for hyperthermia. Dantrolene has been reported to be useful for some individuals with severe muscle rigidity and a NMS-like presentation.

### MOOD STABILIZERS

Lithium toxicity may occur with relatively small overdoses. Overdose situations may occur with deliberate overdose, or with clinical situations that reduce renal clearance (eg, diuretic drugs). Mild lithium intoxication may present as fine tremor, sedation, and GI complaints such as diarrhea or nausea. Individuals with more serious intoxication will exhibit hyper-reflexia, course tremor, changes in consciousness, agitation, ataxia, and myoclonus. EKG abnormalities may also occur. Symptoms of lithium toxicity may occur at "therapeutic" blood levels (0.6-1.5 mEq/L) in some vulnerable patient populations such as the elderly, but generally present at serum lithium levels >2 mEq/L in most individuals. Treatment involves basic assessment/supportive measures described above. Hemodialysis may be beneficial and effective in lithium overdose, and should generally be continued until lithium concentration is <1 mEq/L 8 hours after dialysis.

Carbamazepine overdose may be associated with cardiac abnormalities such as tachycardia and prolonged Q-T interval, along with sedation, ataxia, nystagmus, dysarthria, GI disturbance, seizures, and coma. Cardiac monitoring is particularly important along with basic supportive measures. Activated charcoal may also be of particular benefit.

Valproate is generally far less problematic in overdose compared to either lithium or carbamazepine. Patients may present with GI distress, mental status change, cardiac abnormalities, or liver damage. Basic supportive measures should be followed. Activated charcoal may be particularly helpful.

### SEDATIVES/ANXIOLYTICS

Benzodiazepines, commonly used in clinical settings for management of anxiety, agitation, or insomnia, are less problematic in overdose compared to older sedatives, such as barbiturates. Diazepam doses >1000 mg have been reported to have been taken without significant toxicity, and most cases of overdose with oral benzodiazepines alone are nonfatal in outcome. However, benzodiazepines combined with alcohol or other sedatives may be associated with severe respiratory depression, coma, and death. Symptoms of benzodiazepine toxicity include sedation, slurred speech, ataxia, hypotension, and respiratory depression. Zolpidem overdose appears to present clinically like benzodiazepine overdose. Management includes basic assessment/support. Polydrug ingestion should be considered where clinical presentation is severe or complicated. Flumazenil, a benzodiazepine antagonist, given at a dose of 1-5 mg may be beneficial in cases of pure benzodiazepine overdose, although it has been reported to potentially complicate the clinical situation when multiple drugs have been ingested.

Overdose of opiates may be associated with respiratory depression, pulmonary edema, seizure, cardiac abnormalities, and coma. In early/mild toxicity, the individual may present with urinary retention, itching, muscle spasm, fever, leukocytosis, and hyperamylasemia. Pinpoint pupils are usually, although not always, observed. Naloxone, a narcotic antagonist, reverses opiate overdoses, and should be administered in cases where opiate overdose is suspected, ingestion history is unknown, or in cases of mixed overdosage. Naloxone 0.4-2 mg may be given intravenously, intramuscularly, or subcutaneously depending on patient's clinical status and access available. As naloxone may induce vomiting, comatose patients should be intubated. Although patients may improve rapidly with naloxone, the drug has a short half-life, and may need to be readministered, thus, close clinical monitoring is crucial.

### ANTICHOLINERGICS

Toxicity is characterized by disorientation, slurred speech, ataxia, psychosis, agitation, seizures, and possibly coma. As with most delirium-type presentations, hallucinations tend to be visual, and delusions tend to be fragmented and paranoid in type. Physical symptoms include dilated pupils, hyperpyrexia, tachycardia, dry mouth, constipation, urinary retention, and hypertension. Psychotropic drugs associated with anticholinergic toxicity in overdose include anticholinergics, antipsychotics, and tricyclic antidepressants (see the Antiparkinsonian Agents Comparison Chart *on page 705*). Management of anticholinergic toxicity may include administration of physostigmine 2 mg I.V. given over several minutes, which quickly reverses anticholinergic symptoms. Physostigmine is metabolized rapidly, and readministration of slow I.V. push may need to occur every several hours until the toxicity resolves. Physostigmine should not be given to individuals with cardiac abnormalities or cardiovascular or peripheral vascular disease. In addition to physostigmine, basic supportive measures (eg, cardiac monitoring and fluid maintenance) are used as indicated.

### STIMULANTS

Individuals who overdose on amphetamine-type psychotropic medications may exhibit agitation, irritability, psychosis, and seizures. Physical symptoms include dilated pupils, tachycardia, hypertension, hyperpyrexia, GI disturbance, and arrhythmia. In addition to basic supportive measures, as toxicity resolves, the patient may require management of severe behavioral symptoms. Generally, low doses of antipsychotic medication are safe and effective in treating the psychosis associated with stimulant toxicity. Benzodiazepines may also be used and are preferred by some clinicians. For hyperthermia, cooling measures such as cooling blankets may be helpful.

## VIOLENCE

Violent and agitated behavior creates an emergency situation due to potential risk to patients, bystanders, and healthcare staff. Patients with both nonpsychiatric and psychiatric disorders presenting to emergency rooms may exhibit violent or agitated behavior. It has been reported that up to 80% of teaching hospital emergency rooms experience patient assault of staff members. The initial task in managing a potentially violent individual is to assess for signs of impending violence such as verbal or physical threats, presence of objects that may be used as weapons, signs of substance intoxication, and level of agitation or psychiatric symptoms such as psychosis. Patients who are a potential risk of harm to self or others should be placed in a protective environment. Police or security assistance is often essential, and a calm show of overwhelming force may commonly lead to abandonment of threatening behavior by the patient. The use of physical restraints may be necessary for continued agitated or violent behavior if other less restrictive measures are ineffective, and prompt pharmacotherapy of underlying psychiatric or medical disorders should be initiated. A reassuring, safe, and low stimulation environment is optimum. In some acutely agitated individuals, rapid tranquilization and the use of antipsychotics and benzodiazepines to control severely disruptive behavior is indicated. If violent, agitated patients are unable to take oral medications, many clinicians use a high potency I.M. antipsychotic such as haloperidol 2.5-5 mg I.M. and an injectable benzodiazepine such as lorazepam 0.5-1 mg I.M. to quickly sedate the patient and stabilize disruptive behavior. Patients at risk for acute extrapyramidal symptoms may receive a concomitant anticholinergic such as benztropine 1 mg I.M. The antipsychotic plus benzodiazepine combination may be repeated every 30-60 minutes, if needed, with antipsychotic dosage

## PSYCHIATRIC EMERGENCIES *(Continued)*

generally not exceeding haloperidol 20 mg/day, or the benzodiazepine may be given alternating with the antipsychotic. Rapid tranquilization should not be confused with rapid neuroleptization, a procedure that was used in the past where patients were treated with 'mega' doses of neuroleptic, and were placed at risk of severe neurological side effects. If patients are able to take oral medications, antipsychotic options are increased to include atypical antipsychotics such as risperidone, olanzapine, or quetiapine. Benzodiazepines may also be given orally (eg, diazepam 5-10 mg). For nonpsychotic patients, some clinicians utilize benzodiazepine monotherapy (eg, lorazepam 1-2 mg orally every 1-4 hours).

For the long-term management of individuals with chronic or intermittent aggression, there are a variety of interventions including psychotherapy, treatment of underlying psychiatric illness if present, and pharmacotherapies that target aggressive behaviors. Drugs that may diminish aggressive behavior include mood-stabilizers such as lithium, valproate, and carbamazepine. Antidepressants such as the SSRIs and trazodone may be useful as well as buspirone, and atypical antipsychotics such as clozapine.

## NEUROLEPTIC MALIGNANT SYNDROME

Neuroleptic malignant syndrome (NMS) is a condition characterized by progressive worsening (over 24-72 hours) of muscle rigidity, changes in consciousness, and autonomic instability. Symptoms of autonomic instability include sweating, fever, flushing, tachycardia, and labile blood pressure. Additionally, the white blood count (WBC) and creatine phosphokinase (CPK) may be elevated. Severe CPK elevation may be associated with renal failure. True NMS is a medical emergency. Fortunately, NMS is relatively rare, occurring in <1% of patients on conventional antipsychotics. NMS appears to be extremely rare with atypical antipsychotics. Over 60% of cases of NMS occur during the first 2 weeks of antipsychotic therapy, with strongest risk factors being male gender and previous history of NMS. Mortality ranges from 4% to 22%. Management consists of early diagnosis, immediate discontinuation of antipsychotic drugs, symptomatic treatment, including I.V. hydration and antipyretics. Close monitoring of clinical status/vital signs is essential. Bromocriptine at dosages of 5 mg 3-4 times/day or dantrolene at dosages of 1-3 mg/kg/day may be beneficial in acute NMS.

## CATATONIA

Catatonia is a syndrome associated with a variety of medical disorders such as encephalopathy and ketoacidosis, and a variety of psychiatric disorders such as schizophrenia and serious mood disorders. Catatonia produces cataplexy and waxy flexibility, mutism, intermittent agitation, and resistance to movement and/or instructions. There exists a lethal form of catatonia in which patients experience hyperthermia, rigidity, rhabdomyolysis, and autonomic instability. As its name implies, lethal catatonia has high mortality if untreated.

Patients with suspected catatonia should have a thorough medical evaluation to identify and make appropriate interventions for treatable medical disorders. In cases where no medical etiology can be identified, patients are generally treated in inpatient psychiatric settings. I.V. amobarbital sodium (50 mg/minute for a total dose up to 300 mg) may be used to assist in obtaining history from psychiatric patients with catatonia. However, amobarbital is not effective in treating catatonia as its effects are short-lived and there may be risk of respiratory depression. More recently, it has been demonstrated that parenteral or oral lorazepam is helpful in catatonia and may more safely facilitate the patient's ability to give a history. Lethal catatonia may improve with antipsychotics although most rapid treatment of catatonia generally occurs with ECT.

## ACUTE EXTRAPYRAMIDAL SYNDROMES

### ACUTE DYSTONIAS

Acute dystonias are uncomfortable, involuntary muscle spasms of the face, neck, trunk, or extremities associated with antipsychotic treatment. Dystonias occur in 10% to 15% of patients on conventional antipsychotic medications, usually in the first several weeks of treatment. Acute dystonias are much rarer with atypical antipsychotic medications. Manifestations of acute dystonia include facial grimacing, tongue twisting, dysarthria and/or dysphagia, eye deviation, neck twisting (torticollis), and back spasm (opisthotonos). Acute laryngospasm may be life-threatening. Most prominent risk factors for acute dystonia include male gender, history of acute extrapyramidal symptoms, and adolescence. When dystonia occurs, intramuscular anticholinergic medication (eg, diphenhydramine 50 mg I.M. or benztropine 2 mg I.V.) usually brings rapid symptom reduction. Subsequently, the patient should receive maintenance anticholinergic/antiparkinsonian medication (eg, benztropine 1-2 mg twice daily). Laryngospasm requires immediate I.V. treatment (eg, diphenhydramine 25-50 mg I.V.).

When initiating conventional antipsychotic agents in those patients with strong risk factors for developing acute dystonias, it is reasonable to begin prophylactic anticholinergic treatment. For elderly patients, due to increased risk of anticholinergic toxicity and potential adverse effects on cognitive status, it is usually best to avoid prophylactic anticholinergic medication. Tolerance often develops to dystonic effects over the first month of treatment, and need for maintenance anticholinergic medication should be reassessed at that point.

### AKATHISIA

Akathisia is a subjective feeling of restlessness seen in 20% to 40% of patients on typical antipsychotic medications. Patients may appear agitated, with frequent pacing and inability to keep their legs still. As with all acute extrapyramidal adverse effects, akathisia is significantly less common with atypical antipsychotic agents. Primary management is to lower antipsychotic dosage, or switch antipsychotic agents to either an atypical antipsychotic or to a typical agent with lower dopamine-blocking potency. Medication management of symptoms of akathisia include benzodiazepines such as clonazepam 1 mg twice daily, or alternatively benztropine 1-2 mg/day. Recognition and management of akathisia is important as the condition can be extremely stressful to patients, and there is a danger of misdiagnosis if the agitation of akathisia is mistakenly attributed to worsening of psychotic symptoms.

## DRUG-INDUCED PARKINSONISM

Antipsychotic medication-associated parkinsonism is characterized by rigidity, bradykinesia, masked facies, drooling, and tremor. While not strictly an emergency, the disabling symptoms occur subacutely within the first month of therapy on 10% to 15% of patients on typical antipsychotics. Drug-induced parkinsonism is significantly less common with atypical antipsychotics. Strongest risk factors for parkinsonism are female gender and older age. Treatment is with antiparkinsonian agents such as trihexyphenidyl 2 mg twice daily or benztropine 1-2 mg twice daily. Some tolerance may develop to parkinsonian effects. Alternatively, reduction or resolution of parkinsonian symptoms may be achieved by decreasing antipsychotic medication dosage, switching to a lower potency typical agent, or switching to an atypical agent (see Antiparkinsonian Agents *on page 705*).

# SPECIAL POPULATIONS

## THE ELDERLY

Elderly individuals make up more than 10% of the U.S. population, and the proportion of elderly individuals is expected to increase substantially over the next 30 years, as demographics of the population changes. It is well known that the elderly are commonly prescribed medications in general, and psychotropic medications are frequently used. When prescribing psychotropic medication in elderly individuals, clinicians are faced with a multitude of challenges. Compared to younger individuals, these include:

1. Elderly individuals generally have reduced capacity to metabolize drugs.
2. Elderly individuals are generally more sensitive to medication-associated side effects.
3. Occurrence of medication-associated side effects in the elderly are more likely to lead to complications (eg, falls and hip fracture).
4. Elderly individuals are more likely to be on concomitant medication for medial illness, thus increasing risk of drug-drug interactions.
5. Elderly individuals are more likely to have psychosocial problems (eg, inability to drive to clinic appointments) that potentially complicate treatment.

For most major psychiatric conditions, such as schizophrenia, depression, and bipolar disorder, medication treatments in older adults generally follow similar guidelines as with younger populations with the caveat that drug dosing and speed of titration are likely to be slower and lower, and that side effect profile of the drug is likely to be a greater consideration than with younger individuals. Treatment of behavioral symptoms associated with medical conditions or with dementia are generally focused upon the presenting psychiatric symptoms. If possible, agitation or disruptive behavior should be managed with medications other than neuroleptics (eg, trazodone in low doses, buspirone, or low-dose anticonvulsants).

With the antipsychotic medications, there is evidence to suggest that the atypical antipsychotics may be preferential in older populations as the elderly appear to have greater sensitivity to some forms of extrapyramidal adverse effects associated with antipsychotic medication. With the antidepressant medications, although TCA and related compounds have been proven to be effective in elderly depressed individuals, the elderly are more likely to experience cardiac symptoms, orthostasis, and possible anticholinergic toxicity compared to younger individuals. The cyclic compounds, nortriptyline and desipramine, may be less likely to have cardiovascular side effects among this class of drugs in the elderly. The SSRI antidepressants are widely used in geriatric individuals due to their relative benign side-effect profile. Some clinicians prefer shorter-acting SSRIs (eg, paroxetine, sertraline), with no active metabolite for use in the elderly. Antidepressants from drug classes such as venlafaxine and bupropion are known to be effective in the elderly, again generally at lower dosing (typically 1/3 to 1/2 dose) compared to younger individuals. In elderly depressed patients, ECT may be particularly efficacious.

When using mood stabilizers in elderly populations, similar principles as with other psychotropics apply. Lithium may be particularly problematic in the elderly, as CNS intoxication is more likely, and could potentially be confused with dementia when subacute toxicity occurs. Lithium levels should be closely monitored, and low blood levels (<0.5 mEq/L) may be effective.

Use of stimulant medications has a specific role in the elderly individual with refractory depression, or in situations where severe psychomotor retardation and inability to care for basic physical needs due to depressive illness occur. Low doses of methylphenidate (<20 mg) may be effective in obtaining relatively rapid relief for these individuals. ECT may also be particularly helpful in severely depressed elderly individuals.

Use of sedative/anxiolytic medications in the elderly population is common, and fraught with complications. Although benzodiazepines are generally the safest and most effective medication for management of anxiety or agitation, they may, at times, be associated with motor incoordination, excessive sedation, and cognitive impairments. General guidelines include use of lowest effective dose for short periods of time. Care should be taken to ensure that medication dosing is not inadvertently increased or missed, thereby leading to excessive CNS sedation or alternatively, withdrawal symptoms. Sedatives such as opiates and barbiturates should be avoided in the elderly for most situations.

Anticholinergic medication in the elderly may be associated with anticholinergic toxicity and with a more chronic cognitive impairment. Use of psychotropic drugs with high anticholinergic activity should be avoided, if possible, in older adults. If anticholinergics must be prescribed, dosing should be adjusted to lowest effective dose. See the Antiparkinsonian Agents Comparison Chart *on page 705.*

Acetylcholinesterase inhibitors have recently become studied and introduced as beneficial to cognition for individuals with mild/moderate Alzheimer's disease. These agents work by blocking acetylcholinesterase and enhancing cholinergic functioning. Clinical trials show improved neuropsychological functioning on these agents in patients with Alzheimer's disease compared to placebo.

Tacrine, the first FDA-approved drug in this category, may be associated with hepatotoxicity and elevated liver functions, thus regular monitoring of hepatic function is indicated with tacrine. Due to its more benign safety profile, another compound, donepezil, is generally utilized as a first-line agent for treatment of cognitive symptoms in Alzheimer's disease. Rivastigmine, another compound in this class, has recently received FDA approval. Adverse effects associated with donepezil include GI complaints and insomnia. Additional compounds under investigation in this class of medications include metrifonate, galantamine, long-acting physostigmine, epstatigmine, huperzine, and velnacrine. It is likely that some of these compounds may receive FDA approval in the very near future. At this time, no medications are available which effectively reverse dementing illness.

# CHILDREN AND ADOLESCENTS

The use of psychotropic medications in children is a consideration when severe behavioral symptoms and functional impairment have not responded to nonpharmacologic interventions. The clinician must complete a careful diagnostic evaluation which encompasses psychiatric, medical, neurological, social, and educational aspects of the child's clinical status. Two important considerations which undoubtedly influence clinician prescribing of psychotropic medications in children are that there is a paucity of studies and literature data on use of psychotropics in mentally ill children, and most psychotropics are not FDA approved for use in child populations. Additionally, data on impact of psychotropic medication on the long-term development of children is extremely limited. In spite of these issues, psychotropic medication may be extremely helpful for some children and may substantially improve quality of life for the child and his/her family.

As a general rule, the pharmacokinetics of psychotropics in child/adolescent populations are similar to adults. Initial work-up should include comprehensive assessment of general medical health and medication treatment must take into account the unique clinical profile of the child. Most children metabolize drugs fairly rapidly and thus, half-life of psychotropic medication may be shorter for children than for adults. In children, psychotropic medication dose should be started at a very low dose and slowly increased as tolerated to lowest effective dosage.

## STIMULANTS

The best studied class of psychotropic drugs in children are the stimulants; see the Stimulant Agents Comparison Chart *on page 728*. These are primarily used for attention-deficit hyperactivity disorder (ADHD), a condition found in approximately 5% of school-age children. In up to 15% of children with ADHD, the condition may persist into adolescence and adulthood. Symptoms of ADHD include inattentiveness, high distractibility, impulsivity, and hyperactivity. Schoolwork and interpersonal relationships are often impaired. Stimulants used in ADHD are methylphenidate, D-amphetamine, and pemoline. Approximately 70% of child patients have improvement in ADHD symptoms on stimulants. Most common potential adverse effects include anorexia, insomnia, and irritability. Long-term use may be associated with decreased growth. Methylphenidate and dextroamphetamine are short-acting compounds with rapid onset of action. Methylphenidate is started at 5 mg twice daily and may be increased up to 60 mg/day in divided doses. Dextroamphetamine is started at 2.5 mg twice daily and is increased to a maximum of 40 mg/day in divided doses (twice daily to 4 times/day). Pemoline is a longer-acting compound, with a starting dose of 18.75 mg/day and a maximum daily dose of 112.5 mg/day given once daily. Use of pemoline is often more problematic due to increased risk of hepatic failure and need for regular hepatic function monitoring. Growth should be carefully monitored for children on stimulants. In cases of ADHD persisting into adolescence/adulthood, many clinicians recommend continued stimulant medication therapy.

## ANTIDEPRESSANTS

Antidepressants are used by clinicians for a variety of clinical conditions in children. These include mood disorders, ADHD, enuresis, tic disorders, and anxiety disorders. Much of the data on use of antidepressant agents in children suggests a less robust response to medications in children as compared to adults. However, these findings may be due to methodological problems in research. Side effects are similar to those seen in adults. SSRI antidepressants are preferred by some clinicians for the treatment of depression, OCD, and anxiety as they have less cardiac, anticholinergic, and sedative effects compared to TCA antidepressants. SSRI doses in OCD may be higher than those needed for depression. TCA and antidepressants may be effective for enuresis and tic disorder, however, EKG baseline assessment and regular follow-up monitoring are recommended. There is limited data available on use of novel antidepressants such as venlafaxine and bupropion in children. Blood pressure and cardiac status must be monitored with venlafaxine. Bupropion has been reported to worsen tic disorder in some vulnerable patients, and is associated with a somewhat greater risk of seizures. MAOIs are generally problematic for children due to dietary restrictions.

## MOOD STABILIZERS

Mood stabilizers may be prescribed for children with severe behavioral symptoms associated with bipolar disorder, refractory unipolar mood disorder, or severely aggressive/violent behavior. Lithium is the best studied mood stabilizer in child/adolescent populations. Children have generally increased renal clearance of lithium, and may require larger doses than adults. The usual starting dose of lithium is 10-30 mg/kg in divided doses. There are no clearly established serum level guidelines, although many clinicians utilize similar target guidelines (0.6-0.8 mEq/L) as is indicated in adults. Adverse effects are generally similar to those seen in adults. Long-term effects of lithium therapy in children are unknown.

There is far less data available on the use of carbamazepine and valproate in children. Carbamazepine has been reported to be effective in conduct disorder. Dosage range of carbamazepine in children is 10-50 mg/kg/day in divided doses and the range for valproate is 15-60 mg/kg/day in divided doses. Although children may metabolize anticonvulsants more rapidly than adults, liver functions should be monitored as hepatotoxicity may occur in very young children (particularly with valproate).

## ANXIOLYTICS

Anxiolytics, primarily benzodiazepines and buspirone, have been reported to be useful in some children and adolescents with mental illness/severe behavioral symptoms. High-potency benzodiazepines such as clonazepam (0.01-0.04 mg/kg) have been reported to be beneficial in severe childhood anxiety disorders and in Tourette's disorder. Adverse effects are similar to those seen in adults, primarily sedation and possible disinhibition. Buspirone may have a particular role in the management of disruptive or aggressive behavior in children with developmental disorders.

## SPECIAL POPULATIONS *(Continued)*

### ANTIPSYCHOTICS

Antipsychotics have been reported to be beneficial in children with psychosis and those with autism. Clinicians may also prescribe antipsychotic medication, particularly haloperidol or pimozide to children with Tourette's disorder who do not respond to other treatments. As with adult patients, child patients taking antipsychotic drugs are potentially likely to develop extrapyramidal adverse effects, including tardive dyskinesia. Anticholinergic drugs will reduce acute extrapyramidal symptoms although use of atypical antipsychotic agents may be particularly efficacious in psychotic children and are likely to be associated with fewer extrapyramidal symptoms compared to typical antipsychotics. Psychotic children, like psychotic adults, are more likely to experience improvement in positive symptoms (hallucinations, delusions, etc) compared to negative symptoms (apathy, poor social functioning, etc). The novel antipsychotic drug clozapine has been reported to be effective in treatment-resistant schizophrenia in adolescents.

### OTHER DRUGS

Clonidine, an alpha$_2$-agonist has been reported to be beneficial in children with Tourette's disorder, in ADHD, and in managing severe aggression. Sedation is a common side effect associated with clonidine use. For this reason, clonidine may also be used to manage the insomnia associated with stimulant medication use.

Beta-blockers, particularly propranolol, may be beneficial in childhood aggression, Tourette's disorder, or self-harm behaviors. Dose range is approximately 1-5 mg/kg/day. Sedation and/or hypotension may occur, and beta-blockers should not be prescribed to children with asthma as bronchospasm may occur in some individuals.

The synthetic compound antidiuretic hormone, desmopressin, is prescribed by some clinicians for enuresis. Desmopressin is administered by intranasal spray and suppresses urine production for approximately 8 hours. Headaches and GI disturbance may be seen as adverse effects in some patients, although it is well tolerated by most children.

# MENTALLY RETARDED PATIENTS

Mental retardation (MR) is a disorder characterized by below-average intellectual functioning and impaired adaptive skills with onset before age 18. MR may occur with coexisting medical or psychiatric disorder. Scoring on intelligence quotient (IQ) assessment is approximately 70 or below and degree of level of MR is categorized in DSM-IV as mild, moderate, severe, or profound. Additionally, the category borderline intellectual functioning, outside the MR range, refers to an IQ in the 71-84 range. MR is associated with a wide variety of disorders (eg, Down syndrome and Fragile X syndrome) and multiple psychosocial factors. The prevalence of MR is approximately 1% in the general population, with men more commonly affected than women. Individuals with milder forms of MR may not be recognized and diagnosed until the individual begins school. Individuals with MR may experience behavioral symptoms that impair daily functioning and interpersonal relationships, such as emotional lability, hyperactivity, or aggression/disruptive behavior. Rates of other psychiatric disorders are increased in individuals with MR. Generally, treatment interventions for behavioral symptoms in individuals with MR should be focused on target symptoms (eg, self-injurious behaviors) when there is no clearly identified comorbid psychiatric diagnosis, or should be disorder focused when a specific comorbid psychiatric diagnosis is identified (eg, bipolar disorder). Optimum management includes education for the patient and family, adaptive skills training, and psychotherapy which may include behavioral, cognitive, or group therapies. Pharmacologic treatments may be indicated when severe behavioral symptoms do not respond to psychosocial interventions. In general, individuals with MR who have comorbid psychiatric conditions should receive the same pharmacologic treatments for the psychiatric disorder as would be indicated in non-MR individuals. Behavioral syndromes that may often require pharmacologic intervention in individuals with MR include aggressive behavior (eg, explosive rage), and repetitive stereotypical behaviors (eg, hand flapping). Drugs used by many clinicians to treat aggressive behavioral include lithium, anticonvulsants (eg, carbamazepine or valproate), buspirone, and beta-blockers (eg, nadolol or propranolol). Lithium has been the best-studied drug treatment for aggression and is often prescribed by clinicians treating MR populations. Additionally, bipolar disorder may often present atypically in individuals with MR and, thus, lithium or anticonvulsants are the treatment of choice in these instances. Anticonvulsants may be an ideal choice for individuals with aggressive behaviors, mental retardation, and coexisting seizure disorder. Buspirone at dosages up to 60 mg/day may benefit individuals with mild to moderately aggressive behavior. Beta-blockers may be useful, but clinicians must assess for development of hypotension or bradycardia, particularly during initial drug titration. The antipsychotic drugs (eg, haloperidol), generally decrease repetitive stereotypical behaviors, but individuals with MR appear to be at greater risk of developing tardive dyskinesia, and these drugs should be used very cautiously. The newer atypical antipsychotic medications may be particularly beneficial in individuals with MR and psychosis.

## SPECIAL POPULATIONS *(Continued)*

# MEDICALLY ILL PATIENTS

Individuals with medical illness may require pharmacologic management of a wide variety of behavioral symptoms including depression, psychosis, or agitation/aggression. It has been reported that up to 65% of medical inpatients have psychiatric disorders, most commonly anxiety, depression, and disorientation. Some psychiatric syndromes are caused by medical disorders (see Secondary Mental Disorders *on page 616*) while other psychiatric syndromes may be associated with medications used to treat medical conditions (eg, steroids for autoimmune conditions) or neurological conditions (eg, antiparkinsonian drugs). Individuals with primary psychiatric illness such as schizophrenia often have worsening of psychiatric symptoms when stressed by medical illness. Individuals with medical illness are often older, and may have greater risk of adverse effects from both psychotropic and nonpsychotropic medications. Additionally, some medical illnesses and the intended medications required to treat the medical illness may impose substantially modified prescribing regimens for psychotropic medications.

General guidelines in prescribing psychotropic medications in the medically ill include the following:

1. Evaluate possible role of existing medical conditions in causing behavioral symptoms (eg, hypothyroidism causing or contributing to depressive symptoms).
2. Prescribe psychotropic drugs with least potential for drug-drug interactions and adverse effects based on patient drug regimen and unique patient clinical status. An example of this may be avoidance of TCA antidepressants in individuals with cardiac conduction delays and/or those taking cardiac antiarrhythmic drugs. The role of the consulting psychiatrist or pharmacist may be particularly beneficial in medical settings where collaborative information on drug-drug interactions and likely adverse effects of psychotropic medications on specific patients will promote optimum pharmacologic management.
3. Initiate low dosage of psychotropic medication, titrate slowly, and establish lowest effective dosage.
4. Reassess dosage requirements periodically. This is particularly important for medications with possible adverse effects associated with long-term use such as antipsychotics. Although some psychotropics are often continued long-term in medically ill individuals (eg, antidepressants in some patients), in other situations, psychotropic usage may be temporary (eg, benzodiazepines in most patients) and should be discontinued as clinically indicated.

Specific issues concerning use of the major psychotropic drug categories with medically ill patients include the following:

1. **ANTIDEPRESSANTS**

   a. ***SSRI Antidepressants***

   Most common adverse effects of SSRIs include nausea, nervousness, weight change, insomnia, sedation, excessive sweating, headaches, and sexual dysfunction. These may be worsened in the presence of medical illness. Hematologic side effects of SSRIs (rare) may include easy bruisability/platelet dysfunction. Fluvoxamine and sertraline may interact with warfarin in some patients due to cytochrome interactions.

   b. ***Tricyclic and Related Compounds (TCAs)***

   TCAs often have anticholinergic side effects including dry mouth, constipation, urinary retention, and blurred vision, as well as sedative and hypotensive effects. The tricyclic and tetracycline drugs have class 1A antiarrhythmic activity on the cardiac system, and may potentially exacerbate heart block or ventricular arrhythmias. Cytochrome interactions may lead to increased carbamazepine levels. When used with oral hypoglycemics, TCAs may lead to hypoglycemia. Because of the multitude of side effects, most clinicians prefer to use SSRIs as opposed to TCAs in the medically ill.

   c. ***Bupropion***

   Bupropion is generally well tolerated in the medically ill, although cytochrome interactions may have clinical effects, such as decreased bupropion levels when used with carbamazepine. Due to possible risk of seizures, bupropion should not be used in individuals with seizure disorders or eating disorders.

   d. ***Nefazodone***

   Nefazodone is also generally well tolerated in the medically ill. Care must be taken when used with some benzodiazepines (alprazolam, triazolam, clonazepam) as benzodiazepine levels may be elevated. There may be cardiac abnormalities when used with pimozide or cisapride (withdrawn from the market July, 2000).

   e. ***Mirtazapine***

   Mirtazapine appears generally well tolerated in the medically ill. Primary adverse effects include sedation and weight gain. There have been isolated reports of agranulocytosis associated with mirtazapine, and patients with underlying infection/neutropenia may be difficult to monitor in this respect.

   f. ***Venlafaxine***

   Venlafaxine is generally well tolerated in the medically ill. Primary concern is blood pressure monitoring, as venlafaxine may cause a dose-related sustained increase in diastolic blood pressure.

   g. ***Monoamine Oxidase Inhibitors (MAOIs)***

   MAOIs may be associated with hypertensive crisis or serotonin syndrome. MAOIs should not be used with TCAs or SSRIs. MAOIs in combination with Demerol® or fentanyl may be associated with life-threatening serotonin syndrome.

   h. ***Stimulants***

   Amphetamines and related compounds are sometimes used to treat depression in the medically ill. Primary adverse effects, which may be more problematic in the medically ill, include elevated blood pressure and tachycardia. Pemoline is generally not used in the medically ill due to potential liver dysfunction associated with this compound.

2. **ANXIOLYTICS, SEDATIVE/HYPNOTICS**

a. ***Benzodiazepines***

Benzodiazepines are widely used and generally safe, when used appropriately, in the medically ill. Most common adverse effects are sedation and motor incoordination. Respiratory depression may occur with higher doses, and is a concern in individuals with pulmonary disease, CNS depression, or myasthenia gravis. Benzodiazepines which are short-acting and lack active metabolites, such as lorazepam, oxazepam, and temazepam, are preferred by many clinicians who treat medically ill patients.

b. ***Nonbenzodiazepines***

Buspirone is generally well tolerated in the medically ill, although dizziness and drowsiness are possible adverse effects. The newer hypnotics, zaleplon and zolpidem, are also generally well tolerated, although possible adverse effects include sedation, dizziness, and disorientation.

3. **MOOD STABILIZERS**

a. ***Lithium***

Adverse effects associated with lithium include effects on cardiac rhythm (T wave flattening, first degree A-V block, sinus node dysfunction), hypothyroidism, tremor, polyuria, polydipsia, excessive thirst, and diarrhea/nausea. Because of its narrow therapeutic index, risk of toxicity is fairly high. Because of these adverse effects, lithium is generally not a mood stabilizer of choice in the medically ill, particularly in those with renal disease.

b. ***Valproate***

Valproate appears to have no major cardiovascular adverse effects. Most common adverse effects include sedation, nausea, and vomiting. Patients with liver dysfunction should be monitored closely. There have been isolated cases of valproate-associated pancreatitis, and individuals with underlying GI illness should be treated cautiously. Valproate has been reported to increase the unbound fraction of warfarin up to 32% in patients on anticoagulants.

c. ***Gabapentin***

Gabapentin is generally very well tolerated in the medically ill. It is excreted by the kidneys, and thus should be dose-adjusted in individuals with renal impairment.

4. **ANTIPSYCHOTICS**

a. Among the typical antipsychotics, high potency agents such as haloperidol are generally preferred for the medically ill as they have a lower incidence of anticholinergic and autonomic adverse effects. Many clinicians utilize haloperidol in delirious medically ill patients as a first-line agent. Extrapyramidal symptoms may be a concern however, particularly in the elderly, and dosages should be kept low. Typical antipsychotics have quinidine-like properties on heart conduction. Thioridazine may be associated with prolonged $QT_c$ and should be used cautiously, particularly with calcium channel blockers.

Atypical antipsychotics have less propensity for extrapyramidal symptoms, but may be associated with sedation, orthostasis, and weight gain. Clozapine may cause tachycardia in some patients, and due to its 1% risk of agranulocytosis, is generally not used in individuals with significant neutropenia.

## SPECIAL POPULATIONS *(Continued)*

# PREGNANT AND BREAST-FEEDING PATIENTS

The treatment of psychiatric illness in women who are pregnant or lactating poses a variety of clinical challenges. The effects of psychotropic medication on pregnant women has not been well studied for the most part, and currently the FDA has not approved any psychotropic drug for use during pregnancy. In spite of this, clinicians and patients may need to address the issue as some psychiatric disorders tend to be more prevalent in women of childbearing years (eg, mood disorders), or psychiatric illness may be more likely to flare-up during pregnancy (eg, obsessive-compulsive disorder), or appear in the postpartum period (postpartum depression). When possible, as long as clinical outcome is not compromised, all medications, including psychotropic drugs, should be avoided during pregnancy and lactation. Nonpharmacologic treatments, such as psychotherapy, should be utilized as appropriate, to avoid or reduce use of psychotropic medications. Close coordination between the patient, the psychiatrist, and the obstetrician will improve monitoring and optimize clinical outcome. In some women, the risks of avoiding or discontinuing psychotropic medication outweigh the risks of medication treatment. These include situations where patient self-care, or ability to follow prenatal care instructions are impaired due to psychiatric illness. Suicidal or impulsive behaviors may severely compromise mother or child outcomes and should be given serious attention. A general goal of treatment is to limit risk of psychiatric symptom worsening or relapse while minimizing fetal risk.

Assessment of risk during pregnancy ideally begins before conception, when the patient is seen for initial evaluation or routine outpatient treatment. Family planning should be addressed and risks of psychotropic medication on pregnancy outcome may be discussed. Women with milder illness who plan on becoming pregnant may elect to discontinue psychotropic medication. Patients with severe mood or anxiety disorders, or with schizophrenia may need to continue medication, as a number of reports have suggested that relapse rates are increased in these patients when medication is discontinued. Issues such as comorbid substance abuse, cigarette smoking, nutrition, and use of other on psychotropic medications should also be addressed.

Major fetal organ formation occurs during the first 12 weeks of gestation. Teratogenesis refers to the organ malformation or behavioral abnormality resulting from medication exposure during this period. The baseline incidence of congenital malformations in the U.S. is approximately 2%. Medications are considered teratogenic if they are associated with a significant increase in malformations/abnormalities over the baseline rates. Perinatal syndromes are physical or behavioral symptoms noted shortly after birth. These appear to be related to medication use during or soon after time of birth, and are generally limited in duration. Exposure to a teratogen before 2 weeks gestation (corresponding to the time prior to the first missed menses) does not usually lead to teratogenesis as the fetal placenta (the link between maternal and fetal circulation) is not yet formed during this period. Miscarriage at this time may not be recognized as a pregnancy, but may be reported as a heavier than usual period.

Women may have unplanned pregnancies while on psychotropic medications. Almost 50% of pregnancies are unplanned and up to 35% of pregnant women in industrialized countries take psychotropic medications. Rather than abruptly discontinuing all psychotropic medication, the clinician should evaluate the indications and potential adverse effect of each drug and determine risk of untreated psychiatric disorder compared to risks of drug continuation (possibly at reduced dosage).

Some subgroups of women are at increased risk for postpartum psychiatric illness. Women with previous major depressive episodes have a 30% risk of depressive relapse, while women who have bipolar disorders have a 50% risk of depressive relapse. Women with history of postpartum psychosis have a 70% risk of illness relapse after delivery. Some clinicians advocate mood stabilizers or antidepressant medication prophylaxis in women at high risk of postpartum mood disorders. In these cases, medication may be initiated either prior to delivery or in the early postpartum period.

The decision to use psychotropic medications during lactation is complex, as factors which determine infant exposure and response to maternal psychotropic medication are understudied and not completely known. Medications taken during pregnancy, use of other nonpsychotropic medications, and cigarette smoking all significantly complicate assessment of effect of psychotropic medication on infants during breast-feeding. As with pregnancy, the decision to utilize psychotropic medications during lactation must be a collaborative process between patients and their clinicians.

Finally, some clinicians advocate the use of ECT (see Mood Disorders *on page 600* ) in pregnant or lactating patients with severe psychiatric illness. ECT may be particularly helpful in emergency situations such as mania or postpartum psychosis.

General guidelines for use of psychotropic drugs during pregnancy/lactation include the following:

1. Use medications for which some data exist, and which suggest **relative** safety.
2. If possible, utilize medication which has proven good response for that particular patient.
3. Utilize monotherapy first; additional medications should be introduced cautiously.
4. Utilize lowest effective dosage.
5. Encourage good prenatal/postnatal care including avoidance of alcohol, tobacco, or other substances of abuse as well as minimizing (as appropriate) nonpsychotropic and over-the-counter medications.
6. Utilize adjunctive nonpharmacologic treatments (such as psychotherapy) as needed and available.
7. When assessing risk, consider all involved (mother, baby, others) who may be affected by treatment decisions.

The following text reviews effects of selected classes of psychotropic medications during pregnancy and lactation.

## ANTIDEPRESSANTS

The majority of data available on use of antidepressants in pregnancy/lactation involve the tricyclic antidepressants (TCAs). A combined 500,000 births have been examined, with the data available on over 400 cases of first trimester TCA treatment. Currently, the studies do not consistently suggest an increased risk of congenital malformations associated with first trimester TCA exposure. There have been case reports of perinatal syndromes after TCA exposure including withdrawal symptoms in neonates (seizures, irritability) and anticholinergic related symptoms (urinary retention, bowel obstruction). Behavioral abnormalities have been reported during the first 30 days of life, although long-term sequelae have not been reported.

There have been case reports of apparent TCA accumulations with subsequent toxicity symptoms in neonates, while other reports suggest good tolerability and no adverse effects in neonates whose mothers took TCAs.

The serotonin selective inhibitors (SSRIs) are the most widely utilized antidepressant types, however, less data is available on these drugs during pregnancy/lactation compared to the TCAs. Among the SSRIs, the largest body of data is available on fluoxetine, the first available SSRI in the U.S. Seventeen hundred fluoxetine-exposed children have been evaluated. Overall, no increased risk of major congenital malformations, compared to that seen in the general population, has been reported. Although, one study reported an apparent increased risk of prematurity and early postnatal complications, this report was limited by methodological difficulties. Data on use of paroxetine in first trimester pregnancy showed no congenital malformation in 63 infants although interpretation is limited based on small sample size.

Minimal data is available on the effects of SSRIs on lactation. Most case reports documented no adverse effects on nursing infants, although there are reports of symptoms of toxicity (irritability, decreased sleep, vomiting), apparently associated with fluoxetine accumulation in neonates.

There are very few reports on effects of fetal or neonatal exposure to other antidepressant types/classes. The monoamine oxidase inhibitors (MAOIs) appear to be associated with a higher risk of congenital malformations in infants exposed to these drugs *in utero*. MAOIs would also generally not be a desirable choice for lactating women due to the potential for hypertensive crisis and the need for dietary constraints. It is anticipated that more data on use in pregnancy will become available in the future on other newer antidepressants such as nefazodone and venlafaxine.

Based on the available data, many clinicians first choose an SSRI or tricyclic antidepressant (particularly those least likely to cause orthostatic hypotension), when the decision is made to medicate a depressed pregnant patient. If clinically possible, medication dose should be reduced before delivery to minimize risk of neonatal withdrawal. Breast-fed infants should be closely observed for signs of toxicity.

## ANTIPSYCHOTICS

The data on the risks of fetal exposure to neuroleptics is based on reviews of large numbers of patients in U.S. and European populations. High potency conventional antipsychotic agents (eg, haloperidol) do not appear to be associated with increased risk of congenital malformations. However, available reports suggest increased risk of congenital abnormalities in neonates exposed to low potency conventional neuroleptics (eg, chlorpromazine). Case reports exist on perinatal syndromes associated with neuroleptic therapy, although these symptoms (restlessness, tremor, hypertonicity) are generally transient.

Data on antipsychotic medication use during lactation is limited to case reports which suggest that the pharmacokinetics of psychotropic medication excretion are complex and influenced by a variety of factors such as infant maturity and metabolic capacity. There have been reports that low potency phenothiazines may be associated with lethargy and drowsiness in some breast-fed babies and these infants should be closely monitored.

A report on an infant exposed to clozapine during lactation suggested that clozapine may accumulate in breast milk, possibly due to high lipid solubility.

The limited reports on high potency antipsychotics used during lactation also suggest that haloperidol may accumulate in breast milk, but this may not necessarily lead to clinically significant exposure. As with psychotropic use during pregnancy, the decision to utilize psychotropic drugs during lactation should be a careful and collaborative decision between patients and their clinicians.

## MOOD STABILIZERS

Lithium has been associated with cardiac malformations, specifically, Ebstein's anomaly when used during the first trimester of pregnancy. Since the 1970s, when this association was initially reported, the actual risk estimate has been reduced. Currently, it is believed that risk of Ebstein's anomaly in first trimester lithium exposed infants is 10-20 times greater than the general population. Other adverse effects which may be associated with lithium during later pregnancy include cyanosis and hypertonicity, termed "floppy baby syndrome." Conversely, there are reports of lithium being utilized safely in later pregnancy. The use of lithium has been generally discouraged during lactation.

Studies on use of anticonvulsants in pregnancy have been primarily based on women with epilepsy, where occurrence of birth malformations may be increased compared to the general population. Although data is limited and may be complicated by the effects of epilepsy, anticonvulsants appear to be associated with increased birth defects when used in pregnancy. Valproate has been associated with neural tube defects, with risk estimates of 1% to 3%. Carbamazepine has been associated with a neural tube defect rate of 1%.

In contrast to the pregnancy data, both valproate and carbamazepine are considered compatible with breast-feeding by the American Academy of Pediatrics. There have been isolated reports of transient cholestatic hepatitis/liver enzyme elevation in breast-fed infants exposed to carbamazepine. Valproate has a low transmission into breast milk. As with all psychotropic drugs used during lactation, effect on long-term outcome is unknown and should be approached cautiously.

## ANXIOLYTICS

Most data on anxiolytic use of pregnancy exists for the benzodiazepines. Although there has been concern for the last two decades that benzodiazepine use during the first trimester is associated with increased risk of cleft palate, there are recent conflicting studies that suggest risk may be

## SPECIAL POPULATIONS *(Continued)*

minimally, or not at all increased. As these studies are limited in methodological design, it cannot be stated that benzodiazepines may be safely used, and many clinicians do not advocate their use in early pregnancy.

Perinatal exposure to benzodiazepines have been associated with decreased Apgar scores, hypertonicity, and impaired thermoregulation. Some clinicians taper anxiolytic medication during pregnancy at around the time of birth in order to minimize perinatal effects.

Although there are multiple reports of no apparent adverse effects on breast-fed infants whose mothers were on benzodiazepines, there have been contrasting reports of drug accumulation and subsequent toxicity (CNS depression) in infants.

### AGENTS USED TO TREAT EXTRAPYRAMIDAL SYMPTOMS (EPS)

Data on use of agents to treat extrapyramidal symptoms during pregnancy are extremely limited. There have been reports of anticholinergic agents during pregnancy being associated with increased risk of birth malformations. Dopamine agonists (eg, amantadine) may also be associated with higher rates of pregnancy complications. While beta-blocking agents (eg, atenolol) appear to be relatively safe in pregnancy, the effect of propranolol on maternal heart rate is greater than in nonpregnant women. Prophylactic treatment for extrapyramidal symptoms during pregnancy is not generally recommended, and efforts to utilize lowest effective dose of antipsychotic medication should be made.

There are case reports of neonatal syndromes associated with anticholinergic compounds, although these appear to be generally transient.

Use of anti-EPS agents during lactation has been poorly studied, although low potency antipsychotic agents (with greater anticholinergic activity) are generally less well tolerated than agents with less anticholinergic activity.

# DSM-IV CLASSIFICATION

Used with permission from the American Psychiatric Association, *Diagnostic and Statistical Manual of Mental Disorders,* 4th ed, Washington, DC: American Psychiatric Association, 1994, 13-24,6,7.

## AXIS I AND II CATEGORIES AND CODES

An ellipsis (...) is used in the names of certain disorders to indicate that the name of a specific mental disorder or general medical condition should be inserted when recording the name.

An "x" appearing in a diagnostic code indicates that a specific code number is required.

If criteria are currently met, one of the following severity specifiers may be noted after the diagnosis:

- Mild
- Moderate
- Severe

If criteria are no longer met, one of the following specifiers may be noted:

- In partial remission
- In full remission
- Prior history
- NOS = Not otherwise specified

## AXIS I: CLINICAL DISORDERS; OTHER CONDITIONS THAT MAY BE A FOCUS OF CLINICAL ATTENTION

Axis I is for reporting all the various disorders or conditions in the Classification except for the Personality Disorders and Mental Retardation (which are reported on Axis II). The major groups of disorders to be reported on Axis I are listed in the box. Also reported on Axis I are Other Conditions That May Be a Focus of Clinical Attention.

**AXIS I**
**Clinical Disorders**
**Other Conditions That May Be a Focus of Clinical Attention**

Disorders Usually First Diagnosed in Infancy, Childhood, or Adolescence (excluding Mental Retardation, which is diagnosed on Axis II)
Delirium, Dementia, and Amnestic and Other Cognitive Disorders
Mental Disorders Due to a General Medical Condition
Substance-Related Disorders
Schizophrenia and Other Psychotic Disorders
Mood Disorders
Anxiety Disorders
Somatoform Disorders
Factitious Disorders
Dissociative Disorders
Sexual and Gender Identity Disorders
Eating Disorders
Sleep Disorders
Impulse-Control Disorders Not Elsewhere Classified
Adjustment Disorders
Other Conditions That May Be a Focus of Clinical Attention

## AXIS II: PERSONALITY DISORDERS; MENTAL RETARDATION

Axis II is for reporting Personality Disorders and Mental Retardation. It may also be used for noting prominent maladaptive personality features and defense mechanisms. The listing of Personality Disorders and Mental Retardation on a separate axis ensures that consideration will be given to the possible presence of Personality Disorders and Mental Retardation that might otherwise be overlooked when attention is directed to the usually more florid Axis I disorders. The coding of Personality Disorders on Axis II should not be taken to imply that their pathogenesis or range of appropriate treatment is fundamentally different from that for the disorders coded on Axis I. The disorders to be reported on Axis II are listed in the box.

**AXIS II**
**Personality Disorders**
**Mental Retardation**

Paranoid Personality Disorder
Schizoid Personality Disorder
Schizotypal Personality Disorder
Antisocial Personality Disorder
Borderline Personality Disorder
Histrionic Personality Disorder
Narcissistic Personality Disorder
Avoidant Personality Disorder
Dependent Personality Disorder
Obsessive-Compulsive Personality Disorder
Personality Disorder Not Otherwise Specified
Mental Retardation

## DSM-IV CLASSIFICATION *(Continued)*

# DISORDERS USUALLY FIRST DIAGNOSED IN INFANCY, CHILDHOOD, OR ADOLESCENCE

### MENTAL RETARDATION

**Note:** These are coded on Axis II.

| | |
|---|---|
| 317 | Mild Mental Retardation |
| 318.0 | Moderate Mental Retardation |
| 318.1 | Severe Mental Retardation |
| 318.2 | Profound Mental Retardation |
| 319 | Mental Retardation, Severity Unspecified |

### LEARNING DISORDERS

| | |
|---|---|
| 315.00 | Reading Disorder |
| 315.1 | Mathematics Disorder |
| 315.2 | Disorder of Written Expression |
| 315.9 | Learning Disorder NOS |

### MOTOR SKILLS DISORDER

| | |
|---|---|
| 315.4 | Development Coordination Disorder |

### COMMUNICATION DISORDERS

| | |
|---|---|
| 315.31 | Expressive Language Disorder |
| 315.32 | Mixed Receptive-Expressive Language Disorder |
| 315.39 | Phonological Disorder |
| 307.0 | Stuttering |
| 307.9 | Communication Disorder NOS |

### PERVASIVE DEVELOPMENTAL DISORDERS

| | |
|---|---|
| 299.00 | Autistic Disorder |
| 299.80 | Rett's Disorder |
| 299.10 | Childhood Disintegrative Disorder |
| 299.80 | Asperger's Disorder |
| 299.80 | Pervasive Developmental Disorder NOS |

### ATTENTION-DEFICIT AND DISRUPTIVE BEHAVIOR DISORDERS

| | |
|---|---|
| 314.xx | Attention-Deficit/Hyperactivity Disorder |
| .01 | Combined Type |
| .00 | Predominantly Inattentive Type |
| .01 | Predominantly Hyperactive-Impulsive Type |
| 314.9 | Attention-Deficit/Hyperactivity Disorder NOS |
| 312.xx | Conduct Disorder |
| .81 | Childhood-Onset Type |
| .82 | Adolescent-Onset Type |
| .89 | Unspecified Onset |
| 313.81 | Oppositional Defiant Disorder |
| 312.9 | Disruptive Behavior Disorder NOS |

### FEEDING AND EATING DISORDERS OF INFANCY OR EARLY CHILDHOOD

| | |
|---|---|
| 307.52 | Pica |
| 307.53 | Rumination Disorder |
| 307.59 | Feeding Disorder of Infancy or Early Childhood |

### TIC DISORDERS

| | |
|---|---|
| 307.23 | Tourette's Disorder |
| 307.22 | Chronic Motor or Vocal Tic Disorder |
| 307.21 | Transient Tic Disorder |

Specify if: Single Episode/Recurrent

| | |
|---|---|
| 307.20 | Tic Disorder NOS |

## ELIMINATION DISORDERS

| | |
|---|---|
| ___.__ | Encopresis |
| 787.6 | With Constipation and Overflow Incontinence |
| 307.7 | Without Constipation and Overflow Incontinence |
| 307.6 | Enuresis (Not Due to a General Medical Condition) |

Specify type: Nocturnal Only/Diurnal Only/Nocturnal and Diurnal

## OTHER DISORDERS OF INFANCY, CHILDHOOD, OR ADOLESCENCE

309.21 Separation Anxiety Disorder
Specify if: Early Onset
313.23 Selective Mutism
313.89 Reactive Attachment Disorder of Infancy or Early Childhood
Specify type: Inhibited Type/Disinhibited Type
307.3 Stereotypic Movement Disorder
Specify if: With Self-Injurious Behavior
313.9 Disorder of Infancy, Childhood, or Adolescence NOS

# DELIRIUM, DEMENTIA, AND AMNESTIC AND OTHER COGNITIVE DISORDERS

## DELIRIUM

| | |
|---|---|
| 293.0 | Delirium Due to ... [Indicate the General Medical Condition] |
| ___.__ | Substance Intoxication Delirium (refer to Substance-Related Disorders for substance-specific codes) |
| ___.__ | Substance Withdrawal Delirium (refer to Substance-Related Disorders for substance-specific codes) |
| ___.__ | Delirium Due to Multiple Etiologies (code each of the specific etiologies) |
| 780.09 | Delirium NOS |

## DEMENTIA

290.xx Dementia of the Alzheimer's Type, With Early Onset (also code 331.0 Alzheimer's disease on Axis III)]
.10 Uncomplicated
.11 With Delirium
.12 With Delusions
.13 With Depressed Mood
Specify if: With Behavioral Disturbance
290.xx Dementia of the Alzheimer's Type, With Late Onset (also code 331.0 Alzheimer's disease on Axis III)
.0 Uncomplicated
.3 With Delirium
.20 With Delusions
.21 With Depressed Mood
Specify if: With Behavioral Disturbance
290.xx Vascular Dementia
.40 Uncomplicated
.41 With Delirium
.42 With Delusions
.43 With Depressed Mood
Specify if: With Behavioral Disturbance
294.1 Dementia Due to HIV Disease (also code 042 HIV infection on Axis III)
294.1 Dementia Due to Head Trauma (also code 854.00 head injury on Axis III)
294.1 Dementia Due to Parkinson's Disease (also code 332.0 Parkinson's disease on Axis III)
294.1 Dementia Due to Huntington's Disease (also code 333.4 Huntington's disease on Axis III)
290.10 Dementia Due to Pick's Disease (also code 331.1 Pick's disease on Axis III)
290.10 Dementia Due to Creutzfeldt-Jakob Disease (also code 046.1 Creutzfeldt-Jakob disease on Axis III)
294.1 Dementia Due to ... [Indicate the General Medical Condition not listed above] (also code the general medical condition on Axis III)
___.__ Substance-Induced Persisting Dementia (refer to Substance-Related Disorders for substance-specific codes)
___.__ Dementia Due to Multiple Etiologies (code each of the specific etiologies)
294.8 Dementia NOS

## AMNESTIC DISORDERS

294.0 Amnestic Disorder Due to ... [Indicate the General Medical Condition]
Specify if: Transient/Chronic
___.__ Substance-Induced Persisting Amnestic Disorder (refer to Substance-Related Disorders for substance-specific codes)
294.8 Amnestic Disorder NOS

## DSM-IV CLASSIFICATION *(Continued)*

### OTHER COGNITIVE DISORDERS

294.9 Cognitive Disorder NOS

## MENTAL DISORDERS DUE TO A GENERAL MEDICAL CONDITION NOT ELSEWHERE CLASSIFIED

293.89 Catatonic Disorder Due to ... [Indicate the General Medical Condition]
310.1 Personality Change Due to ... [Indicate the General Medical Condition]
Specify type: Labile Type/Disinhibited Type/Aggressive Type/Apathetic Type/Paranoid Type/Other Type/Combined Type/Unspecified Type
293.9 Mental Disorder NOS Due to ... [Indicate the General Medical Condition]

## SUBSTANCE-RELATED DISORDERS

[a]The following specifiers may be applied to Substance Dependence:

With Physiological Dependence/Without Physiological Dependence

Early Full Remission/Early Partial Remission

Sustained Full Remission/ Sustained Partial Remission

On Agonist Therapy/In a Controlled Environment

The following specifiers apply to Substance-Induced Disorders as noted:

[I]With Onset During Intoxication/[W]With Onset During Withdrawal

### ALCOHOL-RELATED DISORDERS

___ **Alcohol Use Disorders**
303.90 Alcohol Dependence[a]
305.00 Alcohol Abuse
___ **Alcohol-Induced Disorders**
303.00 Alcohol Intoxication
291.81 Alcohol Withdrawal
Specify if: With Perceptual Disturbances
291.0 Alcohol Intoxication Delirium
291.0 Alcohol Withdrawal Delirium
291.2 Alcohol-Induced Persisting Dementia
291.1 Alcohol-Induced Persisting Amnestic Disorder
291.x Alcohol-Induced Psychotic Disorder
.5 With Delusions[I,W]
.3 With Hallucinations[I,W]
291.89 Alcohol-Induced Mood Disorder[I,W]
291.89 Alcohol-Induced Anxiety Disorder[I,W]
291.89 Alcohol-Induced Sexual Dysfunction[I]
291.89 Alcohol-Induced Sleep Disorder[I,W]
291.9 Alcohol-Related Disorder NOS

### AMPHETAMINE (or Amphetamine-Like) - Related Disorders

___ **Amphetamine Use Disorders**
304.40 Amphetamine Dependence[a]]
305.70 Amphetamine Abuse
___ **Amphetamine-Induced Disorders**
292.89 Amphetamine Intoxication
Specify if: With Perceptual Disturbances
292.0 Amphetamine Withdrawal
292.81 Amphetamine Intoxication Delirium
292.xx Amphetamine-Induced Psychotic Disorder
.11 With Delusions[I]
.12 With Hallucinations[I]
292.84 Amphetamine-Induced Mood Disorder[I,W]
292.89 Amphetamine-Induced Anxiety Disorder[I]
292.89 Amphetamine-Induced Sexual Dysfunction[I]
292.89 Amphetamine-Induced Sleep Disorder[I,W]
292.9 Amphetamine-Related Disorder NOS

## CAFFEINE-RELATED DISORDERS

___ **Caffeine-Induced Disorders**

305.90 Caffeine Intoxication
292.89 Caffeine-Induced Anxiety Disorder[I]
292.89 Caffeine-Induced Sleep Disorder[I]
292.9 Caffeine-Related Disorder NOS

## CANNABIS-RELATED DISORDERS

___ **Cannabis Use Disorders**

304.30 Cannabis Dependence[a]
305.20 Cannabis Abuse

___ **Cannabis-Induced Disorders**

292.89 Cannabis Intoxication
Specify if: With Perceptual Disturbance
292.81 Cannabis Intoxication Delirium
292.xx Cannabis-Induced Psychotic Disorder
.11 With Delusions[I]
.12 With Hallucinations[I]
292.89 Cannabis-Induced Anxiety Disorder[I]
292.9 Cannabis-Related Disorder NOS

## COCAINE-RELATED DISORDERS

___ **Cocaine Use Disorders**

304.20 Cocaine Dependence[a]
305.60 Cocaine Abuse

___ **Cocaine-Induced Disorders**

292.89 Cocaine Intoxication
Specify if: With Perceptual Disturbance
292.0 Cocaine Withdrawal
292.81 Cocaine Intoxication Delirium
292.xx Cocaine-Induced Psychotic Disorder
.11 With Delusions[I]
.12 With Hallucinations[I]
292.84 Cocaine-Induced Mood Disorder[I,W]
292.89 Cocaine-Induced Anxiety Disorder[I,W]
292.89 Cocaine-Induced Sexual Dysfunction[I]
292.89 Cocaine-Induced Sleep Disorder[I,W]
292.9 Cocaine-Related Disorder NOS

## HALLUCINOGEN-RELATED DISORDERS

___ **Hallucinogen Use Disorders**

304.50 Hallucinogen Dependence[a]
305.30 Hallucinogen Abuse

___ **Hallucinogen-Induced Disorders**

292.89 Hallucinogen Intoxication
292.89 Hallucinogen Persisting Perception Disorder (Flashbacks)
292.81 Hallucinogen Intoxication Delirium
292.xx Hallucinogen-Induced Psychotic Disorder
.11 With Delusions[I]
.12 With Hallucinations[I]
292.84 Hallucinogen-Induced Mood Disorder[I]
292.89 Hallucinogen-Induced Anxiety Disorder[I]
292.9 Hallucinogen-Related Disorder NOS

## INHALANT-RELATED DISORDERS

___ **Inhalant Use Disorders**

304.60 Inhalant Dependence[a]
305.90 Inhalant Abuse

___ **Inhalant-Induced Disorders**

292.89 Inhalant Intoxication
292.81 Inhalant Intoxication Delirium
292.82 Inhalant-Induced Persisting Dementia
292.xx Inhalant-Induced Psychotic Disorder
.11 With Delusions[I]
.12 With Hallucinations[I]

## DSM-IV CLASSIFICATION *(Continued)*

292.84 Inhalant-Induced Mood Disorder[I]
292.89 Inhalant-Induced Anxiety Disorder[I]
292.9 Inhalant-Related Disorder NOS

## NICOTINE-RELATED DISORDERS

___ **Nicotine Use Disorders**
305.10 Nicotine Dependence[a]
___ **Nicotine-Induced Disorders**
292.0 Nicotine Withdrawal
292.9 Nicotine-Related Disorder NOS

## OPIOID-RELATED DISORDERS

___ **Opioid Use Disorders**
304.00 Opioid Dependence[a]
305.50 Opioid Abuse
___ **Opioid-Induced Disorders**
292.89 Opioid Intoxication
Specify if: With Perceptual Disturbances
292.0 Opioid Withdrawal
292.81 Opioid Intoxication Delirium
292.xx Opioid-Induced Psychotic Disorder
.11 With Delusions[I]
.12 With Hallucinations[I]
292.84 Opioid-Induced Mood Disorder[I]
292.89 Opioid-Induced Sexual Dysfunction[I]
292.89 Opioid-Induced Sleep Disorder[I,W]
292.9 Opioid-Related Disorder NOS

## PHENCYCLIDINE (or Phencyclidine-Like)-RELATED DISORDERS

___ **Phencyclidine Use Disorders**
304.60 Phencyclidine Dependence[a]
305.90 Phencyclidine Abuse
___ **Phencyclidine-Induced Disorders**
292.89 Phencyclidine Intoxication
Specify if: With Perceptual Disturbances
292.81 Phencyclidine Intoxication Delirium
292.xx Phencyclidine-Induced Psychotic Disorder
.11 With Delusions[I]
.12 With Hallucinations[I]
292.84 Phencyclidine-Induced Mood Disorder[I]
292.89 Phencyclidine-Induced Anxiety Disorder[I]
292.9 Phencyclidine-Related Disorder NOS

## SEDATIVE-, HYPNOTIC-, OR ANXIOLYTIC-RELATED DISORDERS

___ **Sedative, Hypnotic, or Anxiolytic Use Disorders**
304.10 Sedative, Hypnotic, or Anxiolytic Dependence[a]
305.40 Sedative, Hypnotic, or Anxiolytic Abuse
___ **Sedative-, Hypnotic-, or Anxiolytic-Induced Disorders**
292.89 Sedative, Hypnotic, or Anxiolytic Intoxication
292.0 Sedative, Hypnotic, or Anxiolytic Withdrawal
Specify if: With Perceptual Disturbances
292.81 Sedative, Hypnotic, or Anxiolytic Intoxication Delirium
292.81 Sedative, Hypnotic, or Anxiolytic Withdrawal Delirium
292.82 Sedative-, Hypnotic-, or Anxiolytic-Induced Persisting Dementia
292.83 Sedative-, Hypnotic-, or Anxiolytic-Induced Persisting Amnestic Disorder
292.xx Sedative-, Hypnotic-, or Anxiolytic-Induced Psychotic Disorder
.11 With Delusions[I,W]
.12 With Hallucinations[I,W]
292.84 Sedative-, Hypnotic-, or Anxiolytic-Induced Mood Disorder[I,W]
292.89 Sedative-, Hypnotic-, or Anxiolytic-Induced Anxiety Disorder[W]
292.89 Sedative-, Hypnotic-, or Anxiolytic-Induced Sexual Dysfunction[I]
292.89 Sedative-, Hypnotic-, or Anxiolytic-Induced Sleep Disorder[I,W]
292.9 Sedative-, Hypnotic-, or Anxiolytic-Related Disorder NOS

## POLYSUBSTANCE-RELATED DISORDER

304.80 Polysubstance Dependence[a]

## OTHER (or Unknown) SUBSTANCE-RELATED DISORDERS

**___ Other (or Unknown) Substance Use Disorders**

304.90 Other (or Unknown) Substance Dependence[a]
305.90 Other (or Unknown) Substance Abuse

**___ Other (or Unknown) Substance-Induced Disorders**

292.89 Other (or Unknown) Substance Intoxication
Specify if: With Perceptual Disturbances
292.0 Other (or Unknown) Substance Withdrawal
Specify if: With Perceptual Disturbances
292.81 Other (or Unknown) Substance-Induced Delirium
292.82 Other (or Unknown) Substance-Induced Persisting Dementia
292.83 Other (or Unknown) Substance-Induced Persisting Amnestic Disorder
292.xx Other (or Unknown) Substance-Induced Psychotic Disorder
.11 With Delusions[I,W]
.12 With Hallucinations[I,W]
292.84 Other (or Unknown) Substance-Induced Mood Disorder[I,W]
292.89 Other (or Unknown) Substance-Induced Anxiety Disorder[I,W]
292.89 Other (or Unknown) Substance-Induced Sexual Dysfunction[I]
292.89 Other (or Unknown) Substance-Induced Sleep Disorder[I,W]
292.9 Other (or Unknown) Substance-Related Disorder NOS

# SCHIZOPHRENIA AND OTHER PSYCHOTIC DISORDERS

295.xx Schizophrenia
The following Classification of Longitudinal Course applies to all subtypes of Schizophrenia:
Episodic With Interepisode Residual Symptoms
(specify if: With Prominent Negative Symptoms)/Episodic With No Interepisode Residual Symptoms/Continuous (specify if: With Prominent Negative Symptoms)
Single Episode In Partial Remission
(specify if: With Prominent Negative Symptoms)/Single Episode In Full Remission
Other or Unspecified Pattern
.30 Paranoid Type
.10 Disorganized Type
.20 Catatonic Type
.90 Undifferentiated Type
.60 Residual Type
295.40 Schizophreniform Disorder
Specify if: Without Good Prognostic Features/With Good Prognostic Features
295.70 Schizoaffective Disorder
Specify type: Bipolar Type/Depressive Type
297.1 Delusional Disorder
Specify type: Erotomanic Type/Grandiose Type/Jealous Type/Persecutory Type/Somatic Type/Mixed Type/Unspecified Type
298.8 Brief Psychotic Disorder
Specify if: With Marked Stressor(s)/Without Marked Stressor(s)/With Postpartum Onset
297.3 Shared Psychotic Disorder
293.xx Psychotic Disorder Due to ... [Indicate the General Medical Condition]
.81 With Delusions
.82 With Hallucinations
___.__ Substance-Induced Psychotic Disorder
(Refer to Substance-Related Disorders for substance-specific codes)
Specify if: With Onset During Intoxication/With Onset During Withdrawal
298.9 Psychotic Disorder NOS

# MOOD DISORDERS

Code current state of Major Depressive Disorder or Bipolar I Disorder in fifth digit:

1 = Mild
2 = Moderate
3 = Severe Without Psychotic Features
4 = Severe With Psychotic Features
Specify: Mood-Congruent Psychotic Features/Mood-Incongruent Psychotic Features
5 = In Partial Remission
6 = In Full Remission
0 = Unspecified

The following specifiers apply (for current or most recent episode) to Mood Disorders as noted:

## DSM-IV CLASSIFICATION *(Continued)*

[a]Severity/Psychotic/Remission Specifiers
[b]Chronic
[c]With Catatonic Features
[d]With Melancholic Features
[e]With Atypical Features
[f]With Postpartum Onset

The following specifiers apply to Mood Disorders as noted:
[g]With or Without Full Interepisode Recovery
[h]With Seasonal Pattern
[i]With Rapid Cycling

### DEPRESSIVE DISORDERS

296.xx Major Depressive Disorder,
.2x Single Episode[a,b,c,d,e,f]
.3x Recurrent[a,b,c,d,e,f,g,h]
300.4 Dysthymic Disorder
Specify if: Early Onset/Late Onset
Specify: With Atypical Features
311 Depressive Disorder NOS

### BIPOLAR DISORDERS

296.xx Bipolar I Disorder,
.0x Single Manic Episode[a,c,f]
Specify if: Mixed
.40 Most Recent Episode Hypomanic[g,h,i]
.4x Most Recent Episode Manic[a,c,f,g,h,i]
.6x Most Recent Episode Mixed[a,c,f,g,h,i]
.5x Most Recent Episode Depressed[a,b,c,d,e,f,g,h,i]
.7 Most Recent Episode Unspecified[g,h,i]
296.89 Bipolar II Disorder[a,b,c,d,e,f,g,h,i]
Specify (current or most recent episode):
Hypomanic/Depressed
301.13 Cyclothymic Disorder
296.80 Bipolar Disorder NOS
293.83 Mood Disorder Due to ... [Indicate the General Medical Condition]
Specify type: With Depressive Features/With Major Depressive-Like Episode/With Manic Features/With Mixed Features
___.__ Substance-Induced Mood Disorder (refer to Substance-Related Disorders for substance-specific codes)
Specify type: With Depressive Features/With Manic Features/With Mixed Features
Specify if: With Onset During Intoxication/With Onset During Withdrawal
296.90 Mood Disorder NOS

## ANXIETY DISORDERS

300.01 Panic Disorder Without Agoraphobia
300.21 Panic Disorder With Agoraphobia
300.22 Agoraphobia Without History of Panic Disorder
300.29 Specific Phobia
Specify type: Animal Type/Natural Environment Type/Blood-Injection-Injury Type/Situational Type/Other Type
300.23 Social Phobia
Specify if: Generalized
300.3 Obsessive-Compulsive Disorder
Specify if: With Poor Insight
309.81 Post-traumatic Stress Disorder
Specify if: Acute/Chronic
Specify if: With Delayed Onset
308.3 Acute Stress Disorder
300.02 Generalized Anxiety Disorder
293.84 Anxiety Disorder Due to ... [Indicate the General Medical Condition]
Specify if: With Generalized Anxiety/With Panic Attacks/With Obsessive-Compulsive Symptoms
___.__ Substance-Induced Anxiety Disorder (refer to Substance-Related Disorders for substance-specific codes)
Specify if: With Generalized Anxiety/With Panic Attacks/With Obsessive-Compulsive Symptoms/With Phobic Symptoms
Specify if: With Onset During Intoxication/With Onset During Withdrawal
300.00 Anxiety Disorder NOS

## SOMATOFORM DISORDERS

300.81 Somatization Disorder
300.82 Undifferentiated Somatoform Disorder
300.11 Conversion Disorder
Specify type: With Motor Symptom or Deficit/With Sensory Symptom or Deficit/With Seizures or Convulsions/With Mixed Presentation
307.xx Pain Disorder
.80 Associated With Psychological Factors
.89 Associated With Both Psychological Factors and a General Medical Condition
Specify if: Acute/Chronic
300.7 Hyperchondriasis
Specify if: With Poor Insight
300.7 Body Dysmorphic Disorder
300.82 Somatoform Disorder NOS

## FACTITIOUS DISORDERS

300.xx Factitious Disorder
.16 With Predominantly Psychological Signs and Symptoms
.19 With Predominantly Physical Signs and Symptoms
.19 With Combined Psychological and Physical Signs and Symptoms
300.19 Factitious Disorder NOS

## DISSOCIATIVE DISORDERS

300.12 Dissociative Amnesia
300.13 Dissociative Fugue
300.14 Dissociative Identity Disorder
300.6 Depersonalization Disorder
300.15 Dissociative Disorder NOS

## SEXUAL AND GENDER IDENTITY DISORDERS

### SEXUAL DYSFUNCTION

The following specifiers apply to all primary Sexual Dysfunctions:
Lifelong Type/Acquired Type
Generalized Type/Situational Type
Due to Psychological Factors/Due to Combined Factors

___ **Sexual Desire Disorders**
302.71 Hypoactive Sexual Desire Disorder
302.79 Sexual Aversion Disorder
___ **Sexual Arousal Disorders**
302.72 Female Sexual Arousal Disorder
302.72 Male Erectile Disorder
___ **Orgasmic Disorders**
302.73 Female Orgasmic Disorder
302.74 Male Orgasmic Disorder
302.75 Premature Ejaculation
___ **Sexual Pain Disorders**
302.76 Dyspareunia (Not Due to a General Medical Condition)
306.51 Vaginismus (Not Due to a General Medical Condition)
___ **Sexual Dysfunction Due to a General Medical Condition**
625.8 Female Hypoactive Sexual Desire Disorder Due to ... [Indicate the General Medical Condition]
608.89 Male Hypoactive Sexual Desire Disorder Due to ... [Indicate the General Medical Condition]
607.84 Male Erectile Disorder Due to ... [Indicate the General Medial Condition]
625.0 Female Dyspareunia Due to ... [Indicate the General Medial Condition]
608.89 Male Dyspareunia Due to ... [Indicate the General Medial Condition]
625.8 Other Female Sexual Dysfunction Due to ... [Indicate the General Medial Condition]
608.89 Other Male Sexual Dysfunction Due to ... [Indicate the General Medial Condition]
___.__ Substance-Induced Sexual Dysfunction (refer to Substance-Related Disorders for substance-specific codes)
Specify if: With Impaired Desire/With Impaired Arousal/With Impaired Orgasm/With Sexual Pain
Specify if: With Onset During Intoxication
302.70 Sexual Dysfunction NOS

## DSM-IV CLASSIFICATION *(Continued)*

### PARAPHILIAS

302.4 Exhibitionism
302.81 Fetishism
302.89 Frotteurism
302.2 Pedophilia
Specify if: Sexually Attracted to Males/Sexually Attracted to Females/Sexually Attracted to Both
Specify if: Limited to Incest
Specify type: Exclusive Type/Nonexclusive Type
302.83 Sexual Masochism
302.84 Sexual Sadism
302.3 Transvestic Fetishism
Specify if: With Gender Dysphoria
302.82 Voyeurism
302.9 Paraphilia NOS

### GENDER IDENTITY DISORDERS

302.xx Gender Identity Disorder
.6 in Children
.85 in Adolescents or Adults
Specify if: Sexually Attracted to Males/Sexually Attracted to Females/Sexually Attracted to Both/Sexually Attracted to Neither
302.6 Gender Identity Disorder NOS
302.9 Sexual Disorder NOS

## EATING DISORDERS

307.1 Anorexia Nervosa
Specify type: Restricting Type; Binge-Eating/Purging Type
307.51 Bulimia Nervosa
Specify type: Purging Type/Nonpurging Type
307.50 Eating Disorder NOS

## SLEEP DISORDERS

### PRIMARY SLEEP DISORDERS

___ **Dyssomnias**
307.42 Primary Insomnia
307.44 Primary Hypersomnia
Specify if: Recurrent
347 Narcolepsy
780.59 Breathing-Related Sleep Disorder
307.45 Circadian Rhythm Sleep Disorder
Specify type: Delayed Sleep Phase Type/Jet Lag Type/Shift Work Type/Unspecified Type
307.47 Dyssomnia NOS
___ **Parasomnias**
307.47 Nightmare Disorder
307.46 Sleep Terror Disorder
307.46 Sleepwalking Disorder
307.47 Parasomnia NOS

### SLEEP DISORDERS RELATED TO ANOTHER MENTAL DISORDER

307.42 Insomnia Related to ... [Indicate the Axis I or Axis II Disorder]
307.44 Hypersomnia Related to ... [Indicate the Axis I or Axis II Disorder]

### OTHER SLEEP DISORDERS

780.xx Sleep Disorder Due to ... [Indicate the Axis I or Axis II Disorder]
.52 Insomnia Type
.54 Hypersomnia Type
.59 Parasomnia Type
.59 Mixed Type
___.__ Substance-Induced Sleep Disorder (refer to Substance-Related Disorders for substance-specific codes)
Specify type: Insomnia Type/Hypersomnia Type/Parasomnia Type/Mixed Type
Specify if: With Onset During Intoxication/With Onset During Withdrawal

## IMPULSE-CONTROL DISORDERS NOT ELSEWHERE CLASSIFIED

| | |
|---|---|
| 312.34 | Intermittent Explosive Disorder |
| 312.32 | Kleptomania |
| 312.33 | Pyromania |
| 312.31 | Pathological Gambling |
| 312.39 | Trichotillomania |
| 312.30 | Impulse-Control Disorder NOS |

## ADJUSTMENT DISORDERS

| | |
|---|---|
| 309.xx | Adjustment Disorder |
| .0 | With Depressed Mood |
| .24 | With Anxiety |
| .28 | With Mixed Anxiety and Depressed Mood |
| .3 | With Disturbance of Conduct |
| .4 | With Mixed Disturbance of Emotions and Conduct |
| .9 | Unspecified |

Specify if: Acute/Chronic

## PERSONALITY DISORDERS

**Note:** These are coded on Axis II.

| | |
|---|---|
| 301.0 | Paranoid Personality Disorder |
| 301.20 | Schizoid Personality Disorder |
| 301.22 | Schizotypal Personality Disorder |
| 301.7 | Antisocial Personality Disorder |
| 301.83 | Borderline Personality Disorder |
| 301.50 | Histrionic Personality Disorder |
| 301.81 | Narcissistic Personality Disorder |
| 301.82 | Avoidant Personality Disorder |
| 301.6 | Dependent Personality Disorder |
| 301.4 | Obsessive-Compulsive Personality Disorder |
| 301.9 | Personality Disorder NOS |

## OTHER CONDITIONS THAT MAY BE A FOCUS OF CLINICAL ATTENTION

### PSYCHOLOGICAL FACTORS AFFECTING MEDICAL CONDITION

316 ... [Specified Psychological Factor] Affecting
... [Indicate the General Medical Condition]
Choose name based on nature of factors:
Mental Disorder Affecting Medical Condition
Psychological Symptoms Affecting Medical Condition
Personality Traits or Coping Style Affecting Medical Condition
Maladaptive Health Behaviors Affecting Medical Condition
Stress-Related Physiological Response Affecting Medical Condition
Other or Unspecified Psychological Factors Affecting Medical Condition

### MEDICATION-INDUCED MOVEMENT DISORDERS

| | |
|---|---|
| 332.1 | Neuroleptic-Induced Parkinsonism |
| 333.92 | Neuroleptic Malignant Syndrome |
| 333.7 | Neuroleptic-Induced Acute Dystonia |
| 333.99 | Neuroleptic-Induced Acute Akathisia |
| 333.82 | Neuroleptic-Induced Tardive Dyskinesia |
| 333.1 | Medication-Induced Postural Tremor |
| 333.90 | Medication-Induced Movement Disorder NOS |

### OTHER MEDICATION-INDUCED DISORDER

| | |
|---|---|
| 995.2 | Adverse Effects of Medication NOS |

## DSM-IV CLASSIFICATION *(Continued)*

### RELATIONAL PROBLEMS

| | |
|---|---|
| V61.9 | Relational Problem Related to a Mental Disorder or General Medical Condition |
| V61.20 | Parent-Child Relational Problem |
| V61.10 | Partner Relational Problem |
| V61.8 | Sibling Relational Problem |
| V62.81 | Relational Problem NOS |

### PROBLEMS RELATED TO ABUSE OR NEGLECT

| | |
|---|---|
| V61.21 | Physical Abuse of Child (code 99.54 if focus of attention is on victim) |
| V61.21 | Sexual Abuse of Child (code 995.53 if focus of attention is on victim) |
| V61.21 | Neglect of Child (code 995.52 if focus of attention is on victim) |
| ___.__ | Physical Abuse of Adult (682) |
| V61.12 | (if by partner) |
| V62.83 | (if by person other than partner) (code 995.81 if focus of attention is on victim) |
| ___.__ | Sexual Abuse of Adult (682) |
| V61.12 | (if by partner) |
| V62.83 | (if by person other than partner) (code 995.83 if focus of attention is on victim) |

### ADDITIONAL CONDITIONS THAT MAY BE A FOCUS OF CLINICAL ATTENTION

| | |
|---|---|
| V15.81 | Noncompliance With Treatment |
| V65.2 | Malingering |
| V71.01 | Adult Antisocial Behavior |
| V71.02 | Child or Adolescent Antisocial Behavior |
| V62.89 | Borderline Intellectual Functioning |

**Note:** This is coded on Axis II

| | |
|---|---|
| 780.9 | Age-Related Cognitive Decline |
| V62.82 | Bereavement |
| V62.3 | Academic Problem |
| V62.2 | Occupational Problem |
| 313.82 | Identity Problem |
| V62.89 | Religious or Spiritual Problem |
| V62.4 | Acculturation Problem |
| V62.89 | Phase of Life Problem |

## ADDITIONAL CODES

| | |
|---|---|
| 300.9 | Unspecified Mental Disorder (nonpsychotic) |
| V71.09 | No Diagnosis or Condition on Axis I |
| 799.9 | Diagnosis or Condition Deferred on Axis I |
| V71.09 | No Diagnosis on Axis II |
| 799.9 | Diagnosis Deferred on Axis II |

## MULTIAXIAL SYSTEM

| | |
|---|---|
| **Axis I** | Clinical Disorders<br>Other Conditions That May Be a Focus of Clinical Attention |
| **Axis II** | Personality Disorders<br>Mental Retardation |
| **Axis III** | General Medical Conditions |
| **Axis IV** | Psychosocial and Environmental Problems |
| **Axis V** | Global Assessment of Functioning |

# APPENDIX TABLE OF CONTENTS

## THERAPY RECOMMENDATIONS



## TOXICOLOGY



## MISCELLANEOUS

# ABBREVIATIONS, ACRONYMS, AND SYMBOLS

| Abbreviation | From | Meaning |
|---|---|---|
| aa, aa | ana | of each |
| AA | | Alcoholics Anonymous |
| ac | ante cibum | before meals or food |
| ad | ad | to, up to |
| a.d. | aurio dextra | right ear |
| ADHD | | attention-deficit/hyperactivity disorder |
| ADLs | | activities of daily living |
| ad lib | ad libitum | at pleasure |
| AIMS | | Abnormal Involuntary Movement Scale |
| a.l. | aurio laeva | left ear |
| AM | ante meridiem | morning |
| amp | | ampul |
| amt | | amount |
| aq | aqua | water |
| aq. dest. | aqua destillata | distilled water |
| ARDS | | adult respiratory distress syndrome |
| a.s. | aurio sinister | left ear |
| ASAP | | as soon as possible |
| a.u. | aures utrae | each ear |
| BDI | | Beck Depression Inventory |
| bid | bis in die | twice daily |
| bm | | bowel movement |
| bp | | blood pressure |
| BPRS | | Brief Psychiatric Rating Scale |
| BSA | | body surface area |
| c | cong | a gallon |
| c̄ | cum | with |
| cal | | calorie |
| cap | capsula | capsule |
| CBT | | cognitive behavioral therapy |
| cc | | cubic centimeter |
| CGI | | Clinical Global Impression |
| cm | | centimeter |
| comp | compositus | compound |
| cont | | continue |
| CRF | | chronic renal failure |
| CT | | computed tomography |
| d | dies | day |
| d/c | | discontinue |
| dil | dilue | dilute |
| disp | dispensa | dispense |
| div | divide | divide |
| DSM-IV | | Diagnostic and Statistical Manual |
| DTs | | delirium tremens |
| dtd | dentur tales doses | give of such a dose |
| ECT | | electroconvulsive therapy |
| EEG | | electroencephalogram |
| elix, el | elixir | elixir |
| emp | | as directed |
| EPS | | extrapyramidal side effects |
| ESRD | | end stage renal disease |
| et | et | and |
| ex aq | | in water |
| f, ft | fac, fiat, fiant | make, let be made |
| FDA | | Food and Drug Administration |
| g | gramma | gram |
| GA | | Gamblers Anonymous |
| GAD | | generalized anxiety disorder |
| GAF | | Global Assessment of Functioning Scale |
| GABA | | gamma-aminobutyric acid |
| GERD | | gastroesophageal reflux disease |
| gr | granum | grain |
| gtt | gutta | a drop |
| GVHD | | graft vs host disease |
| h | hora | hour |
| HAM-A | | Hamilton Anxiety Scale |
| HAM-D | | Hamilton Depression Scale |
| hs | hora somni | at bedtime |
| HSV | | herpes simplex virus |
| I.M. | | intramuscular |

## ABBREVIATIONS, ACRONYMS, AND SYMBOLS *(Continued)*

| Abbreviation | From | Meaning |
|---|---|---|
| I.V. | | intravenous |
| kcal | | kilocalorie |
| kg | | kilogram |
| L | | liter |
| LAMM | | L-α-acetyl methadol |
| liq | liquor | a liquor, solution |
| M | misce | mix |
| M | | molar |
| MADRS | | Montgomery Asberg Depression Rating Scale |
| MAOIs | | monoamine oxidase inhibitors |
| mcg | | microgram |
| MDEA | | 3,4-methylene-dioxy amphetamine |
| m. dict | more dictor | as directed |
| MDMA | | 3,4-methylene-dioxy methamphetamine |
| mEq | | milliequivalent |
| mg | | milligram |
| mixt | mixtura | a mixture |
| mL | | milliliter |
| mm | | millimeter |
| mM | | millimolar |
| MMSE | | Mini-Mental State Examination |
| MPPP | | l-methyl-4-proprionoxy-4-phenyl pyridine |
| MR | | mental retardation |
| MRI | | magnetic resonance imaging |
| NF | | National Formulary |
| NMS | | neuroleptic malignant syndrome |
| no. | numerus | number |
| noc | nocturnal | in the night |
| non rep | non repetatur | do not repeat, no refills |
| NPO | | nothing by mouth |
| O, Oct | octarius | a pint |
| OCD | | obsessive-compulsive disorder |
| o.d. | oculus dexter | right eye |
| o.l. | oculus laevus | left eye |
| o.s. | oculus sinister | left eye |
| o.u. | oculo uterque | each eye |
| PANSS | | Positive and Negative Symptom Scale |
| pc, post cib | post cibos | after meals |
| PCP | | phencyclidine |
| per | | through or by |
| PM | post meridiem | afternoon or evening |
| P.O. | per os | by mouth |
| P.R. | per rectum | rectally |
| prn | pro re nata | as needed |
| PTSD | | post-traumatic stress disorder |
| pulv | pulvis | a powder |
| q | | every |
| qad | quoque alternis die | every other day |
| qd | | every day |
| qh | quiaque hora | every hour |
| qid | quater in die | four times a day |
| qod | | every other day |
| qs | quantum sufficiat | a sufficient quantity |
| qs ad | | a sufficient quantity to make |
| qty | | quantity |
| qv | quam volueris | as much as you wish |
| REM | | rapid eye movement |
| Rx | recipe | take, a recipe |
| rep | repetatur | let it be repeated |
| $\bar{s}$ | sine | without |
| sa | secundum artem | according to art |
| sat | sataratus | saturated |
| S.C. | | subcutaneous |
| sig | signa | label, or let it be printed |
| sol | solutio | solution |
| solv | | dissolve |
| sos | si opus sit | if there is need |
| $\overline{ss}$ | semis | one-half |
| SSRIs | | selective serotonin reuptake inhibitors |
| stat | statim | at once, immediately |

| Abbreviation | From | Meaning |
|---|---|---|
| STD | | sexually transmitted disease |
| supp | suppositorium | suppository |
| syr | syrupus | syrup |
| tab | tabella | tablet |
| tal | | such |
| TCA | | tricyclic antidepressant |
| TD | | tardive dyskinesia |
| tid | ter in die | three times a day |
| tr, tinct | tincture | tincture |
| trit | | triturate |
| tsp | | teaspoonful |
| ung | unguentum | ointment |
| USAN | | United States Adopted Names |
| USP | | United States Pharmacopeia |
| u.d., ut dict | ut dictum | as directed |
| v.o. | | verbal order |
| VZV | | varicella zoster virus |
| w.a. | | while awake |
| x3 | | 3 times |
| x4 | | 4 times |
| YBOC | | Yale Brown Obsessive-Compulsive Scale |
| YMRS | | Young Mania Rating Scale |

# APOTHECARY/METRIC EQUIVALENTS

## Approximate Liquid Measures

Basic equivalent: 1 fluid ounce = 30 mL

Examples:

| | | | |
|---|---|---|---|
| 1 gallon | 3800 mL | 1 gallon | 128 fluid ounces |
| 1 quart | 960 mL | 1 quart | 32 fluid ounces |
| 1 pint | 480 mL | 1 pint | 16 fluid ounces |
| 8 fluid oz | 240 mL | 15 minims | 1 mL |
| 4 fluid oz | 120 mL | 10 minims | 0.6 mL |

## Approximate Household Equivalents

| | | | |
|---|---|---|---|
| 1 teaspoonful | 5 mL | 1 tablespoonful | 15 mL |

## Weights

Basic equivalents:

| | | | |
|---|---|---|---|
| 1 oz | 30 g | 15 gr | 1 g |

Examples:

| | | | |
|---|---|---|---|
| 4 oz | 120 g | 1 gr | 60 mg |
| 2 oz | 60 g | 1/100 gr | 600 mcg |
| 10 gr | 600 mg | 1/150 gr | 400 mcg |
| 7½ gr | 500 mg | 1/200 gr | 300 mcg |
| 16 oz | 1 lb | | |

## Metric Conversions

Basic equivalents:

| | | | |
|---|---|---|---|
| 1 g | 1000 mg | 1 mg | 1000 mcg |

Examples:

| | | | |
|---|---|---|---|
| 5 g | 5000 mg | 5 mg | 5000 mcg |
| 0.5 g | 500 mg | 0.5 g | 500 mcg |
| 0.05 g | 50 mg | 0.05 mg | 50 mcg |

## Exact Equivalents

| | | | | | |
|---|---|---|---|---|---|
| 1 g | = | 15.43 gr | 0.1 mg | = | 1/600 gr |
| 1 mL | = | 16.23 minims | 0.12 mg | = | 1/500 gr |
| 1 minim | = | 0.06 mL | 0.15 mg | = | 1/400 gr |
| 1 gr | = | 64.8 mg | 0.2 mg | = | 1/300 gr |
| 1 pint (pt) | = | 473.2 mL | 0.3 mg | = | 1/200 gr |
| 1 oz | = | 28.35 g | 0.4 mg | = | 1/150 gr |
| 1 lb | = | 453.6 g | 0.5 mg | = | 1/120 gr |
| 1 kg | = | 2.2 lbs | 0.6 mg | = | 1/100 gr |
| 1 qt | = | 946.4 mL | 0.8 mg | = | 1/80 gr |
| | | | 1 mg | = | 1/65 gr |

## Solids*

| | | |
|---|---|---|
| ¼ grain | = | 15 mg |
| ½ grain | = | 30 mg |
| 1 grain | = | 60 mg |
| 1½ grains | = | 90 mg |
| 5 grains | = | 300 mg |
| 10 grains | = | 600 mg |

*Use exact equivalents for compounding and calculations requiring a high degree of accuracy.

# AVERAGE WEIGHTS AND SURFACE AREAS

## Average Weight and Surface Area of Preterm Infants, Term Infants, and Children

| Age | Average Weight (kg)* | Approximate Surface Area ($m^2$) |
|---|---|---|
| **Weeks Gestation** | | |
| 26 | 0.9-1 | 0.1 |
| 30 | 1.3-1.5 | 0.12 |
| 32 | 1.6-2 | 0.15 |
| 38 | 2.9-3 | 0.2 |
| 40 (term infant at birth) | 3.1-4 | 0.25 |
| **Months** | | |
| 3 | 5 | 0.29 |
| 6 | 7 | 0.38 |
| 9 | 8 | 0.42 |
| **Year** | | |
| 1 | 10 | 0.49 |
| 2 | 12 | 0.55 |
| 3 | 15 | 0.64 |
| 4 | 17 | 0.74 |
| 5 | 18 | 0.76 |
| 6 | 20 | 0.82 |
| 7 | 23 | 0.90 |
| 8 | 25 | 0.95 |
| 9 | 28 | 1.06 |
| 10 | 33 | 1.18 |
| 11 | 35 | 1.23 |
| 12 | 40 | 1.34 |
| **Adults** | 70 | 1.73 |

*Weights from age 3 months and older are rounded off to the nearest kilogram.

# BODY SURFACE AREA OF ADULTS AND CHILDREN

### Calculating Body Surface Area in Children

In a child of average size, find weight and corresponding surface area on the boxed scale to the left; or, use the nomogram to the right. Lay a straightedge on the correct height and weight points for the child, then read the intersecting point on the surface area scale.

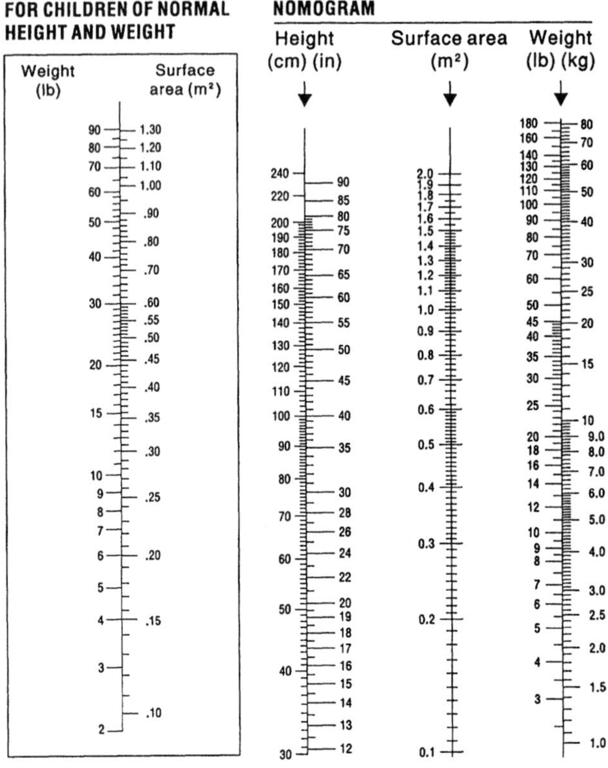


**BODY SURFACE AREA FORMULA**
**(Adult and Pediatric)**

$$BSA\ (m^2) = \sqrt{\frac{Ht\ (in) \times Wt\ (lb)}{3131}} \text{ or, in metric: } BSA\ (m^2) = \sqrt{\frac{Ht\ (cm) \times Wt\ (kg)}{3600}}$$

References

Lam TK and Leung DT, "More on Simplified Calculation of Body Surface Area," *N Engl J Med*, 1988, 318(17):1130 (Letter).

Mosteller RD, "Simplified Calculation of Body Surface Area", *N Engl J Med*, 1987, 317(17):1098 (Letter).

# IDEAL BODY WEIGHT CALCULATION

**Adults** (18 years and older) (IBW is in kg)

| | | |
|---|---|---|
| IBW (male) | = | 50 + (2.3 x height in inches over 5 feet) |
| IBW (female) | = | 45.5 + (2.3 x height in inches over 5 feet) |

**Children** (IBW is in kg; height is in cm)

a. 1-18 years
   $IBW = \frac{(height^2 \times 1.65)}{1000}$

b. 5 feet and taller
   IBW (male) = 39 + (2.27 x height in inches over 5 feet)
   IBW (female) = 42.2 + (2.27 x height in inches over 5 feet)

# MILLIEQUIVALENT AND MILLIMOLE CALCULATIONS & CONVERSIONS

## DEFINITIONS & CALCULATONS

### Definitions

| | | |
|---|---|---|
| mole | = | gram molecular weight of a substance (aka molar weight) |
| millimole (mM) | = | milligram molecular weight of a substance (a millimole is 1/1000 of a mole) |
| equivalent weight | = | gram weight of a substance which will combine with or replace one gram (one mole) of hydrogen; an equivalent weight can be determined by dividing the molar weight of a substance by its ionic valence |
| milliequivalent (mEq) | = | milligram weight of a substance which will combine with or replace one milligram (one millimole) of hydrogen (a milliequivalent is 1/1000 of an equivalent) |

### Calculations

| | | |
|---|---|---|
| moles | = | $\frac{\text{weight of a substance (grams)}}{\text{molecular weight of that substance (grams)}}$ |
| millimoles | = | $\frac{\text{weight of a substance (milligrams)}}{\text{molecular weight of that substance (milligrams)}}$ |
| equivalents | = | moles x valence of ion |
| milliequivalents | = | millimoles x valence of ion |
| moles | = | $\frac{\text{equivalents}}{\text{valence of ion}}$ |
| millimoles | = | $\frac{\text{milliequivalents}}{\text{valence of ion}}$ |
| millimoles | = | moles x 1000 |
| milliequivalents | = | equivalents x 1000 |

**Note:** Use of equivalents and milliequivalents is valid only for those substances which have fixed ionic valences (eg, sodium, potassium, calcium, chlorine, magnesium bromine, etc). For substances with variable ionic valences (eg, phosphorous), a reliable equivalent value cannot be determined. In these instances, one should calculate millimoles (which are fixed and reliable) rather than milliequivalents.

## MILLIEQUIVALENT CONVERSIONS

To convert mg/100 mL to mEq/L the following formula may be used:

$$\frac{\text{(mg/100 mL) x 10 x valence}}{\text{atomic weight}} = \text{mEq/L}$$

To convert mEq/L to mg/100 mL the following formula may be used:

$$\frac{\text{(mEq/L) x atomic weight}}{\text{10 x valence}} = \text{mg/100 mL}$$

To convert mEq/L to volume of percent of a gas the following formula may be used:

$$\frac{\text{(mEq/L) x 22.4}}{10} = \text{volume percent}$$

## MILLIEQUIVALENT AND MILLIMOLE CALCULATIONS & CONVERSIONS *(Continued)*

### Valences and Atomic Weights of Selected Ions

| Substance | Electrolyte | Valence | Molecular Wt |
|---|---|---|---|
| Calcium | $Ca^{++}$ | 2 | 40 |
| Chloride | $Cl^{-}$ | 1 | 35.5 |
| Magnesium | $Mg^{++}$ | 2 | 24 |
| Phosphate | $HPO_4^{--}$(80%) | 1.8 | 96* |
| pH = 7.4 | $H_2PO_4^{-}$(20%) | 1.8 | 96* |
| Potassium | $K^{+}$ | 1 | 39 |
| Sodium | $Na^{+}$ | 1 | 23 |
| Sulfate | $SO_4^{--}$ | 2 | 96* |

*The molecular weight of phosphorus only is 31, and sulfur only is 32.

### Approximate Milliequivalents — Weights of Selected Ions

| Salt | mEq/g Salt | Mg Salt/mEq |
|---|---|---|
| Calcium carbonate ($CaCO_3$) | 20 | 50 |
| Calcium chloride ($CaCl_2 - 2H_2O$) | 14 | 73 |
| Calcium gluconate (Ca gluconate$_2$ – $1H_2O$) | 4 | 224 |
| Calcium lactate (Ca lactate$_2$ – $5H_2O$) | 6 | 154 |
| Magnesium sulfate ($MgSO_4$) | 16 | 60 |
| Magnesium sulfate ($MgSO_4 - 7H_2O$) | 8 | 123 |
| Potassium acetate (K acetate) | 10 | 98 |
| Potassium chloride (KCl) | 13 | 75 |
| Potassium citrate ($K_3$ citrate – $1H_2O$) | 9 | 108 |
| Potassium iodide (KI) | 6 | 166 |
| Sodium bicarbonate ($NaHCO_3$) | 12 | 84 |
| Sodium chloride (NaCl) | 17 | 58 |
| Sodium citrate ($Na_3$ citrate – $2H_2O$) | 10 | 98 |
| Sodium iodine (NaI) | 7 | 150 |
| Sodium lactate (Na lactate) | 9 | 112 |

## CORRECTED SODIUM

Corrected $Na^+$ = measured $Na^+$ + [1.5 x (glucose - 150 divided by 100)]

**Note:** Do not correct for glucose <150.

## WATER DEFICIT

Water deficit = 0.6 x body weight [1 - (140 divided by $Na^+$)]

**Note: Body weight** is estimated weight in kg when fully hydrated; **$Na^+$** is serum or plasma sodium. Use corrected $Na^+$ if necessary. Consult medical references for recommendations for replacement of deficit.

## TOTAL SERUM CALCIUM CORRECTED FOR ALBUMIN LEVEL

[(Normal albumin - patient's albumin) x 0.8] + patient's measured total calcium

## ACID-BASE ASSESSMENT

**Henderson-Hasselbalch Equation**

$$pH = 6.1 + \log (HCO_3^- / (0.03)(pCO_2))$$

**Alveolar Gas Equation**

$PiO_2$ = $FiO_2$ x (total atmospheric pressure – vapor pressure of $H_2O$ at 37°C)
= $FiO_2$ x (760 mm Hg – 47 mm Hg)

$PaO_2$ = $PiO_2 - PaCO_2 / R$

Alveolar/arterial oxygen gradient = $PAO_2 - PaO_2$

Normal ranges:

| | |
|---|---|
| Children | 15-20 mm Hg |
| Adults | 20-25 mm Hg |

where:

| | | |
|---|---|---|
| $P_iO_2$ | = | Oxygen partial pressure of inspired gas (mm Hg) (150 mm Hg in room air at sea level) |
| $FiO_2$ | = | Fractional pressure of oxygen in inspired gas (0.21 in room air) |
| $PAO_2$ | = | Alveolar oxygen partial pressure |
| $PaCO_2$ | = | Alveolar carbon dioxide partial pressure |
| $PaO_2$ | = | Arterial oxygen partial pressure |
| R | = | Respiratory exchange quotient (typically 0.8, increases with high carbohydrate diet, decreases with high fat diet) |

### Acid-Base Disorders

Acute metabolic acidosis (<12 h duration):

$$PaCO_2 \text{ expected} = 1.5\ (HCO_3^-) + 8 \pm 2$$

or

$$\text{expected change in pCO} = (1\text{-}1.5) \times \text{change in } HCO_3^-$$

Acute metabolic alkalosis (<12 h duration):

$$\text{expected change in } pCO_2 = (0.5\text{-}1) \times \text{change in } HCO_3^-$$

Acute respiratory acidosis (<6 h duration):

$$\text{expected change in } HCO_3^- = 0.1 \times pCO_2$$

Acute respiratory acidosis (>6 h duration):

$$\text{expected change in } HCO_3^- = 0.4 \times \text{change in } pCO_2$$

Acute respiratory alkalosis (<6 h duration):

$$\text{expected change in } HCO_3^- = 0.2 \times \text{change in } pCO_2$$

Acute respiratory alkalosis (>6 h duration):

$$\text{expected change in } HCO_3^- = 0.5 \times \text{change in } pCO_2$$

## ACID-BASE EQUATION

$H^+$ (in mEq/L) = (24 x $PaCO_2$) divided by $HCO_3^-$

## Aa GRADIENT

Aa Gradient [(713)($FiO_2$ - ($PaCO_2$ divided by 0.8))] - $PaO_2$

| | | |
|---|---|---|
| Aa gradient | = | alveolar-arterial oxygen gradient |
| $FiO_2$ | = | inspired oxygen (expressed as a fraction) |
| $PaCO_2$ | = | arterial partial pressure carbon dioxide (mm Hg) |
| $PaO_2$ | = | arterial partial pressure oxygen (mm Hg) |

## OSMOLALITY

**Definition:** The summed concentrations of all osmotically active solute particles.

Predicted serum osmolality =

2 $Na^+$ + glucose (mg/dL) / 18 + BUN (mg/dL) / 2.8

The normal range of serum osmolality is 285-295 mOsm/L

## MILLIEQUIVALENT AND MILLIMOLE CALCULATIONS & CONVERSIONS *(Continued)*

Differential diagnosis of increased serum osmolal gap (>10 mOsm/L)

Medications and toxins
- Alcohols (ethanol, methanol, isopropanol, glycerol, ethylene glycol)
- Mannitol
- Paraldehyde

**Calculated Osm**

Osmolal gap = measured Osm - calculated Osm

0 to +10: Normal
>10: Abnormal
<0: Probable lab or calculation error

## BICARBONATE DEFICIT

$HCO_3^-$ deficit = (0.4 x wt in kg) x ($HCO_3^-$ desired – $HCO_3^-$ measured)

**Note:** In clinical practice, the calculated quantity may differ markedly from the actual amount of bicarbonate needed or that which may be safely administered.

## ANION GAP

**Definition:** The difference in concentration between unmeasured cation and anion equivalents in serum.

Anion gap = $Na^+ - Cl^- + HCO_3^-$
(The normal anion gap is 10-14 mEq/L)

**Differential Diagnosis of Increased Anion Gap Acidosis**

Organic anions
- Lactate (sepsis, hypovolemia, seizures, large tumor burden)
- Pyruvate
- Uremia
- Ketoacidosis (β-hydroxybutyrate and acetoacetate)
- Amino acids and their metabolites
- Other organic acids

Inorganic anions
- Hyperphosphatemia
- Sulfates
- Nitrates

**Differential Diagnosis of Decreased Anion Gap**

Organic cations
- Hypergammaglobulinemia

Inorganic cations
- Hyperkalemia
- Hypercalcemia
- Hypermagnesemia

Medications and toxins
- Lithium

Hypoalbuminemia

## RETICULOCYTE INDEX

(% retic divided by 2) x (patients Hct divided by normal Hct) or (% retic divided by 2) x (patient's Hgb divided by normal Hgb)

Normal index: 1.0
Good marrow response: 2.0-6.0

# POUNDS/KILOGRAMS CONVERSION

**1 pound = 0.45359 kilograms**
**1 kilogram = 2.2 pounds**

| lb | = | kg | lb | = | kg | lb | = | kg |
|---|---|---|---|---|---|---|---|---|
| 1 | | 0.45 | 70 | | 31.75 | 140 | | 63.50 |
| 5 | | 2.27 | 75 | | 34.02 | 145 | | 65.77 |
| 10 | | 4.54 | 80 | | 36.29 | 150 | | 68.04 |
| 15 | | 6.80 | 85 | | 38.56 | 155 | | 70.31 |
| 20 | | 9.07 | 90 | | 40.82 | 160 | | 72.58 |
| 25 | | 11.34 | 95 | | 43.09 | 165 | | 74.84 |
| 30 | | 13.61 | 100 | | 45.36 | 170 | | 77.11 |
| 35 | | 15.88 | 105 | | 47.63 | 175 | | 79.38 |
| 40 | | 18.14 | 110 | | 49.90 | 180 | | 81.65 |
| 45 | | 20.41 | 115 | | 52.16 | 185 | | 83.92 |
| 50 | | 22.68 | 120 | | 54.43 | 190 | | 86.18 |
| 55 | | 24.95 | 125 | | 56.70 | 195 | | 88.45 |
| 60 | | 27.22 | 130 | | 58.91 | 200 | | 90.72 |
| 65 | | 29.48 | 135 | | 61.24 | | | |

# TEMPERATURE CONVERSION

**Celsius to Fahrenheit = (°C x 9/5) + 32 = °F**
**Fahrenheit to Celsius = (°F -32) x 5/9 = °C**

| °C | = | °F | °C | = | °F | °C | = | °F |
|---|---|---|---|---|---|---|---|---|
| 100.0 | | 212.0 | 39.0 | | 102.2 | 36.8 | | 98.2 |
| 50.0 | | 122.0 | 38.8 | | 101.8 | 36.6 | | 97.9 |
| 41.0 | | 105.8 | 38.6 | | 101.5 | 36.4 | | 97.5 |
| 40.8 | | 105.4 | 38.4 | | 101.1 | 36.2 | | 97.2 |
| 40.6 | | 105.1 | 38.2 | | 100.8 | 36.0 | | 96.8 |
| 40.4 | | 104.7 | 38.0 | | 100.4 | 35.8 | | 96.4 |
| 40.2 | | 104.4 | 37.8 | | 100.1 | 35.6 | | 96.1 |
| 40.0 | | 104.0 | 37.6 | | 99.7 | 35.4 | | 95.7 |
| 39.8 | | 103.6 | 37.4 | | 99.3 | 35.2 | | 95.4 |
| 39.6 | | 103.3 | 37.2 | | 99.0 | 35.0 | | 95.0 |
| 39.4 | | 102.9 | 37.0 | | 98.6 | 0 | | 32.0 |
| 39.2 | | 102.6 | | | | | | |

# CREATININE CLEARANCE ESTIMATING METHODS IN PATIENTS WITH STABLE RENAL FUNCTION

These formulas provide an acceptable estimate of the patient's creatinine clearance **except** in the following instances.

- Patient's serum creatinine is changing rapidly (either up or down).
- Patients are markedly emaciated.

In above situations, certain assumptions have to be made.

- In patients with rapidly rising serum creatinines (ie, >0.5-0.7 mg/dL/day), it is best to assume that the patient's creatinine clearance is probably <10 mL/minute.
- In emaciated patients, although their actual creatinine clearance is less than their calculated creatinine clearance (because of decreased creatinine production), it is not possible to easily predict how much less.

**Infants**

**Estimation of creatinine clearance using serum creatinine and body length** (to be used when an adequate timed specimen cannot be obtained). **Note:** This formula may not provide an accurate estimation of creatinine clearance for infants younger than 6 months of age and for patients with severe starvation or muscle wasting.

$Cl_{cr} = K \times L/S_{cr}$

where:

$Cl_{cr}$ = creatinine clearance in mL/minute/1.73 $m^2$
K = constant of proportionality that is age specific

| Age | K |
|---|---|
| Low birth weight ≤1 y | 0.33 |
| Full-term ≤1 y | 0.45 |
| 2-12 y | 0.55 |
| 13-21 y female | 0.55 |
| 13-21 y male | 0.70 |

L = length in cm
$S_{cr}$ = serum creatinine concentration in mg/dL

**Reference**

Schwartz GJ, Brion LP, and Spitzer A, "The Use of Plasma Creatinine Concentration for Estimating Glomerular Filtration Rate in Infants, Children, and Adolescents," *Pediatr Clin North Amer,* 1987, 34(3):571-90.

**Children** (1-18 years)

Method 1: (Traub SL and Johnson CE, "Comparison of Methods of Estimating Creatinine Clearance in Children," *Am J Hosp Pharm,* 1980, 37(2):195-201)

$$Cl_{cr} = \frac{0.48 \times (\text{height}) \times BSA}{S_{cr} \times 1.73}$$

where

BSA = body surface area in $m^2$
$Cl_{cr}$ = creatinine clearance in mL/min
$S_{cr}$ = serum creatinine in mg/dL
Height = in cm

Method 2: Nomogram (Traub SL and Johnson CE, "Comparison of Methods of Estimating Creatinine Clearance in Children," *Am J Hosp Pharm*, 1980, 37(2):195-201)

**Children 1-18 Years**

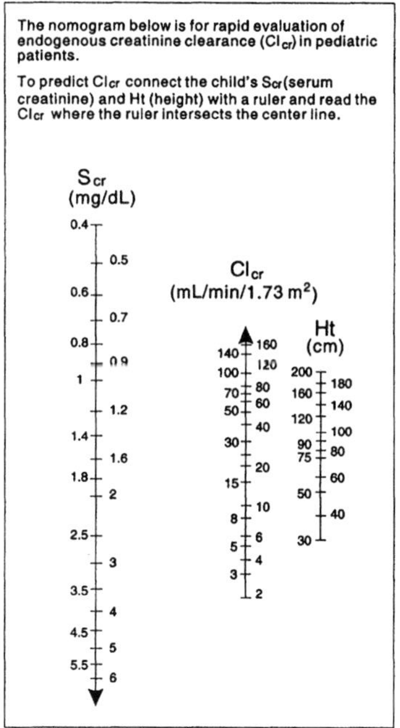

The nomogram below is for rapid evaluation of endogenous creatinine clearance ($Cl_{cr}$) in pediatric patients.
To predict $Cl_{cr}$ connect the child's $S_{cr}$ (serum creatinine) and Ht (height) with a ruler and read the $Cl_{cr}$ where the ruler intersects the center line.
$S_{cr}$ (mg/dL)
$Cl_{cr}$ (mL/min/1.73 m$^2$)
Ht (cm)


**Adults** (18 years and older)

(Cockcroft DW and Gault MH, "Prediction of Creatinine Clearance From Serum Creatinine," *Nephron*, 1976, 16(1):31-41)

Estimated creatinine clearance ($Cl_{cr}$):
(mL/min)

$$\text{Male} = \frac{(140 - \text{age})\ \text{IBW (kg)}}{72 \times \text{serum creatinine}}$$

$$\text{Female} = \text{estimated } Cl_{cr} \text{ male} \times 0.85$$

**Note:** The use of the patient's ideal body weight (IBW) is recommended for the above formula except when the patient's actual body weight is less than ideal. Use of the IBW is especially important in obese patients.

# RENAL FUNCTION TESTS

**Endogenous creatinine clearance vs age** (timed collection)

Creatinine clearance (mL/min/1.73 m$^2$) = ($Cr_u V/Cr_s T$) (1.73/A)

where:

| | | |
|---|---|---|
| $Cr_u$ | = | urine creatinine concentration (mg/dL) |
| V | = | total urine collected during sampling period (mL) |
| $Cr_s$ | = | serum creatinine concentration (mg/dL) |
| T | = | duration of sampling period (min) (24 h = 1440 min) |
| A | = | body surface area (m$^2$) |

Age-specific normal values

| | |
|---|---|
| 5-7 d | 50.6 ± 5.8 mL/min/1.73 m$^2$ |
| 1-2 mo | 64.6 ± 5.8 mL/min/1.73 m$^2$ |
| 5-8 mo | 87.7 ± 11.9 mL/min/1.73 m$^2$ |
| 9-12 mo | 86.9 ± 8.4 mL/min/1.73 m$^2$ |
| ≥18 mo | |
| male | 124 ± 26 mL/min/1.73 m$^2$ |
| female | 109 ± 13.5 mL/min/1.73 m$^2$ |
| Adults | |
| male | 105 ± 14 mL/min/1.73 m$^2$ |
| female | 95 ± 18 mL/min/1.73 m$^2$ |

**Note:** In patients with renal failure ($Cl_{cr}$ <25 mL/min), creatinine clearance may be elevated over GFR because of tubular secretion of creatinine.

**Calculation of Creatinine Clearance From a 24-Hour Urine Collection**

Equation 1:

$$Cl_{cr} = \frac{(U) \times (V)}{P}$$

| | | |
|---|---|---|
| $Cl_{cr}$ | = | creatinine clearance |
| U | = | urine concentration of creatinine |
| V | = | total urine volume in the collection |
| P | = | plasma creatinine concentration |

Equation 2:

$$Cl_{cr} = \frac{\text{(total urine volume [mL]) x (urine Cr concentration [mg/dL])}}{\text{(serum creatinine [mg/dL]) x (time of urine collection [minutes])}}$$

Occasionally, a patient will have a 12- or 24-hour urine collection done for direct calculation of creatinine clearance. Although a urine collection for 24 hours is best, it is difficult to do since many urine collections occur for a much shorter period. A 24-hour urine collection is the desired duration of urine collection because the urine excretion of creatinine is diurnal and thus the measured creatinine clearance will vary throughout the day as the creatinine in the urine varies. When the urine collection is less than 24 hours, the total excreted creatinine will be affected by the time of the day during which the collection is performed. A 24-hour urine collection is sufficient to be able to accurately average the diurnal creatinine excretion variations. If a patient has 24 hours of urine collected for creatinine clearance, equation 1 can be used for calculating the creatinine clearance. To use equation 1 to calculate the creatinine clearance, it will be necessary to know the duration of urine collection, the urine collection volume, the urine creatinine concentration, and the serum creatinine value that reflects the urine collection period. In most cases, a serum creatinine concentration is drawn anytime during the day, but it is best to have the value drawn halfway through the collection period.

### Amylase/Creatinine Clearance Ratio*

$$\frac{\text{Amylase}_u \times \text{creatinine}_p}{\text{Amylase}_p \times \text{creatinine}_u} \times 100$$

u = urine; p = plasma

### Serum BUN/Serum Creatinine Ratio

Serum BUN (mg/dL:serum creatinine (mg/dL))

Normal BUN:creatinine ratio is 10-15

BUN:creatinine ratio >20 suggests prerenal azotemia (also seen with high urea-generation states such as GI bleeding)

BUN:creatinine ratio <5 may be seen with disorders affecting urea biosynthesis such as urea cycle enzyme deficiencies and with hepatitis.

### Fractional Sodium Excretion

Fractional sodium secretion (FENa) = $Na_uCr_s/Na_sCr_u$ x 100%

where:

| | | |
|---|---|---|
| $Na_u$ | = | urine sodium (mEq/L) |
| $Na_s$ | = | serum sodium (mEq/L) |
| $Cr_u$ | = | urine creatinine (mg/dL) |
| $Cr_s$ | = | serum creatinine (mg/dL) |

FENa <1% suggests prerenal failure

FENa >2% suggest intrinsic renal failure

(for newborns, normal FENa is approximately 2.5%)

**Note:** Disease states associated with a falsely elevated FENa include severe volume depletion (>10%), early acute tubular necrosis and volume depletion in chronic renal disease. Disorders associated with a lowered FENa include acute glomerulonephritis, hemoglobinuric or myoglobinuric renal failure, nonoliguric acute tubular necrosis and acute urinary tract obstruction. In addition, FENa may be <1% in patients with acute renal failure **and** a second condition predisposing to sodium retention (eg, burns, congestive heart failure, nephrotic syndrome).

### Urine Calcium/Urine Creatinine Ratio (spot sample)

Urine calcium (mg/dL): urine creatinine (mg/dL)

Normal values <0.21 (mean values 0.08 males, 0.06 females)

Premature infants show wide variability of calcium:creatinine ratio, and tend to have lower thresholds for calcium loss than older children. Prematures without nephrolithiasis had mean Ca:Cr ratio of 0.75 ± 0.76. Infants with nephrolithiasis had mean Ca:Cr ratio of 1.32 ± 1.03 (Jacinto, et al, *Pediatrics*, Vol 81, p 31.)

### Urine Protein/Urine Creatinine Ratio (spot sample)

| $P_u/Cr_u$ | Total Protein Excretion (mg/m²/d) |
|---|---|
| 0.1 | 80 |
| 1 | 800 |
| 10 | 8000 |

where:

$P_u$ = urine protein concentration (mg/dL)

$Cr_u$ = urine creatinine concentration (mg/dL)

# ANGIOTENSIN-RELATED AGENTS

## Comparisons of Indications and Adult Dosages

| Drug | Hypertension | CHF | Renal Dysfunction | Dialyzable | Tablet Strengths (mg) |
|---|---|---|---|---|---|
| Benazepril | 20-80 mg qd<br>qd-bid<br>Maximum: 80 mg qd | Not FDA approved | $Cl_{cr}$ <30 mL/min: 5 mg/day initially<br>Maximum: 40 mg qd | Yes | Tablets<br>5, 10, 20, 40 |
| Candesartan† | 8-32 mg qd<br>qd-bid<br>Maximum: 32 mg qd | Not FDA approved | No adjustment necessary | No | Tablets<br>4, 8, 16, 32 |
| Captopril | 25-150 mg qd<br>bid-tid<br>Maximum: 450 mg qd | 6.25-100 mg tid<br>Maximum: 450 mg qd | $Cl_{cr}$ 10-50 mL/min: 75% of usual dose<br>$Cl_{cr}$ <10 mL/min: 50% of usual dose | Yes | Tablets<br>12.5, 25, 50, 100 |
| Enalapril | 5-40 mg qd<br>qd-bid<br>Maximum: 40 mg qd | 2.5-20 mg bid<br>Maximum: 20 mg bid | $Cl_{cr}$ 30-80 mL/min: 5 mg/day initially<br>$Cl_{cr}$ <30 mL/min: 2.5 mg/day initially | Yes | Tablets<br>2.5, 5, 10, 20 |
| (Enalaprilat*) | (0.625 mg, 1.25 mg, 2.5 mg<br>q6h<br>Maximum: 5 mg q6h) | (Not FDA approved) | $Cl_{cr}$ <30 mL/min: 0.625 mg) | (Yes) | (2.5 mg/2 mL vial) |
| Eprosartan† | 400-800 mg qd<br>qd-bid | Not FDA approved | No dosage adjustment necessary | Unknown | Tablets<br>400, 600 |
| Fosinopril | 10-40 mg qd<br>Maximum: 80 mg qd | 10-40 mg qd | No dosage reduction necessary | Not well dialyzed | Tablets<br>10, 20 |
| Irbesartan† | 150 mg qd<br>Maximum: 300 mg qd | Not FDA approved | No dosage reduction necessary | No | Tablets<br>75, 150, 300 |
| Lisinopril | 10-40 mg qd<br>Maximum: 80 mg qd | 5-20 mg qd | $Cl_{cr}$ 10-30 mL/min: 5 mg/day initially<br>$Cl_{cr}$ <10 mL/min: 2.5 mg/day initially | Yes | Tablets<br>5, 10, 20, 40 |
| Losartan† | 25-100 mg qd or bid | Not FDA approved | No adjustment needed | No | Tablets<br>25, 50 |
| Moexipril | 7.5-30 mg qd<br>qd-bid<br>Maximum: 30 mg qd | Not FDA approved | $Cl_{cr}$ <30 mL/min: 3.75 mg/day initially<br>Maximum: 15 mg/day | Unknown | Tablets<br>7.5, 15 |
| Perindopril | 4-16 mg qd | 4 mg qd<br>(Not FDA approved) | $Cl_{cr}$ 30-60 mL/min: 2 mg qd<br>$Cl_{cr}$ 15-29 mL/min: 2 mg qod<br>$Cl_{cr}$ <15 mL/min: 2 mg on dialysis days | Yes | Tablets<br>2, 4, 8 |
| Quinapril | 10-80 mg qd<br>qd-bid | 5-20 mg bid | $Cl_{cr}$ 30-60 mL/min: 5 mg/day initially<br>$Cl_{cr}$ <10 mL/min: 2.5 mg qd initially | Not well dialyzed | Tablets<br>5, 10, 20, 40 |
| Ramipril | 2.5-20 mg qd<br>qd-bid | 2.5-20 mg qd | $Cl_{cr}$ <40 mL/min: 1.25 mg/day<br>Maximum: 5 mg qd | Unknown | Capsules<br>1.25, 2.5, 5 |
| Telmisartan† | 20-80 mg qd | Not FDA approved | No dosage reduction necessary | No | Tablets<br>40, 80 |
| Trandolapril | 2-4 mg qd<br>maximum: 8 mg/d<br>qd-bid | Not FDA approved | $Cl_{cr}$ <30 mL/min: 0.5 mg/day initially | No | Tablets<br>1 mg, 2 mg, 4 mg |
| Valsartan† | 80-160 mg qd | Not FDA approved | Decrease dose only if $Cl_{cr}$ <10 mL/min | No | Capsules<br>80, 160 |

*Enalaprilat is the only available ACEI in a parenteral formulation.

†Angiotensin II antagonist

Dosage is based on 70 kg adult with normal hepatic and renal function.

## Comparative Pharmacokinetics

| Drug | Prodrug | Lipid Solubility | Absorption (%) | Serum $t_{1/2}$ (h) | Serum Protein Binding (%) | Elimination | Onset of Hypotensive Action (h) | Peak Hypotensive Effects (h) | Duration of Hypotensive Effects (h) |
|---|---|---|---|---|---|---|---|---|---|
| Benazepril | Yes | No data | 37 | 10-12 | >95 | Primarily renal, some biliary | 0.5-1 | 0.5-1 | 24 |
| Benazeprilat | | | | | | | | | |
| Captopril | No | Not very lipophilic | 75 | <2 | 25-30 | Metabolism to disulfide, then renally | 0.25-0.5 | 0.5-1.5 | 6-12 |
| Enalapril | Yes | Lipophilic | 60 (53-73) | 1.3 | 50-60 | Renal | 1 | 4-6 | 24 |
| Enalaprilat | | | | 11 | | | 0.25 | 3-4 | ~6 |
| Fosinopril | Yes | Very lipophilic | 36 | 12 | >95 | Renal 50% Hepatic 50% | 1 | ~3 | 24 |
| Fosinoprilat | | | | | | | | | |
| Lisinopril | No | Very hydrophilic | 25 (6-60) | 12 | 0 | Renal | 1 | ~7 | 24 |
| Moexipril | Yes | No data | | 2-9 | ≥50 | Urine 13% Feces 53% | 1 | | 24 |
| Perindopril | Yes | | 65-95 | 1.5-3 | 10-20 | Hepatic/Renal | | 1 | |
| Perindoprilat | | | | 25-30 | 60 | | | 3-4 | |
| Quinapril | Yes | No data | 60 | 0.8 | 97 | Renal 61% Hepatic 37% | 1 | 1 | 24 |
| Quinaprilat | | | | 2 | | | | | |
| Ramipril | Yes | Somewhat lipophilic | 50-100 | 1-2 | 73 | Renal | 1-2 | 1 | 24 |
| Ramiprilat | | | | 13-17 | 56 | | | | |
| Trandolapril | Yes | Very lipophilic | 10-70 | 0.6-1.1 | 80 | Hepatic/Renal | 0.5 | 2-4 | ≥24 |
| Trandolaprilat | | | 40-60 | 16-24 | 94 | | | | |

# ANTICHOLINERGIC EFFECTS OF COMMON PSYCHOTROPICS

| Drug | Atropine Equivalence Factor* | Common Daily Dose (mg) | Atropine Equivalent (mg/dose) |
|---|---|---|---|
| **ANTICHOLINERGICS** | | | |
| Benztropine | 0.849 | 2 | 1.70 |
| Diphenhydramine | 0.011 | 50 | 0.55 |
| Trihexyphenidyl | 0.828 | 5 | 4.14 |
| **NEUROLEPTICS** | | | |
| Chlorpromazine | 0.030 | 500 | 15.00 |
| Clozapine | 0.125 | 500 | 62.50 |
| Fluphenazine | 0.001 | 25 | 0.03 |
| Haloperidol | 0.000 | 20 | 0.00 |
| Loxapine | 0.005 | 150 | 0.75 |
| Mesoridazine | 0.025 | 150 | 3.75 |
| Molindone | 0.000 | 150 | 0.00 |
| Perphenazine | 0.001 | 32 | 0.03 |
| Thioridazine | 0.104 | 300 | 31.20 |
| Thiothixene | 0.001 | 40 | 0.04 |
| Trifluoperazine | 0.003 | 25 | 0.08 |
| **ANTIDEPRESSANTS** | | | |
| Amitriptyline | 0.121 | 150 | 18.15 |
| Amoxapine | 0.002 | 150 | 0.30 |
| Desipramine | 0.011 | 150 | 1.65 |
| Doxepin | 0.026 | 150 | 3.90 |
| Fluoxetine | 0.001 | 20 | 0.02 |
| Imipramine | 0.024 | 150 | 3.60 |
| Maprotiline | 0.004 | 150 | 0.60 |
| Nortriptyline | 0.015 | 75 | 1.13 |
| Trazodone | 0.000 | 100 | 0.00 |

*Anticholinergic effects of 1 mg of drug in equivalent mg of atropine.

## FREQUENTLY PRESCRIBED DRUGS FOR THE ELDERLY

| Drug* | Atropine Equivalent | Common Dose | Anticholinergic Drug Level (ng/mL of atropine equivalents) |
|---|---|---|---|
| Captopril | 1.5 | 75 | 0.02 |
| Cimetidine | 344 | 400 | 0.86 |
| Codeine | 9.9 | 90 | 0.11 |
| Digoxin | 0.03 | 0.125 | 0.25 |
| Dipyridamole | 24.8 | 225 | 0.11 |
| Dyazide | 2 | 25/37.5 | 0.08 |
| Furosemide | 8.8 | 40 | 0.22 |
| Isosorbide dinitrate | 9 | 60 | 0.15 |
| Nifedipine | 6.6 | 30 | 0.22 |
| Prednisolone | 11 | 20 | 0.55 |
| Ranitidine | 33 | 150 | 0.22 |
| Theophylline | 176 | 400 | 0.44 |
| Warfarin | 0.6 | 5 | 0.12 |

*At a $10^{-8}$ M concentration.

Adapted from Tune L, Carr S, Hoag E, et al, "Anticholinergic Effects of Drugs Commonly Prescribed for the Elderly: Potential Means for Assessing Risk of Delirium," *Am J Psychiatry*, 1992, 149(10):1393-4.

# ANTICONVULSANTS BY SEIZURE TYPE

| Seizure Type | Age | Commonly Used | Alternatives |
|---|---|---|---|
| Primarily generalized tonic-clonic seizures | 1-12 mo | Carbamazepine<br>Phenytoin<br>Phenobarbital | Valproate |
| | 1-6 y | Carbamazepine<br>Phenytoin<br>Phenobarbital | Valproate |
| | 6-11 y | Carbamazepine | Valproate<br>Phenytoin<br>Phenobarbital<br>Lamotrigine† |
| Primarily generalized tonic-clonic seizures with absence or with myoclonic seizures | 1 mo - 18 y | Valproate | Phenytoin‡<br>Phenobarbital‡<br>Carbamazepine‡ |
| Absence seizures | Any age | Ethosuximide | Valproate<br>Clonazepam<br>Diamox<br>Lamotrigine† |
| Myoclonic seizures | Any age | Valproate<br>Clonazepam | Phenytoin†<br>Phenobarbital† |
| Tonic and atonic seizures | Any age | Valproate | Phenytoin†<br>Clonazepam<br>Phenobarbital† |
| Partial seizures | 1-12 mo | Phenobarbital | Carbamazepine<br>Phenytoin |
| | 1-6 y | Carbamazepine | Phenytoin<br>Phenobarbital<br>Valproate†<br>Lamotrigine†<br>Oxcarbazepine (4-6 y)<br>Gabapentin |
| | 6-18 y | Carbamazepine | Lamotrigine<br>Phenytoin<br>Phenobarbital<br>Oxcarbazepine (6-16 y)<br>Tiagabine<br>Topiramate<br>Valproate† |
| Infantile spasms | | Corticotropin (ACTH) | Prednisone†<br>Valproate†<br>Clonazepam†<br>Diazepam† |

†Not FDA approved for this indication.

‡Phenytoin, phenobarbital, carbamazepine will not treat absence seizures. Addition of another anticonvulsant (ie, ethosuximide) would be needed.

# ANTIDEPRESSANT AGENTS

## Comparison of Usual Dosage, Mechanism of Action, and Adverse Effects of Antidepressants

| Drug | Initial Dose | Usual Dosage (mg/d) | Dosage Forms | Adverse Effects | | | | | | Comments |
|---|---|---|---|---|---|---|---|---|---|---|
| | | | | ACH | Drowsiness | Orthostatic Hypotension | Cardiac Arrhythmias | GI Distress | Weight Gain | |
| **TRICYCLIC ANTIDEPRESSANTS & RELATED COMPOUNDS**** | | | | | | | | | | |
| Amitriptyline (Elavil®, Enovil®) | 25-75 mg qhs | 100-300 | T, I | 4+ | 4+ | 4+ | 3+ | 1 | 4+ | Also used in chronic pain, migraine, and as a hypnotic |
| Amoxapine (Asendin®) | 50 mg bid | 100-400 | T | 2+ | 2+ | 2+ | 2+ | 0 | 2+ | May cause EPS |
| Clomipramine* (Anafranil®) | 25-75 mg qhs | 100-250 | C | 4+ | 4+ | 2+ | 3+ | 1+ | 4+ | Approved for OCD |
| Desipramine (Norpramin®) | 25-75 mg qhs | 100-300 | T | 1+ | 2+ | 2+ | 2+ | 0 | 1+ | Blood levels useful for therapeutic monitoring |
| Doxepin (Adapin®, Sinequan®) | 25-75 mg qhs | 100-300 | C, L | 3+ | 4+ | 2+ | 2+ | 0 | 4+ | |
| Imipramine (Janimine®, Tofranil®) | 25-75 mg qhs | 100-300 | T, C, I | 3+ | 3+ | 4+ | 3+ | 1+ | 4+ | Blood levels useful for therapeutic monitoring |
| Maprotiline (Ludiomil®) | 25-75 mg qhs | 100-225 | T | 2+ | 3+ | 2+ | 2+ | 0 | 2+ | |
| Nortriptyline (Aventyl®, Pamelor®) | 25-50 mg qhs | 50-150 | C, L | 2+ | 2+ | 1+ | 2+ | 0 | 1+ | Blood levels useful for therapeutic monitoring |
| Protriptyline (Vivactil®) | 15 mg qAM | 15-60 | T | 2+ | 1+ | 2+ | 3+ | 0 | 0 | |
| Trimipramine (Surmontil®) | 25-75 mg qhs | 100-300 | C | 4+ | 4+ | 3+ | 3+ | 0 | 4+ | |
| **SELECTIVE SEROTONIN REUPTAKE INHIBITORS††** | | | | | | | | | | |
| Citalopram (Celexa™) | 20 mg qAM | 20-60 | T | 0 | 0 | 0 | 0 | 3+§ | 0 | CYP2D6 inhibitor |
| Fluoxetine (Prozac®, Sarafem™) | 10-20 mg qAM | 20-80 | C, L, T | 0 | 0 | 0 | 0 | 3+§ | 0 | CYP2D6, 2C19, and 3A3/4 inhibitor |
| Fluvoxamine (Luvox®)* | 50 mg qhs | 100-300 | T | 0 | 0 | 0 | 0 | 3+§ | 0 | Contraindicated with astemizole, cisapride, terfenadine, CYP1A2, 2C19, and 3A3/4 inhibitors |
| Paroxetine (Paxil™) | 10-20 mg qAM | 20-50 | T, L | 1+ | 1+ | 0 | 0 | 3+§ | 1+ | CYP2D6 inhibitor |
| Sertraline (Zoloft™) | 25-50 mg qAM | 50-150 | T | 0 | 0 | 0 | 0 | 3+§ | 0 | CYP2D6 inhibitor |
| **DOPAMINE-REUPTAKE BLOCKING COMPOUNDS** | | | | | | | | | | |
| Bupropion (Wellbutrin®, Wellbutrin SR®, Zyban®) | 100 mg tid IR 150 mg for 3-7 days, then 150 mg bid SR | 300-450† | T | 0 | 0 | 0 | 1+ | 1+ | 0 | Contraindicated with seizures, bulimia, and anorexia; low incidence of sexual dysfunction |
| **SEROTONIN/NOREPINEPHRINE REUPTAKE INHIBITORS***** | | | | | | | | | | |
| Venlafaxine (Effexor®, Effexor-XR®) | 25 mg bid-tid IR 37.5 mg qd XR | 75-375 | T | 1+ | 1+ | 0 | 1+ | 3+§ | 0 | High-dose is useful to treat refractory depression |
| **5HT2 RECEPTOR ANTAGONIST PROPERTIES** | | | | | | | | | | |
| Nefazodone (Serzone®) | 100 mg bid | 300-600 | T | 1+ | 1+ | 0 | 0 | 1+ | 0 | Contraindicated with astemizole, cisapride, and terfenadine; caution with triazolam and alprazolam; low incidence of sexual dysfunction |
| Trazodone (Desyrel®) | 50 mg tid | 150-600 | T | 0 | 4+ | 3+ | 1+ | 1+ | 2+ | |
| **NORADRENERGIC ANTAGONIST** | | | | | | | | | | |
| Mirtazapine (Remeron®) | 15 mg qhs | 15-45 | T | 1+ | 3+ | 0 | 0 | 0 | 3+ | Dose >15 mg/d less sedating, low incidence of sexual dysfunction |
| **MONOAMINE OXIDASE INHIBITORS** | | | | | | | | | | |
| Phenelzine (Nardil®) | 15 mg tid | 15-90 | T | 2+ | 2+ | 2+ | 1+ | 1+ | 3+ | Diet must be low in tyramine; avoid concurrent sympathomimetics and other antidepressants |
| Tranylcypromine (Parnate®) | 10 mg bid | 10-60 | T | 2+ | 1+ | 2+ | 1+ | 1+ | 2+ | |

**IMPORTANT NOTE: A 1-week supply taken all at once in a patient receiving the maximum dose can be fatal.

*** Do not use with sibutramine; relatively safe in overdose.

Key: N = norepinephrine; S = serotonin; ACH = anticholinergic effects (dry mouth, blurred vision, urinary retention, constipation); 0 - 4+ = absent or rare - relatively common.
T= Tablet, L = Liquid, I = Injectable, C = Capsule

*Not approved by FDA for depression. Approved for OCD.

†Not to exceed 150 mg/dose to minimize seizure risk for IR and 200 mg/dose for SR.

††Flat dose response curve, headache, nausea, and sexual dysfunction are common side effects for SSRIs

§Nausea is usually mild and transient.

# ANTIPARKINSONIAN AGENTS

| Generic Name | Brand Name | Formulation | Dosage Range (mg/day) | Relative Oral Potency |
|---|---|---|---|---|
| | | **ANTICHOLINERGIC** | | |
| Benztropine | Cogentin®* | Tablet: 0.5 mg, 1 mg, 2 mg<br>Injection: 1 mg/mL (2 mL ampul) | 1-6 | 2 |
| Biperiden | Akineton® | Tablet: 2 mg<br>Injection: 5 mg/mL (1 mL ampul) | 2-8 | 2 |
| Orphenadrine | Norflex® | Tablet: 100 mg<br>Tablet, sustained release: 100 mg<br>Injection: 30 mg/mL (2 mL, 10 mL) | 50-400 | 50 |
| | | **ANTIHISTAMINIC** | | |
| Diphenhydramine | Benadryl®* | Capsule: 25 mg, 50 mg<br>Elixir: 12.5 mg/5 mL (4 oz, 8 oz, 16 oz bottle)<br>Injection: 10 mg/mL (10 mL, 30 mL); 50 mg/mL (1 mL, 10 mL)<br>Syrup: 12.5 mg/5 mL<br>Tablet: 25 mg, 50 mg | 25-300 | 25 |
| Ethopropazine | Parsidol® | Tablet: 10 mg, 50 mg | 100-400 | 50 |
| Procyclidine | Kemadrin® | Tablet: 5 mg | 7.5-20 | 5 |
| Trihexyphenidyl | Artane®* | Capsule: 5 mg<br>Tablet: 2 mg, 5 mg<br>Elixir: 2 mg/5 mL | 2-15 | 5 |
| | | **DOPAMINERGIC** | | |
| Amantadine | Symmetrel®*, Symadine® | Tablet: 100 mg<br>Syrup: 50 mg/5 mL (16 oz bottle) | 100-400 | N/A |

*Available in generic form.

# ANTIPSYCHOTIC AGENTS

| Antipsychotic Agent | Dosage Forms | I.M./P.O. Potency | Equiv. Dosages (approx) (mg) | Usual Adult Daily Maint. Dose (mg) | Sedation (Incidence) | Extrapyramidal Side Effects | Anticholinergic Side Effects | Cardiovascular Side Effects |
|---|---|---|---|---|---|---|---|---|
| Chlorpromazine (Thorazine®) | Cap, Conc, Inj, Supp, Syr, Tab | 4:1 | 100 | 200-1000 | High | Moderate | Moderate | Moderate/high |
| Chlorprothixine* (Taractan®) | | | 100 | 75-600 | High | Moderate | Moderate | Moderate |
| Clozapine (Clozaril®)* | Tab | | 50 | 75-900 | High | Very Low | High | High |
| Fluphenazine (Prolixin®, Permitil®) | Conc, Elix, Inj, Tab | 2:1 | 2 | 0.5-40 | Low | High | Low | Low |
| Haloperidol (Haldol®) | Conc, Inj, Tab | 2:1 | 2 | 1-15 | Low | High | Low | Low |
| Loxapine (Loxitane®) | Cap, Conc, Inj | | 10 | 25-250 | Moderate | Moderate | Low | Low |
| Mesoridazine (Serentil®) | Inj, Liq, Tab | 3:1 | 50 | 30-400 | High | Low | High | Moderate |
| Molindone (Moban®)† | Conc, Tab | | 15 | 15-225 | Low | Moderate | Low | Low |
| Olanzapine (Zyprexa™) | Tab | | 4 | 5-20 | Moderate/ High | Low | Moderate/High | Moderate/High |
| Perphenazine (Trilafon®) | Conc, Inj, Tab | | 10 | 16-64 | Low | Moderate | Low | Low |
| Pimozide (Orap™)‡ | Tab | | 2 | 1-20 | Moderate | High | Moderate | Low |
| Promazine (Sparine®) | Inj, Tab | | 200 | 40-1000 | Moderate | Moderate | High | Moderate |
| Quetiapine (Seroquel®) | Tab | | 80 | 75-750 | Moderate | Very Low | Moderate | Moderate |
| Risperidone (Risperdal®)# | Sol, Tab | | 1 | 1-16 | Low/ Moderate | Low | Low | Low |
| Thioridazine (Mellaril®)§ | Conc, Susp, Tab | | 100 | 200-800 | High | Low | High | Moderate/high |
| Thiothixene (Navane®) | Cap, Conc, Inj, Powder for inj | 4:1 | 4 | 5-40 | Low | High | Low | Low/moderate |
| Trifluoperazine (Stelazine®) | Conc, Inj, Tab | | 5 | 2-40 | Low | High | Low | Low |

NA = not available

*Withdrawn from market

## COMMENTS:

*Clozapine (Clozaril®): <1% incidence of agranulocytosis; weekly-biweekly CBC required

†Molindone (Moban®): May cause less weight gain

‡Pimozide (Orap®): Contraindicated with macrolide antibiotics, azole antifungals, protease inhibitors, nefazodone, zileuton, CYP3A inhibitors

#Risperidone (Risperdal®): Target dose: ≤6 mg/day

§Thioridazine (Mellaril®): May cause irreversible retinitis; pigmentosis at doses >800 mg/day; prolongs QTc

# ATYPICAL ANTIPSYCHOTICS*

| Drug | DR EPS | PROL | TD | ACH | SZ | OH | LFTs | SED | WT GAIN | NMS | AGRAN | TX REFR | DOSING |
|---|---|---|---|---|---|---|---|---|---|---|---|---|---|
| Clozapine (Clozaril®) | No | No | No | High | DD | High | Low | High | High | Yes | Yes | Yes | Initiate at 12.5 mg once or twice daily; increase 25-50 mg/d as tolerated; target: 300-500 mg given in 2-4 divided daily dose; range: 50-900 mg/d |
| Risperidone (Risperdal®) | Yes | Yes | Yes | Very low | Low | Mild | Very low | Moderate | Moderate | Yes | Yes** | No | Initiate 1 mg bid; target: 4-6 mg/d; range: 0.5-16 mg given in 1-2 divided daily doses |
| Olanzapine (Zyprexa®) | Yes | No | Yes | Moderate | Low | Moderate | Low | Moderate | Mod-High | Yes | Yes** | No | Initiate at 5-10 mg/d; increase by 5 mg/d at intervals of 1 week to target dose of 10-20 mg/d; range: 2.5-20 g given in 1-2 divided daily doses |
| Quetiapine (Seroquel®) | Maybe | No | ? | Moderate | Low | Moderate | Low | Moderate | Moderate | Yes | No | No | Initiate at 25 mg bid; increase by 50-100 mg/d as tolerated; target dose: 300-600 mg/d; range: 75-750 mg given in 2-3 divided daily doses |

*Defined as 1) decrease or no EPS at doses producing antipsychotic effect; 2) minimum or no increase in prolactin; 3) decrease in both positive and negative symptoms of schizophrenia.

**Case reports

DR EPS = dose related extrapyramidal symptoms

PROL = sustained prolactin elevation (may cause amenorrhea, galactorrhea, gynecomastia, impotence)

TD = tardive dyskinesia

ACH = anticholinergic side effects (dry mouth, blurred vision, constipation, urinary hesitancy)

SZ = seizures

OH = orthostatic hypotension (blood pressure drops upon standing)

LFTs = increase in liver function tests

SED = sedation

WT GAIN = weight gain

NMS = neuroleptic malignant syndrome

AGRAN = agranulocytosis (without white blood cells to fight infection)

TX REFR = treatment refractory

DOSING = initiation dose, target dose, and dosage range

DD = dose dependent

# BENZODIAZEPINES

| Agent | Dosage Forms | Relative Potency | Peak Blood Levels (oral) (h) | Protein Binding (%) | Volume of Distribution (L/kg) | Major Active Metabolite | Half-Life (parent) (h) | Half-Life* (metabolite) (h) | Usual Initial Dose | Adult Oral Dosage Range |
|---|---|---|---|---|---|---|---|---|---|---|
| **ANXIOLYTIC** | | | | | | | | | | |
| Alprazolam (Xanax®) | Tab | 0.5 | 1-2 | 80 | 0.9-1.2 | No | 12-15 | — | 0.25-0.5 tid | 0.75-4 mg/d |
| Chlordiazepoxide (Librium®) | Cap, Powd for inj, Tab | 10 | 2-4 | 90-98 | 0.3 | Yes | 5-30 | 24-96 | 5-25 mg tid-qid | 15-100 mg/d |
| Diazepam (Valium®) | Gel, Inj, Sol, Tab | 5 | 0.5-2 | 98 | 1.1 | Yes | 20-80 | 50-100 | 2-10 mg bid-qid | 4-40 mg/d |
| Halazepam (Paxipam®) | Tab | 20 | | | | Yes | 14 | 50-100 | 20-40 mg tid-qid | 80-160 mg/d |
| Lorazepam (Ativan®)** | Inj, Sol, Tab | 1 | 1-6 | 88-92 | 1.3 | No | 10-20 | — | 0.5-2 mg tid-qid | 2-4 mg/d |
| Oxazepam (Serax®) | Cap, Tab | 15-30 | 2-4 | 86-99 | 0.6-2 | No | 5-20 | — | 10-30 mg tid-qid | 30-120 mg/d |
| Prazepam (Centrax®) | Cap, Tab | 10 | | | | Yes | 1.2 | 30-100 | 10 mg tid | 30 mg/d |
| **SEDATIVE/HYPNOTIC** | | | | | | | | | | |
| Estazolam (ProSom™) | Tab | 0.3 | 2 | 93 | — | No | 10-24 | — | 1 mg qhs | 1-2 mg |
| Flurazepam (Dalmane®) | Cap | 5 | 0.5-2 | 97 | — | Yes | Not significant | 40-114 | 15 mg qhs | 15-60 mg |
| Quazepam (Doral®) | Tab | 5 | 2 | 95 | 5 | Yes | 25-41 | 28-114 | 15 mg qhs | 7.5-15 mg |
| Temazepam (Restoril®) | Cap | 5 | 2-3 | 96 | 1.4 | No | 10-40 | — | 15-30 mg qhs | 15-30 mg |
| Triazolam (Halcion®) | Tab | 0.1 | 1 | 89-94 | 0.8-1.3 | No | 2.3 | — | 0.125-0.25 qhs | 0.125-0.25 mg |
| **MISCELLANEOUS** | | | | | | | | | | |
| Clonazepam (Klonopin™) | Tab | 0.25-0.5 | 1-2 | 86 | 1.8-4 | No | 18-50 h | — | 0.5 mg tid | 1.5-20 mg/d |
| Clorazepate (Tranxene®) | Cap, Tab | 7.5 | 1-2 | 80-95 | — | Yes | Not significant | 50-100 h | 7.5-15 mg bid-qid | 15-60 mg |
| Midazolam (Versed®) | Inj | | 0.4-0.7† | 95 | 0.8-6.6 | No | 2-5 h | — | NA | |

* = significant metabolite.

**Reliable bioavailability when given I.M.

† = I.V. only.

NA = not available.

# BETA-BLOCKERS

## Beta-Blockers Comparison

| Agent | Adrenergic Receptor Blocking Activity | Lipid Solubility | Protein Bound (%) | Half-Life (h) | Bioavailability (%) | Primary (Secondary) Route of Elimination | Indications | Usual Dosage |
|---|---|---|---|---|---|---|---|---|
| Acebutolol (Sectral®) | $beta_1$ | Low | 15-25 | 3-4 | 40<br>7-fold* | Hepatic (renal) | Hypertension, arrhythmias | P.O.: 400-1200 mg/d |
| Atenolol (Tenormin®) | $beta_1$ | Low | <5-10 | 6-9† | 50-60<br>4-fold* | Renal (hepatic) | Hypertension, angina pectoris, acute MI | P.O.: 50-200 mg/d;<br>I.V.: 5 mg x 2 doses |
| Betaxolol (Kerlone®) | $beta_1$ | Low | 50-55 | 14-22 | 84-94 | Hepatic (renal) | Hypertension | P.O.: 10-20 mg/d |
| Bisoprolol (Zebeta®) | $beta_1$ | Low | 26-33 | 9-12 | 80 | Renal (hepatic) | Hypertension, heart failure | P.O.: 2.5-5 mg |
| Carteolol (Cartrol™) | $beta_1$<br>$beta_2$ | Low | 20-30 | 6 | 80-85 | Renal | Hypertension | P.O.: 2.5-10 mg/d |
| Esmolol (Brevibloc®) | $beta_1$ | Low | 55 | 0.15 | NA<br>5-fold* | Red blood cell | Supraventricular tachycardia, sinus tachycardia | I.V. infusion: 25-300 mcg/kg/min |
| Labetalol (Trandate®, Normodyne®) | $alpha_1$<br>$beta_1$<br>$beta_2$ | Moderate | 50 | 5.5-8 | 18-30<br>10-fold* | Renal (hepatic) | Hypertension | P.O.: 200-2400 mg/d;<br>I.V.: 20-80 mg at 10-min intervals up to a maximum of 300 mg **or** continuous infusion of 2 mg/min |
| Metoprolol (Lopressor®) | $beta_1$ | Moderate | 10-12 | 3-7 | 50<br>10-fold* | Hepatic (renal) | Hypertension, angina pectoris, acute MI | P.O.: 100-450 mg/d<br>I.V.: AMI: 15 mg in divided doses<br>I.V.: AFIB: 2.5-5 mg at 5-min intervals for a total of 15 mg |
| Metoprolol (long-acting) | | | | | 77 | | | |
| Nadolol (Corgard®) | $beta_1$<br>$beta_2$ | Low | 25-30 | 20-24 | 30<br>5-8 fold* | Renal | Hypertension, angina pectoris | P.O.: 40-320 mg/d |
| Penbutolol (Levatol™) | $beta_1$<br>$beta_2$ | High | 80-98 | 5 | ≅100 | Hepatic (renal) | Hypertension | P.O.: 20-80 mg/d |
| Pindolol (Visken®) | $beta_1$<br>$beta_2$ | Moderate | 57 | 3-4† | 90<br>4-fold* | Hepatic (renal) | Hypertension | P.O.: 20-60 mg/d |
| Propranolol (Inderal®, various) | $beta_1$<br>$beta_2$ | High | 90 | 3-5† | 30<br>20-fold* | Hepatic | Hypertension, angina pectoris, arrhythmias | P.O.: 40-80 mg/d;<br>I.V.: Reflex tachycardia: 1-10 mg |
| Propranolol long-acting (Inderal-LA®) | $beta_1$<br>$beta_2$ | High | 90 | 9-18 | 20-30 fold* | Hepatic | Hypertropic subaortic stenosis, prophylaxis (post-MI) | P.O.: 180-240 mg/d |
| Sotalol (Betapace®) | $beta_1$<br>$beta_2$ | Low | 0 | 12 | 90-100 | Renal | Ventricular arrhythmias/ tachyarrhythmias | P.O. 160-320 mg/d |
| Timolol (Blocadren®) | $beta_1$<br>$beta_2$ | Low to moderate | <10 | 4 | 75<br>7-fold* | Hepatic (renal) | Hypertension, prophylaxis (post-MI) | P.O.: 20-60 mg/d<br>P.O.: 20 mg/d |

Dosage is based on 70 kg adult with normal hepatic and renal function

**Note:** All $beta_1$ selective agents will inhibit $beta_2$ receptors at higher doses.

*Interpatient variations in plasma levels.

†Half-life increased to 16-27 h in creatinine clearance of 15-35 mL/min and >27 h in creatinine clearances <15 mL/min.

## Selected Properties of Beta-Adrenergic Blocking Drugs

| Drug | Relative $Beta_1$ Selectivity | Beta-Blockade Potency Ratio* | ISA | MSA |
|---|---|---|---|---|
| Acebutolol | + | 0.3 | + | + |
| Atenolol | + | 1 | – | – |
| Betaxolol | + | | 0 | + |
| Bisoprolol | + | | 0 | 0 |
| Carteolol | – | | ++ | 0 |
| Esmolol | + | 0.02 | – | – |
| Labetalol | – | | 0 | 0 |
| Metoprolol | + | 1 | – | – |
| Nadolol | – | 2-9 | – | – |
| Penbutolol | – | | +++ | + |
| Pindolol | – | 6 | ++ | + |
| Propranolol | – | 1 | – | ++ |
| Sotalol | – | 0.3 | – | – |
| Timolol | – | 6 | – | – |

*Propranolol = 1 ISA = intrinsic sympathomimetic activity,
MSA = membrane stabilizing activity.

# CALCIUM CHANNEL BLOCKING AGENTS

| | Amlodipine | Bepridil | Diltiazem | Felodipine | Isradipine | Nicardipine | Nifedipine | Nisoldipine | Verapamil |
|---|---|---|---|---|---|---|---|---|---|
| Bioavailability (%) | 60-65 | 59 | 40 | 15 | 15-24 | 35 | 60-75 | 5 | 20-35 |
| Protein binding (%) | 95-98 | >99 | 77-85 | 99 | 95 | 95 | 95 | >99 | 83-92 |
| Half-life | 35-50 h | 24 h | 3.5-6 h (5-7 h in sustained released preparations) | 10-16 h | 8 h | 2-4 h | 2-5 h | 7-12 h | Oral: One dose: 2.8-7.4 h<br>Rep dose: 4.5-12 h<br>I.V. (biphasic)<br>Short phase: 4 min<br>Long phase: 2-5 h |
| Onset of action | — | 60 min | Oral: 60 min | 2-5 h | 120 min | 20 min | Oral: 10-20 min | — | Oral: 30 min<br>I.V.: 1-5 min |
| Peak | 6-12 h | 2-3 h | Oral: 2-3 h | 2-4 h | 1.5 h | 0.5-2 h | Oral: 0.5-6 h | 6-12 h | Oral: 1-2.2 h<br>Oral, ext release: 5-7 h<br>I.V.: 2 h |
| Duration of action | 24 h | — | Ext release: 12 h<br>Tablet: 6-8 h | 24 h | — | 8 h | 12-24 h | — | Oral, ext release: 24 h<br>Tablet: 8-10 h<br>I.V.: 2 h |
| Elimination | Renal; fecal | Renal | Biliary/renal: 96%-98% (2%-4% unchanged) | Renal: 70%<br>Biliary: 30% | Renal | Renal: 60%<br>Biliary/fecal 35% | Renal: 80%<br>Biliary/fecal 20% | Renal | Renal: 70%<br>Biliary/fecal: 9%-16% |
| Solubility in water | — | — | Yes | — | — | Slightly | No | — | Yes |
| Maximum tolerated dosage (adult) | 250 mg | — | 12 g | — | — | 600 mg (standard)<br>2160 mg (sustained) | 900 mg | — | 16 g (standard)<br>9.6 g (sustained) |
| Therapeutic dose | 5-10 mg/day | 200-400 mg/day | 30-60 mg tid or qid for standard 180-400 mg daily for sustained release | 2-10 mg/day | 5-20 mg/day | 20-40 mg tid for standard 30-60 mg bid for sustained release | 10-40 mg tid or qid for standard 90-180 mg once daily for sustained release | 20-60 mg/day | 80-160 mg qid for standard 120-240 mg once daily for sustained release |
| Actions<br>contractility | 0 | ↓ | ↓ | 0/† | 0 | ↓ | ↑ | 0 | ↓↓ |
| heart rate | 0 | ↓ | ↓ | ↑ | +/– | ↑ | ↑ | +/– | ↓ |
| cardiac output | 0 | 0 | ↑ | ↑ | ↑ | ↑↑ | ↑ | 0 | ↓↑ |
| peripheral vascular resistance | ↓↓ | ↓ | ↓ | ↓↓ | ↓↓↓ | ↓↓↓ | ↓↓↓ | ↓↓↓ | ↓↓ |

ND = no data in humans. ++ = most frequent; + = less frequent; – = rare; 0 = no effect.

# CORTICOSTEROIDS

## Systemic Equivalencies

| Glucocorticoid | Pregnancy Category | Approximate Equivalent Dose (mg) | Routes of Administration | Relative Anti-inflammatory Potency | Relative Mineralo-corticoid Potency | Protein Binding (%) | Half-life Plasma (min) | Half-life Biologic (h) |
|---|---|---|---|---|---|---|---|---|
| **SHORT-ACTING** | | | | | | | | |
| Cortisone | D | 25 | P.O., I.M. | 0.8 | 2 | 90 | 30 | 8-12 |
| Hydrocortisone | C | 20 | I.M., I.V. | 1 | 2 | 90 | 80-118 | 8-12 |
| **INTERMEDIATE-ACTING** | | | | | | | | |
| Methylprednisolone* | — | 4 | P.O., I.M., I.V. | 5 | 0 | — | 78-188 | 18-36 |
| Prednisolone | B | 5 | P.O., I.M., I.V., intra-articular, intradermal, soft tissue injection | 4 | 1 | 90-95 | 115-212 | 18-36 |
| Prednisone | B | 5 | P.O. | 4 | 1 | 70 | 60 | 18-36 |
| Triamcinolone* | C | 4 | P.O., I.M., intra-articular, intradermal, intrasynovial, soft tissue injection | 5 | 0 | — | 200+ | 18-36 |
| **LONG-ACTING** | | | | | | | | |
| Betamethasone | C | 0.6-0.75 | P.O., I.M., intra-articular, intradermal, intrasynovial, soft tissue injection | 25 | 0 | 64 | 300+ | 36-54 |
| Dexamethasone | C | 0.75 | P.O., I.M., I.V., intra-articular, intradermal, soft tissue injection | 25-30 | 0 | — | 110-210 | 36-54 |
| **MINERALOCORTICOID** | | | | | | | | |
| Fludrocortisone | C | — | P.O. | 10 | 125 | 42 | 210+ | 18-36 |

*May contain propylene glycol as an excipient in injectable forms.

## Topical

| Steroid | | Vehicle |
|---|---|---|
| **VERY HIGH POTENCY** | | |
| 0.05% | Augmented betamethasone dipropionate | Ointment |
| 0.05% | Clobetasol propionate | Cream, ointment |
| 0.05% | Diflorasone diacetate | Ointment |
| 0.05% | Halobetasol propionate | Cream, ointment |
| **HIGH POTENCY** | | |
| 0.1% | Amcinonide | Cream, ointment, lotion |
| 0.05% | Betamethasone dipropionate, augmented | Cream |
| 0.05% | Betamethasone dipropionate | Cream, ointment |
| 0.1% | Betamethasone valerate | Ointment |
| 0.05% | Desoximetasone | Gel |
| 0.25% | Desoximetasone | Cream, ointment |
| 0.05% | Diflorasone diacetate | Cream, ointment |
| 0.2% | Fluocinolone acetonide | Cream |
| 0.05% | Fluocinonide | Cream, ointment, gel |
| 0.1% | Halcinonide | Cream, ointment |
| 0.5% | Triamcinolone acetonide | Cream, ointment |
| **INTERMEDIATE POTENCY** | | |
| 0.025% | Betamethasone benzoate | Cream, gel, lotion |
| 0.05% | Betamethasone dipropionate | Lotion |
| 0.1% | Betamethasone valerate | Cream |
| 0.1% | Clocortolone pivalate | Cream |
| 0.05% | Desoximetasone | Cream |
| 0.025% | Fluocinolone acetonide | Cream, ointment |
| 0.05% | Flurandrenolide | Cream, ointment, lotion, tape |
| 0.005% | Fluticasone propionate | Ointment |
| 0.05% | Fluticasone propionate | Cream |
| 0.1% | Hydrocortisone butyrate† | Ointment, solution |
| 0.2% | Hydrocortisone valerate† | Cream, ointment |
| 0.1% | Mometasone furoate† | Cream, ointment, lotion |
| 0.025% | Triamcinolone acetonide | Cream, ointment, lotion |
| 0.1% | Triamcinolone acetonide | Cream, ointment, lotion |
| **LOW POTENCY** | | |
| 0.05% | Alclometasone dipropionate† | Cream, ointment |
| 0.05% | Desonide | Cream |
| 0.01% | Dexamethasone | Aerosol |
| 0.04% | Dexamethasone | Aerosol |
| 0.1% | Dexamethasone sodium phosphate | Cream |
| 0.01% | Fluocinolone acetonide | Cream, solution |
| 0.25% | Hydrocortisone† | Lotion |
| 0.5% | Hydrocortisone† | Cream, ointment, lotion, aerosol |
| 0.5% | Hydrocortisone acetate† | Cream, ointment |
| 1% | Hydrocortisone acetate† | Cream, ointment |
| 1% | Hydrocortisone | Cream, ointment, lotion, solution |
| 2.5% | Hydrocortisone | Cream, ointment, lotion |

†Not fluorinated.

# GLAUCOMA DRUG THERAPY

| Ophthalmic Agent | Reduces Aqueous Humor Production | Increases Aqueous Humor Outflow | Average Duration of Action | Strengths Available |
|---|---|---|---|---|
| **Cholinesterase Inhibitors*** | | | | |
| Demecarium | No data | Significant | 7 d | 0.125%-0.25% |
| Echothiophate | No data | Significant | 2 wk | 0.03%-0.25% |
| Isoflurophate | No data | Significant | 2 wk | 0.025% |
| Physostigmine | No data | Significant | 24 h | 0.25% |
| **Direct-Acting Cholinergic Agents** | | | | |
| Carbachol | Some activity | Significant | 8 h | 0.75%-3% |
| Pilocarpine | Some activity | Significant | 5 h | 0.5%, 1%, 2%, 3%, 4% |
| **Sympathomimetics** | | | | |
| Dipivefrin | Some activity | Moderate | 12 h | 0.1% |
| Epinephrine | Some activity | Moderate | 18 h | 0.25%-2% |
| **Beta-Blockers** | | | | |
| Betaxolol | Significant | Some activity | 12 h | 0.5% |
| Carteolol | Yes | No | 12 h | 1% |
| Levobetaxolol | Significant | No data | 12 h | 0.5% |
| Levobunolol | Significant | Some activity | 18 h | 0.5% |
| Metipranolol | Significant | Some activity | 18 h | 0.3% |
| Timolol | Significant | Some activity | 18 h | 0.25%, 0.5% |
| **Carbonic Anhydrase Inhibitors** | | | | |
| Acetazolamide | Significant | No data | 10 h | 250 mg tab, 500 mg cap |
| Brinzolamide | Yes | No data | 8 h | 1% |
| Dorzolamide | Yes | No | 8 h | 2% |
| Methazolamide | Significant | No data | 14 h | 50 mg |
| **Prostaglandin Agonist** | | | | |
| Latanoprost | | Yes | 8-12 h | 0.005% |

*All miotic drugs significantly affect accommodation.

# HALLUCINOGENIC DRUGS

## Principal Pharmacological Properties of Hallucinogenic Drugs

| Drug; Chemical Structure | Duration of Acute Effect (h) | pKa | Route of Metabolism/ Excretion | Half-Life | Protein Binding (%) | $V_d$ (L/kg) | Urine Screen Positive for | Duration of Psychotropic Effects | Doses of Abuse | Fatal Dose |
|---|---|---|---|---|---|---|---|---|---|---|
| Phencyclidine (PCP); arylcyclohexylamine | 4-6 | 8.5 | Hepatic/urine | 1 h | 65 | 6.2-0.3 | 2 wk | Up to 1 mo | 1-9 mg | 1 mg/kg |
| Cocaine; tropane alkaloid | 0.5 | 5.6 | Plasma hydrolysis* | 48-75 min | 9-90 | 1.2-1.9 | 4 days (benzoylecgonine) | ≤5-7 d | 20-200 mg (intranasally) | 1-1.2 g |
| Cannabis; monoterpenoid | 0.5-3 | 10.6 | Hepatic hydroxylation | 25-57 h | 97-99 | 10 | Up to 4 d | ≤6 h | 5-15 mg THC | |
| LSD; indole alkylamine | 0.7-8 | 7.8 | Hepatic hydroxylation | 2.5 h | | 0.27 | 5 d | May last for days | 100-300 mcg | 0.2 mg/kg |
| Psilocybin; tryptamine | 0.5-6 | | | | | | Not detected | 12 h | 20-100 mushrooms | 5-15 mg of psilocybin |
| Mescaline; phenylalkylamine | 4.6 | Not known | Hepatic/urine† | 6 h | None | Not known | | 12 h | 5 mg/kg | 20 mg/kg |
| Morphine; alkaloid/ derivative of opium | 4-5 | 8.05 | Glucuronidation/ urine | 1.9-3.1 h | 35 | 3.2 | 48 h | ≤6 h | 2-20 mg | Variable – dependent on tolerance, nontolerant fatal dose is 120 mg orally or 30 mg parenterally |
| Heroin; diacetylmorphine | 3.4 | 7.6 | Hepatic‡ | 3-20 min | 40 | 25 | ~40 h | ≤6 h | 2.2 mg | Variable – dependent on tolerance |
| Amphetamine; β-(phenylisopropyl)-amine | Variable | 9.93 | Hepatic§ | 12 h¶ | 16-20 | 3-6 | 2-4 d | Delusions may remain for months | 100-1000 mg/d | Variable – dependent on tolerance |

*By serum cholinesterase.

†60% excreted unchanged.

‡Converted to morphine.

§Converted to phenylacetone.

¶Urine pH-dependent.

Reprinted with permission from Leikin JB, Krantz AJ, Zell-Kanter M, et al, "Clinical Features and Management of Intoxication Due to Hallucinogenic Drugs," *Med Toxicol Adverse Drug Exp*, 1989, 4(5):328.

# HYPOGLYCEMIC DRUGS & THIAZOLIDINEDIONE INFORMATION

## Contraindications to Therapy and Potential Adverse Effects of Oral Antidiabetic Agents

| | Sulfonylureas/ Meglitinide | Metformin | Acarbose/ Miglitol | Pioglitazone/ Rosiglitazone |
|---|---|---|---|---|
| **CONTRAINDICATIONS** | | | | |
| Insulin dependency | A | A | A* | |
| Pregnancy/lactation | A | A | A | |
| Hypersensitivity to the agent | A | A | A | A |
| Hepatic impairment | R | A | R | A |
| Renal impairment | R | A | R | |
| Congestive heart failure | | A | | R |
| Chronic lung disease | | A | | |
| Peripheral vascular disease | | A | | |
| Steroid-induced diabetes | R | R | | |
| Inflammatory bowel disease | | A | A | |
| Major recurrent illness | R | A | | |
| Surgery | R | A | | |
| Alcoholism | R | A | | A |
| **ADVERSE EFFECTS** | | | | |
| Hypoglycemia | Yes | No | No | No |
| Body weight gain | Yes | No | No | Yes |
| Hypersensitivity | Yes | No | No | No |
| Drug interactions | Yes | No | No | Yes/No |
| Lactic acidosis | No | Yes | No | No |
| Gastrointestinal disturbances | No | Yes | Yes | No |

*Can be used in conjunction with insulin. A = absolute; R = relative.

## Comparative Pharmacokinetics

| Drug | Duration of Action (h) | Dose and Frequency (mg) | Metabolism |
|---|---|---|---|
| **Sulfonylureas – First Generation Agents** | | | |
| Acetohexamide | 12-24 | 250-1500 bid | Hepatic (60%) with active metabolite |
| Chlorpropamide | 24-72 | 100-500 qd | Renal excretion (30%) and hepatic metabolism with active metabolites |
| Tolazamide | 10-24 | 100-1000 qd or bid | Hepatic with active metabolites |
| Tolbutamide | 6-24 | 500-3000 qd-tid | Hepatic |
| **Sulfonylureas – Second Generation Agents** | | | |
| Glimepiride | 24 | 1-4 mg qd | Hepatic |
| Glipizide | 12-24 | 2.5-40 qd or bid | Hepatic |
| Glipizide GITS | 24 | 5-10 qd | Hepatic |
| Glyburide | 16-24 | 1.25-20 qd or bid | Hepatic with active metabolites |
| **Meglitinides** | | | |
| Repaglinide | <4 hours (single dose) | 0.4-4 mg administered with meals 2, 3, or 4 times/day | Hepatic to inactive metabolites |

## Comparative Thiazolidinedione Pharmacokinetics

| Parameter | Pioglitazone (Actos®) | Rosiglitazone (Avandia®) |
|---|---|---|
| **Absorption** | Food slightly delays but does not alter the extent of absorption | Absolute bioavailability is 99%<br>Food ↓ $C_{max}$ and delays $T_{max}$, but not change in AUC |
| **$C_{max}$** | 156-342 ng/mL | – |
| **$T_{max}$** | 2 hours | 1 hour |
| **Distribution** | 0.63 ± 0.41 L/kg | 17.6 L |
| **Plasma Protein Binding** | >99% to serum albumin | 99.8% to serum albumin |
| **Metabolism** | Extensive liver metabolism by hydroxylation and oxidation. Some metabolites are pharmacologically active<br><br>CYP2C8 and CYP3A4 metabolism | Extensive metabolism via N-demethylation and hydroxylation with no unchanged drug excreted in the urine<br><br>CYP2C8 and some CYP2C9 metabolism |
| **Excretion** | Urine (15% to 30%) and bile | Urine (64%) and feces (23%) |
| **Half-life** | 3-6 hours (pioglitazone)<br>16-24 hours (pioglitazone and metabolites) | 3.15-3.59 hours |
| **Effect of Hemodialysis** | Not removed | Not removed |

(Package inserts: Actos®, 1999; Avandia®, 1999; Rezulin®, 1999; Plosker, 1999.)

## Approved Indications for Thiazolidinedione Derivatives

| Indication | Pioglitazone (Actos®) | Rosiglitazone (Avandia®) |
|---|---|---|
| **Monotherapy** | | |
| | X | X |
| **Combination Therapy - Dual Therapy** | | |
| Combination with sulfonylureas | X | X |
| Combination therapy with Glucophage® (metformin) | X | X |
| Combination therapy with insulin | X | – |
| **Combination Therapy - Triple Therapy** | | |
| Combination therapy with sulfonylureas and Glucophage® (metformin) | – | – |

(Package inserts: Actos®, 1999; Avandia®, 1999; Rezulin®, 1999.)

## Comparative Lipid Effects

| Parameter | Pioglitazone (Actos®) | Rosiglitazone (Avandia®) |
|---|---|---|
| **LDL** | No significant change | ↑ up to 12.1% |
| **HDL** | ↑ up to 13% | ↑ up to 18.5% |
| **Total Cholesterol** | No significant change | ↑ |
| **Total Cholesterol/HDL Ratio** | – | – |
| **LDL/HDL Ratio** | – | No change |
| **Triglycerides** | ↓ up to 28% | Variable effects |

(Package inserts: Actos®, 1999; Avandia®, 1999; Rezulin®, 1999; Plosker, 1999)

# LAXATIVES, CLASSIFICATION AND PROPERTIES

| Laxative | Onset of Action | Site of Action | Mechanism of Action |
|---|---|---|---|
| **SALINE** | | | |
| Magnesium citrate (Citroma®) Magnesium hydroxide (Milk of Magnesia) | 30 min to 3 h | Small and large intestine | Attract/retain water in intestinal lumen increasing intraluminal pressure; cholecystokinin release |
| Sodium phosphate/ biphosphate enema (Fleet® Enema) | 2-15 min | Colon | |
| **IRRITANT/STIMULANT** | | | |
| Cascara Casanthranol Senna (Senokot®) | 6-10 h | Colon | Direct action on intestinal mucosa; stimulate myenteric plexus; alter water and electrolyte secretion |
| Bisacodyl (Dulcolax®) tablets, suppositories | 15 min to 1 h | Colon | |
| Castor oil | 2-6 h | Small intestine | |
| Cascara aromatic fluid extract | 6-10 h | Colon | |
| **BULK-PRODUCING** | | | |
| Methylcellulose Psyllium (Metamucil®) Malt soup extract (Maltsupex®) Calcium polycarbophil (Mitrolan®, FiberCon®) | 12-24 h (up to 72 h) | Small and large intestine | Holds water in stool; mechanical distention; malt soup extract reduces fecal pH |
| **LUBRICANT** | | | |
| Mineral oil | 6-8 h | Colon | Lubricates intestine; retards colonic absorption of fecal water; softens stool |
| **SURFACTANTS/STOOL SOFTENER** | | | |
| Docusate sodium (Colace®) Docusate calcium (Surfak®) Docusate potassium (Dialose®) | 24-72 h | Small and large intestine | Detergent activity; facilitates admixture of fat and water to soften stool |
| **MISCELLANEOUS AND COMBINATION LAXATIVES** | | | |
| Glycerin suppository | 15-30 min | Colon | Local irritation; hyperosmotic action |
| Lactulose (Cephulac®) | 24-48 h | Colon | Delivers osmotically active molecules to colon |
| Docusate/casanthranol (Peri-Colace®) | 8-12 h | Small and large intestine | Casanthranol – mild stimulant; docusate – stool softener |
| Polyethylene glycol-electrolyte solution (GoLYTELY®) | 30-60 min | Small and large intestine | Nonabsorbable solution which acts as an osmotic agent |
| Sorbitol 70% | 24-48 h | Colon | Delivers osmotically active molecules to colon |

# LIPID-LOWERING AGENTS

## Effects on Lipoproteins

| Drug | Total Cholesterol (%) | LDLC (%) | HDLC (%) | TG (%) |
|---|---|---|---|---|
| Bile-acid resins | ↓20-25 | ↓20-35 | → | ↑5-20 |
| Fibric acid derivatives | ↓10 | ↓10 (↑) | ↑10-25 | ↓40-55 |
| HMG-CoA RI (statins) | ↓15-35 | ↓20-40 | ↑2-15 | ↓7-25 |
| Nicotinic acid | ↓25 | ↓20 | ↑20 | ↓40 |
| Probucol | ↓10-15 | ↓<10 | ↓30 | → |

## Comparative Dosages of Agents Used to Treat Hyperlipidemia

| Antilipemic Agent* | Usual Daily Dose | Average Dosing Interval |
|---|---|---|
| **Fibric Acid Derivatives** | | |
| Clofibrate | 2000 mg | qid |
| Gemfibrozil | 1200 mg | bid |
| **Miscellaneous Agents** | | |
| Niacin | 6 g | tid |
| **Bile Acid Sequestrants** | | |
| Colestipol | max: 30 g | bid |
| Cholestyramine | max: 24 g | tid-qid |

Dosage is based on 70 kg adult with normal hepatic and renal function.

## Recommended Liver Function Monitoring for HMG-CoA Reductase Inhibitors

| Agent | Initial and After Elevation in Dose | 6 Weeks* | 12 Weeks* | Semiannually |
|---|---|---|---|---|
| Atorvastatin | x | x | x | x |
| Cerivastatin | x | x | x | x |
| Fluvastatin | x | x | x | x |
| Lovastatin | x | x | x | x |
| Pravastatin | x | | x | |
| Simvastatin | x | | | x |

*After initiation of therapy or any elevation in dose.

# LIQUID COMPATIBILITY

## Liquid Compatibility with Antipsychotics and Mood Stabilizers

| Drug | Vehicle | | | | | | | | | | | |
|---|---|---|---|---|---|---|---|---|---|---|---|---|
| | Water | Saline | Milk | Coffee | Tea | Apple juice | Grape juice | Grapefruit juice | Orange juice | Prune juice | Cola | 7-Up/Sprite |
| Carbamazepine* | C | C | | | | | | | | | | |
| Lithium | C | C | C | C | C | X | C | C | C | C | C | C |
| Valproate | C | C | | | | | | | | | X | X |
| Chlorpromazine* | C | C | C | U | U | X | X | C | C | U | U | C |
| Fluphenazine | C | C | C | X | X | X | | C | C | C | X | X |
| Haloperidol | C | X | X | X | X | C | X | X | C | | C | |
| Loxapine | | | | C | | | | C | C | | C | C |
| Mesoridazine | C | | | | | | C | C | C | | | |
| Risperidone | C | C | C | C | X | | | | C | | X | |
| Thioridazine | C | C | X | X | X | X | X | C | C | X | X | C |
| Thiothixene | C | | C | X | X | X | | C | C | C | X | |
| Trifluoperazine | C | C | C | U | C | X | X | C | C | C | C | C |

C = Compatible; X - Incompatible; U = Conflicting Data; Blank = No Data

* Carbamazepine is not compatible with chlorpromazine

# MOOD STABILIZERS

| Generic Name (Brand Name) | Dosage Forms | Half-Life (h) | Usual Dose | Therapeutic Range | Comments |
|---|---|---|---|---|---|
| Lithium (Eskalith®; Lithane®; Lithobid®; Lithonate®; Lithotabs®) | T, C, L | 18-24 | 600-1800 mg/day | 0.5-1.5 mEq/L* | Nausea, tremor, polydipsia, and polyuria common; may cause hypothyroidism with chronic use; FDA approved for bipolar disorder |
| Carbamazepine (Epitol®; Tegretol®; Tegretol-XR®) | T, L | 15-50 initial<br>8-20 chronic | 600-1800 mg/day | N/A | Nausea, headache, dizziness, and sedation common; blood levels >12 mcg/mL associated with toxicity; enzyme inducer |
| Valproate (Depakene®; Depakote®) | T, C, L | 5-20 | 1-3 g/day | 50-125 μg/mL* | Nausea, sedation, diarrhea, and tremor are common; also indicated for migraine prophylaxis; loading dose: 20 mg/kg PO; monitor LFTs if using combination anticonvulsants; FDA approved for mania |
| Gabapentin (Neurontin®) | C | 5-6 | 500-3600 mg/day | N/A | Renally eliminated |
| Lamotrigine (Lamictal®) | T | 24 | 100-500 mg/day | N/A | May have antidepressant and mood-stabilizing effects |
| Topiramate (Topamax®), Topamax® Sprinkle) | T, C | 21 | 400-1600 mg/day | N/A | May be associated with weight loss |

T = Tablet, C = Capsule, L = Liquid

N/A = Correlation between serum concentration and clinical response have not been established.

* = Obtain blood level 12 hours after the last dose in the evening

# NARCOTIC AGONISTS

## Comparative Pharmacokinetics

| Drug | Onset (min) | Peak (h) | Duration (h) | Half-Life (h) | Average Dosing Interval (h) | | Equianalgesic Doses* (mg) | |
|---|---|---|---|---|---|---|---|---|
| | | | | | Median | Range | I.M. | Oral |
| Alfentanil | Immediate | ND | ND | 1-2 | — | — | ND | NA |
| Buprenorphine | 15 | 1 | 4-8 | 2-3 | | | 0.4 | — |
| Butorphanol | I.M.: 30-60<br>I.V.: 4-5 | 0.5-1 | 3-5 | 2.5-3.5 | 3 | (3-6) | 2 | — |
| Codeine | P.O.: 30-60<br>I.M.: 10-30 | 0.5-1 | 4-6 | 3-4 | 3 | (3-6) | 120 | 200 |
| Fentanyl | I.M.: 7-15<br>I.V.: Immediate | ND | 1-2 | 1.5-6 | 1 | (0.5-2) | 0.1 | NA |
| Hydrocodone | ND | ND | 4-8 | 3.3-4.4 | 6 | (4-8) | ND | ND |
| Hydromorphone | P.O.: 15-30 | 0.5-1 | 4-6 | 2-4 | 4 | (3-6) | 1.5 | 7.5 |
| Levorphanol | P.O.: 10-60 | 0.5-1 | 4-8 | 12-16 | 6 | (6-24) | 2 | 4 |
| Meperidine | P.O./I.M./S.C.: 10-15<br>I.V.: ≤5 | 0.5-1 | 2-4 | 3-4 | 3 | (2-4) | 75 | 300 |
| Methadone | P.O.: 30-60<br>I.V.: 10-20 | 0.5-1 | 4-6 (acute)<br>>8 (chronic) | 15-30 | 8 | (6-12) | 10 | 20 |
| Morphine | P.O.: 15-60<br>I.V.: ≤5 | P.O./I.M./<br>S.C.: 0.5-1<br>I.V.: 0.3 | 3-6 | 2-4 | 4 | (3-6) | 10 | 60† (acute)<br>30 (chronic) |
| Nalbuphine | I.M.: 30<br>I.V.: 1-3 | 1 | 3-6 | 5 | | — | 10 | — |
| Naloxone‡ | 2-5 | 0.5-2 | 0.5-1 | 0.5-1.5 | | — | — | — |
| Oxycodone | P.O.: 10-15 | 0.5-1 | 4-6 | 3-4 | 4 | (3-6) | NA | 30 |
| Oxymorphone | 5-15 | 0.5-1 | 3-6 | | | | 1 | 10§ |
| Pentazocine | 15-20 | 0.25-1 | 3-4 | 2-3 | 3 | (3-6) | | |
| Propoxyphene | P.O.: 30-60 | 2-2.5 | 4-6 | 3.5-15 | 6 | (4-8) | ND | 130¶-200# |
| Remifentanil | 1-3 | <0.3 | 0.1-0.2 | 0.15-0.3 | — | — | ND | ND |
| Sufentanil | 1.3-3 | ND | ND | 2.5-3 | — | — | 0.02 | NA |

ND = no data available. NA = not applicable.

*Based on acute, short-term use. Chronic administration may alter pharmacokinetics and decrease the oral parenteral dose ratio. The morphine oral-parenteral ratio decreases to ~ 1.5-2.5:1 upon chronic dosing.

†Extensive survey data suggest that the relative potency of I.M.:P.O. morphine of 1:6 changes to 1:2-3 with chronic dosing.

‡Narcotic antagonist

§Rectal.

¶HCl salt.

#Napsylate salt.

## Comparative Pharmacology

| Drug | Analgesic | Antitussive | Constipation | Respiratory Depression | Sedation | Emesis |
|---|---|---|---|---|---|---|
| **Phenanthrenes** | | | | | | |
| Codeine | + | +++ | + | + | + | + |
| Hydrocodone | + | +++ | | + | | |
| Hydromorphone | ++ | +++ | + | ++ | + | + |
| Levorphanol | ++ | ++ | ++ | ++ | ++ | + |
| Morphine Sulfate | ++ | +++ | ++ | ++ | ++ | ++ |
| Oxycodone | ++ | +++ | ++ | ++ | ++ | ++ |
| Oxymorphone | ++ | + | ++ | +++ | | +++ |
| **Phenylpiperidines** | | | | | | |
| Alfentanil | ++ | | | ++ | +++ | ++ |
| Fentanyl | ++ | | | | +++ | + |
| Meperidine | ++ | + | + | ++ | + | |
| Remifentanil | ++ | | | ++ | +++ | ++ |
| Sufentanil | +++ | | | ++ | +++ | ++ |
| **Diphenylheptanes** | | | | | | |
| Methadone | ++ | ++ | ++ | ++ | + | + |
| Propoxyphene | + | | | + | + | + |
| **Agonist/Antagonist** | | | | | | |
| Buprenorphine | ++ | N/A | +++ | +++ | ++ | ++ |
| Butorphanol | ++ | N/A | +++ | +++ | ++ | + |
| Dezocine | ++ | | + | ++ | + | ++ |
| Nalbuphine | ++ | N/A | +++ | +++ | ++ | ++ |
| Pentazocine | ++ | N/A | + | ++ | ++ or stimulation | ++ |

# NONBENZODIAZEPINE ANXIOLYTICS & HYPNOTICS

| Drug | Dosage Forms | Initial Dose | Usual Dosage Range | Onset | Half-Life | Comments |
|---|---|---|---|---|---|---|
| Buspirone | T | 7.5 mg bid | 30-60 mg/d | 30 min to 1.5 h | 2-3 h | Do not use for alcohol or benzodiazepine withdrawal; no sedation or dependence; do not use PRN; use 4 weeks for full therapeutic effect |
| Chloral hydrate | C, R, S | 500 mg to 1 g qhs | 500 mg to 2 g/d | 30 min | 8-11 h | GI irritating; tolerance to hypnotic effect develops rapidly |
| Diphenhydramine | Soln, C, T, Crm, Lot, S, E | 25-50 mg qhs | 25-200 mg/d | 1-3 h | 2-8 h | Anticholinergic; max hypnotic dose: 50 mg/d |
| Hydroxyzine | T, C, L, I, S | 25-100 mg qid | 100-600 mg/d | 30 min | 3-7 h | Anticholinergic |
| Propranolol | T, C, Soln, I | 10 mg tid | 80-160 mg/d | 1-2 h | 4-6 h | Useful for physical manifestations of anxiety (increased heart rate, tremor); second-line agent |
| Zaleplon | C | 5-10 mg qhs | 5-20 mg qhs | 30 min | 1 h | Do not use for alcohol or benzodiazepine withdrawal |
| Zolpidem | T | 10 mg qhs | 10 mg qhs | 30 min | 2.5 h | Do not use for alcohol or benzodiazepine withdrawal |

R = rectal suppository; S = syrup; T = tablet; C = capsule; L = liquid; Crm = cream; Inj = injection; Lot = lotion; E = elixir; Soln = solution

# NONSTEROIDAL ANTI-INFLAMMATORY AGENTS

## Comparative Dosages and Pharmacokinetics

| Drug | Maximum Recommended Daily Dose (mg) | Time to Peak Levels (h)* | Half-life (h) |
|---|---|---|---|
| **Propionic Acids** | | | |
| Fenoprofen (Nalfon®) | 3200 | 1-2 | 2-3 |
| Flurbiprofen (Ansaid®) | 300 | 1.5 | 5.7 |
| Ibuprofen | 3200 | 1-2 | 1.8-2.5 |
| Ketoprofen (Orudis®) | 300 | 0.5-2 | 2-4 |
| Naproxen (Naprosyn®) | 1500 | 2-4 | 12-15 |
| Naproxen sodium (Anaprox®) | 1375 | 1-2 | 12-13 |
| Oxaprozin | 1800 | 3-5 | 42-50 |
| **Acetic Acids** | | | |
| Diclofenac sodium delayed release (Voltaren®) | 225 | 2-3 | 1-2 |
| Diclofenac potassium immediate release (Cataflam®) | 200 | 1 | 1-2 |
| Etodolac (Lodine®) | 1200 | 1-2 | 7.3 |
| Indomethacin (Indocin®) | 200 | 1-2 | 4.5 |
| Indomethacin SR | 150 | 2-4 | 4.5-6 |
| Ketorolac (Toradol®) | I.M.: 120†<br>P.O.: 40 | 0.5-1 | 3.8-8.6 |
| Sulindac (Clinoril®) | 400 | 2-4 | 7.8 (16.4)‡ |
| Tolmetin (Tolectin®) | 2000 | 0.5-1 | 1-1.5 |
| **Fenamates (Anthranilic Acids)** | | | |
| Meclofenamate (Meclomen®) | 400 | 0.5-1 | 2 (3.3)§ |
| Mefenamic acid (Ponstel®) | 1000 | 2-4 | 2-4 |
| **Nonacidic Agent** | | | |
| Nabumetone (Relafen®) | 2000 | 3-6 | 24 |
| **Oxicam** | | | |
| Piroxicam (Feldene®) | 20 | 3-5 | 30-86 |
| **Cox-2 Inhibitors** | | | |
| Celecoxib (Celebrex®) | 400 | 3 | 11 |
| Rofecoxib (Vioxx®) | 50 | 2-3 | 17 |

Dosage is based on 70 kg adult with normal hepatic and renal function.

*Food decreases the rate of absorption and may delay the time to peak levels.

†150 mg on the first day.

‡Half-life of active sulfide metabolite.

§Half-life with multiple doses.

# PHARMACOKINETICS OF SELECTIVE SEROTONIN-REUPTAKE INHIBITORS (SSRIs)

| SSRI | Half-life (h) | Metabolite Half-life | Peak Plasma Level (h) | % Protein Bound | Bioavailability (%) | Initial Dose |
|---|---|---|---|---|---|---|
| Citalopram | 35 | N/A | 4 | 80 | 80 | 20 mg qAM |
| Fluoxetine | Initial: 24-72<br>Chronic: 96-144 | Norfluoxetine:<br>4-16 days | 6-8 | 95 | 72 | 10-20 mg qAM |
| Fluvoxamine | 16 | N/A | 3 | 80 | 53 | 50 mg qhs |
| Paroxetine | 21 | N/A | 5 | 95 | >90 | 10-20 mg qAM |
| Sertraline | 26 | N-desmethyl-sertraline:<br>2-4 days | 5-8 | 98 | — | 25-50 qAM |

# PROTEASE INHIBITORS

## Comparison of Currently Available Protease Inhibitors

| | **Saquinavir Invirase® Roche** | **Ritonavir Norvir® Abbott** | **Indinavir Crixivan® Merck** | **Nelfinavir Viracept® Agouron** |
|---|---|---|---|---|
| Dosage | 600 mg tid | 600 mg bid | 800 mg q8h | 750 mg tid |
| Dosage strength/ form | 200 mg capsule | 100 mg capsule<br>600 mg/7.5 mL oral solution | 200 mg capsule<br>400 mg capsule | 250 mg tablets<br>50 mg/g powder |
| Number/full dose | 3 capsules (9/day full dose) | 6 capsules (12/day full dose) | 2 (400 mg) capsules (6/day full dose) | 3 tablets (9/day full dose) powder |
| Volume/full dose | NA | 7.5 mL (15 mL/day full dose) | NA | Variable, oral powder 50 mg/g may be reconstituted with a small amount of water, milk, formula, soy formula, soy milk, or dietary supplements |
| Relation to food | Take on a full stomach, within 2 hours of a high fat meal if possible (eg, 48 g protein, 60 g carbohydrate, 57 g fat; 1006 Kcal) (Administration of saquinavir on an empty stomach dramatically reduces the drug's absorption) | Take with food if possible. The taste of the oral solution may be improved by mixing with chocolate milk, Ensure®, or Advera®. If the solution is mixed to improve the taste, it must be taken within 1 hour of mixing. | Take on an empty stomach with water 1 hour before or 2 hours after a meal. May be administered with other liquids such as skim milk, juice, coffee, or tea, or with a light meal. (Ingestion of Crixivan® with a meal high in calories, fat, and protein reduces the drug's absorption.) At least 1.5 L of liquids should be taken during the course of 24 hours to ensure adequate hydration and minimize potential side effect of nephrolithiasis. | Take with food. Maximum plasma concentrations and AUC were 2- to 3-fold higher under fed conditions compared to fasting. Meals contained 517-719 Kcal with 153-313 Kcal derived from fat. |
| Dosage initiation/ adjustments (also see drug interactions) | In combination therapy, dose adjustment of the nucleoside analogue should be based on the drug's toxicity profile. Lower doses of saquinavir are not recommended due to poor bioavailability. | Dose escalation may provide relief of nausea when initiating therapy.*<br>Begin at no <300 mg bid and increase by 100 mg bid increments up to 600 mg bid. | Reduce the dose to 600 mg q8h in mild-to-moderate hepatic insufficiency due to cirrhosis. Patients who experience nephrolithiasis may interrupt or discontinue therapy (eg, 1-3 days) during the acute episode. | If a dose is missed, take the dose as soon as possible and return to normal schedule. Do not double the next dose. Pharmacokinetics in patients with hepatic or renal insufficiency have not been studied. However, <2% of nelfinavir is excreted in the urine so the impact of renal impairment is minimal. Caution when administering in patients with hepatic impairment. |
| Storage requirements | Room temperature, tightly closed bottle | Store capsules in the refrigerator at all time and protect from light.<br>Store oral solution in the refrigerator until dispensed. Refrigeration by the patient of the oral solution is recommended but not required if used within 30 days. Store in original container. Avoid exposure to excessive heat. | Room temperature, tightly closed bottle. Capsules are sensitive to moisture and should be dispensed and stored in the original container. The desiccant should remain in the original bottle. | Room temperature; tablets and oral powder.<br>Oral powder mixed with liquids, water, milk, formula, etc, should be used within 6 hours. |
| Combination or monotherapy | Combination use only | Combination and monotherapy use | Combination and monotherapy use | Combination use only |
| Route of metabolism | Cytochrome P-450, specifically CYP3A4 isoenzyme | Cytochrome P-450 (CYP3A >> 2D6 >> 2C > 1A2) | Cytochrome P-450, specifically CYP3A4 isoenzyme | Cytochrome P-450 (CYP3A) |
| Adverse effects *(most frequently reported –* ***check with your physician for complete information****)* | Diarrhea, abdominal discomfort, and nausea | Asthenia, diarrhea, nausea, vomiting, circumoral paresthesia, taste perversion, peripheral paresthesia | Nephrolithiasis, asymptomatic hyperbilirubinemia, nausea, abdominal pain | Diarrhea, nausea, flatulence; diarrhea can usually be controlled with nonprescription drugs, such as Imodium® to slow GI motility |

*Patients initiating combination regimens with Norvir® and nucleoside analogues may improve GI tolerance by initiating Norvir® alone and subsequently adding nucleosides before completing 2 weeks of Norvir® monotherapy.

Adapted from *The Protease Inhibitors Backgrounder*, Office of Special Health Issues and Division of Antiviral Drug Products, Food and Drug Administration, revised December 1997.

## Medications That Should NOT Be Used With Protease Inhibitors

| Drug Category | Saquinavir Invirase® Roche | Ritonavir Norvir® Abbott | Indinavir Crixivan® Merck | Nelfinavir Viracept® Agouron | Potential Alternatives (these alternatives may not be therapeutically equivalent) |
|---|---|---|---|---|---|
| Analgesic | — | Meperidine (Demerol®)<br>Piroxicam (Feldene®)<br>Propoxyphene (Darvon, others) | — | — | Acetaminophen (Tylenol®, others)<br>Aspirin (Bayer®, others)<br>Oxycodone (Percocet®, others) |
| Cardiovascular (antiarrhythmic) | — | Amiodarone (Cordarone®)<br>Encainide (Enkaid®)<br>Flecainide (Tambocor™)<br>Propafenone (Rythmol®)<br>Quinidine (various) | — | — | Very limited clinical experience |
| Cardiovascular (calcium channel blocker) | — | Bepridil (Vascor®) | — | — | Very limited clinical experience |
| Antimycobacterial | Rifampin (Rifadin®, others) | Rifabutin (Mycobutin®) | Rifampin (Rifadin®, others) | Rifampin (Rifadin®, others) | Alternatives for rifabutin (Mycobutin®):<br>clarithromycin (Biaxin™)<br>ethambutol (Myambutol®) |
| Ergot alkaloid (vasoconstrictor) | Dihydroergotamine (D.H.E. 45®) ergotamine (various) | Dihydroergotamine (D.H.E. 45®) ergotamine (various) | Dihydroergotamine (D.H.E. 45®) ergotamine (various) | Dihydroergotamine (D.H.E. 45®) ergotamine (various) | — |
| Cold and allergy (antihistamine) | Astemizole (Hismanal®)<br>Terfenadine (Seldane®) | Astemizole (Hismanal®)<br>Terfenadine (Seldane®) | Astemizole (Hismanal®)<br>Terfenadine (Seldane®) | Astemizole (Hismanal®)<br>Terfenadine (Seldane®) | Loratadine (Claritin®) |
| Gastrointestinal | Cisapride (Propulsid®) | Cisapride (Propulsid®) | Cisapride (Propulsid®) | Cisapride (Propulsid®) | Very limited clinical experience |
| Psychotropic (antidepressant) | — | Bupropion (Wellbutrin®) | — | — | Fluoxetine (Prozac®)<br>Desipramine (Norpramin®) |
| Psychotropic (neuroleptic) | — | Clozapine (Clozaril®)<br>Pimozide (Orap®) | — | — | Very limited clinical experience |
| Psychotropic (sedative/hypnotic) | Midazolam (Versed®)<br>Triazolam (Halcion®) | Clorazepate (Tranxene®)<br>Diazepam (Valium®)<br>Estazolam (ProSom®)<br>Flurazepam (Dalmane®)<br>Midazolam (Versed®)<br>Triazolam (Halcion®)<br>Zolpidem (Ambien®) | Midazolam (Versed®)<br>Triazolam (Halcion®) | Midazolam (Versed®)<br>Triazolam (Halcion®) | Temazepam (Restoril®)<br>Lorazepam (Ativan®) |

Adapted from *The Protease Inhibitors Backgrounder*, Office of Special Health Issues and Division of Antiviral Drug Products, Food and Drug Administration, revised December 1997.

## PROTEASE INHIBITORS *(Continued)*

### Effects of Protease Inhibitors and Other Commonly Used Medications as Determined by Drug Interaction Studies

Dosage adjustments should be determined by a physician.

| Drug | Saquinavir Invirase® Roche | Recommend | Ritonavir Norvir® Abbott | Recommend | Indinavir Crixivan® Merck | Recommend | Nelfinavir Viracept® Agouron | Recommend |
|---|---|---|---|---|---|---|---|---|
| **ANTIFUNGALS** | | | | | | | | |
| Fluconazole (Diflucan®) | No studies have been conducted – no data available | — | Fluconazole increases ritonavir AUC* by 15% | No dosage adjustment necessary | Fluconazole decreases indinavir AUC by 19% ±33% | No dosage adjustment necessary | — | — |
| Ketoconazole (Nizoral®) | Ketoconazole increases saquinavir AUC and $C_{max}$ 3-fold | No dosage adjustment necessary when ketoconazole 200 mg qd and saquinavir 600 mg tid are given | No studies have been conducted – no data available | — | Ketoconazole increases indinavir AUC levels by 68% ± 48% | Reduce indinavir to 600 mg q8h | Ketoconazole increased nelfinavir AUC levels by 35% | No dosage adjustment necessary |
| **ANTIMYCOBACTERIALS** | | | | | | | | |
| Clarithromycin (Biaxin™) | No studies have been conducted – no data available | — | Clarithromycin AUC increases by 77% Rifabutin AUC increases 4-fold Rifabutin metabolite (25-0-desacetyl) AUC increases 35-fold | Dosage adjustment to patient with renal impairment is necessary | Increase indinavir AUC by 29% ± 42% and increases clarithromycin AUC by 53% ± 36% | No dosage adjustment necessary | — | — |
| Rifabutin (Mycobutin®) | Rifabutin decreases saquinavir levels by 40% | If rifabutin therapy is warranted, consider alternative drugs | — | Coadministration of ritonavir and rifabutin is contraindicated | Rifabutin AUC increases by 204% ± 142% | Reduce rifabutin to half the standard dose | Rifabutin AUC increases by 207% | Reduce rifabutin to half the standard dose |
| Rifampin (Rifadin®, others) | Rifampin increases saquinavir levels by 80% | Rifampin and saquinavir should not be administered concomitantly | Rifampin increases ritonavir levels by 35% | No dosage adjustment necessary | Rifampin decreases AUC of saquinavir by approximately 80% | Rifampin and indinavir should not be administered concomitantly | Rifampin decreases nelfinavir by approximately 82% | Rifampin and nelfinavir should not be administered concomitantly |
| **NNRTIs** | | | | | | | | |
| Delavirdine | 5-fold increase in saquinavir AUC | Limited safety and no efficacy data from combination; monitor ALT/AST frequently | No evidence of interaction at doses of DLV 400-600 mg bid and ritonavir 300 mg bid | No safety and efficacy data from this combination | Increase in indinavir plasma concentrations | Dose reduction of indinavir to 600 mg tid should be considered; no safety and efficacy data from this combination | — | — |
| Nevirapine† | 27% decrease in saquinavir AUC | No safety and efficacy data from this combination | 11% decrease in ritonavir AUC (0- to 12-hour) | No safety data from this combination | 28% decrease in indinavir AUC (0- to 8-hour) | Dose adjustment of indinavir 1000 mg q8h should be considered; no safety and efficacy data from this combination | — | — |
| Oral contraceptives | No studies have been conducted – no data available | — | Ethinyl estradiol AUC decreases by 40% | Dosage increase or alternative contraceptive measures should be considered | Ortho-Novum® 1/35 decreases ethinyl estradiol 24% ± 17% and norethindrone by 26% ± 14% | No dosage adjustment necessary | Ovcon® 35 decreases ethinyl estradiol by 47% and norethindrone by 18% | Alternate or additional contraceptive measures should be used |
| **PROTEASE INHIBITORS** | | | | | | | | |
| Indinavir | — | — | — | — | — | — | 83% increase in nelfinavir AUC and 51% increase in indinavir AUC | No safety and efficacy data from this combination |
| Nelfinavir | 18% increase in nelfinavir AUC and 392% increase in saquinavir AUC with soft gelatin formulation of saquinavir | No dose adjustment is needed with hard gelatin formulation of saquinavir; dose adjustments unknown for soft gelatin formulation; safety and efficacy not established | 152% increase in nelfinavir AUC and very little change in ritonavir AUC | Safety and efficacy of this combination has not been established | 83% increase in nelfinavir AUC and 51% increase in indinavir AUC | Safety and efficacy of this combination has not been established | — | — |
| Ritonavir | 20-fold increase in steady-state dose-normalized saquinavir concentration with ritonavir doses of 400 or 600 mg bid | Currently under study; safety and efficacy has not been established | — | — | — | — | 152% increase in nelfinavir AUC and very little change in ritonavir AUC | No safety and efficacy data from this combination |
| Saquinavir | — | — | 20-fold increase in steady-state dose-normalized saquinavir concentration with ritonavir doses of 400 or 600 mg bid | Currently under study – safety and efficacy has not been established | — | — | 18% increase in nelfinavir AUC and 392% increase in saquinavir AUC with soft gelatin formulation of saquinavir | No dose adjustment is needed with hard gelatin formulation of saquinavir; dose adjustments unknown for soft gelatin formulation; safety and efficacy not established |

## Effects of Protease Inhibitors and Other Commonly Used Medications as Determined by Drug Interaction Studies *(continued)*

| Drug | Saquinavir Invirase® Roche | Recommend | Ritonavir Norvir® Abbott | Recommend | Indinavir Crixivan® Merck | Recommend | Nelfinavir Viracept® Agouron | Recommend |
|---|---|---|---|---|---|---|---|---|
| | | | | OTHER | | | | |
| | Ritonavir markedly increases saquinavir plasma levels (see ritonavir) | Safety of this interaction has not been established | Desipramine (Norpramin®, others) AUC increase by 145% | Dosage reduction should be considered | Grapefruit juice decreases indinavir levels by 26% | — | — | — |
| | — | — | >20-fold increase in saquinavir AUC | Safety of this interaction has not been established | — | — | — | — |
| | — | — | Theophylline (Theo-Dur®, others) AUC decreases by 43% | Dosage increase may be required | — | — | — | — |
| | — | — | Tobacco decreases ritonavir AUC by 18% | — | — | — | — | — |

*AUC – Area under the curve is a measurement of plasma concentration levels.

†Letter from Roxane Laboratories, Inc, May 23, 1997.

Adapted from *The Protease Inhibitors Backgrounder*, Office of Special Health Issues and Division of Antiviral Drug Products, Food and Drug Administration, revised December 1997.

# STIMULANT AGENTS USED FOR ADHD

| Generic Name (Brand Name) | Dosage | Formulations | Comments |
|---|---|---|---|
| Amphetamine (Various) | 2.5-5 mg/d, increase by 2.5-5 mg/wk; maximum dose: 40 mg/d | Tablet: 5 mg, 10 mg | Also used for narcolepsy and exogenous obesity |
| Amphetamine and Dextroamphetamine (Adderall®) | 2.5-5 mg qAM, increase by 2.5-5 mg/wk; maximum dose: 40 mg/d on bid schedule | Tablet: 5 mg, 10 mg, 20 mg, 30 mg | Also used for narcolepsy |
| Dextroamphetamine* (Dexedrine®) | 2.5-5 mg qAM, increase by 2.5-5 mg/wk; maximum dose: 40 mg/d | Elixir: 5 mg/5 mL (16 oz bottle)<br>Tablet: 5 mg, 10 mg<br>Spansules, sustained release: 5 mg, 10 mg, 15 mg | Avoid evening doses; monitor growth; also used for narcolepsy and exogenous obesity |
| Dextromethamphetamine (Desoxyn®) | 2.5-5 mg qd-bid, increase by 5 mg/wk until optimum response is achieved, usually 20-25 mg/d | Tablet: 5 mg<br>Tablet, slow release: 5 mg, 10 mg, 15 mg | |
| Methylphenidate* (Ritalin®; Ritalin SR®) | 2.5-5 mg before breakfast or lunch; increase by 5-10 mg/d at weekly intervals; maximum dose: 60 mg/d | Tablet: 5 mg, 10 mg, 20 mg<br>Tablet, slow release: 20 mg | |
| Pemoline (Cylert®) | 37.5 mg qAM, increase by 18.75 mg/d at weekly intervals; usual range: 56.25-75 mg/d; maximum dose: 112.5 mg/d | Tablet: 18.75 mg, 37.5 mg, 75 mg<br>Tablet, chewable: 37.5 mg | See Warnings in Pemoline monograph |

*Available in generic form

# SULFONAMIDE DERIVATIVES

The following table lists commonly prescribed drugs which are either sulfonamide derivatives or are structurally similar to sulfonamides. Please note that the list may not be all inclusive.

## Commonly Prescribed Drugs

| Classification | Specific Drugs |
|---|---|
| Antimicrobial Agents | Mafenide acetate (Sulfamylon®)<br>Silver sulfadiazine (Silvadene®)<br>Sodium sulfacetamide (Sodium Sulamyd®)<br>Sulfadiazine<br>Sulfamethizole<br>Sulfamethoxazole (ie, Bactrim™ and co-trimoxazole)<br>Sulfisoxazole (Gantrisin®) |
| Diuretics, Carbonic Anhydrase Inhibitors | Acetazolamide (Diamox®)<br>Dichlorphenamide (Daranide®)<br>Methazolamide (Neptazane®) |
| Diuretics, Loop | Bumetanide (Bumex®)<br>Furosemide (Lasix®)<br>Torsemide (Demadex®) |
| Diuretics, Thiazide | Bendroflumethiazide<br>Benzthiazide<br>Chlorothiazide (Diuril®)<br>Chlorthalidone (Hygroton®)<br>Cyclothiazide (Anhydron®)<br>Hydrochlorothiazide (Dyazide®, HydroDIURIL®, Maxzide®)<br>Hydroflumethiazide<br>Indapamide (Lozol®)<br>Methyclothiazide (Enduron®)<br>Metolazone (Diulo®, Zaroxolyn®)<br>Polythiazide<br>Quinethazone<br>Trichlormethiazide |
| Hypoglycemic Agents, Oral | Acetohexamide (Dymelor®)<br>Chlorpropamide (Diabinese®)<br>Glipizide (Glucotrol®)<br>Glyburide (DiaBeta®, Micronase®)<br>Tolazamide (Tolinase®)<br>Tolbutamide (Orinase®) |
| Other Agents | Sulfasalazine (Azulfidine®) |

# CYTOCHROME P-450 ENZYMES AND DRUG METABOLISM

## Background

There are five distinct groups of enzymes which account for the majority of drug metabolism in humans. These enzymes "families", known as isoenzymes, are localized primarily in the liver. The nomenclature of this system has been standardized. Isoenzyme families are identified as a cytochrome (CYP prefix), followed by their numerical designation (eg, 1A2).

Enzymes may be inhibited (slowing metabolism through this pathway) or induced (increased in activity or number). Individual drugs metabolized by a specific enzyme are identified as substrates for the isoenzyme. Considerable effort has been expended in recent years to classify drugs metabolized by this system as either an inhibitor, inducer, or substrate of a specific isoenzyme. It should be noted that a drug may demonstrate complex activity within this scheme, acting as an inhibitor of one isoenzyme while serving as a substrate for another.

By recognizing that a substrate's metabolism may be dramatically altered by concurrent therapy with either an inducer or inhibitor, potential interactions may be identified and addressed. For example, a drug which inhibits CYP1A2 is likely to block metabolism of theophylline (a substrate for this isoenzyme). Because of this interaction, the dose of theophylline required to maintain a consistent level in the patient should be reduced when an inhibitor is added. Failure to make this adjustment may lead to supratherapeutic theophylline concentrations and potential toxicity.

This approach does have limitations. For example, the metabolism of specific drugs may have primary and secondary pathways. The contribution of secondary pathways to the overall metabolism may limit the impact of any given inhibitor. In addition, there may be up to a tenfold variation in the concentration of an isoenzyme across the broad population. In fact, a complete absence of an isoenzyme may occur in some genetic subgroups. Finally, the relative potency of inhibition, relative to the affinity of the enzyme for its substrate, demonstrates a high degree of variability. These issues make it difficult to anticipate whether a theoretical interaction will have a clinically relevant impact in a specific patient.

The details of this enzyme system continue to be investigated, and information is expanding daily. However, to be complete, it should be noted that other enzyme systems also influence a drug's pharmacokinetic profile. For example, a key enzyme system regulating the absorption of drugs is the p-glycoprotein system. Recent evidence suggests that some interaction originally attributed to the cytochrome system may, in fact, have been the result of inhibition of this enzyme.

The following tables represent an attempt to detail the available information with respect to isoenzyme activities. Within certain limits, they may be used to identify potential interactions. Of particular note, an effort has been made in each drug monograph to identify involvement of a particular isoenzyme in the drug's metabolism. These tables are intended to supplement the limited space available to list drug interactions in the monograph. Consequently, they may be used to define a greater range of both actual and potential drug interactions.

## DRUGS CAUSING INHIBITORY AND INDUCTIVE INTERACTION

| INHIBITORY (Enhancement of Interacting Drug Effect) | | INDUCTIVE (Impairment of Interacting Drug Effect) |
|---|---|---|
| Amiodarone (Cordarone®) | Itraconazole | Anticonvulsants |
| Cimetidine (Tagamet®) | Ketoconazole | Chronic ethanol use |
| Contraceptives, oral | Neuroleptics | Cigarette smoking |
| Erythromycin | Psoralen dermatologics | Rifampin (Rifadin®, Rimactane®) |
| Ethanol intoxication | Quinidine | |
| Fluconazole | Quinolone antibiotics | |
| Isoniazid (Laniazid®, Nydrazid®) | SSRIs | |
| | Tricyclic antidepressants | |

## LOW THERAPEUTIC INDEX DRUGS

**Hepatic Oxidation (Cytochrome P-450 Mediated Clearance)**

Antiarrhythmic drugs
Anticoagulants, oral
Anticonvulsants
Antineoplastic/immunosuppressive drugs
Theophylline

# CYTOCHROME P-450 ENZYMES AND RESPECTIVE METABOLIZED DRUGS

## CYP1A2

### Substrates

Acetaminophen
Acetanilid
Alosetron
Aminophylline
Amitriptyline (demethylation)
Antipyrine
Apomorphine
Betaxolol
Caffeine
Chlorpromazine
Clomipramine (demethylation)
Clozapine
Cyclobenzaprine (demethylation)
Desipramine (demethylation)
Diazepam
Estradiol
Fluvoxamine
Grepafloxacin
Haloperidol (minor)
Imipramine (demethylation)
Levobupivacaine
Levopromazine
Maprotiline
Methadone
Metoclopramide
Mirtazapine (hydroxylation)
Nortriptyline
Olanzapine (demethylation, hydroxylation)
Ondansetron
Phenacetin
Phenothiazines
Pimozide (minor)
Propafenone
Propranolol
Riluzole
Ritonavir
Ropinirole
Ropivacaine
Tacrine
Tamoxifen
Theophylline
Thioridazine
Thiothixene
Trifluoperazine
Verapamil
Warfarin (R-warfarin, minor pathway)
Zileuton
Zopiclone

### Inducers

Carbamazepine
Charbroiled foods
Cigarette smoke
Cruciferous vegetables (cabbage, Brussels sprouts, broccoli, cauliflower)
Moricizine
Nicotine
Omeprazole
Phenobarbital
Phenytoin
Primidone
Rifampin
Ritonavir

### Inhibitors

Anastrozole
Cimetidine
Ciprofloxacin
Citalopram (weak)
Clarithromycin
Diethyldithiocarbamate
Diltiazem
Enoxacin
Entacapone (high dose)
Erythromycin
Ethinyl estradiol
Fluvoxamine
Fluoxetine (high dose)
Grapefruit juice
Isoniazid
Ketoconazole
Levofloxacin
Mexiletine
Mibefradil
Norfloxacin
Paroxetine (high dose)(weak)
Ritonavir
Sertraline (weak)
Tacrine
Tertiary TCAs
Zileuton

## CYP2A6

### Substrates

Dexmedetomidine
Letrozole
Montelukast
Nicotine
Ritonavir
Tamoxifen

### Inhibitors

Diethyldithiocarbamate
Entacapone (high dose)
Letrozole
Ritonavir
Tranylcypromine

## CYP2B6

### Substrates

Antipyrine
Bupropion (hydroxylation)
Cyclophosphamide
Ifosfamide
Nicotine
Orphenadrine
Tamoxifen

### Inhibitors

Diethyldithiocarbamate
Orphenadrine

## CYTOCHROME P-450 ENZYMES AND DRUG METABOLISM *(Continued)*

### CYP2C
### (Specific isozyme has not been identified)

**Substrates**

Antipyrine
Carvedilol
Clozapine (minor)
Mestranol
Mephobarbital
Tamoxifen
Ticrynafen

**Inducers**

Carbamazepine
Phenobarbital
Phenytoin
Primidone
Rifampin
Sulfinpyrazone

**Inhibitors**

Isoniazid
Ketoconazole
Ketoprofen

### CYP2C8

**Substrates**

Carbamazepine
Diazepam
Diclofenac
Ibuprofen
Mephobarbital
Naproxen (5-hydroxylation)
Omeprazole
Paclitaxel
Pioglitazone
Retinoic acid
Rosiglitazone
Tolbutamide
Warfarin (S-warfarin)

**Inducers**

Carbamazepine
Phenobarbital
Phenytoin
Primidone
Rifampin

**Inhibitors**

Anastrozole
Omeprazole

### CYP2C9

**Substrates**

Alosetron
Amitriptyline (demethylation)
Celecoxib
Dapsone
Diclofenac
Flurbiprofen
Fluvastatin
Glimepiride
Hexobarbital
Ibuprofen
Imipramine (demethylation)
Indomethacin
Irbesartan
Losartan
Mefenamic acid
Metronidazole
Mirtazapine
Montelukast
Naproxen (5-hydroxylation)
Phenytoin
Piroxicam
Quetiapine (minor pathway)
Ritonavir
Rosiglitazone (minor)
Sildenafil citrate
Tenoxicam
Tetrahydrocannabinol
Tolbutamide
Torsemide
Warfarin (S-warfarin)
Zafirlukast (hydroxylation)
Zileuton

**Inducers**

Carbamazepine
Fluconazole
Fluoxetine
Phenobarbital
Phenytoin
Rifampin

**Inhibitors**

Amiodarone
Anastrozole
Chloramphenicol
Cimetidine
Diclofenac
Disulfiram
Entacapone (high dose)
Flurbiprofen
Fluoxetine
Fluvastatin
Fluvoxamine (potent)
Isoniazid
Ketoconazole (weak)
Ketoprofen
Metronidazole
Omeprazole
Phenylbutazone
Ritonavir
Sertraline
Sulfamethoxazole-trimethoprim
Sulfaphenazole
Sulfinpyrazone
Sulfonamides
Troglitazone
Valproic acid
Warfarin (R-warfarin)
Zafirlukast

### CYP2C18

**Substrates**

Dronabinol
Naproxen
Omeprazole
Piroxicam
Proguanil
Propranolol
Retinoic acid
Warfarin

### Inducers

- Carbamazepine
- Phenobarbital
- Phenytoin
- Rifampin

### Inhibitors

- Cimetidine

## CYP2C19

### Substrates

- Amitriptyline (demethylation)
- Apomorphine
- Barbiturates
- Carisoprodol
- Citalopram
- Clomipramine (demethylation)
- Desmethyldiazepam
- Diazepam (N-demethylation, minor pathway)
- Divalproex sodium
- Hexobarbital
- Imipramine (demethylation)
- Lansoprazole
- Mephenytoin
- Mephobarbital
- Moclobemide
- Olanzapine (minor)
- Omeprazole
- Pantoprazole
- Pentamidine
- Phenytoin
- Proguanil
- Propranolol
- Ritonavir
- Tolbutamide
- Topiramate
- Valproic acid
- Warfarin (R-warfarin)

### Inducers

- Carbamazepine
- Phenobarbital
- Phenytoin
- Rifampin

### Inhibitors

- Cimetidine
- Citalopram (weak)
- Entacapone (high dose)
- Felbamate
- Fluconazole
- Fluoxetine
- Fluvoxamine
- Isoniazid
- Ketoconazole (weak)
- Letrozole
- Omeprazole
- Oxcarbazepine
- Proguanil
- Ritonavir
- Sertraline
- Teniposide
- Tolbutamide
- Topiramate
- Tranylcypromine
- Troglitazone

## CYP2D6

### Substrates

- Amitriptyline (hydroxylation)
- Amphetamine
- Betaxolol
- Bisoprolol
- Brofaromine
- Bufurolol
- Captopril
- Carvedilol
- Cevimeline
- Chlorpheniramine
- Chlorpromazine
- Cinnarizine
- Clomipramine (hydroxylation)
- Clozapine (minor pathway)
- Codeine (hydroxylation, o-demethylation)
- Cyclobenzaprine (hydroxylation)
- Cyclophosphamide
- Debrisoquin
- Delavirdine
- Desipramine
- Dexfenfluramine
- Dextromethorphan (o-demethylation)
- Dihydrocodeine
- Diphenhydramine
- Dolasetron
- Donepezil
- Doxepin
- Encainide
- Fenfluramine
- Flecainide
- Fluoxetine (minor pathway)
- Fluphenazine
- Halofantrine
- Haloperidol (minor pathway)
- Hydrocodone
- Hydrocortisone
- Hydroxyamphetamine
- Imipramine (hydroxylation)
- Labetalol
- Loratadine
- Maprotiline
- m-Chlorophenylpiperazine (m-CPP)
- Meperidine
- Methadone
- Methamphetamine
- Metoclopramide
- Metoprolol
- Mexiletine
- Mianserin
- Mirtazapine (hydroxylation)
- Molindone
- Morphine
- Nortriptyline (hydroxylation)
- Olanzapine (minor, hydroxymethylation)
- Ondansetron
- Orphenadrine
- Oxycodone
- Papaverine
- Paroxetine (minor pathway)
- Penbutolol
- Pentazocine
- Perhexiline
- Perphenazine
- Phenformin
- Pindolol
- Promethazine
- Propafenone
- Propranolol
- Quetiapine
- Remoxipride
- Risperidone
- Ritonavir (minor)
- Ropivacaine
- Selegiline
- Sertindole
- Sertraline (minor pathway)
- Sparteine
- Tamoxifen
- Thioridazine
- Tiagabine
- Timolol
- Tolterodine
- Tramadol
- Trazodone
- Trimipramine
- Tropisetron
- Venlafaxine (o-desmethylation)
- Yohimbine

### Inhibitors

- Amiodarone
- Celecoxib
- Chloroquine
- Chlorpromazine
- Cimetidine
- Citalopram
- Clomipramine
- Codeine
- Delavirdine
- Desipramine
- Dextropropoxyphene
- Diltiazem
- Doxorubicin
- Entacapone (high dose)
- Fluoxetine
- Fluphenazine
- Fluvoxamine
- Haloperidol
- Labetalol
- Lobeline
- Lomustine
- Methadone
- Mibefradil
- Moclobemide
- Norfluoxetine
- Paroxetine
- Perphenazine
- Propafenone
- Quinacrine
- Quinidine
- Ranitidine
- Risperidone (weak)
- Ritonavir
- Sertindole
- Sertraline (weak)
- Thioridazine
- Valproic acid
- Venlafaxine (weak)
- Vinblastine
- Vincristine
- Yohimbine

## CYTOCHROME P-450 ENZYMES AND DRUG METABOLISM *(Continued)*

### CYP2E1

#### Substrates

- Acetaminophen
- Acetone
- Aniline
- Benzene
- Caffeine
- Chlorzoxazone
- Clozapine
- Dapsone
- Dextromethorphan
- Enflurane
- Ethanol
- Halothane
- Isoflurane
- Isoniazid
- Methoxyflurane
- Nitrosamine
- Ondansetron
- Phenol
- Ritonavir
- Sevoflurane
- Styrene
- Tamoxifen
- Theophylline
- Venlafaxine

#### Inducers

- Ethanol
- Isoniazid

#### Inhibitors

- Diethyldithiocarbamate (disulfiram metabolite)
- Dimethyl sulfoxide
- Disulfiram
- Entacapone (high dose)
- Ritonavir

### CYP3A3/4

#### Substrates

- Acetaminophen
- Alfentanil
- Alosetron
- Alprazolam**
- Amiodarone
- Amitriptyline (minor)
- Amlodipine
- Anastrozole
- Androsterone
- Antipyrine
- Apomorphine
- Astemizole**
- Atorvastatin
- Benzphetamine
- Bepridil
- Bexarotene
- Bromazepam
- Bromocriptine
- Budesonide
- Bupropion (minor)
- Buspirone
- Busulfan
- Caffeine
- Cannabinoids
- Carbamazepine
- Cevimeline
- Cerivastatin
- Chlorpromazine
- Cimetidine
- Cisapride**
- Citalopram
- Clarithromycin
- Clindamycin
- Clomipramine
- Clonazepam
- Clozapine
- Cocaine
- Codeine (demethylation)
- Cortisol
- Cortisone
- Cyclobenzaprine (demethylation)
- Cyclophosphamide
- Cyclosporine
- Dapsone
- Dehydroepiandrostendione
- Delavirdine
- Desmethyldiazepam
- Dexamethasone
- Dextromethorphan (minor, N-demethylation)
- Diazepam (minor; hydroxylation, N-demethylation)
- Digitoxin
- Diltiazem
- Disopyramide
- Docetaxel
- Dofetilide (minor)
- Dolasetron
- Donepezil
- Doxorubicin
- Doxycycline
- Dronabinol
- Enalapril
- Erythromycin
- Estradiol
- Ethinyl estradiol
- Ethosuximide
- Etoposide
- Exemestene
- Felodipine
- Fentanyl
- Fexofenadine
- Finasteride
- Fluoxetine
- Flutamide
- Glyburide
- Granisetron
- Halofantrine
- Haloperidol
- Hydrocortisone
- Hydroxyarginine
- Ifosfamide
- Imipramine
- Indinavir
- Isradipine
- Itraconazole
- Ketoconazole
- Lansoprazole (minor)
- Letrozole
- Levobupivicaine
- Lidocaine
- Loratadine
- Losartan
- Lovastatin
- Methadone
- Mibefradil
- Miconazole
- Midazolam
- Mifepristone
- Mirtazapine (N-demethylation)
- Montelukast
- Navelbine
- Nefazodone
- Nelfinavir**
- Nevirapine
- Nicardipine
- Nifedipine
- Niludipine
- Nimodipine
- Nisoldipine
- Nitrendipine
- Omeprazole (sulfonation)
- Ondansetron
- Oral contraceptives
- Orphenadrine
- Paclitaxel
- Pantoprazole
- Pimozide**
- Pioglitazone
- Pravastatin
- Prednisone
- Progesterone
- Proguanil
- Propafenone
- Quercetin
- Quetiapine
- Quinidine
- Quinine
- Repaglinide
- Retinoic acid
- Rifampin
- Risperidone
- Ritonavir**
- Salmeterol
- Saquinavir
- Sertindole
- Sertraline
- Sibutramine##
- Sildenafil citrate
- Simvastatin
- Sirolimus
- Sufentanil
- Tacrolimus
- Tamoxifen
- Temazepam
- Teniposide
- Terfenadine**
- Testosterone
- Tetrahydrocannabinol
- Theophylline
- Tiagabine
- Tolterodine
- Toremifene
- Trazodone
- Tretinoin
- Triazolam**
- Troglitazone
- Troleandomycin
- Venlafaxine (N-demethylation)
- Verapamil
- Vinblastine
- Vincristine
- Warfarin (R-warfarin)
- Yohimbine
- Zaleplon
- Zatoestron
- Zileuton
- Ziprasidone
- Zolpidem**
- Zonisamide

#### Inducers

- Carbamazepine
- Dexamethasone
- Glucocorticoids
- Griseofulvin
- Nafcillin
- Nelfinavir
- Nevirapine
- Oxcarbazepine
- Phenobarbital
- Phenylbutazone
- Phenytoin
- Primidone
- Progesterone
- Rifabutin
- Rifampin
- Rofecoxib (mild)
- St John's wort
- Sulfadimidine
- Sulfinpyrazone
- Troglitazone

## Inhibitors

Amiodarone
Anastrozole
Azithromycin
Cannabinoids
Cimetidine
Clarithromycin**
Clotrimazole
Cyclosporine
Danazol
Delavirdine
Dexamethasone
Diethyldithiocarbamate
Diltiazem
Dirithromycin
Disulfiram
Entacapone (high dose)
Erythromycin**
Ethinyl estradiol
Fluconazole (weak)
Fluoxetine (weak)
Fluvoxamine**
Gestodene
Grapefruit juice
Haloperidol
Indinavir
Isoniazid
Itraconazole**
Ketoconazole**
Metronidazole
Mibefradil**
Miconazole (moderate)
Nefazodone**
Nelfinavir
Nevirapine
Norfloxacin
Norfluoxetine
Omeprazole (weak)
Oxiconazole
Paroxetine (weak)
Propoxyphene
Quinidine
Quinine**
Quinupristin and dalfopristin
Ranitidine
Ritonavir**
Saquinavir
Sertindole
Sertraline
Troglitazone
Troleandomycin
Valproic acid (weak)
Verapamil
Zafirlukast
Zileuton

# CYP3A5-7

## Substrates

Cortisol
Ethinyl estradiol
Lovastatin
Nifedipine
Quinidine
Terfenadine
Testosterone
Triazolam
Vinblastine
Vincristine

## Inducers

Phenobarbital
Phenytoin
Primidone
Rifampin

## Inhibitors

Clotrimazole
Ketoconazole
Metronidazole
Miconazole
Troleandomycin

****Contraindications:**
Terfenadine, astemizole, cisapride, and triazolam contraindicated with nefazodone
Pimozide contraindicated with macrolide antibiotics
Alprazolam and triazolam contraindicated with ketoconazole and itraconazole
Terfenadine, astemizole, and cisapride contraindicated with fluvoxamine
Terfenadine contraindicated with mibefradil, ketoconazole, erythromycin, clarithromycin, troleandomycin
Ritonavir contraindicated with triazolam, zolpidem, astemizole, rifabutin, quinine, clarithromycin, troleandomycin
Mibefradil contraindicated with astemizole
Nelfinavir contraindicated with rifabutin

##Do not use with SSRIs, sumatriptan, lithium, meperidine, fentanyl, dextromethorphan, or pentazocine within 2 weeks of an MAOI.

## References


Baker GB, Urichuk CJ, and Coutts RT, "Drug Metabolism and Metabolic Drug-Drug Interactions in Psychiatry," *Child Adolescent Psychopharm News (Suppl)*.

DeVane CL, "Pharmacogenetics and Drug Metabolism of Newer Antidepressant Agents," *J Clin Psychiatry*, 1994, 55(Suppl 12):38-45.

*Drug Interactions Analysis and Management. Cytochrome (CYP) 450 Isozyme Drug Interactions*, Vancouver, WA: Applied Therapeutics, Inc, 523-7.

Ereshefsky L, "Drug-Drug Interactions Involving Antidepressants: Focus on Venlafaxine," *J Clin Psychopharmacol*, 1996, 16(3 Suppl 2):375-535.

Ereshefsky L, *Psychiatr Annal*, 1996, 26:342-50.

Fleishaker JC and Hulst LK, "A Pharmacokinetic and Pharmacodynamic Evaluation of the Combined Administration of Alprazolam and Fluvoxamine," *Eur J Clin Pharmacol*, 1994, 46(1):35-9.

Flockhart DA, et al, *Clin Pharmacol Ther*, 1996, 59:189.

Ketter TA, Flockhart DA, Post RM, et al, "The Emerging Role of Cytochrome P-450 3A in Psychopharmacology," *J Clin Psychopharmacol*, 1995, 15(6):387-98.

Michalets EL, "Update: Clinically Significant Cytochrome P-450 Drug Interactions," *Pharmacotherapy*, 1998, 18(1):84-112.

Nemeroff CB, DeVane CL, and Pollock BG, "Newer Antidepressants and the Cytochrome P450 System," *Am J Psychiatry*, 1996, 153(3):311-20.

Pollock BG, "Recent Developments in Drug Metabolism of Relevance to Psychiatrists," *Harv Rev Psychiatry*, 1994, 2(4):204-13.

Richelson E, "Pharmacokinetic Drug Interactions of New Antidepressants: A Review of the Effects on the Metabolism of Other Drugs," *Mayo Clin Proc*, 1997, 72(9):835-47.

Riesenman C, "Antidepressant Drug Interactions and the Cytochrome P450 System: A Critical Appraisal," *Pharmacotherapy*, 1995, 15(6 Pt 2):84S-99S.

Schmider J, Greenblatt DJ, von Moltke LL, et al, "Relationship of *In Vitro* Data on Drug Metabolism to *In Vivo* Pharmacokinetics and Drug Interactions: Implications for Diazepam Disposition in Humans," *J Clin Psychopharmacol*, 1996, 16(4):267-72.

Slaughter RL, *Pharm Times*, 1996, 7:6-16.

Watkins PB, "Role of Cytochrome P450 in Drug Metabolism and Hepatotoxicity," *Semin Liver Dis*, 1990, 10(4):235-50.

# PERSPECTIVES ON THE SAFETY OF HERBAL MEDICINES

**By Mark Blumenthal**

Adapted from Leikin JB and Paloucek FP, *Poisoning and Toxicology Compendium*, Hudson, OH: Lexi-Comp, Inc, 1998.

With the rapid expansion of consumers' use of herb and phytomedicines in the U.S., the issue of documenting their safety and toxicological concerns becomes more compelling for healthcare professionals. Numerous organizations in the U.S. and in Europe have initiated measures to monitor the quality, safety, and efficacy of these natural products through the publication of official and quasi-official or unofficial monographs.

Such groups include, but are not limited to, the United States Pharmacopeia (official) which has begun to prepare and publish information monographs on botanicals as part of its USP Drug Information System, as well as the German Commission E (official), which is explained below. Also, in the international arena, the World Health Organization (WHO) (quasi-official) has prepared 25 monographs on widely used medicinal plants, and the European Scientific Cooperative on Phytotherapy (ESCOP) (quasi-official) has published 50 therapeutic monographs on medicinal plants used in the European community. A new organization in the U.S., the American Herbal Pharmacopoeia, has begun to produce extensive peer-reviewed monographs (unofficial) on popular botanicals. The monographs produced by all of these organizations contain therapeutic guidelines for the use of the botanical medicines that are based on extensive reviews of the historical, scientific, and medical literature on the respective herb.[1] In England, the British Herbal Medicine Association has published an unofficial Compendium dealing with therapeutic parameters on 84 leading medicinal plants,[2] while a group of pharmacists at the University of London have published a guidebook on herbs for health professionals with a particular emphasis on safety issues.[3]

Numerous articles and books have been published in the past few years dealing with issues of toxicity of botanicals (see footnotes and references). A review of the literature on the safety of herbal medicines was written by Professor Norman R. Farnsworth, Research Professor of Pharmacognosy and Senior University Scholar at the University of Illinois at Chicago.[4] In the "Relative Safety of Herbal Medicines," Farnsworth notes that safety issues are always a relative concept and that the safety and toxicity of botanicals must be seen through the perspective of their totality of use when compared to conventional foods and drugs. The paper "is intended to highlight major types of problems that need to be taken into consideration when developing regulatory guidelines with suggestions for overcoming these difficulties."[4]

In reviewing the side effects and/or toxic reactions to herbal medicines, Farnsworth states, "Based on published reports, side effects or toxic reactions associated with herbal medicines in any form are rare."[4] This could be due to the fact that herbal medicines are generally safe, that adverse reactions following their use are underreported, or because the side effects are of such a nature that reporting them is not done (ie, such as minor allergic reactions).

"It is a rare instance when "advanced" herbal medicines are reported to produce adverse effects in humans. The reason for this is most likely due to the fact that products of this type are produced and marketed in Europe, where firms producing these products are more advanced in the area of quality control, and most either have research programs or support research on their products. Thus, most of the adverse effects reported for herbal medicines are associated with "crude drugs" or powered forms of plant material (ie, not "advanced", at least in-so-far as one can determine from the scientific literature)."[4]

Farnsworth reviews various categories of herbal toxicity: allergic reactions, herbs containing normal toxic substances (eg, pyrrolizidine alkaloids, aristolochic acid, phorbol esters), herbal medicines found toxic due to mislabeling, herbal medicines found toxic due to the intentional addition on unnatural toxic substances (eg, some Asian patent medicines), as well as various incidents of unexplained toxic effects associated with herbs (eg, hepatotoxicity associated with chaparral, *Larrea tridentata*, and germander, *Teucrium chamaedrys*. He concludes that "herbal medicines do not present a major problem with regard to toxicity based on a survey of the scientific literature. In fact, of all classes of substances reported to cause toxicities of sufficient magnitude to be reported in the United States, plants are the least problematic."[4]

With increased use of herbal dietary supplements by an estimated 60 million adult Americans in 1996, reports of adverse reactions have not risen at a corresponding rate. Plant exposure adverse reactions reported to the American Association of Poison Control Centers (AAPCC) do not indicate an alarming increase of herb-related adverse reactions.[5,6] A 1990 report from AAPCC indicated that most plant-related adverse reaction reports pertained to toxic houseplants, hot peppers, pokeweed, and poison ivy and not commercial herbal products.[5]

## STANDARDIZING COMMON NAMES FOR IDENTITY

In 1992, the American Herbal Products Association, the leading organization representing about 200 herb manufacturing and marketing companies, published *Herbs of Commerce*, a compilation of about 550 of the most popular herbs used in commercial herb products.[7] This publication contains the uniform common names and any synonyms, cross-referenced to the accepted botanical name (Latin binomial) and possible binomial synonyms. The primary intention of this publication was to develop uniformity in the way herb ingredients are labeled on commercial herb products, thereby allowing health professionals the opportunity to be able to gain access to reliable information within a reasonable period of time in the event of an adverse reaction. One problem that had previously plagued the herb industry was that without some general uniformity in common names, several different products from various manufacturers could conceivably contain the same ingredient(s), each under a different common name. This could create difficulty for a pharmacist at a poison control center or a nurse or physician at an emergency room who is attempting to find antidote directions for a patient who is experiencing an adverse reaction, presumably related to the ingestion of a commercial herbal product.

The Dietary Supplement Health and Education Act of 1994 (DSHEA) now requires that all labels of herbal products sold as dietary supplements contain both the common and Latin scientific names, as well as the plant part(s) used in the product. This will also assist health professionals in determining the nature of ingredients to research appropriate measures in the event of an adverse reaction.

## AHPA BOTANICAL SAFETY HANDBOOK RATING SYSTEM

In order to help standardize the labeling of commercial herb products with respect to safety issues, the American Herbal Products Association (AHPA) has published the *American Herbal Product Association's Botanical Safety Handbook* (BSH), a listing of over 600 herbs and botanical products sold in the U.S. market with a rating of the relative safety of each herb. This compilation of safety data is based on 29 authoritative general references plus additional references (eg, clinical studies, toxicological and pharmacological studies, case reports, etc) for each botanical. The Dietary Supplement Health and Education Act of 1994 (DSHEA) now permits manufacturers of herbal products to give detailed directions for the use of these products, including specific warnings, side effects, contraindications, and related safety data to help ensure safe and responsible use by consumers, as well as to offer guidance to health professionals. The BSH encourages the standardization of the safety of herbal products by creating four classes of herbs with respect to their relative safety/potential toxicity:

Class 1: Herbs which, when used appropriately, can be consumed safely without specific use restrictions.

Class 2: Herbs for which the following use restrictions apply:

- 2a: For external use only
- 2b: Not to be used during pregnancy. No other use restrictions apply, unless noted.
- 2c: Not to be used while nursing. No other use restrictions apply, unless noted.
- 2d: Other specific use restrictions, as noted.

Class 3: Herbs for which significant data exists to recommend the following labeling: "To be used only under the supervision of an expert qualified in the appropriate use of this substance." Labeling must include proper use information, dosage, contraindications, potential adverse effects, drug interactions, and any other relevant information related to the safe use of this substance.

Class 4: Herbs for which insufficient data is available for classification.

The authors of the BSH acknowledge a number of limitations in the scope of BSH. Namely, they did not include safety concerns that may arise from any of the following conditions:

- Excessive consumption of an herbal preparation; the safety data relates to consumption of herbs at relatively normal levels.
- Safety or toxicity concerns based on isolated constituents; individual phytochemical constituents of an herb (eg, plant-derived pharmaceutical drugs) are not considered herbs or phytomedicines, and thus, they were not included.
- Toxicity data based solely upon intravenous or intraperitoneal administration; only oral consumption and/or topical application was considered, as I.V. and I.P. administration is not consistent with self-selected herbal dietary supplements in the U.S. nor the limited use of herbs by healthcare practitioners in the U.S.
- Traditional Chinese medicine and Ayurvedic contraindications. (The authors limited their scope not to include these areas because they are often based on traditional, energetically-based systems that do not correspond directly to the Western pharmacological classifications.)
- Gastrointestinal disturbances; these are so common with use of many pharmacologically active agents that it seemed unreasonable to include them here, unless there is a real possibility that serious GI disturbances are predictable.
- Potential drug interactions; only those drug interactions that are relatively well documented are included (eg, those documented by Commission E).
- Idiosyncratic reactions; obviously, there is no way to predict this type of problem.
- Allergic reactions; unless a pattern of allergic reactions are well documented, there is always a possibility that sensitive individuals may react to any herb, conventional food, or pharmaceutical drug.
- Contact dermatitis; limited for same reasons as allergic reactions above.
- Well known toxic plants which are not found in trade (eg, *Aconitum napellus*, *Colchicum autumnale*, *Conium maculatum*, *Datura* spp, *Hyoscyamus niger*, *Strychnos nux-vomica*, etc)
- Essential oils
- Herbal products to which chemically-defined active substances, including chemically-defined isolated constituents of an herb, have been added.
- Environmental factors, additives, or contaminants

## PERSPECTIVES ON THE SAFETY OF HERBAL MEDICINES *(Continued)*

## GERMAN COMMISSION E MONOGRAPHS

In 1978, the German government established the Commission E, a special expert panel of physicians, pharmacists, pharmacologists, toxicologists, epidemiologists, and other professionals who are familiar with the vast body of historical and scientific literature dealing with herbs and medicinal plants. The Commission E has reviewed over 300 herbs and herbal combinations that have been sold as medicines in Germany and has assessed their safety according to what has been termed by Dr Varro E. Tyler, Emeritus Dean and Professor of Pharmacognosy at Purdue University, as a "doctrine of absolute certainty" regarding their safety. However, the Commission has determined that the efficacy of herbs can be evaluated according to a "doctrine of reasonable certainty." That is, assessment of efficacy does not necessarily require new clinical studies if there is sufficient scientific evidence in the chemical, toxicological, pharmacological, and/or clinical and epidemiological literature to document the traditional historical use of the product as a nonprescription medicine. In Germany, herbal products are sold in pharmacies and are routinely prescribed by physicians and recommended by pharmacists, both of which are required to study phytomedicine (plant medicine) in medical or pharmacy school. The Commission E publishes the results of its evaluations in the form of monographs in the German government's version of the *Federal Register.*

Commission E has published about 435 monographs and revisions. About 200 of the 300 herb and herb combinations were approved as drugs; the remaining third were either too toxic to be used safely or adequate scientific evidence was lacking to document a positive claim. The Commission E monographs are intended to be used as package inserts to give health professionals and consumers proper guidance in using herbal drugs. They include approved use(s), contraindications (if any are known), side effects (if known), interactions with other drugs (if known), specified dosage or dosage range (based on particular types of galenical formulations), mode of application, duration of administration, and specific pharmacological actions determined as a result of pharmacological and/or experimental research. The entire body of Commission E monographs has been translated from German into English by the American Botanical Council and is available for the first time in a complete book so that health professionals and consumers can obtain specific therapeutic information on the appropriate and responsible use of many herbal products.

**Herbs Contraindicated During Lactation According to German Commission E**

| | |
|---|---|
| Aloe (*Aloe vera*) | Kava kava root (*Piper methysticum*) |
| Basil (*Ocimum basillcum*) | Petasite root (*Pefasites* spp) |
| Buckthorn bark and berry (*Rhamnus frangula, R. cathartica*) | Indian snakeroot (*Rauwolfia serpentina*) |
| Cascara sagrada (*Rhamnus purshiana*) | Rhubarb root (*Rheum palmatum*) |
| Coltsfoot leaf (*Tussilago farfara*) | Senna (*Cassia senna*) |
| Combinations of senna, peppermint oil and caraway oil | |

**Herbs Contraindicated During Pregnancy According to German Commission E**

| | |
|---|---|
| Aloe (*Aloe vera*) | Combination of senna, peppermint oil, and caraway oil |
| Autumn crocus (*Colchicum autumnale*) | Ginger root (*Zingiber officinale*)* |
| Black cohosh root (*Cimicifuga racemosa*) | Indian snakeroot (*Rauwolfia serpentina*) |
| Buckthorn bark and berry (*Rhamnus frangula, R. cathartica*) | Juniper berry (*Juniperus comunis*) |
| Cascara sagrada bark (*Rhamnus purshiana*) | Kava kava root (*Piper methysticum*) |
| Chaste tree fruit (*Vitex agnus-castus*) | Licorice root (*Glycyrrhiza glabra*) |
| Cinchona bark (*Cinchona* spp) | Marsh tea (*Ledum palustre*) |
| Cinnamon bark (*Cinnamomum zeylanicum*) | Mayapple root (*Podophyllum peltatum*) |
| Coltsfoot leaf (*Tussliago farfara*) | Petasite root (*Petasites* spp) |
| Echinacea purpurea herb (*Echinacea purpurea*) | Rhubarb root (*Rheum palmatum*) |
| Fennel oil (*Foeniculum vulgare*) | Sage leaf (*Salvia officinalis*) |
| Combination of licorice, peppermint, and chamomile | Senna (*Cassia senna*) |
| Combination of licorice, primrose, marshmallow, and anise | |

*A subsequent review of the clinical literature could find no basis for the contraindication of ginger, a common spice, during pregnancy (Fulder and Tenne, 1996).

Adapted from Blumenthal M, Goldberg A, Gruenwald J, et al, *German Commission E Monographs: Therapeutic Monographs on Medicinal Plants for Human Use*, Austin, TX: American Botanical Council, 1997.

**Summary of Herb-Drug Interactions as Noted by the German Commission E**

This table shows the herbal drug and information on possible antagonistic or synergistic interactions it may have with conventional pharmaceutical medicines. In most instances, this information has been abbreviated and modified from the original section "Interactions With Other Drugs" in the Commission E monographs.

**Aloe** – Chronic use/abuse can increase loss of serum potassium, thereby potentiating cardiac glycosides and antiarrhythmic agents. Potassium deficiency can be increased by simultaneous use of thiazide diuretics, corticosteroids, and licorice root. (**Note:** Similar data applies to all other approved stimulant laxatives: cascara sagrada bark, buckthorn bark and berry, rhubarb root, and senna leaf. Also, reader should note that the aloe is "drug aloe" (made from the inner leaf) not the aloe gel from which numerous drinks are made and marketed in the U.S. Ingestion of aloe gel does not produce a significant laxative effect nor does it produce the drug interactions noted here.)

**Belladonna leaf and root** – Increased anticholinergic effect by tricyclic antidepressants, amantadine, and quinidine.

**Bromelain** – Increased tendency for bleeding with simultaneous administration of anticoagulants and inhibitors of thrombocytic aggregation. Increased plasma and urine levels of tetracyclines.

**Buckthorn bark/berry** – Chronic use/abuse can increase loss of serum potassium thus potentiating cardiac glycosides and antiarrhythmic agents. Potassium deficiency can be increased by simultaneous use of thiazide diuretics, corticosteroids, and licorice root.

**Bugle weed** – None known. No simultaneous administration of thyroid preparations. Interferes with diagnostic procedures with radioactive isotopes.

**Cascara sagrada bark** – Chronic use/abuse can increase loss of serum potassium thus potentiating cardiac glycosides and antiarrhythmic agents. Potassium deficiency can be increased by simultaneous use of thiazide diuretics, corticosteroids, and licorice root.

**Chaste tree fruits** – Interactions unknown. Animal experiments show evidence of dopaminergic effect; therefore, a reciprocal weakening of the effect can occur in cases of ingestion of dopamine-receptor antagonists.

**Cinchona bark** – Increases the effect of anticoagulants if given simultaneously.

**Cola nut** – Strengthening of the action of psychoaneleptic drugs and caffeine-containing beverages.

**Ephedra** – In combination with cardiac glycosides or halothane: disturbance or heart rhythm; with guanethidine: enhancement of the sympathomimetic effect; with MAO-inhibitors: greatly raising the sympathomimetic action of ephedrine; with secale alkaloid derivatives or oxytocin: development of hypertension.

**Eucalyptus leaf and oil** – None known for leaf. Oil induces liver enzymes system involved in detoxification process so effects of other drugs can be weakened and/or shortened.

**Flaxseed** – Mucilage may negatively affect absorption of other drugs.

**Henbane leaf** – Enhancement of anticholinergic action by tricyclic antidepressants, amantadine, antihistamines, phenothiazines, procainamide, and quinidine.

**Indian snakeroot** – These drugs taken with Indian snakeroot produce the following reactions: Digitalis glycosides – bradycardia; barbiturates – mutual potentiation; levodopa – reduced effectiveness but undesired extra pyramidal motor symptoms can be increased; sympathomimetics (eg, cough/cold medications and appetite suppressants) – initial strong blood pressure increase.

**Kava kava rhizome** – Possible potentiation of effectiveness for substances acting on CNS (eg, alcohol, barbiturates, and psychopharmacological agents).

**Licorice root** – Potassium loss due to other drugs (eg, thiazide diuretics, can be increased, resulting in increased sensitivity to digitalis glycosides).

**Lily-of-the-valley herb** – Increased effectiveness and side effects of simultaneously administered quinidine, calcium, saluretics, laxatives, and extended therapy with glucocorticoids.

**Marshmallow leaf/root** – None known. **Note:** Absorption of other drugs taken simultaneously may be delayed.

**Niauli oil** – High cineol content causes induction of enzymes involved in liver detoxification so effect of other drugs can be reduced and/or shortened.

**Oak bark** – Absorption of alkaloids and other alkaline drugs may be reduced or inhibited.

**Pheasant's eye herb** – Enhanced effectiveness and side effects of simultaneous intake of quinidine, calcium, saluretics, laxatives, and extended therapy with glucocorticoids.

**Psyllium seed, blonde, Psyllium seed husk, blonde** – Intestinal absorption of other medication taken at the same time may be delayed. Possible reduction of insulin dosage in insulin-dependent diabetics.

**Scopolia root** – Increased effectiveness of simultaneously administered tricyclic antidepressants, amantadine, and quinidine.

**Senna fruit/leaf** – Chronic use/abuse can increase loss of serum potassium, thereby potentiating cardiac glycosides and antiarrhythmic agents. Potassium deficiency can be increased by simultaneous use of thiazide diuretics, corticosteroids, and licorice root.

**Squill** – Increased effectiveness and side effects by simultaneously administered quinidine, calcium, saluretics, laxatives, and extended therapy with glucocorticoids.

**Uva ursi leaf** – Should not be administered with any substances which cause acidic urine as this reduces the antibacterial effect.

**White willow bark** – Because of the bark's active constituents, interactions like those encountered with salicylates may arise, although there was no case of this reported in the scientific literature.

**Yeast, medicinal** – Simultaneous intake of MAO inhibitors can cause an increase in blood pressure.

Adapted from Blumenthal M, Goldberg A, Gruenwald J, et al, *German Commission E Monographs: Therapeutic Monographs on Medicinal Plants for Human Use*, Austin, TX: American Botanical Council, 1997.

## PERSPECTIVES ON THE SAFETY OF HERBAL MEDICINES *(Continued)*

### Conventional Drugs and Other Substances That May Interact With Herbal Drugs Approved by the German Commission E

| Drug/Substance | Commission E Herbal Drug |
|---|---|
| Alcohol | Kava kava rhizome |
| Alkaline drugs | Oak bark |
| Alkaloids | Oak bark |
| Amantadine | Belladonna leaf and root<br>Henbane leaf<br>Pheasant's eye herb<br>Scopolia root |
| Antiarrhythmic agents | Aloe<br>Buckthorn bark/berry<br>Cascara sagrada bark<br>Senna fruit/leaves |
| Anticoagulants | Bromelain<br>Cinchona |
| Antihistamines | Henbane leaf |
| Barbiturates | Indian snakeroot<br>Kava kava rhizome |
| Caffeine-containing beverages | Cola |
| Calcium | Lily-of-the-valley<br>Pheasant's eye herb<br>Squill |
| Cardiac glycosides | Aloe<br>Buckthorn bark/berry<br>Cascara sagrada bark<br>Ephedra<br>Senna fruit/leaves |
| Corticosteroids | Aloe<br>Buckthorn bark/berry<br>Cascara sagrada bark<br>Senna fruit/leaves |
| CNS depressants | Kava kava<br>Melatonin<br>Valerian |
| Digitalis glycosides | Indian snakeroot<br>Licorice root |
| Dopamine receptor agonists | Chaste tree fruits (shown in animal experiments only) |
| Glucocorticoids | Lily-of-the-valley<br>Pheasant's eye herb<br>Squill |
| Guanethidine | Ephedra |
| Halothane | Ephedra |
| Laxatives | Lily-of-the-valley<br>Pheasant's eye herb<br>Squill |
| Levodopa | Indian snakeroot |
| Licorice root | Aloe<br>Buckthorn bark/berry<br>Cascara sagrada bark<br>Senna fruit/leaves |
| Lithium | Agave<br>Begolia<br>Borage<br>Broom<br>Buchu<br>Burdock<br>Calamus<br>Celery<br>Chicory<br>Dandelion<br>Ephedra<br>Foxglove<br>Guarana<br>Horsetail<br>Juniper<br>Lovage<br>Mate (yerba mate)<br>Onion<br>Saw palmetto<br>Uva ursi<br>Windflower |
| MAO inhibitors | Ephedra<br>Medicinal yeast |
| Oxytocin | Ephedra |
| Phenothiazines | Henbane leaf |
| Procainamide | Henbane leaf |
| Psychoaneleptic drugs | Cola |
| Psychopharmacological agents | Kava kava rhizome |
| Quinidine | Belladonna leaf and root<br>Henbane leaf<br>Lily-of-the-valley<br>Pheasant's eye herb<br>Scopolia root<br>Squill |

**Conventional Drugs and Other Substances That May Interact With Herbal Drugs Approved by the German Commission E** *(continued)*

| Drug/Substance | Commission E Herbal Drug |
|---|---|
| Radioactive isotopes | Bugle weed |
| Saluretics | Lily-of-the-valley<br>Pheasant's eye herb<br>Squill |
| Secale alkaloid derivatives | Ephedra |
| Sympathomimetics | Indian snakeroot |
| Tetracycline | Bromelain |
| Thiazide diuretics | Aloe<br>Buckthorn bark/berry<br>Cascara sagrada bark<br>Licorice root<br>Senna fruit/leaves |
| Thyroid preparations | Bugle weed |
| Thrombocytic aggregation inhibitors | Bromelain |
| Tricyclic antidepressants | Belladonna leaf and root<br>Henbane leaf<br>Scopolia root |
| Urine-acidifying agents | Uva ursi leaf |

Adapted from Blumenthal M, Goldberg A, Gruenwald J, et al, *German Commission E Monographs: Therapeutic Monographs on Medicinal Plants for Human Use*, Austin, TX: American Botanical Council, 1997.

## Footnotes

1. Blumenthal M, "Herbal Monographs Initiated by Numerous Groups: WHO, USP, ESCOP, ABC, and AHP All Working Towards Similar Goals," *HerbalGram*, 1997, 40:30-7.
2. Bradley P, *British Herbal Compendium*, Vol 1, Bournemouth, England: British Herbal Medical Association, 1992.
3. Newell CA, Anderson LA, and Philippson JD, *Herbal Medicines: A Guide for Healthcare Professionals*, London, England: The Pharmaceutical Press, 1996.
4. Farnsworth NR, "The Relative Safety of Herbal Medicines," *HerbalGram*, 1993, 29:36A-H
5. McCaleb RS, "Food Ingredient Safety Evaluation," *Food Drug Law J*, 1992, 47:657-63.
6. Soloway R, *Personal Communication*, July 21, 1997.
7. Foster S, *Herbs of Commerce*, Austin, TX: American Herbal Products Association, 1992.

## References


Blumenthal M, Goldberg A, Gruenwald J, et al, *German Commission E Monographs: Therapeutic Monographs on Medicinal Plants for Human Use*, Austin, TX: American Botanical Council, 1997.

D'Arcy PF, "Adverse Reactions and Interactions With Herbal Medicines: Part 1. Adverse Reactions," *Adverse Drug Reaction Toxicol Rev*, 1991, 10(4):189-208.

D'Arcy PF, McEmay JC, and Welling PG, *Mechanisms of Drug Interactions*, New York, NY: Springer-Verlag, 1996.

DeSmet PA, "Health Risks of Herbal Remedies," *Drug Saf*, 1995, 13(2):81-93.

DeSmet PA, Keller K, Hansel R, et al, *Adverse Effects of Herbal Drugs*, Vol 3, New York, NY: Springer-Verlag, 1997.

DeSmet PA, Keller K, Hansel R, et al, *Adverse Effects of Herbal Drugs*, Vol 2, New York, NY: Springer-Verlag, 1993.

DeSmet PA, Keller K, Hansel R, et al, *Adverse Effects of Herbal Drugs*, Vol 1, New York, NY: Springer-Verlag.

Ernst E and DeSmet PA, "Risks Associated With Complementary Therapies," *Meyler's Side Effects of Drugs*, 13th ed, Dukes MN ed, New York, NY: Elsevier Science, 1996.

Fulder S and Tenne M, "Ginger as an Antinausea Remedy in Pregnancy: The Issue of Safety," *HerbalGram*, 1996, 36:47-50.

Keller K, "Therapeutic Use of Herbal Drugs and Their Potential Toxicity, Problems and Results of the Revision of Herbal Medicines in the EEC," *Proceedings of the 3rd International Conference on Pharmacopoeias and Quality Control of Drugs*, Rome, November, 1992, published in Bologna, Fondazione Rhone-Poulenc Rorer per le Scienze Mediche, 1993.

McGuffin M, Hobbs C, Upton R, et al, *American Herbal Product Association's Botanical Safety Handbook: Guidelines for the Safe Use and Labeling for Herbs of Commerce*, Boca Raton, FL: CRC Press, 1997.

Siegers CP, "Anthranoid Laxatives and Colorectal Cancer," *Trends in Pharmaceutical Science*, 1992, 13:229-31.

# NATURAL PRODUCTS, HERBALS, AND DIETARY SUPPLEMENTS

Adapted from Wynn RL, Meiller TF, and Crossley HL, *Drug Information Handbook for Dentistry,* 4th ed, Hudson, OH: Lexi-Comp, Inc, 1998.

Medical problem: " I have a toothache."
2000 BC response: "Here, eat this root."
1000 AD: "That root is heathen; here, say this prayer."
1850 AD: "That prayer is superstitious; here, drink this potion."
1940 AD: "That potion is snake oil; here, swallow this pill."
1985 AD: "That pill is ineffective; here, take this new antibiotic."
2000 AD: "That antibiotic is artificial; here, eat this root."

*– Adapted from an anonymous Internet communication*

## INTRODUCTION

For centuries, Eastern and Western civilizations have attributed a large number of medical uses to plants and herbs. Over time, modern scientific methodologies have emerged from some of these remedies. Conversely, some of these agents have fallen into less popularity as more medical knowledge has evolved. In spite of this dichotomy, herbal and natural therapies for treatment of common medical ailments have become exceedingly popular. In America, people consistently seek out natural products that may be able to offset some perceived ailment or may assist in the prevention of an ailment. One area that has consistently drawn patients interested in herbal or natural remedies has been the area of weight loss. There are numerous systemic considerations when some of the natural products that have been attributed weight loss powers are utilized. Many of these products are sold under the blanket of dietary supplements and, therefore, avoid some of the more stringent Food and Drug Administration legislation. In 1994, that legislation was modified to include herbs, vitamins, minerals, and amino acids that may be taken as dietary supplements and that information must be available to patients taking them. The real concern, however, lies in the fact that health claims need not be approved by the FDA, but the advertisements must include a disclaimer saying that the product has not yet been fully evaluated. Claims of medicinal use/value are often drawn from popular use, not necessarily from scientific studies. The safety, however, when these agents are taken in combination with other prescription drugs is of concern and medical risk might result. Many of these natural products may have real medicinal value but caution on the part of the clinician is prudent. It is impossible within this chapter to cover all of the popular natural products. The chapter, therefore, has been limited to brief reviews of some of the most popular dietary supplements, herbs, and natural remedies currently being used by patients you might treat and what we know about the effects of some of these agents on the body's various systems. An extensive reading list is provided.

## TOP 20 MOST POPULAR NATURAL PRODUCTS

### ALFALFA

Alfalfa has been touted as a natural laxative, an antifungal, a liver detoxifier, a diuretic, and a food additive useful in treating kidney stones and urinary infections. Alfalfa is an important animal feed worldwide and its chemical constituents are well known. However, studies have concluded that alfalfa contains nothing of significant therapeutic value in the amounts generally recommended. The seed contains L-canabanine which has been implicated in pancytopenia in humans and may induce systemic lupus in monkeys. Allergic reactions have been provoked in some users.

### ALOE VERA

Products derived from this plant have been used for centuries. Aloe is popularly used as a cure-all and it has been advertised for use in treating acne, burns, and minor wounds. Although the FDA does not recognize the uses of aloe for the treatment of any specific condition, there is evidence to suggest that fresh aloe gel is an effective agent in wound healing. Data to support these claims are inconclusive, however, and the use of aloe by patients should not interfere with care.

### BILBERRY

Bilberry, also known as blueberry, is recommended by herbalists for use in connection with vascular and blood disorders and in treating varicose veins, thromboses, diarrhea, and angina. Preliminary studies have indicated that bilberry may have some benefit in aiding visual acuity, however, there is little clinical evidence to support the widespread usage. Potential interactions with over-the-counter prescription medications are unknown at this time.

### CAYENNE

Most cooks know of the chemical cayenne that is the active ingredient in chili pepper and lends itself to the strong taste of this herb. Cayenne has been known for many years to stimulate digestion and to promote sweating; sometimes assisting, therefore, in reducing fever. Cayenne contains an ingredient known as capsaicin which is the active ingredient in many over-the-counter and prescription forms of cream to treat arthritis. Capsaicin appears to alter the action of the compound associated with pain, the mechanism of which has not been completely studied.

### CHAMOMILE

This agent is often found in the form of dried leaves that can be used to create a tea. The tea is taken internally and has been recommended by naturalists as a cure for stomach pain, menstrual discomfort, and stress. Chamomile teas appear to have some unknown mechanism of immune activation, perhaps due to the presence of flavonoids in the compound.

**CRANBERRY**
Cranberry has been used for centuries as an agent to assist in treatment of urinary tract infections. Cranberry juices contain a pH-altering chemical which may be of use in treating these infections. It is now thought that the cranberry actually prevents bacteria from adhering to the lining of the bladder and urinary tract. Again, this agent is rich in flavonoids, citric acids, and vitamin C.

**ECHINACEA**
Echinacea is reported to have uses for treatment of colds, flu, bacterial and fungal infections, and even cancer. AIDS patients are sometimes advised by their peers to take echinacea. To date, pharmacological components and their actions on the human body are unclear. However, complex polysaccharides are found in the agent and seem to hold some promise as compounds for immunostimulation. In general, echinacea appears to be relatively safe but clinical information is lacking.

**EPHEDRA**
Also known as ma-huang, ephedra has been used in China for more than 4000 years to treat symptoms of upper respiratory infections and asthma. Ephedra can be used as a nasal decongestant and has recently gained new popularity as a weight loss product. This agent, when used in combination with St John's Wort, apparently has effects on serotonin levels similar to the drug fenfluramine which was recently taken off the market. This combination of drugs has been known as natural fen-phen. Ephedra has also been recommended as an aphrodisiac.

**FEVERFEW**
Feverfew has a long history of use in traditional and cult medicine as a treatment for fever, headache, and menstrual irregularities. More recently, it has been suggested for migraine headaches, arthritis, and insect bites. Be aware that patients may self-medicate with feverfew in an effort to treat migraine headaches. One study of commercially available feverfew products has found that there is a lactone present that appears to have some activity. However, there are no long-term toxicology studies to indicate or refute this claim.

**GARLIC**
Garlic and related products have been used for thousands of years. It is generally considered by herbalists and naturalists as a cure-all. When garlic is crushed, it produces allicin which possesses some antibiotic, antiplatelet, anticholesterol properties. In addition, other sulfur-containing compounds are found in garlic and these produce some antithrombotic properties. For the most part, the consumption of moderate amounts of garlic is harmless. Large doses, however, are likely to stimulate heartburn and gastric or intestinal disorders.

**GINGER**
Ginger has been taken for centuries due to its calming effects on an upset stomach. The stem of the rhizome from a tropical plant has been used to make the ginger root. Today it is widely used for morning sickness, seasickness, and motion sickness. Ginger may have some effect on cholesterol levels although further study is necessary. The presence of essential oils in ginger may be the active ingredients in this agent.

**GINKGO BILOBA**
Ginkgo supplements are claimed by herbalists to help with the aging process and with mental acuity. The most popular of these agents is used as an extract to promote improved blood flow to a portion of the body. Clinical research has not proven that these claims are or are not true.

**GINSENG**
Ginseng is commonly used as a substance to support general good health and has also been marketed in some countries as an aphrodisiac. As with the majority of herbal agents, there are few clinical studies. However, commercial products vary widely and the clinician may be aware that ginseng could produce some side effects.

**GREEN TEA**
Green tea has been widely used in Asia to treat numerous ailments. This tea is derived from leaves and delicate leaf buds of an evergreen bush. It is thought that green tea has some antioxidant effect, as well as containing compounds and flavonoids as with many of the other herbs.

**KAVA**
Kava is one of the most popular herbs on today's market. It is extracted from a root and is used to promote sleep and relaxation in anxious patients. This agent appears to be extremely safe, however, the full effect of the active ingredient know as kavalactones, is unknown. They appear to have an effect on the neural transmitter activity in the central nervous system.

**LICORICE**
Licorice has been used for centuries to treat intestinal disorders and stomach distress. There appears to be some activity of licorice on patients who suffer from mild preulcerous conditions in the GI tract. Again, the flavonoids appear to be an active component.

**PSYLLIUM**
Psyllium has been used by herbalists and natural product advocates to promote regular intestinal function, primarily as an agent to assist in constipation and in GI distress.

## NATURAL PRODUCTS, HERBALS, AND DIETARY SUPPLEMENTS *(Continued)*

### ST JOHN'S WORT

St John's wort has become popular in the treatment of depression, anxiety, and even in AIDS. While some of the constituents seem to show a minimal amount of antidepressant activity, other components may suggest that St John's wort is ineffective in treating these illnesses.

### SAW PALMETTO

Saw palmetto was an official drug used for a variety of ailments, mainly associated with urogenital disorders. It has actually been shown to have some efficacy in managing benign prostate hypertrophy. The drug, however, has not yet passed any of the rigid FDA requirements prior to being able to substantiate this claim.

### VALERIAN

Valerian has, for centuries, made claims of being a natural tranquilizer, a relaxant for pain and muscle spasms, as well as promoting restful sleep. Be aware that some patients may be drawn to use valerian in an effort to reduce TMD dysfunction or muscle pain.

Herbalists have often used these natural products singularly or in combination to achieve a therapeutic effect. Some of the natural agents have been combined for assisted weight loss or for reduction of more serious ailments such as high blood pressure or cardiovascular disease. One such combination recommends ephedra and St John's wort as a "natural fen-phen". These agents are not directly related to fenfluramine, but are thought to also act on serotonin levels in the brain. Be aware that there are some known interactions of these agents with drug therapies that may be used. However, our knowledge is extremely limited in this extent.

## EFFECTS ON CENTRAL NERVOUS SYSTEM

**(Aconite, Ginseng, Xanthine derivatives)**

Aconite and hawthorn have potentially sedating effects, and aconite also contains various alkaloids and traces of ephedrine. Some documented central nervous system (CNS) effects of aconite include sedation, vertigo, and incoordination. Hawthorn has been reported to exert a depressive effect on the CNS leading to sedation.

Ginseng, ma-huang, and xanthine derivatives can exert a stimulant effect on the central nervous system. Some of the CNS effects of ginseng include nervousness, insomnia, and euphoria. The action of ma-huang is due to the presence of ephedrine and pseudoephedrine. Ma-huang exerts a stimulant action on the CNS similar to decongestant/weight loss products (Dexatrim®, etc) thus causing nervousness, insomnia, and anxiety. Kola nut, green tea, guarana, and yerba mate contain varying amounts of caffeine, a xanthine derivative. Stimulant properties exerted by these herbs are expected to be comparable to those of caffeine, including insomnia, nervousness, and anxiety.

Products containing aconite and hawthorn should be used with caution in patients with known history of depression, vertigo, or syncope. Ginseng or xanthine derivatives should be avoided in patients with history of insomnia or anxiety. Use of natural products with these components may contribute to a worsening of a patient's pre-existing medical condition. Patients taking CNS-active medications should avoid or use extreme caution when using preparations containing any of the above components. These components may interact directly or indirectly with CNS-active medications causing an increase or decrease in overall effect.

# HERBALS THAT MAY ALTER METABOLISM AND GI ABSORPTION OF DRUGS

| Herbal Medications That May Alter Metabolism | Herbals Medications That May Alter GI Absorption |
|---|---|
| Virginia snakeroot, Serpenteria (*Aristolochia serpenteria*) | California buckeye (*Aesculus californica*) |
| Indian root, Raiz del indio (*Aristolochia watson* | Ohio buckeye (*Aesculus glabra*) |
| Sagebrush (*Artemisia tridentata*) | Horse chestnut (*Aesculus hippocastanum*) |
| Common barberry (*Berberis vulgaris*) | Aloe |
| Button bush (*Cephalanthus*) | Uva, ursi, mananzanita, bearberry (*Arctostaphylos*) |
| Greater celandine (*Chelidonium*) | Cayenne, African bird peppers (*Capsicum*) |
| Balmony, turtlehead (*Chelone*) | Sodium copper chlorophyllin, chlorophyll |
| Fringetree (*Chionanthus*) | Mormon tea, American ephedra, canutillo (*Ephedra viridis*) |
| Wahoo, Burning bush (*Euonymus*) | Rhamnus frangula, buckthorn |
| Goldenseal (*Hydrastis*) | Maravilla (*Mirabilis multifulorum*) |
| Blue flag (*Iris versicolor*) | Wager ash, hop tree (*Ptelea*) |
| Voronicastrum, Culver's root (*Leptandra*) | California buckthorn (*Rhamnus californica*) |
| Oregon grape, Algerita (*Mahonia*) | Buckthorn (*Rhamnus frangula*) |
| American mandrake (*Podophyllum*) | Cascara sagrada (*Rhamnus purshiana*) |
| | Senna |
| | Yucca |

# NATURAL/HERBAL PRODUCTS

| Herb | Use(s) | Administration | Adverse Effects | Clinical Considerations |
|---|---|---|---|---|
| **ALOE** | External: Burns/sunburn, wounds, skin irritation, antimicrobial, moisturizer<br>Internal: Laxative, general healing | External: Aloe vera gel, applied liberally<br>Internal: Aloe vera juice (not recommended, but if used, no more than 1 quart/day should be consumed) | External: Contact dermatitis<br>Internal: Painful intestinal contractions | External: May delay healing of deep, vertical (surgical wounds)<br>Internal: Loss of intestinal potassium with resulting decrease in serum potassium which may potentiate effects of cardiac glycosides and antiarrhythmics; decreased serum potassium is potentiated by concurrent use of thiazides, steroids, licorice, and other potassium-wasting drugs; avoid if pregnant |
| **BILBERRY** | Eye disorders (including day and night vision), cataracts, macular degeneration, diabetic retinopathy | 20-40 mg 3 times/day (calculated as anthocyanidin); bilberry tea | None reported | Inhibits platelet aggregation (monitor patients on antiplatelet drugs and warfarin); lowers blood glucose (monitor patients with diabetes mellitus) |
| **CAYENNE** | External: Pain disorders, including shingle, stump pain, diabetic neuropathy, cluster headache, osteoarthritis, and rheumatoid arthritis<br>Internal: Stomach protectant, thermogenesis | External: 0.025% to 0.075% capsaicin-containing preparation 4 times/day<br>Internal: Liberally or as tolerated in diet | External: Initial transient, local burning<br>Internal: Stomach upset, diarrhea, burning during bowel movements | Remove cayenne from hands with vinegar; eat bananas to decrease GI irritation from ingesting cayenne; protects stomach against NSAID damage by stimulating GI secretions of mucus if given 30 minutes before NSAID; reduces platelet aggregation and increases fibrinolytic activity; monitor patients on antiplatelet drugs and warfarin |
| **CHAMOMILE** | Antispasmodic: Upset stomach and indigestion<br>Sedative: Sleep, nerve calming<br>Anti-inflammatory: Skin problems and muscle stiffness | Tea or compress: Steep 2 tsp of fresh or dried flowers in 1 pint boiling water for 20 minutes; drink 3-4 cups/day | Hypersensitivity: Sneezing, dermatitis, and anaphylaxis; large amounts may cause GI upset | May be ingested regularly for accumulation and subsequent effect; potential for delaying concomitant drug absorption from the gut |
| **DONG QUAI** | Amenorrhea, dysmenorrhea, and menopause (especially hot flashes) | Powdered root or tea: 1-2 g 3 times/day<br>Tincture (1:5): 1 teaspoonful 3 times/day<br>Fluid extract: 1 mL (1/4 teaspoonful) 3 times/day | Sunburn from *Angelica archangelica* sp.; decreases blood pressure; possible CNS stimulation | Some species are phototoxic, resulting in rash or extreme sunburn (phototoxicity may be useful in patients with psoriasis); possible synergism with calcium channel blockers; inhibits platelet aggregation (monitor warfarin patients) |
| **ECHINACEA** | General infectious conditions from virus, bacteria, and *Candida* sp.; influenza, colds, upper respiratory tract infections, and urogenital infections; also snake bites | Fluid extract (1:1): 1-2 mL 3 times/day (1/4-1/2 teaspoonful)<br>Solid extract (6.5:1): 300 mg 3 times/day | Tingling sensation on tongue; fever from freshly pressed juice; cross-sensitivity in patients allergic to sunflower seeds | Continual use not recommended; avoid in patients with autoimmune disease (eg, rheumatoid arthritis and lupus) or leukemia |
| **FEVERFEW** | Prophylactic for migraine headache; relieves fever and arthritis | 25-100 mg dry powdered leaf capsules (standardized to 0.25-0.5 mg parthenolide)/day or 2-3 leaves/day | Aphthous ulcers may result from chewing leaves | May take 4-6 months to see an effect; do not discontinue abruptly; reduces platelet aggregation and increased fibrinolytic activity (monitor patients on antiplatelet drugs and warfarin); avoid in pregnant women (uterine stimulant) and children <2 years |
| **GARLIC** | Broad spectrum antimicrobial; lowers blood pressure and serum cholesterol | 10 mg of allicin or a total allicin potential of 4000 mcg/day or 1 clove (4 g) of fresh garlic/day | Generally nontoxic but may cause GI irritation | Inhibits platelet aggregation and increases fibrinolytic activity (monitor patients on antiplatelet drugs and warfarin); increased serum insulin levels which may decreased blood glucose (monitor blood glucose) |
| **GINGER** | Motion sickness, morning sickness, postoperative nausea, arthritis, muscular pain, and migraine headache | Powdered ginger root: Nausea and vomiting: 250 mg 4 times/day<br>Arthritis: 125-1000 mg 4 times/day | GI discomfort with high doses (>6 g) if taken on an empty stomach | Inhibits platelet aggregation (monitor patients on antiplatelet drugs and warfarin; increased calcium uptake by heart muscle, may alter calcium channel blocker effect; fresh ginger root may yield better results: 1-2 g of powder = approximately 1/4-inch slice |
| **GINKGO** | Vascular insufficiency resulting in short-term memory loss, vertigo, headache, and tinnitus; depression, intermittent claudication, early Alzheimer's disease, senility, diabetic retinopathy | 40 mg 3-4 times/day; use standardized leaf extract containing 24% ginkgo heterosides | Rare with ginkgo biloba extract; most common are GI discomfort and headache | Response may be seen in 2-3 weeks, but take consistently for 12 weeks to improve prospects of positive clinical outcome |
| **GINSENG** (Panax; American, Chinese, Korean) | Antifatigue, antistress, regulates blood pressure (dose dependent), enhances immune function, menopausal symptoms, general adaptogen | Take 1-3 times/day; use product standardized to provide 10 mg of ginsenoside and Rg1:Rb2 ratio of 1:2 | Breast tenderness in women; nervousness and excitation that decreased with continued use or decreased dose; generally low toxicity from high-quality, standardized product | Use cyclically with 2 weeks on, followed by 2 weeks off; decreased platelet adhesiveness (monitor patients taking anticoagulants); variable effects on INR; high doses may inhibit immune function in early stages of infection; hypoglycemia effect (monitor patients with diabetes) |
| **GINSENG** (Siberian) | Adaptogen, antistress, lowers serum cholesterol, decreases blood pressure (increases blood pressure if low), decreases anginal symptoms, increases sense of well being, chronic fatigue syndrome, immune system booster | Take 1-3 times/day; 2-4 mL fluid extract (1:1) or 100-200 mg solid extract (20:1) containing 0.1% eleutheroside E | High doses (>4.5-6 mL 3 times/day) may induce insomnia, irritability, and anxiety; skin eruptions, diarrhea; headache; hypertension; pericardial pain in rheumatic heart patients | Estrogenic effect - do not use any form of ginseng during pregnancy; same clinical considerations as for panax ginseng |
| **GOLDEN SEAL** | Bacterial and fungal infections of the mucous membranes, GI infections that cause diarrhea, liver cirrhosis, inflamed gallbladder, and eye infections | 250-500 mg 3 times/day; use product standardized to contain 8% to 12% berberine | Do not use during pregnancy, nausea, vomiting; CNS stimulant; may interfere with colon's ability to manufacture B vitamins | Use in conjunction with standard antimicrobial therapy; hypoglycemic effect (monitor patients with diabetes); prophylactic use for traveler's diarrhea (give 1 week before, during, and 1 week after travel); use for no longer than 2 months at a time |
| **HAWTHORN** | Atherosclerosis, high blood pressure, mild-to-moderate CHF, rheumatoid arthritis, and periodontal disease | Take 3 times/day: 1-2 mL hawthorn fluid extract (1:)<br>Standardized on procyanidine: 1-1.5 g freeze-dried hawthorn berries | None reported with low doses; high doses may induce hypotension and sedation | Increases body's utilization of vitamin C; inhibits angiotensin-converting enzyme (ACE) and may result in decreased dose requirement of ACE inhibitor drug; potentiates cardiac glycosides resulting in decrease in dose requirements; may take up to 2 weeks to see an effect; do not discontinue abruptly |
| **LaPACHO** (Pau d'arco) | Used to treat bacterial, fungal, viral, and parasitic infections, especially intestinal and vaginal candidiasis | Standardized to provide 1.5-2 g of lapachol/day as a tea or extract | None reported from whole bark | Purchase standardized product from reputable companies, as many products contain no active ingredients (lapachol or quinones) |

| Herb | Use(s) | Administration | Adverse Effects | Clinical Considerations |
|---|---|---|---|---|
| **LICORICE** | Internal: Glycyrrhetinic acid (GA): Antiviral for cold symptoms and HSV-1, PMS, Addison's disease, inflammation<br>External: GA, eczema, canker sore, HSV | Fluid extract (1:1): 2-4 mL<br>Solid extract (4:1): 250-500 mg<br>DGL for peptic ulcer disease: 2-4 380 mg chewable tables 20 minutes before meals | Lethargy to quadriplegia; aldosterone-like effects (increased sodium and water retention; decreased potassium and hypertension with >100 mg/day for more than 6 weeks) | Aldosterone-like effects may be prevented with high potassium/low sodium diet; avoid in patients with hypertension, renal or liver failure, cardiovascular disease, or current cardiac glycoside therapy; potentiates the action of prednisone and prednisolone and increases levels of endogenous corticosteroids; also potentiates topical steroids |
| **MILK THISTLE** | Liver disease, including cirrhosis and chronic hepatitis; gallstones, psoriasis, liver protectant from toxins (eg, death cup mushroom) | 140 mg silymarin 3 times/day, or 100-200 mg of phosphatidylcholine-bound silymarin twice daily | Possible loose stools as result of increased bile flow; mild allergic reaction | Prevent loose stools by ingesting psyllium and oat bran; phosphatidylcholine-bound silymarin is more effective |
| **PEPPERMINT** | Internal: Irritable bowel syndrome (IBS)<br>External: Symptoms of common cold, arthritis, and other musculoskeletal problems | Tea: 1-2 tsp dried leaves in 1 cup water<br>Enteric-coated capsules: 1-2 capsules (0.2 mL/capsule) 3 times/day for IBS<br>Topical: 3-4 times/day | Internal: Skin rash, heart burn, muscle tremor<br>External: Contact dermatitis | May potentiate esophageal reflex by relaxing esophageal sphincter; caution in patients with hiatal hernia<br>External: Avoid concomitant use of topical menthols and heating pads (increases likelihood of contact dermatitis) |
| **ST JOHN'S WORT** | Mild to moderate depression, anxiety, antiviral | 300 mg 3 times/day of standardized 0.3% hypericin extract; take with meals | Rare in humans, possibility of photosensitivity with higher doses | Take with food to prevent GI upset; avoid concomitant use with SSRIs; avoid foods and drugs that interact with MAOIs, including cheese, wine, beer, levodopa, and 5-hydroxytyptophan |
| **SAW PALMETTO** | Benign prostatic hyperplasia (BPH) | 160 mg twice daily of standardized fat-soluble saw palmetto extract containing 85% to 95% fatty acids and sterols | Low, headache reported | Effect seen in patients in 4-6 weeks; no demonstrated effect on serum prostate-specific antigen levels; antiestrogen effect, avoid during pregnancy and in patients with breast cancer |
| **VALERIAN** | Sedative to treat insomnia; treatment of anxiety and stress | 150-300 mg of valerian extract (0.8% valeric acid) 30-45 minutes before bedtime | Rare morning drowsiness, headache, excitability, uneasiness, cardiac disturbances | Usually reduces morning sleepiness; may potentiate effects of other CNS depressants; decrease caffeine intake and daytime naps and increase exercise to improve results |

# REFERENCE VALUES FOR ADULTS

## Automated Chemistry (CHEMISTRY A)

| Test | Values | Remarks |
|---|---|---|
| **SERUM PLASMA** | | |
| Acetone | Negative | |
| Albumin | 3.2-5 g/dL | |
| Alcohol, ethyl | Negative | |
| Aldolase | 1.2-7.6 IU/L | |
| Ammonia | 20-70 mcg/dL | Specimen to be placed on ice as soon as collected |
| Amylase | 30-110 units/L | |
| Bilirubin, direct | 0-0.3 mg/dL | |
| Bilirubin, total | 0.1-1.2 mg/dL | |
| Calcium | 8.6-10.3 mg/dL | |
| Calcium, ionized | 2.24-2.46 mEq/L | |
| Chloride | 95-108 mEq/L | |
| Cholesterol, total | ≤220 mg/dL | Fasted blood required – normal value affected by dietary habits<br>This reference range is for a general adult population |
| HDL cholesterol | 40-60 mg/dL | Fasted blood required – normal value affected by dietary habits |
| LDL cholesterol | 65-170 mg/dL | LDLC calculated by Friewald formula... which has certain inaccuracies and is invalid at trig levels >300 mg/dL |
| $CO_2$ | 23-30 mEq/L | |
| Creatine kinase (CK) isoenzymes | | |
| CK-BB | 0% | |
| CK-MB (cardiac) | 0%-3.9% | |
| CK-MM (muscle) | 96%-100% | |
| CK-MB levels must be both ≥4% and 10 IU/L to meet diagnostic criteria for CK-MB positive result consistent with myocardial injury. | | |
| Creatine phosphokinase (CPK) | 8-150 IU/L | |
| Creatinine | 0.5-1.4 mg/dL | |
| Ferritin | 13-300 ng/mL | |
| Folate | 3.6-20 ng/dL | |
| GGT (gamma-glutamyltranspeptidase) | | |
| male | 11-63 IU/L | |
| female | 8-35 IU/L | |
| GLDH | To be determined | |
| Glucose (2-h postprandial) | Up to 140 mg/dL | |
| Glucose, fasting | 60-110 mg/dL | |
| Glucose, nonfasting (2-h postprandial) | 60-140 mg/dL | |
| Hemoglobin $A_{1c}$ | 8 | |
| Hemoglobin, plasma free | <2.5 mg/100 mL | |
| Hemoglobin, total glycosylated (Hb $A_1$) | 4%-8% | |
| Iron | 65-150 mcg/dL | |
| Iron binding capacity, total (TIBC) | 250-420 mcg/dL | |
| Lactic acid | 0.7-2.1 mEq/L | Specimen to be kept on ice and sent to lab as soon as possible |
| Lactate dehydrogenase (LDH) | 56-194 IU/L | |
| Lactate dehydrogenase (LDH) isoenzymes | | |
| $LD_1$ | 20%-34% | |
| $LD_2$ | 29%-41% | |
| $LD_3$ | 15%-25% | |
| $LD_4$ | 1%-12% | |
| $LD_5$ | 1%-15% | |
| Flipped $LD_1/LD_2$ ratios (>1 may be consistent with myocardial injury) particularly when considered in combination with a recent CK-MB positive result | | |
| Lipase | 23-208 units/L | |
| Magnesium | 1.6-2.5 mg/dL | Increased by slight hemolysis |
| Osmolality | 289-308 mOsm/kg | |
| Phosphatase, alkaline | | |
| adults 25-60 y | 33-131 IU/L | |
| adults 61 y or older | 51-153 IU/L | |
| infancy-adolescence | Values range up to 3-5 times higher than adults | |
| Phosphate, inorganic | 2.8-4.2 mg/dL | |
| Potassium | 3.5-5.2 mEq/L | Increased by slight hemolysis |
| Prealbumin | >15 mg/dL | |
| Protein, total | 6.5-7.9 g/dL | |

## Automated Chemistry (CHEMISTRY A) *(continued)*

| Test | Values | Remarks |
|---|---|---|
| SGOT (AST) | <35 IU/L (20-48) | |
| SGPT (ALT) (10-35) | <35 IU/L | |
| Sodium | 134-149 mEq/L | |
| Transferrin | >200 mg/dL | |
| Triglycerides | 45-155 mg/dL | Fasted blood required |
| Urea nitrogen (BUN) | 7-20 mg/dL | |
| Uric acid | | |
| male | 2.0-8.0 mg/dL | |
| female | 2.0-7.5 mg/dL | |
| **CEREBROSPINAL FLUID** | | |
| Glucose | 50-70 mg/dL | |
| Protein | | |
| adults and children | 15-45 mg/dL | CSF obtained by lumbar puncture |
| newborn infants | 60-90 mg/dL | |
| On CSF obtained by cisternal puncture: About 25 mg/dL | | |
| On CSF obtained by ventricular puncture: About 10 mg/dL | | |
| **Note:** Bloody specimen gives erroneously high value due to contamination with blood proteins | | |
| **URINE** | | |
| **(24-hour specimen is required for all these tests unless specified)** | | |
| Amylase | 32-641 units/L | The value is in units/L and **not** calculated for total volume |
| Amylase, fluid (random samples) | | Interpretation of value left for physician, depends on the nature of fluid |
| Calcium | Depends upon dietary intake | |
| Creatine | | |
| male | 150 mg/24 h | Higher value on children and during pregnancy |
| female | 250 mg/24 h | |
| Creatinine | 1000-2000 mg/24 h | |
| Creatinine clearance (endogenous) | | |
| male<br>female | 85-125 mL/min<br>75-115 mL/min | A blood sample must accompany urine specimen |
| Glucose | 1 g/24 h | |
| 5-hydroxyindoleacetic acid | 2-8 mg/24 h | |
| Iron | 0.15 mg/24 h | Acid washed container required |
| Magnesium | 146-209 mg/24 h | |
| Osmolality | 500-800 mOsm/kg | With normal fluid intake |
| Oxalate | 10-40 mg/24 h | |
| Phosphate | 400-1300 mg/24 h | |
| Potassium | 25-120 mEq/24 h | Varies with diet; the interpretation of urine electrolytes and osmolality should be left for the physician |
| Sodium | 40-220 mEq/24 h | |
| Porphobilinogen, qualitative | Negative | |
| Porphyrins, qualitative | Negative | |
| Proteins | 0.05-0.1 g/24 h | |
| Salicylate | Negative | |
| Urea clearance | 60-95 mL/min | A blood sample must accompany specimen |
| Urea N | 10-40 g/24 h | Dependent on protein intake |
| Uric acid | 250-750 mg/24 h | Dependent on diet and therapy |
| Urobilinogen | 0.5-3.5 mg/24 h | For qualitative determination on random urine, send sample to urinalysis section in Hematology Lab |
| Xylose absorption test | | |
| children | 16%-33% of ingested xylose | |
| adults | >4 g in 5 h | |
| **FECES** | | |
| Fat, 3-day collection | <5 g/d | Value depends on fat intake of 100 g/d for 3 days preceding and during collection |
| **GASTRIC ACIDITY** | | |
| Acidity, total, 12 h | 10-60 mEq/L | Titrated at pH 7 |

## REFERENCE VALUES FOR ADULTS *(Continued)*

### BLOOD GASES

| | Arterial | Capillary | Venous |
|---|---|---|---|
| pH | 7.35-7.45 | 7.35-7.45 | 7.32-7.42 |
| $pCO_2$ (mm Hg) | 35-45 | 35-45 | 38-52 |
| $pO_2$ (mm Hg) | 70-100 | 60-80 | 24-48 |
| $HCO_3$ (mEq/L) | 19-25 | 19-25 | 19-25 |
| $TCO_2$ (mEq/L) | 19-29 | 19-29 | 23-33 |
| $O_2$ saturation (%) | 90-95 | 90-95 | 40-70 |
| Base excess (mEq/L) | -5 to +5 | -5 to +5 | -5 to +5 |

### HEMATOLOGY

#### Complete Blood Count

| Age | Hgb (g/dL) | Hct (%) | RBC (mill/mm$^3$) | RDW |
|---|---|---|---|---|
| 0-3 d | 15.0-20.0 | 45-61 | 4.0-5.9 | <18 |
| 1-2 wk | 12.5-18.5 | 39-57 | 3.6-5.5 | <17 |
| 1-6 mo | 10.0-13.0 | 29-42 | 3.1-4.3 | <16.5 |
| 7 mo to 2 y | 10.5-13.0 | 33-38 | 3.7-4.9 | <16 |
| 2-5 y | 11.5-13.0 | 34-39 | 3.9-5.0 | <15 |
| 5-8 y | 11.5-14.5 | 35-42 | 4.0-4.9 | <15 |
| 13-18 y | 12.0-15.2 | 36-47 | 4.5-5.1 | <14.5 |
| Adult male | 13.5-16.5 | 41-50 | 4.5-5.5 | <14.5 |
| Adult female | 12.0-15.0 | 36-44 | 4.0-4.9 | <14.5 |

| Age | MCV (fL) | MCH (pg) | MCHC (%) | Plts (x 10$^3$/mm$^3$) |
|---|---|---|---|---|
| 0-3 d | 95-115 | 31-37 | 29-37 | 250-450 |
| 1-2 wk | 86-110 | 28-36 | 28-38 | 250-450 |
| 1-6 mo | 74-96 | 25-35 | 30-36 | 300-700 |
| 7 mo to 2 y | 70-84 | 23-30 | 31-37 | 250-600 |
| 2-5 y | 75-87 | 24-30 | 31-37 | 250-550 |
| 5-8 y | 77-95 | 25-33 | 31-37 | 250-550 |
| 13-18 y | 78-96 | 25-35 | 31-37 | 150-450 |
| Adult male | 80-100 | 26-34 | 31-37 | 150-450 |
| Adult female | 80-100 | 26-34 | 31-37 | 150-450 |

#### WBC and Diff

| Age | WBC (x 10$^3$/mm$^3$) | Segs | Bands | Lymphs | Monos |
|---|---|---|---|---|---|
| 0-3 d | 9.0-35.0 | 32-62 | 10-18 | 19-29 | 5-7 |
| 1-2 wk | 5.0-20.0 | 14-34 | 6-14 | 36-45 | 6-10 |
| 1-6 mo | 6.0-17.5 | 13-33 | 4-12 | 41-71 | 4-7 |
| 7 mo to 2 y | 6.0-17.0 | 15-35 | 5-11 | 45-76 | 3-6 |
| 2-5 y | 5.5-15.5 | 23-45 | 5-11 | 35-65 | 3-6 |
| 5-8 y | 5.0-14.5 | 32-54 | 5-11 | 28-48 | 3-6 |
| 13-18 y | 4.5-13.0 | 34-64 | 5-11 | 25-45 | 3-6 |
| Adults | 4.5-11.0 | 35-66 | 5-11 | 24-44 | 3-6 |

| Age | Eosinophils | Basophils | Atypical Lymphs | No. of NRBCs |
|---|---|---|---|---|
| 0-3 d | 0-2 | 0-1 | 0-8 | 0-2 |
| 1-2 wk | 0-2 | 0-1 | 0-8 | 0 |
| 1-6 mo | 0-3 | 0-1 | 0-8 | 0 |
| 7 mo to 2 y | 0-3 | 0-1 | 0-8 | 0 |
| 2-5 y | 0-3 | 0-1 | 0-8 | 0 |
| 5-8 y | 0-3 | 0-1 | 0-8 | 0 |
| 13-18 y | 0-3 | 0-1 | 0-8 | 0 |
| Adults | 0-3 | 0-1 | 0-8 | 0 |

Segs = segmented neutrophils    Lymphs = lymphocytes    Bands = band neutrophils    Monos = monocytes

#### Erythrocyte Sedimentation Rates and Reticulocyte Counts

Sedimentation rate, Westergren:
Children: 0-20 mm/hour
Adult male: 0-15 mm/hour
Adult female: 0-20 mm/hour

Sedimentation rate, Wintrobe:
Children: 0-13 mm/hour
Adult male: 0-10 mm/hour
Adult female: 0-15 mm/hour

Reticulocyte count:
Newborns: 2%-6%
1-6 mo: 0%-2.8%
Adults: 0.5%-1.5%

# ANTIPSYCHOTIC MEDICATION GUIDELINES

Appropriate indications for use of antipsychotic medications are outlined in the Health Care Finance Administration's Omnibus Reconciliation Act (OBRA) of 1987. These regulations require that antipsychotics be used to treat specific conditions (listed below) and not solely for behavior control.

**Approved indications include:**

- acute psychotic episode
- atypical psychosis
- brief reactive psychosis
- delusional disorder
- Huntington's disease
- psychotic mood disorder (including manic depression and depression with psychotic features)
- schizo-affective disorder
- schizophrenia
- schizophrenic form disorder
- Tourette's disease
- short-term (7 days) for hiccups, nausea, vomiting, or pruritus
- organic mental syndrome with psychotic or agitated features:
  - behaviors are quantitatively and objectively documented
  - behaviors must be **persistent**
  - behaviors are not caused by preventable reasons
  - patient presents a danger to self or others
  - continuous crying or screaming if this impairs functional status
  - psychotic symptoms (hallucinations, paranoia, delusions) which cause resident distress or impaired functional capacity

"Clinically contraindicated" means that a resident with a "specific condition" who has had a history of recurrence of psychotic symptoms (eg, delusions, hallucinations) which have been stabilized with a maintenance dose of an antipsychotic drug without incurring significant side effects (eg, tardive dyskinesia) **should not receive gradual dose reductions**. In residents with organic mental syndromes (eg, dementia, delirium), "clinically contraindicated" means that a gradual dose reduction has been attempted **twice** in 1 year and that attempt resulted in the return of symptoms for which the drug was prescribed to a degree that a cessation in the gradual dose reduction, or a return to previous dose levels was necessary.

If the medication is being used outside the guidelines, the physician must provide justification why the continued use of the drug and the dose of the drug is clinically appropriate.

Antipsychotics should not be used if one or more of the following is/are the **only** indication:

- wandering
- poor self care
- restlessness
- impaired memory
- anxiety
- depression (without psychotic features)
- insomnia
- unsociability
- indifference to surroundings
- fidgeting
- nervousness
- uncooperativeness
- agitated behaviors which do **not** represent danger to the resident or others

Selection of an antipsychotic agent should be based on the side effect profile since all antipsychotic agents are equally effective at equivalent doses. Coadministration of two or more antipsychotics does not have any pharmacological basis or clinical advantage and increases the potential for side effects. See Antipsychotic Agents table in Comparison Charts.

## ANTIPSYCHOTIC MEDICATION GUIDELINES *(Continued)*

## DOSING GUIDELINES

1. Daily dosages should be equal to or less than those listed below, unless documentation exists to support the need for higher doses to maintain or improve functional status.

| Generic | Brand | Daily Dose for Patients With Organic Mental Syndrome |
|---|---|---|
| Chlorpromazine | Thorazine® | 75 mg |
| Clozapine | Clozaril® | 50 mg |
| Fluphenazine | Prolixin® | 4 mg |
| Haloperidol | Haldol® | 4 mg |
| Loxapine | Loxitane® | 10 mg |
| Mesoridazine | Serentil® | 25 mg |
| Molindone | Moban® | 10 mg |
| Olanzapine | Zyprexa® | 5 mg |
| Perphenazine | Trilafon® | 8 mg |
| Pimozide | Orap™ | 4 mg |
| Prochlorperazine | Compazine® | 10 mg |
| Promazine | Sparine® | 150 mg |
| Quetiapine | Seroquel® | 100 mg |
| Risperidone | Risperdal® | 2 mg |
| Thioridazine | Mellaril® | 75 mg |
| Thiothixene | Navane® | 7 mg |
| Trifluoperazine | Stelazine® | 8 mg |

2. The dose of prochlorperazine may be exceeded for short-term (up to 7 days) for treatment of nausea and vomiting. Residents with nausea and vomiting secondary to cancer or cancer chemotherapy can also be treated with higher doses for longer periods of time.

3. The residents must receive adequate monitoring for significant side effects such as tardive dyskinesia, postural hypotension, cognitive-behavioral impairment, akathisia, and parkinsonism.

4. Gradual dosage reductions are to be attempted twice in 1 year if prescribed for OMS. If symptoms for which the drug has been prescribed return and both reduction attempts have proven unsuccessful, the physician may indicate further reductions are clinically contraindicated.

5. "Clinically contraindicated" means that a resident **need not undergo** a "gradual dose reduction" or "behavioral interventions" if:

   - The resident has a "specific condition" and has a history of recurrence of psychotic symptoms (eg, delusions, hallucinations), which have been stabilized with a maintenance dose of an antipsychotic drug without incurring significant side effects.

   - The resident has organic mental syndrome (now called "delirium, dementia, and amnestic and other cognitive disorders" by DSM IV) and has had a gradual dose reduction attempted **twice** in 1 year and that attempt resulted in the return of symptoms for which the drug was prescribed to a degree that a cessation in the gradual dose reduction, or a return to previous dose reduction was necessary.

   - The resident's physician provides a justification why the continued use of the drug and the dose of the drug is clinically appropriate. This justification should include: a) a diagnosis, but not simply a diagnostic label or code, but the description of symptoms, b) a discussion of the differential psychiatric and medical diagnosis (eg, why the resident's behavioral symptom is thought to be a result of a dementia with associated psychosis and/or agitated behaviors, and not the result of an unrecognized painful medical condition or a psychosocial or environmental stressor), c) a description of the justification for the choice of a particular treatment, or treatments, and d) a discussion of why the present dose is necessary to manage the symptoms of the resident. This information need not necessarily be in the physician's progress notes, but must be a part of the resident's clinical record.

Examples of evidence that would support a justification of why a drug is being used outside these guidelines but in the best interests of the resident may include, but are not limited to the following.

1. A physician's note indicating for example, that the dosage, duration, indication, and monitoring are clinically appropriate, **and the reasons why they are clinically appropriate**; this note should demonstrate that the physician has carefully considered the risk/benefit to the resident in using drugs outside the guidelines.
2. A medical or psychiatric consultation or evaluation (eg, Geriatric Depression Scale) that confirms the physician's judgment that use of a drug outside the guidelines is in the best interest of the resident.
3. Physician, nursing, or other health professional documentation indicating that the resident is being monitored for adverse consequences or complications of the drug therapy.
4. Documentation confirming that previous attempts at dosage reduction have been unsuccessful.
5. Documentation (including MDS documentation) showing resident's subjective or objective improvement, or maintenance of function while taking the medication.
6. Documentation showing that a resident's decline or deterioration is evaluated by the interdisciplinary team to determine whether a particular drug, or a particular dose, or duration of therapy, may be the cause.
7. Documentation showing why the resident's age, weight, or other factors would require a unique drug dose or drug duration, indication, or monitoring.
8. Other evidence you may deem appropriate.

# ANXIOLYTIC/HYPNOTIC USE IN LONG-TERM CARE FACILITIES

One of the regulations regarding medication use in long-term care facilities concerns "unnecessary drugs." The regulation states, "Each resident's drug regimen must be free from unnecessary drugs." Recently, the Health Care Financing Administration (HCFA) issued the final interpretive guidelines on this regulation. The following is a summary of these guidelines as they pertain to anxiolytic/hypnotic agents.

## A. Long-Acting Benzodiazepines

Long-acting benzodiazepine drugs should not be used in residents unless an attempt with a shorter-acting drug has failed. If they are used, the doses must be no higher than the listed dose, unless higher doses are necessary for maintenance or improvement in the resident's functional status. Daily use should be less then 4 continuous months unless an attempt at a gradual dose reduction is unsuccessful. Residents on diazepam for seizure disorders or for the treatment of tardive dyskinesia are exempt from this restriction. Residents on clonazepam for bipolar disorder, tardive dyskinesia, nocturnal myoclonus, or seizure disorder are also exempt. Residents on long-acting benzodiazepines should have a gradual dose reduction at least twice within 1 year before it can be concluded that the gradual dose reduction is "clinically contraindicated."

| Generic | Brand | Maximum Daily Geriatric Dose (mg) |
|---|---|---|
| Chlordiazepoxide | Librium® | 20 |
| Clonazepam | Klonopin™ | 1.5 |
| Clorazepate | Tranxene® | 15 |
| Diazepam | Valium® | 5 |
| Flurazepam | Dalmane® | 15 |
| Halazepam | Paxipam® | 40 |
| Quazepam | Doral® | 7.5 |

## B. Benzodiazepine or Other Anxiolytic/Sedative Drugs

Anxiolytic/sedative drugs should be used for purposes other than sleep induction only when other possible causes of the resident's distress have been ruled out and the use results in maintenance or improvement in the resident's functional status. Daily use should not exceed 4 continuous months unless an attempt at gradual dose reduction has failed. Anxiolytics should only be used for generalized anxiety disorder, dementia with agitated states that either endangers the resident or others, or is a source of distress or dysfunction; panic disorder or symptomatic anxiety associated with other psychiatric disorders. The dose should not exceed those listed below unless a higher dose is needed as evidenced by the resident's response. Gradual dosage reductions should be attempted at least twice within 1 year before it can be concluded that a gradual dose reduction is "clinically contraindicated."

### Short-Acting Benzodiazepines

| Generic | Brand | Maximum Daily Geriatric Dose (mg) |
|---|---|---|
| Alprazolam | Xanax® | 0.75 |
| Estazolam* | ProSom® | 0.5 |
| Lorazepam | Ativan® | 2 |
| Oxazepam | Serax® | 30 |

*Primarily used as a hypnotic agent.

### Other Anxiolytic and Sedative Drugs

| Generic | Brand | Maximum Daily Geriatric Dose (mg) |
|---|---|---|
| Chloral hydrate | Noctec®, etc | 750 |
| Diphenhydramine | Benadryl® | 50 |
| Hydroxyzine | Atarax®, Vistaril® | 50 |

**Note:** Chloral hydrate, diphenhydramine, and hydroxyzine are not necessarily drugs of choice for treatment of anxiety disorders. HCFA lists them only in the event of their possible use.

## C. Drugs Used for Sleep Induction

Drugs for sleep induction should only be used when all possible reasons for insomnia have been ruled out (ie, pain, noise, caffeine). The use of the drug must result in the maintenance or improvement of the resident's functional status. Daily use of a hypnotic should not exceed 10 consecutive days unless an attempt at a gradual dose reduction is unsuccessful. The dose should not exceed those listed below unless a higher dose has been deemed necessary. Gradual dose reductions should be attempted at least three times within 6 months before it can be concluded that a gradual dose reduction is "clinically contraindicated."

### Hypnotic Drugs

| Generic | Brand | Daily Geriatric Dose (mg) |
|---|---|---|
| Alprazolam* | Xanax® | 0.25 |
| Chloral hydrato | Nootco® | 500 |
| Diphenhydramine | Benadryl® | 25 |
| Estazolam | ProSom™ | 0.5 |
| Hydroxyzine | Atarax®, Vistaril® | 50 |
| Lorazepam* | Ativan® | 1 |
| Oxazepam* | Serax® | 15 |
| Temazepam | Restoril® | 7.5 |
| Triazolam | Halcion® | 0.125 |
| Zaleplon | Sonata® | 5 |
| Zolpidem | Ambien® | 5 |

*Not officially indicated as a hypnotic agent.

**Note:** Chloral hydrate, diphenhydramine, and hydroxyzine are not necessarily drugs of choice for sleep disorders. HCFA lists them only in the event of their possible use.

## D. Miscellaneous Hypnotic/Sedative/Anxiolytic Drugs

The initiation of the following medications should not occur in any dose in any resident. Residents currently using these drugs or residents admitted to the facility while using these drugs should receive gradual dose reductions. Newly admitted residents should have a period of adjustment before attempting reduction. Dose reductions should be attempted at least twice within 1 year before it can be concluded that it is "clinically contraindicated."

### Examples of Barbiturates

| Generic | Brand |
|---|---|
| Amobarbital | Amytal® |
| Amobarbital/Secobarbital | Tuinal® |
| Butabarbital | Butisol Sodium® |
| Combinations | Fiorinal®, etc |
| Pentobarbital | Nembutal® |
| Secobarbital | Seconal™ |

### Miscellaneous Hypnotic/Sedative/Anxiolytic Agents

| Generic | Brand |
|---|---|
| Ethchlorvynol | Placidyl® |
| Glutethimide | Doriden® |
| Meprobamate | Equanil®, Miltown® |
| Methyprylon | Noludar® |
| Paraldehyde | Paral® |

# FEDERAL OBRA REGULATIONS RECOMMENDED MAXIMUM DOSES

## Antidepressants

| Drug | Brand Name | Usual Max Daily Dose for Age ≥65 | Usual Max Daily Dose |
|---|---|---|---|
| Amitriptyline | Elavil® | 150 mg | 300 mg |
| Amoxapine | Asendin® | 200 mg | 400 mg |
| Desipramine | Norpramin® | 150 mg | 300 mg |
| Doxepin | Adapin®, Sinequan® | 150 mg | 300 mg |
| Imipramine | Tofranil® | 150 mg | 300 mg |
| Maprotiline | Ludiomil® | 150 mg | 300 mg |
| Nortriptyline | Aventyl®, Pamelor® | 75 mg | 150 mg |
| Protriptyline | Vivactil® | 30 mg | 60 mg |
| Trazodone | Desyrel® | 300 mg | 600 mg |
| Trimipramine | Surmontil® | 150 mg | 300 mg |

## Antipsychotics

| Drug | Brand Name | Usual Max Daily Dose for Age ≥65 | Usual Max Daily Dose | Daily Oral Dose for Residents With Organic Mental Syndromes |
|---|---|---|---|---|
| Chlorpromazine | Thorazine® | 800 mg | 1600 mg | 75 mg |
| Clozapine | Clozaril® | 25 mg | 450 mg | 50 mg |
| Fluphenazine | Prolixin® | 20 mg | 40 mg | 4 mg |
| Haloperidol | Haldol® | 50 mg | 100 mg | 4 mg |
| Loxapine | Loxitane® | 125 mg | 250 mg | 10 mg |
| Mesoridazine | Serentil® | 250 mg | 500 mg | 25 mg |
| Molindone | Moban® | 112 mg | 225 mg | 10 mg |
| Perphenazine | Trilafon® | 32 mg | 64 mg | 8 mg |
| Promazine | Sparine® | 50 mg | 500 mg | 150 mg |
| Risperidone | Risperdal® | 1 mg | 6 mg | 4 mg |
| Thioridazine | Mellaril® | 400 mg | 800 mg | 75 mg |
| Thiothixene | Navane® | 30 mg | 60 mg | 7 mg |
| Trifluoperazine | Stelazine® | 40 mg | 80 mg | 8 mg |
| Triflupromazine | Vesprin® | 100 mg | 20 mg | – |

## Anxiolytics*

| Drug | Brand Name | Usual Daily Dose for Age ≥65 | Usual Daily Dose for Age ≤65 |
|---|---|---|---|
| Alprazolam | Xanax® | 2 mg | 4 mg |
| Chlordiazepoxide | Librium® | 40 mg | 100 mg |
| Clorazepate | Tranxene® | 30 mg | 60 mg |
| Diazepam | Valium® | 20 mg | 60 mg |
| Halazepam | Paxipam® | 80 mg | 160 mg |
| Lorazepam | Ativan® | 3 mg | 6 mg |
| Meprobamate | Miltown® | 600 mg | 1600 mg |
| Oxazepam | Serax® | 60 mg | 90 mg |
| Prazepam | Centrax® | 30 mg | 60 mg |

***Note:** HCFA-OBRA guidelines strongly urge clinicians not to use barbiturates, glutethimide, and ethchlorvynol due to their side effects, pharmacokinetics, and addiction potential in the elderly. Also, HCFA discourages use of long-acting benzodiazepines in the elderly.

## Hypnotics (Should not be used for more than 10 continuous days*)

| Drug | Brand Name | Usual Max Single Dose for Age ≥65 | Usual Max Single Dose |
|---|---|---|---|
| Alprazolam | Xanax® | 0.25 mg | 1.5 mg |
| Amobarbital | Amytal® | 105 mg | 300 mg |
| Butabarbital | Butisol® | 100 mg | 200 mg |
| Chloral hydrate | Noctec® | 750 mg | 1500 mg |
| Chloral hydrate | Various | 500 mg | 1000 mg |
| Diphenhydramine | Benadryl® | 25 mg | 50 mg |
| Ethchlorvynol | Placidyl® | 500 mg | 1000 mg |
| Flurazepam | Dalmane® | 15 mg | 30 mg |
| Glutethimide | Doriden® | 500 mg | 1000 mg |
| Halazepam | Paxipam® | 20 mg | 40 mg |
| Hydroxyzine | Atarax® | 50 mg | 100 mg |
| Lorazepam | Ativan® | 1 mg | 2 mg |
| Oxazepam | Serax® | 15 mg | 30 mg |
| Pentobarbital | Nembutal® | 100 mg | 200 mg |
| Secobarbital | Seconal® | 100 mg | 200 mg |
| Temazepam | Restoril® | 15 mg | 30 mg |
| Triazolam | Halcion® | 0.125 mg | 0.5 mg |

***Note:** HCFA-OBRA guidelines strongly urge clinicians not to use barbiturates, glutethimide, and ethchlorvynol due to their side effects, pharmacokinetics, and addiction potential in the elderly. Also, HCFA discourages use of long-acting benzodiazepines in the elderly and also discourages the use of diphenhydramine and hydroxyzine.

# HCFA GUIDELINES FOR UNNECESSARY DRUGS IN LONG-TERM CARE FACILITIES

**Procedures: §483.25(1)(1)**

Consider drug therapy "unnecessary" only after determining that the facility's use of the drug is:

- in excessive dose (including duplicate drug therapy)
- for excessive duration
- without adequate monitoring
- without adequate indications of use
- in the presence of adverse consequences which indicate the dose should be reduced or discontinued, or
- any combination of the reasons above

Allow the facility the opportunity to provide a rationale for the use of drugs prescribed outside the preceding guidelines. The facility may not justify the use of a drug prescribed outside the proceeding guidelines solely on the basis of "the doctor ordered it." This justification would render the regulation meaningless. The rationale must be based on sound risk-benefit analysis of the resident's symptoms and potential adverse effects of the drug.

Examples of evidence that would support a justification of why a drug is being used outside these guidelines but in the best interests of the resident may include, but are not limited to:

- a physician's note indicating for example, that the dosage, duration, indication, and monitoring are clinically appropriate, **and the reasons why they are clinically appropriate**; this note should demonstrate that the physician has carefully considered the risk/benefit to the resident in using drugs outside the guidelines

- a medical or psychiatric consultation or evaluation (eg, geriatric depression scale) that confirms the physician's judgment that use of a drug outside the guidelines is in the best interest of the resident

- physician, nursing, or other health professional documentation indicating that the resident is being monitored for adverse consequences or complications of the drug therapy

- documentation confirming that previous attempts at dosage reduction have been unsuccessful

- documentation (including MDS documentation) showing resident's subjective or objective improvement, or maintenance of function while taking the medication

- documentation showing that a resident's decline or deterioration is evaluated by the interdisciplinary team to determine whether a particular drug, or a particular dose, or duration of therapy, may be the cause

- documentation showing why the resident's age, weight, or other factors would require a unique drug dose or drug duration, indication, monitoring, and

- other evidence the survey team may deem appropriate

If the survey team determines that there is a deficiency in the use of antipsychotics, cite the facility under either the "unnecessary drug" regulation or the "antipsychotic drug" regulation, but not both.

**NOTE:** The unnecessary drug criterion of "adequate indications for use" does not simply mean that the **physician's order** must include a reason for using the drug (although such order writing is encouraged). It means that the **resident** lacks a valid clinical reason for use of the drug as evidenced by the survey team's evaluation of some, but not necessarily all, of the following: resident assessment, plan of care, reports of significant change, progress notes, laboratory reports, professional consults, drug orders, observation and interview of the resident, and other information.

# PHARMACOTHERAPY OF URINARY INCONTINENCE

| Incontinence Type | Drug Class | Drug Therapy | Adverse Effects and Precautions | Comments |
|---|---|---|---|---|
| Urge incontinence | Anticholinergic agents | Oxybutynin (2.5-5 mg bid-qid), propantheline (7.5-30 mg at least tid), dicyclomine (10-20 mg tid) | Dry mouth, visual disturbances, constipation, dry skin, confusion | Anticholinergics are the first-line drug therapy (oxybutynin is preferred); propantheline is a second-line therapy |
| | Tricyclic antidepressants (TCAs) | Imipramine, desipramine, nortriptyline (25-100 mg/day) | Anticholinergic effects (as above), orthostatic hypotension, and cardiac dysrhythmia | TCAs are generally reserved for patients with an additional indication (eg, depression, neuralgia) at an initial dose of 10-25 mg 1-3 times/day |
| Stress incontinence | Alpha-adrenergic agonists | Phenylpropanolamine (PPA) in sustained-release form (25-100 mg bid), pseudoephedrine (15-60 mg tid) | Anxiety, insomnia, agitation, respiratory difficulty, sweating, cardiac dysrhythmia, hypertension, tremor; should not be used in obstructive syndromes and/or hypertension | PPA (preferred) or pseudoephedrine are first-line therapy for women with no contraindication (notably hypertension) |
| Stress or combined urge/ stress incontinence | Estrogen replacement agents | Conjugated estrogens (0.3-0.625 mg/day orally or 1 g vaginal cream at bedtime) | Should not be used if suspected or confirmed breast or endometrial cancer, active or past thromboembolism with past oral contraceptive, estrogen, or pregnancy; headache, spotting, edema, breast tenderness, possible depression | Estrogen (oral or vaginal) is an adjunctive therapy for postmenopausal women as it augments alpha-agonists such as PPA or pseudoephedrine |
| | | | Give progesterone with estrogen if uterus is present; pretreatment/ periodic mammogram, gynecologic, breast exam advised | Progestin (eg, medroxyprogesterone 2.5-10 mg/day) continuously or intermittently |
| | Imipramine (10-25 mg tid) | | May worsen cardiac conduction abnormalities, postural hypotension, anticholinergic effects | Combined oral or vaginal estrogen and PPA in postmenopausal women if single drug is inadequate; imipramine is an alternative therapy when first-line therapy is inadequate |
| Overflow | Alpha-adrenergic antagonists | Terazosin (1 mg at bedtime with first dose in supine position and increase by 1 mg every 4 days to 5 mg/day) | Postural hypotension, dizziness, vertigo, heart palpitations, edema, headache, anticholinergic effects | Possible benefit in men with obstructive symptoms of benign prostatic hyperplasia; monitor postural vital signs with first dose/each dose increase; may worsen female stress incontinence |
| | | Doxazosin (1 mg at bedtime with first dose in supine position and increase by 1 mg every 7-14 days to 5 mg/day) | Same as terazosin (may be smaller incidence of hypotension) | Same as terazosin |

"Urinary Incontinence," *Clinical Practice Guideline*, 1996, American Medical Directors Association, reprinted with permission. For more information call 1-800-876-2632.

# SERUM DRUG CONCENTRATIONS COMMONLY MONITORED: GUIDELINES

| Drug | When to Sample | Therapeutic Concentration* | Usual Half-Life | Steady State (Ideal Sampling Time) | Potentially Toxic Concentration* |
|---|---|---|---|---|---|
| **ANTIBIOTICS** | | | | | |
| Gentamicin<br>Tobramycin | 30 min after 30 min infusion<br>Trough: <0.5 h before next dose | Peak: 4-10 mcg/mL<br>Trough: <2.0 mcg/mL | 2 h | 15 h | Peak: >12 mcg/mL<br>Trough: >2 mcg/mL |
| Amikacin | | Peak: 20-35 mcg/mL<br>Trough: <8 mcg/mL | 2 h | 15 h | Peak: >35 mcg/mL<br>Trough: >8 mcg/mL |
| Vancomycin | Peak: 1 h after 1 h infusion<br>Trough: <0.5 h before next dose | Peak: 30-40 mcg/mL<br>Trough: 5-10 mcg/mL | 6-8 h | 24 h | Peak: >80 mcg/mL<br>Trough: >13 mcg/mL |
| **ANTICONVULSANTS** | | | | | |
| Ethosuximide | Trough: Just before next oral dose | 40-100 mcg/mL | 30-60 h | 10-13 d | >100 mcg/mL |
| Gabapentin | | | 5-6 h | | |
| Phenobarbital | Trough: Just before next dose | 15-40 mcg/mL | 40-120 h | 20 d | >40 mcg/mL |
| Phenytoin<br>Free phenytoin | Trough: Just before next dose<br>Draw at same time as total level | 10-20 mcg/mL<br>1-2 mcg/mL | Concentration dependent | 5-14 d | >20 mcg/mL |
| Primidone | Trough: Just before next dose (**Note:** Primidone is metabolized to phenobarb, order levels separately) | 5-12 mcg/mL | 10-12 h | 5 d | >12 mcg/mL |
| **BRONCHODILATORS** | | | | | |
| Aminophylline (I.V.) | 18-24 h after starting or changing a maintenance dose given as a constant infusion | 10-20 mcg/mL | Nonsmoking adults: 8 h<br>Smoking adults: 4 h | 2 d | >20 mcg/mL |
| Theophylline (P.O.) | Peak: Not recommended<br>Trough: Just before next dose | 10-20 mcg/mL | 4-8 h | 2 d | >20 mcg/mL |
| **CARDIOVASCULAR AGENTS** | | | | | |
| Digitoxin | Peak: Not necessary<br>Trough: Prior to dose | 20-35 ng/mL | 7-8 days | 5 wk | >45 ng/mL |
| Digoxin | Trough: Just before next dose (levels drawn earlier than 6 h after a dose will be artificially elevated) | 0.5-2 ng/mL | 36 h | 5 d | >2 ng/mL |
| Lidocaine | Steady-state levels are usually achieved after 6-12 h | 1.2-5.0 mcg/mL | 1.5 h | 5-10 h | >6 mcg/mL |
| Procainamide | Trough: Just before next oral dose<br>I.V.: 6-12 h after infusion started<br>Combined procainamide plus NAPA | 4-10 mcg/mL<br>NAPA: 6-10 h<br>5-30 mcg/mL | Procain: 2.7-5 h<br>>30 (NAPA + procain) | 20 h | >10 mcg/mL |
| Quinidine | Trough: Just before next oral dose | 2-5 mcg/mL | 6 h | 24 h | >10 mcg/mL |
| **PSYCHOTROPIC AGENTS** | | | | | |
| Amitriptyline plus nortriptyline | 12 hours after the last dose | 100-250 ng/mL | Amitriptyline: 9-25 h<br>Nortriptyline: 28-31 h | 4-8 d | >500 ng/mL |
| Carbamazepine | 12 hours after the last dose | 4-12 mcg/mL<br>4-8 mcg/mL in combination with other anticonvulsants | 15-20 h | 7-12 d | >12 mcg/mL |
| Desipramine | 12 hours after the last dose | 125-160 ng/mL | 12-54 h | 3-11 d | >300 ng/mL |
| Imipramine plus desipramine | 12 hours after the last dose | 150-300 ng/mL | 9-24 h | 2-5 d | >500 ng/mL |
| Lithium | 12 hours after the last dose | 0.6-1.2 mEq/mL (acute) | 18-20 h | 2-7 d | >3 mEq/mL |
| Nortriptyline | 12 hours after the last dose | 50-150 ng/mL | 28-31 h | 4-19 d | >500 ng/mL |
| Valproic acid | 12 hours after the last dose | 50-100 mcg/mL | 5-20 h | 4 d | >150 mcg/mL |
| **OTHER AGENT** | | | | | |
| Cyclosporine | Trough: Just before next dose or 12-18 h after oral dose | Months post-transplant:<br>Plasma: 50-150 ng/mL<br>Whole blood: 150-450 ng/mL | 17-40 h | Variable<br>5 half-lives | >400 ng/mL |

*Due to methodology differences, reference ranges may vary from laboratory to laboratory; check with the laboratory service used for their appropriate levels.

# PEDIATRIC ALS ALGORITHMS

## Bradycardia

**Fig. 1:** Pediatric bradycardia decision tree. ABCs indicates airway, breathing, and circulation; ALS, advanced life support; E.T., endotracheal; I.O., intraosseous; and I.V., intravenous.

Used with permission: Emergency Cardiac Care Committee and Subcommittees, American Heart Association, "Guidelines for Cardiopulmonary Resuscitation and Emergency Care, IV: Pediatric Advanced Life Support," *JAMA*, 1992, 268:2262-75.

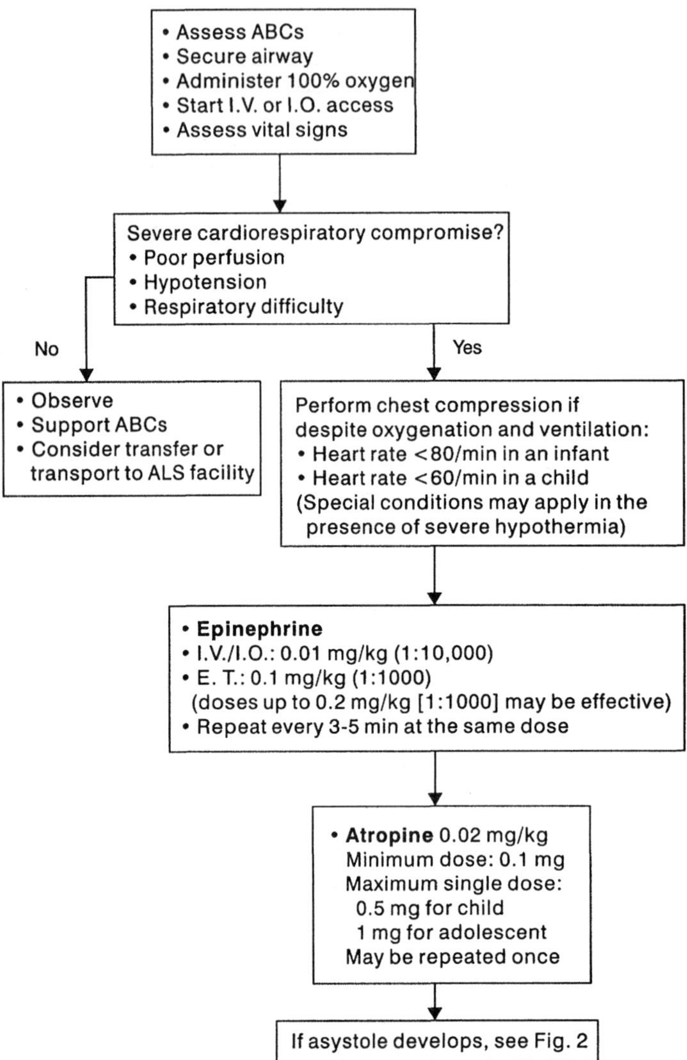

# Asystole and Pulseless Arrest

**Fig. 2:** Pediatric asystole and pulseless arrest decision tree. CPR indicates cardiopulmonary resuscitation; E.T., endotracheal; I.O., intraosseous; and I.V., intravenous.

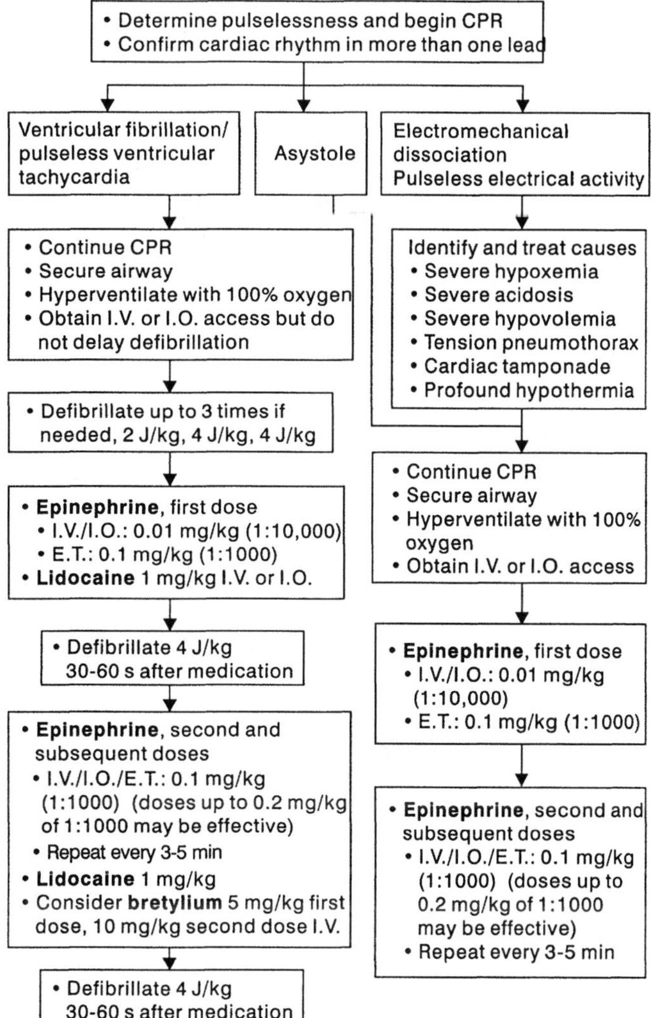

# ADULT ACLS ALGORITHMS

## Emergency Cardiac Care

**Fig. 1**: Universal algorithm for adult emergency cardiac care (ECC)

Used with permission: Emergency Cardiac Care Committee and Subcommittees, American Heart Association, "Guidelines for Cardiopulmonary Resuscitation and Emergency Care, III: Adult Advanced Cardiac Life Support," *JAMA*, 1992, 268:2199-2241.

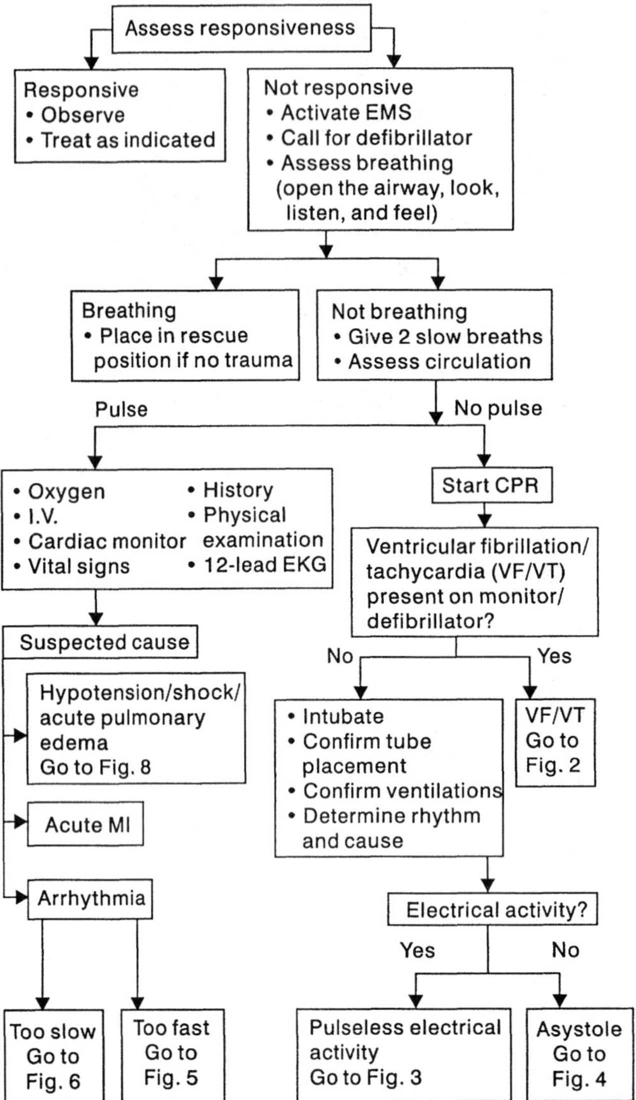

# V. Fib and Pulseless V. Tach

**Fig. 2:** Adult algorithm for ventricular fibrillation and pulseless ventricular tachycardia (VF/VT)

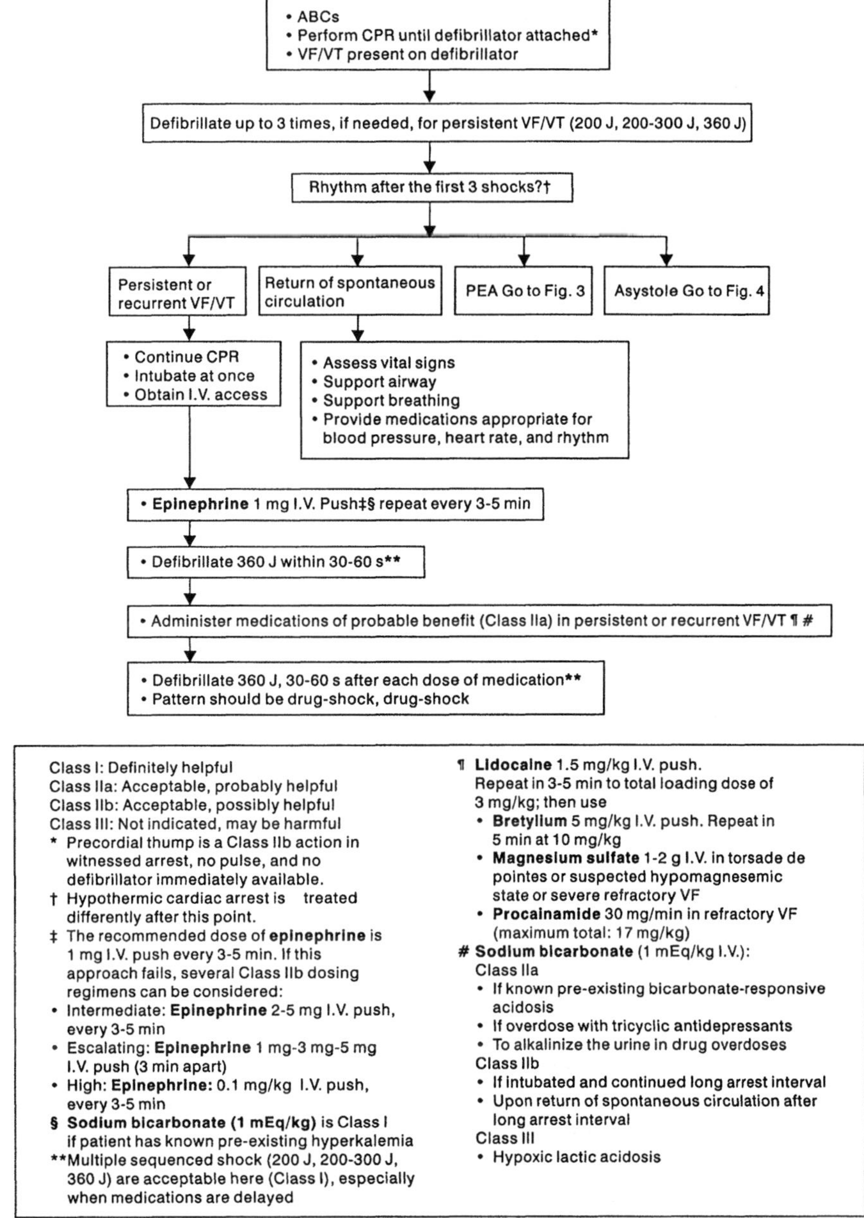


Class I: Definitely helpful
Class IIa: Acceptable, probably helpful
Class IIb: Acceptable, possibly helpful
Class III: Not indicated, may be harmful

* Precordial thump is a Class IIb action in witnessed arrest, no pulse, and no defibrillator immediately available.

† Hypothermic cardiac arrest is treated differently after this point.

‡ The recommended dose of **epinephrine** is 1 mg I.V. push every 3-5 min. If this approach fails, several Class IIb dosing regimens can be considered:
- Intermediate: **Epinephrine** 2-5 mg I.V. push, every 3-5 min
- Escalating: **Epinephrine** 1 mg-3 mg-5 mg I.V. push (3 min apart)
- High: **Epinephrine:** 0.1 mg/kg I.V. push, every 3-5 min

§ **Sodium bicarbonate (1 mEq/kg)** is Class I if patient has known pre-existing hyperkalemia

**Multiple sequenced shock (200 J, 200-300 J, 360 J) are acceptable here (Class I), especially when medications are delayed

¶ **Lidocaine** 1.5 mg/kg I.V. push. Repeat in 3-5 min to total loading dose of 3 mg/kg; then use
- **Bretylium** 5 mg/kg I.V. push. Repeat in 5 min at 10 mg/kg
- **Magnesium sulfate** 1-2 g I.V. in torsade de pointes or suspected hypomagnesemic state or severe refractory VF
- **Procainamide** 30 mg/min in refractory VF (maximum total: 17 mg/kg)

\# **Sodium bicarbonate** (1 mEq/kg I.V.):

Class IIa
- If known pre-existing bicarbonate-responsive acidosis
- If overdose with tricyclic antidepressants
- To alkalinize the urine in drug overdoses

Class IIb
- If intubated and continued long arrest interval
- Upon return of spontaneous circulation after long arrest interval

Class III
- Hypoxic lactic acidosis

Used with permission: Emergency Cardiac Care Committee and Subcommittees, American Heart Association, "Guidelines for Cardiopulmonary Resuscitation and Emergency Care, III: Adult Advanced Cardiac Life Support," *JAMA*, 1992, 268:2199-2241.

## ADULT ACLS ALGORITHMS *(Continued)*

# Pulseless Electrical Activity

**Fig. 3:** Adult algorithm for pulseless electrical activity (PEA) (electromechanical dissociation [EMD]).

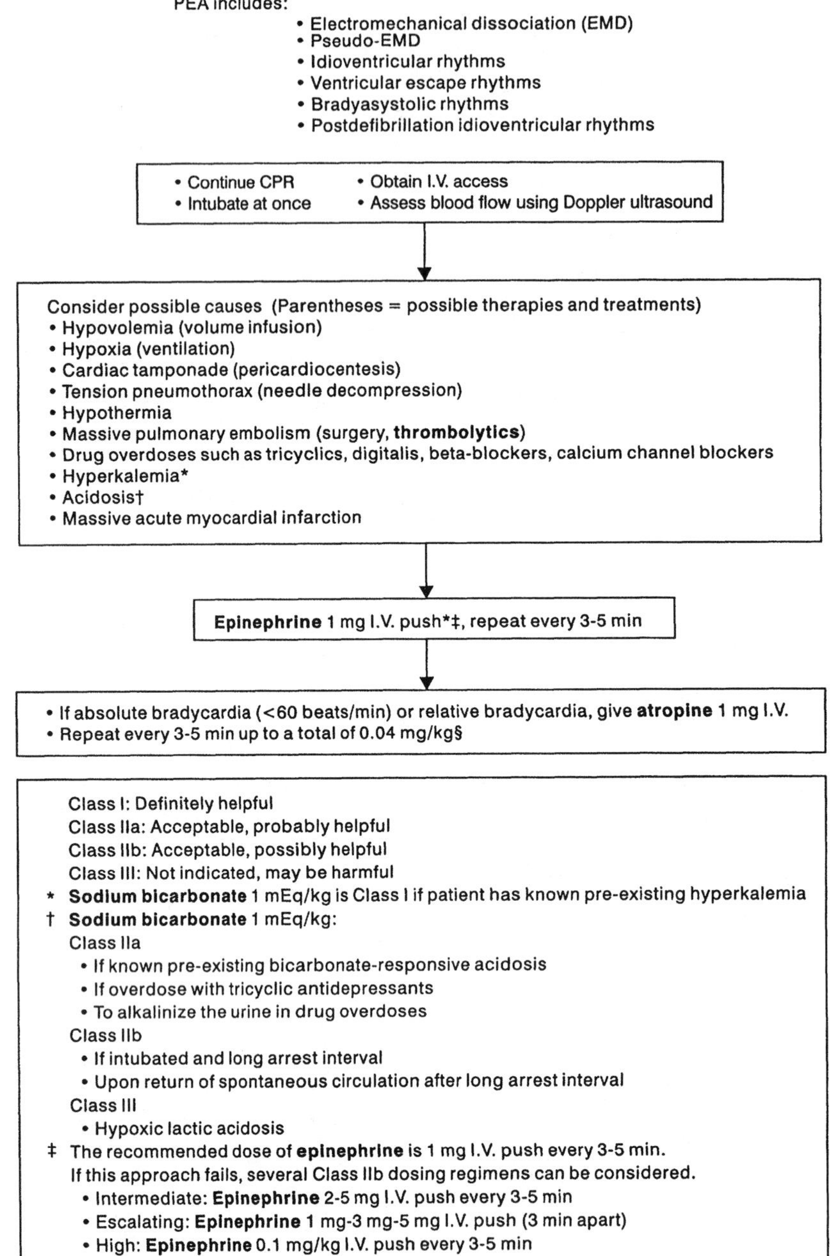

PEA includes:
• Electromechanical dissociation (EMD)
• Pseudo-EMD
• Idioventricular rhythms
• Ventricular escape rhythms
• Bradyasystolic rhythms
• Postdefibrillation idioventricular rhythms
• Continue CPR
• Intubate at once
• Obtain I.V. access
• Assess blood flow using Doppler ultrasound
Consider possible causes (Parentheses = possible therapies and treatments)
• Hypovolemia (volume infusion)
• Hypoxia (ventilation)
• Cardiac tamponade (pericardiocentesis)
• Tension pneumothorax (needle decompression)
• Hypothermia
• Massive pulmonary embolism (surgery, thrombolytics)
• Drug overdoses such as tricyclics, digitalis, beta-blockers, calcium channel blockers
• Hyperkalemia*
• Acidosis†
• Massive acute myocardial infarction
Epinephrine 1 mg I.V. push*‡, repeat every 3-5 min
• If absolute bradycardia (<60 beats/min) or relative bradycardia, give atropine 1 mg I.V.
• Repeat every 3-5 min up to a total of 0.04 mg/kg§


Class I: Definitely helpful
Class IIa: Acceptable, probably helpful
Class IIb: Acceptable, possibly helpful
Class III: Not indicated, may be harmful

* **Sodium bicarbonate** 1 mEq/kg is Class I if patient has known pre-existing hyperkalemia

† **Sodium bicarbonate** 1 mEq/kg:

Class IIa
- If known pre-existing bicarbonate-responsive acidosis
- If overdose with tricyclic antidepressants
- To alkalinize the urine in drug overdoses

Class IIb
- If intubated and long arrest interval
- Upon return of spontaneous circulation after long arrest interval

Class III
- Hypoxic lactic acidosis

‡ The recommended dose of **epinephrine** is 1 mg I.V. push every 3-5 min.
If this approach fails, several Class IIb dosing regimens can be considered.
- Intermediate: **Epinephrine** 2-5 mg I.V. push every 3-5 min
- Escalating: **Epinephrine** 1 mg-3 mg-5 mg I.V. push (3 min apart)
- High: **Epinephrine** 0.1 mg/kg I.V. push every 3-5 min

§ Shorter **atropine** dosing intervals are possibly helpful in cardiac arrest (Class IIb)

Used with permission: Emergency Cardiac Care Committee and Subcommittees, American Heart Association, "Guidelines for Cardiopulmonary Resuscitation and Emergency Care, III: Adult Advanced Cardiac Life Support," *JAMA*, 1992, 268:2199-2241.

# Asystole

**Fig. 4:** Adult asystole treatment algorithm.

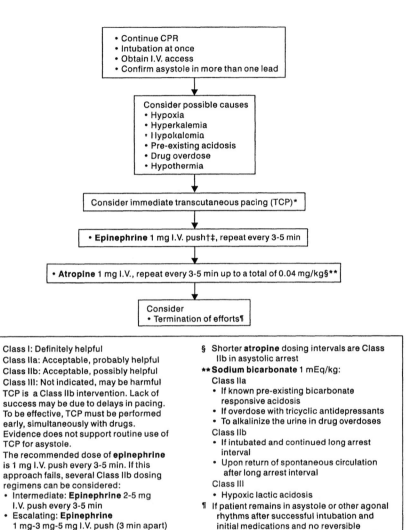

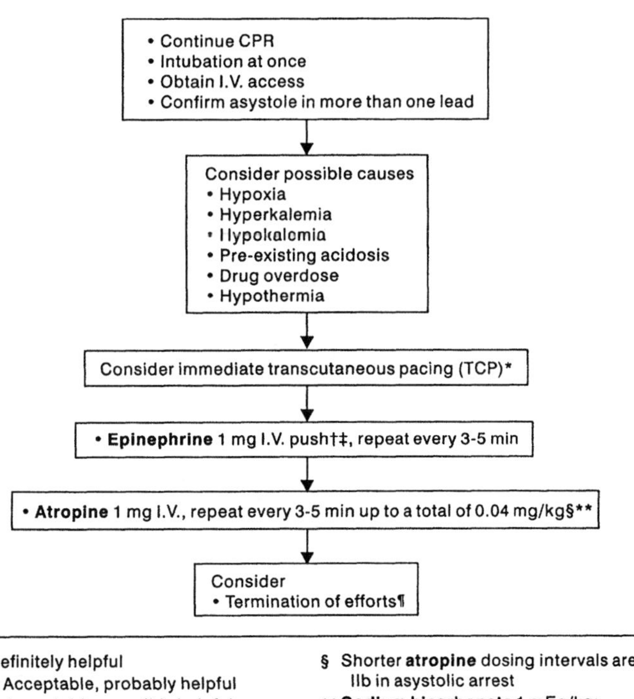

• Continue CPR
• Intubation at once
• Obtain I.V. access
• Confirm asystole in more than one lead
Consider possible causes
• Hypoxia
• Hyperkalemia
• Hypokalemia
• Pre-existing acidosis
• Drug overdose
• Hypothermia
Consider immediate transcutaneous pacing (TCP)*
• Epinephrine 1 mg I.V. push†‡, repeat every 3-5 min
• Atropine 1 mg I.V., repeat every 3-5 min up to a total of 0.04 mg/kg§**
Consider
• Termination of efforts¶


Class I: Definitely helpful
Class IIa: Acceptable, probably helpful
Class IIb: Acceptable, possibly helpful
Class III: Not indicated, may be harmful

* TCP is a Class IIb intervention. Lack of success may be due to delays in pacing. To be effective, TCP must be performed early, simultaneously with drugs. Evidence does not support routine use of TCP for asystole.

† The recommended dose of **epinephrine** is 1 mg I.V. push every 3-5 min. If this approach fails, several Class IIb dosing regimens can be considered:
- Intermediate: **Epinephrine** 2-5 mg I.V. push every 3-5 min
- Escalating: **Epinephrine** 1 mg-3 mg-5 mg I.V. push (3 min apart)
- High: **Epinephrine** 0.1 mg/kg I.V. push Every 3-5 min

**Sodium bicarbonate** 1 mEq/kg is Class I

‡ if patient has known pre-existing hyperkalemia

§ Shorter **atropine** dosing intervals are Class IIb in asystolic arrest

** **Sodium bicarbonate** 1 mEq/kg:

Class IIa
- If known pre-existing bicarbonate responsive acidosis
- If overdose with tricyclic antidepressants
- To alkalinize the urine in drug overdoses

Class IIb
- If intubated and continued long arrest interval
- Upon return of spontaneous circulation after long arrest interval

Class III
- Hypoxic lactic acidosis

¶ If patient remains in asystole or other agonal rhythms after successful intubation and initial medications and no reversible causes are identified, consider termination of resuscitative efforts by a physician. Consider interval since arrest.

## ADULT ACLS ALGORITHMS *(Continued)*

# Tachycardia

**Fig. 5:** Adult tachycardia algorithm.

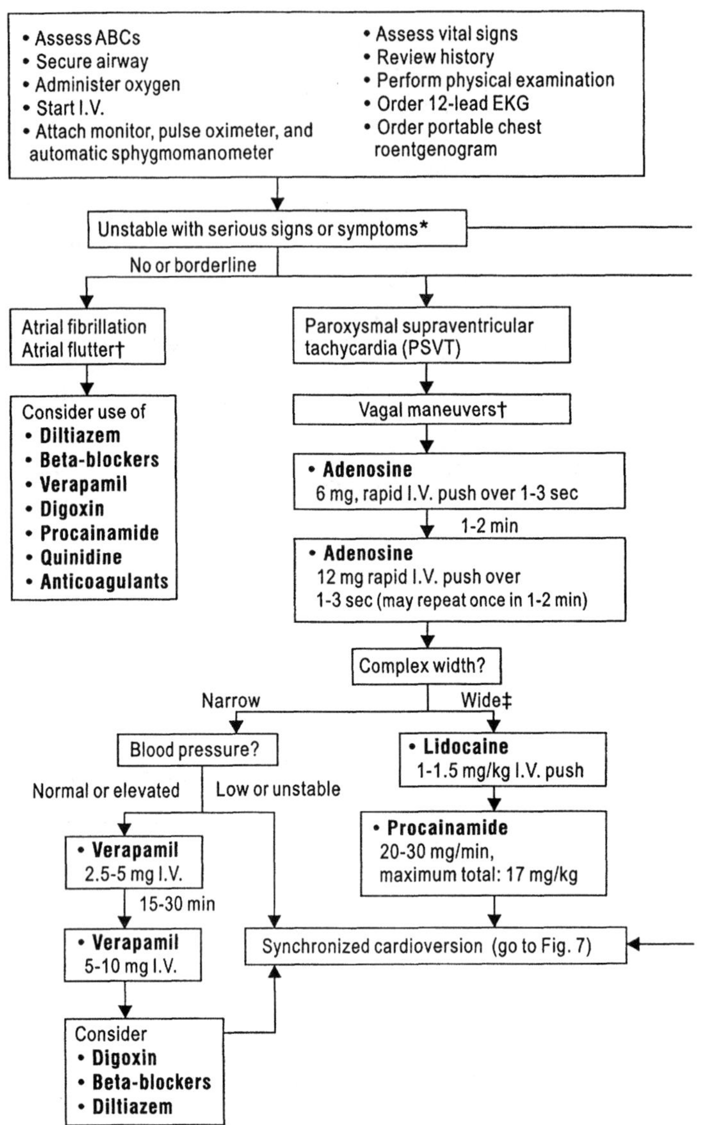

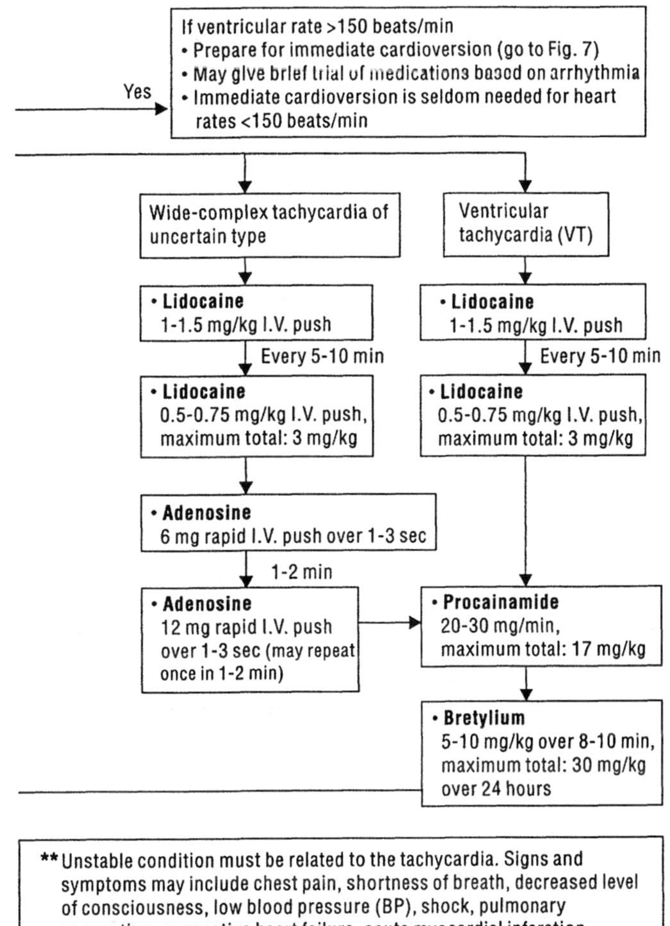
If ventricular rate >150 beats/min
• Prepare for immediate cardioversion (go to Fig. 7)
• May give brief trial of medications based on arrhythmia
• Immediate cardioversion is seldom needed for heart rates <150 beats/min
Yes
Wide-complex tachycardia of uncertain type
Ventricular tachycardia (VT)
• Lidocaine 1-1.5 mg/kg I.V. push
Every 5-10 min
• Lidocaine 0.5-0.75 mg/kg I.V. push, maximum total: 3 mg/kg
• Adenosine 6 mg rapid I.V. push over 1-3 sec
1-2 min
• Adenosine 12 mg rapid I.V. push over 1-3 sec (may repeat once in 1-2 min)
• Lidocaine 1-1.5 mg/kg I.V. push
Every 5-10 min
• Lidocaine 0.5-0.75 mg/kg I.V. push, maximum total: 3 mg/kg
• Procainamide 20-30 mg/min, maximum total: 17 mg/kg
• Bretylium 5-10 mg/kg over 8-10 min, maximum total: 30 mg/kg over 24 hours

** Unstable condition must be related to the tachycardia. Signs and symptoms may include chest pain, shortness of breath, decreased level of consciousness, low blood pressure (BP), shock, pulmonary congestion, congestive heart failure, acute myocardial infarction.

† Carotid sinus pressure is contraindicated in patients with carotid bruits; avoid ice water immersion in patients with ischemic heart disease.

‡ If the wide-complex tachycardia is known with certainty to be PSVT and BP is normal/elevated, sequence can include **verapamil.**

Used with permission: Emergency Cardiac Care Committee and Subcommittees, American Heart Association, "Guidelines for Cardiopulmonary Resuscitation and Emergency Care, III: Adult Advanced Cardiac Life Support," *JAMA*, 1992, 268:2199-2241.

## ADULT ACLS ALGORITHMS *(Continued)*

# Bradycardia

**Fig. 6:** Adult bradycardia algorithm (with the patient not in cardiac arrest).

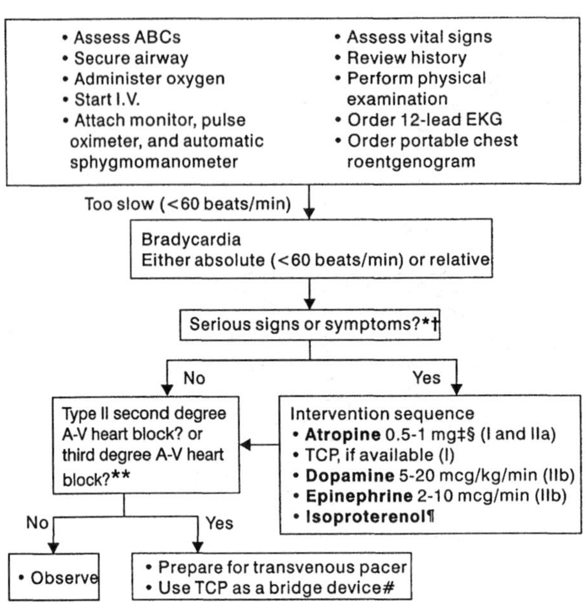


* Serious signs or symptoms must be related to the slow rate. Clinical manifestations include: Symptoms (chest pain, shortness of breath, decreased level of consciousness), and Signs (low BP, shock, pulmonary congestion, CHF, acute MI)

† Do not delay TCP while awaiting I.V. access or for **atropine** to take effect if patient is symptomatic.

‡ Denervated transplanted hearts will not respond to **atropine**. Go at once to pacing, **catecholamine** infusion, or both.

§ **Atropine** should be given in repeat doses in 3-5 min up to a total of 0.04 mg/kg. Consider shorter dosing intervals in severe clinical conditions. It has been suggested that atropine should be used with caution in atrioventricular (A-V) block at the His-Purkinje level (type II A-V block and new third degree block with wide QRS complexes) (Class IIb).

** Never treat third degree heart block plus ventricular escape beats with **lidocaine.**

¶ **Isoproterenol** should be used, if at all, with extreme caution. At low doses it is Class IIb (possibly helpful); at higher doses it is Class III (harmful).

\# Verify patient tolerance and mechanical capture. Use analgesia and sedation as needed.

# Electrical Conversion

**Fig. 7:** Adult electrical cardioversion algorithm (with the patient not in cardiac arrest).

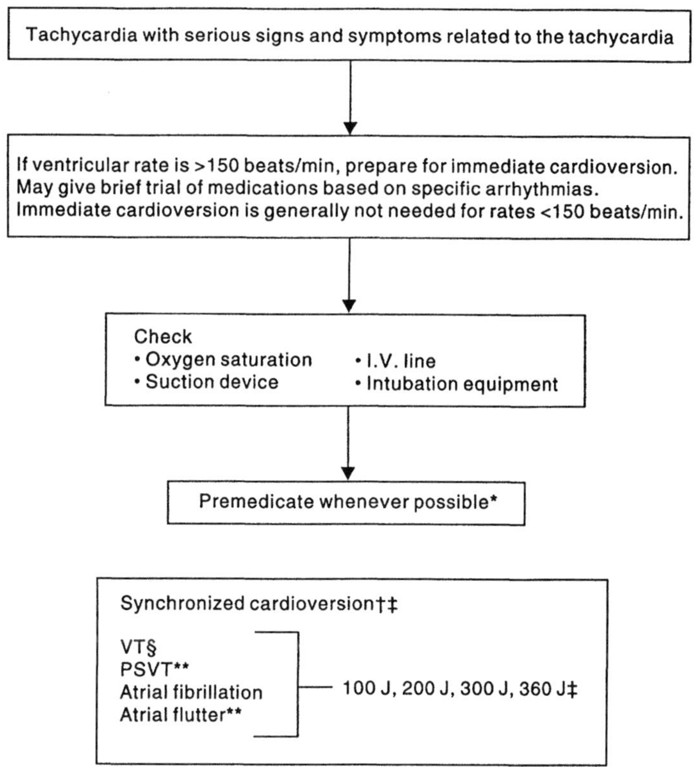
Tachycardia with serious signs and symptoms related to the tachycardia
If ventricular rate is >150 beats/min, prepare for immediate cardioversion. May give brief trial of medications based on specific arrhythmias. Immediate cardioversion is generally not needed for rates <150 beats/min.
Check
• Oxygen saturation
• I.V. line
• Suction device
• Intubation equipment
Premedicate whenever possible*
Synchronized cardioversion†‡
VT§
PSVT**
Atrial fibrillation
Atrial flutter**
100 J, 200 J, 300 J, 360 J‡

* Effective regimens have included a sedative (eg, **diazepam, midazolam barbiturates, etomidate, ketamine, methohexital**) with or without an analgesic agent (eg, **fentanyl, morphine, meperidine**). Many experts recommend anesthesia if service is readily available.

† Note possible need to resynchronize after each cardioversion.

‡ If delays in synchronization occur and clinical conditions are critical, go to immediate unsynchronized shocks.

§ Treat polymorphic VT (irregular form and rate) like VF: 200 J, 200-300 J, 360 J.

** PSVT and atrial flutter often respond to lower energy levels (start with 50 J).

Used with permission: Emergency Cardiac Care Committee and Subcommittees, American Heart Association, "Guidelines for Cardiopulmonary Resuscitation and Emergency Care, III: Adult Advanced Cardiac Life Support," *JAMA*, 1992, 268:2199-2241.

## ADULT ACLS ALGORITHMS *(Continued)*

# Hypotension, Shock

**Fig. 8:** Adult algorithm for hypotension, shock, and acute pulmonary edema.

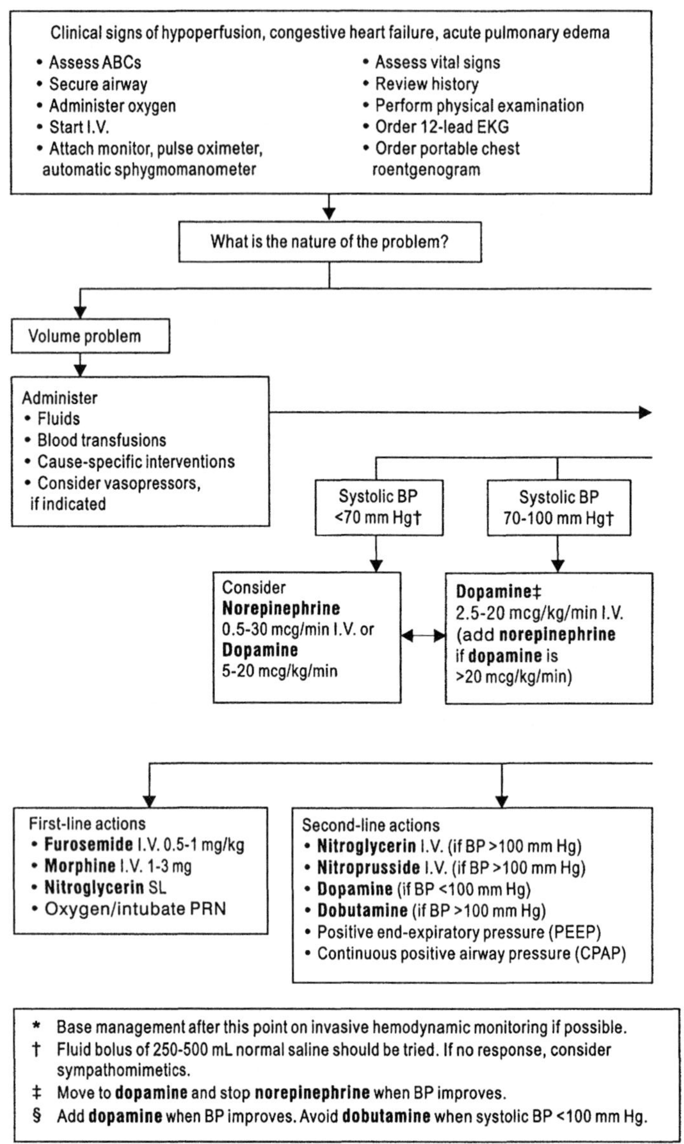


* Base management after this point on invasive hemodynamic monitoring if possible.
† Fluid bolus of 250-500 mL normal saline should be tried. If no response, consider sympathomimetics.
‡ Move to **dopamine** and stop **norepinephrine** when BP improves.
§ Add **dopamine** when BP improves. Avoid **dobutamine** when systolic BP <100 mm Hg.

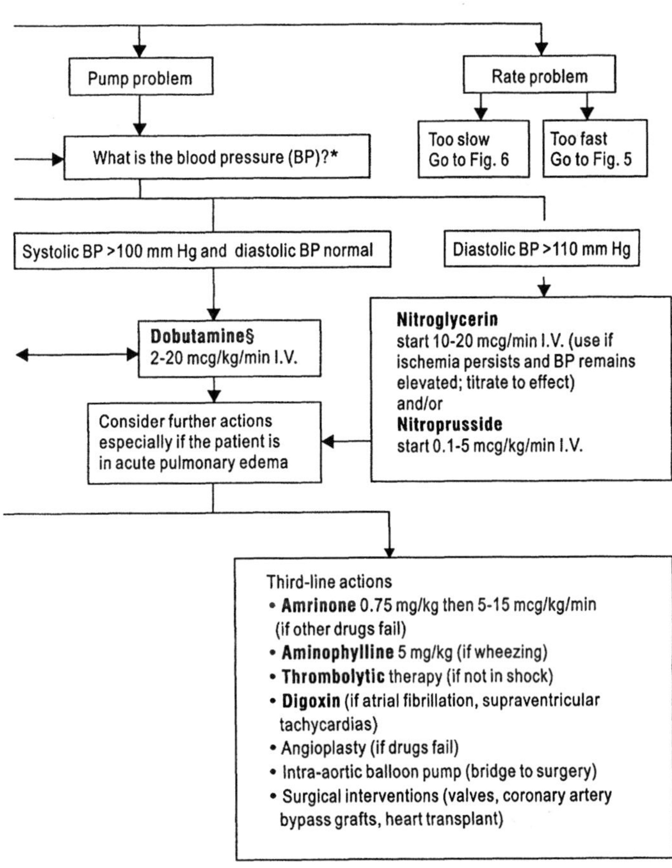
Pump problem
Rate problem
What is the blood pressure (BP)?*
Too slow
Go to Fig. 6
Too fast
Go to Fig. 5
Systolic BP >100 mm Hg and diastolic BP normal
Diastolic BP >110 mm Hg
Dobutamine§
2-20 mcg/kg/min I.V.
Nitroglycerin
start 10-20 mcg/min I.V. (use if ischemia persists and BP remains elevated; titrate to effect)
and/or
Nitroprusside
start 0.1-5 mcg/kg/min I.V.
Consider further actions especially if the patient is in acute pulmonary edema
Third-line actions
• Amrinone 0.75 mg/kg then 5-15 mcg/kg/min (if other drugs fail)
• Aminophylline 5 mg/kg (if wheezing)
• Thrombolytic therapy (if not in shock)
• Digoxin (if atrial fibrillation, supraventricular tachycardias)
• Angioplasty (if drugs fail)
• Intra-aortic balloon pump (bridge to surgery)
• Surgical interventions (valves, coronary artery bypass grafts, heart transplant)

# ADDICTION TREATMENTS

| | |
|---|---|
| Bupropion SR (Zyban®) | Smoking cessation:<br>Initiate at 150 mg every morning for 3 days. If tolerated, increase to 150 mg twice daily on day 4 of dosing. Should be an interval of at least 8 hours between successive doses. Target quit date after at least 1 week of treatment. Trial may be up to 12 weeks. Contraindicated in patients with seizures, anorexia, or bulimia. |
| Clonidine (Catapres®) | Alcohol, nicotine, opioid withdrawal:<br>Initiate 0.1 mg 2-3 times/day |
| Disulfiram (Antabuse®) | Sobriety:<br>125-500 mg/day; patients must be free of alcohol for at least 12 hours prior to initiation. Contraindicated with metronidazole and alcohol (including cough syrups). |
| Levomethadyl (Orlaam®) | Narcotic dependence:<br>Initiate at 20-40 mg 3 times/week |
| Methadone (Dolophine®) | Narcotic dependence:<br>15-60 mg every 6-8 hours; can only be initiated in approved treatment programs |
| Naltrexone (ReVia®) | Alcohol and narcotic dependence:<br>Initiate 25-50 mg/day; patient should be free of opioid for 7-10 days prior to initiation |
| Nicotine gum | Smoking cessation:<br>1-2 pieces/hour; maximum: 30 pieces/day (2 mg/piece). If high tobacco use, give DS (4 mg/piece); maximum: 20/day |
| Nicotine nasal spray | Smoking cessation:<br>1 spray in each nostril once or twice per hour; maximum: 80 sprays |
| Nicotine patches | Smoking cessation:<br>One patch daily for 8 weeks |

# ASTHMA

## NATIONAL ASTHMA EDUCATION AND PREVENTION PROGRAM

## EXPERT PANEL REPORT II: GUIDELINES FOR THE DIAGNOSIS AND MANAGEMENT OF ASTHMA

**February 1997**

### Stepwise Approach for Managing Asthma in Adults and Children >5 Years of Age: Classify Severity

### Goals of Asthma Treatment

- Prevent chronic and troublesome symptoms (eg, coughing or breathlessness in the night, in the early morning, or after exertion)
- Maintain (near) "normal" pulmonary function
- Maintain normal activity levels (including exercise and other physical activity)
- Prevent recurrent exacerbations of asthma and minimize the need for emergency department visits or hospitalizations
- Provide optimal pharmacotherapy with minimal or no adverse effects
- Meet patients' and families' expectations of and satisfaction with asthma care

### Clinical Features Before Treatment*

| Symptoms** | Nighttime Symptoms | Lung Function |
|---|---|---|
| | **STEP 4: Severe Persistent** | |
| •Continual symptoms<br>•Limited physical activity<br>•Frequent exacerbations | Frequent | •$FEV_1$/PEF ≤60% predicted<br>•PEF variability >30% |
| | **STEP 3: Moderate Persistent** | |
| •Daily symptoms<br>•Daily use of inhaled short-acting $beta_2$-agonist<br>•Exacerbations affect activity<br>•Exacerbations ≥2 times/week; may last days | >1 time/week | •$FEV_1$/PEF >60% - 80% predicted<br>•PEF variability >30% |
| | **STEP 2: Mild Persistent** | |
| •Symptoms >2 times/week but <1 time/day<br>•Exacerbations may affect activity | >2 times/month | •$FEV_1$/PEF ≥80% predicted<br>•PEF variability 20% - 30% |
| | **STEP 1: Mild Intermittent** | |
| •Symptoms ≤2 times/week<br>•Asymptomatic and normal PEF between exacerbations<br>•Exacerbations brief (from a few hours to a few days); intensity may vary | ≤2 times/month | •$FEV_1$/PEF ≥80% predicted<br>•PEF variability ≤20% |

*The presence of one of the features of severity is sufficient to place a patient in that category. An individual should be assigned to the most severe grade in which any feature occurs. The characteristics noted in this figure are general and may overlap because asthma is highly variable. Furthermore, an individual's classification may change over time.

**Patients at any level of severity can have mild, moderate, or severe exacerbations. Some patients with intermittent asthma experience severe and life-threatening exacerbations separated by long periods of normal lung function and no symptoms.

## ASTHMA *(Continued)*

### Stepwise Approach for Managing Asthma in Adults and Children >5 Years of Age: Treatment

(Preferred treatments are in **bold** print)

| Long-Term Control | Quick Relief | Education |
|---|---|---|
| | **STEP 4: Severe Persistent** | |
| Daily medications:<br>• **Anti-inflammatory: Inhaled corticosteroid (high dose)**<br>AND<br>• Long-acting bronchodilator: Either **long-acting inhaled beta$_2$-agonist**, sustained-release theophylline, or long-acting beta$_2$-agonist tablets<br>AND<br>• Corticosteroid tablets or syrup long term (2 mg/kg/day, generally do not exceed 60 mg per day). | • Short-acting bronchodilator: **Inhaled beta$_2$-agonists** as needed for symptoms.<br>• Intensity of treatment will depend on severity of exacerbation; see "Managing Exacerbations"<br>• Use of short-acting inhaled beta$_2$-agonists on a daily basis, or increasing use, indicates the need for additional long-term control therapy. | Steps 2 and 3 actions plus:<br>• Refer to individual education/counseling |
| | **STEP 3: Moderate Persistent** | |
| Daily medication:<br>• Either<br>— **Anti-inflammatory: Inhaled corticosteroid (medium dose)**<br>OR<br>— **Inhaled corticosteroid (low-medium dose)** and add a long-acting bronchodilator, especially for nighttime symptoms: Either **long-acting inhaled beta$_2$-agonist**, sustained-release theophylline, or long-acting beta$_2$-agonist tablets.<br>• If needed<br>— Anti-inflammatory: **Inhaled corticosteroids (medium-high dose) AND**<br>— **Long-acting bronchodilator,** especially for nighttime symptoms; either **long-acting inhaled beta$_2$-agonist,** sustained release theophylline, or long-acting beta$_2$-agonist tablets. | • Short-acting bronchodilator: **Inhaled beta$_2$-agonists** as needed for symptoms.<br>• Intensity of treatment will depend on severity of exacerbation; see "Managing Exacerbations."<br>• Use of short-acting inhaled beta$_2$-agonists on a daily basis, or increasing use, indicates the need for additional long-term control therapy. | Step 1 actions plus:<br>• Teach self-monitoring<br>• Refer to group education if available<br>• Review and update self-management plan |
| | **STEP 2: Mild Persistent** | |
| One daily medication:<br>• **Anti-inflammatory:** Either **inhaled corticosteroid** (low doses) or **cromolyn or nedocromil** (children usually begin with a trial of cromolyn or nedocromil).<br>• Sustained-release theophylline to serum concentration of 5-15 mcg/mL is an alternative, but not preferred, therapy. Zafirlukast or zileuton may also be considered for patients ≥12 years of age, although their position in therapy is not fully established. | • Short-acting bronchodilator: **Inhaled beta$_2$-agonists** as needed for symptoms.<br>• Intensity of treatment will depend on severity of exacerbation; see "Managing Exacerbations."<br>• Use of short-acting inhaled beta$_2$-agonists on a daily basis, or increasing use, indicates the need for additional long-term control therapy. | Step 1 actions plus:<br>• Teach self-monitoring<br>• Refer to group education if available<br>• Review and update self-management plan |
| | **STEP 1: Mild Intermittent** | |
| No daily medication needed. | • Short-acting bronchodilator: **Inhaled beta$_2$-agonists** as needed for symptoms.<br>• Intensity of treatment will depend on severity of exacerbation; see "Managing Exacerbations"<br>• Use of short-acting inhaled beta$_2$-agonists more than 2 times/week may indicate the need to initiate long-term control therapy | • Teach basic facts about asthma<br>• Teach inhaler/spacer/holding chamber technique<br>• Discuss roles of medications<br>• Develop self-management plan<br>• Develop action plan for when and how to take rescue actions, especially for patients with a history of severe exacerbations<br>• Discuss appropriate environmental control measures to avoid exposure to known allergens and irritants |

**↓ Step down**
Review treatment every 1-6 months; a gradual stepwise reduction in treatment may be possible.

**↑Step up**
If control is not maintained, consider step up. First, review patient medication technique, adherence, and environmental control (avoidance of allergens or other factors that contribute to asthma severity.)

**Notes:**

- **The stepwise approach presents general guidelines to assist clinical decision making; it is not intended to be a specific prescription. Asthma is highly variable; clinicians should tailor specific medication plans to the needs and circumstances of individual patients.**
- Gain control as quickly as possible; then decrease treatment to the least medication necessary to maintain control. Gaining control may be accomplished by either starting treatment at the step most appropriate to the initial severity of the condition or starting at a higher level of therapy (eg, a course of systemic corticosteroids or higher dose of inhaled corticosteroids).
- A rescue course of systemic corticosteroids may be needed at any time and at any step.
- Some patients with intermittent asthma experience severe and life-threatening exacerbations separated by long periods of normal lung function and no symptoms. This may be especially common with exacerbations provoked by respiratory infections. A short course of systemic corticosteroids is recommended.
- At each step, patients should control their environment to avoid or control factors that make their asthma worse (eg, allergens, irritants); this requires specific diagnosis and education.

## Stepwise Approach for Managing Infants and Young Children (≤5 Years of Age) With Acute or Chronic Asthma Symptoms

| Long-Term Control | Quick Relief |
|---|---|
| **STEP 4: Severe Persistent** | |
| Daily anti-inflammatory medicine<br>• High-dose inhaled corticosteroid with spacer/holding chamber and face mask<br>• If needed, add systemic corticosteroids 2 mg/kg/day and reduce to lowest daily or alternate-day dose that stabilizes symptoms | • Bronchodilator as needed for symptoms (see step 1) up to 3 times/day |
| **STEP 3: Moderate Persistent** | |
| Daily anti-inflammatory medication. Either:<br>• Medium-dose inhaled corticosteroid with spacer/holding chamber and face mask<br>OR<br>Once control is established:<br>• Medium-dose inhaled corticosteroid and nedocromil<br>OR<br>• Medium-dose inhaled corticosteroid and long-acting bronchodilator (theophylline) | • Bronchodilator as needed for symptoms (see step 1) up to 3 times/day |
| **STEP 2: Mild Persistent** | |
| Daily anti-inflammatory medication. Either:<br>• Cromolyn (nebulizer is preferred; or MDI) or nedocromil (MDI only) tid-qid<br>• Infants and young children usually begin with a trial of cromolyn or nedocromil<br>OR<br>• Low-dose inhaled corticosteroid with spacer/holding chamber and face mask | • Bronchodilator as needed for symptoms (see step 1) |
| **STEP 1: Mild Intermittent** | |
| No daily medication needed | • Bronchodilator as needed for symptoms <2 times/week. Intensity of treatment will depend upon severity of exacerbation (see "Managing Exacerbations"). Either:<br>— Inhaled short-acting beta$_2$-agonist by nebulizer or face mask and spacer/holding chamber<br>OR<br>— Oral beta$_2$-agonist for symptoms<br>• With viral respiratory infection:<br>— Bronchodilator q4-6h up to 24 hours (longer with physician consult) but, in general, repeat no more than once every 6 weeks<br>— Consider systemic corticosteroid if current exacerbation is severe<br>OR<br>Patient has history of previous severe exacerbations |

**↓ Step Down**
Review treatment every 1-6 months. If control is sustained for at least 3 months, a gradual stepwise reduction in treatment may be possible.

**↑ Step Up**
If control is not achieved, consider step up. But first: review patient medication technique, adherence, and environmental control (avoidance of allergens or other precipitant factors)

**Notes:**

- **The stepwise approach presents guidelines to assist clinical decision making. Asthma is highly variable; clinicians should tailor specific medication plans to the needs and circumstances of individual patients.**
- Gain control as quickly as possible; then decrease treatment to the least medication necessary to maintain control. Gaining control may be accomplished by either starting treatment at the step most appropriate to the initial severity of their condition or by starting at a higher level of therapy (eg, a course of systemic corticosteroids or higher dose of inhaled corticosteroids).
- A rescue course of systemic corticosteroid (prednisolone) may be needed at any time and step.
- In general, use of short-acting beta$_2$-agonist on a daily basis indicates the need for additional long-term control therapy.
- It is important to remember that there are very few studies on asthma therapy for infants.
- Consultation with an asthma specialist is recommended for patients with moderate or severe persistent asthma in this age group. Consultation should be considered for all patients with mild persistent asthma.

## ASTHMA *(Continued)*

### Management of Asthma Exacerbations: Home Treatment*

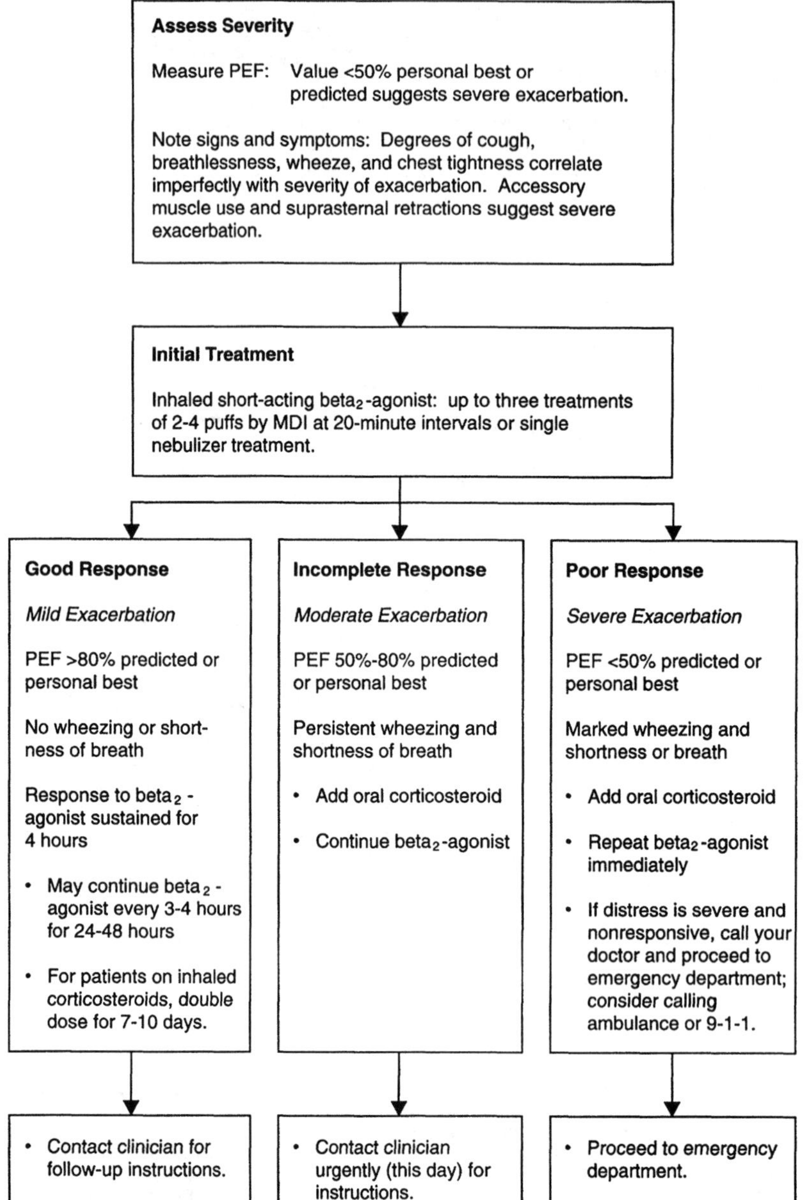

Assess Severity
Measure PEF: Value <50% personal best or predicted suggests severe exacerbation.
Note signs and symptoms: Degrees of cough, breathlessness, wheeze, and chest tightness correlate imperfectly with severity of exacerbation. Accessory muscle use and suprasternal retractions suggest severe exacerbation.
Initial Treatment
Inhaled short-acting beta2-agonist: up to three treatments of 2-4 puffs by MDI at 20-minute intervals or single nebulizer treatment.
Good Response
Mild Exacerbation
PEF >80% predicted or personal best
No wheezing or shortness of breath
Response to beta2-agonist sustained for 4 hours
• May continue beta2-agonist every 3-4 hours for 24-48 hours
• For patients on inhaled corticosteroids, double dose for 7-10 days.
Incomplete Response
Moderate Exacerbation
PEF 50%-80% predicted or personal best
Persistent wheezing and shortness of breath
• Add oral corticosteroid
• Continue beta2-agonist
Poor Response
Severe Exacerbation
PEF <50% predicted or personal best
Marked wheezing and shortness or breath
• Add oral corticosteroid
• Repeat beta2-agonist immediately
• If distress is severe and nonresponsive, call your doctor and proceed to emergency department; consider calling ambulance or 9-1-1.
• Contact clinician for follow-up instructions.
• Contact clinician urgently (this day) for instructions.
• Proceed to emergency department.


*Patients at high risk of asthma-related death should receive immediate clinical attention after initial treatment. Additional therapy may be required.

## Management of Asthma Exacerbations: Emergency Department and Hospital-Based Care

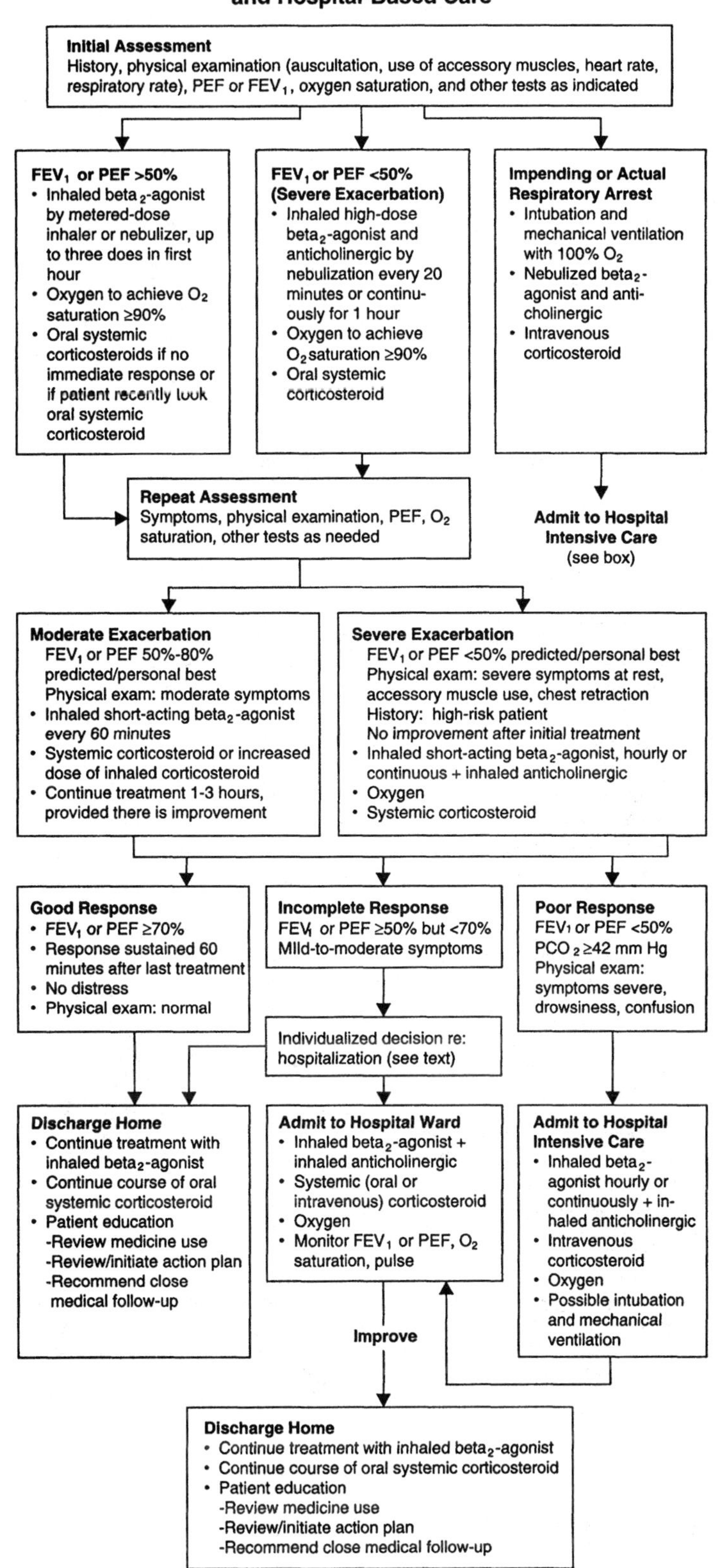

**Initial Assessment**
History, physical examination (auscultation, use of accessory muscles, heart rate, respiratory rate), PEF or $FEV_1$, oxygen saturation, and other tests as indicated
**$FEV_1$ or PEF >50%**
• Inhaled beta$_2$-agonist by metered-dose inhaler or nebulizer, up to three does in first hour
• Oxygen to achieve $O_2$ saturation ≥90%
• Oral systemic corticosteroids if no immediate response or if patient recently took oral systemic corticosteroid
**$FEV_1$ or PEF <50% (Severe Exacerbation)**
• Inhaled high-dose beta$_2$-agonist and anticholinergic by nebulization every 20 minutes or continuously for 1 hour
• Oxygen to achieve $O_2$ saturation ≥90%
• Oral systemic corticosteroid
**Impending or Actual Respiratory Arrest**
• Intubation and mechanical ventilation with 100% $O_2$
• Nebulized beta$_2$-agonist and anticholinergic
• Intravenous corticosteroid
**Repeat Assessment**
Symptoms, physical examination, PEF, $O_2$ saturation, other tests as needed
**Admit to Hospital Intensive Care**
(see box)
**Moderate Exacerbation**
$FEV_1$ or PEF 50%-80% predicted/personal best
Physical exam: moderate symptoms
• Inhaled short-acting beta$_2$-agonist every 60 minutes
• Systemic corticosteroid or increased dose of inhaled corticosteroid
• Continue treatment 1-3 hours, provided there is improvement
**Severe Exacerbation**
$FEV_1$ or PEF <50% predicted/personal best
Physical exam: severe symptoms at rest, accessory muscle use, chest retraction
History: high-risk patient
No improvement after initial treatment
• Inhaled short-acting beta$_2$-agonist, hourly or continuous + inhaled anticholinergic
• Oxygen
• Systemic corticosteroid
**Good Response**
• $FEV_1$ or PEF ≥70%
• Response sustained 60 minutes after last treatment
• No distress
• Physical exam: normal
**Incomplete Response**
$FEV_1$ or PEF ≥50% but <70%
Mild-to-moderate symptoms
**Poor Response**
$FEV_1$ or PEF <50%
$PCO_2$ ≥42 mm Hg
Physical exam: symptoms severe, drowsiness, confusion
Individualized decision re: hospitalization (see text)
**Discharge Home**
• Continue treatment with inhaled beta$_2$-agonist
• Continue course of oral systemic corticosteroid
• Patient education
-Review medicine use
-Review/initiate action plan
-Recommend close medical follow-up
**Admit to Hospital Ward**
• Inhaled beta$_2$-agonist + inhaled anticholinergic
• Systemic (oral or intravenous) corticosteroid
• Oxygen
• Monitor $FEV_1$ or PEF, $O_2$ saturation, pulse
**Admit to Hospital Intensive Care**
• Inhaled beta$_2$-agonist hourly or continuously + inhaled anticholinergic
• Intravenous corticosteroid
• Oxygen
• Possible intubation and mechanical ventilation
Improve
**Discharge Home**
• Continue treatment with inhaled beta$_2$-agonist
• Continue course of oral systemic corticosteroid
• Patient education
-Review medicine use
-Review/initiate action plan
-Recommend close medical follow-up

## ASTHMA *(Continued)*

# ESTIMATED COMPARATIVE DAILY DOSAGES FOR INHALED CORTICOSTEROIDS

### Adults

| Drug | Low Dose | Medium Dose | High Dose |
|---|---|---|---|
| Beclomethasone dipropionate<br>42 mcg/puff<br>84 mcg/puff | 168-504 mcg<br>(4-12 puffs — 42 mcg)<br>(2-6 puffs — 84 mcg) | 504-840 mcg<br>(12-20 puffs — 42 mcg)<br>(6-10 puffs — 84 mcg) | >840 mcg<br>(>20 puffs — 42 mcg)<br>(>10 puffs — 84 mcg) |
| Budesonide Turbuhaler<br>200 mcg/dose | 200-400 mcg<br>(1-2 inhalations) | 400-600 mcg<br>(2-3 inhalations) | >600 mcg<br>(>3 inhalations) |
| Flunisolide<br>250 mcg/puff | 500-1000 mcg<br>(2-4 puffs) | 1000-2000 mcg<br>(4-8 puffs) | >2000 mcg<br>(>8 puffs) |
| Fluticasone<br>MDI: 44, 110, 220 mcg/puff<br><br><br>DPI: 50, 100, 250 mcg/dose | 88-264 mcg<br>(2-6 puffs — 44 mcg)<br>or<br>(2 puffs — 110 mcg)<br>(2-6 inhalations — 50 mcg) | 264-660 mcg<br>(2-6 puffs — 110 mcg)<br><br><br>(3-6 inhalations — 100 mcg) | >660 mcg<br>(>6 puffs — 110 mcg)<br>or<br>(>3 puffs — 220 mcg)<br>(>6 inhalations — 100 mcg) |
| Triamcinolone acetonide<br>100 mcg/puff | 400-1000 mcg<br>(4-10 puffs) | 1000-2000 mcg<br>(10-20 puffs) | >2000 mcg<br>(>20 puffs) |

### Children

| Drug | Low Dose | Medium Dose | High Dose |
|---|---|---|---|
| Beclomethasone dipropionate<br>42 mcg/puff<br>84 mcg/puff | 84-336 mcg<br>(2-8 puffs) | 336-672 mcg<br>(8-16 puffs) | >672 mcg<br>(>16 puffs) |
| Budesonide Turbuhaler<br>200 mcg/dose | 100-200 mcg | 200-400 mcg<br>(1-2 inhalations — 200 mcg) | >400 mcg<br>(>2 inhalations — 200 mcg) |
| Flunisolide<br>250 mcg/puff | 500-750 mcg<br>(2-3 puffs) | 1000-1250 mcg<br>(4-5 puffs) | >1250 mcg<br>(>5 puffs) |
| Fluticasone<br>MDI: 44, 110, 220 mcg/puff<br><br><br>DPI: 50, 100, 250 mcg/dose | 88-176 mcg<br>(2-4 puffs — 44 mcg)<br><br><br>(2-4 inhalations — 50 mcg) | 176-440 mcg<br>(4-10 puffs — 44 mcg)<br>or<br>(2-4 puffs — 110 mcg)<br>(2-4 inhalations — 100 mcg) | >440 mcg<br>(>4 puffs — 110 mcg)<br><br><br>(>4 inhalations — 100 mcg) |
| Triamcinolone acetonide<br>100 mcg/puff | 400-800 mcg<br>(4-8 puffs) | 800-1200 mcg<br>(8-12 puffs) | >1200 mcg<br>(>12 puffs) |

**Notes:**

- **The most important determinant of appropriate dosing is the clinician's judgment of the patient's response to therapy.** The clinician must monitor the patient's response on several clinical parameters and adjust the dose accordingly. The stepwise approach to therapy emphasizes that once control of asthma is achieved, the dose of mediation should be carefully titrated to the minimum dose required to maintain control, thus reducing the potential for adverse effect.
- The reference point for the range in the dosages for children is data on the safety on inhaled corticosteroids in children, which, in general, suggest that the dose ranges are equivalent to beclomethasone dipropionate 200-400 mcg/day (low dose), 400-800 mcg/day (medium dose), and >800 mcg/day (high dose).
- Some dosages may be outside package labeling.
- Metered-dose inhaler (MDI) dosages are expressed as the actuator dose (the amount of drug leaving the actuator and delivered to the patient), which is the labeling required in the United States. This is different from the dosage expressed as the valve dose (the amount of drug leaving the valve, all of which is not available to the patient), which is used in many European countries and in some of the scientific literature. Dry powder inhaler (DPI) doses (eg, Turbuhaler) are expressed as the amount of drug in the inhaler following activation.

# ESTIMATED CLINICAL COMPARABILITY OF DOSES FOR INHALED CORTICOSTEROIDS

Data from *in vitro* and in clinical trials suggest that the different inhaled corticosteroid preparations are not equivalent on a per puff or microgram basis. However, it is not entirely clear what implications these differences have for dosing recommendations in clinical practice because there are few data directly comparing the preparations. Relative dosing for clinical comparability is affected by differences in topical potency, clinical effects at different doses, delivery device, and bioavailability. The Expert Panel developed recommended dose ranges for different preparations based on available data and the following assumptions and cautions about estimating relative doses needed to achieve comparable clinical effect.

- **Relative topical potency using human skin blanching**
  - The standard test for determining relative topical anti-inflammatory potency is the topical vasoconstriction (MacKenzie skin blanching) test.
  - The MacKenzie topical skin blanching test correlates with binding affinities and binding half-lives for human lung corticosteroid receptors (see table below) (Dahlberg, et al, 1984; Hogger and Rohdewald 1994).
  - The relationship between relative topical anti-inflammatory effect and clinical comparability in asthma management is not certain. However, recent clinical trials suggest that different in vitro measures of anti-inflammatory effect is not certain. However, recent clinical trials suggest that different in vitro measures of anti-inflammatory effect correlate with clinical efficacy (Barnes and Pedersen 1993; Johnson 1996; Kamada, et al, 1996; Ebden, et al, 1986; Leblanc, et al, 1994; Gustaffson, et al, 1993; Lundback, et al, 1993; Barnes, et al, 1993; Fabbri, et al, 1993; Langdon and Capsey, 1994; Ayres, et al, 1995; Rafferty, et al, 1985; Bjorkander, et al, 1982, Stiksa, et al, 1982; Willey, et al, 1982.)

| Medication | Topical Potency (Skin Blanching)* | Corticosteroid Receptor Binding Half-Life | Receptor Binding Affinity |
|---|---|---|---|
| Beclomethasone dipropionate (BDP) | 600 | 7.5 hours | 13.5 |
| Budesonide (BUD) | 980 | 5.1 hours | 9.4 |
| Flunisolide (FLU) | 330 | 3.5 hours | 1.8 |
| Fluticasone propionate (FP) | 1200 | 10.5 hours | 18.0 |
| Triamcinolone acetonide (TAA) | 330 | 3.9 hours | 3.6 |

*Numbers are assigned in reference to dexamethasone, which has a value of "1" in the MacKenzie test.

- **Relative doses to achieve similar clinical effects**
  - Clinical effects are evaluated by a number of outcome parameters (eg, changes in spirometry, peak flow rates, symptom scores, quick-relief beta$_2$-agonist use, frequency of exacerbations, airway responsiveness).
  - The daily dose and duration of treatment may affect these outcome parameters differently (eg, symptoms and peak flow may improve at lower doses and over a shorter treatment time than bronchial reactivity) (van Essen-Zandvliet, et al, 1992; Haahtela, et al, 1991)
  - Delivery systems influence comparability. For example, the delivery device for budesonide (Turbuhaler) delivers approximately twice the amount of drug to the airway as the MDI, thus enhancing the clinical effect (Thorsson, et al, 1994); Agertoft and Pedersen, 1993).
  - Individual patients may respond differently to different preparations, as noted by clinical experience.
  - Clinical trials comparing effects in reducing symptoms and improving peak expiratory flow demonstrate:
  - BDP and BUD achieved comparable effects at similar microgram doses by MDI (Bjorkander, et al, 1982; Ebden, et al, 1986; Rafferty, et al, 1985).
  - BDP achieved effects similar to twice the dose of TAA on a microgram basis.

# CLOZAPINE-INDUCED SIDE EFFECTS

## INCIDENCE AND MANAGEMENT

| Effect | Incidence | Management |
|---|---|---|
| Sedation & fatigue | 35% | Initiate split dosing with long-term goal to administer twice daily with larger portion at bedtime (appears to be dose-dependent). For chronic sedation, consider an empiric trial of methylphenidate 5-20 mg/day. |
| Sialorrhea | 25% | Clozapine may affect the swallowing mechanism; behavioral approach may be best. Consider lowering the dose. Pharmacological management consists of clonidine 0.1-0.9 mg/day (monitor blood pressure) or benztropine 0.5-2 mg/day (monitor for increased anticholinergic side effects). |
| Weight gain | 35% | Diet and exercise best. No pharmacological agent shown to be consistently useful; one study showed the addition of quetiapine to clozapine minimized weight gain; consider lowering dose. |
| Urinary incontinence | 25% | If patient receiving co-pharmacy with typical antipsychotic, consider discontinuing; pharmacological management consists of ephedrine 25-150 mg/d, oxybutynin 5 mg tid, or desmopressin. |
| Tachycardia | 25% | Dose dependent. Beta-blocker; atenolol 50 mg/d or propranolol 10 mg tid (adjust for rate) |
| Constipation | 20% | Discontinue other medications with anticholinergic activity, if possible. May need chronic psyllium and/or docusate. |
| Seizures | 4% | Dose dependent. Valproic acid/valproate; initiate at 250 mg tid or 500 mg bid and titrate to serum level of at least 50 mcg/mL |
| Agranulocytosis | 1% | Stop drug. Do not rechallenge. Consider filgrastim (G-CSF) or sargramostim (GM-CSF) during acute recovery phase. |

# DEPRESSION

## Medications That May Precipitate Depression

| | |
|---|---|
| Anticancer agents | Vinblastine, vincristine, interferon, procarbazine, asparaginase, tamoxifen, cyproterone |
| Anti-inflammatory & analgesic agents | Indomethacin, pentazocine, phenacetin, phenylbutazone |
| Antimicrobial agents | Cycloserine, ethambutol, sulfonamides, select gram-negative antibiotics |
| Cardiovascular/antihypertensive agents | Clonidine, digitalis, diuretics, guanethidine, hydralazine, indapamide, methyldopa, prazocin, procainamide, propranolol, reserpine |
| CNS agents | Alcohol, amantadine, amphetamine & derivatives, barbiturates, benzodiazepines, chloral hydrate, carbamazepine, cocaine, haloperidol, L-dopa, phenothiazines, succinimide derivatives |
| Hormonal agents | ACTH, corticosteroids, estrogen, melatonin, oral contraceptives, progesterone |
| Miscellaneous | Cimetidine, disulfiram, organic pesticides, physostigmine |

## Medical Disorders & Psychiatric Disorders Associated With Depression

| | |
|---|---|
| Endocrine diseases | Acromegaly, Addison's disease, Cushing's disease, diabetes mellitus, hyperparathyroidism, hypoparathyroidism, hyperthyroidism, hypothyroidism, insulinoma, pheochromocytoma, pituitary dysfunction |
| Deficiency states | Pernicious anemia, severe anemia, Wernicke's encephalopathy |
| Infections | Encephalitis, fungal infections, meningitis, neurosyphilis, influenza, mononucleosis, tuberculosis, AIDS |
| Collagen disorders | Rheumatoid arthritis |
| Systemic lupus erythematosus | |
| Metabolic disorders | Electrolyte imbalance, hypokalemia, hyponatremia, hepatic encephalopathy, Pick's disease, uremia, Wilson's disease |
| Cardiovascular disease | Cerebral arteriosclerosis, chronic bronchitis, congestive heart failure, emphysema, myocardial infarction, paroxysmal dysrhythmia, pneumonia |
| Neurologic disorders | Alzheimer's disease, amyotrophic lateral sclerosis, brain tumors, chronic pain syndrome, Creutzfeldt-Jakob disease, Huntington's disease, multiple sclerosis, myasthenia gravis, Parkinson's disease, poststroke, trauma (postconcussion) |
| Malignant disease | Breast, gastrointestinal, lung, pancreas, prostate |
| Psychiatric disorders | Alcoholism, anxiety disorders, eating disorders, schizophrenia |

# DIABETES MELLITUS TREATMENT

## INSULIN-DEPENDENT DIABETES MELLITUS

Treatment goals that emphasize glycemic control have been recommended by the American Diabetes Association (see table).

### Glycemic Control for People With Diabetes

| Biochemical Index | Nondiabetic | Goal | Action Suggested |
|---|---|---|---|
| Preprandial glucose | <115 | 80-120 | <80<br>>140 |
| Bedtime glucose (mg/dL) | <120 | 100-140 | <100<br>>160 |
| Hb $A_{1C}$ (%) | <8 | <7 | >8 |

These values are for nonpregnant individuals. Action suggested depends on individual patient circumstances, Hb $A_{1C}$ referenced to a nondiabetic range of 4% to 6% (mean 5%, SD 0.5%).

### Effect on Glycemic Control of Oral Hypoglycemic Agents as Monotherapy

| Agent | Fasting Blood Glucose | Postprandial Blood Glucose | $HbA_{1c}$ |
|---|---|---|---|
| Precose® (acarbose)<br>25-100 g 3 times/day | -25 mg/dL | -49 mg/dL | -0.44% to -0.74% |
| Glucophage® (metformin)<br>Up to 2500 mg/day | -52 mg/dL | – | -1.4% |
| Amaryl® (glimepiride)<br>1-8 mg/day | -60 mg/dL | – | -1.5% to 2% |
| Diaβeta/Micronase (glyburide)<br>1.25-20 mg/day | | | |
| Glynase PresTab® (glyburide)<br>0.75-12 mg/day | | | |
| Prandin® (repaglinide)<br>0.25-4 mg 3 times/day | -31 to -.82 mg/dL | -48 mg/dL | -0.6% to -1.9% |

(Package inserts: Diaβeta®, 1997; Glynase PresTab®, 1999; Micronase®, 1999; Prandin®, 1997; Goldberg, 1999)

**Pharmacological Algorithm for Treatment of Type 2 Diabetes**
**(Patients inadequately controlled with diet and exercise)**

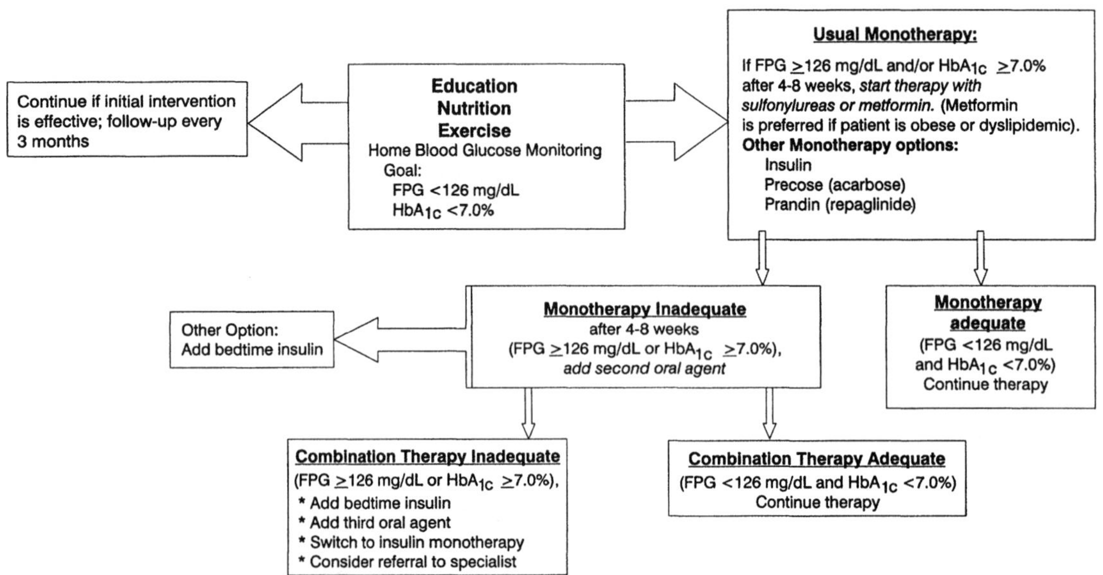


Modified from DeFronzo RA, "Pharmacological Treatment for Type 2 Diabetes Mellitus," *Ann Intern Med*, 1999, 131:281-303.

# EPILEPSY

## Antiepileptic Drugs for Children and Adolescents by Seizure Type and Epilepsy Syndrome

| Seizure Type or Epilepsy Syndrome | First Line Therapy | Alternatives |
|---|---|---|
| Partial seizures (with or without secondary generalization) | Carbamazepine | Valproate, phenytoin, gabapentin, lamotrigine, vigabatrin, phenobarbital, primidone; consider clonazepam, clorazepate, acetazolamide |
| Generalized tonic-clonic seizures | Valproate or carbamazepine | Phenytoin, phenobarbital, primidone; consider clonazepam |
| Childhood absence epilepsy | | |
| Before 10 years of age | Ethosuximide or Valproate | Methsuximide, acetazolamide, clonazepam, lamotrigine |
| After 10 years of age | Valproate | Ethosuximide, methsuximide, acetazolamide, clonazepam, lamotrigine; consider adding carbamazepine, phenytoin, or phenobarbital for generalized tonic-clonic seizures if valproate not tolerated |
| Juvenile myoclonic epilepsy | Valproate | Phenobarbital, primidone, clonazepam; consider carbamazepine, phenytoin, methsuximide, acetazolamide |
| Progressive myoclonic epilepsy | Valproate | Valproate plus clonazepam, phenobarbital |
| Lennox-Gastaut and related syndromes | Valproate | Clonazepam, phenobarbital, lamotrigine, ethosuximide, felbamate; consider methsuximide, ACTH or steroids, pyridoxine, ketogenic diet |
| Infantile spasms | ACTH or steroids | Valproate; consider clonazepam, vigabatrin (especially with tuberous sclerosis), pyridoxine |
| Benign epilepsy of childhood with centrotemporal spikes | Carbamazepine or valproate | Phenytoin; consider phenobarbital, primidone |
| Neonatal seizures | Phenobarbital | Phenytoin; consider clonazepam, primidone, valproate, pyridoxine |

Adapted from Bourgeois BFD, "Antiepileptic Drugs in Pediatric Practice," *Epilepsia*, 1995, 36 (Suppl 2):S34-S45.

# *HELICOBACTER PYLORI* TREATMENT

**Multiple Drug Regimens for the Treatment of *H. pylori* Infection**

| Drug | Dosages* | Duration of Therapy |
|---|---|---|
| $H_2$-receptor antagonist | Any one given at appropriate dose | 4 weeks |
| *plus* | | |
| Bismuth subsalicylate | 525 mg 4 times/day | 2 weeks |
| *plus* | | |
| Metronidazole | 250 mg 4 times/day | 2 weeks |
| *plus* | | |
| Tetracycline | 500 mg 4 times/day | 2 weeks |
| Ranitidine bismuth citrate | 400 mg twice daily | 2 weeks |
| *plus* | | |
| Clarithromycin | 500 mg twice daily | 2 weeks |
| *plus* | | |
| Amoxicillin | 1000 mg twice daily | 2 weeks |
| Ranitidine bismuth citrate | 400 mg twice daily | 2 weeks |
| *plus* | | |
| Clarithromycin | 500 mg twice daily | 2 weeks |
| *plus* | | |
| Metronidazole | 500 mg twice daily | 2 weeks |
| Ranitidine bismuth citrate | 400 mg twice daily | 2 weeks |
| *plus* | | |
| Clarithromycin | 500 mg twice daily | 2 weeks |
| *plus* | | |
| Tetracycline | 500 mg twice daily | 2 weeks |
| Proton pump inhibitor | Lansoprazole 30 mg twice daily<br>Omeprazole 20 mg twice daily | 2 weeks |
| *plus* | | |
| Clarithromycin | 500 mg twice daily | 2 weeks |
| *plus* | | |
| Amoxicillin | 1000 mg twice daily | 2 weeks |
| Proton pump inhibitor | Lansoprazole 30 mg twice daily<br>Omeprazole 20 mg twice daily | 2 weeks |
| *plus* | | |
| Clarithromycin | 500 mg twice daily | 2 weeks |
| *plus* | | |
| Metronidazole | 500 mg twice daily | 2 weeks |
| Proton pump inhibitor | Lansoprazole 30 mg once daily<br>Omeprazole 20 mg once daily | 2 weeks |
| *plus* | | |
| Bismuth | 525 mg 4 times/day | 2 weeks |
| *plus* | | |
| Metronidazole | 500 mg 3 times/day | 2 weeks |
| *plus* | | |
| Tetracycline | 500 mg 4 times/day | 2 weeks |

From Howden CS and Hunt RH, "Guidelines for the Management of *Helicobacter pylori* Infection," *AJG*, 1998, 93:2336.

# HYPERLIPIDEMIA

(*JAMA*, 1993, 269(23):3015-23)

### Risk Status Based on Presence of CHD Risk Factors Other Than Low-Density Lipoprotein Cholesterol*

**Positive Risk Factors**

Male ≥45 y

Female ≥55 y or premature menopause without estrogen replacement therapy

Family history of premature CHD (definite myocardial infarction or sudden death before 55 y of age in father or other male first-degree relative, or before 65 y of age in mother or other female first-degree relative)

Current cigarette smoking

Hypertension (blood pressure ≥140/90 mm Hg†, or taking antihypertensive medication)

Low HDL cholesterol (<35 mg/dL† [0.9 mmol/L])

Diabetes mellitus

**Negative Risk Factor‡**

High HDL cholesterol (≥60 mg/dL [1.6 mmol/L])

*High risk, defined as a net of two or more coronary heart disease (CHD) risk factors, leads to more vigorous intervention, shown in Figures 1 and 2. Age (defined differently for men and women) is treated as a risk factor because rates of CHD are higher in the elderly than in the young, and in men than in women of the same age. Obesity is not listed as a risk factor because it operates through other risk factors that are included (hypertension, hyperlipidemia, decreased high-density lipoprotein [HDL] cholesterol, and diabetes mellitus), but it should be considered a target for intervention. Physical inactivity is similarly not listed as a risk factor, but it too should be considered a target for intervention, and physical activity is recommended as desirable for everyone. High risk due to coronary or peripheral atherosclerosis is addressed directly in Figure 3.

†Confirmed by measurements on several occasions.

‡If the HDL cholesterol level is ≥60 mg/dL (1.6 mmol/L), subtract one risk factor (because high HDL cholesterol levels decrease CHD risk)

### Initial Classification Based on Total Cholesterol and HDL Cholesterol Levels*

| Cholesterol Level | | Initial Classification |
|---|---|---|
| **Total Cholesterol** | | |
| <200 mg/dL | (5.2 mmol/L) | Desirable blood cholesterol |
| 200-239 mg/dL | (5.2-6.2 mmol/L) | Borderline-high blood cholesterol |
| ≥240 mg/dL | (6.2 mmol/L) | High blood cholesterol |
| **HDL Cholesterol** | | |
| <35 mg/dL | (0.9 mmol/L) | Low HDL cholesterol |

*HDL indicated high-density lipoprotein.

## Summary of the Second Report of the National Cholesterol Education Program (NCEP) Expert Panel on Detection, Evaluation, and Treatment of High Blood Cholesterol in Adults (Adult Treatment Panel II)

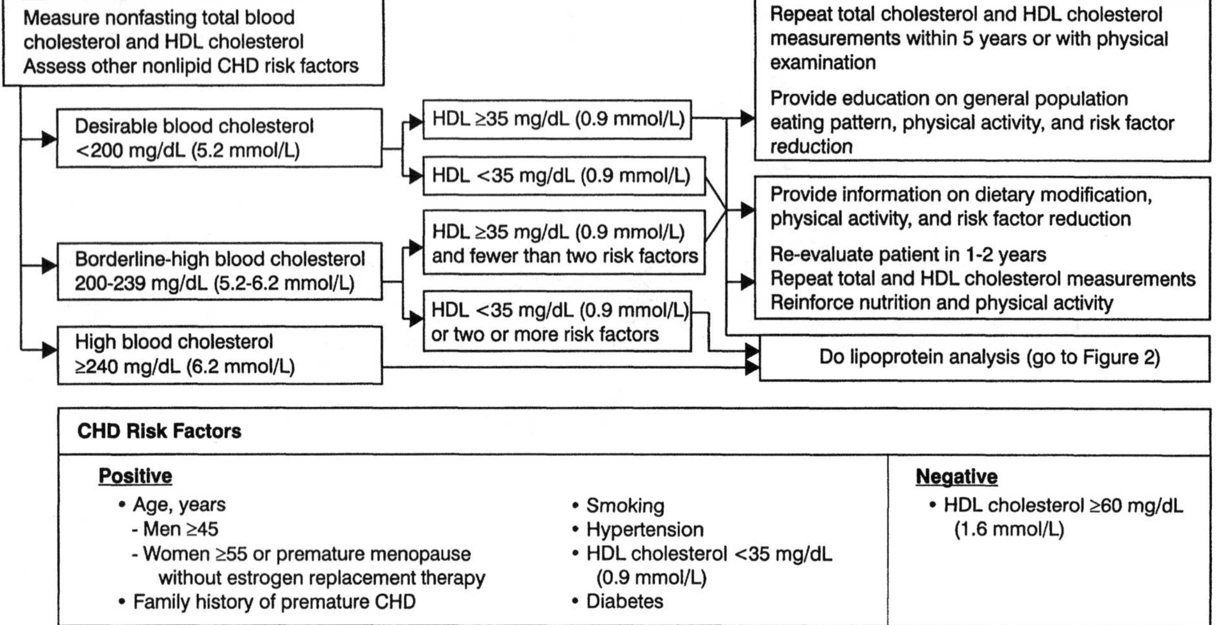


**CHD Risk Factors**

| Positive | | Negative |
|---|---|---|
| • Age, years<br>- Men ≥45<br>- Women ≥55 or premature menopause without estrogen replacement therapy<br>• Family history of premature CHD | • Smoking<br>• Hypertension<br>• HDL cholesterol <35 mg/dL (0.9 mmol/L)<br>• Diabetes | • HDL cholesterol ≥60 mg/dL (1.6 mmol/L) |

**Fig. 1** - Primary prevention in adults **without** evidence of coronary heart disease (CHD). Initial classification is based on total cholesterol and high-density lipoprotein (HDL) cholesterol levels.

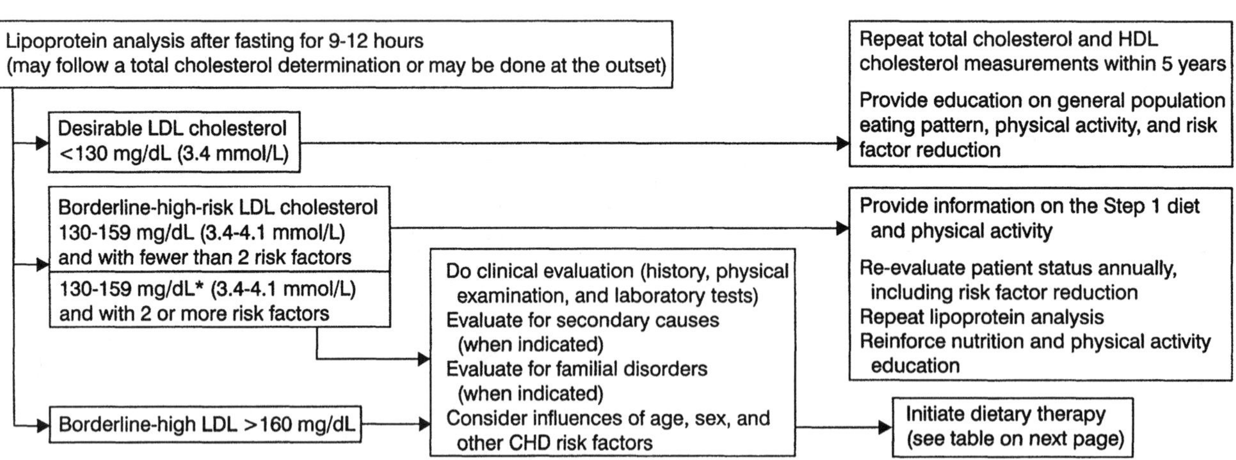


* On the basis of the average of two determinations. If the first two LDL cholesterol test results differ by more than 30 mg/dL (0.7 mmol/L), a third test result should be obtained within 1-8 weeks and the average value of the three tests used.

**Fig. 2** - Primary prevention in adults **without** evidence of coronary heart disease (CHD). Subsequent classification is based on low-density lipoprotein (LDL ) cholesterol level.

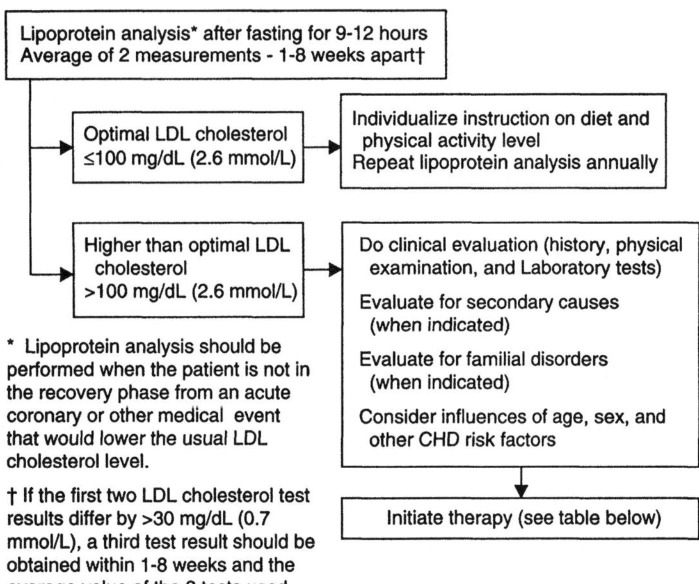
Lipoprotein analysis* after fasting for 9-12 hours
Average of 2 measurements - 1-8 weeks apart†
Optimal LDL cholesterol
≤100 mg/dL (2.6 mmol/L)
Individualize instruction on diet and physical activity level
Repeat lipoprotein analysis annually
Higher than optimal LDL cholesterol
>100 mg/dL (2.6 mmol/L)
Do clinical evaluation (history, physical examination, and Laboratory tests)
Evaluate for secondary causes (when indicated)
Evaluate for familial disorders (when indicated)
Consider influences of age, sex, and other CHD risk factors
Initiate therapy (see table below)
* Lipoprotein analysis should be performed when the patient is not in the recovery phase from an acute coronary or other medical event that would lower the usual LDL cholesterol level.
† If the first two LDL cholesterol test results differ by >30 mg/dL (0.7 mmol/L), a third test result should be obtained within 1-8 weeks and the average value of the 3 tests used.

**Fig. 3** - Secondary prevention in adults **with** evidence of coronary heart disease (CHD). Classification is based on low-density lipoprotein (LDL) cholesterol level.

## Treatment Decisions Based on LDL Cholesterol Level*

| Patient Category | Initiation Level | LDL Goal |
|---|---|---|
| **Dietary Therapy** | | |
| Without CHD and with fewer than two risk factors | ≥160 mg/dL (4.1 mmol/L) | <160 mg/dL (4.1 mmol/L) |
| Without CHD and with two or more risk factors | ≥130 mg/dL (3.4 mmol/L) | <130 mg/dL (3.4 mmol/L) |
| With CHD | >100 mg/dL (2.6 mmol/L) | ≤100 mg/dL (2.6 mmol/L) |
| **Drug Treatment** | | |
| Without CHD and with fewer than two risk factors | ≥190 mg/dL (4.9 mmol/L) | <160 mg/dL (4.1 mmol/L) |
| Without CHD and with two or more risk factors | ≥160 mg/dL (4.1 mmol/L) | <130 mg/dL (3.4 mmol/L) |
| With CHD | ≥130 mg/dL (3.4 mmol/L) | ≤100 mg/dL (2.6 mmol/L) |

*LDL: low-density lipoprotein; CHD: coronary heart disease

## Classification of Serum Triglyceride Levels

| Classification | Serum Triglyceride Concentration |
|---|---|
| Normal | ≤200 mg/dL |
| Borderline-high | 200-400 mg/dL |
| High | 400-1000 mg/dL |
| Very high | >1000 mg/dL |

## NCEP Stepped Approach for Dietary Modification

| Nutrient | Step 1 Diet (% total kcal) | Step 2 Diet (% total kcal) |
|---|---|---|
| Total fat | <30 | <30 |
| saturated | <10 | <7 |
| polyunsaturated | Up to 10 | Up to 10 |
| monounsaturated | 10-15 | 10-15 |
| Carbohydrates | 50-60 | 50-60 |
| Protein | 10-20 | 10-20 |
| Cholesterol | <300 mg/d | <200 mg/d |
| Total calories | qs to maintain desirable wt | qs to maintain desirable wt |

# HYPERTENSION

The optimal blood pressure for adults is <120/80 mm Hg. Consistent systolic pressure ≥140 mm Hg or a diastolic pressure ≥90 mm Hg, in the absence of a secondary cause, define hypertension. Hypertension affects approximately 25% (50 million people) of the United States population. Of those patients on antihypertensive medication, only one in four patients have their blood pressure controlled (<140/90 mm Hg). Recent mortality rates for stroke and heart disease, in which hypertension is an antecedent, remain unchanged. The prevention, detection, evaluation, and treatment of high blood pressure is therefore paramount for each person and for all healthcare providers.

The Sixth Report of the Joint National Committee (JNC VI) is an excellent reference and guide for the treatment of hypertension (*Arch Intern Med*, 1997, 157:2413-46). Hypertension is classified in stages for adults (see Table 1).

**Table 1. Adult Classification of Blood Pressure**

| Category | Systolic (mm Hg) | | Diastolic (mm Hg) |
|---|---|---|---|
| Optimal | <120 | and | <80 |
| Normal | <130 | and | <85 |
| High normal | 130-139 | or | 85-89 |
| Hypertension | | | |
| Stage 1 | 140-159 | or | 90-99 |
| Stage 2 | 160-179 | or | 100-109 |
| Stage 3 | ≥180 | or | ≥110 |
| Isolated systolic | ≥140 | and | <90 |

Adapted from the Sixth Report of the Joint National Committee on Prevention, Detection, Evaluation, and Treatment of High Blood Pressure, NIH Publication No. 98-4080, November 1997.

**Table 2. Normal Blood Pressure in Children**

| Age (y) | Girls' SBP/DBP (mm Hg) | | Boys' SBP/DBP (mm Hg) | |
|---|---|---|---|---|
| | 50th Percentile for Height | 75th Percentile for Height | 50th Percentile for Height | 75th Percentile for Height |
| 1 | 104/58 | 105/59 | 102/57 | 104/58 |
| 6 | 111/73 | 112/73 | 114/74 | 115/75 |
| 12 | 123/80 | 124/81 | 123/81 | 125/82 |
| 17 | 129/84 | 130/85 | 136/87 | 138/88 |

SBP = systolic blood pressure.
DBP = diastolic blood pressure.
Adapted from the report by the NHBPEP Working Group on Hypertension Control in Children and Adolescents.

Initial follow up of adult patients is based on office blood pressure recordings (see Table 3).

**Table 3. Blood Pressure Screening and Follow-up**

| Initial Screening BP (mm Hg) | | Follow-up Recommended |
|---|---|---|
| Systolic | Diastolic | |
| <130 | <85 | Recheck in 2 years |
| 130-139 | 85-89 | Recheck in 1 year |
| 140-159 | 90-99 | Confirm within 2 months |
| 160-179 | 100-109 | Evaluate/treatment within 1 month |
| ≥180 | ≥110 | Evaluate/treatment immediately or within 1 week |

Adapted from the Sixth Report of the Joint National Committee on Prevention, Detection, Evaluation, and Treatment of High Blood Pressure, NIH Publication No. 98-4080, November 1997.

Based on these initial assessments, treatment strategies for patients with hypertension are stratified based on their blood pressure and their risk group classification (see Table 4).

**Table 4. Blood Pressure and Risk Stratification**

| Blood Pressure Stages | Risk Group A (no RF or TOD) | Risk Group B (≥1 RF, not including diabetes, no TOD) | Risk Group C (TOD and/or diabetes regardless of RF) |
|---|---|---|---|
| High normal (130-139/85-89 mm Hg) | Lifestyle modification | Lifestyle modification | Drug therapy* and lifestyle modification |
| Stage 1 (140-159/90-99 mm Hg) | Lifestyle modification (up to 12 mo) | Lifestyle modification (up to 6 mo)† | Drug therapy and lifestyle modification |
| Stages 2 and 3 (≥160/≥100 mm Hg) | Drug therapy and lifestyle modification | Drug therapy and lifestyle modification | Drug therapy and lifestyle modification |

*For those with heart failure, renal insufficiency, or diabetes.

†For patients with multiple risk factors, consider starting both drug and lifestyle modification together.

RF = risk factor.

TOD = target-organ disease.

Adapted from the Sixth Report of the Joint National Committee on Prevention, Detection, Evaluation, and Treatment of High Blood Pressure, NIH Publication No. 98-4080, November 1997.

Patients in Risk **Group A** have no risk factors; **Group B**, at least one risk factor (other than diabetes), and no cardiovascular disease or target organ disease (see Table 5); **Group C**, have cardiovascular disease or diabetes or target organ disease (see Table 5). Risk factors include smoking, dyslipidemia, diabetes, age >60 years, male gender, postmenopausal women, and family history of cardiovascular disease (cardiovascular event in first degree female relatives <65 years and in first degree male relatives <55 years).

**Table 5. Target-Organ Disease**

| Organ System | Manifestation |
|---|---|
| Cardiac | Clinical, EKG, or radiologic evidence of coronary artery disease; prior MI, angina, post-CABG; left ventricular hypertrophy (LVH); left ventricular dysfunction or cardiac failure |
| Cerebrovascular | Transient ischemic attack or stroke |
| Peripheral vascular | Absence of pulses in extremities (except dorsalis pedis), claudication, aneurysm |
| Renal | Serum creatinine ≥130 μmol/L (1.5 mg/dL); proteinuria (≥1+); microalbuminuria |
| Retinopathy | Hemorrhages or exudates, with or without papilledema |

Adapted from the Sixth Report of the Joint National Committee on Prevention, Detection, Evaluation, and Treatment of High Blood Pressure, NIH Publication No. 98-4080, November 1997.

Treatment of hypertension should be individualized. Lower blood pressures should be achieved for patients with diabetes or renal disease. A treatment algorithm (see following page) may be used to select specific antihypertensives based on specific or compelling indications. Special consideration for starting combination therapy should be made in each patient. Starting drug therapy at a low dose and titrating upward if blood pressure is not controlled is recommended. The benefit of these strategies is to minimize the occurrence of adverse effects while achieving optimal blood pressure control. One caveat for starting at a low dose and then titrating upward is that patients and clinicians must commit to well-timed follow-up so that blood pressure is controlled in a timely manner. Lifestyle modification and risk reduction should be begun and continued throughout treatment.

## HYPERTENSION *(Continued)*

### HYPERTENSION TREATMENT ALGORITHM

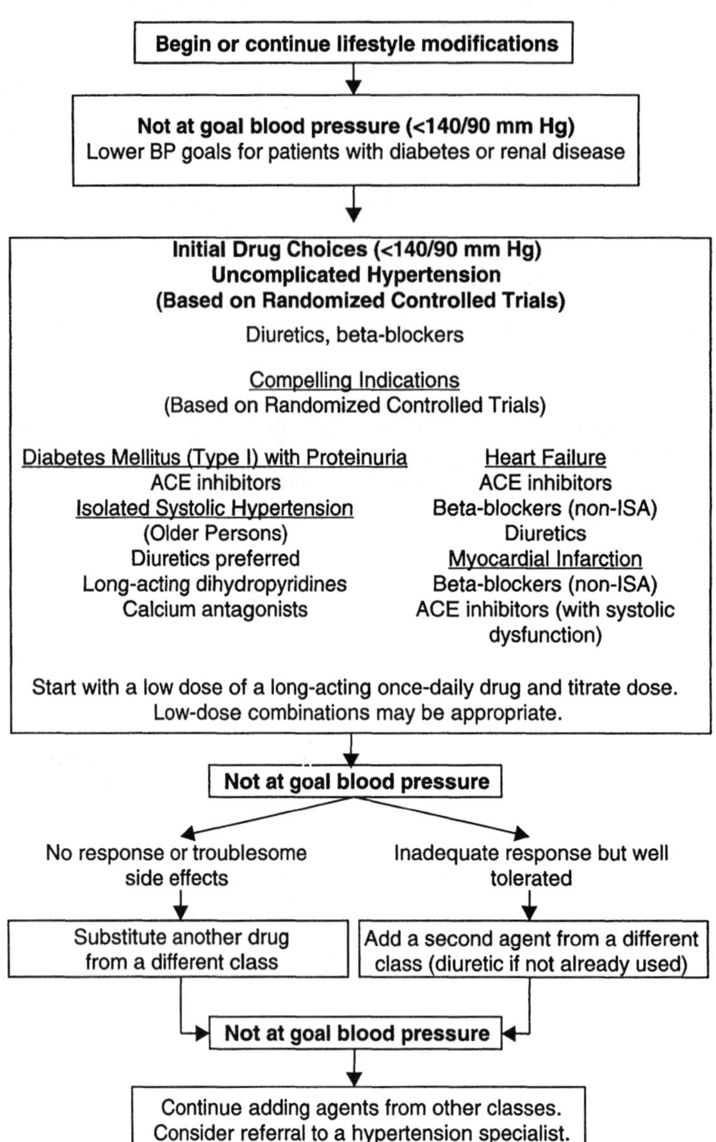


Adapted from *Arch Intern Med*, 1998, 157:2450.

## COMBINATION THERAPY IN THE TREATMENT OF HYPERTENSION

Important concerns in treating hypertension are the efficacy and side effects of therapy. In the past, progressive increases in dosage of a single drug were used to improve blood pressure control. Historically (based on the Joint National Committee [JNC] recommendations), the maximum doses of recommended drugs have decreased from those proposed in earlier JNC reports.

More recently, the concept of combination therapy has begun to gain increasing favor. This is reflected most clearly in the report of the Sixth Joint National Committee on Detection, Evaluation, and Treatment of High Blood Pressure (JNC VI). Specifically, JNC VI endorses the use of low doses of two antihypertensive drugs in fixed-dose combinations as a possible route for initial treatment of hypertension. This recommendation extends earlier JNC V recognition that combining drugs with different modes of action may allow smaller doses of drugs to be used to achieve control, and minimize the potential for dose-dependent side effects.

Combination therapy thus constitutes the use of an additional antihypertensive medication before the first therapeutic agent is necessarily at maximum dose, or the use of two agents in low doses at the onset of antihypertensive treatment. The rationale, background, and experience with combination therapy are nicely reviewed in Kaplan NM and Sever PS, "Combination Therapy: A Key to Comprehensive Patient Care," *Am J Hyperten*, 1997, 10(7 part 2):127S and by Moser M and Black HR, "The Role of Combination Therapy in the Treatment of Hypertension," *Am J Hyperten*, 11:73S-8S).

Fundamental to the combination therapy approach are the following considerations.

- Drugs with different and complementary mechanisms of action may often produce synergistic reductions in blood pressure, classically evident in the use of diuretics and ACE inhibitors.
- Low doses of a single drug are less likely to induce side effects.
- More than 50% of all hypertensive patients will need more than one drug to achieve blood pressure control.

In effect, this therapeutic strategy allows exploitation of the steepest part of the antihypertensive dose response curve, achieving synergistic or additive therapeutic benefit while limiting potential for side effects. Disadvantages include first, the need to take two drugs, often resulting in taking two separate tablets. It is important to ensure that both therapeutic preparations have equivalent durations of action. Second, the cost of separate products may exceed that of increased doses of a single medication.

In mitigation, fixed-dose combinations of antihypertensive preparations are available with recent options, including Lexxel® (calcium channel blocker and ACE inhibitor), Hyzaar® (angiotensin receptor blocker and hydrochlorothiazide), Capozide® (ACE inhibitor and hydrochlorothiazide), and Ziac® (beta-blocker and hydrochlorothiazide). These combinations help address cost and convenience issues in combination therapy.

## COMPELLING INDICATIONS FOR SPECIFIC THERAPIES

| Indication | Drug Therapy |
|---|---|
| **Compelling Indications Unless Contraindicated** | |
| Diabetes mellitus (type I) with proteinuria | ACEI |
| Heart failure | ACEI, diuretics, BB (carvedilol, metoprolol XL/CR, bisoprolol, hydralazine + isosorbide dinitrate) |
| Isolated systolic hypertension (older patients) | Diuretics (preferred), CCB (long-acting) |
| Myocardial infarction | Beta-blockers (non-ISA), ACEI (with systolic dysfunction) |
| High-risk patients (CVD plus risk factors) | ACEI (ramipril) |
| **May Have Favorable Effects on Comorbid Conditions** | |
| Angina | Beta-blockers, CCB (long-acting) |
| Atrial tachycardia and fibrillation | Beta-blockers, CCB (non-DHP) |
| Cyclosporine-induced hypertension (caution with the dose of cyclosporine) | CCB |
| Diabetes mellitus (types I and II) with proteinuria | ACEI (preferred), CCB |
| Diabetes mellitus (type II) | Low-dose diuretics (≤25 mg HCTZ) |
| Dyslipidemia | Alpha-blockers |
| Essential tremor | Beta-blockers (noncardioselective) |
| Heart failure | Losartan, candesartan |
| Hyperthyroidism | Beta-blockers |
| Migraine | Beta-blockers (noncardioselective), CCB (long-acting) (non-DHP) |
| Myocardial infarction (non-Q-wave with normal systolic function and no edema) | Diltiazem, verapamil (long-acting) |
| Osteoporosis | Thiazides |
| Preoperative hypertension | Beta-blockers |
| Prostatism (BPH) | Alpha-blockers |
| Renal insufficiency (caution in renovascular hypertension and creatinine ≥265.2 mmol/L [3 mg/dL]) | ACEI |
| **May Have Unfavorable Effects on Comorbid Conditions*** | |
| Bronchospastic disease | Beta-blockers† |
| Depression | Beta-blockers, central alpha-agonists, reserpine† |
| Diabetes mellitus (types I and II) | Beta-blockers, high-dose diuretics |
| Dyslipidemia | Beta-blockers (non-ISA), diuretics (high-dose) |
| Gout | Diuretics |
| Second or third degree heart block | Beta-blockers†, CCB (non-DHP)† |
| Heart failure | Beta-blockers (with high ISA), CCB (except amlodipine, felodipine) |
| Liver disease | Labetalol hydrochloride, methyldopa† |
| Peripheral vascular disease | Beta-blockers |
| Pregnancy | ACEI†, angiotensin II receptor blockers† |
| Renal insufficiency | Potassium-sparing agents |
| Renovascular disease | ACEI, angiotensin II receptor blockers |

ACEI indicates angiotensin-converting enzyme inhibitors; BPH, benign prostatic hyperplasia; CCB, calcium antagonists; DHP, dihydropyridine; ISA, intrinsic sympathomimetic activity; MI, myocardial infarction; and non-CS, noncardioselective.

Conditions and drugs are listed in alphabetical order.

*These drugs may be used with special monitoring unless contraindicated.

†Contraindicated.

## HYPERTENSION AND PREGNANCY

The report of the NHBPEP Working Group on High Blood Pressure in Pregnancy permits continuation of drug therapy in women with chronic hypertension (**except for ACE inhibitors**). In addition, angiotensin II receptor blockers should not be used during pregnancy. In women with chronic hypertension with diastolic levels ≥100 mm Hg (lower when end organ damage or underlying renal disease is present) and in women with acute hypertension when levels are ≥105 mm Hg, the following agents are suggested (see table).

| Suggested Drug | Comments |
|---|---|
| Central alpha-agonists | Methyldopa (C) is the drug of choice recommended by the NHBPEP Working Group. |
| Beta-blockers | Atenolol (C) and metoprolol (C) appear to be safe and effective in late pregnancy. Labetalol (C) also appears to be effective (alpha- and beta-blockers). |
| Calcium antagonists | Potential synergism with magnesium sulfate may lead to precipitous hypotension. (C) |
| ACE inhibitors, angiotensin II receptor blockers | Fetal abnormalities, including death, can be caused, and these drugs **should not** be used in pregnancy. (D) |
| Diuretics | Diuretics (C) are recommended for chronic hypertension if prescribed before gestation or if patients appear to be salt-sensitive. They are not recommended in pre-eclampsia. |
| Direct vasodilators | Hydralazine (C) is the parenteral drug of choice based on its long history of safety and efficacy. (C) |

Adapted from Sibai and Lindheimer. There are several other antihypertensive drugs for which there are very limited data. The U.S. Food and Drug Administration classifies pregnancy risk as follows: C = adverse effects in animals; no controlled trials in humans; use if risk appears justified; D = positive evidence of fetal risk. ACE = angiotensin-converting enzyme.

# TOXIDROMES

## Management of Overdoses

| Toxin | Vital Signs | Mental Status | Symptoms | Physical Exam | Laboratories |
|---|---|---|---|---|---|
| Acetaminophen | Normal | Normal | Anorexia, nausea, vomiting | RUQ tenderness, jaundice | Elevated LFTs |
| Cocaine | Hypertension, tachycardia, hyperthermia | Anxiety, agitation, delirium | Hallucinations | Mydriasis, tremor, diaphoresis, seizures, perforated nasal septum | EKG abnormalities, increased CPK |
| Cyclic antidepressants | Tachycardia, hypotension, hyperthermia | Decreased, including coma | Confusion, dizziness | Mydriasis, dry mucous membranes, distended bladder, decreased bowel sounds, flushing, seizures | Long QRS complex, cardiac dysrhythmias |
| Iron | Early: Normal; Late: Hypotension, tachycardia | Normal; lethargic if hypotensive | Nausea, vomiting, diarrhea, abdominal pain, hematemesis | Abdominal tenderness | Heme + stool and vomit, metabolic acidosis, EKG and x-ray findings, elevated serum iron (early); child: hyperglycemia, leukocytosis |
| Opioids | Hypotension, bradycardia, hypoventilation, hypothermia | Decreased, including coma | Intoxication | Miosis, absent bowel sounds | Abnormal ABGs |
| Salicylates | Hyperventilation, hyperthermia | Agitation; lethargy, including coma | Tinnitus, nausea, vomiting, confusion | Diaphoresis, tender abdomen | Anion gap metabolic acidosis, respiratory alkalosis, abnormal LFTs, and coagulation studies |
| Theophylline | Tachycardia, hypotension, hyperventilation, hyperthermia | Agitation, lethargy, including coma | Nausea, vomiting. diaphoresis, tremor, confusion | Seizures, arrhythmias | Hypokalemia, hyperglycemia, metabolic acidosis, abnormal EKG |

## Examples of Toxidromes

| Toxidromes | Pattern | Example of Drugs | Treatment Approach |
|---|---|---|---|
| Anticholinergic | Fever, ileus, flushing, tachycardia, urinary retention, inability to sweat, visual blurring, and mydriasis. Central manifestations include myoclonus, choreoathetosis, toxic psychosis with lilliputian hallucinations, seizures, and coma. | Antihistamines<br>Baclofen<br>Benztropine<br>Jimson weed<br>Methylpyroline<br>Phenothiazines<br>Propantheline<br>Tricyclic antidepressants | Physostigmine for life-threatening symptoms only; may predispose to arrhythmias |
| Cholinergic | Characterized by salivation, lacrimation, urination, defecation, gastrointestinal cramps, and emesis ("sludge"). Bradycardia and bronchoconstriction may also be seen. | Carbamate<br>Organophosphates<br>Pilocarpine | • Atropine<br>• Pralidoxime for organophosphate insecticides |
| Extrapyramidal | Choreoathetosis, hyper-reflexia, trismus, opisthotonos, rigidity, and tremor | Haloperidol<br>Phenothiazines | • Diphenhydramine<br>• Benztropine |
| Hallucinogenic | Perceptual distortions, synthesis, depersonalization, and derealization | Amphetamines<br>Cannabinoids<br>Cocaine<br>Indole alkaloids<br>Phencyclidine | Benzodiazepine |
| Narcotic | Altered mental status, unresponsiveness, shallow respirations, slow respiratory rate or periodic breathing, miosis, bradycardia, hypothermia | Opiates<br>Dextromethorphan<br>Pentazocine<br>Propoxyphene | Naloxone |
| Sedative/ Hypnotic | Manifested by sedation with progressive deterioration of central nervous system function. Coma, stupor, confusion, apnea, delirium, or hallucinations may accompany this pattern. | Anticonvulsants<br>Antipsychotics<br>Barbiturates<br>Benzodiazepines<br>Ethanol<br>Ethchlorvynol<br>Fentanyl<br>Glutethimide<br>Meprobamate<br>Methadone<br>Methocarbamol<br>Opiates<br>Quinazolines<br>Propoxyphene<br>Tricyclic antidepressants | • Naloxone<br>• Flumazenil; usually not recommended due to increased risk of seizures<br>• Urinary alkalinization (barbiturates) |

## TOXIDROMES *(Continued)*

### Examples of Toxidromes *(continued)*

| Toxidromes | Pattern | Example of Drugs | Treatment Approach |
|---|---|---|---|
| Seizuregenic | May mimic stimulant pattern with hyperthermia, hyper-reflexia, and tremors being prominent signs | Anticholinergics<br>Camphor<br>Chlorinated hydrocarbons<br>Cocaine<br>Isoniazid<br>Lidocaine<br>Lindane<br>Nicotine<br>Phencyclidine<br>Strychnine<br>Xanthines | • Antiseizure medications<br>• Pyridoxine for isoniazid<br>• Extracorporeal removal of drug (ie, lindane, camphor, xanthines)<br>• Physostigmine for anticholinergic agents |
| Serotonin | Confusion, myoclonus, hyper-reflexia, diaphoresis, tremor, facial flushing, diarrhea, fever, trismus | Clomipramine<br>Fluoxetine<br>Isoniazid<br>L-tryptophan<br>Paroxetine<br>Phenelzine<br>Sertraline<br>Tranylcypromine<br>Drug combinations include:<br>• MAO inhibitors with L-tryptophan<br>• Fluoxetine or meperidine<br>• Fluoxetine with carbamazepine or sertraline<br>• Clomipramine and moclobemide<br>• Trazadol and buspirone<br>• Paroxetine and dextromethorphan | Withdrawal of drug/benzodiazepine |
| Solvent | Lethargy, confusion, dizziness, headache, restlessness, incoordination, derealization, depersonalization | Acetone<br>Chlorinated hydrocarbons<br>Hydrocarbons<br>Naphthalene<br>Trichloroethane<br>Toluene | Avoid catecholamines |
| Stimulant | Restlessness, excessive speech and motor activity, tachycardia, tremor, and insomnia — may progress to seizure. Other effects noted include euphoria, mydriasis, anorexia, and paranoia. | Amphetamines<br>Caffeine (xanthines)<br>Cocaine<br>Ephedrine/pseudoephedrine<br>Methylphenidate<br>Nicotine<br>Phencyclidine | Benzodiazepines |
| Uncoupling of oxidative phosphylation | Hyperthermia, tachypnea, diaphoresis, metabolic acidosis (usually) | Aluminum phosphide<br>Aspirin/salicylates<br>2,4-Dichlorophenol<br>Di-n-Butyl phthalate<br>Dinitrophenols<br>Dinitro-cresols<br>Hexachlorobutadiene<br>Phosphorus<br>Pentachlorophenol<br>Tin (?)<br>Zinc phosphide | Sodium bicarbonate to treat metabolic acidosis<br>Patient cooling techniques<br>Avoidance of atropine or salicylate agents<br>Hemodialysis may be required for acidosis treatment |

From Nice A, Leikin JB, Maturen A, et al, "Toxidrome Recognition to Improve Efficiency of Emergency Urine Drug Screens," *Ann Emerg Med*, 1988, 17(7):676-80.

# BREAST-FEEDING

## Toxins/Drugs to Be Avoided During Breast-Feeding

Acebutolol
Aloe (*Aloe vera*)
Alprazolam
Amantadine
5-Aminosalicylic acid
Amiodarone
Amphetamine
Anthraquinones (laxatives)
Antineoplastic agents*
Atenolol
Atropine
Azathioprine
Basil (*Oaknum basillcum*)
Betaxolol
Bismuth subsalicylate
Bromides
Bromocriptine
Buckthorn bark and berry
Buflomedill
Calciferol
Carisoprodol
*Cascara sagrada*
Chloral hydrate
Chloramphenicol
Chlordane
Chlordiazepoxide
Chlorpromazine
Chlorthalidone
Cimetidine
Clemastine
Clonidine
Cocaine
Colchicine
Coltsfoot leaf
Copper-64 (50 hours)
Cyclophosphamide
Cyclosporine
Cyproheptadine
Danazol
Danthron
Donepezil
Dexfenfluramine
Dexrazoxane
Diazepam
Dieldrin
Dihydrotachysterol
Diphenhydramine
Diuretics
Donepezil
Doxorubicin
Dyphylline
Ergotamine
Ethanol
Ethylene dichloride
Famciclovir (Penciclovir)
Fluconazole
Fluorescein
Fluoxetine
Gallium-67 (14 days*)†
Gold salts
Guanfacine
Heptachlor
Heroin
Hexachlorobenzene
Hexachlorophene
Hydroxyurea
Indian snakeroot (*Rauwolfia serpentina*)
Indium-111 isotope (20 hours*)
Iodides (especially potassium iodide)
Iodine-123 (36 hours*)
Iodine-125 (12 days*)†
Iodine-131 (14 days*)†
Isoniazid
Ivermectin
Kava kava rhizome/root
Ketorolac
Lead (venous blood lead levels >35 mcg/dL)
Lindane
Lithium
Lovastatin
Marijuana (dronabinol)
Maté (Paraguay tea)
Meperidine
Mepindolol
Meprobamate
Mercaptopurine
Mercury
Methotrexate
Methimazole
Metoclopramide
Metronidazole (discontinue breast-feeding for 1 day)
Mifepristone
Minocycline
Moricizine
Nadolol
Nicergoline
Nicotine
Olanzapine
Opiates
Organochlorines
Oxprenolol
Perchloroethylene
Petasite root
Phencyclidine
Phenindione
Phenobarbital
Phenolphthalein
Piperazine
Piroxicam
Polychlorinated/polybrominated biphenyls
Povidone-iodine
Prazepam
Prednisone (>20 mg/day)
Primidone
Proguanil
Propofol
Quinolone antibiotics
Radioactive diagnostic and therapeutic agents
Ranitidine
Reserpine
Retinoids
Riluzole
Rhubarb root
Salicylate (>1 g)
Selegiline
Senna (*Cassia senna*)
Sertraline
Sodium isotope (4 days*)
Sotalol
Strontium chloride (Sr 89)
Sulfasalazine
Technetium-99m (1-3 days†)
Tetracycline
Theophylline (sustained release)
Thiouracil
Tilidine
Timolol
Tinidazole (discontinue breast-feeding for 1 day)
Tocainide
Zipeprol

*Antineoplastic agents, in general, with the possible exception of azathioprine (75-100 mg/day) with close infant monitoring.

†Duration of radioactivity excretion in breast milk.

Breast-feeding should be discontinued if the following radioisotopes are utilized: $^{131}$I-HSA, $^{125}$I-HSA, $^{125}$I-fibrinogen, Na-$^{131}$I, $^{67}$Ga-citrate, $^{75}$Se-methionine, sodium $^{32}$P phosphate, and chromic $^{32}$P phosphate.

# CONTROLLED SUBSTANCES – USES AND EFFECTS

| Drugs | CSA Schedules | Trade or Other Names | Medical Uses | Physical Dependence | Psychological Dependence | Tolerance | Duration (hours) | Usual Method |
|---|---|---|---|---|---|---|---|---|
| **NARCOTICS** | | | | | | | | |
| Heroin | I | Diacetylmorphine, Horse, Smack | None in U.S; analgesic, antitussive | High | High | Yes | 3-6 | Injected, sniffed, smoked |
| Morphine | II | Duramorph, MS-Contin, Roxanol, Oramorph SR | Analgesic | High | High | Yes | 3-6 | Oral, smoked, injected |
| Codeine | II, III, V | Tylenol w/ codeine, Empirin w/codeine, Robitussin A-C, Fiorinal w/ codeine, APAP w/codeine | Analgesic, antitussive | Moderate | Moderate | Yes | 3-6 | Oral, injected |
| Hydrocodone | II, III | Tussionex, Vicodin, Hycodan, Lorcet | Analgesic, antitussive | High | High | Yes | 3-6 | Oral |
| Hydromorphone | II | Dilaudid | Analgesic | High | High | Yes | 3-6 | Oral, injected |
| Oxycodone | II | Percodan, Percocet, Tylox, Roxicet, Roxicodone | Analgesic | High | High | Yes | 4-5 | Oral |
| Methadone and LAAM | I, II | Dolophine, Methadone, Levo-alpha-acetylmethadol, levomethadyl acetate | Analgesic, treatment of dependence | High | High | Yes | 12-72 | Oral, injected |
| Fentanyl and analogs | I, II | Innovar, Sublimaze, Alfenta, Sufenta, Duragesic | Analgesic, adjunct to anesthesia, anesthetic | High | High | Yes | 0.1-72 | Injected, transdermal patch |
| Other narcotics | II, III, IV, V | Percodan, Percocet, Tylox, Opium, Darvon, Talwin[2], Buprenorphine, Meperidine (Pethidine), Demerol | Analgesic, antidiarrheal | High-low | High-low | Yes | Variable | Oral, injected |
| **Possible Effects:** Euphoria; drowsiness; respiratory depression; constricted pupils; nausea | | | | | | | | |
| **Effects of Overdose:** Slow and shallow breathing; clammy skin; convulsions; coma; possible death | | | | | | | | |
| **Withdrawal Symptoms:** Watery eyes; runny nose; yawning; loss of appetite; irritability; tremors; panic; cramps; nausea; chills and sweating | | | | | | | | |
| **DEPRESSANTS** | | | | | | | | |
| Chloral hydrate | IV | Noctec Somnos, Felsules | Hypnotic | Moderate | Moderate | Yes | 5-8 | Oral |
| Barbiturates | II, III, IV | Amytal, Fiorinal, Nembutal, Seconal, Tuinal, Phenobarbital, Pentobarbital | Anesthetic, anticonvulsant, sedative, hypnotic, veterinary euthanasia agent | High-moderate | High-moderate | Yes | 1-16 | Oral, injected |
| Benzodiazepines | IV | Ativan, Dalmane, Diazepam, Librium, Xanax, Serax, Valium, Tranxene, Verstran, Versed, Halcion, Paxipam, Restoril | Antianxiety, sedative, anticonvulsant, hypnotic | Low | Low | Yes | 4-8 | Oral, injected |
| Glutethimide | II | Doriden | Sedative, hypnotic | High | Moderate | Yes | 4-8 | Oral |
| Other depressants | I, II, III, IV | Equanil, Miltown, Noludar, Placidyl, Valmid, Methaqualone | Antianxiety, sedative, hypnotic | Moderate | Moderate | Yes | 4-8 | Oral |
| **Possible Effects:** Slurred speech; disorientation; drunken behavior without odor of alcohol | | | | | | | | |
| **Effects of Overdose:** Shallow respiration; clammy skin; dilated pupils; weak and rapid pulse; coma; possible death | | | | | | | | |
| **Withdrawal Symptoms:** Anxiety; insomnia; tremors; delirium; convulsions; possible death | | | | | | | | |
| **STIMULANTS** | | | | | | | | |
| Cocaine[1] | II | Coke, Flake, Snow, Crack | Local anesthetic | Possible | High | Yes | 1-2 | Sniffed, smoked, injected |
| Amphetamine/ methamphetamine | II | Biphetamine, Desoxyn, Dexedrine, Obetrol, Ice | Attention deficit disorder, narcolepsy, weight control | Possible | High | Yes | 2-4 | Oral, injected, smoked |
| Methylphenidate | II | Ritalin | Attention deficit disorder, narcolepsy | Possible | High | Yes | 2-4 | Oral, injected |

| Drugs | CSA Schedules | Trade or Other Names | Medical Uses | Physical Dependence | Psychological Dependence | Tolerance | Duration (hours) | Usual Method |
|---|---|---|---|---|---|---|---|---|
| Other stimulants | I, II, III, IV | Adipex, Didrex, Ionamin, Melfiat, Plegine, Captagon, Sanorex, Tenuate, Tepanil, Prelu-2, Preludin | Weight control | Possible | High | Yes | 2-4 | Oral, injected |
| **Possible Effects:** Increased alertness; excitation; euphoria; increased pulse rate and blood pressure; insomnia; loss of appetite | | | | | | | | |
| **Effects of Overdose:** Agitation; increased body temperature; hallucinations; convulsions; possible death | | | | | | | | |
| **Withdrawal Symptoms:** Apathy; long periods of sleep; irritability; depression; disorientation | | | | | | | | |
| **CANNABIS** | | | | | | | | |
| Marijuana | I | Pot, Acapulco gold, Grass, Reefer, Sinsemilla, Thai sticks | None | Unknown | Moderate | Yes | 2-4 | Smoked, oral |
| Tetrahydro-cannabinol | I, II | THC, Marinol | Antinauseant | Unknown | Moderate | Yes | 2-4 | Smoked, oral |
| Hashish and hashish oil | I | Hash, Hash oil | None | Unknown | Moderate | Yes | 2-4 | Smoked, oral |
| **Possible Effects:** Euphoria; relaxed inhibitions; increased appetite; disorientation | | | | | | | | |
| **Effects of Overdose:** Fatigue; paranoia; possible psychosis | | | | | | | | |
| **Withdrawal Symptoms:** Occasional reports of insomnia; hyperactivity; decreased appetite | | | | | | | | |
| **HALLUCINOGENS** | | | | | | | | |
| LSD | I | Acid, Microdot | None | None | Unknown | Yes | 8-12 | Oral |
| Mescaline and peyote | I | Mescal, Buttons, Cactus | None | None | Unknown | Yes | 8-12 | Oral |
| Amphetamine variants | I | 2,5-DMA, STP, MDA, MDMA, Ecstasy, DOM, DOB | None | Unknown | Unknown | Yes | Variable | Oral, injected |
| Phencyclidine and analogs | I, II | PCE, PCPy, TCP, PCP, Hog, Loveboat, Angel dust | None | Unknown | High | Yes | Days | Oral, smoked |
| Other hallucinogens | I | Bufotenine, Ibogaine, DMT, DET, Psilocybin, Psilocyn | None | None | Unknown | Possible | Variable | Smoked, oral, injected, sniffed |
| **Possible Effects:** Illusions and hallucinations; altered perception of time and distance | | | | | | | | |
| **Effects of Overdose:** Longer; more intense "trip" episodes; psychosis; possible death | | | | | | | | |
| **Withdrawal Symptoms:** Unknown | | | | | | | | |
| **ANABOLIC STEROIDS** | | | | | | | | |
| Testosterone (Cypionate, Enanthate) | III | Depo-testosterone, Delatestryl | Hypogonadism | Unknown | Unknown | Unknown | 14-28 days | Injected |
| Nandrolone (Decanoate, Phenpropionate) | III | Nortestosterone, Durabolin, Deca-durabolin, Deca | Anemia, breast cancer | Unknown | Unknown | Unknown | 14-21 days | Injected |
| Oxymetholone | III | Anadrol-50 | Anemia | Unknown | Unknown | Unknown | 24 | Oral |
| **Possible Effects:** Virilization; acne; testicular atrophy; gynecomastia; aggressive behavior; edema | | | | | | | | |
| **Effects of Overdose:** Unknown | | | | | | | | |
| **Withdrawal Symptoms:** Possible depression | | | | | | | | |

[1]Designated a narcotic under the CSA.

[2]Not designated a narcotic under the CSA.

Adapted from the U.S. Department of Justice Drug Enforcement Administration, *Drugs of Abuse*, 1996, with permission.

# DISCONTINUATION OF PSYCHOTROPIC\DRUGS

## Withdrawal Symptoms and Recommendations

| Drug | Withdrawal Symptoms | Recommendations |
|---|---|---|
| Amantadine | Neuroleptic malignant syndrome, drug-induced catatonia | In Parkinson's disease, dosage should be reduced gradually in order to prevent exacerbation of symptoms |
| Antipsychotics | Nausea, emesis, anorexia, diarrhea, rhinorrhea, diaphoresis, myalgia, paresthesia, anxiety, agitation, restlessness, insomnia | Reinitiate antipsychotic[1] |
| Benzodiazepines | Rebound symptoms, tachycardia, insomnia, tremor, seizures, psychosis | Taper dose slowly or switch to benzodiazepine with a long half-life at a high affinity (preferable) for the GABA benzodiazepine receptor site |
| Benztropine | Nervousness, craving, restlessness, depression, poor concentration, nausea, vomiting, headache, blurred vision, malaise | Dosage should be reduced gradually to prevent sudden increase in adverse symptoms; half-life of benztropine is 24 hours |
| Biperiden | Anxiety, depression, motor agitation, hallucinations, physical complaints | When discontinuing an antidyskinetic, taper gradually to avoid a rebound of adverse symptoms |
| Bromocriptine | Recurrence of symptoms, galactorrhea | No definitive information available on dosage reduction; however, when initiating therapy, begin with low dose and increase gradually (2.5 mg every 14-28 days for Parkinson's and 3-7 days for other indications) to prevent development of side effects |
| Diphenhydramine | Recurrence of insomnia, increased daytime restlessness, irritability, excessive blinking, increased defecation (rebound cholinergic reaction) | No specific recommendations reported |
| Levodopa | Confusion, fever, seizure activity, hyper-rigidity, profuse diaphoresis, tachycardia, tachypnea, muscle enzyme elevation | Gradually reduce dose to avoid the neuroleptic malignant-like syndrome (NLMLS); after discontinuation, dantrolene and/or bromocriptine have been used in patients with evident NLMLS to decrease fever and avoid a potentially lethal complication |
| Pergolide | Hallucinations, confusion, paranoid ideation, worsening parkinsonism symptoms | No recommendations reported |
| SSRIs | Dizziness, light-headedness, insomnia, fatigue, anxiety, agitation, nausea, headache, sensory disturbances | Restart SSRI or another antidepressant with a similar pharmacologic profile[2] |
| TCAs | Malaise, myalgia, anergy, diaphoresis, rhinitis, paresthesia, headache, nausea, vomiting, diarrhea, anorexia, insomnia, irritability, depressed mood | Administer antimuscarinic agents |
| Trihexyphenidyl | Anxiety, tachycardia, orthostatic hypotension, deterioration of sleep quality, extrapyramidal symptoms, deterioration of psychotic symptomatology, life-threatening respiratory difficulties | Reduce dose gradually to avoid withdrawal symptoms or an increase in psychotic symptoms |

1. Dilsaver SC and Alessi NE, "Antipsychotic Withdrawal Symptoms: Phenomenology and Pathophysiology," *Acta Psychiatr Scand*, 1988, 77(3):241-6.
2. Zajecka J, Tracy KA, and Mitchell S, "Discontinuation Symptoms After Treatment with Serotonin Reuptake Inhibitors: A Literature Review," *J Clin Psychiatry*, 1997, 58(7):291-7.

# DRUGS THAT MAY CAUSE PHOTOSENSITIVITY REACTIONS

| Drug | Comments |
|---|---|
| Alprazolam | |
| Amantadine | Single case report, confirmed with patch test |
| Amiodarone | Incidence may be as high as 76%; usually occurs within first 4 months of use of the drug |
| Amoxapine | |
| Benzocaine | Two cases; not confirmed in another study |
| Benzodiazepines | Two well-documented cases (alprazolam, chlordiazepoxide) |
| Carbamazepine | Photoallergic reaction; incidence is about 0.1%; **even reported with UVA light from a photocopier** |
| Chlordiazepoxide | |
| Chloroquine | An incidence of 0.3% in one large study |
| Clomipramine | Photoallergy confirmed in one case |
| Coal tar | Causes stinging and burning ("coal smart") within minutes of sun exposure, sometimes followed by hives; avoid sunlight for 24-72 hours after application |
| Corticosteroids | Two reports |
| Dacarbazine | Well-documented; a burning sensation may occur in 36% |
| Dantrolene | |
| Dapsone | Two reports |
| Diazepam | |
| Diltiazem | Two reports |
| Diphenhydramine | One case reported with oral and one with topical use |
| Estazolam | |
| Fluoxetine | |
| Griseofulvin | Rare reaction, but well-documented |
| Haloperidol | |
| Isocaboxazid | |
| Loxapine | |
| Maprotiline | |
| Methotrexate | May enhance sunburn if given up to 3 days after sun exposure |
| Minoxidil | One case report |
| Nifedipine | Four cases reported |
| Nonsteroidal anti-inflammatory drugs | Low potential for phototoxic reactions; reported with ibuprofen, aspirin, indomethacin, piroxicam, and naproxen |
| Paroxetine | |
| Pentobarbital | |
| Phenelzine | |
| Phenothiazines | Reported with many drugs in this class, frequency may be highest with chlorpromazine; as high as 3% |
| Promethazine | |
| Psoralens | Symptoms within 6-12 hours, peak at 48 hours |
| Pyrazinamide | Red-brown discoloration on sun-exposed skin |
| Quinine or quinidine | Photoallergic reaction; cross-sensitivity between these two agents. Note: Quinine found in nonprescription drugs for leg cramps. |
| Quinolones | Reported with ciprofloxacin, lomefloxacin, ofloxacin, nalidixic acid; incidence may be as high as 10% |
| Retinoids | Increased tendency to sunburn noted in 25% to 50% of those taking etretinate and 5% taking isotretinoin |
| Secobarbital | |
| Selegiline | |
| Sertraline | |
| Sulfonamides | Reported with oral, topical, and ophthalmic use; low potential with silver sulfadiazine |
| Sulfonylureas | Three cases reported with three different agents in this class |
| Sunscreens | Such reactions have been well-documented after exposure to aminobenzoic acid derivatives (eg, Presun®, Tropical Blend®), avobenzone (eg, Shade UVA Guard®), benzophenones (eg, Bain de Soleil®), cinnamates (eg, Bullfrog®, Coppertone®), homosalates (eg, Coppertone®, Tropical Blend®), and methyl anthranilate (eg, Hawaiian Tropic®, Neutrogena®) |
| Tetracyclines | Phototoxic; incidence with minocycline may be lowest |
| Thiazide diuretics | Very uncommon, suggesting photoallergic reactions |
| Trazodone | |
| Triamterene | Single case |
| Tricyclic derivatives | |
| Trimethoprim | Single case |

Adapted with permission from Allen JE, "Drug-Induced Photosensitivity," *Clin Pharm*, 1993, 12(8):580-7.

Used with permission from *New Developments in Medicine & Drug Therapy*, Glenview, IL: Physicians & Scientists Publishing Co, Inc, 1994.

# FOOD-DRUG INTERACTIONS, KEY SUMMARY

| Drug | Food | Interaction |
|---|---|---|
| Acetaminophen | Watercress | Decreased levels of oxidative metabolites (mercapturate) of acetaminophen |
| Aspirin<br>Azithromycin<br>Captopril<br>Didanosine<br>Fosfomycin<br>Isoniazid<br>Mercaptopurine<br>Methotrexate<br>Methyldopa<br>Penicillin G and V<br>Phenobarbital<br>Propantheline<br>Rifampin<br>Riluzole<br>Tetracycline<br>Valsartan | Any food | Decreased absorption |
| Carbamazepine<br>Cefuroxime<br>Hydralazine<br>Lithium<br>Metoprolol | Any food | Increased absorption |
| Cyclosporine | Many foods | Decreased absorption |
| Acitretin<br>Albendazole<br>Atovaquone<br>Beta-carotene<br>Cyclosporine<br>Etretinate<br>Griseofulvin<br>Halofantrine<br>Isotretinoin<br>Mefenamic acid<br>Phenytoin<br>Vitamin A<br>Vitamin D<br>Vitamin E<br>Vitamin K | Dietary fat | Increased absorption |
| Biphosphonates (ie, etidronate, alendronate, tiludronate) | Foods with high mineral content (ie, milk) | Reduced absorption |
| Griseofulvin | High-fat meal | Faster absorption; increased serum levels by 50% |
| Misoprostol | High-fat meal | Reduced peak by delaying absorption |
| Pilocarpine (tablets)<br>Zidovudine | High-fat meal | Reduced absorption |
| Cyclosporine<br>Felodipine<br>Nifedipine<br>Nimodipine<br>Nisoldipine<br>Nitrendipine<br>Verapamil | Grapefruit juice (naringen) | Increased absorption; increased oral bioavailability |
| Caffeine | Grapefruit juice (naringen) | Possibly prolongs caffeine's half-life |
| Coumarin | Grapefruit juice (naringen) | Delayed urinary excretion of 7-hydroxy-coumarin |
| Midazolam (oral) | Grapefruit juice (naringen) | Delayed absorption; increased bioavailability |
| Quinidine | Grapefruit juice (naringen) | Delayed absorption of quinidine; inhibits metabolism of quinidine |
| Terfenadine | Grapefruit juice (naringen) | Increases terfenadine bioavailability (can increase Q-T interval on EKG); increased absorption |
| Erythromycin stearate | Any food | Increased or decreased absorption |
| Furosemide | Any food | Decreased rate of absorption, potentially decreasing effect |
| Mercaptopurine | Any food | Decreased bioavailability by 30% |
| Isoniazid | Tuna, mackerel, salmon (dark meat fish) | Increased risk for scombroid fish poisoning |
| Levodopa | High-protein diet | Decreased absorption |
| Digoxin<br>Lovastatin | High fiber meal | Decreased absorption |

| Drug | Food | Interaction |
|---|---|---|
| Lithium | Sodium | Enhanced elimination requiring higher doses |
| Methyldopa | Iron | Reduced absorption |
| MAO inhibitors<br>Phenelzine<br>Procarbazine<br>Tranylcypromine | High-protein foods that have undergone aging, fermentation, pickling, smoking; aged cheeses, red wines, pods of broad beans, fava beans; bananas, raisins, avocados; caffeine-containing drinks, beer, ale, chocolate | Elevated blood pressure |
| Phenobarbital | High doses of vitamin $B_6$ (pyridoxine) and folic acid | Decreased absorption |
| Levodopa | Vitamin $B_6$ (pyridoxine) | Reduces blood level |
| Diprafenone<br>Felodipine<br>Hydralazine<br>Metoprolol<br>Nitrofurantoin<br>Propranolol | Any food | Increased bioavailability |
| Phenobarbital<br>Phenytoin<br>Theophylline<br>Warfarin | Charcoal-broiled foods | Increased metabolism requiring higher doses |
| Ketoconazole | Acidic beverages (pH <2.5, ie, Coca-Cola Classic®) | Increased absorption |
| Phenytoin | Most foods<br>Pudding | Absorption increased by 25%<br>Absorption decreased by 50% |
| Quinolones (eg, ciprofloxacin)<br>Minocycline<br>Tetracycline | Iron, calcium, aluminum, zinc, magnesium (eg, dairy products) | Decreased absorption |
| Quinidine | High salt (>400 mEq/day) | Increased first-pass hepatic elimination |
| Warfarin | Diets rich in vitamin K such as cauliflower, spinach, broccoli, turnip greens, liver, beans, rice, pork, fish, and some cheeses | Antagonism of effect |

Reprinted with permission from Saltiel E, "Food-Drug Interactions," *New Developments in Medicine & Drug Therapy*, Glenview, IL: Physicians & Scientists Publishing Co, Inc, 1994, 3(4):61.

D'Arcy PF, "Nutrient-Drug Interactions," *Adverse Drug React Toxicol Rev*, 1995, 14(4):233-54.

# HEMATOLOGIC ADVERSE EFFECTS OF DRUGS

| Drug | Red Cell Aplasia | Thrombocytopenia | Neutropenia | Pancytopenia | Hemolysis |
|---|---|---|---|---|---|
| Acetazolamide | | + | + | + | |
| Allopurinol | | | + | | |
| Amiodarone | + | | | | |
| Amphotericin B | | | | + | |
| Amrinone | | ++ | | | |
| Asparaginase | | +++ | +++ | +++ | ++ |
| Barbiturates | | + | | + | |
| Benzocaine | | | | | ++ |
| Captopril | | | ++ | | + |
| Carbamazepine | | ++ | + | | |
| Cephalosporins | | | + | | ++ |
| Chloramphenicol | | + | ++ | +++ | |
| Chlordiazepoxide | | | + | + | |
| Chloroquine | | + | | | |
| Chlorothiazides | | ++ | | | |
| Chlorpropamide | + | ++ | + | ++ | + |
| Chlortetracycline | | | | + | |
| Chlorthalidone | | | + | | |
| Cimetidine | | + | ++ | + | |
| Codeine | | + | | | |
| Colchicine | | | | + | |
| Cyclophosphamide | | +++ | +++ | +++ | + |
| Dapsone | | | | | +++ |
| Desipramine | | ++ | | | |
| Digitalis | | + | | | |
| Digitoxin | | ++ | | | |
| Erythromycin | | + | | | |
| Estrogen | | + | | + | |
| Ethacrynic acid | | | + | | |
| Fluorouracil | | +++ | +++ | +++ | + |
| Furosemide | | + | + | | |
| Gold salts | + | +++ | +++ | +++ | |
| Heparin | | ++ | | + | |
| Ibuprofen | | | + | | + |
| Imipramine | | | ++ | | |
| Indomethacin | | + | ++ | + | |
| Isoniazid | | + | | + | |
| Isosorbide dinitrate | | | | | + |
| Levodopa | | | | | ++ |
| Meperidine | | + | | | |
| Meprobamate | | + | + | + | |
| Methimazole | | | ++ | | |
| Methyldopa | | ++ | | | +++ |
| Methotrexate | | +++ | +++ | +++ | ++ |
| Methylene blue | | | | | + |
| Metronidazole | | | + | | |
| Mirtazapine | | | + | | |
| Nalidixic acid | | | | | + |
| Naproxen | | | | + | |
| Nitrofurantoin | | | ++ | | + |
| Nitroglycerine | | + | | | |
| Penicillamine | | ++ | + | | |
| Penicillins | | + | ++ | + | +++ |
| Phenazopyridine | | | | | +++ |
| Phenothiazines | | + | ++ | +++ | + |
| Phenylbutazone | | + | ++ | +++ | + |
| Phenytoin | | ++ | ++ | ++ | + |
| Potassium iodide | | + | | | |
| Prednisone | | + | | | |
| Primaquine | | | | | +++ |
| Procainamide | | | + | | |
| Procarbazine | | + | ++ | ++ | + |
| Propylthiouracil | | + | ++ | + | + |
| Quinidine | | +++ | + | | |
| Quinine | | +++ | + | | |
| Reserpine | | + | | | |

| Drug | Red Cell Aplasia | Thrombocytopenia | Neutropenia | Pancytopenia | Hemolysis |
|---|---|---|---|---|---|
| Rifampicin | | ++ | + | | +++ |
| Spironolactone | | | + | | |
| Streptomycin | | + | | + | |
| Sulfamethoxazole with trimethoprim | | | + | | |
| Sulfonamides | + | ++ | ++ | ++ | ++ |
| Sulindac | + | + | + | + | |
| Tetracyclines | | + | | | + |
| Thioridazine | | | ++ | | |
| Tolbutamide | | ++ | + | ++ | |
| Triamterene | | | | | + |
| Valproate | + | + | | | |
| Vancomycin | | | + | | |

+ = rare or single reports.

++ = occasional reports.

+++ = substantial number of reports.

Adapted from D'Arcy PF and Griffin JP, eds, *Iatrogenic Diseases*, New York, NY: Oxford University Press, 1986, 128-30.

# LABORATORY DETECTION OF DRUGS

| Agent | Time Detectable in Urine* |
|---|---|
| Alcohol | 12-24 h |
| Amobarbital | 2-4 d |
| Amphetamine | 2-4 d |
| Butalbital | 2-4 d |
| Cannabinoids | |
| Occasional use | 2-7 d |
| Regular use | 30 d |
| Cocaine (benzoylecgonine) | 12-72 h |
| Codeine | 2-4 d |
| Chlordiazepoxide | 30 d |
| Diazepam | 30 d |
| Dilaudid® | 2-4 d |
| Ethanol | 12-24 h |
| Heroin (morphine) | 2-4 d |
| Hydromorphone | 2-4 d |
| Librium® | 30 d |
| Marijuana | |
| Occasional use | 2-7 d |
| Regular use | 30 d |
| Methamphetamine | 2-4 d |
| Methaqualone | 2-4 d |
| Morphine | 2-4 d |
| Pentobarbital | 2-4 d |
| Phencyclidine (PCP) | |
| Occasional use | 2-7 d |
| Regular use | 30 d |
| Phenobarbital | 30 d |
| Quaalude® | 2-4 d |
| Secobarbital | 2-4 d |
| Valium® | 30 d |

*The periods of detection for the various abused drugs listed above should be taken as estimates since the actual figures will vary due to metabolism, user, laboratory, and excretion.

Chang JY, "Drug Testing and Interpretation of Results," *Pharmchem Newsletter*, 1989, 17:1.

# SEROTONIN SYNDROME

## Diagnostic Criteria for Serotonin Syndrome

- Recent addition or dosage increase of any agent increasing serotonin activity or availability (usually within 1 day).
- Absence of abused substances, metabolic infectious etiology, or withdrawal.
- No recent addition or dosage increase of a neuroleptic agent prior to onset of signs and symptoms.
- Presence of three or more of the following: Altered mental status (seen in 40% of patients, primarily confusion or hypomania); agitation; tremor (50% incidence); shivering; diarrhea; hyperreflexia (pronounced in lower extremities; myoclonus (50% incidence); ataxia or incoordination; fever (50% incidence; temperature >105°F associated with grave prognosis); diaphoresis

## Drugs (as Single Causative Agent) Which Can Induce Serotonin Syndrome

Specific serotonin reuptake inhibitors (SSRI)
MDMA (Ectasy)
Clomipramine

## Drug Combinations Which Can Induce Serotonin Syndrome*

Alprazolam – Clomipramine

Bromocriptine – Levodopa/carbidopa

Buspirone – Trazodone

Citalopram – Moclobemide

Clomipramine – Clorgiline

Clomipramine – Lithium

Clomipramine – Monoamine oxidase inhibitor

Dihydroergotamine – Sertraline

Dihydroergotamine – Amitriptyline

Fentanyl – Sertraline

Fluoxetine – Carbamazepine

Fluoxetine – Lithium

Fluoxetine – Remoxipride

Fluoxetine – Tryptophan

Lithium – Fluvoxamine

Lithium – Paroxetine

Lysergic acid diethylamide (LSD) – Fluoxetine

Moclobemide – Citalopram

Moclobemide – Clomipramine

Moclobemide – Fluoxetine

Moclobemide – Pethidine

Monoamine oxidase inhibitor – Dextromethorphan

Monoamine oxidase inhibitor – Fluoxetine

Monoamine oxidase inhibitor – Fluvoxamine

Monoamine oxidase inhibitor – Meperidine

Monoamine oxidase inhibitor – Sertraline

Monoamine oxidase inhibitor – Tricyclic antidepressants

Monoamine oxidase inhibitor – Tryptophan

Monoamine oxidase inhibitor – Venlafaxine

Nefazodone – Paroxetine

Nortriptyline – Trazodone

Paroxetine – Dextromethorphan

Paroxetine – Dihydroergotamine

Paroxetine – Trazodone

Phenelzine – Trazodone – Dextropropoxyphene

S-adenosylmethionine – Clomipramine

Sertraline – Amitriptyline

St John's wort – Selective serotonin reuptake inhibitors

Sumatriptan – Sertraline

Tranylcypromine – Clomipramine

Tramadol – Sertraline

Trazodone – Lithium – Amitriptyline

Trazodone – Fluoxetine

Valproic acid – Nefazodone

Venlafaxine – Tranylcypromine

Venlafaxine – Selegiline

*When administered within 2 weeks of each other.

## SEROTONIN SYNDROME *(Continued)*

### Guidelines for Treatment of Serotonin Syndrome

Therapy is primarily supportive with intravenous crystalloid solutions utilized for hypotension and cooling blankets for mild hyperthermia. Norepinephrine is the preferred vasopressor. Chlorpromazine (25 mg I.M.) or dantrolene sodium (1 mg/kg I.V. – maximum dose 10 mg/kg) may have a role in controlling fevers, although there is no proven benefit. Benzodiazepines are the first-line treatment in controlling rigors and thus, limiting fever and rhabdomyolysis, while clonazepam may be specifically useful in treating myoclonus. Endotracheal intubation and paralysis may be required to treat refractory muscular contractions. Tachycardia or tremor can be treated with beta-blocking agents; although due to its blockade of 5-HTIA receptors, the syndrome may worsen. Serotonin blockers such as diphenhydramine (50 mg I.M.), cyproheptadine (adults: 4-8 mg every 2-4 hours up to 0.5 mg/kg/day; children: up to 0.25 mg/kg/day), or chlorpromazine (25 mg I.M.) have been used with variable efficacy. Methysergide (2-6 mg/day) and nitroglycerin (I.V. infusion of 2 mg/kg/minute with lorazepam) also has been utilized with variable efficacy in case reports. It appears that cyproheptadine is most consistently beneficial.

Recovery seen within 1 day in 70% of cases; mortality rate is about 11%.

### References

Gitlin MJ, "Venlafaxine, Monoamine Oxidase Inhibitors, and the Serotonin Syndrome," *J Clin Psychopharmacol*, 1997, 17:66-7.

Heisler MA, Guidery JR, and Arnecke B, "Serotonin Syndrome Induced by Administration of Venlafaxine and Phenelzine," *Ann Pharmacother*, 1996, 30:84.

Hodgman MJ, Martin TG, and Krenzelok EP, "Serotonin Syndrome Due to Venlafaxine and Maintenance Tranylcypromine Therapy," *Hum Exp Toxicol*, 1997, 16:14-7.

John L, Perreault MM, Tao T, et al, "Serotonin Syndrome Associated With Nefazodone and Paroxetine," *Ann Emerg Med*, 1997, 29:287-9.

LoCurto MJ, "The Serotonin Syndrome," *Emerg Clin North Am*, 1997, 15(3):665-75.

Martin TG, "Serotonin Syndrome," *Ann Emerg Med*, 1996, 28:520-6.

Mills K, "Serotonin Toxicity: A Comprehensive Review for Emergency Medicine," *Top Emerg Med*, 1993, 15:54-73.

Mills KC, "Serotonin Syndrome: A Clinical Update," *Crit Care Clin*, 1997, 13(4):763-83.

Nisijima K, Shimizu M, Abe T, et al, "A Case of Serotonin Syndrome Induced by Concomitant Treatment With Low-Dose Trazodone, and Amitriptyline and Lithium," *Int Clin Psychopharmacol*, 1996, 11:289-90.

Sobanski T, Bagli M, Laux G, et al, "Serotonin Syndrome After Lithium Add-On Medication to Paroxetine," *Pharmacopsychiatry*, 1997, 30:106-7.

Sporer, "The Serotonin Syndrome: Implicated Drugs, Pathophysiology and Management," *Drug Safety*, 1995, 13(2):94-104.

Sternbach H, "The Serotonin Syndrome," *Am J Psychiatry*, 1991, 146:705-7.

Van Berkum MM, Thiel J, Leikin JB, et al, "A Fatality Due to Serotonin Syndrome," *Medical Update for Psychiatrists*, 1997, 2:55-7.

# TABLETS THAT CANNOT BE CRUSHED OR ALTERED

There are a variety of reasons for crushing tablets or capsule contents prior to administering to the patient. Patients may have nasogastric tubes which do not permit the administration of tablets or capsules; an oral solution for a particular medication may not be available from the manufacturer or readily prepared by pharmacy; patients may have difficulty swallowing capsules or tablets; or mixing of powdered medication with food or drink may make the drug more palatable.

Generally, medications which should not be crushed fall into one of the following categories.

- **Extended-Release Products.** The formulation of some tablets is specialized as to allow the medication within it to be slowly released into the body. This is sometimes accomplished by centering the drug within the core of the tablet, with a subsequent shedding of multiple layers around the core. Wax melts in the GI tract. Slow-K® is an example of this. Capsules may contain beads which have multiple layers which are slowly dissolved with time.
- **Medications Which Are Irritating to the Stomach.** Tablets which are irritating to the stomach may be enteric-coated which delays release of the drug until the time when it reaches the small intestine. Enteric-coated aspirin is an example of this.
- **Foul-Tasting Medication.** Some drugs are quite unpleasant to taste so the manufacturer coats the tablet in a sugar coating to increase its palatability. By crushing the tablet, this sugar coating is lost and the patient tastes the unpleasant tasting medication.
- **Sublingual Medication.** Medication intended for use under the tongue should not be crushed. While it appears to be obvious, it is not always easy to determine if a medication is to be used sublingually. Sublingual medications should indicate on the package that they are intended for sublingual use.
- **Effervescent Tablets.** These are tablets which, when dropped into a liquid, quickly dissolve to yield a solution. Many effervescent tablets, when crushed, lose their ability to quickly dissolve.

## Recommendations

1. It is not advisable to crush certain medications.
2. Consult individual monographs prior to crushing capsule or tablet.
3. If crushing a tablet or capsule is contraindicated, consult with your pharmacist to determine whether an oral solution exists or can be compounded.

| Drug Product | Dosage Forms | Reasons/Comments |
|---|---|---|
| Accutane® | Capsule | Mucous membrane irritant |
| Actifed 12® Hour | Capsule | Slow release† |
| Acutrim® | Tablet | Slow release |
| Adalat® CC | Tablet | Slow release |
| Aerolate® SR, JR, III | Capsule | Slow release*† |
| Allerest® 12-Hour | Tablet | Slow release |
| Artane® Sequels® | Capsule | Slow release*† |
| Arthritis Bayer® Time Release | Capsule | Slow release |
| A.S.A.® Enseals® | Tablet | Enteric-coated |
| Atrohist® Plus | Tablet | Slow release* |
| Atrohist® Sprinkle | Capsule | Slow release |
| Azulfidine® EN-tabs® | Tablet | Enteric-coated |
| Baros | Tablet | Effervescent tablet¶ |
| Bayer® Aspirin, low adult 81 mg strength | Tablet | Enteric-coated |
| Bayer® Aspirin, regular strength 325 mg caplet | Tablet | Enteric-coated |
| Bayer® Aspirin, regular strength EC caplet | Tablet | Enteric-coated |
| Betachron E-R® | Capsule | Slow release |
| Betapen®-VK | Tablet | Taste†† |
| Biohist® LA | Tablet | Slow release♦ |
| Bisacodyl | Tablet | Enteric-coated‡ |
| Bisco-Lax® | Tablet | Enteric-coated‡ |
| Bontril® Slow-Release | Capsule | Slow release |
| Breonesin® | Capsule | Liquid filled§ |
| Brexin® L.A. | Capsule | Slow release |
| Bromfed® | Capsule | Slow release† |
| Bromfed-PD® | Capsule | Slow release† |
| Calan® SR | Tablet | Slow release♦ |
| Cama® Arthritis Pain Reliever | Tablet | Multiple compressed tablet |
| Carbiset-TR® | Tablet | Slow release |
| Cardizem® | Tablet | Slow release |

# TABLETS THAT CANNOT BE CRUSHED OR ALTERED *(Continued)*

| Drug Product | Dosage Forms | Reasons/Comments |
|---|---|---|
| Cardizem® CD | Capsule | Slow release* |
| Cardizem® SR | Capsule | Slow release* |
| Carter's Little Pills® | Tablet | Enteric-coated |
| Ceftin® | Tablet | Taste<br>**Note:** Use suspension for children |
| Charcoal Plus® | Tablet | Enteric-coated |
| Chloral Hydrate | Capsule | **Note:** Product is in liquid form within a special capsule† |
| Chlorpheniramine Maleate Time Release | Capsule | Slow release |
| Chlor-Trimeton® Repetab® | Tablet | Slow release† |
| Choledyl® SA | Tablet | Slow release† |
| Cipro™ | Tablet | Taste†† |
| Claritin-D® | Tablet | Slow release |
| Codimal-L.A.® | Capsule | Slow release |
| Codimal-L.A.® Half | Capsule | Slow release |
| Colace® | Capsule | Taste†† |
| Comhist® LA | Capsule | Slow release* |
| Compazine® Spansule® | Capsule | Slow release† |
| Congess SR, JR | Capsule | Slow release |
| Contac® | Capsule | Slow release* |
| Cotazym-S® | Capsule | Enteric-coated* |
| Covera-HS™ | Tablet | Slow release |
| Creon® 10 Minimicrospheres™ | Capsule | Enteric-coated* |
| Creon® 20 | Capsule | Enteric-coated* |
| Cytospaz-M® | Capsule | Slow release |
| Cytoxan® | Tablet | **Note:** Drug may be crushed, but maker recommends using injection |
| Dallergy® | Capsule | Slow release† |
| Dallergy-D® | Capsule | Slow release |
| Dallergy-JR® | Capsule | Slow release |
| Deconamine® SR | Capsule | Slow release† |
| Deconsal® II | Tablet | Slow release |
| Deconsal® Sprinkle® | Capsule | Slow release* |
| Defen L.A.® | Tablet | Slow release♦ |
| Demazin® Repetabs® | Tablet | Slow release† |
| Depakene® | Capsule | Slow-release-mucous membrane irritant† |
| Depakote® | Capsule | Enteric-coated |
| Desoxyn® Gradumets® | Tablet | Slow release |
| Desyrel® | Tablet | Taste†† |
| Dexatrim® Max Strength | Tablet | Slow release |
| Dexedrine® Spansule® | Capsule | Slow release |
| Diamox® Sequels® | Capsule | Slow release |
| Dilatrate-SR® | Capsule | Slow release |
| Disobrom® | Tablet | Slow release |
| Disophrol® Chronotab® | Tablet | Slow release |
| Dital® | Capsule | Slow release |
| Donnatal® Extentab® | Tablet | Slow release† |
| Donnazyme® | Tablet | Enteric-coated |
| Drisdol® | Capsule | Liquid filled§ |
| Drixoral® | Tablet | Slow release† |
| Drixoral® Sinus | Tablet | Slow release |
| Dulcolax® | Tablet | Enteric-coated‡ |
| Dynabac® | Tablet | Enteric-coated |
| Easprin® | Tablet | Enteric-coated |
| Ecotrin® | Tablet | Enteric-coated |
| E.E.S.® 400 | Tablet | Enteric-coated† |
| Efidac/24® | Tablet | Slow release |
| Efidac® 24 Chlorpheniramine | Tablet | Slow release |
| E-Mycin® | Tablet | Enteric-coated |
| Endafed® | Capsule | Slow release |
| Entex® LA | Tablet | Slow release† |
| Equanil® | Tablet | Taste†† |
| Eryc® | Capsule | Enteric-coated* |
| Ery-Tab® | Tablet | Enteric-coated |
| Erythrocin Stearate | Tablet | Enteric-coated |
| Erythromycin Base | Tablet | Enteric-coated |
| Eskalith CR® | Tablet | Slow release |
| Exgest® LA | Tablet | Slow release |
| Fedahist® Timecaps® | Capsule | Slow release† |
| Feldene® | Capsule | Mucous membrane irritant |
| Feocyte | Tablet | Slow release |
| Feosol® | Tablet | Enteric-coated† |
| Feosol® Spansule® | Capsule | Slow release*† |
| Feratab® | Tablet | Enteric-coated† |
| Fero-Grad 500® | Tablet | Slow release |
| Fero-Gradumet® | Tablet | Slow release |

| Drug Product | Dosage Forms | Reasons/Comments |
|---|---|---|
| Ferralet S.R.® | Tablet | Slow release |
| Feverall™ Sprinkle Caps | Capsule | Taste* **Note:** Capsule contents intended to be placed in a teaspoonful of water or soft food. |
| Fumatinic® | Capsule | Slow release |
| Gastrocrom® | Capsule | **Note:** Contents should be dissolved in water for administration. |
| Geocillin® | Tablet | Taste |
| Glucotrol® XL | Tablet | Slow release |
| Gris-PEG® | Tablet | **Note:** Crushing may result in precipitation of larger particles. |
| Guaifed® | Capsule | Slow release |
| Guaifed®-PD | Capsule | Slow release |
| Guaifenex® LA | Tablet | Slow release♦ |
| Guaifenex® PSE | Tablet | Slow release♦ |
| GuaiMAX-D® | Tablet | Slow release |
| Humibid® DM | Tablet | Slow release |
| Humibid® DM Sprinkle | Capsule | Slow release* |
| Humibid® LA | Tablet | Slow release |
| Humibid® Sprinkle | Capsule | Slow release* |
| Hydergine® LC | Capsule | **Note:** Product is in liquid form within a special capsule† |
| Hydergine® Sublingual | Tablet | Sublingual route† |
| Hytakerol® | Capsule | Liquid filled§† |
| Iberet® | Tablet | Slow release† |
| Iberet-500® | Tablet | Slow release† |
| ICAPS® Plus | Tablet | Slow release |
| ICAPS® Time Release | Tablet | Slow release |
| Ilotycin® | Tablet | Enteric-coated |
| Imdur™ | Tablet | Slow release♦ |
| Inderal® LA | Capsule | Slow release |
| Inderide® LA | Capsule | Slow release |
| Indocin® SR | Capsule | Slow release*† |
| Ionamin® | Capsule | Slow release |
| Isoptin® SR | Tablet | Slow release |
| Isordil® Sublingual | Tablet | Sublingual form• |
| Isordil® Tembid® | Tablet | Slow release |
| Isosorbide Dinitrate Sublingual | Tablet | Sublingual form• |
| Isosorbide Dinitrate SR | Tablet | Slow release |
| K+ 8® | Tablet | Slow release† |
| K+ 10® | Tablet | Slow release† |
| Kaon-Cl® 6.7 | Tablet | Slow release† |
| Kaon-Cl® 10 | Tablet | Slow release† |
| K+ Care® ET | Tablet | Effervescent tablet†¶ |
| K-Lease® | Capsule | Slow release*† |
| Klor-Con® | Tablet | Slow release† |
| Klor-Con/EF® | Tablet | Effervescent tablet†¶ |
| Klorvess® | Tablet | Effervescent tablet†¶ |
| Klotrix® | Tablet | Slow release† |
| K-Lyte® | Tablet | Effervescent tablet¶ |
| K-Lyte®/Cl | Tablet | Effervescent tablet¶ |
| K-Lyte DS® | Tablet | Effervescent tablet¶ |
| K-Tab® | Tablet | Slow release† |
| Levsinex® Timecaps® | Capsule | Slow release |
| Lexxel® | Tablet | Slow release |
| Lodrane LD® | Capsule | Slow release* |
| Mag-Tab® SR | Tablet | Slow release |
| Mestinon® | Tablet | Slow release† |
| Mi-Cebrin® | Tablet | Enteric-coated |
| Mi-Cebrin® T | Tablet | Enteric-coated |
| Micro-K® | Capsule | Slow release*† |
| Monafed® | Tablet | Slow release |
| Monafed® DM | Tablet | Slow release |
| Motrin® | Tablet | Taste†† |
| MS Contin® | Tablet | Slow release† |
| Muco-Fen-LA® | Tablet | Slow release♦ |
| Naldecon® | Tablet | Slow release† |
| Naprelan® | Tablet | Slow release |
| Nasatab LA® | Tablet | Slow release |
| Niaspan® | Tablet | Slow release |
| Nico-400® | Capsule | Slow release |
| Nicobid® | Capsule | Slow release |
| Nitro-Bid® | Capsule | Slow release* |
| Nitroglyn® | Capsule | Slow release* |
| Nitrong® | Tablet | Sublingual route• |
| Nitrostat® | Tablet | Sublingual route• |
| Nolamine® | Tablet | Slow release |
| Nolex® LA | Tablet | Slow release |
| Norflex® | Tablet | Slow release |

## TABLETS THAT CANNOT BE CRUSHED OR ALTERED *(Continued)*

| Drug Product | Dosage Forms | Reasons/Comments |
|---|---|---|
| Norpace CR® | Capsule | Slow release form within a special capsule |
| Novafed® A | Capsule | Slow release |
| Ondrox® | Tablet | Slow release |
| Optilets-500® | Tablet | Enteric-coated |
| Optilets-M-500® | Tablet | Enteric-coated |
| Oragrafin® | Capsule | **Note:** Product is in liquid form within a special capsule |
| Ordrine® SR | Capsule | Slow release |
| Oramorph SR™ | Tablet | Slow release† |
| Ornade® Spansule® | Capsule | Slow release |
| OxyContin® | Tablet | Slow release |
| Pabalate® | Tablet | Enteric-coated |
| Pabalate-SF® | Tablet | Enteric-coated |
| Pancrease® | Capsule | Enteric-coated* |
| Pancrease® MT | Capsule | Enteric-coated* |
| Panmycin® | Capsule | Taste |
| Papaverine Sustained Action | Capsule | Slow release |
| Pathilon® Sequels® | Capsule | Slow release* |
| Pavabid® Plateau® | Capsule | Slow release* |
| PBZ-SR® | Tablet | Slow release† |
| Pentasa® | Capsule | Slow release |
| Perdiem® | Granules | Wax coated |
| Permitil® Chronotab® | Tablet | Slow release† |
| Phazyme® | Tablet | Slow release |
| Phazyme® 95 | Tablet | Slow release |
| Phenergan® | Tablet | Taste††† |
| Phyllocontin® | Tablet | Slow release |
| Plendil® | Tablet | Slow release |
| Pneumomits® | Tablet | Slow release♦ |
| Polaramine® Repetabs® | Tablet | Slow release† |
| Posicor® | Tablet | Mucus membrane irritant |
| Prelu-2® | Capsule | Slow release |
| Prevacid® | Capsule | Slow release |
| Prilosec™ | Capsule | Slow release |
| Pro-Banthine® | Tablet | Taste |
| Procainamide HCl SR | Tablet | Slow release |
| Procanbid® | Tablet | Slow release |
| Procardia® | Capsule | Delays absorption§# |
| Procardia XL® | Tablet | Slow release<br>**Note:** AUC is unaffected. |
| Profen® II | Tablet | Slow release♦ |
| Profen LA® | Tablet | Slow release♦ |
| Pronestyl-SR® | Tablet | Slow release |
| Proscar® | Tablet | **Note:** Crushed tablets should not be handled by women who are pregnant or who may become pregnant |
| Proventil® Repetabs® | Tablet | Slow release† |
| Prozac® | Capsule | Slow release* |
| Quibron-T/ SR® | Tablet | Slow release† |
| Quinaglute® Dura-Tabs® | Tablet | Slow release |
| Quinidex® Extentabs® | Tablet | Slow release |
| Quin-Release® | Tablet | Slow release |
| Respa-1st® | Tablet | Slow release♦ |
| Respa-DM® | Tablet | Slow release♦ |
| Respa-GF® | Tablet | Slow release♦ |
| Respahist® | Capsule | Slow release* |
| Respaire® SR | Capsule | Slow release |
| Respbid® | Tablet | Slow release |
| Ritalin-SR® | Tablet | Slow release |
| Robimycin® Robitab® | Tablet | Enteric-coated |
| Rondec-TR® | Tablet | Slow release† |
| Roxanol SR™ | Tablet | Slow release† |
| Ru-Tuss® DE | Tablet | Slow release |
| Sinemet CR® | Tablet | Slow release♦ |
| Singlet for Adults® | Tablet | Slow release |
| Slo-bid™ Gyrocaps® | Capsule | Slow release* |
| Slo-Niacin® | Tablet | Slow release |
| Slo-Phyllin GG® | Capsule | Slow release† |
| Slo-Phyllin® Gyrocaps® | Capsule | Slow release*† |
| Slow FE® | Tablet | Slow release† |
| Slow FE® With Folic Acid | Tablet | Slow release |
| Slow-K® | Tablet | Slow release† |
| Slow-Mag® | Tablet | Slow release |
| Sorbitrate SA® | Tablet | Slow release |
| Sorbitrate® Sublingual | Tablet | Sublingual route |
| Sparine® | Tablet | Taste†† |

| Drug Product | Dosage Forms | Reasons/Comments |
|---|---|---|
| S-P-T | Capsule | **Note:** Liquid gelatin thyroid suspension. |
| Sudafed® 12-Hour | Capsule | Slow release† |
| Sudal® 60/500 | Tablet | Slow release |
| Sudal® 120/600 | Tablet | Slow release |
| Sudafed® 12-Hour | Tablet | Slow release† |
| Sudex® 60/500 | Tablet | Slow release♦ |
| Sustaire® | Tablet | Slow release† |
| Syn™-Rx | Tablet | Slow release |
| Syn™-Rx DM | Tablet | Slow release |
| Tavist-D® | Tablet | Multiple compressed tablet |
| Teczam® | Tablet | Slow release |
| Tegretol XR® | Tablet | Slow release |
| Teldrin® | Capsule | Slow release* |
| Tessalon® Perles | Capsule | Slow release |
| Theo-24® | Tablet | Slow release† |
| Theobid® Duracaps® | Capsule | Slow release*† |
| Theoclear® L.A | Capsule | Slow release† |
| Theochron® | Tablet | Slow release |
| Theo-Dur® | Tablet | Slow release†♦ |
| Theolair SR® | Tablet | Slow release† |
| Theo-Sav® | Tablet | Slow release♦ |
| Theo-Time® SR | Tablet | Slow release |
| Theovent® | Capsule | Slow release† |
| Theo-X® | Tablet | Slow release |
| Thorazine® Spansule® | Capsule | Slow release |
| Toprol XL® | Tablet | Slow release♦ |
| Touro A&H® | Capsule | Slow release* |
| Touro Ex® | Tablet | Slow release♦ |
| Touro LA® | Tablet | Slow release♦ |
| T-Phyl® | Tablet | Slow release |
| Trental® | Tablet | Slow release |
| Triaminic® | Tablet | Enteric-coated† |
| Triaminic®-12 | Tablet | Slow release† |
| Triaminic® TR | Tablet | Multiple compressed tablet† |
| Trilafon® Repetabs® | Tablet | Slow release† |
| Tri-Phen-Chlor® Time Release | Tablet | Slow release |
| Tri-Phen-Mine® SR | Tablet | Slow release |
| TripTone® Caplets | Tablet | Slow release |
| Tuss-LA® | Tablet | Slow release |
| Tylenol® Extended Relief Caplets | Tablet | Slow release |
| ULR-LA® | Tablet | Slow release |
| Uni-Dur® | Tablet | Slow release |
| Uniphyl® | Tablet | Slow release |
| Verelan® | Capsule | Slow release* |
| Volmax® | Tablet | Slow release† |
| Wellbutrin® | Tablet | Anesthetize mucus membrane |
| Wygesic® | Tablet | Taste |
| ZORprin® | Tablet | Slow release |
| Zyban™ | Tablet | Slow release |
| Zymase® | Capsule | Enteric-coated |

*Capsule may be opened and the contents taken without crushing or chewing; soft food such as applesauce or pudding may facilitate administration; contents may generally be administered via nasogastric tube using an appropriate fluid, provided entire contents are washed down the tube.

†Liquid dosage forms of the product are available; however, dose, frequency of administration, and manufacturers may differ from that of the solid dosage form.

‡Antacids and/or milk may prematurely dissolve the coating of the tablet.

§Capsule may be opened and the liquid contents removed for administration.

††The taste of this product in a liquid form would likely be unacceptable to the patient; administration via nasogastric tube should be acceptable.

¶Effervescent tablets must be dissolved in the amount of diluent recommended by the manufacturer.

#If the liquid capsule is crushed or the contents expressed, the active ingredient will be, in part, absorbed sublingually.

•Tablets are made to disintegrate under the tongue.

♦Tablet is scored and may be broken in half without affecting release characteristics.

Adapted from Mitchell JF and Pawlicki KS, "Oral Solid Dosage Forms That Should Not Be Crushed: 1998 Revision," *Hosp Pharm*, 1994, 29(7):666-75.

# TERATOGENIC RISKS OF PSYCHOTROPIC MEDICATIONS

| Drug | Risk Category | Possible Effects |
|---|---|---|
| | | **ANXIOLYTICS** |
| Benzodiazepines | D | "Floppy baby," withdrawal, cleft lip |
| Buspirone | B | Unknown |
| Hypnotic benzodiazepines | X | Decreased intrauterine growth |
| | | **ANTIDEPRESSANTS** |
| MAOIs | C | Rare fetal malformations; rarely used in pregnancy due to hypertension |
| SSRIs | C | Increased perinatal complications |
| TCAs | C/D | Fetal tachycardia, fetal withdrawal, fetal anticholinergic effects, urinary retention, bowel obstruction |
| | | **ANTIPARKINSONIAN** |
| Amantadine | C | Increase in pregnancy complications |
| Benztropine | C | Increase in minor malformations |
| Diphenhydramine | B | Oral clefts |
| Procyclidine | C | Increase in minor malformations |
| Trihexyphenidyl | C | Increase in minor malformations |
| | | **ANTIPSYCHOTICS** |
| Conventional | C | Rare anomalies, fetal jaundice, fetal anticholinergic effects at birth |
| Atypical, clozapine | B | Unknown |
| Atypical, risperidone, quetiapine, olanzapine | C | Unknown |
| | | **MOOD STABILIZERS** |
| Carbamazepine | D | Neural tube defects, minor anomalies |
| Lithium | D | Behavioral effects, Epstein's anomaly |
| Valproate | D | Neural tube defects |

Pregnancy Categories: A = Controlled studies show no risk to humans; B = no evidence of risk in humans, but adequate human studies may not have been performed; C = risk cannot be ruled out; D = positive evidence of risk to humans, risk may be outweighed by potential benefit; X = contraindicated in pregnancy.

TCA = tricyclic antidepressant; MAOI = monoamine oxidase inhibitor; SSRI = selective serotonin reuptake inhibitor

# TYRAMINE CONTENT OF FOODS

| Food | Allowed | Minimize Intake | Not Allowed |
|---|---|---|---|
| Beverages | Milk, decaffeinated coffee, tea, soda | Chocolate beverage, caffeine-containing drinks, clear spirits | Acidophilus milk, beer, ale, wine, malted beverages |
| Breads/cereals | All except those containing cheese | None | Cheese bread and crackers |
| Dairy products | Cottage cheese, farmers or pot cheese, cream cheese, ricotta cheese, all milk, eggs, ice cream, pudding (except chocolate) | Yogurt (limit to 4 oz per day) | All other cheeses (aged cheese, American, Camembert, cheddar, Gouda, gruyere, mozzarella, parmesan, provolone, romano, Roquefort, stilton |
| Meat, fish, and poultry | All fresh or frozen | Aged meats, hot dogs, canned fish and meat | Chicken and beef liver, dried and pickled fish, summer or dry sausage, pepperoni, dried meats, meat extracts, bologna, liverwurst |
| Starches — potatoes/rice | All | None | Soybean (including paste) |
| Vegetables | All fresh, frozen, canned, or dried vegetable juices except those not allowed | Chili peppers, Chinese pea pods | Fava beans, sauerkraut, pickles, olives, Italian broad beans |
| Fruit | Fresh, frozen, or canned fruits and fruit juices | Avocado, banana, raspberries, figs | Banana peel extract |
| Soups | All soups not listed to limit or avoid | Commercially canned soups | Soups which contain broad beans, fava beans, cheese, beer, wine, any made with flavor cubes or meat extract, miso soup |
| Fats | All except fermented | Sour cream | Packaged gravy |
| Sweets | Sugar, hard candy, honey, molasses, syrups | Chocolate candies | None |
| Desserts | Cakes, cookies, gelatin, pastries, sherbets, sorbets | Chocolate desserts | Cheese-filled desserts |
| Miscellaneous | Salt, nuts, spices, herbs, flavorings, Worcestershire sauce | Soy sauce, peanuts | Brewer's yeast, yeast concentrates, all aged and fermented products, monosodium glutamate, vitamins with Brewer's yeast |

# PHARMACOLOGIC CATEGORY INDEX

(Continued)

(Continued)

## LOCAL ANESTHETIC (Continued)



## LOCAL ANESTHETIC, INJECTABLE



## LOW MOLECULAR WEIGHT HEPARIN



## LUNG SURFACTANT



## LUTEINIZING HORMONE-RELEASING HORMONE ANALOG



## MAGNESIUM SALT



## MAST CELL STABILIZER



## MISCELLANEOUS PRODUCT



## MONOCLONAL ANTIBODY



## MUCOLYTIC AGENT



## NEURAMINIDASE INHIBITOR



## NEUROMUSCULAR BLOCKER AGENT, DEPOLARIZING



## NEUROMUSCULAR BLOCKER AGENT, NONDEPOLARIZING



## NONSTEROIDAL ANTI-INFLAMMATORY AGENT (NSAID)



## NONSTEROIDAL ANTI-INFLAMMATORY AGENT (NSAID), CYCLOOXYGENASE 2 INHIBITOR



## NUTRITIONAL SUPPLEMENT



## OPHTHALMIC AGENT, ANTIGLAUCOMA



## OPHTHALMIC AGENT, MIOTIC



## OPHTHALMIC AGENT, MYDRIATIC



## OPHTHALMIC AGENT, OSMOTIC



## OPHTHALMIC AGENT, TOXIN



## OPHTHALMIC AGENT, VASOCONSTRICTOR



## OPHTHALMIC AGENT, VISCOELASTIC



## OPHTHALMIC AGENT, MISCELLANEOUS



## OTIC AGENT, CERUMENOLYTIC



## OVULATION STIMULATOR



## OXYTOCIC AGENT



## PEDICULOCIDE



## PHOSPHATE BINDER

## TYROSINE HYDROXYLASE INHIBITOR



## URICOSURIC AGENT



## URINARY TRACT PRODUCT



## VACCINE



## VASOCONSTRICTOR



## VASODILATOR



## VASOPRESSIN ANALOG, SYNTHETIC



## VESICANT



## VITAMIN



## VITAMIN A DERIVATIVE



## VITAMIN D ANALOG



## VITAMIN, FAT SOLUBLE



## VITAMIN, TOPICAL



## VITAMIN, WATER SOLUBLE



## XANTHINE OXIDASE INHIBITOR

# ALPHABETICAL INDEX

# INTERNATIONAL BRAND NAME INDEX

The following countries are included in this index and are abbreviated as follows:

Austria (Austria)
Australia (Astral)
Belgium (Belg)
Brazil (Bra)
Canada (Can)
Denmark (Den)
France (Fr)
Germany (Ger)
Ireland (Irl)
Italy (Ital)
Japan (Jpn)
Mexico (Mex)
Monaco (Mon)
Netherlands (Neth)
Norway (Norw)
Portugal (Por)
South Africa (S. Afr)
Spain (Spain)
Sweden (Swed)
Switzerland (Switz)
United Kingdom (UK)
United States (USA)

Frubiase Calcium *see* Calcium Carbonate (Ger) . . . 84
Frubilurgyl *see* Chlorhexidine Gluconate (Ger) . . . 111
Frubizin *see* Cetylpyridinium (Ger) . . . 106
Frubizin Forte *see* Cetylpyridinium and Benzocaine (Ger) . . . 106
Frumax *see* Furosemide (UK) . . . 243
Frusehexal *see* Furosemide (Astral) . . . 243
Frusetic *see* Furosemide (UK) . . . 243
Frusid *see* Furosemide (UK) . . . 243
Frusol *see* Furosemide (UK) . . . 243
FS Shampoo *see* Fluocinolone (USA) . . . 231
FUDR *see* Floxuridine (USA) . . . 227
Fugerel *see* Flutamide (Astral, Austria, Ger) . . . 236
Fugoa N *see* Phenylpropanolamine (Ger, Switz) . . . 440
Fulcin *see* Griseofulvin (Astral, Austria, Bra, Den, Irl, Ital, Neth, Norw, Por, S. Afr, Spain, Swed, Switz, UK) . . . 255
Fulcine *see* Griseofulvin (Fr) . . . 255
Fulcin S *see* Griseofulvin (Ger) . . . 255
Fulcro *see* Fenofibrate (Ital) . . . 220
Fulgram *see* Norfloxacin (Ital) . . . 399
Fulixan *see* Diflorasone (Spain) . . . 168
Fulvicin *see* Griseofulvin (Can) . . . 255
Fulvicina *see* Griseofulvin (Spain) . . . 255
Fulvicin P/G *see* Griseofulvin (USA) . . . 255
Fulvicin-U/F *see* Griseofulvin (USA) . . . 255
Fulvina P/G *see* Griseofulvin (Mex) . . . 255
Fumafer *see* Ferrous Fumarate (Fr) . . . 223
Fumarenid *see* Furosemide (Ger) . . . 243
Fumasorb [OTC] *see* Ferrous Fumarate (USA) . . . 223
Fumerin [OTC] *see* Ferrous Fumarate (USA) . . . 223
Fungarest *see* Ketoconazole (Spain) . . . 302
Fungata *see* Fluconazole (Austria, Ger) . . . 227
Fungederm *see* Clotrimazole (UK) . . . 135
Fungibacid *see* Tioconazole (Ger) . . . 550
Fungiderm *see* Clotrimazole (Ger) . . . 135
Fungiderm *see* Miconazole (Ital) . . . 364
Fungidermo *see* Clotrimazole (Spain) . . . 135
Fungilonga *see* Ciclopirox (Spain) . . . 122
Funginazol *see* Miconazole (Spain) . . . 364
Fungiquim *see* Miconazole (Mex) . . . 364
Fungireduct *see* Nystatin (Ger) . . . 402
Fungisdin *see* Miconazole (Spain) . . . 364
Fungistat *see* Terconazole (Mex) . . . 536
Fungistat Dual *see* Terconazole (Mex) . . . 536
Fungisten *see* Clotrimazole (Norw) . . . 135
Fungivin *see* Griseofulvin (Norw) . . . 255
Fungizid *see* Clotrimazole (Ger) . . . 135
Fungizone *see* Amphotericin B (Conventional) (USA) . . . 41
Fungo *see* Miconazole (Astral) . . . 364
Fungo-Hubber *see* Ketoconazole (Spain) . . . 302
Fungoid Creme *see* Miconazole (USA) . . . 364
Fungoid Solution *see* Clotrimazole (USA) . . . 135
Fungoid Tincture *see* Miconazole (USA) . . . 364
Fungoral *see* Ketoconazole (Bra, Norw, Swed) . . . 302
Fungotox *see* Clotrimazole (Switz) . . . 135
Fungowas *see* Ciclopirox (Spain) . . . 122
Fungur M *see* Miconazole (Ger) . . . 364
Furabid *see* Nitrofurantoin (Neth) . . . 396
Furacin *see* Nitrofurazone (Astral, Bra, Ital, S. Afr, Spain, UK) . . . 396
Furacine *see* Nitrofurazone (Belg, Neth) . . . 396
Furacin-Sol *see* Nitrofurazone (Ger) . . . 396
Furacin Topical *see* Nitrofurazone (USA) . . . 396
Furadantin *see* Nitrofurantoin (Astral, Austria, Ger, Irl, Ital, Norw, S. Afr, Swed, UK, USA) . . . 396
Furadantina *see* Nitrofurantoin (Mex, Por) . . . 396
Furadantine *see* Nitrofurantoin (Belg, Fr, Switz) . . . 396
Furadantine MC *see* Nitrofurantoin (Neth) . . . 396
Furadoine *see* Nitrofurantoin (Fr) . . . 396
Furanthril *see* Furosemide (Ger) . . . 243
Furantoina *see* Nitrofurantoin (Spain) . . . 396
Furasept *see* Nitrofurazone (S. Afr) . . . 396
Furedan *see* Nitrofurantoin (Ital) . . . 396
Furese *see* Furosemide (Den) . . . 243
Furex *see* Nitrofurazone (S. Afr) . . . 396
Furil *see* Nitrofurantoin (Ital) . . . 396
Furix *see* Furosemide (Den, Norw, Swed) . . . 243
Furo *see* Furosemide (Ger) . . . 243
Furobactina *see* Nitrofurantoin (Spain) . . . 396
furo-basan *see* Furosemide (Switz) . . . 243
Furobeta *see* Furosemide (Ger) . . . 243
Furodrix *see* Furosemide (Switz) . . . 243
Furomed *see* Furosemide (Ger) . . . 243
Furon *see* Furosemide (Austria) . . . 243
Furonet *see* Furosemide (Den) . . . 243
Furophen Tc *see* Nitrofurantoin (Neth) . . . 396
Furo-Puren *see* Furosemide (Ger) . . . 243
Furorese *see* Furosemide (Ger) . . . 243
Furosal *see* Furosemide (Ger) . . . 243
Furoscand *see* Furosemide (Swed) . . . 243
Furosemix *see* Furosemide (Fr) . . . 243
Furoside *see* Furosemide (Can) . . . 243
Furosifar *see* Furosemide (Switz) . . . 243
Furotyrol *see* Furosemide (Austria) . . . 243
Furoxona Gotas *see* Furazolidone (Mex) . . . 242
Furoxona Tabletas *see* Furazolidone (Mex) . . . 242
Furoxone *see* Furazolidone (Astral, Ital, S. Afr, USA) . . . 242
Fursemida *see* Furosemide (Bra) . . . 243
Fursol *see* Furosemide (Switz) . . . 243
Fusid *see* Furosemide (Ger, Neth) . . . 243
Fustaren Retard *see* Diclofenac (Mex) . . . 163
Fuxen *see* Naproxen (Mex) . . . 384
Fuxol *see* Furazolidone (Mex) . . . 242
FX Passage *see* Magnesium Sulfate (Austria, Ger) . . . 331
Fynnon Calcium Aspirin *see* Aspirin (UK) . . . 49
G-1 *see* Butalbital Compound and Acetaminophen (USA) . . . 80
Gabbroral *see* Paromomycin (Belg, Ital) . . . 421
Gabitril *see* Tiagabine (Astral, Austria, Den, Fr, Irl, UK, USA) . . . 547
Gabrilen *see* Ketoprofen (Ger) . . . 302
Gabroral *see* Paromomycin (Spain) . . . 421
Galactoquin *see* Quinidine (Austria, Ger) . . . 485
Galantase *see* Lactase (Jpn, S. Afr) . . . 305
Galcodine *see* Codeine (UK) . . . 137
Galecin *see* Clindamycin (Mex) . . . 128
Galedol *see* Diclofenac (Mex) . . . 163
Galenamet *see* Cimetidine (Irl, UK) . . . 123
Galenamox *see* Amoxicillin (Irl, UK) . . . 38
Galfer *see* Ferrous Fumarate (Irl, UK) . . . 223
Galidrin *see* Ranitidine Hydrochloride (Mex) . . . 488
Galmax *see* Ursodiol (Ital) . . . 577
Galotam *see* Ampicillin and Sulbactam (Spain) . . . 43
Galprofen *see* Ibuprofen (UK) . . . 280
Galpseud *see* Pseudoephedrine (Irl, UK) . . . 478
Galpseud Plus *see* Chlorpheniramine and Pseudoephedrine (UK) . . . 114
Gamadiabet *see* Acetohexamide (Spain) . . . 17
Gamalat *see* Aluminum Hydroxide, Magnesium Hydroxide, and Simethicone (Bra) . . . 28
Gambex *see* Lindane (S. Afr) . . . 318
Gamikal *see* Amikacin (Mex) . . . 30
Gamimune N *see* Immune Globulin, Intravenous (USA) . . . 284
Gammadin *see* Povidone-Iodine (Ital) . . . 456
Gammagard *see* Immune Globulin, Intravenous (USA) . . . 284
Gammagard S/D *see* Immune Globulin, Intravenous (USA) . . . 284
Gamma Glob Antihepa B *see* Hepatitis B Immune Globulin (Spain) . . . 266
Gammaglob Antihep B *see* Hepatitis B Immune Globulin (Spain) . . . 266
Gammaprotect *see* Hepatitis B Immune Globulin (Ger) . . . 266
Gammar-P I.V. *see* Immune Globulin, Intravenous (USA) . . . 284
Gammatet *see* Tetracycline (S. Afr) . . . 537
Gammistin *see* Brompheniramine (Ital) . . . 73
Ganite *see* Gallium Nitrate (USA) . . . 245
Ganor *see* Famotidine (Ger) . . . 218
Gantanol *see* Sulfamethoxazole (Can, USA) . . . 524
Gantaprim *see* Co-Trimoxazole (Ital) . . . 142
Gantrim *see* Co-Trimoxazole (Ital) . . . 142
Gantrisin *see* Sulfisoxazole (Astral, USA) . . . 526
Gaopathyl *see* Aluminum Hydroxide and Magnesium Hydroxide (Fr) . . . 28
Gaoptol *see* Timolol (Mon) . . . 549
Gaosedal Codeine *see* Acetaminophen and Codeine (Fr) . . . 14
Garacol *see* Gentamicin (Neth) . . . 248
Garalen *see* Gentamicin (Mex) . . . 248
Garalone *see* Gentamicin (Por) . . . 248
Garamicina *see* Gentamicin (Bra, Mex) . . . 248
Garamycin *see* Gentamicin (Astral, Can, Den, Neth, Norw, S. Afr, Swed, Switz, UK) . . . 248
Garamycin Injection *see* Gentamicin (USA) . . . 248
Garamycin Ophthalmic *see* Gentamicin (USA) . . . 248
Garamycin Topical *see* Gentamicin (USA) . . . 248
Garanil *see* Captopril (Spain) . . . 89
Garatec *see* Gentamicin (Can) . . . 248
Gardan P *see* Acetaminophen (Ger) . . . 14
Gardenal *see* Phenobarbital (Belg, Bra, Fr, S. Afr, Spain, UK) . . . 435
Gardenale *see* Phenobarbital (Ital) . . . 435
Gargocetil *see* Cetylpyridinium (Bra) . . . 106
Garia *see* Fluocinonide (Spain) . . . 231
Garoin *see* Phenytoin With Phenobarbital (S. Afr) . . . 443
Garranil *see* Captopril (Spain) . . . 89
Garze Disinfettanti alla Pomata Betadine *see* Povidone-Iodine (Ital) . . . 456
Gas Ban [OTC] *see* Calcium Carbonate and Simethicone (USA) . . . 85
Gas-Ban DS [OTC] *see* Aluminum Hydroxide, Magnesium Hydroxide, and Simethicone (USA) . . . 28
Gasec *see* Omeprazole (Por) . . . 404
Gaspiren *see* Omeprazole (Bra) . . . 404
Gas Relief *see* Simethicone (USA) . . . 512
Gaster *see* Cromolyn Sodium (Ital) . . . 142
Gaster *see* Famotidine (Jpn) . . . 218
Gastopride *see* Famotidine (Por) . . . 218
Gastracol *see* Aluminum Hydroxide (Switz) . . . 28
Gastral *see* Sucralfate (Spain) . . . 521
Gastralka *see* Aluminum Hydroxide and Magnesium Hydroxide (S. Afr) . . . 28
Gastran *see* Aluminum Hydroxide, Magnesium Hydroxide, and Simethicone (Bra) . . . 28
Gastrax *see* Nizatidine (Ger) . . . 398
Gastrec *see* Ranitidine Hydrochloride (Mex) . . . 488
Gastrese LA *see* Metoclopramide (UK) . . . 360
Gastribien *see* Aluminum Hydroxide and Magnesium Trisilicate (Spain) . . . 28
Gastricalm *see* Magaldrate (Belg) . . . 330
Gastridin *see* Famotidine (Ital) . . . 218
Gastridina *see* Ranitidine Hydrochloride (Por) . . . 488
Gastrifam *see* Famotidine (Por) . . . 218
Gastrimagal *see* Magaldrate (Ger) . . . 330
Gastrimut *see* Omeprazole (Spain) . . . 404
Gastrion *see* Famotidine (Spain) . . . 218
Gastripan *see* Magaldrate (Ger) . . . 330
Gastrium *see* Omeprazole (Bra) . . . 404
Gastrobid Continus *see* Metoclopramide (Irl, UK) . . . 360
Gastrobitan *see* Cimetidine (Norw) . . . 123
Gastrobon *see* Magaldrate (S. Afr) . . . 330
Gastrocaps A *see* Aluminum Hydroxide (Ger) . . . 28
Gastrocolon *see* Metoclopramide (S. Afr) . . . 360
Gastrocrom Oral *see* Cromolyn Sodium (USA) . . . 142
Gastrodine *see* Cimetidine (Bra) . . . 123
Gastrodomina *see* Famotidine (Spain) . . . 218
Gastroflat *see* Simethicone (Bra) . . . 512
Gastroflux *see* Metoclopramide (UK) . . . 360
Gastrofrenal *see* Cromolyn Sodium (Ital, Spain) . . . 142
Gastrogel *see* Aluminum Hydroxide, Magnesium Hydroxide, and Simethicone (Bra) . . . 28
Gastrogel *see* Sucralfate (Ital, Switz) . . . 521
Gastro H2 *see* Cimetidine (Spain) . . . 123
Gastrolav *see* Ranitidine Hydrochloride (Por) . . . 488
Gastroloc *see* Omeprazole (Ger) . . . 404
Gastromax *see* Metoclopramide (UK) . . . 360
Gastromet *see* Cimetidine (Ital) . . . 123
Gastromol *see* Magaldrate (Spain) . . . 330
Gastron *see* Loperamide (S. Afr) . . . 324
Gastronerton *see* Metoclopramide (Austria, Ger) . . . 360
Gastropeache Susp *see* Aluminum Hydroxide and Magnesium Hydroxide (Spain) . . . 28
Gastropect *see* Kaolin and Pectin (S. Afr) . . . 300
Gastropen *see* Famotidine (Spain) . . . 218
Gastroplus *see* Aluminum Hydroxide, Magnesium Hydroxide, and Simethicone (Bra) . . . 28
Gastroprotect *see* Cimetidine (Ger) . . . 123
Gastrosan *see* Aluminum Hydroxide and Magnesium Hydroxide (Spain) . . . 28
Gastrosed *see* Hyoscyamine (USA) . . . 279
Gastrosil *see* Metoclopramide (Austria, Ger, Switz) . . . 360
Gastrostad *see* Magaldrate (Ger) . . . 330
Gastro-Stop *see* Loperamide (Astral) . . . 324
Gastro-Tablinen *see* Metoclopramide (Ger) . . . 360
Gastrotat *see* Metoclopramide (S. Afr) . . . 360
Gastrotem *see* Metoclopramide (Ger) . . . 360
Gastro-Timelets *see* Metoclopramide (Austria, Den, Ger, Switz) . . . 360
Gastrotranquil *see* Metoclopramide (Ger) . . . 360
Gastrotrop *see* Metoclopramide (Ger) . . . 360
Gastroulcerina *see* Aluminum Hydroxide and Magnesium Trisilicate (Spain) . . . 28
Gasulsol *see* Aluminum Hydroxide and Magnesium Trisilicate (Can) . . . 28
Gasva *see* Aluminum Hydroxide and Magnesium Trisilicate (Can) . . . 28
Gas-X *see* Simethicone (Can) . . . 512
Gas-X [OTC] *see* Simethicone (USA) . . . 512
Gatinar *see* Lactulose (Spain, Switz) . . . 306
Gaviscon-2 Tablet [OTC] *see* Aluminum Hydroxide and Magnesium Trisilicate (USA) . . . 28
Gaviscon Liquid [OTC] *see* Aluminum Hydroxide and Magnesium Carbonate (USA) . . . 28
Gaviscon Prevent *see* Cimetidine (Can) . . . 123
Gaviscon Tablet [OTC] *see* Aluminum Hydroxide and Magnesium Trisilicate (USA) . . . 28
Gaviz *see* Aluminum Hydroxide and Magnesium Carbonate (Bra) . . . 28
Gaviz *see* Aluminum Hydroxide and Magnesium Trisilicate (Bra) . . . 28
GBH *see* Lindane (Can) . . . 318

# NOTES

# NOTES

# NOTES

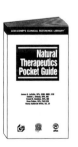

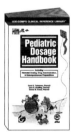

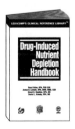

# Other titles offered by

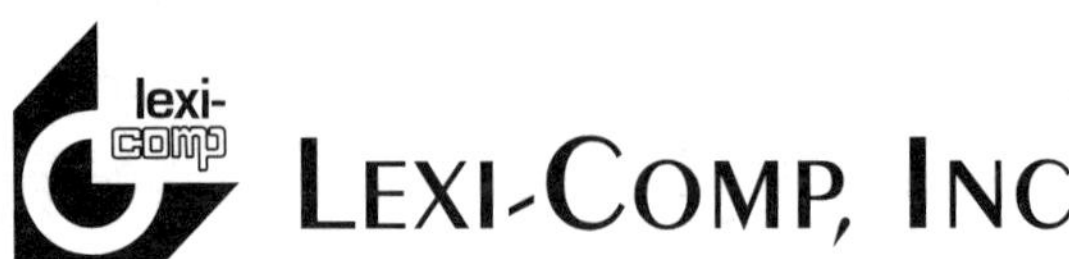


### DRUG INFORMATION HANDBOOK FOR PHYSICIAN ASSISTANTS

by Michael J. Rudzinski, RPA-C, RPh; J. Fred Bennes, RPA, RPh

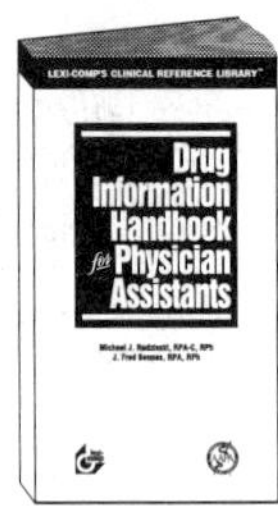

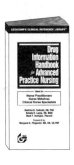


This comprehensive and easy-to-use handbook covers over 3600 drugs and also includes monographs on commonly used herbal products. There are up to 24 key fields of information per monograph, such as Pediatric And Adult Dosing With Adjustments for Renal/hepatic Impairment, Labeled And Unlabeled Uses, Pregnancy & Breast-feeding Precautions, and Special PA issues. Brand (U.S. and Canadian) and generic names are listed alphabetically for rapid access. It is fully cross-referenced by page number and includes alphabetical and pharmacologic indices.

### DRUG INFORMATION HANDBOOK FOR CARDIOLOGY

by Bradley G. Phillips, PharmD; Virend K. Somers, MD, Dphil

An ideal resource for physicians, pharmacists, nurses, residents, and students. This handbook was designed to provide the most current information on cardio-vascular agents and other ancillary medications.

- Each monograph includes information on Special Cardiovascular Considerations and I.V. to Oral Equivalency
- Alphabetically organized by brand and generic name
- Appendix contains information on Hypertension, Anticoagulation, Cytochrome P-450, Hyperlipidemia, Antiarrhythmia, and Comparative Drug Charts
- Special Topics/Issues include Emerging Risk Factors for Cardiovascular Disease, Treatment of Cardiovascular Disease in the Diabetic, Cardiovascular Stress Testing, and Experimental Cardiovascular Therapeutic Strategies in the New Millenium, and much more . . .

### DRUG INFORMATION HANDBOOK FOR ADVANCED PRACTICE NURSING

by Beatrice B. Turkoski, RN, PhD; Brenda R. Lance, RN, MSN; Mark F. Bonfiglio, PharmD

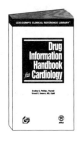


This handbook was designed specifically to meet the needs of Nurse Practitioners, Clinical Nurse Specialists, Nurse Midwives and graduate nursing students. The handbook is a unique resource for detailed, accurate information, which is vital to support the advanced practice nurse's role in patient drug therapy management.

A concise introductory section reviews topics related to Pharmacotherapeutics.

Over 4750 U.S., Canadian, and Mexican medications are covered in the 1055 monographs. Drug data is presented in an easy-to-use, alphabetically organized format covering up to 46 key points of information. Monographs are cross-referenced to an Appendix of over 230 pages of valuable comparison tables and additional information. Also included are two indices, Pharmacologic Category and Controlled Substance, which facilitate comparison between agents.

### DRUG INFORMATION HANDBOOK FOR ONCOLOGY

by Dominic A. Solimando, Jr, MA; Linda R. Bressler, PharmD, BCOP; Polly E. Kintzel, PharmD, BCPS, BCOP; Mark C. Geraci, PharmD, BCOP

Presented in a concise and uniform format, this book contains the most comprehensive collection of oncology-related drug information available. Organized like a dictionary for ease of use, drugs can be found by looking up the *brand or generic name*!

This book contains 253 monographs, including over 1100 Antineoplastic Agents and Ancillary Medications.

It also contains up to 33 fields of information per monograph including Use, U.S. Investigational, Bone Marrow/Blood Cell Transplantation, Vesicant, Emetic Potential. A Special Topics Section, Appendix, and Therapeutic Category & Key Word Index are valuable features to this book, as well.

### DRUG INFORMATION HANDBOOK FOR NURSING

by Beatrice B. Turkoski, RN, PhD; Brenda R. Lance, RN, MSN; Mark F. Bonfiglio, PharmD

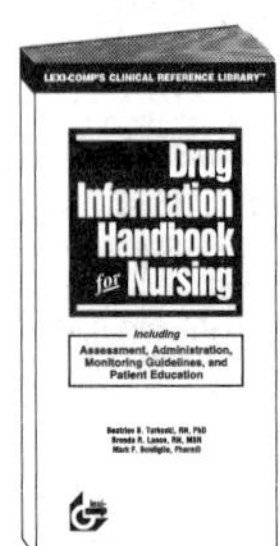

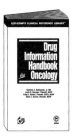


Registered Professional Nurses and upper-division nursing students involved with drug therapy will find this handbook provides quick access to drug data in a concise easy-to-use format.

Over 4750 U.S., Canadian, and Mexican medications are covered with up to 43 key points of information in each monograph. The handbook contains basic pharmacology concepts and nursing issues such as patient factors that influence drug therapy (ie, pregnancy, age, weight, etc) and general nursing issues (ie, assess-ment, administration, monitoring, and patient education). The Appendix contains over 220 pages of valuable information.

### ANESTHESIOLOGY & CRITICAL CARE DRUG HANDBOOK

by Andrew J. Donnelly, PharmD; Francesca E. Cunningham, PharmD; and Verna L. Baughman, MD

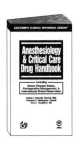


Containing over 512 generic medications with up to 25 fields of information presented in each monograph. This handbook also contains the following Special Issues and Topics: Allergic Reaction, Anesthesia for Cardiac Patients in Noncardiac Surgery, Anesthesia for Obstetric Patients in Nonobstetric Surgery, Anesthesia for Patients With Liver Disease, Chronic Pain Management, Chronic Renal Failure, Conscious Sedation, Perioperative Management of Patients on Antiseizure Medication, and Substance Abuse and Anesthesia.

The Appendix includes Abbreviations & Measurements, Anesthesiology Information, Assessment of Liver & Renal Function, Comparative Drug Charts, Infectious Disease-Prophylaxis & Treatment, Laboratory Values, Therapy Recommendations, Toxicology information, *and much more.*

**To order call toll free anywhere in the U.S.: 1-800-837-LEXI (5394)**
**Outside of the U.S. call: 330-650-6506 or online at www.lexi.com**

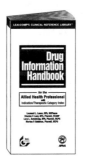

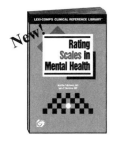

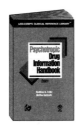

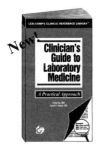

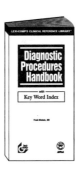

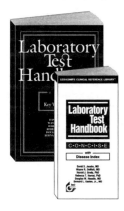

# Other titles offered by

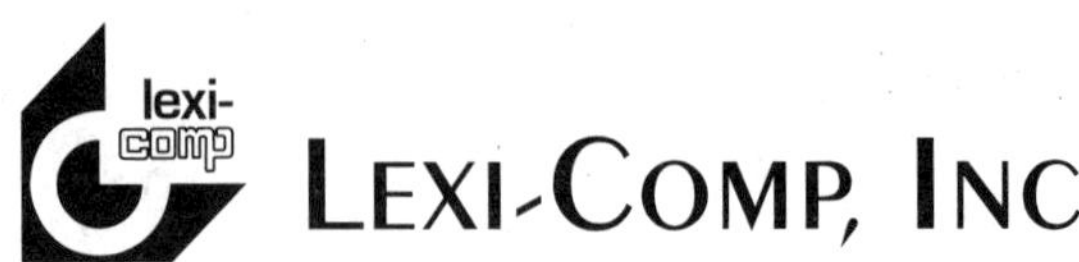


### *DRUG INFORMATION HANDBOOK FOR DENTISTRY*

(International edition available) by Richard L. Wynn, BSPharm, PhD; Timothy F. Meiller, DDS, PhD; and Harold L. Crossley, DDS, PhD

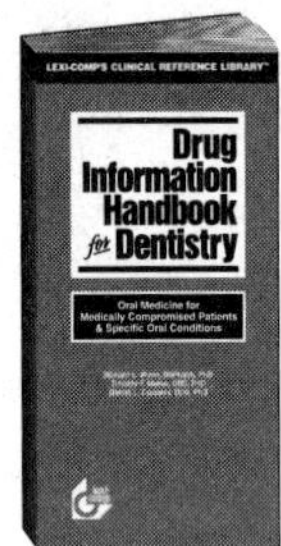


This handbook presents dental management and therapeutic considerations in medically compromised patients. Issues covered include oral manifestations of drugs, pertinent dental drug interactions, and dosing of drugs in dental treatment.

Selected oral medicine topics requiring therapeutic intervention include managing the patient with acute or chronic pain including TMD, managing the patient with oral bacterial or fungal infections, current therapeutics in periodontal patients, managing the patient receiving chemotherapy or radiation for the treatment of cancer, managing the anxious patient, managing dental office emergencies, and treatment of common oral lesions.

### *ORAL SOFT TISSUE DISEASES*

byJ. Robert Newland, DDS, MS; Timothy F. Meiller, DDS, PhD; Richard L. Wynn, BSPharm, PhD; Harold L.Crossley, DDS, PhD

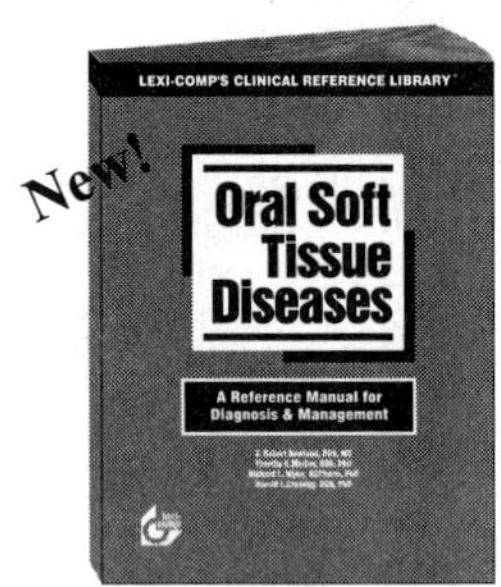


Designed for all dental professionals as an easy reference to assist in the diagnosis and management of oral soft tissue diseases.

Easy-to-use, tabbed sections:

1.) Diagnosis process: obtaining a history, examining the patient, establishing a differential diagnosis, selecting appropriate diagnostic tests, interpreting the results, etc. 2.) White lesions 3.) Red lesions 4.) Blistering-sloughing lesions 5.) Ulcerated lesions 6.) Pigmented lesions 7.) Papillary lesions 8.) Soft tissue swelling (Each lesion is illustrated with a color representative photograph) 9.) Specific medications to treat oral soft tissue diseases.

### *CLINICIAN'S ENDODONTIC HANDBOOK*

by Thom C. Dumsha, MS, DDS; James L. Gutmann, DDS, FACD, FICD

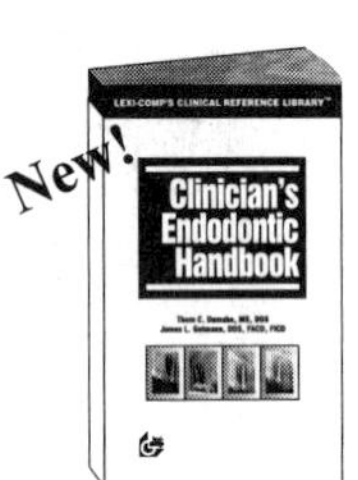


Designed for all general practice dentists.

- A quick reference addressing current endodontics
- Easy to use format and alphabetical index
- Latest techniques, procedures, and materials
- Root canal therapy: Why's and Why Nots
- A guide to diagnosis and treatment of endodontic emergencies
- Facts and rationale behind treating endodontically-involved teeth
- Straight-forward dental trauma management information
- Pulpal Histology, Access Openings, Bleaching, Resorption, Radiology, Restoration, and Periodontal / Endodontic Complications
- Frequently Asked Questions (FAQ) section and "Clinical Note" sections throughout.

### *DENTAL OFFICE MEDICAL EMERGENCIES*

by Timothy F. Meiller, DDS, PhD; Richard L. Wynn, BSPharm, PhD; Ann Marie McMullin, MD; Cynthia Biron, RDH, EMT, MA; Harold L. Crossley, DDS, PhD

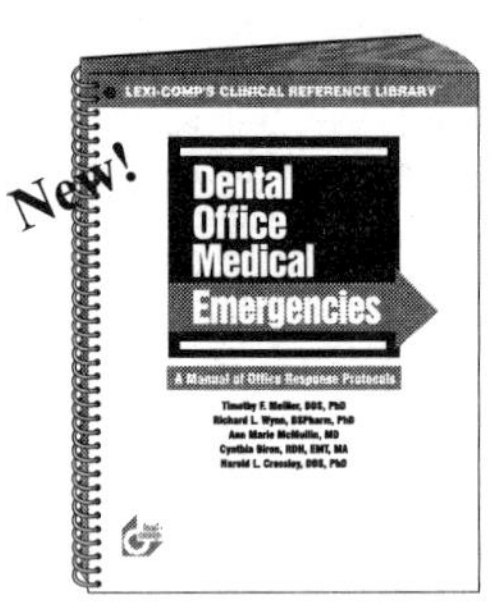


Designed specifically for general dentists during times of emergency. A tabbed paging system allows for quick access to specific crisis events. Created with urgency in mind, it is spiral bound and drilled with a hole for hanging purposes.

- Basic Action Plan for Stabilization
- Loss of Consciousness / Respiratory Distress / Chest Pain
- Allergic / Drug Reactions
- Altered Sensation / Changes in Affect
- Management of Acute Bleeding
- Office Preparedness / Procedures and Protocols

### *DRUG INFORMATION HANDBOOK FOR THE CRIMINAL JUSTICE PROFESSIONAL*

by Marcelline Burns, PhD; Thomas E. Page, MA; and Jerrold B. Leikin, MD

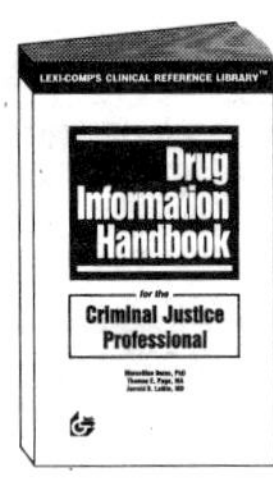


Compiled and designed for police officers, law enforcement officials, and legal professionals who are in need of a reference which relates to information on drugs, chemical substances, and other agents that have abuse and/or impairment potential. Contains over 450 medications, agents, and substances. Each monograph is presented in a consistent format and contains up to 33 fields of information including Scientific Name, Commonly Found In, Abuse Potential, Impairment Potential, Use, When to Admit to Hospital, Mechanism of Toxic Action, Signs & Symptoms of Acute Overdose, Drug Interactions, Warnings/Precautions, and Reference Range. There are many diverse chapter inclusions as well as a glossary of medical terms for the layman along with a slang street drug listing. The Appendix contains Chemical, Bacteriologic, and Radiologic Agents - Effects and Treatment; Controlled Substances - Uses and Effects; Medical Examiner Data; Federal Trafficking Penalties, *and much more.*

### *POISONING & TOXICOLOGY COMPENDIUM*

by Jerrold B. Leikin, MD and Frank P. Paloucek, PharmD

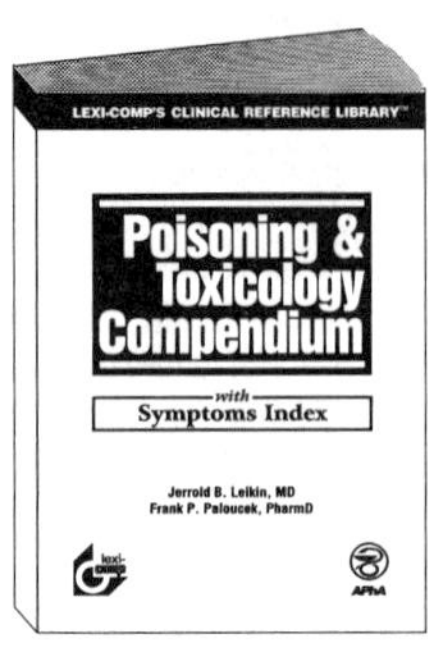


A six-in-one reference wherein each major entry contains information relative to one or more of the other sections. This handbook offers comprehensive concisely-stated monographs covering 645 medicinal agents, 256 nonmedicinal agents, 273 biological agents, 49 herbal agents, 254 laboratory tests, 79 antidotes, and 222 pages of exceptionally useful appendix material.

A truly unique reference that presents signs and symptoms of acute overdose along with considerations for overdose treatment. Ideal reference for emergency situations.

**To order call toll free anywhere in the U.S.: 1-800-837-LEXI (5394)**
**Outside of the U.S. call: 330-650-6506 or online at www.lexi.com**